Bailey & Scott's

DIAGNOSTIC
MICROBIOLOGY

Fifteenth Edition

PATRICIA M. TILLE, PhD, MLS(ASCP), AHI(AMT), FACSc
Chair of Microbiology Advisory Committee;
Editor in Chief IJBLS; International Federation of
Biomedical Laboratory Science
Graduate Program Director/Faculty
Medical Laboratory Science
University of Cincinnati
Cincinnati, Ohio

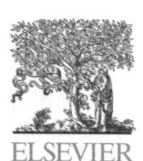

ELSEVIER

Elsevier
3251 Riverport Lane
St. Louis, Missouri 63043

Notice

Practitioners and researchers must always rely on their own experience and knowledge in evaluating and using any information, methods, compounds or experiments described herein. Because of rapid advances in the medical sciences, in particular, independent verification of diagnoses and drug dosages should be made. To the fullest extent of the law, no responsibility is assumed by Elsevier, authors, editors or contributors for any injury and/or damage to persons or property as a matter of products liability, negligence or otherwise, or from any use or operation of any methods, products, instructions, or ideas contained in the material herein.

Previous editions copyrighted 2017, 2014, 2007, 2002, 1998, 1994, 1990, 1986, 1982, 1978, 1974, 1970, 1966, 1962.

International Standard Book Number: 978-0-323-68105-6

Content Strategist: Heather Bays-Petrovic
Director, Content Development: Laurie Gower
Content Development Specialist: Betsy McCormac
Publishing Services Manager: Catherine Jackson
Health Content Management Specialist: Kristine Feeherty
Design Direction: Bridget Hoette

Printed in India

Last digit is the print number: 9   8   7   6   5   4   3   2

Working together to grow libraries in developing countries

www.elsevier.com • www.bookaid.org

Life is fleeting, but you must always remember friends, colleagues, and family. I will always thank my husband, David, and our children, Chrissy, Malissa, D.J., and Katie, along with their significant others. I would be remiss if I did not mention the seven little "smiles" that bring daily joy to our lives: Aedan, Milan Jr., Julia, Maja, Jayce, Riley, and Mila!

Lastly, no endeavor such as this would continue to evolve from one edition to the next without the insightful comments and input from numerous professional users and students. Thank you for your dedication, hard work, and humor.

This edition was created during a time of great unrest and challenges in the medical field, with the world facing the COVID-19 pandemic. I myself was struck with the virus and hospitalized for a period. I can say firsthand that the care and compassion of the health care workers was amazing, from physical, occupational, and respiratory therapy; nursing staff; phlebotomists; and laboratory professionals. They all came together to ensure the best care!

This edition is dedicated to all the essential workers who keep the country going and the health care professionals who continue to save lives as we battle this formidable viral adversary! To all the lives lost, may you rest in peace and know that the knowledge developed during the pandemic continues to save more lives every day!

Reviewers

Shari Batson, BSc, ART(Microbiology)
Professor
Health Sciences
St. Lawrence College
Kingston, Ontario, Canada

Jimmy L. Boyd, MS/MHS, MLS(ASCP)^CM
Program Director/Department Chair (Tenured)
Medical Laboratory Sciences
Arkansas State University-Beebe
Beebe, Arkansas

Lisa K. Cremeans, MMDS, MLS(ASCP)^CM, SM^CM, MB^CM
Assistant Professor
Department of Allied Health Sciences
Division of Clinical Laboratory Science
The University of North Carolina at Chapel Hill
Chapel Hill, North Carolina

Guyla Corbett Evans, PhD, MLS(ASCP)^CMSC^CM
Clinical Assistant Professor
Clinical Laboratory Science
East Carolina University
Greenville, North Carolina

Kathleen J. Fennema, BS, MT(ASCP)
Clinical Laboratory Scientist
Infectious Diseases Diagnostic Laboratory (Mycology and Parasitology Section)
University of Minnesota Medical Center (M Health)
Minneapolis, Minnesota

Michele G. Harms, MS, MLS(ASCP)
Program Director
Medical Laboratory Science Program
UPMC Chautauqua Hospital
Jamestown, New York

Janet Hudzicki, PhD, MLS(ASCP)^CM, SM(ASCP)^CM
Associate Professor
Department of Clinical Laboratory Sciences
KU Medical Center
The University of Kansas
Kansas City, Kansas

Cynthia Kaufman, MS, MT(ASCP)SM
Assistant Clinical Professor
Department of Pathology and Laboratory Medicine
Indiana University School of Medicine
Indianapolis, Indiana

Louise Millis, MS, MLS(ASCP)^CM
MLS Certification
Associate Professor of Biology and MLS Program Director
Department of Biology
St. Cloud State University
St. Cloud, Minnesota

Mathumathi Rajavel, PhD
Associate Professor
Medical Technology Program
School of Computer, Mathematical and Natural Sciences
Morgan State University
Baltimore, Maryland

Katherine M. Steele, MPH, MLS(ASCP)^CM
Assistant Clinical Professor
Pathology and Laboratory Medicine
Indiana University School of Medicine
Indianapolis, Indiana

Contributors

Hassan A. Aziz, PhD, MSc
Associate Dean for Academic, Faculty, and Student Affairs
College of Health Professions
Professor
Clinical Laboratory Science
The University of Tennessee Health Science Center
Memphis, Tennessee
  Chapter 34: Legionella
  Chapter 77: Quality in the Clinical Microbiology
    Laboratory
  Chapter 78: Infection Control
  Chapter 79: Sentinel Laboratory Response to Bioterrorism

Erin Barger, BS MLS, MA Education
Medical Technologist
Microbiology
UC Health
Cincinnati, Ohio
  Chapter 21: Pseudomonas, Burkholderia, and Similar
    Organisms
  Chapter 25: Vibrio, Aeromonas, Plesiomonas shigelloides,
    and *Chromobacterium violaceum*

**Janice Conway-Klaassen, PhD, MLS(ASCP)^{CM},
  SM^{CM}, FACSc**
Director
Medical Laboratory Sciences
University of Minnesota
Minneapolis, Minnesota
  Chapter 46: Overview of the Methods and Strategies in
    Parasitology
  Chapter 48: Blood and Tissue Protozoa

April Harkins, PhD, MT(ASCP)
Associate Professor and Department Chair
Clinical Laboratory Science
Marquette University
Milwaukee, Wisconsin
  Chapter 60: Dematiaceous (Melanized) Molds
  Chapter 61: Atypical and Parafungal Agents

Stephanie Jacobson, MS, MLS(ASCP)^{CM}
MLS Upward Mobility Online Instructor
Medical Laboratory Science
South Dakota State University
Brookings, South Dakota;
Microbiologist
Laboratory
Monument Health
Rapid City, South Dakota
  Chapter 15: Bacillus and Similar Organisms
  Chapter 16: Listeria, Corynebacterium, and Similar
    Organisms
  Chapter 17: Erysipelothrix, Lactobacillus, and Similar
    Organisms
  Chapter 47: Intestinal Protozoa
  Chapter 49: Protozoa From Other Body Sites
  Chapter 50: Intestinal Nematodes
  Chapter 51: Tissue Nematodes
  Chapter 52: Blood and Tissue Filarial Nematodes
  Chapter 53: Intestinal Cestodes
  Chapter 54: Tissue Cestodes
  Chapter 55: Intestinal Trematodes
  Chapter 56: Liver and Lung Trematodes
  Chapter 57: Blood Trematodes

James March Mistler, MS
Program Director/Lecturer
Department of Medical Laboratory Science
University of Massachusetts Dartmouth
North Dartmouth, Massachusetts
  Chapter 39: Neisseria and *Moraxella catarrhalis*

Meghan May, PhD, MS
Associate Professor
Biomedical Sciences
University of New England
Biddeford, Maine
  Chapter 44: Cell Wall–Deficient Bacteria: *Mycoplasma*
    and *Ureaplasma*

Caterina Miraglia, DC, MLS(ASCP)^{CM}
Assistant Professor
Medical Laboratory Science
University of Massachusetts Dartmouth
North Dartmouth, Massachusetts
   Chapter 45: The Spirochetes

Nicholas M. Moore, PhD
Assistant Professor
Department of Medical Laboratory Science and Pathology
Assistant Director
Division of Clinical Microbiology
Rush University Medical Center
Chicago, Illinois
   Chapter 10: Principles of Antimicrobial Action and Resistance
   Chapter 11: Laboratory Methods and Strategies for Antimicrobial Susceptibility Testing
   Chapter 20: Acinetobacter, Stenotrophomonas, and Other Organisms
   Chapter 62: The Yeasts and Yeastlike Organisms
   Chapter 63: Antifungal Susceptibility Testing, Therapy, and Prevention

Rodney E. Rohde, PhD, MS, BS
Chair and Professor
Clinical Laboratory Science
Associate Dean for Research
College of Health Professions
Associate Director for Translational Health Research Initiative
Texas State University
San Marcos, Texas;
Associate Adjunct Professor of Biology
Department of Biology
Austin Community College
Austin, Texas
   Chapter 8: Nucleic Acid–Based Analytic Methods for Microbial Identification and Characterization
   Chapter 13: Staphylococcus, Micrococcus, and Similar Organisms
   Chapter 35: Brucella
   Chapter 37: Francisella
   Chapter 44: Cell Wall–Deficient Bacteria: *Mycoplasma* and *Ureaplasma*
   Chapter 64: Overview of the Methods and Strategies in Virology
   Chapter 65: Viruses in Human Disease

Frank Scarano, PhD, MS, BA, AAS
Professor
Medical Laboratory Science
University of Massachusetts Dartmouth
Dartmouth, Massachusetts
   Chapter 28: Eikenella corrodens and Similar Organisms
   Chapter 29: Pasteurella and Similar Organisms

Tim Southern, MS, PhD, D(ABMM)
Laboratory Director
South Dakota Public Health Laboratory
South Dakota Department of Health
Pierre, South Dakota
   Chapter 12: Overview of Bacterial Identification Methods and Strategies
   Chapter 19: Enterobacterales
   Chapter 43: Obligate Intracellular and Nonculturable Bacterial Agents

Shannon Weigum, BA, MS, PhD
Associate Professor
Department of Biology
Materials Science, Engineering, and Commercialization Program
Texas State University
San Marcos, Texas
   Chapter 8: Nucleic Acid–Based Analytic Methods for Microbial Identification and Characterization
   Chapter 64: Overview of the Methods and Strategies in Virology
   Chapter 65: Viruses in Human Disease

Preface

This, the fifteenth edition of *Bailey & Scott's Diagnostic Microbiology*, is the third edition that I have had the great pleasure to edit and author with some amazing colleagues. The dynamics of infectious disease trends, along with the technical developments available for diagnosing, treating, and controlling these diseases, continues to present major challenges in the laboratory and medical care. In meeting these challenges, the primary goal for the fifteenth edition is to provide an updated and reliable reference text for practicing clinical microbiologists and technologists, while also presenting this information in a format that supports the educational efforts of all those responsible for preparing others for a career in diagnostic microbiology. The text retains the traditional information needed to develop a solid, basic understanding of diagnostic microbiology while integrating the dynamic expansion of molecular diagnostics and advanced techniques such as matrix-assisted laser desorption time-of-flight mass spectrometry.

We have kept the favorite features and made adjustments in response to important critical input from users of the text. The succinct presentation of each organism group's key laboratory, clinical, epidemiologic, and therapeutic features in tables and figures has been kept and updated. Regarding content, the major changes reflect the changes that the discipline of diagnostic microbiology continues to experience. Also, although the grouping of organisms into sections according to key features (e.g., Gram reaction, catalase or oxidase reaction, growth on MacConkey agar) has remained, changes regarding the genera and species discussed in these sections have been made. These changes, along with changes in organism nomenclature, were made to accurately reflect the changes that have occurred, and continue to occur, in taxonomy. Also, throughout the text, the content has been enhanced with new photographs and artistic drawings. Finally, although some classic methods for bacterial identification and characterization developed over the years (e.g., catalase, oxidase, Gram stain) still play a critical role in today's laboratory, others have given way to commercial identification systems. We realize that in a textbook such as this, a balance is needed for practicing and teaching diagnostic microbiology; our selection of identification methods that received the most detailed attention may not always meet the needs of both groups. However, we have tried to be consistent in selecting those methods that reflect the most current and common practices of today's clinical microbiology laboratories, along with those that present historical information required within an educational program.

Finally, in terms of organization, the fifteenth edition is similar in many aspects to the fourteenth edition, but some changes have been made. Various instructor ancillaries, specifically geared for the fifteenth edition, are available on the Evolve website, including an expanded test bank, updated PowerPoints, a laboratory manual with answers, review questions with answer key, and an electronic image collection. Student resources include a laboratory manual, review questions, online case studies, and online procedures.

We sincerely hope that clinical microbiology practitioners and educators find *Bailey & Scott's Diagnostic Microbiology*, fifteenth edition, to be a worthy and useful tool to support their professional activities.

Acknowledgments

I would like to acknowledge the help of my colleagues at Elsevier who guided me through this project: Kristine Feeherty, Health Content Management Specialist, and Betsy McCormac, Content Development Specialist.

Patricia M. Tille

Contents

1

Microbial Taxonomy

OBJECTIVES

1. Define classification, identification, species, genus, type genus, and binomial nomenclature.
2. Properly use binomial nomenclature in the identification of microorganisms, including syntax, capitalization, and punctuation.
3. Identify a microorganism's characteristics as either phenotypic or genotypic.
4. Define polyphasic taxonomy and chemotaxonomic methods and how they are being applied to the classification of microorganisms.
5. Describe how the classification, naming, and identification of organisms play a role in diagnostic microbiology in the clinical setting.

The science of **taxonomy** is a systematic process applied to all living entities, providing a consistent means to classify, name (nomenclature), and identify organisms. This consistency allows biologists worldwide to use a common label for every organism studied within the multitude of biologic disciplines. The common language of taxonomy minimizes confusion about organisms' names, physiology, and biologic relatedness. Taxonomy is important in the **phylogeny** (the evolutionary history of organisms) and scientific study of all living things in virtually every biologic discipline, including microbiology.

As a result of the advances in molecular biology, traditional taxonomy based on genotypic, phenotypic, and phylogenetic or evolutionary relationships currently encompasses a multifaceted analysis of **epigenetic** (variations in gene expression not caused by nucleic acid sequence similarities or differences) and **chemotaxonomic methods**. This method of classification or **polyphasic taxonomy** provides a more detailed but very complex analysis of the current classification system using ribosomal ribonucleic acid (rRNA) sequences, whole genome sequences, epigenetics, and mass spectrometry (MS). The "gold standard" for classification of bacterial species has historically been based on deoxyribonucleic acid (DNA) including DNA hybridization (DDH) patterns and 16S rRNA gene (16S rDNA) sequence homology. With the implementation of next generation sequencing, a more detailed analysis of organism

genomes including the average nucleotide identity (ANI), multilocus phylogenetic, and genome-to-genome distance (GGD) analysis permit the resolution of microorganisms from closely related subspecies to specific species. Not all parameters clearly delineate each organism to the species level. In other words, some characteristics may strengthen the organization of the genus, and some may be useful at the species level. Species identification techniques have distinct variations in cutoff values or thresholds for the differentiation of organisms at the genus and species levels. The comparative thresholds indicate the likelihood that two genomes are from the same organism (Table 1.1). When using a single sequence such as the 16S rRNA, the possibility of gene transfer may also affect genotypic classification. Although 16S rRNA sequences are evolutionarily highly conserved, ANI evaluates multiple coding regions across an entire genome, making the genomic analysis more detailed and accurate. Finally, lateral gene transfer among organisms, particularly bacteria, creates difficulty in the classification of organisms according to phenotypic traits or biochemical traits and genotypic criteria such as DNA G + C content, which has historically been the hallmark of diagnostic microbiology. Molecular methods have provided a means for identifying the historical core genomes used in classification and species identification. However, it is important to recognize that phenotypic expression and classification of organisms will continue to be compounded by the variation in genomes as a result of gene transfer among organisms.

In addition to more advanced genomic analysis, **chemotaxonomic methods** are more frequently being applied to the identification and classification of microorganisms. These methods include protein studies, fatty acid analysis, and cell wall composition. MS and matrix-assisted laser desorption ionization time-of-flight mass spectrometry (MALDI-TOF MS) use the separation and analysis of high-abundance proteins and peptides for the classification and identification of bacterial isolates. Techniques such as rapid evaporative ionization mass spectrometry (REIMS) are able to identify molecules and create images of tissues and microorganisms from laboratory growth medium. This polyphasic analysis beyond genomics provides a mechanism to use the MS data in conjunction with the genomic analysis and phenotypic characteristics to identify and classify organisms, as well as monitor biochemical therapies in complex disease states.

TABLE 1.1   Identification Criteria and Characteristics for Microbial Classification

Criteria	Characteristics
Phenotypic	
Macroscopic morphology	The microbial growth patterns on artificial media as observed when inspected with the unaided eye. Examples include the size, texture, and pigmentation of bacterial colonies.
Microscopic morphology	The size, shape, intracellular inclusions, cellular appendages, and arrangement of cells when observed with the aid of microscopic magnification.
Staining characteristics	The ability of an organism to reproducibly stain a particular color with the application of specific dyes and reagents. Staining is used in conjunction with microscopic morphology for bacterial identification. For example, the Gram stain for bacteria is a critical criterion for differential identification.
Environmental requirements	The ability of an organism to grow at various temperatures, in the presence of oxygen and other gases, at various pH levels, or in the presence of other ions and salts, such as NaCl.
Nutritional requirements	The ability of an organism to use various carbon and nitrogen sources as nutritional substrates when grown under specific environmental conditions.
Resistance profiles	The exhibition of a characteristic inherent resistance to specific antibiotics, heavy metals, or toxins.
Antigenic properties	The profiles of microorganisms established by various serologic and immunologic methods to determine relatedness among various microbial groups.
Subcellular properties	Molecular constituents of the cell that are typical of a particular taxon, or organism group, as established by various analytic methods. Some examples include cell wall components, components of the cell membrane, and enzymatic content of the microbial cell.
Chemotaxonomic properties	The chemical constituents of the cell, such as the structure of teichoic acids, fatty acid analysis, and protein profiles, as determined by analytical methods.
Genotypic	
DNA base composition ratio	DNA comprises four bases (guanine, cytosine, adenine, and thymine). The extent to which the DNA from two organisms is made up of cytosine and guanine (i.e., G + C content) relative to their total base content can be used as an indicator of relatedness or lack thereof. For example, an organism with a G + C content of 50% is not closely related to an organism with a G + C content of 25%.
Nucleic acid (DNA and RNA) base sequence characteristics, including those determined by hybridization assays	The order of bases along a strand of DNA or RNA is known as the **base sequence**. The extent to which sequences are **homologous** (similar) between two microorganisms can be determined directly or indirectly by various molecular methods. The degree of similarity in the sequences may be a measure of the degree of organism relatedness, specifically, the rRNA sequences that remain stable in comparison to the genome as a whole.
Average nucleotide identity (ANI)	This method analyses multiple coding sequences in a microorganism's genome to determine the average nucleotide identity using genome sequencing and computer algorithms. The relatedness of microorganisms is accurate at 95%–96% threshold for organism identification.
Genome-to-Genome Distance (GGD)	This is a computerized calculation that uses inference by in-silico genome comparisons eliminating the limitations and errors associated with wet-lab techniques. Organisms are related with a GGD threshold score of 70% or greater.

DNA, Deoxyribonucleic acid; *RNA,* ribonucleic acid; *rRNA,* ribosomal RNA.

As technology improves, the classification and identification of organisms will undoubtedly continue to evolve along with the changes in the populations of organisms. In diagnostic microbiology, classification, nomenclature, and identification of microorganisms play a central role in providing an accurate, timely diagnosis and monitoring the management of infectious disease. A brief, detailed discussion of the major components of taxonomy is important for a basic understanding of bacterial identification and application to diagnostic microbiology.

Classification

Classification is a method for organizing microorganisms into groups or **taxa** based on similar morphologic, physiologic, and genetic traits. The hierarchical classification system consists of the following taxa:
- Domains (Bacteria, Archaea, and Eukarya)
- Kingdom (contains similar divisions or phyla; most inclusive taxa)
- Phylum (contains similar classes; equivalent to the Division taxa in botany)

- Class (contains similar orders)
- Order (contains similar families)
- Family (contains similar genera)
- Genus (contains similar species)
- Species (specific epithet; lowercase Latin adjective or noun; most exclusive taxa)

Bacteria or **prokaryotes** (prenucleus) are separated into two domains, the Bacteria and the Archaea (ancient bacteria). The Bacteria contain the environmental prokaryotes (blue green or cyanobacteria) and the heterotrophic medically relevant bacteria. The Archaea are environmental isolates that live in extreme habitats such as high salt concentrations, jet fuel, or high temperatures. The third domain, Eukarya, *eukaryotes* (true nucleus), also contains medically relevant organisms, including fungi and parasites.

There are several other taxonomic sublevels below the domains, as noted previously; however, the typical application of organism classification in the diagnostic microbiology laboratory primarily uses the taxa beginning at the family designation.

Family

A **family** encompasses a group of organisms that may contain multiple genera and consists of organisms with a common attribute. The name of a family is formed by adding the suffix -aceae to the root name of one of the group's genera, called the **type genus;** for example, the *Streptococcaceae* family type genus is *Streptococcus.* One exception to the rule in microbiology is Enterobacterales; it is named after the "enteric" group of bacteria rather than the type species *Escherichia coli.* Bacterial (prokaryotic)-type species or strains are determined according to guidelines published by the International Committee for the Systematics of Prokaryotes (ICSP) in The International Code of Nomenclature of Prokaryotes (ICNP). This code provides the guidelines for linking nomenclature, classification, and characterization of organisms using the physiologic, biochemical, genetic, and phenotypic traits of organisms. Microorganism type species should be described in detail using diagnostic and comparable methods that are reproducible, and all authentic strains must be available for further analysis.

Genus

Genus (plural, genera), the next taxon, contains different species that have several important features in common. Each species within a genus differs sufficiently to maintain its status as an individual species. Placement of a species within a particular genus is based on various genetic and phenotypic characteristics shared among the species.

Microorganisms do not possess the multitude of physical features exhibited by higher organisms such as plants and animals. For instance, they rarely leave any fossil record, and they exhibit a tremendous capacity to intermix genetic material among seemingly unrelated species and genera. For these reasons, confidently establishing a microorganism's relatedness in higher taxa beyond the genus level is difficult. Although grouping similar genera into common families and similar families into common orders is used for classification of plants and animals, these higher taxa designations (i.e., division, class, and order) are not useful for classifying bacteria.

Species

Species (abbreviated as **sp.**, singular, or **spp.**, plural) is the most basic of the taxonomic groups and can be defined as a collection of bacterial strains that share common physiologic and genetic features and differ notably from other microbial species. Occasionally, taxonomic subgroups within a species, called **subspecies,** are recognized. Furthermore, designations such as **biotype, serotype,** or **genotype** may be given to groups below the subspecies level that share specific but relatively minor characteristics. For example, *Klebsiella pneumoniae* and *Klebsiella oxytoca* are two distinct species within the genus *Klebsiella. Serratia odorifera* biotype 2 and *Treponema pallidum* subsp. *pallidum* are examples of a biotype and a subspecies designation. A biotype is considered the same species with the same genetic makeup but displays differential physiologic characteristics. Subspecies do not display significant enough divergence to be classified as a biotype or a new species. Although these subgroups may have some taxonomic importance, their usefulness in diagnostic microbiology is limited.

Nomenclature

Nomenclature is the naming of microorganisms according to established rules and guidelines set forth in the ICNP. It provides the accepted labels by which organisms are universally recognized. Because genus and species are the groups commonly used by microbiologists, the discussion of rules governing microbial nomenclature is limited to these two taxa. In this **binomial** (two name) system of nomenclature, every organism is assigned a genus and a species of Latin or Greek derivation. Each organism has a scientific "label" consisting of two parts: the genus designation, in which the first letter is always capitalized, and the species designation, in which the first letter is always lowercase. The two components are used simultaneously and are printed in italics or underlined in script. For example, the streptococci include *Streptococcus pneumoniae, Streptococcus pyogenes, Streptococcus agalactiae,* and *Streptococcus bovis,* among others. Alternatively, the name may be abbreviated by using the uppercase form of the first letter of the genus designation followed by a period (.) and the full species name (e.g., *S. pneumoniae, S. pyogenes, S. agalactiae,* and *S. bovis*). Finally, when discussing a single specific organism, the species may be designated using sp., and a group of species within the genus using spp. (e.g., *Staphylococcus* sp. and *Staphylococcus* spp.). Frequently an informal designation (e.g., staphylococci, streptococci, enterococci) may be used to label a particular group of organisms. These designations are not capitalized or italicized.

As more information is gained regarding organism classification and identification, a particular species may be moved to a different genus or assigned a new genus name. The rules and criteria for these changes are beyond the scope of this chapter, but such changes are documented in the *International Journal of Systemic and Evolutionary Microbiology*. Published nomenclature may be found at http://www.bacterio.net for bacteria, http://www.ictvonline.org for viruses, http://www.iapt-taxon.org/nomen/main.php for fungi, and http://www.iczn.org for parasites. It is important to note that the fungi and parasite lists are difficult to maintain and may not reflect the current validity at the time of review. In the diagnostic laboratory, changes in nomenclature are phased in gradually so that physicians and laboratorians have ample opportunity to recognize that a familiar pathogen has been given a new name. This is usually accomplished by using the new genus designation while continuing to provide the previous designation in parentheses; for example, *Stenotrophomonas (Xanthomonas) maltophilia* or *Burkholderia (Pseudomonas) cepacia*.

Identification

Microbial identification is the process by which a microorganism's key features are delineated. Once those features have been established, the profile is compared with those of other previously characterized microorganisms. The organism can then be assigned to the most appropriate taxa and can be given appropriate genus and species names; both are essential aspects of taxonomy in diagnostic microbiology and the management of infectious disease (Box 1.1).

Identification Methods

A wide variety of methods and criteria are used to establish a microorganism's identity. These methods can be separated into either of two general categories: genotypic or phenotypic characteristics. **Genotypic characteristics** relate to an organism's genetic makeup, including the nature of the organism's genes and constituent nucleic acids (see Chapter 2 for more information about microbial genetics). **Phenotypic characteristics** are based on features beyond the genetic level, including both readily observable characteristics and features that may require extensive analytic procedures to be detected. Examples of characteristics used as criteria for bacterial identification and classification are provided in Table 1.1. Modern microbial taxonomy uses a combination of several methods to characterize microorganisms thoroughly to classify and name each organism.

Although the criteria and examples in Table 1.1 are given in the context of microbial identification for classification purposes, the principles and practices of classification parallel the approaches used in diagnostic microbiology for the identification and characterization of microorganisms encountered in the clinical setting. Fortunately, because of the previous efforts and accomplishments of microbial taxonomists, microbiologists do not have to use several burdensome classification

---

• BOX 1.1   Role of Taxonomy in Diagnostic Microbiology

- Establishes and maintains records of key characteristics of clinically relevant microorganisms
- Facilitates communication among technologists, microbiologists, physicians, and scientists by assigning universal names to clinically relevant microorganisms. This is essential for:
  - Establishing an association of particular diseases or syndromes with specific microorganisms
  - Epidemiology and tracking outbreaks
  - Accumulating knowledge regarding the management and outcome of diseases associated with specific microorganisms
  - Establishing patterns of resistance to antimicrobial agents and recognition of changing microbial resistance patterns
  - Understanding the mechanisms of antimicrobial resistance and detecting new resistance mechanisms exhibited by microorganisms
  - Recognizing new and emerging pathogenic microorganisms
  - Recognizing changes in the types of infections or diseases caused by characteristic microorganisms
  - Revising and updating available technologies for the development of new methods to optimize the detection and identification of infectious agents and the detection of resistance to antiinfective agents (microbial, viral, fungal, and parasitic)
  - Developing new antiinfective therapies (microbial, viral, fungal, and parasitic)

---

and identification schemes to identify infectious agents. Instead, microbiologists use key phenotypic and genotypic features on which to base their identification to provide clinically relevant information in a timely manner (Chapter 12). This should not be taken to mean that the identification of all clinically relevant organisms is easy and straightforward. This is also not meant to imply that microbiologists can identify or recognize only organisms that have already been characterized and named by taxonomists. Indeed, the clinical microbiology laboratory is well recognized as the place where previously unknown or uncharacterized infectious agents are initially encountered, and as such it has an ever-increasing responsibility to be the source of information and reporting for emerging etiologies of infectious disease.

ⓔ Visit the Evolve site for a complete list of procedures, review questions and answers, and case studies.

Bibliography

Bennett J, Dolin R, Blaser M: *Principles and practice of infectious diseases*, ed 9, Philadelphia, 2015, Elsevier-Saunders.

Bhandari V, Naushad HS, Gupta RS: Protein based molecular markers provide reliable means to understand prokaryotic phylogeny and support darwinian mode of evolution, *Front Cell Infect Microbiol* 2:98, 2012.

Brock TD, Madigan M, Martinko J, et al.: *Biology of microorganisms*, Englewood Cliffs, NJ, 2009, Prentice Hall.

Clark AE, Kaleta EJ, Arora A, Wolk DM: Matrix-assisted laser desorption ionization time-of-flight mass spectrometry: a fundamental shift in the routine practice of clinical microbiology, *Clin Microbiol Rev* 26:547–603, 2013.

Cleary J, Sanchez L: *Large scale MALDI-T of imaging of metabolites from filamentous fungi*, Billerica MA, 2018, Ebook Bruker Daltonics Inc.

Dworkin M, Falkow S, Rosenberg E, et al.: *The prokaryotes: a handbook on the biology of bacteria: ecophysiology, isolation, identification, applications* (Vol. 1–4). New York, 2006, Springer.

Figueras M, Beaz-Hidalgo R, Hossain MJ, Liles MR: Taxonomic affiliation of new genomes should be verified using average nucleotide identity and multilocus phylogenetic analysis, *Genome Announc* 2(6):e00927–e01014, 2014, https://doi.org/10.1128/genomeA.00927-14.

Golf O, Strittmatter N, Karancsi T, et al.: Rapid evaporative ionization mass spectrometry imaging platform for direct mapping from bulk tissue and bacterial growth media, *Anal Chem* 87:2527–2534, 2015.

Jorgensen J, Pfaller M, Carroll K, et al.: *Manual of clinical microbiology*, ed 11, Washington, DC, 2015, ASM Press.

Kook JK, Park SN, Lim YK, et al.: Genome-based reclassification of fusobacterium nucleatum subspecies at the species level, *Curr Microbiol* 74:1137–1147, 2017.

Martins MD, Machado-de-Lima NM, Branco LHZ: Polyphasic approach using multilocus analyses supports the establishment of the new aerophytic cyanobacterial genus *Pycnacronema (Coleofas ciculaceae, Oscillatoriales)*, *J Phycol* 55:146–159, 2018, https://doi.org/10.1111/jpy.12805.

Mohr KI, Wolf C, Nübel U, et al.: A polyphasic approach leads to seven new species of cellulose decomposing genus sorangium, *Sorangium ambruticinum* sp. *nov., sorangium arenae* sp. *nov., sorangium bulgaricum* sp. *nov., sorangium dawidii* sp. *nov, sorangium kjenyense* sp. *nov., sorangium orientale* sp. *nov.* and *sorangium richenbachii* sp. *nov, Int J Syst Evol Microbiol* 68:3576–3586, 2018.

Parker CT, Tindall BJ, Garrity GM: International code of nomenclature for prokaryotes, *Int J Syst Evol Microbiol* 69:S1–S111, 2019, Available at http://ijs.microbiologyresearch.org/content/journal/ijsem/10.1099/ijsem.0.000778#tab9.

2

Bacterial Genetics, Metabolism, and Structure

Microbial genetics, metabolism, and structure are the keys to microbial viability and survival. These processes involve numerous pathways that are widely varied, often complicated, and frequently interactive. Essentially, survival requires nutrients and energy to fuel the synthesis of materials necessary to grow, propagate, and carry out other metabolic processes (Fig. 2.1). Although the goal of survival is the same for all organisms, the strategies microorganisms use to accomplish this vary substantially.

Knowledge regarding genetic, metabolic, and structural characteristics of microorganisms provides the basis for understanding almost every aspect of diagnostic microbiology, including:

- The mechanisms by which microorganisms cause disease
- The development and implementation of techniques for microbial detection, cultivation, identification, and characterization

- Antimicrobial action and resistance
- The development and implementation of tests for the detection of antimicrobial resistance
- Potential strategies for disease therapy and control of microorganisms

Microorganisms vary significantly in their genomic and metabolic pathways and therefore structure. A detailed consideration of these differences is beyond the scope of this textbook. Therefore, a generalized description of bacterial systems is used as a model to discuss microbial physiology and structure. Information regarding characteristics of fungi, parasites, and viruses can be found in subsequent chapters for each specific taxonomic group.

Bacterial Genetics

Genetics, the process of heredity and variation, is the starting point from which all other cellular pathways, functions, and structures originate. The ability of a microorganism to maintain viability, adapt, multiply, and cause disease is determined by the organism's genetic composition. The three major aspects of microbial genetics that require discussion include:

- The structure and organization of genetic material
- Replication and expression of genetic information
- The mechanisms by which genetic information is altered and exchanged among bacteria

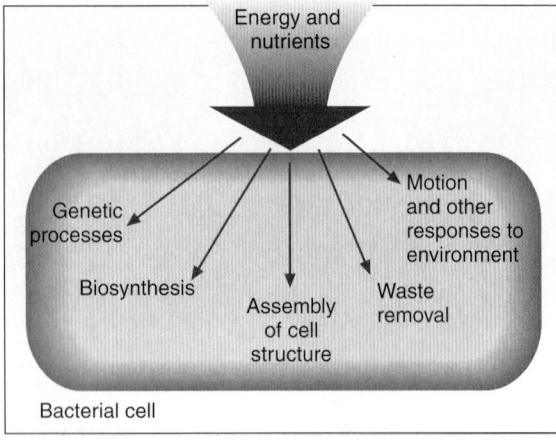

• **Fig. 2.1** General overview of bacterial cellular processes.

Nucleic Acid Structure and Organization

For all living entities, hereditary information resides or is encoded in nucleic acids. The two major classes of nucleic acids are **deoxyribonucleic acid (DNA),** which is the most common macromolecule that encodes genetic information, and **ribonucleic acid (RNA).** In some forms, RNA encodes genetic information for various viruses; in other forms, RNA plays an essential role in several of the genetic processes in prokaryotic and eukaryotic cells, including the regulation and transfer of information. Prokaryotic, or prenuclear, organisms do not have membrane-bound organelles, and the cells' genetic material is therefore not enclosed in a nucleus. Eukaryotic, or "true nucleus," organisms have the genetic material enclosed in a nuclear envelope.

Nucleotide Structure and Sequence

DNA consists of deoxyribose sugars connected by phosphodiester bonds (Fig. 2.2A). The bases that are covalently linked to each deoxyribose sugar are the key to the **genetic code** within the DNA molecule. The four nitrogenous bases

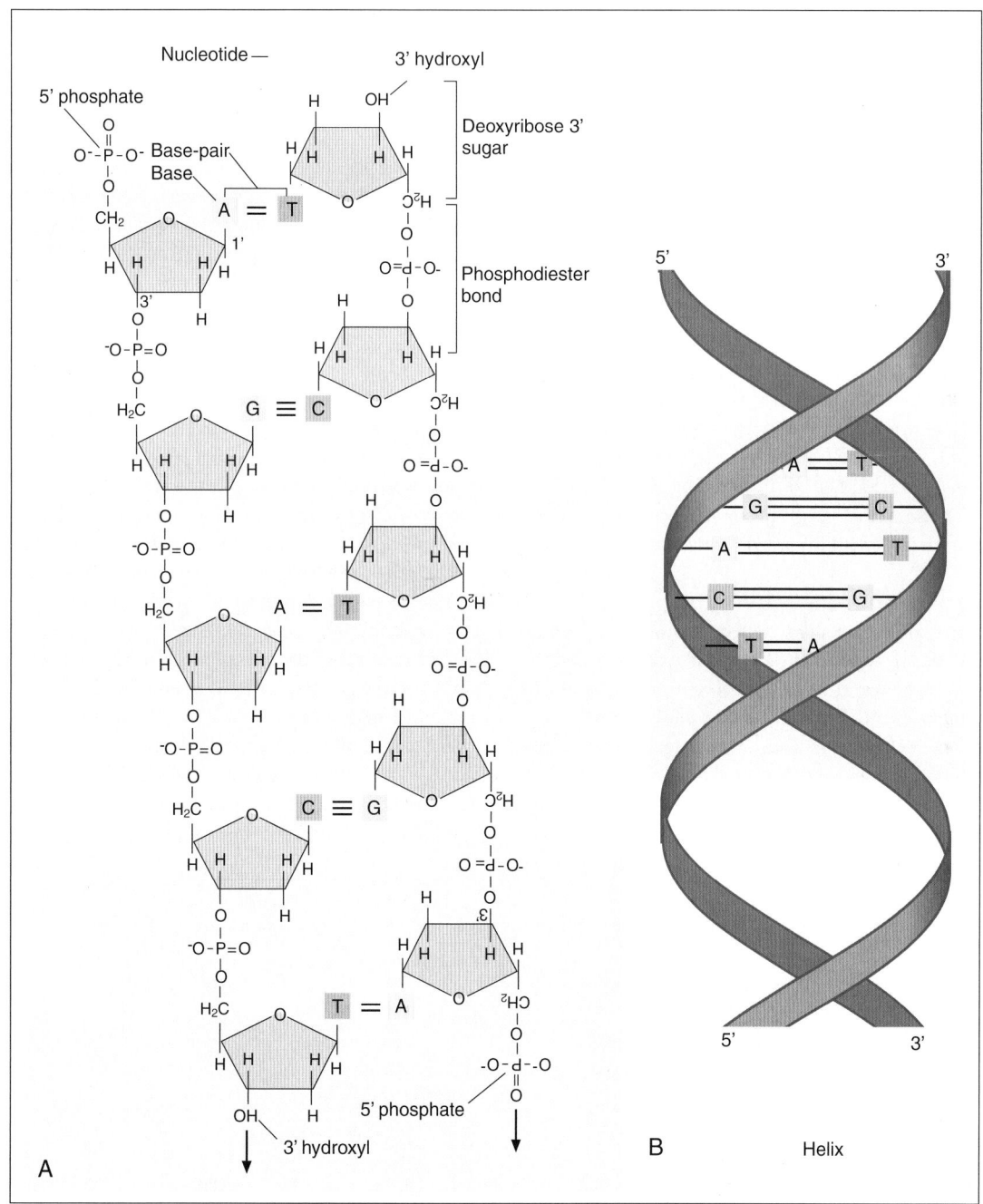

• **Fig. 2.2** (A) Molecular structure of deoxyribonucleic acid (DNA) depicting nucleotide structure, phosphodiester bonds connecting nucleotides, and complementary base pairing (*A,* adenine; *T,* thymine; *G,* guanine; *C,* cytosine) between antiparallel nucleic acid strands. (B) 5′ and 3′ antiparallel polarity and double-helix configuration of DNA.

include two **purines**, adenine (A) and guanine (G), and the two **pyrimidines**, cytosine (C) and thymine (T) (Fig. 2.3). In RNA, uracil replaces thymine. The combined sugar, phosphate, and a base form a single unit referred to as a **nucleotide** (adenosine triphosphate [ATP], guanine triphosphate [GTP], cytosine triphosphate [CTP], and thymine triphosphate [TTP] or uridine triphosphate [UTP]). DNA and RNA are nucleotide polymers (i.e., chains or strands), and the order of bases along a DNA or RNA strand is known as the **base sequence.** This sequence provides the information that codes for the proteins that will be synthesized by microbial cells; that is, the sequence is the genetic code.

Deoxyribonucleic Acid Molecular Structure

The intact DNA molecule is composed of two nucleotide polymers. Each strand has a 5′ (prime) phosphate and a 3′ (prime) hydroxyl terminus (Fig. 2.2A). The two strands run **antiparallel,** with the 5′ of one strand opposed to the 3′ terminal of the other. The strands are also complementary. This adherence to A-T and G-C base pairing results in a double-stranded DNA (dsDNA) molecule (double helix). The two antiparallel single strands of DNA form a "twisted ladder" structure (Fig. 2.2B). In addition, the dedicated base pairs (bp) provide the format for consistent replication and expression of the genetic code. In contrast to DNA, which carries the genetic code, RNA rarely exists as a double-stranded molecule. There are four major types of RNA (**messenger RNA [mRNA], transfer RNA [tRNA], and ribosomal RNA [rRNA]**) along with a variety of **noncoding RNA (ncRNA)** molecules such as microRNA (miRNA) that play key roles in posttranscriptional regulation of gene expression.

Genes and the Genetic Code

A DNA sequence that encodes a specific product (RNA or protein) is defined as a **gene.** Thousands of genes in an organism encode messages or blueprints for the production of one or more proteins and RNA products that play essential metabolic roles in the cell. All the genes in an organism comprise the organism's **genome.** The genome of a microorganism includes the chromosomes and the **mobilome** (extrachromosomal mobile genetic elements). The size of a gene and an entire genome are usually expressed in the number of bp present (e.g., kilobases [103 bases], megabases [106 bases]).

Certain genes are widely distributed among various organisms, whereas others are limited to a particular species. In addition, the base pair sequence for individual genes may be highly conserved (i.e., show limited sequence differences among different organisms) or be widely variable. As discussed in Chapter 8, these similarities and differences in genetic content and sequences are the basis for the development of molecular methods used to detect, identify, and characterize microorganisms.

Chromosomes

The genome is organized into discrete elements known as **chromosomes.** The set of genes within a given chromosome is arranged in a linear fashion, but the number of genes per chromosome is variable. Similarly, although the number of chromosomes per cell is consistent for a given species, this number varies considerably among species. For example, human cells contain 23 pairs (i.e., diploid) of chromosomes, whereas bacteria contain a single, unpaired (i.e., haploid) chromosome.

Bacteria are classified as prokaryotes; therefore the chromosome is not located in a membrane-bound organelle (i.e., **nucleus**). The bacterial chromosome contains the genes essential for viability and exists as a double-stranded, closed, circular macromolecule. The molecule is extensively folded and twisted (i.e., supercoiled) to fit within the confined space of the bacterial cell. The linearized, unsupercoiled chromosome of the bacterium *Escherichia coli* is approximately 130 μm long, but it fits within a cell 1 × 3 μm; this attests to the extreme compact structure of the supercoiled bacterial chromosome. For genes in the compacted chromosome to be expressed and replicated, unwinding or relaxation of the molecule is required.

In contrast to the bacterial chromosome, the chromosomes of parasites and fungi number more than one per cell, are linear, and are housed within a membrane-bound organelle (the nucleus) of the cell. This difference is a major criterion for classifying bacteria as prokaryotes and fungi and parasites as eukaryotes. The genetic makeup of a virus may consist of DNA or RNA contained within a protein coat rather than a cell.

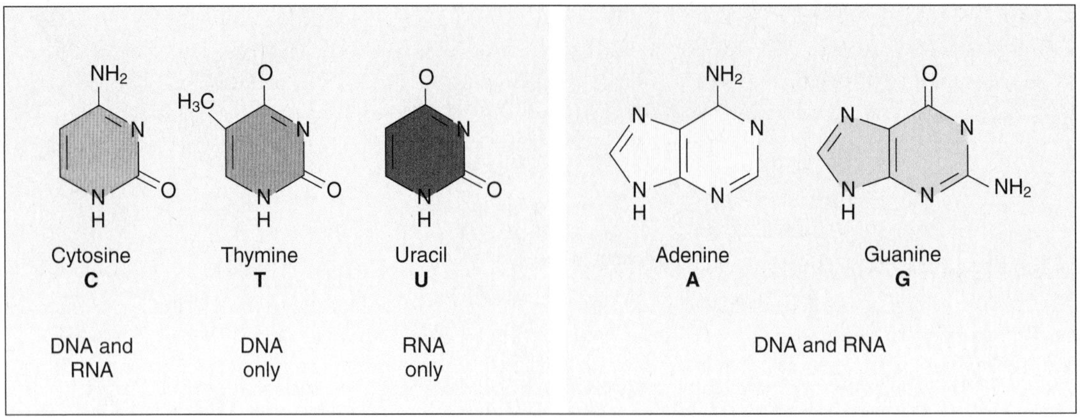

• **Fig. 2.3** Molecular structure of nucleic acid bases. *DNA*, Deoxyribonucleic acid; *RNA*, ribonucleic acid. Pyrimidines: cytosine, thymine, and uracil. Purines: adenine and guanine.

Nonchromosomal Elements (Mobilome)

Although the bacterial chromosome represents the majority of a cell's genome, not all genes are confined to the chromosome. Many genes may also be located on **plasmids** and **transposable elements.** Both of these extrachromosomal elements are able to replicate and encode information for the production of various cellular products. Many of these elements replicate by integration into the host chromosome, whereas others, referred to as **episomes,** are capable of replication independently of the host chromosome. Although considered part of the bacterial genome, they are not as stable as the chromosome and may be lost during cellular replication, often without any detrimental effects on the viability of the cell.

Plasmids exist as double-stranded, closed, circular, autonomously replicating extrachromosomal genetic elements ranging in size from 1 to 2 kilobases up to 1 megabase or more. The number of plasmids per bacterial cell varies extensively, and each plasmid is composed of several genes. Some genes encode products that mediate plasmid replication and transfer between bacterial cells, whereas others encode products that provide a specialized function, such as a determinant of antimicrobial resistance or a unique metabolic process. Unlike most chromosomal genes, plasmid genes do not usually encode for products essential for viability. Plasmids, in whole or in part, may also become incorporated into the chromosome.

Transposable elements are pieces of DNA that move from one genetic element to another, from plasmid to chromosome or vice versa. Unlike plasmids, many are unable to replicate independently and do not exist as separate entities in the bacterial cell. The two types of transposable elements are the **simple transposon** or **insertion sequence (IS)** and the **composite or complex transposon.** Insertion sequences are limited to containing the genes that encode information required for movement from one site in the genome to another. Composite transposons are cassettes (grouping of genes) flanked by insertion sequences. The internal gene embedded in the IS encodes for an accessory function, such as antimicrobial resistance. Plasmids and transposable elements coexist with chromosomes in the cells of many bacterial species. These extrachromosomal elements play a key role in the exchange of genetic material throughout the bacterial microbiosphere, including genetic exchange among clinically relevant bacteria.

DNA Replication

Replication

Bacteria multiply by **binary fission** (a form of cell division), resulting in the production of two daughter cells from one parent cell. As part of this process, the genome must be replicated and each daughter cell receives an identical copy of functional DNA. **Replication** is a complex process mediated by various enzymes, such as DNA polymerase and cofactors; replication must occur quickly and accurately. For descriptive purposes, replication may be considered in four stages (Fig. 2.4):

1. Unwinding or relaxation of the chromosome's super-coiled DNA
2. Separation of the complementary strands of the parental DNA. Each strand may serve as a **template** (i.e., pattern) for synthesis of new DNA strands, referred to as **semiconservative replication**
3. Synthesis of the new (i.e., daughter) DNA strands
4. Termination of replication, releasing two identical chromosomes, one for each daughter cell

Relaxation of supercoiled chromosomal DNA is required, which permits the enzymes and cofactors involved in replication access to the DNA molecule at the site where the replication process will originate (i.e., origin of replication). The **origin of replication** (a specific sequence of approximately 300 bp) is recognized by several initiation proteins, followed by the separation of the complementary strands of parental DNA. Each parental strand serves as a template for the synthesis of a new complementary daughter strand. The site of active replication is referred to as the **replication fork;** two bidirectional forks are involved in the replication process. Each replication fork moves through the parent DNA molecule in opposite directions as a bidirectional process. Activity at each replication fork involves different cofactors and enzymes, with **DNA polymerase** playing a central role. Using each parental strand as a template, DNA polymerase adds nucleotide bases to each growing daughter strand in a sequence that is complementary to the base sequence of the template (parent) strand. The complementary bases of each strand are then held together by hydrogen bonding between nucleotides and the hydrophobic nature of the nitrogenous bases. The new nucleotides can be added only to the 3′ hydroxyl end of the growing strand. The synthesis for each daughter strand occurs in the 5′ to 3′ direction.

Termination of replication occurs when the replication forks meet. The result is two complete chromosomes, each containing two complementary strands, one of parental origin and one newly synthesized daughter strand. Although the time required for replication can vary among bacteria, the process generally takes approximately 20 to 40 minutes in rapidly growing bacteria such as *E. coli.* The replication time for a particular bacterial strain can vary depending on environmental conditions, such as the availability of nutrients or the presence of toxic substances (e.g., antimicrobial agents).

Expression of Genetic Information

Gene **expression** is the processing of information encoded in genetic elements (i.e., chromosomes, plasmids, and transposons) that results in the production of biochemically functional molecules, including RNA and proteins. The overall process of gene expression is composed of two steps, **transcription** and **translation.** Gene expression

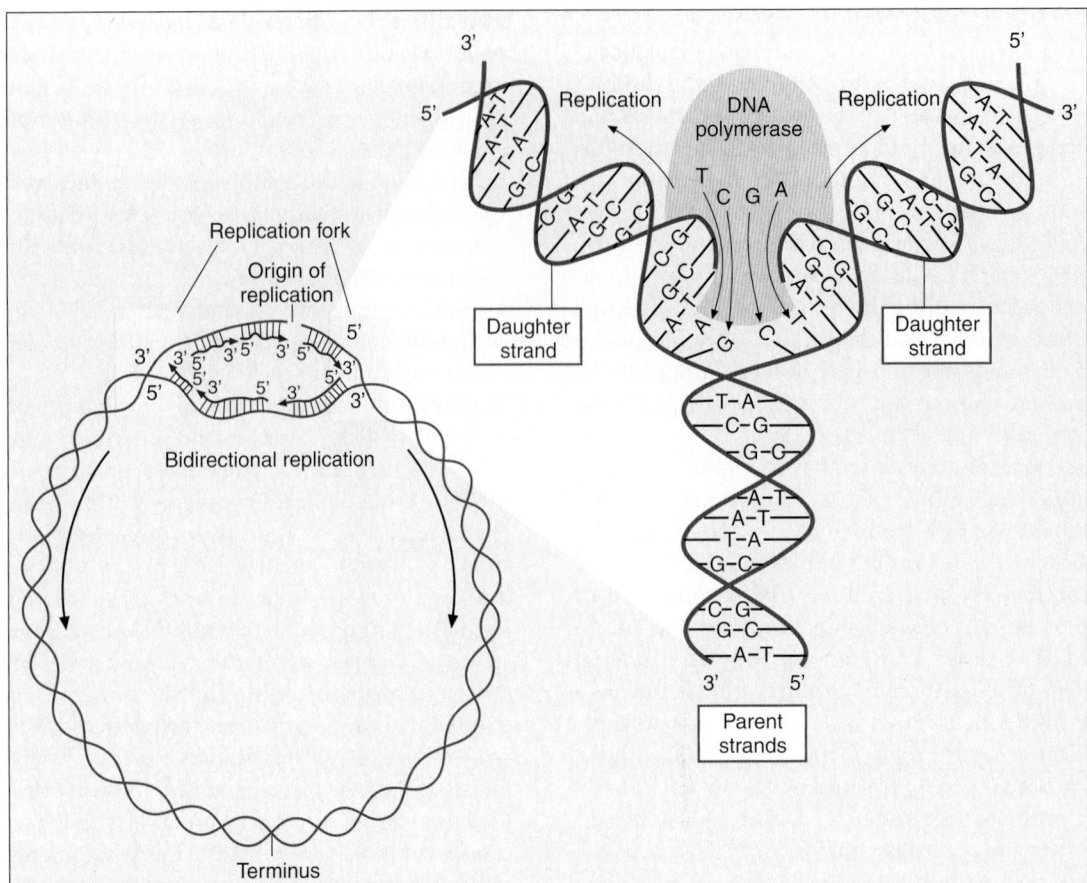

• **Fig. 2.4** Bacterial deoxyribonucleic acid (DNA) replication with bidirectional movement of two replication forks from the origin of replication. Each parent strand serves as a template for production of a complementary daughter strand and, eventually, two identical chromosomes.

requires various components, including a DNA template representing a single gene or cluster of genes, various enzymes and cofactors, and RNA molecules of specific structure and function.

Transcription

Gene expression begins with transcription. During transcription the DNA base sequence of the gene (i.e., the genetic code) is converted into an mRNA molecule that is complementary to the gene's DNA sequence (Fig. 2.5). Usually only one of the two DNA strands (**sense strand**) encodes for a functional gene product. This same strand is the template for mRNA synthesis.

RNA polymerase is the enzyme central to the transcription process. The enzyme is composed of four protein subunits and a sigma (σ) factor. **Sigma factors** are required for the RNA polymerase to identify the appropriate site on the DNA template where transcription of mRNA is initiated. This initiation site is also known as the **promoter sequence**. The remainder of the enzyme functions to unwind the dsDNA at the promoter sequence and use the DNA strand as a template to sequentially add ribonucleotides (ATP, GTP, UTP, and CTP) to form the growing mRNA strand.

Transcription proceeds in a 5′ to 3′ direction. However, in mRNA, the TTP of DNA is replaced with UTP. TTP

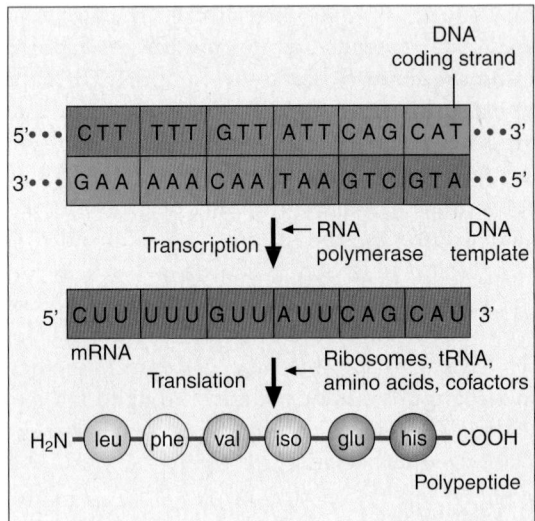

• **Fig. 2.5** Overview of gene expression components: transcription for production of messenger ribonucleic acid (mRNA) and translation for production of a polypeptide (protein). *DNA,* Deoxyribonucleic acid; *RNA,* ribonucleic acid; *tRNA,* transfer RNA.

contains thymine, and UTP contains uracil. Both molecules contain a heterocyclic ring and are classified as pyrimidines. During synthesis and modification of these molecules, a portion of the molecules are dehydroxylated, forming a

2′-deoxynucleotide monophosphate. The dehydroxylated uracil monophosphate (dUMP) is then methylated, forming dehydroxylated thymine monophosphate (dTMP). After phosphorylation, thymine is found only in the final state as deoxythymidine and therefore cannot be incorporated into an RNA molecule. Synthesis of the single-stranded mRNA product ends when specific nucleotide base sequences on the DNA template are encountered. Termination of transcription may be facilitated by a rho (a prokaryotic protein) cofactor or an intrinsic termination sequence. Both of these mechanisms disrupt the mRNA-RNA polymerase template DNA complex.

In bacteria, the mRNA molecules that result from the transcription process are **polycistronic;** that is, they encode for several gene products. Polycistronic mRNA may encode several genes whose products (proteins) are involved in a single or closely related cellular function. When a cluster of genes is under the control of a single promoter sequence, the gene group is referred to as an **operon.**

The transcription process not only produces mRNA but also tRNA, rRNA, and regulatory non coding (ncRNA) molecules. All types of RNA molecules have key roles in protein synthesis. To initiate transcription, accessory factors are needed to localize the RNA polymerase to the promoter upstream of the coding sequence. In bacteria, the σ factor binds to the RNA polymerase and recognizes the gene-specific promotor. In some bacteria a small regulatory RNA (sRNA), 6S RNA, binds the sigma factor to repress transcription in the late stationary phase of bacterial growth. The 6S RNA binds and forms a bulge or loop. The loop serves as an RNA-dependent site for RNA synthesis. The RNA synthesized from the loop is referred to as pRNA. When sufficient pRNA is produced, it causes the 6S RNA to detach from the promotor, permitting transcription to continue.

Transfer RNA (tRNA) binds to the A site in the ribosome and delivers the appropriate amino acid during elongation. However, tRNAs exist in many more diverse forms than once believed. In bacteria, the initiation codon codes for an N-formylmethionine. This modified amino acid is never placed inside the coding sequence of a bacterial protein. In other words, there are two forms of tRNA that are produced in bacteria that are cable of carrying methionine. One is the initiator tRNA^Met and the other is the elongation tRNA^Met. The elongation tRNA^Met binds to the A site of the ribosome, whereas the initiation tRNA^Met is capable of binding only to the P site within the ribosome. The binding of the elongation-specific tRNA is controlled by transcription elongation factor 1.

Ribosomal RNA, specifically the 16S rRNA, has historically been associated with classification of organisms based on evolutionary relatedness. The 16S rRNA is present in all organisms and is responsible for catalyzing the peptidyl transferase reaction during protein synthesis. A very small portion of the molecule is capable of undergoing genetic changes without deleterious effects to the transcription process, providing a means to monitor the evolutionary development of bacterial species.

In addition to the differences in tRNA specificity, bacteria have developed numerous mechanisms to regulate gene transcription and respond to the environment, including transcriptional and posttranscriptional regulation. Many sensory and regulatory RNA molecules have now been identified that serve as RNA thermosensors and riboswitches. These molecules may undergo structural alterations during temperature changes or serve as antisense RNAs and sRNAs that bind to either nucleic acid–binding proteins modulating their activity or directly to mRNA sequences to suppress and alter gene expression. This reversible regulation is clearly evident in the expression of virulence genes in many known pathogens including *E. coli, Shigella* spp., and *Yersinia* spp. The global changes of RNA expression within the transcriptome of a pathogenic bacteria allows the organism to rapidly adjust to changes in the environment associated with temperature, ionic conditions, oxygen conditions, pH, calcium, iron, and other metals to maintain growth and survival.

Translation

The next phase in gene expression, translation, involves protein synthesis. Through this process the genetic code in mRNA molecules is translated into specific amino acid sequences that are responsible for protein structure and function (Fig. 2.5).

The process of protein translation requires the use of a genetic alphabet or code. The code consists of triplets of nucleotide bases, referred to as **codons;** each codon encodes for a specific amino acid. Because there are 64 different codons for 20 amino acids, an amino acid can be encoded by more than one codon (Table 2.1). Each codon is specific for a single amino acid. The codon sequences in mRNA direct which amino acids are added and in what order. Translation ensures that proteins with proper structure and function are produced. Errors in the process can result in aberrant proteins that are nonfunctional, emphasizing the need for translation to be well controlled and accurate.

To accomplish the task of translation, intricate interactions between mRNA, tRNA, and rRNA are required. Sixty different standard types of tRNA molecules are responsible for transferring different amino acids from intracellular locations to the site of protein synthesis. These molecules, which have a structure that resembles an inverted *t*, contain one **anticodon** (sequence recognition site) for binding to specific codons (3-base sequences) on the mRNA molecule (Fig. 2.6). A second site binds specific amino acids, the building blocks of proteins. Each amino acid is joined to a specific tRNA molecule through the enzymatic activity of aminoacyl-tRNA synthetases. Transfer RNA molecules use the codons of the mRNA molecule as the template for precisely delivering a specific amino acid for polymerization. This process occurs in **ribosomes**, which are compact nucleoproteins, composed of rRNA and proteins. They are central to translation, assisting with the coupling of all required components and controlling the translational process.

TABLE 2.1 The Genetic Code as Expressed by Triplet-Base Sequences of Messenger Ribonucleic Acid[a]

Codon	Amino Acid	Codon	Amino Acid	Codon	Amino Acid	Codon	Amino Acid
UUU	Phenylalanine	CUU	Leucine	GUU	Valine	AUU	Isoleucine
UUC	Phenylalanine	CUC	Leucine	GUC	Valine	AUC	Isoleucine
UUG	Leucine	CUG	Leucine	GUG	Valine	AUG (start)[b]	Methionine
UUA	Leucine	CUA	Leucine	GUA	Valine	AUA	Isoleucine
UCU	Serine	CCU	Proline	GCU	Alanine	ACU	Threonine
UCC	Serine	CCC	Proline	GCC	Alanine	ACC	Threonine
UCG	Serine	CCG	Proline	GCG	Alanine	ACG	Threonine
UCA	Serine	CCA	Proline	GCA	Alanine	ACA	Threonine
UGU	Cysteine	CGU	Arginine	GGU	Glycine	AGU	Serine
UGC	Cysteine	CGC	Arginine	GGC	Glycine	AGC	Serine
UGG	Tryptophan	CGG	Arginine	GGG	Glycine	AGG	Arginine
UGA	None (stop signal)	CGA	Arginine	GGA	Glycine	AGA	Arginine
UAU	Tyrosine	CAU	Histidine	GAU	Aspartic	AAU	Asparagine
UAC	Tyrosine	CAC	Histidine	GAC	Aspartic	AAC	Asparagine
UAG	None (stop signal)	CAG	Glutamine	GAG	Glutamic	AAG	Lysine
UAA	None (stop signal)	CAA	Glutamine	GAA	Glutamic	AAA	Lysine

[a]The codons in deoxyribonucleic acid (DNA) are complementary to those given here. Thus U is complementary to the A in DNA, C is complementary to G, G to C, and A to T. The nucleotide on the left is at the 5′ end of the triplet.
[b]AUG codes for N-formylmethionine at the beginning of messenger ribonucleic acid (mRNA) in bacteria.
Modified from Brock TD, Madigan M, Martinko J, et al., eds. *Biology of Microorganisms*. Upper Saddle River, NJ: Prentice Hall; 2009.

Translation, diagrammatically shown in Fig. 2.6, involves three steps: **initiation, elongation,** and **termination.** After termination, bacterial proteins often undergo posttranslational modifications as a final step in protein synthesis.

Initiation begins with the association of ribosomal subunits, mRNA, formylmethionine (f-met) tRNA (carrying the initial amino acid of the protein to be synthesized), and various initiation factors (Fig. 2.6A). Assembly of the complex begins at a specific 3- to 9-base sequence (Shine-Dalgarno sequence) on the mRNA approximately 10 bp upstream of the AUG start codon. After the initial complex has been formed, addition of individual amino acids begins.

Elongation involves tRNAs and a host of elongation factors that mediate the addition of amino acids in a specific sequence dictated by the codon on the mRNA molecule (Fig. 2.6B and C and Table 2.1). As the mRNA molecule threads through the ribosome in a 5′ to 3′ direction, peptide bonds are formed between adjacent amino acids, still bound by their respective tRNA molecules in the peptide (P) and acceptor (A) sites of the ribosome. During the process, the forming peptide is moved to the P site, and the 5′ tRNA is released from the exit (E) site. This movement vacates the A site, which contains the codon specific for the next amino acid, so that the incoming tRNA–amino acid can join the complex (Fig. 2.6C).

Because multiple proteins encoded on an mRNA strand can be translated at the same time, multiple ribosomes may be simultaneously associated with one mRNA molecule. Such an arrangement is referred to as a **polysome;** its appearance resembles a string of pearls.

Termination, the final step in translation, occurs when the ribosomal A site encounters a stop or non sense codon that does not specify an amino acid (i.e., a "stop signal"; Table 2.1). At this point, the protein synthesis complex disassociates and the ribosomes are available for another round of translation. After termination, most proteins must undergo modification, such as folding or enzymatic trimming, so that protein function, transportation, or incorporation into various cellular structures can be accomplished. This process is referred to as **posttranslational modification.**

Regulation and Control of Gene Expression

The vital role that gene expression and protein synthesis play in the survival of cells dictates that bacteria judiciously

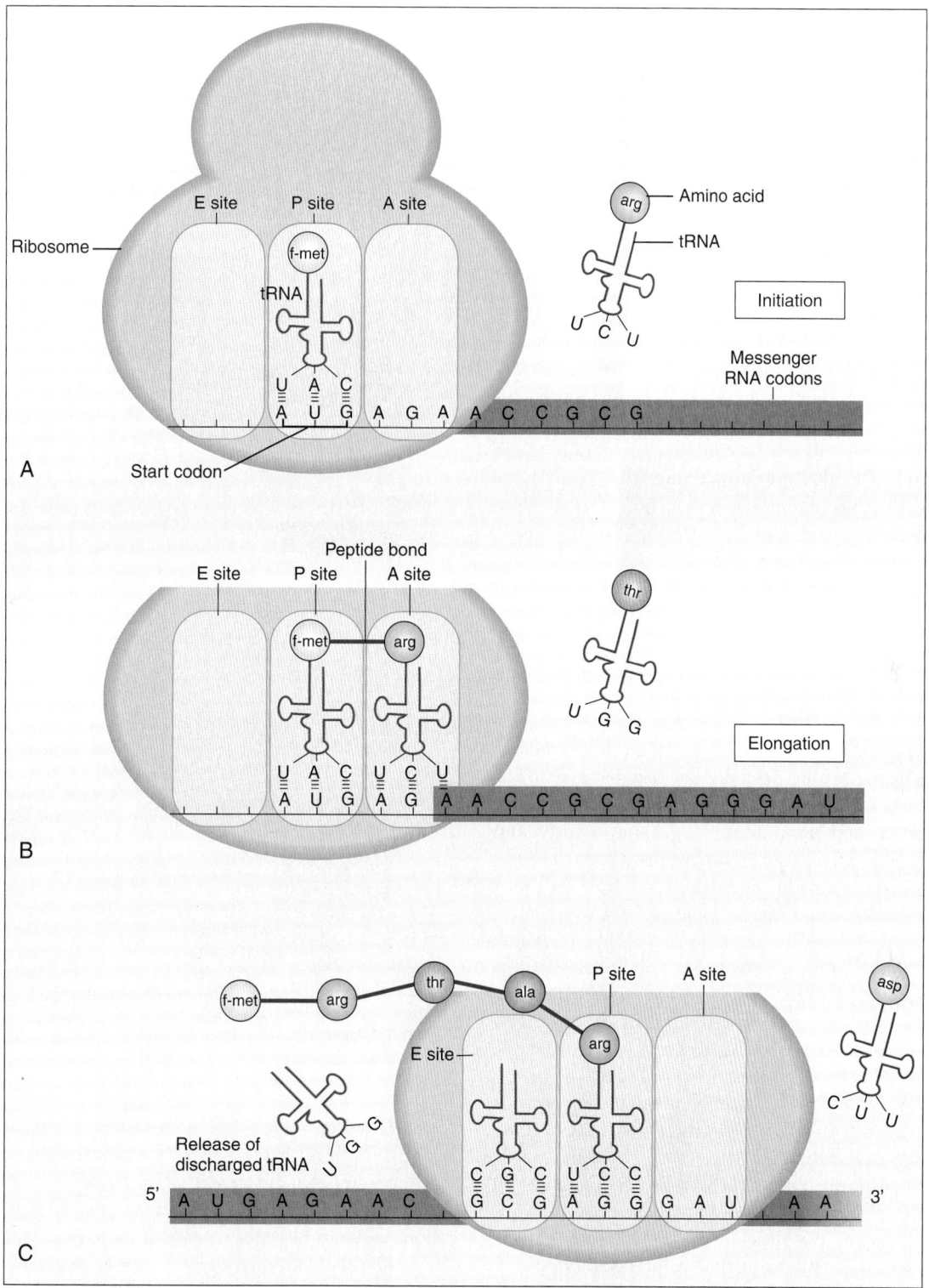

• **Fig. 2.6** Overview of translation in which messenger ribonucleic acid (mRNA) serves as the template for the assembly of amino acids into polypeptides. The three steps include initiation (A), elongation (B and C), and termination (not shown). *tRNA,* transfer RNA.

control these processes. The cell must regulate gene expression and control the activities of gene products so that a physiologic balance is maintained. Regulation and control are also key factors. These are highly complex mechanisms by which single-cell organisms are able to respond and adapt to environmental challenges, regardless of whether the challenges occur naturally or result from medical intervention (e.g., antibiotics).

Regulation occurs at one of three levels of information transfer from the gene expression and protein synthesis pathway: **transcriptional, translational,** or **posttranslational.** The most common is transcriptional regulation. Because direct interactions with genes and their ability to be transcribed to mRNA are involved, transcriptional regulation is also referred to as **genetic control.** Genes that encode enzymes involved in **anabolic** processes (biosynthesis) and genes that encode enzymes for **catabolic** processes (biodegradation) are examples of genetic control.

In general, genes that encode anabolic enzymes for the synthesis of particular products are **repressed** (i.e., are not transcribed and therefore are not expressed) in the presence of the gene end product. This strategy prevents waste and overproduction of products that are already present in sufficient supply. In this system, the product acts as a corepressor that forms a complex with a repressor molecule. In the absence of corepressor product (i.e., gene product), transcription occurs (Fig. 2.7A). When present in sufficient quantity, the product forms a complex with the repressor. The complex then binds to a specific base region of the gene sequence known as the **operator region** (Fig. 2.7B). This binding blocks RNA polymerase progression from the promoter sequence and inhibits transcription. As the supply of product (corepressor) dwindles, an insufficient amount remains to form a complex with the repressor. The operator region is no longer bound to the repressor molecule. Transcription of the genes for the anabolic enzymes commences and continues until a sufficient supply of end product is again available.

In contrast to repression, genes that encode catabolic enzymes are usually **induced;** that is, transcription occurs when the substrate to be degraded by enzymatic action is present. Production of degradative enzymes in the absence of substrates would be a waste of cellular energy and resources. When the substrate is absent in an inducible system, a repressor binds to the operator sequence of the DNA and blocks transcription of the gene for the degradative enzyme (Fig. 2.7C). In the presence of an inducer, which often is the target substrate for degradation, a complex is formed between the inducer and the repressor that results in the release of the repressor from the operator site, allowing transcription of the genes encoding the specific catabolic enzyme (Fig. 2.7D).

Certain genes are not regulated; that is, they are not under the control of inducers or repressors. These genes are referred to as **constitutive.** Because they usually encode for products that are essential for viability under almost all growth and environmental conditions, these genes are continuously expressed. In addition, not all regulation occurs at the genetic level (i.e., transcriptional regulation). For example, the production of some enzymes may be controlled at the protein synthesis (i.e., translational) level. The activities of other enzymes that have already been synthesized may be regulated at a posttranslational level; that is, certain catabolic or anabolic metabolites may directly interact with enzymes either to increase or to decrease their enzymatic activity.

Among different bacteria and even different genes in the same bacterium, the mechanisms by which inducers and corepressors are involved in gene regulation vary widely. Furthermore, bacterial cells have mechanisms to detect

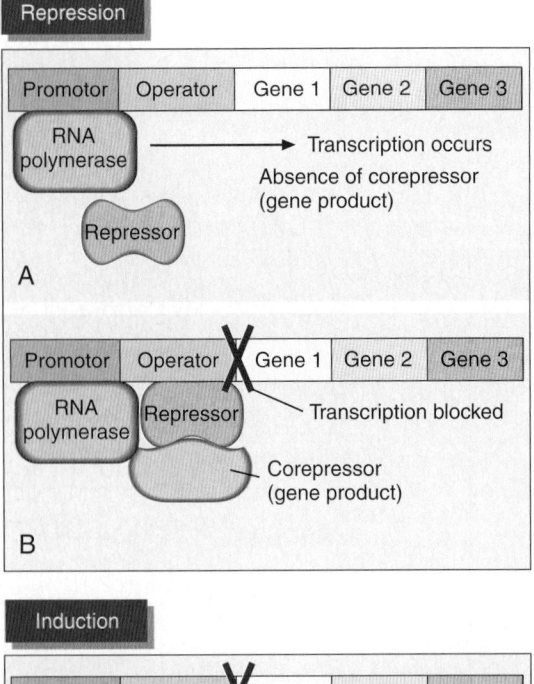

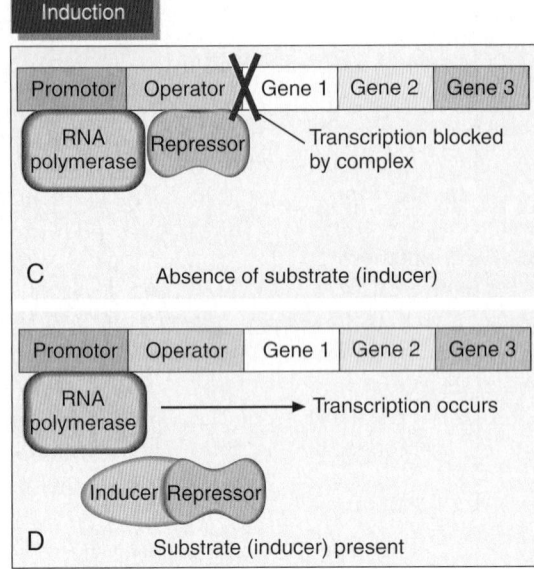

• **Fig. 2.7** Transcriptional control of gene expression. (A and B) Gene repression. (C and D) Induction. *RNA,* Ribonucleic acid.

environmental changes. These changes can generate signals that interact with the gene expression mechanism, ensuring that appropriate products are made in response to the environmental change. In addition, several complex interactions between different regulatory systems are found within a single cell. Such diversity and interdependence are necessary components of metabolism that allow an organism to respond to environmental changes in a rapid, well-coordinated, and appropriate way.

Genetic Exchange and Diversity

In eukaryotic organisms, genetic diversity is achieved by sexual reproduction, which allows for the mixing of genomes through genetic exchange. Bacteria multiply by simple binary cell division in which two identical daughter cells result by division of one parent cell. Each daughter cell receives the full genetic complement contained in the original parent cell. This process does not allow for the mixing of genes from other cells and leaves no means of achieving genetic diversity among bacterial progeny. Without genetic diversity and change, the essential ingredients for evolution are lost. However, microorganisms have been on earth for billions of years, and microbiologists have witnessed their ability to change as a result of exposure to chemicals (i.e., antibiotics) and environmental conditions (i.e., temperature or oxygenation). It is evident that these organisms are fully capable of evolving and altering their genetic composition.

Genetic alterations and diversity in bacteria are accomplished by three basic mechanisms: **mutation, genetic recombination,** and **genetic exchange,** with or without recombination. Throughout diagnostic microbiology and infectious diseases, there are numerous examples of the effect these genetic alteration and exchange mechanisms have on clinically relevant bacteria and the management of the infections they cause.

Mutation

Mutation is defined as an alteration in the original nucleotide sequence of a gene or genes within an organism's genome (i.e., a change in the organism's genotype). This alteration may involve a single DNA base in a gene, an entire gene, or several genes. Mutational changes in the sequence may arise spontaneously, perhaps by an error made during DNA replication. Alternatively, mutations may be induced by **mutagens** (i.e., chemical or physical factors) in the environment or by biologic factors, such as the introduction of foreign DNA into the cell. Alterations in the DNA base sequence can result in changes in the base sequence of mRNA during transcription. This, in turn, can affect the types and sequences of amino acids that will be incorporated into the protein during translation.

Depending on the site and extent of the mutation, various outcomes may affect the physiologic functions of the organism. For example, a mutation may be so devastating that it is lethal to the organism; therefore the mutation "dies" along with the organism. In another instance, the mutation may be silent so that no changes are detected in the organism's **phenotype** (i.e., observable properties). Alternatively, the mutation may result in a noticeable alteration in the organism's phenotype, and the change may provide the organism with a survival advantage. This outcome, in Darwinian terms, is the basis for prolonged survival and evolution. Nonlethal mutations are considered stable if they are passed on from one generation to another as an integral part of the cell's genotype (i.e., genetic composition). In addition, genes that have undergone stable mutations may also be transferred to other bacteria by one of the mechanisms of genetic exchange. In other instances, the mutation may be lost as a result of cellular repair mechanisms capable of restoring the original genotype and phenotype, or it may be lost spontaneously during subsequent cycles of DNA replication.

Genetic Recombination

Besides mutations, bacterial genotypes can be altered through **recombination.** In this process, a segment of DNA originating from one bacterial cell (i.e., the donor) enters a second bacterial cell (i.e., the recipient) and is exchanged with a DNA segment of the recipient's genome. This is also referred to as **homologous recombination,** because the pieces of DNA that are exchanged usually have extensive homology or similarities in their nucleotide sequences. Recombination involves a number of binding proteins, with the bacterial recombinase protein (RecA) playing a central role (Fig. 2.8A). RecA is capable of binding single-stranded DNA (ssDNA) to the complementary dsDNA, providing a mechanism for DNA repair and recombination to occur. After recombination, the recipient DNA consists of one original, unchanged strand and a second strand from the donor DNA fragment that has been recombined.

Recombination is a molecular event that occurs frequently in many varieties of bacteria, including most of the clinically relevant species, and it may involve any portion of the organism's genome. However, the recombination event may go unnoticed unless the exchange of DNA results in a distinct alteration in the phenotype. Nonetheless, recombination is a major means by which bacteria may achieve genetic diversity.

Genetic Exchange

An organism's ability to undergo recombination depends on the acquisition of "foreign" DNA from a donor cell. The three mechanisms by which bacteria physically exchange DNA are **transformation, transduction,** and **conjugation.**

Transformation

Transformation involves recipient cell uptake of naked (free) DNA released into the environment when another bacterial cell (i.e., the donor) dies and undergoes lysis (Fig. 2.8B). This genomic DNA exists as fragments in the environment. Certain bacteria are able to take up naked DNA from their surroundings; that is, they are able to undergo transformation. Such bacteria are said to be **competent.** Among the bacteria that cause human infections, competence is a characteristic commonly associated with members of the genera *Haemophilus, Streptococcus,* and *Neisseria.*

Once the donor DNA, usually as a single strand, gains access to the interior of the recipient cell, recombination with the recipient's homologous DNA can occur. The mixing of DNA between bacteria via transformation and recombination plays a major role in the development of antibiotic resistance and in the dissemination of genes that encode factors essential to an organism's ability to cause disease. In addition, genetic exchange by transformation is not limited to organisms of the same species, thus allowing important characteristics to be disseminated to a greater variety of medically important bacteria.

Transduction

Transduction is a second mechanism by which DNA from two bacteria may come together in one cell, thus allowing for recombination (Fig. 2.8C). This process is mediated

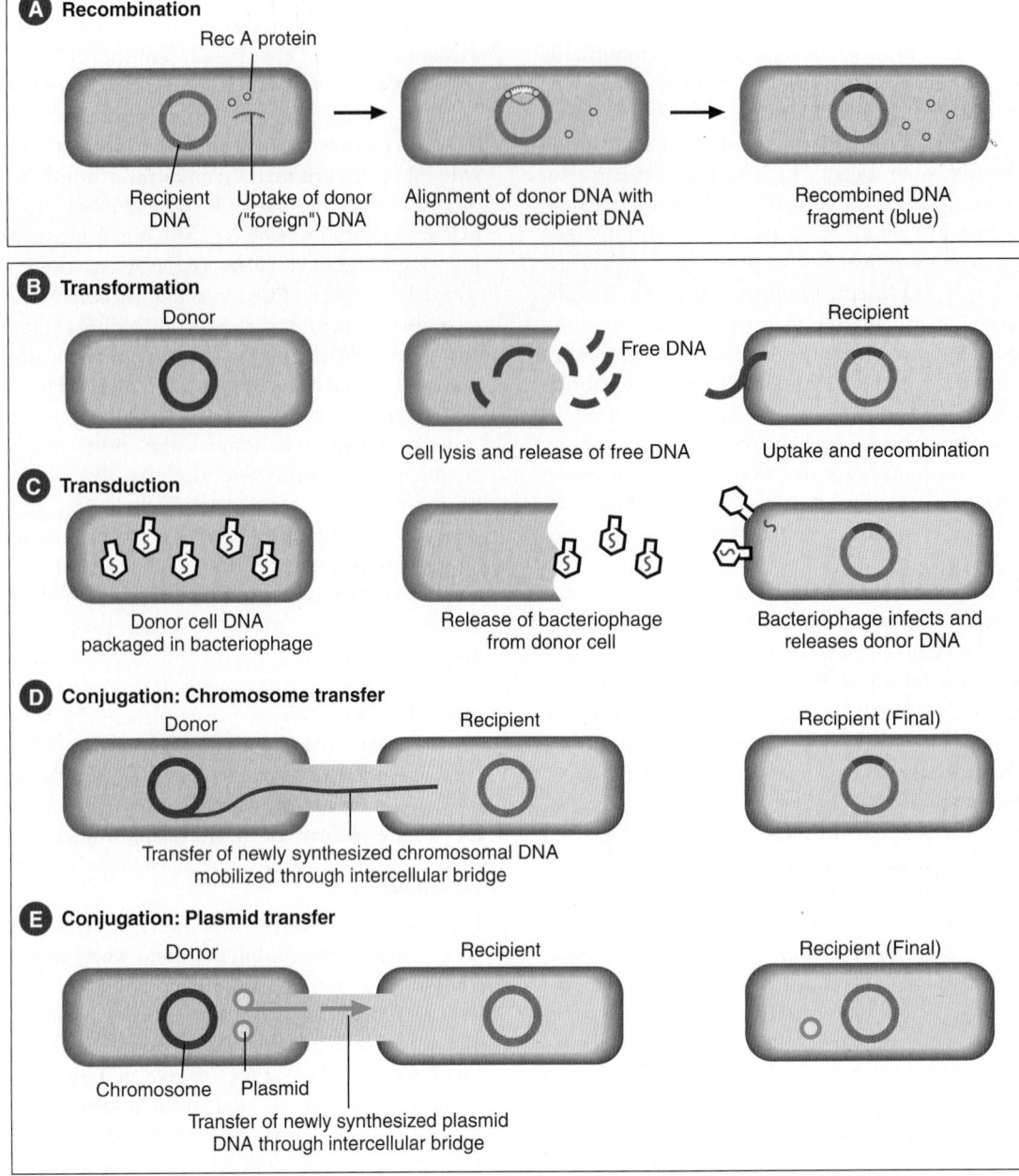

• **Fig. 2.8** (A) Genetic recombination. The mechanisms of genetic exchange between bacteria are transformation (B), transduction (C), and conjugational transfer of chromosomal (D) and plasmid (E) deoxyribonucleic acid *(DNA)*.

through viruses capable of infecting bacteria (i.e., **bacteriophages**). In their "life cycle," these viruses integrate their DNA into the bacterial cell's chromosome, where viral DNA replication and expression occur. When the production of viral products is complete, viral DNA is excised (cut) from the bacterial chromosome and packaged within a protein coat. The excision process is not always accurate, resulting in the removal of genetic material that contains both the bacterial and viral DNA. The newly formed recombinant virion (virus particle), along with the additional multiple virions, is released when the infected bacterial cell lyses.

The bacterial DNA may be randomly incorporated with viral DNA (**generalized transduction**), or it may be incorporated along with specific adjacent viral DNA (**specialized transduction**). In generalized transduction, the viral DNA is inserted randomly into any area of the bacterial genome. However, in specialized transduction, the virus inserts into particular genes in an organism based on sequence specificity and resulting in a higher frequency of genetic material in those regions being transferred through recombination. In either case, when the virus infects another bacterial cell, it releases its DNA, which includes the previously incorporated bacterial donor DNA. The newly infected cell is then the recipient of donor DNA introduced by the bacteriophage, and recombination between DNA from two different cells occurs.

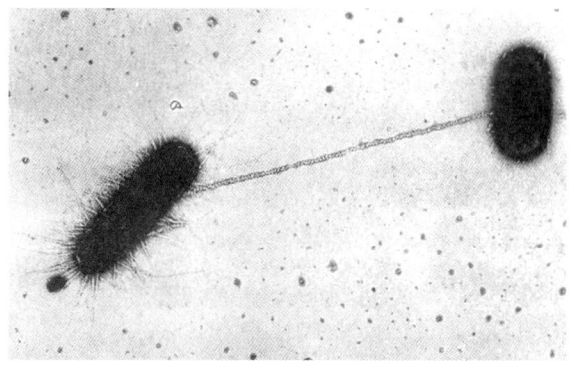

• **Fig. 2.9** Photomicrograph of an *Escherichia coli* sex pilus between a donor and a recipient cell. (From Brock TD, Madigan M, Martinko J, et al, eds. *Biology of Microorganisms.* Upper Saddle River, NJ: Prentice Hall; 2009.)

Conjugation

The third mechanism of DNA exchange between bacterial cells is conjugation. This process involves cell-to-cell contact and requires mobilization of the donor bacterium's chromosome or other mobile genetic element. The nature of intercellular contact is not well characterized in all bacterial species capable of conjugation. However, in *E. coli,* contact is mediated by a sex pilus (Fig. 2.9). The sex pilus originates from the donor and establishes a conjugative bridge that serves as the conduit for DNA transfer from donor to recipient cell. With intercellular contact established, mobilization of the genetic element is undertaken and involves DNA synthesis. One new DNA strand is produced by the donor and is passed to the recipient (Fig. 2.8D). The amount of DNA transferred depends on how long the cells are able to maintain contact, but usually only portions of the donor molecule are transferred. In any case the newly introduced DNA is then available to recombine with the recipient's genome.

In addition to chromosomal DNA, genes encoded in extrachromosomal genetic elements, such as plasmids and transposons, may be transferred by conjugation (Fig. 2.8E). Not all plasmids are capable of conjugative transfer, but for those that are, the donor plasmid usually is replicated so that the donor retains a copy of the plasmid transferred to the recipient. (See the discussion of the F plasmid in the section Cellular Appendages, later in the chapter.) Plasmid DNA may also become incorporated into the host cell's chromosome.

In contrast to plasmids, most transposons do not exist independently in the cell. Except when they are moving from one location to another, many transposons must be incorporated into the chromosome, plasmids, or both. These elements are often referred to as "jumping genes" because of their ability to change location within and even between the genomes of bacterial cells. **Transposition** is the process by which these genetic elements excise from one genomic location and insert into another. Transposons carry genes that have products that help to mediate the transposition process, in addition to genes that encode for other accessory characteristics, such as antimicrobial resistance.

Homologous recombination between the genes of plasmids or transposons and the host bacterium's chromosomal DNA may occur.

Plasmids and transposons play a key role in genetic diversity and the dissemination of genetic information among bacteria. Many characteristics that significantly alter the activities of clinically relevant bacteria are encoded and disseminated on these elements. Furthermore, as shown in Fig. 2.10, the variety of strategies that bacteria can use to mix and match genetic elements provides them with a tremendous capacity to genetically adapt to environmental changes, including those imposed by human medical practices. A good example of this is the emergence and widespread dissemination of resistance to antimicrobial agents among clinically important bacteria. Bacteria have used their capacity for disseminating genetic information to establish resistance to many of the commonly prescribed antibiotics. (See Chapter 10 for more information about antimicrobial resistance mechanisms.)

Bacterial Metabolism

Fundamentally, bacterial metabolism involves all the cellular processes required for the organism's survival and replication. Familiarity with bacterial metabolism is essential to understand bacterial interactions with human host cells, the mechanisms bacteria use to cause disease, and the basis of diagnostic microbiology (i.e., the tests and strategies used for laboratory identification of infectious organisms). Because metabolism is an extensive and complicated topic, this section focuses on processes typical of medically relevant bacteria.

For the sake of clarity, metabolism is discussed in terms of four primary, but interdependent, processes: fueling, biosynthesis, polymerization, and assembly (Fig. 2.11).

Fueling

Fueling is considered the utilization of metabolic pathways involved in the acquisition of nutrients from the environment, production of precursor metabolites, and energy production.

Acquisition of Nutrients

Bacteria use various strategies for obtaining essential nutrients from the external environment and transporting these substances into the cell's interior. For nutrients to be internalized, they must cross the bacterial cell wall and membrane. These complex structures help to protect the cell from environmental insults, maintain intracellular equilibrium, and transport substances into and out of the cell. Although some key nutrients (e.g., water, oxygen, and carbon dioxide) enter the cell by simple diffusion across the cell membrane, the uptake of other substances is controlled by membrane-selective permeability; still other substances use specific transport mechanisms.

Active transport is among the most common methods used for the uptake of nutrients such as certain sugars, most

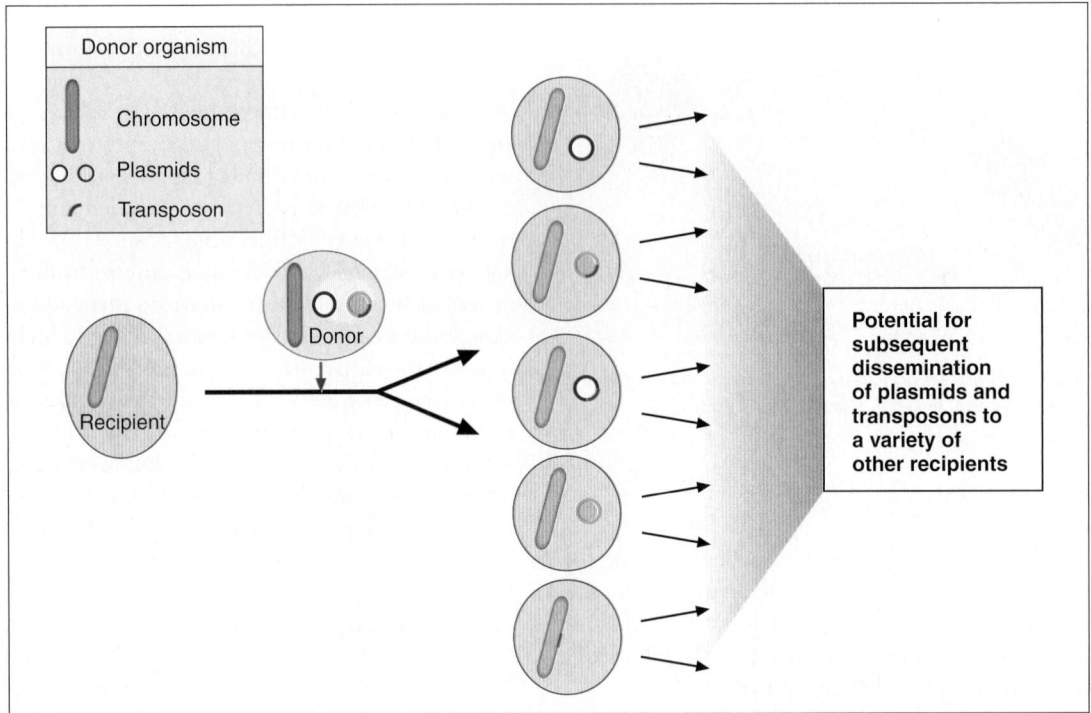

• **Fig. 2.10** Pathways for bacterial dissemination of plasmids and transposons, together and independently.

amino acids, organic acids, and many inorganic ions. The mechanism, driven by an energy-dependent pump, involves carrier molecules embedded in the membrane portion of the cell structure. These carriers combine with the nutrients, transport them across the membrane, and release them inside the cell. Group translocation is another transport mechanism that requires energy but differs from active transport in that the nutrients being transported undergo chemical modification. Many sugars, purines, pyrimidines, and fatty acids are transported by this mechanism.

Production of Precursor Metabolites

Once inside the cell, many nutrients serve as the raw materials from which precursor metabolites for subsequent biosynthetic processes are produced. These metabolites, listed in Fig. 2.11, are produced through two central pathways: the Embden-Meyerhof-Parnas (EMP) pathway (glycolysis) and the tricarboxylic acid (TCA) cycle. The two major pathways and their relationship to one another are shown in Fig. 2.12; not shown are the alternative pathways (e.g., the Entner-Doudoroff and the pentose phosphate pathway) that play key roles in redirecting and replenishing the precursors as they are used in subsequent processes. The Entner-Doudoroff pathway catalyzes the degradation of gluconate and glucose. The gluconate is phosphorylated, dehydrated, and converted into pyruvate and glyceraldehyde, leading to ethanol production. Alternatively, the pentose phosphate pathway uses glucose to produce reduced nicotinamide adenine dinucleotide phosphate (NADPH), pentoses, and tetroses for biosynthetic reactions such as nucleoside and amino acid synthesis.

The production efficiency of a bacterial cell resulting from these precursor-producing pathways can vary substantially, depending on the growth conditions and availability of nutrients. This is an important consideration because the accurate identification of medically important bacteria has traditionally depended on methods that measure the presence of products and byproducts of these metabolic pathways.

Energy Production

The third type of fueling pathway is one that produces the energy required for nearly all cellular processes, including nutrient uptake and precursor production. Energy production is accomplished by the breakdown of chemical substrates (i.e., chemical energy) through the degradative process of catabolism coupled with oxidation-reduction reactions. In this process, the energy source molecule (i.e., substrate) is oxidized as it donates electrons to an electron-acceptor molecule, which is then reduced. The transfer of electrons is mediated through carrier molecules, such as nicotinamide-adenine-dinucleotide (NAD^+) and nicotinamide-adenine-dinucleotide-phosphate ($NADP^+$). The energy released by the oxidation-reduction reaction is transferred to phosphate-containing compounds, where high-energy phosphate bonds are formed. ATP is the most common of such molecules. The energy contained in this compound is eventually released by the hydrolysis of ATP under controlled conditions. The release of this chemical energy, coupled with enzymatic activities, specifically catalyzes each biochemical reaction in the cell and drives cellular reactions.

Precursor metabolites

- Glucose 6-phosphate
- Fructose 6-phosphate
- Pentose 5-phosphate
- Erythrose 4-phosphate
- 3-Phosphoglycerate
- Phosphoenolpyruvate
- Pyruvate
- Acetyl CoA
- α-Ketoglutarate
- Succinyl CoA
- Oxaloacetate

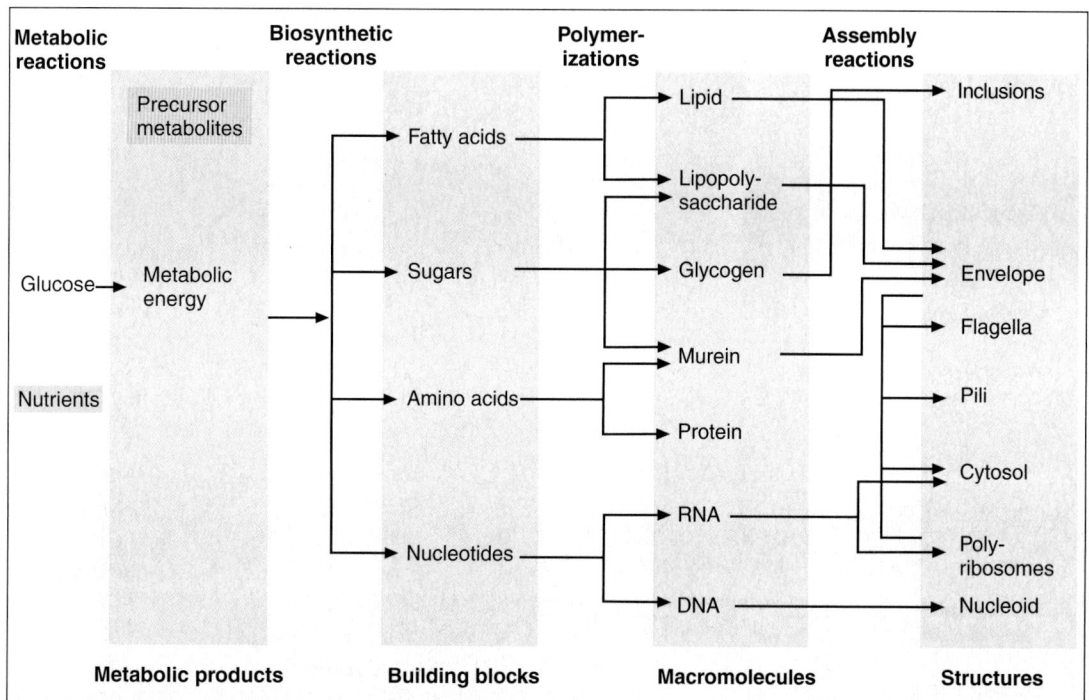

Nutrients

- Gases
  Carbon dioxide (CO_2)
  Oxygen (O_2)
  Ammonia (NH_3)
- Organic compounds, including amino acids
- Water (H_2O)
- Nitrate (NO_3^-)
- Phosphate (PO_4^{3-})
- Hydrogen sulfide (H_2S)
- Sulfate (SO_4^{2-})
- Potassium ($K+$)
- Magnesium (Mg^{2+})
- Calcium (Ca^{2+})
- Sodium (Na^+)
- Iron (Fe^{3+})
  Organic iron complexes

• **Fig. 2.11** Overview of bacterial metabolism, which includes the processes of fueling, biosynthesis, polymerization, and assembly. *CoA,* Coenzyme A; *DNA,* deoxyribonucleic acid; *RNA,* ribonucleic acid. (Modified from Niedhardt FC, Ingraham JL, Schaechter M, eds. *Physiology of the Bacterial Cell: A Molecular Approach.* Sunderland, MA: Sinauer Associates; 1990.)

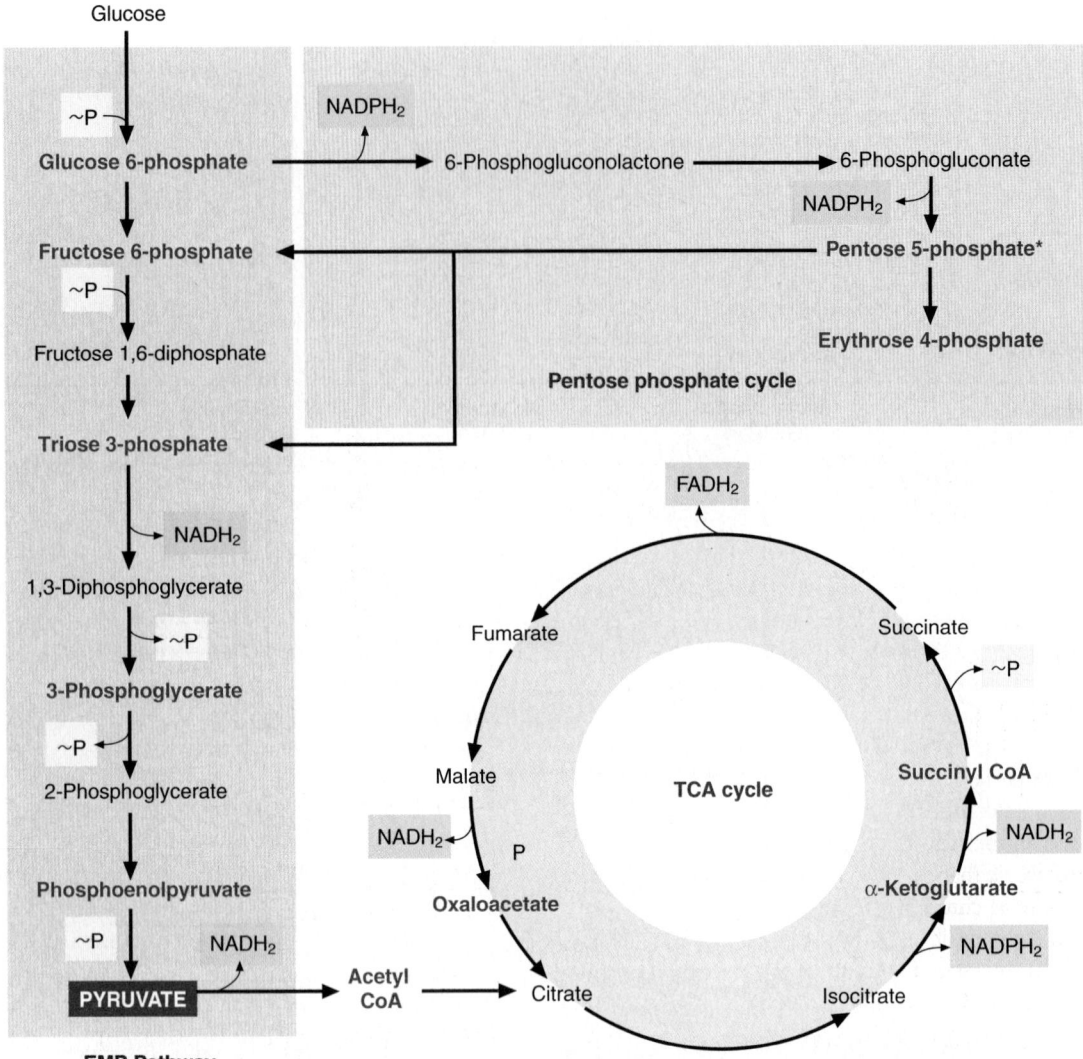

EMP Pathway

• **Fig. 2.12** Overview of the central metabolic pathways (Embden-Meyerhof-Parnas [EMP], the tricarboxylic acid [TCA] cycle, and the pentose phosphate shunt). Precursor metabolites (Fig. 2.11) that are produced are highlighted in *red;* production of energy in the form of adenosine triphosphate *(~P)* by substrate-level phosphorylation is highlighted in *yellow;* and reduced carrier molecules for transport of electrons used in oxidative phosphorylation are highlighted in *green*. (Modified from Niedhardt FC, Ingraham JL, Schaechter M, eds. *Physiology of the Bacterial Cell: A Molecular Approach.* Sunderland, MA: Sinauer Associates; 1990.)

The two general mechanisms for ATP production in bacterial cells are **substrate-level phosphorylation** and electron transport, also referred to as **oxidative phosphorylation.** In substrate-level phosphorylation, high-energy phosphate bonds produced by the central pathways are donated to adenosine diphosphate (ADP) to form ATP directly from the substrate as opposed to generation via the electron transport chain (Fig. 2.12). In addition, pyruvate, a primary intermediate in the central pathways, serves as the initial substrate for several other pathways to generate ATP by substrate-level phosphorylation. These other pathways constitute **fermentative metabolism,** which does not require oxygen and produces various end products, including alcohols, acids, carbon dioxide, and hydrogen. The specific fermentative pathways and the end products produced vary with different bacterial species. Detection of these products is an important basis for laboratory identification of bacteria. (See Chapter 7 for more information on the biochemical basis for bacterial identification.)

Oxidative Phosphorylation

Oxidative phosphorylation involves an electron transport system that conducts a series of electron transfers from reduced carrier molecules such as $NADH_2$, $NADPH_2$, and $FADH_2$ (flavin adenine dinucleotide), produced in the central pathways (Fig. 2.12), to a terminal electron acceptor. The energy produced by the series of oxidation-reduction reactions is used to generate ATP from ADP. When oxidative phosphorylation uses oxygen as the terminal electron acceptor, the process is known as **aerobic respiration. Anaerobic respiration** refers to processes that use final electron acceptors other than oxygen.

A knowledge of which mechanisms bacteria use to generate ATP is important for designing laboratory protocols for cultivating and identifying these organisms. For example, some bacteria depend solely on aerobic respiration and are unable to grow in the absence of oxygen (**strictly aerobic bacteria**). Others can use either aerobic respiration or fermentation, depending on the availability of oxygen (**facultative anaerobic bacteria**). For still others, oxygen is absolutely toxic (**strictly anaerobic bacteria**).

Biosynthesis

The fueling reactions essentially bring together all the raw materials needed to initiate and maintain all other cellular processes. The production of precursors and energy is accomplished through catabolic processes and the degradation of substrate molecules. The three remaining pathways for biosynthesis, polymerization, and assembly depend on anabolic metabolism. In **anabolic metabolism,** precursor compounds are joined for the creation of larger molecules (polymers) required for assembly of cellular structures (Fig. 2.11).

Biosynthetic processes use the precursor products in dozens of pathways to produce a variety of building blocks, such as amino acids, fatty acids, sugars, and nucleotides (Fig. 2.11). Many of these pathways are highly complex and interdependent, whereas other pathways are completely independent. In many cases the enzymes that drive the individual pathways are encoded on a single mRNA molecule that has been transcribed from contiguous genes in the bacterial chromosome (i.e., an operon).

As previously mentioned, bacterial genera and species vary extensively in their biosynthetic capabilities. Knowledge of these variations is necessary to determine the optimal conditions for growing organisms under laboratory conditions. For example, some organisms may not be capable of synthesizing an essential amino acid necessary as a building block for proteins. Without the ability to synthesize the amino acid, the bacterium must obtain the building block from the environment. Thus, if the organism is cultivated in the microbiology laboratory, the amino acid must be provided in the artificial culture medium.

Polymerization and Assembly

Various anabolic reactions assemble (polymerize) the building blocks into macromolecules, including lipids, lipopolysaccharides, polysaccharides, proteins, and nucleic acids. This synthesis of macromolecules is driven by energy and enzymatic activity in the cell. Similarly, energy and enzymatic activities also drive the assembly of various macromolecules into the component structures of the bacterial cell. Cellular structures are the product of all the genetic and metabolic processes discussed.

Structure and Function of the Bacterial Cell

Based on key characteristics, all cells are classified into two basic types: prokaryotic and eukaryotic. Although these two cell types share many common features, they have important differences in terms of structure, metabolism, and genetics.

Eukaryotic and Prokaryotic Cells

Among clinically relevant organisms, **bacteria** are single-cell prokaryotic microorganisms. **Fungi** and **parasites** are single-cell or multicellular eukaryotic organisms, as are plants and all higher animals. **Viruses** are dependent on host cells for survival and therefore are not considered cellular organisms but rather infectious agents. **Prions,** which are abnormal infectious proteins, are also not considered living cells.

A notable characteristic of eukaryotic cells, such as parasites and fungi, is the presence of membrane-enclosed organelles that have specific cellular functions. Examples of these organelles and their respective functions include:

- Endoplasmic reticulum—process and transport proteins
- Golgi body—modification of substances and transport throughout the cell, including internal delivery of molecules, and exocytosis or secretion of other molecules
- Mitochondria—generate energy (ATP)
- Lysosomes—provide an environment for controlled enzymatic degradation of intracellular substances
- Nucleus—provide a membrane enclosure for chromosomes

In addition, eukaryotic cells have an infrastructure, or **cytoskeleton**, which provides support for cellular structure, organization, and movement. The cytoskeleton in eukaryotic cells also plays an essential role in immunology by mediating phagocytosis for the removal of foreign materials from the host, including bacteria, fungi, and viral agents.

Prokaryotic cells, such as bacteria, do not contain organelles. All functions take place in the cytoplasm or cytoplasmic membrane of the cell. Prokaryotic and eukaryotic cell types differ considerably at the macromolecular level, including protein synthesis machinery, chromosomal organization, and gene expression. One notable structure present only in prokaryotic bacterial cells is a **cell wall** composed of **peptidoglycan.** This structure has an immeasurable effect on the practice of diagnostic bacteriology and the management of bacterial diseases.

Bacterial Morphology

Most clinically relevant bacterial species range in size from 0.25 to 1 µm in width and 1 to 3 µm in length, thus requiring microscopy for visualization (see Chapter 6 for more information on microscopy). Just as bacterial species and genera vary in their metabolic processes, their cells also vary in size, morphology, and cell-to-cell arrangements and in the chemical composition and structure of the cell wall. The bacterial cell wall differences provide the basis for the **Gram stain,** a fundamental staining technique used in bacterial identification schemes. This staining procedure separates almost all medically relevant bacteria into two general types: **gram-positive** bacteria, which stain a deep blue or purple, and **gram-negative** bacteria, which stain a pink to red (Fig. 6.3). This simple

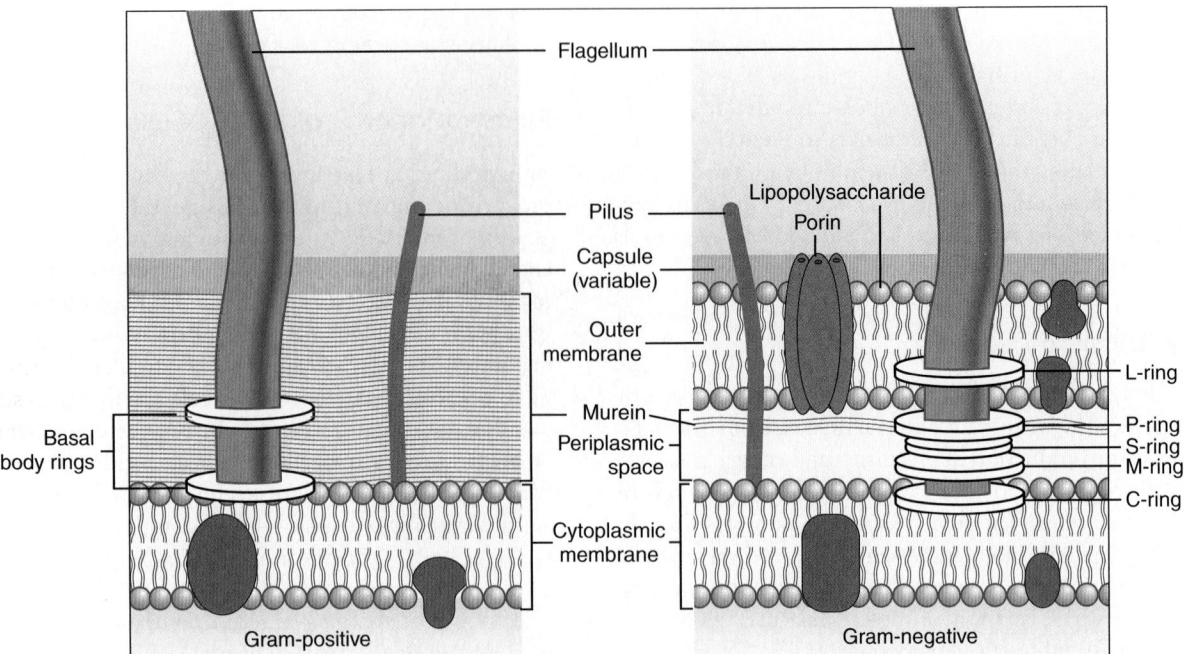

• **Fig. 2.13** General structures of the gram-positive and gram-negative bacterial cell envelopes. The outer membrane and periplasmic space are present only in the envelope of gram-negative bacteria. In addition to porins, bacterial membranes contain additional proteins involved in stabilizing the layers of the cellular structure, adherence, or sorting and reacting to chemical signals. The murein layer is substantially more prominent in gram-positive envelopes. (Modified from Niedhardt FC, Ingraham JL, Schaechter M, eds. *Physiology of the Bacterial Cell: A Molecular Approach.* Sunderland, MA: Sinauer Associates; 1990.)

but important color distinction is the result of differences in the constituents of bacterial cell walls that influence the cell's ability to retain differential dyes after treatment with a decolorizing agent.

Common bacterial cellular morphologies include **cocci** (circular), **coccobacilli** (ovoid), and **bacilli** (rod shaped), as well as **fusiform** (pointed end), curved, or spiral shapes. Cellular arrangements are also noteworthy. Cells may characteristically occur singly, in pairs, or grouped as tetrads, clusters, or in chains (see Fig. 6.4 for examples of bacterial staining and morphologies). The determination of the Gram stain reaction and the cell size, morphology, and arrangement are essential aspects of bacterial identification.

Bacterial Cell Components

Bacterial cell components can be divided into those that make up the outer cell structure and its appendages (**cell envelope**) and those associated with the cell's interior. It is important to note that the cellular structures work together to function as a complex and integrated unit.

Cell Envelope

As shown in Fig. 2.13, the outermost structure, the cell envelope, comprises:

- An outer membrane (in gram-negative bacteria only)
- A cell wall composed of the peptidoglycan macromolecule (also known as the murein layer)

- Periplasm (in gram-negative bacteria only)
- The cytoplasmic or cell membrane, which encloses the cytoplasm

Outer Membrane

Outer membranes, which are found only in gram-negative bacteria, function as the cell's initial barrier to the environment. These membranes serve as the primary permeability barriers to hydrophilic and hydrophobic compounds and contain essential enzymes and other proteins located in the periplasmic space. The membrane is a bilayered structure composed of lipopolysaccharide, which gives the surface of gram-negative bacteria a net negative charge. The outer membrane also plays a significant role in the ability of certain bacteria to cause disease.

Scattered throughout the lipopolysaccharide macromolecules are protein structures called **porins.** These water-filled structures control the passage of nutrients and other solutes, including antibiotics, through the outer membrane. The number and types of porins vary with bacterial species. These differences can substantially influence the extent to which various substances pass through the outer membranes of different bacteria. In addition to porins, other proteins (murein lipoproteins) facilitate the attachment of the outer membrane to the next internal layer in the cell envelope, the cell wall, and may serve as adhesions for attachment to a host cell or as transporters.

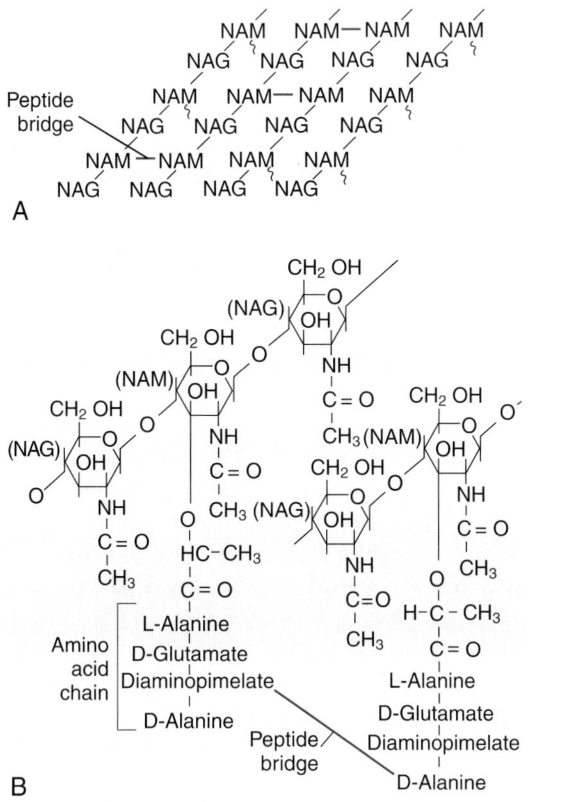

```
        NAM   NAM─NAM   NAM
         NAG  NAG   NAG   NAG
Peptide    NAM   NAM─NAM   NAM
bridge      NAG   NAG  NAG   NAG
       NAM─NAM   NAM   NAM
        NAG  NAG   NAG  NAG
 A
```

• **Fig. 2.14** Peptidoglycan sheet (A) and subunit (B) structure. Multiple peptidoglycan layers compose the murein structure, and different layers are extensively cross-linked by peptide bridges. Note that amino acid chains are only derived from NAM. *NAG,* N-acetylglucosamine; *NAM,* N-acetylmuramic acid. (Modified from Saylers AA, Whitt DD. *Bacterial Pathogenesis: A Molecular Approach.* Washington, DC: American Society for Microbiology Press; 2010.)

Cell Wall (Murein Layer)

The cell wall, also referred to as the peptidoglycan, or **murein layer,** is an essential structure found in nearly all clinically relevant bacteria. This structure gives the bacterial cell shape and strength to withstand changes in environmental osmotic pressures that would otherwise result in cell lysis. The murein layer protects against mechanical disruption of the cell and offers some barrier to the passage of larger substances. Because this structure is essential for the survival of bacteria, its synthesis and structure are often the primary target for the development and design of several antimicrobial agents.

The structure of the cell wall is unique and is composed of disaccharide-pentapeptide subunits. The disaccharides N-acetylglucosamine and N-acetylmuramic acid are the alternating sugar components (moieties) with the amino acid chain linked to N-acetylmuramic acid molecules (Fig. 2.14). Polymers of these subunits cross-link to one another by means of peptide bridges to form peptidoglycan sheets. In turn, layers of these sheets are cross-linked with one another, forming a multilayered, cross-linked structure of considerable strength. Referred to as the **murein sacculus,** or sack, this peptidoglycan structure surrounds the entire cell.

A notable difference between the cell walls of gram-positive and gram-negative bacteria is the substantially thicker peptidoglycan layer in gram-positive bacteria (Fig. 2.13). In addition, the cell wall of gram-positive bacteria contains **teichoic acids** (i.e., glycerol or ribitol phosphate polymers combined with various sugars, amino acids, and amino sugars). Some teichoic acids are linked to N-acetylmuramic acid, and others (e.g., lipoteichoic acids) are linked to the next underlying layer, the **cellular** or **cytoplasmic membrane.** Other bacteria (e.g., *Mycobacteria*) have waxy substances within the murein layer, such as mycolic acids. Mycolic acids make the cells more refractory to toxic substances, including acids. Bacteria with mycolic acid in the cell wall require unique staining procedures and growth media in the diagnostic laboratory.

Periplasmic Space

The **periplasmic space** typically is found only in gram-negative bacteria (whether it is present in gram-positive organisms is a subject of debate). The periplasmic space is bounded by the internal surface of the outer membrane and the external surface of the cellular membrane. This area, which contains the murein layer, consists of gel-like substances that assist in the capture of nutrients from the environment. This space also contains several enzymes involved in the degradation of macromolecules and detoxification of environmental solutes, including antibiotics that enter through the outer membrane.

Cytoplasmic (Inner) Membrane

The **cytoplasmic** (inner) **membrane** is present in both gram-positive and gram-negative bacteria and is the deepest layer of the cell envelope. The cytoplasmic membrane is heavily laced with various proteins, including a number of enzymes vital to cellular metabolism. The cell membrane serves as an additional osmotic barrier and is functionally similar to the membranes of several eukaryotic cellular organelles (e.g., mitochondria, Golgi complexes, lysosomes). The cytoplasmic membrane functions include:

• Transport of solutes into and out of the cell
• Housing of enzymes involved in outer membrane synthesis, cell wall synthesis, and the assembly and secretion of extracytoplasmic and extracellular substances
• Generation of chemical energy (i.e., ATP)
• Cell motility
• Mediation of chromosomal segregation during replication
• Housing of molecular sensors that monitor chemical and physical changes in the environment

Cellular Appendages

In addition to the components of the cell envelope, cellular appendages (i.e., capsules, fimbriae, and flagella) are associated with or proximal to this portion of the cell. The presence of these appendages, which can play a role in the mediation of infection and in laboratory identification, varies among bacterial species and even among strains within the same species.

The **capsule** is immediately exterior to the murein layer of gram-positive bacteria and the outer membrane of gram-negative bacteria. The capsule is composed of high-molecular-weight polysaccharides, the production of which may depend on the environment and growth conditions surrounding the bacterial cell. The capsule does not function as an effective permeability barrier or add strength to the cell envelope, but it does protect bacteria from attack by components of the human immune system. The capsule also facilitates and maintains bacterial colonization of biologic (e.g., teeth) and inanimate (e.g., prosthetic heart valves) surfaces through the formation of "slime layers" or biofilms. Both **slime layers** and **biofilms** imply the presence of an extracellular polymer matrix that varies in composition and structure in different organisms. A biofilm may consist of a monomicrobic or polymicrobic group of bacteria housed in a complex biochemical matrix. This extracellular matrix stabilizes the cell to protect the organism from hydrodynamic forces in the host and plays a protective role against biocides and agents of the host's immune system. (See Chapter 3 for further discussion of microbial biofilms.)

Fimbriae, or **pili,** are hairlike, proteinaceous structures that extend from the cell membrane into the external environment; some may be up to 2 μm long. Fimbriae may serve as adhesins that help bacteria attach to animal host cell surfaces, often as the first step in establishing infection. In addition, a pilus may be referred to as a **sex pilus;** this structure, which is well characterized in the gram-negative bacillus *E. coli,* serves as the conduit for the passage of DNA from the donor to the recipient during conjugation. The sex pilus is present only in cells that produce a protein referred to as the **F factor.** F-positive cells initiate mating or conjugation only with F-negative cells, thereby limiting the conjugative process to cells capable of transporting genetic material through the hollow sex pilus.

Flagella are complex structures, mostly composed of the protein flagellin, that are intricately embedded in the cell envelope. These structures are responsible for bacterial motility. Although not all bacteria are motile, motility plays an important role in survival and the ability of bacteria to cause disease. Depending on the bacterial species, a single flagellum may be located at one end of the cell (**monotrichous flagella**), a group of flagella may be located at one end of the cell (**lophotrichous flagella**), a single flagellum may reside at both ends of the cell (**amphitrichous flagella**), or the entire cell surface may be covered with flagella (**peritrichous flagella**). The flagellum acts as a rotary motor containing a complex set of rings that act as bushings to control cellular movement. Gram-negative flagella are equipped with a basal body structure that contains five rings, the L-ring that is embedded in the lipid bilayer, the P-ring in the periplasmic space, a smaller S-ring (stator ring) attached to the M-ring or motor ring, and the C-ring, which anchors the entire complex to the cell. Because gram-positive organisms have a much more stable complex cellular structure because of the thick layer of peptidoglycan, the flagella contain only two basal body rings: One is embedded in the peptidoglycan layer, which is very stable, and the second is embedded in the cell membrane.

Cell Interior

Those structures and substances that are bound internally by the cytoplasmic membrane compose the cell interior and include the cytosol, polysomes, inclusions, nucleoid, plasmids, and endospores.

The **cytosol,** where nearly all other functions not conducted by the cell membrane occur, contains thousands of enzymes and is the site of protein synthesis. The cytosol has a granular appearance caused by the presence of many polysomes (mRNA complexed with several ribosomes during translation and protein synthesis) and inclusions (i.e., storage reserve granules). The number and nature of the inclusions vary depending on the bacterial species and the nutritional state of the organism's environment. Two common types of granules include glycogen, a storage form of glucose, and polyphosphate granules, a storage form for inorganic phosphates. These granules may be microscopically visible in bacteria stained with specific dyes.

Unlike eukaryotic chromosomes, the bacterial chromosome is not enclosed within a membrane-bound nucleus. Instead the bacterial chromosome exists as a **nucleoid** in which the highly coiled DNA is intermixed with RNA, polyamines, and various proteins that lend structural support. At times, depending on the stage of cell division, more than one chromosome may be present per bacterial cell. Plasmids are the other genetic elements that exist independently in the cytosol, and their numbers may vary from none to several hundred per bacterial cell.

The final bacterial structure to be considered is the **endospore.** Under adverse physical and chemical conditions or when nutrients are scarce, some bacterial genera (*Bacillus* and *Clostridium* spp.) are able to form spores (i.e., sporulate). Sporulation involves substantial metabolic and structural changes in the bacterial cell. Essentially, the cell transforms from an actively metabolic and growing state to a dormant state, with a decrease in cytosol and a concomitant increase in the thickness and strength of the cell envelope. The endospore remains in a dormant state until favorable conditions for growth are again encountered. This survival tactic is demonstrated by a number of clinically relevant bacteria and complicates thorough sterilization of materials and food for human use.

ⓔ Visit the Evolve site for a complete list of procedures, review questions, and case studies.

Bibliography

Aguilar C, Mano M, Eulalio A: MicroRNAs at the host-bacteria interface: host defense and bacterial offense, *Trends Microbiol* 27:206–218, 2019, https://doi.org/10.1016/j.tim.2018.10.011.

Bennett J, Dolin R, Blaser M: *Principles and practice of infectious diseases,* ed 8, Philadelphia, PA, 2015, Elsevier-Saunders.

Brock TD, Madigan M, Martinko J, et al.: *Biology of microorganisms*, Upper Saddle River, NJ, 2009, Prentice Hall.

Goodrich JA, Kugel JF: From bacteria to humans, chromatin to elongation, and activation to repression: the expanding roles of noncoding RNAs in regulating transcription, *Crit Rev Biochem Mol Biol* 44:3–15, 2009.

Joklik WK, Willett H, Amos B, et al.: *Zinsser microbiology*, Norwalk, CT, 1992, Appleton & Lange.

Krebs JE, Goldstein ES, Kilpatrick ST: *Lewin's genes X*, Sandbury, MA, 2011, Jones and Bartlett Learning.

Martinez JL, Coque TM, Lanza VF, de la Cruz F, Baquero F: Genomic and metagenomic technologies to explore the antibiotic resistance mobilome, *Ann NY Acad Sci* 1388:26–41, 2017.

Moat AG, Foster JW: *Microbial physiology*, New York, 2002, Wiley-Liss.

Neidhardt FC, Ingraham JL, Schaecter M, editors: *Physiology of the bacterial cell: a molecular approach*, Sunderland, MA, 1990, Sinauer Associates.

Nuss AM, Heroven AK, Waldmann B, et al.: Transcriptomic profiling of *Yersinia pseudotuberculosis* reveals programming of the Crp regulon by temperature and uncovers Crp as a master regulator of small RNAs, *PLoS Genet* 11:1–26, 2015.

Ryan KJ, editor: *Sherris medical microbiology: an introduction to infectious diseases*, Norwalk, CT, 2003, McGraw-Hill Medical.

Saylers AA, Wilson BA, Whitt DD, Winkler ME: *Bacterial pathogenesis: a molecular approach*, Washington, DC, 2010, American Society for Microbiology Press.

Schomburg D, Gerhard M: *Biochemical pathways: an atlas of biochemistry and molecular biology*, ed 2, New York, 2012, Wiley.

Stortchevoi A, Varshney U, RajBhandary UL: Common location of determinants in initiator transfer RNAs for initiator-elongator discrimination in bacteria and in eukaryotes, *J Biol Chem* 278(20):17672, 2003.

Zhurina MV, Gannesen AV, Zdorovenko EL, Plakunov VK: Composition and functions of the extracellular polymer matrix of bacterial biofilms, *Microbiology* 83:713–722, 2014.

3

Host-Microorganism Interactions

OBJECTIVES

1. List the various reservoirs (environments) that facilitate host-microorganism interactions.
2. Define direct versus indirect transmission, and provide examples of each.
3. Define and differentiate the interactions between the host and microorganism, including colonization, infection, microbiota, microbiome, pathogens, opportunistic pathogens, and nosocomial (health care–acquired or –associated) and community-acquired infection.
4. List and describe the components involved in specific versus nonspecific immune defenses, including inflammation, phagocytosis, antibody production, and cellular responses.
5. Identify elements involved in the two arms of the immune system: humoral and cell-mediated immunity.
6. Provide specific examples of disease prevention strategies, including preventing transmission, controlling reservoirs, and minimizing risk of exposure.
7. Differentiate between bacterial endotoxins and exotoxins, and provide examples of each.
8. Given a patient history of an infectious process, identify and differentiate a sign versus a symptom.
9. Define and differentiate between an acute infectious process and one that is chronic and/or latent.
10. Describe the three major steps in the formation of a microbial biofilm, and list the advantages of biofilm formation to the microorganism and the disadvantages to the infected host.

Interactions between humans and microorganisms are exceedingly complex and far from being completely understood. The interactions between these two living entities plays an important role in the practice of diagnostic microbiology and in the management of infectious disease. Understanding these interactions is necessary for establishing methods to isolate specific microorganisms from patient specimens and for developing effective treatment strategies. This chapter provides the framework for understanding the various aspects of host-microorganism interactions. Box 3.1 lists a variety of terms and definitions associated with host-microorganism interactions.

Host-microorganism interactions should be viewed as bidirectional in nature. Humans use the abilities and natural products of microorganisms in various settings, including the food and fermentation industry, as biologic insecticides for agriculture; to genetically engineer a multitude of products; and even for biodegrading industrial waste. However, microbial populations share the common goal of survival with humans, using their relationship with humans for food, shelter, and dissemination, and they have been successful at achieving those goals. Which participant in the relationship is the user and which is the used is a fine and intricate balance of nature. This is especially true when considering the microorganisms most closely associated with humans and human disease.

In 2008, the National Institutes of Health initiated a project referred to as the *Human Microbiome Project* (http://commonfund.nih.gov/hmp/index). The human **microbiome** consists of microorganisms that are present in and on the human body at any given time without causing harm. Phase I (2008–2012) of the microbiome project focused on four major goals:

(1) identify and characterize a core human microbiome in healthy individuals, both male and female;

(2) determine whether changes in the human microbiome correlate with health and disease;

(3) develop new technology and bioinformatic tools to manage the project data; and

(4) address the ethical, legal, and social implications associated with the microbiome project.

Interestingly, the study has elucidated that the microbiome complex ecosystem varies significantly across the body and between individuals. Analysis of the human microbiome has demonstrated that it is clearly an emergent property. One hundred and thirteen females were examined for the presence of microorganisms at 18 body sites and 129 males at 15 body sites (excluding vaginal collections). The data demonstrated that dependent on the body site, both low diversity of microorganisms and a high diversity of microorganisms correlates with the development of disease. Phase I also examined the relationships between the microbiome and characteristics of the host, including age, body mass index, and available medical history. The second phase of the project, the *Integrative Human Microbiome Project*, has begun to analyze data from phase I and apply it to host interactions in healthy and disease states. Established in 2014, Phase II focuses on three major areas: (1) the vaginal

• BOX 3.1 Definitions of Selected Epidemiologic Terms

- **Carrier:** A person who harbors the etiologic agent but shows no apparent signs or symptoms of infection or disease
- **Common source:** A single source or reservoir from which an etiologic agent responsible for an epidemic or outbreak originates
- **Community-associated infection:** Infection acquired in an activity or group that is not in a health care setting or environment.
- **Disease incidence:** The number of new diseases or infected persons in a population
- **Disease prevalence:** The percentage of diseased persons in a given population at a particular time
- **Endemic:** A disease constantly present at some rate of occurrence in a particular location
- **Epidemic:** A larger-than-normal number of diseased or infected individuals in a particular location
- **Etiologic agent:** A microorganism responsible for causing infection or infectious disease
- **Health care–associated infection:** Infections acquired as a result of a short- or long-term admission into a health care facility
- **Iatrogenic:** Infection acquired as a result of a medical procedure.
- **Microbiome:** An individual's microbiologic environment, present in or on the human host
- **Mode of transmission:** The means by which etiologic agents are brought in contact with the human host (e.g., infected blood, contaminated water, insect bite)

- **Morbidity:** The state of disease and its associated effects on the host
- **Morbidity rate:** The incidence of a particular disease state
- **Mortality:** Death resulting from disease
- **Mortality rate:** The incidence in which a disease results in death
- **Nosocomial infection:** Infection for which the etiologic agent was acquired in a hospital or long-term health care center or facility
- **Outbreak:** A larger than normal number of diseased or infected individuals that occurs over a relatively short period
- **Pandemic:** An epidemic that spans the world
- **Reservoir:** The origin of the etiologic agent or location from which it disseminates (e.g., water, food, insects, animals, other humans)
- **Strain typing:** Laboratory-based characterization of etiologic agents designed to establish their relatedness to one another during a particular outbreak or epidemic
- **Surveillance:** Any type of epidemiologic investigation that involves data collection for characterizing circumstances surrounding the incidence or prevalence of a particular disease or infection
- **Vector:** A living entity (animal, insect, or plant) that transmits the etiologic agent
- **Vehicle:** A nonliving entity that is contaminated with the etiologic agent and as such is the mode of transmission for that agent

microbiome associated with pregnancy and preterm birth; (2) gastrointestinal microbiome and the development of inflammatory bowel disease; and (3) microbiome and the development of type 2 diabetes. Undoubtedly, this research will continue to evolve and potentially provide insight into the characterization, risk, and prevention of disease. The relationship between host and microorganism is ultimately associated with the variation and balance of the normal human microbiome and the appearance of a potentially infectious agent.

The complex relationships between the human host and medically relevant microorganisms are demonstrated in the sequential steps associated with microbe-host interactions and the subsequent development of infection and disease. The stages of interaction include (1) the physical encounter between the host and microorganism; (2) colonization or survival of the microorganism on an internal (gastrointestinal, respiratory, or genitourinary tract) or external (skin) surface of the host; (3) microbial entry, invasion, and dissemination to deeper tissues and organs of the human body; and (4) resolution or outcome.

The Encounter Between Host and Microorganism

The Human Host's Perspective

Because microorganisms are ubiquitous in nature, human encounters are inevitable, but the means of encounter vary widely. Which microbial population and the mechanism of

exposure are often direct consequences of a person's activity or behaviors. Certain activities carry different risks for an encounter. There is a wide spectrum of activities and situations over which a person may or may not have absolute control. For example, acquiring salmonellosis because one fails to cook the holiday turkey thoroughly is avoidable, whereas contracting tuberculosis living in conditions of extreme poverty and overcrowding may be unavoidable. The role that human activities play in the encounter between humans and microorganisms cannot be overstated. Most of the crises associated with infectious disease are preventable or can be greatly reduced with changes in human behavior and living conditions.

Microbial Reservoirs and Transmission

Humans encounter microorganisms when they enter or are exposed to the same environment in which the microbial agents live or when the infectious agents are brought to the human host by indirect means. The environment or place of origin of the infecting agent is the **reservoir.** As shown in Fig. 3.1, microbial reservoirs include humans, animals, water, food, air, and soil. The human host may acquire microbial agents by various means or **modes of transmission.** The mode of transmission is direct when the host directly contacts the microbial reservoir and is indirect when the host encounters the microorganism by an intervening agent of transmission.

The agents of transmission that bring the microorganism from the reservoir to the host may be a living entity, such as

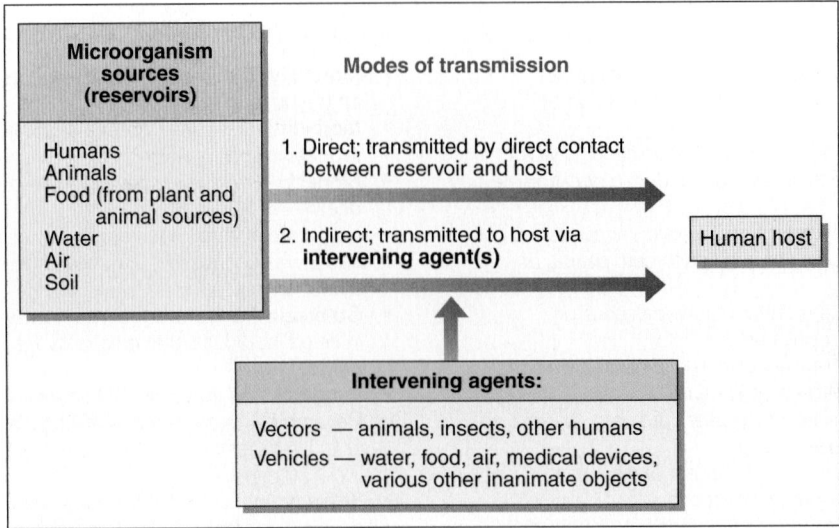

• **Fig. 3.1** Summary of microbial reservoirs and modes of transmission to humans.

an insect, in which case they are called **vectors,** or they may be a nonliving entity, referred to as a **vehicle** or **fomite.** In addition, some microorganisms may have a single mode of transmission, whereas others may spread by various methods. From a diagnostic microbiology perspective, knowledge about an infectious agent's mode of transmission is often important for determining optimal specimens for isolation of the organism and for implementing precautions that minimize the risk of laboratory or health care–associated infections (HAIs) (see Chapters 4, 78, and 79 for more information regarding laboratory safety, infection control, and sentinel laboratory responses, respectively).

Human and Microbe Interactions

Humans play a substantial role as microbial reservoirs. In fact, the passage of a neonate from the sterile environment of the mother's womb through the birth canal, which is heavily colonized with various microbial agents, is a primary example of one human directly (i.e., **direct transmission**) acquiring a microorganism from another human serving as the reservoir. This is the mechanism that newborns first encounter microbial agents. Other examples in which humans serve as the microbial reservoir include the acquisition of streptococcal pharyngitis through touching; hepatitis through blood transfusions; gonorrhea, syphilis, and acquired immunodeficiency syndrome (AIDS) through sexual contact; and tuberculosis and the common cold through aerosolized droplets associated with coughing or sneezing. **Indirect transmission** can occur when microorganisms from one individual contaminate a vehicle of transmission, such as water (e.g., cholera), that is then ingested by another person. In the medical setting, indirect transmission of microorganisms from one human host to another by means of a medical procedure (i.e., **iatrogenic**) and contaminated medical devices helps to disseminate infections in hospitals. Hospital-acquired, health care–associated, or long-term care–associated infections are considered **nosocomial**

infections. Health care–associated infections (HAIs) include exposure in a variety of settings and not confined to in-patient care in a health care institution. These exposures occur during field containment or transportation of infectious agents as well as in daily contact with infected patients in clinics. In addition, HAIs are not limited to health care professionals and patients, but also include visitors, support staff, and students.

In addition, humans are routinely exposed to infectious agents through participation in activities and events throughout their daily lives. These activities include direct and indirect transmission of infectious agents in community settings. These infections are considered **community-associated (CA) infections.**

Animals as Microbial Reservoirs

Infectious agents from animal reservoirs are transmissible directly to humans through an animal bite (e.g., rabies) or indirectly through the bite of insect vectors that feed on both animals and humans (e.g., Lyme disease and Rocky Mountain spotted fever). Animals may also transmit infectious agents by acquiring them from or depositing them in water and food supplies. For example, beavers heavily colonized with parasites can cause infection of the human gastrointestinal tract. These parasites may be encountered and subsequently acquired when stream water is contaminated by the beaver and is used by a vacationing camper. Alternatively, animals used for human food carry numerous bacteria (e.g., *Salmonella* and *Campylobacter*) that, if not destroyed through appropriate cooking during preparation, can cause severe gastrointestinal illness.

Many other infectious diseases can be encountered through direct or indirect animal contact, and information regarding a patient's exposure to animals is often a key component in the diagnosis of these infections. Some microorganisms primarily infect animal populations and on occasion accidentally encounter and infect humans. When a human infection results from such an encounter, it is a **zoonotic infection.** More specifically, if the human infection is a result of regular interaction with animals for food production, the infection is **livestock-associated.**

Insects as Vectors

The most common role of insects (arthropods) in the transmission of infectious disease is as vectors rather than as reservoirs. A variety of arthropods can transmit viral, parasitic, and bacterial disease from animals to humans, whereas others transmit microorganisms between human hosts without an intermediate animal reservoir. Malaria, a deadly disease, is a prime example of an infectious disease maintained in the human population by the feeding and survival of an insect vector, the mosquito. Still other arthropods may themselves be agents of disease. These include organisms such as lice and scabies spread directly between humans and cause skin irritations but do not penetrate the body. Because they are able to survive on the skin of the host without gaining access to internal tissues, they are **ectoparasites** (Chapter 46). In addition, nonfungal infections may result when microbial agents in the environment, such as endospores, are introduced mechanically through the bite of a vector, scratch, or other penetrating wound.

The Environment as a Microbial Reservoir

The soil and natural environmental debris are reservoirs for countless types of microorganisms. It is not surprising that these also serve as reservoirs for microorganisms that can cause infection in humans. Many of the fungal agents (see Part V: Mycology) are acquired by inhalation of soil and dust particles containing microorganisms (e.g., San Joaquin Valley fever). Other, nonfungal infections (e.g., tetanus endospores) may result when microbial agents in the environment are introduced into the human body by a penetrating wound.

The Microorganism's Perspective

Clearly, numerous activities can result in human encounters with microorganisms. Because humans are engaged in all of life's complex activities, the tendency is to perceive the microorganism as having a passive role in the encounter process. However, this assumption is a gross oversimplification.

Microorganisms are driven by survival, and the environment of the reservoirs they occupy must allow their metabolic and genetic needs to be fulfilled. Reservoirs can be inhabited by hundreds or thousands of different microorganisms. Yet human encounters with the reservoirs, either directly or indirectly, do not result in all microorganisms establishing an association with the human host. Although some microorganisms have evolved strategies that do not require a human host to ensure survival, others have included humans to a lesser or greater extent as part of their survival tactics. These organisms often have mechanisms that enhance their chances for a human encounter.

Depending on factors associated with both the human host and the microorganism involved, the encounter may have a beneficial, disastrous, or inconsequential effect on each of the participants.

Microorganism Colonization of Host Surfaces

The Host's Perspective

Once a microbe is in contact with a human host, the outcome of the encounter depends on what happens during each step of the interaction, beginning with **colonization.** The human host's role in microbial colonization, defined as the persistent survival of microorganisms on a surface of the human body, is dictated by the defenses that protect vital internal tissues and organs against microbial invasion. The first defenses are the external and internal body surfaces that are in direct contact with the external environment and are the anatomic regions where the microorganisms will initially encounter the human host. These surfaces include:

- Skin (including the conjunctival epithelium covering the eye)
- Mucous membranes lining the mouth or oral cavity, the respiratory tract, the gastrointestinal tract, and the genitourinary tract

Because body surfaces are always present and provide protection against all microorganisms, skin and mucous membranes are constant and **nonspecific defense mechanisms.** As is discussed later in this text, other protective mechanisms are produced in response to the presence of microbial agents (inducible defenses), and some are directed specifically at particular microorganisms (**specific defense mechanisms**).

Skin and Skin Structures

Skin serves as a physical and chemical barrier to microorganisms; its protective characteristics are summarized in Table 3.1 and Fig. 3.2. The acellular, outermost layer of the skin, along with the tightly packed cellular layers underneath, provides an impenetrable physical barrier to all microorganisms, unless damaged. In addition, these layers continuously shed, thus dislodging bacteria that have attached to the outer layers. The skin is also a dry and cool environment, which is incompatible with the growth requirements of many microorganisms that thrive in a warm, moist environment.

The follicles and glands of the skin produce various natural antibacterial substances, including sebum and sweat. However, many microorganisms can survive the conditions of the skin. These bacteria, or the skin microbiome, are **skin colonizers,** and they often produce substances that may be toxic and inhibit the growth of more harmful microbial agents. The skin human microbiome differs among healthy individuals more than any other body site. Beneath the outer layers of skin are various host cells that protect against organisms that breach the surface barriers. These cells, collectively known as **skin-associated lymphoid tissue,**

TABLE 3.1	Protective Characteristics of the Skin and Skin Structures
Skin Structure	**Protective Activity**
Outer (dermal) layers	• Act as a physical barrier to microbial penetration • Remove attached bacteria through sloughing of the outer layers • Provide dry, acidic, and cool conditions that limit bacterial growth
Hair follicles, sweat glands, sebaceous glands	• Produce acids, alcohols, and toxic lipids that limit bacterial growth
Eyes/conjunctival epithelium	• Flushing action of tears: removes microorganisms • Lysozyme in tears: destroys the bacterial cell wall • Mechanical blinking of the eyelid: removes microorganisms
Skin-associated lymphoid tissue	• Mediates specific and nonspecific protection mechanisms against microorganisms that penetrate the outer tissue layers

TABLE 3.2	Protective Characteristics of Mucous Membranes
Mucous Membrane	**Protective Activity**
Mucosal cells	• Rapid sloughing for bacterial removal • Tight intercellular junctions: prevent bacterial penetration

Goblet cells	• Mucus production: protective lubrication of cells; bacterial trapping; contains specific antibodies with specific activity against bacteria
	• Provision of antibacterial substances to mucosal surface:
	  • Lysozyme (degrades bacterial cell wall)
	  • Lactoferrin (competes for bacterial iron supply)
	  • Lactoperoxidase (production of substances toxic to bacteria)

Mucosa-associated lymphoid tissue	• Mediates specific responses against bacteria that penetrate the outer layer

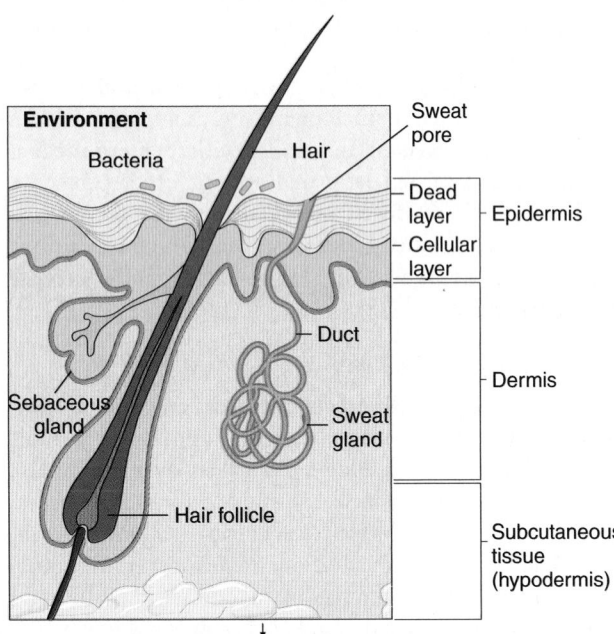

• **Fig. 3.2** Skin and skin structures.

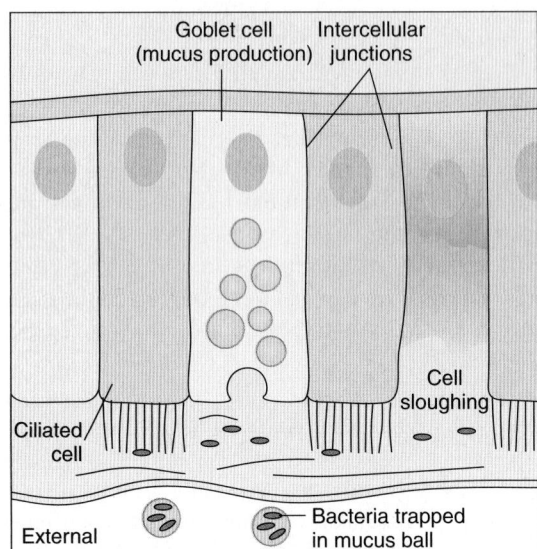

• **Fig. 3.3** General features of mucous membranes, highlighting the protective features such as ciliated cells, mucus production, tight intercellular junctions, and cell sloughing.

mediate specific and nonspecific responses directed at controlling microbial invaders.

Mucous Membranes

Because cells that line the respiratory tract, gastrointestinal tract, and genitourinary tract are involved in numerous functions besides protection, they are not covered with a hardened, acellular layer. However, the cells that compose these membranes still exhibit various protective characteristics (Table 3.2 and Fig. 3.3).

General Protective Characteristics

Mucus is a major protective component of the membranes. This substance serves to trap bacteria before they can reach the outer surface of the cells, lubricates the cells to prevent damage that promotes microbial invasion, and contains specific chemical (i.e., antibodies) and nonspecific antibacterial substances. In addition to the chemical properties and physical movement of the mucus and trapped microorganisms mediated by ciliary action, rapid cellular shedding and tight intercellular connections provide effective barriers to infection. As is the case with the skin, specific cell clusters,

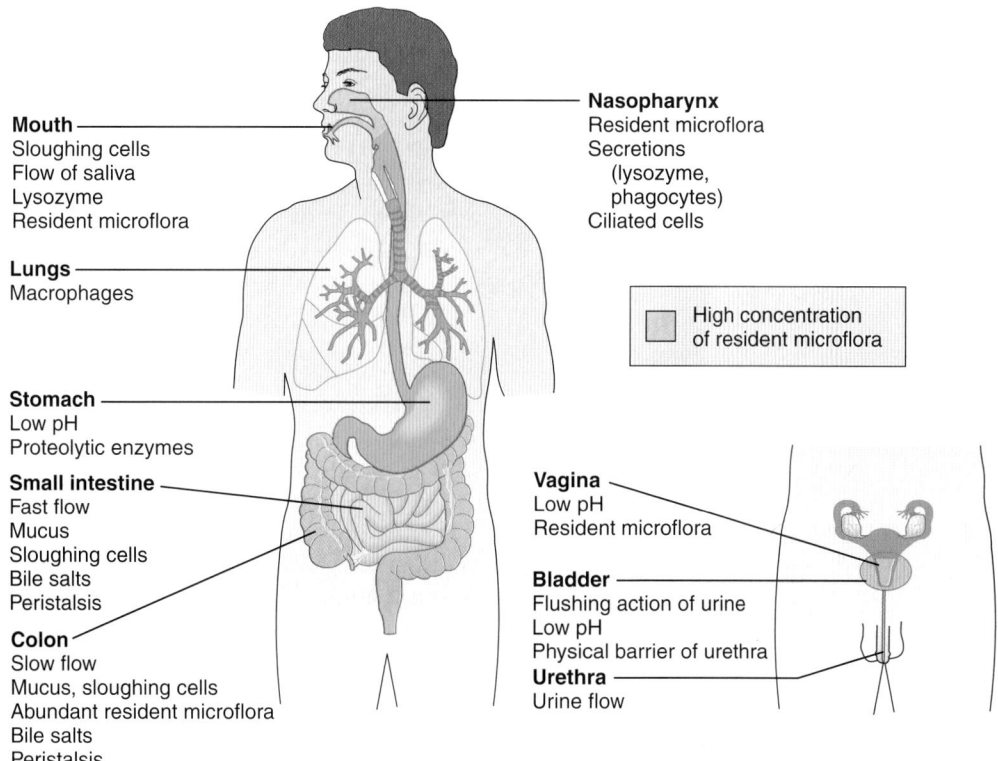

Mouth
Sloughing cells
Flow of saliva
Lysozyme
Resident microflora

Lungs
Macrophages

Stomach
Low pH
Proteolytic enzymes

Small intestine
Fast flow
Mucus
Sloughing cells
Bile salts
Peristalsis

Colon
Slow flow
Mucus, sloughing cells
Abundant resident microflora
Bile salts
Peristalsis

Nasopharynx
Resident microflora
Secretions
  (lysozyme,
  phagocytes)
Ciliated cells

☐ High concentration
  of resident microflora

Vagina
Low pH
Resident microflora

Bladder
Flushing action of urine
Low pH
Physical barrier of urethra
Urethra
Urine flow

• **Fig. 3.4** Protective characteristics associated with the mucosal linings of different internal body surfaces.

known as **mucosa-associated lymphoid tissue,** exist below the outer cell layer and mediate specific protective mechanisms against microbial invasion.

Specific Protective Characteristics

Besides the general protective properties of mucosal cells, the mucosal linings throughout the body have characteristics specific to each anatomic site (Fig. 3.4).

The mouth, or **oral cavity,** is protected by the flow of saliva that physically carries microorganisms away from cell surfaces and contains antibacterial substances, such as antibodies (immunoglobulin A [IgA]) and **lysozyme** that participate in the destruction of bacterial cells. The mouth is heavily colonized with protective microorganisms that produce substances that hinder successful invasion by harmful organisms.

In the gastrointestinal tract, the low pH and proteolytic (protein-digesting) enzymes of the stomach prevent the growth of many microorganisms. In the small intestine, bile salts provide protection that disrupts bacterial membranes, and by peristaltic movement and the fast flow of intestinal contents, which hinder microbial attachment to mucosal cells. Although the large intestine also contains bile salts, the movement of bowel contents is slower, permitting a higher concentration of microbial agents the opportunity to attach to the mucosal cells and inhabit the gastrointestinal tract. As in the oral cavity, the high concentration of normal microbial inhabitants in the large bowel also contributes significantly to protection.

In the upper respiratory tract, nasal hairs keep out large airborne particles that may contain microorganisms. The cough-sneeze reflex significantly contributes to the removal of potentially infective agents. The cells lining the trachea contain **cilia** (hairlike cellular projections) that move microorganisms trapped in mucus upward and away from the delicate cells of the lungs (Fig. 3.3) by the **mucociliary escalator.** These barriers are so effective that only inhalation of particles smaller than 2 to 3 μm have a chance of reaching the lungs.

In the female urogenital tract, the vaginal lining and the cervix are protected by colonization with normal microbial inhabitants and a low pH. A thick mucus plug in the cervical opening is a substantial barrier that keeps microorganisms from ascending and invading the delicate tissues of the uterus, uterine tubes, and ovaries. The anterior urethra of males and females is colonized with microorganisms, and a stricture at the urethral opening provides a physical barrier that, combined with a low urine pH and the flushing action of urination, protects against bacterial invasion of the bladder, ureters, and kidneys.

The Microorganism's Perspective

As previously discussed, microorganisms that inhabit many surfaces of the human body (Fig. 3.4) are referred to as **colonizers, normal flora, normal microbiota,** and collectively as the **human microbiome.** Some are **transient colonizers** because they are able to survive, but do not multiply, on the surface and frequently shed with the host cells. Others, called **resident microbiota,** not only survive but also thrive and multiply; their presence is more persistent.

The body's microbiota varies considerably with anatomic location. For example, environmental conditions, such as temperature and oxygen availability, differ considerably between the nasal cavity and the small bowel. Only microorganisms with the metabolic capability to survive under the physiologic conditions of the anatomic location are inhabitants of those particular body surfaces.

Knowledge of the microbiota of the human body is extremely important in diagnostic microbiology, especially for determining the clinical significance of microorganisms isolated from patient specimens. Organisms considered normal microbiota are often in clinical specimens. This may be a result of contamination of normally sterile specimens during the collection process or because the colonizing organism is actually involved in the infection. Microorganisms considered as normal colonizers of the human body and the anatomic locations they colonize are addressed in Part VII.

Microbial Colonization

Colonization may be the last step in the establishment of a long lasting, mutually beneficial (i.e., commensal) or harmless relationship between a colonizer and the human host. Alternatively, colonization may be the first step in the process for the development of infection and disease. Whether colonization results in a harmless or damaging infection depends on the characteristics of the host and the microorganism. In either case, successful initial colonization depends on the microorganism's ability to survive the conditions first encountered on the host surface (Box 3.2).

To avoid the dryness of the skin, organisms often seek moist areas of the body, including hair follicles, sebaceous (oil or **sebum**) and sweat glands, skin folds, underarms, the genitals or anus, the face, the scalp, and areas around the mouth. Microbial penetration of mucosal surfaces is mediated when an organism embedded in food particles survives oral and gastrointestinal conditions or is contained within airborne particles to aid survival in the respiratory tract. Microorganisms also exhibit metabolic capabilities that assist in their survival. For example, the ability of staphylococci to thrive in relatively high salt concentrations enhances their survival in and among the sweat glands of the skin.

Besides surviving the host's physical and chemical conditions, colonization also requires that microorganisms **attach** and **adhere** to host surfaces (Box 3.2). Attachment can be particularly challenging in places such as the mouth and bowel, in which the surfaces are frequently flushed with passing fluids. Pili, the rodlike projections of bacterial envelopes; various molecules (e.g., adherence proteins and adhesins); and biochemical complexes (e.g., biofilm) work together to enhance attachment of microorganisms to the host cell surface. Biofilm is discussed in more detail later in this chapter. (For more information concerning the structure and functions of pili, see Chapter 2.)

In addition, microbial motility with flagella allows organisms to move around and actively seek optimum conditions. Finally, because no single microbial species is a lone colonizer, successful colonization also requires that a microorganism be able to coexist with other microorganisms.

Microorganism Entry, Invasion, and Dissemination

The Host's Perspective

In most instances, to establish infection, microorganisms must **penetrate** or circumvent the host's physical barriers (i.e., skin or mucosal surfaces); overcoming these defensive barriers depends on both host and microbial factors. When these barriers are broken, numerous other host defensive strategies activate.

Disruption of Surface Barriers

Any situation that disrupts the physical barrier of the skin and mucosa, alters the environmental conditions (e.g., loss of stomach acidity or dryness of the skin), changes the functioning of surface cells, or alters the normal microbiota facilitates the penetration of microorganisms past the barriers and into deeper host tissues. Disruptive factors may vary from accidental or intentional (medical) trauma resulting in surface destruction to the use of antibiotics that remove normal, protective, colonizing microorganisms (Box 3.3). A number of these factors are a result of a medical intervention or procedure.

Responses to Microbial Invasion of Deeper Tissue

Once an organism circumvents surface barriers, the host responds to a microbial presence in the underlying tissue in various ways. Some of these responses are nonspecific, because they occur regardless of the type of invading organism; other responses are more specific and involve the host's immune system. Both nonspecific and specific host responses are critical if the host is to survive. Without them, microorganisms would multiply and invade vital tissues and organs, resulting in severe damage to the host.

• BOX 3.3 Factors That Contribute to the Disruption of the Skin and Mucosal Surface

Trauma
- Penetrating wounds
- Abrasions
- Burns (chemical and fire)
- Surgical wounds
- Needle sticks

Inhalation
- Noxious or toxic gases
- Particulate matter
- Smoking

Implantation of Medical Devices
Other Diseases
- Malignancies
- Diabetes
- Previous or simultaneous infections
- Alcoholism and other chemical dependencies

Childbirth
Overuse of Antibiotics

Nonspecific Responses

Some nonspecific responses are biochemical; others are cellular. Biochemical factors remove essential nutrients, such as iron, from tissues so that it is unavailable for use by invading microorganisms. Cellular responses are central to tissue and organ defenses, and the primary cells responsible are **phagocytes.**

Phagocytes

Phagocytes are cells that ingest and destroy bacteria and other foreign particles. The types of phagocytes are polymorphonuclear leukocytes, also known as **neutrophils (PMNs), monocytes** (circulating mononuclear white blood cells) or **macrophages (mononuclear white blood cells found in tissue),** and **dendritic cells.** Phagocytes ingest bacteria by a process known as **phagocytosis** and engulf them in a membrane-lined structure called a **phagosome** (Fig. 3.5). The phagosome fuses with a second structure, the **lysosome.** When the lysosome, which contains toxic chemicals and destructive enzymes, combines with the phagosome, the bacteria that are trapped within the **phagolysosome** are neutralized and destroyed. This destructive process occurs inside membrane-lined structures to prevent the noxious substances contained within the phagolysosome from destroying the phagocyte itself. This is evident during the course of rampant infections when thousands of phagocytes exhibit "sloppy" ingestion of the microorganisms and toxic substances spill from the cells, damaging the surrounding host tissue.

The two major phagocytes, PMNs and mononuclear cells, differ in viability and anatomic distribution. PMNs develop in the bone marrow and spend their short lives (usually a day

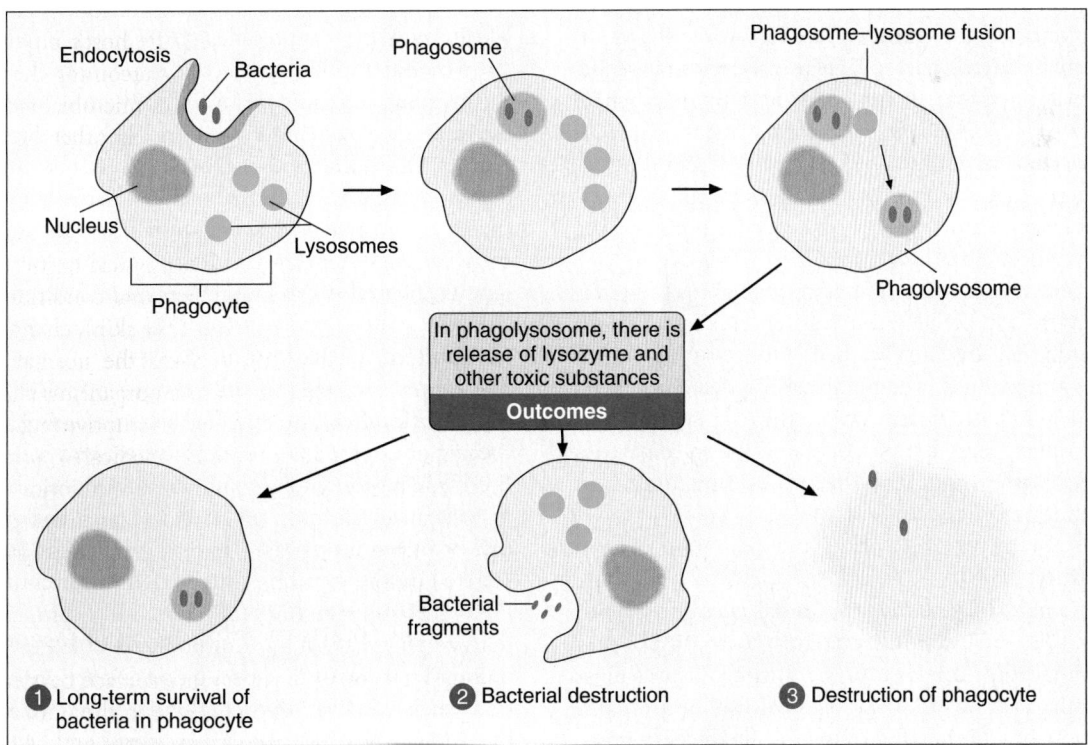

• **Fig. 3.5** Overview of phagocyte activity and possible outcomes of phagocyte-bacterial interactions.

TABLE 3.3	Components of Inflammation
Component	**Functions**
Phagocytes (poly-morphonuclear neutrophils [PMNs], dendritic cells, and monocytes)	• Ingest and destroy microorganisms
Complement system (coordinated group of serum proteins)	• Attracts phagocytes to the site of infection (chemotaxis) • Helps phagocytes to recognize and bind to bacteria (opsonization) • Directly kills gram-negative bacteria (membrane attack complex)
Coagulation system (wide variety of proteins and other biologically active compounds)	• Attracts phagocytes to the site of infection • Increases blood and fluid flow to the site of infection • Walls off the site of infection, physically inhibiting the spread of microorganisms
Cytokines (proteins secreted by macrophages and other cells)	• Multiple effects that enhance the activities of many different cells essential to nonspecific and specific defensive responses

or less) circulating in blood and tissues. Widely dispersed in the body, PMNs usually are the first cells on the scene of bacterial invasion. Mononuclear cells (**monocytes**) also develop in the bone marrow. When deposited in tissue or at a site of infection, monocytes transform into mature macrophages. In the absence of infection, macrophages usually reside in specific organs, such as the spleen, lymph nodes, liver, or lungs, where they live for days to several weeks, awaiting encounters with invading bacteria. In addition to the ingestion and destruction of bacteria, macrophages play an important role in mediating immune system defenses (see Specific Responses—The Immune System later in this chapter).

In addition to the inhibition of microbial proliferation by phagocytes and biochemical substances such as lysozyme, microorganisms are "washed" from tissues during the flow of lymph fluid. The fluid carries infectious agents through the lymphatic system, where they are deposited in tissues and organs (e.g., lymph nodes and the spleen) heavily populated with phagocytes. This process functions as an efficient filtration system.

Inflammation

Because microbes may survive the initial encounters with phagocytes (Fig. 3.5), the inflammatory response plays an extremely important role as a primary mechanism against microbial survival and proliferation in tissues and organs. Inflammation has both cellular and biochemical components that interact in various complex ways (Table 3.3).

The **complement system** is composed of a coordinated group of proteins activated by the immune system because of the presence of invading microorganisms. On activation of this system, a cascade of biochemical events occurs that attracts (**chemotaxis**) and enhances the activities of phagocytes. Because PMNs and macrophages are widely dispersed throughout the body, signals attract and concentrate these cells at the point of invasion, and serum complement proteins provide many of these signals. **Cytokines** are chemical substances, or proteins secreted by a cell, that have effects on the activities of other cells. Cytokines draw more phagocytes toward the infection and activate the maturation of monocytes to macrophages.

Additional protective functions of the complement system is enhanced by hemostasis, which works to increase blood flow to the area of infection and can effectively wall off the infection through the production of clots and barriers composed of cellular debris.

The manifestations of **inflammation** are readily evident and are familiar to most adults; they include the following:
- Swelling—caused by an increased flow of fluid and cells to the affected body site
- Redness—results from vasodilation of blood vessels and increased blood flow at the infection site
- Heat—results from increased cellular metabolism and energy production in the affected area
- Pain—caused by tissue damage and pressure on nerve endings from an increased flow of fluid and cells

On a microscopic level, the presence of phagocytes at the infection site is an important observation in diagnostic microbiology. Microorganisms associated with these host cells are frequently identified as the cause of a particular infection.

Specific Responses—The Immune System

The immune system provides the human host with the ability to mount a specific protective response to the presence of the invading microorganism. In addition to this specificity, the immune system has a "memory." When a microorganism is encountered a second or third time, an immune-mediated defensive response is immediately available. However, nonspecific (i.e., phagocytes, inflammation) and specific (i.e., the immune system) host defensive systems are interdependent in their efforts to limit the spread of infection.

Components of the Immune System

The central molecule of the immune response is the antibody. **Antibodies,** also referred to as **immunoglobulins,** are specific glycoproteins produced by **plasma cells** (activated B cells) in response to the presence of a molecule recognized as foreign to the host (referred to as an **antigen**). In the case of infectious diseases, antigens are chemicals or toxins secreted by the invading microorganism or components of the organism's structure and are usually composed of proteins or polysaccharides. Antibodies circulate in the plasma or liquid portion of the host's blood and are present in secretions such as saliva. These molecules have two active areas: the antigen-binding site (**Fab region**) and the phagocyte and complement binding sites (**Fc region**) (Fig. 3.6).

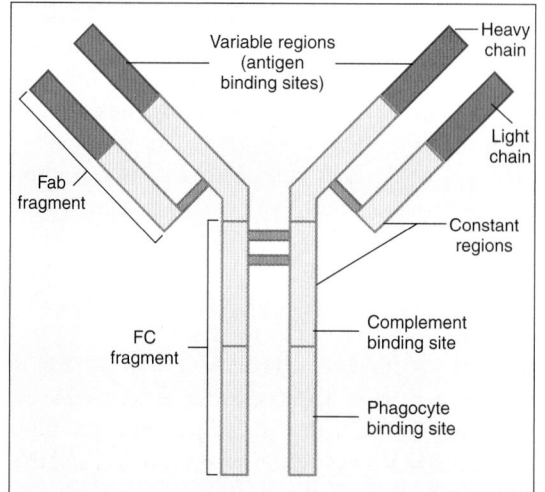

• **Fig. 3.6** General structure of the immunoglobulin G (IgG)-class antibody molecule.

Five major classes or **isotypes** of antibody exist: IgG, IgA, IgM, IgD, and IgE. Each class has distinctive molecular configurations. **IgM** is the largest and first antibody produced when an invading microorganism is encountered in the host; production of the most abundant antibody, **IgG,** follows. IgG consists of four subclasses, IgG1 to IgG4, that have variations in their constant regions resulting in different effector functions related to phagocytosis, complement activation, and antibody-dependent cell-mediated cytotoxicity. **IgA** is secreted in various body fluids (e.g., saliva and tears) and primarily protects body surfaces lined with mucous membranes. IgA also includes subclasses: IgA1 is predominantly located in the blood stream, and IgA2, which is more resistant to proteolytic cleavage, is located predominantly in secretions. Increased **IgE** is associated with parasitic infections and allergies. **IgD** is attached to the surface of specific immune system cells and is involved in the regulation of antibody production. As is discussed in Chapter 9, the ability to measure specific antibody production is a valuable tool for the laboratory diagnosis of infectious diseases.

Regarding the cellular components of the immune response, there are three major types of cells: **B lymphocytes (B cells), T lymphocytes (T cells),** and **natural killer cells (NK cells)** (Box 3.4). B lymphocytes originate from stem cells and develop into B cells in the bone marrow before being widely distributed to lymphoid tissues throughout the body. These cells primarily function as antibody producers (plasma cells). T lymphocytes also originate from bone marrow stem cells, but they mature in the thymus and either directly destroy infected cells (cytotoxic T cells, TC or CTLs) or work with B cells (**helper T cells, TH**) to regulate antibody production. **Regulatory T cells (Tregs)** suppress autoimmune responses by other T lymphocytes and mediate immune tolerance. NK cells are a subset of T cells. There are different types of NK cells, with the most prevalent referred to as **invariant natural killer T (NKT) cells.** NKT cells develop in the thymus from the same precursor cells as other T lymphocytes. NKT cells have a limited repertoire of T-cell receptors that respond to synthetic, bacterial, and fungal glycolipids. NKT cells are activated by the release of cytokines during viral infections. Each of the three cell types is strategically located in lymphoid tissue throughout the body to maximize the chances of encountering invading microorganisms that the lymphatic system drains from the site of infection.

Two Branches of the Immune System

The immune system provides immunity through two main branches:

- **Antibody-mediated immunity,** or **humoral immunity**
- **Cell-mediated immunity,** or **cellular immunity**

Antibody-mediated immunity involves the activities of B cells and the production of antibodies. When a B cell encounters a microbial antigen, the cell is activated and initiates a series of events. These events are mediated by helper T cells and the release of cytokines. Cytokines mediate **clonal expansion** and the number of B cells capable of recognizing the antigen increases. Cytokines also activate the maturation of B cells into plasma cells that produce antibodies specific for the antigen. The process results in the production of B memory cells (Fig. 3.7). **B memory cells** remain quiescent in the body until a second (anamnestic) or subsequent exposure to the original antigen occurs. With secondary exposure, the B memory cells are preprogrammed

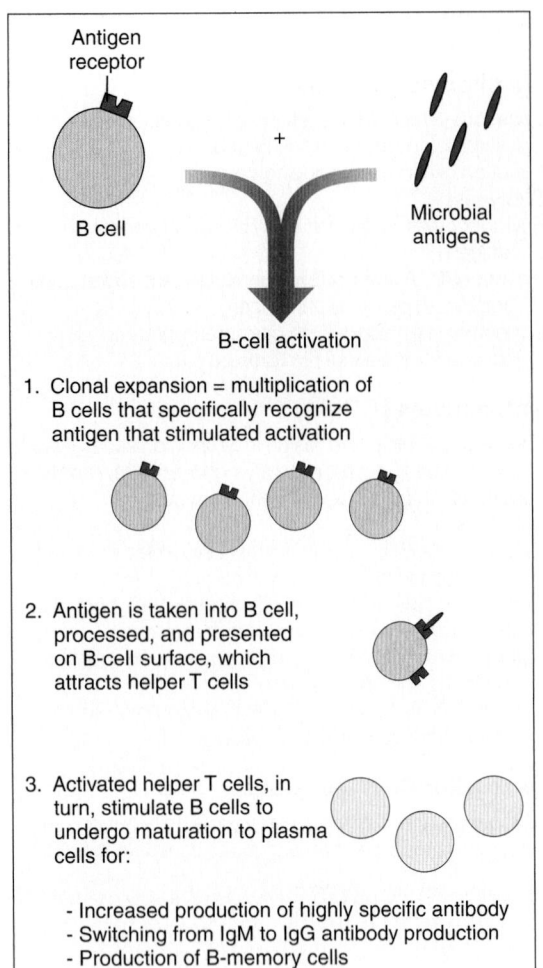

Antigen receptor

B cell

+

Microbial antigens

B-cell activation

1. Clonal expansion = multiplication of B cells that specifically recognize antigen that stimulated activation

2. Antigen is taken into B cell, processed, and presented on B-cell surface, which attracts helper T cells

3. Activated helper T cells, in turn, stimulate B cells to undergo maturation to plasma cells for:

- Increased production of highly specific antibody
- Switching from IgM to IgG antibody production
- Production of B-memory cells

• **Fig. 3.7** Overview of B-cell activation, which is central to antibody-mediated immunity.

to produce specific antibodies immediately upon encountering the original antigen.

Antibodies protect the host in a number of ways:

- Helping phagocytes to ingest and kill microorganisms through a coating mechanism, referred to as **opsonization**
- Neutralizing microbial toxins that are detrimental to host cells and tissues
- Promoting bacterial clumping (**agglutination**) that facilitates clearing from the infection site
- Inhibiting bacterial motility
- **Viral neutralization;** blocking the virus from entering the host cell
- Combining with microorganisms to activate the complement system and inflammatory response

Because a population of activated specific B cells is a developmental process that results from exposure to microbial antigens, antibody production is delayed when the host is first exposed to an infectious agent. This delay in the **primary antibody response** underscores the importance of nonspecific response defenses, such as inflammation, that work to hold the invading organisms in check while antibody production begins. This also emphasizes the

importance of B memory cell production. By virtue of this memory, any subsequent exposure or **secondary antibody response** to the same microorganism results in rapid production of protective antibodies avoiding the delays characteristic of the primary exposure.

Some antigens, such as bacterial capsules and outer membranes, activate B cells to produce antibodies without the intervention of helper T cells. However, this activation does not result in the production of B memory cells, and subsequent exposure to the same bacterial antigens does not result in a rapid host memory response.

The primary cells involved in cell-mediated immunity are T lymphocytes (cytotoxic T cells) that recognize and destroy human host cells infected with microorganisms. This function is extremely important for the destruction and elimination of infecting microorganisms. Cytotoxic T cells activated during the primary immune response also form a subset of memory T cells that are able to respond quickly to a subsequent infection from a previously encountered pathogen. Some pathogens (e.g., viruses, tuberculosis, some parasites, and fungi) are able to survive in host cells, protected from antibody interaction. Antibody-mediated immunity targets microorganisms outside human cells, whereas cell-mediated immunity targets microorganisms inside human cells. However, in many instances, these two branches of the immune system overlap and work together.

Like B cells, T cells must become activated in order to be effective. T-cell activation occurs through interactions with other cells that process microbial antigens and present them on their surface (e.g., macrophages, dendritic cells, and B cells). The responses of activated T cells are very different and depend on the subtype of T cell (Fig. 3.8). Activated helper T cells work with B cells for antibody production (Fig. 3.7) and facilitate inflammation by releasing cytokines. Cytotoxic T cells directly interact with and destroy host cells containing microorganisms or other infectious agents, such as viruses. The activated T cell subset, helper or cytotoxic cells, are controlled by an extremely complex series of biochemical pathways and genetic diversity within the **major histocompatibility complex (MHC).** MHC molecules are present on cells and form a complex with the antigen to present them to the T cells. The two primary classes of major histocompatibility molecules are **MHC I** and **MHC II.** MHC I molecules are located on every nucleated cell in the body and are predominantly responsible for the recognition of **endogenous proteins** expressed from within the cell. MHC II molecules are located on specialized cell types, including macrophages, dendritic cells, and B cells, for the presentation of extracellular molecules or **exogenous proteins.**

In summary, the host presents a spectrum of challenges to invading microorganisms, from physical barriers, including the skin and mucous membranes, to the interactive cellular and biochemical components of inflammation and the immune system. All these systems work together to minimize microbial invasion and prevent damage to vital tissues and organs resulting from the presence of infectious agents.

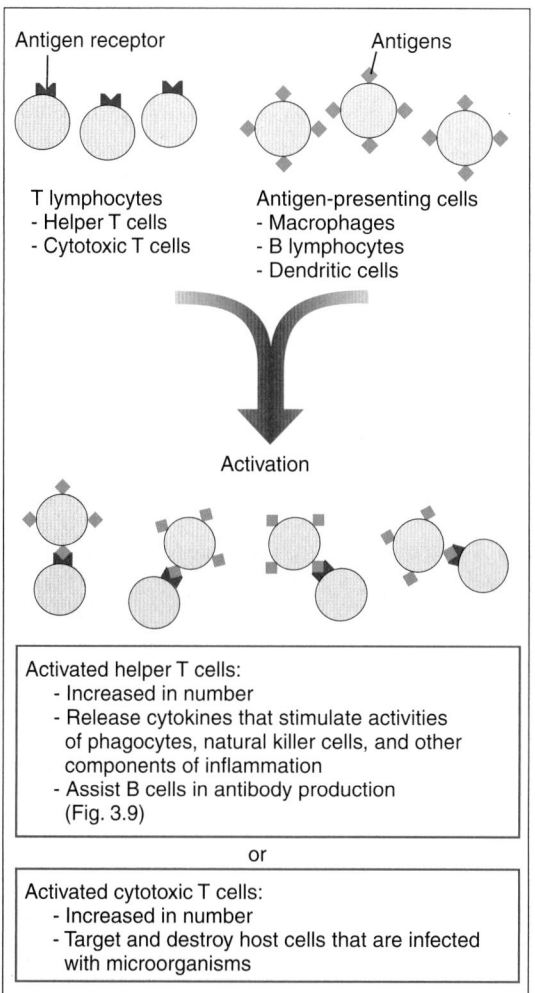

Antigen receptor

Antigens

T lymphocytes
- Helper T cells
- Cytotoxic T cells

Antigen-presenting cells
- Macrophages
- B lymphocytes
- Dendritic cells

Activation

Activated helper T cells:
- Increased in number
- Release cytokines that stimulate activities of phagocytes, natural killer cells, and other components of inflammation
- Assist B cells in antibody production (Fig. 3.9)

or

Activated cytotoxic T cells:
- Increased in number
- Target and destroy host cells that are infected with microorganisms

• **Fig. 3.8** Overview of T-cell activation, which is central to cell-mediated immunity.

The Microorganism's Perspective

Given the complexities of the human host's defense systems, it is no wonder that microbial strategies designed to survive these systems are equally complex.

Colonization and Infection

Many surfaces on the human body are colonized with a wide variety of microorganisms or microbiota without apparent detriment. In contrast, an **infection** involves the growth and multiplication of microorganisms that result in damage to the host. The extent and severity of the damage depend on many factors, including the microorganism's ability to cause disease, the site of the infection, and the general health of the individual infected. **Disease** results when the infection produces notable changes in human physiology associated with damage or loss of function to one or more of the body's organ systems.

Pathogens and Virulence

Microorganisms that cause infections or disease are considered **pathogens,** and the characteristics that enable

them to cause disease are referred to as **virulence factors.** Most virulence factors protect the organism against host attack or mediate damaging effects on host cells. The terms **pathogenicity** and **virulence** reflect the degree to which a microorganism is capable of causing disease. Pathogenicity specifically refers to the organism's ability to cause disease, whereas virulence refers to the measure or degree of pathogenicity of an organism. An organism of high pathogenicity is very likely to cause disease, whereas an organism of low pathogenicity is much less likely to cause infection. When disease does occur, highly virulent organisms often severely damage the human host. The degree of severity decreases with diminishing virulence of the microorganism.

Because host factors play a role in the development of infectious diseases, the distinction between a **pathogenic** and **nonpathogenic** organism and colonizer is not always clear. For example, many organisms that colonize the skin usually do not cause disease (i.e., exhibit low pathogenicity) under normal circumstances. However, when damage to the skin occurs (Box 3.3) or when the skin is disrupted in some other way, these organisms can gain access to deeper tissues and establish an infection.

Organisms that cause infection when one or more of the host's defense mechanisms are disrupted or malfunction are known as **opportunistic pathogens,** and the infections they cause are referred to as **opportunistic infections.** On the other hand, several pathogens known to cause serious infections can be part of an individual's microbiome (i.e., **carriers**) and never cause disease. However, the same organism can cause life-threatening infection when transmitted to other individuals. The reasons for these inconsistencies are not fully understood, but such widely different results undoubtedly involve complex interactions between microorganism and human. Recognizing and separating a pathogenic from a nonpathogenic organism present one of the greatest challenges in interpreting diagnostic microbiology laboratory results.

Microbial Virulence Factors

Virulence factors provide microorganisms with the capacity to avoid host defenses and damage host cells, tissues, and organs in a number of ways. Some virulence factors are specific for certain pathogenic genera, species, or strains of a microorganism, and substantial differences exist in the way bacteria, viruses, parasites, and fungi cause disease. Knowledge of a microorganism's capacity to cause specific types of infections plays a major role in the development of diagnostic microbiology procedures used for isolating and identifying microorganisms. (See Part VII for more information regarding diagnosis by organ system.)

Attachment

Whether humans encounter microorganisms in the air, through ingestion, or by direct contact, the first step of infection and disease development, a process referred to as **pathogenesis,** is microbial **attachment** to a surface (exceptions being instances in which the organisms are directly introduced by trauma or other means into deeper tissues).

Many of the microbial factors that facilitate attachment of pathogens are the same as those used by nonpathogenic colonizers (Box 3.2). Most pathogenic organisms are not part of the normal human microbiota, and attachment to the host requires that they outcompete the microbiota for a place on the body's surface. Medical interventions, such as the overuse of antimicrobial agents, result in the destruction of the normal microbiota, creating a competitive advantage for the invading pathogenic organism.

Invasion

Once surface attachment has been secured, microbial **invasion** into subsurface tissues and organs (i.e., infection) is accomplished by disruption of the skin and mucosal surfaces by several mechanisms (Box 3.3) or by the direct action of an organism's virulence factors. Some microorganisms produce factors that force **mucosal surface phagocytes (M cells)** to ingest them and then release them unharmed into the tissue below the surface. Other organisms, such as staphylococci and streptococci, are not so subtle. These organisms produce an array of enzymes (e.g., hyaluronidases, nucleases, collagenases) that hydrolyze host proteins and nucleic acids, destroying host cells and tissues. This destruction allows the pathogen to "burrow" through minor openings in the outer surface of the skin and into deeper tissues. Once a pathogen has penetrated the body, it uses a variety of strategies to survive attack by the host's inflammatory and immune responses. Alternatively, some pathogens cause disease at the site of attachment without further penetration. For example, in diseases such as diphtheria and whooping cough, the bacteria produce toxic substances that destroy surrounding tissues. The organisms generally do not penetrate the mucosal surface they inhabit.

Survival Against Inflammation

If a pathogen is to survive, the action of the phagocytes and the complement components of inflammation must be avoided or controlled (Box 3.5). Some organisms, such as *Streptococcus pneumoniae,* a common cause of bacterial pneumonia and meningitis, avoid phagocytosis by producing a large capsule that inhibits the phagocytic process. Other pathogens may not be able to avoid phagocytosis but are not effectively destroyed once internalized and are able to survive within phagocytes. This is the case for *Mycobacterium tuberculosis,* the bacterium that causes tuberculosis. Still other pathogens use toxins and enzymes to attack and destroy phagocytes before the phagocytes attack and destroy them.

The defenses offered by the complement system depend on a series of biochemical reactions triggered by specific microorganism molecular structures. Therefore microbial avoidance of complement activation requires that the infecting agent either mask its activating molecules (e.g., via production of a capsule that covers bacterial surface antigens)

• BOX 3.5 Microbial Strategies for Surviving Inflammation

Avoid Killing by Phagocytes (Polymorphonuclear Leukocytes)

- Producing a capsule, thereby inhibiting phagocytes' ability to ingest them
- Antigenic variation, changing surface antigens to limit the number of cells recognized by the immune system

Avoid Phagocyte-Mediated Killing

- Inhibiting phagosome-lysosome fusion
- Being resistant to destructive agents (e.g., lysozyme) released by lysosomes
- Actively and rapidly multiplying within a phagocyte
- Releasing toxins and enzymes that damage or kill phagocytes

Avoid Effects of the Complement System

- Using a capsule to hide surface molecules that would otherwise activate the complement system, including the formation of a complex protein polysaccharide matrix (biofilm)
- Producing substances that inhibit the processes involved in complement activation
- Producing substances that destroy specific complement proteins

---

or produce substances (e.g., enzymes) that disrupt critical biochemical components of the complement pathway.

Any single microorganism may possess numerous virulence factors, and several may be expressed simultaneously. For example, while trying to avoid phagocytosis, an organism may also secrete other enzymes and toxins that destroy and penetrate tissue and produce other factors designed to interfere with the immune response. Microorganisms may also use host systems to their own advantage. For example, the lymphatic and circulatory systems used to carry monocytes and lymphocytes to the site of infection may serve to disperse the organism throughout the body.

Survival Against the Immune System

Microbial strategies to avoid the defenses of the immune system are outlined in Box 3.6. Again, a pathogen can use more than one strategy to avoid immune-mediated defenses, and microbial survival does not necessarily require devastation of the immune system. The pathogen may merely need to "buy" time to reach a safe area in the body or to be transferred to the next susceptible host. In addition, microorganisms can avoid much of the immune response if they do not penetrate the surface layers of the body. This strategy is the hallmark of diseases caused by microbial toxins.

Microbial Toxins

Toxins are biochemically active substances released by microorganisms that have a particular effect on host cells. Microorganisms use toxins to establish infections and multiply within the host. Alternatively, a pathogen may be restricted to

- Rapid invasion and multiplication resulting in damage to the host before the immune response can be fully activated, or organism's virulence is so great that the immune response is insufficient
- Invasion and destruction of cells involved in the immune response
- Survival in host cells and avoiding detection by the immune system
- Masking the organism's antigens with a capsule or biofilm so that an immune response is not activated
- Altering the expression and presentation of antigens so that the immune system is constantly fighting a primary encounter (i.e., the memory of the immune system is neutralized)
- Production of enzymes (proteases) that directly destroy or inactivate antibodies

• BOX 3.7 Summary of Bacterial Toxins

Endotoxins
- General toxin common to almost all gram-negative bacteria
- Composed of the lipopolysaccharide portion of cell envelope
- Released when a gram-negative bacterial cell is destroyed
  - Effects on host include:
    - Disruption of clotting, causing clots to form throughout the body (i.e., disseminated intravascular coagulation [DIC])
    - Fever
    - Activation of complement and immune systems
    - Circulatory changes that lead to hypotension, shock, and death

Exotoxins
- Most commonly associated with gram-positive bacteria
- Produced and released by living bacteria; do not require bacterial death for release
- Specific toxins target specific host cells; the type of toxin varies with the bacterial species
- Some kill host cells and help spread bacteria in tissues (e.g., enzymes that destroy key biochemical tissue components or specifically destroy host cell membranes)
- Some destroy or interfere with specific intracellular activities (e.g., interruption of protein synthesis, interruption of internal cell signals, or interruption of the neuromuscular system)

a particular body site from which toxins are released to cause systemic damage throughout the body. Toxins also can cause human disease in the absence of the pathogens that produced them. This common mechanism of food poisoning involves ingestion of preformed bacterial toxins (present in the food at the time of ingestion) and is referred to as **intoxication,** a notable example of which is botulism.

Endotoxin and **exotoxin** are the two general types of bacterial toxins (Box 3.7). Endotoxin is a component of the cellular structure of gram-negative bacteria and can have

devastating effects on the body's metabolism, the most serious being endotoxic shock, which often results in death. The effects of exotoxins produced by gram-positive bacteria tend to be more limited and specific than the effects of gram-negative endotoxin. The activities of exotoxins range from enzymes produced by many staphylococci and streptococci that augment bacterial invasion by damaging host tissues and cells to highly specific activities (e.g., diphtheria toxin inhibits protein synthesis, and cholera toxin interferes with host cell signals). Examples of other highly active and specific toxins are those that cause botulism and tetanus by interfering with neuromuscular functions.

Genetics of Virulence: Pathogenicity Islands

Many virulence factors are encoded in genomic regions of pathogens known as **pathogenicity islands (PAIs).** These mobile genetic elements contribute to the change and spread of virulence factors among bacterial populations of a variety of species. These genetic elements are believed to have evolved from lysogenic bacteriophages and plasmids and are spread by horizontal gene transfer (see Chapter 2 for information about bacterial genetics). PAIs typically comprise one or more virulence-associated genes and "mobility" genes (i.e., integrases and transposases) that mediate movement between various genetic elements (e.g., plasmids and chromosomes) and among different bacterial strains. In essence, PAIs facilitate the dissemination of virulence capabilities among bacteria in a manner similar to the mechanism diagramed in Fig. 2.10; this also facilitates dissemination of antimicrobial resistance genes (Chapter 10). PAIs are widely disseminated among medically important bacteria. For example, PAIs have been identified as playing a role in virulence for each of the following organisms:

Helicobacter pylori
Pseudomonas aeruginosa
Shigella spp.
Yersinia spp.
Vibrio cholerae
Salmonella spp.
Escherichia coli (enteropathogenic, enterohemorrhagic or serotoxigenic, verotoxigenic, uropathogenic, enterotoxigenic, enteroinvasive, enteroaggregative, meningitis-sepsis associated; Chapter 19)
Neisseria spp.
Bacteroides fragilis
Listeria monocytogenes
Staphylococcus aureus
Streptococcus spp.
Enterococcus faecalis
Clostridioides difficile

Biofilm Formation

Microorganisms typically exist as a group or community of organisms capable of adhering to each other or to other surfaces. A variety of bacterial pathogens, along with other microorganisms, are capable of forming biofilms, such as *S. aureus, P. aeruginosa, Aggregatibacter* spp., *Salmonella* spp.,

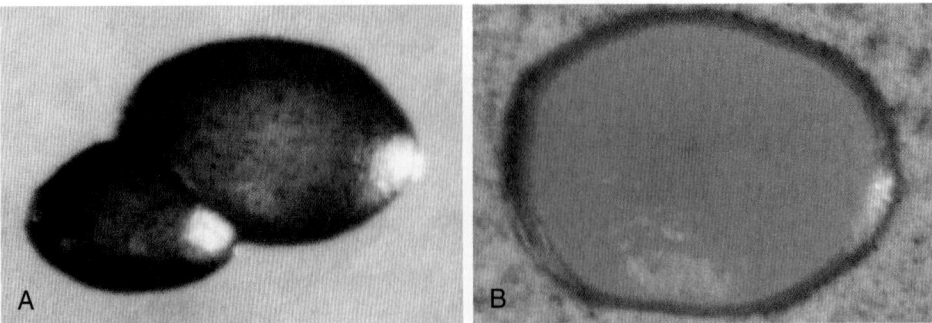

• **Fig. 3.9** (A) Biofilm forming isolate of *Staphylococcus aureus* cultivated on Congo red agar. Biofilm production results in the formation of a black precipitate. (B) Non–biofilm-producing strain of *S. aureus* cultivated on Congo red agar.

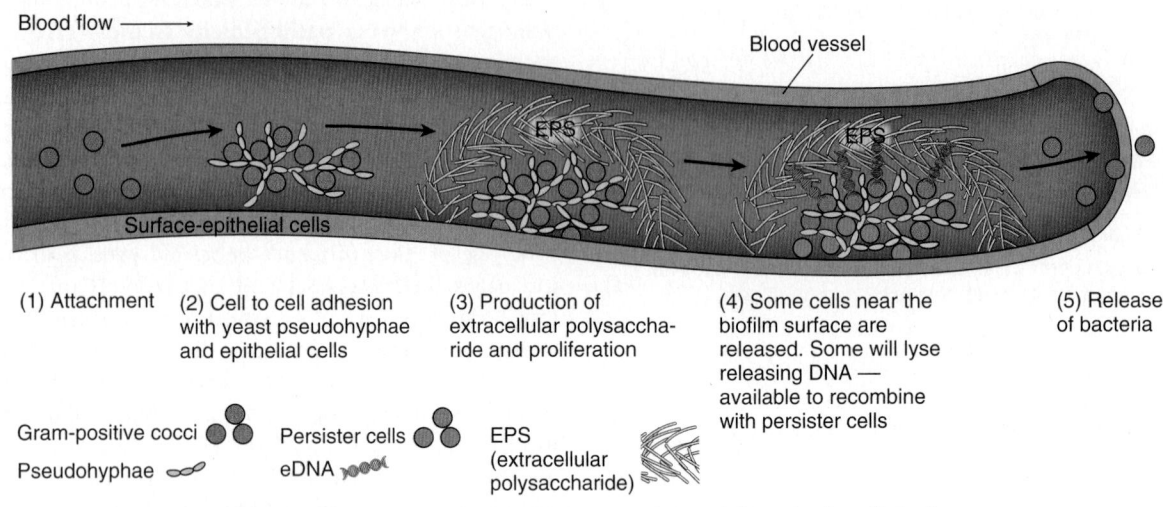

• **Fig. 3.10** Overview of biofilm formation, maturation, and dissemination of infection.

Citrobacter koseri, and *Candida albicans.* A biofilm is an accumulation of microorganisms embedded in a complex matrix composed of proteins, polysaccharides, extracellular DNA (eDNA), and other molecules. Pathogenic microorganisms use the formation of biofilm to adhere to implants and prosthetic devices. For example, health care–related infections with *Staphylococcus* spp. (Fig. 3.9) associated with implants have become more prevalent. Biofilm-forming strains have a much more complex antibiotic resistance profile, indicating failure of the antibiotic to penetrate the polysaccharide layer. In addition, some of the cells in a **sessile** or stationary biofilm may experience nutrient deprivation and therefore exist in a slow-growing or starved state (i.e., **persister cells**), displaying reduced susceptibility to antimicrobial agents. These organisms also have demonstrated a differential gene expression compared with their **planktonic** or free-floating counterparts. The biofilm-forming communities are able to adapt and respond to changes in their environment, similar to a multicellular organism.

Biofilms may form from the accumulation of a single microorganism (**monomicrobic aggregation**) or from the accumulation of numerous species (**polymicrobic aggregation**). The initial stage in biofilm formation begins with the synthesis of

an extracellular polymer matrix accompanied by aggregation and recognition. This process is facilitated by the formation of polysaccharides, proteins, and eDNA. The formation of the biofilm protects the organism from desiccation, forms a barrier against toxic compounds, and prevents the loss of protective organic and inorganic molecules. Once the initial biofilm has developed, a process of maturation of the biofilm occurs, which takes approximately 4 to 6 hours, depending on the growth rate of the microorganism. This includes the complex formation of a three-dimensional architecture, including pores and channels within the polymer matrix. During biofilm accumulation, the cells reach a critical mass that result in the alteration in metabolism and gene expression in the persister cells. This is accomplished through a mechanism of signaling between cells or organisms through chemical signals or inducer molecules, such as acyl homoserine lactone (AHL) in gram-negative bacteria or oligopeptides in gram-positive bacteria. These signals are capable of interspecies and intraspecies communication. In addition, the formation of a complex polymicrobial biofilm provides favorable conditions for the exchange of genetic information and horizontal gene transfer. Fig. 3.10 provides an overview of biofilm formation, maturation, and seeding that results in further dissemination and infection.

Microbial biofilm formation is important to many disciplines, including environmental science, industry, and public health. Biofilm formation affects the efficient treatment of wastewater; it is essential for the effective production of beer, which requires aggregation of yeast cells; and it affects bioremediation for toxic substances such as oil. It has been reported that approximately 65% of hospital-associated infections are associated with biofilm formation. Box 3.8 provides an overview of pathogenic organisms associated with biofilm formation in human infections.

Outcome and Prevention of Infectious Diseases

Outcome of Infectious Diseases

Given the complexities of host defenses and microbial virulence, it is not surprising that the factors determining

---

• **BOX 3.8** **Biofilms and Human Infections**

These pathogenic organisms have been associated with biofilm formation in human infections.
- *Acinetobacter* spp.
- *Aeromonas* spp.
- *Candida albicans*
- *Citrobacter* spp.
- Coagulase-negative staphylococci
- *Cronobacter* spp.
- *Enterobacter* spp.
- *Enterococcus* spp.
- *Escherichia coli*
- *Klebsiella* spp.
- *Listeria monocytogenes*
- *Proteus* spp.
- *Pseudomonas aeruginosa*
- *Serratia* spp.
- *Staphylococcus aureus*
- *Streptococcus* spp.
- *Listeria monocytogenes*

Not intended to be an all-inclusive list.

---

outcome between these two living entities are also complicated. Outcome depends on the state of the host's health, the virulence of the pathogen, and whether the host can clear the pathogen before infection and disease cause irreparable harm or death (Fig. 3.11).

The time from exposure to an infectious agent and the development of a disease or infection depends on host and microbial factors. Infectious processes that develop quickly are referred to as **acute infections,** and those that develop and progress slowly, sometimes over a period of years, are known as **chronic infections.** Some pathogens, particularly certain viruses, can be clinically silent inside the body without any noticeable effect on the host before suddenly causing a severe and acute infection. During the silent phase, the infection is said to be **latent.** Again, depending on host and microbial factors, acute, chronic, or latent infections can result in any of the outcomes detailed in Fig. 3.11.

Medical intervention can help the host to fight the infection but usually is not instituted until after the host is aware that an infectious process is underway. The clues that an infection is occurring are known as the signs and symptoms of disease and result from host responses (e.g., inflammatory and immune responses) to the action of microbial virulence factors (Box 3.9). **Signs** are measurable indications or physical observations, such as an increase in body temperature (fever) or the development of a rash or swelling. **Symptoms** are indictors as described by the patient, such as headache, aches, fatigue, and nausea. The signs and symptoms reflect the stages of infection. In turn, the stages of infection generally reflect the stages in host-microorganism interactions (Fig. 3.12).

Whether medical procedures contribute to controlling or clearing an infection depends on key factors, including:
- The severity of the infection, which is determined by the host and microbial interactions already discussed
- Accuracy in diagnosing the pathogen or pathogens causing the infection

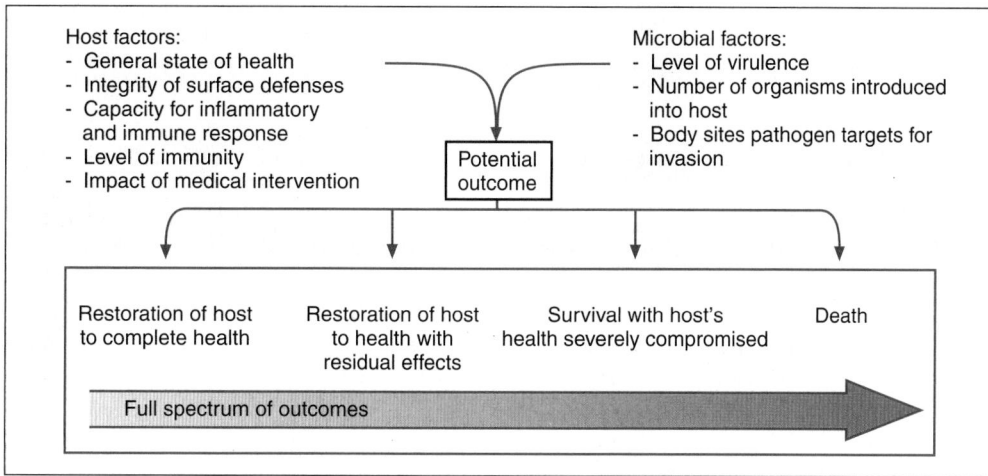

• **Fig. 3.11** Possible outcomes of infections and infectious diseases.

- Whether the patient receives appropriate treatment for the infection (which depends on accurate diagnosis)

Prevention of Infectious Diseases

The treatment of an infection is often difficult and not always successful. Because much of the damage may already have been done before appropriate medical intervention is provided, the microorganisms gain too much of a "head start." Another strategy for combating infectious diseases is to stop infections before they start (i.e., disease prevention). As discussed at the beginning of this chapter, the first step in any host-microorganism relationship is the encounter and exposure to the infectious agent. Therefore, strategies to prevent disease involve interrupting or minimizing the risk of infection when exposures occur. As outlined in Box 3.10, interruption of encounters may be accomplished

by preventing transmission of the infecting agents and by controlling or destroying reservoirs of human pathogens. Interestingly, most of these measures do not really involve medical practices but rather social practices and policies.

Immunization

Medical strategies exist for minimizing the risk of disease development when exposure to infectious agents occurs. One of the most effective methods is **vaccination,** also referred to as **immunization.** This practice

---

• **BOX 3.9** **Signs and Symptoms of Infection and Infectious Diseases**

- General or localized aches and pains
- Headache
- Fever
- Fatigue
- Swollen lymph nodes
- Rashes
- Redness and swelling
- Cough and sneezes
- Congestion of nasal and sinus passages
- Sore throat
- Nausea and vomiting
- Diarrhea

• **BOX 3.10** **Strategies for Preventing Infectious Diseases**

Preventing Transmission

- Avoid direct contact with infected persons or take protective measures when direct contact will occur (e.g., wear gloves, wear condoms).
- Block the spread of airborne microorganisms by wearing masks or isolating persons with infections transmitted by air.
- Use sterile medical techniques.

Controlling Microbial Reservoirs

- Sanitation and disinfection
- Sewage treatment
- Food preservation
- Water treatment
- Control of pests and insect vector populations

Minimizing Risk Before or Shortly After Exposure

- Immunization or vaccination
- Cleansing and use of antiseptics
- Prophylactic use of antimicrobial agents

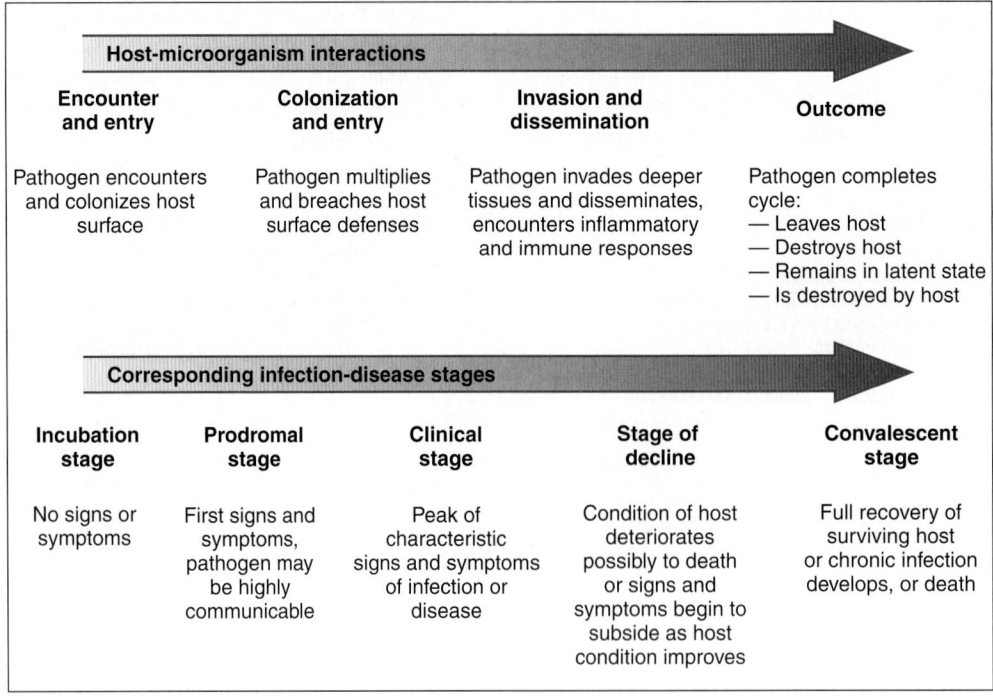

• **Fig. 3.12** Host-microorganism interactions and stages of infection or disease.

takes advantage of the specificity and memory of the immune system. The two basic approaches to immunization are **active immunization** and **passive immunization.** With active immunization, modified antigens from pathogenic microorganisms are introduced into the body and cause an immune response. If or when the host encounters the pathogen in nature, the memory of the immune system ensures minimal delay in the immune response, thus affording strong protection. With passive immunization, antibodies against a particular pathogen that have been produced in one host are transferred to a second host, where they provide temporary protection. The passage of maternal antibodies to the newborn is a key example of natural passive immunization. Active immunity is generally longer lasting, because the immunized host's own immune response has been activated. However, for complex reasons, naturally acquired active immunity has had limited success for relatively few infectious diseases, necessitating the development of vaccines. Successful immunization has proven effective against many infectious diseases, including diphtheria, whooping cough (pertussis), tetanus, influenza, polio, smallpox, measles, hepatitis, and certain *S. pneumoniae* and *Haemophilus influenzae* infections.

Prophylactic antimicrobial therapy, the administration of antibiotics when the risk of developing an infection is high, is another common medical intervention for preventing infection.

Epidemiology

To prevent infectious diseases, information is required regarding the sources of pathogens, the mode of transmission to and among humans, human risk factors for encountering the pathogen and developing infection, and factors that contribute to good and bad outcomes resulting from the exposure. **Epidemiology** is the science that characterizes these aspects of infectious diseases and monitors the effect diseases have on public health. Fully characterizing the circumstances associated with the acquisition and dissemination of infectious diseases gives researchers a better chance of preventing and eliminating the diseases. In addition, many epidemiologic strategies developed for use in public health systems also apply in long-term care facilities (e.g., nursing homes, hospitals, assisted-living centers) for the control of HAI infections (i.e., nosocomial infections; for more information on infection control, see Chapter 79).

The field of epidemiology is broad and complex. Diagnostic microbiology laboratory personnel and epidemiologists often work closely to investigate problems. Familiarity with certain epidemiologic terms and concepts is important (Box 3.1).

Because the central focus of epidemiology is on tracking and characterizing infections and infectious diseases, this field depends heavily on diagnostic microbiology. Epidemiologic investigations cannot proceed unless researchers first know the **etiologic** or **causative agents.** Therefore the procedures and protocols used in diagnostic microbiology to detect, isolate, and characterize human pathogens are essential for patient care and also play a central role in epidemiologic studies focused on disease prevention and the general improvement of public health. In fact, microbiologists who work in clinical laboratories are often the first to recognize patterns that suggest potential outbreaks or epidemics.

ⓔ Visit the Evolve site for a complete list of procedures, review questions, and case studies.

Bibliography

Akondy RS, Fitch M, Edupuganti S, et al.: Origin and differentiation of human memory CD8 T cells after vaccination, *Nature* 552:362–367, 2017.

Bennett J, Dolin R, Blaser M: *Principles and practice of infectious diseases*, 9th ed., Philadelphia, PA, 2020, Elsevier Saunders.

Brock TD, Madigan M, Martinko J, et al.: *Biology of microorganisms*, Upper Saddle River, NJ, 2009, Prentice Hall.

Carroll KC, Pfaller MA, Landry ML, et al.: *Manual of clinical microbiology*, 12th ed., Washington D.C., 2019, ASM.

Ding T, Scholoss PD: Dynamics and associations of microbial community types across the human body, *Nature* 509:357–360, 2014.

Dobrindt U: Genomic islands in pathogenic and environmental microorganisms, *Nat Rev Microbiol* 2:414–424, 2002.

Engleberg NC, DiRita V, Dermody TS: *schaechter's mechanisms of microbial disease*, Baltimore, MD, 2007, Lippincott Williams & Wilkins.

Hu T, Gimferrer I, Alberola-Ila J: Control of early stages in invariant natural killer T-cell development, *Immunology* 134:1–7, 2011.

Huttenhower C, Gevers D, Knight R, et al.: Structure, function and diversity of the Healthy Human Microbiome, *Nature* 486:207–214, 2012.

Karunakaran E, Mukherjee J, Ramalingam B, Biggs CA: Biofilmology: a multidisciplinary review of the study of microbial biofilms, *Appl Microbiol Biotechnol* 90:1869–1881, 2011.

Lister JL, Horswill AR: *Staphylococcus aureus* biofilms: recent developments in biofilm dispersal, *Front Cell Infect Microbiol* 4:178, 2014.

Manandhar S, Singh A, Varma A, et al.: Evaluation of methods to detect in vitro biofilm formation by staphylococcal clinical isolates, *BMC Res Notes* 11:714, 2018.

Simões LC, Lemos M, Pereira AM, et al.: Persister cells in a biofilm treated with a biocide, *Biofouling* 27(4):403–411, 2011.

Murray PR, editor: *Medical microbiology*, 5th ed., St Louis, MO, 2008, Mosby.

Schmidt H, Hensel M: Pathogenicity islands in bacterial pathogenesis, *Clin Microbiol Rev* 17:14–56, 2004.

Vaishnavi C, Samanta J, Kochhar R: Characterization of biofilms in biliary stents and potential factors involved in occlusion, *World J Gastroenterol* 24:112–123, 2018.

Vidarsson G, Dekkers G, Rispens T: IgG subclasses and allotypes: from structure to effector functions, *Front Immunol* 5:520, 2014.

Youngblood B, Hale JS, Kissick HT, et al.: Effector CD8 T cells dedifferentiate into long-lived memory cells, *Nature* 552:404–409, 2017.

Zhurina MV, Gannesen AV, Zdorovenko EL, Plakunov VK: Composition and functions of the extracellular polymer matrix of bacterial biofilms, *Microbiology* 83:713–722, 2014.

4

Laboratory Safety

OBJECTIVES

1. Define and differentiate sterilization, disinfection, decontamination, and antiseptic.
2. List the factors that influence the effectiveness of disinfectants in the microbiology laboratory.
3. Describe the methods used for the disposal of hazardous waste, including physical and chemical methods, and the material and/or organisms effectively eliminated by each method.
4. Define a chemical hygiene plan and describe the purpose of the methods and items that are elements of the plan, including proper labeling of hazardous materials, training programs, and safety data sheets (SDS).
5. Name the four types of fire extinguishers and the specific flammables that each is effective in controlling.
6. Describe the process of Standard Precautions in the microbiology laboratory, including handling of infectious materials, personal hygiene, use of personal protective equipment (PPE), handling sharp objects, and hand-washing procedures.
7. Define Biosafety Levels 1 through 4, including the precautions required for each and type of facility; identify a representative organism for each.
8. Outline the basic guidelines for packing and shipping infectious substances.
9. Describe the management and response required during a biologic or chemical exposure incident in the laboratory.

Microbiology laboratory safety practices were first published in 1913. They included admonitions such as the necessity to (1) wear gloves, (2) wash hands after working with infectious materials, (3) disinfect all instruments immediately after use, (4) use water to moisten specimen labels rather than the tongue, (5) disinfect all contaminated waste before discarding, and (6) report to appropriate personnel all accidents or exposures to infectious agents.

These guidelines are still incorporated into safety programs in the diagnostic microbiology laboratory. Safety programs have been expanded to include the proper handling of biologic hazards encountered in processing patient specimens and handling infectious microorganisms that include standard precautions and transmission-based precautions, engineering and work place controls and risk assessment; fire and electrical safety; the safe handling, storage, and disposal of chemicals and radioactive substances; and techniques for safely lifting or moving heavy objects. In areas of the country prone to natural disasters (e.g., earthquakes, hurricanes, snowstorms), safety programs include disaster preparedness plans that outline the steps to take in an emergency. Although all microbiologists are responsible for their own health and safety, the institution and supervising personnel are required to provide safety training to familiarize microbiologists with known hazards in the workplace and to prevent exposure. Infection control is also a vital part of laboratory safety and is discussed in detail in Chapter 78.

Laboratory safety is considered an integral part of overall laboratory services, and federal law in the United States mandates preemployment safety training, followed by quarterly safety in-services. Safety training regulations are enforced by the United States Department of Labor Occupational Safety and Health Administration (OSHA). Regulations and requirements may vary based on the type of laboratory and updated regulations. It is recommended that the laboratory review these requirements as outlined by OSHA (www.osha.gov).

Microbiologists should be knowledgeable, properly trained, and equipped with the proper protective materials, engineering, and working controls while performing duties in the laboratory. Investigation of the causes of accidents indicates that unnecessary exposures to infectious agents occur when individuals become sloppy in performing their duties or when they deviate from standardized safety precautions.

TABLE 4.1 Classification Scheme of Items Requiring Sterilization or Disinfection

Classification	Description	Items	Methods
Critical items	Pose a high risk of infection if contaminated with infectious agents.	Surgical instruments Cardiac and urinary catheters Implants Ultrasound probes used in sterile body cavities	Purchased as sterilized Heat-sensitive objects: ethylene oxide, hydrogen peroxide gas plasma Chemical: glutaraldehyde, stabilized hydrogen peroxide with or without peracetic acid in specific concentrations
Semi-critical items	Generally items that are exposed to the mucous membranes or nonintact skin. These items should be free of all infectious agents including vegetative bacteria, fungi, and viruses.	Respiratory therapy and anesthesia equipment, endoscopes, laryngoscope blades, esophageal manometry probes, cystoscopes, anorectal manometry catheters, and diaphragm fitting rings.	Glutaraldehyde, hydrogen peroxide, ortho-phthaladehyde, hydrogen peroxide with peracetic acid
Non-critical items	Items that contact intact skin but not mucous membranes.	Noncritical patient care items such as bedpans, blood pressure cuffs, computers, crutches etc. Noncritical environmental surfaces: bed rails, bedside tables, patient furniture, and floors.	

Adapted from Centers for Disease and Control Guideline for Disinfection and Sterilization in Healthcare Facilities; https://www.cdc.gov/infectioncontrol/pdf/guidelines/disinfection-guidelines.pdf

Sterilization, Disinfection, and Decontamination

The Guideline for Disinfection and Sterilization in Healthcare Facilities provides evidence-based recommendations for all cleaning, disinfection, and sterilization of medical devices and the healthcare environment (Table 4.1). Equipment and services associated with patient care and the healthcare environment are all subject to regulations and recommendations for the level of sterilization and/or disinfection based on the risk of infection to the patient. These items as well as considerations for disinfection in the ambulatory care and home care environment are included in Chapter 78.

Sterilization is a process that kills all forms of microbial life, including bacterial endospores. **Disinfection** is a process that destroys pathogenic organisms, but not necessarily all microorganisms, endospores, or prions. However, some disinfectants will kill endospores with prolonged exposure times (3 to 12 hours). These disinfectants are **chemical sterilants. Decontamination** is the removal of pathogenic microorganisms so items are safe to handle or dispose of. Many factors limit the success or degree of sterilization, disinfection, or decontamination in a health care setting, such as organic load (organisms and other contaminating materials such as blood or body fluids), the type of organisms present, the concentration and exposure time to the germicide, the physical and chemical nature of the object or surface (hinges, cracks, rough or smooth surfaces), temperature, pH, humidity,

and presence of a biofilm. These processes may be accomplished by a variety of physical or chemical methods.

Methods of Sterilization

The physical methods of sterilization include:
- Incineration
- Moist heat
- Dry heat
- Filtration
- Ionizing (gamma) radiation
- Chemicals (ethylene oxide [EtO] gas, hydrogen peroxide gas plasma, vaporized hydrogen peroxide, and other liquid chemicals)

Incineration is a method of treating infectious waste. Hazardous material is literally burned to ashes at temperatures of 870°C to 980°C. Incineration is the safest method to ensure that no infective materials remain in samples or containers when disposed. Prions (infective proteins) are not eliminated using conventional methods. Therefore incineration is recommended. Toxic air emissions and the presence of heavy metals in ash have limited the use of incineration in the United States.

Moist heat (steam under pressure) is used to sterilize biohazardous trash and heat-stable objects; an **autoclave** is used for this purpose. An autoclave is essentially a large pressure cooker. Moist heat in the form of saturated steam under one atmosphere (15 pounds per square inch [psi]) of pressure causes the irreversible denaturation of enzymes and structural proteins. The most commonly used steam

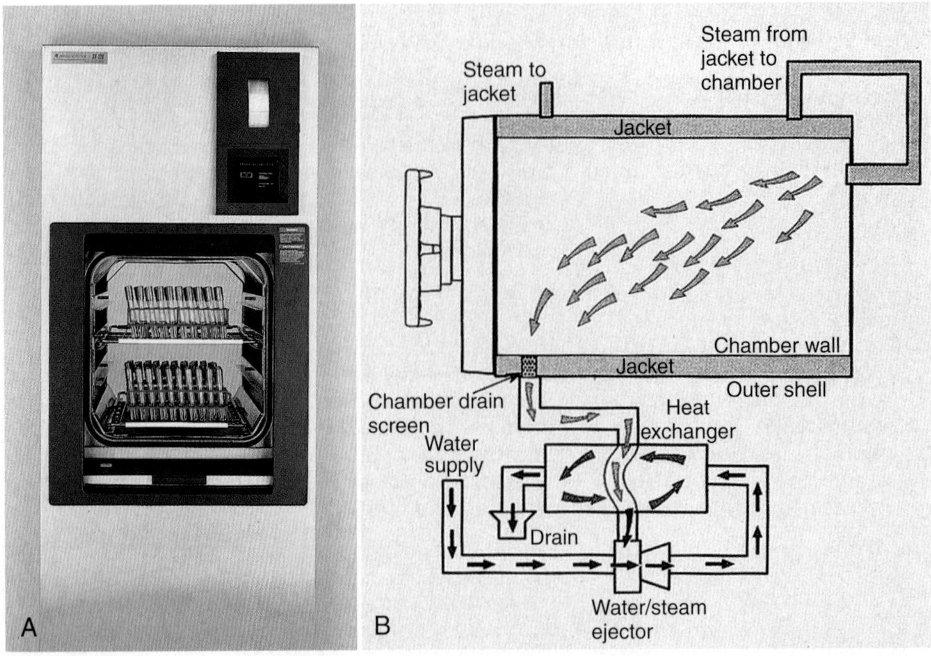

• **Fig. 4.1** Gravity displacement type of autoclave. (A) Typical Eagle Century Series sterilizer for laboratory applications. (B) Typical Eagle 3000 sterilizer piping diagram. The arrows show the entry of steam into the chamber and the displacement of air. (Courtesy AMSCO International, a subsidiary of STERIS Corp., Mentor, Ohio.)

sterilizer in the microbiology laboratory is the gravity displacement autoclave (Fig. 4.1). Steam enters at the top of the sterilizing chamber; because steam is lighter than air, it displaces the air in the chamber and forces it out the bottom through the drain vent. The two common sterilization temperatures are 121°C and 132°C. Biologic waste that includes broth or solid media is usually autoclaved for 30 minutes at 121°C in a displacement sterilizer or 4 minutes at 132°C in a prevacuum sterilizer. Infectious medical waste containing body fluids or blood, on the other hand, is often sterilized at 132°C for 30 to 60 minutes to allow penetration of the steam throughout the waste and the displacement of air trapped inside the autoclave bag. Prions require a much more extensive sterilization process. Several options are recommended for the removal of prions from surgical instruments or other laboratory materials contaminated with high-risk tissue such as brain, spinal cord, and eye tissue. There are four methods for sterilization: (1) autoclave at 134°C for 18 minutes in a prevacuum sterilizer; (2) autoclave at 132°C for 1 hour in a gravity displacement sterilizer; (3) immerse in 1 N sodium hydroxide for 1 hour, remove and rinse with water, then autoclave at 121°C in a gravity displacement or 134°C in a prevacuum sterilizer for 1 hour; or (4) immerse in 1 N sodium hydroxide for 1 hour and heat in a gravity displacement at 121°C for 30 minutes, then clean and subject to routine equipment sterilization. Moist heat is the fastest and simplest physical method of sterilization.

Dry heat requires longer exposure times (1.5 to 3 hours) and higher temperatures than moist heat (160° to 180°C). Dry heat ovens are used to sterilize items such as glassware, oil, petrolatum, or powders. **Filtration** is the method of choice for antibiotic solutions, toxic chemicals, radioisotopes, vaccines, and carbohydrates, which are all heat sensitive. Filtration of liquids is accomplished by pulling the solution through a cellulose acetate or cellulose nitrate membrane with a vacuum. Filtration of air is accomplished using high-efficiency particulate air (HEPA) filters designed to remove organisms larger than 0.3 µm from isolation rooms, operating rooms, and biologic safety cabinets (BSCs). Although considered a method of sterilization, filtration simply removes microorganisms and particles larger than the pore size; smaller particles will not be removed using this method. The ionizing radiation used in microwaves and radiograph machines is composed of short-wavelength and high-energy gamma rays. Ionizing radiation is used for sterilizing disposables such as plastic syringes, catheters, or gloves before use. The most common chemical sterilant is EtO, which is used in gaseous form for sterilizing heat-sensitive objects. The main disadvantages of EtO use are the lengthy cycle times and the potential health hazards it produces. Vapor-phase hydrogen peroxide (an oxidizing agent) has been used to sterilize HEPA filters in BSCs, metals, and nonmetal devices such as medical instruments (e.g., scissors). There are no toxic byproducts produced using vapor-phase hydrogen peroxide. Hydrogen peroxide gas plasma is another method that uses hydrogen peroxide and generates plasma by exciting the gas in an enclosed chamber under deep vacuum with the use of radiofrequency or microwave energy.

Methods of Disinfection

Physical Methods of Disinfection

The three physical methods of disinfection are:

- Boiling at 100°C for 15 minutes, which kills vegetative bacteria
- Pasteurizing at 70°C for 30 minutes, which kills food pathogens without damaging the nutritional value or flavor
- Using nonionizing radiation such as ultraviolet (UV) light

UV rays are long wavelength and low energy. They do not penetrate well, and organisms must have direct surface exposure, such as the working surface of a BSC, for this form of disinfection to work.

Chemical Methods of Disinfection

Chemical disinfectants comprise many classes, including:

- Alcohols
- Aldehydes
- Halogens (chlorine and chlorine compounds)
- Peracetic acid
- Hydrogen peroxide
- Quaternary ammonium compounds
- Phenolics

Chemicals used to destroy all life are called **chemical sterilants,** or **biocides;** however, these same chemicals, when used for shorter periods, act as disinfectants. Disinfectants used on living tissue (skin) are called **antiseptics.**

Resistance to disinfectants varies with the type of infectious agent. Prions are the most resistant, followed by bacterial endospores (such as *Bacillus* spp.); mycobacteria (acid-fast bacilli); nonenveloped viruses (e.g., poliovirus); fungi; vegetative (nonsporulating) bacteria (e.g., gram-negative rods); and enveloped viruses (e.g., herpes simplex virus), which are the most susceptible to the action of disinfectants. The Environmental Protection Agency (EPA) registers chemical disinfectants used in the United States and requires manufacturers to specify the activity level of each compound at the working dilution. Therefore, microbiologists who must recommend appropriate disinfectants should check the manufacturer's cut sheets (product information) for the classes of infectious agents that will be killed. Generally, the time necessary for killing infectious agents increases in direct proportion to the microbial load or bioburden (number of organisms). In the clinical environment, the bioburden generally contains multiple types of infectious agents; it is important to ensure that the exposure time is adequate to kill the most resistant agents within the sample. Organic material such as blood, pus, or mucus also affects killing of the infectious agents by inactivating the chemical disinfectant or preventing contact between the chemical and the infectious agent. The organic material should be mechanically removed before chemical sterilization to decrease the microbial load. This is analogous to removing dried food from utensils before placing them in a dishwasher, and it is important for cold sterilization of instruments such as bronchoscopes.

The type of water and its concentration in a solution are also important. Hard water may reduce the rate of killing of microorganisms. In addition, **60% to 90% ethyl or isopropyl alcohol solution** (volume/volume) is optimally bactericidal, virucidal, fungicidal, and mycobactericidal, because the increased ability of water (H_2O) to hydrolyze bonds in protein molecules makes the killing of microorganisms more effective. Ethyl or isopropyl alcohol is nonsporicidal (does not kill endospores) and evaporates quickly. Therefore, its use is limited to the skin as an antiseptic or on thermometers and injection vial rubber septa as a disinfectant.

Stabilized hydrogen peroxide has demonstrated bactericidal, virucidal, sporicidal, and fungicidal activities. Commercially available 3% hydrogen peroxide has been used as a disinfectant on inanimate surfaces.

The most common disinfectant in the United States is hypochlorite solutions (NaOCl), 5.25% to 6.15%, referred to as **household bleach.** The disinfecting capability of bleach is bactericidal, virucidal, fungicidal, mycobactericidal, and sporicidal. It is inexpensive and its effectiveness is not decreased based on the quality of the water used in the solution preparation. One disadvantage is that hypochlorite may cause minor ocular, oropharyngeal, and esophageal irritation if an individual is exposed to high concentrations without proper ventilation. It is also corrosive to metals in high concentrations, discolors fabrics, and can produce a toxic gas if improperly mixed with ammonia or acid in other cleaning agents. The Centers for Disease Control and Prevention (CDC) recommends that tabletops be cleaned after blood spills with a 1:10 dilution of bleach.

Because of their irritating fumes, the aldehydes (formaldehyde and glutaraldehyde) are generally not used as surface disinfectants. Glutaraldehyde, which is sporicidal (kills endospores) in 3 to 10 hours, is used for medical equipment such as bronchoscopes because it does not corrode lenses, metal, or rubber. Ortho-phthaladehyde (OPA) has similar effects as glutaraldehyde including the ability to kill endospores. OPA has several advantages over glutaraldehyde. It is considered more stable, requires no activation, does not require exposure monitoring, and is not known to irritate the eyes and nasal passages. Peracetic acid (0.23%) combined with hydrogen peroxide (1.0%) is effective in the presence of organic material and has been used for the surface sterilization of surgical instruments. The use of glutaraldehyde, OPA, or peracetic acid is called **cold sterilization.**

Quaternary ammonium compounds are used to disinfect bench tops or other surfaces in the laboratory. However, high water hardness and gross contamination with organic materials, such as blood, may inactivate heavy metals or quaternary ammonium compounds, thus limiting their utility. They are most often used on noncritical surfaces such as floors, furniture, and walls.

Finally, phenolics are derivatives of carbolic acid (phenol). Two phenol derivatives commonly included in hospital disinfectants are *ortho*-phenylphenol and *ortho*-benzyl-*para*-chlorophenol. These products are generally considered bactericidal, fungicidal, virucidal, and tuberculocidal, but not sporicidal. The addition of detergent results in a product that cleans and disinfects at the same time, and at concentrations of 2% to 5%, these products are used for cleaning bench tops.

Antiseptics

In addition to decontamination of inanimate objects or surfaces, personal laboratory safety and preparation of patients for invasive procedures require the use of an antiseptic. A variety of antiseptics are used to prepare a patient's skin for blood draws or other invasive procedures. Ethyl alcohol solutions, as previously indicated, are considered bactericidal, virucidal, fungicidal, and mycobactericidal. Iodine is prepared either as a tincture with alcohol or as an iodophor coupled to a neutral polymer (e.g., povidone-iodine or poloxamer-iodine). Both iodine compounds are widely used antiseptics. In fact, 70% ethyl alcohol, followed by an iodophor, is the most common combination used for skin disinfection before drawing blood specimens for culture or surgery. Iodophors have also been used as disinfectants for hard surfaces but at higher concentrations.

Superoxidized water (SOW), 144 mg/L of hypochlorous acid and chlorine, requires preparation onsite prior to use. The antiseptic is exposed to sodium chloride through a semipermeable membrane and production of oxycholine ions is completed using electrolysis. The solution has proven to be an economical alternative to expensive antiseptics and has been used as a treatment option for the cleaning of chronic wounds prior to administration of antibiotics. The solution may also be used for hand washing as well as a potential disinfectant for equipment and surfaces in the health care setting.

Because mercury is toxic to the environment, heavy metals containing mercury are no longer recommended. An eye drop solution containing 1% silver nitrate was placed in the eyes of newborns to prevent infections with *Neisseria gonorrhoeae*. Silver nitrate, however, is no longer manufactured in the United States. The current chemical treatment is either an ointment containing erythromycin or povidone-iodide.

The most important point to remember when working with biocides, antiseptics, or disinfectants is to prepare a working solution of the compound exactly according to the manufacturer's package insert. Many individuals believe that if the manufacturer says to dilute 1:200, they will get a stronger product if they dilute it 1:10. However, the ratio of water to active ingredient may be critical, and if sufficient water is not added, the chemical for surface disinfection may not be effective.

Chemical Safety

The OSHA Hazard Communication Standard provides for institutional educational practices to ensure that all laboratory personnel have a thorough working knowledge of the

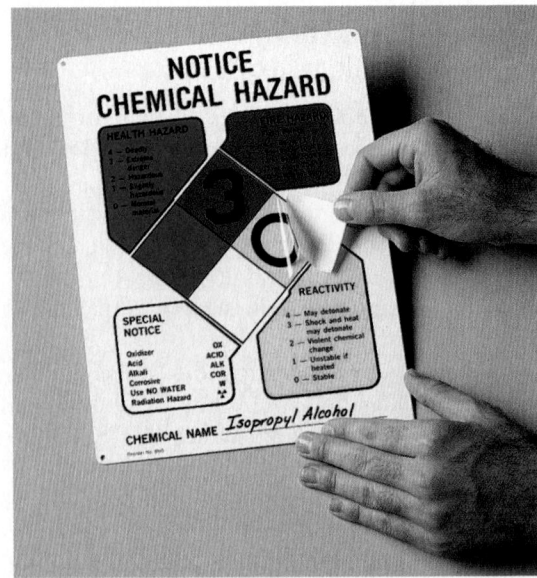

• **Fig. 4.2** National Fire Protection Association diamond indicating a chemical hazard. This information can be customized (as shown here for isopropyl alcohol) by applying the appropriate self-adhesive polyester numbers to the corresponding color-coded hazard area. (Courtesy Lab Safety Supply, Janesville, Wisconsin.)

hazards of the chemicals with which they work. This standard has also been called the "employee right to know." It mandates that all hazardous chemicals in the workplace be identified and clearly marked with a National Fire Protection Association (NFPA) label stating the health risks, such as **carcinogen** (cause of cancer), mutagen (cause of mutations in deoxyribonucleic acid [DNA] or ribonucleic acid [RNA]), or **teratogen** (cause of birth defects), and the hazard class, for example, **corrosive** (harmful to mucous membranes, skin, eyes, or tissues), **poisonous, flammable,** or **oxidizing** (Fig. 4.2).

Each laboratory should have a **chemical hygiene plan** that includes guidelines on proper labeling of chemical containers, manufacturers' **safety data sheets (SDSs, formerly Material Safety Data Sheets [MSDSs]),** and the written chemical safety training and retraining programs. Hazardous chemicals must be inventoried annually. In addition, laboratories are required to maintain a file of every chemical they use and a corresponding SDS. The manufacturer provides the SDS for every hazardous chemical; some manufacturers also provide letters for nonhazardous chemicals, such as saline, so that these can be included with the other SDSs. The SDSs are required to present the information in a consistent 16-section format. The sections in the SDS include:

- Identification
- Chemical name, recommended uses and the name, address, and telephone number of manufacturer or supplier
- Hazard(s) identification
- Classification of the chemical (e.g., flammable, health hazard, etc.), precautionary statements, hazard symbols or pictures related to the risks, and any other hazards or unknown components included in the chemical.

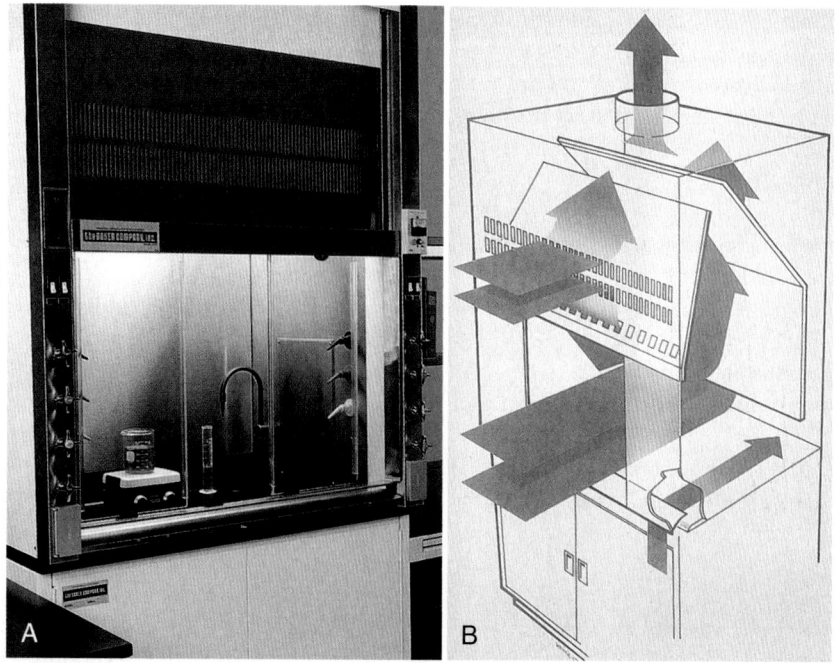

• **Fig. 4.3** Fume hood schematics. *Arrows* indicate airflow through the cabinet to the outside vent. (Courtesy the Baker Co., Sanford, Maine.)

- Composition/information on ingredients
- Specific chemical substances or mixtures
- First-aid measures
- Instructions based on exposure, symptoms, or effects of exposure and recommended follow-up treatment or medical care
- Firefighting measures
- Accidental release measures
- Containment, evacuation, and cleanup procedures
- Handling and storage
- Exposure controls and personal protection
- Engineering controls and PPE and procedures
- Physical and chemical properties
- Stability and reactivity
- Toxicological information
- Routes of transmission and exposure, effects of that exposure, symptoms and numerical measures related to toxicity such as lethal dose or exposure time
- Ecological information (nonmandatory)
- Environmental impact statement
- Disposal considerations (nonmandatory)
- Transport information (nonmandatory)
- Shipping and transportation regulations and requirements
- Regulatory information (nonmandatory)
- Any regional and national regulatory specifications associated with agencies such as OSHA, Department of Transportation, Environmental Protection Agency, or Consumer Product Safety Commission
- Other information
- Date of preparation or revision of SDS

Employees should become familiar with the location and organization of SDS files in the laboratory so that they know where to look in the event of an emergency.

Fume hoods (Fig. 4.3) are provided in the laboratory to prevent inhalation of toxic fumes. Fume hoods protect against chemical odor by exhausting air to the outside, but they are not HEPA-filtered to trap pathogenic microorganisms. It is important to remember that a biosafety cabinet (discussed later in the chapter) is not a fume hood.

Work with toxic or noxious chemicals should always be performed while wearing nitrile gloves, in a fume hood or while wearing a fume mask. Spills should be cleaned up using a fume mask, gloves, impervious (impenetrable to moisture) apron, and goggles. Acid and alkaline, flammable, and radioactive spill kits are available to assist in rendering any chemical spills harmless.

Fire Safety

Fire safety is an important component of the laboratory safety program. Each laboratory is required to post fire evacuation plans that are essentially blueprints for finding the nearest exit in case of fire. Fire drills conducted quarterly or annually, depending on local laws, ensure that all personnel know what to do in case of fire. Exit paths should always remain clear of obstructions, and employees should be trained to use fire extinguishers. The local fire department is often an excellent resource for training in the types and use of fire extinguishers.

Type A fire extinguishers are used for trash, wood, and paper; type B extinguishers are used for chemical fires; and type C extinguishers are used for electrical fires. Combination type ABC extinguishers are found in most laboratories so that personnel need not worry about which extinguisher to reach for in case of a fire. However, type C extinguishers, which contain carbon dioxide (CO_2) or another dry chemical to smother flames, are also used, because this type of extinguisher does not damage equipment.

The important actions in case of fire and the order in which to perform tasks can be remembered with the acronym RACE:

1. **R**escue any injured individuals.
2. **A**ctivate the fire alarm.
3. **C**ontain (smother) the fire, if feasible (close fire doors).
4. **E**xtinguish the fire, if possible.

If you are able to extinguish the fire, it is important to follow four basic steps: PASS.

1. **P**ull the pin—to release the operating handle.
2. **A**im—toward the base of the flames at the ignition and fuel source.
3. **S**queeze—the handle to release the contents.
4. **S**weep—side to side across the base of the flame to extinguish the fire.

Electrical Safety

Electrical cords should be checked regularly for fraying and replaced when necessary. All plugs should be the three-prong, grounded type. All sockets should be checked for electrical grounding and leakage at least annually. No extension cords should be used in the laboratory.

Handling of Compressed Gases

Compressed gas cylinders (CO_2, anaerobic gas mixture) contain pressurized gases and must be properly handled and secured. When leaking cylinders have fallen, tanks have become missiles, resulting in loss of life and destruction of property. Therefore, gas tanks should be properly chained and stored in well-ventilated areas. The metal cap, which is removed when the regulator is installed, should always be in place when a gas cylinder is not in use. Cylinders should be transported chained to special dollies.

Biosafety

Individuals are exposed in various ways to health care–associated infections, transporting specimens and in public areas such as elevators or cafeterias, by:

- Rubbing the eyes or nose with contaminated hands
- Inhaling aerosols produced during centrifugation, mixing with a vortex, or spills of liquid cultures
- Accidentally ingesting microorganisms by putting pens or fingers in the mouth
- Receiving percutaneous inoculation (i.e., through puncture from an accidental needle stick)
- Manipulating or opening bacterial cultures in liquid media or on plates, creating potentially hazardous aerosols, outside of a biosafety hood
- Failure to wash hands upon leaving the restroom or other public areas before entering the laboratory

Risks from a microbiology laboratory may extend to adjacent laboratories and to the families of those who work in the microbiology laboratory. For example, Blaser and Feldman noted that 5 of 31 individuals who contracted typhoid fever from proficiency testing specimens did not work in a microbiology laboratory. Two patients were family members of a microbiologist who had worked with *Salmonella enteric* subsp. *enterica* Typhi, two were students whose afternoon class was in the laboratory where the organism had been cultured that morning, and one worked in an adjacent chemistry laboratory.

In the clinical microbiology laboratory, shigellosis, salmonellosis, tuberculosis, brucellosis, and hepatitis are commonly acquired laboratory infections. Additional infections have been reported from agents such as *Coxiella burnetii*, *Francisella tularensis*, *Trichophyton mentagrophytes*, and *Coccidioides immitis*. Viral agents transmitted through blood and body fluids cause many health care–associated infections in non–microbiology laboratory workers and in health care workers in general. These include hepatitis B virus (HBV), hepatitis C virus (HCV), hepatitis D virus (HDV), and human immunodeficiency virus (HIV). Laboratory-associated infection is not a new phenomenon, but data are based primarily on voluntary reporting. Therefore, such incidents are widely underreported because of fears of repercussions associated with such events.

Exposure Control Plan

The laboratory director and supervisor are legally responsible for ensuring that an **Exposure Control Plan** has been implemented and that the mandated safety guidelines are followed. The plan identifies tasks that are hazardous to employees and promotes employee safety through use of the following:

- Employee education and orientation
- Appropriate disposal of hazardous waste
- Standard (formerly Universal) Precautions
- Engineering controls and safe work practices, as well as appropriate waste disposal and use of BSCs
- PPE, such as laboratory coats, shoe covers, gowns, gloves, and eye protection (goggles, face shields)
- A post-exposure plan for investigating all accidents and a plan to prevent recurrences

Employee Education and Orientation

Each institution should have a safety manual that is reviewed by all employees and a safety officer who is knowledgeable about the risks associated with health care–associated infections. The safety officer should provide orientation for new employees and quarterly continuing education updates for all personnel. Initial training and all retraining should be documented in writing.

This training should include all items in the laboratory exposure control plan as well as fire, chemical, hazardous materials management (use, storage, and disposal), and blood borne pathogens.

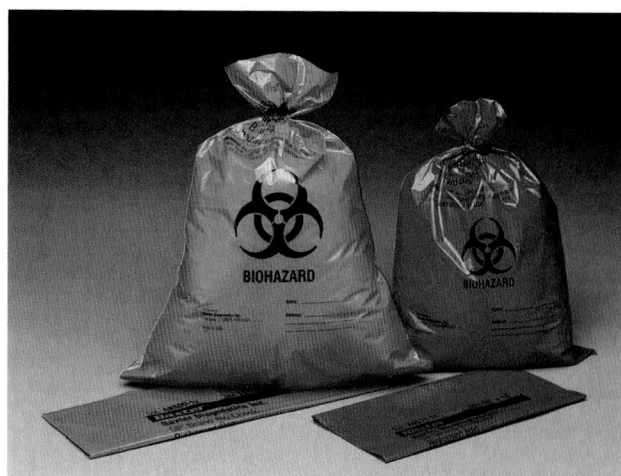

• **Fig. 4.4** Autoclave bags. (Courtesy Allegiance Healthcare, McGaw Park, Illinois.)

Disposal of Hazardous Waste

All materials contaminated with potentially infectious agents must be decontaminated before disposal. These include unused portions of patient specimens, patient cultures, stock cultures of microorganisms, and disposable sharp instruments, such as glass microscope slides, glass or plastic tubes, scalpels, syringes, and needles. It is recommended that syringes with needles not be accepted in the laboratory; staff members should be required to submit capped syringes to the laboratory. Infectious waste may be decontaminated by use of an autoclave, incinerator, or any one of several alternative waste-treatment methods. Some state or local municipalities permit urine and feces to be carefully poured into a sanitary sewer. Infectious waste from microbiology laboratories is usually autoclaved on site or sent for incineration.

Infectious waste (agar plates, plastic tubes, and reagent bottles) should be placed into two leak-proof, plastic bags for sturdiness (Fig. 4.4); this is known as **double bagging.** Sharp objects, including pipettes, microscope slides, broken glass, glass tubes or bottles, scalpels, and needles, are placed in sharps containers (Fig. 4.5), then autoclaved or incinerated.

Standard Precautions

The CDC guidelines known as **Standard Precautions (previously Universal Precautions)** require that blood and body fluids from every patient be treated as potentially infectious. The essentials of Standard Precautions and safe laboratory work practices are as follows:

• Do not eat, drink, smoke, or apply cosmetics (including lip balm).
• Do not insert or remove contact lenses.
• Do not bite nails or chew on pens.
• Do not mouth-pipette.
• Limit access to the laboratory to trained personnel only.

• Assume all patients are infectious for all blood-borne pathogens.
• Use appropriate barrier precautions to prevent skin and mucous membrane exposure, including wearing gloves at all times and masks, goggles, gowns, or aprons if splash or droplet formation is a risk.
• Thoroughly wash hands and other skin surfaces after removing gloves and immediately after any contamination.
• Take special care to prevent injuries with sharp objects, such as needles and scalpels.

Standard Precautions should be followed for handling blood and body fluids, including all secretions and excretions submitted to the microbiology laboratory (e.g., serum, semen, all sterile body fluids, saliva from dental procedures, and vaginal secretions). Standard Precautions applies to blood and all body fluids, except sweat. Practice of Standard Precautions by health care workers handling all patient material lessens the risks associated with such specimens.

Among the Standard Precautions, hand washing is one of the single most useful techniques to prevent the transmission and acquisition of infection in a health care setting. Hand washing using running water with plain or antimicrobial soaps does not disrupt the normal microbiota but has demonstrated a reduction in transient microorganisms and viral agents. Studies have indicated that effective hand washing with plain soap versus antimicrobial products are both equally efficient and directly correlates with the duration of the hand washing. All personnel should wash their hands with soap and water after removing gloves, after handling infectious material, and before leaving the laboratory area. When hand washing is not available, waterless alcohol-based (60% to 62%) products provide a rapid and convenient means of controlling transmission of many organisms. These alcohol-based products have been used worldwide to control infections and restrict the transmission of pathogens. However, some pathogens such as *Enterococcus faecium* have now become tolerant or resistant to these products. Alcohol-based products are also not useful when hands are soiled or contaminated with other organic material such as blood and body fluids.

Mouth-pipetting is strictly prohibited. Mechanical devices must be used for drawing all liquids into pipettes. Eating, drinking, and applying cosmetics are strictly forbidden in work areas. Food and drink must be stored in refrigerators in areas separate from the work area.

All health care workers should follow Standard Precautions whether working inside or outside the laboratory. When collecting specimens outside the laboratory, individuals should follow these guidelines:

• Wear gloves and a laboratory coat.
• Deal carefully with needles and lancets.
• Discard sharps in an appropriate, puncture-resistant container.
• Never recap needles by hand, if necessary, special safety devices are available. (Needles are available with built-in safety devices to prevent accidental needle sticks).

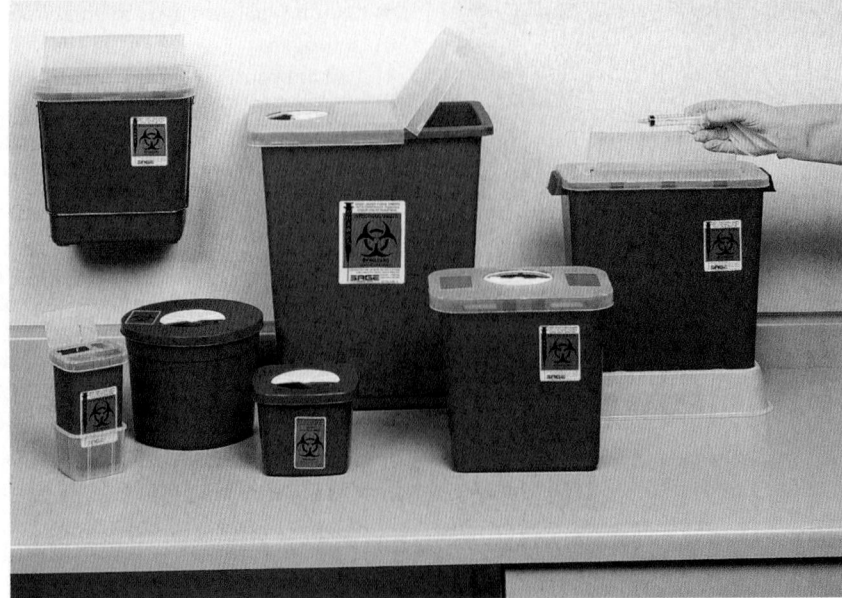

• **Fig. 4.5** Sharps containers. (Courtesy Lab Safety Supply, Janesville, Wisconsin.)

Laboratory Design and Engineering Controls

Laboratory Environment

Microbiology laboratory environments are classified according to the **Biosafety Level (BSL)** of the classification of microorganisms or risk groups that are approved for testing in the laboratory. The BSL determines the design of the laboratory environment; procedures, access, and laboratory safety controls are based on the potential for transmission of the infectious agents to prevent laboratory-acquired infections and exposure to others. The laboratory should be designed to facilitate a one-way workflow from initial specimen handling of biologically contaminated specimens to areas where pure cultures and additional testing is performed to prevent cross-contamination of specimens. The BSL should be prominently displayed on laboratory doors to restrict access, and the biohazard symbol should be displayed on any equipment (refrigerators, incubators, centrifuges) that contains infectious material The air-handling system of a microbiology laboratory should move air from lower- to higher-risk areas, never the reverse. Ideally, the microbiology laboratory should be under negative pressure, and air should not be recirculated. The selected use of the appropriate BSC for procedures that generate infectious aerosols is critical to laboratory safety.

The microbiology laboratory poses many hazards to unsuspecting and untrained people; therefore, access should be limited to employees and other necessary personnel (biomedical engineers, housekeepers). Visitors, especially young children, should be discouraged. Certain areas of high risk, such as the mycobacteriology and virology laboratories, should be closed to visitors. Custodial personnel should be trained to discriminate among the waste containers, dealing only with those that contain noninfectious material. Care

should be taken to prevent insects from infesting any laboratory area. Mites, for example, can crawl over the surface of media, carrying microorganisms from colonies on a plate to other areas. Houseplants can also serve as a source of insects and should be excluded from the laboratory environment. A pest control program should be in place to control rodents and insects.

Biological Safety Levels

The *Biosafety in Microbiological and Biomedical Laboratories Manual* published by the CDC serves as a reference for laboratory design, work-practice and environmental controls, personnel requirements, disposal, and personnel according to the relative risks of working with various biologic agents. The risk assessment used to determine the recommended Biological Safety Level is based on the characterization of the agent in the following categories:

1. Route of transmission—direct exposure, inoculation, ingestion, or inhalation
2. Infective dose—amount of organism required to cause an infection.
3. Stability in the environment—temperature, desiccation, decontamination, or sterilization of surfaces.
4. Host range—human, insects (vectors), animals
5. Endemic nature—indigenous versus exotic non-indigenous; wild type versus genetically modified agents.

The manual is available on the CDC website (www.cdc.gov/biosafety/publications/bmbl5/BMBL.pdf).

Biosafety Level 1 (BSL-1) agents include those that have no known potential for infecting healthy adult individuals and are well defined and characterized. These agents are used in laboratory teaching exercises for undergraduate students, secondary educational training, and teaching laboratories for students in microbiology. Precautions for working with BSL-1 agents include standard good laboratory technique such as hand washing, but do not require the use of engineering or work practice controls that are considered **primary** or **secondary barriers.** BSL levels and practices are summarized in Table 4.2.

BSL-2 agents are those most commonly being sought in clinical specimens and used in diagnostic, teaching, and other laboratories. BSL-2 precautions are sufficient for the handling of clinical specimens suspected of harboring any indigenous pathogens that pose moderate risk of infection. Specimens expected to contain prions (PrPSc), abnormal proteins associated with neurodegenerative diseases, including spongiform encephalitis, should be handled using BSL-2 procedures. This level of safety includes the principles outlined previously, provided the potential for splash or aerosol is low. If splash or aerosol is probable, the use of primary containment equipment is recommended, as are limiting access to the laboratory during working procedures, training laboratory personnel in handling pathogenic agents, direction by competent supervisors, and performing aerosol-generating procedures in a BSC.

BSL-3 procedures have been recommended for the handling of material suspected of harboring organisms unlikely to be encountered in a routine clinical laboratory. However, although rarely encountered in a routine clinical laboratory, agents included in this group may be identified or utilized in a clinical, diagnostic, teaching, research, or production facility. These precautions, in addition to those undertaken for BSL-2 agents, consist of laboratory design and engineering controls that contain potentially dangerous material by careful control of air movement and the requirement that personnel wear protective clothing and gloves. Those working with BSL-3 agents should have baseline sera specimens stored for comparison with acute sera that can be drawn in the event of unexplained illness. BSL-3 organisms are primarily transmitted by infectious aerosol.

BSL-4 agents are exotic agents that are considered high risk and cause life-threatening disease. Personnel and all materials must be decontaminated before leaving the facility, and all procedures are performed under maximum containment (special protective clothing, class III BSC). There are two general types of BSL-4 facilities, a cabinet laboratory that utilizes a BSC-3 and a suit laboratory where employees wear a positive-pressure-supplied air-protective suit. Most of the facilities that deal with BSL-4 agents are public health or research laboratories. As mentioned, BSL-4 agents pose life-threatening risks and are transmitted via aerosols; in addition, no vaccine or therapy is available for these organisms.

Biologic Safety Cabinets

A BSC is a device that encloses a workspace in such a way as to protect workers from aerosol exposure to infectious disease agents. Either air that contains the infectious material is sterilized, by heat, ultraviolet light, or, most commonly, by passage through a HEPA filter that removes most particles

larger than 0.3 μm in diameter. These cabinets are designated as class I through III, according to the effective level of biologic containment. **Class I cabinets** allow room (unsterilized) air to pass into the cabinet and around the area and material within, sterilizing only the air to be exhausted (Fig. 4.6). They have negative pressure, may be ventilated to the outside or exhausted to the work area, and are usually operated with an open front.

Class II cabinets sterilize air that flows over the infectious material, as well as air to be exhausted. The air flows in "sheets," which serve as barriers to particles from outside the cabinet and direct the flow of contaminated air into the filters (Fig. 4.7). Such cabinets are called **vertical laminar flow BSCs. Class II cabinets** have a variable sash opening through which the operator gains access to the work surface. Depending on their inlet flow velocity and the percent of air that is HEPA filtered and recirculated, class II cabinets are further differentiated into type A or B. A class IIA cabinet is self-contained, and 70% of the air is recirculated into the work area. The exhaust air in class IIB cabinets is discharged outside the building. A class IIB cabinet is selected if radioisotopes, toxic chemicals, or carcinogens will be used.

Because they are completely enclosed and have negative pressure, **Class III cabinets** afford the most protection to the worker. Air coming into and going out of the cabinet is filter sterilized, and the infectious material within is handled with rubber gloves that are attached and sealed to the cabinet (Fig. 4.8).

Most hospital clinical microbiology laboratory scientists use class IIA or IIB cabinets. Routine inspection and documentation of adequate function of these cabinets are critical factors in an ongoing quality assurance program. It is important to the proper operation of laminar flow cabinets that an open area of 3 feet around the cabinet be maintained during operation of the air-circulating system; this ensures that infectious material is directed through the HEPA filter. BSCs must be certified initially, whenever moved more than 18 inches, and annually thereafter.

Personal Protective Equipment

OSHA regulations require that health care facilities provide employees with all **personal protective equipment (PPE)** necessary to protect them from hazards encountered during the course of work (Fig. 4.9). PPE usually includes plastic shields or goggles to protect workers from droplets, disposal containers for sharp objects, trays in which to carry smaller hazardous items (e.g., culture tubes), handheld pipetting devices, impervious gowns, laboratory coats, disposable gloves, masks, safety carriers for centrifuges (especially those used in the acid fast bacteriology [AFB] laboratory), and HEPA respirators.

HEPA respirators are required for all health care workers, including phlebotomists, who enter the rooms of patients with tuberculosis, as well as workers who clean up spills of pathogenic microorganisms (Chapter 78). All respirators should be fit-tested for each individual so that each person

TABLE 4.2 **Laboratory Biosafety Levels**

Biosafety Level	Risk Group	Representative Organisms	BSC	Primary Barriers	Secondary Barriers	Additional Practices
BSL-1	Agents not associated with disease in healthy individuals. Low individual and community risk.	*Bacillus subtilis* *Naegleria gruberi* Exempt organisms according to NIH guidelines.	None	None	General good laboratory practice, handwashing.	Limit laboratory access. Decontamination procedures in addition, surfaces that are easily cleaned, non-porous.
BSL-2	Agents associated with disease that is preventable and treatable and disease is not considered serious. Moderate individual and low community risk.	Broad spectrum, indigenous moderate risk agents. Representative agents include: HIV Hepatitis B virus *Salmonella* spp. *Toxoplasmosis* sp.	BSC-2 or other primary barrier when procedures may produce aerosols or splash.	Primary BSC-2 as indicated or other equipment that prevents aerosolization during manipulation such as enclosed centrifuge safety cups. Requires the use of PPE as appropriate.	Same as above In addition, waste decontamination and disposal of contaminated sharps. Laboratory decontamination procedures and practices. Eye wash station. Pest management program.	Same as above. Biohazard symbol posted on entrance. Immunization requirements and medical surveillance for exposure for personnel. Specific personnel training requirements. Biosafety manual including incident and exposure procedures.
BSL-3	Agents associated with serious or lethal disease and where it may be preventable and treatable. High individual risk and low community risk.	Indigenous or exotic agents with potential respiratory transmission. Representative agents include: *Mycobacterium tuberculosis,* St. Louis encephalitis virus, *Coxiella burnetii* Mold stages of systemic fungi and organisms grown in quantities greater than found in clinical specimens.	BSC-2 or 3	Same as above and all equipment should be enclosed for laboratory manipulations such as the use of a gas-tight aerosol generation chamber. PPE is solid-front or wrap around, scrub suits or coveralls that are not removed from the laboratory.	Same as above and the addition of ventilation requirements that minimize release of infectious aerosols from the laboratory. Separated from the main laboratory with self-closing doors; all windows must be sealed. Access limited using an anteroom to prevent exchange with outside areas of the laboratory	Same as above. Serum samples of personnel routinely checked for seroconversion comparisons to monitor exposure.
BSL-4	Agents highly likely to cause serious or lethal disease and is not generally known to be preventable or treatable. High individual and community risk.	Dangerous and exotic agents. Representative agents include Marburg virus or Congo-Crimean hemorrhagic fever.	BSC-3 or in a full-body, air-supplied positive pressure personnel suite	Same as above.	Same as above, with specialized zone ventilation systems. Laboratory is generally a separate building. Items are processed through a fumigation chamber or airlock system.	Same as above. Personnel decontamination procedures included such as showering or chemical treatment. Log of all personnel or items entering and leaving laboratory. Generally includes complex waste management procedures.

BSC, Biologic safety cabinet; *HIV,* human immunodeficiency virus; *NIH,* National Institutes of Health; *PPE,* personal protective equipment.
Adapted from information included in the United States Department of Health and Human Services, Centers for Disease and Control. Biosafety in Microbiological and Biomedical Laboratories. 5th ed. Washington, DC: US Government Printing Office; 2009. Accessed January 13, 2019.

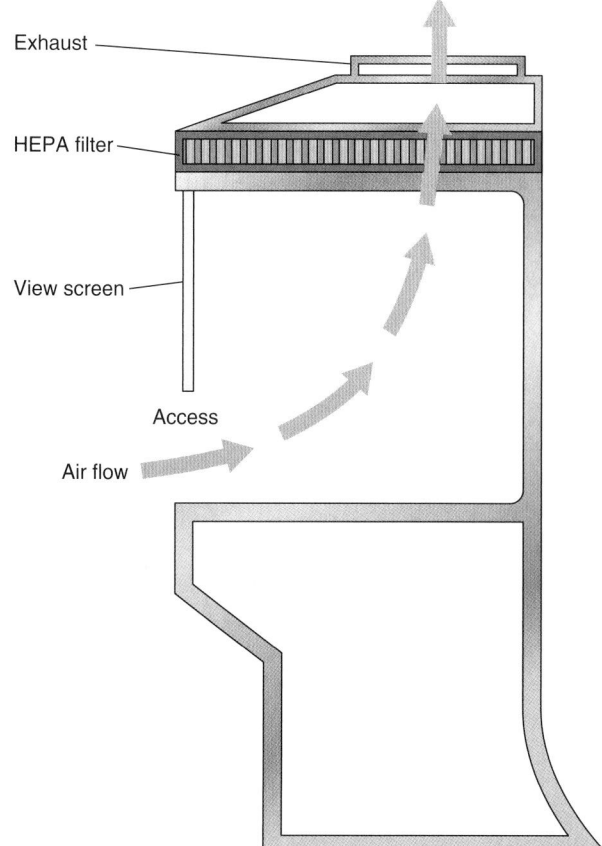

• **Fig. 4.6** Schematic of Class I biologic safety cabinet. Room air flows into the cabinet and is circulated out through a high-efficiency particulate air (HEPA) filter and the exhaust portals.

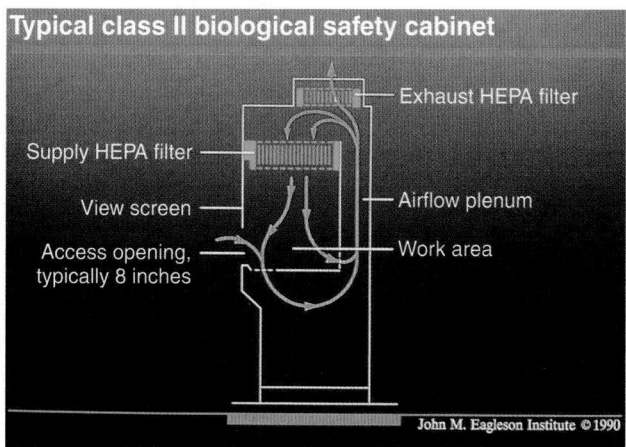

• **Fig. 4.7** Schematic of a Class II biologic safety cabinet indicating the airflow. Air is pulled into the cabinet and circulated through an airflow plenum through two levels of HEPA filter prior to exiting through the exhaust portals. (Courtesy the Baker Co., Sanford, Maine.)

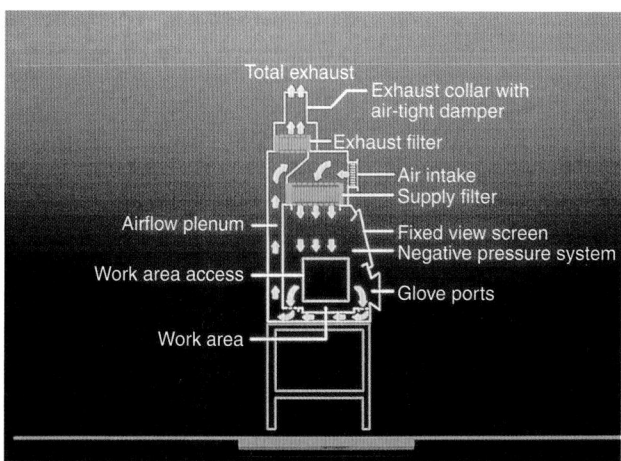

• **Fig. 4.8** Schematic of a Class III biologic safety cabinet with arrows showing airflow through cabinet. The cabinet is self-contained providing the maximum amount of protection to the laboratory from any aerosolized particles. (Courtesy the Baker Co., Sanford, Maine.)

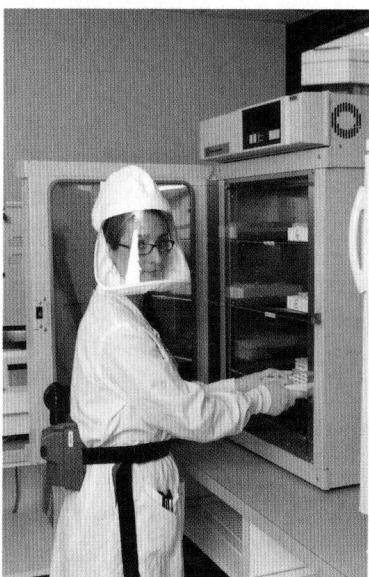

• **Fig. 4.9** Personal protective equipment. A microbiologist wearing a laboratory coat, gloves, and hood with a shield attached to a HEPA filter pack with a high efficiency particulate air system.

is assured that his or hers is working properly. Men must shave their facial hair to achieve a tight fit. Respirators are evaluated according to guidelines of the National Institute for Occupational Safety and Health (NIOSH), a branch of the CDC. N95 or P100 disposable masks are commonly used in the clinical laboratory and are available from a variety of manufacturers.

Microbiologists should wear laboratory coats over their uniform scrubs or street clothes, and these coats should be removed before leaving the laboratory. Most exposures to blood-containing fluids occur on the hands or forearms, so gowns with closed wrists or forearm covers and gloves that cover all potentially exposed skin on the arms are most beneficial. Most laboratories utilize disposable gowns and lab coats. If the laboratory protective clothing becomes contaminated with body fluids or potential pathogens, it should be removed and disposed of in the biohazard waste. If washable laboratory attire is provided, the institution or a uniform agency should clean laboratory coats; it is no longer permissible for microbiologists to launder their own coats. Obviously, laboratory workers who plan to enter an area of the hospital where patients at special risk of acquiring

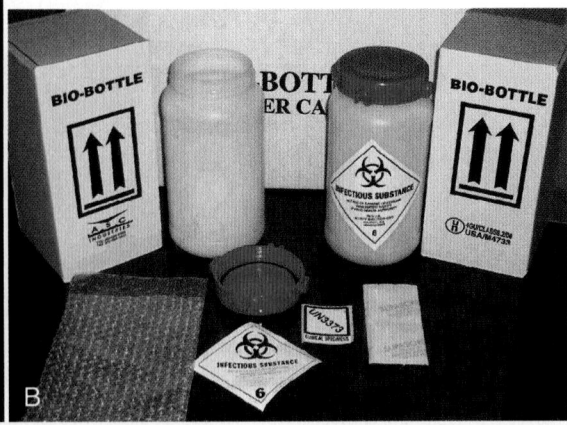

• **Fig. 4.10** (A) The Bio-Pouch (lower right) is made of laminated, low-density polyethylene, which is virtually unbreakable. (B) The Bio-Bottle is made of high-density polyethylene and is used as the secondary container. This packaging is used for both types of infectious substances. (Courtesy Air Sea Containers, Miami, Florida.)

infection are present (e.g., intensive care units, the nursery, operating rooms, or areas in which immunosuppressive therapy is being administered) should take every precaution to cover their uniform scrubs or street clothes with clean or sterile protective clothing appropriate to the area. Special impervious protective clothing is advisable for certain activities, such as working with radioactive substances or caustic chemicals. Solid-front gowns are indicated for those working with specimens being cultured for mycobacteria. Unless large-volume spills of potentially infectious material are anticipated, impervious laboratory gowns are not necessary in most microbiology laboratories.

Postexposure Control

All laboratory accidents and potential exposures must be reported to the supervisor and safety officer, who will immediately arrange to send the individual to employee health or an outside occupational health physician. Immediate medical care is of foremost importance; investigation of the accident should take place after the employee has received appropriate care. If the accident is a needle stick injury, for example, the patient should be identified and the risk of the laboratorian acquiring a blood-borne infection should be assessed. The investigation helps the physician determine the need for prophylaxis, such as hepatitis B virus immunoglobulin (HBIG) or an HBV booster immunization in the event of exposure to hepatitis B. The physician also is able to discuss the potential for disease transmission to family members, such as after exposure to a patient with *Neisseria meningitidis.* Postexposure prophylaxis should be administered, and additional sera should be collected at intervals of 6 weeks, 3 months, and 6 months for HIV testing. Finally, the safety committee, or at least the laboratory director and safety officer, should review the events of the accident to determine whether it could have been prevented and to delineate measures to prevent future accidents. The

investigation of the accident and corrective action should be documented in an incident report.

Mailing Biohazardous Materials

The requirements for packaging and shipping biologic materials, dangerous goods, or infectious substances are highly regulated by the Department of Transportation in the United States along with the International Air Transport Association (IATA) and the International Civil Aviation Organization (IACO). Infectious substances now are classified as category A, B, or C organisms. A category A specimen is an infectious substance capable of causing disease in healthy humans and animals. Category B includes infectious substances that are not included in category A. Only the category A organisms or specimens listed in Table 4.1 must be shipped as dangerous goods. If the laboratory director is unsure whether a patient has symptoms of a category A agent, it is prudent to ship the specimen as an infectious substance rather than a biologic substance. Fig. 4.10A shows triple packaging for diagnostic, clinical, or infectious substances in a pouch; Fig. 4.10B shows triple packaging for diagnostic, clinical, or infectious substances in a rigid bottle. Packaging instructions are available in the annual IATA regulations under section 620 (dangerous goods). All air and ground shippers, such as the US Postal Service (USPS), the US Department of Transportation (DOT), and Federal Express (FedEx), have adopted IATA standards.

Training in the proper packing and shipping of infectious material is a key feature of the regulations. Every institution that ships infectious materials, whether a hospital or physician office laboratory (POL), is required to have appropriately trained individuals; training may be obtained through carriers, package manufacturers, and special safety training organizations. The **shipper** is the individual (institution) ultimately responsible for safe and appropriate packaging. Any fines or penalties are the shipper's responsibility.

Infectious specimens or isolates should be wrapped with absorbent material and placed inside a plastic biohazard bag, called a **primary receptacle.** The primary receptacle is then inserted into a secondary container, most often a watertight, hard plastic mailer. The secondary container is capped and placed inside an outer, tertiary container that protects it from physical and water damage (Fig. 4.10B). A label on the outer box confirms that the packaging meets all the required standards. The package must be labeled with a specific hazard label as an infectious substance. A packing list and a Shippers Declaration for Dangerous Goods Form must accompany the air bill or ground form. Diagnostic or clinical specimens are packaged similarly.

The shipper should note that some carriers have additional requirements for coolant materials, such as ice, dry ice, or liquid nitrogen. Because the shipper is liable for appropriate packaging, it is best to check with individual carriers in special circumstances and update the instructions yearly when the new IATA Dangerous Goods Regulations are published. IATA regulations can be found at the website www.iata.org. International importation or exportation of biologic agents requires a permit from the CDC. Information on importing and exporting a variety of materials may be found at http://www.cdc.gov/laboratory/specimen-submission/shipping-packing.html.

ⓔ Visit the Evolve site for a complete list of procedures, review questions, and case studies.

Bibliography

Bennett J, Dolin R, Blaser M: *Principles and practice of infectious diseases*, ed 9, Philadelphia, PA, 2020, Elsevier Saunders.

Blaser MJ, Feldman RA: Acquisition of typhoid fever from proficiency testing specimens, *N Engl J Med* 303:1481, 1980.

Carroll KC, Pfaller MA, Landry ML, et al.: *Manual of clinical microbiology*, ed 12, Washington, DC, 2019, ASCM Press.

Centers for Disease Control and Prevention: *Guideline for Disinfection and Sterilization in Healthcare Facilities.* 2008, revised edition February 2017. Available at: https://www.cdc.gov/infectioncontrol/pdf/guidelines/disinfection-guidelines.pdf.

Centers for Disease Control and Prevention: Guidelines for safe work practices in human and animal medical diagnostic laboratories, *Morb Mortal Wkly Rep* 61:1–101, 2012. Accessed 13 January 2019.

Eftekharizadeh F, Dehnavieh R, Hekmat SN, et al.: Health technology assessment on superoxidized water for treatment of chronic wounds, *Med J Islam Repub Iran* 30:384, 2016.

Fleming DO, Hunt DL: *Biological safety: principles and practices*, ed 3, Washington, DC, 2000, ASM Press.

Occupational Safety and Health Administration: *Hazard Communication Standard: Safety Data Sheets: 29 CFR Part 1910, 1200(g)*, Revised, 2012.

Pidot SJ, Gao W, Buultjens AH, et al.: Increasing tolerance of hospital *Enterococcus faecium* to handwash alcohols, *Sci Transl Med* 10(452), 2018. https://doi.org/10.1126/scitranslmed.aar6115.

United States Department of Health and Human Services, Centers for Disease and Control: *Biosafety in microbiological and biomedical laboratories*, ed 5, Washington, DC, 2009, US Government Printing Office. Accessed 13 January 2019.

5

Specimen Management

OBJECTIVES

1. State four critical parameters that should be monitored in the laboratory from specimen collection to set up and describe the effects each may have on the quality of the laboratory results (e.g., false negatives or positives, inadequate specimen type, incorrect sample).
2. Identify the proper or improper labeling of a specimen, and determine the adequacy of a specimen given a patient scenario.
3. Define and differentiate backup broth, nutritive media, and differential and selective media.
4. Describe the oxygenation states (atmospheric conditions) associated with anaerobic and aerotolerant, facultative anaerobic, aerobic, and microaerobic (microaerophilic and capnophilic) organisms. Provide an example for each.
5. Determine specimen acceptability and the proper procedure for rejection or recollection.
6. List the critical parameters associated with the reporting of direct and indirect organism detection.

Microbiologists work in public health laboratories, hospital laboratories, reference or independent laboratories, and physician office laboratories (POLs). The current trend in the diagnostic setting is changing the landscape of laboratory services. Many health care systems are consolidating microbiology to a single laboratory. This creates a potential for an increase in the time between specimen collection and processing. The result may be a delay in reporting critical results and compromised integrity of the specimen.

Depending on the level of service and type of testing at each facility, in general, a microbiologist will perform one or more of the following functions:

- Cultivation (growth), identification, and antimicrobial susceptibility testing of microorganisms
- Direct detection of infecting organisms by microscopy
- Direct detection of specific products of infecting organisms using chemical, immunologic, or molecular techniques
- Detection of antibodies produced by the patient in response to an infecting organism (serology)

This chapter presents an overview of the issues involved with infectious disease diagnostic testing. Many of these issues are covered in detail in separate chapters.

General Concepts for Specimen Collection and Handling

Specimen collection and transportation are critical considerations because the results generated by the laboratory are limited by the quality and condition of the specimen upon arrival in the laboratory. Specimens should be obtained to preclude or minimize the possibility of introducing contaminating microorganisms that are not involved in the infectious process and can either interfere with the growth of or outgrow the pathogen. This is a particular problem, for example, in specimens collected from mucous membranes that are already colonized with an individual's endogenous or "normal" microbiota; these organisms are usually contaminants but may also be opportunistic pathogens. For example, the throats of hospitalized patients on ventilators may be colonized with *Klebsiella pneumoniae*; although *K. pneumoniae* is not usually involved in cases of community-acquired pneumonia, it can cause a hospital-acquired respiratory infection in this subset of patients. Using special techniques that bypass areas containing normal microbiota when feasible (e.g., covered-brush bronchoscopy in critically ill patients with pneumonia) prevents many problems associated with false-positive results. Likewise, careful skin preparation before procedures, such as blood cultures and spinal taps, decreases the chance that organisms normally present on the skin will contaminate the specimen.

Appropriate Collection Techniques

Specimens should be collected during the **acute** (early) **phase** of an illness (or within 2 to 3 days for viral infections) and before antimicrobials, antifungals, or antiviral medications are administered, if possible. Swabs generally are poor specimens if tissue or needle aspirates can be obtained. It is the microbiologist's responsibility to provide clinicians with a collection manual or instruction cards listing optimal specimen collection techniques and transport information. Information for the nursing staff and clinicians should include the following:

- Safety considerations
- Selection of the appropriate anatomic site and specimen
- Collection instructions, including the type of swab or transport medium

- Transportation instructions, including time and temperature constraints
- Labeling instructions, including patient demographic information (minimum of two patient identifiers)
- Special instructions, such as patient preparation
- Sterile versus nonsterile collection devices
- Minimal acceptable quality and recommended quantity

Instructions should be written so that specimens collected by the patient (e.g., urine, sputum, or stool) are handled properly. Most urine or stool collection kits contain instructions in several languages, but nothing substitutes for a concise set of verbal instructions. Similarly, when distributing kits for sputum collection, the microbiologist should be able to explain to the patient the difference between spitting in a cup (saliva) and producing good lower respiratory secretions from a deep cough (sputum). General collection information is shown in Table 5.1. An in-depth discussion of each type of specimen is found in Part VII.

Specimen Transport

Ideally, most specimens should be transported to the laboratory within 2 hours of collection. There are instances where the time from collection to laboratory processing should not exceed 15 minutes if not refrigerated or placed in specific transport media (Table 5.2). All specimen containers should be leak-proof, and the specimens should be transported within sealable, leak-proof plastic bags with a separate section for paperwork; resealable bags or bags with a permanent seal are common for this purpose. Bags should be marked with a biohazard label (Fig. 5.1). Many microorganisms are susceptible to environmental conditions such as the presence of oxygen (anaerobic bacteria), changes in temperature (*Neisseria meningitidis*), or changes in pH (*Shigella*). Thus the use of special preservatives or temperature-controlled or holding media for the transportation of specimens is important to ensure organism viability (survival).

Specimen Preservation

Preservatives, such as **boric acid** for urine or **polyvinyl alcohol (PVA)** and **buffered formalin** for stool for ova and parasite (O&P) examination, are designed to maintain the appropriate colony counts (urines) or the integrity of trophozoites and cysts (O&P), respectively. Other transport or holding media maintain the viability of microorganisms present in a specimen without supporting the growth of the organisms. This maintains the organisms in a state of suspended animation so that no organism overgrows another or dies out. **Stuart's medium** and **Amie's medium** are two common holding media. Sometimes charcoal is added to these media to absorb fatty acids present in the specimen that could result in pH changes in the media and the killing of fastidious (fragile) organisms such as *Neisseria gonorrhoeae* or *Bordetella pertussis*.

Anticoagulants are used to prevent clotting of specimens such as blood, bone marrow, and synovial fluid because microorganisms will otherwise be bound up in the clot. The type and concentration of anticoagulant are very important because many organisms are inhibited by some of these chemicals. **Sodium polyanethol sulfonate (SPS)** at a concentration of 0.025% (w/v) is usually used because *Neisseria* spp. and some anaerobic bacteria are particularly sensitive to higher concentrations. Because the ratio of specimen to SPS is so important, it is necessary to have both large (adult-size) and small (pediatric-size) tubes available, so organisms in small amounts of bone marrow or synovial fluid are not overwhelmed by the concentration of SPS. SPS is also included in blood culture collection systems. Heparin is also a commonly used anticoagulant, especially for viral cultures, although it may inhibit the growth of gram-positive bacteria and yeast. Citrate, ethylenediaminetetraacetic acid (EDTA), or other anticoagulants should not be used for microbiology because their efficacy has not been demonstrated for most organisms. It is the microbiologist's job to make sure media containing the appropriate anticoagulant is used for each procedure. The laboratory generally should not specify a color ("yellow-top") tube for collection without specifying the anticoagulant (SPS) because at least one popular brand of collection tube (Vacutainer, Becton, Dickinson and Company) has a yellow-top tube with either SPS or trisodium citrate/citric acid/dextrose (ACD); ACD is not appropriate for use in microbiology.

Specimen Storage

If specimens cannot be processed as soon as they are received, they must be stored (Table 5.1). Several storage methods are used (refrigerator temperature [4°C], ambient [room] temperature [22–25°C], body temperature [35–37°C], and freezer temperature [either –20°C or –70°C]), depending on the type of transport media (if applicable) and the etiologic (infectious) agents suspected. Urine, stool, viral specimens, sputa, swabs, and foreign devices such as catheters should be stored at 4°C. Serum for serologic studies may be frozen for up to 1 week at –20°C, and tissues or specimens for long-term storage should be frozen at –70°C.

Specimen Labeling

Specimens should be labeled with the patient's name, identifying number (hospital or sample number), birth date, date and time of collection, source, and the initials of the individual that collected the sample. Enough information must be provided on the specimen label so that the specimen can be matched with the test requisition when it is received in the laboratory.

Specimen Requisition

The specimen (or test) requisition is an order form that is sent to the laboratory along with a specimen. Often the

TABLE 5.1 Collection, Transport, Storage, and Processing of Specimens Commonly Submitted to a Microbiology Laboratory[a]

Specimen	Container	Patient Preparation	Special Instructions	Transportation to Laboratory	Storage Before Processing	Primary Plating Media	Anaerobic Media	Direct Examination	Comments
Abscess (Also Lesion, Wound, Pustule, Ulcer)									
Superficial	Recommend E-swab transport system or aerobic swab moistened with Stuart's or Amie's medium	Wipe area with sterile saline or 70% alcohol.	Aspirate or tissue are preferred if possible, pass swab deeply into the lesion along leading edge of wound.	≤2 h	24 h/RT	BA, CA, Mac, CNA optional	BBA, LKV, BBE	Gram	Contamination of surface material may introduce normal microbiota. Add CNA if smear suggests mixed gram-positive and gram-negative flora.
Deep	Anaerobic transporter; ≥1 mL if sample	Wipe area with sterile saline or 70% alcohol.	Aspirate material from wall or excise tissue.	≤2 h	24 h/RT	BA, CA, Mac, CNA	BBA, LKV, BBE	Gram	Wash any granules and "emulsify" in saline.
Blood									
	Blood culture media set (aerobic and anaerobic bottle) Disinfect the container with 70% isopropyl alcohol or chlorhexidine, wait 30 s	Disinfect venipuncture site with chlorhexidine-alcohol.	Draw blood at time of febrile episode; draw two sets from right and left arms; do not draw more than four sets in a 24-h period; draw ≥20 mL/set (adults) or 1-20 mL/set (pediatric) depending on patient's weight; or per manufacturer's instructions.	Within 2 h/RT	≤2 h/RT Must be incubated at 37°C on receipt in laboratory.	Blood culture bottles, aerobic; consider isolator tubes fungi and other intracellular agents.	Blood culture bottles, anaerobic.	Direct Gram stain from positive blood culture bottles.	C or BCYE if *F. tularensis* is suspected. Other considerations: brucellosis, tularemia, cell wall–deficient bacteria, leptospirosis, or AFB; blood cultures should be collected before administration of antibiotics when possible.

Bone Marrow Aspirate

Specimen	Device	Preparation	Collection	Transport	Storage	Media	Anaerobic media	Stain	Comments
Bone marrow	Blood culture bottles or 1.5 mL lysis-centrifugation tube	Puncture site prepared by primary care provide for surgical incision.		≤24 h, RT if in culture bottle or tube	24 h, RT	BA, CA May use blood culture bottles if volume is sufficient.	BBA		Isolator tubes for the detection of *Brucella* and intracellular bacteria.

Body Fluids

Specimen	Device	Preparation	Collection	Transport	Storage	Media	Anaerobic media	Stain	Comments
Amniotic, abdominal, ascites (peritoneal), bile, joint (synovial), pericardial, pleural	Sterile, screw-cap tube or anaerobic transporter or direct inoculation into blood culture bottles, or capped syringe	Disinfect skin with iodine preparation before aspirating specimen.	Needle aspiration	≤15 min	<24 h/RT: Pericardial fluid and other fluids for fungal cultures. <25 h/4°C: Incubate blood culture bottles at 37°C on receipt in laboratory. <24 h/4°C: Pericardial fluid and fluids for fungal cultures.	May use an aerobic and anaerobic blood culture bottle set for body fluids. BA, CA, thio, CNA, Mac	BBA, BBE, LKV	Gram	May need to concentrate by centrifugation or filtration—stain and culture sediment.
Bone	Sterile, screw-cap container	Disinfect skin before surgical procedure.	Take sample from affected area for biopsy.	Immediately/RT	Plate as soon as received.	BA, CA, Mac, thio	BBA, BBE, LKV	Gram	May need to homogenize.

Cerebrospinal Fluid (CSF)

Specimen	Device	Preparation	Collection	Transport	Storage	Media	Anaerobic media	Stain	Comments
	Sterile, screw-cap tube	Disinfect skin with iodine or chlorhexidine before aspirating specimen.	Consider rapid testing (e.g., Gram stain; cryptococcal antigen).	≤15 min RT Never refrigerate for bacteriology.	<24 h/RT Except for viruses, which can be held at 4°C for up to 3 days.	BA, CA (Routine) BA, CA, Mac, thio (shunt)		Gram—best sensitivity by cytocentrifugation (may also want to do AO if cytocentrifuge not available).	If only 1 tube, submit to microbiology first to avoid contamination; otherwise tube 2. Add thio for CSF collected from shunt. Recommended to also collect blood culture.

Continued

TABLE 5.1 Collection, Transport, Storage, and Processing of Specimens Commonly Submitted to a Microbiology Laboratory—cont'd

Specimen	Container	Patient Preparation	Special Instructions	Transportation to Laboratory	Storage Before Processing	Primary Plating Media	Anaerobic Media	Direct Examination	Comments
Ear									
Inner	Sterile, screw-cap tube or anaerobic transporter	Clean ear canal with mild soap solution.	Aspirate material behind drum with syringe if eardrum intact; use flexible shaft swab to collect material from ruptured eardrum.	≤ 2 h	24 h/RT	BA, CA (add thio if prior antimicrobial therapy)	BBA	Gram	Add anaerobic culture plates for tympanocentesis specimens.
External	Wound or E-swab transport system or aerobic swab moistened with Stuart's or Amie's medium	Wipe away crust with sterile saline.	Firmly rotate swab in outer canal.	≤2 h/RT	24 h/4°C	BA, CA, Mac		Gram	
Eye									
Conjunctiva	Direct culture inoculation to BA and Choc; or E-swab transport system		Sample both eyes; use separate swabs pre-moistened with sterile saline.	Plates ≤15 min, RT Swabs ≤2 h/RT	24 h/RT	BA, CA		Gram, AO, histologic stains (e.g., Giemsa)	Other considerations: Chlamydia trachomatis, viruses, and fungi.
Aqueous/vitreous fluid	Sterile, screw-cap tube	Prepare eye for needle aspiration.		≤15 min/RT	<24 h/RT Set up immediately on receipt.	BA, CA		Gram/AO	Other considerations: fungal media; some anesthetics may be inhibitory to some organisms.
Corneal scrapings	Bedside inoculation of BHI 10%	Clinician should instill local anesthetic before collection.		≤15 min/RT	<24 h/RT Must be incubated at 28°C (SDA) or 37°C (everything else) on receipt in laboratory.	BHI 10% Sheep blood, C, SDA with antibiotics		Gram/AO The use of 10-mm frosted ring slides assists with location of specimen because of the size of the specimen.	Other considerations: Acanthamoeba spp., herpes simplex virus and other viruses, Chlamydia trachomatis, and fungi.

Foreign Bodies

Specimen	Container	Collection	Notes	Transport	Storage	Media	Stain	Other considerations
IUD	Sterile, screw-cap container	Disinfect skin before removal.		≤15 min/RT	Plate as soon as received.	Thio		
IV catheters, pins	Sterile, screw-cap container	Disinfect skin with alcohol before removal.	Do not culture Foley catheters; IV catheters are cultured quantitatively by rolling the segment back and forth across agar with sterile forceps four times; ≥15 colonies are associated with clinical significance.	≤15 min/RT	Plate as soon as received, if possible; store <2 h/4°C.	BA, Thio, prosthetic valves		

GI Tract

Specimen	Container	Collection	Notes	Transport	Storage	Media	Stain	Other considerations
Gastric wash or lavage	Sterile, screw-cap tube	Collect in early AM before patient eats or gets out of bed.	Most gastric aspirates are on infants or for AFB.	≤15 min/RT	<24 h/4°C Must be neutralized with sodium bicarbonate within 1 h of collection.	BA, CA, Mac, HE, CNA, EB	Gram/AO	Other considerations: AFB.
Gastric biopsy	Sterile, screw-cap tube with transport media		Rapid urease test or culture for *Helicobacter pylori*.	<1 h/RT	24 h/4°C	Skirrow, BA; BBA	H&E stain optional; immunostaining.	Other considerations: urea breath test; antigen test (*H. pylori*).

Continued

TABLE 5.1 Collection, Transport, Storage, and Processing of Specimens Commonly Submitted to a Microbiology Laboratory—cont'd

Specimen	Patient Preparation	Container	Special Instructions	Transportation to Laboratory	Storage Before Processing	Primary Plating Media	Anaerobic Media	Direct Examination	Comments
Rectal swab		Swab placed in enteric transport medium	Insert swab, 1–1.5 in past anal sphincter; feces should be visible on swab.	≤2 h/RT	<24 h/RT	BA, Mac, HE, Campy, EB		Methylene blue for fecal leukocytes.	Optional: Mac-sorbitol, chromogenic agar, Shiga toxin testing. Other considerations: *Vibrio* (TCBS), *Yersinia enterocolitica* (CIN), *Escherichia coli* O157:H7, *N. gonorrhoeae*, *Shigella*, *Campylobacter*, herpes simplex virus and carriage of group B streptococci.
Stool (feces) routine culture		Clean, leak-proof container; transfer feces to enteric transport medium (Cary-Blair-holding medium)	Routine culture should include *Salmonella*, *Shigella*, and *Campylobacter*; specify *Vibrio*, *Aeromonas*, *Plesiomonas*, *Yersinia*, *Escherichia coli* O157:H7, if needed.	Within 24 h/ RT in holding media Unpreserved ≤1 h/RT	24 h/4°C <48 h/RT or 4°C	BA, Mac., HE, Campy, EB;		Methylene blue for fecal leukocytes; optional: Shiga toxin testing.	Optional: Mac-sorbitol, chromogenic agar, Shiga-toxin testing. See considerations in previous rectal swabs. Do not perform routine stool cultures for patients whose length of stay in the hospital exceeds 3 days and whose admitting diagnosis was not diarrhea; these patients should be tested for *Clostridiodes difficile*.
Clostridiodes difficile		Sterile, leak-proof container		≤1 h, RT 1–24 h, 4°C	2 days, 4°C for culture or nucleic acid detection	CCFA			Nucleic acid testing is more sensitive than culture. Patients should be passing ≥3 liquid or soft stools per 24 hours without having received laxatives.

Organism/Specimen	Container/Transport Device	Transport Time/Temperature	Media	Comments
Escherichia coli O157:H7 or other Shiga-toxin producing serotypes	Sterile leak-proof container, or Cary-Blair holding medium	≤1 h, RT unpreserved; ≤24 h, RT or 4°C in swab transport system	Mac-sorbitol; <24 h, 4°C unpreserved	Shiga toxin EIA and nucleic acid testing are more sensitive than culture. Bloody or liquid stools collected following 6 days of onset of symptoms yield more positives. Serotyping for O and H antigens.
O&P	O&P transporters (e.g., 10% formalin and PVA)	Wait 5–10 days minimum (up to 2 weeks) if patient has received antiparasitic compounds, barium, iron, Kaopectate, metronidazole, Milk of Magnesia, Pepto-Bismol, or tetracycline. Collect three specimens every other day at a minimum for outpatients; hospitalized patients (inpatients) should have a daily specimen collected for 3 days; specimens from inpatients hospitalized more than 3 days should be discouraged.	Indefinitely/RT	Fresh nonpreserved liquid specimens should be examined within 30 min of passage; semiformed within 1 hour of passage. Specimen in fixatives, 24 h/RT. Fresh liquid specimen should be examined for the presence of motile organisms.

Genital Tract

Female

Specimen	Container/Transport Device	Transport Time/Temperature	Media	Comments
Bartholin cyst	Anaerobic transporter	≤2 h/RT; 24 h/RT	BA, CA, Mac, TM, CNA; BBA, LKV, BBE; Gram	Disinfect skin with iodine preparation before collection.

Continued

TABLE 5.1 Collection, Transport, Storage, and Processing of Specimens Commonly Submitted to a Microbiology Laboratory—cont'd

Specimen	Container	Patient Preparation	Special Instructions	Transportation to Laboratory	Storage Before Processing	Primary Plating Media	Anaerobic Media	Direct Examination	Comments
Cervix	Swab moistened with Stuart's or Amie's medium	Remove mucus before collection of specimen.	Do not use lubricant on speculum; use viral/chlamydial transport medium, if necessary; swab deeply into endocervical canal.	≤2 h/RT	24 h/RT	BA, CA, TM		Gram	
Cul-de-sac fluid	Anaerobic transporter		Submit aspirate.	<2 h/RT	24 h/RT	BA, CA, Mac, TM, CNA	BBA, LKV, BBE	Gram	
Endometrium	Anaerobic transporter		Surgical biopsy or transcervical aspirate via sheathed catheter.	≤2 h/RT	24 h/RT	BA, CA, Mac, TM, CNA	BBA, LKV, BBE	Gram	
Products of conception	Sterile tube or anaerobic transport system		If no discharge can be obtained, wash periurethral area with povidone-iodine soap; rinse with water. Insert swab 2–4 cm into urethra, rotate for 2 s	≤2 h/RT	24 h/RT	BA, CA, Mac, TM, CNA	BBA, LKV, BBE		
Urethra	Swab moistened with Stuart's or Amie's medium	Collect 1 hour after patient's last urination. Remove exudate from urethral opening.	Collect discharge by massaging urethra against pubic symphysis or insert flexible swab 2–4 cm into urethra and rotate swab for 2 s; collect at least 1 h after patient has urinated.	≤2 h/RT	24 h/RT	TM		Gram	Other considerations: chlamydia, mycoplasma.

	Transport Device	Patient Preparation	Specimen Collection	Transport Time/Temp	Transport Time/Temp	Media	Comments	Stain	Comments
Vagina	Swab moistened with Stuart's or Amie's medium	Remove exudate.	Swab secretions and mucous membrane of vagina. If a smear is also required, use a second swab.	≤2 h/RT	24 h/RT	BA, TM	Culture is not recommended for the diagnosis of bacterial vaginosis; inoculate selective medium for group B streptococcus (LIM broth) if indicated for vaginal/rectal screen in pregnant women.	Gram	Examine Gram stain for bacterial vaginosis, especially white blood cells, clue cells, gram-positive rods indicative of *Lactobacillus*, and curved, gram-negative rods indicative of *Mobiluncus* spp. Subculture Group B streptococcus enrichment broth to chromogenic screening agar, or use broth for nucleic acid testing.
Male or female genital lesion	Swab transport		Remove surface of the lesion with sterile scalpel; rub base of lesion with a sterile swab.	≤2 h/RT	24 h/RT				
H. ducreyi						CA with vancomycin (3µg/Ml)		Gram	Gram stain resembling a "school of fish."
Male									
Prostate	Swab moistened with Stuart's or Amie's medium or sterile, screw-cap tube	Clean urethral meatus with soap and water and massage the prostate through the rectum.	Collect secretions on swab or in tube.	≤2 h/RT for swab; immediately if in tube/RT	24 h/RT for swab; plate secretions immediately if in tube	BA, CA, Mac, TM, CNA, BBA, LKV, BBE		Gram	

Continued

TABLE 5.1 Collection, Transport, Storage, and Processing of Specimens Commonly Submitted to a Microbiology Laboratory—cont'd

Specimen	Container	Patient Preparation	Special Instructions	Transportation to Laboratory	Storage Before Processing	Primary Plating Media	Anaerobic Media	Direct Examination	Comments
Urethra	Swab moistened with Stuart's or Amie's medium		Insert flexible swab 2–4 cm into urethra and rotate for 2 s or collect discharge.	≤2 h/RT	24 h/RT	TM		Gram	Other considerations: chlamydia, mycoplasma.

Hair, Nails, or Skin Scrapings (for Fungal Culture)

Specimen	Container	Patient Preparation	Special Instructions	Transportation to Laboratory	Storage Before Processing	Primary Plating Media	Anaerobic Media	Direct Examination	Comments
	Clean, screw-top tube	Nails or skin: wipe with 70% alcohol	Hair: collect hairs with intact shaft. Nails: send clippings of affected area. Skin: scrape skin at leading edge of lesion.	Within 72 h/RT	Indefinitely/RT	SDA, IMAcg, SDAcg		CW	

Respiratory Tract

Lower

Specimen	Container	Patient Preparation	Special Instructions	Transportation to Laboratory	Storage Before Processing	Primary Plating Media	Anaerobic Media	Direct Examination	Comments
BAL, BB, BW or endotracheal aspirate	Sterile, screw-top container		Anaerobic culture appropriate only if sheathed (protected) catheter used.	≤2 h/RT	24 h/4°C	BA, CA, Mac, CNA	BBA, LKV (only acceptable for protected bronchoscopic brushing in anaerobic transport).	Gram and other special stains as requested (e.g., Legionella DFA, acid-fast stain).	Other considerations: quantitative culture for BAL, AFB, Legionella (BCYE), Nocardia, Mycoplasma, Pneumocystis, Cytomegalovirus.
Sputum	Sterile, screw-top container	Have patient brush teeth and then rinse or gargle with water before collection.	Have patient collect from deep cough; specimen should be examined for suitability for culture by Gram stain; induced sputa on pediatric or uncooperative patients may be watery because of saline nebulization.	≤2 h/RT	<24 h/4°C	BA, CA, Mac, Cystic fibrosis patients, add BCSA/, OFPBL, Mannitol salt and IMA		Gram and other special stains as requested (e.g., Legionella DFA, acid-fast stain)	Other considerations: AFB, Nocardia, Legionella (BCYE).

Upper

Source	Device	Collection	Transport	Storage	Media	Additional media	Gram	Other considerations
Nasopharynx	Swab moistened with Stuart's or Amie's medium	Insert flexible swab through nose into posterior nasopharynx and rotate for 5 s; specimen of choice for *Bordetella pertussis*.	≤15 min, RT without transport media ≤2 h/RT using transport media	24 h/RT	BA, CA			Other considerations: add special media for *Corynebacterium diphtheria* (cystine-tellurite or Loeffler's medium), pertussis, *Chlamydia*, and *Mycoplasma*.
Nasal	Swab transport	Premoisten swab with sterile saline; insert approximately 1–2 cm into nares; rotate against nasal mucosa.	≤2 h/RT	24 h/RT	B, chromogenic agar for MRSA screening			
Pharynx (throat)	Swab moistened with Stuart's or Amie's medium Swab dry with or without silica gel for *S. pyogenes* and *C. diphtheriae*	Swab posterior pharynx and tonsils	≤2 h/RT	24 h/RT	BA or SSA			Other considerations: add special media for *C. diphtheria* (cystine-tellurite or Loeffler's medium), *Neisseria gonorrhoeae*, and epiglottis (*Haemophilus influenzae*)

Tissue

Source	Device	Collection	Transport	Storage	Media	Additional media	Gram	Other considerations
Collected during surgery or biopsy procedure	Anaerobic transporter or sterile, screw-cap tube	Disinfect skin.	≤15 min/RT	24 h/RT	BA, CA, Mac, CNA, Thio;	BBA, LKV, BBE	Gram	May need to homogenize.

Urine

Source	Device	Collection	Transport	Storage	Other considerations
Male and female voided for nucleic acid detection	Sterile tube or transport medium provided by manufacturer		Unpreserved ≤2 h, RT; ≤24 h, 4°C	Specified by manufacturer	*Chlamydia* and *N. gonorrhoeae* detection.

Continued

TABLE 5.1 Collection, Transport, Storage, and Processing of Specimens Commonly Submitted to a Microbiology Laboratory—cont'd

Specimen	Container	Patient Preparation	Special Instructions	Transportation to Laboratory	Storage Before Processing	Primary Plating Media	Anaerobic Media	Direct Examination	Comments
Clean-voided midstream (CVS)	Sterile, screw-cap container Containers that include a variety of chemical urinalysis preservatives may also be used.	Females: clean area with soap and water, then rinse with water; hold labia apart and begin voiding in commode; after several mL have passed, collect midstream. Males: clean glans with soap and water, then rinse with water; retract foreskin; begin voiding in commode; after several mL have passed, collect midstream.		Preserved ≤24 h/RT Unpreserved ≤1/2 h/RT	24 h/4°C	BA, Mac Optional: chromogenic agar		Check for pyuria, Gram stain not recommended	Plate quantitatively at 1:1000; consider plating quantitatively at 1:100 if patient is a female of childbearing age with white blood cells and possible acute urethral syndrome.
Straight catheter (in and out)	Sterile, screw-cap container or urine transport tube with boric acid preservative	Clean urethral area (soap and water) and rinse (water).	Insert catheter into bladder; allow first 15 mL to pass; then collect remainder.	Unpreserved ≤1/2 h/RT Preserved ≤ 24 h/RT	24 h/4°C	BA, Mac Optional: chromogenic agar		Gram or check for pyuria	Plate quantitatively at 1:100 and 1:1000. Culture of Foley catheters is not recommended.
Suprapubic aspirate	Sterile, screw-cap container or anaerobic transporter	Disinfect skin.	Needle aspiration above the symphysis pubis through the abdominal wall into the full bladder.	Immediately/RT	Plate as soon as received	BA, Mac, CNA Thio	BBA, LKV, BBE	Gram or check for pyuria	Plate quantitatively at 1:100 and 1:1000.

AFB, Acid-fast bacilli; *AM,* morning; *AO,* acridine orange stain; *BA,* blood agar; *BAL,* bronchial alveolar lavage; *BB,* bronchial brush; *BBA,* brucella blood agar; *BBE, Bacteroides* bile esculin agar; *BCSA, B. cepacia* selective agar; *BCYE,* buffered charcoal-yeast extract agar; *BHI,* brain heart infusion agar; *BW,* bronchial wash; *CA,* chocolate agar; *CCFA,* cycloserine-cefoxitin-fructose agar; *Campy,* selective *Campylobacter* agar; *CIN,* cefsulodin-Igrasan-novobiocin agar; *CNA,* Columbia agar with colistin and nalidixic acid; *CW,* calcofluor white stain; *DFA,* direct fluorescent antibody stain; *EB,* enrichment broth; *GC, Neisseria gonorrhoeae; GI,* gastrointestinal; *Gram,* Gram stain; *H&E,* hematoxylin and eosin; *HE,* Hektoen enteric agar; *IMA,* inhibitory mold agar; *IMAcg,* inhibitory mold agar with chloramphenicol and gentamicin; *IUD,* intrauterine device; *LKV,* laked blood agar with kanamycin and vancomycin; *Mac,* MacConkey agar; *Mac-S,* MacConkey-sorbitol; *OFPBL,* oxidative-fermentative polymyxin B-bacitracin-lactose-agar; *O&P,* ova and parasite examination; *PVA,* polyvinyl alcohol; *RT,* room temperature; *SDA,* Sabouraud dextrose agar; *SDAcg,* Sabouraud dextrose agar with cycloheximide and gentamicin; *SPS,* sodium polyanethol sulfonate; *SSA,* group A *streptococcus* selective agar; *thio,* thioglycollate broth; *TM,* Thayer-Martin agar.

*aSpecimens for viruses, chlamydia, and mycoplasma are usually submitted in appropriate transport media at 4°C to stabilize respective microorganisms.

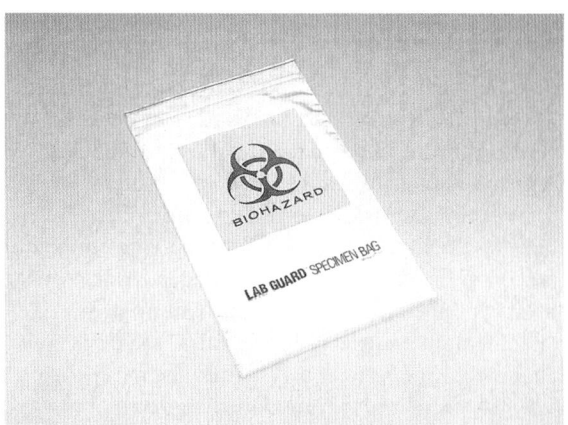

• **Fig. 5.1** Specimen bag with biohazard label, separate pouch for paperwork, and self-seal. (Courtesy Allegiance Healthcare Corp., McGaw Park, IL.)

requisition is a hard (paper) copy of the physician's orders and the patient's demographic information (e.g., name and hospital number). Sometimes, however, if a hospital information system offers computerized order entry, the requisition is transported to the laboratory electronically. The requisition should contain as much information as possible regarding the patient history and diagnosis. This information helps the microbiologist work up the specimen and determine which organisms are significant in the culture. A complete requisition should include the following:
• The patient's name
• Hospital identification number
• Age and date of birth
• Sex
• Collection date and time
• Ordering physician
• Exact nature and source of the specimen
• Diagnosis (may be ICD-10-CM code)
• Current antimicrobial therapy

Rejection of Unacceptable Specimens

Criteria for specimen rejection should be set up and distributed to all clinical practitioners. In general, specimens are unacceptable if any of the following conditions apply:
• The information on the label does not match the information on the requisition or the specimen is not labeled at all (the patient's name or the source of the specimen is different).
• The specimen has been transported at the improper temperature.
• The specimen has not been transported in the proper medium (e.g., specimens for anaerobic bacteria submitted in aerobic transports).
• The quantity of specimen is insufficient for testing (the specimen is considered quantity-not-sufficient [QNS]).
• The specimen is leaking.
• The specimen transport time exceeds the recommended postcollection to set-up time or the specimen is not preserved.

• The specimen was received in a fixative (formalin), which, in essence, kills any microorganism present.
• The specimen has been received for anaerobic culture from a site known to have anaerobes as part of the normal microbiota (vagina, mouth).
• The specimen is dried.
• Processing the specimen would produce information of questionable medical value (e.g., Foley catheter tip).

It is important to always talk to the requesting physician or another member of the health care team before discarding unacceptable specimens. This is particularly important if the specimen was collected using an invasive technique such as a surgical biopsy and collection of a new specimen would be difficult or impossible. In these cases, mislabeling of a specimen or requisition may be corrected by having the person who collected the specimen and filled out the paperwork come to the laboratory and correct the problem; a mislabeled specimen or requisition should not be identified over the telephone. However, correction of mislabeled specimens must be completed at the discretion of the laboratory's standard operating procedures. It is often necessary to do the best possible job on a less than optimal specimen if it would be impossible to collect the specimen again because the patient is taking antibiotics, the tissue was collected at surgery, or the patient would have to undergo a second invasive procedure (bone marrow or spinal tap). A notation regarding improper collection should be added to the final report in this instance because only the primary caregiver is able to determine the validity of the results.

Specimen Processing

Depending on the site of testing (hospital, independent laboratory, physician's office laboratory) and how the specimens are transported to the laboratory (in-house, courier, or driver), microbiology samples may arrive in the laboratory in large numbers or as single tests. Although batch processing may be possible in large independent laboratories, hospital testing is typically performed as specimens arrive. Surgical specimens or specimens from a patient in the emergency room should be processed immediately for any direct testing orders such as Gram staining or nucleic acid testing, prior to the administration of antibiotics. When multiple specimens arrive at the same time, priority should be given to those that are most critical, such as cerebrospinal fluid (CSF), tissue, blood, and sterile fluids. Urine, throat, sputa, stool, or wound drainage specimens can be saved for later. On arrival in the laboratory, the time and date received should be recorded. Acid-fast, viral, and fungal specimens are usually batched for processing. When a specimen is received with multiple requests but the amount of specimen is insufficient to do all of them, the microbiologist should call the clinician to prioritize the testing. Any time a laboratory staff member contacts the physician or nurse, the conversation and agreed-upon information should be documented to ensure proper follow-up.

Gross Examination of Specimen

All processing should begin with a gross examination of the specimen. Areas with blood or mucus should be located and sampled for culture and direct examination. Stool should be examined for evidence of barium (i.e., chalky white color), which would preclude O&P examination. Notations should be made on the handwritten or electronic work card regarding the status of the specimen (e.g., bloody, cloudy, clotted) so that if more than one person works on the sample, the results of the gross examination are available for consultation.

Direct Microscopic Examination

All appropriate specimens should have a **direct microscopic examination** (smear of the primary specimen). The direct examination serves several purposes. First, the quality of the specimen can be assessed; for example, sputa can be rejected that represents saliva and not lower respiratory tract secretions by quantitation of white blood cells or squamous epithelial cells present in the specimen. Second, the microbiologist and clinician can be given an early indication of what may be wrong with the patient (e.g., 4+ gram-positive cocci in clusters in an exudate). Third, the work-up of the specimen can be guided by comparing what grows in culture to what was seen on the original smear. A situation in which three different **morphotypes** (cellular types) are seen on direct Gram stain but only two grow in culture, for example, alerts the microbiologist to the fact that the third organism may be an anaerobic bacterium. If there were more than three organisms on the culture plate that were not visible on Gram stain, this would indicate possible contamination. Gram stains are often also layered with cells and debris. Organisms that appear on the surface of white blood cells actually may be ingested organisms that are no longer viable or capable of growth. It is imperative that the Gram stain results and specimen culture correlate to the type of specimen to ensure that accurate information is provided to the clinician.

Direct examinations are usually not performed on throat, nasopharyngeal, or stool specimens because of the presence of abundant normal microbiota but are indicated from most other sources.

The most common stain in bacteriology is the Gram stain, which helps the clinician visualize rods, cocci, white blood cells, red blood cells, or squamous epithelial cells present in the sample. The most common direct fungal stains are KOH (potassium hydroxide), PAS (periodic-acid Schiff), GMS (Grocott's methenamine silver stain), and calcofluor white. Although rarely used in the clinical laboratory, the most common direct acid-fast stain is the Kinyoun modification (cold method) of the Ziehl-Neelsen (hot method) procedure. Chapter 6 describes the use of microscopy in clinical diagnosis in more detail.

Selection of Culture Media

Primary culture media are divided into several categories. The first is **nutritive media,** such as blood agar. Nutritive media support the growth of a wide range of nonfastidious microorganisms and are considered nonselective because, theoretically, the growth of most organisms is supported. Nutritive media can also be differential, in that microorganisms can be distinguished on the basis of certain growth characteristics evident on the medium. Blood agar is considered both a nutritive and differential medium because it differentiates organisms based on whether they are alpha (α)-, beta (β)-, or gamma (γ)-hemolytic (Fig. 5.2). **Selective media** support the growth of one group of organisms but not another by adding antimicrobials, dyes, alcohol, or other inhibitory chemicals to a particular medium. MacConkey agar, for example, contains the dye crystal violet, which inhibits gram-positive organisms. Columbia agar with colistin and nalidixic acid (CNA) is a selective medium for gram-positive organisms because the antimicrobials colistin and nalidixic acid inhibit gram-negative organisms. Selective media can also be differential media if, in addition to their inhibitory activity, they differentiate between groups of organisms. MacConkey agar, for example, differentiates between lactose-fermenting and nonfermenting gram-negative rods by the color of the colonial growth (pink or clear, respectively); this is shown in Fig. 5.3. Fastidious organisms are organisms that require specific nutritional or environmental conditions to enhance their growth. Chocolate agar is considered an **enrichment media** that is used in most routine cultures for the enhancement of growth for commonly isolated fastidious organisms such as *Haemophilus* spp. In some cases (sterile body fluids, tissues, or deep abscesses in a patient receiving antimicrobial therapy), **backup broth** (also called supplemental or enrichment broth) medium is inoculated, along with primary solid (agar) media, so small numbers of organisms present may be detected; this allows detection of anaerobes in aerobic cultures and organisms that may be damaged by either previous or concurrent antimicrobial therapy. Thioglycollate (thio) broth, brain-heart infusion broth (BHIB), and tryptic soy broth (TSB) are common backup broths.

Selection of media to inoculate for any given specimen is usually based on the organisms most likely to be involved in the disease process at the particular site of infection. For example, in determining what to set up for a CSF specimen, one considers the most likely pathogens that cause meningitis (*Streptococcus pneumoniae, Haemophilus influenzae, Neisseria meningitidis, Escherichia coli*, group B streptococcus) and selects media that will support the growth of these organisms (blood and chocolate agar at a minimum). Likewise, if a specimen is collected from a source likely to be contaminated with normal microbiota—for example, an anal fistula (an opening of the surface of the skin near the anus that may communicate with the rectum)—the laboratorian might want to add a selective medium, such as CNA, to suppress gram-negative bacteria and allow gram-positive bacteria and yeast to be recovered.

In addition to primary plating media, chromogenic agars are now available for a variety of organisms that

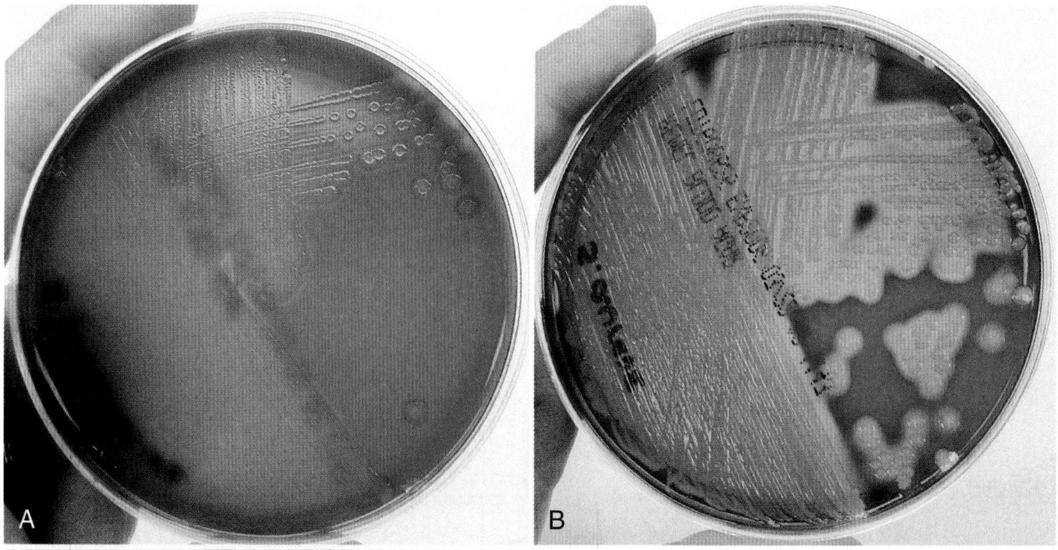

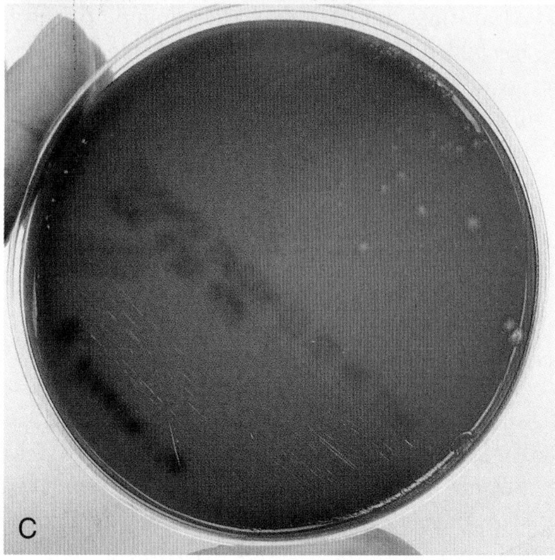

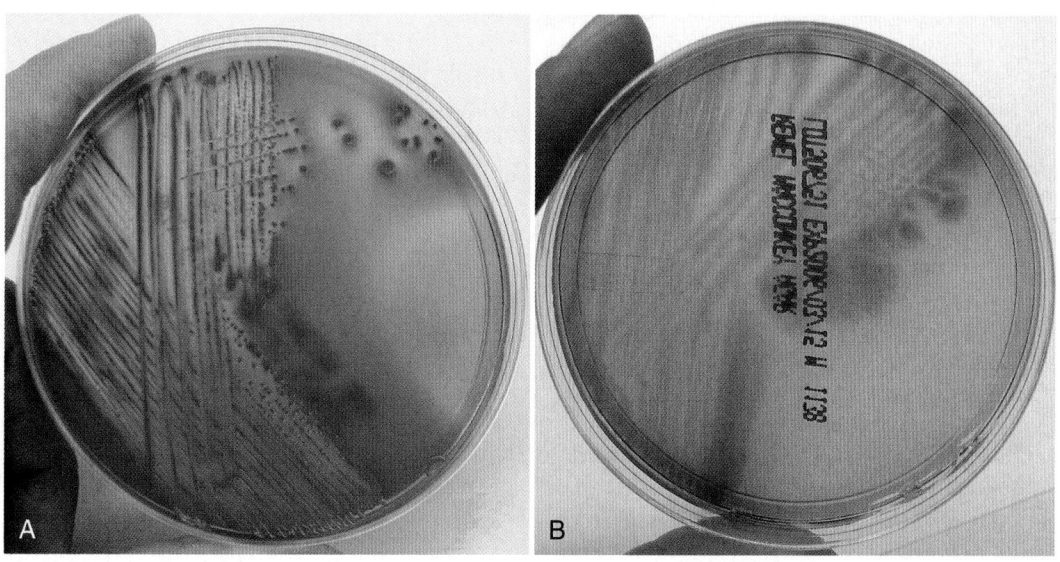

• **Fig. 5.2** Examples of various types of hemolysis on blood agar. (A) *Streptococcus pneumoniae* showing alpha (α)-hemolysis (i.e., greening around colony). (B) *Staphylococcus aureus* showing beta (β)-hemolysis (i.e., clearing around colony). (C) *Enterococcus faecalis* showing gamma (γ)-hemolysis (i.e., no hemolysis around colony).

• **Fig. 5.3** MacConkey agar. (A) *Escherichia coli*, a lactose fermenter. (B) *Pseudomonas aeruginosa*, a nonlactose fermenter.

produce pigmented colonies based on the genus or species of a particular group of bacteria or yeast. These media are often used for screening specimens for pathogens, such as methicillin-resistant *Staphylococcus aureus* (MRSA), vancomycin-resistant enterococci (VRE), and *Candida* species, to name a few.

Routine primary plating media and direct examinations for specimens commonly submitted to the microbiology laboratory are shown in Table 5.1. Samples received on swab should be plated to the least inhibitory media first, followed by additional media prior to making a smear for Gram staining. Chapter 7 on bacterial cultivation reemphasizes the strategies for selection and the use of bacterial media.

Specimen Preparation

Many specimens require some form of initial treatment before inoculation onto primary plating media. Such procedures include **homogenization,** grinding of bone, or mincing of tissue; concentration by centrifugation or filtration of large volumes of sterile fluids, such as ascites (peritoneal) or pleural (lung) fluids; or decontamination of respiratory specimens, such as those for legionellae or mycobacteria. Traditional fiber swab specimens have an internal mattress core that can trap organisms and may be vortexed (mixed) in 0.5 to 1 mL of saline or broth for 10 to 20 seconds to dislodge material from the fibers. Flocked swabs contain no mattress core. The fibers are designed to ionically bind the negative charges on the surface of cells (Copan Diagnostics, Murrieta, CA). Some flocked swabs come in liquid media; the specimen can be mixed in the original container by vortexing prior to inoculating media and preparing a direct smear.

Inoculation on Solid Media

Specimens can be inoculated (plated) onto solid media either quantitatively by a dilution procedure or by means of a **quantitative loop** or **semiquantitatively** using an ordinary inoculating loop. Urine cultures and tissues from burn victims are plated quantitatively; everything else is usually plated semiquantitatively. Plates inoculated for quantitation are usually streaked with a 1:100 or 1:1000 loop. Plates inoculated for semiquantitation are usually streaked out in four quadrants. A variety of automated medium inoculators are also available. Detailed methods for streaking solid media are provided in Chapter 7, Fig. 7.9. Semiquantitation is referred to as **streaking for isolation** because the microorganisms present in the specimen are successively diluted out as each quadrant is streaked until finally each morphotype is present as a single colony. Numbers of organisms present can subsequently be graded as 4+ (many, heavy growth) if growth is out to the fourth quadrant, 3+ (moderate growth) if growth is out to the third quadrant, 2+ (few or light growth) if growth is in the second quadrant, and 1+ (rare) if growth is in the first quadrant. This tells the clinician the relative numbers of different organisms present in the specimen; such semiquantitative information is usually sufficient for the physician to be able to treat the patient.

Incubation Conditions

Inoculated media are incubated under various temperatures and environmental conditions, depending on the organisms suspected—for example, 25° to 30°C for fungi and 35° to 37°C for most bacteria, viruses, and acid-fast bacillus. A number of different environmental conditions exist. **Aerobes** grow in ambient air, which contains 21% oxygen (O_2) and a small amount (0.03%) of carbon dioxide (CO_2). Anaerobes usually cannot grow in the presence of O_2, and the atmosphere in anaerobe jars, bags, or chambers is composed of 5% to 10% hydrogen (H_2), 5% to 10% CO_2, 80% to 90% nitrogen (N_2), and 0% O_2. **Aerotolerant** microorganisms are anaerobes that do not use oxygen but are not killed by a small amount. **Microaerobic** refers to both capnophilic and microaerophilic organisms. Capnophiles, such as *Haemophilus influenzae* and *Neisseria gonorrhoeae*, require increased concentrations of CO_2 (5% to 10%) and approximately 15% O_2. This atmosphere can be achieved by a candle jar (3% CO_2) or a CO_2 incubator, chamber, or bag. **Microaerophiles** (*Campylobacter jejuni, Helicobacter pylori*) grow under reduced O_2 (5% to 10%) and increased CO_2 (8% to 10%). This environment can also be obtained in specially designed chambers, jars, or bags. Both anaerobic and microaerobic environments may be produced using an automated microprocessor-controlled system, such as the Advanced Axonomat, to create the desired atmospheric balance of gases required for specific organismal growth (Advanced Instruments, Norwood, MA). More detailed information is included in Chapter 40.

Specimen Work-Up

One of the most important functions that a microbiologist performs is deciding what is clinically relevant regarding specimen work-up. Considerable judgment is required to decide what organisms to look for and report. It is essential to recognize what constitutes **indigenous (normal) microbiota** and what constitutes a potential pathogen. Indiscriminate identification, susceptibility testing, and reporting of normal microbiota can contribute to the unnecessary use of antibiotics and the potential emergence of resistant organisms. Because organisms that are clinically relevant to identify and report vary by source, the microbiologist should know which organisms cause disease at various sites. Part VII contains a detailed discussion of these issues.

Extent of Identification Required

As health care continues to change, one of the most problematic issues for microbiologists is the extent of culture work-up. Microbiologists still rely heavily on definitive identification, although shortcuts, including the use of limited

TABLE 5.2 Common Transport Media

Media	Description
Amies transport media	Recovery of aerobic and anaerobic bacteria
Amies transport media with charcoal	Recovery of aerobic and anaerobic bacteria; charcoal neutralized bacterial toxins and other inhibitory substances, maintains pH
Anaerobic transport media	Numerous commercial systems available; recovery of anaerobes, and microaerobic bacteria
Cary-Blair	Recovery of enteric pathogens
Formalin (5%–10%), PVA (poly-vinyl alcohol), SAF (sodium acetate-acetic acid-formalin), Total-Fix, Eco-Fix	Recovery of gastrointestinal parasites; some may be acceptable for immunoassays
Stuart's transport media	Recovery of bacteria
Universal transport media	Recovery of chlamydia, mycoplasmas and ureaplasmas and viruses

identification procedures in some cases, are becoming commonplace in most clinical laboratories. Careful application of knowledge of the significance of various organisms in specific situations and thoughtful use of limited approaches will keep microbiology testing cost-effective and the laboratory's workload manageable, while providing for optimum patient care.

Complete identification of a blood culture isolate, such as *Clostridium septicum* as opposed to a genus identification of *Clostridium* spp., will alert the clinician to the possibility of malignancy or other disease. At the same time, a presumptive identification of *Escherichia coli* if a gram-negative, spot indole-positive rod is recovered with appropriate colony morphology on MacConkey agar (flat, lactose-fermenting colony that is precipitating bile salts) is probably permissible from an uncomplicated urinary tract infection. In the final analysis, culture results should always be compared with the suspected diagnosis. The clinician should be encouraged to supply the microbiologist with all pertinent information (e.g., recent travel history, pet exposure, pertinent radiograph findings) so that the microbiologist can use the information to interpret culture results and plan appropriate strategies for work-up.

Communication of Laboratory Findings

To fulfill their professional obligation to the patient, microbiologists must communicate their findings to those health care professionals responsible for treating the patient. This task is not as easy as it may seem. This is nicely illustrated in

a study in which a group of physicians was asked whether they would treat a patient with a sore throat given two separate laboratory reports—that is, one that stated "many group A streptococci" and one that stated "few group A streptococci." Although group A streptococcus (*Streptococcus pyogenes*) is considered significant in any numbers in a symptomatic individual, the physicians said that they would treat the patient with many organisms but not the one with few organisms. Thus, although a pathogen (group A streptococcus) was isolated in both cases, one word on the report (either many or few) made a difference in how the patient would be treated.

In communicating with the physician, the microbiologist can prevent confusion and misunderstanding by not using jargon or abbreviations and by providing reports with clear-cut conclusions. The microbiologist should not assume that the clinician is fully familiar with laboratory procedures or the latest microbial taxonomic schemes. Thus, when appropriate, interpretive statements should be included in the written report along with the specific results. One example would be the addition of a statement such as "suggests contamination at collection" when more than three organisms are isolated from a clean-voided midstream urine specimen.

Laboratory newsletters should be used to provide physicians with material such as details of new procedures, nomenclature changes, and changes in usual antimicrobial susceptibility patterns of frequently isolated organisms. This last information, discussed in more detail in Chapter 11, is very useful to clinicians when selecting empiric therapy. **Empiric therapy** is based on the physician determining the most likely organism causing a patient's clinical symptoms and then selecting an antimicrobial that, in the past, has worked against that organism in a particular hospital or geographic area. Empiric therapy is used to initiate treatment following a direct testing method such as a Gram stain or nucleic acid test before the results of the patient's culture are known and may be critical to the patient's well-being in cases of life-threatening illnesses.

Positive findings should be communicated to the clinician in a timely manner, and all verbal reports should be followed by written confirmation of results. Results should be generated electronically in the **laboratory information system (LIS).**

Critical (Panic) Values

Certain **critical results** must be communicated to the clinician immediately. Each clinical microbiology laboratory, in consultation with its medical staff, should prepare a list of these so-called "panic values." Common panic values include the following:
- Positive blood cultures
- Positive spinal fluid Gram stain or culture
- *Streptococcus pyogenes* (group A streptococcus) in a surgical wound
- Gram stain suggestive of gas gangrene (large boxcar-shaped gram-positive rods)

- Blood smear positive for malaria
- Positive cryptococcal antigen test
- Positive acid-fast stain
- Detection of a select agent (e.g., *Brucella*) or other significant pathogen (e.g., *Legionella*, vancomycin-resistant *S. aureus*, or other antibiotic-resistant organisms as outlined by the facility and infection control policies)

Expediting Results Reporting: Computerization

Laboratories process information using an LIS or laboratory information system. Many LIS systems are, in turn, interfaced with a **hospital information system (HIS)**. Between the HIS and LIS, most functions involved in ordering and reporting laboratory tests can be handled electronically. Order entry, patient identification, and specimen identification can be handled using the same type of bar coding that is commonly used in supermarkets. The LIS also takes care of result reporting and supervisory verification of results, stores quality control data, allows easy test inquiries, and assists in test management reporting by storing, for example, the number of positive, negative, and unsatisfactory specimens. LIS systems are capable of interfacing (communicating) with microbiology instruments to automatically download

(transfer) and store data regarding positive cultures or antimicrobial susceptibility results. Results of individual organism **antibiograms** (patterns) can then be retrieved monthly so hospital-wide susceptibility patterns can be studied for the emergence of resistant organisms or other epidemiologic information. LIS systems can be interfaced with printers or electronic facsimile machines (faxes) as well as accessed through smartphones or tablets for quick and easy reporting and information retrieval, further improving the quality of patient care.

ⓔ Visit the Evolve site for a complete list of procedures, review questions, and case studies.

Bibliography

Bennett J, Dolin R, Blaser M: *Principles and practice of infectious diseases*, ed 9, Philadelphia, PA, 2020, Elsevier Saunders.

Carroll KC, Pfaller MA, Landry ML, et al.: *Manual of clinical microbiology*, ed 12, Washington, DC, 2019, ASM Press.

Daley P, Castricianao S, Chernesky M, Smiej M: Comparison of flocked and rayon swabs for collection of respiratory epithelial cells from uninfected volunteers and symptomatic patients, *J Clin Microbiol* 44:2265, 2006.

Leber AL: Collection, transport, and manipulation of clinical specimens. In Leber AL, ed: *Clinical microbiology procedures handbook*, ed 4, Washington, DC, 2016, ASM Press.

6

Role of Microscopy

OBJECTIVES

1. Explain the role of microscopy in the identification of etiologic agents, including bacteria, fungi, viruses, and parasites.
2. List the four major types of microscopic techniques available for diagnostic evaluation in the clinical laboratory, explain their basic principles, and list a clinical application for each.
3. Define the three main principles of light microscopy, magnification, resolution, and contrast.
4. List the staining techniques used to aid in the visualization of bacteria, explain the chemical principle and limitations for each, and provide an example of a clinical application for each stain. Include the following stains: Gram stain, the Kinyoun stain, the Ziehl-Neelsen stain, the calcofluor white stain, the Acridine orange stain, and the Auramine-Rhodamine stain.
5. Explain the chemical principle for fluorescent dyes in microscopy, and list two examples used in the clinical laboratory.
6. Describe the purpose and method for Kohler illumination.

The basic flow of procedures involved in the laboratory diagnosis of infectious diseases is as follows:

1. Direct examination of patient specimens for the presence of etiologic agents
2. Growth and cultivation or nucleic acid direct detection of the agents from the specimens
3. Analysis of the cultivated organisms to establish their identification, confirm identification from direct techniques, and other pertinent characteristics such as susceptibility to antimicrobial agents

For some infectious agents, this process may also include measuring the patient's immune response to the infectious agent.

Despite the direct detection of nucleic acids in clinical specimens, microscopy remains useful in the clinical laboratory. Direct detection by molecular testing does not provide information, such as the relative amount of normal microbiota to pathogens in a sample or whether

or not the patient is colonized or infected. In addition, direct molecular detection of microorganisms can remain positive even after the organisms are no longer viable within the patient. Finally, direct molecular detection does not provide any information related to specimen quality, and although capable of detecting some antibiotic resistant markers, they cannot predict antimicrobial susceptibility patterns. Microscopy remains an important, highly complex, diagnostic technique in the clinical laboratory.

Microscopy is used for the detection of microorganisms directly in clinical specimens and for the characterization of organisms grown in culture (Box 6.1). **Microscopy** is defined as the use of a microscope to magnify (i.e., visually enlarge) objects too small to be visualized with the naked eye so that their characteristics are readily observable. Because most infectious agents cannot be detected with the unaided eye, microscopy plays a pivotal role in the laboratory. Microscopes and microscopic methods vary. Those of primary use in diagnostic microbiology include bright-field (light) microscopy, phase contrast, fluorescent, and dark-field microscopy.

The method used to process patient specimens is dictated by the type and body source of the specimen (Part VII). Regardless of the method used, some portion of the specimen usually is reserved for microscopic examination. Specific stains or dyes applied to the specimen, combined with particular methods of microscopy, can detect etiologic agents in a rapid, relatively inexpensive, and productive way. Microscopy also plays a key role in the characterization of organisms that have been cultivated in the laboratory (for more information regarding the cultivation of bacteria, see Chapter 7).

The types of microorganisms to be detected, identified, and characterized determine the most appropriate types of microscopy to use. Table 6.1 outlines the basic types of microscopy and their relative utility for each of the four major types of infectious agents. **Bright-field microscopy** (also known as light microscopy) has the widest use and application within the clinical microbiology laboratory. **Fluorescence microscopy** has been used for specific detection of infectious agents. In some cases, fluorescent microscopy has been replaced with highly sensitive methods for the direct detection of organisms using nucleic acid methods. **Dark-field** and **electron microscopes** are not typically found within a clinical laboratory and are predominantly used in reference or research settings. Because of advances in technology, all types of microscopy are available in formats that take advantage of virtual or digital imaging for the acquisition and transmission of images. The microorganisms that can be detected or identified by each microscopic method also depends on the methods used to highlight the microorganisms and their key characteristics. This enhancement is usually achieved using various dyes or stains.

• BOX 6.1   Applications of Microscopy in Diagnostic Microbiology

- Rapid preliminary organism identification by direct visualization in patient specimens
- Rapid final identification of certain organisms by direct visualization in patient specimens
- Detection of different organisms present in the same specimen
- Detection of organisms not easily cultivated in the laboratory
- Evaluation of patient specimens for the presence of cells indicative of inflammation (i.e., phagocytes) or contamination (i.e., squamous epithelial cells)
- Determination of an organism's clinical significance; bacterial contaminants usually are not present in patient specimens at sufficiently high numbers (×105 cells/mL) to be seen by light microscopy
- Preculture information about which organisms might be expected to grow so that appropriate cultivation or direct detection methods are used
- Determination of which tests and methods should be used for the identification and characterization of cultivated organisms
- A method for investigating unusual or unexpected laboratory test results

---

Bright-Field (Light) Microscopy

Principles of Light Microscopy

For bright-field (light) microscopy, visible light is passed through the specimen and then through a series of lenses that bend the light in a manner that results in a magnification of the organisms present in the specimen (Fig. 6.1). The total magnification achieved is the product of the lenses used.

Magnification

In most light microscopes, the objective lens, which is closest to the specimen, magnifies objects 100× (times), and the ocular lens, which is nearest the eye, magnifies 10×. Using these two lenses in combination (**total magnification**), organisms in the specimen are magnified 1000× their actual size when viewed through the ocular lens. Objective lenses of lower magnification are available so that those of 10×, 20×, and 40× magnification power can provide total magnifications of 100×, 200×, and 400×, respectively. Magnification of 1000× allows for the visualization of fungi, most parasites, and most bacteria, but it is not sufficient for observing viruses, which require magnification of 100,000× or more (see "Electron Microscopy" in this chapter).

Resolution

To optimize visualization, other factors besides magnification must be considered. **Resolution,** defined as the extent to which detail in the magnified object is maintained, is also essential. Without it, everything would be magnified as an indistinguishable blur. Therefore, **resolving power,** which is the closest distance between two objects that, when magnified, still allows the two objects to be distinguished from each other, is extremely important. The resolving power of light microscopes allows bacterial cells to be distinguished from one another but usually does not allow bacterial structures, internal or external, to be detected.

To achieve the level of resolution desired with 1000× magnification, oil immersion must be used in conjunction with light microscopy. Immersion oil has specific optical and viscosity characteristics designed for use in microscopy. **Immersion oil** is used to fill the space between the objective lens and the glass slide onto which the specimen has been affixed. When light passes from a material of one refractive index to a

---

TABLE 6.1   Microscopy for Diagnostic Microbiology

Organism Group	Bright-Field Microscopy	Digital Microscopy	Fluorescence Microscopy	Phase-Contrast Microscopy	Dark-Field Microscopy
Bacteria	+	+	+	+	±
Fungi	+	+	+	+	−
Parasites	+	+	+	+	−
Viruses	−	+	+	−	−

+, Commonly used; ±, limited use; −, rarely used.

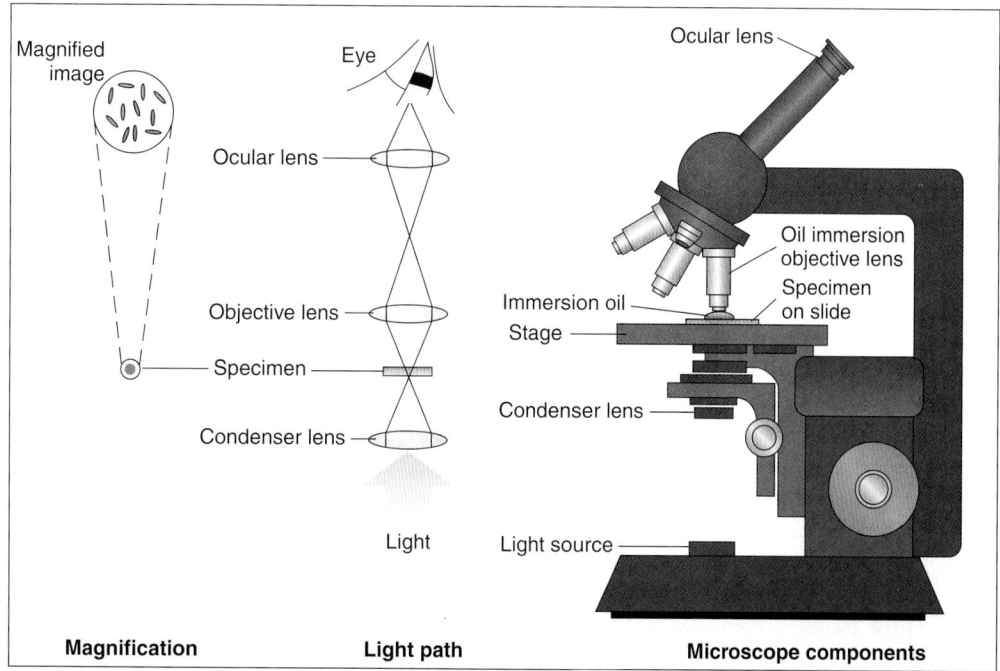

Magnified image

Eye

Ocular lens

Objective lens

Specimen

Condenser lens

Light

Magnification

Light path

Ocular lens

Oil immersion objective lens

Immersion oil

Specimen on slide

Stage

Condenser lens

Light source

Microscope components

• **Fig. 6.1** Principles of bright-field (light) microscopy. (Modified from Atlas RM. *Principles of Microbiology*. St. Louis: Mosby; 2006.)

material with a different refractive index, as from glass to air, the light bends. Light of different wavelengths bends at different angles, creating a less distinct, distorted image. Placing immersion oil with the same refractive index as glass between the objective lens and the cover slip or slide decreases the number of refractive surfaces the light must pass through during microscopy. The oil enhances resolution by preventing light rays from dispersing and changing wavelength after passing through the specimen. A specific objective lens, the **oil immersion lens**, is designed for use with oil; this lens provides 100× magnification on light microscopes.

Lower magnifications (i.e., 100× or 400×) may be used to locate specimen samples in certain areas on a microscope slide or to observe microorganisms such as fungi and parasites. The 1000× magnification provided by the combination of ocular and oil immersion lenses is required for optimal detection and characterization of bacteria.

Contrast

The third key component to light microscopy is **contrast**, which is needed to make objects stand out from the background. Because microorganisms are essentially transparent because of their microscopic dimensions and high water content, they cannot be easily detected among the background materials and debris in patient specimens. Lack of contrast is also a problem for the microscopic examination of microorganisms grown in culture. Contrast is most commonly achieved by staining techniques that highlight organisms and allow them to be differentiated from one another and from background material and debris. In the absence of staining, the simplest way to improve contrast is to reduce the diameter of the microscope aperture diaphragm,

increasing contrast at the expense of the resolution. Setting the controls for bright-field microscopy requires a procedure referred to as setting the Kohler illumination (Evolve Procedure 6.1). A properly set-up microscope will display a clear image that is evenly illuminated without glare.

Direct and Indirect Smears

Staining methods are either used directly with patient specimens or are applied to preparations made from microorganisms grown in culture. A **direct smear** is a preparation of the primary clinical sample received in the laboratory for processing. A direct smear provides a mechanism to identify the number and type of cells present in a specimen, including white blood cells, epithelial cells, and predominant organism type. Occasionally an organism may grow in a culture that was not seen in the direct smear. There is a variety of potential reasons for this, including the possibility that a slow-growing organism was present, the patient was receiving antibiotic treatment to prevent growth of the organism, the specimen was not processed appropriately and the organisms are no longer viable, or the organism requires special media for growth. Preparation of an **indirect smear** indicates that the primary sample has been processed in culture and the smear contains organisms obtained after purification or growth on artificial media. Indirect smears may include preparation from solid or semisolid media or broth. Care should be taken to ensure the smear is not too thick when preparing the slide from solid media. In addition, smears from a liquid broth should not be diluted. Liquid broth cultures result in smears that more clearly and accurately represent the native cellular morphology and arrangement compared with smears from solid media. Details of specimen processing are presented throughout Part VII, and in most instances, the preparation of every specimen includes the application of some portion of the specimen to a clean glass slide (i.e., "smear" preparation) for subsequent microscopic evaluation.

Generally, specimen samples are placed on the slide using a swab or a direct smear that contains patient material or by using a pipette into which liquid specimen has been aspirated (Fig. 6.2). Material to be stained is dropped (if liquid), rolled (if on a swab), or spread (if on a loop) onto the surface of a clean, dry, glass slide. To prevent contamination of culture media, once a swab has touched the surface of a nonsterile slide, it should not be used for subsequently inoculating media.

For staining microorganisms grown in culture or an indirect smear, a sterile loop or needle may be used to transfer a small amount of growth from a solid medium to the surface of the slide. This material is emulsified in a drop of sterile water or saline on the slide. For small amounts of growth that might become lost in even a drop of saline, a sterile wooden applicator stick can be used to touch the growth; this material is then rubbed directly onto the slide, where it can be easily seen. The material placed on the slide to be stained is allowed to air-dry and is affixed to the slide by placing it on a slide warmer (60°C) for at least 10 minutes or by flooding it with 95% methanol for 1 minute. Smears should be air-dried completely before heat fixing to prevent the distortion of cell shapes before staining. To examine organisms grown in liquid medium, an aspirated sample of the broth culture is applied to the slide, air-dried, and fixed before staining.

A **squash** or **crush prep** may be used for a tissue, bone marrow aspirate, or other aspirated sample. The aspirate may be placed in the anticoagulant ethylenediaminetetraacetic acid (EDTA) tube and inverted several times to mix the contents. This prevents clotting of the aspirated material. To prepare the slide, a drop of the aspirate is placed on a slide and a second slide is gently placed on top; the two slides are pressed together, crushing or squashing any particulate

matter. The two slides are then gently slid or pulled apart using a horizontal motion and air-dried before staining.

A **cytocentrifugation,** or concentration of a sterile body fluid such as cerebral spinal fluid (CSF), enhances the ability to identify cells in a specimen that may contain small numbers of microorganisms. In a cytocentrifuge, the hydraulic forces of the liquid cause the fluid to move away from the sediment, which is then collected on an absorbent material, leaving the particulate matter and cellular debris in the center of the microscope slide. The slide may then be stained for microscopy. A fresh or well-preserved specimen and the absence of interfering material are the two primary factors that affect the quality of the preparation using a cytocentrifuge. If the specimen is too old, the biologic cells may have disintegrated, resulting in high protein content or background material. If the sample contains numerous cells, such as in a bloody spinal tap, the organisms may be indistinguishable from the background material.

Smear preparation varies depending on the type of specimen being processed (see the chapters in Part VII that discuss specific specimen types) and on the staining methods to be used. Nonetheless, the general rule for smear preparation is that sufficient material must be applied to the slide so that the chances for detecting and distinguishing microorganisms are maximized. At the same time, the application of excessive material that could interfere with the passage of light through the specimen or that could distort the details of microorganisms must be avoided. Finally, the staining methods used to visualize the contents of the smear are dictated by which microorganisms are suspected in the specimen.

Staining Techniques

As listed in Table 6.1, light microscopy has applications for bacteria, fungi, and parasites. However, the stains used for these microbial groups differ extensively. Those primarily designed for examination of parasites and fungi by light microscopy are discussed in Chapters 46 and 58, respectively. The stains for microscopic examination of bacteria, the Gram stain, and the acid-fast stains are discussed here.

Gram Stain

The Gram stain is the principal stain used for microscopic examination of bacteria and is one of the most important bacteriologic techniques within the microbiology laboratory. Gram staining provides a mechanism for the rapid presumptive identification of pathogens, and it gives important clues related to the quality of a specimen and whether bacterial pathogens from a specific body site are considered normal microbiota colonizing the site or the actual cause of infection. Nearly all clinically important bacteria can be detected using this method, the only exceptions being those organisms that exist almost exclusively within host cells (e.g., chlamydia), those that lack a cell wall (e.g., mycoplasma and ureaplasma), and those of insufficient dimension to be resolved by light microscopy (e.g., spirochetes). First devised by Hans Christian Gram during the late nineteenth century,

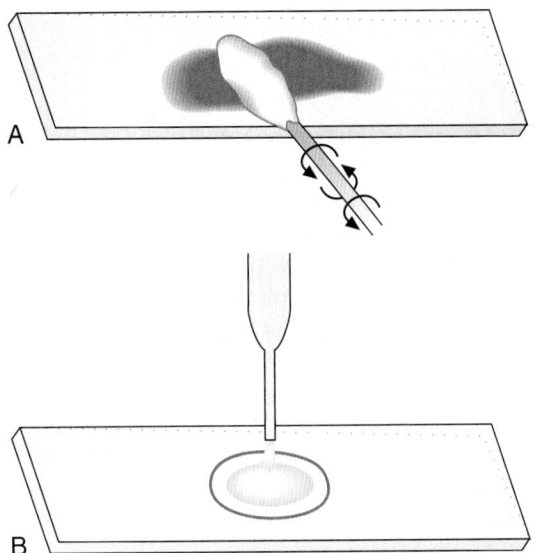

• **Fig. 6.2** Smear preparations by swab roll (A) and pipette deposition (B) of a patient specimen on a glass slide.

the Gram stain can be used to divide most bacterial species into two large groups: those that take up the basic dye, crystal violet (i.e., gram-positive bacteria), and those that allow the crystal violet dye to wash out easily with the decolorizer alcohol or acetone (i.e., gram-negative bacteria). Therefore, the Gram stain is considered a **differential stain**, based on the chemical differentiation of organisms as a result of the structural chemical components of the organism's cell wall.

Procedure Overview

Although modifications of the classic Gram stain that involve changes in reagents and timing do exist, the principles and results are the same for all modifications. The classic Gram stain procedure entails fixing clinical material to the surface of the microscope slide, either by heating or by using methanol. Methanol fixation preserves the morphology of host cells, as well as bacteria, and is especially useful for examining bloody specimens. Slides are overlaid with 95% methanol for 1 minute; the methanol is allowed to run off, and the slides are air-dried before staining. After fixation, the first step in the Gram stain is the application of the **primary stain**, crystal violet (CV). A **mordant**, Gram's iodine (I), is applied after the crystal violet to chemically

bond the alkaline dye to the iodine, forming a CV-I complex and cross-linking the complex in the bacterial cell wall. The **decolorization** step distinguishes gram-positive from gram-negative cells. Therefore, after decolorization, organisms that stain gram-positive retain the crystal violet, and those that are gram-negative are cleared of crystal violet. Addition of the **secondary stain** or **counterstain** safranin will then stain the colorless gram-negative bacteria pink or red (Fig. 6.3). See Evolve Procedure 6.2 for detailed methodology, expected results, and limitations.

Principle

The difference in composition between gram-positive cell walls, which contain thick peptidoglycan with numerous teichoic acid cross-linkages, and gram-negative cell walls, which consist of a thinner layer of peptidoglycan and an outer lipid bilayer that is dehydrated during decolorization, accounts for the Gram staining differences between these two major groups of bacteria. Presumably, the extensive teichoic acid cross-links contribute to the ability of gram-positive organisms to resist alcohol decolorization. Although the gram-positive organisms may take up the counterstain, their purple appearance will not be altered.

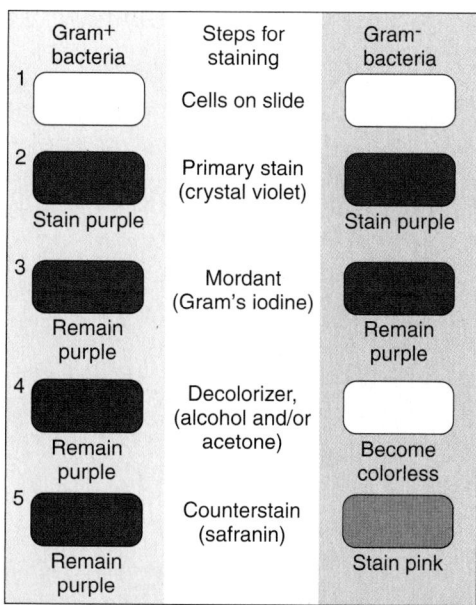

Gram+ bacteria	Steps for staining	Gram- bacteria
1	Cells on slide	1
2 — Stain purple	Primary stain (crystal violet)	2 — Stain purple
3 — Remain purple	Mordant (Gram's iodine)	3 — Remain purple
4 — Remain purple	Decolorizer, (alcohol and/or acetone)	4 — Become colorless
5 — Remain purple	Counterstain (safranin)	5 — Stain pink

1 Fix material on slide with methanol or heat. If slide is heat fixed, allow it to cool to the touch before applying stain.
2 Flood slide with crystal violet (*purple*) and allow it to remain on the surface without drying for 10 to 30 seconds. Rinse the slide with tap water, shaking off all excess.
3 Flood the slide with iodine to increase affinity of crystal violet and allow it to remain on the surface without drying for twice as long as the crystal violet was in contact with the slide surface (20 seconds of iodine for 10 seconds of crystal violet, for example). Rinse with tap water, shaking off all excess.
4 Flood the slide with decolorizer for 10 seconds or less (optimal decolorization depends on chemical used) and rinse off immediately with tap water. Repeat this procedure until the blue dye no longer runs off the slide with the decolorizer. Thicker smears require more prolonged decolorizing. Rinse with tap water and shake off excess.
5 Flood the slide with counterstain and allow it to remain on the surface without drying for 30 seconds. Rinse with tap water and gently blot the slide dry with paper towels or bibulous paper or air dry. For delicate smears, such as certain body fluids, air drying is the best method.
6 Examine microscopically under an oil immersion lens at 1000x for phagocytes, bacteria, and other cellular material.

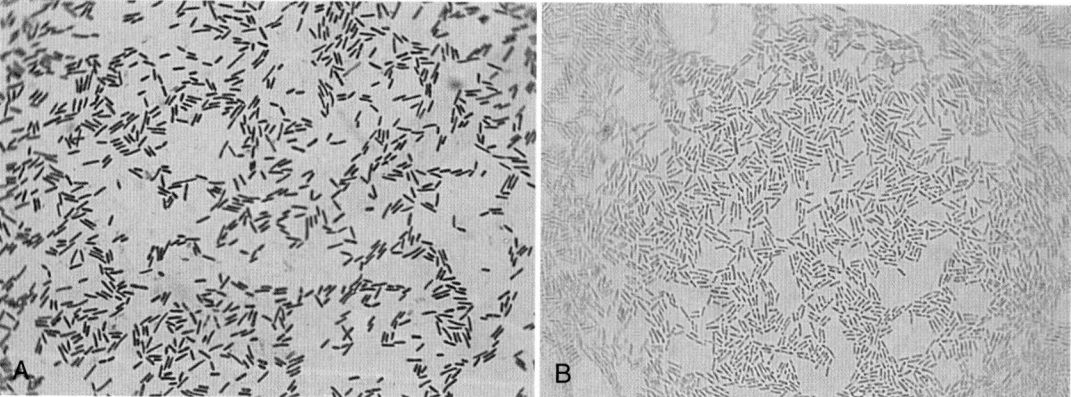

• **Fig. 6.3** Gram stain procedures and principles. (A) Gram-positive bacteria observed under oil immersion appear purple. (B) Gram-negative bacteria observed under oil immersion appear pink. (Modified from Atlas RM. *Principles of Microbiology*. St. Louis: Mosby; 2006.)

Gram-positive organisms that have lost cell wall integrity because of antibiotic treatment, dead or dying cells, or the action of autolytic enzymes may allow the crystal violet to wash out with the decolorizing step and may appear gram-variable, with some cells staining pink and others staining purple. However, for identification purposes, these organisms are considered to be gram-positive. On the other hand, gram-negative bacteria rarely, if ever, retain crystal violet (i.e., appear purple) if the staining procedure has been properly performed. Host cells, such as red and white blood cells (phagocytes), allow the crystal violet stain to wash out with decolorization and should appear pink on smears that have been correctly prepared and stained.

Gram Stain Examination (Direct Smear)

Once stained, the smear is examined using the low power or 40Xobjective (400X magnification). The microbiologist should scan the slide looking for white blood cells, epithelial cells, and larger organisms such as fungi or parasites. Next, the smear should be examined using the oil immersion or 100× objective (1000× magnification) lens. When clinical material is Gram stained (e.g., the direct smear), the slide is evaluated for the presence of bacterial cells as well as the Gram reactions, morphologies (e.g., cocci or bacilli), and arrangements (e.g., chains, pairs, clusters) of the cells (Fig. 6.4). This information often provides a preliminary diagnosis regarding the infectious agents and frequently is used to direct initial therapies for the patient.

Direct smears should also be examined for the presence of inflammatory cells (e.g., phagocytes) that are key indicators of an infectious process. Noting the presence of other host cells, such as squamous epithelial cells in respiratory specimens, is also helpful, because the presence of these cells may indicate contamination with organisms and cells from the oral cavity (for more information regarding the interpretation of respiratory smears, see Chapter 69). Observing background tissue debris and proteinaceous material, which generally stain gram-negative, also provides helpful information. For example, the presence of such material indicates that specimen material was adequately affixed to the slide. The absence of bacteria or inflammatory cells on a smear is a true negative and not likely the result of loss of specimen during staining (Fig. 6.5). Other ways that Gram stain evaluations of how direct smears are used are discussed throughout the chapters of Part VII, which deal with infections of specific body sites.

Several examples of Gram stains of direct smears are provided in Fig. 6.6. Whatever is observed is also recorded and is used to produce a laboratory report for

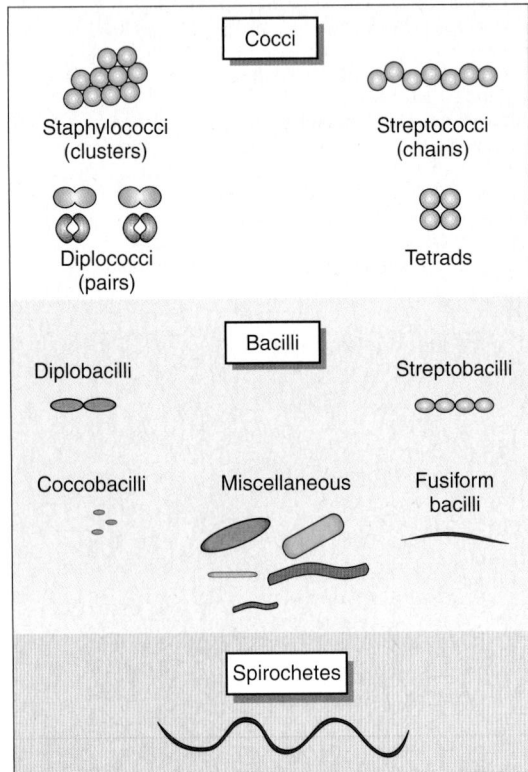

• **Fig. 6.4** Examples of common bacterial cellular morphologies, Gram staining reactions, and cellular arrangements.

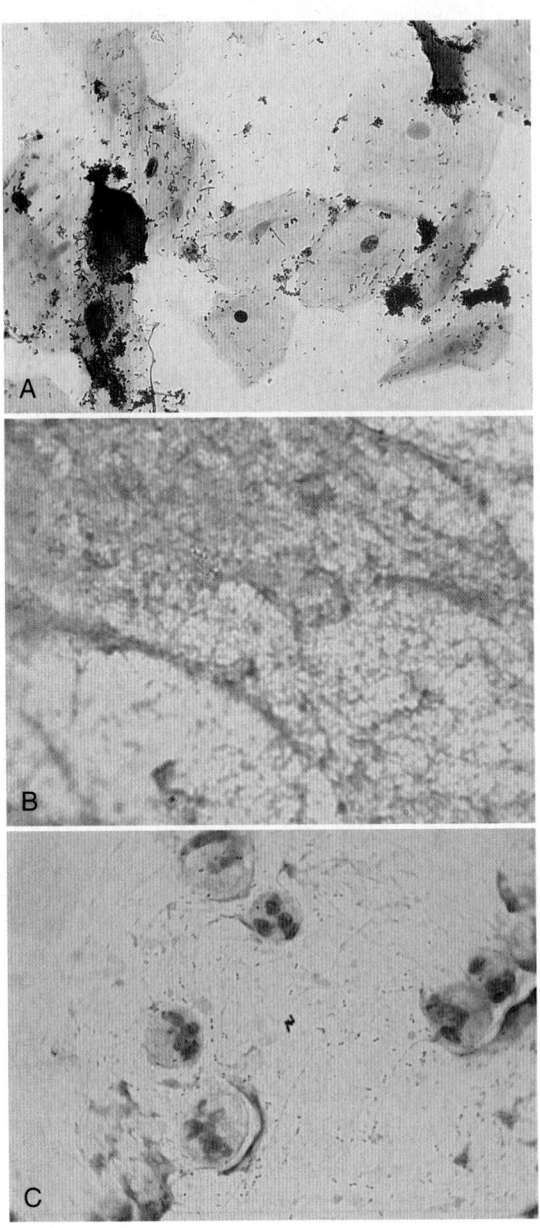

• **Fig. 6.5** Gram stains of direct smears showing squamous cells and bacteria (A), proteinaceous debris (B), and proteinaceous debris with polymorphonuclear leukocytes and bacteria (C).

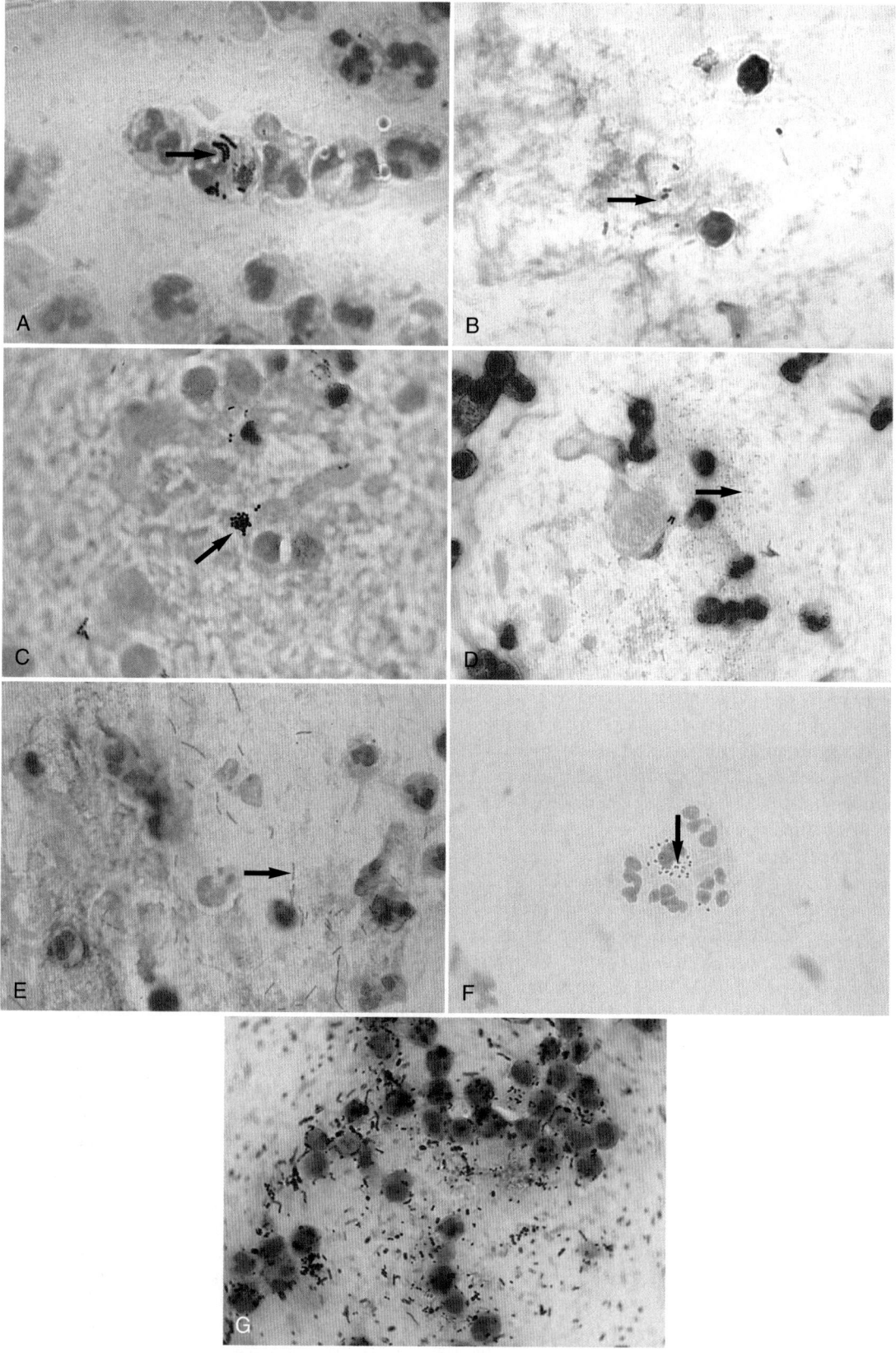

• **Fig. 6.6** Gram stain of direct smears showing polymorphonuclear leukocytes, proteinaceous debris, and bacterial morphologies (*arrows*), including gram-positive cocci in chains (A), gram-positive cocci in pairs (B), gram-positive cocci in clusters (C), gram-negative coccobacilli (D), gram-negative bacilli (E), gram-negative diplococci (F), and mixed gram-positive and gram-negative morphologies (G).

the physician. The report typically includes the following (Evolve Procedure 6.2):

- The presence and type of host cells.
- The Gram reactions, morphologies (e.g., cocci, bacilli, coccobacilli), and arrangement of bacterial cells present; prominent morphotypes indicating an infectious microorganism are important to note. It is also important to differentiate contaminating microorganisms or microbiota that would be confusing to the clinician and of little to no diagnostic value. Note: Reporting the absence of bacteria and host cells can be equally important.
- Optionally, the relative amounts of bacterial cells (e.g., rare, few, moderate, many) in direct smears should be reported. However, it is important to remember that to visualize bacterial cells by light microscopy, a minimum concentration of 105 cells per 1 mL of specimen is required. This is a large number of bacteria for any normally sterile body site, and to describe the quantity as rare or few based on microscopic observation may be understating their significance in a clinical specimen. On the other hand, noting the relative amounts seen on direct smear may be useful laboratory information to correlate smear results with the amount of growth observed subsequently from cultures.
- Direct correlation to the type of specimen, whether or not the specimen was collected from a sterile or nonsterile site, the presence of inflammatory cells, and the expected pathogens are critical to the microscopic evaluation of Gram reactions. Gram stain evaluations are discussed throughout the chapters of Part VII that deal with infections of specific body sites.

Although Gram stain evaluation of direct smears is routinely used to aid in the diagnosis of bacterial infections, unexpected but significant findings of other infectious etiologies may be detected and cannot be ignored. For example, fungal cells and elements generally stain gram-positive, but they may take up the crystal violet poorly and appear gram-variable (e.g., both pink and purple) or gram-negative. Because infectious agents besides bacteria may be detected by Gram stain, any unusual cells or structures observed on the smear should be evaluated further before being dismissed as unimportant (Fig. 6.7).

Gram Stain of Bacteria Grown in Culture (Indirect Smear)

The Gram stain also plays a key role in the identification of bacteria grown in culture. Similar to direct smears, indirect smears prepared from bacterial growth are evaluated for the bacterial cells' Gram reactions, morphologies, and arrangements (see Fig. 6.4). If growth from more than one specimen is to be stained on the same slide, a wax pencil may be used to create divisions. The smear results will be used to determine subsequent testing for identifying and characterizing the organisms isolated from the patient specimen.

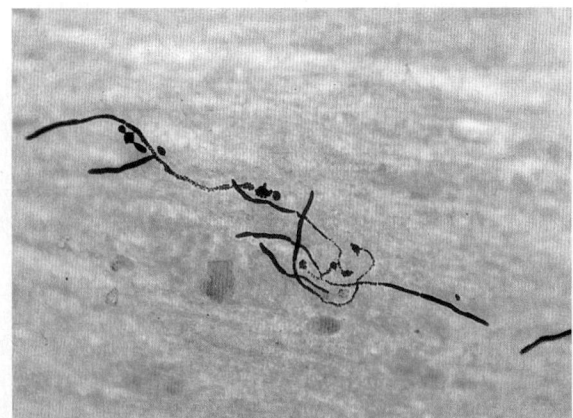

• **Fig. 6.7** Gram stains of direct smears can reveal infectious etiologies other than bacteria, such as the yeast *Candida tropicalis*.

Acid-Fast Stains

The acid-fast stain is the other commonly used stain for light-microscopic examination of bacteria.

Principle

Similar to the Gram stain, the **acid-fast stain** is specifically designed for a subset of bacteria whose cell walls contain long-chain fatty (**mycolic**) acids and is considered a differential stain. Mycolic acids render the cells resistant to decolorization with acid alcohol decolorizers. These bacteria are referred to as acid-fast. Although these organisms may stain slightly or poorly as gram-positive, the acid-fast stain takes full advantage of the waxy content of the cell walls to maximize detection. Mycobacteria are the most commonly encountered acid-fast bacteria, typified by *Mycobacterium tuberculosis,* the etiologic agent of tuberculosis. Bacteria lacking cell walls fortified with mycolic acids cannot resist decolorization with acid alcohol and are categorized as being non–acid-fast, a trait typical of most other clinically relevant bacteria. However, some degree of acid-fastness is a characteristic of a few non-mycobacterial bacteria, such as *Nocardia* spp., and coccidian parasites, such as *Cryptosporidium* spp.

Procedure Overview

The classic acid-fast staining method, Ziehl-Neelsen, is depicted in Fig. 6.8 and outlined in Evolve Procedure 6.3. The procedure requires heat to allow the primary stain (carbolfuchsin) to enter the waxy, mycolic acid-containing cell wall. A modification of this procedure, the Kinyoun acid-fast method (Evolve Procedure 6.4), does not require the use of heat or boiling water, minimizing safety concerns during the procedure. Because of a higher concentration of phenol in the primary stain solution, heat is not required for the intracellular penetration of carbolfuchsin. This modification is referred to as the "cold" method. When the acid-fast–stained smear is read with 1000× magnification, acid-fast–positive organisms stain red. Depending on the type of counterstain used (e.g., methylene blue or malachite green),

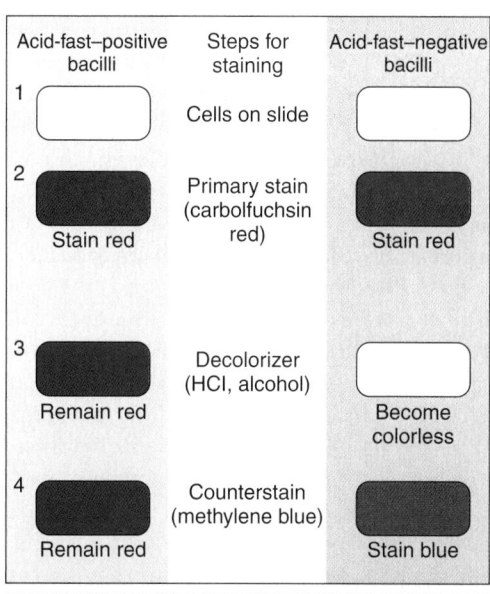

Acid-fast–positive bacilli	Steps for staining	Acid-fast–negative bacilli
1	Cells on slide	
2 Stain red	Primary stain (carbolfuchsin red)	Stain red
3 Remain red	Decolorizer (HCl, alcohol)	Become colorless
4 Remain red	Counterstain (methylene blue)	Stain blue

1 Fix smears on heated surface (60°C for at least 10 minutes).

2 Flood smears with carbolfuchsin (primary stain) and heat to almost boiling by performing the procedure on an electrically heated platform or by passing the flame of a Bunsen burner underneath the slides on a metal rack. The stain on the slides should steam. Allow slides to sit for 5 minutes after heating; do not allow them to dry out. Wash the slides in distilled water (note: tap water may contain acid-fast bacilli). Drain off excess liquid.

3 Flood slides with 3% HCl in 95% ethanol (decolorizer) for approximately 1 minute. Check to see that no more red color runs off the surface when the slide is tipped. Add a bit more decolorizer for very thick slides or those that continue to "bleed" red dye. Wash thoroughly with water and remove the excess.

4 Flood slides with methylene blue (counterstain) and allow to remain on surface of slides for 1 minute. Wash with distilled water and stand slides upright on paper towels to air dry. Do not blot dry.

5 Examine microscopically (see **A** and **B** below), screening at 400× magnification and confirm all suspicious (i.e., red) organisms at 1000× magnification using an oil-immersion lens.

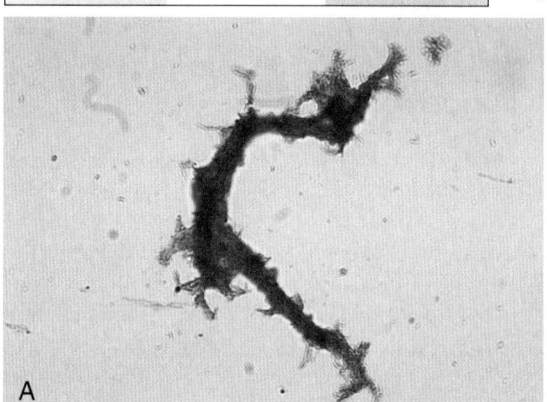
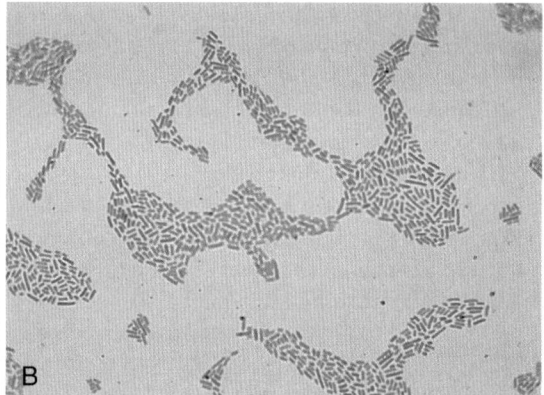

• **Fig. 6.8** The Ziehl-Neelsen acid-fast stain procedures and principles. (A) Acid-fast positive bacilli. (B) Acid-fast negative bacilli. (Modified from Atlas RM. *Principles of Microbiology.* St. Louis: Mosby; 2006.)

other microorganisms, host cells, and debris stain a blue to blue-green color (Figs. 6.8 and 6.9).

As with the Gram stain, the acid-fast stain is used to detect acid-fast bacteria (e.g., mycobacteria) directly in clinical specimens and provide preliminary identification information for suspicious bacteria grown in culture. Because mycobacterial infections are much less common than infections caused by other non–acid-fast bacteria, the acid-fast stain is only performed on specimens from patients highly suspected of having a mycobacterial infection. That is, Gram staining is a routine part of most bacteriology procedures, whereas acid-fast staining is reserved for specific situations. Similarly, the acid-fast stain is applied to bacteria grown in culture when mycobacteria are suspected based on other growth characteristics (for more information regarding the identification of mycobacteria, see Chapter 42). Because of the development of nucleic acid–based testing for the identification of organisms that are difficult to cultivate in the laboratory, such as acid-fast microorganisms, this technique is no longer widely available in many clinical laboratories.

Phase-Contrast Microscopy

Instead of using a stain to achieve the contrast necessary for observing microorganisms, altering microscopic techniques to enhance contrast offers another approach. **Phase-contrast microscopy** does not use a fixed smear preparation, but instead is used to view organisms and other cells in a wet preparation or **wet mount.** A wet mount preparation may consist of a nonviscous liquid such as urine or a sample suspended in sterile saline, such as a vaginal sample. Phase-contrast microscopy uses beams of light passing through the specimen that are partially deflected by the different densities or thicknesses (i.e., refractive indices) of the microbial cells or cell structures in the specimen. The greater the refractive index of an object, the more the beam of light is slowed, which results in decreased light intensity. These differences in light intensity translate into differences that provide contrast. Phase microscopy translates differences in phases within the specimen into differences in light intensities that result in contrast among objects within the specimen being observed.

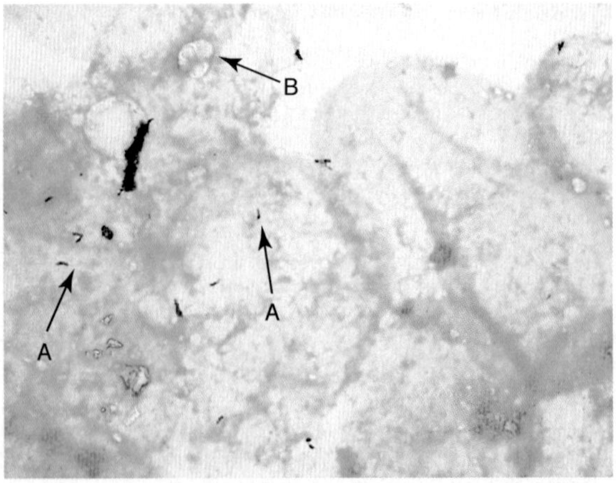

• **Fig. 6.9** Acid-fast stain of direct smear to show acid-fast bacilli staining deep red *(arrow A)* and non–acid-fast bacilli and host cells staining blue with the counterstain methylene blue *(arrow B).*

Smear preparations and permanent staining are used to visualize cellular structures from nonliving or dead microorganisms. Because staining is not part of phase contrast microscopy, this method offers the advantage of allowing observation of viable microorganisms. The method is not commonly used in diagnostic microbiology, but it is used to identify medically important fungi grown in culture (for more information regarding the use of phase-contrast microscopy for fungal identification, see Chapter 58, and for parasitic identification, see Chapter 46).

Fluorescent Microscopy

Principle of Fluorescent Microscopy

Certain dyes, called **fluorophores** or **fluorochromes,** can be raised to a higher energy level after absorbing ultraviolet (excitation) light. When the dye molecules return to their normal, lower energy state, they release excess energy in the form of visible (fluorescent) light. This process is called **fluorescence,** and microscopic methods have been developed to exploit the enhanced contrast and detection that this phenomenon provides.

Fig. 6.10 diagrams the principle of fluorescent microscopy in which the excitation light is emitted from above (**epifluorescence**). An excitation filter passes light of the desired wavelength to excite the fluorochrome that has been used to stain the specimen. A barrier filter in the objective lens prevents the excitation wavelengths from damaging the eyes of the observer. When observed through the ocular lens, fluorescing objects appear brightly lit against a dark background.

The color of the fluorescent light depends on the dye and light filters used. For example, use of the fluorescent dyes acridine orange, auramine, and fluorescein isothiocyanate (FITC) require blue excitation light, exciter filters that select for light in the 450- to 490-λ wavelength range, and a barrier filter for 515-λ. Calcofluor white, on the other hand, requires violet excitation light, an exciter filter that selects for

light in the 355- to 425-λ wavelength range, and a barrier filter for 460-λ. Which dye is used often depends on which organism is suspected and the fluorescent method used. The intensity of the contrast obtained with fluorescent microscopy is an advantage it has over the use of chromogenic dyes (e.g., the crystal violet and safranin of the Gram stain) and light microscopy. The disadvantage of fluorescent microscopy results from photobleaching or quenching of the fluorophore over time. **Photobleaching,** or fading, is the permanent loss of fluorescence because of chemical damage to the fluorochrome. **Quenching** is a result of the transfer of the light energy to nearby molecules in the sample such as free radicals, salts of heavy metals, or halogens. Quenching may be alleviated by adding chemical scavengers to the mounting fluid. Storing fluorescent slides in a dark container and refrigerated at 2°C to 8°C will decrease the loss of fluorescence over time. Digital photography is frequently used to maintain permanent records for fluorescent microscopy.

Staining Techniques for Fluorescent Microscopy

Based on the composition of the fluorescent stain reagents, fluorescent staining techniques may be divided into two general categories: fluorochroming, in which a fluorescent dye or fluorophore is used alone, and **immunofluorescence,** in which fluorescent dyes have been linked (conjugated) to specific antibodies. The principal differences between these two methods are outlined in Fig. 6.11.

Fluorochroming

In fluorochroming, a direct chemical interaction occurs between the fluorescent dye or fluorophore and a component of the bacterial cell; this interaction is the same as occurs with the stains used in light microscopy. The difference is that the use of a fluorescent dye enhances contrast and amplifies the observer's ability to detect stained cells tenfold greater than would be observed by light microscopy. For example, a minimum concentration of at least 105 organisms per milliliter of specimen is required for visualization by light microscopy, whereas by fluorescent microscopy, that number decreases to 104 per milliliter. The most common fluorochroming methods used in diagnostic microbiology include acridine orange, auramine-rhodamine, and calcofluor white.

Acridine Orange

The fluorochrome acridine orange binds to nucleic acid. This staining method (Evolve Procedure 6.5) can be used to confirm the presence of bacteria in blood cultures when Gram stain results are difficult to interpret or when the presence of bacteria is highly suspected but none are detected using light microscopy. Because acridine orange stains all nucleic acids, it is nonspecific. All microorganisms and nucleic acid–containing host cells will stain and give a bright orange fluorescence. Although this stain can be used to enhance detection, it does

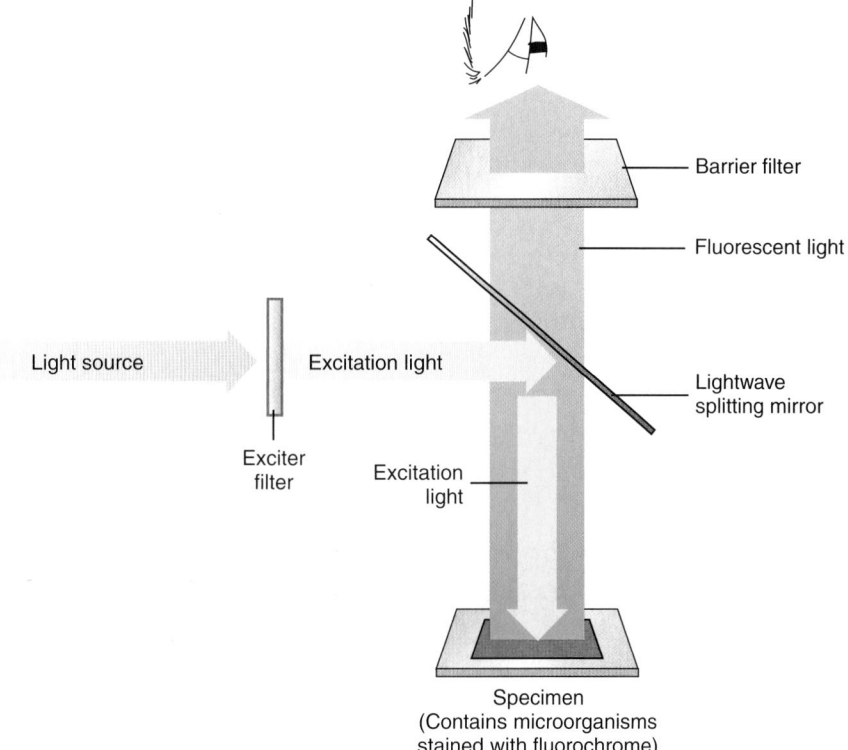

• **Fig. 6.10** Principle of fluorescent microscopy. Microorganisms in a specimen are stained with a fluorescent dye. On exposure to excitation light, organisms are visually detected by the emission of fluorescent light by the dye with which they have been stained (i.e., fluorochroming) or "tagged" (i.e., immunofluorescence).

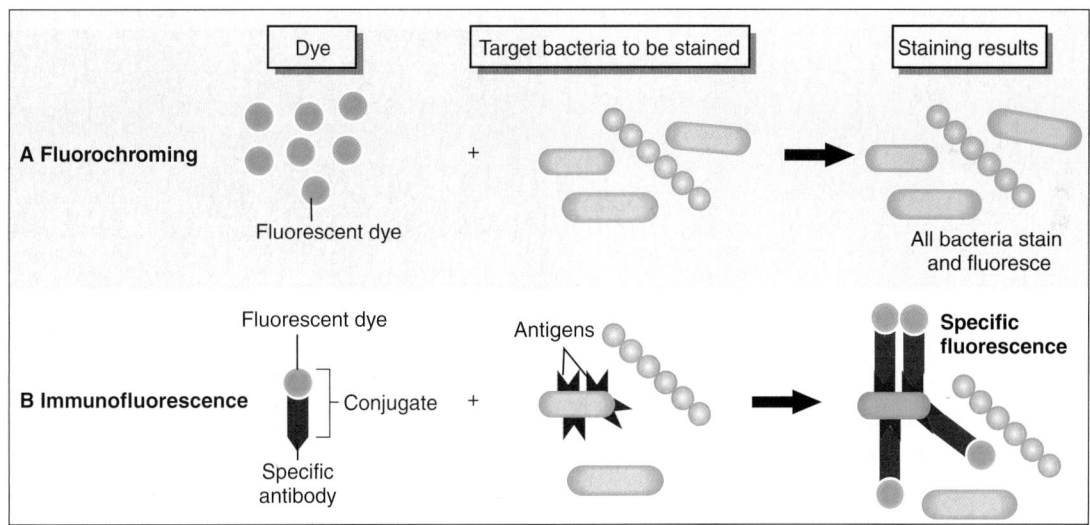

• **Fig. 6.11** Principles of fluorochroming and immunofluorescence. Fluorochroming (A) involves nonspecific staining of any bacterial cell with a fluorescent dye. Immunofluorescence (B) uses antibodies labeled with fluorescent dye (i.e., a conjugate) to specifically stain a particular bacterial species.

not discriminate between gram-negative and gram-positive bacteria. The stain is also used for the detection of cell wall–deficient bacteria (e.g., mycoplasmas) grown in cultures that are incapable of retaining the dyes used in the Gram stain (Fig. 6.12; Evolve Procedure 6.5).

Auramine-Rhodamine

The waxy mycolic acids in the cell walls of mycobacteria have an affinity for the fluorochromes auramine and rhodamine. As shown in Fig. 6.13, these dyes will nonspecifically bind to nearly all mycobacteria. The mycobacterial cells appear

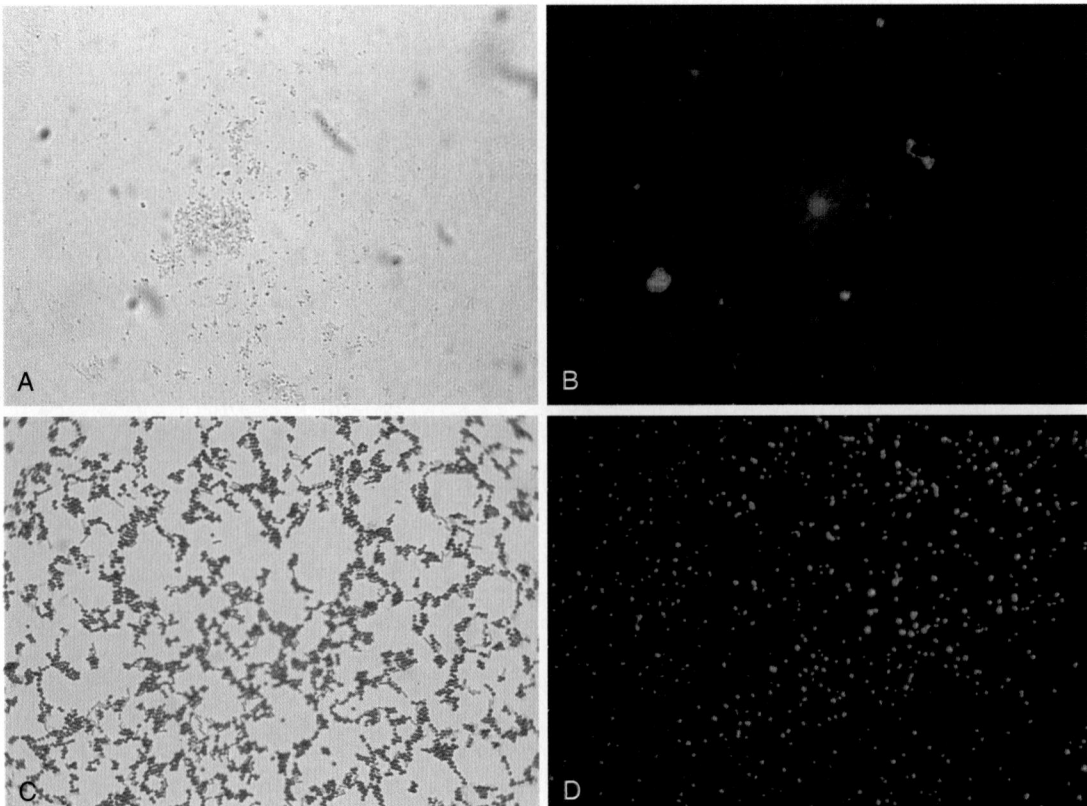

Fig. 6.12 Comparison of acridine orange fluorochroming and Gram stain. Gram stain of mycoplasma demonstrates the inability to distinguish cell wall–deficient organisms from amorphous gram-negative debris (A). Staining the same specimen with acridine orange confirms the presence of nucleic acid–containing organisms (B). Gram stain distinguishes between gram-positive and gram-negative bacteria (C), but all bacteria stain the same with the nonspecific acridine orange dye (D).

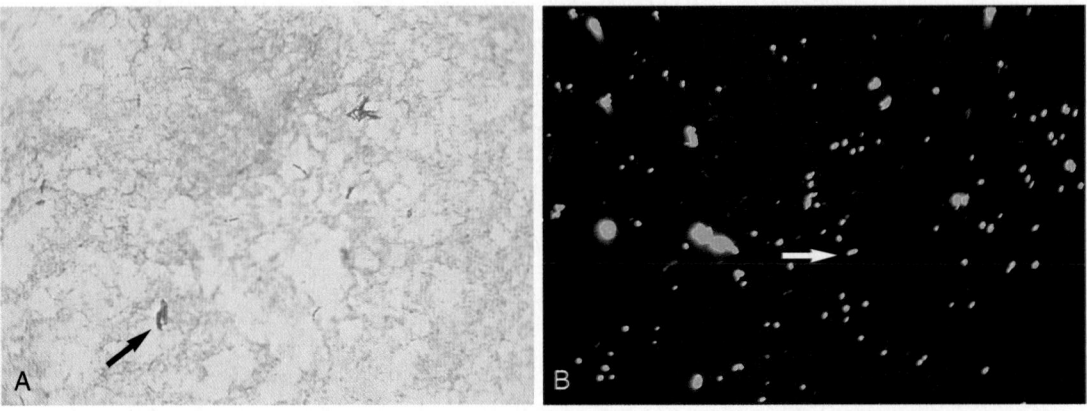

• **Fig. 6.13** Comparison of the Ziehl-Neelsen–stained (A) and auramine-rhodamine–stained (B) *Mycobacterium* spp. *(arrows).*

bright yellow or orange against a greenish background. This fluorochroming method can be used to enhance the detection of mycobacteria directly in patient specimens and for the initial characterization of cells grown in culture.

Calcofluor White

The cell walls of fungi will bind the stain calcofluor white, which greatly enhances fungal visibility in tissue and other specimens. Calcofluor white binds to cells that are composed of chitin or cellulose. This fluorochrome is commonly used

to directly detect fungi in clinical material and to observe subtle characteristics of fungi grown in culture (for more information regarding the use of calcofluor white for the laboratory diagnosis of fungal infections, see Chapter 58). Calcofluor white may also be used to visualize some parasites such as microsporidia.

Immunofluorescence

As discussed in Chapter 3, antibodies are molecules that have high specificity for interacting with microbial antigens.

Antibodies specific for an antigen characteristic of a particular microbial species will only combine with that antigen. When antibodies are conjugated (chemically linked) to a fluorescent dye, the resulting dye-antibody conjugate can be used to detect, or "tag," specific microbial agents (Fig. 6.11). When "tagged," the microorganisms become readily detectable by fluorescent microscopy. Thus, immunofluorescence combines the amplified contrast provided by fluorescence with the specificity of antibody-antigen binding.

This method is used to directly examine patient specimens for bacteria that are difficult or slow to grow (e.g., *Legionella* spp. and *Chlamydia trachomatis*) or to identify organisms already grown in culture. FITC, which emits an intense, apple green fluorescence, is the fluorochrome commonly used for conjugation to antibodies (Fig. 6.14). Immunofluorescence can also be used in virology (Chapter 64) and to some extent in parasitology (Chapter 46).

Fluorescent in situ hybridization using peptide nucleic acid probes is a powerful technique used in the clinical laboratory and is discussed in further detail in Chapter 8.

Two additional types of microscopy, dark-field microscopy and electron microscopy, are not commonly used to diagnose infectious diseases. However, because of their importance in the detection and characterization of certain microorganisms, they are discussed here.

Dark-Field Microscopy

Dark-field microscopy is similar to phase-contrast microscopy in that it involves the alteration of microscopic technique rather than the use of dyes or stains to achieve contrast. By the dark-field method, the condenser does not allow light to pass directly through the specimen but directs the light to hit the specimen at an oblique angle (Fig. 6.15A). Only light that hits objects, such as microorganisms in the specimen, will be deflected upward into the objective lens for visualization. All other light that passes through the specimen will miss the objective, thus making the background a dark field.

This method has the greatest utility for detecting certain bacteria directly in patient specimens that, because of their thin dimensions, cannot be seen by light microscopy and, because of their physiology, are difficult to grow in culture. Dark-field microscopy is used to detect spirochetes, the most notorious of which is the bacterium *Treponema pallidum*, the causative agent of syphilis (for more information regarding spirochetes, see Chapter 45). As shown in Fig. 6.15B, spirochetes viewed using dark-field microscopy will appear extremely bright against a black field. The use of dark-field microscopy is confined to specialized research laboratories. Dark-field microscopy in diagnostic clinical microbiology has been replaced with serologic techniques for the diagnosis of syphilis.

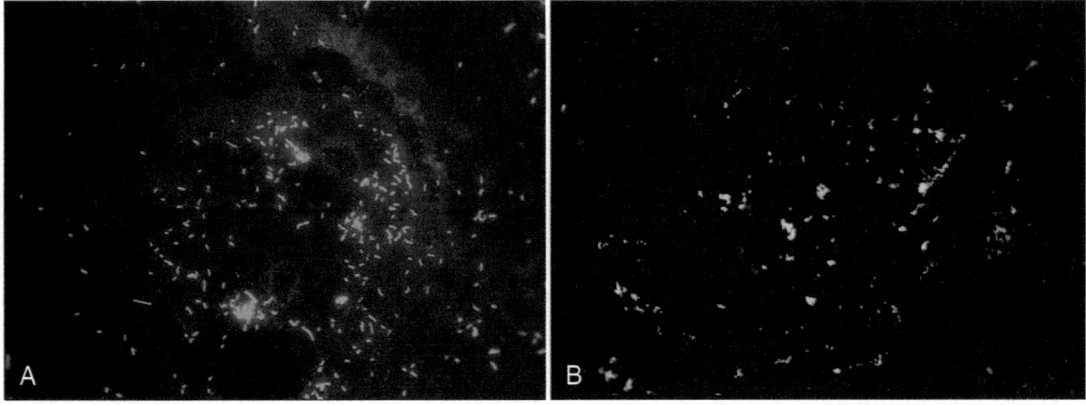

• **Fig. 6.14** Immunofluorescence stains of *Legionella* spp. (A) and *Bordetella pertussis* (B) used for identification.

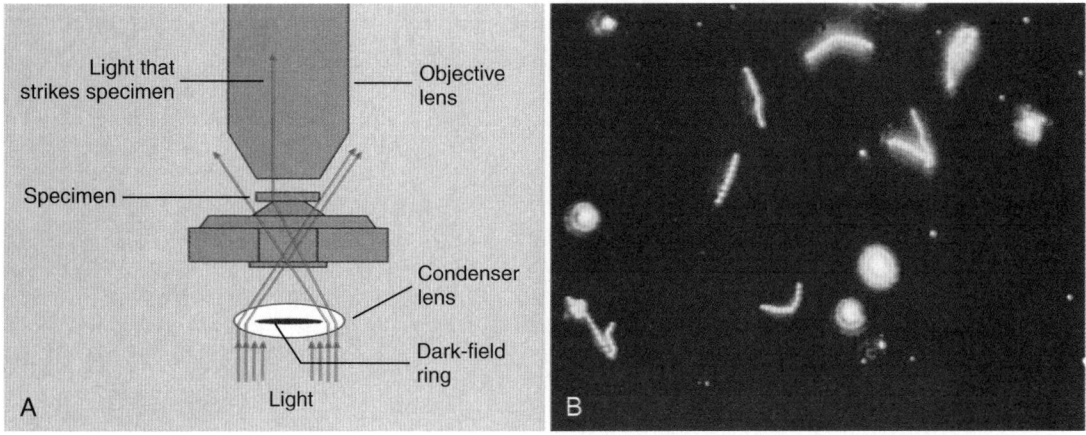

• **Fig. 6.15** Dark-field microscopy. Principal (A) and dark-field photomicrograph showing the tightly coiled characteristics of the spirochete *Treponema pallidum* (B). (From Atlas RM. *Principles of Microbiology*. St. Louis: Mosby; 2006.)

Digital Automated Microscopy

Automation in **digital microscopy** using sophisticated software and unique technology now permits laboratories to acquire microscopic digital images of Gram stains using a web-based interface. This interface allows images using a fully automated microscope to be viewed on a single screen (COPAN, Murieta, CA, and MetaSystems GmbH, Boston, MA). Digital imaging, including scanning entire slides, provides an opportunity for standardization, cost reductions, quality improvement, and increased efficiency.

Digital or virtual microscopy can greatly aid departments, college programs, and professional organizations in the delivery of quality cost-effective microscopy training. An additional tool that now allows whole slide imaging is available, enabling the viewer to track the slide on x- and y-axes, very much like using a standard microscope. Several technologies provide mobile device viewers for virtual microscopy.

Digital Holographic Microscopy

Digital holographic microscopy (DHM) has been used to visualize bacteria in aqueous environments without the loss of resolution in samples one millimeter thick. This is approximately 100-fold greater resolution than most bright-field microscopes. Although currently under development, this technique has the potential to improve the identification of low concentrations of organisms in clinical samples.

ⓔ Visit the Evolve site for a complete list of procedures, review questions, and case studies.

Bibliography

Atlas RM: *Principles of microbiology*, St Louis, 2006, Mosby.

Bedrossian M, Barr C, Lindensmith CA, Nealson K, Nadeau JL: Quantifying microorganisms at low concentrations using digital holographic microscopy, *J Vis Exp* (129), 2017.

Carroll KC, Pfaller MA, Landry ML, et al.: *Manual of clinical microbiology*, ed 12, Washington, DC, 2019, ASM.

Hamilton PW, Wang Y, McCullough SJ: Virtual microscopy and digital pathology in training and education, *APMIS* 120:305–315, 2012.

Hanna MG, Reuter VE, Hameed MR, et al.: Whole slide image equivalency and efficiency study: experience at a large academic center, *Mod Pathol* 32:916–928, 2019, https://doi.org/10.1038/s41379-019-0205-0.

Lenhoff A: Digital imaging: transformative new technology, *MLO Med Lab Obs* 47:32, 2015.

Stokes BO: Principles of cytocentrifugation, *Lab Med* 7:434–437, 2004.

7

Overview of Conventional Cultivation and Systems for Identification

OBJECTIVES

1. Define bacterial cultivation and list the three most important purposes for bacterial cultivation.
2. Define bacterial media; list the four general types of media and explain the general biochemical principle for each type.
3. List the environmental conditions that are crucial in supporting bacterial *in vitro* growth and explain how each factor is controlled and monitored.
4. Explain the most common bacterial streaking technique, the principle associated with the technique, and how colonies are enumerated using this technique.
5. Identify the key criteria used in characterizing and reporting bacterial culture growth pertaining to the phenotypic results; differentiate genotypic and phenotypic characteristics.
6. Describe the importance of using colony morphology, Gram staining, and site of infection to identify a potential pathogenic microorganism.
7. Explain the use and chemical principle of the following enzymatic tests used in preliminary bacterial identification: catalase test, oxidase test, urease test, indole test, PYR test, and hippurate hydrolysis.
8. Define and differentiate bacterial susceptibility and resistance; give an example of how these are used to assist in the identification of bacteria.
9. Describe the steps required to develop "rapid" identification schemes and explain how these differ from conventional schemes.
10. List the four basic identification components common to all commercially available biochemical multitest systems.
11. Explain the basic principle of matrix-assisted laser desorption ionization time-of-flight mass spectrometry (MALDI-TOF MS) for the identification of microorganisms.
12. List the limitations associated with organism identification using MALDI-TOF MS.
13. Explain the use and limitations of genotypic systems for the identification of infectious agents.

for definitive confirmation, identification, and characterization, including sensitivity testing. This chapter presents the various principles and methods required for microorganism identification and cultivation.

Organism Identification

As previously described in Chapter 6, a direct Gram stain (DGS) provides the clinician with preliminary information regarding the likely presence or absence of a pathogen based on the cellular morphology, quantitation, cellular arrangement, and microscopic structure of the organisms observed. In addition, information regarding the presence, type, and quantity of inflammatory cells or other cellular material may alert the clinician to the source or etiologic agent of the infection if the organism cannot be visualized. After the laboratorian reviews, the preliminary information provided by a DGS, the specimen or patient sample is then processed for identification by either a **phenotypic method** as described in this chapter, **genotypic method** (nucleic acid–based) (Chapter 8), **immunologic method** (Chapter 9), or a combination of methods.

Principles of Bacterial Cultivation

This section focuses on the principles and practices of bacterial cultivation, which has three main purposes:
- To grow and isolate bacteria present in a clinical specimen
- To determine which of the bacteria that grow are most likely causing infection and which are likely contaminants or colonizers (normal microbiota)
- To obtain sufficient growth of clinically relevant bacteria for confirmation, identification, characterization, and susceptibility testing

Cultivation is the process of growing microorganisms in culture by taking bacteria from the infection site (i.e., the *in vivo* environment) by specimen collection and growing the organisms in the artificial environment of the laboratory (i.e., the *in vitro* environment). Once grown in culture, most bacterial populations are observed without microscopy and are present in sufficient quantities

D irect laboratory methods such as microscopy and nucleic acid detection provide preliminary information about the bacteria and fungi involved in an infection, but microorganism growth is usually required for laboratory identification or confirmation procedures to be performed.

The successful transition from the *in vivo* to the *in vitro* environment requires that the nutritional and environmental growth requirements of bacterial pathogens be met. The environmental transition is not necessarily easy for bacteria. *In vivo* they are utilizing various complex metabolic and physiologic pathways developed for survival on or within the human host. Then, relatively suddenly, they are exposed to the artificial *in vitro* environment of the laboratory. The bacteria must adjust to survive and multiply. The survival of the organism depends on the availability of essential nutrients and appropriate environmental conditions.

Although growth conditions can be met for most known bacterial pathogens, the needs of certain clinically relevant bacteria are not sufficiently understood to allow for development of *in vitro* laboratory growth conditions. Examples include *Treponema pallidum* (the causative agent of syphilis) and *Mycobacterium leprae* (the causative agent of leprosy). Additional identification systems such as immunologic or genotypic methods must be used to identify these organisms in a clinical specimen. If an organism is not identifiable through alternate methods, the clinician must rely on the patient signs and symptoms to determine the likely cause of the patient's illness and an appropriate treatment option.

Nutritional Requirements

As discussed in Chapter 2, bacteria have numerous nutritional needs that include different gases, water, various ions, vitamins, minerals, nitrogen (peptones or casein), nutrients (meat and plant infusions), sources for carbon, and energy. The source for carbon and energy is commonly supplied in carbohydrates (e.g., sugars and their derivatives) and proteins.

General Concepts of Culture Media

In the laboratory, nutrients are incorporated into culture media on or in which bacteria are grown. If a culture medium meets a bacterial cell's growth requirements, then that cell will multiply to sufficient numbers to allow visualization by the unaided eye. Of course, bacterial growth

after inoculation also requires that the medium be placed in optimal environmental conditions.

Because different pathogenic bacteria have different nutritional needs, various types of culture media have been developed for use in diagnostic microbiology. For certain bacteria, the needs are relatively complex, and exceptional media components must be used for growth. Bacteria with special nutritional or environmental requirements are said to be **fastidious.** Alternatively, the nutritional needs of most clinically important bacteria are relatively basic and straightforward. These bacteria are considered **nonfastidious.**

Phases of Growth Media

Growth media are primarily used in two phases: either **broth** (liquid) or **agar** (solid). In some instances (e.g., certain blood culture methods), a **biphasic medium** that contains both a liquid and a solid phase, or a **semi-solid media** (e.g., thioglycollate broth) that contains a small percentage of agar may be used.

In **broth media,** nutrients are dissolved in water, and bacterial growth is indicated by a change in the broth's appearance from clear to turbid (cloudy). The **turbidity,** or cloudiness, of the broth results from light deflected by bacteria present in the culture (Fig. 7.1). More growth indicates a higher cell density and greater turbidity. At least 106 bacteria per milliliter of broth are needed for turbidity to be detected with the unaided eye. Some broths may also contain a pH indicator, such as phenol red, that may change color in the presence of bacterial metabolites rather than relying solely on the growth of the organism.

In addition to amount of growth present, the location of growth within the broth, such as the thioglycollate broth, provides an indication of the type of organism present based on oxygen requirements. Strict anaerobes will grow at the bottom of the broth tube, whereas aerobes will grow near the surface. Microaerophilic organisms require oxygen and will grow slightly below the surface where oxygen concentrations are lower than atmospheric concentrations. In addition, microaerobic organisms do not utilize the oxygen and include facultative anaerobes and aerotolerant organisms that grow throughout the medium, because they are unaffected by the variation in oxygen content.

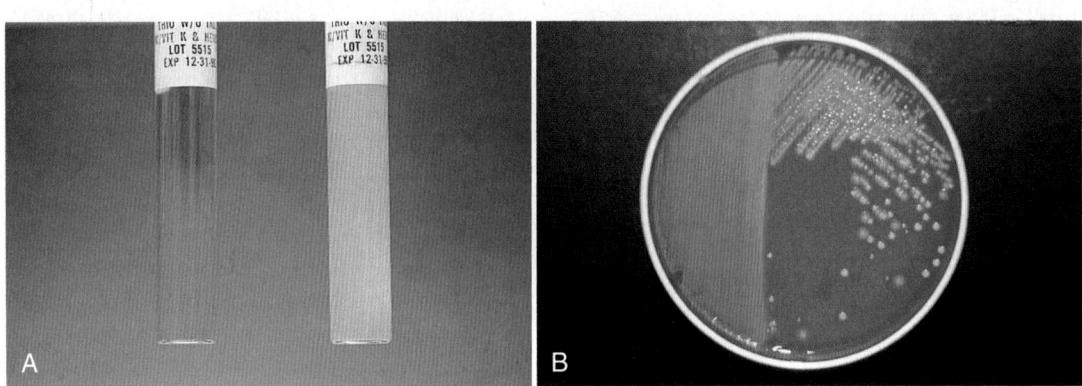

• **Fig. 7.1** (A) Clear broth indicating no bacterial growth *(left)*, and turbid broth indicating bacterial growth *(right)*. (B) Individual bacterial colonies growing on the agar surface after incubation.

A solid medium is a combination of a solidifying agent and the nutrients and water. **Agar,** the most common solidifying agent, has the unique property of melting at high temperatures (≥95°C) and solidifying after the temperature falls below 50°C. The addition of agar allows a solid medium to be prepared by heating to an extremely high temperature, which is required for sterilization. The media is then cooled to 55°C to 60°C for distribution into petri dishes. On further cooling, the agar-containing medium forms a stable solid gel. The petri dish containing the agar is an agar plate. Solid media may also be placed in tubes; a tube with a flat surface is an **agar deep** and a tube with a slanted surface is an **agar slant.** Different agar media usually are identified according to the major nutritive components of the medium (e.g., sheep blood agar [BA], bile esculin agar, xylose-lysine-deoxycholate [XLD] agar).

With appropriate incubation conditions, each bacterial cell inoculated onto the agar medium surface will proliferate to sufficiently large numbers to be observable with the unaided eye (Fig. 7.1). Theoretically, the resulting bacterial population is considered to be derived from a single bacterial cell and is known as a **pure colony.** In other words, all bacterial cells within a single colony are the same genus and species, having identical genetic and phenotypic characteristics (are derived from a single clone). Pure cultures are required for subsequent procedures used to identify and characterize bacteria. The ability to select pure (individual) colonies is one of the first and most important steps required for bacterial identification and characterization.

Media Classifications and Functions

Media are categorized according to their function and use. In diagnostic bacteriology, there are four general categories of media: enrichment, nutritive, selective, and differential.

Enrichment media contain specific nutrients required for the growth of particular bacterial pathogens that may be present alone or with other bacterial species in a patient specimen. This media type is used to enhance the growth of a particular bacterial pathogen from a mixture of organisms by providing specific nutrients for the organism's growth. One example of such a medium is buffered charcoal–yeast extract agar (BCYE), which provides L-cysteine and other nutrients required for the growth of *Legionella pneumophila,* the causative agent of Legionnaire disease (Fig. 7.2).

Enrichment media also includes specialized enrichment broths used to enhance the growth of organisms present in low numbers. Broths may be used to ensure growth of an organism when no organisms grow on solid media after initial specimen inoculation. Broths used to ensure growth of organisms that do not grow on solid media, and that do not contain specific nutrients to enhance the growth of microorganisms, are referred to as **back-up broths.** Back-up broths, or **enrichment broths,** that contain specific nutrients and may include selective properties to prevent the growth of contaminating organisms often include thioglycollate for the isolation of anaerobes, LIM (Todd Hewitt broth containing colistin and nalidixic acid [NA]) broth for selective enrichment of group B streptococci, and gram-negative (GN) broth for the selective enrichment of enteric GN organisms.

Nutritive media contain nutrients that support growth of most nonfastidious organisms without giving any particular organism a growth advantage. Nutrient media include tryptic soy agar and nutrient agar plates for bacteria, or Sabouraud's dextrose agar for fungi. **Selective media** contain one or more agents that are inhibitory to all organisms except those "selected" by the specific growth condition or chemical. In other words, these media select for the growth of certain bacteria to the disadvantage of others. Inhibitory agents used for this purpose include dyes, bile salts, alcohols, acids, and antibiotics. An example of a selective medium is phenylethyl alcohol (PEA) agar with 5% sheep blood, which inhibits the growth of aerobic and facultatively anaerobic GN rods and allows gram-positive cocci to grow (Fig. 7.3). Selective and inhibitory chemicals included within nutritive media prevent the overgrowth of normal microbiota or contaminating organisms that would prevent the identification of pathogenic organisms. However, the use of selective media does not ensure that the inhibited organisms are not present in small quantity and may simply be too small to see. In addition, prolonged incubation of selective media may result in dehydration or evaporation of the selective agent, permitting contaminating organisms to grow.

Differential media employ some factor (or factors) that allows colonies of one bacterial species or type to exhibit certain metabolic or culture characteristics that can be used to distinguish them from other bacteria growing on the same agar plate. One commonly used differential medium is MacConkey agar (MAC), which differentiates between GN bacteria that can and cannot ferment the sugar lactose (Fig. 7.4).

Of importance, many media used in diagnostic bacteriology provide more than one function. For example, MAC is both differential and selective, or a **combination media,** because the media will not allow most gram-positive

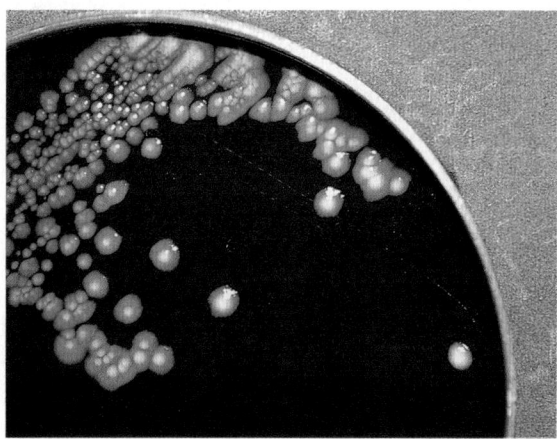

• **Fig. 7.2** Growth of *Legionella pneumophila* on the enrichment medium buffered charcoal–yeast extract agar, used specifically to grow this bacterial genus.

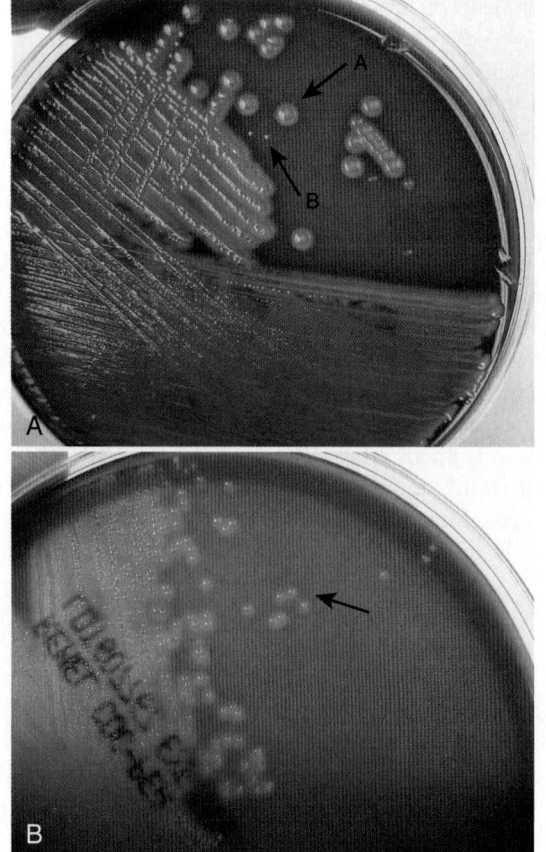

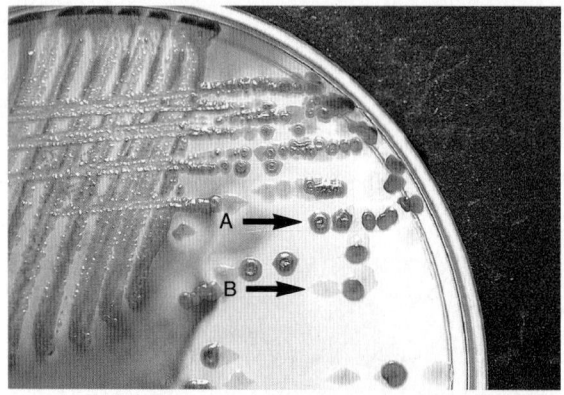

• **Fig. 7.3** (A) Heavy mixed growth of the gram-negative bacillus *Escherichia coli (arrow A)* and the gram-positive coccus *Enterococcus* spp. *(arrow B)* on the nonselective medium sheep blood agar (SBA). (B) The selective medium SBA containing phenylethyl-alcohol with 5% sheep blood only allows the enterococci to grow *(arrow)*.

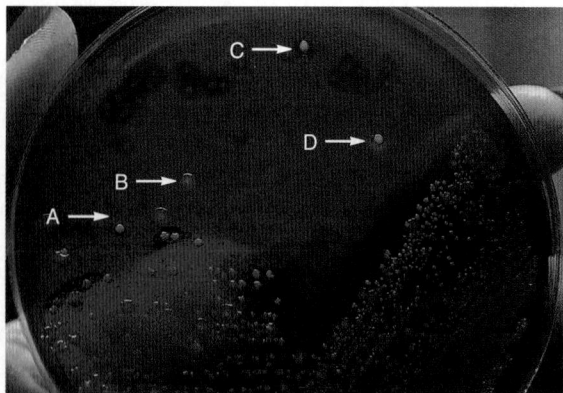

• **Fig. 7.5** Different colony morphologies exhibited on sheep blood agar by various bacteria, including alpha-hemolytic streptococci *(arrow A)*, gram-negative bacilli *(arrow B)*, beta-hemolytic streptococci *(arrow C)*, and *Staphylococcus aureus (arrow D)*.

patterns of the organisms, as indicated in Fig. 5.2. Fig. 7.5 shows differential hemolytic patterns of various organisms.

Summary of Artificial Media for Routine Bacteriology

Various broth and agar media that have enrichment, selective, or differential capabilities and are used frequently for routine bacteriology are listed alphabetically in Table 7.1. Anaerobic bacteriology (Part III, Section 13), mycobacteriology (Part III, Section 14), and mycology (Chapter 58) use similar media strategies; details regarding these media are provided in the appropriate chapters.

Of the dozens of available media, those commonly used for routine diagnostic bacteriology are summarized in this discussion. It is important to note that different diagnostic microbiology laboratories use different algorithms and combinations of media for the primary isolation and characterization of microorganisms. Part VII discusses representative media used to culture bacteria from various clinical specimens. Similarly, other chapters throughout Part III discuss representative media used to identify and characterize specific organisms.

Blood Agar

Most bacteriology specimens are inoculated to BA plates, because this medium supports growth for all but the most fastidious clinically significant bacteria. In addition, the colony morphologies that commonly encounter bacteria exhibited on this medium are familiar to most clinical microbiologists. The medium consists of a base containing a protein source (e.g., tryptones), soybean protein digest (containing a slight amount of natural carbohydrate), sodium chloride, agar, and 5% sheep blood. Rabbit or horse blood may also be used for the characterization of organisms such as *Haemophilus* spp. that are incapable of growth on sheep BA.

Certain bacteria produce extracellular enzymes that lyse red blood cells in the agar (**hemolysis**). This activity can result in complete clearing of the red blood cells around the bacterial colony (**beta-hemolysis**) or in only partial lysis of the cells to produce a greenish discoloration around the colony

• **Fig. 7.4** Differential capabilities of MacConkey agar as gram-negative bacilli capable of fermenting lactose appear deep purple *(arrow A)*, whereas those not able to ferment lactose appear light pink or relatively colorless *(arrow B)*.

bacteria to grow; it is differential based on fermentation of lactose as previously described. Another example is sheep BA. This is the most commonly used nutritive medium for diagnostic bacteriology, because it allows most nonfastidious organisms to grow. However, this agar is also differential, because the appearance of colonies produced by certain bacterial species is distinguishable based on the hemolytic

TABLE 7.1   Plating Media for Routine Bacteriology

Medium	Components/Comments	Primary Purpose
Bile esculin agar (BEA)	Nutrient agar base with ferric citrate. Hydrolysis of esculin imparts a brown color to medium; sodium deoxycholate inhibits many bacteria.	Differential isolation and presumptive identification of group D streptococci and non-group D enterococci, and Enterobacterales, *Klebsiella, Enterobacter* and *Serratia,* from other enteric bacteria. Can also be used for differentiation of *Listeria monocytogenes.*
Bile esculin azide agar with vancomycin	Contains azide to inhibit gram-negative bacteria, vancomycin to select for resistant gram-positive bacteria, and bile esculin to differentiate enterococci from other vancomycin-resistant bacteria that may grow	Selective and differential for cultivation of vancomycin-resistant enterococci from clinical and surveillance specimens
Blood agar (BA)	Trypticase soy agar, *Brucella* agar, or beef heart infusion with 5% sheep blood. Rabbit blood or horse blood may be used for the characterization of hemolytic strains of *Haemophilus* spp.	Cultivation of nonfastidious microorganisms, determination of hemolytic reactions
Bordet-Gengou agar	Potato-glycerol–based medium enriched with 15%–20% defibrinated blood; contaminants inhibited by methicillin (final concentration of 2.5 μm/mL)	Isolation of *Bordetella pertussis* (small, smooth, pearl-like colonies with a narrow zone of hemolysis), *Bordetella parapertussis (*brown colonies with a green-black coloration on the reverse side), and *Bordetella bronchiseptica* (brown, medium sized colonies with a rough, pitted surface).
Brain-heart infusion agar or broth	Dextrose, pork brain, and heart dehydrated infusions	Cultivation of fastidious and nonfastidious organisms
Brilliance agar	Organism-specific nutrient base, selective supplements and chromogenic substrate. Brilliance CRE Brilliance ESBL Brilliance methicillin-resistant *Staphylococcus aureus* (MRSA) Brilliance Salmonella agar Brilliance UTI agar Brilliance UTI Clarity agar Brilliance VRE agar	This medium is specific for the organism that is intended for isolation. The formulas include media for the presumptive identification of carbapenem-resistant *E. coli, Klebsiella, Enterobacter, Serratia,* and *Citrobacter* (KESC); ESBL is used for the detection of extended-spectrum β-lactamase producing organisms; MRSA is used for screening for methicillin-resistant *Staphylococcus aureus;* Salmonella agar is used for the presumptive identification of *Salmonella* spp.; UTI/UTI Clarity are used for the presumptive identification and differentiation of *Enterococcus* spp., *E. coli, Proteus, Morganella,* and *Providencia* spp.; VRE is used for the identification of vancomycin-resistant *Enterococcus faecalis* and *Enterococcus faecalis.*
Buffered charcoal–yeast extract agar (BCYE)	Yeast extract, agar, charcoal, and salts supplemented with L-cysteine HCl, ferric pyrophosphate, ACES buffer, and alpha-ketoglutarate	Enrichment for *Legionella* spp. Supports the growth of *Francisella* and *Nocardia* spp.
Buffered charcoal–yeast extract (BCYE) agar with antibiotics	BCYE supplemented with polymyxin B, vancomycin, and ansamycin to inhibit gram-negative bacteria, gram-positive bacteria, and yeast, respectively	Enrichment and selection for *Legionella* spp.
Burkholderia cepacia selective agar	Bile salts, gentamicin, ticarcillin, polymyxin B, peptone, yeast extract	For recovery of *B. cepacia* from cystic fibrosis patients
Campy-blood agar	Contains vancomycin (10 mg/L), trimethoprim (5 mg/L), polymyxin B (2500 U/L), amphotericin B (2 mg/L), and cephalothin (15 mg/L) in a *Brucella* agar base with sheep blood	Selective for *Campylobacter* spp.

Continued

TABLE 7.1 **Plating Media for Routine Bacteriology—cont'd**

Medium	Components/Comments	Primary Purpose
Campylobacter thioglycollate broth	Thioglycollate broth supplemented with increased agar concentration and antibiotics cephalothin, vancomycin, trimethoprim, amphotericin B, and polymyxin B. Contains sodium sulfite and sodium thioglycolate to protect cells from damage.	Selective holding or transport medium for recovery of *Campylobacter* spp.
CDC[a] anaerobe 5% sheep blood agar	Tryptic soy broth with phenyl-ethyl alcohol, 5% sheep blood, and added nutrients yeast extract, vitamin K$_1$, hemin, and cystine.	Improved growth of fastidious, obligate, slow-growing anaerobes
Cefoperazone, vancomycin, amphotericin (CVA) medium	Blood-supplemented enrichment medium containing cefoperazone, vancomycin, and amphotericin to inhibit growth of most gram-negative bacteria, gram-positive bacteria, and yeast, respectively	Selective medium for isolation of *Campylobacter* spp.
Cefsulodin-irgasan-novobiocin (CIN) agar	Peptone base with yeast extract, mannitol, and bile salts; supplemented with cefsulodin, irgasan, and novobiocin; neutral red and crystal violet indicators	Selective for *Yersinia* spp.; may be useful for isolation of *Aeromonas* spp.
Chocolate agar	Peptone base, enriched with solution of 2% hemoglobin or IsoVitaleX (BD BBL™ Becton Dickenson, Sparks MD)	Cultivation of fastidious microorganisms such as *Haemophilus* spp., *Brucella* spp., and pathogenic *Neisseria* spp.
Chromogenic media	Organism-specific nutrient base, selective supplements, and chromogenic substrate	Designed to optimize growth and differentiate a specific type of organism; routinely used in the identification of *Acinetobacter,* extended-spectrum β-lactamase and carbapenemase producing organisms, *E. coli, Listeria monocytogenes, Enterococcus* spp., *Pseudomonas aeruginosa, Salmonella* spp., shiga toxin-producing *E. coli, E. coli* O157-H7, group B streptococcus, *Vibrio* spp., *Yersinia enterocolitica,* yeasts, MRSA, and a variety of other organisms
Columbia colistin-nalidixic acid (CNA) agar	Columbia agar base with 10 mg colistin per liter, 15 mg nalidixic acid per liter, and 5% sheep blood	Selective isolation of gram-positive cocci
Cystine-tellurite blood agar	Infusion agar base with 5% sheep blood; reduction of potassium tellurite by *Corynebacterium diphtheriae* produces dark grey to black colonies	Isolation of *Corynebacterium diphtheriae*
Eosin methylene blue (EMB) agar (Levine)	Peptone base containing lactose; eosin Y and methylene blue as indicators	Isolation and differentiation of lactose-fermenting and non–lactose-fermenting enteric bacilli
Gram-negative broth (GN)	Peptone-base broth with glucose and mannitol; sodium citrate and sodium deoxycholate act as inhibitory agents	Selective (enrichment) liquid medium for enteric pathogens *Salmonella* and *Shigella* spp.
Hektoen enteric (HE) agar	Peptone-base agar with bile salts, lactose, sucrose, salicin, and ferric ammonium citrate; indicators include bromothymol blue and acid fuchsin	Differential, selective medium for the isolation and differentiation of *Salmonella* and *Shigella* spp. from other GN enteric bacilli
LIM broth	Modification of Todd-Hewitt broth; peptones, slats and dextrose with yeast extract for additional enrichment. Contains colistin and nalidixic acid to inhibit GN bacteria	Enriched, selective media for the isolation of cultivation of *Streptococcus agalactiae.*
Loeffler medium	Dextrose, egg-and-beef serum, infusion from heart muscle and digest of animal tissue	Isolation and growth of *Corynebacterium* spp.
MacConkey agar	Peptone base with lactose; gram-positive organisms inhibited by crystal violet and bile salts; neutral red as indicator	Isolation and differentiation of lactose fermenting and non–lactose-fermenting enteric bacilli

TABLE 7.1   Plating Media for Routine Bacteriology—cont'd

Medium	Components/Comments	Primary Purpose
MacConkey sorbitol agar	A modification of MacConkey agar in which lactose has been replaced with D-sorbitol as the primary carbohydrate	For the selection and differentiation of *E. coli* O157:H7 in stool specimens
Mannitol salt agar	Peptone base, mannitol, and phenol red indicator; salt concentration of 7.5% inhibits most bacteria	Selective differentiation of staphylococci
New York City (NYC) agar	Peptone agar base with cornstarch, supplemented with yeast dialysate, 3% hemoglobin, and horse plasma; antibiotic supplement includes vancomycin (2 μg/mL), colistin (5.5 μg/mL), amphotericin B (1.2 μg/mL), and trimethoprim (3 μg/mL)	Isolation and cultivation of pathogenic *Neisseria* spp. also supports the growth of *Ureaplasma urealyticum* and some *Mycoplasma* spp.
Phenylethyl alcohol (PEA) agar with or without blood	Nutrient agar base; PEA inhibits growth of GN organisms. May add moxalactam and lithium chloride for additional selection	Selective isolation of aerobic gram-positive cocci and bacilli and anaerobic gram-positive cocci. This agar should not be used for observation of hemolytic reactions.
Regan Lowe	Charcoal agar supplemented with horse blood, cephalexin, and amphotericin B	Enrichment and selective medium for isolation of *Bordetella pertussis* and *Bordetella parapertussis.*
Selenite broth	Peptone-base broth; sodium selenite toxic for most Enterobacterales	Enrichment and isolation of *Salmonella* spp.
Skirrow agar	Peptone and soy protein–base agar with lysed horse blood; vancomycin inhibits gram-positive organisms; polymyxin B and trimethoprim inhibit most GN organisms	Selective for *Campylobacter* spp.
Streptococcal selective agar (SSA)	Contains crystal violet, colistin, and trimethoprim-sulfamethoxazole in 5% sheep blood agar base	Selective for *Streptococcus pyogenes* and *Streptococcus agalactiae*
Tetrathionate broth	Peptone-base broth; iodine and potassium iodide, bile salts, and sodium thiosulfate inhibit gram-positive organisms and Enterobacterales	Selective for *Salmonella* and *Shigella* spp., except *Salmonella enterica* Typhi and *Arizona* spp. from fecal and urine specimens.
Thayer-Martin agar (TM) (modified Thayer Martin [MTM])	Blood agar base enriched with hemoglobin and supplement B; contaminating organisms inhibited by colistin, nystatin, vancomycin, and trimethoprim	Selective for *N. gonorrhoeae* and *N. meningitidis.* Supports the growth of *Francisella* and *Brucella* spp.
Thioglycollate broth	Pancreatic digest of casein, soy broth, and glucose enrich growth of most microorganisms; includes reducing agents thioglycollate, cystine, and sodium sulfite; semisolid medium with a low concentration of agar reducing oxygen diffusion in the medium	Supports growth of anaerobes, aerobes, microaerophilic, and fastidious microorganisms
Thiosulfate citrate–bile salts (TCBS) agar	Peptone base agar with yeast extract, oxgall (bile), sodium cholate, citrate, sucrose, ferric citrate, and sodium thiosulfate; thymol blue and bromothymol blue act as indicators.	Selective and differential for *Vibrio cholerae* and *Vibrio parahaemolyticus*
Todd-Hewitt broth supplemented with antibiotics (LIM)	Supplemented with nalidixic acid and gentamicin or colistin for greater selectivity; thioglycollate and agar reduce redox potential.	Selection and enrichment for *Streptococcus agalactiae* in female genital specimens
Trypticase soy broth (TSB)	All-purpose basal broth that can support the growth of many nonfastidious organisms or when supplemented with additional nutrients, it is used to cultivate fastidious microorganisms.	Basal back-up broth or enrichment broth used for subculturing various bacteria from primary agar plates

[a]Media was originally formulated by the Centers for Disease Control or CDC.
CRE, Carbapenemase-resistant Enterobacterales; *ESBL,* extended spectrum beta-lactamase; *UTI,* urinary tract infection; *VRE,* vancomycin-resistant enterococci.

(**alpha-hemolysis**). Other bacteria have no effect on the red blood cells, and no halo is produced around the colony (**gamma-hemolysis** or nonhemolytic). Microbiologists often use colony morphology and the degree or absence of hemolysis as criteria for determining what additional steps will be necessary for identification of a bacterial isolate. To read the hemolytic reaction on a BA plate accurately, the technologist must hold the plate up to the light and observe the plate with the light coming from behind (i.e., transmitted light).

Hemolysis, similar to lactose fermentation, relies on the production of an extracellular enzyme resulting in the lysis or partial lysis of the red blood cells. Variations in the production of the hemolysins or extracellular enzymes by the organisms may result in a different hemolytic pattern than is expected based on initial Gram stain and growth characteristics. It is important for the microbiologist to carefully consider the organism identification in conjunction with additional growth characteristics and biochemical reactions.

Brain-Heart Infusion

Brain-heart infusion (BHI) is a nutritionally rich medium used to grow fastidious and nonfastidious microorganisms, either as a broth or as an agar, with or without added blood. Key ingredients include infusion from several animal tissue sources, added peptone (protein), phosphate buffer, and a small concentration of dextrose. The carbohydrate provides a readily accessible source of energy for many bacteria. BHI broth is often used as a major component of the media developed for culturing a patient's blood for bacteria (Chapter 67), for establishing bacterial identification, and for certain tests to determine bacterial susceptibility to antimicrobial agents (Chapter 10).

Chocolate Agar

Chocolate agar is an enriched agar that is essentially the same as BA except that during preparation the red blood cells are lysed when added to molten agar base. The cell lysis provides for the release of intracellular nutrients such as heme, **hemin ("X" factor),** into the agar for utilization by fastidious bacteria. Red blood cell lysis gives the medium the chocolate-brown color from which the agar gets its name. The most common bacterial pathogens that require this enriched medium for growth include *Neisseria gonorrhoeae,* the causative agent of gonorrhea, and *Haemophilus influenzae,* which cause infections usually involving the respiratory tract and middle ear. Neither of these organisms are able to grow on sheep BA.

Columbia Colistin-Nalidixic Acid With Blood

Columbia agar base is a nutritionally rich formula containing three peptone sources and 5% defibrinated (whole blood with fibrin removed to prevent clotting) sheep blood. This supportive medium can also be used to help differentiate bacterial colonies based on the hemolytic reactions they produce. **Columbia colistin-nalidixic acid (CNA)** refers to the antibiotics colistin (C) and NA that are added to the medium to suppress the growth of most GN organisms while allowing gram-positive bacteria to grow, thus conferring a selective property to this medium. Colistin disrupts the cell membranes of GN organisms, and nalidixic aid blocks DNA replication in susceptible organisms.

Eosin Methylene Blue Agar, Levine

Eosin methylene blue agar (EMB) is used as a primary selective and differential agar. This medium contains eosin Y and methylene blue dye to inhibit the growth of gram-positive bacteria and allows many types of GN bacilli to grow. Bacterial fermentation of lactose appears as dark purple to black, or with a green metallic sheen. Non–lactose-fermenters, such as *Shigella* spp., remain colorless and translucent. Fermentation of lactose is a biochemical property of microorganisms. The differentiation of microorganisms on EMB relies on the expression of the pathway for the fermentation of lactose. Some organisms are considered slow fermenters and may not demonstrate a positive fermentation reaction in the first 24 hours of growth. Interpretation of this media may be difficult to the untrained microbiologist. This is due to the subtle difference in color change in slow lactose fermenters in comparison to the color of the media. Caution should be used in the application and interpretation of this reaction when characterizing microorganisms for identification.

Gram-Negative Broth

A selective broth, GN broth is used for the cultivation of gastrointestinal pathogens (i.e., *Salmonella* spp. and *Shigella* spp.) from stool specimens and rectal swabs. The broth contains several active ingredients, including sodium citrate and sodium deoxycholate (a bile salt) that inhibit gram-positive organisms and the early multiplication of GN, nonenteric pathogens. The broth also contains mannitol as the primary carbon source. Mannitol is the favored energy source for many enteric pathogens, but it is not widely used by other nonpathogenic enteric organisms. To optimize its selective nature, GN broth should be subcultured 6 to 8 hours after initial inoculation and incubation. After this time, the nonenteric pathogens begin to overgrow the pathogens that may be present in very low numbers.

Hektoen Enteric Agar

Hektoen enteric (HE) agar contains bile salts and dyes (bromothymol blue and acid fuchsin) to selectively slow the growth of most nonpathogenic GN bacilli found in the gastrointestinal tract while allowing *Salmonella* spp. and *Shigella* spp. to grow. The medium is also differential, because many nonenteric pathogens that do grow will appear as orange to salmon-colored colonies. This colonial appearance results from the organism's ability to ferment the lactose, sucrose, or salicin in the medium, resulting in the production of acid, which lowers the medium's pH and causes a color change in the pH indicator bromothymol blue. *Salmonella* spp. and *Shigella* spp. do not ferment these carbon compounds, so no color change occurs, and their colonies maintain the original blue-green color of the medium. As an additional differential characteristic, the medium contains ferric ammonium citrate, an indicator for the detection of H_2S; so that H_2S-producing organisms, such as *Salmonella* spp., can be visualized as colonies exhibiting a black precipitate (Fig. 7.6).

MacConkey Agar

MAC is frequently used as the primary selective and differential agar for the isolation and differentiation of GN bacilli. This medium contains crystal violet dye to inhibit the growth of gram-positive bacteria and fungi. The pH indicator, neutral red, provides this medium with a differential capacity. Bacterial fermentation of lactose results in acid production, which decreases the pH of the medium and causes the neutral red indicator to give bacterial colonies a pink to red color. Non–lactose-fermenters, such as *Shigella* spp., remain colorless and translucent (Fig. 7.4). Caution should be used in the application and interpretation of this reaction when characterizing microorganisms for identification.

Phenylethyl Alcohol Agar

Phenylethyl alcohol (PEA) agar is essentially sheep BA that is supplemented with PEA to inhibit the growth of GN bacteria. The 5% sheep blood in PEA provides nutrients for common gram-positive cocci such as *enterococci, streptococci*, and *staphylococci* (Fig. 7.3). Although it contains sheep blood, PEA agar should not be used in the interpretation of hemolytic reactions.

Modified Thayer-Martin Agar

Modified Thayer-Martin (MTM) agar is an enrichment and selective medium for the isolation of *N. gonorrhoeae,* the causative agent of gonorrhea, and *Neisseria meningitidis,* a life-threatening cause of meningitis from specimens containing mixed microbiota. The enrichment portion of the medium includes peptone starch, amino acids, glucose, nucleotides, and the chocolatized blood, and the addition of antibiotics provides a selective capacity. The glucose and agar concentrations are lower than the original Thayer-Martin agar, which improves growth of the fastidious organisms. The antibiotic trimethoprim is added to inhibit *Proteus* spp., which tend to swarm over the agar surface and mask the detection of

individual colonies of the pathogenic *Neisseria* spp. Additional antibiotics may be included in other formulas including colistin to inhibit other GN bacteria, vancomycin to inhibit gram-positive bacteria, and nystatin to inhibit yeast. A further modification, **Martin-Lewis agar,** substitutes ansamycin for nystatin and has a higher concentration of vancomycin.

Thioglycollate Broth

Thioglycollate broth is the back-up broth or semisolid media most frequently used in diagnostic bacteriology. The broth contains many nutrient factors, including casein, yeast and beef extracts, and vitamins, to permit the growth of most medically important bacteria. Other nutrient supplements, an oxidation-reduction indicator (resazurin), dextrose, vitamin K_1, and hemin have been used to modify the basic thioglycollate formula. In addition, this medium contains 0.075% agar to prevent convection currents from carrying atmospheric oxygen throughout the broth. This agar supplement and the presence of thioglycolic acid, which acts as a reducing agent to create an anaerobic environment deeper in the tube, allow anaerobic bacteria to grow.

GN facultatively anaerobic bacilli (i.e., those that can grow in the presence or absence of oxygen) generally produce diffuse, even growth throughout the broth, whereas gram-positive cocci demonstrate flocculation or clumps. Strict aerobic bacteria (i.e., require oxygen for growth), such as *Pseudomonas* spp., tend to grow toward the surface of the broth, whereas strict anaerobic bacteria (i.e., those that cannot grow in the presence of oxygen) grow at the bottom of the broth (Fig. 7.7). Although the medium provides a means to potentially identify atmospheric growth conditions,

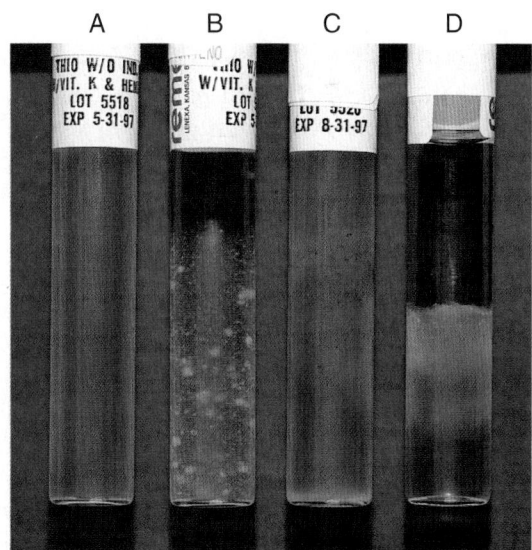

• **Fig. 7.7** Growth characteristics of various bacteria in thioglycollate broth. (A) Facultatively anaerobic gram-negative bacilli (i.e., those that grow in the presence or absence of oxygen) grow throughout the broth. (B) Gram-positive cocci exhibit flocculation. (C) Strictly aerobic organisms (i.e., those that require oxygen for growth), such as *Pseudomonas aeruginosa,* grow toward the top of the broth. (D) Strictly anaerobic organisms (i.e., those that do not grow in the presence of oxygen) grow in the bottom of the broth.

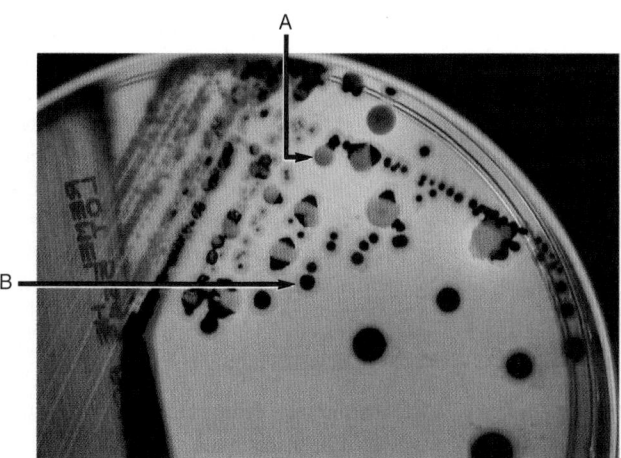

• **Fig. 7.6** Differential capabilities of Hektoen enteric agar for lactose-fermenting, gram-negative bacilli (e.g., *Escherichia coli*, arrow A) and H_2S producers (e.g., *Salmonella* spp., arrow B).

this property is not typically reportable, and therefore the medium is not considered a differential medium in the clinical laboratory.

Xylose-Lysine-Deoxycholate Agar

As with HE agar, **xylose-lysine-deoxycholate (XLD) agar** is selective and differential for *Shigella* spp. and *Salmonella* spp. The salt, sodium deoxycholate, inhibits many GN bacilli that are not enteric pathogens and inhibits gram-positive organisms. A phenol red indicator in the medium detects increased acidity from carbohydrate (i.e., lactose, xylose, and sucrose) fermentation. Enteric pathogens, such as *Shigella* spp., do not ferment these carbohydrates, so their colonies remain colorless (i.e., the same approximate pink to red color of the uninoculated medium). Even though they often ferment xylose, colonies of *Salmonella* spp. are also colorless on XLD because of the decarboxylation of lysine, which results in a pH increase that causes the pH indicator to turn red. These colonies often exhibit a black center that results from *Salmonella* spp. producing H$_2$S. Several nonpathogenic microorganisms ferment one or more of the sugars and produce yellow colonies (Fig. 7.8).

Preparation of Artificial Media

Nearly all media are commercially available as ready-to-use agar plates or tubes of broth. If media are not purchased, laboratory personnel can prepare agars and broths using dehydrated powders that are reconstituted in water (distilled or deionized) according to the manufacturers' recommendations. Generally, media are reconstituted by dissolving a specified amount of media powder, which usually contains all necessary components, in water. Boiling is often required to dissolve the powder, but specific manufacturers' instructions printed in media package inserts should be followed exactly. The pH of the media may be adjusted prior to sterilization or after with sterile acid or base solutions based on the formula of the media. Most media require sterilization so that only bacteria from patient specimens will grow and not contaminants from water or the powdered media. Broth media are distributed to individual tubes before sterilization. Agar media are usually sterilized in large flasks or bottles capped with either plastic screw caps or plugs before being placed in an autoclave.

Media Sterilization

The timing of autoclave sterilization should start from the moment the temperature reaches 121°C and usually requires a minimum of 15 minutes. Once the sterilization cycle is completed, molten agar is allowed to cool to approximately 50°C before being distributed to individual petri plates ($\approx$20 to 25 mL of molten agar per plate). If other ingredients are to be added (e.g., supplements such as sheep blood or specific vitamins, nutrients, or antibiotics), they should be incorporated when the molten agar has cooled, just before distribution to plates.

Delicate media components that cannot withstand steam sterilization by autoclaving (e.g., serum, certain carbohydrate

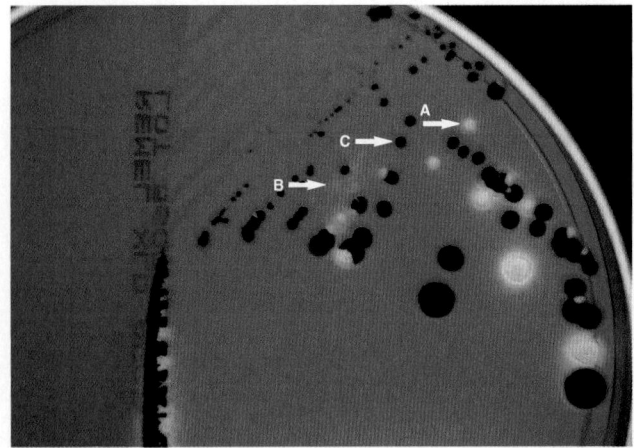

• **Fig. 7.8** Differential capabilities of xylose-lysine-deoxycholate agar for lactose-fermenting, gram-negative bacilli (e.g., *Escherichia coli*, *arrow A*), non–lactose-fermenters (e.g., *Shigella* spp., *arrow B*), and H$_2$S producers (e.g., *Salmonella* spp., *arrow C*).

solutions, certain antibiotics, and other heat-labile substances) can be sterilized at lower temperatures (116°C to 118°C) or by membrane filtration to prevent decomposition or the formation of toxic compounds that would interfere with growth of the microorganisms. Passage of solutions through membrane filters with pores ranging in size from 0.2 to 0.45 µm in diameter will not remove viruses but does effectively remove most bacterial and fungal contaminants. Finally, all media, whether purchased or prepared, must be subjected to stringent quality control (for more information regarding quality control see Chapter 77).

Cell Cultures

Although most bacteria grow readily on artificial media, certain pathogens require factors provided by living cells. These bacteria are obligate intracellular parasites that require viable host cells for propagation. Although all viruses are obligate intracellular parasites, chlamydiae, rickettsiae, and rickettsiae-like organisms are bacterial pathogens that require living cells for cultivation.

The cultures for growth of these bacteria comprise layers of living cells growing on the surface of a solid matrix such as the inside of a glass tube or the bottom of a plastic flask. The presence of bacterial pathogens within the cultured cells is detected by specific changes in the cells' morphology. Alternatively, nucleic acid detection or detection using specific stains composed of antibody conjugates may be used to detect bacteria within the cells. Cell cultures may also detect certain bacterial toxins (e.g., *Clostridioses difficile* cytotoxin). Cell culture maintenance and inoculation is addressed in Chapter 65.

Environmental Requirements

Optimizing the environmental conditions to support the most robust growth of clinically relevant bacteria is as important as meeting the organisms' nutritional needs for *in vitro* cultivation. The four most critical environmental factors to consider include the percentage of oxygen and carbon dioxide (CO_2), temperature, pH, and moisture content of the medium.

Oxygen and Carbon Dioxide Concentration

Most clinically relevant bacteria are aerobic, facultatively anaerobic, or strictly anaerobic. Aerobic bacteria use oxygen as a terminal electron acceptor and grow well in ambient air. Most clinically significant aerobic organisms are actually facultatively anaerobic, being able to grow in the presence (i.e., aerobically) or absence (i.e., anaerobically) of oxygen. However, some bacteria, such as *Pseudomonas* spp., members of the *Neisseriaceae* family, *Brucella* spp., *Bordetella* spp., and *Francisella* spp., are strictly aerobic and cannot grow in the absence of oxygen. Other aerobic bacteria require low levels of oxygen ($\approx 20\%$ or less) and are referred to as being microaerophilic. Anaerobic bacteria are unable to use oxygen as an electron acceptor, but some **aerotolerant** strains do not use the oxygen but will grow slowly and poorly in the presence of oxygen. Oxygen is inhibitory or lethal for strictly anaerobic bacteria.

In addition to oxygen, the availability of CO_2 is important for growth of certain bacteria. Organisms that grow best with higher CO_2 concentrations (i.e., reduced oxygen $\leq 15\%$ and 5% to 10% CO_2) than is provided in ambient air are considered **capnophilic.**

Temperature

Bacterial pathogens generally multiply best at temperatures similar to those of internal human host tissues and organs. Cultivation of most medically relevant bacteria use incubators with temperatures maintained at 35°C to 37°C. An incubation temperature of 30°C (i.e., the approximate temperature of the body's surface), on the other hand, may be preferable for fungal organisms and some bacteria.

Recovery of certain organisms can be enhanced by incubation at other temperatures. For example, the gastrointestinal pathogen *Campylobacter jejuni* is able to grow at 42°C. Incubation at this temperature is used as a **temperature enrichment** procedure. Other bacteria, such as *Listeria monocytogenes* and *Yersinia enterocolitica,* are able to grow at 4°C to 43°C but grow optimally between 20° and 40°C. **Cold enrichment** has been used to enhance the recovery of these organisms in the laboratory.

pH

The pH scale is a measure of the hydrogen ion concentration in the environment, with a pH value of 7.0 being neutral. Values less than 7 indicate the environment is acidic; values greater than 7 indicate alkaline conditions. Most clinically relevant bacteria prefer a near-neutral pH range, from 6.5 to 7.5. Commercially prepared media are buffered in this range, and checking the pH is rarely necessary.

Moisture

Water is provided as a major constituent of both agar and broth media. However, when media are incubated at the temperatures used for bacterial cultivation, a large portion of water content can be lost by evaporation. Loss of water from media can be deleterious to bacterial growth in two ways: (1) less water is available for essential bacterial metabolic pathways and (2) with a loss of water, there is a relative increase in the solute concentration of the media. An increased solute concentration can osmotically shock the bacterial cell and cause lysis. In addition, increased atmospheric humidity enhances the growth of certain bacterial species. For these reasons, measures such as sealing agar plates or using humidified incubators ($\geq 70\%$) ensure appropriate moisture levels are maintained throughout the incubation period.

Methods for Providing Optimal Incubation Conditions

Incubators provide the environmental conditions required for cultivating microorganisms. The conditions of incubators can be altered to accommodate different types of organisms. This section focuses on the incubation of routine bacteriology cultures. Conditions for growing anaerobic bacteria (Part III, Section 13), mycobacteria (Part III, Section 14), fungi (Chapter 58), and viruses (Chapter 64) are covered in other areas of the text.

Once inoculated with patient specimens, most media are placed in incubators with temperatures maintained between 35°C and 37°C and humidified atmospheres that contain 5% to 10% CO_2. Some media that contain pH indicators cannot be placed in CO_2 incubators. The presence of CO_2 will acidify the media, causing the pH indicator to change color and thereby disrupt the differential properties of the media (e.g., HE agar and MAC). Incubators containing room air may be used for some media, but the lack of increased CO_2 may hinder the growth of certain bacteria.

Various atmosphere-generating systems are commercially available and are used instead of CO_2-generating incubators. For example, a self-contained culture medium and a compact CO_2-generating system can be used for culturing fastidious organisms such as *N. gonorrhoeae*. A tablet of sodium bicarbonate is dissolved by the moisture created within an airtight plastic bag and releases sufficient CO_2 to support growth of the pathogen.

Finally, the duration of incubation required for obtaining good bacterial growth depends on the organisms being cultured. Most bacteria encountered in routine bacteriology will grow within 24 to 48 hours. Certain anaerobic bacteria may require longer incubation, and mycobacteria frequently take weeks before detectable growth occurs.

Bacterial Cultivation

The process of bacterial cultivation involves the use of optimal artificial media and incubation conditions to isolate and identify the bacterial etiologies of an infection as rapidly and as accurately as possible.

Isolation of Bacteria From Specimens

The cultivation of bacteria from infections at various body sites is accomplished by inoculating processed specimens directly onto artificial media. Representative media are summarized in Table 7.1. Incubation conditions are selected for their ability to support the growth of the bacteria most likely to be involved in the infectious process.

To enhance the growth, isolation, and selection of etiologic agents, specimen inocula are usually spread over the surface of plates in a standard pattern so that individual bacterial colonies are obtained, and semiquantitative analysis can be performed. A standardized semiquantitative streaking technique is illustrated in Fig. 7.9. Using this method, the relative numbers of organisms in the original specimen can be estimated based on the growth of colonies past the original area of inoculation. To enhance isolation of bacterial colonies, the loop should be flamed for sterilization between the streaking of each subsequent quadrant.

Streaking plates inoculated with a measured amount of specimen, such as when a calibrated loop is used to quantify colony-forming units (CFUs) in urine cultures, is accomplished by spreading the inoculum down the center of the plate. Without flaming the loop, the plate is then streaked side to side across the initial inoculum to evenly distribute the growth on the plate (Fig. 7.10). This facilitates counting colonies by ensuring that individual bacterial cells will be well dispersed over the agar surface. Typically, a calibrated loop of 1 µL is used for urine cultures. However, if a lower count of bacteria may be present, such as a suprapubic aspiration, a 10 µL loop may be needed to identify the lower count of organisms. The number of colonies identified on the plate is multiplied by the dilution factor to determine the number of CFUs per millimeter in the original specimen (103 for a 1 µL loop and 102 for a 10 µL loop). In addition, to standardize the interpretation of colony count, laboratories should have guidelines for the reporting of organisms based on the number and types of organisms present. A sample standardized method is outlined in Evolve Procedure 73.1.

In addition to manual streaking, automated instrumentation is available that provides a standardized specimen processing and media inoculation. The specimen is associated with the liquid phase or more accurately released from the swab into the transport media efficiently. The liquid-based specimen enables an automated system to retrieve the sample, inoculate a microscope slide or a smear, and inoculate a variety of media efficiently and effectively.

Evaluation of Colony Morphologies

The initial evaluation of colony morphologies on the primary plating media is extremely important. Laboratorians can provide physicians with early preliminary information regarding the patient's culture results. This information is also important for deciding how to proceed for definitive organism identification and characterization. Initial interpretation of the **primary culture** growth on selective, differential, or enriched media provides critical results to ensure rapid and proper treatment of the patient. The initial interpretation of the specimen cultivation, or **primary plate reading,** is used to correlate the growth of the organism on a variety of media in conjunction with the direct Gram stain results when included in the initial set-up of the specimen in the microbiology laboratory. For example, a sputum sample previously reported on a DGS as gram-positive diplococci in the presence of many polymorphonuclear cells (PMNs) should demonstrate growth on sheep BA as alpha-hemolytic, translucent, umbilicate colonies that also grow on chocolate agar but fail to grow on MAC, which is inhibitory to gram-positive organisms. A skilled microbiologist should recognize this as the characteristic presentation of *Streptococcus pneumoniae,* a common pathogen associated with bacterial pneumonia.

Type of Media Supporting Bacterial Growth

As previously discussed, different media are used to recover particular bacterial pathogens. In other words, the media selected for growth is a clue to the type of organism isolated (e.g., growth on MAC indicates the organism is most likely a GN bacillus). Yeast and some gram-positive *cocci* are capable of limited growth on MAC. The incubation conditions that support growth may also be a preliminary indicator of which bacteria have been isolated (e.g., aerobic versus anaerobic bacteria).

Relative Quantities of Each Colony Type

The predominance of a bacterial isolate is often used as one of the criteria, along with direct smear results, organism virulence, and the body site from which the culture was obtained, for establishing the organism's clinical significance. Several methods are used for semiquantitation of bacterial quantities, including many, moderate, few, or a numerical designation (4+, 3+, 2+, 1+) based on the number of colonies identified in each streak area (Table 7.2).

Colony Characteristics

Noting key features of a bacterial colony is important for any bacterial identification; success or failure of subsequent identification procedures often depends on the accuracy of these observations. Criteria frequently used to characterize bacterial growth (**colony morphology**) include the following:

- Colony size (usually measured in millimeters or described in relative terms such as <1 mm, pinpoint; 1 to 2 mm, small; 2 to 3 mm, medium; >3 mm, large)
- Colony pigmentation (e.g., white, buff, yellow)
- Colony shape (includes form, elevation, and margin of the colony [Fig. 7.11])
- Colony density or opacity (e.g., transparent—clear, translucent—nearly clear, frosted appearance, iridescent—changes color when light is reflected as the plate is tipped or moved)
- Colony surface texture: smooth, glistening (shiny), rough (dull)

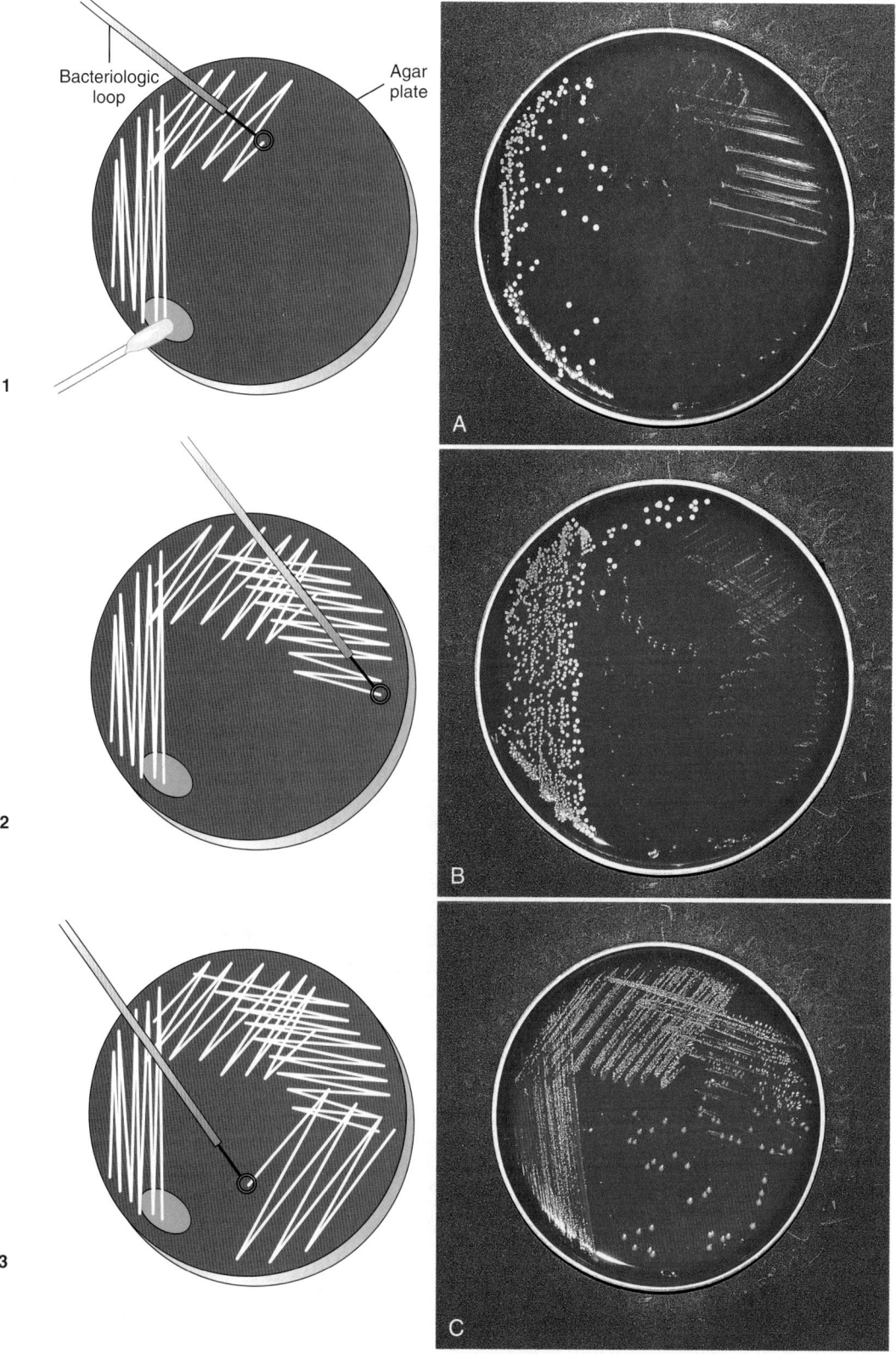

• **Fig. 7.9** Dilution streak technique for isolation and semiquantitation of bacterial colonies. (A) Actual plates show sparse, or 1+, bacterial growth that is limited to the first quadrant. (B) Moderate, or 2+, bacterial growth that extends to the second quadrant. (C) Heavy, or 3+ to 4+, bacterial growth that extends to the fourth quadrant.

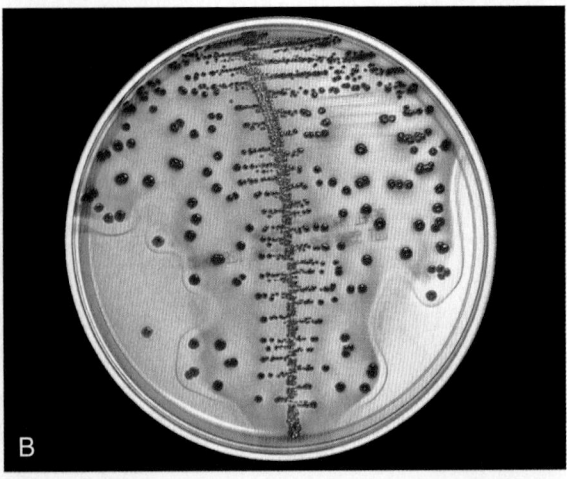

Streak pattern

Liquid specimen of inoculum

A

B

• **Fig. 7.10** (A) Streaking pattern using a calibrated loop for enumeration of bacterial colonies grown from a liquid specimen such as urine. (B) An actual plate shows well-isolated and dispersed bacterial colonies for enumeration obtained with the calibrated loop streaking technique.

TABLE 7.2	Semiquantitation Grading Procedure for Bacterial Isolates on Growth Media			
	Number of Colonies Visible in Each Quadrant			
Score	1 (Initial Quadrant)	2	3	4
1+	Less than 10			
2+	Less than 10	Less than 10		
3+	Greater than 10	Greater than 10	Less than 10	
4+	Greater than 10	Greater than 10	Greater than 10	Greater than 5

Note: This is a general guideline. Individual laboratories may vary in the methods used for quantitation.

- Colony consistency: butyrous (buttery), friable (brittle and breaks apart), viscous (sticks to the loop), mucoid (slimy and strings from the loop)
- Changes in agar media resulting from bacterial growth (e.g., hemolytic pattern on BA, changes in color of pH indicators, pitting of the agar surface; Figs. 7.3 through 7.8)

Odor is not typically considered a reportable colonial morphologic feature. However, some organisms produce distinct odors. It is important to note that smelling colonies of unknown organisms is not recommended, to avoid potential laboratory-acquired respiratory infections. In addition, pigmentation may not be clearly visible on the culture media. To clearly visualize pigmentation, a sterile white swab may be used. Take the swab and pick up a small amount of the colony to determine the pigmentation. This allows the microbiologist to visualize the actual pigment of the colony and not a reflection of color from the base of the agar media.

Many of these criteria are somewhat subjective, and the adjectives and descriptive terms used may vary among different laboratories. Regardless of the terminology used, laboratory protocol for bacterial identification begins with agreed-upon colony description of the commonly encountered pathogens.

Although careful determination of colony appearance is important, it is unwise to place total confidence on colony morphology for preliminary identification. Bacteria of one species may exhibit colony characteristics that are indistinguishable from those of many other species. In addition, bacteria of the same species exhibit morphologic diversity. For example, certain colony characteristics may be typical of a given species, but different strains of that species may have different morphologies.

Indirect Gram Stain and Subcultures

Isolation of individual colonies during cultivation is important for examining morphologies and characteristics and necessary for timely performance of indirect Gram stains and subcultures.

The Gram stain and microscopic evaluation of cultured bacteria are used along with colony morphology to decide which identification steps are needed. To prevent confusion, organisms from a single colony are stained. In other cases, staining may not be necessary, because growth on a particular selective agar provides dependable evidence of the organism's Gram stain morphology (e.g., GN bacilli essentially are the only clinically relevant bacteria that grow well on MAC).

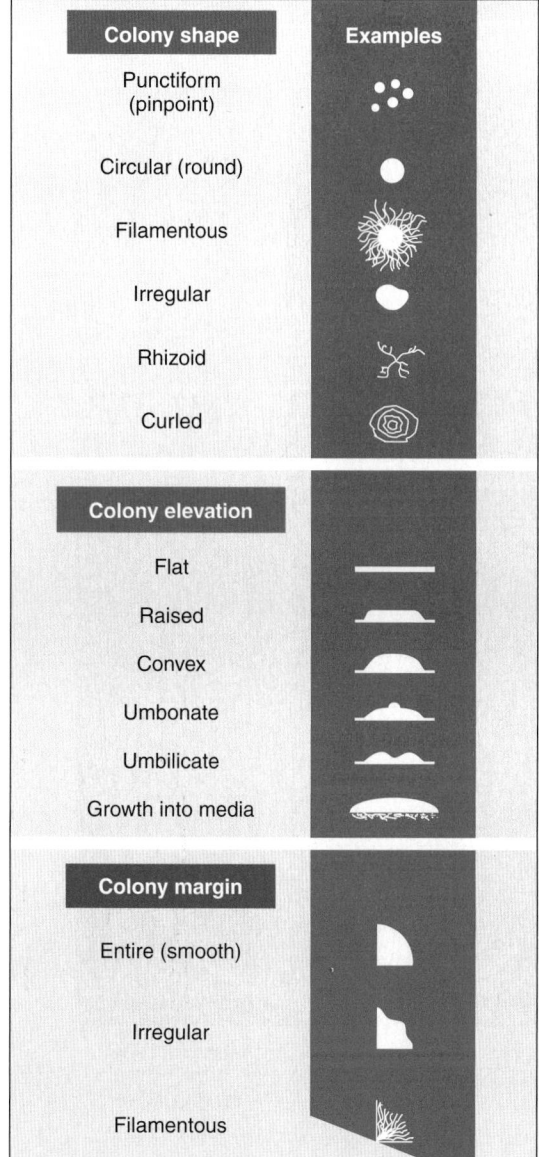

Colony shape	Examples
Punctiform (pinpoint)	
Circular (round)	
Filamentous	
Irregular	
Rhizoid	
Curled	

Colony elevation	
Flat	
Raised	
Convex	
Umbonate	
Umbilicate	
Growth into media	

Colony margin	
Entire (smooth)	
Irregular	
Filamentous	

• **Fig. 7.11** Colony morphologic features and descriptive terms for commonly encountered bacterial colonies.

After characterization of growth on primary plating media, all subsequent procedures for definitive identification require the use of pure cultures (i.e., cultures containing one strain of a single species). If sufficient inocula for testing can be obtained from the primary media, a **subculture** is not necessary, except as a precaution to obtain more of the etiologic agent if needed and to ensure that a pure inoculum has been used for subsequent tests (i.e., a "purity" check). However, frequently the primary media do not yield sufficient amounts of bacteria in pure culture and a subculture step is required (Fig. 7.12).

Using a sterile loop, a portion of an isolated colony is taken and transferred to the surface of a suitable enrichment medium and incubated under conditions optimal for the organism. When making transfers for subculture, it is beneficial to flame the inoculating loop between streaks to each area on the agar surface. This prevents over-inoculation of

the subculture media and ensures individual colonies will be obtained. Once a pure culture is available in a sufficient amount, an inoculum for subsequent identification procedures can be prepared.

Principles of Identification

Microbiologists use various methods to identify organisms cultivated from patient specimens. Although many of the principles and issues associated with bacterial identification discussed in this chapter are generally applicable to most clinically relevant bacteria, specific information regarding particular organism groups is covered in the appropriate chapters in Part III.

The importance of accurate bacterial identification cannot be overstated and is central to diagnostic bacteriology issues, including the following:

- Determining the clinical significance of a particular pathogen (e.g., is the isolate a pathogen, a contaminant, or normal microbiota.)
- Guiding physician care of the patient through presumptive and final identification methods
- Determining whether laboratory testing for detection of antimicrobial resistance is warranted
- Determining the type of antimicrobial therapy that is appropriate
- Determining whether the antimicrobial susceptibility profiles are unusual or aberrant for a particular bacterial species
- Determining whether the infecting organism is a risk for other patients in the hospital, the public, or laboratory workers (i.e., is the organism one that may pose problems for infection control, public health, or laboratory safety?)
- Collecting epidemiologic data to monitor the control and transmission of organisms

The identification of a bacterial isolate requires analysis of information gathered from laboratory tests that provide characteristic profiles of bacteria. The tests and the order in which they are used for organism identification are an **identification scheme** or **workup** of the organism. Identification schemes can be classified into one of two categories: (1) those based on genotypic characteristics of bacteria and (2) those based on phenotypic characteristics. Certain schemes rely on both genotypic and phenotypic characteristics. In addition, some tests, such as the Gram stain, are an integral part of many schemes used for identifying a wide variety of bacteria, whereas other tests may only be used in the identification scheme for a single species.

Organism Identification Using Genotypic Criteria

Genotypic identification methods involve characterization of some portion of a bacterium's genome using molecular methods for DNA or RNA analysis. This usually involves detecting the presence of a gene, or a part

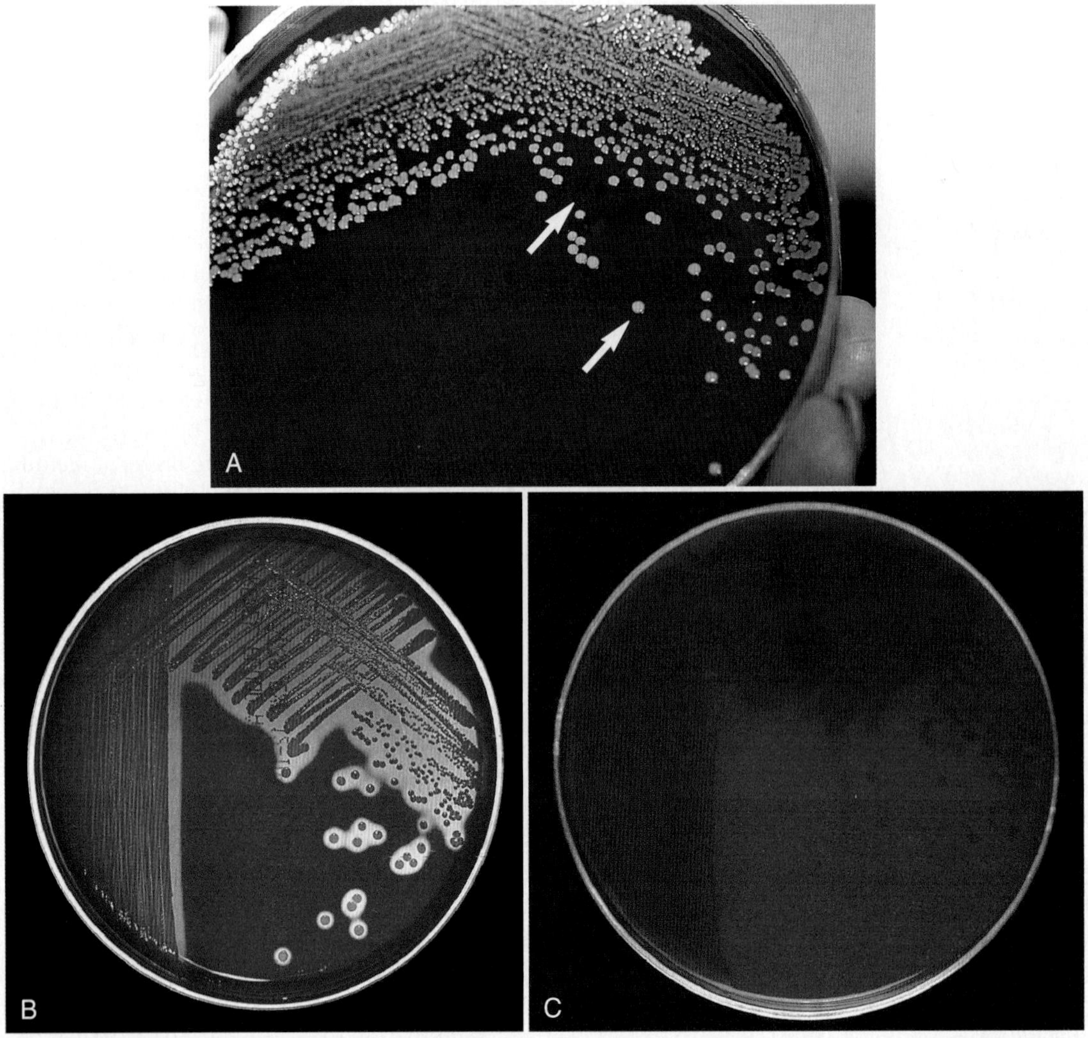

• **Fig. 7.12** (A) Mixed bacterial culture on sheep blood agar *(arrows)*. (B) Pure culture of *Staphylococcus aureus* (β-hemolysis is evident). (C) *Streptococcus pneumoniae* (α-hemolytic).

thereof, or an RNA product that is specific for a particular organism. In principle, the presence of a specific gene or a particular nucleic acid sequence unique to the organism is interpreted as identification of the organism. Sequencing of the specific DNA or RNA target sequence provides definitive identification. The most common conserved DNA target sequence used to identify bacteria is the 16s rRNA gene (16s ribosomal DNA). In some microorganisms, the 16s rRNA gene is highly conserved within the genus and additional DNA sequencing of a subsequent gene is required to identify specific species within the group. Genotypic identification is highly specific and sensitive. **Specificity** refers to the percentage of patients without disease that will test negative for the presence of the organism. **Sensitivity** indicates the percentage of patients in whom the organism is present who actually test positive. The DNA sequence is then compared to reference sequences available in public or private databases. The sample nucleotide match and mismatches are then converted and reported as a percent identity score. The acceptable percent identity for an organism is dependent

on the target sequence and the microorganism (for more information regarding molecular methods, see Chapter 8).

Organism Identification Using Phenotypic Criteria

Phenotypic criteria are observable physical or metabolic characteristics of bacteria—that is, identification is through analysis of gene products rather than through the genes themselves. The phenotypic approach is the classic approach to bacterial classification and identification, as previously discussed in Chapter 1. Other characterizations are based on the antigenic makeup of the organisms and involve techniques based on antigen-antibody interactions (for more information regarding immunologic diagnosis of infectious diseases, see Chapter 9). Phenotypic characterizations used in diagnostic bacteriology are based on methods that establish a bacterial isolate's morphology and metabolic capabilities. Phenotypic criteria include the following:

• Microscopic morphology and staining characteristics
• Macroscopic (colony) morphology

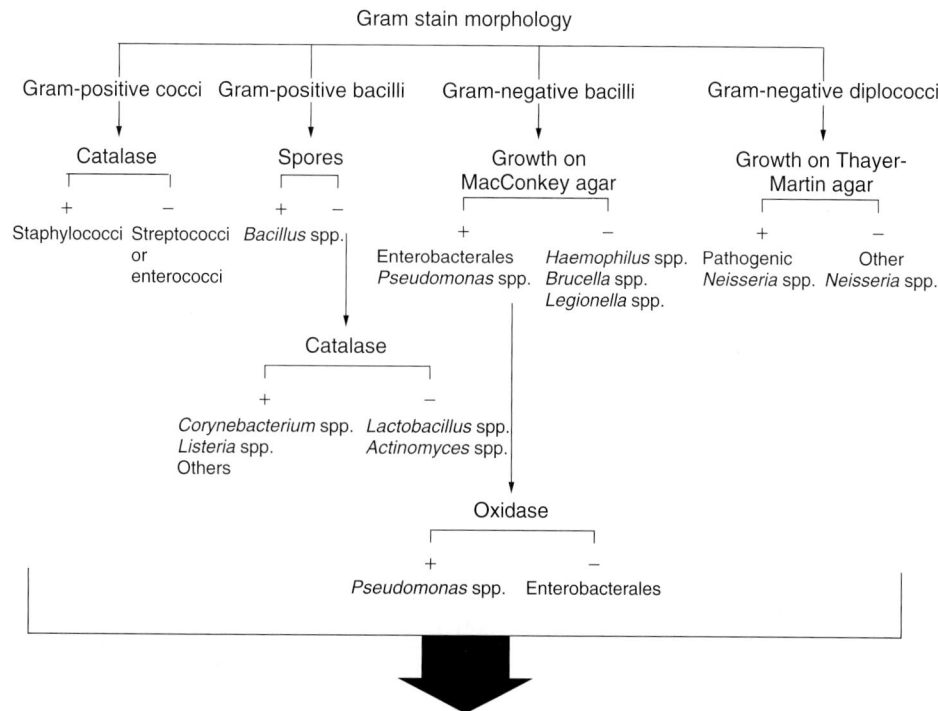

Gram stain morphology

Gram-positive cocci — Catalase
+ Staphylococci
− Streptococci or enterococci

Gram-positive bacilli — Spores
+ *Bacillus* spp.
− Catalase
+ *Corynebacterium* spp. *Listeria* spp. Others
− *Lactobacillus* spp. *Actinomyces* spp.

Gram-negative bacilli — Growth on MacConkey agar
+ Enterobacterales *Pseudomonas* spp. — Oxidase
+ *Pseudomonas* spp.
− Enterobacterales
− *Haemophilus* spp. *Brucella* spp. *Legionella* spp.

Gram-negative diplococci — Growth on Thayer-Martin agar
+ Pathogenic *Neisseria* spp.
− Other *Neisseria* spp.

Selection and performance of appropriate definitive bacterial identification schemes or systems

• **Fig. 7.13** Example of a bacterial identification scheme (not applicable to anaerobic organisms).

- Environmental requirements for growth
- Resistance or susceptibility to antimicrobial agents
- Nutritional requirements and metabolic capabilities
- Biochemical reactions including enzymatic reactions or chemical profiles
- Protein expression patterns (e.g., matrix-assisted laser desorption ionization time-of-flight mass spectrometry [MALDI-TOF MS])

Microscopic Morphology and Staining Characteristics

Microscopic evaluation of bacterial cellular morphology, as facilitated by the Gram stain or other enhancing methods discussed in Chapter 6, provides basic and important information that supports identification schemes and strategies. Most clinically relevant bacteria can be microscopically divided into four distinct Gram stain groups: gram-positive cocci, gram-negative diplococci, gram-positive bacilli, and gram-negative bacilli (Fig. 7.13). Some bacterial species are morphologically indistinct and are described as "GN coccobacilli," "gram-variable bacilli," or pleomorphic (i.e., exhibiting various shapes). Still other morphologies include curved rods and spirals.

Even without staining, examination of a wet preparation of bacterial colonies under oil immersion (1000× magnification) can provide clues as to possible identity. For example, a wet preparation prepared from a translucent, alpha-hemolytic colony on blood agar may reveal cocci in chains, a strong indication that the bacteria are probably streptococci. In addition, the presence of yeast, whose colonies can closely mimic bacterial colonies but

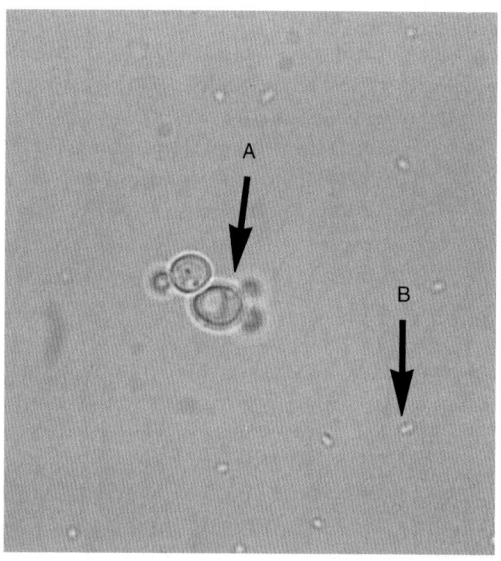

• **Fig. 7.14** Microscopic examination of a wet preparation demonstrates the size difference between most yeast cells, such as those of *Candida albicans* (arrow A), and bacteria, such as *Staphylococcus aureus* (arrow B).

whose cells are generally much larger, can be determined (Fig. 7.14).

In most instances, schemes for final identification are based on the cellular morphologies and staining characteristics of bacteria. To illustrate, an abbreviated identification flowchart for commonly encountered bacteria is shown in Fig. 7.13 (more detailed identification schemes are presented throughout Part III); this flowchart illustrates how microorganisms' microscopic morphology is integrated into identification schemes based on the organism's nutritional requirements and metabolic capabilities.

Macroscopic (Colony) Morphology

Evaluation of colony morphology includes considering colony size, shape, color (pigment), opacity, surface texture and consistency, and any changes that colony growth produces in the surrounding agar medium (e.g., hemolysis of blood in BA plates). A characteristic odor can support an identification of an organism such as *Pseudomonas aeruginosa,* which is described as having a fruity or grapelike smell. (Note: Smelling plates in a clinical setting can be dangerous and is strongly discouraged.)

Although these characteristics usually are not sufficient for establishing a final or definitive identification, the information gained provides preliminary information necessary for determining what identification procedures should follow. However, it is unwise to place too much confidence on colony morphology alone for preliminary identification of isolates. Microorganisms often grow as colonies whose appearance is not that different from many other species, especially if the colonies are relatively young (i.e., <14 hours old). Unless the colony morphology is distinctive or the growth occurs on a particular selective medium, other characteristics must be included in the identification scheme.

Environmental Requirements for Growth

Environmental conditions required for growth can be used to supplement other identification criteria. However, as with colony morphologies, this information alone is not sufficient for establishing a final identification. The ability to grow in particular incubation atmospheres frequently provides insight about the organism's potential identity. For example, organisms growing only in the bottom of a tube containing thioglycollate broth are not likely to be strictly aerobic bacteria, thus eliminating these types of bacteria from the list of identification possibilities. Similarly, anaerobic bacteria can be discounted in the identification schemes for organisms that grow on BA plates incubated in an ambient atmosphere. An organism's requirement, or preference, for increased carbon dioxide concentrations can provide hints for the identification of bacteria such as *S. pneumoniae, H. influenzae,* and *N. gonorrhoeae.*

In addition to atmosphere, the ability to survive or thrive in temperatures that exceed or are well below the normal body temperature of 37°C may be helpful for organism identification. The growth of *C. jejuni* at 42°C and the ability of *Yersinia enterocolitica* to survive at 0°C are two examples in which temperature enrichment can be used to identify an organism.

Resistance or Susceptibility to Antimicrobial Agents

The ability of an organism to grow in the presence of certain antimicrobial agents or specific toxic substances is widely used to establish preliminary identification. This is accomplished by using agar media supplemented with inhibitory substances or antibiotics (Table 7.1) or by directly measuring an organism's resistance to antimicrobial agents that may be used to treat infections (for more information regarding antimicrobial susceptibility testing, see Chapter 11).

As discussed earlier in this chapter, most clinical specimens are inoculated to several media, including some selective or differential agars. The first clue to identification of an isolated colony is the nature of the media on which the organism is growing. For example, with rare exceptions, only GN bacteria grow well on MAC. Alternatively, other agar plates, such as Columbia agar with CNA, support the growth of gram-positive organisms and inhibit the growth of most GN bacilli. Chocolate agar will support the growth of all aerobic microorganisms including the fastidious *Neisseria* spp.; the antibiotic-supplemented Modified-Thayer-Martin formulation will almost exclusively support the growth of the pathogenic species *N. meningitidis* and *N. gonorrhoeae* while inhibiting other species within the genus.

Directly testing a bacterial isolate's susceptibility to a particular antimicrobial agent may be a very useful part of an identification scheme. Many gram-positive bacteria (with a few exceptions, such as certain *Enterococcus* spp., *Lactobacillus* spp., *Leuconostoc* spp., and *Pediococcus* spp.) are susceptible to vancomycin, an antimicrobial agent that acts on the bacterial cell wall. In contrast, most clinically important GN bacteria are resistant to vancomycin. Susceptibility to vancomycin can be used to help establish the organism's Gram "status." Any zone of inhibition around a vancomycin-impregnated disk after overnight incubation is usually indicative of a gram-positive bacterium (Fig. 7.15). It is important to understand that with the increasing use of antibiotics to treat serious infections, some gram-positive organisms have acquired mechanisms of resistance to vancomycin. With few exceptions (e.g., certain *Chryseobacterium* spp., *Moraxella* spp., or *Acinetobacter* spp. isolates may be vancomycin susceptible), truly GN bacteria are resistant to vancomycin. Conversely, most GN bacteria are susceptible

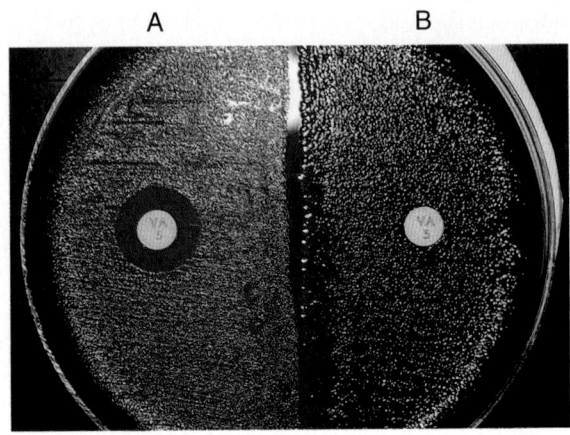

• **Fig. 7.15** (A) Zone of growth inhibition around the 5-μg vancomycin disk is indicative of a gram-positive bacterium. (B) The gram-negative organism is not inhibited by this antibiotic, and growth extends to the edge of the disk.

to the antibiotics colistin or polymyxin, whereas gram-positive bacteria are typically resistant to these agents.

Nutritional Requirements and Metabolic Capabilities

Determining the nutritional and metabolic capabilities of a bacterial isolate is the traditional approach used for determining the genus and species of an organism. The methods available for making these determinations share many commonalties but also have some important differences. In general, all methods use a combination of tests to establish the enzymatic capabilities of a given bacterial isolate as well as the isolate's ability to grow or survive in the presence of certain inhibitors (e.g., salts, surfactants, toxins, and antibiotics).

Establishing Enzymatic Capabilities

As discussed in Chapter 2, enzymes are the driving force in bacterial metabolism. Because enzymes are genetically encoded, the enzymatic content of an organism is a direct reflection of the organism's genetic makeup, which, in turn, is specific for individual bacterial species.

Types of Enzyme-Based Tests

In diagnostic bacteriology, **enzyme-based tests** are designed to measure the presence of a specific enzyme or a complete metabolic pathway that may contain several different enzymes. Although the specific tests most useful for the identification of particular bacteria are discussed in Part III, some examples of tests commonly used to characterize bacteria are reviewed here.

Single Enzyme Tests

Several tests are commonly used to determine the presence of a single enzyme. These tests usually provide rapid results because they can be performed on organisms already grown in culture. These tests are easy to perform, interpret, and often play a key role in the identification scheme. Although most **single enzyme tests** do not yield sufficient information to provide species identification, they are used extensively to determine which subsequent identification steps should be followed. For example, the catalase test can provide pivotal information and is commonly used in schemes for gram-positive identifications. The oxidase test is of comparable importance in identification schemes for GN bacteria (Fig. 7.13).

Catalase Test

The enzyme **catalase** catalyzes the release of water and oxygen from hydrogen peroxide ($2H_2O_2$ + catalase d $2H_2O$ + O_2); its presence is determined by direct analysis of a bacterial culture (Procedure 12.9). The rapid production of bubbles (effervescence) when bacterial growth is mixed with a hydrogen peroxide solution is interpreted as a positive test (i.e., the presence of catalase). Failure to produce effervescence or weak effervescence is interpreted as negative. If the bacterial inoculum is inadvertently contaminated with red blood cells when the test inoculum is collected from a

BA plate, weak production of bubbles may occur, but this should not be interpreted as a positive test.

Because the catalase test is key to the identification scheme of many gram-positive organisms, interpretation must be completed carefully. For example, most staphylococci are catalase-positive, whereas streptococci and enterococci are negative; similarly, the catalase reaction differentiates *L. monocytogenes* and corynebacteria (catalase-positive) from other Gram-positive, non–spore-forming bacilli (Fig. 7.13).

Oxidase Test

Cytochrome oxidase participates in electron transport and in the nitrate metabolic pathways of certain bacteria. Testing for the presence of oxidase can be performed by flooding bacterial colonies on the agar surface with 1% **tetramethyl-p-phenylenediamine dihydrochloride.** Alternatively, a sample of the bacterial colony can be rubbed onto filter paper impregnated with the reagent (Procedure 12.34). A positive reaction is indicated by the development of a purple color. If an iron-containing wire is used to transfer growth, a false-positive reaction may result; therefore, platinum wire or wooden sticks are recommended. Certain organisms may show slight positive reactions after the initial 10 seconds have passed; such results are not considered definitive.

The test is initially used for differentiating between groups of GN bacteria. Among the commonly encountered GN bacilli, Enterobacterales, *Stenotrophomonas maltophilia,* and *Acinetobacter* spp. are oxidase-negative, whereas many other bacilli, such as *Pseudomonas* spp. and *Aeromonas* spp., are positive (Fig. 7.13). The oxidase test is also a key reaction for the identification of *Neisseria* spp. (oxidase-positive).

Indole Test

Bacteria that produce the enzyme **tryptophanase** are able to degrade the amino acid tryptophan into pyruvic acid, ammonia, and indole. **Indole** is detected by combining with an indicator, aldehyde ([4-dimethylamino] benzaldehyde, 37% hydrochloric acid, and amyl alcohol, also referred to as Kovac's reagent), which results in the formation of a pink to red color (Procedure 12.21). Spot indole contains p-dimethylaminocinnamaldehyde (DMACA), 37% hydrochloric acid, and deionized water, which results in the formation of a blue color. This test is used in numerous identification schemes, especially to presumptively identify *Escherichia coli* in conjunction with microscopic and macroscopic colony morphology.

L-pyroglutamyl-aminopeptidase Test

The enzyme **L-pyroglutamyl-aminopeptidase (PYR)** hydrolyzes the substrate L-pyrrolidonyl-β-naphthylamide to produce a beta-naphthylamine. When the beta-naphthylamine combines with a cinnamaldehyde reagent, a bright red color is produced (Procedure 12.37). The PYR test is particularly helpful in identifying gram-positive cocci such as *Streptococcus pyogenes* and *Enterococcus* spp., which test positive, whereas other streptococci test negative.

Tests for the Presence of Metabolic Pathways

Several identification schemes are based on determining what metabolic pathways an organism uses and the substrates processed by these pathways. In contrast to single enzyme tests, these pathways may involve several interactive enzymes. The presence of a product resulting from these interactions is measured in the testing system. Assays for metabolic pathways can be classified into three general categories: **carbohydrate oxidation and fermentation, amino acid degradation,** and **single substrate utilizations.**

Oxidation and Fermentation Tests

As discussed in Chapter 2, bacteria use various metabolic pathways to produce biochemical building blocks and energy. For most clinically relevant bacteria, this involves utilization of carbohydrates (e.g., sugar or sugar derivatives) and protein substrates. Determining whether substrate utilization is an oxidative or fermentative process is important for the identification of several different bacteria.

Oxidative processes require oxygen; fermentative ones do not. The clinical laboratory determines how an organism utilizes a substrate by observing whether acid byproducts are produced in the presence or absence of oxygen (**fermentation**). In most instances, the presence of acid byproducts is detected by a change in the pH indicator incorporated into the medium. The color changes that occur in the presence of acid depend on the type of pH indicator used.

Oxidation-fermentation determinations are usually accomplished using a special semisolid medium (oxidative-fermentative [O-F] medium) that contains low concentrations of peptone and a single carbohydrate substrate such as glucose. The organism to be identified is inoculated into two glucose O-F tubes, one of which is then overlaid with mineral oil as a barrier to oxygen. Common pH indicators used for O-F tests, and the color changes they undergo with acidic conditions, include bromocresol purple, which changes from purple to yellow; Andrade's acid fuchsin indicator, which changes from pale yellow to pink; phenol red, which changes from red to yellow; and bromothymol blue, which changes from green to yellow.

As shown in Fig. 7.16, when acid production is detected in both tubes, the organism is identified as a glucose fermenter and oxidizer. If acid is only detected in the open, aerobic tube, the organism is characterized as a glucose oxidizer. As a third possibility, some bacteria do not use glucose as a substrate, no acid is detected in either tube and the organism is considered asaccharolytic (a noncarbohydrate utilizer). The glucose fermentative or oxidative capacity is generally used to separate organisms into major groups (e.g., Enterobacterales are fermentative; *Pseudomonas* spp. are oxidative). However, the utilization pattern for several other carbohydrates (e.g., lactose, sucrose, xylose, and maltose) is often needed to help identify an organism's genus and species.

Amino Acid Degradation

Determining the ability of bacteria to produce enzymes that either deaminate, dihydrolyze, or decarboxylate certain amino acids is often used in identification schemes. The amino acid substrates most often tested include lysine, tyrosine, ornithine, arginine, and phenylalanine. (The indole test for tryptophan cleavage is presented earlier in this chapter.)

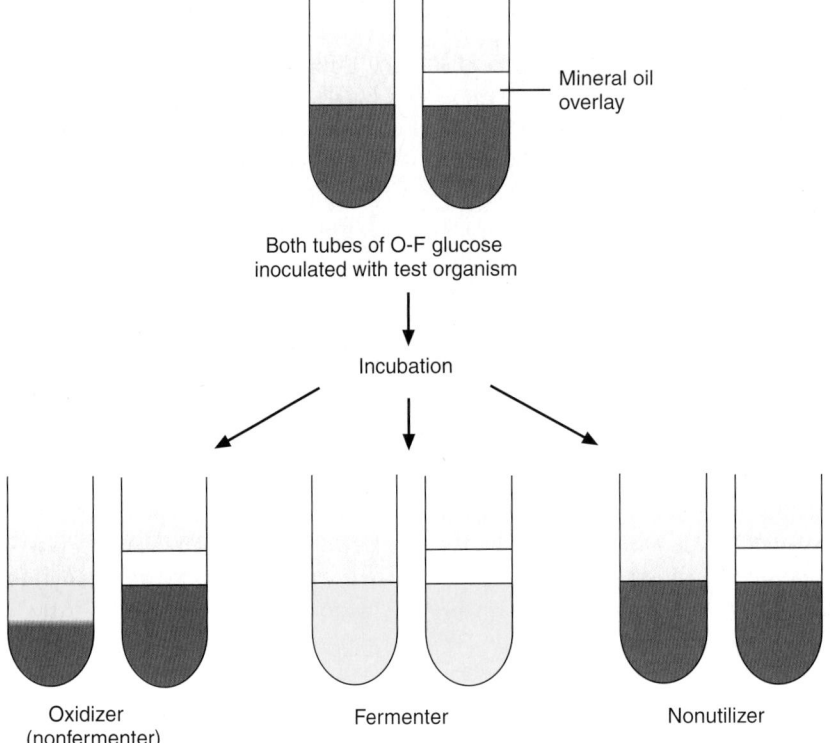

• **Fig. 7.16** Principle of glucose oxidative-fermentation *(O-F)* test. Fermentation patterns shown in O-F tubes include examples of oxidative, fermentative, and nonutilizing bacteria.

Decarboxylases cleave the carboxyl group from amino acids so that amino acids are converted into amines; lysine is converted to cadaverine, and ornithine is converted to putrescine. Because amines increase medium pH, they are readily detected by color changes in a pH indictor indicative of alkalinity. **Decarboxylation** is an anaerobic process that requires an acid environment for activation. The most common medium used for this test is Moeller decarboxylase base that contains glucose, the amino acid substrate of interest (i.e., lysine, ornithine, or arginine), and a pH indicator.

Organisms are inoculated into the tube medium, which is then overlaid with mineral oil to ensure anaerobic conditions (Chapter 12). Early during incubation, bacteria utilize the glucose and produce acid, resulting in a yellow coloration of the pH indicator. Organisms that can decarboxylate the amino acid then begin to attack the substrate and produce the amine product, which increases the pH and changes the indicator back from yellow to purple (if bromcresol purple is the pH indicator used; red if phenol red is the indicator). After overnight incubation, a positive test is indicated by a purple color, and a negative test (i.e., lack of decarboxylase activity) is indicated by a yellow color. With each amino acid tested, a control tube of the glucose-containing broth base without amino acid is inoculated. The standard's (control) color is compared with that of the tube containing the amino acid after incubation.

Because it is a two-step process, the breakdown of arginine is more complicated than that of lysine or ornithine. Arginine is first dihydrolyzed to citrulline, which is subsequently converted to ornithine. Ornithine is then decarboxylated to putrescine, which results in the same pH indicator changes as just outlined for the other amino acids.

Unlike decarboxylation, **deamination,** the cleavage of the amine group from an amino acid, occurs in air. Deamination of the amino acid phenylalanine results in the presence of the product (phenylpyruvic acid). Phenylpyruvic acid is detected by the addition of 10% ferric chloride, which results in the development of a green color. An agar slant medium, **phenylalanine deaminase agar (PDA),** is commercially available for this test.

Lysine iron agar medium is a combination medium used for the identification of decarboxylation and deamination in a single tube. Dextrose is incorporated in the medium in a limited concentration of 0.1%. The organism is then stabbed into the media approximately within 3 mm of the bottom of the tube. When removing the inoculating needle from the stab, the slant of the medium is streaked. Organisms capable of dextrose fermentation will produce acid, resulting in a yellow butt. Organisms that decarboxylate lysine will produce alkaline products that will return the yellow color to the original purple color of the medium. Hydrogen sulfide–positive organisms produce gas that reacts with iron salts, ferrous sulfate, and ferric ammonium citrate in the media, producing a black precipitate. It is important to note that *Proteus* spp. are capable of deaminating lysine in the presence of oxygen, resulting in a red color change on the slant of the medium.

Single Substrate Utilization

Whether an organism can grow in the presence of a single nutrient or carbon source provides useful identification information. Such tests entail inoculating organisms to a medium that contains a single source of nutrition (e.g., citrate, malonate, or acetate) and, after incubation, observing the medium for growth. Growth is determined by observing the presence of bacterial colonies or by using a pH indicator to detect the products of metabolic activity.

Establishing Inhibitor Profiles

The ability of a bacterial isolate to grow in the presence of one or more inhibitory substances can provide valuable identification information. Examples regarding the use of inhibitory substances are presented earlier in this chapter.

In addition to the information gained from using inhibitory media or antimicrobial susceptibility testing, other more specific tests may be incorporated into bacterial identification schemes. Because most of these tests are used to identify a particular group of bacteria, their protocols and principles are discussed in the appropriate chapters in Part III. A few examples of such tests include the following:

- Growth in the presence of various NaCl concentrations (identification of *Enterococcus* spp. and *Vibrio* spp.)
- Susceptibility to optochin and bile solubility (identification of *S. pneumoniae*)
- Ability to hydrolyze esculin in the presence of bile (identification of *Enterococcus* spp. in combination with NaCl)
- Ethanol survival (identification of *Bacillus* spp.)

Principles of Phenotypic Identification Schemes

As shown in Fig. 7.13, growth characteristics, microscopic morphologies, and single-test results are used to categorize most bacterial isolates into general groups. However, the definitive identification to species requires use of schemes designed to produce metabolic or protein profiles of the organisms. Biochemical phenotypic identification systems usually consist of four major components:

- Selection and inoculation of a set (i.e., battery) of specific metabolic substrates and growth inhibitors
- Incubation to allow substrate utilization to occur or to allow growth inhibitors to act
- Determination of metabolic activity that occurred during incubation
- Analysis of metabolic profiles and comparison with established profile databases for known bacterial species to establish definitive identification

Selection and Inoculation of Identification Biochemical Test Battery

The number and types of tests that are selected for inclusion in a biochemical test battery depends on various factors, including the type of bacteria to be identified, the clinical significance of the bacterial isolate, and the availability of reliable testing methods.

Type of Bacteria to Be Identified

Certain organisms have such unique features that relatively few tests are required to establish identity. For example, *Staphylococcus aureus* is essentially the only major pathogen that is a gram-positive cocci that appears microscopically in large clusters, macroscopically is generally yellow to golden, β-hemolytic on BA, is catalase-positive, and produces coagulase. This information would be sufficient to presumptively identify the organism as *S. aureus*. Confirmation of the identification would follow with a metabolic profile test battery or other identification method. In contrast, identification of most clinically relevant GN bacilli, such as those of the Enterobacterales order requires establishing metabolic profiles using a biochemical test battery or other identification system in order to identify the genus and species of the microorganism.

Clinical Significance of the Bacterial Isolate

Although a relatively large number of tests may be required to identify a particular bacterial species, the decision to identify the isolate depends on the specimen source, the amount of organism present, and the presence of additional bacterial species. For instance, if a GN bacillus is mixed with five other bacterial species in a urine culture, it is likely to be a contaminant. In this setting, multiple tests to establish species identity are not warranted and should not routinely be performed. However, if this same organism is isolated in pure culture from cerebrospinal fluid, the full battery of tests required for definitive identification should be performed.

Availability of Reliable Testing Methods

Because of an increasing population of immunocompromised patients and the increasing multitude of complicated medical procedures, the isolation of uncommon or unusual bacteria is occurring more frequently. Because of the unusual nature exhibited by some of these bacteria, reliable testing methods and identification criteria may not be established in most clinical laboratories. In these instances, only the genus of the organism may be identified (e.g., *Bacillus* spp.), or identification may not go beyond a description of the organism's microscopic morphology (e.g., gram-positive pleomorphic bacilli, or gram-variable branching organism). When such bacteria are encountered and are thought to be clinically significant, they should be sent to a reference laboratory whose personnel are experienced in identifying unusual organisms.

Although the number of tests included in an identification battery may vary and different identification systems may require various inoculation techniques, the one common feature of all systems is the requirement for inoculation with a pure culture. Inoculation with a mixture of bacteria produces mixed and often uninterpretable results. To expedite identification, cultivation strategies (described earlier in this chapter) should focus on obtaining pure cultures as soon as possible. Furthermore, **positive** and **negative controls** should be run in parallel with most identification systems as a check for purity of the culture used to inoculate the system.

Incubation for Substrate Utilization

The time required to obtain bacterial identification depends heavily on the length of incubation needed before the test result is available. In turn, the duration of incubation depends on whether the test is measuring metabolic activity that requires bacterial growth or whether the assay is measuring the presence of a particular enzyme or cellular product that can be detected without the need for bacterial growth.

Conventional Identification

Because the **generation time** (i.e., the time required for a bacterial population to double) for most clinically relevant bacteria is 20 to 30 minutes, **growth-based tests** usually require hours of incubation before the presence of an end product can be measured. Many conventional identification schemes require 18 to 24 hours of incubation, or longer, before the tests can be accurately interpreted. Although the conventional approach has been the standard for most bacterial identification schemes, the desire to produce results and identifications in a more rapid fashion has resulted in the development of rapid identification strategies.

Rapid Identification

In the context of diagnostic bacteriology, the term "rapid" is relative. A **rapid method** is one that provides a result the same day that the test was inoculated. Alternatively, the definition may be more precise, whereby rapid (10 minutes or less) or **quick test** (1 to 4 hours) is used to describe tests that provide results within 4 hours of inoculation. It is important to note that rapid identification still requires overnight incubation of culture media to provide pure-culture isolates from the primary specimen.

Two general approaches have been developed to obtain more rapid identification results. One is to vary the conventional testing approach by decreasing the test substrate medium volume and increasing the concentration of bacteria in the inoculum. Several conventional methods, such as carbohydrate fermentation profiles, use this strategy for more rapid results.

The second approach uses unique or unconventional substrates. Particular substrates are chosen based on their ability to detect enzymatic activity at all times. That is, detection of the enzyme does not depend on multiplication of the organism (i.e., this is not a growth-based test), so delays caused by depending on bacterial growth are minimized. The catalase, oxidase, and PYR tests discussed previously are examples of such tests, but many others are available as part of commercial testing batteries.

Still other rapid identification schemes are based on antigen-antibody reactions, such as latex agglutination tests, that are commonly used to quickly and easily identify certain β-hemolytic streptococci and *S. aureus* (for more information regarding these test formats, see Chapter 9).

Matrix-Assisted Laser Desorption Ionization Time of Flight Mass Spectrometry

Matrix-assisted laser desorption ionization time of flight mass spectrometry (MALDI-TOF MS) is an advanced chemical technique that uses laser excitation to ionize chemical functional groups that are included in the proteins of an organism. MALDI-TOF MS significantly reduces turnaround time and identification rates, while at the same time reducing the cost of consumables in the microbiology laboratory (Fig. 7.17). Identification of microorganisms is approximately 3 minutes per isolate compared to 1 to 1.5 days using conventional biochemical identification systems. Following isolation on primary culture media, the organism is either applied directly onto a plate from a pure culture, in an on-plate formic acid preparation, or prepared as an ethanol-formic acid protein extract before application. The sample is then mixed with a chemical matrix (Procedure 7.1). The laser is applied to the sample, and the matrix absorbs the energy, transferring heat to the sample proteins and creating ions; this is essentially the desorption and ionization process. These ions are then separated in a **flight tube.** The lighter the ions, the faster they will travel in the tube. The ions are measured using a detector, and a protein spectrum for the specific organism is created as a mass spectrum using the mass-to-charge ratio and signal intensity. The proteins that are detected efficiently would include small relatively abundant proteins such as ribosomal proteins (Fig. 7.18). This new organism protein profile is then compared with other

organisms included in a computerized database. Commercially available MALDI-TOF MS systems, including MALDI Biotyper (Bruker Daltonics Inc, Fremont, CA) (Fig. 7.17) and Vitek MS (bioMérieux, Etoile, France) (Fig. 7.19) are used for the clinical identification of microorganisms including bacteria, fungi, and viruses. The range of organisms that can be identified using MALDI-TOF MS is limited to the size of the proprietary database. The technique is also limited to the identification of organisms from pure colony isolation and is not useful on specimens containing contaminating microbiota or multiple species. Additional disadvantages associated with laboratory technique include smearing between organisms on the testing plate, the amount of organism spotted on the target, the homogeneity of the smear and failure to properly clean the plates before each subsequent use. As long as the quality of the technical process is maintained, results are generally reproducible. Additional errors may include variation in the composition of the solvent and matrix, culture conditions, the organism's biologic variation, and poorly developed quality-control strategies. Further information and the application of MALDI-TOF MS in the identification of specific microorganisms is provided in Parts III and V.

Detection of Metabolic Activity

The accuracy of an identification scheme heavily depends on the ability to reliably detect whether a bacterial isolate has utilized the substrates composing the identification battery. The sensitivity and strength of the detection signal can also contribute to how rapidly results are available. No matter how quickly an organism may metabolize

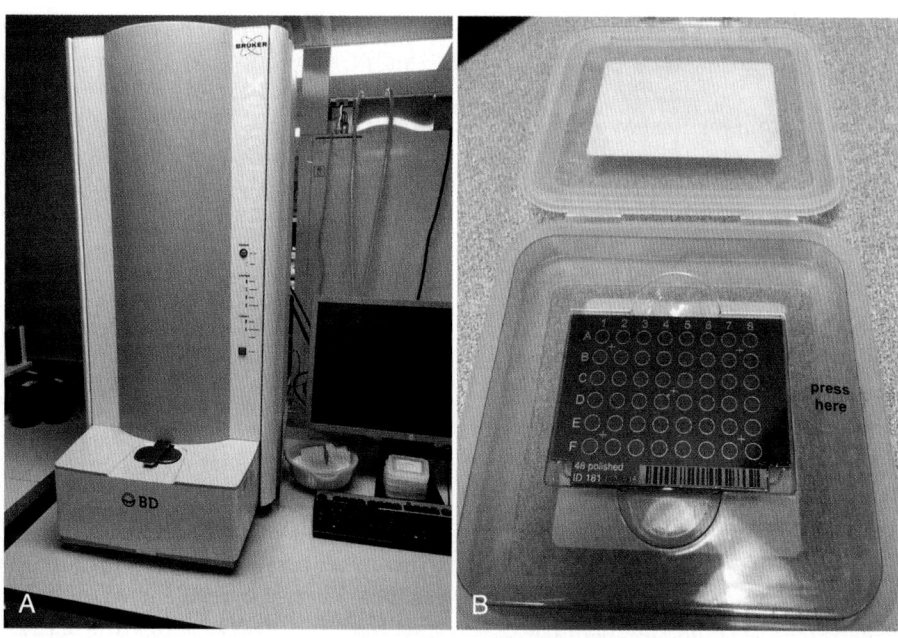

• **Fig. 7.17** (A) Matrix-assisted laser desorption ionization time of flight mass spectrometry. (B) A colony from a primary culture plate is transferred to a "spot" on a target plate. Cells are then treated with formic acid on the target plate and dried and then a matrix is added. The plate is placed into the mass spectrometer for analysis, and a mass spectrum is generated and compared with the database, providing an identification of the organism. (Photos courtesy Cory Gunderson, Avera Regional Laboratory, Sioux Falls, SD.)

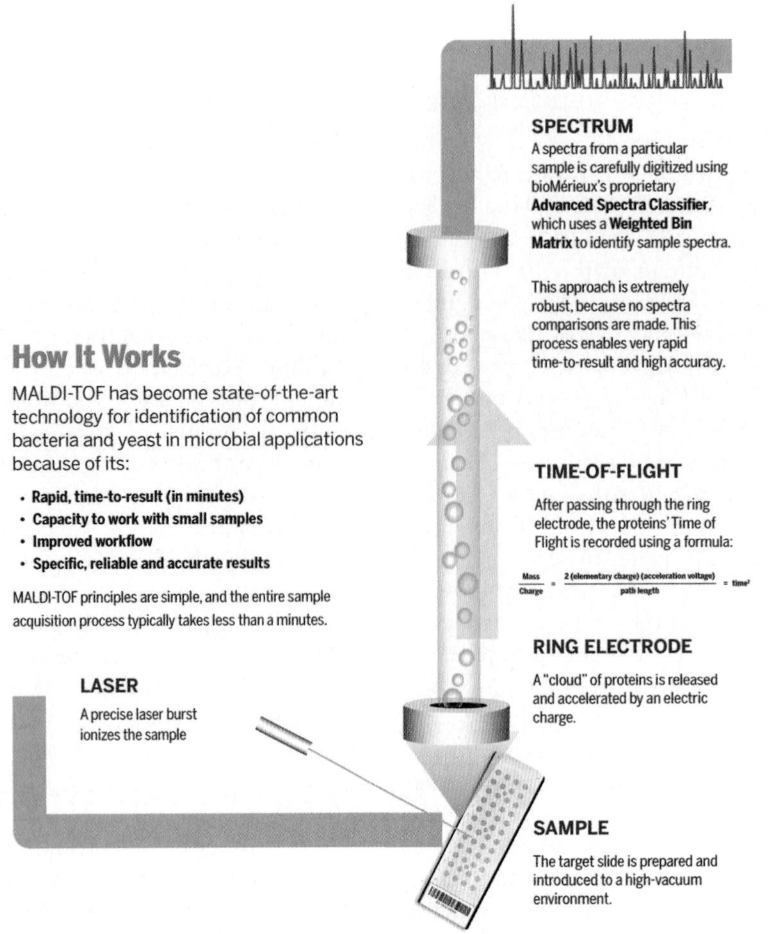

How It Works

MALDI-TOF has become state-of-the-art technology for identification of common bacteria and yeast in microbial applications because of its:

- Rapid, time-to-result (in minutes)
- Capacity to work with small samples
- Improved workflow
- Specific, reliable and accurate results

MALDI-TOF principles are simple, and the entire sample acquisition process typically takes less than a minutes.

LASER

A precise laser burst ionizes the sample

SPECTRUM

A spectra from a particular sample is carefully digitized using bioMérieux's proprietary **Advanced Spectra Classifier**, which uses a **Weighted Bin Matrix** to identify sample spectra.

This approach is extremely robust, because no spectra comparisons are made. This process enables very rapid time-to-result and high accuracy.

TIME-OF-FLIGHT

After passing through the ring electrode, the proteins' Time of Flight is recorded using a formula:

$$\frac{Mass}{Charge} = \frac{2\ (elementary\ charge)\ (acceleration\ voltage)}{path\ length} = time^2$$

RING ELECTRODE

A "cloud" of proteins is released and accelerated by an electric charge.

SAMPLE

The target slide is prepared and introduced to a high-vacuum environment.

• **Fig. 7.18** How it works! Matrix-assisted laser desorption ionization time of flight basic principle of operation and acquisition of the organisms' spectrum. (Image provided by bioMérieux, Inc., St. Louis, MO.)

a particular substrate, if the products are slowly or weakly detected, the ultimate production of results will still be "slow."

Detection strategies for determining the products of different metabolic pathways use colorimetry, fluorescence, or turbidity.

Colorimetry

Several identification systems measure color change (**colorimetry**) to detect the presence of metabolic products. Frequently the color change is produced using pH indicators included in the media. Depending on the byproducts measured and the testing method, additional reagents may need to be added to the reaction before the results are interpreted. An alternative to the use of pH indicators is the oxidation-reduction potential indicator tetrazolium violet. Organisms are inoculated into wells that contain a single, utilizable carbon source. Metabolism of that substrate generates electrons that reduce the tetrazolium violet, producing a purple color (positive reaction) that can be spectrophotometrically detected. In a third approach, the substrates themselves may be chromogenic so that when they are "broken down" by the organism, the altered substrate produces a color.

Some commercial systems use a miniaturized modification of conventional biochemical batteries, with the color change being detectable with the unaided eye. Alternatively, in certain automated systems, a photoelectric cell measures the change in the wavelength of light transmitted through miniaturized growth cuvettes or wells, thus eliminating the need for direct visual interpretation by laboratory personnel. In addition, a complex combination of dyes and filters may be used to enhance and broaden the scope of substrates and color changes that can be used in such systems. These combinations hasten identification and increase the variety of organisms that can be reliably identified.

Fluorescence

There are two basic strategies for using fluorescence to measure metabolic activity. In one approach, substrate-fluorophore complexes are used. If a bacterial isolate processes the substrate, the fluorophore is released and assumes a fluorescent configuration. Alternatively, pH changes resulting from metabolic activity can be measured by changes in fluorescence of certain fluorophore markers. In these pH-driven, fluorometric reactions, pH changes result either in the fluorophore becoming fluorescent or, in other instances, fluorescence being quenched or lost. To detect fluorescence, ultraviolet light of appropriate

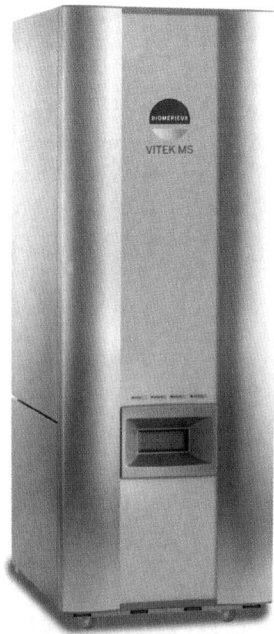

• **Fig. 7.19** bioMérieux vitek MS (MALDI-TOF) identification system. (Image provided by bioMérieux, Inc., St. Louis, MO.)

wavelength is focused on the reaction mixture and a special kind of photometer, a fluorometer, measures fluorescence.

Turbidity

Turbidity measurements are not commonly used for bacterial identifications but do have widespread application for determining growth in the presence of specific growth inhibitors, including antimicrobial agents, and for detecting bacteria present in certain clinical specimens.

Turbidity is the ability of particles in suspension to refract and deflect light rays passing through the suspension such that the light is reflected back into the eyes of the observer. The optical density (OD), a measurement of turbidity, is determined in a **spectrophotometer.** This instrument compares the amount of light that passes through the suspension (the percent transmittance) with the amount of light that passes through a control suspension without particles. A photoelectric sensor, or **photometer,** converts the light that impinges on its surface to an electrical impulse, which can be quantified. A second type of turbidity measurement is obtained by **nephelometry,** or light scatter. In this case, the photometers are placed at angles to the suspension, and the scattered light, generated by a laser or incandescent bulb is measured. The amount of light scattered depends on the number and size of the particles in suspension.

Analysis of Metabolic Profiles

The **metabolic profile** obtained with a particular bacterial isolate is essentially the phenotypic fingerprint, or signature, of that organism. Typically, the profile is recorded as a series of pluses (+) for positive reactions and minuses (–) for negative or nonreactions (Fig. 7.20). Although this profile by itself provides little information, powerful data systems can

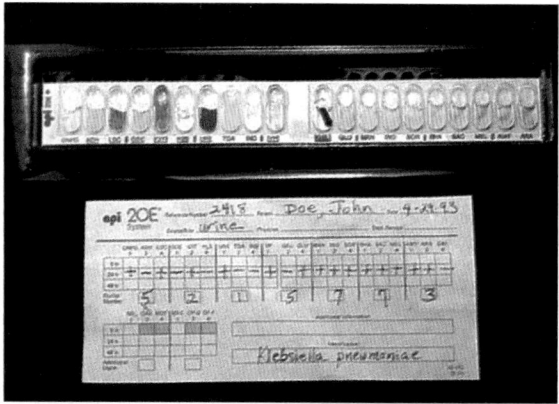

• **Fig. 7.20** Example of converting a metabolic profile to an octal profile for bacterial identification. *ONPG,* Orthonitrophenyl galactoside.

compare the profile with an extensive identification database to establish the identity of that specific isolate.

Identification Databases

Reference databases are available for clinical use. These databases are maintained by manufacturers of identification systems and are based on the continuously updated taxonomic status of clinically relevant bacteria. Although microbiologists typically do not establish and maintain their own databases, an overview of the general approach provides background information.

The first step in developing a database is to accumulate many bacterial strains of the same species. Each strain is inoculated to an identical battery of metabolic tests to generate a positive-negative test profile. The cumulative results of each test are expressed as a percentage of each genus or species that possesses that characteristic. For example, suppose that 100 different known *E. coli* strains and 100 known *Shigella* spp. strains are tested in four biochemicals, yielding the results illustrated in Table 7.3. In reality, many more strains and tests would be performed. However, the principle—to generate a database for each species that contains the percentage probability for a positive result with each test in the battery—is the same.

Manufacturers develop databases for each of the identification systems they produce for diagnostic use (e.g., Enterobacterales, gram-positive cocci, nonfermentative GN bacilli). Because the data are based on organism "behavior" in a particular commercial system, the databases cannot and should not be applied to interpret profiles obtained by other testing methods.

Furthermore, most databases are established with the assumption that the isolate to be identified has been appropriately characterized using adjunctive tests. For example, if a *S. aureus* isolate is mistakenly tested using a system for identification of Enterobacterales, the database will not identify the gram-positive cocci, because the results obtained will only be compared with data available for enteric bacilli. This underscores the importance of accurately performing preliminary tests and observations, such as colony and Gram stain morphologies, before selecting a particular identification battery.

Use of the Database to Identify Unknown Isolates

Once a metabolic profile has been obtained with a bacterial isolate of unknown identity, the profile must be converted to a numeric code that will facilitate comparison of the unknown organism's phenotypic fingerprint with the appropriate database.

To exemplify this step in the identification process, a binary code conversion system that uses the numerals 0 and 1 to represent negative and positive metabolic reactions, respectively, is used as an example (although other strategies are now used). As shown in Fig. 7.20, using binary code conversion, a 21-digit binomial number (e.g., 101100001001101111010, as read from top to bottom in the figure) is produced from the test result. This number is then used in an octal code conversion scheme to produce a mathematic number (octal profile [Fig. 7.20]). The octal profile number is used to generate a numerical profile distinctly related to a specific bacterial species. As shown in Fig. 7.20, the octal profile for the unknown organism is 5144572. This profile would then be compared with database profiles to determine the most likely identity of the organism. In this example, the octal profile indicates the unknown organism is *E. coli*.

Confidence in Identification

Once metabolic profiles have been translated into numeric scores, the probability that a correct correlation with the database has been made must be established—that is, how confident the laboratorian can be that the identification is correct. This is accomplished by establishing the percentage probability, which is usually provided as part of most commercially available identification database schemes.

For example, unknown organism X is tested against the four biochemicals listed in Table 7.3 and yields results as follows: lactose (+), sucrose (+), indole (−), and ornithine (+). Based on the results of each test, the percentage of known strains in the database that produced positive results are used to calculate the percentage probability that strain X is a member of one of the two genera (*Escherichia* or *Shigella*) given in the example (Table 7.4). Therefore, if 91% of *Escherichia* spp. are lactose-positive (Table 7.3), the probability that X is a species of *Escherichia* based on lactose alone is 0.91. If 38% of *Shigella* spp. are indole positive (Table 7.3), then the probability that X is a species of *Shigella* based on indole alone is 0.62 (1.00 [all *Shigella*] − 0.38 [percent positive *Shigella*] = 0.62 [percent of all *Shigella* that are indole negative]). The probabilities of the individual tests are then multiplied to achieve a calculated likelihood that X is one of these two genera. In this example, X is more likely to be a species of *Escherichia,* with a probability of 357:1 (1 divided by 0.0028; Table 7.4). This is still a very unlikely probability for correct identification, but only four parameters were tested, and the indole result was atypical. As more parameters are added to the formula, the importance of just one test decreases, and the overall pattern prevails.

With many organisms being tested for 20 or more reactions, computer-generated databases provide the probabilities. As more organisms are included in the database, the genus and species designations and probabilities become more precise. In addition, with more profiles in a database, the unusual patterns can be more readily recognized and, in some cases, new or unusual species may be discovered.

The most common commercial suppliers of multicomponent identification systems are driven by patent information technology and data management systems that automatically provide analysis and outcome of the metabolic process and identification.

Commercial Identification Systems and Automation

Advantages and Examples of Commercial System Designs

Commercially available identification systems have replaced compilations of conventional test media and

TABLE 7.3   Generation and Use of Genus-Identification Database Probability: Percentage of Positive Reactions for 100 Known Strains

Organism	Biochemical Parameter			
	Lactose	Sucrose	Indole	Ornithine
Escherichia spp.	91	49	99	63
Shigella spp.	1	1	38	20

TABLE 7.4   Generation and Use of Genus-Identification Database Probability: Probability That Unknown Strain X Is a Member of a Known Genus Based on Results of Each Individual Parameter Tested

Organism	Biochemical Parameter			
	Lactose	Sucrose	Indole	Ornithine
X	+	+	−	+
Escherichia spp.	0.91	0.49	0.01	0.63
Shigella spp.	0.01	0.01	0.62	0.20

Probability that X is *Escherichia* = 0.91 × 0.49 × 0.01 × 0.63 = 0.002809.
Probability that X is *Shigella* = 0.01 × 0.01 × 0.62 × 0.20 = 0.000012.

substrates prepared in-house for bacterial identification. This replacement has mostly come about because the design of commercial systems has continuously evolved to maximize the speed and optimize the convenience with which all four identification components can be achieved. Because laboratory workload has increased and the qualified workforce continues to decrease, conventional methodologies have had difficulty competing with the advantages of convenience and updated databases offered by commercial systems.

Some of the simplest multitest commercial systems consist of a conventional format that can be inoculated once to yield more than one result. By combining reactants, for example, one substrate can be used to determine indole and nitrate results; indole and motility results; motility, indole, and ornithine decarboxylase; or other combinations. Alternatively, conventional tests have been assembled in smaller volumes and packaged so that they can be inoculated easily with one manipulation instead of several. When used in conjunction with a computer-generated database, species identifications are made relatively easily.

Another approach is to have substrates dried in plastic cupules that are arranged in series on strips into which a suspension of the test organism is placed (Fig. 7.21). For some of these systems, use of a heavy inoculum or use of substrates with a utilization that is not dependent on extended bacterial multiplication allows results to be available after 4 to 6 hours of incubation.

Still other identification battery formats have been designed to more fully automate several aspects of the identification process. One example is the use of "cards" that are substantially smaller than most microtiter trays or cupule strips (Fig. 7.21). Analogous to the microtiter tray format, these cards contain dried substrates in tiny wells that are suspended upon inoculation.

Commercial systems are often categorized as either automated or manual. Various aspects of an identification system can be automated, and these usually include, in whole or in part, specimen processing, the inoculation steps, the incubation, the preliminary plate reading and the reading of biochemical tests, and the analysis of results. Automated specimen processing includes agitation, centrifugation, and using sediment for inoculation. Automated systems are capable of producing smears and sorting primary culture media into CO_2 or aerobic atmospheres. Following placement in the appropriate incubator, the automated systems monitor growth on individual plates using digital imaging. Computer workstations are used to view images to select colonies for identification and characterization without removing the culture plates from the incubator. The automated systems permit the laboratory to determine algorithms for the automatic discard of growth or no-growth cultures, as well as the simultaneous comparison of multiple cultures from a single patient. The advantages of automation in the microbiology laboratory include the ability to standardize and process liquid-based

	Test/ substrate	Test results (− or +)	Binary code conversion (0 or 1)	Octal value	Octal score	Octal triplet total	Octal profile
1	ONPG	+	1	× 1	1		
2	Arginine dihydrolase	−	0	× 2	0	5	
3	Lysine decarboxylase	+	1	× 4	4		
4	Ornithine decarboxylase	+	1	× 1	1		
5	Citrate utilization	−	0	× 2	0	1	
6	H₂S production	−	0	× 4	0		
7	Urea hydrolysis	−	0	× 1	0		
8	Tryptophane deaminase	−	0	× 2	0	4	
9	Indole production	+	1	× 4	4		
10	VP test	−	0	× 1	0		
11	Gelatin hydrolysis	−	0	× 2	0	4	
12	Glucose fermentation	+	1	× 4	4		5144572 (E. coli)
13	Mannitol fermentation	+	1	× 1	1		
14	Inositol fermentation	−	0	× 2	0	5	
15	Sorbitol fermentation	+	1	× 4	4		
16	Rhamnose fermentation	+	1	× 1	1		
17	Sucrose fermentation	+	1	× 2	2	7	
18	Melibiose fermentation	+	1	× 4	4		
19	Amygdalin fermentation	−	0	× 1	0		
20	Arabinose fermentation	+	1	× 2	2	2	
21	Oxidase production	−	0	× 4	0		

Octal code conversion* spans Octal value, Octal score, Octal triplet total, Octal profile.

*As derived from API 20E (bioMérieux, Inc.) for identification of Enterobacterales.

• **Fig. 7.21** Biochemical test panel. The test results obtained with the substrates in each cupule are recorded, and an organism identification code is calculated by octal code conversion on the form provided. The octal profile obtained then is matched with an extensive database to establish organism identification. *ONPG,* Orthonitrophenyl galactoside; *VP, Voges Proskauer.* (API; bioMérieux, Inc., St. Louis, MO.)

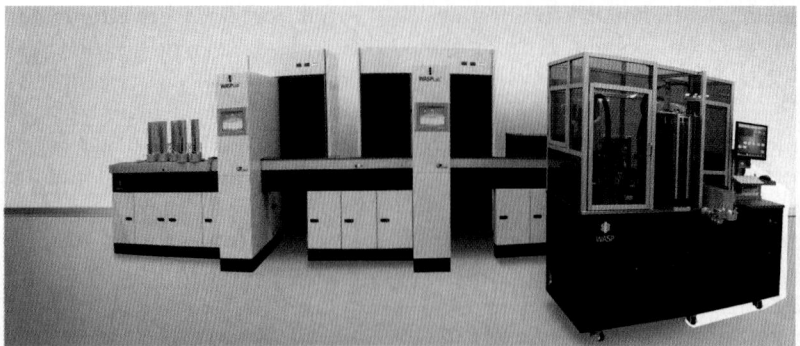

• **Fig. 7.22** Copan WASPLab™ microbiology system. (Photo courtesy of Beckman Coulter, Inc.; Brea, CA.)

specimens. The Copan WASPLab™ Microbiology System is a customizable specimen processor that sets up the cultures, incubates them, and produces high-quality images for review (Fig. 7.22). A variety of samples such as tissues, bone, and catheter tips cannot be processed in an automated system. Furthermore, regardless of the lack or level of automation, the selection of a cultivation and identification system ultimately depends on system accuracy and reliability, whether the system meets the needs of the laboratory, and limitations imposed by laboratory financial resources. Microbiology laboratory automation has demonstrated an average reduction in staffing needs equivalent to 1.2 FTE (full time equivalent).

Despite the technological advances of automated specimen processing, plating, and identification systems, non-automated platforms, kits, and assays are still needed for complex specimens, unusual pathogens, or fastidious organisms that fail to grow. In addition, some clinical isolates of microorganisms may produce a biofilm or be too viscous for the automated instrument, resulting in a failed attempt at identification. The complexity of microbial identification, despite automation, still requires the knowledge and understanding of the microorganism's physiology, genomics, and growth characteristics, as well as laboratory testing methods, identification schemes, and limitations in order to correlate automated results and reactions to ensure proper patient care and treatment.

ⓔ Visit the Evolve site for a complete list of procedures, review questions, and case studies.

Bibliography

Alatoom AA, Cunningham SA, Ihde SM, Mandrekar J, Patel R: Comparison of direct colony method versus extraction method for identification of Gram-positive cocci by use of Bruker Biotype matrix-assisted laser desorption ionization-time of flight mass spectrometry, *J Clin Microbiol* 49:2868, 2011.

Bourbeau PP, Ledeboer NA: Automation in clinical microbiology, *J Clin Microbiol* 51:1658, 2013.

Brink B: *Urease test protocol*, 2013, American Society for Microbiology, Available at: http://www.microbelibrary.org/library/laboratory+test/3223-urease-test-protocol. Accessed 6 July 2015.

Carroll KC, Pfaller MA, Landry ML, et al.: *Manual of clinical microbiology*, ed 12, Washington, DC, 2019, ASM.

Saffert RT, Cunningham SA, Ihde SM, Jobe KE, Mandrekar J, Patel R: Comparison of bruker biotyper matrix-assisted laser desorption ionization-time of flight mass spectrometer to BD phoenix automated microbiology system for identification of gram-negative bacilli, *J Clin Microbiol* 49:887, 2011.

8

Nucleic Acid–Based Analytic Methods for Microbial Identification and Characterization

OBJECTIVES

1. Explain the importance of molecular testing methods in the microbiology laboratory. List the three categories of molecular testing methods and provide a brief explanation of the methodology for each type.
2. Identify at least three factors affecting nucleic acid sample integrity during collection and transport of a molecular specimen.
3. Construct a flow chart describing the workflow and basic steps involved in a nonamplified nucleic acid hybridization method; include the key reagents or components involved and the products for each step.
4. Repeat the flow chart for an amplified hybridization method as indicated in objective 3.
5. Identify the key differences in a nonamplified and amplified nucleic acid hybridization method.
6. Define the characteristics required to design a nucleic acid hybridization probe for the detection of a specific viral or bacterial strain versus detection of a broad category of microorganism.
7. List at least three different functional types of hybridization probe reporter molecules used in nucleic acid–based tests; classify each as either direct or indirect and rank the sensitivity, from lowest to highest, for each type.
8. Predict the melting temperature of a deoxyribonucleic acid (DNA)/DNA hybridized duplex.
9. Explain how the melting temperature of a probe or primer would be affected by a single nucleotide mutation on a target nucleic acid sequence.
10. Explain the methodology for peptide nucleic acid fluorescence *in situ* hybridization (PNA FISH) and provide an example of a clinical application.
11. Compare and contrast the advantages, disadvantages, and outcomes of the three types of nucleic acid extraction techniques.
12. Outline the three major steps in polymerase chain reaction (PCR) and describe the critical parameters of each step, including reagents, temperature, time, and interfering substances.
13. Define reverse transcription polymerase chain reaction (RT-PCR); explain how and why it is used and the methodology that differentiates it from a traditional PCR test.
14. Explain real-time PCR and list the four potential advantages this procedure has over conventional PCR.
15. Describe the benefits and drawbacks of isothermal amplification versus conventional PCR. Identify clinical settings where isothermal methods would be most appropriate.
16. List the factors that limit multiplex capacity in PCR and propose a method or technique to overcome these challenges.
17. Describe how restriction endonucleases are used in epidemiologic applications and strain typing in molecular diagnostics.
18. Define pulsed-field gel electrophoresis (PFGE) and restriction fragment length polymorphism (RFLP) and state an application for each.

The principles of bacterial cultivation and identification discussed in Chapter 7 focus on phenotypic and advanced methods for identification including MALDI-TOF and the use of genotypic systems. The identification and characterization of microorganisms in the laboratory rely on a combination of phenotypic and genotypic techniques. Phenotypic methods use readily observable bacterial traits and characteristics to aid in the identification and characterization of bacterial species. Genotypic techniques rely on the nucleic acid make-up of the organisms. Both types of methods provide information for the detailed identification and characterization of microorganisms, and both have limitations. No single methodology can be used to identify all of the potential infectious microorganisms that are important in the clinical laboratory. Some of the notable limitations associated with the use of phenotypic methods include:

- Inability or an extensive delay in cultivation and identification of fastidious or slowly growing bacteria
- Inability to maintain viability of certain pathogens during transport of specimens to the laboratory
- Lack of reliable and specific methods to identify certain organisms grown *in vitro*
- Use of considerable time and other resources to identify and confirm the presence of pathogens in specimens using culture-based methods

Molecular methods used to identify organisms in the diagnostic microbiology laboratory offer alternatives to the culture-based, phenotypic strategies discussed in Chapter 7 and have evolved to overcome several of the aforementioned limitations. Molecular methods involve the detection and manipulation of nucleic acids (deoxyribonucleic acid [DNA] and ribonucleic acid [RNA]), allowing microbial genes to be examined directly (i.e., genotypic methods) rather than by analysis of their products, such as enzymes, other proteins, and toxins, or identifiable characteristics of organism growth (i.e., phenotypic methods). Because nucleic acids are essential for the viability of all infectious agents, molecular methods are adaptable for the detection of viral, fungal, and parasitic pathogens, in addition to bacterial microorganisms. Key applications of molecular diagnostics in clinical microbiology include the qualitative and quantitative detection of pathogenic organisms in patient specimens, microbial identity testing after culture, negative validation testing, and genotyping for antimicrobial drug resistance. However, as with phenotypic methods, molecular methods also have limitations that include:

- The level of assay specificity and sensitivity; although multiplex assays can be used for the identification of pathogens in clinical syndromes, they are less sensitive than monoplex methods.
- Potential for contamination and false positive results due to environmental and clinical factors.
- Level of complexity for the implementation of advanced testing methodologies and shortage of trained personnel.
- Discriminatory properties; some organisms cannot be fully identified to the species level based on the lack of information and genetic relatedness in the sequences used for characterization.
- Cost of the testing is prohibitory for many laboratories and is increasing health care costs for the patient and insurer.
- Lack of standardization in extraction methods, nucleic acid targets, and specimens across platforms and manufacturer's or laboratory developed tests.
- Overuse in some instances for routine diagnostic testing in lieu of culture-based methods has had a detrimental effect on public health information and epidemiological studies needed to monitor the development of novel strains and antibiotic susceptibility patterns.

In the past several decades, the use of molecular testing in the clinical laboratory has dramatically expanded with the availability of lower-cost instrumentation, automated systems that enable high-throughput testing, and an increasing menu of commercially available reagents and kits for pathogen detection. More recently, fully automated multiplex systems have emerged to detect 20+ pathogens from a single specimen within a few hours or less. With the evolution of these technologies and the high-content information provided, molecular techniques have become a mainstay in the detection and diagnosis of infectious diseases in an attempt to enhance, or even replace, many of the phenotypic methods once widely used in the clinical laboratory. Advancements in molecular methods including whole genome sequencing continue to evolve. These techniques provide the identification and characterization of single microbial pathogens and can be used to characterize polymicrobial populations of organisms on the human body referred to as the microbiome (Chapter 3).

This chapter discusses the general principles, techniques, and applications of molecular diagnostics in the clinical laboratory. It is intended to be an overview; additional methods are included in upcoming chapters.

Overview of Nucleic Acid–Based Methods

Molecular diagnostic tests are based on the consistent and somewhat predictable nature of DNA and RNA; therefore, a basic knowledge regarding the structure of nucleic acids and their composition is essential for understanding nucleic acid-based methods. A review of the section Nucleic Acid Structure and Organization in Chapter 2 is recommended.

The nucleic acid–based methods included in this chapter are classified into one of three categories: (1) **hybridization,** (2) **amplification,** and (3) **sequencing** and **enzymatic digestion** of nucleic acids. Considerations for specimen collection, transport, and initial processing before nucleic acid–based testing is also discussed.

Specimen Collection and Transport

Proper specimen collection, transport, and processing are essential in all areas of the diagnostic laboratory to ensure accurate results. Nucleic acids for molecular testing can be isolated from bacterial, parasitic, viral, and fungal pathogens found in a wide variety of specimen types from virtually any anatomic site, such as blood, urine, sputum, swabs, and tissues. The quality and quantity of the specimen is essential to obtaining an accurate result and must be matched to the molecular diagnostic technique that is clinically relevant in relationship to the patient's disease state.

Unlike traditional culture, nucleic acid–based testing does not always require the detection of viable or intact organisms. However, maintaining the integrity of the nucleic acids within the sample is of utmost importance, because DNA and RNA are inherently sensitive to degradation by endogenous nucleases present in specimens. Factors that may affect the integrity of the sample include specimen type, specimen collection device, and timing of collection and transport, and storage conditions. For example, plastic swabs are recommended for collection of bacteria, viruses, and mycoplasmas from mucosal membranes. The organisms are more easily removed from the plastic shafts than from other materials such as wooden shafts or wire. This provides an increase in nucleic acid yield, thereby increasing analytical sensitivity of the molecular test. In addition, calcium alginate swabs with aluminum shafts have been reported to interfere with the amplification of nucleic acids. Most molecular test kits include transport containers that contain liquid fixatives, nuclease inhibitors, and/or lysing agents to improve nucleic acid isolation and improve yield from specimens that contain cellular debris or other contaminants. In molecular diagnostics, it is essential that the specimen be collected and stored in the recommended container or medium as indicated by the manufacturer of each individual assay.

Nucleic Acid Hybridization Methods

Hybridization methods are based on the ability of two nucleic acid strands with **complementary** base sequences to bond specifically with each other and form a double-stranded molecule, also called a **duplex** or **hybrid.** This duplex formation is driven by the hydrophobic structure and hydrogen bonding pattern of the nucleotides, which ensure that, in DNA, the base adenine always bonds to thymine (A = T; two hydrogen bonds), whereas the bases guanine and cytosine (G ≡ G; three hydrogen bonds) always form a bonding pair (Fig. 2.2). In RNA, the same base pairing rules follow for guanine and cytosine, but uracil replaces thymine to form a base pair with adenine (A = U).

To identify the presence of an organism suspected of causing disease, hybridization assays rely upon duplex formation between two nucleic acid strands; one strand (the **probe**) consists of a reporter-labeled nucleic acid molecule that is complementary to a nucleic acid target of a suspected pathogen. The carefully designed and pre-synthesized probe is mixed with nucleic acids purified from the patient specimen (**target** nucleic acids). If nucleic acids from the suspected pathogen are present in the patient specimen, a DNA duplex will form between the probe and target molecule, resulting in a positive hybridization signal (Fig. 8.1). A negative hybridization test result indicates that the organism being

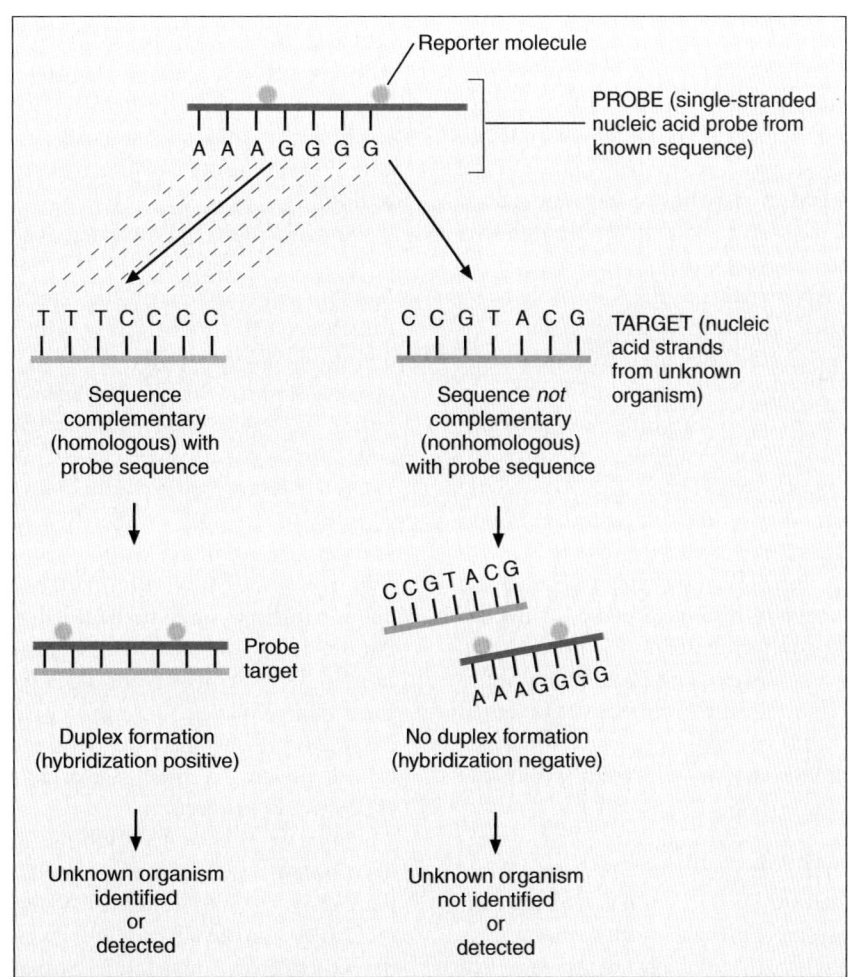

• **Fig. 8.1** Principles of nucleic acid hybridization. Identification of an unknown organism is established by positive hybridization (i.e., duplex formation) between a nucleic acid strand from the known sequence (i.e., the probe) and a target nucleic acid strand from the organism to be identified. Failure to hybridize indicates lack of homology between the probe and the target nucleic acid.

tested for is either not present or below the **limit of detection** for the hybridization test.

Single-stranded nucleic acid probes may be either RNA or DNA; therefore, DNA-DNA, DNA-RNA, and even RNA-RNA duplexes may form depending on the specific design of the hybridization assay. Hybridization assays may be classified as either nonamplified or amplified. A nonamplified assay requires four basic steps: selection of a probe, preparation (purification) of the test sample (nucleic acid), hybridization, and signal detection. Amplified assays include an additional step, whereby initial hybridization is followed by target amplification, and then by signal detection. As such, amplified assays are inherently more sensitive than nonamplified assays and, when optimized, can detect as few as one copy of a specific nucleic acid sequence in the specimen.

Hybridization Steps and Components

The basic steps in a hybridization assay include:
1. Production and labeling of single-stranded nucleic acid probe
2. Preparation of single-stranded target nucleic acid
3. Mixture and hybridization of target and probe nucleic acid
4. Detection of hybridization

Production and Labeling of Nucleic Acid Probe

In keeping with the requirement of **complementarity** for hybridization, the probe design (i.e., probe length and the sequence of nucleic acid bases) depends on the sequence of the intended target nucleic acid. Most clinically relevant pathogen sequences are known. Probes can be designed to recognize unique species/strain-specific sequences using public sequence databases such as the National Center for Biotechnology Information (NCBI) and custom primer design tools from companies like Integrated DNA Technologies (IDT). Furthermore, since similarities between base sequences in DNA/RNA are an indication of evolutionary relationships among organisms (i.e., homology) hybridization probes can be designed to recognize common sequences using highly conserved genes/regions to identify closely related microorganisms. For example, if a probe is to be used to recognize only gram-positive bacteria, its nucleic acid sequence must be complementary to a nucleic acid sequence common only to gram-positive bacteria and not to gram-negative bacteria. Nucleic acid probes can be designed to identify a particular bacterial genus or species, a virulence factor, or an antibiotic-resistance gene present within the genome of a given species.

Historically, probes were produced through a labor-intensive process involving recombinant DNA and cloning techniques with the nucleic acid sequence of interest. DNA and RNA probes are now chemically synthesized, modified, and purified with extreme high fidelity and yield by many commercial vendors at a relatively low cost. The base sequence of potential target genes, sequence patterns, or gene fragments for probe design are easily accessed using online sequence databases (e.g., GENBANK, National Center for Biological Information). Although probes may be hundreds to thousands of bases long, **oligonucleotide probes** (i.e., those 15 to 50 bases long) usually are sufficient for detection of most clinically relevant targets. Other considerations in probe design include stability during storage (i.e., shelf life), formation of secondary structures, melting temperature, and tendency to self-hybridize. In short, the design and production of nucleic acid probes is relatively easy but remains critical to the overall success and accuracy of nucleic acid–based assays.

In addition to probe design, all hybridization tests must have a means to detect or measure the hybridization reaction, directly or indirectly. This is accomplished with the use of a **reporter molecule** attached directly to the single-stranded nucleic acid probe. Common reporter molecules include radioactive isotopes (e.g., 32P, 3H, 125I, or 35S), biotin-avidin, digoxigenin, a variety of fluorescent molecules, or chemiluminescent compounds (Fig. 8.2).

Radioactive labels are directly incorporated into the nucleic acid molecules during probe synthesis. With the use of radioactively labeled probes, hybridization is detected by the emission of radioactivity from the probe-target complex (Fig. 8.2A). Quantification of the complexes may be achieved through scintillation counting or densitometry. Although this is a highly sensitive method for detecting hybridization, the requirements for radioactive training, monitoring, licensing, and disposal of radioactive waste have limited the use of radioactive labeling in the diagnostic setting.

Nonradioactive alternatives for labeling nucleic acid probes involve the covalent attachment of a reporter molecule to the probe using a chemical coupling reaction. Attachment of biotin (i.e., "biotinylation") enables the detection of target-probe duplexes using a biotin-binding protein, avidin, which is conjugated to an enzyme, such as horseradish peroxidase. When a chromogenic substrate is added, the enzyme catalyzes a chemical reaction, producing a colored product that can be detected visually or spectrophotometrically (Fig. 8.2B). Biotin labels are classified as indirect because of the requirement for a secondary biotin-avidin–enzyme complex formation for detection. Variations on this **indirect enzyme-based detection** scheme include the use of digoxigenin-labeled probes, in which hybridization is detected using antidigoxigenin antibodies conjugated to an enzyme. Successful duplex formation means the enzyme is present; therefore, with the addition of a chromogenic substrate a color change or development is interpreted as positive hybridization.

Fluorescent and chemiluminescent reporter molecules have become widely used in molecular diagnostics rather than enzyme-based reporters. Chemiluminescent reporter molecules can be chemically linked directly (i.e., **direct detection**) to the nucleic acid probe without using a conjugated protein or antibody. These molecules (e.g., acridinium or isoluminol) emit light during hybridization between the chemiluminescent-labeled probe and target nucleic acid.

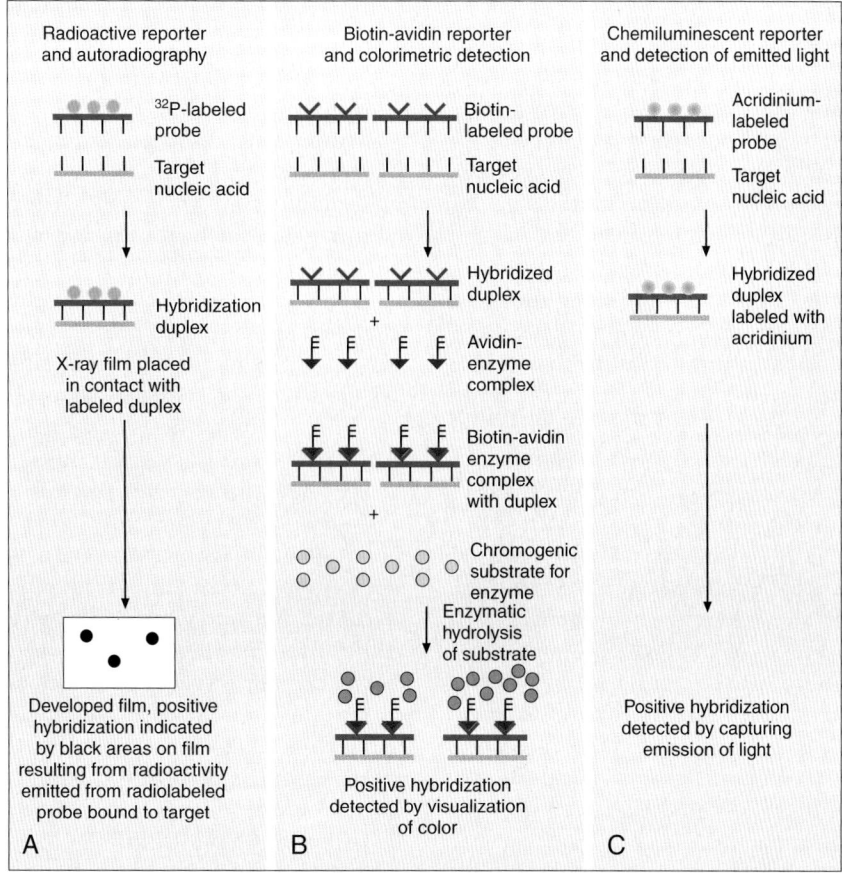

• **Fig. 8.2** (A) Reporter molecule labeling of nucleic acid probes and principles of hybridization detection. Use of probes labeled with a radioactive reporter, with hybridization detected by autoradiography. (B) Probes labeled with a biotin-avidin reporter, with hybridization detected by a colorimetric assay. (C) Probes labeled with a chemiluminescent reporter (i.e., acridinium), with hybridization detected by a luminometer to detect emitted light.

The light is detected using a luminometer (Fig. 8.2C). Fluorescent labels and fluorometric reporter groups (e.g., fluorescein, rhodamine, or proprietary dyes such as the Alexa-Fluor series) are also considered direct nucleic acid probes and are available in a range of wavelengths and colors.

These methods have also enabled the detection of multiple nucleic acid targets using a cocktail of probes, each attached to a different fluorophore whose excitation and emission wavelengths are spectrally separated. This process, known as **multiplexing,** increases the number of pathogens that can be detected simultaneously in a single reaction. Direct probe hybridization assays generally have poor analytical sensitivity in comparison to amplified probe techniques. Therefore, direct hybridization assays are generally used in clinical situations where the number of organisms are large.

Preparation of Target Nucleic Acid

Because hybridization is dependent on complementary binding between the probe and target, the target nucleic acid must be present as a single strand and the base sequence integrity must be maintained. Failure to meet these requirements can result in negative hybridization reactions (i.e.,

false-negative results) due to target degradation, insufficient target yield, and/or the presence of interfering substances such as organic chemicals.

Because the relatively rigorous procedures needed to release nucleic acids from the target microorganism can be deleterious to the DNA/RNA molecule's structure, obtaining the target nucleic acid and maintaining its appropriate conformation and sequence can be challenging. The steps in target preparation vary, depending on the organism source and the nature of the environment from which the target organism is being prepared (laboratory culture media; fresh clinical specimens, such as bodily fluids, tissue, stool, or mucosal swabs; fixed or preserved clinical material). Generally, target preparation involves enzymatic and/or chemical destruction of the tissue and microbial envelope to release target nucleic acids, the removal of contaminating molecules such as cellular components (protein), stabilization of the target nucleic acid to preserve structural integrity, and, if the target is DNA, denaturation to a single strand, which is necessary for binding the complementary nucleic acid. Nucleic acid extraction procedures are optimized to ensure a high degree of purity, integrity, and yield of the desired nucleic acid.

Two primary physical methods are available for nucleic acid extraction: **liquid-phase extraction** and **solid-phase extraction.** Nucleic acid extractions via the liquid-phase may be classified as **organic** or **nonorganic extractions.** Organic extractions employ phenol, chloroform, or isoamyl alcohol to disrupt the cellular membranes, denature, and remove proteins. After chemical treatment with the organic solution, the mixture is centrifuged, which results in the separation or phasing of the cellular material layered over the top of the organic molecules and waste along the bottom of the tube. The **aqueous phase,** containing the desired nucleic acid, is then extracted from the **organic phase,** and the resulting nucleic acid is precipitated using a buffered solution. Nonorganic extractions rely on protein precipitations and nucleic acid precipitations without the use of organic chemicals. Cell membranes and proteins are denatured with a detergent, and the proteins are precipitated with a salt solution. Nonorganic extractions are primarily used in clinical laboratories because they are fast, are easy, and do not require the disposal of hazardous organic materials.

Solid-phase extractions use solid support columns constructed of fibrous or silica matrices, magnetic beads, or chelating agents to bind the nucleic acids. After impurities are removed, the nucleic acids are chemically released and recovered for analysis or amplification. Solid-phase extractions are typically simpler than liquid-phase extractions, requiring less sample volume and providing for ease of operation, processing of large batches, high reproducibility, and adaptability to automation.

Regardless of extraction method chosen, DNA isolation tends to not be as technically demanding as RNA extraction. RNA may be degraded rapidly by the presence of RNase enzymes. **RNase enzymes** are very stable, ubiquitous in the environment, and elevated in certain tissues, such as the placenta, liver, and some tumors. The inadvertent introduction of RNase enzymes into specimens during RNA purification will result in low or no RNA yield and render the molecular test invalid. To minimize RNA degradation, a dedicated laboratory space, or clean bench isolation chamber is recommended for RNA manipulation. RNase-free reagents, water, pipette tips, etc., must be used. **Guanidinium isothiocyanate** can be used to denature and inactivate RNase enzymes to preserve nucleic acid samples but must be removed before most downstream hybridization reactions. Additional clean-up steps may be needed such as buffer exchange or size-exclusion chromatography.

Mixture and Hybridization of Target and Probe

Designs for mixing target and probe nucleic acids are discussed later, but some general concepts regarding the hybridization reaction require consideration.

The ability of the probe to bind the correct target depends on the extent of base sequence identity between the two nucleic acid strands and the environment in which the probe and target are brought together. Environmental conditions set the **stringency** for a hybridization reaction,

and the degree of stringency can determine the outcome of the reaction. Hybridization stringency is most affected by:

- Salt concentration in the hybridization buffer (stringency increases as salt concentration decreases)
- Temperature (stringency increases as temperature increases)
- Concentration of destabilizing agents (stringency increases with increasing concentrations of formamide or urea)

With greater stringency, a higher degree of base-pair complementarity is required between the probe and target to obtain successful hybridization (i.e., less tolerance for deviations in base sequence). Under less stringent conditions, strands with less base-pair complementarity (i.e., strands with a higher number of mismatched base pairs within the sequence) may still hybridize. Therefore, as stringency increases, the specificity of hybridization increases and as stringency decreases, specificity decreases. For example, under high stringency a probe specific for a target sequence in *Streptococcus pneumoniae* may only bind to the target prepared from this species (high specificity), but under low stringency the same probe may also bind to targets from closely related streptococcal species (lower specificity). Therefore, to ensure accuracy in hybridization, reaction conditions must be carefully controlled.

Detection of Hybridization

The method of detecting hybridization depends on the reporter molecule used for labeling the probe nucleic acid and on the hybridization format (Fig. 8.2). Traditionally, hybridization probes used radioactively labeled reporters and visualized after the reaction mixture was exposed to radiographic film (i.e., **autoradiography**). Today, hybridization with nonradioactively labeled probes is preferred with detection achieved via colorimetry, fluorescence, or **chemiluminescence,** and quantified using spectrophotometer, fluorometer, or luminometer instruments, respectively. The more commonly used nonradioactive detection systems (e.g., digoxigenin, chemiluminescence, fluorescence) are able to detect approximately 10^4 target nucleic acid sequences per nonamplified hybridization reaction.

Hybridization Formats

Hybridization reactions can be performed using either a liquid or solid support format.

Liquid Format

In the liquid format, probe and target nucleotide strands are placed in a liquid reaction mixture that is constantly but gently shaken to facilitate molecular collisions and duplex formation; hybridization occurs substantially faster than with a solid support format. However, before duplex formation can be detected, the hybridized labeled probes must be separated from the unbound or nonhybridized probes (i.e., "background noise"). Separation methods include enzymatic digestion (e.g., S1 nuclease) of single-stranded probes and precipitation of hybridized duplexes, use of hydroxyapatite or charged magnetic microparticles that preferentially bind duplexes, or chemical destruction of the reporter molecule (e.g., acridinium dye) attached to the nonhybridized probe nucleic acid. After the duplexes have been "purified" from the reaction mixture and the background noise minimized, hybridization detection can proceed by the method appropriate for the type of reporter molecule used to label the probe. Several direct solution-phase methods are available to detect microorganisms such as *Chlamydia trachomatis, Neisseria gonorrhoeae,* and *Streptococcus pyogenes* (Figs. 8.3 and 8.4).

Solid Support Format

Either the probe or target nucleic acids may be attached to a solid support matrix and still be capable of forming hybridized duplexes with complementary strands. Common solid support materials/formats include filter hybridizations, southern or northern hybridizations, sandwich hybridizations, and *in situ* hybridizations.

Filter (membrane) hybridization has several variations that are collectively referred to as "dot blots." Here the target sample, which can be purified DNA, the microorganism containing the target DNA, or the clinical specimen containing the microorganism of interest, is affixed to a membrane material with high binding capacity (e.g.,

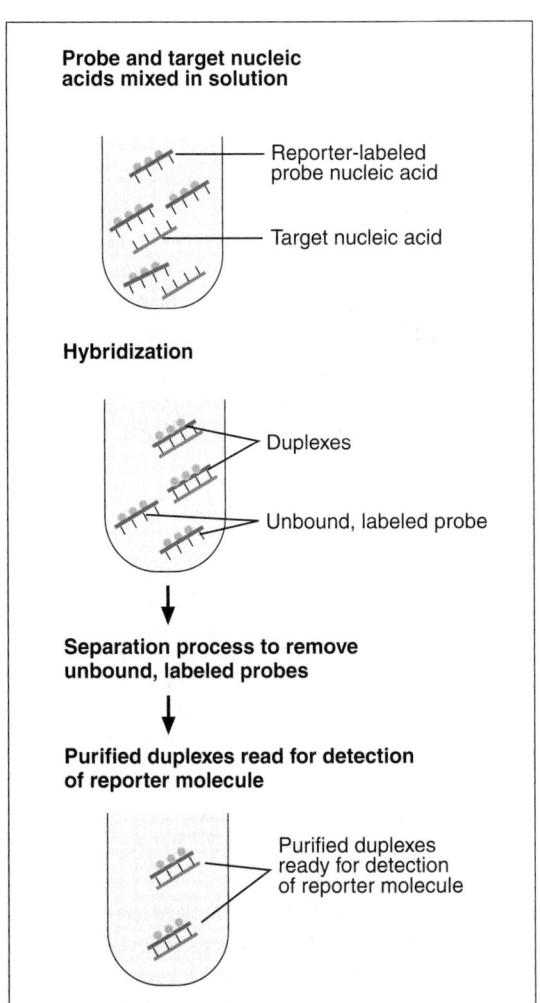

• **Fig. 8.3** Principle of the solution hybridization format.

nitrocellulose or nylon fiber filters). To identify specimens, samples are usually oriented on the membrane using a template or grid. The membrane is chemically treated, causing release of the target DNA from the microorganism and denaturing the nucleic acid to single strands. The membrane is then submerged in a solution containing the labeled nucleic acid probe and incubated (typically for 30 minutes to several hours), allowing hybridization to occur. After a series of incubations and washings to remove unbound probe, the membrane is processed for detection of duplexes (Fig. 8.5A). An advantage of this method is that a single membrane can hold several samples for exposure to the same probe. Disadvantages of this method include lengthy incubation and washing periods, the significant hands-on time needed, and the limited quantitative capacity.

Southern hybridization is another method that uses membranes as the solid support. In this instance the nucleic acid target is purified from the organisms and digested with specific enzymes to produce several fragments of various sizes (Fig. 8.5B) (also see Enzymatic Digestion and Electrophoresis of Nucleic Acids later in this chapter). The nucleic acid fragments, which carry a net negative charge, are subjected to an electrical field, forcing them to migrate through an agarose gel matrix (i.e., **gel electrophoresis**). Because fragments of different sizes migrate through the porous agarose at different rates, they can be separated by molecular size and kilobase length. When electrophoresis is complete, the nucleic acid fragments are stained, typically with the fluorescent dye **ethidium bromide** or other less-toxic stains, so that fragment "banding patterns" can be visualized on exposure of the gel to ultraviolet (UV) light. For southern hybridization, the target nucleic acid bands are transferred from the electrophoretic gel to a membrane that is then submerged in a buffer solution, allowing for hybridization of the nucleic acid probe. After hybridization, the membrane is analyzed to detect and quantify the specific target nucleic acid fragment using the probe signal. The complexity, time, and labor intensity of this procedure precludes its common use in the clinical diagnostic laboratory.

With **sandwich hybridizations,** two probes are used. One unlabeled probe is attached to the solid support, and "captures" the target nucleic acid from the sample to be tested via hybridization. The presence of this duplex is then detected using a second, labeled probe that is specific for another region of the target sequence (Fig. 8.5C). Sandwiching the target between two probes decreases nonspecific reactions but requires a greater number of processing and washing steps. For such formats, plastic microtiter wells coated with probes have replaced filters as the solid support material, thereby facilitating the automation and high-throughput testing of a large number of specimens.

In Situ Hybridization

In situ **hybridization** (*in situ* meaning "in place" or "in position") allows a pathogen to be identified from a specimen using the patient's cells or tissues as the solid support phase. Tissue specimens thought to be infected with a

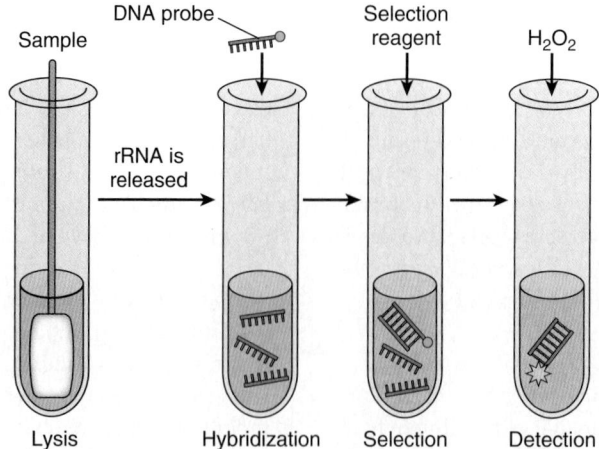

• **Fig. 8.4** The GEN-PROBE Group A streptococcus direct test uses nucleic acid solution hybridization for the qualitative detection of Group A streptococcal ribosomal RNA *(rRNA)* from throat swabs. (Adapted from teaching materials, courtesy Jim Flanigan, American Society for Clinical Laboratory Science.)

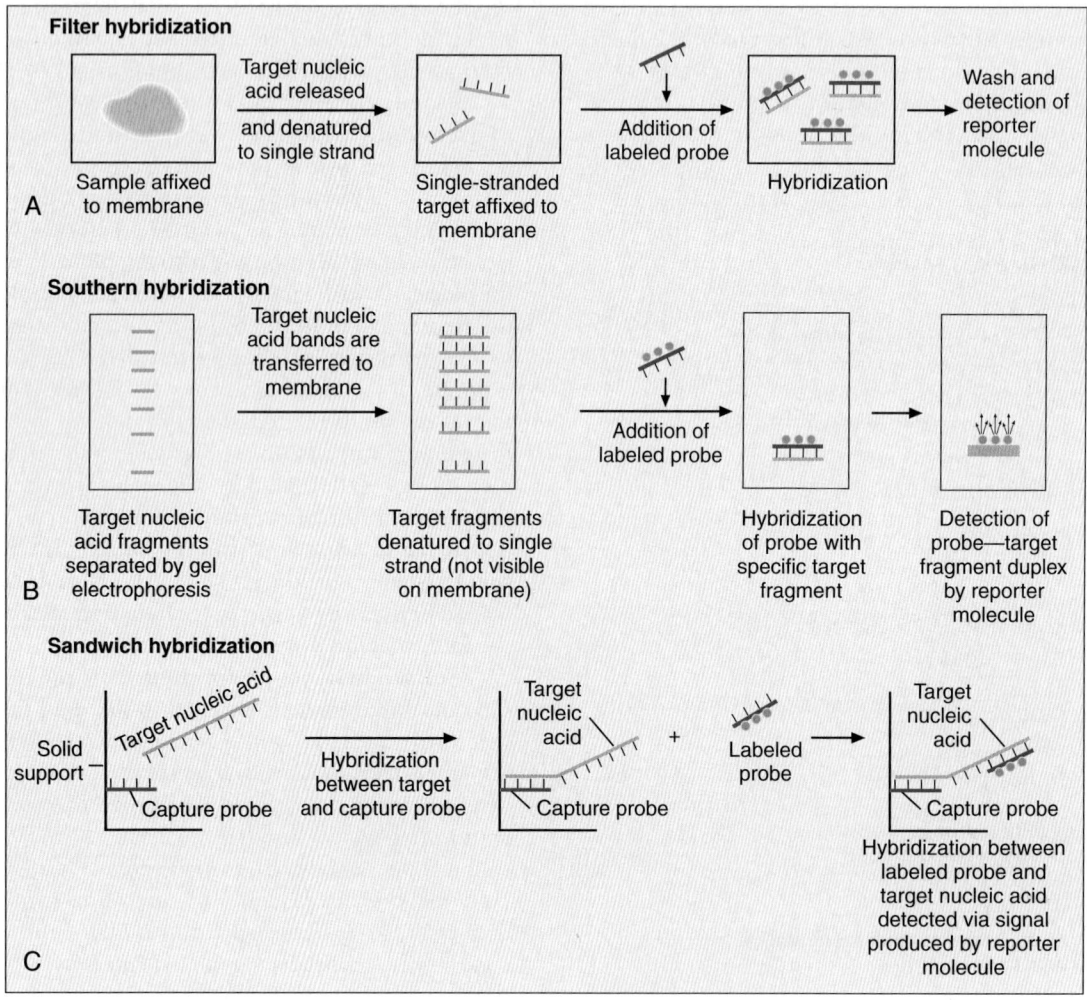

• **Fig. 8.5** Principle of solid support hybridization formats. (A) Filter hybridization. (B) Southern hybridization. (C) Sandwich hybridization.

particular pathogen are processed in a manner that maintains the structural integrity of the tissue and cells, yet allows the nucleic acid of the pathogen to be accessed *in situ* and denatured to a single strand with the base sequence intact for hybridization with the pathogen-specific probe.

When the probe is attached to a fluorescent molecule, this hybridization technique is known as **fluorescence *in situ* hybridization (FISH).** Although the processing steps can be technically demanding, this method can be extremely informative, because it combines the power of molecular diagnostics with the additional information provided through histopathologic examination.

Peptide Nucleic Acid Fluorescence *In Situ* Hybridization

A variant of the FISH method replaces standard DNA or RNA nucleic acids with a synthetic **peptide nucleic acid (PNA) probe.** PNAs are synthetic nucleic acids that have unique chemical characteristics in which the negatively charged sugar-phosphate backbone of DNA is replaced by a neutral polyamide backbone (Fig. 8.6). Individual nucleotide bases can be attached to this neutral backbone, which then allows the PNA probe to hybridize with complementary nucleic acid targets according to the standard base pairing rules (A-T/U; C-G). However, because of the synthetic structure of the backbone, PNA probes have improved hybridization characteristics, providing faster and more specific results than traditional DNA/RNA probes. In addition, because these probes are not degraded by nucleases and proteases, they offer a longer shelf life in diagnostic applications.

An example of *in vitro* diagnostic PNA FISH assays that are approved by the US Food and Drug Administration (FDA) is one available from AdvanDx (Woburn, MA). These kits can be used to directly identify *Staphylococcus aureus,* coagulase-negative staphylococci, *Pseudomonas aeruginosa, Klebsiella pneumoniae,* and *Candida albicans* and to differentiate *Enterococcus faecalis* from other enterococci in blood cultures. In brief, a drop from a positive blood culture bottle is added to a slide containing a drop of fixative solution. After fixation, the fluorescent-labeled PNA probe is added and allowed to hybridize with purified RNA from a patient specimen; the slides are then washed and air dried. After the addition of a mounting medium and a coverslip, the slides are examined under a fluorescent microscope using a special filter set. Identification is based on the presence of bright green, fluorescent-staining organisms (Fig. 8.7A and B). For negative results, only slightly red-stained background material is observed (Fig. 8.7C and D). Collectively, these methods have demonstrated high sensitivity and specificity for pathogen detection.

Hybridization With Signal Amplification

To increase the sensitivity of hybridization assays, methods have been developed to amplify the probe signal (i.e., **signal amplification**) without amplification of the target sequence. For example, one commercially available kit uses genotype-specific RNA probes in a cocktail to detect either a high-risk or a low-risk human papillomavirus (HPV) DNA in clinical specimens (Chapter 65). Essentially, sensitivity of HPV detection by hybridization is increased by multimeric layering of reporter molecules, increasing their number on an antibody directed toward DNA-RNA hybrids using chemiluminescence; thus sensitivity of detection is enhanced by virtue of greater signal produced (i.e., chemiluminescence) for each antibody bound to the target hybrids.

Molecular diagnostic methods that use signal amplification include **branched DNA (bDNA), hybrid capture,**

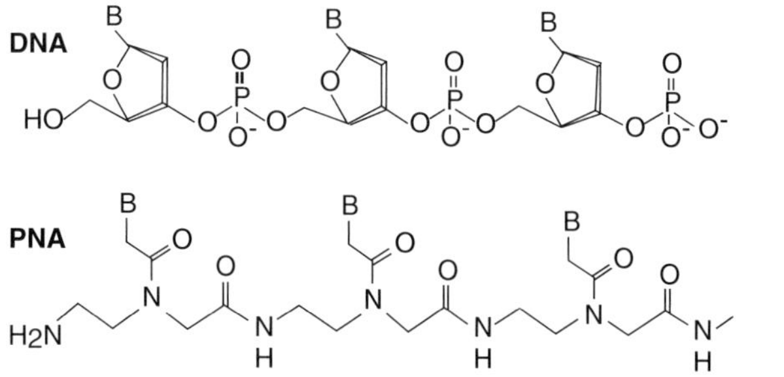

• **Fig. 8.6** Peptide nucleic acid probes. The structure of deoxyribonucleic acid *(DNA)* is compared with the structure of a synthetic peptide nucleic acid *(PNA)* probe; the chemical modification of DNA allows for greater sensitivity and specificity of the PNA probes compared with the DNA probes. (Courtesy AdvanDx, Woburn, MA.)

and cleavase-invader or **isothermal** (constant temperature) cycling probe technology. In bDNA, a target-specific probe is attached to a substrate such as a microtiter well. The complementary target is captured by hybridization to the capture probe. In addition, the assay may contain a second set of target-specific probes in solution that will also bind to the target to increase the capture of the target and enhance binding to the anchored probes attached to the substrate. Washing of the complexed target and probes removes any unbound nucleic acids. An amplifier molecule added to the assay will then bind to the target-probe complexes. The amplifier molecule is designed similar to a tree trunk, with multiple branches extending from the trunk. The multiple branches are modified with a reporter molecule, such as an enzyme substrate that will emit light after addition of the enzyme, producing a characteristic emission of light that indicates the presence of bound target nucleic acid.

Nonspecific hybridization may also occur using bDNA as previously discussed for general hybridization techniques. In bDNA methods, nonspecific hybridization of the probes or nontarget sequences present in the sample may lead to an amplification of the background. **Isocytidine (isoC)** and **isoguanosine (isoG)** have been used to reduce background. These chemically altered isomers can be incorporated into the bDNA probes and will base pair with each other, but not with the naturally occurring cytosine and guanosine. This reduces the potential for background signal and increases the detection limits without reducing specificity.

Hybrid capture differs from bDNA assays in that the hybridization occurs in solution using nucleic acid–specific probes followed by a bound universal capture antibody. Here, the target nucleic acid is denatured, separating double-stranded DNA molecules. The denatured nucleic acids are then hybridized with a target-specific RNA probe. The DNA-RNA hybrids are captured with an anti-hybrid antibody that contains a chemiluminescent reporter molecule (i.e., alkaline phosphatase). The light emitted is then measured using a luminometer. Varieties of hybrid capture assays are FDA-approved for the detection of *C. trachomatis, N. gonorrhoeae,* and HPV (Qiagen, Germantown, MD).

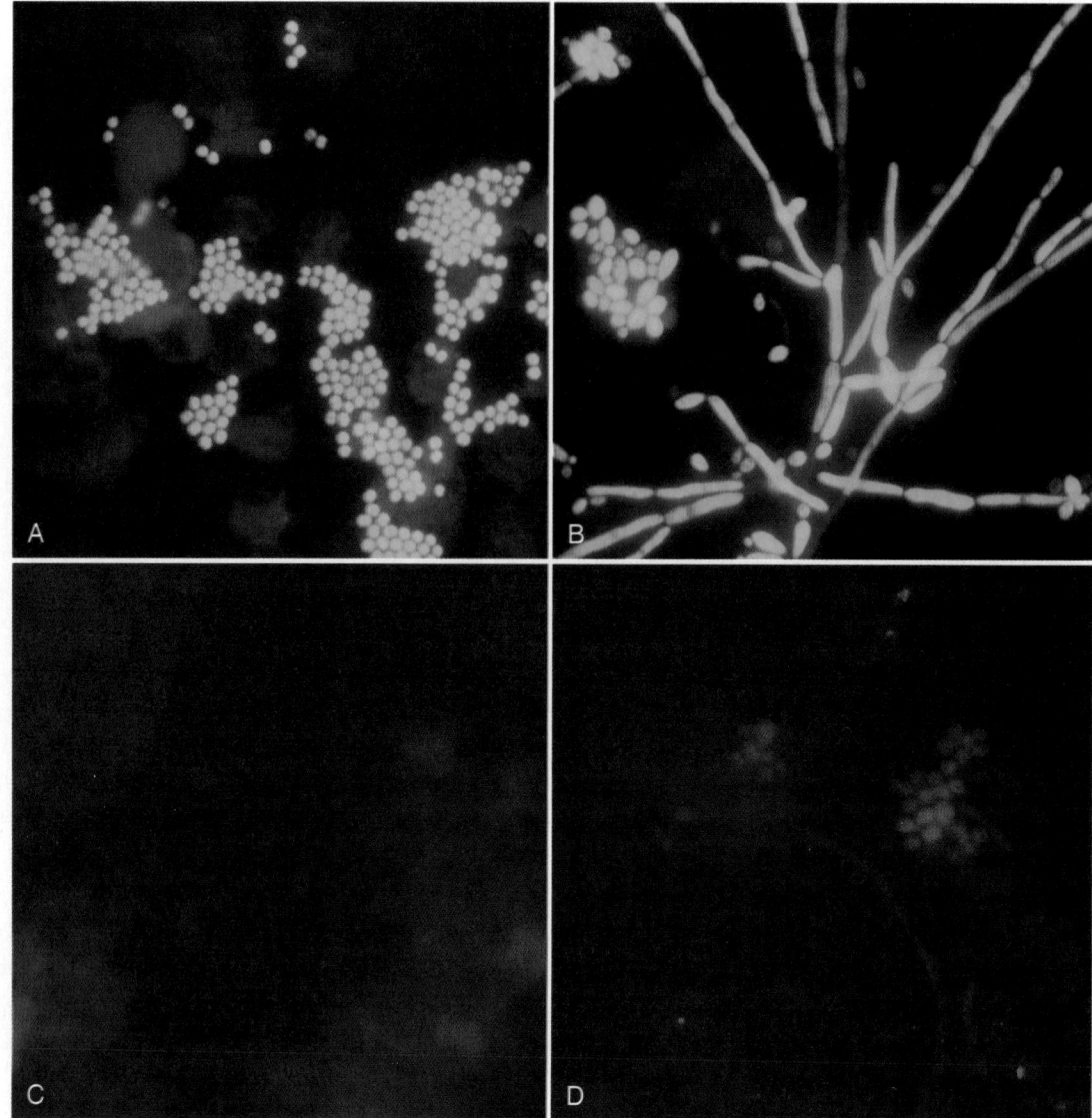

• **Fig. 8.7** Using a fluorescent-tagged peptide nucleic acid (PNA) probe in conjunction with fluorescence *in situ* hybridization (FISH), *Staphylococcus aureus* (A), or *Candida albicans* (B) can be directly identified in blood cultures. A drop from the positive blood culture bottle is added to a slide containing a drop of fixative solution, which keeps the cells intact. After fixation, the appropriate fluorescent-labeled PNA probe is added. The PNA probe penetrates the microbial cell wall and hybridizes to the ribosomal RNA (rRNA). Slides are examined under a fluorescent microscope. If the specific target is present, bright green, fluorescent-staining organisms are present. Blood cultures negative for either *S. aureus* (C) or *C. albicans* (D) by PNA FISH technology are shown for comparison. (Courtesy AdvanDx, Woburn, MA.)

Cleavase-invader technology (Hologic, Bedford, MA) uses the enzymatic cleavage of a DNA structure by a specific DNA polymerase referred to as **cleavase.** The method uses two probes that hybridize to the target sequence. The signal probe hybridizes to the specific target, followed by the invader probe that will dislodge the 5′ end of the signal probe. The cleavase then enzymatically removes the free, dangling 5′ region of the signal probe. This product then becomes the invader probe for the subsequent hybridization and detection reaction. This is accomplished using a fluorescent energy transfer (FRET) probe that includes a reporter molecule and a **quencher molecule.** The specific chemical design of a probe using FRET is discussed in more detail later in this chapter. The FRET probe is designed so that the two fluorescent molecules, the reporter and quencher, are incorporated into the probe. As long as the probe remains intact, the quencher prevents the release of a high fluorescent signal by the reporter. Once the cleaved product from the first reaction is released, it becomes the invader probe, and the reporter molecule is cleaved from the quencher, resulting in a fluorescent signal. This technology relies on the hybridization and formation of the initial probe-target duplex for the formation of substrate for the cleavase. Without the formation of the specific hybridization structure, there is no cleaving of the probe and no secondary reaction occurs, indicating the target is not present.

Similar to the invader technology, **cycling probe technology** uses a DNA-RNA combination probe that includes a fluorescent reporter and a quencher molecule. The probe is designed with an RNA sequence in the center of two flanking DNA sequences that contain the reporter and quencher molecules. Using the appropriate denaturing and hybridization conditions, the probe hybridizes to the single-stranded DNA target. Once hybridized, **RNase H,** a highly specific RNA degrading enzyme that is active only in the presence of DNA-RNA hybrids, cleaves or degrades the RNA portion of the probe. This reaction releases the two flanking DNA regions of the probe, separating the quencher molecule from the reporter molecule and resulting in a fluorescent signal. As the reaction continues, additional probes will bind, become degraded, and the fluorescent signal will increase over time. As with the previous signal-enhancing methods, the presence of the target leads to the formation of a specific structure and activation of the signal, indicating a positive reaction. While often used alone, signal amplification strategies may be coupled with target amplification methods, discussed in the next section, to further improve assay sensitivity and detection limits.

Amplification Methods—Polymerase Chain Reaction–Based

Although hybridization methods are highly specific for organism detection and identification, they are limited by their sensitivity; that is, without sufficient target nucleic acid (large numbers of organisms) in the reaction, false-negative results can occur. Hybridization methods may require "amplifying" of a target nucleic acid by growing target organisms in enrichment broths prior to detection. The requirement for growth enrichment greatly diminishes the potential of molecular diagnostics to provide faster detection and identification of the organism. Undoubtedly, it has been the development of sequence-specific **amplification techniques** that do not rely on organism multiplication that have unlocked the true potential of molecular diagnostics for rapid, highly specific and sensitive detection of clinically relevant microorganisms. For purposes of discussion, amplification methods are divided into two major categories: methods that use polymerase chain reaction (PCR) technology, and methods that are not PCR-based.

Overview of Polymerase Chain Reaction and Derivations

The most widely used target nucleic acid amplification method is the **PCR.** This method combines the principles of complementary nucleic acid hybridization with those of nucleic acid replication applied repeatedly through numerous cycles. This method is able to exponentially amplify a single copy of a nucleic acid target, undetectable by standard hybridization methods, to 107 or more copies in a relatively short period. This provides ample target that can be readily detected by a variety of existing methods.

Conventional PCR involves as few as 20 to 50 repetitive cycles, with each cycle comprising three sequential reactions: **denaturation** of the target nucleic acid, primer **annealing** (i.e., hybridizing) to single-stranded target nucleic acid, and **extension** of the primer-target duplex.

Extraction and Denaturation of the Target Nucleic Acid

For PCR, nucleic acid is first **extracted** (released) from the organism or a clinical sample using heat, chemical, or enzymatic methods. As discussed earlier in this chapter, numerous liquid-phase and solid-phase methods are available to accomplish this task, including a variety of commercially available kits that extract total nucleic acids or either DNA/RNA, depending on the specific target of interest. Other commercially available kits are designed to extract nucleic acids from specific types of clinical specimens, such as blood or tissues. Most recently, automated instruments employing magnetic beads or other solid-phase extraction methods and fluid dispensing robotics (such as the Roche MagNa Pure 96, Beckman Coulter SPRI-TE nucleic acid extractor, and Qiagen QIAcube/QIAsymphony product lines) have been introduced to extract nucleic acid from various sources. These automated instruments streamline the molecular diagnostic workflow and significantly increase throughput for nucleic acid–based testing.

Once extracted, nucleic acids are added to the **reaction mix** containing all the necessary components for PCR (primers, nucleotides, covalent ions, buffer, and enzymes) and placed into a thermal cycler to undergo amplification (Fig. 8.8). Before PCR begins, the target nucleic acid must be in the single-stranded conformation so that the second reaction, primer annealing, can occur. Denaturation to a single strand, which is not necessary for RNA targets, is accomplished by heating to 94°C (Fig. 8.8).

Primer Annealing

Primers are short, single-stranded sequences of nucleic acid (i.e., oligonucleotides usually 20 to 30 nucleotides long) selected to hybridize specifically to a particular nucleic acid target, essentially functioning like hybridization probes described above but without the inclusion of a reporter molecule. As noted for hybridization tests, the abundance of available gene sequence data allows for the design of primers specific for a number of microbial pathogens and their virulence or antibiotic resistance genes. Thus, primer nucleotide sequences are designed to match the intended unique nucleotide sequence target that may include genus-specific genes, species-specific genes, genes encoding virulence factors, or antibiotic-resistance genes.

Unlike hybridization probes, PCR primers are designed in pairs that flank the target sequence of interest (Fig. 8.8). When the primer pair is mixed with the denatured target DNA, one primer anneals to a specific site at one end of the target sequence and the other primer anneals to a specific site at the opposite end of the other, complementary target strand. Usually primers are designed to amplify an internal target nucleic acid sequence ranging between 50 and 1000 base pairs; however, longer sequences (>5kb) can be amplified using commercially available polymerases other than *Taq* (described below). The annealing process is typically conducted at 50°C to 58°C or higher but is optimized according to the nucleic acid sequences of the primers and the target based upon the predicted melting temperature.

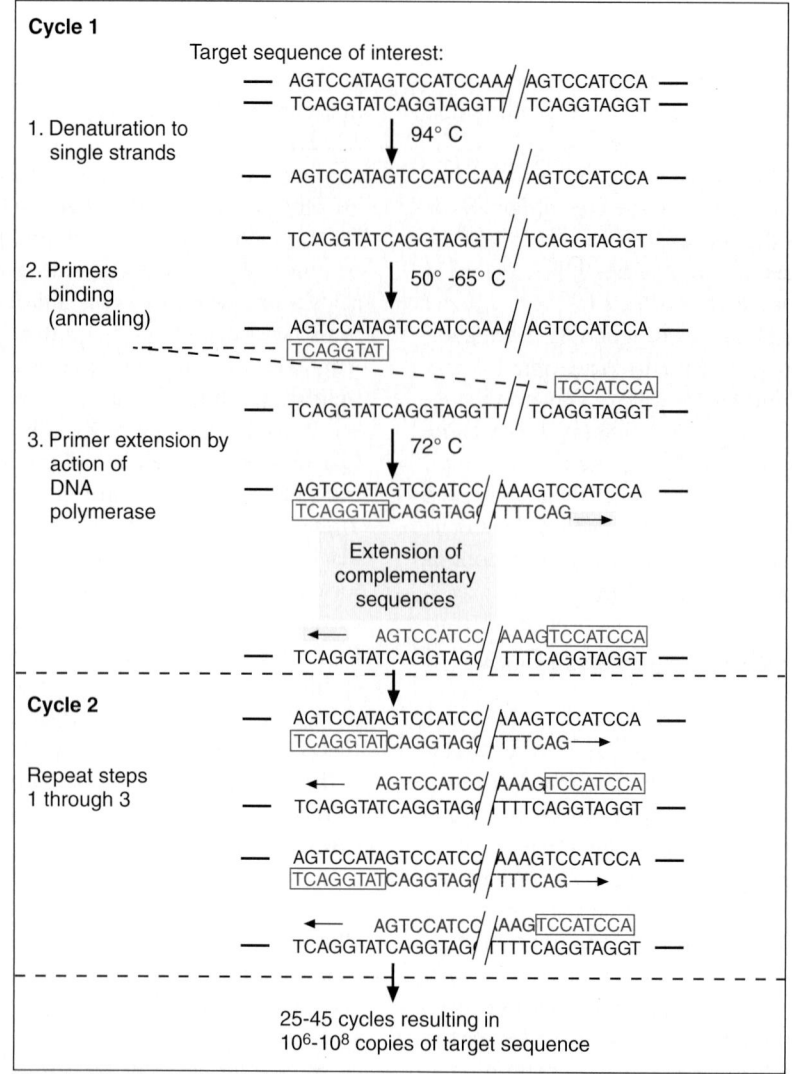

• **Fig. 8.8** Overview of a polymerase chain reaction. The target sequence is denatured to single strands, primers specific for each target strand sequence are added, and deoxyribonucleic acid *(DNA)* polymerase catalyzes the addition of deoxynucleotides to extend and produce new strands complementary to each of the target sequence strands (cycle 1). In cycle 2, both double-stranded products of cycle 1 are denatured and subsequently serve as targets for more primer annealing and extension by DNA polymerase. After 25 to 30 cycles, at least 107 copies of target DNA may be produced. (Modified from Ryan KJ, Champoux JJ, Drew WL, et al. *Sherris Medical Microbiology: An Introduction to Infectious Diseases.* Norwalk, CT: McGraw-Hill; 1994.)

The nucleic acid sequence (e.g., composition of A, C, T, and G nucleotides) of the primer determines the **melting temperature (Tm) or annealing temperature in the reaction.** The Tm is defined as the temperature at which 50% of the primers, or in the case of a hybridization assay, the probe, are annealed to the specific target sequence. Because of the complementary binding of nucleotides, the melting temperature may be determined for a known nucleotide sequence. The melting temperature is calculated according to a simple formula:

$$2 \times (A + T) + 4 \times (G + C)$$

Primer pairs should be optimally designed to anneal within 1 to 5 degrees of each other to maintain the specificity of the amplification reaction. Specificity decreases when the annealing temperature is farther away or lower than the actual Tm of the primers.

Extension of the Primer-Target Duplex

Annealing of the primers to the target DNA sequences provides the necessary structure that DNA polymerase enzyme needs to add nucleotides to the 3′ **terminus** (end) of each primer and extend the DNA sequence complementary to the full-length target template (Fig. 8.9), mimicking nucleic acid replication and generating a new double-stranded molecule. **Taq polymerase,** derived from the thermophilic bacteria *Thermus aquaticus,* is the enzyme commonly used for **primer extension,** which occurs at 72°C. This enzyme is used because of its ability to function efficiently at elevated temperatures and to withstand the denaturing temperature

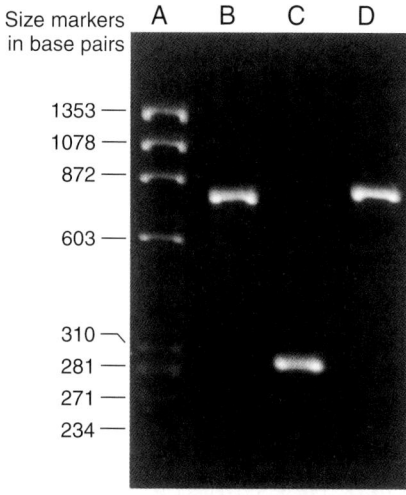

• **Fig. 8.9** Use of ethidium bromide–stained agarose gels to determine the size of polymerase chain reaction (PCR) amplicons for identification. Lane A shows molecular-size markers, with the marker sizes indicated in base pairs. Lanes B, C, and D contain PCR amplicons typical of the enterococcal vancomycin-resistance genes *vanA* (783 kb), *vanB* (297 kb), and *vanC1* (822 kb), respectively.

of 94°C through several amplification cycles. Enzymes from other thermophilic bacteria that can be used in PCR include *Pyrococcus furiosus* (Pfu polymerase), *Thermococcus litoralis* (Wind or Tli polymerase or Vent polymerase), and *Thermus thermophilus* (Tth polymerase). The choice of a specific polymerase typically depends on the nature/size of the template and the type of amplification reaction being performed.

The three reaction steps in PCR occur in the same tube containing the mixture of target nucleic acid, primers, components to optimize polymerase activity (i.e., buffer, cation [MgCl$_2$], and salt), and **deoxynucleotides (dNTPs).** To minimize the time lag required to alter the reaction temperature between denaturation, annealing, and extension over several cycles, automated programmable **thermal cyclers** are used. These cyclers hold the reaction vessel and carry the PCR mixture through each reaction step at the precise temperature and for the optimal duration.

As shown in Fig. 8.8, for each target DNA originally present in the PCR mixture, two double-stranded fragments containing the target sequence are produced after one cycle. At the beginning of the second cycle of PCR, denaturation produces four templates to which the primers will anneal. After extension at the end of the second cycle, there will be four double-stranded fragments containing target nucleic acid. Therefore, with completion of each cycle, there is a doubling or logarithmic increase in the concentration of amplified target nucleic acids.

Although it is possible to detect a single copy of a pathogen's target gene in a sample or patient specimen by PCR technology, detection is dependent on the ability of the primers to locate and anneal to the single target copy, and on optimization of the PCR conditions. The presence of PCR inhibitors in some biological matrices also increases the DNA copy number needed for accurate amplification.

Nonetheless, PCR has proven to be a powerful amplification technique to enhance the sensitivity of molecular diagnostic tests.

Detection of Polymerase Chain Reaction Products

The specific PCR amplification product containing the target nucleic acid of interest is referred to as the **amplicon.** Because PCR produces an amplicon in substantial quantities, any of the basic methods previously described for detecting hybridization can be adopted for detecting specific amplicons. Detection involves using a labeled probe specific for the target sequence in the amplicon. Therefore, solution or solid-phase formats may be used with reporter molecules that generate radioactive, colorimetric, fluorometric, or chemiluminescent signals. Probe-based detection of amplicons serves two purposes: it allows visualization of the PCR product, and it provides specificity by ensuring that the amplicon is the target sequence of interest and not the result of nonspecific amplification.

When the reliability of PCR for a particular amplicon has been well established, hybridization-based detection may not be necessary; confirming the presence of the correct-size amplicon may be sufficient. This is commonly accomplished by subjecting a portion of the PCR mixture, after amplification, to gel electrophoresis. After electrophoresis, the gel is stained to visualize the amplicon and, using **molecular weight–size markers,** the presence of amplicons of appropriate size (the size of the target sequence amplified depends on the primers selected for PCR) is confirmed (Fig. 8.9).

Derivations of the Polymerase Chain Reaction Method

The powerful amplification capacity of PCR has prompted the development of several modifications that enhance the utility of this methodology, particularly in the diagnostic setting. Specific examples include multiplex PCR, nested PCR, quantitative PCR, reverse transcription PCR (RT-PCR), arbitrary primed PCR, digital PCR, and PCR for nucleotide sequencing.

Multiplex PCR is a method by which more than one primer pair is included in the PCR mixture. This approach offers a couple of notable advantages. For one, it enables inclusion of internal amplification controls. For example, one primer pair can be directed at sequences present in all clinically relevant bacteria (i.e., the control or universal primers), and the second primer pair can be directed at a sequence specific for the particular organism/gene of interest (i.e., the test primers). The control amplicon should always be detectable after PCR; absence of the internal control indicates that PCR conditions were not met; the test is invalid and must be repeated. When the control amplicon is detected, absence of the test amplicon can be more confidently interpreted to indicate the absence of target nucleic acid in the specimen rather than a failure of the PCR assay (Fig. 8.10).

The most obvious advantage of multiplex PCR is the ability to search for different targets in a single reaction. Primer pairs directed at sequences specific for different organisms or genes

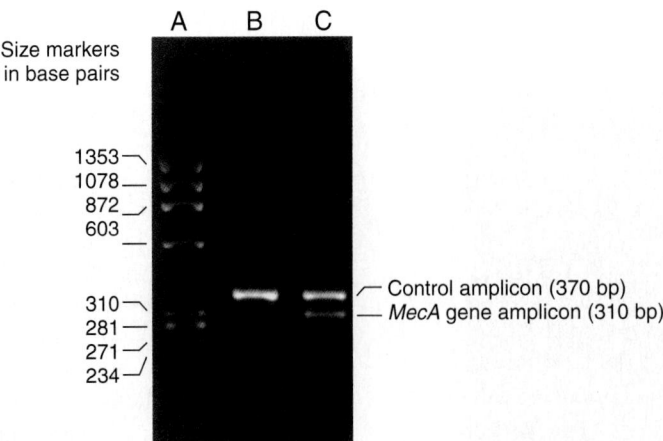

Size markers in base pairs

1353
1078
872
603

310 — Control amplicon (370 bp)
281 — MecA gene amplicon (310 bp)
271
234

• **Fig. 8.10** Ethidium bromide–stained gels containing amplicons produced by multiplex polymerase chain reaction (PCR). Lane A shows molecular-size markers, with the marker sizes indicated in base pairs. Lanes B and C show amplicons obtained with multiplex PCR consisting of control primers and primers specific for the staphylococcal methicillin-resistance gene *mecA*. The presence of only the control amplicon (370 bp) in Lane B indicates that PCR was successful, but the strain on which the reaction was performed did not contain *mecA*. Lane C shows both the control and the *mecA* (310 bp) amplicons, indicating that the reaction was successful and that the strain tested carries the *mecA* resistance gene.

can be combined in a single assay, avoiding the use of multiple reaction vessels, thereby minimizing the volume of specimen/reagents required and the total turnaround time. In addition, multiplex PCR can provide more clinically relevant information to health care providers through detection of co-infections and by eliminating potential disease-causing pathogens, which elicit similar symptoms. Respiratory and gastroenteritis panels targeting up to 20 pathogens each are currently the most widely used multiplex PCR assays in clinical microbiology (Fig. 8.11). A limitation of multiplex PCR is that mixing different primers can cause some interference in the amplification process. For instance, amplification of a high-copy analyte may utilize a disproportionate amount of the reaction components, and thereby impair or prevent amplification of a low-copy analyte within the same reaction. Optimizing multiplex PCR conditions can be challenging, especially as the number of primer pairs increases within the assay, which increases the potential for primer-primer interactions that can generate nonspecific amplification products and negatively impact sensitivity. In addition, as more true targets are amplified, the ability to differentiate between the amplicons becomes challenging and additional detection/separation techniques may be needed, such as bead-based or spatial microfluidic arrays.

Nested PCR involves the sequential use of two primer sets. The first set is used to amplify a target sequence. The amplicon obtained is used as the target sequence for a second amplification using primers internal to those of the first amplicon. The advantage of this approach is extreme sensitivity and confirmed specificity without the need to use probes. Because production of the second amplicon requires the presence of the first amplicon, production of the second amplicon automatically verifies the accuracy of the first amplicon. The problem encountered with nested PCR is that the procedure requires open manipulations of amplified DNA that is readily, albeit inadvertently, aerosolized and capable of contaminating other reaction vials.

Arbitrary primed PCR uses short (random) primers not specifically complementary to a particular sequence of a target DNA. Although these primers are not specifically directed, their short sequence ($\approx$10 nucleotides) ensures that they randomly anneal to multiple sites in a chromosomal sequence. Upon cycling, the multiple annealing sites result in the amplification of multiple fragments of different sizes. Theoretically, strains with similar nucleotide sequences have similar annealing sites and thus produce amplified fragments (i.e., amplicons) of similar sizes. Therefore, by comparing fragment migration patterns after agarose gel electrophoresis, the examiner can judge strains or isolates to be the same, similar, or unrelated.

The PCR methods discussed thus far have focused on amplification of a DNA target. **Reverse transcription PCR (RT-PCR)** amplifies an RNA target. Because many clinically important viruses have genomes composed of RNA rather than DNA (e.g., the human immunodeficiency virus [HIV], hepatitis C virus), the ability to amplify RNA greatly facilitates laboratory-based diagnostic testing for these infectious agents. Reverse transcription includes a unique initial step that requires the use of the enzyme **reverse transcriptase** to direct the synthesis of DNA from the viral RNA template, usually within 30 minutes. Once the DNA has been produced, routine PCR technology is applied to obtain amplification.

Real-time homogenous kinetic quantitative PCR (qPCR) is an approach that combines the power of PCR for the detection and identification of infectious agents with the ability to quantitate the actual number of targets present in the clinical specimen. When the amplification products are detected as they are generated following each amplification cycle, qPCR is said to occur in "real time" as described in detail below. This technology has arguably been the most significant advancement for molecular diagnostics to date, with many FDA-approved diagnostic

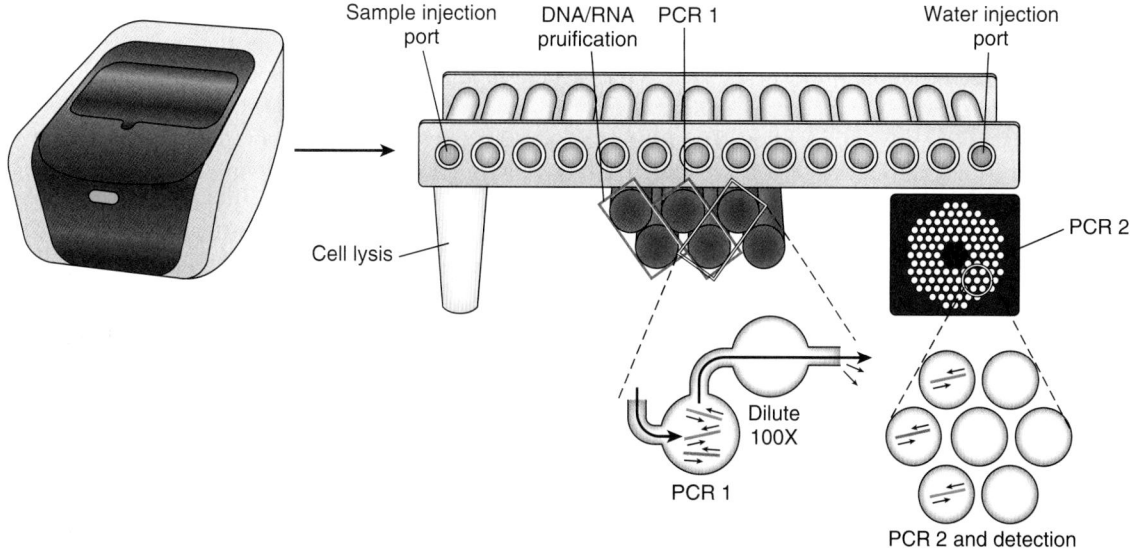

• **Fig. 8.11** The BioFire FilmArray Multiplex polymerase chain reaction (PCR) system integrates sample preparation, extraction, amplification, detection, and analysis. The multiplex system can simultaneously identify viruses, bacteria, parasites, yeasts, and antimicrobial genes in patient samples. (Adapted from teaching materials, courtesy Jim Flanigan, American Society for Clinical Laboratory Science.)

systems utilizing qPCR methodology. The ability to quantitate "infectious burden" adds significant clinical value toward understanding the disease state, establishing the prognosis of certain infections, and monitoring the effectiveness of antibiotic or antiviral therapy (e.g., quantifying HIV or hepatitis C viral loads in patients is critical for evaluating therapeutic efficacy and monitoring disease progression). **Digital PCR (dPCR)** is a real-time or endpoint quantitative method that performs traditional PCR in separate, nanoliter-sized droplets. In comparison to traditional PCR, where multiple target sequence copies are amplified in a single-reaction cuvette or well, digital PCR separates individual nucleic acids or oligonucleotide fragments from a single specimen into thousands of separate droplets (20,000 or more) using a water-in-oil emulsion microfluidic technique such that each droplet will either contain no molecule or a single target molecule. Following PCR amplification, each droplet generates a negative or positive reaction signal; therefore, the quantitation of the amplification is achieved by counting the droplets that contain a positive amplified product. Since quantitation is not based on exponential amplification in comparison with the starting quantity of the target, errors associated with rate of amplification changes that are affected by interfering substances and the use of a standard curve (described in the melting curve analysis in this chapter) can be minimized or eliminated. dPCR also provides a possible resolution for the detection of infectious agents or pathogens that are present in very low numbers in biologic samples.

Real-Time Polymerase Chain Reaction

In principle, real-time amplification is accomplished in the same manner as previously described for conventional PCR-based assays in which denaturation of double-stranded nucleic acid and primer annealing and extension (elongation) are performed in repetitive cycles. It is the detection process that discriminates real-time PCR from conventional PCR assays. In **real-time PCR** assays, accumulation of amplicon is monitored during synthesis using fluorescence that increases as new amplicons are made. Monitoring of amplified target is made possible by labeling of the primers, oligonucleotide probes (oligoprobes), or amplicons with molecules capable of fluorescing (known as **fluorophores**). These labels produce a change in fluorescent signal intensity that is measured by an optical instrument after their direct interaction with or hybridization to the amplicon.

Currently, a range of fluorescent chemistries are used for amplicon detection; the more commonly used chemistries can be divided into two categories: (1) those that involve the nonspecific binding of a fluorescent dye to double-stranded DNA (e.g., SYBR Green I) and (2) fluorescent oligonucleotide probes that bind specifically to the target of interest. SYBR Green I chemistry is based on the binding of SYBR Green I to a site referred to as the **minor groove** (where the strand backbones of DNA are closer together on one side of the helix than on the other), which is present in all double-stranded DNA. Once bound, fluorescence of this dye increases more than 100-fold. Therefore, as the amount of double-stranded amplicon increases, the fluorescent signal or output increases proportionally and can be measured by the instrument during the elongation stage of amplification. A major disadvantage of this detection strategy is that the signal cannot discriminate between specific and nonspecific amplified products without additional melting curve analysis, as described in more detail later.

The second category of real-time PCR detection chemistries can be further subdivided based upon the type of fluorescent molecules used in the PCR reaction and include (1)

hydrolysis and **hybridization probes** (e.g., TaqMan, and Molecular Beacons), (2) **primer probes** (Scorpions and Angler), and (3) **nucleic acid analog probes** (PNAs). The diversity of unique probe chemistries in each of these categories has dramatically increased within the last 15 years, but not all have found their way into the clinical arena. Fig. 8.12 highlights some of the most commonly used approaches to detect amplicons in real-time PCR. Hybridization probes, as previously described, are tagged with two light-sensitive molecules (a fluorophore and quencher pair, or two fluorophores) that interact only at very close spatial distances. In the presence of a quencher, which absorbs the excitation energy of the fluorescent dye, sufficient amounts of fluorescence are possible only after cleavage of the probe (hydrolysis probes) or during hybridization of a hairpin oligonucleotide with a stem-loop structure, known as a **molecular beacon,** to the amplicon (Fig. 8.12A and B). Alternatively, two fluorescent dyes whose excitation and emission spectra overlap can be attached to two oligonucleotides (**dual hybridization probes**), which both bind to the amplicon, allowing for the fluorescence excitation energy of one dye to be transferred to the second dye, generating a fluorescent emission signal that is detected by the qPCR instrument only when the two fluorophores are in close proximity (i.e., bound to their complementary targets located adjacent to each other on the amplicon) (Fig. 8.12C). This energy transfer between the two fluorescent dyes is known as **Förster resonance energy transfer (FRET)**. In both cases, fluorescence is evident only after a new amplicon is generated, thereby facilitating the monitoring of the progression of the reaction in real time.

Other PCR probes consist of a primer-probe oligonucleotide construct that combines the PCR primer and detection probe into a single molecule. One of these primer-probes, known as a **scorpion probe,** involves attaching the 5′ end of the PCR primer directly to a molecular-beacon style probe (Fig 8.12D). This effectively limits primer extension to the 3′ end. After extension, the probe hybridizes to the newly synthesized DNA, releasing the influence of the quencher from the fluorophore and increasing the fluorescence signal. Nearly all of the probe designs can also be synthesized using nucleic acid analogs, such as PNAs, to increase their stability and binding efficiency. Additional information regarding unique real-time PCR detection chemistries is available from Navarro et al., "Real-time PCR detection chemistries" (2015).

Real-time automated instruments that combine target nucleic acid amplification with qualitative or quantitative measurement of amplified product are commercially available. These instruments are noteworthy for four reasons:

1. The instruments combine thermal cycling for target DNA amplification with the ability to detect amplified target with fluorescently labeled probes as the hybrids are formed (i.e., detection of amplicon in real time).
2. Both amplification and product detection can be accomplished in one reaction vessel without opening the vessel (a "**closed system**"), the major concern of cross-contamination of samples with amplified products.
3. The instruments are able to measure amplified product (amplicon) as it is made and quantitate the amount of product, thereby determining the number of copies of target in the original specimen.
4. The time required to complete a real-time PCR assay is significantly reduced compared with conventional PCR-based assays, chiefly by monitoring reaction dynamics in real time and thereby eliminating the need for postreaction analyses (e.g., gel electrophoresis).

Several instruments (also referred to as **platforms**) are available for amplification in conjunction with real-time detection of PCR-amplified products (Fig. 8.13). Although not an exhaustive list, each instrument has unique features that permit some flexibility, such that a clinical laboratory can fulfill its specific needs in terms of specimen throughput, number of targets simultaneously detected, detection format, and time to results. Nevertheless, all instruments have amplification (i.e., thermal cycling) capability, as well as an excitation or light source, an emission detection source, and a computer interface to monitor the formation of amplified product. In addition, some real-time PCR instruments (e.g., LightCycler; Roche Diagnostics, Indianapolis, IN) can detect multiple targets (multiplex PCR) by using different probes labeled with specific fluorescent dyes, each with unique emission spectra.

Some real-time PCR instruments also have the ability to perform melting curve analysis. This type of analysis of amplified products confirms the origin (i.e., specificity) of the amplified product and/or identifies nonspecific products. Melting curve analysis can be performed with assays using hybridization probes and molecular beacons but not hydrolysis probes, because hydrolysis probes are destroyed during the amplification process. For simplicity, this discussion focuses on SYBR Green I–based melting curve analyses. The underlying basis of melting curve analysis lies in the ability to denature (i.e., split the strands) the double-stranded DNA amplicon upon heating (referred to as **melting** or denaturation), thereby eliminating the fluorescence. The melting temperature (Tm), as previously described for primers, is the temperature at which the DNA denatures into two strands ("melts") and is dependent on the nucleotide composition of the molecule (stretches of double-stranded DNA with more cytosines and guanines require more heat [energy] to break the three hydrogen bonds between these two bases, in contrast to adenine and thymidine base pairing, which has only two hydrogen bonds). Because the Tm of the amplicon is specific for the target sequence, dependent primarily on base composition, amplification products can be confirmed as correct by the melting characteristics or Tm. Of significance, the Tm can also be used to distinguish base pair differences (e.g., genotypes, mutations, or polymorphisms) in target DNA, thus forming the basis for many genetic testing assays, because base pair mismatches resulting from mutations alter the Tm.

In real-time PCR, melting curve analysis is performed once amplification is completed. The temperature of the reaction vessel is lowered to approximately 50 degrees, and

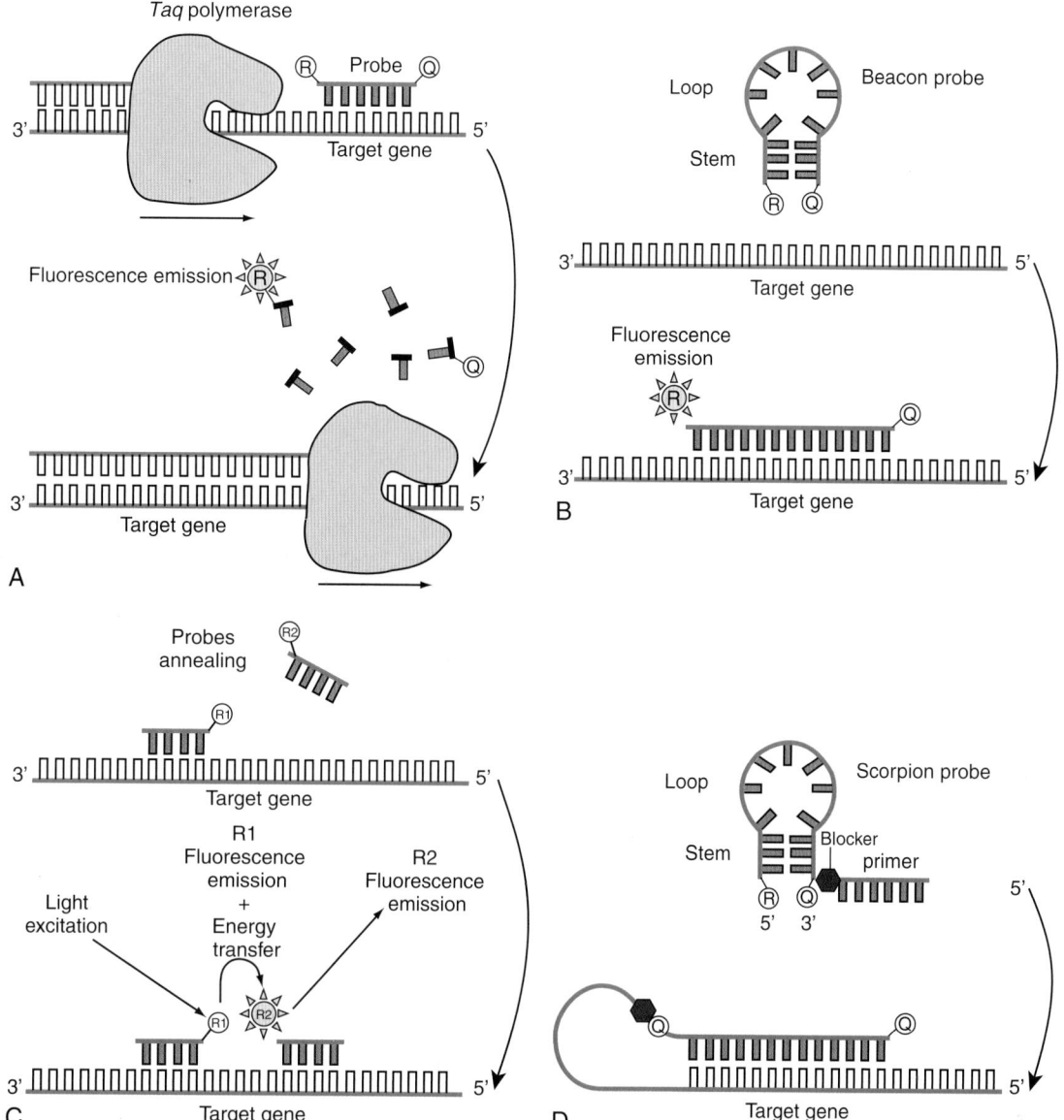

• **Fig. 8.12** Fluorogenic probes (probes with an attached fluorophore, a fluorescent molecule that can absorb light energy and then be elevated to an excited state and released as fluorescence in the absence of a quencher) commonly used for detection of amplified product in real-time polymerase chain reaction *(PCR)* assays. (A) Hydrolysis probe. In addition to the specific primers for amplification, an oligonucleotide probe with a reporter fluorescent dye *(R)* and a quencher dye *(Q)* at its 5′ and 3′ ends, respectively, is added to the reaction mix. During the extension phase, the quencher (the molecule that can accept energy from a fluorophore and then dissipate the energy, resulting in no fluorescence when the two dyes are close to each other *(a)*. Once amplification occurs and the fluorogenic probe binds to the amplified product, the bound probe is degraded by the 5′–3′ exonuclease activity of Taq polymerase; therefore, quenching is no longer possible, and fluorescence is emitted and then measured *(b)*. (B) Molecular beacon. Molecular beacons are hairpin-shaped molecules with an internally quenched fluorophore that fluoresces once the beacon probe binds to the amplified target and the quencher is no longer in proximity to the fluorophore. These probes are designed such that the loop portion of the molecule is a sequence complementary to the target of interest (a). The "stem" portion of the beacon probe is formed by the annealing of complementary arm sequences on the respective ends of the probe sequence. In addition, a fluorescent moiety (R) and a quencher moiety (Q) at opposing ends of the probe are attached (a). The stem portion of the probe keeps the fluorescent and quencher moieties in proximity to one another, quenching the fluorescence of the fluorophore. When it encounters a target molecule with a complementary sequence, the molecular beacon undergoes a spontaneous conformational change that forces the stem apart, thereby causing the fluorophore and quencher to move away from each other and leading to restoration of fluorescence (b). (C), Fluorescent resonant energy transfer (FRET) or hybridization probes. Two different hybridization probes are used, one carrying a fluorescent reporter moiety at its 3′ end (designated R1) and the other carrying a fluorescent dye at its 5′ end (designated R2) (a). These two oligonucleotide probes are designed to hybridize to an amplified deoxyribonucleic acid (DNA) target in a head-to-tail arrangement in very close proximity to one another. The first dye (R1) is excited by a filtered light source and emits a fluorescent light at a slightly longer wavelength. Because the two dyes are so close to each other, the energy emitted from R1 excites R2 (attached to the second hybridization probe), which emits fluorescent light at an even longer wavelength (b). This energy transfer is referred to as FRET. Selection of an appropriate detection channel on the instrument allows the intensity of light emitted from R2 to be filtered and measured. (Modified from Mocellin S, Rossi CR, Pilati P, et al. Quantitative real-time PCR: a powerful ally in cancer research. *Trends Mol Med.* 2003;9:189.) (D) Scorpion probe. A scorpion probe consists of a molecular beacon-style hairpin DNA that is directly linked to the 5′ end of the PCR primer through a blocker. The blocker prevents extension of the PCR primer from the 5′ end. After extension of the primer from the 3′ end by DNA polymerase, the loop region of the probe that is complementary to the target DNA sequence is able to hybridize to the newly synthesized DNA, thereby increasing the distance between the fluorophore and quencher pair. The increased distance relieves the quenching effect on the fluorophore, resulting in an increase in fluorescence emission that is detectable by the real-time PCR instrument. (Modified from Maurin M. Real-time PCR as a diagnostic tool for bacterial diseases. *Expert Rev Mol Diagn.* 2012;12:7.)

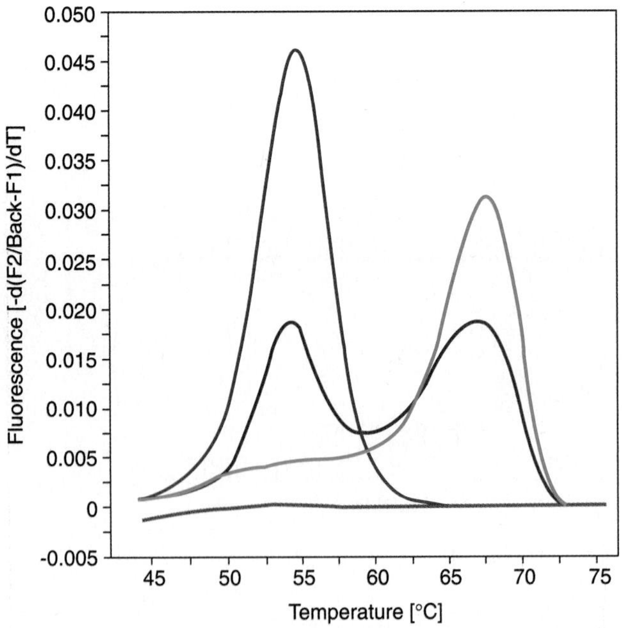

• **Fig. 8.13** Melting curve analyses performed using the LightCycler HSV1/2 Detection Kit. Deoxyribonucleic acid (DNA) was extracted and subjected to real-time polymerase chain reaction (PCR) using the LightCycler to detect the presence of herpes simplex virus (HSV) DNA. After amplification, melting curve analysis was performed in which amplified product was cooled to below 55°C, and the temperature then was raised slowly. The Tm is the temperature at which half of the DNA is single stranded and is specific for the sequence of the particular DNA product. The specific melting temperature is determined at 640 nm (channel F2 on the cycler) for the clinical samples and the positive and negative controls. For illustration purposes, melting curve analyses are "overlaid" relative to one another in this fig for three clinical samples and the HSV-1 and HSV-2 positive or "template" control. The clinical specimens containing HSV-1 DNA *(red line)* or HSV-2 *(green line)* result in a melting peak at 54°C or 67°C, respectively (the Tms). The LightCycler positive or template control containing HSV-1 and HSV-2 DNA, displayed as a *purple line,* shows two peaks at 54°C and 67°C, respectively. The clinical sample that is negative *(brown line)* for both HSV-1 and HSV-2 shows no peaks.

the reaction temperature is slowly raised with concomitant measurements of fluorescence at regular intervals. As the amplicon reaches its melting temperature and the DNA strands split apart, the SYBR Green I dye will dissipate from the DNA molecule, resulting in a marked decrease in fluorescent signal. Similar approaches to melting curve analysis are used for hybridization probes and molecular beacons as described in Fig. 8.13.

Finally, real-time PCR assays also have the ability to quantitate the amount of target in a clinical sample. For quantitative analysis, amplification curves are evaluated. As previously discussed, amplification is monitored either through the fluorescence of double-stranded DNA–specific dyes (e.g., SYBR Green 1) or by sequence-specific probes; thus during amplification, a curve is generated. During real-time PCR, there are at least three distinct phases for these curves: (1) an initial **lag phase** in which no amplicon is detected, (2) an **exponential phase** of amplification, and (3) a **plateau phase.** The number of targets in the original specimen can be determined with precision when the number of cycles needed for the signal

to achieve an arbitrary **threshold** (the portion of the curve where the signal begins to increase exponentially or logarithmically) is determined. This segment of the real-time PCR cycle is within the linear amplification portion of the reaction where conditions are optimal and fluorescence accumulates in proportion to the amplicon.

With most instrument analyses, the value used for quantitative measurement is the PCR cycle number in which the fluorescence reaches a threshold value of 10 times the standard deviation of baseline fluorescence emission; this cycle number is referred to as the **threshold cycle (CT), crossing point (CP),** or **cycle of quantification (CQ)** and is inversely proportional to the starting amount of target present in the clinical sample (Mackay, 2004). In other words, this value is the cycle number in which the fluorescent signal rises above background (the threshold value previously defined) and is dependent on the amount of target nucleic acid in the original sample. Thus to quantitate the target in a clinical specimen, a **standard curve** is generated in which known amounts of target are prepared and then subjected to real-time PCR, in parallel with the clinical sample containing an unknown amount of target. A standard curve is generated using the CT values for each of the known amounts of target amplified. By taking the CT value of the clinical specimen and extrapolating from the standard curve, the amount of target in the original sample can be determined (Fig. 8.14). Advances in instrumentation have resulted in the development of platforms that incorporate various PCR methods in high throughput formats that allow the detection of multiple organisms but also multiple samples simultaneously (Fig. 8.15). Quantitative nucleic acid methods are used to monitor response to therapy, detect the development of drug resistance, and predict disease progression.

The introduction of commercially available **analyte-specific reagents (ASRs)** followed the introduction of real-time PCR. ASRs represent a new regulatory approach by the FDA in which reagents in this broad category (e.g., antibodies; specific receptor proteins; ligands; oligonucleotides, such as DNA or RNA probes or primers; and many reagents used in **laboratory developed tests [LDT])** can be used in multiple diagnostic applications. ASR-labeled reagents carry the "For Research Use Only" label, and the manufacturer is prohibited from promoting any applications for these reagents or providing recipes for using the reagents. Because rulings vary on a state-by-state basis, laboratory supervisors should check into Medicare reimbursement before developing and introducing an ASR assay. A laboratory designated as high complexity according to the Clinical Laboratory Improvement Amendment (CLIA) must take full responsibility for developing, validating, and offering the diagnostic assay using these reagents. This regulation essentially allows new diagnostic methods to become available more quickly, particularly methods targeted toward smaller patient populations. It is important to note that because good manufacturing practices are mandated, ASRs provide more standardized products for the performance of amplification assays. ASRs are available for a number of organisms.

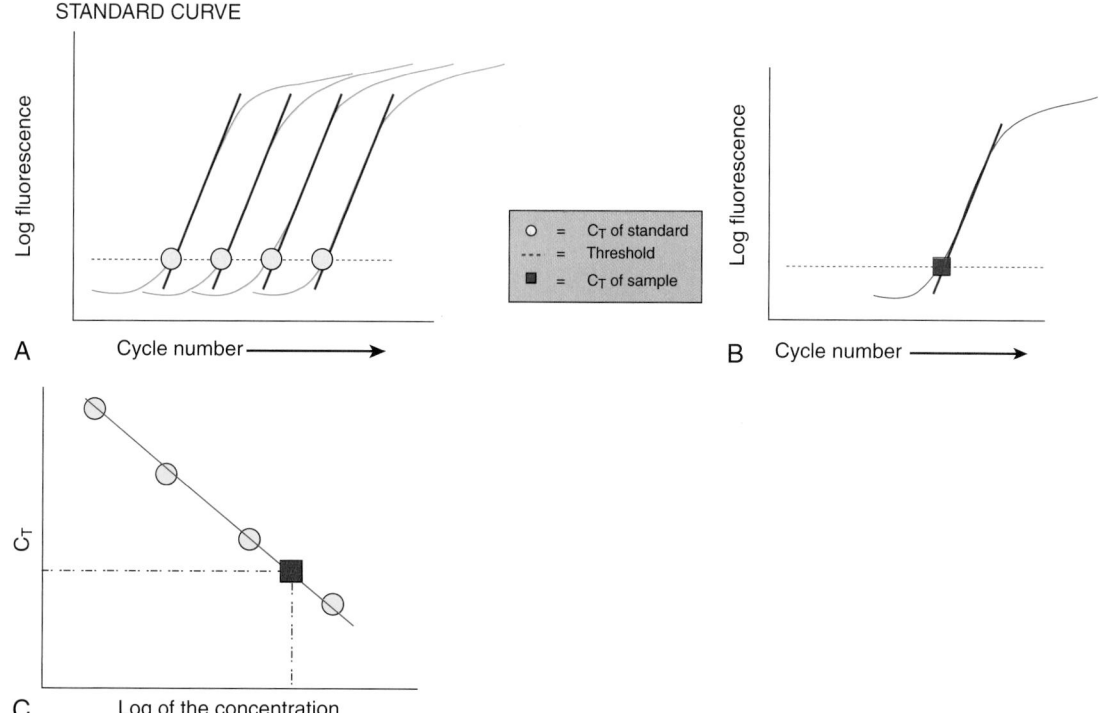

STANDARD CURVE

• **Fig. 8.14** Quantitation using real-time polymerase chain reaction. (A) In the example, four samples containing known amounts of target are amplified by real-time polymerase chain reaction (PCR). The inverse log of their fluorescence is plotted against the cycle number and their respective C_T is determined; the fewer the number of targets, the greater the C_T value. (B) Similarly, the clinical specimen is also amplified by real-time PCR, and its C_T value is determined. (C) The log of the nucleic acid concentration and the respective C_T value for each specimen containing a known amount of target or nucleic acid are plotted to generate a standard curve. Knowing the C_T value of the clinical specimen allows the concentration of target in the original sample to be determined.

Amplification Methods: Non–Polymerase Chain Reaction–Based

Although PCR was developed first and numerous PCR-based assays are available, rapid, sensitive, and specific detection of infectious agents by nucleic acid amplification can be achieved by a number of methods other than PCR. These amplification formats can be divided into two broad categories: those that amplify the signal used to detect the target nucleic acid and those that directly amplify the target nucleic acid but are not PCR based.

Coupled Target and Signal (Probe) Amplification

As previously described regarding signal amplification, the Invader technology can also be considered a probe amplification assay. In other words, the amplified product or signal no longer contains the target nucleic acid sequence. The Invader assay (Hologic, Bedford, MA) is an isothermal system that can be used to amplify DNA or RNA. Invader chemistry has been incorporated into a new Invader PLUS system that combines a PCR reaction followed by an invader reaction, yielding a coupled target and signal amplification strategy that improves the detection of nucleic acids present in low copy numbers in the initial specimen.

Isothermal (Constant Temperature) Amplification

Many isothermal amplification techniques have been developed to eliminate the need for the rapid heating and cooling cycles found in PCR-based techniques. **Loop-mediated isothermal amplification (LAMP)** uses four primers and proceeds using a constant temperature coupled to a strand displacement reaction. This technology was developed by the Eiken Chemical Company (Tokyo, Japan). In addition to LAMP, other isothermal methods have been developed that also use strand displacement for amplification. **Strand displacement** requires four primers, two for each strand of the parent double helix. One primer binds downstream of the other. The downstream primer contains a restriction endonuclease site on the 5′ tail. DNA polymerase I (exonuclease deficient) extends from both primers and incorporates a modified nucleotide (2′-deoxyadenosine 5′-O-[1-thiotriphosphate]). During the extension, the newly synthesized strand that is extended from the downstream primer is displaced by the new molecule that is being synthesized by the second primer that is upstream or outside of the first primer. A subsequent set of primers is then capable of binding to the new strand, producing additional amplification product. This amplification product is used in the second stage of the amplification. In the second step of the reaction, the restriction endonuclease nicks the 5′ end of the original

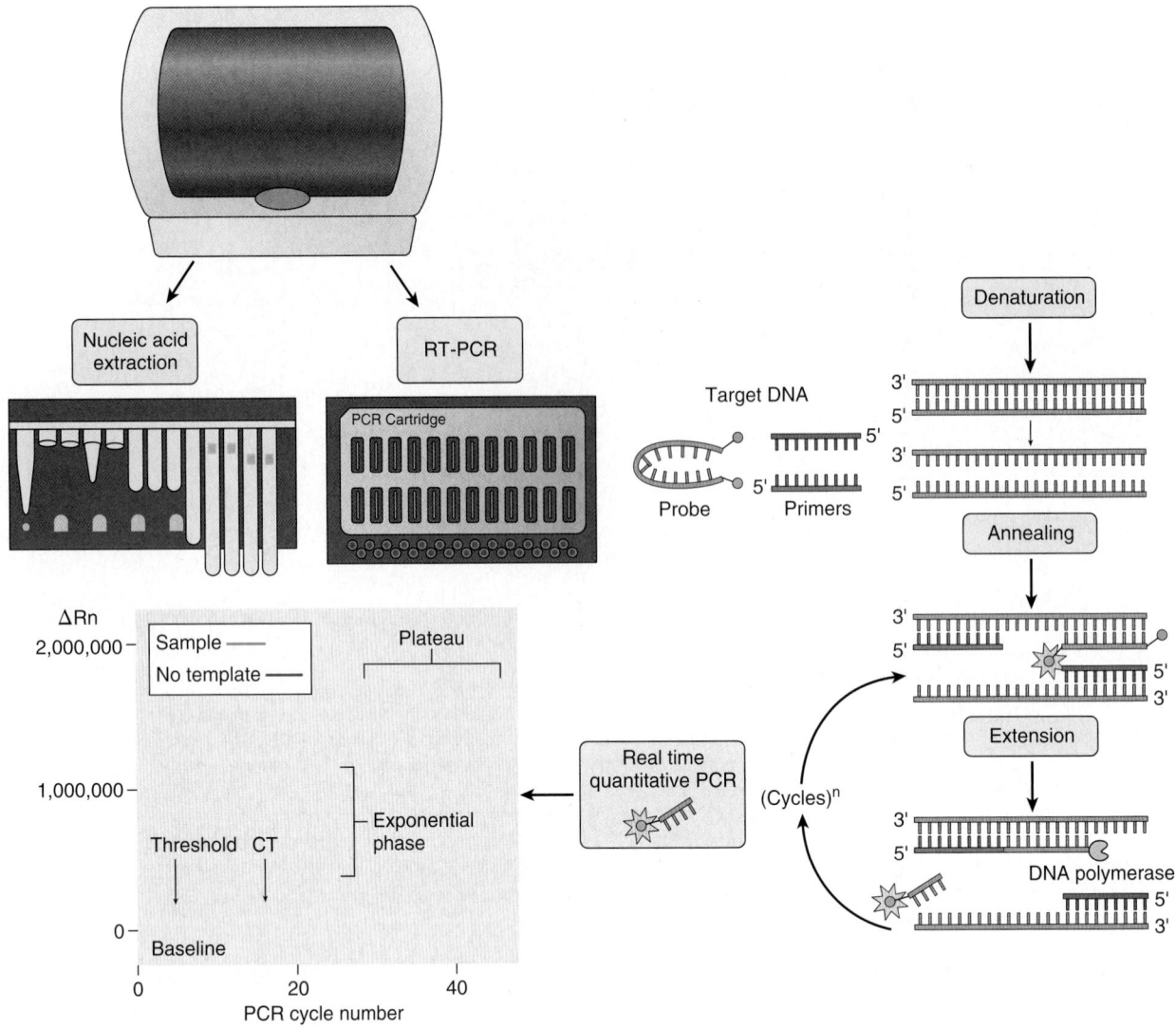

• **Fig. 8.15** BD Max system provides lysis and extraction with pre-filled reagent strips, capable of running multiple specimen types and assays in a single run, producing highly sensitive and specific results using real-time polymerase chain reaction *(PCR)* technology (14). Free fluorescent probe released by DNA polymerase during strand amplification is continuously measured until a threshold level of fluorescence *(Ct)* is achieved, triggering a positive test result. (Adapted from teaching materials, courtesy Jim Flanigan, American Society for Clinical Laboratory Science.)

downstream primer that is incorporated into the displaced strand. The complementary strand cannot be nicked, because the modified nucleotide that has been incorporated into the strand blocks restriction digestion, and the restriction site therefore is inactive. Once the restriction site has been cleaved, a new double-strand region that contains the primer/probe provides for a new cycle of amplification.

Additional isothermal amplifications include **nucleic acid sequence–based amplification (NASBA)** and **transcription-mediated amplification (TMA).** Both methods are used for the isothermal amplification of RNA and have clinical utility for the amplification of viral RNA, identification of *Mycobacterium* spp. antibiotic resistance, and detection of bacteria. The assays use a reverse transcriptase (RT) to copy the target RNA into a **complementary DNA molecule (cDNA).** Either RNase H or an RT molecule with

RNase activity degrades the RNA molecule in the RNA-DNA hybrid. The remaining cDNA molecule is replicated into double-stranded DNA molecules by the DNA polymerase activity of the polymerase (i.e., T7 bacteriophage RNA polymerase). The RT uses a promoter that was incorporated into the cDNA engineered into the primer for the first amplification of the cDNA. The RT then transcribes antisense RNA molecules from the cDNA molecules. The resulting antisense RNA amplicons then continue the cycle for increased amplification of the target sequence.

A relatively new **helicase-dependent amplification (HDA)** method uses DNA helicase, rather than heat, to separate double-stranded DNA molecules to generate single-stranded templates for amplification. Once separated, single-stranded DNA binding proteins stabilize the single strands to allow binding of the PCR primers. DNA polymerase extends the primers, and the newly synthesized DNA duplexes serve as templates for further amplification cycles. HDA reactions are typically performed at 60°C and can be used to amplify targets present in complex matrices, such as crude bacterial lysates or blood. Another isothermal technique, **recombinase polymerase amplification (RPA),** employs the enzyme recombinase to catalyze the hybridization of the PCR primer with its complementary target sequence. This method first requires formation of the primer-recombinase complex, which then scans the dsDNA target looking for a homologous sequence. Once the sequence is located, the recombinase enzyme facilitates separation of the dsDNA and hybridization of the primer before elongation is completed by DNA polymerase. The newly synthesized strand displaces the old strand and serves as a template for the next amplification cycle. RPA is rapid and sensitive but often suffers from high background signals. Some of the non–PCR-based technologies that have been successfully used to detect infectious agents are included in Table 8.1. As with PCR, these assays are able to amplify DNA and RNA targets, have multiplex capabilities, and may be qualitative or quantitative. To learn more about these alternative target amplification methods, refer to additional reading and articles authored by Ginocchio (2004), Yan et al. (2014), and Zhao et al. (2015).

Nicking Endonuclease Amplification

The detection of influenza A and B in respiratory specimens is available in a CLIA-waived point-of-care (POC) platform referred to as nicking endonuclease amplification reaction (NEAR). The assay is an isothermal process that uses a double-stranded template that is nicked by an enzyme that denatures the template. There is a T1 primer complexed to the enzyme that binds to the recognition site for extension of the template. A second T2 primer binds, is extended, and displaces the first primer. This creates a double stranded molecule. The nicked primers provide the means for recycling and repeat amplification.

Postamplification End-Point Analysis

While real-time techniques enable amplification and detection concurrently, there are a variety of postamplification analysis methods that are used to provide additional clinical information critical to pathogen identification and characterization.

Nucleic Acid Electrophoresis

Traditional postamplification analysis is performed via **gel electrophoresis,** which uses an electric current, a buffer, and a porous matrix of agarose or polyacrylamide to separate nucleic acid molecules according to size. As the electric current is applied to the system, the negatively charged nucleic acids will migrate through the gel matrix toward the positive pole or anode within the chamber. Electrophoresis may use a horizontal or vertical gel apparatus or a small tube (i.e., capillary) system. **Capillary electrophoresis** uses a thin glass silica capillary tube for faster separation and detection using fluorescent detection. Agarose is a polysaccharide polymer that is

TABLE 8.1 | **Non–Polymerase Chain Reaction–Based Nucleic Acid Amplification Methods**

Amplification Method	Method Overview	Additional Comments
Nucleic acid sequence-based amplification (NASBA)	1. Isothermal amplification achieved through coordination of three enzymes (avian myeloblastosis, RNase H, T7 RNA polymerase) in conjunction with two oligonucleotide primers specific for the target sequence 2. Amplification based on primer extension and ribonucleic acid (RNA) transcription	1. Can be adapted to real-time format using molecular beacons 2. Can develop in-house assays 3. Automated instrumentation is available

Transcription-mediated amplification (TMA)	1. Autocatalytic, isothermal amplification using reverse transcriptase and T7 RNA polymerase and two primers complementary to the target
	2. Exponential extension of RNA (up to 10 billion amplicons within 10 min)
		1. Second-generation TMA assays demonstrate improved removal of interfering substances
		  • Less labor intensive
		  • Uses target capture after sample lysis using an intermediate capture oligomer
		  • TMA performed directly on captured target
		2. Fully automated systems
		3. Instruments handle specimen processing through amplification and detection

Strand displacement amplification (SDA)	1. Isothermal process in which a single-stranded target is first generated 2. Exponential amplification of target	1. Reagents dried in separate disposable microwell strips 2. All assays have internal control to monitor for inhibition 3. Automated system for sample processing

extracted from seaweed. It is relatively inexpensive and easy to use. Polyacrylamide is typically a mixture of acrylamide and a cross-linking methylenebisacrylamide. Polyacrylamide is a more porous or highly cross-linked gel that provides for a higher resolution of smaller fragments and single-stranded molecules. Despite the benefit of the higher resolving power of acrylamide gels, the powder and unpolymerized acrylamide is highly neurotoxic and proper safety precautions should be used during handling.

In addition to various electrophoretic systems and matrices, different buffers may be used for the separation of nucleic acids. The two most common buffering systems include **Tris acetate** or **Tris borate buffers.** Tris borate ethylenediaminetetraacetic acid (EDTA) (TBE, 0.089 M Tris-base, 0.089 boric acid, 0.0020 M EDTA) has a greater buffering capacity. However, TBE has a tendency to precipitate during storage and generates heat during electrophoresis. Excessive heating during electrophoresis can result in distorted patterns and make detection or interpretation of migration patterns difficult. Tris acetate EDTA (TAE, 0.04 M Tris-base, 0.005 M sodium acetate, 0.002 M EDTA) provides for faster migration or separation during electrophoresis. **Denaturing agents** such as detergents, formamide, or urea may be added to the buffers that break hydrogen bonds between the complementary sequences on DNA or RNA molecules that may alter migration patterns.

Sequencing and Enzymatic Digestion of Nucleic Acids

The nucleotide sequence of a microorganism's genome is the blueprint for the organism. Therefore, molecular methods that elucidate some part of a pathogen's genomic sequence provide a powerful tool for diagnostic microbiology. Other methods either used independently or in conjunction with hybridization or amplification procedures can provide nucleotide sequence information to detect, identify, and characterize microorganisms. These methods include nucleic acid sequencing, enzymatic digestion, and electrophoresis of nucleic acids.

Nucleic Acid Sequencing

Nucleic acid sequencing involves methods that determine the exact nucleotide sequence of a single gene or gene fragment obtained from an organism. Recently whole genome sequencing has become available in large research and clinical laboratories for detection of microbial pathogens. Although the technologic details of nucleic acid sequencing are beyond the scope of this text, these techniques are sure to have a powerful impact in the clinical laboratory for some time to come. To illustrate, nucleotide sequences obtained from a microorganism can be compared with an ever-growing gene sequence database for:
- Identifying microbial pathogens and their subtypes
- Detecting and classifying previously unknown human pathogens

- Determining which specific nucleotide changes resulting from mutations are responsible for antibiotic resistance
- Identifying sequences or gene cassettes that have moved from one organism to another
- Establishing the genetic relatedness between isolates of the same species
- Analyzing the balance between the human microbiome and pathogen(s) and the role of their interactions in the development and prevention of infectious disease

Before the development of rapid and automated methods, DNA sequencing was a laborious task only undertaken in the research setting. However, determining the sequence of nucleotides in a segment of nucleic acid from an infectious agent can be accomplished rapidly using an amplified target from the organism and an automated DNA sequencing instrument. As such, identification of microorganisms using PCR in conjunction with automated sequencing is slowly making its way into clinical microbiology laboratories. It is becoming quite clear that combinations of phenotypic and genotypic characterization are most successful in identifying microorganisms for which identification via culture or PCR alone is difficult, such as the speciation of *Nocardia* and mycobacteria. Recently, Applied Biosystems (Thermo Fisher Scientific, Waltham, MA) has introduced MicroSEQ kit-based reagents in conjunction with automated sequencing that allows analysis of a sequence of either the bacterial 16S rRNA gene or the D2 expansion segment region of the nuclear large-subunit rRNA gene of fungi. Of significance, the MicroSEQ sequence libraries contain accurate and rigorously verified sequence data; an important component for successful sequencing in the identification of organisms is an accurate and complete sequence database. In addition, the ability to create customized libraries for specific sequences of interest is possible by the availability of flexible software.

Pyrosequencing

Traditional nucleic acid sequencing is based on chain termination and the addition of a labeled nucleotide (TTP, GTP, ATP, CTP, or UTP) that is then detected using a radiolabeled or fluorescent tag. **Pyrosequencing** is a newer method that incorporates a luminescent signal (generation of a pyrophosphate) when nucleotides are added to the growing nucleic acid strand. The reaction incorporates a sequencing primer that hybridizes to the single-stranded target. The hybrids are incubated with DNA polymerase, ATP sulfurylase, luciferase, and apyrase along with the substrates adenosine-5′-phosphosulfate and luciferin. A single dNTP (deoxynucleotide triphosphate) is added to the reaction. As the polymerase extends the target from the primer, the dNTP is incorporated, releasing a pyrophosphate (PPi). The ATP sulfurylase then converts the PPi to ATP, which drives the conversion of luciferin to oxyluciferin, generating light. The amount of light generated is proportional to the amount of the specific nucleotide incorporated, generating a report or **pyrogram.** The apyrase degrades the ATP and unincorporated dNTPs, turning off the light and regenerating the reaction mixture. The next dNTP is added, repeating the process for each subsequent nucleotide. Pyrosequencing is useful for identifying drug-resistant mutations and for identification of viral, bacterial, or fungal nucleic acids.

Next Generation Sequencing

Next generation sequencing or massive parallel sequencing have greatly increased the ability to identify microorganisms in terms of the amount of sequence produced and decreased cost in comparison to traditional dideoxynucleotide chain termination methods. Various next generation sequencing platforms are available that differ in the sequencing method, read lengths, depths of coverage, run times, total bases per run, sequence accuracy and cost. These platforms are having a direct impact on microbial identification, strain typing, and the detection of rare mutations including drug-resistance in organisms such as HIV-1. Standards and guidelines for nucleic acid sequencing in the clinical laboratory are available from the Clinical and Laboratory Standards Institute (CLSI).

Nucleic Acid and Oligonucleotide Arrays
High-Density Deoxyribonucleic Acid Probes

An alternative to sequencing has been the introduction of the **high-density oligonucleotide probe arrays.** This technology was developed by Affymetrix, Inc. (Santa Clara, CA). The method relies on the hybridization of a fluorescent-labeled nucleic acid target to large sets of oligonucleotides synthesized at precise locations on a miniaturized glass substrate that may include glass or siliconized wafer, referred to as a "chip." The hybridization pattern of the probe to the various oligonucleotides is then used to gain primary structure information about the target (Fig. 8.16). Hybridization high-density microarrays in combination with sequence-independent amplification (PCR) have also been used to identify pathogens. This technology has been applied to a broad range of nucleic acid sequence analysis problems, including pathogen identification and classification, polymorphism detection, and drug-resistant mutations for viruses (e.g., HIV) and bacteria.

Low- to Moderate-Density Arrays

More recently, **low- to moderate-density microarray** platforms have been developed and commercialized that are less expensive than high-density arrays. This has allowed many laboratories to incorporate this new and powerful technology into the daily operations of the diagnostic microbiology laboratory. These microarrays use layered film, gold-plated electrodes, and electrochemical detection or gold nanoparticles for the detection of target sequences. There are currently several FDA-approved platforms available in the United States. These instruments are closed systems and user-friendly, making the detection of nucleic acids relatively simple and free from the hazards of contamination by other circulating nucleic acids or amplification products. In addition, multiplexing capacity continues to increase and expand the capacity for detection of multiple pathogens associated with clinical syndromes, such as gastroenteritis and respiratory conditions.

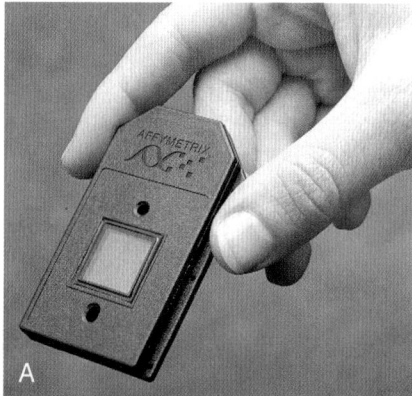

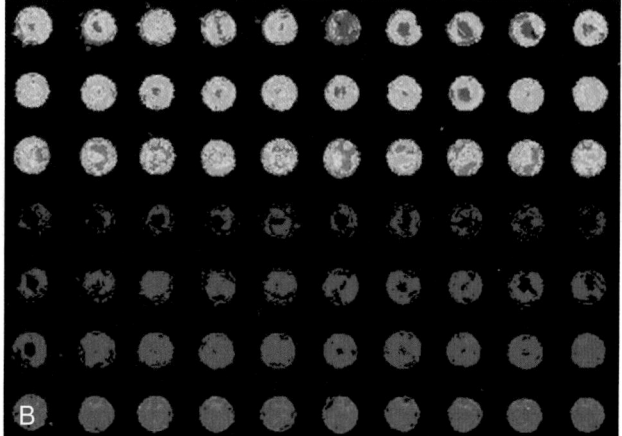

• **Fig. 8.16** Overview of high-density deoxyribonucleic acid probes. High-density oligonucleotide arrays are created using light-directed chemical synthesis that combines photolithography and solid-phase chemical synthesis. Because of this sophisticated process, more than 500 to as many as 1 million different oligonucleotide probes may be formed on a chip; an array is shown in (A). Nucleic acid is extracted from a sample and then hybridized within seconds to the probe array in a GeneChip Fluidics Station. The hybridized array (B) is scanned using a laser confocal fluorescent microscope that looks at each site (i.e., probe) on the chip, and the intensity of hybridization is analyzed using imaging processing software.

Magnetic Resonance

Miniaturized magnetic resonance automation can be used to detect amplified target nucleic acid using supramagnetic nanoparticles coated with nucleic acid probes. The nanoparticles bind to the amplified targets that create clusters altering the magnetic properties of the sample. This changes the single resulting in a positive detection. The FDA approved T2 Magnetic Resonance System or T2MR (Biosystems, Lexington, MA) currently has two panels available for diagnostic use, the bacterial and *Candida* panel. The reported detection limit is significantly lower than other systems that use PCR-based technology (Fig. 8.17).

Enzymatic Digestion and Electrophoresis of Nucleic Acids

Enzymatic digestion and electrophoresis of DNA fragments are not as specific as sequencing or specific amplification assays in identifying and characterizing microorganisms. However, enzyme digestion–electrophoresis procedures still

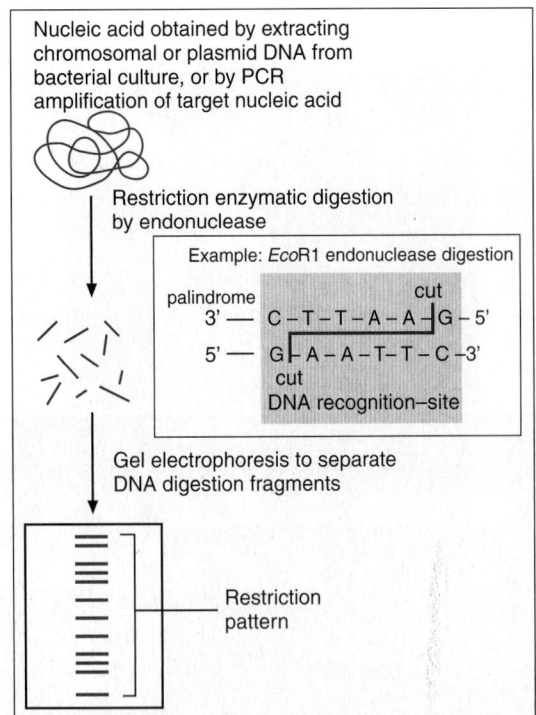

• **Fig. 8.17** Deoxyribonucleic acid (DNA) enzymatic digestion and gel electrophoresis to separate DNA fragments resulting from the digestion. An example of a nucleic acid recognition site and enzymatic cut produced by EcoR1, a commonly used endonuclease, is shown in the inset. PCR, Polymerase chain reaction.

• **Fig. 8.18** Restriction fragment length polymorphisms of vancomycin-resistant *Enterococcus faecalis* isolates in Lanes A through G as determined by pulsed-field gel electrophoresis. All isolates appear to be the same strain.

provide valuable information for the diagnosis and control of infectious diseases.

Enzymatic digestion of DNA is accomplished using any of a number of enzymes known as **restriction endonucleases.** Each specific endonuclease recognizes a specific nucleotide sequence (usually 4 to 8 nucleotides in length), known as the enzyme's **recognition** or **restriction site.** Restriction sites are often **palindromic sequences;** in other words, the two strands have the same sequence, which run antiparallel to one another. Once the recognition site has been located, the enzyme catalyzes the digestion of the nucleic acid strand at that site, causing a break, or cut, in the nucleic acid strand (Fig. 8.18).

The number and size of fragments produced by enzymatic digestion depend on the length of nucleic acid being digested (the longer the strand, the greater the likelihood of more recognition sites and thus more fragments), the nucleotide sequence of the strand being digested (which dictates the number and location of restriction sites), and the particular enzyme used for digestion. For example, enzymatic digestion of a bacterial plasmid whose nucleotide sequence provides several recognition sites for endonuclease A, but only rare sites for endonuclease B, will produce more fragments with endonuclease A. In addition, the size of the fragments produced will depend on the number of nucleotides between each of endonuclease A's recognition sites present on the nucleic acid being digested.

The DNA used for digestion is obtained by various methods. A target sequence may be obtained by amplification via PCR, in which case the length of the DNA to be digested is relatively short (e.g., 50 to 1000 bases). Alternatively, specific procedures may be used to cultivate the organism of interest to large numbers (e.g., 10^{10} bacterial cells) from which plasmid DNA, chromosomal DNA, or total cellular DNA may be isolated and purified for endonuclease digestion.

After digestion, fragments are subjected to agarose gel electrophoresis, which allows them to be separated according to their size differences as previously described for Southern hybridization (Fig. 8.5B). During electrophoresis, all nucleic acid fragments of the same size comigrate as a single band. For many digestions, electrophoresis results in the separation of several different fragment sizes (Fig. 8.19). The nucleic acid bands in the agarose gel are stained with the fluorescent dye ethidium bromide, which allows them to be visualized on exposure to UV light. Stained gels are analyzed by comparing the banding patterns present and photographing them to retain a permanent record of the results (Figs. 8.19 and 8.20).

One variation of this method, known as **ribotyping,** involves enzymatic digestion of chromosomal DNA followed by Southern hybridization using probes for genes that encode ribosomal RNA. Because all bacteria contain ribosomal genes, a hybridization pattern will be obtained with almost any isolate, but the pattern will vary depending on the arrangement of genes in a particular strain or organism's genome. Regardless of the method, the process by which enzyme digestion patterns are analyzed is referred to as **restriction enzyme analysis (REA).** The patterns obtained after gel electrophoresis are referred to as **restriction patterns,** and differences between microorganism restriction patterns are known as restriction fragment length polymorphisms (RFLPs). Because RFLPs reflect differences or similarities in nucleotide sequences, REA methods can be used for organism identification and/or for establishing strain relatedness within the same species (Figs. 8.19 and 8.20).

Applications of Nucleic Acid–Based Methods

Categories for the application of molecular diagnostic microbiology methods are the same as those for conventional, phenotype-based methods:
* Direct detection of microorganisms in patient specimens
* Identification of microorganisms grown in culture
* Characterization of microorganisms beyond basic identification

Nucleic acid–based methods can also be used to validate the result of a negative test using another technique with lower sensitivity, such as rapid diagnostic tests or immunochromatographic "strip" tests.

Direct Detection of Microorganisms

Nucleic acid hybridization and target or probe amplification methods are the molecular techniques most commonly used for direct organism detection in clinical specimens.

Advantages and Disadvantages

When considering the advantages and disadvantages of nucleic acid–based approaches to direct organism detection, a comparison with the current "gold standard" or most

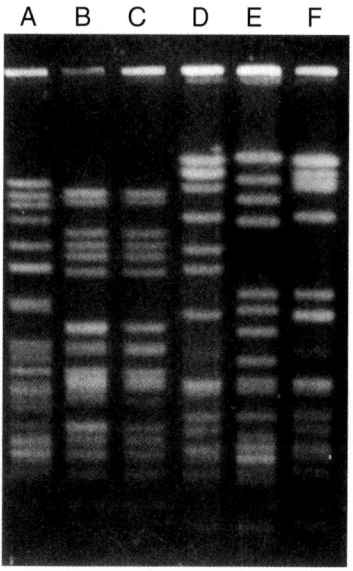

• **Fig. 8.19** Although antimicrobial susceptibility profiles indicated that several methicillin-resistant *Staphylococcus aureus* isolates were the same strain, restriction fragment length polymorphism analysis using pulsed-field gel electrophoresis (Lanes A through F) demonstrates that only isolates B and C were the same.

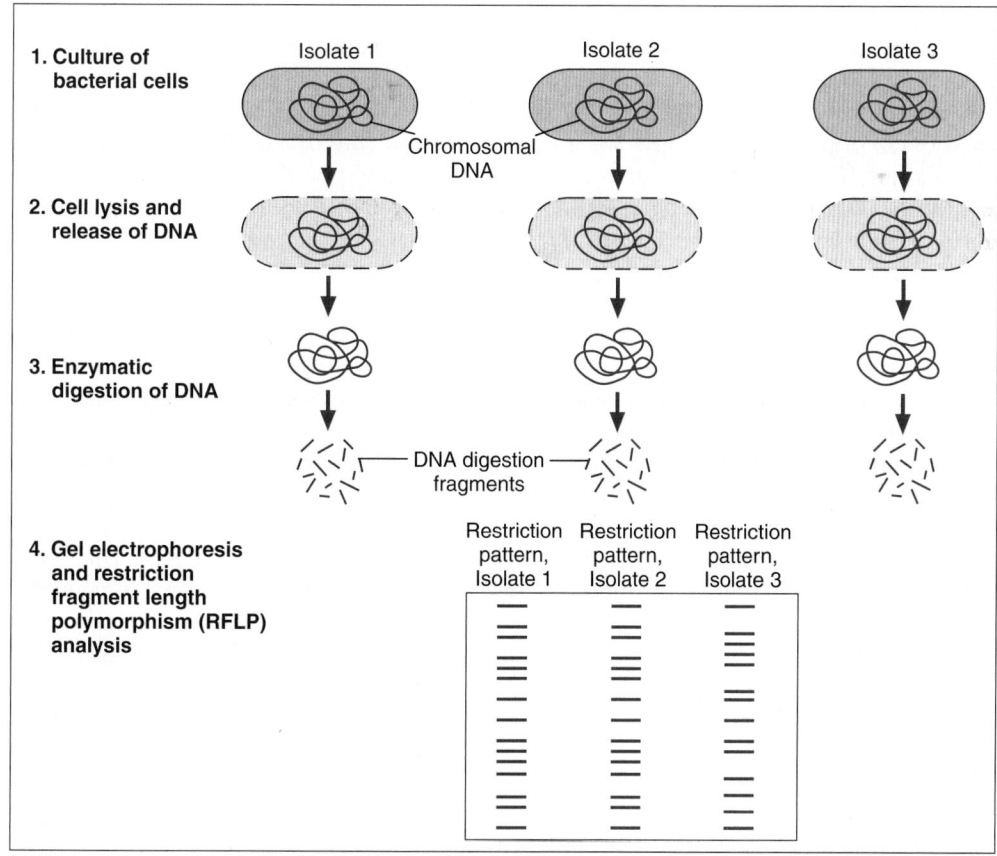

• **Fig. 8.20** Procedural steps for pulsed-field gel electrophoresis.

commonly used conventional methods (i.e., direct smears, culture, and microscopy) is helpful.

Analytical Specificity

Both hybridization and amplification methods are driven by the specificity of a nucleotide sequence for a particular organism, or **analytical specificity.** Therefore, a positive assay indicates the presence of an organism but also provides the organism's identity, potentially precluding the need for follow-up culture. Although molecular methods may not be faster than microscopic smear examinations, the opportunity to prevent the delays associated with a culture can be a substantial advantage.

However, for many infectious agents, detection and identification are only part of the diagnostic requirement. Determination of certain characteristics, such as strain relatedness or resistance to antimicrobial agents, is often an important diagnostic or epidemiologic component that is not possible without the availability of culture. For this reason, most molecular detection methods target organisms for which antimicrobial susceptibility testing is not routinely needed (e.g., *Chlamydia* spp.) or for which reliable cultivation methods are not widely available (e.g., *Ehrlichia* spp.).

The high specificity of molecular techniques also presents a limitation in what can be detected with any one assay; that is, most molecular assays focus on detecting the presence of only one or two potential pathogens. Even if tests for those organisms are positive, the possibility of a mixed infection involving other organisms has not been ruled out. If the tests are negative, other procedures may be needed to determine whether additional pathogens are present. In contrast, smear examination and cultivation procedures can detect and identify a broader selection of possible infectious etiologies. Of importance, a follow-up Gram-stained smear may be necessary to determine the clinical relevance of finding a particular organism upon culture or detection using molecular assays.

However, a number of novel molecular platforms and reagents have recently emerged that greatly expand the spectrum of detectable organisms in any particular specimen.

FDA-cleared gastrointestinal, respiratory, and blood culture panels with the ability to simultaneously detect more than 20 different pathogens are available on the BioFire FilmArray automated system.

Finally, as mentioned throughout this chapter, a concern associated with any amplification-based assay is the possibility for cross contamination between samples or by amplified byproduct. Thus, it is of utmost importance for any laboratory performing these assays to employ measures to prevent false-positive results. Automated and "closed systems" that integrate sample preparation, amplification, and direct detection greatly reduce the potential for contamination.

Analytical Sensitivity

Hybridization-based methods are not completely reliable in directly detecting small numbers of organisms. **Analytical**

sensitivity is defined as the lower limit of organism or nucleic acid concentration for reproducible detection of a pathogen on a specific testing platform. This value can be affected by several factors, including adequacy of specimen collection, assay optimization, interfering substances, and specimen transport and storage. For example, the quantity of target nucleic acid may be insufficient, or the patient specimen may contain substances that interfere with or cross-react in the hybridization and signal-generating reactions. As was discussed with direct hybridization methods, patient specimens may contain substances that interfere with or inhibit amplification reactions such as PCR. Nonetheless, the ability to amplify target or probe nucleic acid to readily detectable levels has provided an invaluable means of overcoming the lack of sensitivity characteristic of most direct hybridization methods. One approach developed by Hologic (Madison, WI) to enhance sensitivity has been to use DNA probes targeted for bacterial ribosomal RNA, of which there are up to 10,000 copies per cell. Essentially, amplification is accomplished by the choice of a target that exists within the cell as multiple copies rather than as a single copy; this may serve to negate the potential effects of interfering substances to preserve the high analytical sensitivity characteristic of tests that target rRNA.

Besides the potential for providing more reliable test results than direct hybridization (i.e., fewer false-negative results), amplification methods have other advantages that include:

- Ability to detect nonviable organisms that are not retrievable by cultivation-based methods
- Ability to detect and identify organisms that cannot be grown in culture or are extremely difficult to grow (e.g., hepatitis B virus, *Mycoplasma* spp., and the agent of Whipple disease)
- More rapid detection and identification of slow-growing organisms (e.g., mycobacteria, certain fungi)
- Ability to detect previously unknown agents directly in clinical specimens by using broad-range primers (e.g., use of primers that anneal to a region of target DNA conserved among all bacteria)
- Ability to quantitate infectious agent burden in patient specimens, an application that has particular importance for managing HIV, cytomegalovirus (CMV), and hepatitis B and hepatitis C infections

Despite these significant advantages, limitations still exist, notably the ability to find only the organisms toward which the primers have been targeted. In addition, no cultured organism is available if subsequent characterization beyond identification is necessary. As with hybridization, the first limitation may eventually be addressed using broad-range amplification methods to screen specimens for the presence of any organism (e.g., bacteria, fungi, viruses, or parasites). Specimens positive by this test would then be processed further for a more specific diagnosis. The second limitation is more difficult to overcome and is one reason culture methods will remain a major part of diagnostic microbiology for some time to come.

An interesting consequence of using highly sensitive amplification methods is the effect on clinical interpretation of results. For example, if a microbiologist detects organisms that are no longer viable, can he or she assume the organisms are or were involved in the infectious process being diagnosed? In addition, amplification may detect microorganisms present in insignificant quantities as part of the patient's normal or transient microbiota, or as an established latent infection, that have nothing to do with the current disease state of the patient.

Finally, as previously mentioned, an underlying complication in the development and application of any direct detection method is that various substances in patient specimens can interfere with the hybridization or amplification reaction, thereby reducing analytical sensitivity. Specimen interference is one of the major issues that must be addressed in the design of any useful direct method for molecular diagnosis of infectious diseases.

Applications for Direct Molecular Detection of Microorganisms

Given their inherent advantages and disadvantages, molecular direct detection methods are most useful when:

- One or two pathogens cause the majority of infections (e.g., *C. trachomatis* and *N. gonorrhoeae* as common agents of genitourinary tract infections)
- Further organism characterization, such as antimicrobial susceptibility testing, is not required for management of the infection (e.g., various viral agents)
- Either no reliable diagnostic methods exist or they are notably suboptimal (e.g., various bacterial, parasitic, viral, and fungal agents)
- Reliable diagnostic methods exist but are slow (e.g., *Mycobacterium tuberculosis*)
- Quantitation of infectious agent burden influences patient management (e.g., HIV quantification for monitoring antiretroviral therapy or AIDS progression)

A variety of commercially available molecular systems and products for the detection and identification of infectious organisms are currently available. These include automated and semiautomated systems, many of which are included throughout this textbook. In addition, many molecular assays have been developed by research laboratories (laboratory-developed tests [LDTs]) associated with academic medical centers. Therefore, direct molecular diagnostic methods based on amplification will continue to expand and enhance our understanding and diagnosis of infectious diseases. However, as with any laboratory method, their ultimate utility and application will depend on accuracy, impact on patient care, advantages over currently available methods, and resources required to establish and maintain their use in the diagnostic setting.

Identification of Microorganisms Grown in Culture

Once organisms are grown in culture, hybridization, amplification, or RFLP analysis may be used to establish identity. Because the target nucleic acid is already amplified via microbial cultivation, sensitivity is not usually a problem for nucleic acid–based identification methods.

In addition, extensive nucleotide sequence data are available for most clinically relevant organisms, providing the required information to produce highly specific probes and primers.

The criteria often considered in comparing nucleic acid–based and conventional methods for microbial identification include speed, accuracy, and cost. For slow-growing organisms, such as mycobacteria and fungi, culture-based identification schemes can take weeks to months to produce a result. Nucleic acid–based methods can identify these microorganisms almost immediately after sufficient inoculum is available, clearly demonstrating a speed advantage over conventional culture-based methods. For example, *Mycobacteria* spp. may take several months to culture and correctly identify using phenotypic methods. However, a nucleic acid–based test is available that specifically amplifies a fragment of the DNA encoding the 16s subunit of the rRNA, a genetic characteristic common to all species of mycobacteria. This provides a screening method to detect the presence of a *Mycobacterium* species within a specimen. This procedure may then be followed by amplification of an insertion sequence (S6110) that is unique and specific for *M. tuberculosis*. Additional species may be identified using the differential restriction digestion patterns for the *hsp65* gene present in all mycobacteria. Historically, phenotypic-based methods used to identify frequently encountered bacteria, such as *S. aureus* and beta-hemolytic streptococci, can usually provide highly accurate results within minutes and are less costly and time-consuming than any currently available molecular method. Rapid, POC tests that use real-time PCR–based methods are commercially available for methicillin-resistant *Staphylococcus aureus* (MRSA) screening of patients upon admission to a long-term care or hospital facility. This technology provides for immediate isolation of carriers, preventing the spread of nosocomial infections throughout the facility.

Although many of the phenotype-based identification schemes are highly accurate and reliable, in some situations phenotypic profiles may yield uncertain identifications. Nucleic acid–based methods are providing an alternative for establishing a definitive or confirmatory organism identification. This is especially true when a common pathogen exhibits unusual phenotypic traits (e.g., optochin-resistant *S. pneumoniae*).

Characterization of Microorganisms Beyond Identification

Situations exist in which characterizing a microbial pathogen beyond identification provides important information for patient management and public health. In such situations, knowledge regarding an organism's virulence, resistance to antimicrobial agents, or relatedness to other strains of the same species can be extremely important. Although various phenotypic methods have been able to provide some of this information, the development of nucleic acid–based testing has greatly expanded the capability to generate this information in the diagnostic setting in a more timely fashion. This is especially true with regard to antimicrobial resistance and strain relatedness among bacteria.

Detection of Antimicrobial Resistance

As are all phenotypic traits, those that render microorganisms resistant to antimicrobial agents are encoded on specific genes (for more information regarding antimicrobial resistance mechanisms, see Chapter 10). Therefore, nucleic acid–based tests can be used to detect the genes encoding the antimicrobial resistance. In many ways, phenotypic methods for resistance detection are reliable and are the primary methods for antimicrobial susceptibility testing (Chapter 11). However, the complexity of emerging resistance mechanisms often challenges the ability of commonly used susceptibility testing methods to "keep up" with the evolving patterns of resistance in a population. As with the nucleic acid–based identification previously described, *Mycobacterium* spp. resistant to rifampin and isoniazid may be readily identified using nucleic acid–based methods by targeting the *rpoB* and *katG* genes.

Methods such as PCR play a role in the detection of certain resistance profiles that may not always be readily detected by phenotypic methods. Two such examples include detection of the *van* genes, which mediate vancomycin resistance among enterococci (Fig. 8.19), and the *mec* gene, which encodes resistance among staphylococci to all currently available drugs of the beta-lactam class (Fig. 8.20). Undoubtedly, conventional and molecular methods will both continue to play key roles in the characterization of microbial resistance to antimicrobial agents.

Investigation of Strain Relatedness and Pulsed-Field Gel Electrophoresis

An important component of recognizing and controlling disease outbreaks inside or outside of a hospital is identification of the reservoir and mode of transmission of the infectious agents involved. Strain typing provides a mechanism for monitoring the spread of drug-resistant pathogens, the evaluation of multiple isolates from a single patient, and differentiation of relapse from a new infection. Epidemiology and infection control measures often require establishing relatedness among the pathogens isolated during an outbreak. For example, if all the microbial isolates thought to be associated with a nosocomial infection outbreak are shown to be identical or at least very closely related, then a common source or reservoir for those isolates must be identified. If the etiologic agents are not the same, other explanations for the outbreak must be investigated (Chapter 79). Because each species of a microorganism comprises an almost limitless number of strains, identification of an organism to the species level is not sufficient for establishing relatedness. **Strain typing,** the process used to establish the relatedness among organisms belonging to the same species, is required.

Although phenotypic characteristics (e.g., biotyping, serotyping, antimicrobial susceptibility profiles) historically

TABLE 8.2	Examples of Methods to Determine Strain Relatedness
Method	**Advantages/Limitations**
Plasmid analysis	Simple to implement but cannot often discriminate because many bacterial species have few or no plasmids
Multilocus enzyme electrophoresis	Provides only an estimate of overall genetic relatedness and diversity (protein-based)
Multilocus sequence typing	Data are electronically portable and used as non–culture-based typing method; labor intensive and expensive
Pulsed-field gel electrophoresis	Highly discriminatory but it is difficult to resolve bands of similar size and interlaboratory reproducibility is limited
Randomly amplified polymorphic deoxyribonucleic acid (DNA)	High discriminatory power but poor laboratory interlaboratory and intralaboratory reproducibility due to short random primer sequences and low polymerase chain reaction (PCR) annealing temperatures
Repetitive sequence–based PCR	*Manual system:* Useful for strain typing, but low rates of interlaboratory reproducibility; suboptimal turnaround times (TATs) for both manual and automated systems *Automated system:* Increased reproducibility and decreased TATs
Ribotyping and PCR ribotyping	Difficult to distinguish among different subtypes
Whole-genome sequencing	Reproducibility, ability to discriminate novel mutations for improved susceptibility testing

have been used to type strains, these methods often are limited by their inability to consistently discriminate between different strains, their labor intensity, or their lack of reproducibility. In contrast, certain molecular methods do not have these limitations and have enhanced strain-typing capabilities. The molecular typing methods either directly compare nucleotide sequences between strains or produce results that indirectly reflect similarities in nucleotide sequences among "outbreak" organisms. Indirect methods usually involve enzymatic digestion and electrophoresis of microbial DNA to enable RFLP analysis.

Several molecular methods have been investigated for establishing strain relatedness (Table 8.2). The method chosen primarily depends on the extent to which the following four criteria proposed by Maslow and colleagues are met:

- **Typeability:** The method's capacity to produce clearly interpretable results with most strains of the bacterial species to be tested
- **Reproducibility:** The method's capacity to repeatedly obtain the same typing profile result with the same bacterial strain
- **Discriminatory power:** The method's ability to produce results that clearly allow differentiation between unrelated strains of the same bacterial species
- **Practicality:** The method should be versatile, relatively rapid, inexpensive, technically simple, and provide readily interpretable results

The last criterion, practicality, is especially important for busy clinical microbiology laboratories that provide support for infection control and hospital epidemiology.

Among the molecular methods used for strain typing, **pulsed-field gel electrophoresis (PFGE)** meets most of Maslow's criteria for a good typing system and is frequently referred to as the microbial typing "gold standard." This method is applicable to most of the commonly encountered bacterial pathogens, particularly those frequently associated with nosocomial infections and outbreaks, such as staphylococci (MRSA), enterococci (vancomycin-resistant enterococci), and gram-negative pathogens, including *Escherichia coli* and *Klebsiella, Enterobacter,* and *Acinetobacter* spp. For these reasons, PFGE has been widely accepted among microbiologists, infection control personnel, and infectious disease specialists as a primary laboratory tool for epidemiology.

PFGE uses a specialized electrophoresis device to separate chromosomal fragments produced by enzymatic digestion of intact bacterial chromosomal DNA. Bacterial suspensions are first embedded in agarose plugs, where they are carefully lysed (lysozyme) to release intact chromosomal DNA; the interfering contaminating proteins are then removed by treating the sample with proteinase K; the DNA is then digested using restriction endonuclease enzymes. Enzymes that have relatively few restriction sites on the genomic DNA are selected so that 10 to 20 DNA fragments ranging in size from 10 to 1000 kb are produced (Fig. 8.20). Because of the large DNA fragment sizes produced, resolution of the banding patterns requires the use of a pulsed electrical field across the agarose gel that subjects the DNA fragments to different voltages from varying angles at different time intervals.

Although comparison and interpretation of RFLP profiles produced by PFGE can be complex, the basic premise is that strains with the same or highly similar digestion profiles share substantial similarities in their nucleotide sequences and therefore are likely to be most closely related.

One example of PFGE application for the investigation of an outbreak is shown in Fig. 8.18. After Sma I endonuclease enzymatic digestion of DNA from seven vancomycin-resistant *E. faecalis* isolates, RFLP profiles show that the resistant isolates are probably the same strain. Such a finding strongly supports the probability of clonal dissemination of

the same vancomycin-resistant strain among the patients from which the organisms were isolated.

The discriminatory advantage that PFGE profiles have over phenotype-based typing methods is demonstrated in Fig. 8.19. Because all six MRSA isolates exhibited identical antimicrobial susceptibility profiles, they were initially thought to be the same strain. However, PFGE profiling established that only isolates B and C were the same.

PFGE can also be used to determine whether a recurring infection in the same patient is due to insufficient original therapy, possibly because of developing antimicrobial resistance during therapy, or to acquisition of a second, more resistant, strain of the same species. Fig. 8.20 shows restriction patterns obtained by PFGE with *S. pneumoniae* isolated from a patient with an unresolved middle ear infection. The PFGE profile of isolate B, which was fully susceptible to penicillin, differs substantially from the profile of isolate C, which was resistant to penicillin. The clear difference in PFGE profiles between the two strains indicates that the patient was most likely reinfected with a second, more resistant, strain. Alternatively, the patient's original infection may have been a mixture of both strains, with the more resistant one being lost during the original culture workup. In any case, this application of PFGE demonstrates that the method not only is useful for investigating outbreaks or strain dissemination involving several patients, it also gives us the ability to investigate questions regarding reinfections, treatment failures, and mixed infections involving more than one strain of the same species.

Automation and Advances in Molecular Diagnostic Instrumentation

Molecular diagnostics has traditionally required extensive hands-on technical expertise to process specimens, extract the nucleic acids, amplify, and detect the target sequence. In addition, the high cost of consumable reagents and instrumentation initially limited molecular diagnostics to large, centralized clinical laboratories, research hospitals, and public health departments. However, technologic advances have rapidly changed the diagnostic microbiology laboratory, making nucleic acid–based testing accessible to the vast majority of clinical labs even in small local and regional hospitals. Traditional amplification instruments are still available (e.g., basic thermal cyclers); however, real-time amplification and detection as well as fully automated closed systems are rapidly replacing these instruments and becoming more widely accessible to small and mid-sized clinical laboratories. This new generation of instruments facilitates the amplification and analysis of numerous samples simultaneously in a single run (e.g., increasing throughput) and reduces the amount of hands-on interaction required (e.g., mixing or adding reagents) with preloaded reagent packs and/or microfluidic components. The overall cost of these automated and semiautomated instruments has also sharply declined in the past few years, making them financially viable in many different clinical settings. These trends toward greater automation, user-friendliness, and reduced cost are expected to continue, making molecular diagnostic testing increasingly available worldwide.

As these technologies continue to evolve, the cost and speed of testing is expected to decline, such that WG-NGS and MS will become routine tests in infectious disease diagnostics.

ⓔ Visit the Evolve site for a complete list of procedures, review questions, and case studies.

Bibliography

Buckingham L: *Molecular diagnostics, fundamentals, methods, and clinical applications*, ed 2, Philadelphia, 2012, FA Davis.

Buller RS: Molecular detection of respiratory viruses, *Clin Lab Med* 33:439–460, 2013.

Caroll KC, Pfaller MA: *Manual of clinical microbiology*, ed 12, Washington, DC, 2019, ASM Press.

Chapin K, Musgnug M: Evaluation of three rapid methods for the direct identification of *Staphylococcus aureus* from positive blood cultures, *J Clin Microbiol* 41:4324–4327, 2003.

Cockerill FR: Application of rapid-cycle real-time polymerase chain reaction for diagnostic testing in the clinical microbiology laboratory, *Arch Pathol Lab Med* 127:1112–1120, 2003.

Drouin R, Dridi W, Samassekou O: DNA Polymerases for PCR Applications. In Polaina J, MacCabe AP, editors: *Industrial enzymes: structure, function and applications*, ed 1, Springer, 2007, pp 379–401.

Fairfax MR, Salimnia H: Diagnostic molecular microbiology: a 2013 snapshot, *Clin Lab Med* 33:787–803, 2013.

Fong WK, Modrusan Z, Mcnevin JP, Marostenmaki J, Zin B, Bekkaoui F: Rapid solid-phase immunoassay for detection of methicillin-resistant *Staphylococcus aureus* using cycling probe technology, *J Clin Microbiol* 38:2525–2529, 2000.

Fontana C, Favaro M, Pellicioni M, Pistoia ES, Favalli C: Use of the MicroSeq 500 16S rRNA gene-based sequencing for identification of bacterial isolates that commercial automated systems failed to identify correctly, *J Clin Microbiol* 43:615–619, 2005.

Forbes BA: Introducing a molecular test into the clinical microbiology laboratory: development, evaluation, and validation, *Arch Pathol Lab Med* 127:1106–1111, 2003.

Ginocchio CC: Life beyond PCR: alternative target amplification technologies for the diagnosis of infectious diseases. Part I, *Clin Microbiol Newsl* 26:121–128, 2004.

Ginocchio CC: Life beyond PCR: alternative target amplification technologies for the diagnosis of infectious diseases. Part II, *Clin Microbiol Newsl* 26:129, 2004.

Goering RV: Molecular strain typing for the clinical laboratory: current application and future direction, *Clin Microbiol Newsl* 22:169–173, 2000.

Haanperä M, Huovinen P, Jalava J: Detection and quantification of macrolide resistance mutations at positions 2058 and 2059 of the 23s rRNA gene by pyrosequencing, *Antimicrob Agents Chemother* 49:457–460, 2005.

Hall L, Wohlfiel S, Roberts GD: Experience with the MicroSeq D2 large-subunit ribosomal DNA sequencing kit for identification of commonly encountered, clinically important yeast species, *J Clin Microbiol* 41:5009–5102, 2003.

Healy M, Huong J, Bittner T, et al.: Microbial DNA typing by automated repetitive-sequenced-based PCR, *J Clin Microbiol* 43:199–207, 2005.

Hindson BJ, Ness KD, Masquelier DA, et al.: High-throughput droplet digital PCR system for absolute quantitation of DNA copy number, *Anal Chem* 83:8604–8610, 2011.

Huang HS, Tsai CL, Chang J, Hsu TC, Lin S, Lee CC: Multiplex PCR system for the rapid diagnosis of respiratory virus infection: systematic review and meta-analysis, *Clin Microbiol Infect* 10:1055–1063, 2018.

Jung C, Chung JW, Kim UO, Kim MH, Park HG: Isothermal target and signaling probe amplification method, based on a combination of an isothermal chain amplification technique and a fluorescence resonance energy transfer cycling probe technology, *Anal Chem* 82:5937–5943, 2010.

Kirchgesser M, von Felten C, Kalin C, et al.: The new MagNa Pure LC 2.0 system: new design and improved performance combined with a proven nucleic acid isolation technique, *Roche Applied Science. Biochemica* 3:20–22, 2008.

Liu J, Kabir F, Manneh J, et al.: Development and assessment of molecular diagnostic tests for 15 enteropathogens causing childhood diarrhoea: a multicentre study, *Lancet Infect Dis* 14:716–724, 2014.

Mackay IM: Real-time PCR in the microbiology laboratory, *Clin Microbiol Infect* 10:190–212, 2004.

Maslow JN, Mulligan ME, Arbeit RD: Molecular epidemiology: application of contemporary techniques to the typing of microorganisms, *Clin Infect Dis* 17:153–162, 1993.

Maurin M: Real-time PCR as a diagnostic tool for bacterial diseases, *Expert Rev Mol Diagn* 12:731–754, 2012.

McGowin CL, Rohde RE, Whitlock GC: Other pathogens of significant public health concern. In Hu P, Hedge M, Lennon PA, editors: *Modern clinical molecular techniques, (New Edition)*. New York, 2012, Springer Press.

McGowin CL, Rohde RE, Redwine G: Molecular diagnosis of sexually transmitted infections: a diverse and dynamic landscape, *Clin Lab Sci* 27:40–42, 2014.

Navarro E, Serrano-Heras G, Castano MJ, Solera J: Real-time PCR detection chemistries, *Clin Chim Acta* 439:231–250, 2015.

Oliveira K, Brecher SM, Durbin A, et al.: Direct identification of *Staphylococcus aureus* from positive blood culture bottles, *J Clin Microbiol* 41:889–891, 2003.

Sexton DJ, Bentz ML, Welsh RM, Litvintseva AP: Evaluation of a new T2 magnetic resonance assay for rapid detection of emergent fungal pathogen *Candida auris* on clinical skin swab samples, *Mycoses* 61(10):786–790, 2018.

Tenover FC, Arbeit RD, Goering RV, et al.: Interpreting chromosomal DNA restriction patterns produced by pulsed-field gel electrophoresis: criteria for bacterial strain typing, *J Clin Microbiol* 33:2233–2239, 1995.

Wang D, Urisman A, Liu YT, et al.: Viral discovery and sequence recovery using DNA microarrays, *PLOS Biol* 1(2):E2, 2003.

Wetmur JG: DNA probes: applications of the principles of nucleic acid hybridization, *Crit Rev Biochem Mol Biol* 26:227–259, 1991.

Yan L, Zhou J, Zheng Y, et al.: Isothermal amplified detection of DNA and RNA, *Mol Biosyst* 10:970–1003, 2014.

Zacharioudakis IM, Zervou FN, Mylonakis E: T2 Magnetic resonance assay: overview of 617 available data and clinical implications, *J Fungi (Basel)* 4(45):1–10, 2018.

Zhao Y, Chen F, Li Q, Wang L, Fan C: Isothermal amplification of nucleic acids, *Chem Rev* 115:12491–12545, 2015.

9

Overview of Immunochemical Methods Used for Organism Detection

OBJECTIVES

1. Define the two categories of human specific immune response, cell mediated and antibody mediated, including the definition of T cells and B cells and their role in the responses.
2. List the five classes of antibodies, define their roles in infectious disease, and explain the three antibody functions.
3. Explain the following serologic tests, considering their clinical applications: direct, indirect and reverse passive agglutination, flocculation tests, immunofluorescent assays, and enzyme immunoassay.
4. Describe a cross reaction, and explain why it occurs and how it may affect antibody testing.
5. In defining hemagglutination and neutralization assays, explain their similarity in testing, along with their disparities.
6. Explain how the difference in the size and structure of the immunoglobulin M (IgM) antibody is important to its activity and function.
7. Explain what the complement fixation test is, and describe the two-step reaction.
8. Explain the principle of the Western blot assay and why it is used as a confirmatory test for some assays.
9. Define a polyclonal antibody and a monoclonal antibody, and explain the difference between the two.
10. Explain how monoclonal antibodies are produced. How has their development affected immunochemical testing?
11. Explain the difference between a direct fluorescent antibody (DFA) test and an indirect fluorescent antibody (IFA) test, and explain how each is used in the clinical laboratory.
12. Explain the function of the hypoxanthine, aminopterin, and thymidine (HAT) medium in hybridoma production.

The diagnosis of an infectious disease by culture and biochemical techniques can be hindered by several factors. These factors include the inability to cultivate an organism on artificial media, such as is the case with *Treponema pallidum*, the agent that causes syphilis, or the fragility of an organism and its subsequent failure to survive transport to the laboratory, such as with respiratory syncytial virus (RSV) and varicella-zoster virus (VZV). Another factor, the fastidious nature of some organisms (e.g., *Leptospira* spp. or *Bartonella* spp.), can result in long incubation periods before growth is evident. In addition, administration of antimicrobial therapy before specimen collection, such as with a patient who has received partial treatment, can impede diagnosis. In these cases, detecting a specific product of the infectious agent in clinical specimens is very important, because this product would not be present in the specimen in the absence of the agent. This chapter provides a basic overview of the immune system and its functions and the direct detection of microorganisms in patient specimens using immunochemical methods and the identification of microorganisms. Specific information and the application of immunochemical methods used for organism identification is included in Parts III through VI of this textbook.

Immunochemical methods are used as diagnostic tools for serodiagnosis of infectious disease. An understanding of how these methods have been adapted for this purpose requires a basic working knowledge of the components and functions of the immune system. **Immunology** is the study of the components and functions of the immune system. The immune system is the body's defense mechanism against invading "foreign" antigens. One of the functions of the immune system is distinguishing "self" from "non-self" (i.e., the proteins or antigens from foreign substances). (Chapter 3 presents a more in-depth discussion of the host's response to foreign substances.) This chapter is intended to provide a brief overview and review of immunology. The complexity and detail required to fully understand immunology and serology are beyond the scope of this text.

Features of the Immune Response

The host, or patient, has physical barriers, such as intact skin and ciliated epithelial cells, and chemical barriers, such as

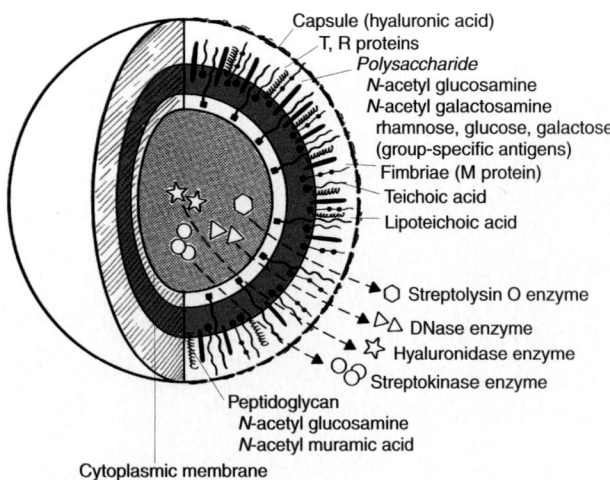

Capsule (hyaluronic acid)
T, R proteins
Polysaccharide
N-acetyl glucosamine
N-acetyl galactosamine
rhamnose, glucose, galactose
(group-specific antigens)
Fimbriae (M protein)
Teichoic acid
Lipoteichoic acid

Streptolysin O enzyme
DNase enzyme
Hyaluronidase enzyme
Streptokinase enzyme

Peptidoglycan
N-acetyl glucosamine
N-acetyl muramic acid

Cytoplasmic membrane

• **Fig. 9.1** Group A streptococci *(Streptococcus pyogenes)* contain many antigenic structural components and produce various antigenic enzymes, each of which may elicit a specific antibody response from the infected host.

oils produced by the sebaceous glands and lysozyme found in tears and saliva, to prevent infections by foreign organisms. In addition, **natural (innate) immunity,** which is not specific, activates chemotaxis, the process that recruits phagocytes to a site of invasion and engulf organisms entering the host. **Acquired active immunity** is the specific response of the host to an infecting organism.

The human specific immune responses are divided into two categories: cell mediated and antibody mediated.

Cell-mediated immune responses are carried out by special lymphocytes of the T-cell (thymus derived) class. T cells proliferate and differentiate into various effector T cells, including cytotoxic and helper cells. **Cytotoxic T (TC) lymphocytes** specifically attack and kill microorganisms or host cells damaged or infected by pathogens. Helper T (TH) lymphocytes promote the maturation of B lymphocytes by producing activator cytokines that induce the B cells to produce antibodies and attach to and kill invading organisms. Although diagnosis of certain diseases may be aided by measuring the cell-mediated immune response to the pathogen, such tests entail skin tests performed by physicians or *in vitro* cell function assays performed by specially trained immunologists. These tests are usually not within the repertoire of clinical microbiology laboratories.

Immunochemical methods use antigens and antibodies as tools to detect microorganisms. Antigens are substances recognized as "foreign" in the human body. Antigens are usually high-molecular-weight proteins or carbohydrates that elicit the production of other proteins, called antibodies, in a human or animal host (Chapter 3). Antibodies attach to the antigens and aid the host in removing the infectious agent. Antigens may be part of the physical structure of the pathogen, such as the bacterial cell wall, or they may be a chemical produced and released by the pathogen, such as an enzyme or a toxin. Each antigen contains a region recognized by the immune system. These regions are antigenic determinants or **epitopes.** Fig. 9.1 shows the

multiple molecules within group A streptococcus *(Streptococcus pyogenes)* that are recognized by the immune system as antigenic.

Specific proteins generated by lymphocytes of the B-cell (bone marrow–derived) class produce antibody-mediated immune responses. These proteins are made in response to the antigens or antigenic determinants of a specific infectious agent. The proteins, immunoglobulins or antibodies, generated in response to the foreign agent demonstrate immunologic function and fold into a globular structure in the active state. Antibodies are either secreted into the blood or lymphatic fluid (and sometimes other body fluids) by plasma cells (activated B lymphocytes), or they remain attached to the surface of the lymphocyte or other cells. Because the cells involved in this category of immune response primarily circulate in the blood, this type of immunity is also called humoral immunity. For purposes of determining whether a patient's body has produced an antibody against a particular infectious agent, the serum (or occasionally the plasma) is examined for the presence of the antibody. The study of the diagnosis of disease by measuring antibody levels in serum is **serology.**

Characteristics of Antibodies

Immunocompetent humans are able to produce antibodies specifically directed against almost all the antigens with which they may come into contact throughout their lifetimes and that the body recognizes as "foreign." Antigens may be part of the physical structure of a pathogen or a chemical produced and released by the pathogen, such as an exotoxin. One pathogen may contain or produce many different antigens that the host recognizes as foreign. Infection with one agent may cause the production of a number of different antibodies. In addition, some antigenic determinants on a pathogen may not be available for recognition by the host until the pathogen has undergone a physical change. For example, until a pathogenic bacterium has been digested by a human polymorphonuclear (PMN) leukocyte, certain antigens deep in the cell wall are not detected by the host immune system. Once the bacterium has been broken down, these new antigens are released and the specific antibodies are produced. For this reason, a patient may produce different antibodies at different times during the course of a single disease. The immune response to an antigen also matures with continued exposure, and the antibodies produced become more specific and more **avid** (able to bind more tightly).

Antibodies function by (1) attaching to the surface of pathogens and making the pathogens more amenable to ingestion by phagocytic cells (**opsonizing antibodies**); (2) binding to and blocking surface receptors for host cells (**neutralizing antibodies**); or (3) attaching to the surface of pathogens and contributing to their destruction by the lytic action of complement (**complement-fixing antibodies**). Routine diagnostic serologic methods are used to measure primarily two antibody classes, immunoglobulin M (IgM)

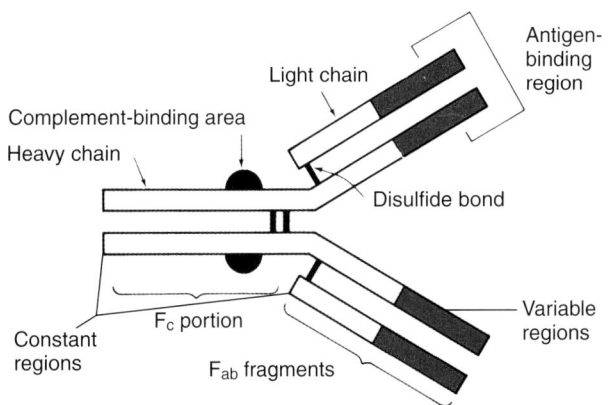

• **Fig. 9.2** Structure of immunoglobulin G. The heavy chains determine the antibody class (IgG, IgA, IgD, IgE, or IgM). The Fab fragment containing the variable regions determines the antibody-binding specificity. The Fc portion (or function cells) binds to various immune cells to activate specific functions in the immune system.

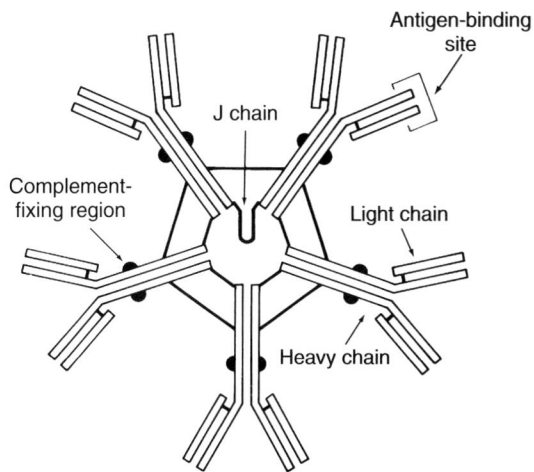

• **Fig. 9.3** Structure of immunoglobulin M.

and immunoglobulin G (IgG); however, antibodies are categorized into five classes: IgG, IgM, immunoglobulin A (IgA), immunoglobulin D (IgD), and immunoglobulin E (IgE). IgA, also referred to as **secretory antibody,** is the predominant class of antibody in saliva, tears, and intestinal secretions. IgD is attached to the surface of B cells and is involved in immune regulations. IgE levels increase in infections caused by several parasites or in response to allergic reactions.

The basic structure of an antibody molecule comprises two mirror images, each composed of two identical protein chains (Fig. 9.2). At the terminal ends of the antibody are the **antigen-binding sites,** or **variable regions,** which specifically attach to the antigen. Depending on the specificity of the antibody, antigens of some similarity, but not total identity, to the inducing antigen may also be bound; this is called a **cross-reaction.** The complement-binding site or **constant region** is found in the center of the molecule in a structure similar for all antibodies of the same class. IgM is produced as a first response to many antigens, although the levels remain high transiently. The presence of IgM usually indicates recent or active exposure to an antigen or infection. In contrast, IgG may persist long after an infection has run its course.

The IgM antibody type (Fig. 9.3) consists of five identical proteins (pentamer), with the basic antibody structures linked at the bases with 10 antigen binding sites on the molecule. IgG consists of one basic antibody molecule (monomer) that has two binding sites. The differences in the size and conformation between these two classes of immunoglobulins result in differences in activities and functions.

Features of the Humoral Immune Response Useful in Diagnostic Testing

Immunocompetent individuals produce both IgM and IgG antibodies in response to most pathogens. In most cases, IgM is produced by a patient after the first exposure

to a pathogen and is no longer detectable within a relatively short period. For serologic diagnostic purposes, it is important to note that IgM is unable to cross the placenta. Any IgM detected in the serum of a newborn must have been produced by the infant and indicates an infection in utero. The larger number of binding sites on IgM molecules provides for more rapid clearance of the offending pathogen, even though each individual antigen-binding site may not be the most efficient for binding to the antigen. Over time, the cells producing IgM switch to production of IgG. IgG is the most prevalent circulating antibody in the human body.

IgG is often more specific for the antigen (i.e., it has higher avidity). IgG has two antigen-binding sites, but it can also bind complement. Complement is a complex series of serum proteins that is involved in modulating several functions of the immune system, including cytotoxic cell death, chemotaxis, and opsonization. When IgG is bound to an antigen, the base of the molecule (Fc portion) is exposed in the environment. Structures on this Fc portion attract and bind the cell membranes of phagocytes, increasing the chances of engulfment and destruction of the pathogen by the host cells. A second exposure to the same pathogen induces a faster and greater IgG response and a much lesser IgM response. Several B lymphocytes retain memory of the pathogen, allowing for a more rapid response and a higher level of antibody production than the primary exposure or response. This enhanced response is called the **anamnestic response.** B-cell memory is not perfect. Occasional clones of memory cells can be stimulated through interaction with an antigen that is similar but not identical to the original antigen. The anamnestic response may be polyclonal and nonspecific. For example, reinfection with cytomegalovirus (CMV) may stimulate memory B cells to produce antibody against Epstein-Barr virus (EBV) (another herpes family virus), which the host encountered previously, in addition to antibody against CMV. The relative humoral responses are diagrammatically represented in Fig. 9.4.

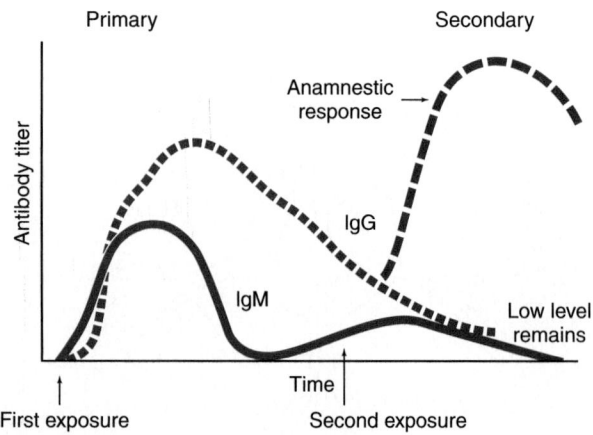

• **Fig. 9.4** Relative humoral response to antigen stimulation over time. *IgG*, Immunoglobulin G, *IgM*, immunoglobulin M.

Interpretation of Serologic Tests

In serology, a change in **antibody titer** is a central concept for the diagnosis and monitoring of disease progression. The titer of antibody is the reciprocal of the highest dilution of the patient's serum in which the antibody is still detectable. Patients with large amounts of antibody have high titers, because antibody is still detectable at very high dilutions of serum. Serum for antibody levels should be drawn during the acute phase of the disease as acute sera (when first suspected) and again during convalescence as convalescent sera (usually at least 2 weeks later). For some infections, such as Legionnaires' disease and hepatitis, titers may not rise until months after the acute infection, or they may never rise. Changes in titer must be carefully correlated with the patient's signs and symptoms of the specific disease or suspected infectious agent.

Patients with intact humoral immunity develop increasing amounts of antibody to a pathogen over several weeks. If it is the patient's first exposure to the pathogenic organism and the specimen has been obtained early enough, no or very low titers of antibody are detected at the onset of disease. In the case of a second exposure, the patient's serum usually contains measurable antibody during the initial phase of the disease, and the antibody level quickly increases because of the anamnestic response. For most pathogens, an increase in the patient's titer of two doubling dilutions (e.g., from a positive result of 1:8 to a positive result of 1:32) is considered to be diagnostic of current infection. This is described as a **fourfold rise in titer.**

For many infections, accurate results used for diagnosis are achieved when acute and convalescent sera are tested concurrently in the same test system. Variables inherent in the procedures and laboratory error can cause a difference of one doubling (or twofold) dilution in the results obtained from the same sample tested concurrently in different laboratories. Unfortunately, a certain proportion of infected patients never demonstrate a rise in titer, necessitating the use of other diagnostic tests. Because the delay inherent in testing paired acute and convalescent

sera results in diagnostic information becoming available too late to affect the initial therapy, increasing numbers of early (IgM) serologic testing assays are being commercially evaluated. Moreover, it is sometimes more realistic to see a fourfold fall in titer between acute and convalescent sera when samples are tested concurrently in the same system. This is a result of the sera being collected late in the course of an infection, when antibodies have already begun to decrease.

The prevalence of antibody to an etiologic agent of disease in the population correlates with the number of people who have been exposed to the agent, not the number who actually develop disease. For most diseases, only a small proportion of infected individuals actually develop symptoms; others develop protective antibodies without experiencing signs and symptoms of the disease whether the individual has developed a true immunity to infection or a secondary reinfection.

Alternatively, depending on the etiologic agent, even low levels of antibody may protect a patient from pathologic effects of disease and not prevent reinfection. For example, a person previously immunized with killed poliovirus vaccine who becomes infected with pathogenic poliovirus experiences multiplication of the virus in the gut and virus entry into the circulation. Damage to the central nervous system is blocked by humoral antibody in the circulation. Moreover, patients may respond to an antigenic stimulus by producing cross-reacting antibodies. These antibodies are nonspecific and may cause misinterpretation of serologic tests.

Table 9.1 provides a brief list of representative serologic tests available for immunodiagnosis of infectious diseases, the specimen required, interpretation of positive and negative test results, and examples of applications of each technique. Because serologic assays are rapidly evolving, this table is not intended to be all-inclusive.

Production of Antibodies for Use in Laboratory Testing

Polyclonal Antibodies

Because an organism contains many different antigens, the host response produces many different antibodies to these antigens; these heterogeneous antibodies are **polyclonal antibodies.** Polyclonal antibodies used in immunodiagnosis are prepared by immunizing animals (usually rabbits, sheep, or goats) with an infectious agent and then isolating and purifying the resulting antibodies from the animal's serum. Antibody idiotype variation is caused by alterations in the nucleotide sequence during antibody production. Individual animals are able to produce different antibodies with different **idiotypes** (antigen binding sites). This variation in antigen-binding sites creates a lack of uniformity in polyclonal antibody reagents and requires continual monitoring and comparisons of different antibody reagent lots for specificity and avidity in any given immunochemical test system.

TABLE 9.1	Noninclusive Overview of Tests Available for Serodiagnosis of Infectious Diseases		
Test	**Sera Needed**	**Interpretation**	**Application**
IgM	Single, acute (collected at onset of illness)	Newborn, positive: in utero (congenital) infection Adult, positive: primary or current infection Adult, negative: no infection or past infection	Newborn: STORCH agents; other organisms Adults: any infectious agent
IgG	Acute and convalescent (collected 2–6 weeks after onset)	Positive: fourfold rise or fall in titer between acute and convalescent sera tested at the same time in the same test system Negative: no current infection or past infection, or patient is immunocompromised and cannot mount a humoral antibody response, or convalescent specimen collected before increase in IgG (Lyme disease, *Legionella* sp.)	Any infectious agent
IgG	Single specimen collected between onset and convalescence	Adult, positive: evidence of infection at some unknown time except in certain cases in which a single high titer is diagnostic (rabies, *Legionella, Ehrlichia* spp.). Newborn, positive: maternal antibodies that crossed the placenta Newborn, negative: patient has not been exposed to microorganism or patient has a congenital or acquired immune deficiency or specimen collected before increase in IgG (Lyme disease or *Legionella* sp.)	Any infectious agent
Immune status evaluation	Single specimen collected at any time	Positive: previous exposure Negative: no exposure	Rubella testing for women of childbearing age, syphilis testing may be required in some states to obtain a marriage license, cytomegalovirus testing for transplant donor and recipient

Ig, Immunoglobulin; *STORCH*, syphilis, *Toxoplasma*, rubella virus, cytomegalovirus, herpes simplex virus.

Monoclonal Antibodies

Monoclonal antibodies are antibodies that are completely characterized and highly specific. The ability to create an immortal cell line that produces large quantities of a monoclonal antibody has revolutionized immunologic testing. Monoclonal antibodies are produced by the fusion of a malignant single antibody-producing myeloma cell with an antibody-producing plasma B cell, forming a **hybridoma cell.** Clones of the hybridoma cells continuously produce specific monoclonal antibodies. One technique for the production of a clone of cells is illustrated in Fig. 9.5.

The process starts with immunization of a mouse with an antigen. The animal responds by producing many antibodies to the epitope (antigenic determinant) injected. The mouse's spleen is removed and emulsified to separate antibody-producing plasma cells. The cells are then placed into individual wells of a microdilution tray. Viability of cells is maintained by fusing them with cells capable of continuously propagating, or immortal cells of a multiple myeloma. A **multiple myeloma** is a disease that produces a malignant tumor containing antibody-producing plasma cells. Myeloma tumor cells used for hybridoma production are deficient in the enzyme hypoxanthine phosphoribosyl

transferase. This defect leads to their inability to survive in a medium containing hypoxanthine, aminopterin, and thymidine (**HAT medium**). However, antibody-producing spleen cells contain the enzyme. Fused hybridoma cells survive in the selective medium and can be recognized by their ability to grow indefinitely. Unfused antibody-producing lymphoid cells die after several multiplications *in vitro* because they are not immortal, and unfused myeloma cells die in the presence of the toxic enzyme substrates. The only surviving cells are true hybrids.

The growth medium supernatant from the microdilution tray wells in which the hybridoma cells are growing is tested for the presence of the desired antibody. Many such cell lines are usually examined before a suitable antibody is identified. The antibody must be specific enough to bind to the individual antigenic determinant to which the animal was exposed, but not so specific that it binds only to the antigen from the particular strain of organism with which the mouse was first immunized. When a good candidate antibody-producing cell is found, the hybridoma cells either are grown in cell culture *in vitro* or are reinjected into the peritoneal cavities of many mice, where the cells multiply and produce large quantities of antibody in the ascitic

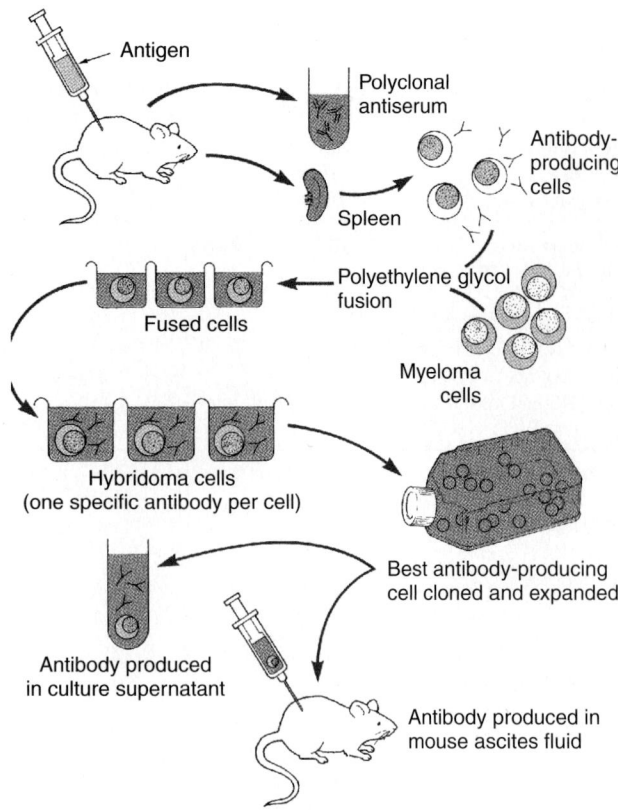

• **Fig. 9.5** Production of a monoclonal antibody.

(peritoneal) fluid. Ascitic fluid can be removed from mice many times during the animals' lifetime, providing a continual supply of antibody formed to the originally injected antigen. Polyclonal and monoclonal antibodies are both used in commercial systems to detect infectious agents.

Immunoglobulin M Clinical Significance

IgM testing is especially helpful for diseases that have nonspecific clinical presentations, such as toxoplasmosis, and for conditions that require rapid therapeutic decisions. For example, rubella infection in pregnant women can lead to congenital defects in the unborn fetus, such as cataracts, glaucoma, mental retardation, and deafness. Pregnant women exposed to rubella virus and develop a mild febrile illness can be tested for the presence of antirubella IgM. In addition, identification of IgM within the amniotic fluid of a pregnant mother is diagnostic of neonatal infection. Because IgG can readily cross the placenta, newborns carry titers of IgG passed from the mother to the fetus during the first 2 to 3 months of life until the infant produces his or her own antibodies. This is the only form of **natural passive immunity.** Accurate serologic diagnosis of infection in neonates requires either demonstration of a rise in titer (which takes time to occur) or the detection of specific IgM directed against the putative agent. Because the IgM molecule does not cross the placental barrier, any IgM would have to be of fetal origin and diagnostic of neonatal infection. Agents that are difficult to culture or those that

adult females would be expected to have encountered during their lifetimes, such as *T. pallidum,* CMV, herpes virus, *Toxoplasma* spp., or rubella virus, are organisms that may cause an infection and elevation of fetal IgM. The names of some of these agents have been grouped together with the acronym **STORCH** (syphilis, *Toxoplasma* spp., rubella, CMV, and herpes). These tests should be ordered separately, depending on the clinical illness of a newborn. However, in many instances, infected babies display no clinical signs or symptoms of infection. Furthermore, in many cases, serologic tests yield false-positive or false-negative results. Multiple considerations, including the patient history and the clinical signs and symptoms, must be included in the serodiagnosis of neonatal infection, and in many cases culture is still the most reliable diagnostic method.

Separating Immunoglobulin M from Immunoglobulin G for Serologic Testing

Several methods have been developed to measure specific IgM in sera that may also contain IgG. In addition to using a labeled antibody specific for IgM as the marker or the IgM capture sandwich assays, the immunoglobulins can be separated from each other by physical means. Centrifugation through a sucrose gradient, performed at very high speeds, has been used in the past to separate IgM, which has a greater molecular weight than IgG.

Other available IgM separation systems use the presence of certain proteins on the surface of staphylococci (protein A) and streptococci (protein G expressed by group C and G streptococci) that bind the Fc portion of IgG. A simple centrifugation step separates the particles and their bound immunoglobulins from the remaining mixture, which contains the bulk of the IgM. Other methods use antibodies to remove IgM from sera containing both IgG and IgM. An added bonus of IgM separation systems is that **rheumatoid factor,** IgM antibodies produced by some patients against their own IgG, often binds to the IgG molecules being removed from the serum. Consequently, these IgM antibodies are removed along with the IgG. Rheumatoid factor can cause nonspecific reactions and interfere with the results in a variety of serologic tests.

Principles of Immunochemical Methods Used for Organism Detection

Numerous immunologic methods are used for the rapid detection of bacteria, fungi, parasites, and viruses in patient specimens and many of the same reagents often can be used to identify these organisms grown in culture. The immunochemical methods are classified in a variety of general categories: **precipitation tests, particle agglutination tests, flocculation, hemagglutination,** immunofluorescence assays, **enzyme immunoassay (EIA),** and variations of each major technique.

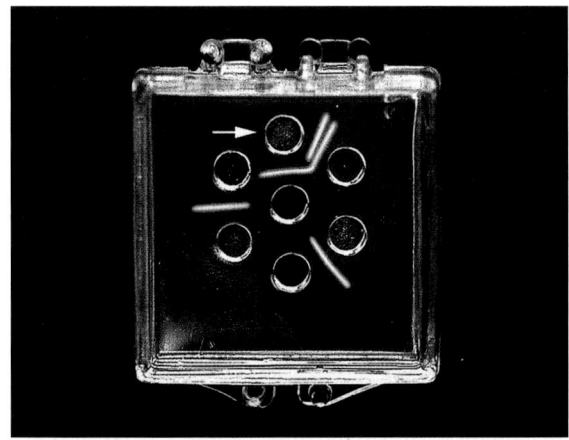

• **Fig. 9.6** Exo-Antigen Identification System (Immuno-Mycologics, Inc., Norman, OK). The center well is filled with a 50X concentrate of an unknown mold. The *arrow* identifies well 1; wells 2 to 6 are shown clockwise. Wells 1, 3, and 5 are filled with anti-*Histoplasma*, anti-*Blastomyces,* and anti-*Coccidioides* reference antisera, respectively. Wells 2, 4, and 6 are filled with *Histoplasma* antigen, *Blastomyces* antigen, and *Coccidioides* antigen, respectively. The unknown organism can be identified as *Histoplasma capsulatum* based on the formation of lines of identity *(arc)* linking the control bands with one or more bands formed between the unknown extract (center well) and the reference antiserum well (well 1).

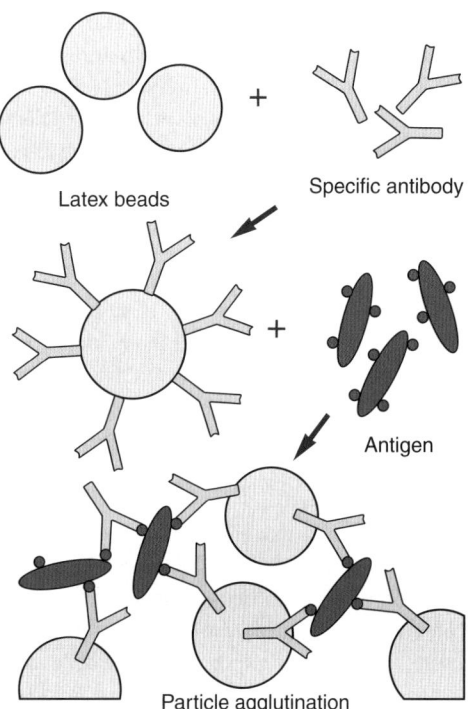

• **Fig. 9.7** Alignment of antibody molecules bound to the surface of a latex particle and latex agglutination reaction.

Precipitation Tests

The classic method of detecting soluble antigen and antibody (i.e., antigen and antibody in solution) is the Ouchterlony method, a double immunodiffusion precipitation method.

Double Immunodiffusion

In the **double immunodiffusion** method (Ouchterlony gel diffusion), small circular wells are cut in an agarose gel, a gelatin-like matrix derived from agar, which is a chemical purified from the cell walls of brown algae. The agarose forms a porous material through which molecules can readily diffuse. For detection of antigens, the patient specimen is placed in a well, and antibody directed against the antigen is placed in the adjacent well. Over 18 to 24 hours, the antigen and antibody diffuse toward each other, producing a visible precipitin band (a lattice structure or visible band) at the point in the gel where the antigen and antibody are in equal proportion (**zone of equivalence**). If the concentration of antibody is significantly higher than that of the antigen, no lattice forms and no precipitation reaction occurs, this is a **prozone effect.** Conversely, if excess antigen prevents lattice formation, resulting in no band formation, the effect is termed **postzone.** Immunodiffusion is used to detect exoantigens produced by the systemic fungi (*Blastomyces dermatitidis, Coccidioides immitis, Coccidioides posadasii, Aspergillus* spp., and *Histoplasma capsulatum*) or specific antibodies (Fig. 9.6).

Single Immunodiffusion

Single immunodiffusion, or Oudin gel diffusion, antibodies are added to a liquid agarose preparation and allowed to solidify in a petri dish, reaction cuvette, or tube. The patient's sample containing the antigen is then added to a test well or added to the top of the gel in a tube and allowed to diffuse. As previously described with double immunodiffusion, when the zone of equivalence is reached, a visible precipitin band is formed, indicating a positive reaction. When a petri dish is used, the assay or **radial immunodiffusion** provides a means of semiquantification of the antigen in the patient's sample. A set of standards containing known concentrations of antigen are also placed in wells within the same agarose plate. The samples diffuse radially from each well. The diameter of the precipitin ring is measured and plotted against the known concentration of the standards, creating a standard curve. The patient's sample ring is also measured, and using the standard curve, the amount of antigen in the sample can be determined.

Although immunodiffusion methods are relatively inexpensive, technically simple to perform, and highly specific, the interpretations are subjective. In addition, the assays demonstrate low sensitivity, making clinical utility questionable. Because of these disadvantages and the time-consuming nature associated with immunodiffusion, use is limited to large reference laboratories and for educational purposes.

Particle Agglutination

Numerous procedures have been developed to detect antigen by means of the agglutination (clumping) of an artificial carrier particle or insoluble matrix, such as a latex bead, with antibody bound to the surface (Fig. 9.7). These assays are classified as **indirect agglutination reactions,** also referred to as **reverse passive agglutination.** In addition, agglutination assays that detect an intact antigen directly on an organism's surface or cell are classified as **direct agglutination assays.** The assays use an inactivated whole organism mixed with patient serum to identify antibodies that indicate exposure to the infectious agent. Specific antibodies bind to surface antigens of the bacteria in a thick suspension and cause the bacteria to clump in visible aggregates. Such antibodies are called **agglutinins,** and the test is referred to as **bacterial agglutination.** Electrostatic and additional chemical interactions influence the formation of aggregates in solutions. Because most bacterial surfaces have a negative charge, they tend to repel each other. Performance of agglutination tests in sterile physiologic saline (0.9% sodium chloride in distilled water), which contains free positive ions, enhances the ability of antibody to cause aggregation of bacteria. Although bacterial agglutination tests can be performed on the surface of plastic-coated reaction cards and in test tubes, tube agglutination tests, despite being more sensitive because a longer incubation period can be used, allowing more antigen and antibody to interact, are rarely used in the modern clinical laboratory.

Examples of bacterial agglutination tests include assays for antibodies to *Francisella tularensis* and *Brucella* spp., which are part of a panel referred to as **febrile agglutinin tests.** Bacterial agglutination tests are often used to diagnose diseases in which the bacterial agent is difficult to cultivate *in vitro.* Diseases diagnosed by this technique include tetanus, yersiniosis, leptospirosis, brucellosis, and tularemia. The reagents necessary to perform many of these tests are commercially available, singly or as complete systems. Because most laboratories are able to culture and identify the causative agent, agglutination tests for diseases, such as typhoid fever, are seldom used today. Furthermore, the typhoid febrile agglutinin test (called the **Widal test**) is often positive in patients with infections caused by other bacteria because of crossreacting antibodies or a previous immunization against typhoid. Appropriate specimens from patients suspected of having typhoid fever should be cultured for the presence of salmonellae.

Whole cells of parasites, including *Plasmodium* spp., *Leishmania* spp., and *Toxoplasma gondii,* have also been used for direct detection of antibody by agglutination. In addition to using the actual infecting bacteria or parasites as the agglutinating particles, certain bacteria may be agglutinated by antibodies produced against another infectious agent. Many patients infected with one of the rickettsiae produce antibodies capable of nonspecifically agglutinating bacteria of the genus *Proteus,* specifically *Proteus vulgaris.* The **Weil-Felix test** detects these cross-reacting antibodies. Because newer, more specific serologic methods of diagnosing rickettsial disease have become more widely available, the use of the *Proteus* agglutinating test is no longer offered in most laboratories.

The results of particle agglutination tests depend on several factors, including the amount and avidity of antigen conjugated to the carrier, the time of incubation with the patient's serum (or other source of antibody), and the microenvironment of the interaction (including pH and protein concentration). In addition, some constituents of body fluids, such as rheumatoid factor or complement, have been found to cause false-positive reactions in latex agglutination systems. To counteract this problem, some agglutination methods require specimens to be pretreated by heating at 56°C or with ethylenediaminetetraacetic acid (EDTA) to inactivate complement proteins before testing. Commercial tests have been developed as systems, complete with their own diluents, controls, and containers. For accurate results, a serologic test kit should be used as a unit, without modification or mixing from another kit. In addition, tests developed for use with cerebrospinal fluid, for example, should not be used with serum unless the package insert or the technical representative has certified such use.

Depending on the procedure, some reactions are reported as positive or negative and other reactions are graded on a 1+ to 4+ scale, with 2+ usually the minimum amount of agglutination visible in a positive sample without the aid of a microscope. Control latex (coated with antibody from the same animal species from which the specific antibody was made) is tested alongside the test latex. If the patient specimen or the culture isolate reacts with both the test and control latex, the test is considered nonspecific and the results are invalid.

Latex tests are very popular in clinical laboratories for detecting antigen to *Cryptococcus neoformans* in cerebrospinal fluid or serum and to confirm the presence of β-hemolytic streptococci from culture plates. Latex tests are continually being developed for a variety of organisms. Some examples of additional latex tests are available for the detection of *Clostridium difficile* toxins A and B, rotavirus, and *Escherichia coli* O157:H7.

Coagglutination

Similar to latex agglutination, **coagglutination** uses antibody bound to a particle to enhance the visibility of the agglutination reaction between antigen and antibody. In this case the particles are killed and treated *Staphylococcus aureus* organisms (Cowan I strain), which contain a large amount of an antibody-binding protein, protein A, in their cell walls. In contrast to latex particles, these staphylococci bind only the base of the heavy chain portion of the antibody, leaving both antigen-binding ends free to form complexes with specific antigen. Several commercial suppliers have prepared coagglutination reagents for identification of streptococci, including Lancefield groups A, B, C, D, F, G, and N; *Streptococcus pneumoniae; Neisseria meningitidis;* and *Haemophilus influenzae* types A to F grown in culture. The coagglutination reaction is highly specific and demonstrates reduced sensitivity in comparison with commercially prepared latex agglutination systems.

Hemagglutination

Hemagglutination is the clumping of red blood cells by either a direct or an indirect mechanism. This type of agglutination reaction is used in immunohematology for blood group typing (direct) or the detection of a red cell antibody (indirect). Hemagglutination is also used in virology. The monospot test is a hemagglutination assay that detects **heterophile** (nonspecific antibodies) produced in the early stages of infection with EBV. More recently, **indirect hemagglutination** assays that use antigen from the infectious agent attached to a latex bead can be used to detect antibodies to human immunodeficiency virus (HIV), *T. pallidum,* and hepatitis viruses (A, B, and C). Another alternate method, termed **hemagglutination inhibition,** that takes advantage of hemagglutinating properties of viruses that cause hemagglutination *in vivo,* combine viral particles, red blood cells, and patient serum. If the patient's serum contains antibodies to the viral agent, hemagglutination is inhibited. In this method, no agglutination is considered a positive reaction. Influenza virus is the most common infectious agent diagnosed using a hemagglutination inhibition assay.

The most widely used indirect assays include the microhemagglutination test for antibody to *T. pallidum* (MHA-TP, so called because it is performed in a microtiter plate), the hemagglutination treponemal test for syphilis (HATTS), the passive hemagglutination tests for antibody to extracellular antigens of streptococci, and the rubella indirect hemagglutination tests, all of which are available commercially. Certain reference laboratories, such as the Centers for Disease Control and Prevention (CDC), also perform indirect hemagglutination tests for antibodies to some clostridia, *Burkholderia pseudomallei, Bacillus anthracis, Corynebacterium diphtheriae, Leptospira* spp., and the agents of several viral and parasitic diseases.

Hemagglutination Inhibition Assays

Many human viruses can bind to surface structures on red blood cells from different species. For example, rubella virus particles can bind to human type O, goose, or chicken erythrocytes and cause agglutination of the red blood cells. Influenza and parainfluenza viruses agglutinate guinea pig, chicken, or human O erythrocytes; many arboviruses agglutinate goose red blood cells; adenoviruses agglutinate rat or rhesus monkey cells; mumps virus binds red blood cells of monkeys; and herpes virus and CMV agglutinate sheep red blood cells. Serologic tests for the presence of antibodies to these viruses exploit the agglutinating properties of the virus particles. Patients' sera treated with kaolin or heparin-magnesium chloride (to remove nonspecific inhibitors of red cell agglutination and nonspecific agglutinins of the red cells) are added to a system containing the suspected virus. If antibodies to the virus are present, they form complexes and block the binding sites on the viral surfaces. When the proper red cells are added to the solution, all of the virus particles are bound by antibody, preventing the virus from agglutinating the red cells. This indicates that the patient's serum is positive for hemagglutination-inhibiting antibodies. As for most serologic procedures, a fourfold increase in the titer is considered diagnostic. The hemagglutination inhibition tests for most agents are performed in reference laboratories. However, rubella antibodies are often detected with this method in routine diagnostic laboratories. Several commercial rubella hemagglutination inhibition test systems are also available.

Flocculation Tests

In contrast to the aggregates formed when particulate antigens bind to specific antibody, the interaction of soluble antigen with antibody may result in the formation of a precipitate, a concentration of fine particles, usually visible only because the precipitated product is forced to remain in a defined space within a matrix. Variations of precipitation and flocculation are widely used for serologic studies.

In flocculation tests, the precipitin product forms macroscopically or microscopically visible clumps. The **Venereal Disease Research Laboratory test,** known as the **VDRL,** is the most widely used flocculation test. Patients infected with pathogenic treponemes, most commonly *T. pallidum,* the agent of syphilis, form an antibody-like protein called **reagin** that binds to the test antigen, cardiolipin-lecithin–coated cholesterol particles, causing the particles to flocculate. Reagin is not a specific antibody directed against *T. pallidum* antigens. The test is highly sensitive but not highly specific. However, it is a good screening test, detecting more than 99% of the cases of secondary syphilis.

The VDRL is the single most useful test available for testing cerebrospinal fluid in cases of suspected neurosyphilis, although it may be falsely positive in the absence of disease. Performance of the VDRL test requires scrupulously clean glassware and attention to detail, including numerous daily quality control checks. In addition, the reagents must be prepared fresh immediately before the test is performed, and patients' sera must be inactivated (complement inactivation) by heating for 30 minutes at 56°C before testing. Because of this complexity, the VDRL has been replaced in many laboratories by a qualitatively comparable test, the **rapid plasma reagin (RPR) test.**

The RPR test is commercially available as a complete system containing positive and negative controls, the reaction card, and the prepared antigen suspension. The antigen, cardiolipin-lecithin–coated cholesterol with choline chloride, also contains charcoal particles to allow for macroscopically visible flocculation. Sera can be tested without heating, and the reaction takes place on the surface of a specially treated cardboard card, which is then discarded (Fig. 9.8). The RPR test is not recommended for testing of cerebrospinal fluid. All procedures are standardized and clearly described in product inserts, and these procedures should be strictly followed. Overall, the RPR appears to be a more specific screening test for syphilis than the VDRL, and it is not as technically complex. Several modifications have been made, such as the use of dyes to enhance visualization of results and the use of automated techniques.

Conditions and infections other than syphilis can cause a patient's serum to yield a positive result in the VDRL or RPR test; these are **biologic false-positive tests.** Autoimmune diseases, such as systemic lupus erythematosus and rheumatic fever, in addition to infectious mononucleosis, hepatitis, pregnancy, and old age, have been known to cause false-positive reactions. The results of screening tests should always be considered presumptive until confirmed with a specific treponemal test.

Neutralization Assays

An antibody that inhibits the infectivity of a virus by blocking the host cell receptor site is a neutralizing antibody. The test serum is mixed with a suspension of infectious viral particles of the virus suspected in a patient's infection. A control suspension of viruses is mixed with normal serum. The viral suspensions are then inoculated into a cell culture system that supports growth of the virus. The control cells display evidence of viral infection. If the patient's serum contains antibody to the virus, that antibody binds the viral particles and prevents them from invading the cells in culture; the antibody has neutralized the "infectivity" of the virus. These tests are technically demanding and time consuming and are generally performed in reference laboratories.

Antibodies to bacterial toxins and other extracellular products that display measurable activities can be tested in a similar fashion. The ability of a patient's serum to neutralize the erythrocyte-lysing capability of streptolysin O, an extracellular enzyme produced by *S. pyogenes* during infection, has been used for many years as a test for identifying a previous streptococcal infection. After

pharyngitis with streptolysin O–producing strains, most patients show a high titer of the antibody to streptolysin O (i.e., antistreptolysin O [ASO] antibody). Streptococci also produce the enzyme deoxyribonuclease B (DNase B) during infections of the throat, skin, or other tissue. A neutralization test that prevents activity of this enzyme, the anti–DNase B test, has also been used extensively as an indicator of recent or previous streptococcal disease. However, the use of particle agglutination tests (latex or indirect hemagglutination) for the presence of antibody to many of the streptococcal enzymes has replaced the use of these neutralization tests in many laboratories.

Complement Fixation Assays

One of the classic methods of demonstrating the presence of antibody in a patient's serum is the **complement fixation (CF) test.** This test consists of two separate systems. The first (the test system) consists of the antigen suspected of causing the patient's disease and the patient's serum. The second (the indicator system) consists of a combination of sheep red blood cells, complement-fixing antibody (IgG) raised against the sheep red blood cells in another animal, and an exogenous source of complement (usually guinea pig serum). When these three components are mixed together in optimum concentrations, the anti–sheep erythrocyte antibody binds to the surface of the red blood cells, and the complement then binds to the antigen-antibody complex, ultimately causing lysis (bursting) of the red blood cells. For this reason the anti–sheep red blood cell antibody is also called **hemolysin.** For the CF test, these two systems are tested in sequence (Fig. 9.9). The patient's serum is first added to the putative antigen; then the limiting amount of complement is added to the solution. If the patient's serum contains antibody to the antigen, the resulting antigen-antibody complexes bind all the complement added. In the next step, the sheep red blood cells and the hemolysin (indicator system) are added. The patient's complement is available to bind to the sheep cell–hemolysin complexes and cause lysis if the complement has not been bound by a complex formed with antibody from the patient's serum. A positive result, meaning the patient has complement-fixing antibodies, is evident by failure of the red blood cells to lyse in the final test system. Lysis of the indicator cells indicates lack of antibody and a negative CF test result.

Although this test requires many manipulations, takes at least 48 hours to complete both stages, and often yields nonspecific results, it has been used for many years to detect many types of antiviral and antifungal antibodies. Many new systems have replaced the CF test, because they demonstrate improved recovery of pathogens or their products and provide more sensitive and less demanding procedures for detecting antibodies, such as particle agglutination, indirect fluorescent antibody (IFA) tests, and enzyme-linked

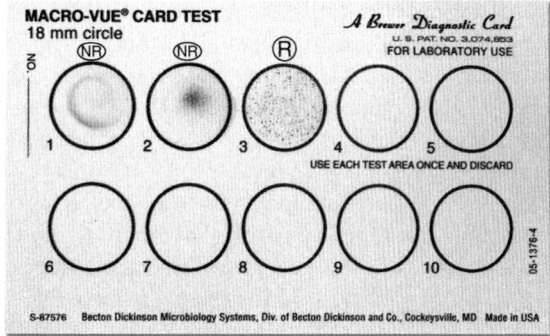

• **Fig. 9.8** MACRO-VUE Rapid Plasma Reagin Card Test. *NR,* Nonreactive (negative test), indicated by a smooth suspension or nondiffuse slight roughness as demonstrated here as a peripheral roughness in well 1 or somewhat centric roughness in well 2; *R,* reactive (positive) test indicated by the diffuse degree of clumping. (Courtesy Becton Dickinson Diagnostic Systems, Sparks, MD.)

immunosorbent assay (ELISA). CF tests remain useful in the diagnosis of unusual infections.

Immunofluorescent Assays

Immunofluorescent assays are frequently used for detecting bacterial and viral antigens in clinical laboratories. In these tests, antigens in the patient specimens are immobilized and fixed onto glass slides with formalin, methanol, ethanol, or acetone. Monoclonal or polyclonal antibodies conjugated (attached) to fluorescent dyes are applied to the specimen. After appropriate incubation, washing, and counterstaining (staining of the background with a nonspecific fluorescent stain such as rhodamine or Evan's blue), the slide is viewed using a microscope equipped with a high-intensity light source (usually halogen) and filters to excite the fluorescent tag. Most kits used in clinical microbiology laboratories use fluorescein isothiocyanate (FITC) as the fluorescent dye. FITC fluoresces a bright apple-green (Fig. 9.10).

Fluorescent antibody tests are performed using either a direct fluorescent antibody (DFA) or an IFA technique (Fig. 9.11). In the DFA technique, FITC is conjugated directly to the specific antibody. In the IFA technique, the antigen-specific antibody is unlabeled, and a second antibody (usually raised against the animal species from which the antigen-specific antibody was harvested) is conjugated to the FITC. The IFA is a two-step, or sandwich, technique. The IFA technique is more sensitive than the DFA method,

although the DFA method is faster because it involves a single incubation.

IFA determination is a widely applied method of detecting diverse antibodies. For these types of tests, the antigen against which the patient makes antibody (e.g., whole *Toxoplasma* organisms or virus-infected tissue culture cells) is fixed to the surface of a microscope slide. The patient's serum is diluted and placed on the slide, covering the area in which antigen was placed. If present in the serum, antibody binds to the specific antigen. Unbound antibody is removed by washing the slide. In the second stage of the procedure, a conjugate of antihuman globulin directed specifically against IgG or IgM and a fluorescent dye (e.g., fluorescein) is placed on the slide. This labeled marker for human antibody binds to the antibody already bound to the antigen on the slide and serves as a detector, indicating binding of the antibody to the antigen when viewed under a fluorescent microscope (Fig. 9.12). Commercially available test kits include slides coated with the antigen, positive and negative control sera, diluent for the patients' sera, and the properly diluted conjugate. As with other commercial products, IFA systems should be used as units, without modification of the manufacturer's instructions. Commercially available IFA tests include those for antibodies to *Legionella* spp., *Borrelia burgdorferi*, *T. gondii*, VZV, CMV, EBV capsid antigen, early antigen and nuclear antigen, herpes simplex virus (HSV) types 1 and 2, rubella virus, *Mycoplasma pneumoniae*, *T. pallidum* (the **fluorescent treponemal antibody absorption test [FTA-ABS]**), and several rickettsiae.

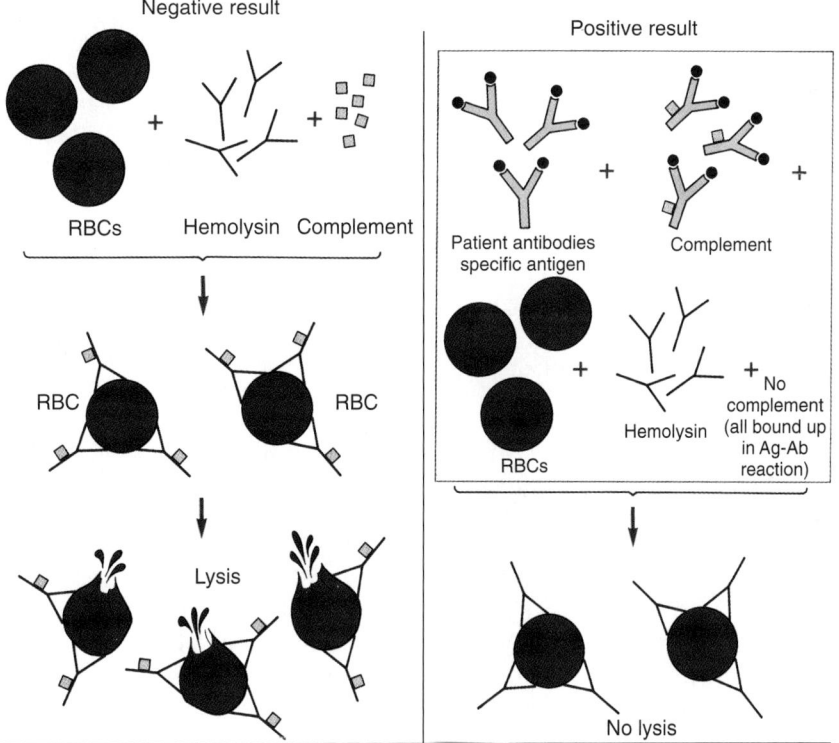

• **Fig. 9.9** Complement fixation test.

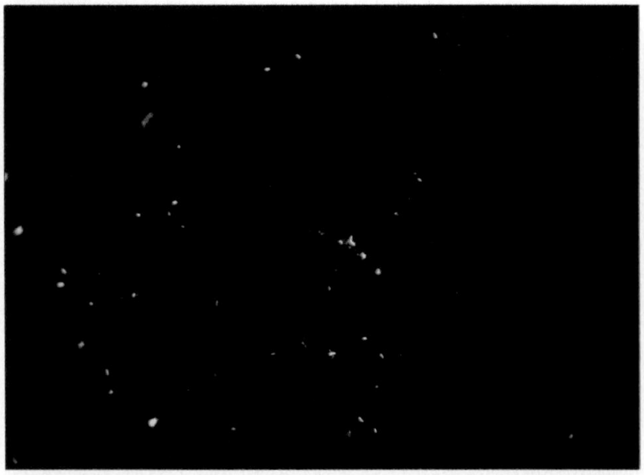

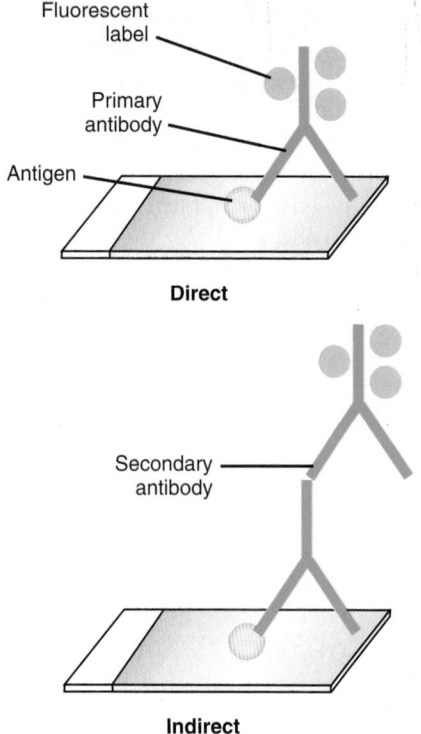

• **Fig. 9.10** *Legionella* (direct) fluorescent test system (Scimedx Corp., Denville, NJ). *Legionella pneumophila* serogroup 1 in sputum.

• **Fig. 9.11** Direct and indirect fluorescent antibody tests for antigen detection.

Most of these tests, if performed properly, give extremely specific and sensitive results. Proper interpretation of IFA tests requires experienced and technically competent technologists. These tests can be performed rapidly and are cost effective.

The major advantage of immunofluorescent microscopy assays is the ability to evaluate the specimen. This is a major factor in tests for the identification of chlamydial elementary bodies or RSV antigens. Microbiologists can discern whether the specimen was collected from the columnar epithelial cells at the opening of the cervix in the case of the *Chlamydia* DFA test or from the basal cells of the nasal epithelium in the case of RSV. Reading immunofluorescent assays requires extensive training and practice for laboratory personnel to become proficient. Finally, fluorescent dyes fade rapidly over time, requiring digital imaging to maintain archives of the results. For this reason, some antibodies have been conjugated to other markers instead of fluorescent dyes. These colorimetric labels use enzymes, such as horseradish peroxidase, alkaline phosphatase, and avidin-biotin, to detect the presence of antigen by converting a colorless substrate to a colored product. The advantage of these tags is that they allow the preparation of permanent mounts, because the reactions do not fade with storage, and visualization does not require a fluorescent microscope.

In clinical specimens, fluorescent antibody tests are commonly used to detect infected cells that harbor *Bordetella pertussis; T. pallidum; Legionella pneumophila; Giardia, Cryptosporidium, Pneumocystis,* and *Trichomonas* spp.; HSV; CMV; VZV; RSV; adenovirus; influenza virus; and parainfluenza virus.

Enzyme Immunoassays

EIA, or **ELISA,** was developed during the 1960s. The basic method consists of antibodies bonded to enzymes; the enzymes remain able to catalyze a reaction, yielding a visually discernible product while attached to the antibodies. Furthermore, the antibody binding sites remain free to react with their specific antigen. The use of enzymes as labels has several advantages. First, the enzyme itself is not changed during activity; it can catalyze the reaction of many substrate molecules, greatly amplifying the reaction and enhancing detection. Second, enzyme-conjugated antibodies are stable and can be stored for a relatively long time. Third, the formation of a colored product allows direct observation of the reaction or automated spectrophotometric reading.

The use of monoclonal antibodies has helped increase the specificity of currently available ELISA systems. New ELISA systems are continually being developed for the detection of etiologic agents or their products. In some instances, such as detection of RSV, HIV, and certain adenoviruses, ELISA systems may even be more sensitive than culture methods.

Solid-Phase Immunoassay

Most ELISA systems developed to detect infectious agents consist of antibody firmly fixed to a solid matrix, either the inside of the wells of a microdilution tray or the outside of a spherical plastic or metal bead or some other solid matrix (Fig. 9.13). Such systems are called **solid-phase immunosorbent assays (SPIAs).** If antigen is present in the specimen, stable antigen-antibody

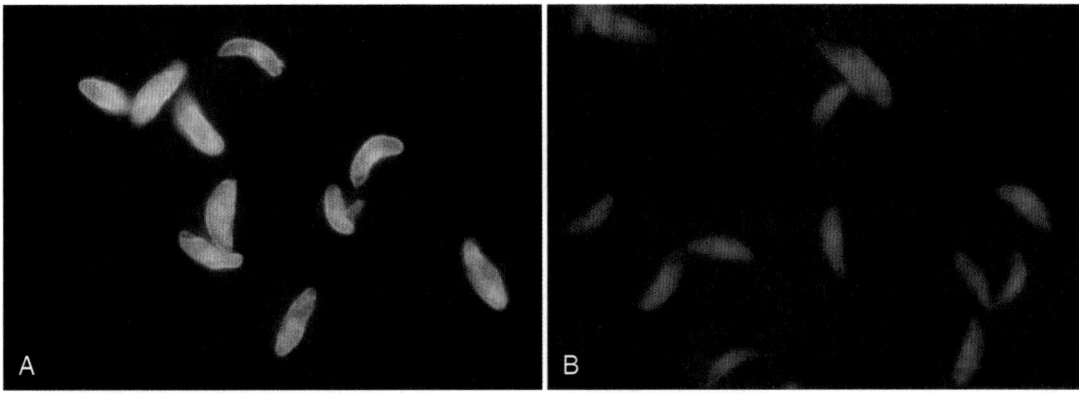

• **Fig. 9.12** Indirect fluorescent antibody tests for *Toxoplasma gondii,* immunoglobulin G antibodies. (A) Positive reaction. (B) Negative reaction. (Courtesy Meridian, Cincinnati, OH.)

complexes form when the sample is added to the matrix. Unbound antigen is thoroughly removed by washing, and a second antibody against the antigen is then added to the system. This antibody has been complexed to an enzyme such as alkaline phosphatase or horseradish peroxidase. If the antigen is present on the solid matrix, it binds the second antibody, forming a sandwich with antigen in the middle. After washing has removed unbound, labeled antibody, the addition and hydrolysis of the enzyme substrate causes the color change and completes the reaction. The visually detectable end point appears wherever the enzyme is present (Fig. 9.14). Because of the expanding nature of the reaction, even minute amounts of antigen (>1 ng/mL) can be detected. These systems require a specific enzyme–labeled antibody for each antigen tested. However, it is simpler to use an indirect assay in which a second, unlabeled antibody binds to the antigen-antibody complex on the matrix. A third antibody, labeled with enzyme and directed against the nonvariable Fc portion of the unlabeled second antibody, can then be used as the detection marker for many different antigen-antibody complexes (Fig. 9.14). ELISA systems are diagnostic tools used for hepatitis Bs (surface) and hepatitis Be (early) antigens and HIV p24 protein, all indicators of early, active, acute infection. However, some of these tests have been replaced with molecular tests that detect the viral nucleic acid. Nucleic acid detection is a more reliable test for the detection of viral replication and an active acute infection.

Membrane-Bound Solid-Phase Enzyme Immunosorbent Assay

The flow-through and large surface area characteristics of nitrocellulose, nylon, and other membranes have been exploited to enhance the speed and sensitivity of ELISA reactions. An absorbent material below the membrane pulls the liquid reactants through the membrane and helps to separate nonreacted components from the antigen-antibody complexes bound to the membrane; washing steps are also simplified. Membrane-bound

SPIA systems are available for several viruses, group A beta-hemolytic streptococci antigen directly from throat swabs, and group B streptococcal antigen in vaginal secretions. In addition to their use in clinical laboratories, these assays are expected to become more prevalent for home testing systems.

Commercial microdilution or solid-phase matrix systems are available to detect antibody specific for hepatitis virus antigens, HSV 1 and 2, RSV, CMV, HIV, rubella virus (both IgG and IgM), mycoplasmas, chlamydiae, *B. burgdorferi, Entamoeba histolytica,* and many other agents.

The introduction of membrane-bound ELISA components has improved sensitivity and ease of use dramatically. Slot-blot and dot-blot assays force the target antigen through a membrane filter, causing it to become fixed in the shape of the hole (a dot or a slot). Several antigens can be placed on one membrane. When test (patient) serum is layered onto the membrane, specific antibodies, if present, bind to the corresponding dot or slot of antigen. Addition of a labeled second antibody and subsequent development of the label allows visual detection of the presence of antibodies based on the pattern of antigen sites. Cassette-based membrane-bound ELISA assays, designed for testing a single serum, can be performed rapidly (often within 10 minutes). Commercial kits to detect antibodies to *Helicobacter pylori, T. gondii,* and some other infectious agents are available.

Antibody capture ELISAs are particularly valuable for detecting IgM in the presence of IgG. Anti-IgM antibodies are fixed to the solid phase. Only IgM antibodies, if present in the patient's serum, are bound. In a second step, specific antigen is added in a sandwich format, and a second antigen-specific labeled antibody is added. Toxoplasmosis, rubella, and other infections are diagnosed using this technology, typically in research settings.

Automated Fluorescent Immunoassays

In automated **fluorescent immunoassays (FIAs)** the antigen is labeled with a compound that fluoresces under the

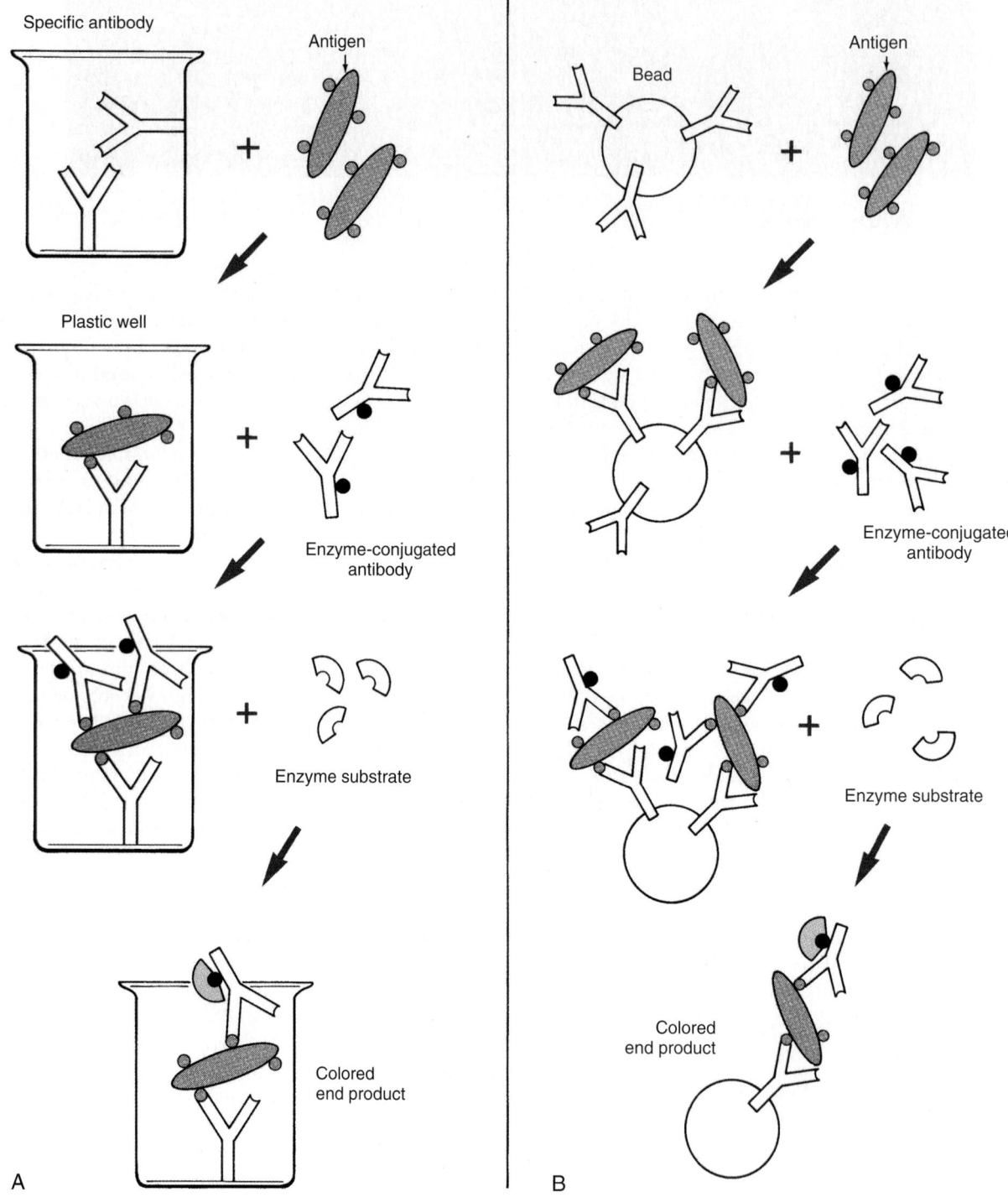

• **Fig. 9.13** Principle of direct solid-phase enzyme immunosorbent assay. (A) The solid phase is the microtiter well. (B) The solid phase is the bead.

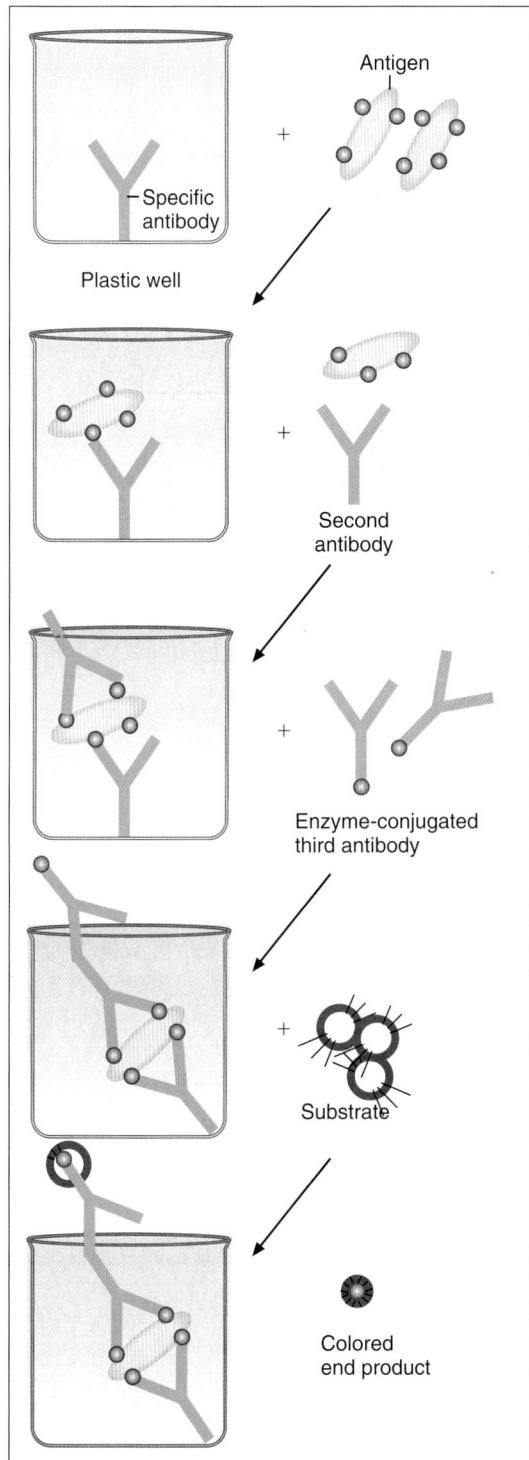

• **Fig. 9.14** of indirect solid-phase enzyme immunosorbent assay.

appropriate light emission source. Binding of patient antibody to a fluorescent-labeled antigen can reduce or quench the fluorescence, or binding can cause fluorescence by allowing conformational change in a fluorescent molecule.

Measurement of fluorescence is a direct measurement of antigen-antibody binding and is not dependent on a second marker, as in ELISA tests. Systems are commercially available to measure antibody developed against numerous infectious agents, as well as against self-antigens (autoimmune antibodies).

Western Blot Immunoassays

Requirements for the detection of very specific antibodies led to the development of the **Western blot immunoassay**. The method is based on the electrophoretic separation of major proteins of an infectious agent in a two-dimensional agarose (first dimension) and acrylamide (second dimension) matrix. A suspension of the organism is mechanically or chemically disrupted, and the solubilized antigen suspension is placed at one end of a polyacrylamide (polymer) gel. Under the influence of an electrical current, the proteins migrate through the gel. Most bacteria or viruses contain several major proteins that can be recognized based on their position in the gel after electrophoresis. Smaller proteins travel faster and migrate farther in the lanes of the gel. The protein bands are transferred from the gel to a nitrocellulose or other type of thin membrane, and the membrane is treated to immobilize the proteins. The membrane is then cut into many thin strips, each carrying the pattern of protein bands. When patient serum is layered over the strip, antibodies bind to each of the protein components represented by a band on the strip. The pattern of antibodies present can be used to determine whether the patient has a current infection or is immune to the agent (Fig. 9.15). Antibodies against microbes with numerous cross-reacting antibodies, such as *T. pallidum, B. burgdorferi,* HSV 1 and 2, and HIV, are identified more specifically using this technology than a single method that is used to identify a single antibody type. For example, the CDC defines an ELISA or immunofluorescence assay as a first line test for Lyme disease antibody, but positive or equivocal results must be confirmed by a Western blot test.

Summary

The immunochemical detection of microorganisms and other infectious agents is continually evolving. This chapter is intended to be a basic overview of some of the more common methods used in the direct detection of infectious agents or antibodies in a patient's serum. Detailed information or application of immunochemical techniques are included in the organism-specific sections in Parts III through VI of this text.

ⓔ Visit the Evolve site for a complete list of procedures, review questions, and case studies.

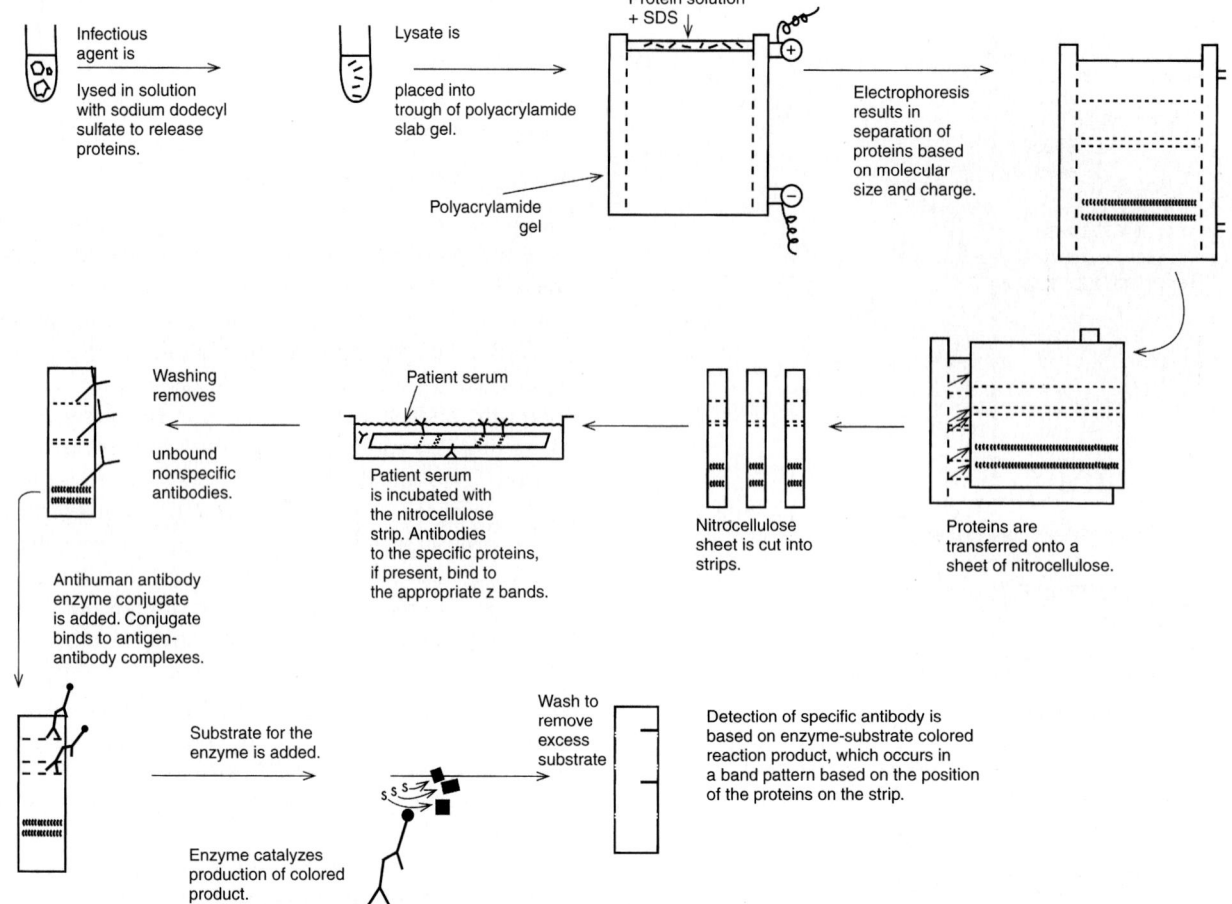

• **Fig. 9.15** Human immunodeficiency virus type 1 (HIV-1) Western blot immunoassay. Samples are characterized as positive, indeterminate, or negative based on the bands found to be present in significant intensity. A positive blot has any two or more of the following bands: p24, gp41, and gp120/160. An indeterminate blot contains some bands but not the definitive ones. A negative blot has no bands present. Lane 16 shows antibodies from a control serum binding to the virus-specific proteins *(p)* and glycoproteins *(gp)* transferred onto the nitrocellulose paper. *SDS*, Sodium dodecyl sulfate. (Courtesy Calypte Biomedical Corp., Pleasanton, CA.)

Bibliography

Benjamini E, Sunshine G, Leskowitz S: *Immunology: a short course*, 6th ed., New York, NY, 1999, Wiley-Liss.

Carroll KC, Pfaller MA, Landry ML, et al.: *Manual of clinical microbiology*, 12th ed., Washington, DC, 2020, ASM Press.

Jesudason MV, Balajii V, Sirisinha S, Sridharan G: Rapid identification of *Burkholderia pseudomallei* in blood culture supernatants by coagglutination assay, *Clin Microbiol Infect* 11:930–933, 2005.

Turgeon L: *Immunology and serology in laboratory medicine*, 6th ed., St Louis, MO, 2018, Elsevier.

Wee EJH, Lau HY, Botella JR, Trau M: Re-purposing bridging flocculation for on-site, rapid, qualitative DNA detection in resource poor settings, *Chem Comm* 51:5828–5831, 2015.

10

Principles of Antimicrobial Action and Resistance

OBJECTIVES

1. List the five general categories of antimicrobial action.
2. Define antibiotic and antimicrobial.
3. Define and differentiate between bactericidal and bacteriostatic agents.
4. Compare and contrast the following terms: biologic versus clinical resistance, environmentally mediated versus microorganism-mediated resistance, and intrinsic versus acquired resistance.
5. Describe the basic structure and chemical principle for the mechanism of beta-lactam antimicrobials.
6. List common beta-lactam antibiotics, and provide an example of a common pathogen susceptible to these agents.
7. Discuss two mechanisms of resistance both gram-positive and gram-negative bacteria use to decrease the effect of beta-lactam antibiotics.
8. Describe the chemical principle for the antimicrobial effects of glycopeptide agents.
9. List common glycopeptides, and provide an example of a common pathogen susceptible to these agents.
10. List examples of cell membrane inhibitors, inhibitors of protein synthesis, inhibitors of deoxyribonucleic acid (DNA) or ribonucleic acid (RNA) synthesis, and metabolic inhibitors. Provide an example of a common pathogen susceptible to each agent listed.
11. List five general mechanisms for antimicrobial resistance and provide at least one example of an antimicrobial agent that is affected by each mechanism.
12. Describe how the spread of antimicrobial resistance affects diagnostic microbiology, including effects on sensitivity testing, therapeutic options, and organism identification.

Medical intervention in an infection primarily involves attempts to eradicate the infecting pathogen using substances that actively inhibit or kill the organism. Some of these substances are obtained and purified from other microbial organisms and are known as **antibiotics.** Others are chemically synthesized. Collectively, these natural and synthesized substances are referred to as

antimicrobial agents. Depending on the type of organisms targeted, these substances can be classified and described as **antibacterial, antifungal, antiparasitic,** or **antiviral agents.**

Because antimicrobial agents play a central role in the control and management of infectious diseases, understanding their mode of action and the mechanisms used by microorganisms to circumvent antimicrobial activity is important. This is especially important because diagnostic laboratories are expected to design and implement tests that measure a pathogen's response to antimicrobial activity (Chapter 11). Much of what is discussed here regarding antimicrobial action and resistance is based on antibacterial agents, but the principles generally apply to almost all antiinfective agents. More information about antiparasitic, antifungal, and antiviral agents can be found in Parts IV, V, and VI, respectively.

Antimicrobial Action

Principles

Several key steps must be completed for an antimicrobial agent to successfully inhibit or kill an infecting microorganism (Fig. 10.1). First, the agent must be in an **active form.** This is ensured through the **pharmacodynamic design** of the drug, which takes into account the route by which the patient receives the agent (e.g., orally, intramuscularly, and intravenously). Second, the antibiotic must be able to achieve sufficient levels or concentrations at the site of infection so that it has a chance to exert an antibacterial effect (i.e., it must be in anatomic approximation with the infecting bacteria). The ability to achieve adequate levels depends on the **pharmacokinetic properties** of the agent, such as rate of absorption, distribution, metabolism, and excretion of the agent's metabolites. Table 10.1 provides examples of various anatomic limitations characteristic of a few commonly used antibacterial agents. Some agents, such as ampicillin and ceftriaxone, achieve therapeutically

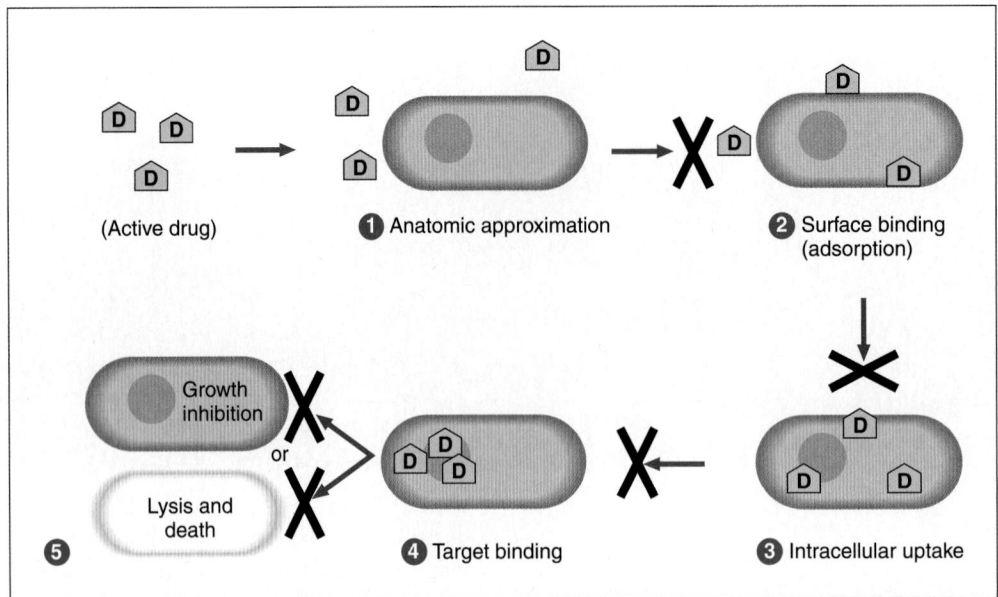

• **Fig. 10.1** The basic steps required for antimicrobial activity and strategic points for bacterial circumvention or interference (X) of antimicrobial action, leading to resistance.

TABLE 10.1	Anatomic Distribution of Some Common Antibacterial Agents		
	Serum or Blood[a]	**Cerebrospinal Fluid**	**Urine**
Ampicillin	+	+	+
Ceftriaxone	+	+	+
Meropenem	+	+	+
Vancomycin	+	±	+
Ciprofloxacin	+	±	+
Gentamicin	+	−	+
Clindamycin	+	−	−
Norfloxacin	−	−	+
Nitrofurantoin	−	−	+

[a]Serum or blood represents a general anatomic distribution.
+, Therapeutic levels generally achievable at that site;
±, therapeutic achievable levels moderate to poor;
−, therapeutic levels generally not achievable at that site.

effective levels in several body sites, whereas others, such as nitrofurantoin and norfloxacin, are limited to the urinary tract. Knowledge of the site of infection can substantially affect the selection of the antimicrobial agent for therapeutic use.

The remaining steps in antimicrobial action relate to direct interactions between the antibacterial agent and the bacterial cell. The antibiotic is attracted to and maintains contact with the cell surface. Because most targets of antibacterial agents are intracellular, uptake of the antibiotic to some location inside the bacterial cell is required. Once the antibiotic has achieved sufficient intracellular

concentration, binding to a specific target occurs. This binding involves molecular interactions between the antimicrobial agent and one or more biochemical components that play an important role in the microorganism's cellular metabolism. Adequate binding of the target results in disruption of cellular processes, leading to cessation of bacterial cell growth and, depending on the antimicrobial agent's mode of action, cell death. Antimicrobial agents that inhibit bacterial growth, but do not kill the organism, are **bacteriostatic agents.** Effectively reducing the growth rate of an organism provides adequate protection in individuals whose immune system is

Generally Bacteriostatic

Chloramphenicol
Erythromycin and other macrolides
Clindamycin
Sulfonamides
Trimethoprim
Tetracyclines
Tigecycline
Linezolid
Quinupristin/dalfopristin

Generally Bactericidal

Aminoglycosides
Beta-lactams
Vancomycin
Daptomycin
Fosfomycin
Tedizolid
Levofloxacin
Rifampin
Metronidazole
Colistin

aThe bactericidal and bacteriostatic nature of an antimicrobial may vary depending on the concentration of the agent used and the bacterial species targeted.

capable of removing the agent of infection. Agents that kill target organisms are **bactericidal** (Box 10.1). Bactericidal agents are more effective against organisms that are more difficult to control in combination with the host's immune system.

The primary goal in the development and design of antimicrobial agents is to optimize a drug's ability to efficiently achieve all steps outlined in Fig. 10.1 while minimizing toxic effects on human cells and physiology. Different antibacterial agents exhibit substantial specificity in terms of their bacterial cell targets (i.e., their **mode of action).** Antimicrobial agents are frequently categorized according to their mode of action.

Mode of Action of Antibacterial Agents

The interior of a bacterial cell has several potential antimicrobial targets. However, the processes or structures most frequently targeted include bacterial cell wall (peptidoglycan [PG] synthesis, the cell membrane, protein synthesis, key metabolic pathways, and nucleic acid synthesis (Table 10.2).

Inhibitors of Cell Wall Synthesis

The bacterial cell wall, also known as the PG or murein layer, plays an essential role in the life of the bacterial cell. This fact, combined with the lack of a similar structure in human cells, has made the cell wall the focus of attention for the development of bactericidal agents that are relatively nontoxic for humans.

Beta-Lactams

Beta-lactam antibiotics have a four-member, nitrogen-containing, beta-lactam ring at the core of their structure (Fig. 10.2). The antibiotics differ in ring structure and attached chemical groups. This drug class comprises the largest group of antibacterial agents, and dozens of derivatives are available for clinical use. Types of beta-lactam agents include penicillins, cephalosporins, carbapenems, and monobactams. The popularity of these agents results from their bactericidal action and lack of toxicity to humans. In addition, their molecular structures can be manipulated to achieve greater activity for wider therapeutic applications.

The beta-lactam ring is the key to the mode of action of these drugs. It is structurally similar to acyl-D-alanyl-D-alanine, the normal substrate required for synthesis of the linear glycopeptide in the bacterial cell wall. The beta-lactam binds the enzyme, inhibiting transpeptidation and cell wall synthesis. Most bacterial cells cannot survive once they have lost the capacity to produce and maintain their PG layer. The enzymes essential for this function are anchored in the cell membrane and are referred to as **penicillin-binding proteins (PBPs).** Bacterial species may have four to six different types of PBPs. The PBPs involved in cell wall cross-linking (i.e., transpeptidases) are often the most critical for survival. When beta-lactams bind to these PBPs, cell wall synthesis is halted. Death results from osmotic instability caused by faulty cell wall synthesis, or binding of the beta-lactam to PBP may trigger a series of events that leads to autolysis and cell death.

Because nearly all clinically relevant bacteria have cell walls, beta-lactam agents act against a broad spectrum of gram-positive and gram-negative bacteria. However, because of differences among bacteria in their PBP content, natural structural characteristics (e.g., the outer membrane present in gram-negative but not gram-positive bacteria), and common antimicrobial resistance mechanisms, the effectiveness of beta-lactams against different types of bacteria can vary widely. Gram-positive bacteria secrete **beta-lactamase** into the environment, whereas beta-lactamases produced by gram-negative bacteria remain in the periplasmic space, providing increased protection from beta-lactam antimicrobials. In addition, any given beta-lactam drug has a specific group or type of bacteria against which it is considered to have the greatest activity. The type of bacteria against which a particular antimicrobial agent does and does not have activity is the drug's **spectrum of activity.** Many factors contribute to an antibiotic's spectrum of activity, and knowledge of this spectrum is key to many aspects of antimicrobial use and laboratory testing.

TABLE 10.2 Summary of Mechanisms of Action for Commonly Used Antibacterial Agents

Antimicrobial Class	Examples (Not Inclusive)	Mechanism of Action	Spectrum of Activity
Beta-lactams Natural Semisynthetic Aminopenicillins Beta-lactam–beta-lactamase inhibitor combination Carbapenems Carbapenems–beta-lactamase inhibitor combination	Penicillin Nafcillin, oxacillin Amoxicillin, ampicillin Ampicillin-sulbactam, amoxicillin-clavu-lanate, piperacillin-tazobactam Imipenem, meropenem Meropenem-vaborbac-tam	Inhibit cell wall synthesis by binding enzymes involved in peptidoglycan (PG) production (i.e., penicillin-binding proteins [PBPs])	Both gram-positive and gram-negative bacteria, but spectrum varies depending on individual antibiotic
Cephalosporins 1st Generation 2nd Generation 3rd Generation 4th Generation 5th Generation Cephalosporin–beta-lactamase inhibitor combination	Cefaclor, cefazolin Cefprozil, cefuroxime Cefixime, cefotaxime, ceftazidime Cefepime Ceftaroline, ceftobiprole Ceftolozane-tazobac-tam, ceftazidime-avibactam		
Aminoglycosides	Gentamicin, tobramy-cin, amikacin, strep-tomycin, kanamycin	Inhibit protein synthesis by binding to 30S ribosomal subunit	Gram-positive and gram-negative bacteria; not anaerobes
Ansamycin (i.e., rifampin)		Inhibits RNA synthesis by binding DNA-dependent, RNA polymerase	Gram-positive and certain gram-negative (e.g., *Neisseria meningitidis*) bacteria
Chloramphenicol		Inhibits protein synthesis by binding to 50S ribosomal subunit	Gram-positive and gram-negative bacteria
Folate pathway inhibitors (e.g., sulfonamides [S3], trim-ethoprim [T])		Interfere with folic acid pathway; S3 binds dihydropteroate syn-thase; T binds dihydrofolate reductase	Gram-positive and many gram-negative bacteria
Fluoroquinolones	Ciprofloxacin, levofloxa-cin, moxifloxacin	Inhibit DNA synthesis by binding DNA gyrase and topoisomer-ase IV	Gram-positive and gram-negative bacteria; spectrum may vary with individual antibiotic
Glycopeptides Lipoglycopeptides	Vancomycin Dalbavancin, orita-vancin, teicoplanin	Inhibit cell wall synthesis by binding to end of PG, interfering with crosslinking	Gram-positive bacteria, includ-ing methicillin-resistant *Staphylococcus aureus*
Glycylglycines	Tigecycline	Inhibition of protein synthesis by binding to 30S ribosomal subunit	Wide spectrum of gram-positive and gram-negative species, including those resistant to tetracycline
Macrolides Lincosamide	Erythromycin, azithro-mycin, clarithromycin Clindamycin	Inhibition of protein synthesis by binding to 50S ribosomal subunit	Most aerobic and anaerobic gram-positive bacteria and atypical bacteria; clindamy-cin primarily for anaerobes
Lipopeptides	Daptomycin	Binding and disruption of cell membrane	Gram-positive bacteria, includ-ing those resistant to beta-lactams and glycopeptides
Nitrofurans	Nitrofurantoin	Exact mechanism uncertain; probable bacterial enzyme tar-gets and direct DNA damage	Gram-positive and gram-negative bacteria; treatment of UTI only

Continued

TABLE 10.2	Summary of Mechanisms of Action for Commonly Used Antibacterial Agents—cont'd		
Antimicrobial Class	**Examples (Not Inclusive)**	**Mechanism of Action**	**Spectrum of Activity**
Oxazolidinones	Linezolid, tedizolid	Bind to 50S ribosomal subunit to interfere with initiation of protein synthesis	Wide variety of gram-positive bacteria, including those resistant to other antimicrobials
Polymyxins	Colistin	Disruption of cell membrane	Gram-negative bacteria
Streptogramins	Quinupristin/dalfopristin	Inhibit protein synthesis by binding to 2 sites on 50S ribosomal subunit	Primarily gram-positive bacteria
Tetracyclines	Doxycycline, tetracycline, minocycline	Inhibits protein synthesis by binding to 30S ribosomal subunit	Gram-positive and gram-negative bacteria and several intracellular bacterial pathogens (e.g., chlamydia)

DNA, Deoxyribonucleic acid; *RNA*, ribonucleic acid; *UTI*, urinary tract infection.

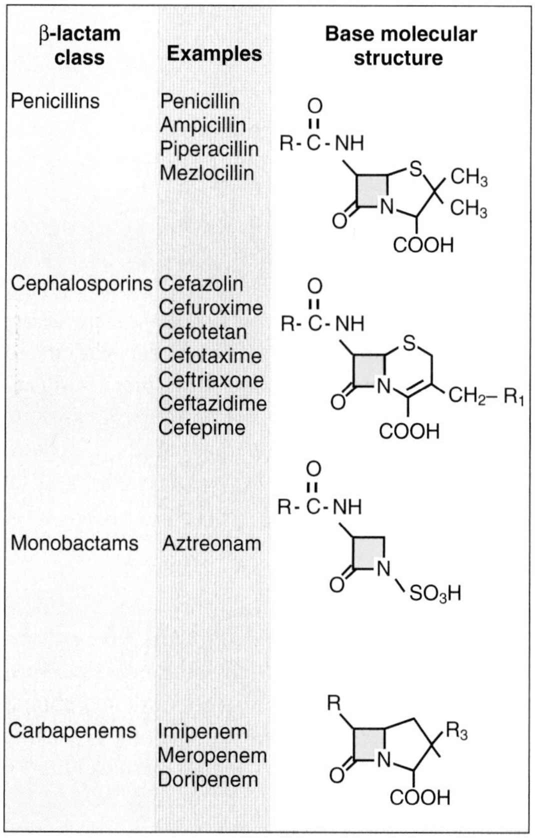

• **Fig. 10.2** Basic structures and examples of commonly used beta-lactam antibiotics. The core beta-lactam ring is highlighted in yellow in each structure. (Modified from Salyers AA, Whitt DD, eds. Bacterial Pathogenesis: A Molecular Approach. Washington, DC: ASM Press; 1994.)

A common mechanism of bacterial resistance to beta-lactams is production of enzymes (i.e., beta-lactamases) that bind and hydrolyze these drugs. Just as there is a variety of beta-lactam antibiotics, there is a variety of beta-lactamases. The beta-lactamases are grouped into four major

categories: classes A, B, C, and D. Classes A and D are **serine beta-lactamases;** class C comprises **cephalosporinases;** and those in class B, which require zinc as a cofactor, are **metallo-beta-lactamases**. Beta-lactamase genes can be located on plasmids or transposons, within an integron, or within the chromosome of the organism. An **integron** is a large cassette region that contains antibiotic resistance genes and the enzyme integrase, which is required for insertion of the cassette from one genetic element to another. In addition, the antimicrobial may be constitutively produced or it may be induced by the presence of a beta-lactam agent.

Of note, over the past decade **carbapenemase-producing Enterobacterales (CPE)** isolates have emerged. The beta-lactamase enzymes they produce belong to group 2f serine carbapenemases (e.g., KPC, SME, IMI, NMC-A, and GES), and MBLs (e.g., VIM, IMP, NDM), or 2d (e.g., OXA-beta-lactamases). These beta-lactamases are encoded on mobile genetic elements (i.e., plasmids) that often harbor resistance genes to other groups of antibiotics, severely limiting therapeutic options. In addition, several bacteria have chromosomally encoded carbepenemases, including *Stenotrophomonas maltophilia, Bacillus anthracis,* and *Bacteroides fragilis.*

Bacteria normally susceptible to beta-lactams have developed several resistance mechanisms against these antimicrobials. Resistance mechanisms include genetic mutations in the PBP coding sequence, altering the structure, and reducing the binding affinity to the drug; genetic recombination, resulting in a PBP structure resistant to binding of the drug; overproduction of normal PBP beyond achievable drug levels capable of inhibiting PBP activity; and acquiring a new genetic coding sequence for PBP from another organism with a lower affinity to the drug. These acquired types of beta-lactam resistance are generally found in gram-positive bacteria.

To circumvent the development of antimicrobial resistance, beta-lactam combinations comprising a beta-lactam

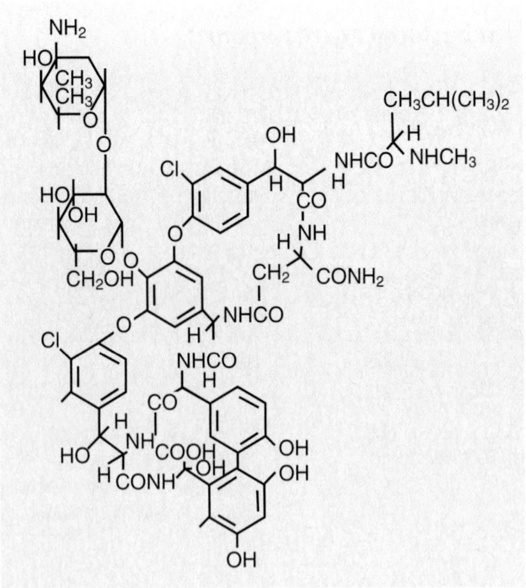

• **Fig. 10.3** Structure of vancomycin, a non–beta-lactam antibiotic that inhibits cell wall synthesis. (Modified from Salyers AA, Whitt DD, eds. *Bacterial Pathogenesis: A Molecular Approach.* Washington, DC: ASM Press; 1994.)

and a beta-lactamase inhibitor have been developed. The beta-lactamase inhibitor blocks the beta-lactamases produced by the bacteria from binding to the beta-lactam ring, thereby allowing the beta-lactam to exert its antimicrobial effect. Examples of these beta-lactam/beta-lactamase–inhibitor combinations are listed in Table 10.2. Such combinations are effective against organisms that produce beta-lactamases bound by the inhibitor. They have little effect on resistance that is mediated by altered PBPs (see Mechanisms of Antibiotic Resistance later in this chapter).

Fosfomycin

Fosfomycin tromethamine is a synthetic, organic phosphonate derivative. It is bactericidal and works by inhibiting cell wall formation by inactivating enol-pyruvyl transferase, the enzyme that catalyzes the first step in the synthesis of PG. Fosfomycin is approved in the United States as a single oral dose for uncomplicated urinary tract infections (UTIs) caused by susceptible strains of *Enterococcus faecalis* and *Escherichia coli*. Outside of the United States, there is documented use of fosfomycin for *Staphylococcus aureus,* including methicillin-resistant *S. aureus,* some coagulase-negative staphylococci, and *Pseudomonas aeruginosa.*

Glycopeptides and Lipoglycopeptides

Glycopeptides are another major class of antibiotics that inhibits bacterial cell wall synthesis by binding to the end of PG, interfering with transpeptidation. This is a different mechanism from that of the beta-lactams, which bind directly to the enzyme. Vancomycin (Fig. 10.3) and teicoplanin are large molecules and function differently from beta-lactam antibiotics. With glycopeptides, the binding interferes with the ability of the PBP enzymes, such as transpeptidases and transglycosylases, to incorporate the precursors into the

growing cell wall. With the cessation of cell wall synthesis, cell growth stops, and death often follows. Because glycopeptides have a different mode of action, resistance to beta-lactam agents by gram-positive bacteria does not generally hinder the activity of glycopeptides. However, because of their relatively large size, they cannot penetrate the outer membrane of most gram-negative bacteria. These agents are not used clinically for infections. Teicoplanin is approved for use throughout the world but is not available in the United States. If vancomycin is used for more than 3 days, the patient should be monitored for renal toxicity by obtaining a blood sample drawn within 30 minutes of the next dose (i.e., **trough level**). To determine efficacy, blood can be drawn 30 minutes after the end of an infusion (i.e., **peak level**), or a single random level can be drawn 6 to 14 hours after the start of the infusion, because the drug should not accumulate.

The **lipoglycopeptides** dalbavancin, oritavancin, and telavancin are structurally similar to vancomycin. These semisynthetic molecules are glycopeptides that contain hydrophobic chemical groups. The change in the molecular structure of lipoglycopeptides provides a mechanism by which they can bind to the bacterial cell membrane, increasing the inhibition of cell wall synthesis. In addition, the lipoglycopeptides increase cell permeability and cause depolarization of the cell membrane potential. These agents also inhibit the transglycosylation process necessary for cell wall synthesis by complexing with the D-alanyl-D-alanine residues. The lipoglycopeptides' spectrum of activity is comparable with that of vancomycin but also includes vancomycin-intermediate *S. aureus* (VISA).

Several other cell wall–active antibiotics have been discovered and developed over the years, but toxicity to the human host has prevented their widespread clinical use. One example is bacitracin, which inhibits the recycling of certain metabolites required for maintaining PG synthesis. Because of potential toxicity, bacitracin is used as a topical antibacterial agent.

Inhibitors of Cell Membrane Function

Lipopeptides

The **lipopeptide** daptomycin exerts its antimicrobial effect by binding to and disrupting the cell membrane of gram-positive bacteria. The drug binds to the cytoplasmic membrane and inserts its hydrophobic tail into the membrane, disrupting the cell membrane and increasing its permeability, which results in cell death. Daptomycin has potent activity against gram-positive cocci, including those resistant to other agents such as beta-lactams and glycopeptides (e.g., methicillin-resistant *S. aureus* [MRSA], multidrug-resistant isolates of staphylococci, pneumococci and streptococci, vancomycin-resistant enterococci [VRE], and vancomycin-resistant *S. aureus* [VRSA]). Because of its large size, daptomycin cannot penetrate the outer membrane of gram-negative bacilli and thus is ineffective. On rare occasions, daptomycin has caused eosinophilic allergic pneumonitis. Telavancin use has been repeatedly associated with nephrotoxicity.

Polymyxins (polymyxin B and E [colistin]) are cyclic lipopeptide agents that disrupt bacterial cell membranes. The polymyxins act as detergents, interacting with phospholipids in the cell membranes to increase permeability. This disruption results in leakage of macromolecules and ions essential for cell survival. Because their effectiveness varies with the molecular makeup of the bacterial cell membrane, polymyxins are not equally effective against all bacteria. Most notably, they are most effective against gram-negative bacteria, whereas activity against gram-positive bacteria tends to be poor. In addition, the emergence of plasmid-mediated polymyxin resistance in gram-negative bacteria is currently a global concern and has compromised the clinical use of this antibiotic. Furthermore, human host cells also have membranes; therefore, polymyxins pose a risk of toxicity. The major side effects are neurotoxicity and nephrotoxicity. Because of these risks, colistin use fell out of favor in the 1970s and 1980s as newer, less-toxic alternatives were being developed by pharmaceutical companies. However, once again, colistin use has resurged over the last decade. Colistin is regarded as a "last resort" antibiotic to treat extremely drug-resistant infections. Most notably, a triple combination regimen of colistin, tigecycline, and meropenem for carbapenemase-producing *Klebsiella pneumoniae* infections has been used quite successfully in severe cases.

Inhibitors of Protein Synthesis

Several classes of antibiotics target bacterial protein synthesis and severely disrupt cellular metabolism. Antibiotic classes that act by inhibiting protein synthesis include aminoglycosides, **macrolide-lincosamide-streptogramins** (MLS group), **ketolides** (e.g., telithromycin) chloramphenicol, tetracyclines, glycylglycines (e.g., tigecycline), and **oxazolidinones** (e.g., linezolid and tedizolid phosphate). Although these antibiotics are generally categorized as protein synthesis inhibitors, the specific mechanisms by which they inhibit protein synthesis differ significantly.

Aminoglycosides

Aminoglycosides (aminoglycosidic aminocyclitol) inhibit bacterial protein synthesis by irreversibly binding to protein receptors on the organism's 30S ribosomal subunit. This process interrupts several steps, including initial formation of the protein synthesis complex, accurate reading of the messenger RNA (mRNA) code, and formation of the ribosomal-mRNA complex. The structure of a commonly used aminoglycoside, gentamicin, is shown in Fig. 10.4. Other aminoglycosides include tobramycin, amikacin, streptomycin, and kanamycin. The spectrum of activity of aminoglycosides includes a wide variety of aerobic gram-negative and certain gram-positive bacteria and *Mycobacterium tuberculosis*. Although the aminoglycosides are active against gram-positive bacteria, they are not recommended for treatment of infections caused by staphylococci due to drug toxicity. Bacterial uptake of aminoglycosides is accomplished by using them in combination with cell wall–active antibiotics, such as beta-lactams or vancomycin. Anaerobic bacteria are

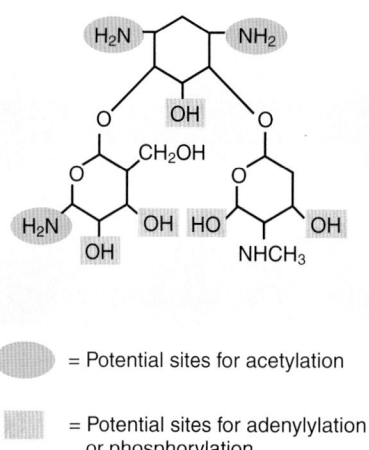

= Potential sites for acetylation

= Potential sites for adenylylation or phosphorylation

• **Fig. 10.4** Structure of the commonly used aminoglycoside gentamicin. Potential sites of modification by adenylating, phosphorylating, and acetylating enzymes produced by bacteria are highlighted. (Modified from Salyers AA, Whitt DD, eds. *Bacterial Pathogenesis: A Molecular Approach.* Washington, DC: ASM Press; 1994.)

unable to uptake these agents intracellularly and are typically not inhibited by aminoglycosides. Levels of aminoglycosides in blood should be monitored during therapy to prevent nephrotoxicity and auditory or vestibular toxicity.

Macrolide-Lincosamide-Streptogramin Group

The most commonly used antibiotics in the MLS group are the **macrolides** (e.g., erythromycin, azithromycin, clarithromycin, and clindamycin, which is a lincosamide). Protein synthesis is inhibited by the antimicrobial reversibly binding to the 23S ribosomal RNA (rRNA) on the bacterial 50S ribosomal subunit and subsequent disruption of the growing peptide chain by blocking of translocation. Macrolides are generally bacteriostatic but may be bactericidal if the infective dose of the organism is low and the drug is used in high concentrations. Primarily because of uptake difficulties associated with the outer membranes of gram-negative bacteria, the macrolides and clindamycin are not effective against most genera of gram-negative organisms. However, they are effective against gram-positive bacteria, mycoplasmas, treponemes, and rickettsiae. Toxicity is generally low with macrolides, although hearing loss and reactions with other medications may occur. They are considered bacteriostatic agents, but some may be bactericidal at high drug concentrations. Fidaxomicin is a newer macrolide antibiotic approved for the treatment of diarrhea due to *Clostridioides (Clostridium) difficile* in adults.

The **lincosamides,** clindamycin and lincomycin (which is not used in the United States and will not be discussed in depth), bind to the 50S ribosomal subunit and prevent elongation by interfering with the peptidyl transfer during protein synthesis. They may exhibit bactericidal or bacteriostatic activity, depending on the bacterial species, size of the inoculum, and drug concentration. Clindamycin is effective against gram-positive cocci. It is often used for treatment of anaerobic gram-positive bacteria and some anaerobic gram-negative bacteria. Warnings regarding increased risk of *C. difficile* colitis after clindamycin therapy are well documented.

Streptogramins are naturally occurring cyclic peptides that enter bacterial cells by passive diffusion and bind irreversibly to the 50S subunit of the bacterial ribosome, which induces a conformational change in the ribosome. The altered ribosome structure interferes with peptide bond formation during protein synthesis, disrupting elongation of the growing peptide. Streptogramins are able to enter most tissues and are effective against gram-positive and some gram-negative organisms. Quinupristin-dalfopristin is a dual streptogramin that targets two sites on the 50S ribosomal subunit. These drugs have low toxicity, with localized phlebitis as the major complication of intravenous infusion, which is reported in approximately 47% of patients.

Ketolides

The **ketolide** group of compounds consists of chemical derivatives of erythromycin A and other macrolides. As such, they act by binding to the 23S rRNA of the 50S ribosomal subunit, inhibiting protein synthesis. The key difference between the only currently available ketolide, telithromycin, and the macrolides is that telithromycin maintains activity against most macrolide-resistant gram-positive organisms and does not induce a common macrolide resistance mechanism (i.e., macrolide-lincosamide-streptogramin-B [MLSB] methylase), the alteration of the ribosomal target. Ketolides are effective against respiratory pathogens and intracellular bacteria. The agents are particularly effective against gram-positive and some gram-negative bacteria, as well as *Mycoplasma, Mycobacteria, Chlamydia,* and *Rickettsia* spp. and *Francisella tularensis.* Ketolides have low toxicity, and their major side effects are gastrointestinal symptoms, including diarrhea, nausea, and vomiting.

Oxazolidinones

The **oxazolidinones** (linezolid and tedizolid) are a class of synthetic antibacterial agents available for clinical use. These synthetic agents inhibit protein synthesis by specifically interacting with the 23S rRNA in the 50S ribosomal subunit, inhibiting 70S initiation complex formation and blocking translation of any mRNA, thereby preventing protein synthesis. These drugs are not expected to be affected by resistance mechanisms that affect other drug classes. Linezolid and tedizolid are effective against most gram-positive bacteria and mycobacteria. They are used to treat infections associated with multidrug-resistant staphylococci including MRSA, streptococci, and multidrug-resistant enterococci or VRE infections in patients who cannot tolerate vancomycin. Toxicity is generally low, and may cause gastrointestinal symptoms, including diarrhea and nausea. In spite of low toxicity for acute use, prolonged use (i.e., more than 4 weeks of therapy) is not recommended due to the risk

for serious hematologic and neurologic toxicity. A serious side effect known as serotonin syndrome can occur when the drug interacts with adrenergic or serotonergic drugs. Based on limited data, tedizolid has less potential compared with linezolid.

Chloramphenicol

Chloramphenicol inhibits the addition of amino acids to the growing peptide chain by reversibly binding to the 50S ribosomal subunit, inhibiting transpeptidation. This antibiotic is highly active against a wide variety of gram-negative and gram-positive bacteria as well as *Chlamydia* spp., *Rickettsia* spp., *Coxiella burnetii,* and *Mycoplasma* spp. Chloramphenicol is also effective against some anaerobic bacteria. However, clinical use is limited because of the severe toxicity, including bone marrow toxicity resulting in serious blood dyscrasias (e.g., aplastic anemia). In addition, acquired resistance can occur in bacteria from a plasmid-encoded chloramphenicol acetyltransferase that inactivates the antibiotic. It is primarily used as an alternative agent for doxycycline.

Tetracyclines

The **tetracyclines** are considered broad-spectrum bacteriostatic antibiotics. They inhibit protein synthesis by binding reversibly to the 30S ribosomal subunit, interfering with the binding of the transfer RNA (tRNA)–amino acid complexes to the ribosome, preventing peptide chain elongation. Tetracyclines have a broad spectrum of activity that includes gram-negative bacteria, gram-positive bacteria, *Mycoplasma* spp., several intracellular bacterial pathogens (e.g., *Chlamydia* and *Rickettsia* spp.), and some protozoa. Many Enterobacterales are currently resistant to tetracyclines, including *E. coli,* and some strains of *Shigella* and *Salmonella. Pseudomonas* spp. are also resistant to tetracyclines. Toxicity includes upper gastrointestinal effects, such as esophageal ulcerations, nausea, vomiting, and epigastric distress. In addition, cutaneous phototoxicity may develop, resulting in disease, including photoallergic immune reactions.

Glycylglycines

Glycylglycine agents are semisynthetic tetracycline derivatives. Tigecycline is the first agent of this class approved for clinical use. Similar to the tetracyclines, tigecycline inhibits protein synthesis by reversibly binding to the 30S ribosomal subunit. However, tigecycline has the advantage of being refractory to the most common tetracycline-resistance mechanisms expressed by gram-negative and gram-positive bacteria. The antibiotic is used to treat complicated intra-abdominal infections, skin infections, and community-associated pneumonia. The most common side effects are nausea, vomiting, and diarrhea. An increase in mortality has been reported in patients that receive tigecycline. The US Food and Drug Administration (FDA) currently recommends that the use of tigecycline be limited to infections when there is no other alternative.

Mupirocin

Mupirocin (pseudomonic acid A) is a topical antibacterial agent synthesized from the fermentation products of *P. fluorescens*. Mupirocin prevents protein synthesis by inhibiting isoleucyl-tRNA synthetase. It is approved for treatment of skin infections caused by staphylococci. There are no reported systemic toxic effects, but mild skin irritation (redness, itching, stinging) have been reported, although these reactions are thought to be attributed to the polyethylene glycol base in the ointment. This agent has been successfully used to decolonize patients with nasal carriage of MRSA but may not be effective in health care–associated infections.

Inhibitors of Nucleic Acid Synthesis

The primary antimicrobial agents that target DNA metabolism are the fluoroquinolones and metronidazole.

Fluoroquinolones

Fluoroquinolones, also often simply referred to as quinolones, are derivatives of nalidixic acid. Commonly used fluoroquinolones include besifloxacin and gatifloxacin (topical use only), ciprofloxacin, delafloxacin, gemifloxacin, levofloxacin, moxifloxacin, norfloxacin (urinary tract only), and ofloxacin. These agents bind to and interfere with DNA gyrase enzymes involved in the regulation of bacterial DNA supercoiling, a process essential for DNA replication, recombination, and repair. The newer fluoroquinolones also inhibit topoisomerase IV. Topoisomerase IV functions very similarly to DNA gyrase, unlinking DNA after replication. The fluoroquinolones are divided into broad-spectrum and narrow-spectrum antibiotics. The broad-spectrum fluoroquinolones are potent bactericidal agents and are used to treat infections associated with gram-negative and gram-positive organisms. The narrow-spectrum fluoroquinolone, nalidixic acid, is not active against infections caused by gram-positive cocci and widespread use has caused an increase in resistance among bacteria, limiting the utility of the drug. Moxifloxacin is the only fluoroquinolone active against anaerobic bacteria. Ciprofloxacin, levofloxacin, and delafloxacin remain the only oral available antibiotics with reliable activity against non-UTIs caused by *P. aeruginosa*. However, the spectrum of activity and toxicity varies with the individual quinolone agent. Postmarketing reports from the FDA warn of tendinitis and rupture of the Achilles tendon associated with fluoroquinolone use in the general population, and the risk is greater in patients older than 60 years, those on concomitant steroid therapy, and transplant recipients. In December 2018, the FDA released a new safety alert warning that systemic fluoroquinolone use can increase the occurrence of aortic dissections or ruptures. Use should be avoided in patients with an existing aortic aneurysm or in patients with increased risk of developing an aneurysm (i.e., patients with hypertension, atherosclerotic vascular disease).

Metronidazole

The exact mechanism of **metronidazole's** antibacterial activity is due to the presence of a nitro group in the chemical structure. The nitro group is reduced by a nitroreductase in the bacterial cytoplasm, generating cytotoxic compounds and free radicals that disrupt the host DNA. Activation of metronidazole requires reduction under conditions of low redox potential, such as anaerobic environments. Therefore this agent is most potent against anaerobic and microaerophilic organisms, notably those that are gram negative. The drug is also effective in the treatment of protozoans, including *Trichomonas* and *Giardia* spp. and *Entamoeba histolytica*. Tinidazole, a second-generation compound, is also approved for treatment of protozoan parasites. Because susceptibility testing is not routinely performed on anaerobes, resistance is likely underreported. An emerging resistance to metronidazole (e.g., *C. [Clostridium] difficile*) is creating difficulties associated with bacterial diagnosis and treatment. Adverse side effects may include headache and mild gastrointestinal symptoms. Interaction with alcohol can lead to a disulfiram-like reaction, including vomiting, flushing, nausea, headache, and hypotension.

Rifamycin

Rifamycins, which include the drug rifampin (also known as rifampicin), are semisynthetic antibiotics that bind to the enzyme DNA-dependent RNA polymerase and inhibit synthesis of RNA. Because rifampin does not effectively penetrate the outer membrane of most gram-negative bacteria, activity against these organisms is decreased compared with gram-positive bacteria. In addition, spontaneous mutation, resulting in the production of rifampin-insensitive RNA polymerases, occurs at a relatively high frequency. Rifampin is typically used in combination with other antimicrobial agents such as isoniazid, pyrazinamide, and ethambutol for the treatment of *M. tuberculosis* infections prior to the completion of susceptibility testing. Rifaximin, a derivative of rifampin, has a broad spectrum of activity against many enteric pathogens. Emerging resistance to rifaximin has been reported in *C. difficile*. Rifampin's side effects include gastrointestinal symptoms and hypersensitivity reactions.

Inhibitors of Other Metabolic Processes

Antimicrobial agents that target bacterial processes other than those already discussed include sulfonamides, trimethoprim, and nitrofurantoin.

Sulfonamides

The bacterial folic acid pathway produces precursors required for DNA synthesis (Fig. 10.5). **Sulfonamides** target and bind to one of the enzymes, dihydropteroate synthase, and disrupt the folic acid pathway. Several different sulfonamide derivatives are available for clinical use. These agents are active against a wide variety of bacteria, including gram-positive and gram-negative (except *P. aeruginosa*) bacteria, actinomycetes, *Chlamydia* spp., *Toxoplasma gondii*, and *Plasmodium* spp. Sulfonamides are moderately toxic, causing vomiting, nausea, and hypersensitivity reactions. Sulfonamides are also antagonistic for several other medications, including warfarin, phenytoin, and oral hypoglycemic agents.

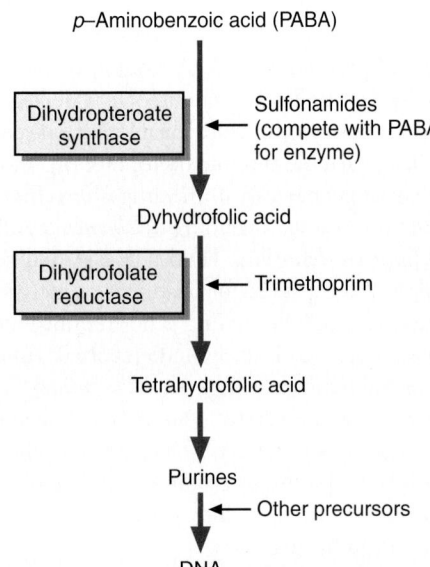

p–Aminobenzoic acid (PABA)

Dihydropteroate synthase ← Sulfonamides (compete with PABA for enzyme)

Dyhydrofolic acid

Dihydrofolate reductase ← Trimethoprim

Tetrahydrofolic acid

Purines

Other precursors

DNA

• **Fig. 10.5** Bacterial folic acid pathway indicating the target enzymes for sulfonamide and trimethoprim activity. (Modified from Katzung BG. *Basic and Clinical Pharmacology.* Norwalk, CT: The McGraw-Hill Companies; 1995.)

Trimethoprim

Like the sulfonamides, **trimethoprim** targets the folic acid pathway. However, it inhibits a different enzyme, dihydrofolate reductase (Fig. 10.5). Trimethoprim is active against several gram-positive and gram-negative species. Frequently, trimethoprim is combined with a sulfonamide (usually sulfamethoxazole) into a single formulation to produce an antibacterial agent that can simultaneously attack two targets in the same folic acid metabolic pathway. This drug combination can enhance activity against various bacteria and may help to prevent the emergence of bacterial resistance to a single agent. Toxicity is typically mild. Adverse side effects include gastrointestinal symptoms and allergic skin rashes. Patients with human immunodeficiency virus (HIV)/acquired immunodeficiency syndrome (AIDS) are more likely to develop side effects than immunocompetent individuals.

Nitrofurantoin

Nitrofurantoin is a synthetic antibiotic that consists of a nitro group on a heterocyclic ring available as an oral suspension or capsule. The mechanism of action of nitrofurantoin is multifaceted. Nitrofurantoin is converted by bacterial nitroreductases to reactive intermediates. These intermediates bind bacterial ribosomal proteins and rRNA, disrupting synthesis of RNA, DNA, and proteins. Nitrofurantoin is approved in the United States to treat complicated and recurrent cystitis caused by *E. coli, S. saprophyticus, S. aureus,* enterococci, *Klebsiella,* and *Enterobacter* spp. Toxicity primarily consists of gastrointestinal symptoms, including diarrhea, nausea, and vomiting. Pulmonary conditions are the most common side effect associated with nitrofurantoin, including irreversible pulmonary fibrosis in patients who take nitrofurantoin longer than 6 months.

Mechanisms of Antibiotic Resistance

Principles

In spite of the tremendous benefits that antibiotics have on the treatment of microbial infections, there is significant global concern regarding the emergence of drug-resistant organisms that fail to respond to antimicrobial regimens.

Successful bacterial resistance to antimicrobial action requires interruption or disturbance of one or more steps essential for effective antimicrobial action (Fig. 10.1). These disturbances or resistance mechanisms can occur as a result of various processes. The end result is partial or complete loss of antibiotic effectiveness. Different aspects of antimicrobial resistance mechanisms discussed include biologic versus clinical antimicrobial resistance, environmentally mediated antimicrobial resistance, and microorganism-mediated antimicrobial resistance.

Biologic Versus Clinical Resistance

The development of bacterial resistance to antimicrobial agents to which they were originally susceptible requires alterations in the cell's physiology or structure. **Biologic resistance** refers to changes that result in observably reduced susceptibility of an organism to a particular antimicrobial agent. When antimicrobial susceptibility has been lost to such an extent that the drug is no longer effective for clinical use, the organism has achieved clinical resistance.

It is important to note that biologic resistance and **clinical resistance** do not necessarily coincide. In fact, because most laboratory methods used to detect resistance focus on detecting clinical resistance, microorganisms may undergo substantial change in their levels of biologic resistance without notice. For example, *Streptococcus pneumoniae,* a common cause of pneumonia and meningitis, was inhibited by penicillin at concentrations of 0.03 μg/mL or less. However, the clinical laboratory focused on detection of strains requiring 2 μg/mL of penicillin or more for inhibition as the defined threshold for resistance required for interference with effective treatment using penicillin. Although no isolates were being detected that required more than 2 μg/mL of penicillin for inhibition, strains were developing biologic resistance that required penicillin concentrations 10 to 50 times higher than 0.03 μg/mL for inhibition.

From a clinical laboratory and public health perspective, it is important to realize that biologic development of antimicrobial resistance is an ongoing process that requires continuous monitoring. Our inability to reliably detect all these processes with current laboratory procedures and criteria should not be misinterpreted as evidence that no changes in biologic resistance are occurring.

Environmentally Mediated Antimicrobial Resistance

Antimicrobial resistance is the result of nearly inseparable interactions involving the drug, the microorganism, and the environment in which they coexist. Characteristics of the antimicrobial agents, other than the mode and spectrum of activity, include important aspects of each drug's pharmacologic attributes. However, these factors are beyond the scope of this text. Microorganism characteristics are discussed in subsequent sections of this chapter (see Microorganism-Mediated Antimicrobial Resistance). The importance of environmental effect on antimicrobial activity cannot be overstated.

Environmentally mediated resistance is defined as resistance directly resulting from physical or chemical characteristics of the environment that either directly alter the antimicrobial agent or alter the microorganism's normal physiologic response to the agent. Examples of environmental factors that mediate resistance include pH, atmosphere, cation concentrations, and thymidine content.

Several antibiotics are affected by the pH in the environment. For instance, the antibacterial activities of erythromycin and aminoglycosides diminish with decreasing pH, whereas the activity of tetracycline decreases with increasing pH.

Aminoglycoside-mediated shutdown of bacterial protein synthesis requires intracellular uptake across the cell membrane. Most of the aminoglycoside uptake is driven through oxidative processes in the cell. In the absence of oxygen, uptake (and hence the activity of the aminoglycoside) is substantially diminished.

Aminoglycoside activity is also affected by the concentration of cations in the environment, such as calcium and magnesium (Ca^2 and Mg^2). This effect is most notable with *P. aeruginosa*. As shown in Fig. 10.1, an important step in antimicrobial activity is the adsorption of the antibiotic to the bacterial cell surface. Aminoglycoside molecules have a net positive charge, and as is true for most gram-negative bacteria, the outer membrane of *P. aeruginosa* has a net negative charge. This electrostatic attraction facilitates attachment of the drug to the surface before internalization and subsequent inhibition of protein synthesis (Fig. 10.6). However, calcium and magnesium cations compete with the aminoglycosides for negatively charged binding sites on the cell surface. If the positively charged calcium and magnesium ions outcompete aminoglycoside molecules for these sites, the amount of the antimicrobial that enters the cell is decreased and antimicrobial activity is diminished. For this reason, aminoglycoside activity against *P. aeruginosa* decreases as environmental cation concentrations increase.

The presence of certain metabolites or nutrients in the environment may also affect antimicrobial activity. For example, enterococci can use thymine and other exogenous folic acid metabolites to circumvent the activities of the sulfonamides and trimethoprim, which are folic acid pathway inhibitors (Fig. 10.5). In essence, if the environment supplies other metabolites for the microorganism, the activities of antibiotics that target pathways for producing those metabolites are greatly reduced, if not entirely lost. In the absence of metabolites, full susceptibility to the antimicrobial may be restored.

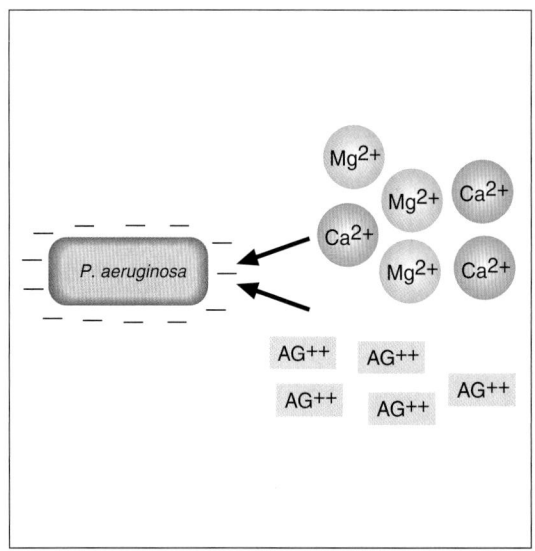

• **Fig. 10.6** Cations (Mg^2 and Ca^2) and aminoglycosides (AG++) compete for the negatively charged binding sites on the outer membrane surface of *P. aeruginosa*. Such competition is an example of the effect that environmental factors (e.g., cation concentrations) can have on the antibacterial activity of aminoglycosides.

Information about environmentally mediated resistance is used to establish standardized testing methods that minimize the effect of environmental factors and for the accurate determination of microorganism-mediated resistance mechanisms (see the following discussion). It is important to note that *in vitro* testing conditions are not established to create the *in vivo* physiology of infection but rather are set to optimize detection of resistance expressed by microorganisms.

Microorganism-Mediated Antimicrobial Resistance

Microorganism-mediated resistance refers to antimicrobial resistance from genetically encoded traits of the microorganism. Organism-based resistance can be divided into two subcategories, intrinsic (or inherent) resistance and acquired resistance.

Intrinsic Resistance

Antimicrobial resistance resulting from the normal genetic, structural, or physiologic state of a microorganism is **intrinsic resistance** (Table 10.3). These resistance factors are often chromosomally encoded in the organism's genome and are not readily transferrable. Such resistance is considered a natural and consistently inherited characteristic associated with the majority of strains in a particular bacterial group, genus, or species. Therefore, this resistance pattern may be predictable and may lead to identification of the organism. Intrinsic resistance profiles are useful for determining which antimicrobial agents should be included in the battery of drugs tested against specific types of organisms. For example, referring to the information in Table 10.3, aztreonam would not be included in antimicrobial batteries tested against gram-positive cocci. Similarly, vancomycin would

TABLE 10.3	Examples of Intrinsic Resistance to Antibacterial Agents	
Natural Resistance	**Mechanism**	
Anaerobic bacteria versus aminoglycosides	Lack of oxidative metabolism to drive uptake of amino-glycosides	
Gram-positive bacteria versus aztreonam (beta-lactam)	Lack of penicillin-binding protein (PBP) targets that bind this beta-lactam antibiotic	
Gram-negative bacteria versus vancomycin	Lack of uptake resulting from inability of vancomycin to penetrate outer membrane	
Pseudomonas aeruginosa versus sulfonamides, trimethoprim, tetracycline, or chloramphenicol	Lack of uptake resulting in ineffective intracellular concentrations of these antimicrobials	
Klebsiella spp. versus ampicillin (a beta-lactam) targets	Production of enzymes (beta-lactamases) that destroy ampicillin before it reaches its PBP target	
Aerobic bacteria versus metronidazole	Inability to anaerobically reduce drug to its active form	
Enterococci versus aminoglycosides	Lack of sufficient oxidative metabolism to drive uptake of aminoglycosides	
Enterococci versus all cephalosporin antibiotics	Lack of PBPs that effectively bind and are inhibited by these beta-lactam agents	
Lactobacilli and *Leuconostoc* spp. versus vancomycin	Lack of appropriate cell wall precursor target to bind vancomycin and inhibit cell wall synthesis	
Stenotrophomonas maltophilia versus imipenem (beta-lactam)	Production of enzymes (beta-lactamases) that destroy imipenem before it reaches PBP targets	

not be routinely tested against gram-negative bacilli. As discussed in Chapter 7, intrinsic resistance profiles are useful markers to aid in the identification of certain bacteria or bacterial groups.

Acquired Resistance

Antimicrobial resistance resulting from altered cellular physiology and structure caused by changes in a microorganism's genetic makeup is **acquired resistance.** Unlike intrinsic resistance, acquired resistance may be a trait associated with specific strains of a particular organism group or species. The presence of this type of resistance in any clinical isolate is unpredictable. This unpredictability is the primary reason laboratory methods are necessary to detect resistance patterns (also known as **antimicrobial susceptibility profiles**) in clinical isolates.

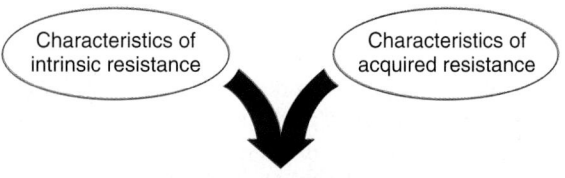

Common pathways of resistance

1. Enzymatic degradation or modification of the antimicrobial agent
2. Decreased uptake or accumulation of the antimicrobial agent
3. Altered antimicrobial target
4. Circumvention of the consequences of antimicrobial action
5. Uncoupling of antimicrobial agent–target interactions and subsequent effects on bacterial metabolism
6. Any combination of mechanisms 1 through 5

• **Fig. 10.7** Overview of common pathways bacteria use to effect antimicrobial resistance.

Because acquired resistance mechanisms are all genetically encoded, the methods for acquisition involve genetic change or exchange. Resistance may be acquired by:
- Successful genetic mutation
- Acquisition of genes from other organisms via gene transfer mechanisms (Chapter 2)
- A combination of mutational and gene transfer events

Common Pathways for Antimicrobial Resistance

Whether resistance is intrinsic or acquired, bacteria share similar pathways or strategies to effect resistance to antimicrobial agents. Of the pathways listed in Fig. 10.7, those that involve enzymatic destruction or alteration of the antimicrobial, decreased intracellular uptake or accumulation of drug, and altered antibiotic target are the most common. One or more of these pathways may be expressed by a single cell avoiding and protecting itself from the action of one or more antimicrobials.

Resistance to Beta-Lactam Antimicrobials

As discussed earlier, bacterial resistance to beta-lactams may be mediated by enzymatic destruction (e.g., beta-lactamases); altered antibiotic targets, resulting in low affinity or decreased binding of antibiotic to the target PBPs; or decreased intracellular uptake or increased cellular efflux of the drug (Table 10.4). All three pathways play an important role in clinically relevant antibacterial resistance, but bacterial destruction of beta-lactams through the production of beta-lactamases is by far the most common method of resistance. Extended spectrum beta-lactamases (ESBLs) are derived from beta-lactamases and confer resistance to both penicillins and cephalosporins; carbapenem hydrolyzing beta-lactamases confer resistance to carbapenems, such

TABLE 10.4   Summary of Resistance Mechanisms for Beta-Lactams, Vancomycin, Aminoglycosides, and Fluoroquinolones

Antimicrobial Class	Resistance Pathway	Specific Mechanism	Examples (Not Inclusive)
Beta-lactams	Enzymatic destruction	Beta-lactamase enzymes destroy beta-lactam ring, thus antibiotic cannot bind to penicillin-binding protein (PBP) and interfere with cell wall synthesis (Fig. 10.8).	Staphylococcal resistance to penicillin; resistance of Enterobacterales and *Pseudomonas aeruginosa* to several penicillins, cephalosporins, carbapenems, and aztreonam
	Altered target	Mutational changes in original PBPs or acquisition of different PBPs that do not bind beta-lactams sufficiently to inhibit cell wall synthesis (Fig. 10.9).	Staphylococcal resistance to methicillin and other available beta-lactams Penicillin and cephalosporin resistance in *S. pneumoniae* and viridans streptococci
	Decreased uptake	Porin channels (through which beta-lactams cross the outer membrane to reach PBPs of gram-negative bacteria) change in number or character so that beta-lactam uptake is substantially reduced (Fig. 10.9).	*P. aeruginosa* resistance to imipenem
Glycopeptides	Altered target	Alteration in the molecular structure of cell wall precursor components decreases binding of vancomycin, allowing cell wall synthesis to continue.	Enterococcal and *Staphylococcus aureus* resistance to vancomycin
	Target overproduction	Excess peptidoglycan.	Vancomycin-intermediate staphylococci
Aminoglycosides	Enzymatic modification	Modifying enzymes alter various sites on the aminoglycoside molecule; thus, ability of drug to bind to ribosome and halt protein synthesis is greatly diminished or lost.	Gram-positive and gram-negative resistance to aminoglycosides
	Decreased uptake	Porin channels (through which aminoglycosides cross the outer membrane to reach ribosomes of gram-negative bacteria) change in number or character so aminoglycoside uptake is substantially diminished.	Aminoglycoside resistance in a variety of gram-negative bacteria
	Altered target	Mutational changes in ribosomal binding sites diminish ability of aminoglycoside to bind sufficiently and halt protein synthesis.	Enterococcal resistance to streptomycin (may also be mediated by enzymatic modifications)
Quinolones	Decreased uptake	Alterations in outer membrane diminish uptake of drug and/or activation of an "efflux" pump that removes quinolones before sufficient intracellular concentrations to inhibit DNA metabolism are achieved.	Gram-negative and staphylococcal (efflux mechanism only) resistance to various quinolones
	Altered target	Changes in DNA gyrase subunits decrease ability of quinolones to bind this enzyme and interfere with DNA processes.	Gram-negative and gram-positive resistance to various quinolones
Macrolides	Efflux	Pumps drug out of cell before target binding.	Various streptococci and staphylococci
	Altered target	Enzymatic alteration of ribosomal target reduces drug binding.	Various streptococci and staphylococci

DNA, Deoxyribonucleic acid; *RNA*, ribonucleic acid.

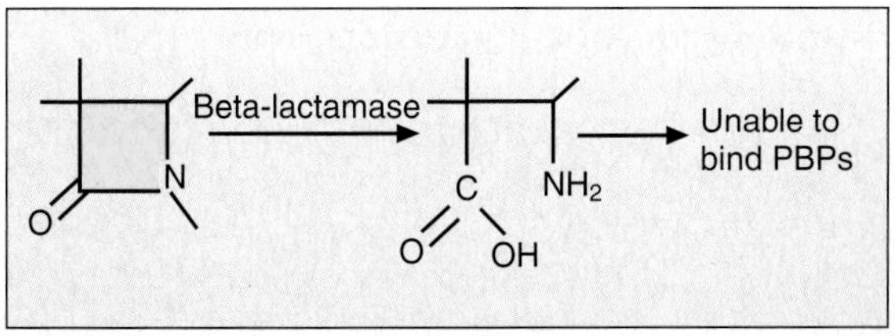

• **Fig. 10.8** Mode of beta-lactamase enzyme activity. The enzyme cleaves the beta-lactam ring, and the molecule can no longer bind to penicillin-binding proteins (PBPs) and is no longer able to inhibit cell wall synthesis. (Modified from Salyers AA, Whitt DD, eds. *Bacterial Pathogenesis: A Molecular Approach.* Washington, DC: ASM Press; 1994.)

as meropenem. Beta-lactamases function by hydrolyzing the beta-lactam ring and the altered structure prevents subsequent effective binding to PBPs; consequently, cell wall synthesis is able to continue (Fig. 10.8).

Staphylococci are the gram-positive bacteria that commonly produce beta-lactamase. Approximately 90% or more of clinical isolates are resistant to penicillin because of enzyme production. Rare isolates of enterococci also produce beta-lactamase. Gram-negative bacteria, including Enterobacterales, *P. aeruginosa,* and *Acinetobacter* spp., produce several different beta-lactamases that mediate resistance to one or more beta-lactam antibiotics.

Although the basic mechanism for beta-lactamase activity shown in Fig. 10.8 is the same for all types of these enzymes, there are distinct differences. For example, beta-lactamases produced by gram-positive bacteria, such as staphylococci, are secreted into the surrounding environment, where the hydrolysis of beta-lactams takes place before the drug can bind to PBPs in the cell membrane (Fig. 10.9). In contrast, beta-lactamases produced by gram-negative bacteria remain intracellular, in the periplasmic space. Here they are strategically positioned to hydrolyze beta-lactams as they traverse the outer membrane through water-filled, protein-lined porin channels (Fig. 10.9). Beta-lactamases also vary in their spectrum of substrates; that is, not all beta-lactams are susceptible to hydrolysis by every beta-lactamase. For example, staphylococcal beta-lactamase can readily hydrolyze penicillin and penicillin derivatives (e.g., ampicillin); however, it cannot effectively hydrolyze many cephalosporins or imipenem.

Various molecular alterations in the beta-lactam structure have been developed to protect the beta-lactam ring against enzymatic hydrolysis. This development has resulted in the production of more effective antimicrobials in this class. For example, oxacillin and nafcillin, closely related to their precursor antimicrobial methicillin, are second-generation derivatives of penicillin that by the nature of their structure are beta-lactamase resistant. These agents are the mainstay of antistaphylococcal therapy. Similar strategies have been applied to develop penicillins and cephalosporins that are more resistant to the variety of beta-lactamases produced by gram-negative bacilli. Even with this strategy, it is important to note that among

common gram-negative bacilli (e.g., Enterobacterales, *P. aeruginosa,* and *Acinetobacter* spp.), the list of molecular types and numbers of beta-lactamases continues to emerge and diverge, thus challenging the effectiveness of currently available beta-lactam agents.

Altered targets also play a key role in clinically relevant beta-lactam resistance (Table 10.4). Through this pathway the organism changes, or acquires from another organism, genes that encode altered cell wall–synthesizing enzymes (i.e., PBPs). These new PBPs continue their function even in the presence of a beta-lactam antibiotic, usually because the beta-lactam lacks sufficient affinity for the altered PBP. This is the mechanism by which staphylococci are resistant to methicillin and all other beta-lactams. MRSA produces an altered PBP designated PBP2a, which is encoded by the gene *mecA*. Because of the decreased binding between beta-lactam agents and PBP2a, cell wall synthesis proceeds. Changes in PBPs are also responsible for ampicillin resistance in *Enterococcus faecium* and in the widespread beta-lactam resistance observed in *S. pneumoniae* and viridans streptococci.

Because gram-positive bacteria do not have outer membranes through which beta-lactams must pass before reaching their PBP targets, decreased uptake is not a pathway for beta-lactam resistance among these bacteria. However, decreased uptake can contribute significantly to beta-lactam resistance in gram-negative bacteria (Fig. 10.9). Changes in the number or characteristics of outer membrane porins through which beta-lactams pass contribute to absolute resistance (e.g., *P. aeruginosa* resistance to imipenem). In addition, porin changes combined with the presence of certain beta-lactamases in the periplasmic space may result in clinical resistance.

Resistance to Glycopeptides

To date, acquired, high-level resistance to vancomycin has been encountered among enterococci, rarely among staphylococci, and not at all among streptococci. The mechanism involves the production of altered cell wall precursors unable to bind vancomycin with sufficient avidity to allow inhibition of PG-synthesizing enzymes. The altered targets are readily incorporated into the cell wall, allowing synthesis to progress (Table 10.4). A second mechanism of resistance to glycopeptides, described only among staphylococci, results in a lower level of resistance. This mechanism is mediated by the overproduction of the PG layer, which binds excessive amounts of the glycopeptide molecule, reducing the ability of the drug to exert its antibacterial effect.

Because enterococci have high-level vancomycin resistance genes and the ability to exchange genetic information, the potential for spread of vancomycin resistance to other gram-positive bacteria poses a serious threat to public health. In fact, the emergence of VRSA clinical isolates has been documented. In all instances, the patients were previously infected or colonized with enterococci.

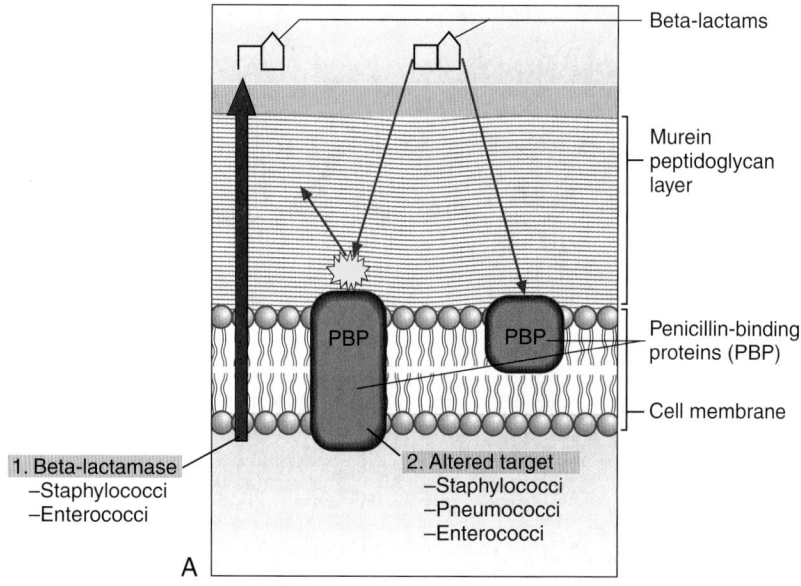

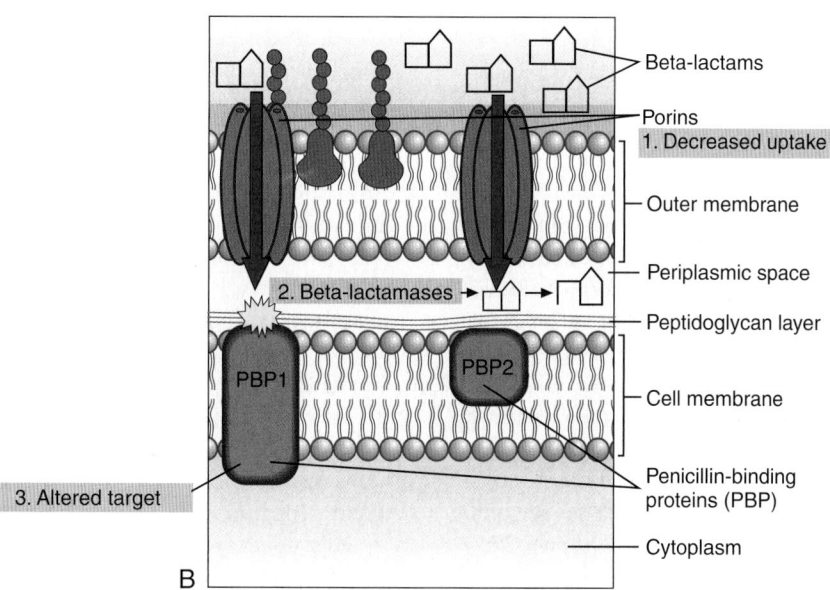

• **Fig. 10.9** Diagrammatic summary of beta-lactam resistance mechanisms for gram-positive (A) and gram-negative (B) bacteria. (A) Among gram-positive bacteria, resistance is mediated by (1) secretion of beta-lactamase that hydrolyzes beta-lactam antibiotic and (2) genetic mutation that produces an altered penicillin-binding protein (PBP) target that beta-lactam antibiotic does not bind. (B) In gram-negative bacteria, resistance can also be mediated by (1) decreased uptake through the outer membrane porin channels, (2) membrane-bound beta-lactamase enzymes that hydrolyze beta-lactam antibiotic, and (3) genetic mutation that produces an altered PBP target that beta-lactam antibiotic does not bind or binds with lesser affinity.

Resistance to Aminoglycosides

Analogous to beta-lactam resistance, aminoglycoside resistance is accomplished by enzymatic, altered target, or decreased uptake pathways (Table 10.4). Gram-positive and gram-negative bacteria produce several different aminoglycoside-modifying enzymes. Three general types of enzymes catalyze one of the following modifications of an aminoglycoside molecule (Fig. 10.4):

• Phosphorylation of hydroxyl groups
• Adenylation of hydroxyl groups
• Acetylation of amine groups

Once an aminoglycoside has been modified, its affinity for binding to the 30S ribosomal subunit may be sufficiently diminished or totally lost, allowing protein synthesis to occur.

Aminoglycosides enter the gram-negative cell by passing through outer membrane porin channels and alterations in those channels can contribute to aminoglycoside resistance among these bacteria. Although some mutations resulting in altered ribosomal targets have been described, this mechanism of resistance is rare in bacteria exposed to common aminoglycosides.

• **BOX 10.2** **Bacterial Resistance Mechanisms for Miscellaneous Antimicrobial Agents**

Chloramphenicol

Enzymatic modification (chloramphenicol acetyltransferase)
Decreased uptake

Tetracyclines

Diminished accumulation (efflux system)
Altered or protected ribosomal target
Enzymatic inactivation

Macrolides (i.e., Erythromycin) and Clindamycin

Altered ribosomal target
Diminished accumulation (efflux system)
Enzymatic modification

Sulfonamides and Trimethoprim

Altered enzymatic targets (dihydropteroate synthase and dihydrofolate reductase for sulfonamides and trimethoprim, respectively) that no longer bind the antibiotic

Rifampin

Altered enzyme (DNA-dependent RNA polymerase) target

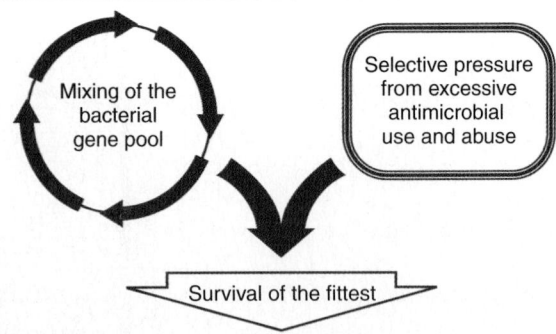

1. Emergence of "new" genes (e.g., methicillin-resistant staphylococci, vancomycin-resistant enterococci)
2. Spread of "old" genes to new hosts (e.g., penicillin-resistant *Neisseria gonorrhoeae*)
3. Mutations of "old" genes resulting in more potent resistance (e.g., β-lactamase–mediated resistance to advanced cephalosporins in *Escherichia coli* and *Klebsiella* spp.)
4. Emergence of intrinsically resistant opportunistic bacteria (e.g., *Stenotrophomonas maltophilia*)

• **Fig. 10.10** Factors contributing to the emergence and dissemination of antimicrobial resistance among bacteria.

Resistance to Quinolones

Components of the gram-negative cellular envelope can limit fluoroquinolone access to the bacterial cell. Other bacteria, notably staphylococci, exhibit a mechanism by which the antimicrobial is actively pumped out of the cell, keeping the intracellular concentration of the antimicrobial below an effective level. This efflux process therefore reduces the intracellular accumulation of the antibiotic rather than decreased uptake. The primary quinolone resistance pathway involves mutational changes in the targeted subunits of the DNA gyrase. With a sufficient number or substantial major changes in molecular structure, the gyrase no longer binds quinolones, allowing DNA replication to continue. Enzymatic degradation or alteration of quinolones has not been described as a resistance pathway. Resistance is most frequently mediated either by a decrease in uptake or in accumulation or by production of an altered target (Table 10.4).

Resistance to Other Antimicrobial Agents

Bacterial resistance mechanisms for other antimicrobial agents involve modifications or derivations of the recurring pathway strategies of enzymatic activity, altered target, decreased uptake, or diminished accumulation (Box 10.2).

Emergence and Dissemination of Antimicrobial Resistance

The resistance pathways that have been discussed are not necessarily newly evolved mechanisms in bacteria. By definition, antibiotics originate from microorganisms. Antibiotic resistance mechanisms have always been part of the evolution of bacteria as a means of survival among antibiotic-producing competitors. However, with the introduction of antibiotics into medical practice, clinically relevant bacteria have adopted resistance mechanisms as part of their survival strategy. Because of the increased use of antimicrobial agents, a "survival of the fittest" strategy has been documented as bacteria adapt to the pressures of antimicrobial attack (Fig. 10.10).

All bacterial resistance strategies are encoded on one or more genes. These resistance genes are readily shared between strains of the same species, between species of different genera, and even between distantly related bacteria. When a resistance mechanism arises, either by mutation or gene transfer, in a particular bacterial strain or species, it is possible for this mechanism to be passed on to other organisms using paths of genetic communication (Fig. 2.10). Resistance may spread to a wide variety of bacteria, and any single organism may acquire multiple genes and become resistant to the full spectrum of available antimicrobial agents. For example, strains of enterococci and *P. aeruginosa* already exist for which there are few effective therapeutic choices. In addition, a gene encoding a single, very potent resistance mechanism may mediate resistance to multiple antimicrobial agents. One such example is the *mecA* gene, which encodes staphylococcal resistance to all but one beta-lactam available for use against these organisms; this leaves vancomycin as the only available and effective cell wall–inhibiting agent. The sole effective beta-lactam for treating MRSA infections, either community-acquired pneumonia or skin and skin structure infections, is ceftaroline fosamil. Ceftaroline is approved for adults and pediatric patients as parenteral therapy.

In summary, antibiotic use, coupled with the formidable repertoire bacteria have for thwarting antimicrobial activity and their ability to genetically share these strategies, drives the ongoing process of emerging resistance (Fig. 10.10). The constant development and spread of antimicrobial resistance is manifested in the emergence of new genes of unknown origin (e.g., methicillin-resistant staphylococci and VRE), the movement of old genes into new bacterial hosts (e.g., penicillin-resistant *Neisseria gonorrhoeae* [PPNG]), mutations in familiar resistance genes that result in greater potency (e.g., beta-lactamase–mediated resistance to cephalosporins in *E. coli* and other Enterobacterales), and the emergence of new pathogens for which the most evident virulence factor is intrinsic or natural resistance to many of the antimicrobial agents used in the hospital setting (e.g., *S. maltophilia*).

Because of the ongoing nature of the emergence and dissemination of resistance, reliable laboratory procedures to detect drug resistance serve as crucial aids to managing patients' infections and as a means of monitoring changing resistance trends among clinically relevant bacteria.

ⓔ Visit the Evolve site for a complete list of procedures, review questions, and case studies.

Bibliography

Bettiol E, Harbarth S: Development of new antibiotics: taking off finally? *Swiss Med Wkly* 145:w14167, 2015.

Carroll KC, Pfaller MA, Landry ML, et al.: *Manual of clinical microbiology*, ed 12, Washington, DC, 2019, ASM.

Garau J: Other antimicrobials of interest in the era of extended-spectrum beta-lactamases: fosfomycin, nitrofurantoin and tigecycline, *Clin Microbiol Infect* 14:198–202, 2008.

Huang SS, Septimus E, Kleinman K, et al.: Targeted versus universal decolonization to prevent ICU infection, *New Engl J Med* 368:2255–2265, 2013.

Kalogeropoulos A, Tsiodras S, Loverdos D, et al.: Eosinophilic pneumonia associated with daptomycin: a case report and a review of the literature, *J Med Case Reports* 5:13, 2011.

Mayers DL: *Antimicrobial drug resistance*, vol. 1. New York, NY, 2009, Springer.

Queenan A, Bush K: Carbapenemases: versatile β-lactamases, *Clin Microbiol Rev* 20:440–458, 2007.

Roberts KD, Azad MAK, Wang J, et al.: Antimicrobial activity and toxicity of the major lipopeptide components of polymyxin B and colistin: last-line antibiotic against multidrug-resistant gram-negative bacteria, *ACS Infect Dis* 1:568–575, 2015.

The Internet Drug Index: www.rxlist.com. Accessed June 22, 2016.

Tsala M, Vourli S, Georgiou PC, et al.: Triple combination of meropenem, colistin and tigecycline was bactericidal in a dynamic model despite mere additive interactions in chequerboard assays against carbapenemase-producing *Klebsiella pneumoniae* isolates, *J Antimicrob Chemother* 74:387–394, 2019.

U.S. Food and Drug Administration: *Drugs*. Available at: www.fda.gov/Drugs/default.htm. Accessed June 22, 2016.

Zhanel GG, Calic D, Schweizer F, et al.: New lipoglycopeptides: a comparative review of dalbavancin, oritavancin, and telavancin, *Drugs* 70:859–886, 2010.

Zhanel GG, Love R, Adam H, et al.: Tedizolid: a novel oxazolidinone with potent activity against multidrug-resistant gram-positive pathogens, *Drugs* 75:253–270, 2015.

11

Laboratory Methods and Strategies for Antimicrobial Susceptibility Testing

OBJECTIVES

1. List the relevant factors considered for control and standardization of antimicrobial susceptibility testing.
2. Explain how antimicrobial agents are selected for testing with regard to specimen source, site of infection, organism identity, and intrinsic resistance.
3. Discuss testing conditions (medium, inoculum density, incubation conditions, incubation duration, controls, and purpose) for the broth dilution, agar dilution, and disk diffusion methods and how results are affected if conditions are not well controlled.
4. Define a McFarland standard and explain how it is used to standardize susceptibility testing.
5. Describe how endpoints are determined for the broth dilution, agar dilution, and disk diffusion methods.
6. Define susceptible (S), intermediate (I), and resistant (R) interpretive categories of antimicrobial susceptibility testing. Also, discuss nuances of the categories of non-susceptible (NS) and susceptible-dose dependent (SDD).
7. Define the minimal inhibitory concentration (MIC) breakpoint and identify the types of testing used to determine an MIC.
8. Define peak and trough levels. Describe the data associated with peak and trough levels and discuss the clinical application.
9. Outline basic principles for agar screens, disk screens, and the D-test for antimicrobial resistance detection in gram-positive bacteria, including methods and clinical use.
10. Explain the principle and purpose of the chromogenic cephalosporinase test. Name bacterial species and clinical situations in which this test may be useful.
11. Compare and contrast molecular methods to detect resistance mechanisms versus traditional phenotypic susceptibility methods, including clinical utility, effectiveness, and specificity.
12. Explain the principles of the minimal bactericidal concentration (MBC), time-kill assay, serum bactericidal test, and synergy test and their clinical usefulness.
13. Contrast drug combination interaction terms: synergy, indifference, and antagonism.
14. Discuss the use of drug susceptibility testing as it relates to the use of predictor drugs (i.e., prototype agents) and organism identification.
15. List criteria for determining when to perform susceptibility testing.
16. Describe the importance of reviewing susceptibility profiles and provide examples of profiles that require further evaluation.

As discussed in Chapter 10, most clinically relevant bacteria are capable of acquiring and expressing resistance to antimicrobial agents commonly used to treat infections. Therefore, once an organism is isolated in the laboratory, characterization frequently includes tests to detect antimicrobial resistance. In addition to identifying the organism, the antimicrobial susceptibility profile is considered the most critical component of the clinical microbiology laboratory report produced for the clinician responsible for the patient's care. The procedures used to produce antimicrobial susceptibility results and detect *in vitro* resistance to antimicrobial agents are **antimicrobial susceptibility testing (AST)** methods. The methods applied for profiling aerobic and facultative anaerobic bacteria are the focus of

this chapter. Strategies for when and how these methods should be applied are also considered. Procedures for AST of clinical isolates of anaerobic bacteria, mycobacteria, and yeasts are discussed in Chapters 40, 42, and 63, respectively.

Goal and Limitations

The primary goal of AST is to determine whether the bacterial isolate expresses resistance to the antimicrobial agents commonly selected for treatment at the site of infection. Because intrinsic resistance is known for most organisms, testing for intrinsic resistance is often not necessary, and organism identification is sufficient. In essence, AST is designed to determine acquired resistance in clinically important organisms for which the antimicrobial susceptibility profile is unpredictable.

Standardization

For laboratory tests to accurately determine organism-based resistance, the potential influence of environmental factors on antibiotic activity should be minimized (refer to Chapter 10 for additional detail). This does not mean that environmental resistance does not play a clinically relevant role; however, the major focus of *in vitro* AST is to measure an organism's expression of resistance. To control the impact of environmental factors, testing conditions for AST are extensively standardized. Standardization serves three important purposes:

- It optimizes bacterial growth conditions so that inhibition of growth can be attributed to the antimicrobial agent that the organism is being tested against and is not the result of limitations of nutrients, temperature, or other environmental conditions.
- It optimizes conditions for maintaining antimicrobial integrity and activity. Failure to inhibit bacterial growth can be attributed to organism-associated resistance mechanisms rather than to environmental drug inactivation.
- It maintains reproducibility and consistency in the resistance profile of an organism, regardless of the microbiology laboratory performing the test.

Standard conditions for AST methods have been established based on numerous laboratory investigations. The procedures, guidelines, and recommendations are published in documents from the Subcommittee on AST of the Clinical and Laboratory Standards Institute (CLSI). The CLSI documents that describe various methods of AST are continuously updated and may be obtained by contacting CLSI, 950 W. Valley Road, Suite 2500, Wayne, PA 19087, or at http://www.clsi.org.

The standardized components of AST include:
- Bacterial inoculum
- Growth medium (typically a Mueller-Hinton base)
  - pH
  - Cation concentration
  - Blood and serum supplements
  - Thymidine content
- Incubation atmosphere
- Incubation temperature
- Incubation duration
- Antimicrobial concentrations

Limitations of Standardization

Although standardization of *in vitro* conditions is essential, the use of standard conditions has some limitations. Most notably, the laboratory test conditions cannot reproduce the *in vitro* environment at the infection site where the antimicrobial agent and bacteria will actually interact. Factors such as the bacterial inoculum, pH, cation concentration, and oxygen tension can differ substantially, depending on the site of infection. Several other important factors play key roles in the patient outcome and are not taken into account by susceptibility testing. Some of these factors include:
- Antibiotic diffusion into tissues and host cells
- Serum protein binding of antimicrobial agents
- Drug interactions and interference
- Host immune response
- Multiple simultaneous illnesses
- Virulence and pathogenicity of infecting bacterium
- Site and severity of infection

Despite these limitations, antimicrobial resistance can substantially alter the rates of morbidity and mortality in infected patients. Early and accurate recognition of resistant bacteria significantly aids the selection of antimicrobial therapy and optimal patient management. *In vitro* AST provides valuable data that are used in conjunction with other diagnostic information to guide patient therapeutic options. As discussed later in this chapter, AST provides the data to track resistance trends among clinically relevant bacteria.

Testing Methods

Principles

Three general methods are available to detect and evaluate antimicrobial susceptibility:
- Methods that directly measure the activity of one or more antimicrobial agents against a bacterial isolate
- Methods that directly detect the presence of a specific resistance mechanism in a bacterial isolate
- Special methods that measure complex antimicrobial-organism interactions

The method used depends on factors such as clinical need, accuracy, and convenience. Given the complexities of antimicrobial resistance patterns, a laboratory may commonly use methods from more than one category.

Methods That Directly Measure Antimicrobial Activity

Methods that directly measure antimicrobial activity involve bringing the antimicrobial agents of interest and the infecting bacterium together in the same *in vitro* environment to determine the effect of the drug on bacterial growth or viability. The level of effect on bacterial growth is measured, and a categorical interpretation that is susceptible, intermediate, or resistant to each agent is reported to the clinician. Direct measures of antimicrobial activity are accomplished using:
- Traditional susceptibility testing methods such as broth dilution, agar dilution, and disk diffusion
- Commercial antimicrobial susceptibility testing (cAST) systems
- Special screens and indicator tests

Conventional Testing Methods: General Considerations

Some general considerations apply to all three methods, including inoculum preparation and selection of antimicrobial agents.

Inoculum Preparation

Properly prepared inocula are the key to any AST method. Inconsistencies in inoculum preparation will lead to poor reproducibility and inaccuracies in susceptibility test results. The two important requirements for correct inoculum preparation are use of a pure culture and use of a standardized inoculum.

Interpretation of results obtained with a mixed culture is not reliable and can delay reporting of results. Pure inocula are obtained by selecting three to five colonies of the same morphology, inoculating them into a broth medium, and allowing the culture to achieve active growth (i.e., midlogarithmic phase), as indicated by observable turbidity in the broth. For most organisms, this requires 3 to 5 hours of incubation. Alternatively, clinical microbiologists may use the direct colony suspension method where three to five colonies 18 to 24 hours of age from an agar plate are suspended in broth or 0.9% saline solution to achieve a turbid suspension.

Use of a standard inoculum is as important as culture purity and is accomplished by comparing the turbidity of the organism suspension with a turbidity standard. **McFarland turbidity standards,** prepared by mixing 1% sulfuric acid and 1.175% barium chloride to obtain a solution with a specific optical density, are commonly used. The 0.5 McFarland standard, which is commercially available, provides an optical density comparable to the density of a bacterial suspension of 1.5×10^8 CFU/mL. Pure cultures are grown or are prepared directly from agar plates to match the turbidity of the 0.5 McFarland standard (Fig. 11.1). The newly inoculated bacterial suspension and McFarland standard are compared by examining turbidity against a dark background. Alternatively, any commercially available instrument capable of measuring turbidity may be used to standardize the inoculum. If the bacterial suspension does not match the standard's turbidity, the suspension must be further diluted or supplemented with more organisms as needed.

Selection of Antimicrobial Agents for Testing

The antimicrobial agents chosen for testing against a particular bacterial isolate are the **antimicrobial battery** or **panel.** A laboratory may use different testing batteries, but the content and application of each battery is based on specific criteria. Although the criteria listed in Box 11.1 influence the selection of the panel's content, the final decision should not be made independently by the laboratory; input from the medical staff (particularly infectious diseases specialists) and pharmacists (e.g., a Pharmacy and Therapeutics committee) is essential.

CLSI annually publishes up-to-date tables listing potential antimicrobial agents in the M100 document

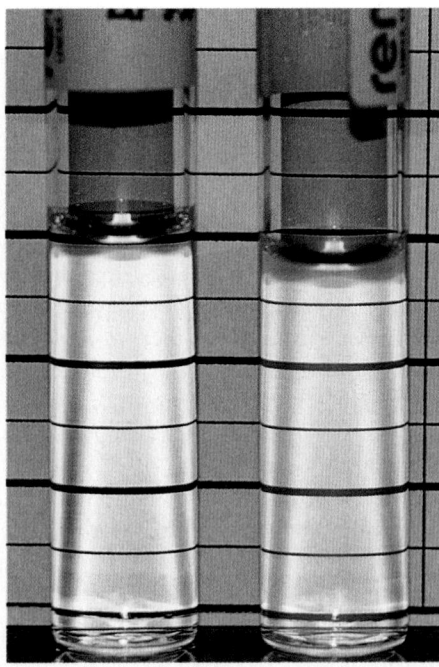

• **Fig. 11.1** Bacterial suspension prepared to match the turbidity of the 0.5 McFarland standard. Matching this turbidity provides a bacterial inoculum concentration of 1 to 2×10^8 CFU/mL. The McFarland standard on the right indicates the correct turbidity required for testing.

recommended for inclusion in batteries for testing against specific organisms or organism groups. Two tables are of particular interest: Table 1A, "Suggested Groupings of Antimicrobial Agents With US Food and Drug Administration (FDA) Clinical Indications That Should Be Considered for Routine Testing and Reporting on Nonfastidious Organisms by Clinical Microbiology Laboratories," and Table 1B, "Suggested Groupings of Antimicrobial Agents With US FDA Clinical Indications That Should Be Considered for Routine Testing and Reporting on Fastidious Organisms by Clinical Microbiology Laboratories." A third table, Table 1C, lists suggested FDA-approved agents for testing and reporting on anaerobic organisms. Because revisions are made annually, laboratory protocols should be reviewed and modified accordingly (see the Bibliography). Further considerations regarding antimicrobials that may be used for a specific organism or group are presented later in this chapter and in various chapters in Part III of this text.

Testing profiles are considered for each of the common organism groupings:

- Enterobacterales
- *Pseudomonas aeruginosa, Burkholderia cepacia,* and *Stenotrophomonas maltophilia*
- *Acinetobacter* spp.
- *Staphylococcus* spp.
- *Enterococcus* spp.
- *Streptococcus* spp. (not including *S. pneumoniae*)
- *Streptococcus pneumoniae*
- *Haemophilus influenzae*
- *Neisseria gonorrhoeae*

Criteria for Antimicrobial Battery Content and Use

Organism Identification or Group

Antimicrobials to which the organism is intrinsically resistant are routinely excluded from the test battery (e.g., vancomycin vs. gram-negative bacilli). Similarly, certain antimicrobials were developed specifically for use against particular organisms, but not against others (e.g., ceftazidime for use against *Pseudomonas aeruginosa* but not against *Staphylococcus aureus*); such agents should be included only in the appropriate battery.

Acquired Resistance Patterns Common to Local Microbial Flora

If resistance to a particular agent is common, the utility of the agent may be sufficiently limited, and routine testing is not warranted. More potent antimicrobials are then included in the test battery. Conversely, more potent agents may not need to be in the test battery if susceptibility to less potent agents is highly prevalent.

Antimicrobial Susceptibility Testing Method Used

Depending on the testing method, some agents do not reliably detect resistance and should not be included in the battery.

Site of Infection

Some antimicrobial agents, such as nitrofurantoin, achieve effective levels only in the urinary tract and should not be included in batteries tested against bacterial isolates from other body sites (i.e., the agent must be able to achieve anatomic approximation; Fig. 11.1).

Availability of Antimicrobial Agents in the Formulary

Antimicrobial test batteries are selected for their ability to detect bacterial resistance to agents used by the medical staff and accessible in the pharmacy.

For other, less frequently encountered fastidious microorganisms, CLSI publishes updates to breakpoints in the M45 document. These organisms include:

- *Abiotrophia* and *Granulicatella*
- *Aerococcus* spp.
- *Aeromonas* spp.
- *Bacillus* spp. (not *B. anthracis*)
- *Campylobacter jejuni* and *C. coli*
- *Corynebacterium* spp.
- *Erysipelothrix rhusiopathiae*
- *Gemella* spp.
- HACEK Group (*Aggregatibacter* spp., *Cardiobacterium* spp., *Eikenella corrodens,* and *Kingella* spp.)
- *Helicobacter pylori*
- *Lactobacillus* spp.
- *Lactococcus* spp.
- *Leuconostoc* spp.
- *Listeria monocytogenes*
- *Moraxella catarrhalis*
- *Pasteurella* spp.
- *Pediococcus* spp.
- *Rothia mucilaginosa*
- *Vibrio* spp. (including *V. cholerae*)

- Potential agents of bioterrorism (*B. anthracis, Yersinia pestis, Burkholderia mallei, B. pseudomallei, Francisella tularensis,* and *Brucella* spp.)

Conventional Testing Methods: Broth Dilution

Broth dilution testing involves challenging the organism of interest with antimicrobial agents in a liquid environment. Each antimicrobial agent is tested using a range of concentrations, commonly expressed as micrograms (μg) of active drug per milliliter (mL) of broth (i.e., μg/mL). The concentration range examined for a particular drug depends on specific criteria, including the safest therapeutic concentration possible in a patient's serum. The concentration range examined often varies between drugs depending on the pharmacologic properties of the antimicrobial agent. In addition, the concentration range may be based on the level of drug required to reliably detect a particular resistance mechanism. In this case, the test concentration for a drug may vary depending on the organism and its associated resistances. For example, to detect clinically significant resistance to cefepime in *S. pneumoniae* in cerebrospinal fluid isolates, the dilution scheme uses a maximum concentration of 2 μg/mL, whereas in nonmeningitis isolates, the maximum concentration used is 4 μg/mL. Moreover, for *Escherichia coli* the required maximum concentration to detect cefepime resistance is 16 μg/mL or higher.

Typically, the range of concentrations examined for each antimicrobial is a series of doubling dilutions (e.g., 128, 64, 32, 16, 8, 4, 2, 1, 0.5, 0.25 μg/mL); the lowest antimicrobial concentration that completely inhibits visible bacterial growth, as detected visually or with an automated or semi-automated method, is recorded as the **minimal inhibitory concentration (MIC)**.

Procedures

The key features of broth dilution testing procedures are shown in Table 11.1. Because changes are made in these procedural recommendations, the CLSI M07 series "Methods for Dilution Antimicrobial Susceptibility Tests for Bacteria That Grow Aerobically," should be consulted annually.

Medium and Antimicrobial Agents. With *in vitro* susceptibility testing methods, certain conditions must be altered when examining fastidious organisms to optimize growth and facilitate expression of bacterial resistance. For example, the Mueller-Hinton preparation is the standard medium used for most broth dilution testing, and conditions in the medium (e.g., pH, cation concentration, thymidine content) are well controlled by commercial manufacturers. However, media supplements or different media are required to obtain good growth and reliable susceptibility profiles for bacteria such as *S. pneumoniae* and *H. influenzae*. For streptococci, Mueller-Hinton agar is supplemented with 5% sheep blood if disk diffusion testing is performed, whereas 2.5% to 5% laked horse blood is used for MIC testing methods. Although staphylococci are not considered fastidious organisms, media supplemented with sodium chloride (NaCl) enhances expression and detection of methicillin-resistant isolates (Table 11.1).

Broth dilution testing is divided into two general categories: **microdilution** (broth microdilution or BMD) and **macrodilution.** The principle of each test is the same; the

TABLE 11.1	Summary of Broth Dilution Susceptibility Testing Conditions			
Organism Groups	Test Medium (Broth)	Inoculum Size (CFU/mL)	Incubation Conditions	Incubation Duration
Enterobacterales	Cation-adjusted Mueller-Hinton broth (CAMHB)	5×10^5	35°C; room air	16–20 h
Staphylococci (to detect methicillin-resistance [meth-R])	CAMHB (plus 2% NaCl)	5×10^5	30°C–35°C; room air	16–20 h (24 h for meth-R)
Streptococcus pneumoniae and other streptococci	CAMHB plus 2%–5% lysed horse blood	5×10^5	35°C; room air	20–24 h
Haemophilus influenzae	*Haemophilus* test medium	5×10^5	35°C; room air	20–24 h
Neisseria meningitidis	CAMHB plus 2.5%–5% lysed horse blood	5×10^5	35°C; 5%–7% carbon dioxide (CO_2)	20–24 h

CFU, Colony-forming units.

only difference is the volume of broth in which the test is performed. For microdilution testing, the total broth volume is 0.05 to 0.1 mL; for macrodilution testing, the broth volumes are usually 1 mL or greater. Because most susceptibility test batteries require testing of several antimicrobials at several different concentrations, the smaller volume used in microdilution allows this to be accomplished in a single microtiter tray (Fig. 11.2).

The need for multiple large test tubes in the macrodilution method makes that technique cumbersome and labor intensive when several bacterial isolates are tested simultaneously. For this reason, macrodilution is rarely used in most clinical laboratories, and subsequent discussion about broth dilution focuses on the microdilution approach.

A key component of broth testing is proper preparation and dilution of the antimicrobial agents into the broth medium. Most laboratories that perform BMD use commercially supplied microdilution panels in which the broth is already supplemented with appropriate antimicrobial concentrations. Antimicrobial preparation and dilution are not commonly carried out in most clinical laboratories. Details of this procedure are outlined in the CLSI M07 document. In most instances, each antimicrobial agent is included in the microtiter trays as a series of doubling two-fold dilutions. To ensure against loss of antibiotic potency, antibiotic microdilution panels are prepared with testing. Since preparation of in-house panels is a labor-intensive practice, panels may be prepared in advance and stored at –20°C or lower and thawed immediately before use. Once thawed the panels should never be refrozen, because substantial loss of antimicrobial action and potency can occur. Alternatively, the antimicrobial agents may be lyophilized or freeze-dried with the medium or drug in each well; upon inoculation with the bacterial suspension, the medium and drug are simultaneously reconstituted to appropriate concentrations. Commercial dried panels are available for routine AST. It is important to follow the manufacturer's recommendations for storage, as well as inoculation, incubation, and interpretation when using commercially purchased panels.

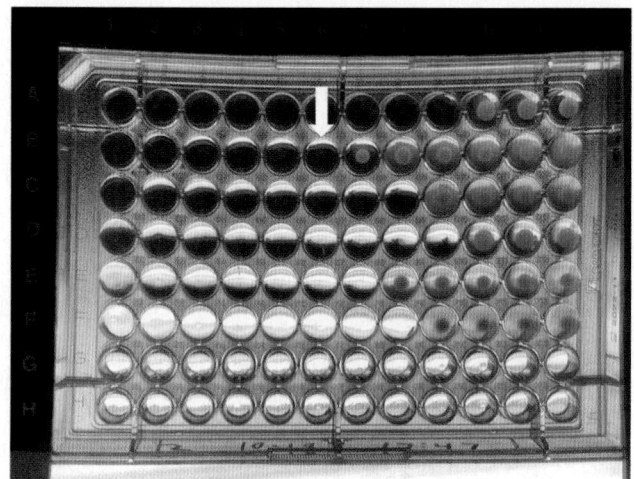

• **Fig. 11.2** Microtiter tray used for broth microdilution testing. In this example, each well in rows A through F contain doubling dilutions of the antimicrobial agent colistin from 128 to 0.125 μg/mL. The final well in each row (column 12) contains medium and the organism without antibiotic (growth control well). The MIC is recorded as the well with no visible growth seen. In row B, the isolate is growing in the presence of colistin in wells 11 (0.125 μg/mL) to well 7, making the MIC well 6 (*arrow*, 4 μg/mL).

Inoculation and Incubation. Standardized bacterial suspensions that match the turbidity of the 0.5 McFarland standard (i.e., 1.5×10^8 CFU/mL) usually serve as the starting point for dilutions ultimately achieving the required final standard bacterial concentration of 5×10^5 CFU/mL in each microtiter well. It is essential to prepare the standard inoculum from a fresh, overnight, pure culture of the test organism. The microdilution panel is inoculated using manual or automated multichannel inoculators calibrated to deliver the precise volume of inoculum to each well in the panel simultaneously.

Inoculated trays are incubated under optimal environmental conditions to optimize bacterial growth without interfering with the antimicrobial activity (i.e., avoiding environmentally mediated results). For the most commonly tested bacteria (e.g., Enterobacterales, *P. aeruginosa*, staphylococci, and enterococci), the environmental condition consists of room air at 35°C (Table 11.1). Fastidious bacteria, such as *H. influenzae* and *N. gonorrhoeae,* require incubation in 5% to 10% carbon dioxide (CO_2). Similarly, incubation durations for some organisms may need to be extended beyond the usual 16 to 20 hours (Table 11.1). However, prolonged incubation times beyond recommended limits should be avoided because antimicrobial deterioration may result in false or elevated resistance patterns. This primary factor limits the ability to perform accurate testing with some slow-growing bacteria.

Reading and Interpretation of Results. After incubation, the microdilution trays are examined for bacterial growth. Each tray should include a growth (i.e., Positive) control that does not contain antimicrobial agent and a sterility (i.e., Negative) control that was not inoculated. Once growth in the growth control and no growth in the sterility control wells have been confirmed, the growth profiles for each antimicrobial dilution can be established, and the MIC determined. The detection of growth in microdilution wells is often augmented through the use of light boxes and reflecting mirrors. When a panel is placed in these devices, bacterial growth, manifested as light to heavy turbidity or a button of growth on the well bottom, is easily visualized (Fig. 11.2). Trailing is a phenomenon in which there is heavy growth at low concentrations followed by significantly reduced growth in subsequent wells tested at higher concentrations. This can manifest in BMD panels as a very small button or slight haze of the broth. Trailing can commonly occur with trimethoprim-sulfamethoxazole, but can also occur in other drug classes as well. This could represent contamination, in which case the purity plate should be carefully examined for pure growth. Skipped wells are a phenomenon in which there is growth at higher concentrations and no growth at one or more of lower concentrations of antibiotic. This can often occur due to errors in pipetting (improper inoculation). A single skipped well in a series can usually be ignored, but for more than one skipped well, testing with the isolate should be repeated.

When the dilution series for each antimicrobial is evaluated, the microdilution well containing the lowest drug concentration that completely inhibits visible bacterial growth is recorded as the MIC. In Fig. 11.2, the arrow indicates that the MIC for colistin is 64 μg/mL. Once the MICs for the antimicrobials in the test battery for an organism have been recorded, they are usually translated into one of three general **interpretive categories,** specifically **susceptible (S), intermediate (I),** or **resistant (R).** In some specific drug/bug combinations, the MIC result may be interpreted as **susceptible dose-dependent (SDD)** (Box 11.2). In some instances, there is only a recognized susceptible interpretation, but clinical data is lacking to provide interpretations of intermediate or resistant. In those instances, organisms that test with an MIC above the susceptible breakpoint are classified as **non-susceptible (NS).** The interpretive criteria for these categories are based on extensive studies that correlate the MIC with serum-achievable levels for each

antimicrobial agent, particular resistance mechanisms, and successful therapeutic outcomes. The interpretive criteria for an array of antimicrobial agents is published in the CLSI M07 series document "Methods for Dilution Antimicrobial Susceptibility Tests for Bacteria That Grow Aerobically (M100 supplements)." For example, using these standards, an isolate of *P. aeruginosa* with an meropenem MIC of less than or equal to 2 μg/mL would be classified as susceptible; an MIC of 4 μg/mL would be classified as intermediate; and an MIC greater than or equal to 8 μg/mL would be classified as resistant to meropenem.

• BOX 11.2 Definitions of Susceptibility Testing Interpretive Categories[a]

Susceptible (S)

Indicates that the antimicrobial agent in question may be an appropriate choice for treating the infection caused by the organism. Bacterial resistance is absent or at a clinically insignificant level.

Susceptible-Dose Dependent (SDD)

This category implies that susceptibility of an isolate is dependent on dosing regimen and that altering dosing (e.g., higher doses, more frequent doses, or both) results in higher drug exposure than the dose that was used to establish the susceptible breakpoint. The concept of SDD has been included within the intermediate category definition. SDD is assigned when doses well above those used to calculate the susceptible breakpoint are approved and used clinically, and where sufficient data to justify the designation exist and have been reviewed.

Intermediate (I)

Indicates a number of possibilities, including:
- The potential utility of the antimicrobial agent in body sites where it may be concentrated (e.g., the urinary tract) or if high concentrations of the drug are used
- Possible effectiveness of the antimicrobial agent against the isolate, but possibly less so than against a susceptible isolate
- Use as an interpretive safety margin to prevent relatively small changes in test results from leading to major swings in interpretive category (e.g., resistant to susceptible or vice versa)

Resistant (R)

Indicates that the antimicrobial agent in question may not be an appropriate choice for treatment, either because the organism is not inhibited with serum-achievable levels of the drug or because the test result highly correlates with a resistance mechanism that indicates questionable successful treatment.

Nonsusceptible (NS)

Used for isolates for which only susceptible interpretive criterion has been established because of the absence or rare occurrences of resistant strains; antimicrobial agents with MICs above or zone diameters below the susceptible breakpoint should be reported as NS. Note: Confirmation of the organism's identification and susceptibility test results should be performed.

[a]Although these definitions are adapted from CLSI guidelines M7-A3 and M100-S25, they are commonly applied to results obtained by various susceptibility testing methods.

TABLE 11.2	Summary of Agar Dilution Susceptibility Testing Conditions			
Organism Groups	**Test Medium (Agar)**	**Inoculum Size (CFU/spot)**	**Incubation Conditions**	**Incubation Duration**
Enterobacterales	Mueller-Hinton Agar (MHA)	1×10^4	35°C; room air	16–20 h
Enterococci (to detect vancomycin-resistance)	MHA (brain-heart infusion with ≥ 6 µg/mL vancomycin)		35°C; room air	24 h
Staphylococci (to detect methicillin-resistance)	MHA plus 2% NaCl		30°–35°C; room air	24 h
Neisseria meningitidis	MHA plus 5% sheep blood	1×10^4	35°C; 5%–7% carbon dioxide (CO_2)	20–24 h
Streptococcus pneumoniae	Agar dilution not recommended; recent studies have not been performed or reviewed by CLSI subcommittee			
Other streptococci	MHA plus 5% sheep blood; recent studies have not been performed or reviewed by CLSI subcommittee	1×10^4	35°C; air, CO_2 may be needed for some isolates	20–24 h
Neisseria gonorrhoeae	GC agar plus cysteine-free supplements	1×10^4	35°C; 5%–7% CO_2	20–24 h

CFU, Colony-forming units; *CLSI,* Clinical and Laboratory Standards Institute.

After the MICs are determined and their respective and appropriate interpretive categories assigned, the laboratory may report the MIC, the categorical interpretation, or both. Because the MIC alone will not provide most physicians with a meaningful interpretation of data, the categorical result with the MIC is reported.

In some settings, the full range of antimicrobial dilutions is not used; only concentrations that separate the categories of susceptible, intermediate, and resistant are used. The specific concentrations that separate or define the different categories are **breakpoints**, and panels that contain these antimicrobial concentrations are **breakpoint panels**. In this case, only interpretive category results are produced; precise MICs are not available, because the full range of dilutions is not tested.

Recently the term **epidemiologic cutoff value (ECV)** has been introduced. The ECV has been proposed for specific bacterial isolates (e.g., *Cutibacterium acnes* and vancomycin) and may signal the emergence or evolution of non-wild-type strains with acquired mechanisms of resistance. The European Committee on Antimicrobial Susceptibility Testing (EUCAST) maintains a large database of MIC and zone diameter distributions for a wide range of antimicrobial and antifungal agents (http://www.eucast.org/mic_distribution s_and_ecoffs/). The CLSI has begun publishing guidance related to calculating and interpreting ECVs in the M100S document in Appendix G. CLSI has published an ECV for colistin with certain species of Enterobacterales because there is no set clinical breakpoint. The colistin ECV is ≤ 2 µg/mL, and isolates with MICs of 2 or less are considered wild type; an isolate with an MIC of ≥ 4 µg/mL is considered non wild type. For example, an *E. coli* isolate with an MIC of 1 µg/mL to colistin is considered wild type. Unlike clinical breakpoints, based on MIC distributions, pharmacokinetic/pharmacodynamics data, and clinical outcomes, the ECV is based on the MIC distribution of the organism.

Conventional Testing Methods: Agar Dilution

With **agar dilution,** the antimicrobial concentrations and organisms to be tested are brought together on an agar-based medium rather than in liquid broth. Each doubling dilution of an antimicrobial agent is incorporated into a single agar plate; therefore, testing of a series of six dilutions of one drug requires the use of six plates, plus one positive growth control plate without an antimicrobial. The standard conditions and media for agar dilution testing are shown in Table 11.2. The surface of each plate is inoculated with 1×10^4 CFU (Fig. 11.3). This method allows examination of one or more bacterial isolates per plate. After incubation the plates are examined for growth; the MIC is the lowest concentration of an antimicrobial agent in agar that completely inhibits visible growth. The same MIC breakpoints and interpretive categories used for broth dilution are applied for interpretation of agar dilution methods. Similarly, test results may be reported as the MICs, the category, or both.

The preparation of agar dilution plates (see the CLSI M07 series document "Methods for Dilution Antimicrobial Susceptibility Tests for Bacteria That Grow Aerobically") is sufficiently labor intensive to preclude use of this method in most clinical laboratories where multiple antimicrobial agents must be tested, even though several isolates may be tested per plate. As with broth dilution, the standard medium is the Mueller-Hinton preparation, but supplements and substitutions are made as needed to facilitate

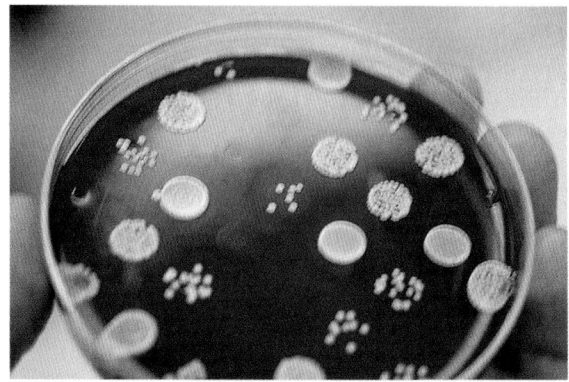

• **Fig. 11.3** Growth pattern on an agar dilution plate. Each plate contains a single concentration of antibiotic. Growth is indicated by a spot on the agar surface. No spot is seen for isolates inhibited by the concentration of antibiotic incorporated into the agar of that particular plate.

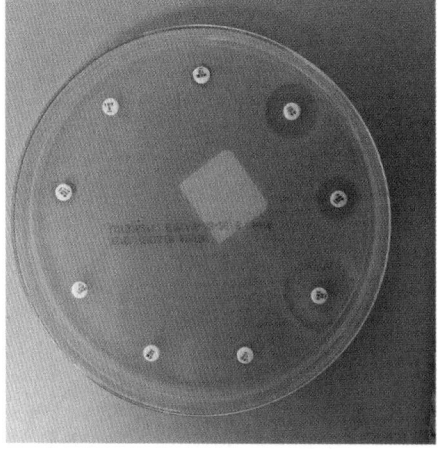

• **Fig. 11.4** Disk diffusion method: antibiotic disks are placed on the agar surface just after inoculation of the surface with the test organism. Zones of growth inhibition around various disks are apparent after 16 to 18 hours of incubation. Zone sizes are measured and used to apply categorical breakpoints.

growth of more fastidious organisms. In fact, one advantage of this method is that it provides a means for determining MICs for *N. gonorrhoeae,* which does not grow sufficiently in broth dilution methods.

Conventional Testing Methods: Disk Diffusion

As more antimicrobial agents were created to treat bacterial infections, limitations of the macrodilution method became apparent. Before microdilution technology became widely available, it was clear that a more practical and convenient method of testing multiple antimicrobial agents against bacterial strains was needed. Out of this need **disk diffusion** testing was developed, emerging from the landmark study by Bauer et al. in 1966. These investigators standardized and correlated the use of antibiotic-impregnated filter paper disks (i.e., antibiotic disks) with MICs using many bacterial strains. The disk diffusion susceptibility test detects antimicrobial resistance by challenging bacterial isolates with antibiotic disks placed on the surface of an agar plate seeded with a lawn of the bacterial isolate being investigated (Fig. 11.4).

When disks containing a known concentration of an antimicrobial agent are placed on the surface of a freshly inoculated plate, the agent immediately begins to diffuse into the agar and establishes a concentration gradient around the paper disk. The highest concentration is closest to the disk. Upon incubation, the bacteria grow on the surface of the plate except where the antibiotic concentration in the gradient around each disk is sufficiently high to inhibit growth. After incubation, the diameter of the zone of inhibition around each disk is measured in millimeters using a caliper (Fig. 11.4).

To establish reference inhibitory zone–size breakpoints to define the susceptible, intermediate, and resistant categories for each antimicrobial agent/bacterial species combination, hundreds of strains are tested. The inhibition zone sizes obtained are then correlated with MICs obtained by broth or agar dilution, and a regression analysis is completed comparing the zone size in millimeters

(mm) against the MIC (Fig. 11.5). As the MICs of the bacterial strains tested increase (i.e., the more resistant bacterial strains), the corresponding inhibition zone sizes (i.e., diameters) decrease. Using Fig. 11.6 to illustrate, horizontal lines are drawn from the MIC-resistant breakpoint and the susceptible MIC breakpoint, 8 µg/mL and 2 µg/mL, respectively. Where the horizontal lines intersect the regression line, vertical lines are drawn to delineate the corresponding inhibitory zone–size breakpoints (in mm). Using this approach, zone size interpretive criteria have been established for most of the commonly tested antimicrobial agents and are published in the CLSI M02 series, "Performance Standards for Antimicrobial Disk Susceptibility Tests."

Procedures

The key features of disk diffusion testing procedures are summarized in Table 11.3; more details and updates are available through CLSI.

Medium and Antimicrobial Agents. The Mueller-Hinton preparation is the standard agar-base medium used for testing most bacterial organisms, although certain supplements and substitutions are required for testing fastidious organisms. In addition to factors such as the pH and cation content, the depth of the agar medium can affect test accuracy and must be carefully controlled. Because antimicrobial agents diffuse in all directions from the surface of the agar plate, the thickness of the agar affects the antimicrobial drug concentration gradient. If the agar is too thick, the antimicrobial agent diffuses down through the agar as well as outward, resulting in smaller zone sizes, which may cause errors in interpretation (e.g., false resistance); if the agar is too thin, the inhibition zones are larger, which may result in a false susceptible interpretation. Most laboratories that perform disk diffusion testing purchase properly prepared and controlled Mueller-Hinton plates from reliable commercial vendors. For more fastidious organisms, an alternative

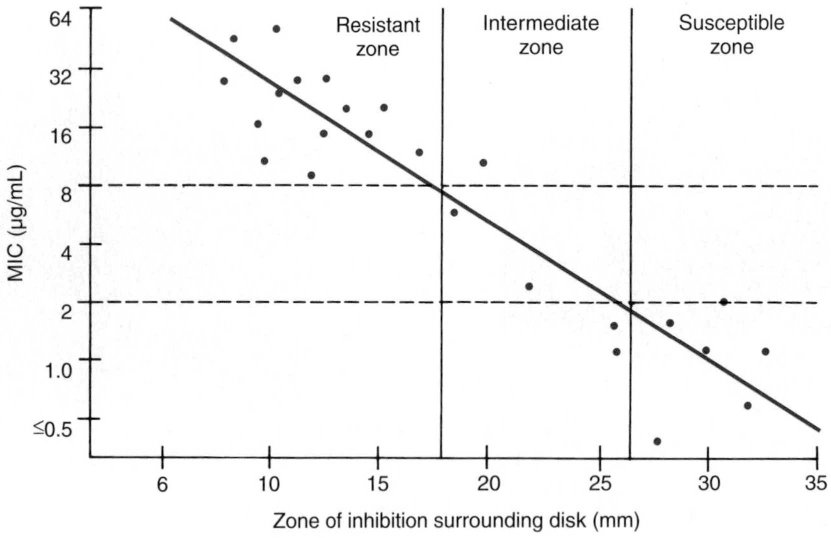

• **Fig. 11.5** Example of a regression analysis plot to establish zone-size breakpoints to define the categorical limits for susceptible, intermediate, and resistant for an antimicrobial agent. In this example, the maximum achievable serum concentration of the antibiotic is 8 μg/mL. Disk inhibition zones less than or equal to 18 mm in diameter indicate resistance; zones greater than or equal to 26 mm in diameter indicate susceptibility; the intermediate category is indicated by zones ranging from 19 to 25 mm in diameter. *MIC,* Minimum inhibitory concentration.

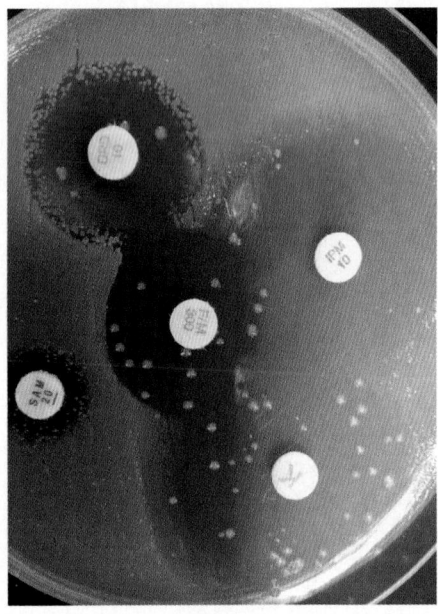

• **Fig. 11.6** A disk diffusion plate inoculated with a mixed culture, as evidenced by the various colonial morphologies appearing throughout the lawn of growth.

medium may be required. For example, when performing AST against an isolate of *H. influenzae,* one must use the *Haemophilus* Test Medium.

The appropriate concentration of drug for each disk is predetermined and set by the FDA. The disks are available from various commercial sources and should be stored at the recommended temperature in a desiccator until use.

Inappropriate storage can lead to deterioration of antimicrobial agents and cause erroneous zone diameters.

To ensure equal diffusion of the drug into the agar, the disks must be placed flat on the surface and firmly applied to ensure adhesion. This is accomplished by using any one of several disk dispensers available through commercial disk manufacturers. With these dispensers, all disks in the test battery are simultaneously delivered to the inoculated agar surface and spaced to minimize the chances for inhibition zone overlap and significant interactions between antimicrobials. In most instances, a maximum of 12 antibiotic disks may be applied to the surface of a single 150-mm Mueller-Hinton agar plate (Fig. 11.4).

Inoculation and Incubation. Before disk placement, the plate surface is inoculated using a swab that has been submerged in a bacterial suspension standardized to match the 0.5 McFarland turbidity standard, equivalent to 1.5×10^8 CFU/mL. The surface of the plate is swabbed in three directions and around the rim of the plate to ensure confluent growth of the inoculum over the entire surface of the agar plate. Within 15 minutes of inoculation, the antimicrobial disks are applied and the plates are inverted for incubation to prevent the accumulation of moisture on the agar surface, which would interfere with the interpretation of test results.

Most organisms are incubated at 35°C in ambient air, but increased CO_2 is used for testing of specific fastidious bacteria (Table 11.3). Similarly, the incubation time may be increased beyond 16 hours to enhance detection of certain resistance patterns (e.g., methicillin resistance in staphylococci and vancomycin resistance in enterococci) and to

TABLE 11.3 Summary of Disk Diffusion Susceptibility Testing Conditions

Organism Groups	Test Medium (Agar)	Inoculum Size (CFU/mL)	Incubation Conditions	Incubation Duration
Enterobacterales	Mueller-Hinton Agar (MHA)	Swab from 1.5×10^8 suspension	35°C; room air	16–18 h
Pseudomonas aeruginosa	MHA	Swab from 1.5×10^8 suspension	35°C; room air	16–18 h
Enterococci	MHA	Swab from 1.5×10^8 suspension	35°C; room air	16–18 h (24 h for vancomycin-R[a])
Staphylococci (to detect methicillin-resistance)	MHA (add 2% NaCl for meth-R)	Swab from 1.5×10^8 suspension	30°–35°C; air (temp >35°C may mask meth-R)	16–18 h (24 h for meth-R and vancomycin-R[a])
Streptococcus pneumoniae and other streptococci	MHA plus 5% sheep blood	Swab from 1.5×10^8 suspension	35°C; 5%–7% carbon dioxide (CO_2)	20–24 h
Haemophilus influenzae	*Haemophilus* test medium	Swab from 1.5×10^8 suspension	35°C; 5%–7% CO_2	16–18 h
Neisseria gonorrhoeae	GC agar plus supplements	Swab from 1.5×10^8 suspension	35°C; 5%–7% CO_2	20–24 h

[a]Methicillin (i.e., oxacillin) and vancomycin zone sizes should be read using transmitted light.
CFU, Colony-forming units.

ensure accurate results for fastidious organisms such as *N. gonorrhoeae.*

The dynamics and timing of antimicrobial agent diffusion required for establishing a concentration gradient, in addition to growth of the organisms over 18 to 24 hours, are critical for reliable results. Incubation of disk diffusion plates beyond the allotted time should be avoided. In general, disk diffusion is not an acceptable method for testing slow-growing organisms requiring extended incubation, such as mycobacteria and anaerobes.

Reading and Interpretation of Results. Before results with individual antimicrobial agent disks are read, the plate is examined to confirm that a confluent lawn of growth has been obtained (Fig. 11.4). If growth between inhibitory zones around each disk is poor and nonconfluent, the test should not be interpreted and must be repeated. The lack of confluent growth may be due to insufficient inoculum. Alternatively, a particular isolate may have undergone mutation, and growth factors supplied by the standard medium are no longer sufficient to support robust growth. In the latter case, medium supplemented with blood and/or incubation in CO_2 may enhance growth. However, caution in interpreting results is required when extraordinary measures are used to obtain good growth and the standard medium recommended for a particular type of organism is not used. Plates must also be examined for purity. Mixed cultures are evident through the appearance of different colony morphologies scattered throughout the lawn of bacteria (Fig. 11.6). AST results in mixed cultures must not be reported, and the bacteria should be isolated for pure growth and testing repeated.

A dark background and reflected light are used to examine disk diffusion diameters (Fig. 11.7). A ruler or caliper can be used to measure the zone diameters for each antimicrobial agent. Certain motile organisms, such as *Proteus* spp., may swarm over the surface of the plate and complicate clear interpretation of zone boundaries. In these cases, the swarming haze is ignored and zone diameters are measured at the point where growth is obviously inhibited. Similarly, hazes of bacterial growth may be observed when testing sulfonamides and trimethoprim, because the organisms may go through several doubling generations before inhibition occurs; the resulting haze of growth should be ignored for interpretation of disk diffusion results with these agents.

In instances not involving swarming organisms or the testing of sulfonamides and trimethoprim, hazes of growth that occur in obvious inhibition zones should not be ignored. In many instances, this is the only way clinically relevant resistance patterns are evident by certain bacterial isolates using the disk diffusion method. Key examples in which this may occur include cephalosporin resistance among several species of Enterobacterales, methicillin resistance in staphylococci, and vancomycin resistance in some enterococci. In fact, the haze produced by some staphylococci and enterococci is best detected using transmitted rather than reflected light. In these cases, the disk diffusion plates are held in front of the light source when reading methicillin- and vancomycin-inhibition zones (Fig. 11.7). Still other significant resistances may appear as individual colonies in an obvious zone of inhibition (Fig. 11.8). When such colonies are seen, purity of the test isolate must be confirmed.

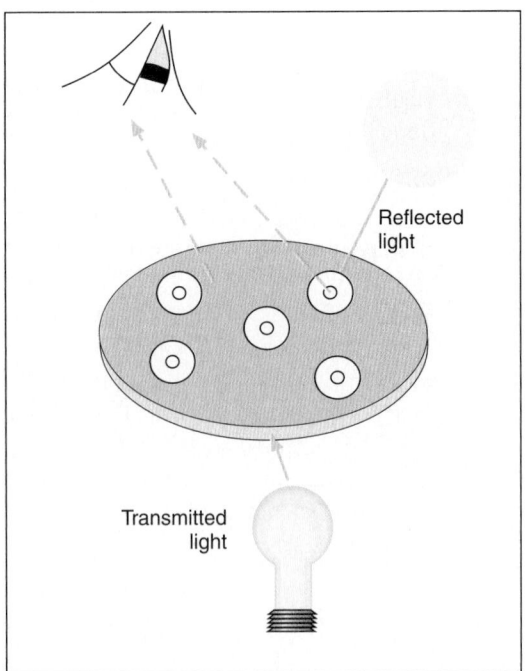

• **Fig. 11.7** Examination of a disk diffusion plate by transmitted and reflected light.

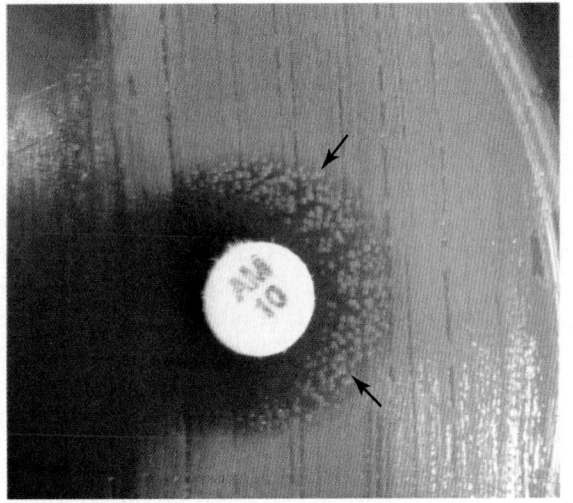

• **Fig. 11.8** Bacterial growth is visible inside the zone of inhibition *(arrows)*. This may indicate inoculation with a mixed culture. However, emergence of resistant mutants of the test isolate is a more likely reason for this growth pattern.

If purity is confirmed, the individual colonies are considered variants or resistant mutants of the same species (e.g., a heteroresistant subpopulation), and the test isolate should be considered resistant.

Once zone diameters have been recorded, interpretive categories are assigned. Interpretive criteria for antimicrobial agent/organism combinations that may be tested by disk diffusion are listed in the annual CLSI-M02 series and M100 supplement (to be used with M02, M07, and M011 documents). The definitions of susceptible, intermediate, and resistant are the same as those used for dilution methods (Box 11.2). For example, using the CLSI interpretive

standards, an *E. coli* isolate that produces an ampicillin zone diameter of 13 mm or less is classified as resistant; if the zone is 14 to 16 mm the isolate is considered intermediate; if the zone is 17 mm or greater the organism is susceptible.

Unlike MICs, zone diameters are used to determine the categorical interpretation, and the diameter values themselves have no clinical utility. When testing is performed by disk diffusion, only the categorical interpretation is reported.

It is very important to report results properly to avoid errors in patient treatment. Despite standardization requirements, the testing method includes significant variability based on organism growth, inoculum, and the interpretation of results. When interpreting results, it is always best to err on the side of reporting an organism as more resistant than more susceptible. An error of reporting a drug as susceptible that is resistant, will result in treatment failure and serious consequences—even death—to the patient.

Advantages and Disadvantages. Two important advantages of the disk diffusion test are convenience and user friendliness. Up to 12 antimicrobial agents can be tested against one bacterial isolate with minimal use of extra materials and devices if set up using a 150 mm diameter agar plate. The selection of and positioning of disks by the user allows for enormous flexibility when preparing test batteries, rather than purchasing panels produced by a device manufacturer. Because the results are generally accurate for commonly encountered bacteria, the disk diffusion technique is still among the most frequently used methods for AST. The major disadvantages of this method are lack of interpretive criteria for organisms not included in Table 11.3 and the inability to provide more precise data (e.g., MIC value) about the level of an organism's resistance or susceptibility. There are also some drugs in which AST cannot be reliably performed using disk diffusion methods, for example, colistin for gram-negative bacteria.

Commercial Antimicrobial Susceptibility Testing Systems

The variety and widespread use of cAST methods reflect the key role resistance detection plays in the responsibilities of clinical microbiology laboratories. In many instances, the commercial methods are variations of the conventional dilution or disk diffusion methods, and their accuracies have been evaluated by comparison of results with those obtained by conventional methods. In addition, many of the media and environmental conditions standardized for conventional methods are maintained with the use of commercial systems. The goal of detecting resistance is the same for all commercial methods, but the principles and practices vary with respect to:

- The format in which bacteria and antimicrobial agents are brought together
- The extent of automation for inoculation, incubation, interpretation, and reporting
- The method used for detection of bacterial growth inhibition

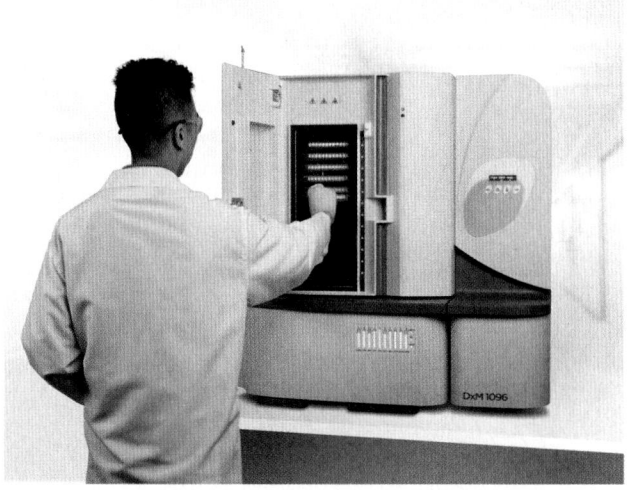

• **Fig. 11.9** Microdilution tray format is used with the MicroScan WalkAway instrument for automated incubation, reading, and interpretation of antimicrobial susceptibility tests. (Courtesy Beckman Coulter, Inc., Brea, CA.)

• The speed with which results are produced
• Accuracy

Accuracy is an extremely important aspect of any susceptibility testing system and is addressed in more detail later in this chapter.

The commercial AST systems available for use in the United States include the Vitek 2 (bioMérieux, Inc., Durham, NC), the MicroScan WalkAway (Beckman Coulter, Inc., Brea, CA) (Fig. 11.9), the Phoenix (BD Diagnostics, Franklin Lakes, NJ), and the Sensititre Aris 2X (Trek Diagnostics Systems, Inc., Oakwood Village, OH). These different systems vary with respect to the extent of automation of inoculum preparation and inoculation, the methods used to detect growth, and the algorithms within the instrument software used to interpret and assign MIC values and categorical interpretations.

The Vitek 2 AST inoculum is automatically introduced by a filling tube into a miniaturized, plastic, 64-well, closed card containing specified concentrations of antimicrobials. Cards are incubated in a temperature-controlled compartment. Optical readings are recorded every 15 minutes to measure the light transmitted through each well, including a growth control well. Algorithmic analysis of the growth kinetics in each well is calculated by the system's software to derive the MIC data. The MIC results are validated with the Advanced Expert System (AES) software, a categorical interpretation is assigned, and the AST results are reported. Resistance detection is enhanced with the sophisticated AES software, which can recognize and report resistance patterns using MICs. In summary, this system facilitates standardized susceptibility testing in a closed environment with validated results and recognition of an organism's antimicrobial resistance mechanism in 6 to 8 hours for most clinically relevant bacteria.

The MicroScan WalkAway system uses the BMD panel format manually inoculated with a multichannel (RENOK) device. Inoculated panels are placed in the WalkAway

system, where they are incubated for the required time, and the growth patterns are automatically recorded and interpreted using the LabPro software. Depending on the microdilution tray used, bacterial growth may be detected using spectrophotometry or fluorometry.

Spectrophotometric analyzed panels require overnight incubation, and the growth patterns can be read manually as described for routine microdilution testing. Fluorometric analysis is based on the degradation of fluorogenic substrates by viable bacteria. The fluorogenic approach can provide susceptibility results in 3.5 to 5.5 hours. Either full dilution schemes or breakpoint panels are available. In addition to speed and facilitation of workflow, the automated systems provide increasingly powerful computer-based data management to evaluate the accuracy of results, manage larger databases, and interface with the pharmacy to improve and advance the utility of AST data. One benefit of the WalkAway over the Vitek or Phoenix is the ability to visually read and interpret AST panels in the event of a system failure.

The Phoenix system provides a convenient, albeit manual, gravity-based inoculation process. Growth is monitored in an automated fashion based on a redox indicator system, with results available in 8 to 12 hours. Supplemental testing (e.g., confirmatory extended-spectrum beta-lactamase [ESBL] test for *E. coli*) is included in each panel, reducing the need for additional or repeat testing. Interpretation of results is augmented by a rules-based data management expert system using the EpiCenter software.

The Sensititre Aris 2X system is a fully automated benchtop system that incorporates an incubation and reading modules. The system capacity is 64 MIC, breakpoint or identification panels. It can be paired with the Sensititre Automated Inoculation Module (AIM) to rapidly inoculate 96-well microtiter plates.

Rapid ID/Antimicrobial Susceptibility Testing Systems

Any clinician caring for a patient will indicate that it is critical for MIC-based AST results to become available as soon as possible. The delay in results is due to the inherent nature of AST methods discussed previously. One new revolutionary system that can deliver same-day MIC-based AST results is the Accelerate Pheno system (Accelerate Diagnostics, Tucson, AZ). The system utilizes an Accelerate PhenoTest BC cartridge and fully automated fluorescence in situ hybridization (FISH) probes to perform bacterial and fungal identification in approximately 2 hours. The MIC testing is performed by morphokinetic cellular analysis using dark field microscopy, which provides susceptibility and interpretation of living cells immobilized on a membrane in the presence of a single concentration of the antimicrobial. Images are recorded every 10 minutes, and the instrument software plots the growth curve, cell divisions, and growth patterns. MIC results are available after approximately 7 hours. A large multicenter trial of this system demonstrated essential agreement and categorical agreement of MIC results of 97.6% and 97.9%, respectively compared to Vitek 2. The system significantly reduces hands-on tech time and decision points in the workup of positive blood cultures. At the time of this writing, only blood culture testing is currently FDA cleared, but other specimen types are being investigated. Use of this system is predicted to have substantial impact and benefits on hospital antimicrobial stewardship programs.

Gradient Diffusion Testing

One method has been developed that combines the convenience of disk diffusion with the ability to generate MIC data. The Etest (bioMérieux, Durham, NC) and Liofilchem (Liofilchem S.r.l, Roseto degli Abruzzi (Te), Italy) use plastic and paper strips, respectively. One side of the strip contains the antimicrobial agent concentration gradient, and the other contains a numeric scale that indicates the drug concentration (Fig. 11.10). Mueller-Hinton plates are inoculated using the same technique as disk diffusion, and the strips are placed on the inoculum lawn. Several strips may be placed radially on the same plate so that multiple antimicrobials may be tested against a single isolate. After overnight incubation, the plate is examined, and the number present at the point where the border of growth inhibition intersects the E-strip is taken as the MIC (Fig. 11.10). The same MIC interpretive criteria used for dilution methods, as provided in CLSI guidelines, are used with gradient strips to assign a categorical interpretation. This method provides a means of producing MIC data in situations in which the level of resistance can be clinically relevant (e.g., penicillin or cephalosporins against *S. pneumoniae*).

Another system (BIOMIC V3, Giles Scientific, Inc., Santa Barbara, CA) is an open platform automated reader that uses a camera to acquire high-resolution images of BMD panels, cAST panels (e.g., MicroScan), agar plates with gradient strips, or disk diffusion testing. Automated zone readings and interpretations are combined with computer software to produce MIC values and to allow data manipulations for detecting unusual resistance profiles and producing antibiogram reports.

Alternative Approaches for Enhancing Resistance Detection

Although the various conventional and commercial antimicrobial susceptibility test methods provide accurate results in most cases, certain clinically relevant resistance mechanisms can be difficult to detect. In these instances, supplemental tests and alternative approaches are needed to ensure reliable detection of resistance. As new and clinically important resistance mechanisms emerge and are recognized, a lag time will occur, during which conventional and commercial methods are being developed to ensure accurate detection of new resistance patterns. During such lag periods, special tests may be used until more conventional or commercial methods become available. Key examples of such alternative approaches are discussed in this section.

Supplemental Testing Methods

Table 11.4 highlights some of the features of supplemental tests that may be used to enhance resistance detection.

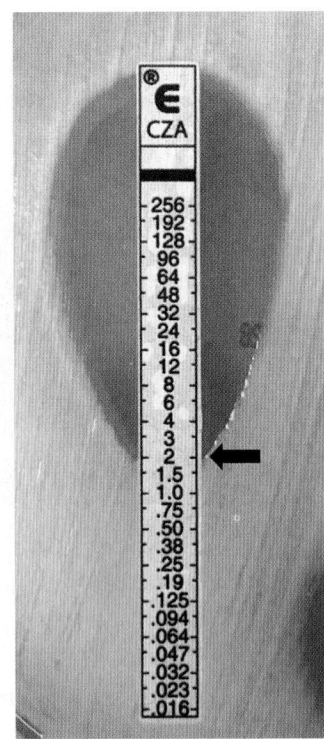

• **Fig. 11.10** The Etest strip (bioMérieux) uses the principle of a predefined antibiotic gradient on a plastic strip to generate a minimum inhibitory concentration (MIC) value. It is processed in the same way as the disk diffusion. After incubation, the MIC is read where the growth/inhibition edge intersects the strip graduated with an MIC scale across half-step dilutions (*arrow*). Results of half-step MICs are commonly rounded up to the next doubling dilution (reported MIC of 1.5 is rounded up to 2 µg/mL). Several antibiotic strips can be tested on a plate.

For certain strains of staphylococci, conventional and commercial systems may have difficulty detecting resistance to oxacillin and related drugs methicillin and nafcillin. The oxacillin agar screen provides a backup test that may be used when other methods provide equivocal or uncertain profiles. Growth on the screen correlates with the presence of oxacillin (or methicillin) resistance, and no growth is strong evidence that an isolate is susceptible. This is important, because strains classified as resistant are considered resistant to all other currently available beta-lactam antibiotics, indicating the need for therapy to include the use of vancomycin. The agar screen plates can be made in-house but are also available commercially (e.g., Remel, Lenexa, KS; BBL, Cockeysville, MD). In addition, other commercial tests are designed to rapidly detect oxacillin resistance. Rapid latex agglutination and immunochromatographic qualitative assays for the detection of penicillin-binding protein 2a (PBP2a) direct from *Staphylococcus aureus* culture isolates as an aid in detecting methicillin-resistant *Staphylococcus aureus* (MRSA) are commercially available. Since 2012, CLSI has recommended the use of 30-µg cefoxitin disks if testing is performed by disk diffusion to improve the detection of *mecA*-mediated resistance in staphylococci. According to this method, cefoxitin zone diameters less than or equal to 21 mm for *S. aureus* and *Staphylococcus lugdunensis* and less than or equal to 24 mm for coagulase-negative staphylococci (CoNS) indicate oxacillin resistance. Disk diffusion testing using cefoxitin is not a reliable method to detect *mecA*-mediated resistance in *Staphylococcus pseudintermedius* or *Staphylococcus schleiferi*. Detection of *mecA*-mediated resistance in *S. aureus* and *S. lugdunensis* can be performed by the broth dilution method. Growth in the presence of 4 μg/mL cefoxitin would indicate oxacillin resistance in these to two staphylococci species. Cefoxitin MIC testing is not recommended with isolates of *S. epidermidis, S. pseudintermedius,* and *S. schleiferi.*

Similarly, reduced staphylococcal susceptibility to vancomycin (i.e., MICs from 4 to 16 μg/mL) can be difficult to detect by disk diffusion and some commercial methods. Although the therapeutic relevance of staphylococci with vancomycin MICs in this range is currently uncertain, the diminished susceptibility is outside the normal MIC range for susceptible strains; therefore this phenotype needs to be detected. The agar screen is essentially the same as for enterococci and is outlined in Table 11.4. Strains that grow on the screen should be tested by BMD to obtain a definitive MIC value.

Similarly, detection of enterococcal resistance to vancomycin can be difficult by some conventional and commercial methods, and the agar screen may be helpful in confirming the resistance pattern (Table 11.4). However, some enterococci that grow on the screening agar are not resistant to vancomycin at clinically relevant levels. MIC testing by the BMD method should be performed. Resistant isolates that are non-motile and non-pigmented can be assumed to have acquired resistance by transfer *vanA* or *vanB* genes, whereas motile, pigmented species such as *Enterococcus gallinarum* and *Enterococcus casseliflavus,* which express intrinsic resistance to vancomycin, are encoded by the *vanC* gene.

Aminoglycosides also play a key role in therapy for serious enterococcal infections, and acquired high-level resistance, which essentially destroys the therapeutic value of these drugs for combination therapy with ampicillin or vancomycin, is not readily detected by conventional methods. Therefore screens using high concentrations of aminoglycosides (Table 11.4) have been developed and are available commercially (e.g., Remel, Lenexa, KS; BBL, Cockeysville, MD).

With emergence of penicillin resistance in *S. pneumoniae,* the penicillin disk diffusion test became insufficiently sensitive to detect subtle but significant changes in susceptibility to penicillin. To address this issue, the oxacillin disk screen described in Table 11.4 is useful with a notable limitation. Organisms identified with zones greater than or equal to 20 mm can be accurately characterized as penicillin susceptible. However, the penicillin susceptibility status of isolates with zones less than 20 mm remains uncertain, and subsequent testing using a MIC test method must be done to determine whether the isolate is susceptible or resistant to penicillin.

With regard to macrolide (e.g., erythromycin, azithromycin, clarithromycin) and lincosamide (e.g., clindamycin) resistance among staphylococci, interpretation of *in vitro* results can be complicated by different underlying mechanisms of resistance with different therapeutic implications. Isolates that produce a profile of resistance to a macrolide (e.g., erythromycin) and susceptibility to clindamycin may result from two different resistance mechanisms. If this profile is the result of the efflux (*msrA* gene) mechanism, the isolate can be considered susceptible to clindamycin. However, if this profile occurs through the inducible macrolide-lincosamide-streptogramin-B (iMLS_B) mechanism, encoded by an erythromycin ribosomal methylase gene that alters the ribosomal target, this can cause bacteria to rapidly become clindamycin-resistant during therapy with this agent. Such strains should be reported as resistant to clindamycin. The D test that is used to distinguish between these two different resistance mechanisms is described in Table 11.4.

Multidrug-resistant organisms remain significant problems for health care facilities. Of particular concern are gram-negative bacilli that are resistant to ESBL and carbapenemase-producing GNB. Screening and confirmatory tests for these resistant phenotypes is described in Tables 3A, 3B, and 3C in M100-S29. In 2010, CLSI reduced the MIC susceptible breakpoints and interpretive criteria for cefazolin, cefotaxime, ceftazidime, ceftizoxime, ceftriaxone, and aztreonam. Using these new interpretive criteria, routine testing for ESBL is no longer required, but some laboratories may continue to perform for epidemiologic or infection control purposes. As there are various mechanisms of carbapenem resistance, it is appropriate for clinical microbiology laboratories to test for carbapenemase production in isolates that are NS to any of the tested carbapenems (e.g., imipenem, meropenem, doripenem, and/or ertapenem). Testing may be warranted in species belonging to the Enterobacterales, *P. aeruginosa,* and *Acinetobacter* spp. depending on the local epidemiology where the microbiology lab is located and where patient samples are referred. Carbapenemase detection can be confirmed using phenotypic or molecular methods. While phenotypic methods are inexpensive, they are less specific overall compared to polymerase chain reaction (PCR) assays. The Xpert Carba-R assay (Cepheid, Sunnyvale, CA) has demonstrated excellent performance characteristics for the identification of *bla*_KPC, *bla*_NDM-1, *bla*_OXA-48, *bla*_VIM, and *bla*_IMP when testing rectal swabs directly or isolated colonies of Enterobacterales, *P. aeruginosa,* or *A. baumannii* species on sheep blood or MacConkey agar.

Predictor Antimicrobial Agents

Another approach that may be used to ensure accuracy in resistance detection is the use of "predictor" antimicrobial agents in the test batteries. The basic premise of this approach is to use antimicrobial agents (**predictor drugs**) that are the most sensitive indicators of certain resistance mechanisms. The profile obtained with such a battery is used to deduce the underlying resistance mechanism. A susceptibility report is produced based on the likely effect the resistance mechanisms would have on the antimicrobials

TABLE
11.4 **Supplemental Methods for Detection of Antimicrobial Resistance**

Test	Purpose (Bacteria/ Antimicrobial-R)	Conditions	Interpretation
Oxacillin agar screen	*Staphylococcus aureus*/penicillinase-resistant penicillins (e.g., oxacillin, methicillin, or nafcillin)	Medium: Mueller-Hinton agar plus 6 μg oxacillin/mL plus 4% NaCl Inoculum: 1 μL or swab from 1.5 × 10^8 standard suspension Incubation: 30°C–35°C 24 h	Growth = resistance No growth = susceptible Read using transmitted light.
Cefoxitin to detect *mecA*-mediated oxacillin resistance	Staphylococci (*S. aureus* and *S. lugdunensis*) and coagulase-negative staphylococci (CoNS)/oxacillin-resistance	Disk diffusion: MHA and 30 μg cefoxitin disk Incubation: 33°C–35°C, 16–18 h: *S. aureus* and *S. lugdunensis*; 24 h: CoNS	16–18 h: *S. aureus* and *S. lugdunensis* ≤21 mm = *mecA* positive; ≥ 22 mm = *mecA* negative 24 h: CoNS, ≤ 24 mm = *mecA* positive; ≥ 25 mm = *mecA* negative
Vancomycin agar screen	Enterococci and staphylococci/vancomycin-resistance	Medium: brain-heart infusion agar plus 6 μg vancomycin/mL Inoculum: spot of 10^5–10^6 CFU Incubation: 35°C, 24 h	Growth = resistance No growth = susceptible Read using transmitted light for staphylococci.
Aminoglycoside screens (high-level aminoglycoside resistance)	Enterococci/high-level resistance to aminoglycosides that would compromise synergy with a cell wall–active agent (e.g., ampicillin or vancomycin)	Medium: brain-heart infusion broth: 500 μg/mL gentamicin; 1000 μg/mL streptomycin Agar: 500 μg/mL gentamicin; 2000 μg/mL streptomycin Inoculum: broth: 5 × 10^5 CFU/mL Agar: 10^6 CFU/spot Incubation: 35°C, 24 h	Growth = resistance No growth = susceptible For streptomycin only, if no growth at 24 h, incubate additional 24 h.
Oxacillin disk screen	*Streptococcus pneumoniae*/penicillin resistance	Medium: Mueller-Hinton agar plus 5% sheep blood plus 1 μg oxacillin disk Inoculum: swab with 1.5 × 10^8 CFU/mL suspension Incubation: 5%–7% CO$_2$, 35°C; 20–24 h	Inhibition zone ≥20 mm: penicillin susceptible Inhibition zone ≤19 mm: penicillin resistant, intermediate, or susceptible; further testing by MIC method required.
D-zone test	*S. aureus, S. lugdunensis,* CoNS, *Streptococcus pneumoniae,* and beta-hemolytic streptococci (e.g., group B)/inducible clindamycin resistance Differentiation of inducible iMLS$_B$ resistance (by *ermA* or *ermC* genes) versus erythromycin resistance by efflux mechanism (i.e., *msrA* gene)	Medium: 5% sheep blood agar or MHA (for staphylococci) or MHA plus 5% sheep blood (for streptococci) Antimicrobials: 15 μg erythromycin (E) and 2 μg clindamycin (Cd) (for staphylococci, space 15–26 mm apart; for streptococci, space 12 mm apart) Incubation: staphylococci: 35°C, air, 16–18 h; streptococci: 35°C, 5% CO$_2$, 20–24 h	Flattening of Cd zone adjacent to E zone to give "D" pattern: inducible clindamycin resistance (i.e., iMLS$_B$ resistance) report as clindamycin-R.
Carba NP confirmatory test	Enterobacterales, *Pseudomonas aeruginosa, Acinetobacter* spp./carbapenem resistance Performs well in detecting KPC, NDH, VIM, IMP, SPM, and SME carbapenemases; ability to detect other carbapenemases may vary.	Colorimetric microtube assay: tube A, solution A without imipenem; tube B, solution B with imipenem Phenol red indicator Inoculum: isolate plus bacterial protein extraction reagent Incubation: 35°C for up to 2 h	Tube A: red or red-orange or tube B: yellow = positive: carbapenemase present. Tube B: red or red-orange = negative: no carbapenemase present.

CFU, Colony-forming units; *MIC,* minimum inhibitory concentration; *MLSB,* macrolide-lincosamide-streptogramin-B.

being considered for therapeutic use. The use of predictor drugs is not a new concept, and this approach has been taken in a number of cases, such as the following:

- Staphylococcal resistance to oxacillin is used to determine and report resistance to all currently available beta-lactams, including penicillins, cephalosporins, and carbapenems.
- Enterococcal high-level gentamicin resistance predicts resistance to nearly all other currently available aminoglycosides, including amikacin, tobramycin, netilmicin, and kanamycin.
- Enterococcal resistance to ampicillin predicts resistance to all penicillin derivatives.

Methods That Directly Detect Specific Resistance Mechanisms

As an alternative to detecting resistance by measuring the effect of antimicrobial presence on bacterial growth, some strategies focus on assaying for the presence of a particular mechanism. When the presence or absence of the mechanism is established, the resistance profile of the organism can be generated without having to test several different antimicrobial agents. The utility of this approach, which can involve phenotypic and genotypic methods, depends on the presence of a particular resistance mechanism as being a sensitive and specific indicator of clinical resistance.

Phenotypic Methods

The most common phenotypic-based assays test for the presence of beta-lactamase enzymes in the clinical bacterial isolate of interest. Less commonly used tests detect the chloramphenicol-modifying enzyme chloramphenicol acetyltransferase (CAT).

Beta-Lactamase Detection

Beta-lactamases play a key role in bacterial resistance to beta-lactam agents, and detection of their presence can provide useful information (Chapter 10). Various assays are available to detect beta-lactamases, but the most useful in clinical laboratories is the chromogenic cephalosporinase test. Beta-lactamases exert their effect by hydrolyzing the beta-lactam ring that prevents the antibiotic from binding to penicillin binding proteins. When a chromogenic cephalosporin (e.g., nitrocefin) is used as the substrate, this process results in a colored product. The Cefinase disk (BD Microbiology Systems, Cockeysville, MD) is an example of a commercially available chromogenic test (Fig. 11.11). A positive test indicates resistance to penicillin, ampicillin, amoxicillin, carbenicillin, and piperacillin.

Useful application of tests to directly detect beta-lactamase production is limited to organisms producing enzymes whose spectrum of activity is known. This also must include the beta-lactams commonly considered for therapeutic eradication of the organism. Examples of useful applications include detection of:

- *Enterococcus* resistance to ampicillin
- *N. gonorrhoeae* resistance to penicillin

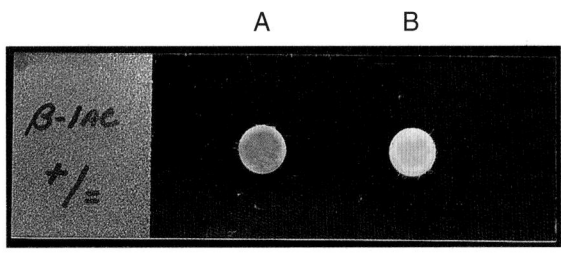

• **Fig. 11.11** The chromogenic cephalosporin test allows direct detection of beta-lactamase production. When the beta-lactam ring of the cephalosporin substrate in the disk is hydrolyzed by the bacterial inoculum, a deep pink color is produced (A). Lack of color production indicates the absence of beta-lactamase (B).

- *H. influenzae* resistance to ampicillin
- *Bacteroides* spp. and other gram-negative anaerobes resistance to penicillin and ampicillin
- Staphylococci resistance to penicillin; if negative do **zone edge test** (disk diffusion with penicillin) to detect penicillin resistance caused by other mechanisms

The actual utility of this approach, even for the organisms listed, is decreasing. As beta-lactamase–mediated resistance has become widespread among *N. gonorrhoeae, H. influenzae,* and staphylococci, other agents not affected by the beta-lactamases have become the therapeutic antimicrobials of choice. Therefore, the need to know the beta-lactamase status of these bacterial species has become less urgent. Whereas several Enterobacterales and *P. aeruginosa* produce beta-lactamases, the effect of these enzymes on the various beta-lactams depends on which enzymes are produced. A positive beta-lactamase assay provides little or no information about which antimicrobial agents are affected. It is recommended that detection of beta-lactam resistance among these organisms be accomplished using conventional and commercial systems that directly evaluate antimicrobial agent/organism interactions.

Penicillin-Binding Protein 2a

Rapid detection of beta-lactam resistance among *S. aureus* is critically important when isolated in clinical specimens. In *S. aureus* and other staphylococci, resistance to beta-lactams is usually conferred by alterations to the penicillin-binding proteins in the bacterial cell wall. **Penicillin-binding protein 2a (PBP2a or PBP2')**, which is encoded by the *mecA* gene, has reduced affinity for beta-lactam antibiotics, allowing cell wall synthesis to continue in the presence of cell wall active agents (beta-lactams). The use of a rapid immunochromatographic lateral flow assay (Alere PBP2a) can be used to detect PBP2a in staphylococci isolated on routine laboratory media. Multiple studies have demonstrated the use and agreement with overnight susceptibility test methods for *S. aureus,* and non–*S. aureus* staphylococcal species including *S. intermedius, S. lugdunensis,* and *S. schleiferi.*

Chloramphenicol Acetyltransferase Detection

Chloramphenicol modification by **CAT** is one mechanism by which bacteria may express resistance to this agent. This, coupled with diminished use of chloramphenicol in today's clinical settings, significantly limits the use of the CAT detection test. Commercial assays provide a convenient method to detect this enzyme. If the CAT is positive, chloramphenicol resistance can be reported, but a negative test result does not rule out resistance mediated by other mechanisms, such as decreased uptake of the drug.

Genotypic Methods

The genes that encode many of the clinically relevant acquired resistance mechanisms are known, as are all or part of their nucleotide sequences. This has allowed for the development of molecular methods involving nucleic acid hybridization and amplification for the study and detection of antimicrobial resistance (for more information on molecular methods for the characterization of bacteria, see Chapter 8). The ability to definitively determine the presence of a particular gene encoding antimicrobial resistance has several advantages, but limitations also exist.

From a research and development perspective, molecular methods can more thoroughly characterize resistance profiles of bacterial collections used to establish and evaluate conventional standards recommended by CLSI.

It has been demonstrated that matrix-assisted laser desorption ionization time-of-flight mass spectrometry (MALDI-TOF MS) can be used to detect beta-lactamases and carbapenemases from isolated colonies with high accuracy compared to phenotypic and PCR-based assays. For carbapenemase detection, for example, a heavy suspension (equivalent to 3.0 McFarland) of gram-negative bacilli is suspended in 20 mM Tris-HCl-20 mM NaCl. A 1mL aliquot of the suspension is centrifuged and the pellet resuspended in 50 µL of a 20 mM Tris-HCl, 0.01% SDS solution with 0.1 mM meropenem and incubated for 2 hours at 35°C. Following centrifugation, 1 µL of the supernatant is spotted to a target slide and mixed with 1 µL of dihydroxybenzoic acid and dried before acquiring the mass spectra. This method relies on the technologists' interpretation of mass spectral patterns and recognition of changes in the pattern that reflect hydrolysis of the antimicrobial that produces characteristic peaks of a specific mass range. These methods are still experimental and for research use only. While this method is promising and could lead to more rapid detection of antimicrobial resistance mechanisms, the extensive modification of an FDA-cleared device, changes in extraction methods, and manual interpretation of mass spectra will inhibit this from being adopted widely until more simplified methods are available. Molecular methods may be directly applied in the clinical setting as an adjunct to investigate and arbitrate equivocal results obtained by phenotypic methods. For example, the clinical importance of accurately detecting methicillin resistance among staphylococci, coupled with the inconsistencies of phenotypic methods, is problematic. In doubtful situations, molecular detection of the *mecA* gene encoding methicillin resistance can be applied to definitively establish an isolate's methicillin resistance. Similarly, doubt raised by equivocal phenotypic results obtained with potentially vancomycin-resistant enterococci can be resolved by establishing the presence and classification of the *van* genes that mediate this resistance.

Although molecular methods have been and will continue to be extremely important in antimicrobial resistance detection, numerous factors still complicate their use beyond supplementing phenotype-based susceptibility testing protocols. These factors include the following:

- Use of probes or oligonucleotides for specific resistance genes. Resistance mediated by divergent genes or different mechanisms could be missed (i.e., the absence of one gene may not guarantee antimicrobial susceptibility).
- Phenotypic resistance to a level that is clinically significant for any one antimicrobial agent may be the result of a culmination of processes that involve enzymatic modification of the antimicrobial, decreased uptake, altered affinity of the drug's target, or some combination of mechanisms (i.e., the presence of one gene does not guarantee resistance).
- The presence of a gene encoding resistance does not provide information about the status of the control genes necessary for expression of resistance; that is, although present, the genes may be silent or nonfunctional, and the organism may not be capable of expressing the resistance encoded by the gene.
- From a clinical laboratory perspective, it may be impractical to adopt molecular methods specific for only a few resistance mechanisms when most susceptibility testing still will be accomplished using phenotypic-based methods. Items to consider before adopting molecular tests may include (but are not limited to) clinical efficacy, space, personnel, and financial management.

Even though adoption of molecular methods for routine AST poses challenges, these methods will continue to enhance detection of antibiotic resistance.

Special Methods for Complex Antimicrobial/ Organism Interactions

Certain *in vitro* tests have been developed to investigate aspects of antimicrobial activity not routinely addressed by routine susceptibility testing procedures. Specifically, these are tests designed to measure bactericidal activity (i.e., bacterial killing) or to measure the antibacterial effect of combination therapy with antimicrobial agents.

These tests are often labor intensive, fraught with technical problems, commonly difficult to interpret, and of uncertain clinical utility. For these reasons, their use should be limited, and they should be performed only if expert microbiology and infectious disease consultants are available.

Bactericidal Tests

Bactericidal tests are designed to determine the ability of antimicrobial agents to kill bacteria. The killing ability of most drugs is already known, and antimicrobials are commonly classified as bacteriostatic or bactericidal agents. However, many variables, including the concentration of antimicrobial agent and the species of targeted organism, can influence this classification. For example, beta-lactams, such as penicillin, typically are bactericidal against most gram-positive cocci but are usually only bacteriostatic against enterococci. If bactericidal tests are clinically appropriate, they should be applied only to evaluate antimicrobials typically considered to be bactericidal (e.g., beta-lactams and vancomycin) and not to agents known to be bacteriostatic (e.g., macrolides).

Situations in which achieving bactericidal activity is of greatest clinical importance include severe and life-threatening infections, infections in immunocompromised patients, and infections in body sites where assistance from the patient's own defenses is minimal (e.g., endocarditis or osteomyelitis). Based on research using animal models and clinical trials in humans, the most effective therapy for these types of infections is often already known. However, occasionally the laboratory may be asked to substantiate that bactericidal activity is being achieved or is achievable. The methods available for this include **minimal bactericidal concentration (MBC) testing, time-kill studies,** and **serum-bactericidal testing (SBT).** Regardless of the method used, the need to interpret the results cautiously, with the understanding of uncertain clinical correlation and the potential for substantial technical artifacts, cannot be overemphasized.

Minimal Bactericidal Concentration

The MBC test involves continuation of conventional broth dilution testing. After incubation and determination of the antimicrobial agent's MIC, an aliquot from each tube or well in the dilution series demonstrating inhibition of visible bacterial growth is subcultured to an enriched agar medium (e.g., sheep blood agar). After overnight incubation, the plates are examined, and the colony forming units (CFUs) determined. With the volume of the aliquot and the number of CFUs obtained, the number of viable cells per milliliter for each antimicrobial dilution can be calculated. This number is compared with the known CFU per milliliter in the original inoculum. The antimicrobial concentration resulting in a 99.9% reduction in CFU per milliliter compared with the organism concentration in the original inoculum is recorded as the MBC.

Although the clinical significance of MBC results is uncertain, this information may be helpful in determining whether treatment failure could be a result of the organism's MBC exceeding the serum-achievable level for the antimicrobial agent. Alternatively, if an antibiotic's MBC is greater than or equal to 32 times higher than its MIC, the organism may be tolerant to the drug. **Tolerance** is a phenomenon most commonly associated with bacterial resistance to beta-lactam antibiotics that reflects an organism's ability to be inhibited, not killed, by an agent that is usually bactericidal. Although the physiologic basis of tolerance has been studied in several bacterial species, the actual clinical relevance of this phenomenon has not been established.

Time-Kill Studies

Another approach to examining bactericidal activity of an antimicrobial agent involves exposing a bacterial isolate to a concentration of antibiotic in a broth medium and measuring the rate of killing over a specified time. In time-kill studies, samples are collected from the antibiotic-broth solution immediately after addition of the inoculum and at regular intervals afterward. Each time-sample is plated to agar plates; after incubation, CFU counts are performed as described for MBC testing. The number of viable bacteria from each sample is plotted over time to determine the rate of killing. Generally, a 1000-fold decrease in the number of viable bacteria in the antibiotic-containing broth after a 24-hour period, compared with the number of bacteria in the original inoculum, is interpreted as bactericidal activity. Although time-kill analysis is used in the research environment to study the *in vitro* activity of antimicrobial agents, the labor intensity and technical specifications of the procedure preclude its use in most clinical microbiology laboratories.

Serum Bactericidal Test (Schlichter Test)

The SBT, also known as the Schlichter test, is analogous to the MIC-MBC test except that the test medium used is the patient's serum containing the therapeutic antimicrobial agents the patient has been receiving. Using the patient's serum to detect bacteriostatic and bactericidal activity allows observation of the antibacterial effect of factors other than the antibiotics (e.g., antibodies and complement).

Two serum samples are required for each test. One is collected just before (within 30 minutes) the patient is to receive the next antimicrobial dose (i.e., **trough specimen**). The other sample is collected after the antimicrobial agent(s) is given when the serum antimicrobial concentration is highest (i.e., **peak specimen**). The appropriate time to collect the peak specimen varies with pharmacokinetic properties of the antimicrobial agents and their route of administration. Peak levels for intravenously, intramuscularly, and orally administered agents are generally obtained 30 to 60 minutes, 60 minutes, and 90 minutes after administration, respectively. The trough and peak samples should be collected for the same dose and tested simultaneously.

Serial twofold dilutions of trough and peak serum samples are prepared and inoculated with the bacterial isolate from the patient (final inoculum of 5×10^5 CFU/mL). Dilutions are incubated overnight. The highest dilution that inhibits visibly detectable growth is the serum-static titer (e.g., 8, 16, and 32). Aliquots of known size are taken from each dilution at or below the **serum-static titer** (i.e., dilutions that inhibited bacterial growth) and are plated on sheep blood agar plates. After incubation, the CFUs per plate are counted, and the serum dilution, resulting in a 99.9% reduction in the CFU/mL compared with the original inoculum, is recorded as the **serum-cidal titer.** For example, if a bacterial isolate showed a serum-static titer of 32, the tubes containing dilutions of 1/2, 1/4, 1/8, 1/16, and 1/32 would be subcultured. If the 1/8 dilution was the highest dilution to yield a 99.9% decrease in CFUs, the serum-cidal titer would be recorded as 8.

The SBT was originally developed to aid in predicting the clinical efficacy of antimicrobial therapy for staphylococcal endocarditis. Peak serum-cidal titers of 32 to 64 or greater have been thought to correlate with a positive clinical outcome. However, even though the test is performed on the patient's serum, many differences go unaccounted for between the *in vitro* test environment and the *in vitro* site of infection. Although the test is used to evaluate whether effective bactericidal concentrations are being achieved, the predictive clinical value for staphylococcal endocarditis or other infections caused by other bacteria remains uncertain. Details regarding the performance of these bactericidal tests are provided in the CLSI document M26-A, "Methods for Determining Bactericidal Activity of Antimicrobial Agents."

Tests for Activity of Antimicrobial Combinations

Therapeutic management of bacterial infections often requires simultaneous use of more than one antimicrobial agent. Some of the reasons for use of multiple therapies include:

- Treating polymicrobial infections caused by organisms with different antimicrobial resistance profiles
- Achieving more rapid bactericidal activity than may be achieved with any single agent
- Achieving bactericidal activity against bacteria for which no single agent is lethal
- Minimizing the emergence of resistant organisms during therapy

Testing the effectiveness of antimicrobial combinations against a single bacterial isolate is **synergy testing.** When combinations are tested, three outcome categories are possible:

- **Synergy:** the activity of the antimicrobial combination is substantially greater than the activity of the single most active drug alone
- **Indifference:** the activity of the combination is no better or worse than the single most active drug alone
- **Antagonism:** the activity of the combination is substantially less than the activity of the single most active drug alone (an interaction to be avoided)

The checkerboard assay and the time-kill assay are two basic methods of synergy testing but are not routinely performed in the clinical laboratory. In the checkerboard method, MIC panels are set up containing two antimicrobial agents serially diluted independently and in combination. After inoculation and incubation, the MICs obtained with the individual agents and the various combinations are recorded. By calculating the MIC ratios obtained with individual and combined agents, the drug combination in question is classified as synergistic, indifferent, or antagonistic.

With the time-kill assay, the same procedure described for testing bactericidal activity is used, except that the killing curve obtained with a single agent is compared with the killing curve obtained with antimicrobial combinations. Synergy is indicated when the combination exhibits killing that is greater by

100-fold or more than the most active single agent tested alone after 24 hours of incubation. Killing rates between the most active agent and the combination that are similar are interpreted as indifference. Antagonism is evident when the combination appears less active than the most active single agent.

The decision to use more than one antimicrobial agent may be based on antimicrobial resistance profiles or identification of particular bacterial pathogens reported by the clinical microbiology laboratory. However, the decision regarding which antimicrobial agents to combine should not rely on the results of complex synergy tests. Most clinically useful antimicrobial combinations have been investigated in a clinical research setting and are well described in the medical literature. These data should be used to guide the decision for combination therapy. The technical difficulties associated with performing and interpreting synergy tests preclude their utility in the diagnostic setting.

Laboratory Strategies for Antimicrobial Susceptibility Testing

The clinical microbiology laboratory is responsible for maximizing the positive impact that AST information can have on the use of antimicrobial agents to treat infectious diseases. However, meeting this responsibility is difficult because of demands for more efficient use of laboratory resources, increasing complexities of important bacterial resistance profiles, and continued expectations for high-quality results. To ensure quality in the midst of dwindling resources and expanding antimicrobial resistance, strategies for AST must be carefully developed. These strategies should target relevance, accuracy, and communication (Fig. 11.12).

Relevance

AST should be performed when sufficient potential exists for providing clinically useful and reliable information about antimicrobial agents appropriate for the bacterial isolate in question. For the sake of relevance, two questions must be addressed:

- When should testing be performed?
- Which antimicrobial agents should be tested?

When to Perform a Susceptibility Test

The first issue that must be resolved is whether AST is appropriate for a particular isolate. Although the answer may not always be clear, the issue must always be addressed. The decision to perform susceptibility testing depends on the following criteria:

- Clinical significance of a bacterial isolate
- Predictability of a bacterial isolate's susceptibility to the antimicrobial agents most commonly used against them, often referred to as the **therapeutic drugs of choice**
- Availability of reliable standardized methods for testing the isolate

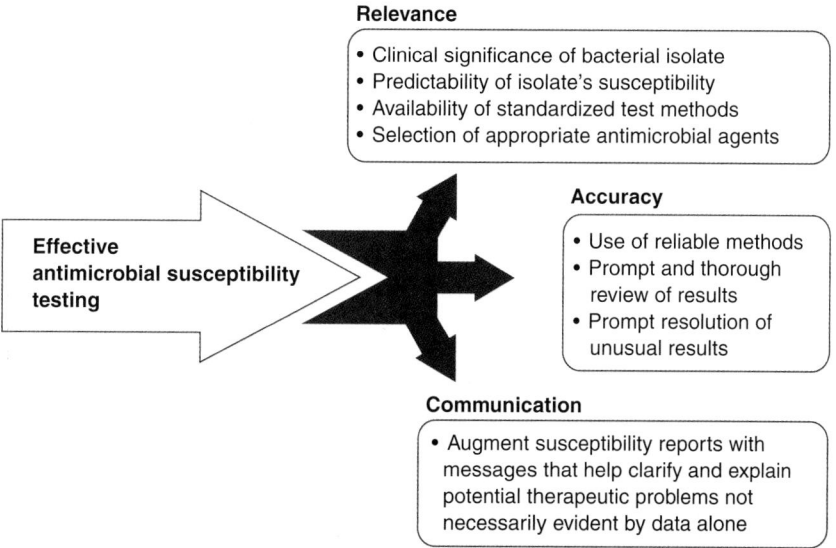

Relevance
- Clinical significance of bacterial isolate
- Predictability of isolate's susceptibility
- Availability of standardized test methods
- Selection of appropriate antimicrobial agents

Effective antimicrobial susceptibility testing

Accuracy
- Use of reliable methods
- Prompt and thorough review of results
- Prompt resolution of unusual results

Communication
- Augment susceptibility reports with messages that help clarify and explain potential therapeutic problems not necessarily evident by data alone

• **Fig. 11.12** Goals of effective antimicrobial susceptibility testing strategies.

Determining Clinical Significance

Performing tests and reporting antimicrobial susceptibility data on clinically insignificant bacterial isolates are a waste of resources and, more importantly, can mislead physicians, who depend on laboratory information to assist in establishing the clinical significance of a bacterial isolate. Useful criteria for establishing the clinical importance of a bacterial isolate include:

- Detection and/or the abundance of the organism on direct Gram stain of a patient's specimen, preferably in the presence of white blood cells, and growth of an organism with the same morphology in culture
- Known ability of the bacterial species isolated to cause infection at the body site from which the specimen was obtained (see Part VII)
- Whether the organism is usually considered either an epithelial or mucosal colonizer or is usually considered a pathogen
- Body site from which the organism was isolated (normally sterile or typically colonized)

Although these criteria are helpful and heavily depend on the capacity of the bacterial species isolated to cause disease, the final designation of clinical significance often still requires dialogue between laboratory professionals and the physicians responsible for the patient's care.

Reporting susceptibility results for organisms with questionable clinical importance may be incorrectly interpreted as an indicator of clinical significance. Using criteria such as those listed should be included in the laboratory's AST strategy.

Predictability of Antimicrobial Susceptibility

If the organisms are clinically significant, then the chances that they could be resistant to the antimicrobial agents commonly used to eradicate them must be determined. Unfortunately, the increasing dissemination of

resistance among clinically relevant bacteria has diminished the number of bacteria for which antimicrobial susceptibility can be confidently predicted based on identification without the need to perform testing. Table 11.5 categorizes many of the commonly encountered bacteria according to the need to perform testing to detect resistance.

Acquired resistance to various antimicrobial agents necessitates that AST be performed on all clinically relevant isolates. For other organisms, such as *H. influenzae* and *N. gonorrhoeae*, resistance to the original drugs of choice has become widespread and more potent antimicrobials—for example, ceftriaxone, for which no resistance has been described—have become the treatments of choice. One notable exception to the widespread emergence of resistance has been the absence of penicillin resistance among beta-hemolytic streptococci. Because susceptibility to penicillin is extremely predictable among these organisms, testing against penicillin provides little, if any, information not already provided by accurate organism identification. However, if the patient cannot tolerate penicillin, then alternative agents, such as erythromycin, should be considered. Because erythromycin resistance among β-hemolytic streptococci has been well documented, susceptibility testing in this instance is required.

The recommendations outlined in Table 11.5 are guidelines and are always being updated. In clinical settings, exceptions will arise that must be considered in consultation with the physician and pharmacist with infectious disease training. These guidelines are designed to provide data on the management of a single patient's infection, but they may not apply when AST is performed to gather surveillance data when monitoring for emerging resistance (see Accuracy and Antimicrobial Resistance Surveillance later in this chapter).

TABLE 11.5	Categorization of Bacteria According to Need for Routine Performance of Antimicrobial Susceptibility Testing[a]
Need for Testing	**Bacteria**
Testing commonly required	Staphylococci *Streptococcus pneumoniae* viridans streptococci[b] Enterococci Enterobacterales *Pseudomonas aeruginosa* *Acinetobacter* spp.
Testing occasionally required[c]	*Haemophilus influenzae* *Neisseria gonorrhoeae* *Moraxella catarrhalis* Anaerobic bacteria
Testing rarely required	Beta-hemolytic streptococci (groups A, B, C, F, and G) *Neisseria meningitidis* *Listeria monocytogenes*

[a]Based on the assumption that the organism is clinically significant. Table includes bacteria for which standardized testing procedures are available, as outlined and recommended by the Clinical and Laboratory Standards Institute (CLSI).
[b]Viridans streptococci require testing when implicated in endocarditis or isolated in pure culture from a normally sterile site with a strong suspicion of being clinically important.
[c]Testing is required if an antimicrobial to which the organisms are frequently resistant is still considered for use (e.g., penicillin for *Neisseria gonorrhoeae*).

Availability of Reliable Susceptibility Testing Methods

If a reliable, standardized method for testing a particular bacterial genus or species does not exist, the ability to produce accurate and meaningful data is substantially compromised. Although standard methods exist for most of the commonly encountered bacteria (Tables 11.1 to 11.3), there do exist clinically relevant bacteria for which standard testing methods do not exist. In these instances, the dilemma stems from the conflict between the laboratorian's desire to contribute in some way by providing data and the lack of confidence in producing interpretable and accurate information.

Many organisms not listed in Table 11.5 grow on the media and under the conditions recommended for testing commonly encountered bacteria. However, the ability to grow and the ability to detect important antimicrobial resistance patterns are not the same thing. For example, the gram-negative bacillus *S. maltophilia* grows extremely well under most susceptibility testing conditions, but the results obtained with beta-lactam antibiotics can vary widely and be seriously misleading. This organism produces potent beta-lactamases that seriously compromise the effectiveness of most beta-lactam agents, yet certain isolates may appear susceptible by standard *in vitro* testing. Even though testing may provide a potential answer, the answer may be incorrect.

Given the uncertainty surrounding the testing of bacteria for which standardized methods are lacking, two approaches

may be used. One is to not perform testing, but rather to provide physicians with information based on clinical studies published in the medical literature about the antimicrobial agents generally accepted as the treatment of choice for the bacterial species in question. This approach should include a consultation with the laboratory medical director and infectious disease specialist. The other option is to provide the information from the literature and perform the test to the best of the laboratory's ability. In this case, results must be accompanied by a disclaimer indicating that testing was performed by a nonstandardized method, and results should be interpreted with caution. When such tests are undertaken, customized antimicrobial batteries, including the agents most commonly used to eradicate the bacterial species of interest, must be communicated to the physician.

Selection of Antimicrobial Agents for Testing

Selection of relevant antimicrobial agents is based on the criteria outlined in Box 11.1. These criteria should be carefully considered when antimicrobial agents are selected to avoid cluttering reports with superfluous information, to minimize the risk of confusing physicians, and to substantially decrease the waste of time and resources in the clinical microbiology laboratory.

Antimicrobial agents that may be considered for inclusion in batteries to be tested against certain bacterial groups are listed in Table 11.6. The list is not exhaustive but is useful for illustrating some points about developing relevant antimicrobial test batteries. For example, with all the penicillins, cephalosporins, and other beta-lactam antibiotics available for testing, only penicillin and cefoxitin (or oxacillin) should be tested against staphylococci. The information acquired with these two agents is sufficient to predict the effectiveness of any other beta-lactam. If an isolate of *S. aureus* tests resistant to cefoxitin, then it is considered resistant to all beta-lactam antibiotics and should be reported as methicillin-resistant *S. aureus*. Similarly, ampicillin can be used independently as an indicator of enterococcal susceptibility to various penicillins, and because of intrinsic resistance, cephalosporins should never be tested against these organisms.

In contrast to the relatively few agents that may be included in testing batteries for gram-positive cocci, several potential choices exist for use against gram-negative bacilli. This is mostly because of the commercial availability of several beta-lactams with similar activities against Enterobacterales and the general inability of one beta-lactam to serve as a reliable predictor drug for other beta-lactams. Although cefazolin is recommended as a predictor drug for oral cephalosporins for urinary tract isolates, an organism resistant to cefazolin may or may not be resistant to cefotetan, and an organism resistant to cefotetan may or may not be resistant to ceftazidime. Thus because of the lack of potential for selecting a predictor drug in these instances, more agents must be

TABLE 11.6 Selection of Antimicrobial Agents for Testing Against Common Bacterial Groups[a]

Antimicrobial Agents	Enterobac-terales	Pseudomonas aeruginosa	Staphylococci	Enterococci	Streptococcus pneumoniae	Viridans streptococci
Penicillins						
Penicillin	–	–	+	–	+	+
Cefoxitin for oxacillin susceptibility	–	–	+	–	–	–
Ampicillin	+	–	–	+	–	–
Piperacillin/tazobactam	+	+	–	–	–	–
Cephalosporins						
Cefazolin	+	–	–	–	–	–
Cefotetan	+	–	–	–	–	–
Ceftriaxone	+	–	–	–	+	+
Ceftazidime	+	+	–	–	–	–
Ceftaroline	+	–	+ (S. aureus only)	–	+	–
Other Beta-Lactams						
Aztreonam	+	+	–	–	–	–
Imipenem	+	+	–	–	±	–
Glycopeptides						
Vancomycin	–	–	+	+	+	+
Aminoglycosides						
Gentamicin	+	+	±	+[b]	–	–
Tobramycin	+	+	–	–	–	–
Amikacin	+	+	–	–	–	–
Quinolones						
Ciprofloxacin	+	+	+	–	+	–
Levofloxacin	+	+	+	–	+	+
Other Agents						
Erythromycin	–	–	+	–	+	+
Clindamycin	–	–	+	–	+	+
Trimethoprim-sulfa-methoxazole	+	–	+	–	+	–, ±
Tigecycline	+	–	+	+	±	+
Daptomycin[c]	–	–	+	+	±	±
Linezolid	–	–	+	+	±	+

[a]Not all available antimicrobial agents are included. Selection recommendation is based on non–urinary tract infections.
[b]Gentamicin testing against enterococci requires use of high-concentration disks or a special screen (Table 11.4).
[c]Daptomycin should not be reported for isolates from the respiratory tract.
+, May be selected for inclusion in testing batteries (not all agents with + need to be selected); ±, may be selected in certain situations; –, selection for testing is not necessary or not recommended.

tested. For example, the spectra of activity of ceftriaxone and cefotaxime are sufficiently similar to allow the use of one in the testing battery.

Many scenarios exist in which the spectrum of activity and other criteria listed in Box 11.1 are considered for the sake of designing the most relevant and useful testing batteries. These criteria should be considered in consultation with the patients' physicians and the pharmacy staff.

Accuracy

Susceptibility testing strategies focused on production of accurate results have two key components:

- Use of methods that produce accurate results
- The application of real-time review of results before reporting

Use of Accurate Methodologies

Because of the complexities of the various resistance mechanisms, no one method, conventional, automated, or molecular, is sufficient for detection of all clinically relevant resistance patterns. The selection of testing methods and careful consideration of how different methods are most effectively used together is necessary to ensure accurate and reliable detection of resistance.

Microbiologists must be aware of the strengths and weaknesses of the primary susceptibility testing methods in the laboratory for detecting relevant resistance patterns and know when adjunct or supplemental testing is necessary. This awareness is accomplished by reviewing studies published in peer-reviewed journals focusing on the performance of antimicrobial testing systems and periodically challenging one's own system with organisms that have been thoroughly characterized with respect to their resistance profiles (e.g., proficiency testing programs). Furthermore, accurate and relevant testing not only means using various conventional methods or even using a mixture of automated, conventional, and screening methods, but also encompasses the potential application of molecular techniques and predictor drugs.

Testing of *S. pneumoniae* provides one example of the need to be aware of testing limitations and the importance of implementing supplemental tests. Not long ago, routine susceptibility testing of *S. pneumoniae* was considered unnecessary. However, with the emergence of beta-lactam resistance, testing has become essential. As the need for testing emerged, the inability of conventional tests, such as penicillin disk diffusion, to detect resistance became apparent. Fortunately, a test that uses the penicillin derivative oxacillin was developed and is widely used as a reliable screen for detecting resistance to penicillin. However, this test is only a screen, because the level of penicillin intermediate resistance (i.e., the MIC) can vary greatly among nonsusceptible isolates, and some strains that appear resistant by the screen may actually be susceptible. Because the level of resistance can affect therapeutic decisions, another method that allows for MIC determinations should be used to test these organisms. In addition, the emergence of cephalosporin resistance requires the use of tests for the detection of resistance to these agents.

Other important examples in which more than one method is required to obtain complete and accurate susceptibility testing data for some organism groups or species include vancomycin-resistant enterococci, MRSA, and ESBL–producing Enterobacterales. In addition, molecular methods may be used in the clinical setting as an important backup resource to investigate and arbitrate equivocal results obtained by phenotypic methods.

However, multiple testing protocols are not routinely necessary for every organism encountered in the clinical laboratory. In most laboratories, one conventional or commercial method is likely to be the mainstay for testing, with additional testing available as a supplement when necessary.

Review of Results

In addition to selecting one or more methods to accurately detect resistance, the strengths and weaknesses of the testing systems must be continuously monitored. This is primarily accomplished by carefully reviewing the susceptibility data produced daily. In the past, establishing and maintaining aggressive and effective monitoring programs have been prohibitively labor intensive. However, the speed and flexibility afforded by computerization of results review and reporting greatly facilitate the administration of such quality assurance programs, even in laboratories with modest resources. Effective computer programs may be a part of the general laboratory information system (or, in some cases, such programs are available through the commercial susceptibility testing system). Because automated expert data review greatly facilitates the review process and enhances data accuracy, this feature should be considered when selecting an AST system.

Susceptibility profiles must be scrutinized manually or with the aid of computers according to what profiles are likely, somewhat likely, somewhat unlikely, and nearly impossible. This awareness not only pertains to profiles exhibited by organisms in a particular institution, but also to those exhibited by clinically relevant bacteria in general. The unusual resistance profiles must be identified and evaluated expeditiously to determine whether they are the result of technical or clerical errors or are truly indicative of an emerging resistance. The urgency of making this determination is twofold. First, if the profile results from laboratory error, it must be corrected and the physician notified so the patient is not subjected to ineffective or inappropriate antimicrobial therapy. Second, if the profile is valid and presents a threat to the patient and to others (e.g., the emergence of vancomycin-resistant staphylococci), immediate notification of infection control and infectious disease personnel is warranted.

Components of Results Review Strategies

Any laboratory strategy for monitoring the accuracy of results and the emergence of resistance must have two components:
- Data review—a mechanism for recognizing new or unusual susceptibility profiles
- Resolution—the application of protocols for determining whether an unusual profile is a result of an error (technical or clerical) or accurately reflects the emergence of a new resistance mechanism

Both components must be integrated into the review process to ensure efficient and timely use of resources.

TABLE 11.7 Examples of Susceptibility Testing Profiles Requiring Further Evaluation

Organism	Susceptibility Profile
All bacterial isolates	Nonsusceptible (NS) results
Staphylococci	Vancomycin intermediate or resistant Clindamycin resistant; erythromycin susceptible Linezolid resistant Daptomycin resistant
Beta-hemolytic streptococci	NS result for ampicillin or penicillin or any other appropriate antimicrobial tested
Streptococcus pneumoniae	NS results for vancomycin or linezolid; fluoroquinolone or meropenem intermediate or resistant
Viridans streptococci	NS results to any or all: vancomycin, daptomycin, ertapenem, linezolid; quinupristin-dalfopristin intermediate or resistant
Enterococci	Vancomycin resistant, high level of aminoglycoside resistance by disk diffusion
Enterococcus faecium	Linezolid resistant
Acinetobacter baumannii	Colistin/polymyxin B and/or carbapenem resistant
Enterobacterales	Gentamicin, tobramycin, and amikacin resistant; any carbapenem intermediate or resistant
Enterobacter/Citrobacter/Serratia/ Morganella/Providencia/Klebsiella	Susceptible to ampicillin or cefazolin
Pseudomonas aeruginosa	Amikacin resistant; gentamicin or tobramycin susceptible; carbapenem resistant
Stenotrophomonas maltophilia	Imipenem susceptible; trimethoprim/sulfamethoxazole intermediate or resistant
Neisseria gonorrhoeae	Ceftriaxone resistant
Neisseria meningitidis	Ampicillin or penicillin resistant; NS result for meropenem

Modified from Courvalin P. Interpretive reading of antimicrobial susceptibility tests. *Am Soc Microbiol News* 2015;58:368; CLSI M100-S25 guideline Appendix A.

Data Review

Recognition of unusual resistance profiles is accomplished by carefully reviewing the daily laboratory susceptibility data. AST systems include expert rules and algorithms to aid the microbiologist in detecting and recognizing patterns of resistance that are unusual for the bug/drug combo, that could represent a testing error or may represent an acquired mechanism of resistance. Examples of unusual susceptibility profiles for gram-positive and gram-negative bacteria are included in Table 11.7. The examples are a mixture of profiles that clearly demonstrate a likely error (i.e., clindamycin-resistant, erythromycin-susceptible staphylococci); profiles that have rarely been encountered but if observed require immediate attention (i.e., vancomycin resistance in staphylococci); and profiles that have been described but may not be common (i.e., imipenem resistance in Enterobacterales).

The data review process for the evaluation of profiles should not be the responsibility of a single person in the laboratory. Furthermore, the process requires checks and balances that do not impede workflow or increase the time required to get the results to the physicians. The way this is established varies, depending on a particular laboratory's division of labor and workflow, but several key aspects must be considered:

- Identification of the organism is essential. Without knowing the organism's identification, it is impossible to determine whether the AST results are unusual.

- Susceptibility results should be analyzed and reported as early in the day as possible. The workflow should allow time for corrective action for errors found during data review so corrected, or substantiated, results are available to physicians as soon as possible.

- Two or more tiers of data review should be used. The first tier is at the bench level, where technologists are simultaneously reading the results and evaluating an organism's AST results for appropriateness. When unusual profiles are identified, the technologist should initiate troubleshooting protocols (see the next section). To prevent release of erroneous and potentially dangerous information, results should not be reported at this point. The second tier is at the level of supervisor or laboratory director. The purpose of review at this level is to answer questions from the bench microbiologists, to take responsibility for the accuracy of results, and to provide guidance for resolution of the unusual profiles.

- The review process must be flexible and continuously updated. Because bacterial capabilities for antimicrobial resistance profiles change, accurate detection of resistance in the laboratory relies on up-to-date knowledge and methods. The list of unusual profiles requires periodic review and updating.

Resolution

The importance of having strategies for resolving unusual profiles cannot be overstated. However, developing detailed procedures for every contingency is not possible or practical. Most resolution strategies should focus on certain general approaches, with supervisor or laboratory director consultation always being among the options available to technologists. Although the steps taken to investigate and resolve an unusual profile often depend on the organism and antibiotics involved, most protocols for resolution should include one or more of the following approaches:

- Review the data for a possible clerical error.
- Verify the susceptibility panel and identification system were inoculated with the same isolate.
- Reexamine the test panel or plate for a reading error (e.g., misreading of actual zone of inhibition).
- Confirm the purity of the inoculum and proper inoculum preparation.
- For commercial systems, determine whether the manufacturer's recommended procedures were followed.
- Establish the accuracy of organism identification.
- Confirm resistance by using a second method or screening test.

Often a quick review of the data recording and interpretation aspects, or purity of culture, will reveal the reason an unusual profile was identified. Other times more extensive testing, perhaps by more than one method, may be needed to establish the validity of an unusual or unexpected resistance profile.

Accuracy and Antimicrobial Resistance Surveillance

Surveillance of antimicrobial resistance involves tracking and carefully reviewing AST data generated by testing the bacteria encountered in a particular institution and in a specific geographic location. This can be generalized to a single hospital or be as specific as a unit or ward within a hospital, especially if there are very complex and unique patient populations. For laboratories that serve a particular institution or group of institutions, the laboratory should publish, at a minimum, an annual antibiogram containing significant pathogens and the associated susceptibility data. CLSI provides guidance in the data compilation and reporting guidelines in the M39-A4 document. These reports provide valuable information for monitoring emerging resistance trends. Such information is also helpful for establishing **empiric therapy** guidelines (i.e., therapy that is instituted before knowledge of the infecting organism's identification or its antimicrobial susceptibility profile), detecting areas of potential inappropriate or excessive antimicrobial use, and contributing data to larger, more extensive national and international surveillance programs.

Data that have been validated through a results review and resolution program not only enhance the reliability of laboratory reports for patient management, but also strengthen the credibility of susceptibility data used for resistance surveillance and antibiogram profiling. Meeting the need for each institution to scrutinize susceptibility profiles daily can be accomplished by establishing a results review and resolution format that ensures the accuracy for patient management, detects emerging resistance patterns quickly, and maintains accuracy of the data included in the summary antibiogram reports.

Communication

Susceptibility testing profiles produced for each bacterial isolate are typically reported to the physician as a listing of the antimicrobial agents, with each agent accompanied by the categorical interpretation of susceptible, intermediate, or resistant. In most instances, this reporting approach is sufficient. However, as resistance profiles and their underlying mechanisms become more varied and complex, laboratory personnel must ensure that the significance of susceptibility data is clearly and accurately communicated to clinicians in a way that optimizes both patient care and antimicrobial use. In many situations, passively communicating the susceptibility data to the physician without adding comments or appropriately amending the reports is no longer sufficient. Moreover, the categories of SDD and nonsusceptible may require conversations between microbiology laboratory professionals, infectious disease physicians, and pharmacy staff members.

For example, MRSA are to be considered cross-resistant to all beta-lactams, but *in vitro* results occasionally may indicate susceptibility to certain cephalosporins, beta-lactam/beta-lactamase inhibitor combinations, or imipenem. Simply reporting these findings without editing such profiles to reflect probable resistance to all beta-lactams would be seriously misleading and could lead to ineffective treatment should one of these agents be prescribed. As another example, serious enterococcal infections often require combination therapy, including both a cell wall–active agent (ampicillin or vancomycin) and an aminoglycoside (i.e., gentamicin). This important information would not be conveyed in a report that simply lists the agents and their interpretive category results. Such an approach can leave the false impression that a "susceptible" result for any single agent indicates that one drug used alone provides appropriate therapy. An explanatory note that clearly states the recommended use of combination therapy should accompany the enterococcal susceptibility report.

To prevent misinterpretations that may result by providing only AST data, strategies must consider organism antimicrobial combinations that may require reporting of supplemental messages to the physician. For example, an isolate of *K. pneumoniae* identified in the blood that has a genotypic test positive for the *bla*KPC gene should contain a message requiring the patient to be placed in contact isolation and that an infectious disease consult is strongly recommended. Consultations with infectious disease specialists and other members of the medical staff are an important part of determining when such messages are needed and what the content should include. Finally, if a laboratory does not have the means to reliably relay these messages, either by computer or by paper, a policy of direct communication with the attending physician by telephone or in person should be established.

(e) Visit the Evolve site for a complete list of procedures, review questions, and case studies.

Bibliography

Arnold AR, Burnham C-AD, Ford BA, et al.: Evaluation of an immunochromatographic assay for rapid detection of penicillin-binding protein 2A in human and animal *Staphylococcus intermedius* group, *Staphylococcus lugdunensis*, and *Staphylococcus schleiferi* clinical isolates, *J Clin Microbiol* 54:745–748, 2016.

Bauer AW, Kirby WM, Sherris JC, et al.: Antibiotic susceptibility testing by a single disc method, *Am J Clin Pathol* 45:493–496, 1966.

Canver MC, Gonzalez MD, Ford BA, et al.: Improved performance of a rapid immunochromatographic assay for detection of PBP2a in non-*Staphylococcus aureus* staphylococcal species, *J Clin Microbiol* 57:e01417–1819, 2019. https://doi.org/10.1128/JCM.01417-18.

CDC Grand Rounds: The growing threat of multidrug-resistant gonorrhea, *MMWR* 62:103–106, 2013.

Charnot-Katsikas A, Tesic V, Love N, et al.: Use of the accelerate pheno system for identification and antimicrobial susceptibility testing of pathogens in positive blood cultures and impact on time to results and workflow, *J Clin Microbiol* 56(1),:e01166-17, 2017.

Clinical and Laboratory Standards Institute: *Methods for determining bactericidal activity of antimicrobial agents: approved guideline M26-A*, Wayne, PA, 1999, CLSI.

Clinical and Laboratory Standards Institute: *Methods for dilution antimicrobial susceptibility testing for bacteria that grow aerobically: M07-A11*, Wayne, PA, 2018, CLSI.

Clinical and Laboratory Standards Institute: *Methods for antimicrobial dilution and disk susceptibility testing of infrequently isolated or fastidious bacteria: M45-A3*, Wayne, PA, 2015, CLSI.

Clinical and Laboratory Standards Institute: *Analysis and presentation of cumulative antimicrobial susceptibility test data: approved guideline—M39-A4*, Wayne, PA, 2014, CLSI.

Clinical and Laboratory Standards Institute: *Performance standards for antimicrobial disk susceptibility testing: M02-A13*, Wayne, PA, 2018, CLSI.

Clinical and Laboratory Standards Institute: *Performance standards for antimicrobial susceptibility testing; 29th information supplement. M100-S29*, Wayne, PA, 2019, CLSI.

Courvalin P: Interpretive reading of antimicrobial susceptibility tests, *Am Soc Microbiol News* 58:368, 1992.

Cunningham SA, Noorle T, Meunier D, et al.: Rapid and simultaneous detection of genes encoding *Klebsiella pneumoniae* carbapenemase (bla_{KPC}) and New Delhi metallo-β-lactamase (bla_{NDM}) in gram-negative bacilli, *J Clin Microbiol* 51:1269–1271, 2013.

Girlich D, Polrel L, Nordmann P: Value of the modified Hodge test for detection of emerging carbapenemases in *Enterobacteriaceae*, *J Clin Microbiol* 50:477–479, 2012.

Hrabák J, Študentová V, Walková R, et al.: Detection of NDM-1, VIM-1, KPC, OXA-48, and OXA-162 carbapenemases by matrix-assisted laser desorption ionization–time of flight mass spectrometry, *J Clin Microbiol* 50:2441–2443, 2012.

Laudano JB: Ceftaroline fosamil: a new broad-spectrum cephalosporin. Review, *J Antimicrob Chemother* 66(Suppl 3):iii11–iii18, 2011.

Moore NM, Cantón R, Carretto E, et al.: Rapid Identification of Five Classes of Carbapenem Resistance Genes Directly from Rectal Swabs by Use of the Xpert Carba-R Assay, *J Clin Microbiol* 55:2268–2275, 2017.

Nordmann P, Poirel L, Dortet L: Rapid detection of carbapenemase-producing *Enterobacteriaceae*, *Emerg Infect Dis* 18(9):1503–1507, 2012. https://doi.org/10.3201/eid1809.120355.

Ohnishi M, Saika T, Hoshira S, et al.: Ceftriaxone-resistant *Neisseria gonorrhoeae*, Japan, *Emerg Infect Dis* 17:148–149, 2011.

Pancholi P, Carroll KC, Buchan BW, et al.: Multicenter Evaluation of the Accelerate PhenoTest BC Kit for Rapid Identification and Phenotypic Antimicrobial Susceptibility Testing Using Morphokinetic Cellular Analysis, *J Clin Microbiol*:e01329-17, 2018.

Papagiannitsis CC, Študentová V, Izdebski R, et al.: Matrix-Assisted Laser Desorption Ionization–Time of Flight Mass Spectrometry Meropenem Hydrolysis Assay with NH4HCO3, a Reliable Tool for Direct Detection of Carbapenemase Activity, *J Clin Microbiol* 53:1731–1735, 2015.

Prabhu K, Rao S, Rao V: Inducible clindamycin resistance in *Staphylococcus aureus* isolated from clinical samples, *J Lab Physicians* 3:25–27, 2011.

Singhal N, Kumar M, Kanaujia PK, Virdi JS: MALDI-TOF mass spectrometry: an emerging technology for microbial identification and diagnosis, *Front Microbiol* 6:791, 2015.

Traczewski MM, Carretto E, Cantón R, et al.: Multicenter evaluation of the Xpert Carba-R assay for detection of carbapenemase genes in gram-negative isolates, *J Clin Microbiol* 56:e00272-18, 2018.

Vasoo S, Cunningham SA, Kohner PC, et al.: Comparison of a novel, rapid chromogenic biochemical assay, the Carba NP test, with the modified Hodge test for detection of carbapenemase-producing gram-negative bacilli, *J Clin Microbiol* 51:3097–3101, 2013.

12

Overview of Bacterial Identification Methods and Strategies

OBJECTIVES

This chapter provides an overview of some of the traditional biochemical methods (rapid and culture based) used to identify microorganisms. Additional tests for specific organisms are included throughout the text. Students and practitioners should use these detailed technical procedures in conjunction with specific chapters in this section to develop a clear understanding of the full laboratory diagnostic process from specimen collection to identification. General objectives for the methods presented in this chapter include the following:

1. State the specific diagnostic purpose for each test methodology.
2. Briefly describe the test principle associated with each test methodology.
3. Outline limitations and explain ways to troubleshoot or report results in the event the test result indicates a false positive or false negative or is equivocal.
4. State the appropriate quality control organisms and results used with each testing procedure.

Rationale for Approaching Organism Identification

Effectively presenting and teaching diagnostic microbiology in a way that is sufficiently comprehensive and yet not excessively cluttered with rare and seldom-needed facts about bacterial species that are uncommonly encountered can be challenging. The chapters included in Part III, Bacteriology, are intended to be comprehensive in terms of the variety of bacterial species presented. However, it is helpful to keep in perspective which taxa are most likely to be encountered in the clinical environment and associated with specific anatomic sites of infection.

Many texts (including this one) provide flow charts containing algorithms or identification schemes for organism workup. Although these are helpful, these flow charts have limitations. In some cases, they may be too general to be helpful; that is, they may lack sufficient detail to be useful for discriminating among key microbial groups and species. In other cases, they may be too esoteric to be of practical use in routine clinical practice. In addition, many other criteria that must be incorporated into the identification process are too complex to be included in most flow charts. Microorganisms are biologically active living things and therefore are able to alter their biochemical activity and expression of that activity under a variety of environmental stresses. Therefore, it is important to note that a flow-chart is limited based on the inability to adjust for inherent organismal variability; thus it is only one of many tools used in the field of diagnostic microbiology.

In addition, as discussed later in this chapter, organism taxonomy and profiles continuously change. Detailed flow charts are at risk of quickly becoming outdated. Furthermore, as is evident throughout the chapters in Part III, diagnostic microbiology is full of exceptions to rules, and flow charts are not constructed in a manner that readily captures many of the important exceptions.

To meet the challenges of bacterial identification processes beyond what can be portrayed in flow charts, the chapters in Part III have been arranged to guide the student and practicing professional through the entire workup of a microorganism, beginning with the microscopic characteristics and initial culture or growth of the isolates from the clinical specimen. In many instances, the first information a microbiologist uses in the identification process is the microscopic characteristics of the organism and the clinical specimen (Chapter 6). This information guides the clinician to initiate immediate therapy for life-threatening infections until additional characterization or organismal identification is complete. In most instances, the microscopic information a microbiologist uses in the identification process is followed by a macroscopic description of the colony, or colony morphology. This includes the type of hemolysis (if any), pigment (if present), size, texture (opaque, translucent, or transparent), adherence to agar, pitting of agar, and many other characteristics (Chapter 7). After careful observation of the colony, the Gram stain or additional microscopy may be used to validate or separate the organism identification into a variety of broad categories based on Gram stain reaction and the cellular morphology of gram-positive or gram-negative bacteria (e.g., gram-positive cocci, gram-negative rods; Chapter 6). For gram-positive organisms, the catalase test should follow the Gram stain, and testing on gram-negative organisms should begin with the oxidase test. These simple tests, plus growth on MacConkey agar if the isolate is a gram-negative rod or coccobacillus, help the microbiologist assign the organism to one of the primary categories (organized here as subsections). Application of the various identification methods and systems outlined in this chapter generate the data and criteria discussed in each chapter for the definitive identification of clinically relevant bacteria. Many of the rapid biochemical or culture-based procedures described in the following chapters can be found in this chapter. However, additional test methods, including nucleic acid–based tests, rapid commercial identification systems, and MALDI-TOF MS are also available for a variety of organisms. In this chapter, each procedure includes a photograph of positive and negative reactions. Chapter 6 includes photographs of some commonly used bacterial stains.

Diagnostic microbiology is centered around the identification of organisms based on common phenotypic and genotypic traits shared with known members of the same genus or family, so microbiologists "play the odds" every day by finding the best biochemical "fit" and assigning the most probable identification. For example, the gram-negative rod *Neisseria animaloris* may be considered with either MacConkey-positive or MacConkey-negative organisms in contrast to other *Neisseria* species, because it grows on MacConkey agar 50% of the time. Therefore, although classified as oxidase-positive, MacConkey-positive, gram-negative bacilli and coccobacilli in this text, it also may appear as an oxidase-positive, MacConkey-negative, gram-negative bacilli and coccobacilli. This example clearly demonstrates the limitations of solely depending on biochemical flow charts for the identification process.

The identification process often can be arduous and a drain on resources. Laboratorians must make every effort to identify only those organisms most likely to be involved in the infection process. To that end, the chapters in Part III have also been designed to provide guidance for determining whether a clinical isolate is relevant and requires full identification. Furthermore, the clinical diagnosis and the source of the specimen can help determine which group of organisms to consider. For example, if a patient has endocarditis or the specimen source is blood and a small, gram-negative rod is observed on Gram stain, the microbiologist should consider a group of gram-negative bacilli known as HACEK (*Haemophilus* spp., *Aggregatibacter* spp., *Cardiobacterium* spp., *Eikenella corrodens,* and *Kingella* spp.). Similarly, if a patient has suffered an animal bite, the microbiologist should think of *Pasteurella* spp. if the isolate is gram negative, *Staphylococcus hyicus* and *Staphylococcus intermedius* if the organism is gram positive. Finally, in consideration of an isolate's clinical relevance, each chapter also provides information on whether antimicrobial susceptibility testing is indicated and, if needed, the way it should be performed.

Future Trends of Organism Identification

Several dynamics are involved in clinical microbiology and infectious diseases that continue to challenge bacterial identification practices. For instance, new species associated with human infections will continue to be discovered, and well-known species may alter their expression of biochemical characteristics, affecting the criteria used to identify them. For these reasons, identification schemes and strategies for both conventional methods and commercial systems must be continually reviewed and updated. Also, although most identification schemes are based on the phenotypic characteristics of bacteria, the use of molecular and other advanced methods (e.g., MALDI-TOF MS, whole genome multilocus sequence typing, and next-generation sequencing) to detect, identify, and characterize bacteria continues to expand and play a greater role in diagnostic microbiology. In addition, phenotypic, molecular, and advanced chemical methods increasingly will become incorporated into simpler automated systems.

Ⓔ Visit the Evolve site for a complete list of procedures, review questions, and case studies.

PROCEDURE 12.1

Acetamide Utilization

Purpose

Differentiate microorganisms based on the ability to use acetamide as the sole source of carbon.

Principle

Bacteria capable of growth on this medium produce the enzyme acylamidase, which deaminates acetamide to release ammonia. The production of ammonia results in an alkaline pH, causing the medium to change color from green to royal blue.

Media: NaCl (5 g), $NH_4H_2PO_4$ (1 g), K_2HPO_4 (1 g), agar (15 g), bromothymol blue indicator (0.8 g) per 1000 mL, acetamide (10 g), pH 6.8. Note: The medium may be an agar (as pictured here) or a broth.

Method

1. Inoculate acetamide slant with a needle using growth from an 18- to 24-h culture. Do not inoculate from a broth culture, because the growth will be too heavy.
2. Incubate aerobically at 35°C to 37°C for up to 4 days. If equivocal, the slant may be reincubated for 2 additional days.

Expected Results

Positive: Deamination of the acetamide, resulting in a blue color (Fig. 12.1A).
Negative: No color change (Fig. 12.1B).

Limitations

Growth without a color change may indicate a positive test result. If further incubation results in no color change, repeat test with less inoculum.

Quality Control

Positive: *Pseudomonas aeruginosa* (ATCC 27853)—growth; blue color
Negative: *Escherichia coli* (ATCC 25922)—no growth; green color

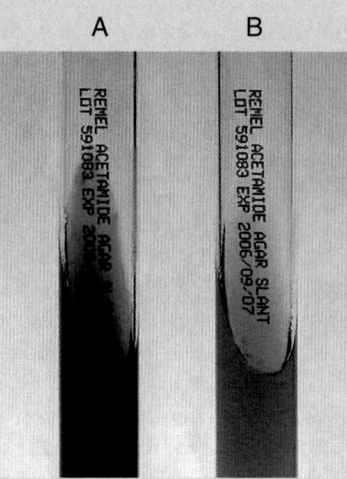

• **Fig. 12.1** Acetamide utilization. (A) Positive. (B) Negative.

PROCEDURE 12.2

Acetate Utilization

Purpose

Differentiate organisms based on ability to use acetate as the sole source of carbon. Generally used to differentiate *Shigella* spp. from *Escherichia coli*.

Principle

This test is used to differentiate an organism capable of using acetate as the sole source of carbon. Organisms capable of using sodium acetate grow on the medium, resulting in an alkaline pH, turning the indicator from green to blue.

Media: $NaC_2H_3O_2$ (2 g); $MgSO_4$ (0.1 g); NaCl (5 g); $NH_4H_2PO_4$ (1 g); agar (20 g); bromothymol blue indicator (0.8 g) per 1000 mL, pH 6.7.

Method

1. With a straight inoculating needle, inoculate acetate slant lightly from an 18- to 24-h culture. Do not inoculate from a broth culture, because the growth will be too heavy.
2. Incubate at 35°C–37°C for up to 7 days.

Expected Results

Positive: Medium becomes alkalinized *(blue)* because of the growth and use of acetate (Fig. 12.2A).
Negative: No growth or growth with no indicator change to blue (Fig. 12.2B).

Limitations

Some strains of *E. coli* may use acetate at a very slow rate or not at all, resulting in a false negative reaction in the identification process.

Quality Control

Positive: *Escherichia coli* (ATCC 25922)—growth; blue
Negative: *Shigella sonnei* (ATCC 25931)—small amount of growth; green

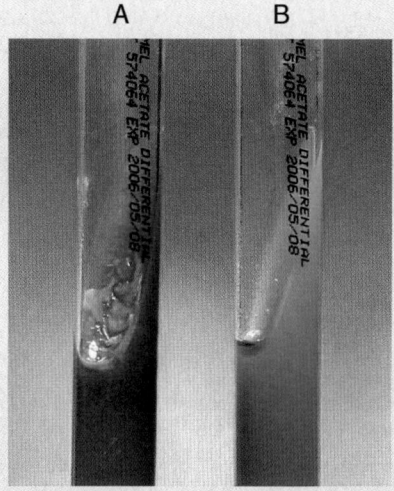

• **Fig. 12.2** Acetate utilization. (A) Positive. (B) Negative.

PROCEDURE 12.3

L-Alanine-7-amido-4-methylcourmarin (Gram-Sure)

Purpose

This test is used in conjunction with the Gram stain to distinguish aerobic gram-positive rods or coccobacilli that may appear gram-negative or gram-variable.

Principle

The compound L-alanine-7-amido-4-methylcourmarin is impregnated in a commercially prepared disk (Remel-Thermo Fisher Scientific, Lenexa, KS). Gram-negative organisms produce an aminopeptidase that is capable of hydrolyzing the reagent in the disk, forming a blue fluorescent compound that is visible under long-wave UV light.

Method

1. Inoculate a pure colony of overnight growth (16–18 h after initial culture) to 0.25 mL of demineralized water in a clean 12 by 75 mm test tube.
2. Place a Gram-Sure disk in the emulsion.
3. Incubate at room temperature for 5–10 min.
4. Observe blue fluorescence by placing the tube under long-wave ultraviolet light.

Expected Results

Aerobic, gram-negative rods and coccobacilli will appear fluorescent or blue.
Aerobic, gram-positive rods and coccobacilli will appear colorless.

Limitations

Obligate anaerobic organisms may fail to give expected results.

Quality Control

Positive: *Escherichia coli* (ATCC 25922)—blue fluorescence (Fig. 12.3A)
Negative: *Staphylococcus aureus* (ATCC 25923)—no fluorescence (Fig. 12.3B)

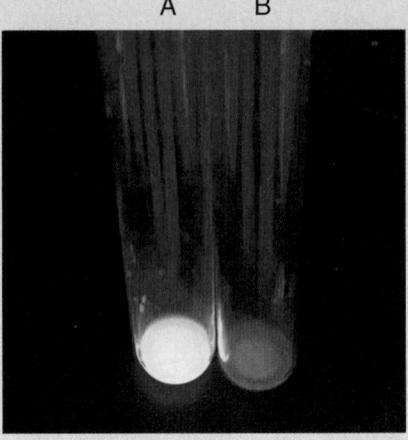

• **Fig. 12.3** L-alanine-7-amido-4-methylcourmarin (Gram-Sure). (A) Positive. (B) Negative.

PROCEDURE 12.4

Bacitracin Susceptibility

Purpose

This test is used for presumptive identification and differentiation of beta-hemolytic group A streptococci (*Streptococcus pyogenes*–susceptible) from other beta-hemolytic streptococci. It is also used to distinguish staphylococci species (resistant) from micrococci (susceptible).

Principle

The antibiotic bacitracin inhibits the synthesis of bacterial cell walls. A disk (TaxoA) impregnated with a small amount of bacitracin (0.04 units) is placed on an agar plate, allowing the antibiotic to diffuse into the medium and inhibit the growth of susceptible organisms. After incubation, the inoculated plates are examined for zones of inhibition surrounding the disks.

Method

1. Using an inoculating loop, streak two or three suspect colonies of a pure culture onto a blood agar plate.
2. Using heated forceps, place a bacitracin disk in the first quadrant (area of heaviest growth). Gently tap the disk to ensure adequate contact with the agar surface.
3. Incubate the plate for 18–24 h at 35°C–37°C in ambient air for staphylococci and in 5% to 10% carbon dioxide (CO_2) for streptococci differentiation.
4. Look for a zone of inhibition around the disk.

Expected Results

Positive: Any zone of inhibition greater than 10 mm; susceptible (Fig. 12.4A).
Negative: No zone of inhibition; resistant (Fig. 12.4B).

Limitations

Performance depends on the integrity of the disk. Proper storage and expiration dates should be maintained.

Quality Control

Positive: *Streptococcus pyogenes* (ATCC19615)—susceptible
   Micrococcus luteus (ATCC10240)—susceptible
Negative: *Streptococcus agalactiae* (ATCC27956)—resistant
   Staphylococcus aureus (ATCC25923)—resistant
   Viridans streptococci—bile insoluble

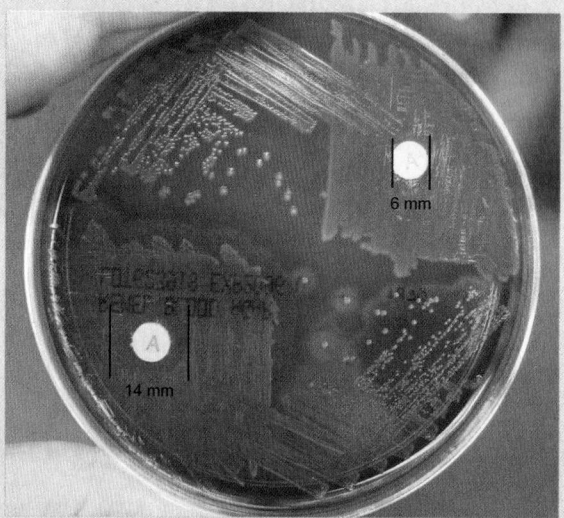

• **Fig. 12.4** Bacitracin (*A disk*) susceptibility. Any zone of inhibition is positive (*Streptococcus pyogenes*); growth up to the disk is negative (*Streptococcus agalactiae*).

PROCEDURE 12.5

Bile Esculin Test

Purpose

This test is used for the presumptive identification of enterococci and organisms in the *Streptococcus bovis* group. The test differentiates enterococci and group D streptococci from non–group D viridans streptococci.

Principle

Gram-positive bacteria other than some streptococci and enterococci are inhibited by the bile salts in this medium. Organisms capable of growth in the presence of 4% bile and able to hydrolyze esculin to esculetin will demonstrate growth. In addition, esculetin reacts with Fe^{3+} and forms a dark brown to black precipitate.

Media: Beef extract (11 g), enzymatic digest of gelatin (34.5 g), esculin (1 g), ox bile (2 g), ferric ammonium citrate (0.5 g), agar (15 g) per 1000 mL, pH 6.6.

Method

1. Inoculate one to two colonies from an 18– 24-h culture onto the surface of the slant.
2. Incubate at 35°C–37°C in ambient air for 48 h.

Expected Results

Positive: Growth and blackening of the agar slant (Fig. 12.5A).
Negative: Growth and no blackening of medium (Fig. 12.5B).
No growth (not shown).

Limitations

Because of nutritional requirements, some organisms may grow poorly or not at all on this medium.

Quality Control

Positive: *Enterococcus faecalis* (ATCC19433)—growth; black precipitate
Negative: *Escherichia coli* (ATCC25922)—growth; no color change
Streptococcus pyogenes (ATCC19615)—no growth; no color change

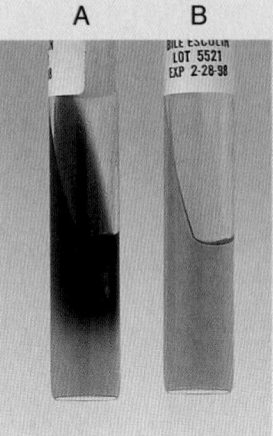

• **Fig. 12.5** Bile esculin agar. (A) Positive. (B) Negative.

PROCEDURE 12.6

Bile Solubility Test

Purpose

This test differentiates *Streptococcus pneumoniae* (positive; soluble) from alpha-hemolytic streptococci (negative; insoluble).

Principle

Bile or a solution of a bile salt (e.g., sodium deoxycholate) rapidly lyses pneumococcal colonies. Lysis depends on the presence of an intracellular autolytic enzyme, amidase. Bile salts lower the surface tension between the bacterial cell membrane and the medium, thus accelerating the organism's natural autolytic process.

Method

1. After 12–24 h of incubation on 5% sheep blood agar, place one to two drops of 10% sodium deoxycholate on a well-isolated colony. *Note*: A tube test is performed with 2% sodium deoxycholate.
2. Gently wash liquid over the colony without dislodging the colony from the agar.
3. Incubate the plate at 35°C–37°C in ambient air for 30 min.
4. Examine for lysis of colony.

Expected Results

Positive: Colony disintegrates; an imprint of the lysed colony may remain in the zone (Fig. 12.6A).
Negative: Intact colonies (Fig. 12.6B).

Limitations

Enzyme activity may be reduced in old cultures. Therefore, negative results with colonies resembling *S. pneumoniae* should be further tested for identification with alternate methods.

Quality Control

Positive: *Streptococcus pneumoniae* (ATCC49619)—bile soluble
Negative: *Enterococcus faecalis* (ATCC29212)—bile insoluble
Viridans streptococci—bile insoluble

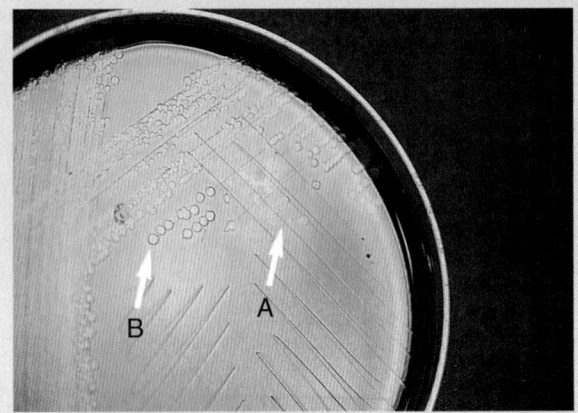

• **Fig. 12.6** Bile solubility (deoxycholate) test. (A) Colony lysed. (B) Intact colony.

PROCEDURE 12.7

Butyrate Disk (Catarrhalis Test)

Purpose

This is a rapid test to detect the enzyme butyrate esterase, to aid identification of *Moraxella catarrhalis*.

Principle

Organisms capable of producing butyrate esterase hydrolyze bromo-chlor-indolyl butyrate. Hydrolysis of the substrate in the presence of butyrate esterase releases indoxyl, which in the presence of oxygen spontaneously forms indigo, a blue to blue-violet color.

Method

1. Remove a disk from the vial and place on a glass microscope slide.
2. Add one drop of reagent-grade water. This should leave a slight excess of water on the disk.
3. Using a wooden applicator stick, rub a small amount of several colonies from an 18–24-h pure culture onto the disk.
4. Incubate at room temperature for up to 5 min.

Expected Results

Positive: Development of a blue color during the 5-min incubation period (Fig. 12.7A).
Negative: No color change (Fig. 12.7B).

Limitations

Incubation longer than 5 min may result in a false-positive reaction.

False-negative reactions may occur if the inoculum is too small. If the organism is negative, repeat with a larger inoculum and follow up with additional methods.

Quality Control

Positive: *Moraxella catarrhalis* (ATCC25240)—formation of blue color
Negative: *Neisseria gonorrhoeae* (ATCC43069)—no color change

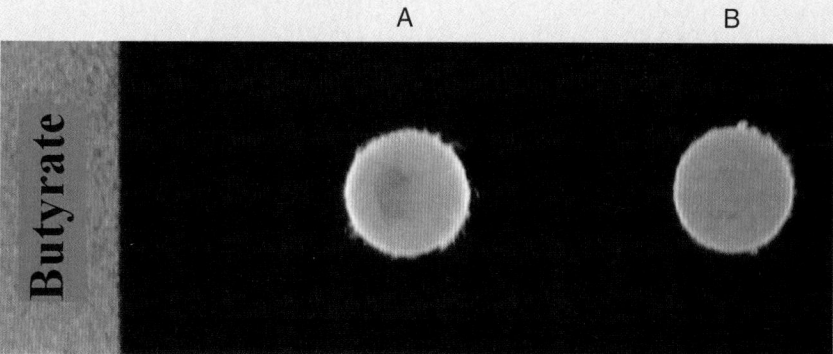

• **Fig. 12.7** Butyrate disk. (A) Positive. (B) Negative.

PROCEDURE 12.8

CAMP Test

Purpose

The Christie, Atkins, and Munch-Peterson (CAMP) test is used to differentiate group B streptococci (*Streptococcus agalactiae*–positive) from other streptococcal species. *Listeria monocytogenes* also produces a positive CAMP reaction.

Principle

Certain organisms (including group B streptococci) produce a diffusible extracellular hemolytic protein (CAMP factor) that acts synergistically with the beta-lysin of *Staphylococcus aureus* to cause enhanced lysis of red blood cells. The group B streptococci are streaked perpendicular to a streak of *S. aureus* on sheep blood agar. A positive reaction appears as an arrowhead zone of hemolysis adjacent to the place where the two streak lines come into proximity.

Method

1. Streak a beta-lysin–producing strain of *S. aureus* down the center of a sheep blood agar plate.
2. Streak test organisms across the plate perpendicular to the *S. aureus* streak within 2 mm. (Multiple organisms can be tested on a single plate.)
3. Incubate overnight at 35°C–37°C in ambient air.

Expected Results

Positive: Enhanced hemolysis is indicated by an arrowhead-shaped zone of beta-hemolysis at the juncture of the two organisms (Fig. 12.8A).
Negative: No enhancement of hemolysis (Fig. 12.8B).

Limitations

A small percentage of group A streptococci may have a positive CAMP reaction. The test should be limited to colonies with the characteristic group B streptococci morphology and narrow-zone beta-hemolysis on sheep blood agar.

Quality Control

Positive: *Streptococcus agalactiae* (ATCC13813)—enhanced arrowhead hemolysis
Negative: *Streptococcus pyogenes* (ATCC19615)—beta-hemolysis without enhanced arrowhead formation

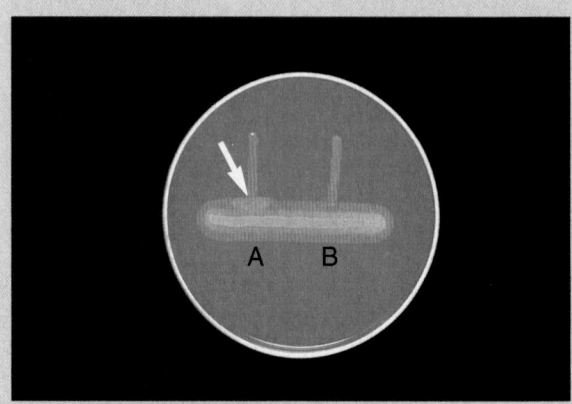

• **Fig. 12.8** Christie, Atkins, and Munch-Peterson test. (A) Positive; *arrowhead* zone of beta-hemolysis (at *arrow*), typical of group B streptococci. (B) Negative; no enhancement of hemolysis.

PROCEDURE 12.9

Catalase Test

Purpose

This test differentiates catalase-positive micrococcal and staphylococcal species from catalase-negative streptococcal species.

Principle

Aerobic and facultative anaerobic organisms produce hydrogen peroxide (H_2O_2) and superoxide radical (O_2-) during normal metabolism. These bacteria have two enzymes that detoxify the products of normal metabolism. One of these enzymes, catalase, is capable of converting hydrogen peroxide to water and oxygen. The presence of the enzyme in a bacterial isolate is evidenced when a small inoculum introduced into hydrogen peroxide (30% for the slide test) causes rapid elaboration of oxygen bubbles. The lack of catalase is evident by a lack of or weak bubble production.

Method

1. Use a loop or sterile wooden stick to transfer a small amount of colony growth to the surface of a clean, dry glass slide.

2. Place a drop of 30% hydrogen peroxide (H_2O_2) onto the medium. (3% can also be used for most organisms.)
3. Observe for the evolution of oxygen bubbles (Fig. 12.9).

Expected Results

Positive: Copious bubbles are produced (Fig. 12.9A).
Negative: No or few bubbles are produced (Fig. 12.9B).

Limitations

Some organisms (enterococci) produce a peroxidase that slowly catalyzes the breakdown of H_2O_2, and the test may appear weakly positive. This reaction is not a truly positive test.

False positives may occur if the sample is contaminated with blood agar.

Quality Control

Positive: *Staphylococcus aureus* (ATCC25923)
Negative: *Streptococcus pyogenes* (ATCC19615)

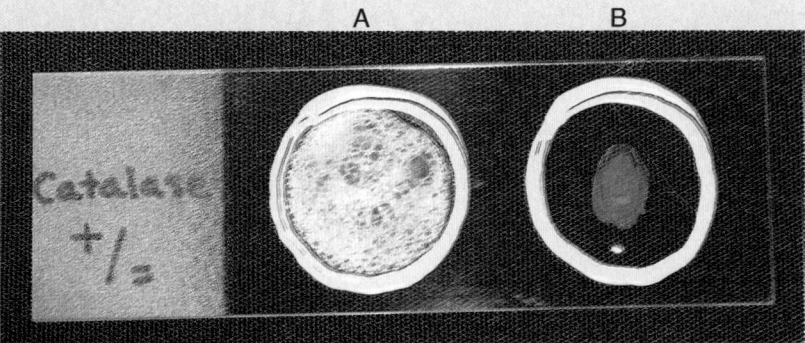

• **Fig. 12.9** Catalase test. (A) Positive. (B) Negative.

PROCEDURE 12.10

Cetrimide Agar

Purpose

This test is primarily used to isolate and purify *Pseudomonas aeruginosa* from contaminated specimens.

Principle

The test is used to determine the ability of an organism to grow in the presence of cetrimide, a toxic substance that inhibits the growth of many bacteria by causing the release of nitrogen and phosphorus, which slows or kills the organism. *P. aeruginosa* is resistant to cetrimide.

Media: Enzymatic digest of gelatin (20 g), $MgCl_2$ (1.4 g), K_2SO_4 (10 g), cetrimide (cetyltrimethylammonium bromide) (0.3 g), agar (13.6), pH 7.2.

Method

1. Inoculate a cetrimide agar slant with one drop of an 18–24-h brain-heart infusion broth culture.
2. Incubate at 35°C–37°C for up to 7 days.
3. Examine the slant for bacterial growth.

Expected Results

Positive: Growth, variation in color of colonies (Fig. 12.10A).
Negative: No growth (Fig. 12.10B).

Limitations

Some enteric organisms will grow and exhibit a weak yellow color in the media. This color change is distinguishable from the production of fluorescein.

Additional testing is necessary to confirm a diagnosis of *P. aeruginosa*.

Quality Control

Positive: *Pseudomonas aeruginosa* (ATCC27853)—growth and color change; yellow-green to blue-green colonies
Negative: *Escherichia coli* (ATCC25922)—no growth and no color change

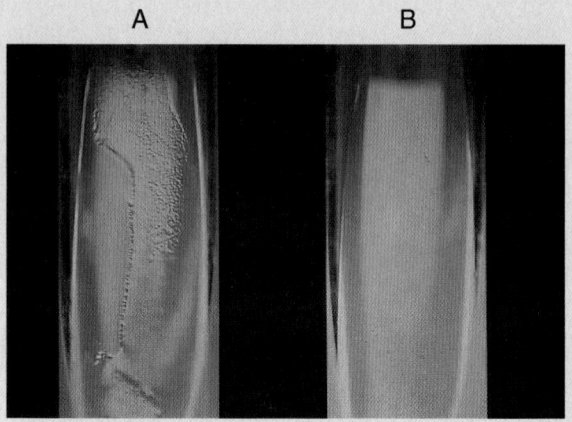

• **Fig. 12.10** Cetrimide agar. (A) Positive. (B) Negative.

PROCEDURE 12.11

Citrate Utilization

Purpose

The purpose of this test is to identify organisms capable of using sodium citrate as the sole carbon source and inorganic ammonium salts as the sole nitrogen source. The test is part of a series referred to as IMViC (indole, methyl red, Voges-Proskauer, and citrate), which is used to differentiate Enterobacterales from other gram-negative rods.

Principle

Bacteria that can grow on this medium produce an enzyme, citrate-permease, capable of converting citrate to pyruvate. Pyruvate can then enter the organism's metabolic cycle for the production of energy. Bacteria capable of growth in this medium use the citrate and convert ammonium phosphate to ammonia and ammonium hydroxide, creating an alkaline pH. The pH change turns the bromothymol blue indicator from green to blue.

Media: $NH_4H_2PO_4$ (1 g), K_2HPO_4 (1 g), NaCl (5 g), sodium citrate (2 g), $MgSO_4$ (0.2 g), agar (15 g), bromothymol blue (0.08 g) per 1000 mL, pH 6.9.

Method

1. Inoculate Simmons citrate agar lightly on the slant by touching the tip of a needle to a colony that is 18–24 h old. Do not inoculate from a broth culture, because the inoculum will be too heavy.
2. Incubate at 35°C–37°C for up to 7 days.
3. Observe for growth and the development of blue color, denoting alkalinization.

Expected Results

Positive: Growth on the medium, with or without a change in the color of the indicator. Growth typically results in the bromothymol blue indicator turning from green to blue (Fig. 12.11A).
Negative: Absence of growth (Fig. 12.11B).

Limitations

Some organisms are capable of growth on citrate and do not produce a color change. Growth is considered a positive citrate utilization test, even in the absence of a color change.

Quality Control

Positive: *Klebsiella aerogenes* (ATCC13048)—growth; blue color
Negative: *Escherichia coli* (ATCC25922)—little to no growth; no color change

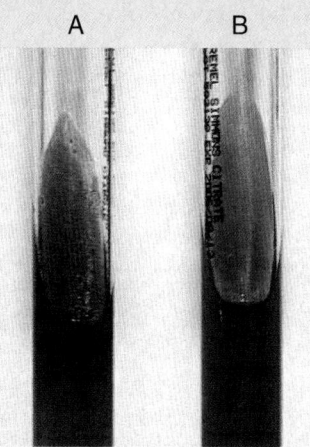

• **Fig. 12.11** Citrate utilization. (A) Positive. (B) Negative.

PROCEDURE 12.12

Coagulase Test

Purpose

The test is used to differentiate *Staphylococcus aureus* (positive) from coagulase-negative staphylococci (negative).

Principle

S. aureus produces two forms of coagulase, bound and free. Bound coagulase, or "clumping factor," is bound to the bacterial cell wall and reacts directly with fibrinogen. This results in precipitation of fibrinogen on the staphylococcal cell, causing the cells to clump when a bacterial suspension is mixed with plasma. The presence of bound coagulase correlates with free coagulase, an extracellular protein enzyme that causes the formation of a clot when *S. aureus* colonies are incubated with plasma. The clotting mechanism involves activation of a plasma coagulase-reacting factor (CRF), which is a modified or derived thrombin molecule, to form a coagulase-CRF complex. This complex in turn reacts with fibrinogen to produce the fibrin clot.

Method

A. Slide Test (Detection of Bound Coagulase or Clumping Factor)
1. Place a drop of coagulase plasma (preferably rabbit plasma with ethylenediaminetetraacetic acid [EDTA]) reagent on the reaction provided by the manufacturer.
2. Place a drop of distilled water or saline next to the drop of plasma in an adjacent reaction well as a negative control.
3. Place a drop of coagulase plasma reagent in a third adjacent reaction well as a positive control.
4. With a loop, straight wire, or wooden stick, emulsify a portion of the isolated colony in the rabbit plasma reagent. Try to create a smooth suspension.
5. Mix well with a wooden applicator stick.
6. With a loop, straight wire, or wooden stick, emulsify a known *Staphylococcus species* in the positive (*Staphylococcus aureus*) and negative (*Staphylococcus epidermidis*) control wells.
7. Mix all samples well with a new wooden applicator stick for each sample.
8. Rock the slide gently for 5–10 s.

Expected Results

Positive: Macroscopic clumping in 10 s or less in coagulated plasma drop positive control, unknown clinical isolate along with no clumping in saline or water drop (Fig. 12.12A, *left side*).
Negative: No clumping in the unknown clinical isolate well as long as the positive and negative controls demonstrate appropriate reactions as described.
Note: All negative slide tests must be confirmed using the tube test (Fig. 12.12B, *right side*).
B. Tube Test (Detection of Free Coagulase)
1. Emulsify several colonies of the unknown clinical isolate in 0.5 mL of rabbit plasma (with EDTA) to give a milky suspension.
2. Repeat the same process with a known positive and negative control organism.

2. Incubate tube at 35°C–37°C in ambient air for 1–4 h.
3. Check for clot formation.

Expected Results

Positive: Clot of any size (Fig. 12.12A, *left side*).
Negative: No clot (Fig. 12.12B, *right side*).

Limitations

Slide Test
Equivocal: Clumping in both the rabbit plasma reagent and water or saline control drops indicate that the organism autoagglutinates and is unsuitable for the slide coagulase test.

Tube Test
1. Test results can be positive at 1–4 h and then revert to negative after 24 h.
2. If negative at 4 h, incubate at room temperature overnight and check again for clot formation.

Quality Control

Positive: *Staphylococcus aureus* (ATCC25923)
Negative: *Staphylococcus epidermidis* (ATCC12228)

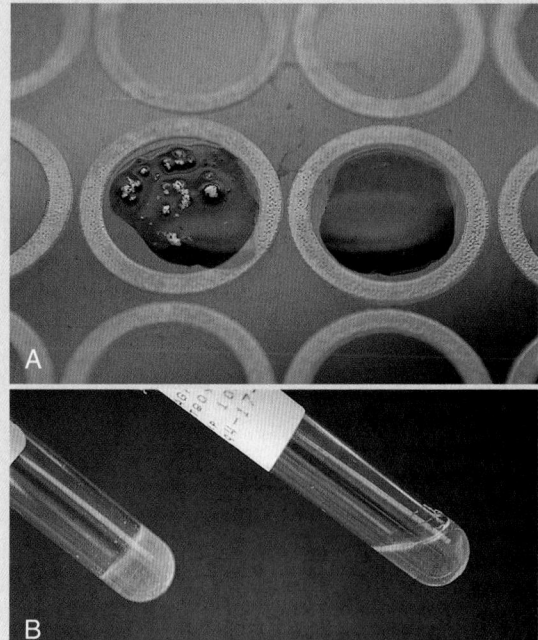

• **Fig. 12.12** Coagulase test. (A) Slide coagulase test for clumping factor. Left side is positive; right side is negative. (B) Tube coagulase test to detect free coagulase. Tube on the left is positive, exhibiting clot. Tube on the right is negative.

PROCEDURE 12.13

Decarboxylase Tests (Moeller's Method)

Purpose

This test is used to differentiate decarboxylase-producing Enterobacterales from other gram-negative rods.

Principle

This test measures the enzymatic ability (decarboxylase) of an organism to decarboxylate (or hydrolyze) an amino acid to form an amine. Decarboxylation, or hydrolysis, of the amino acid results in an alkaline pH and a color change from yellow or orange to purple.

Media: Peptic digest of animal tissue (5 g), beef extract (5 g), bromocresol purple (0.1 g), cresol red (0.005 g), dextrose (0.5 g), pyridoxal (0.005 g), amino acid (10 g), pH 6.0.

Method

A. Glucose-Nonfermenting Organisms
1. Prepare a suspension (McFarland No. 5 turbidity standard) in brain-heart infusion broth from an overnight culture (18–24 h old) growing on 5% sheep blood agar.
2. Inoculate each of the three decarboxylase broths (arginine, lysine, and ornithine) and the control broth (no amino acid) with four drops of broth.
3. Add a 4-mm layer of sterile mineral oil to each tube.
4. Incubate the cultures at 35°C–37°C in ambient air. Examine the tubes at 24, 48, 72, and 96 h.
B. Glucose-Fermenting Organisms
1. Inoculate tubes with one drop of an 18–24-h brain-heart infusion broth culture.
2. Add a 4-mm layer of sterile mineral oil to each tube.
3. Incubate the cultures for 4 days at 35°C–37°C in ambient air. Examine the tubes at 24, 48, 72, and 96 h.

Expected Results

Positive: Alkaline (purple) color change compared with the control tube (Fig. 12.13A).
Negative: No color change or acid (yellow) color in test and control tube. Growth in the control tube.

Limitations

The fermentation of dextrose in the medium causes the acid color change. However, it would not mask the alkaline color

change brought about by a positive decarboxylation reaction (Fig. 12.13B). An uninoculated tube is shown in Fig. 12.13C.

Quality Control

Positive:
  Lysine—*Klebsiella pneumoniae* (ATCC33495)—yellow to purple
  Ornithine—*Klebsiella aerogenes* (ATCC13048)—yellow to purple
  Arginine—*Pseudomonas aeruginosa* (ATCC27853)—yellow to purple
Base Control:
  Positive Glucose Fermenters *Klebsiella pneumoniae* (ATCC27736)—yellow
  Klebsiella aerogenes (ATCC13048)—yellow
Negative:
  Lysine—*Citrobacter freundii* (ATCC331218)—yellow
  Ornithine—*Proteus vulgaris* (ATCC6380)—yellow
  Arginine—*Escherichia coli* (ATCC25922)—yellow

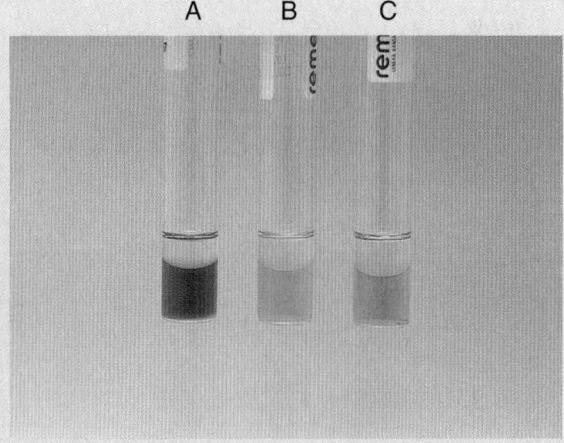

• **Fig. 12.13** Decarboxylase tests (Moeller's Method). (A) Positive. (B) Negative. (C) Uninoculated tube.

PROCEDURE 12.14

Deoxyribonucleic Acid Hydrolysis (DNase Test Agar)

Purpose

This test is used to differentiate organisms based on the production of deoxyribonuclease. It is used to distinguish *Serratia* spp. (positive) from *Enterobacter* spp., *Staphylococcus aureus* (positive) from other species, and *Moraxella catarrhalis* (positive) from *Neisseria* spp.

Principle

The test is used to determine the ability of an organism to hydrolyze deoxyribonucleic acid (DNA). The medium is pale green because of the DNA–methyl green complex. If the organism growing on the medium hydrolyzes DNA, the green color fades and the colony is surrounded by a colorless zone.

Media: Pancreatic digest of casein (10 g), yeast extract (10 g), deoxyribonucleic acid (2 g), NaCl (5 g), agar (15 g), methyl green (0.5 g), pH 7.5.

Method

1. Inoculate the DNase agar with the organism to be tested and streak for isolation.
2. Incubate aerobically at 35°C–37°C for 13–24 h.

Expected Results

Positive: When DNA is hydrolyzed, methyl green is released and combines with highly polymerized DNA at a pH of 7.5, turning the medium colorless around the test organism (Fig. 12.14A and B).

Negative: If no degradation of DNA occurs, the medium remains green (Fig. 12.14C).

Limitations

Agar must be inoculated with a suspension of a young broth culture (4 h old) or an 18–24-h overnight colony in 1–2 mL of saline.

Quality Control

Positive: *Staphylococcus aureus* (ATCC25923)
Negative: *Escherichia coli* (ATCC25922)

Note: Several variations of this media are available that include agarose slants and toluene blue (positive result appears a deep pink) or precipitation of the DNA by flooding with hydrochloric acid resulting in a visible precipitation of the polymerized DNA in the absence of a dye.

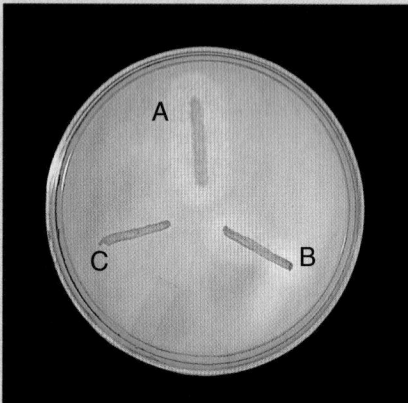

• **Fig. 12.14** Deoxyribonucleic acid hydrolysis. (A) Positive, *Staphylococcus aureus*. (B) Positive, *Serratia marcescens*. (C) Negative, *Escherichia coli*.

PROCEDURE 12.15

Esculin Hydrolysis

Purpose

This test is used for the presumptive identification and differentiation of Enterobacterales.

Principle

This test is used to determine whether an organism is able to hydrolyze the glycoside esculin. Esculin is hydrolyzed to esculetin, which reacts with Fe^{3+} and forms a dark brown to black precipitate.

Media: NaCl (8 g), K_2HPO_4 (0.4 g), KH_2PO_4 (0.1 g), esculin (5 g), ferric ammonium citrate (0.5 g), agar (15 g) per 1000 mL, pH 7.0.

Method

1. Inoculate the medium with one drop of a 24-h broth culture.
2. Incubate at 35°C–37°C for up to 7 days.
3. Examine the slants for blackening and, under the ultraviolet rays of a Wood's lamp, for esculin hydrolysis.

Expected Results

Positive: Blackened medium (Fig. 12.15A), which would also show a loss of fluorescence under the Wood's lamp.
Negative: No blackening and no loss of fluorescence under the Wood's lamp, or slight blackening with no loss of fluorescence under the Wood's lamp. An uninoculated tube is shown in Fig. 12.15B.

Limitations

This medium is a nonselective agar. The bile esculin hydrolysis test presented in Procedure 12.5 is a selective differential method.

Quality Control

Positive: *Enterococcus faecalis* (ATCC29212)
Negative: *Escherichia coli* (ATCC25922)
          Streptococcus pyogenes (ATCC 19615)

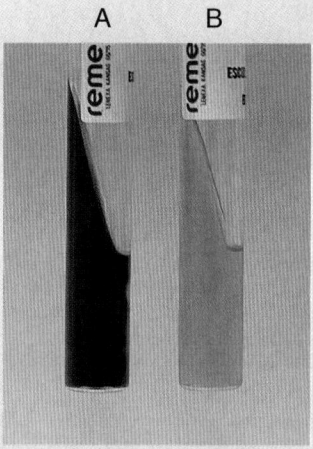

• **Fig. 12.15** Esculin hydrolysis. (A) Positive, blackening of slant. (B) Uninoculated tube.

PROCEDURE 12.16

Fermentation Media

Purpose

Fermentation media are used to differentiate organisms based on their ability to ferment carbohydrates incorporated into the basal medium. Andrade's formula is used to differentiate enteric bacteria from coryneforms, and bromocresol purple is used to distinguish enterococci from streptococci.

Principle

Carbohydrate fermentation is the process microorganisms use to produce energy. Most microorganisms convert glucose to pyruvate during glycolysis; however, some organisms use alternate pathways. A fermentation medium consists of a basal medium containing a single carbohydrate (glucose, lactose, or sucrose) for fermentation. However, the medium may contain various color indicators, such as Andrade's indicator, bromocresol, or others. In addition to a color indicator to detect the production of acid from fermentation, a Durham tube is placed in each tube to capture gas produced by metabolism.

    Basal media: Pancreatic digest of casein (10 g), beef extract (3 g), NaCl (5 g), carbohydrate (10 g), specific indicator (Andrade's indicator [10 mL, pH 7.4] or bromocresol purple [0.02 g, pH 6.8]).

Method

A. Peptone Medium with Andrade's Indicator (for Enterics and Coryneforms)
1. Inoculate each tube with one drop of an 18–24-h brain-heart infusion broth culture.
2. Incubate at 35°C–37°C for up to 7 days in ambient air. *Note*: Tubes are held only 4 days for organisms belonging to Enterobacterales.
3. Examine the tubes for acid (indicated by a pink color) and gas production.
4. Tubes must show growth for the test to be valid. If no growth in the fermentation tubes or control is seen after 24 h of incubation, add one to two drops of sterile rabbit serum per 5 mL of fermentation broth to each tube.

Expected Results

Positive: Indicator change to pink with or without gas formation in Durham tube (Fig. 12.16A, *left* and *middle*).
Negative: Growth, but no change in color. Medium remains clear to straw colored (Fig. 12.16A, *right*).
B. Broth (Brain-Heart Infusion Broth May Be Substituted) with Bromocresol Purple Indicator (for Streptococci and Enterococci)
1. Inoculate each tube with two drops of an 18–24-h brain-heart infusion broth culture.
2. Incubate 4 days at 35°C–37°C in ambient air.
3. Observe daily for a change of the bromocresol purple indicator from purple to yellow (acid).

Expected Results

Positive: Indicator change to yellow (Fig. 12.16B, *left*).
Negative: Growth, but no change in color. Medium remains purple (Fig. 12.16B, *right*).

Limitations

Readings after 24 h may not be reliable if no acid is produced. No color change or a result indicating alkalinity may occur if the organism deaminates the peptone, masking the evidence of carbohydrate fermentation.

Quality Control

Note: Appropriate organisms depend on which carbohydrate has been added to the basal medium. An example is given for each type of medium.
A. Peptone Medium with Andrade's Indicator
Dextrose:
    Positive, with gas: *Escherichia coli* (ATCC25922)
    Positive, no gas: *Shigella flexneri* (ATCC12022)
B. Brain-Heart Infusion Broth with Bromocresol Purple Indicator
Dextrose:
    Positive, with gas: *Escherichia coli* (ATCC25922)
    Negative, no gas: *Moraxella osloensis* (ATCC10973)

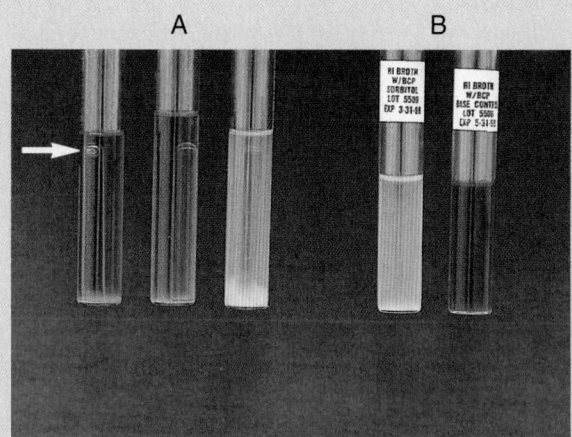

A   B

• **Fig. 12.16** Fermentation media. (A) Peptone medium with Andrade's indicator. The tube on the left ferments glucose with the production of gas (visible as a bubble *[arrow]* in the inverted [Durham] tube); the tube in the middle ferments glucose with no gas production; and the tube on the right does not ferment glucose. (B) Heart infusion broth with bromocresol purple indicator. The tube on the left is positive; the tube on the right is negative.

PROCEDURE 12.17

Flagella Stain (Wet Mount Technique)

Purpose

This technique is used to visualize the presence and arrangement of flagella for the presumptive identification of motile bacterial species.

Principle

Flagella are too thin to be visualized using a bright field microscope with ordinary stains, such as the Gram stain, or a simple stain. A wet mount technique is used for staining bacterial flagella, and it is simple and useful when the number and arrangement of flagella are critical to the identification of species of motile bacteria. The staining procedures require the use of a mordant so that the stain adheres in layers to the flagella, allowing visualization.

Method

1. Grow the organism to be stained at room temperature on blood agar for 16–24 h.
2. Add a small drop of water to a microscope slide.
3. Dip a sterile inoculating loop into sterile water.
4. Touch the loopful of water to the colony margin briefly (this allows motile cells to swim into the droplet of water).
5. Touch the loopful of motile cells to the drop of water on the slide. *Note*: Agitating the loop in the droplet of water on the slide causes the flagella to shear off the cell.
6. Cover the faintly turbid drop of water on the slide with a cover slip. A proper wet mount has barely enough liquid to fill the space under a cover slip. Small air spaces around the edge are preferable.
7. Examine the slide immediately under 40× to 50× magnification for motile cells. If motile cells are not seen, do not proceed with the stain.
8. If motile cells are seen, leave the slide at room temperature for 5–10 min. This allows the bacterial cells time to adhere either to the glass slide or to the cover slip.
9. Gently apply two drops of Ryu flagella stain (available from multiple manufacturers) to the edge of the cover slip. The stain will flow by capillary action and mix with the cell suspension. Small air pockets around the edge of the wet mount are useful in aiding the capillary action.
10. After 5–10 min at room temperature, examine the cells for flagella.
11. Cells with flagella may be observed at 100× (oil) magnification in the zone of optimum stain concentration, about halfway from the edge of the cover slip to the center of the mount.
12. Focusing the microscope on the cells attached to the cover slip rather than on the cells attached to the slide facilitates visualization of the flagella. The precipitate from the stain is primarily on the slide rather than the cover slip.

Expected Results

Observe the slide and note the following:
1. Presence or absence of flagella
2. Number of flagella per cell

3. Location of flagella per cell
   a. Peritrichous (Fig. 12.17A)
   b. Lophotrichous
   c. Polar or monotrichous (Fig. 12.17B)
   d. Amphitrichous
4. Amplitude of wavelength
   a. Short
   b. Long
5. Whether or not "tufted"

Limitations

Even with a specific stain, visualization of flagella requires an experienced laboratory scientist and is not considered an entry-level technique.

Quality Control

Peritrichous: *Escherichia coli*
Polar: *Pseudomonas aeruginosa*
Negative: *Klebsiella pneumoniae*

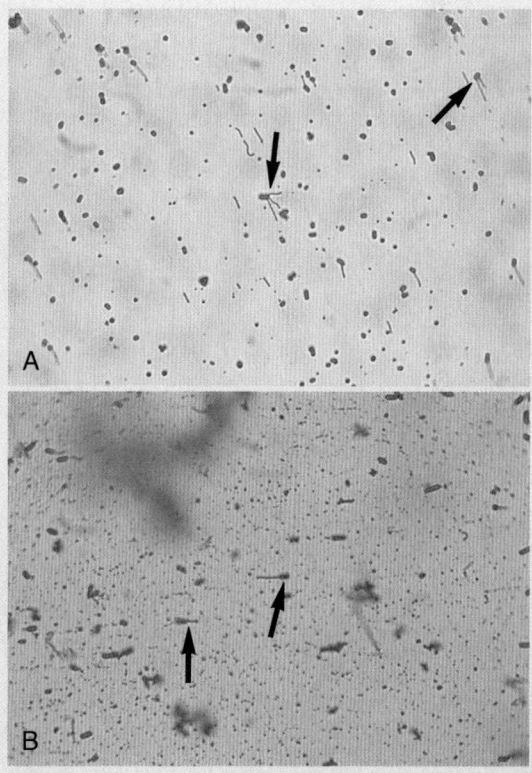

• **Fig. 12.17** Flagella stain (wet mount technique). (A) *Alcaligenes* spp., peritrichous flagella *(arrows)*. (B) *Pseudomonas aeruginosa*, polar flagella *(arrows)*.

PROCEDURE 12.18

Gelatin Hydrolysis

Purpose

The production of gelatinases capable of hydrolyzing gelatin is used as a presumptive test for the identification of various organisms, including *Staphylococcus* spp., Enterobacterales, and some gram-positive bacilli.

Principle

This test is used to determine the ability of an organism to produce extracellular proteolytic enzymes (gelatinases) that liquefy gelatin, a component of vertebrate connective tissue.

Nutrient gelatin medium differs from traditional microbiology media in that the solidifying agent (agar) is replaced with gelatin. When an organism produces gelatinase, the enzyme liquefies the growth medium.

Media: Enzymatic digest of gelatin (5 g), beef extract (3 g), gelatin (120 g) per 1000 mL, pH 6.8.

Method

1. Inoculate the gelatin deep with four to five drops of a 24-h broth culture.
2. Incubate at 35°C–37°C in ambient air for up to 14 days. *Note*: Incubate the medium at 25°C if the organism grows better at 25°C than at 35°C.
3. Alternatively, inoculate the gelatin deep from a 24-h-old colony by stabbing four or five times, 0.5 inch into the medium.
4. Remove the gelatin tube daily from the incubator and place at 4°C to check for liquefaction. Do not invert or tip the tube, because sometimes the only discernible liquefaction occurs at the top of the deep where inoculation occurred.
5. Refrigerate an uninoculated control along with the inoculated tube. Liquefaction is determined only after the control has hardened (gelled).

Expected Results

Positive: Partial or total liquefaction of the inoculated tube (the control tube must be completely solidified) at 4°C within 14 days (Fig. 12.18A).
Negative: Complete solidification of the tube at 4°C (Fig. 12.18B).

Limitations

Some organisms may grow poorly or not at all in this medium.
Gelatin is liquid above 20°C; therefore, determination of results must be completed after refrigeration.

Quality Control

Positive: *Bacillus subtilis* (ATCC9372)
Negative: *Escherichia coli* (ATCC25922)
Uninoculated control tube: Medium becomes solid after refrigeration.

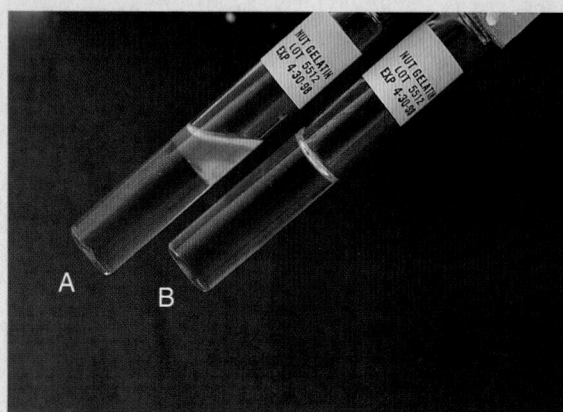

• **Fig. 12.18** Gelatin hydrolysis. (A) Positive; note liquefaction at top of tube. (B) Uninoculated tube.

PROCEDURE 12.19

Growth at 42°C

Purpose

This test is used to differentiate a pyocyanogenic pseudomonad from other *Pseudomonas* spp.

Principle

The test is used to determine the ability of an organism to grow at 42°C. Several *Pseudomonas* spp. have been isolated in the clinical laboratory that are capable of growth at elevated temperatures.

Method

1. Inoculate two tubes of trypticase soy agar (TSA) with a light inoculum by lightly touching a needle to the top of a single 13–24-h-old colony and streaking the slant.
2. Immediately, incubate one tube at 35°C and one at 42°C.
3. Record the presence of growth on each slant after 18–24 h.

Expected Results

Positive: Good growth at both 35°C and 42°C (Fig. 12.19A).
Negative: No growth at 42°C (Fig. 12.19B), but good growth at 35°C.

Quality Control

Positive: *Pseudomonas aeruginosa* (ATCC10145)
Negative: *Pseudomonas fluorescens* (ATCC13525)

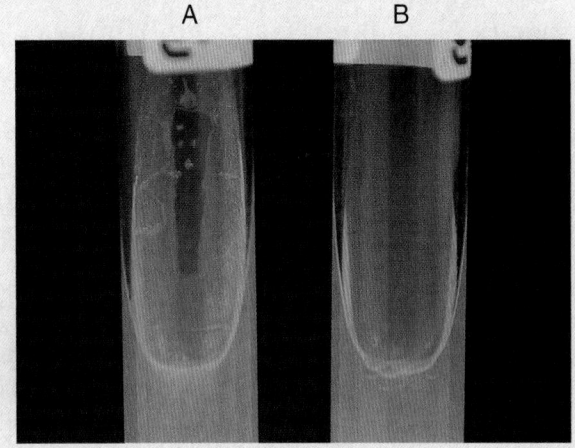

• **Fig. 12.19** Growth at 42°C. (A) Positive; good growth. (B) Negative; no growth.

PROCEDURE 12.20

Hippurate Hydrolysis

Purpose

Production of the enzyme hippuricase is used for the presumptive identification of a variety of microorganisms.

Principle

The products of hydrolysis of hippuric acid by hippuricase include glycine and benzoic acid. Glycine is deaminated by the oxidizing agent ninhydrin, which is reduced during the process. The products of the ninhydrin oxidation react to form a purple-colored product. The test medium must contain only hippurate, because ninhydrin might react with any free amino acids present in growth media or other broths.

Method

1. Add 0.1 mL of sterile water to a 12 by 75 mm plastic test tube.
2. Make a heavy suspension of the organism to be tested.
3. Using heated forceps, place a rapid hippurate disk in the mixture.
4. Cap and incubate the tube for 2 h at 35°C; use of a water bath is preferred.
5. Add 0.2 mL ninhydrin reagent and reincubate for an additional 15–30 min. Observe the solution for the development of a deep purple color.

Expected Results

Positive: Deep purple color (Fig. 12.20A).
Negative: Colorless or slightly yellow pink color (Fig. 12.20B).

Limitations

A false-positive result may occur if incubation with ninhydrin exceeds 30 min.

Quality Control

Positive: *Streptococcus agalactiae* (ATCC12386)
Negative: *Streptococcus pyogenes* (ATCC19615)

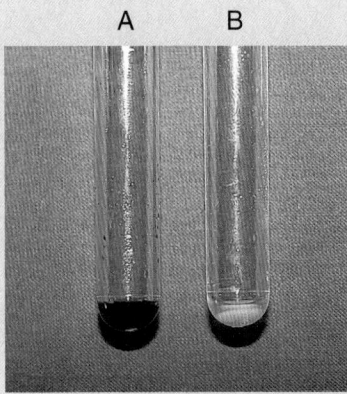

• **Fig. 12.20** Hippurate hydrolysis. (A) Positive. (B) Negative.

PROCEDURE 12.21

Indole Production

Purpose
This test is used to identify organisms that produce the enzyme tryptophanase.

Principle
The test is used to determine an organism's ability to hydrolyze tryptophan to form the compound indole. Tryptophan is present in casein and animal protein. Bacteria with tryptophanase are capable of hydrolyzing tryptophan to pyruvate, ammonia, and indole. Kovac's reagent (dimethylamine-benzaldehyde and hydrochloride), when added to the broth culture, reacts with the indole, producing a red color. An alternative method uses Ehrlich's reagent. Ehrlich's reagent has the same chemicals as the Kovac preparation, but it also contains absolute ethyl alcohol, making it flammable. Ehrlich's reagent is more sensitive for detecting small amounts of indole. (The spot indole test is described in Procedure 12.40)

Media: Casein peptone (10 g), NaCl (5 g), tryptophan (10 g) per 1000 mL.

Method
A. Enterobacterales
1. Inoculate tryptophan broth with one drop from a 24-h brain-heart infusion broth culture.
2. Incubate at 35°C–37°C in ambient air for 48 h.
3. Add 0.5 mL of Kovac's reagent to the broth culture.
B. Other Gram-Negative Bacilli
1. Inoculate tryptophan broth with one drop of a 24-h broth culture.
2. Incubate at 35°C–37°C in ambient air for 48 h.
3. Add 1 mL of xylene to the culture.
4. Shake the mixture vigorously to extract the indole and allow it to stand until the xylene forms a layer on top of the aqueous phase.
5. Add 0.5 mL of Ehrlich's reagent down the side of the tube.

Expected Results
Positive: Pink- to wine-colored ring after addition of appropriate reagent (Fig. 12.21A).

Negative: No color change after addition of the appropriate reagent (Fig. 12.21B).

Limitations
Ehrlich's method may also be used to differentiate organisms under anaerobic conditions.

Quality Control
A. Kovac's Method
Positive: *Escherichia coli* (ATCC25922)
Negative: *Klebsiella pneumoniae* (ATCC13883)
B. Ehrlich's Method
Positive: *Haemophilus influenzae* (ATCC49766)
Negative: *Haemophilus parainfluenza* (ATCC76901)
C. Ehrlich's Method (Anaerobic)
Positive: *Porphyromonas asaccharolytica* (ATCC25260)
Negative: *Bacteroides fragilis* (ATCC25285)

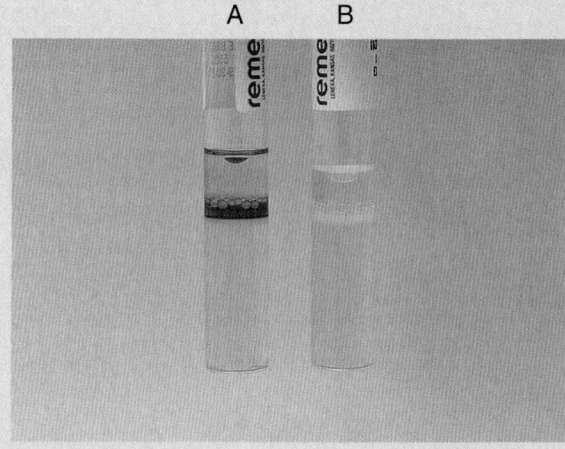

• **Fig. 12.21** Indole production. (A) Positive. (B) Negative.

PROCEDURE 12.22

Leucine Aminopeptidase Test

Purpose

The leucine aminopeptidase (LAP) test is used for the presumptive identification of catalase-negative gram-positive cocci.

Principle

The LAP disk is a rapid test for the detection of the enzyme leucine aminopeptidase. Leucine-beta-naphthylamide–impregnated disks serve as a substrate for the detection of leucine aminopeptidase. After hydrolysis of the substrate by the enzyme, the resulting beta-naphthylamine produces a red color upon addition of cinnamaldehyde reagent.

Method

1. Before incubation, slightly dampen the LAP disk with reagent-grade water. Do not supersaturate the disk.
2. Using a wooden applicator stick, rub a small amount of several colonies of an 18–24-h pure culture onto a small area of the LAP disk.
3. Incubate at room temperature for 5 min.
4. After this incubation period, add one drop of cinnamaldehyde reagent.

Expected Results

Positive: Development of a red color within 1 minute after adding cinnamaldehyde reagent (Fig. 12.22A; swab test is depicted)
Negative: No color change or development of a slight yellow color (Fig. 12.22B).

Limitations

The test result depends on the integrity of the substrate-impregnated disk.

Quality Control

Positive: *Enterococcus faecalis* (ATCC29212)—red color
Negative: *Aerococcus viridans* (ATCC11563)—no color
    change

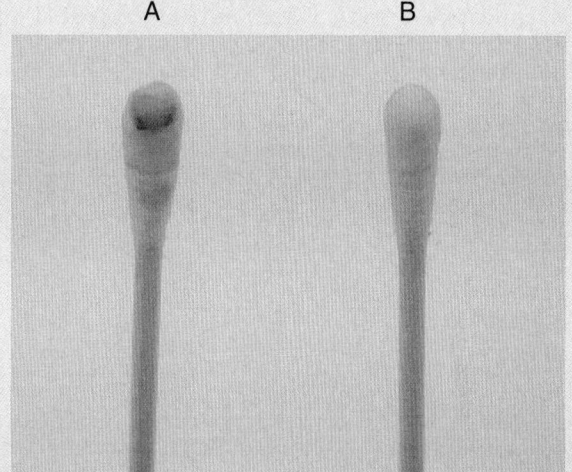

• **Fig. 12.22** Leucine aminopeptidase test. (A) Positive. (B) Negative.

PROCEDURE 12.23

Litmus Milk Medium

Purpose

This test differentiates microorganisms based on various metabolic reactions in litmus milk, including fermentation, reduction, clot formation, digestion, and the formation of gas. Litmus milk is also used to grow lactic acid bacteria.

Principle

This test is used to determine an organism's ability to metabolize litmus milk. Fermentation of lactose is demonstrated when the litmus turns pink because of acid production. If sufficient acid is produced, casein in the milk is coagulated, solidifying the milk. With some organisms, the curd shrinks and whey is formed at the surface. Some bacteria hydrolyze casein, causing the milk to become straw colored and resemble turbid serum. In addition, some organisms reduce litmus, in which case the medium becomes colorless in the bottom of the tube.

Media: Powdered skim milk (100 g), litmus (0.5 g), sodium sulfite (0.5 g) per 1000 mL, pH 6.8.

Method

1. Inoculate with four drops of a 24-h. broth culture.
2. Incubate at 35°C–37°C in ambient air.
3. Observe daily for 7 days for alkaline reaction (litmus turns blue), acid reaction (litmus turns pink), indicator reduction, acid clot, rennet clot, and peptonization. Multiple changes can occur over the observation period.
4. Record all changes.

Quality Control

Fermentation: *Clostridium perfringens* (ATCC13124)—gas production
Acid: *Lactobacillus acidophilus* (ATCC11506)—clot formation
Peptonization: *Pseudomonas aeruginosa* (ATCC27853)—clearing
Appearance of indicator (litmus dye)

Limitations

Litmus media reactions are not specific and should be followed up with additional tests for definitive identification of microorganisms.

Expected Results

APPEARANCE OF INDICATOR (LITMUS DYE)

Color	pH Change to	Record
Pink, mauve (Fig. 12.23A)	Acid	Acid (A)
Blue (Fig. 12.23B)	Alkaline	Alkaline (K)
Purple (identical to uninoculated control) (Fig. 12.23C)	No change	No change

APPEARANCE OF INDICATOR (LITMUS DYE)

Color	pH Change to	Record
White (Fig. 12.23D)	Independent of pH change; result of reduction of indicator	Decolorized

APPEARANCE OF MILK

Consistency of Milk	Occurs When pH Is	Record
Coagulation or clot (Fig. 12.23E)	Acid or alkaline	Clot
Dissolution of clot with clear, grayish, watery fluid and a shrunken, insoluble pink clot (Fig. 12.23F)	Acid	Digestion
Dissolution of clot with grayish, watery fluid and a clear, shrunken, insoluble blue clot	Alkaline	Peptonization

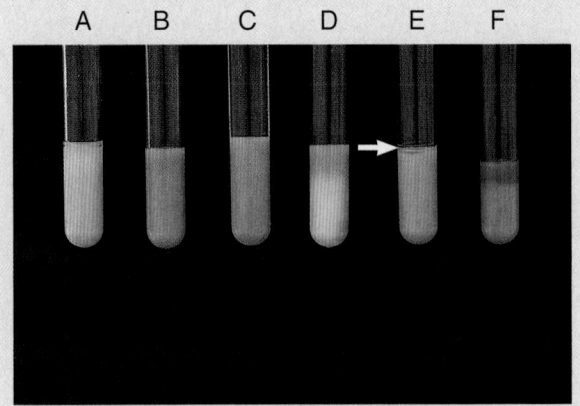

• **Fig. 12.23** Litmus milk. (A) Acid reaction. (B) Alkaline reaction. (C) No change. (D) Reduction of indicator. (E) Clot. (Note separation of clear fluid from clot at arrow.) (F) Peptonization.

PROCEDURE 12.24

Lysine Iron Agar

Purpose

This test is used to differentiate gram-negative bacilli based on decarboxylation or deamination of lysine and the formation of hydrogen sulfide (H_2S).

Principle

Lysine iron agar (LIA) contains lysine, peptones, and a small amount of glucose, ferric ammonium citrate, and sodium thiosulfate. The medium has an aerobic slant and an anaerobic butt. When glucose is fermented, the butt of the medium becomes acidic (yellow). If the organism produces lysine decarboxylase, cadaverine is formed. Cadaverine neutralizes the organic acids formed by glucose fermentation, and the butt of the medium reverts to the alkaline state (purple). If the decarboxylase is not produced, the butt remains acidic (yellow). If oxidative deamination of lysine occurs, a compound is formed that, in the presence of ferric ammonium citrate and a coenzyme, flavin mononucleotide, forms a burgundy color on the slant. If deamination does not occur, the LIA slant remains purple. Bromocresol purple, the pH indicator, is yellow at or below pH 5.2 and purple at or above pH 6.8.

Media: Enzymatic digest of gelatin (5 g), yeast extract (3 g), dextrose (1 g), L-lysine (10 g), ferric ammonium citrate (0.5 g), sodium thiosulfate (0.04 g), bromocresol purple (0.02 g), agar (13.5 g) per 1000 mL, pH 6.7.

Method

1. With a straight inoculating needle, inoculate LIA (Fig. 12.24E) by twice stabbing through the center of the medium to the bottom of the tube and then streaking the slant.
2. Cap the tube tightly and incubate at 35°C–37°C in ambient air for 18–24 h.

Expected Results

Alkaline slant/alkaline butt (K/K)—lysine decarboxylation and no fermentation of glucose (Fig. 12.24A).

Alkaline slant/acid butt (K/A)—glucose fermentation (Fig. 12.24C).

Note: Patterns shown in Fig. 12.24A and C can be accompanied by a black precipitate of ferrous sulfide (FeS), which indicates production of H_2S (Fig. 12.14B).

Red slant/acid butt (R/A)—lysine deamination and glucose fermentation (Fig. 12.24D).

Limitations

Proteus spp. that produce hydrogen sulfide will not blacken the medium. Additional testing, such as triple sugar iron (TSI) agar, should be used as a follow-up identification method.

Quality Control

Alkaline slant and butt: H_2S positive: *Citrobacter freundii* (ATCC8090)

Alkaline slant and butt: *Escherichia coli* (ATCC25922)

Alkaline slant and butt: H_2S positive: *Salmonella enterica* subsp. *enterica* serovar Typhimurium (ATCC14028)

Red slant, acid butt: *Proteus mirabilis* (ATCC12453)

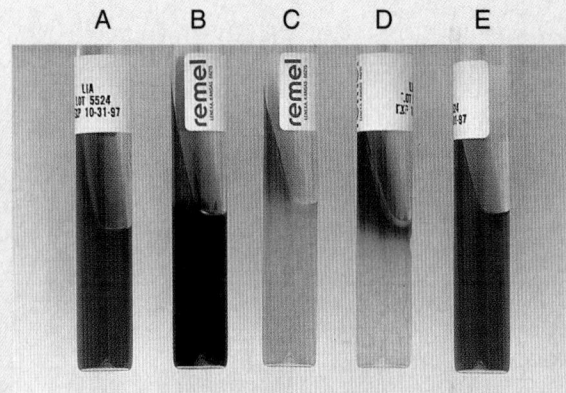

• **Fig. 12.24** Lysine iron agar. (A) Alkaline slant/alkaline butt (K/K). (B) Alkaline slant/alkaline butt, H_2S positive (K/K H_2S+). (C) Alkaline slant/acid butt (K/A). (D) Red slant/acid butt (R/A). (E) Uninoculated tube.

PROCEDURE 12.25

Methyl Red and Voges-Proskauer Tests

Purpose

The combination test methyl red (MR) and Voges-Proskauer (VP) differentiates members of Enterobacterales.

Principle

This test is used to determine the ability of an organism to produce and maintain stable acid end products from glucose fermentation, to overcome the buffering capacity of the system, and to determine the ability of some organisms to produce neutral end products (e.g., 2,3-butanediol or acetoin) from glucose fermentation. The methyl red detects mixed acid fermentation that lowers the pH of the broth. The MR indicator is added after incubation. MR is red at pH 4.4 and yellow at pH 6.2. A clear red is a positive result; yellow is a negative result; and various shades of orange are negative or inconclusive. The VP detects the organism's ability to convert the acid products to acetoin and 2,3-butanediol. Organisms capable of using the VP pathway produce a smaller amount of acid during glucose fermentation and therefore do not produce a color change when the MR indicator is added. A secondary reagent is added, alpha-naphthol, followed by potassium hydroxide (KOH); a positive test result is indicated by a red color complex.

Media: Peptic digest of animal tissue (3.5 g), pancreatic digest of casein (3.5 g), dextrose (5 g), KPO_4 (5 g) per 1000 mL, pH 6.9.

Method

1. Inoculate MRVP broth with one drop from a 24-h brain-heart infusion broth culture.
2. Incubate at 35°C–37°C for a minimum of 48 h in ambient air. Tests should not be made with cultures incubated less than 48 h, because the products build up to detectable levels over time. If results are equivocal at 48 h, repeat the tests with cultures incubated at 35°C–37°C for 4–5 days in ambient air; in such instances, duplicate tests should be incubated at 25°C.
3. Split broth into aliquots for MR test and VP test.
A. Methyl Red (MR Test
1. Add five or six drops of methyl red reagent per 5 mL of broth.
2. Read reaction immediately.

Expected Results

Positive: Bright red color, indicative of mixed acid fermentation (Fig. 12.25A).
Weakly positive: Red-orange color.
Negative: Yellow color (Fig. 12.25B).
B. VP Test (Barritt's Method) for Gram-Negative Rods
1. Add 0.6 mL (6 drops) of solution A (alpha-naphthol) and 0.2 mL (2 drops) of solution B (KOH) to 1 mL of MRVP broth.
2. Shake well after addition of each reagent.
3. Observe for 5 min.

Expected Results

Positive: Red color, indicative of acetoin production (Fig 12.25C).
Negative: Yellow color (Fig 12.25D).

C. VP Test (Coblentz Method) for streptococci
1. Use 24-h growth from a blood agar plate to heavily inoculate 2 mL of MRVP broth.
2. After 6 h of incubation at 35°C in ambient air, add 1.2 mL (12 drops) of solution A (alpha-naphthol) and 0.4 mL (4 drops) solution B (40% KOH with creatine).
3. Shake the tube and incubate at room temperature for 30 min.

Limitations

The MR test should not be read before 48 h, because some organisms will not have produced enough products from the fermentation of glucose.
MR-negative organisms may also not have had sufficient time to convert those products and will appear MR positive.
MRVP testing should be used in conjunction with other confirmatory tests to differentiate organisms among the Enterobacterales.

Quality Control

MR positive/VP negative: *Escherichia coli* (ATCC25922)
MR negative/VP positive: *Klebsiella aerogenes* (ATCC13048)

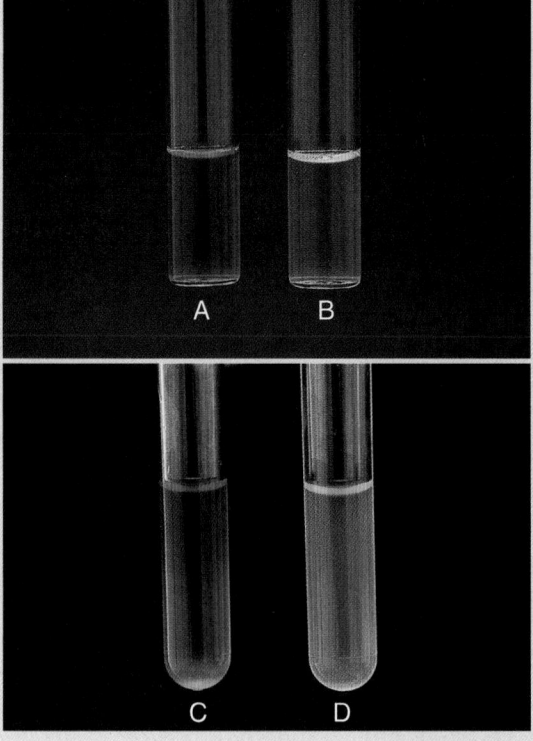

• **Fig. 12.25** Methyl red/Voges-Proskauer tests. (A) Positive methyl red. (B) Negative methyl red. (C) Positive Voges-Proskauer. (D) Negative Voges-Proskauer.

PROCEDURE 12.26

Microdase Test (Modified Oxidase)

Purpose

This test is used to differentiate gram-positive, catalase-positive cocci (micrococci from staphylococci).

Principle

The microdase test is a rapid method to differentiate *Staphylococcus* from *Micrococcus* spp. by detection of the enzyme oxidase. In the presence of atmospheric oxygen, the oxidase enzyme reacts with the oxidase reagent and cytochrome C to form the colored compound, indophenol.

Method

1. Using a wooden applicator stick, rub a small amount of several colonies of an 18- to 24-hour pure culture grown on blood agar onto a small area of the microdase disk. *Note*: Do not rehydrate the disk before use.
2. Incubate at room temperature for 2 min.

Expected Results

Positive: Development of blue to purple-blue color (Fig. 12.26A).
Negative: No color change (Fig. 12.26B).

Limitations

Staphylococci should yield a negative color change, except for *S. sciuri, S. lentus*, and *S. vitellus*.

Quality Control

Positive: *Micrococcus luteus* (ATCC10240)
Negative: *Staphylococcus aureus* (ATCC25923)

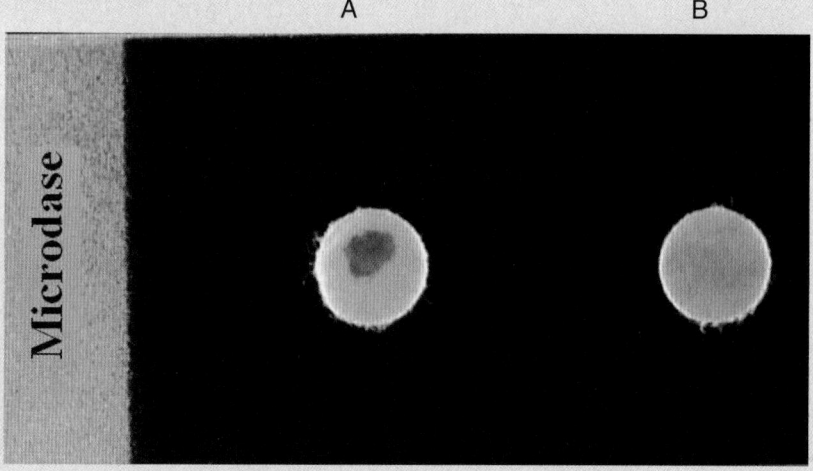

• **Fig. 12.26** Microdase test. (A) Positive. (B) Negative.

PROCEDURE 12.27

Motility Testing

Purpose

These tests are used to determine whether an enteric organism is motile. An organism must have flagella to be motile.

Principle

The inoculum is stabbed into the center of a semisolid agar deep. Bacterial motility is evident by a diffuse zone of growth extending out from the line of inoculation. Some organisms grow throughout the entire medium, whereas others show small areas or nodules that grow out from the line of inoculation.

Media: Enzymatic digest of gelatin (10 g), beef extract (3 g), NaCl (5 g), agar (4 g) per 1000 mL, pH 7.3.

Method

1. Touch a straight needle to a colony of a young (18–24-h) culture growing on agar medium.
2. Stab once to a depth of only 1/3–1/4 inch in the middle of the tube.
3. Incubate at 35°C–37°C and examine daily for up to 7 days.

Expected Results

Positive: Motile organisms will spread out into the medium from the site of inoculation (Fig. 12.27A).
Negative: Nonmotile organisms remain at the site of inoculation (Fig. 12.27B).

Limitations

Some organisms will not display sufficient growth in this medium to make an accurate determination, and additional follow-up testing is required.

Quality Control

Positive: *Proteus vulgaris* (ATCC29905)
Negative: *Klebsiella pneumoniae* (ATCC13883)

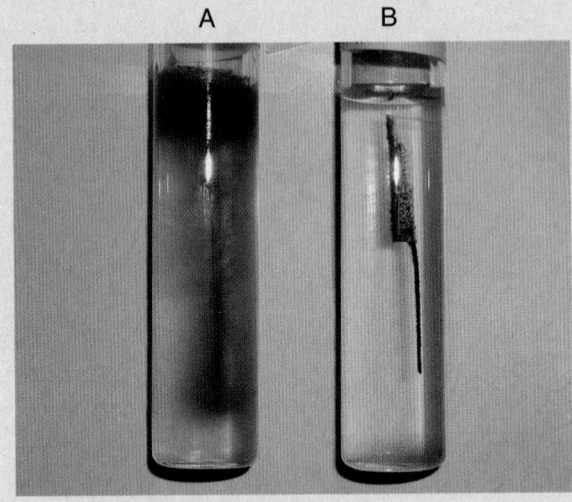

• **Fig. 12.27** Motility test. (A) Positive. (B) Negative.

PROCEDURE 12.28

Lactobacillus MRS Broth

Purpose

This test is used to determine whether an organism forms gas during glucose fermentation. Some *Lactobacillus* spp. and *Leuconostoc* spp. produce gas.

Principle

The MRS broth contains sources of carbon, nitrogen, and vitamins to support the growth of lactobacilli and other organisms. It is a selective medium that uses sodium acetate and ammonium citrate to prevent overgrowth by contaminating organisms. Growth is considered a positive result. A Durham tube may be added to differentiate *Lactobacillus* spp. from *Leuconostoc* spp.

Media: Enzymatic digest of animal tissue (10 g), beef extract (10 g), yeast extract (5 g), dextrose (20 g), $NaC_2H_3O_2$ (5 g), polysorbate 80 (1 g), KH_2PO_4 (2 g), ammonium citrate (2 g), $MgSO_4$ (0.1 g), $MnSO_4$ (0.05 g) per 1000 mL, pH 6.5.

Method

1. Inoculate MRS broth with an 18–24-h culture from agar or broth.
2. Incubate 24–48 h at 35°C–37°C in ambient air.

Expected Results

Positive: *Leuconostoc* spp.—growth; gas production indicated by a bubble in the Durham tube (Fig. 12.28A).
Positive: *Lactobacillus* spp.—growth; no gas production (Fig. 12.28B).
Negative: No growth (not shown).

Quality Control

Positive: *Lactobacillus lactis* (ATCC19435)
Negative: *Escherichia coli* (ATCC25922)

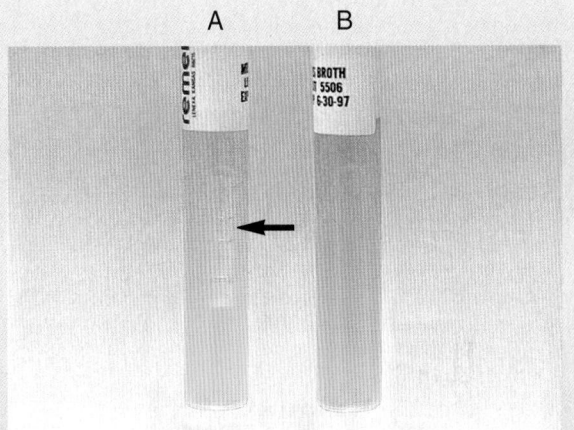

• **Fig. 12.28** MRS broth. (A) Positive; gas production by *Leuconostoc* sp. *(arrow)*. (B) Positive: growth, no gas production by *Lactobacillus* sp.

PROCEDURE 12.29

4-Methylumbelliferyl-β-d-Glucuronide Test

Purpose

This test is used to presumptively identify various genera of Enterobacterales and verotoxin-producing *Escherichia coli*.

Principle

E. coli and other Enterobacterales produce the enzyme β-d-glucuronidase, which hydrolyzes β-d-glucopyranosid-uronic derivatives to aglycons and d-glucuronic acid. The substrate 4-methylumbelliferyl-β-d-glucuronide is impregnated into the disk and is hydrolyzed by the enzyme to yield the 4-methylumbelliferyl moiety, which fluoresces blue under long wavelength ultraviolet light. However, verotoxin-producing strains of *E. coli* do not produce 4-methylumbelliferyl-β-d-glucuronide (MUG) so a negative test result may still indicate the presence of a clinically important strain.

Method

1. Wet the disk with one drop of water.
2. Using a wooden applicator stick, rub a portion of a colony from an 18- to 24-h-old pure culture onto the disk.
3. Incubate at 35°C–37°C in a closed container for up to 2 h.
4. Observe the disk using a 366-nm ultraviolet light.

Expected Results

Positive: Electric blue fluorescence (Fig. 12.29A).
Negative: Lack of fluorescence (Fig. 12.29B).

Limitations

Do not test colonies isolated from media containing dyes (eosin methylene blue [EMB], MacConkey [MAC]), because it may make the interpretation difficult.

Only test on oxidase-positive organisms, because some oxidase-negative organisms naturally fluoresce.

Quality Control

Positive: *Escherichia coli* (ATCC25922)
Negative: *Klebsiella pneumoniae* (ATC13883)

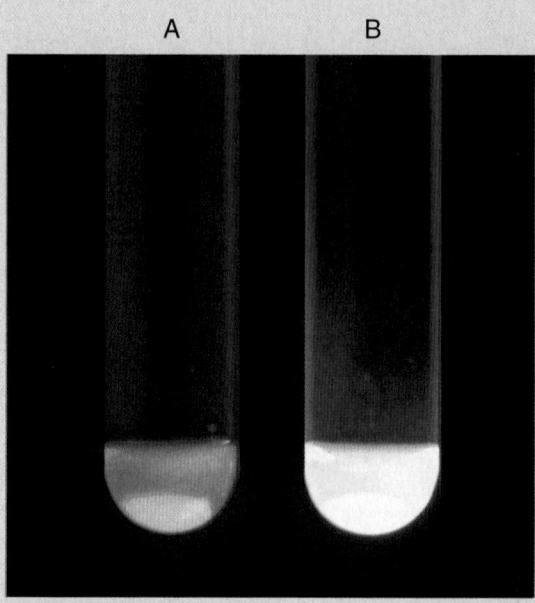

• **Fig. 12.29** 4-Methylumbelliferyl-β-d-glucuronide test. (A) Positive. (B) Negative.

PROCEDURE 12.30

Nitrate Reduction

Purpose

This test is used to determine the ability of an organism to reduce nitrate to nitrite. All members of Enterobacterales reduce nitrate, but some members further metabolize nitrite to other compounds.

Principle

Anaerobic metabolism requires an electron acceptor other than atmospheric oxygen (O_2). Many gram-negative bacteria use nitrate as the final electron acceptor. The organisms produce nitrate reductase, which converts the nitrate (NO_3) to nitrite (NO_2). The reduction of nitrate to nitrite is determined by adding sulfanilic acid and alpha-naphthylamine. The sulfanilic acid and nitrite react to form a diazonium salt. The diazonium salt then couples with the alpha-naphthylamine to produce a red, water-soluble azo dye. If no color change occurs, the organism did not reduce nitrate or reduced it further to NH_3, NO, or N_2O_2. Zinc is added at this point; if nitrate remains, the zinc will reduce the compound to nitrite and the reaction will turn positive, indicating a negative test result for nitrate reduction by the organism. If no color change occurs after the addition of zinc, this indicates that the organism reduced nitrate to one of the other nitrogen compounds previously described. A Durham tube is placed in the broth for two reasons: (1) to detect deterioration of the broth before inoculation, as evidenced by gas formation in the tube, and (2) to identify denitrification by organisms that produce gas by alternate pathways; if gas is formed in the tube before the addition of the color indicator, the test result is negative for nitrate reduction by this method.

Media: Pancreatic digest of gelatin (20 g), KNO_3 (2 g) per 1000 mL.

Method

1. Inoculate nitrate broth with one to two drops from a young broth culture of the test organism.
2. Incubate for 48 h at 35°C–37°C in ambient air (some organisms may require longer incubation for adequate growth). Test these cultures 24 h after obvious growth is detected or after a maximum of 7 days.
3. After a suitable incubation period, test the nitrate broth culture for the presence of gas, reduction of nitrate, and reduction of nitrite according to the following steps:
  a. Observe the inverted Durham tube for the presence of gas, indicated by bubbles inside the tube.
  b. Add five drops each of nitrate reagent solution A (sulfanilic acid) and B (alpha-naphthylamine). Observe for at least 3 min for a red color to develop.
  c. If no color develops, test further with zinc powder. Dip a wooden applicator stick into zinc powder and transfer only the amount that adheres to the stick to the nitrate broth culture to which solutions A and B have been added. Observe for at least 3 min for a red color to develop. Breaking the stick into the tube after the addition of the zinc provides a useful marker for the stage of testing.

Expected Results

The nitrate reduction test is read for the presence or absence of three metabolic products: gas, NO_3, and NO_2. The expected results can be summarized as follows:

Reaction	Gas	Color After Addition of Solutions A and B	Color After Addition of Zinc	Interpretation
$NO_3 \rightarrow NO_2$ (Fig. 12.30A)	None	Red	—	NO_3+, no gas
$NO_3 \rightarrow NO_2$, gas partial non-gaseous end products	None	Red	—	NO_3+, no gas
$NO_3 \rightarrow NO_2$, gaseous end products (Fig. 12.30B)	Yes	Red	—	NO_3+, gas
$NO_3 \rightarrow$ gaseous end product (Fig. 12.30C)	Yes	None	None	NO_3+, NO_2+, gas+ C)
$NO_3 \rightarrow$ non-gaseous end products	None	None	None	NO_3+, NO_2+, no gas
$NO_3 \rightarrow$ no reaction (Fig. 12.30D)	None	None	Red	Negative
Uninoculated tube	None			Uninoculated tube

Limitations

Nitrate reduction is a supportive test for identification of Enterobacterales to the genus level; however, additional follow-up confirmatory testing is required for final identification.

Quality Control

Positive: NO_3+, no gas: *Escherichia coli* (ATCC25922)
Positive: NO_3+, gas: *Pseudomonas aeruginosa* (ATCC17588)
Negative: *Acinetobacter baumannii* (ATCC19606)

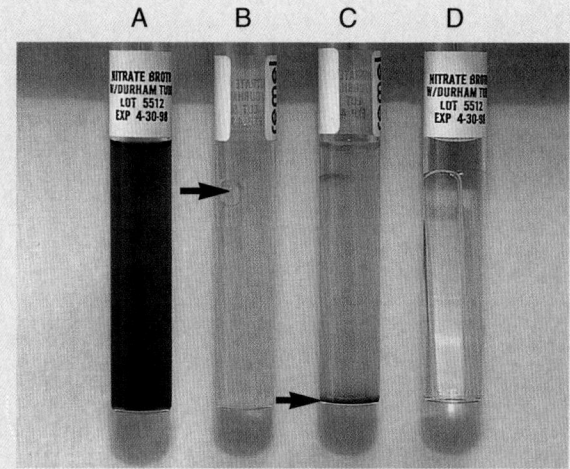

A   B   C   D

• **Fig. 12.30** Nitrate reduction. (A) Positive, no gas. (B) Positive, gas *(arrow)*. (C) Positive, no color after addition of zinc *(arrow)*. (D) Uninoculated tube.

PROCEDURE 12.31

Nitrite Reduction

Purpose

This test is used to determine whether an organism can reduce nitrites to gaseous nitrogen or to other compounds containing nitrogen.

Principle

Microorganisms capable of reducing nitrite to nitrogen do not turn color and do produce gas in the nitrate reduction test (Procedure 12.30). The test does not require the addition of zinc dust.

Media: Brain-heart infusion broth (2 g), pancreatic digest of casein (10 g), peptic digest of animal tissue (5 g), yeast extract (3 g), NaCl (5 g), NaNO$_2$ (0.1 g) per 1000 mL, pH 6.9.

Method

1. Inoculate nitrite broth with one drop from a 24-h broth culture.
2. Incubate for 48 h at 35°C–37°C.
3. Examine 48-h nitrite broth cultures for nitrogen gas in the inverted Durham tube and add five drops each of the nitrate reagents A and B to determine whether nitrite is still present in the medium (reagents A and B are described under the nitrate reduction test in Procedure 12.30).

Expected Results

Positive: No color change to red 2 min after the addition of the reagents; gas production observed in the Durham tube (Fig. 12.31A).

Negative: The broth becomes red after the addition of the reagents. No gas production is observed (Fig. 12.31B).

Limitations

If the broth does not become red and no gas production is observed, zinc dust is added to determine whether the nitrite has not been oxidized to nitrate (thus invalidating the test). If oxidation has occurred, the mixture turns red after the addition of zinc.

Quality Control

Positive: *Proteus mirabilis* (ATCC12453)—colorless; gas production

Negative: *Acinetobacter baumannii* (ATCC19606)—red; no gas production

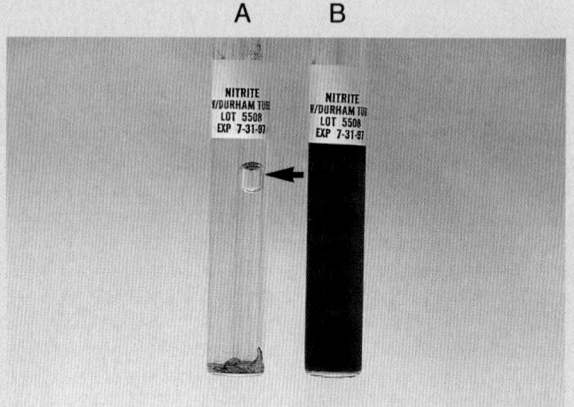

• **Fig. 12.31** Nitrite reduction. (A) Positive, no color change after addition of zinc dust and gas in Durham tube *(arrow)*. (B) Negative.

PROCEDURE 12.32

o-Nitrophenyl-β-D-Galactopyranoside Test

Purpose

This test is used to determine the ability of an organism to produce β-galactosidase, an enzyme that hydrolyzes the substrate o-nitrophenyl-β-D-galactopyranoside (ONPG) to form a visible (yellow) product, ortho-nitrophenol. The test distinguishes late lactose fermenters from non–lactose fermenters of Enterobacterales.

Principle

Lactose fermenters must be able to transport the carbohydrate (β-galactoside permease) and hydrolyze (β-galactosidase) the lactose to glucose and galactose. Organisms unable to produce β-galactosidase may become genetically altered through a variety of mechanisms and be identified as late-lactose fermenters. ONPG enters the cells of organisms that do not produce the permease but are capable of hydrolyzing the ONPG to galactose and a yellow compound, o-nitrophenol, indicating the presence of β-galactosidase.

Media (tube method): Na_2HPO_4 (9.46 g), phenylalanine (4 g), ONPG (2 g), KH_2PO_4 (0.907 g) per 1000 mL, pH 8.0.

Method

1. Aseptically suspend a loop full of organism in 0.85% saline.
2. Place an ONPG disk in the tube.
3. Incubate for 4 h at 37°C in ambient air.
4. Examine tubes for a color change.

Expected Results

Positive: Yellow (presence of β-galactosidase) (Fig. 12.32A).
Negative: Colorless (absence of enzyme) (Fig. 12.32B).

Quality Control

Positive: *Shigella sonnei* (ATCC9290)
Negative: *Salmonella enterica* subsp. *enterica* serovar Typhimurium (ATCC14028)

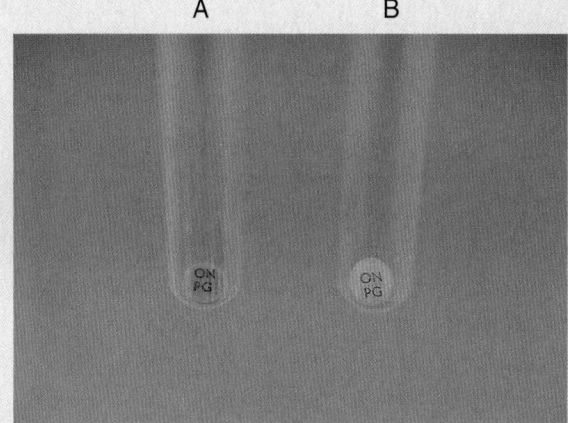

• **Fig. 12.32** o-Nitrophenyl-β-D-galactopyranoside test. (A) Positive. (B) Negative.

PROCEDURE 12.33

Optochin (P disk) Susceptibility Test

Purpose

This test is used to determine the effect of optochin (ethylhydrocupreine hydrochloride) on an organism. Optochin lyses pneumococci (positive test), but alpha-streptococci are resistant (negative test).

Principle

Optochin is an antibiotic that interferes with the ATPase and production of adenosine triphosphate (ATP) in microorganisms. The optochin-impregnated disk (TaxoP) is placed on a lawn of organism on a sheep blood agar plate, allowing the antibiotic to diffuse into the medium. The antibiotic inhibits the growth of a susceptible organism, creating a clearing, or zone of inhibition, around the disk. A zone of 14–16 mm is considered susceptible and presumptive identification for *Streptococcus pneumoniae*.

Method

1. Using an inoculating loop, streak two or three suspect colonies of a pure culture onto half of a 5% sheep blood agar plate.
2. Using heated forceps, place an optochin disk in the upper third of the streaked area. Gently tap the disk to ensure adequate contact with the agar surface.
3. Incubate the plate for 18–24 h at 35°C in 5% CO_2. *Note*: Cultures do not grow as well in ambient air, and larger zones of inhibition occur.
4. Measure the zone of inhibition in millimeters, including the diameter of the disk.

Expected Results

Positive: Zone of inhibition at least 14 mm in diameter with 6-mm disk (Fig. 12.33A).
Negative: No zone of inhibition (Fig. 12.33B).

Limitations

Equivocal: Any zone of inhibition less than 14 mm is questionable for pneumococci; the strain is identified as a pneumococcus with confirmation by a positive bile-solubility test.

Quality Control

Positive: *Streptococcus pneumoniae* (ATCC6305)
Negative: *Streptococcus pyogenes* (ATCC12384)

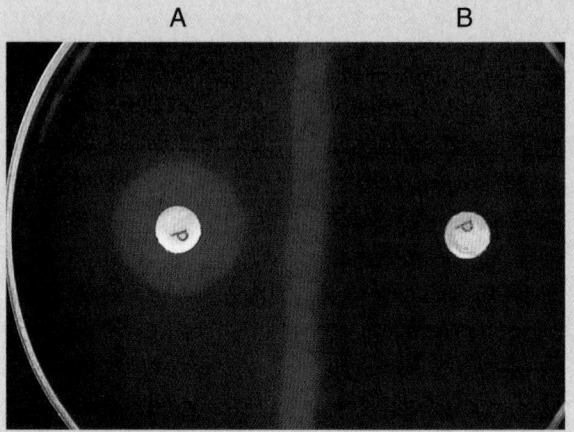

• **Fig. 12.33** Optochin (TaxoP disk) test. (A) *Streptococcus pneumoniae* showing zone of inhibition greater than 14 mm. (B) Alpha-hemolytic *Streptococcus* spp. growing up to the disk.

PROCEDURE 12.34

Oxidase Test (Kovac's Method)

Purpose

This test determines the presence of cytochrome oxidase activity in microorganisms for the identification of oxidase-negative Enterobacterales, differentiating them from other gram-negative bacilli.

Principle

To determine the presence of bacterial cytochrome oxidase using the oxidation of the substrate tetramethyl-p-phenylenediamine dihydrochloride to indophenol, a dark purple–colored end product. A positive test (presence of oxidase) is indicated by the development of a dark purple color. No color development indicates a negative test and the absence of the enzyme.

Method

1. Moisten filter paper with the substrate (1% tetramethyl-p-phenylenediamine dihydrochloride) or select a commercially available paper disk that has been impregnated with the substrate.
2. Use a platinum wire or wooden stick to remove a small portion of a bacterial colony (preferably not more than 24 h old) from the agar surface and rub the sample on the filter paper or commercial disk.
3. Observe the inoculated area of paper or disk for a color change to deep blue or purple (Fig. 12.34) within 10 seconds (timing is critical).

Expected Results

Positive: Development of a dark purple color within 10 seconds (Fig. 12.34A).
Negative: Absence of color (Fig. 12.34B).

Limitations

Using nickel-base alloy wires containing chromium and iron (nichrome) to rub the colony paste onto the filter paper may cause false-positive results.

Quality Control

Positive: *Pseudomonas aeruginosa* (ATCC27853)
Negative: *Escherichia coli* (ATCC25922)

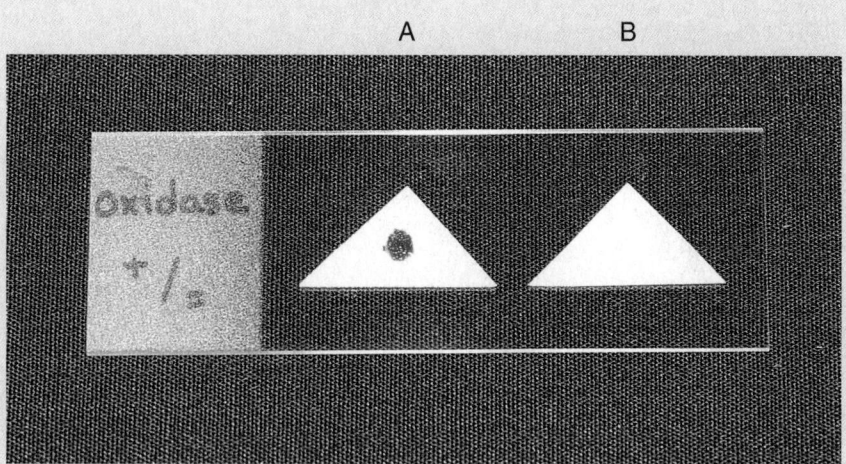

• **Fig. 12.34** Oxidase test. (A) Positive. (B) Negative.

PROCEDURE 12.35

Oxidation and Fermentation of Medium (CDC Method)

Purpose

This test is used to differentiate microorganisms based on the ability to oxidize or ferment specific carbohydrates.

Principle

This test is used to determine whether an organism uses carbohydrate substrates to produce acid byproducts. Nonfermentative bacteria are routinely tested for their ability to produce acid from six carbohydrates (glucose, xylose, mannitol, lactose, sucrose, and maltose). In addition to the six tubes containing carbohydrates, a control tube containing the OF base without carbohydrate is also inoculated. Triple sugar iron (TSI) agar (Procedure 12.41) is also used to determine whether an organism can ferment glucose. OF glucose is used to determine whether an organism ferments (Fig. 12.35A) or oxidizes (Fig. 12.35B) glucose. If no reaction occurs either in the TSI or OF glucose, the organism is considered a non–glucose utilizer (Fig. 12.35C). Hugh and Leifson's formula uses a low peptone-to-carbohydrate ratio and a limiting amount of carbohydrate. The reduced peptone limits the formation of alkaline amines that may mask acid production resulting from oxidative metabolism. Two tubes are required for interpretation of the OF test. Both are inoculated, and one tube is overlaid with mineral oil, producing an anaerobic environment. Production of acid in the overlaid tube results in a color change and is an indication of fermentation. Acid production in the open tube and color change is the result of oxidation.

Media: Pancreatic digest of casein (2 g), glycerol (10.0 mL), phenol red (King method) (0.03 g), agar (3 g) per 1000 mL, pH 7.3.

Method

1. To determine whether acid is produced from carbohydrates, inoculate agar deeps, each containing a single carbohydrate, with bacterial growth from an 18- to 24-h culture by stabbing a needle four to five times into the medium to a depth of 1 cm. Note: Two tubes of OF dextrose are usually inoculated; one is overlaid with either sterile melted petrolatum or sterile paraffin oil to detect fermentation.
2. Incubate the tubes at 35°C–37°C in ambient air for up to 7 days. Note: If screwcap tubes are used, loosen the caps during incubation to allow for air exchange. Otherwise, the control tube and tubes containing carbohydrates that are not oxidized might not become alkaline.

Expected Results

Positive: Acid production (A) is indicated by the color indicator changing to yellow in the carbohydrate-containing deep.

Weak-positive (Aw): Weak acid formation can be detected by comparing the tube containing the medium with carbohydrate with the inoculated tube containing medium with no carbohydrate. Most bacteria that can grow in the OF base produce an alkaline reaction in the control tube. If the color of the medium in a tube containing carbohydrate remains about the same as it was before the medium was inoculated, and if the inoculated medium in the control tube becomes a deeper red (i.e., becomes alkaline), the culture being tested is considered weakly positive, assuming the amount of growth is about the same in both tubes.

Negative: Red or alkaline (K) color in the deep with carbohydrate equal to the color of the inoculated control tube.

No change (NC) or neutral (N): There is growth in the media, but neither the carbohydrate-containing medium nor the control base turns alkaline (red).

Note: If the organism does not grow at all in the OF medium, mark the reaction as no growth (NG).

Limitations

Slow-growing organisms may not produce results for several days.

Quality Control

Note: Appropriate organisms depend on which carbohydrate has been added to the basal medium. Glucose is used as an example.
Fermenter: *Escherichia coli* (ATCC25922)
Oxidizer: *Pseudomonas aeruginosa* (ATCC27853)

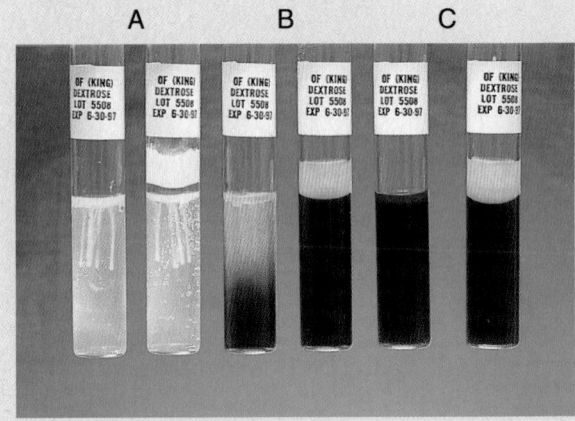

• Fig. 12.35 Oxidation and fermentation medium (CDC method). (A) Fermenter. (B) Oxidizer. (C) Nonutilizer.

PROCEDURE 12.36

Phenylalanine Deaminase Agar

Purpose

This test is used to determine the ability of an organism to oxidatively deaminate phenylalanine to phenylpyruvic acid. The genera *Morganella*, *Proteus*, and *Providencia* can be differentiated from other members of Enterobacterales.

Principle

Microorganisms that produce phenylalanine deaminase remove the amine (NH_2) from phenylalanine. The reaction results in the production of ammonia (NH_3) and phenylpyruvic acid. The phenylpyruvic acid is detected by adding a few drops of 10% ferric chloride; a green-colored complex is formed between these two compounds.

 Media: Phenylalanine (2 g), yeast extract (3 g), NaCl (5 g), Na_3PO_4 (1 g), agar (12 g) per 1000 mL, pH 7.3.

Method

1. Inoculate phenylalanine slant with one drop of a 24-h brain-heart infusion broth.
2. Incubate 18–24 h (or until good growth is apparent) at 35°C–37°C in ambient air with the cap loose.
3. After incubation, add 4–5 drops of 10% aqueous ferric chloride to the slant.

Expected Results

Positive: Green color develops on slant after ferric chloride is added (Fig. 12.36A).

Negative: Slant remains original color after the addition of ferric chloride (Fig. 12.36B).

Quality Control

Positive: *Proteus mirabilis* (ATCC12453)
Negative: *Escherichia coli* (ATCC25922)

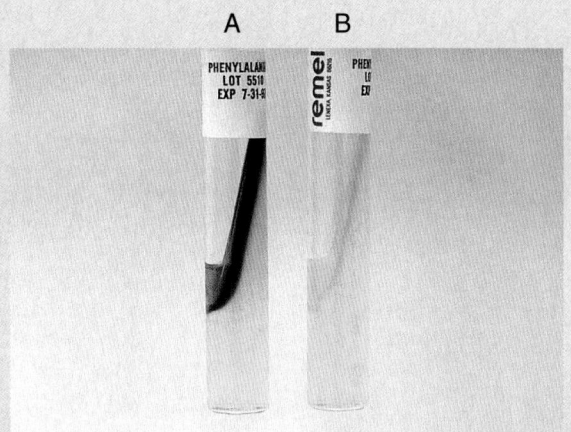

• **Fig. 12.36** Phenylalanine deaminase. (A) Positive. (B) Negative.

PROCEDURE 12.37

L-Pyrrolidonyl Arylamidase Test

Purpose

This test is used for the presumptive identification of group A streptococci (*Streptococcus pyogenes*) and enterococci by the presence of the enzyme L-pyrrolidonyl arylamidase.

Principle

The enzyme L-pyrrolidonyl arylamidase hydrolyzes the L-pyrrolidonyl-β-naphthylamide substrate to produce a β-naphthylamine. The β-naphthylamine can be detected in the presence of N,N-methylamino-cinnamaldehyde reagent by the production of a bright red precipitate.

Method

1. Before inoculation, moisten the disk slightly with reagent-grade water. Do not flood the disk.
2. Using a wooden applicator stick, rub a small amount of several colonies of an 18–24-h pure culture onto a small area of the L-pyrrolidonyl arylamidase (PYR) disk.
3. Incubate at room temperature for 2 min.
4. Add a drop of detector reagent, N,N-dimethylamino-cinnamaldehyde, and observe for a red color within 1 min.

Expected Results

Positive: Bright red color within 5 min (Fig. 12.37A).
Negative: No color change or an orange color (Fig. 12.37B).

Quality Control

Positive: *Enterococcus faecalis* (ATCC29212)
Streptococcus pyogenes (ATCC19615)
Negative: *Streptococcus agalactiae* (ATCC10386)

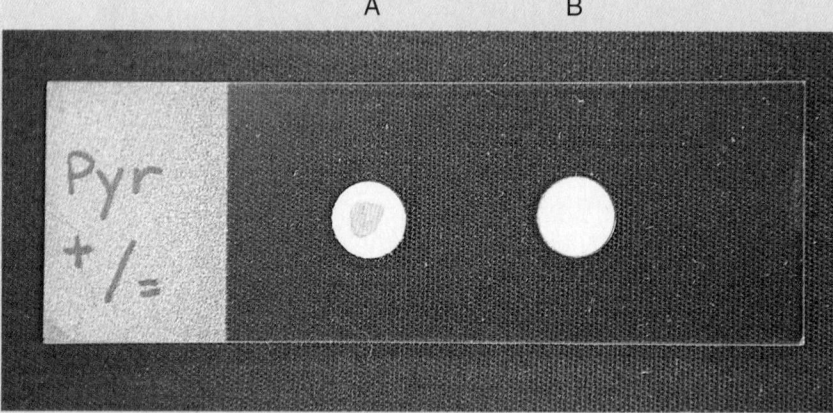

• **Fig. 12.37** L-Pyrrolidonyl arylamidase test. (A) Positive. (B) Negative.

PROCEDURE 12.38

Pyruvate Broth

Purpose

This test is used to determine the ability of an organism to utilize pyruvate. This aids in the differentiation between *Enterococcus faecalis* (positive) and *Enterococcus faecium* (negative).

Principle

Pyruvate broth is a carbohydrate-free, nutrient-limited medium. Pyruvic acid is added to the broth to determine whether the microorganism is able to use pyruvate, resulting in the formation of metabolic acids. Bromothymol blue indicator changes from blue to yellow in the presence of acid as a result of the decrease in pH.

Media: Pancreatic digest of casein (10 g), pyruvic acid, sodium (10 g), yeast extract (5 g), K_2HPO_4 (5 g), NaCl (5 g), bromothymol blue (40 g) per 1000 mL, pH 7.3.

Method

1. Lightly inoculate the pyruvate broth with an 18–24-h culture of the organism from 5% sheep blood agar.
2. Incubate at 35°C–37°C in ambient air for 24–48 h.

Expected Results

Positive: Indicator changes from green to yellow (Fig. 12.38A).
Negative: No color change; yellow-green indicates a weak reaction and should be regarded as negative (Fig. 12.38B).

Quality Control

Positive: *Enterococcus faecalis* (ATCC29212)
Negative: *Streptococcus gallolyticus* (ATCC9809)

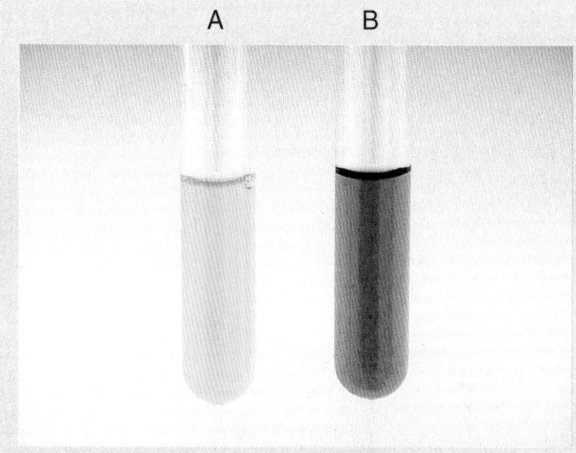

A   B

• **Fig. 12.38** Pyruvate broth. (A) Positive. (B) Negative.

PROCEDURE 12.39

Salt Tolerance Test

Purpose

This test is used to determine the ability of an organism to grow in high concentrations of salt. It is used to differentiate enterococci (positive) from nonenterococci (negative).

Principle

The salt tolerance test is a selective and differential medium. Enterococci are resistant to high salt concentration. A heart infusion broth containing 6.5% NaCl is used as the test medium. This broth also contains a small amount of glucose and bromocresol purple as the indicator for acid production.

Media: Brain-heart infusion (BHI) broth may be used in place of the individual components with the addition of NaCl and indicator dye. Components: Heart digest (10 g), enzymatic digest of animal tissue (10 g), NaCl (65 g), dextrose (1 g), bromocresol purple (0.016 g) per 1000 mL.

Method

1. Inoculate one or two colonies from an 18- to 24-h culture into 6.5% NaCl broth.
2. Incubate the tube at 35°C–37°C in ambient air for 48 h.
3. Check daily for growth.

Expected Results

Positive: Visible turbidity in the broth, with or without a color change from purple to yellow (Fig. 12.39A).
Negative: No turbidity and no color change (Fig. 12.39B).

Quality Control

Positive: *Enterococcus faecalis* (ATCC29212)—growth; color change to yellow
Negative: *Streptococcus gallolyticus* (ATCC9809)—inhibition, as demonstrated by little to no growth; no color change

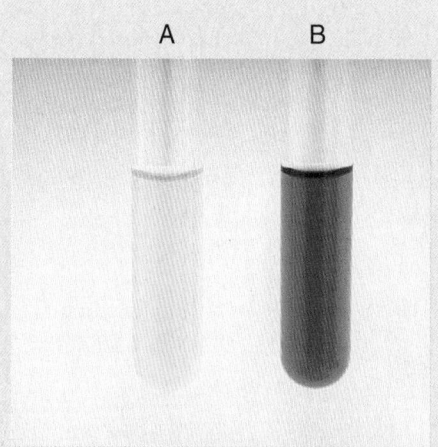

A   B

• **Fig. 12.39** Salt tolerance (6.5% NaCl) test. (A) Positive. (B) Negative.

PROCEDURE 12.40

Spot Indole Test

Purpose

This test is used to determine the presence of the enzyme tryptophanase. It is a rapid method that can be used in lieu of the tube test described in Procedure 12.21.

Principle

Tryptophanase breaks down tryptophan to release indole, which is detected by its ability to combine with certain aldehydes to form a colored compound. For indole-positive bacteria, the blue-green compound formed by the reaction of indole with cinnamaldehyde is easily visualized. The absence of enzyme results in no color production (indole negative).

Method

1. Saturate a piece of filter paper with the 1% paradimethylamino-cinnamaldehyde reagent.
2. Use a wooden stick or bacteriologic loop to remove a small portion of a bacterial colony from the agar surface and rub the sample on the filter paper. Rapid

development of a blue color indicates a positive test result. Most indole-positive organisms turn blue within 30 seconds.

Expected Results

Positive: Development of a blue color within 20 s (Fig. 12.40A).
Negative: No color development or slightly pink color (Fig. 12.40B).

Limitations

The bacterial inoculum should not be selected from MacConkey agar, because the color of lactose-fermenting colonies on this medium can interfere with test interpretation.

Quality Control

Positive: *Escherichia coli* (ATCC25922)
Negative: *Klebsiella pneumoniae* (ATCC13883)

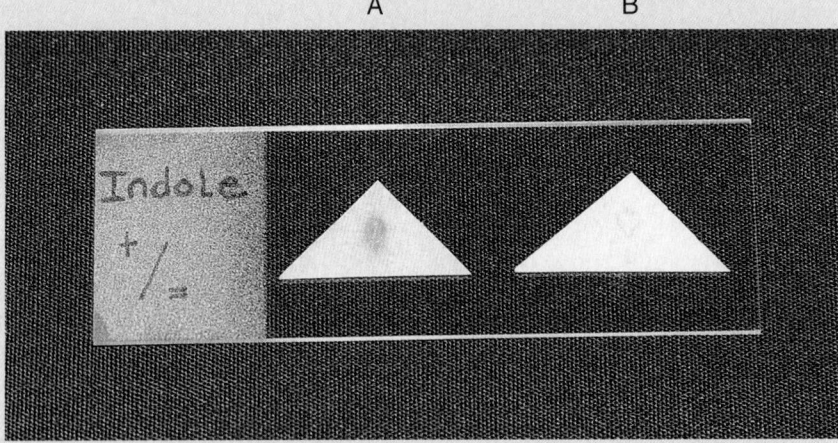

• **Fig. 12.40** Spot indole test. (A) Positive. (B) Negative.

PROCEDURE 12.41

Triple Sugar Iron Agar

Purpose

Triple sugar iron (TSI) agar is used to determine whether a gram-negative rod ferments glucose and lactose or sucrose and forms hydrogen sulfide (H_2S). The test is used primarily to differentiate members of Enterobacterales from other gram-negative rods.

Principle

The composition of TSI is 10 parts lactose: 10 parts sucrose: 1 part glucose and peptone. Phenol red and ferrous sulfate serve as indicators of acidification and H_2S formation, respectively. A glucose-fermenting organism turns the entire medium acidic (yellow) in 8–12 h. The butt remains acidic after the recommended 18–24-h incubation period because of the presence of organic acids resulting from the fermentation of glucose under anaerobic conditions in the butt of the tube. The slant, however, reverts to the alkaline (red) state because of oxidation of the fermentation products under aerobic conditions on the slant. This change is a result of the formation of CO_2 and H_2O and the oxidation of peptones in the medium to alkaline amines. When, in addition to glucose, lactose and/or sucrose are fermented, the large amount of fermentation products formed on the slant neutralizes the alkaline amines and renders the slant acidic (yellow), provided the reaction is read in 18–24 h. Reactions in TSI should not be read beyond 24 hours of incubation, because aerobic oxidation of the fermentation products from lactose and/or sucrose proceeds and the slant eventually reverts to the alkaline state. The formation of CO_2 and hydrogen gas (H_2) is indicated by the presence of bubbles or cracks in the agar or by separation of the agar from the sides or bottom of the tube. The production of H_2S (sodium thiosulfate reduced to H_2S) requires an acidic environment, and reaction with the ferric ammonium citrate produces a blackening of the agar butt in the tube.

Media: Enzymatic digest of casein (5 g), enzymatic digest of animal tissue (5 g), yeast-enriched peptone (10 g), dextrose (1 g), lactose (10 g), sucrose (10 g), ferric ammonium citrate (0.2 g), NaCl (5 g), sodium thiosulfate (0.3 g), phenol red (0.025 g), agar (13.5 g) per 1000 mL, pH 7.3.

Method

1. With a straight inoculation needle, touch the top of a well-isolated colony.
2. Inoculate TSI (Fig. 12.41D) by first stabbing through the center of the medium to the bottom of the tube and then streaking the surface of the agar slant.
3. Leave the cap on loosely and incubate the tube at 35°C–37°C in ambient air for 18–24 h.

Expected Results

Alkaline slant/no change in the butt (K/NC): Glucose, lactose, and sucrose nonutilizer; this may also be recorded as K/K (alkaline slant/alkaline butt) (Fig. 12.41C).

Alkaline slant/acid butt (K/A): Glucose fermentation only.

Acid slant/acid butt (A/A): Glucose, sucrose, and/or lactose fermenter (Fig. 12.41A).

Note: A black precipitate in the butt indicates production of ferrous sulfide and H_2S gas (H_2S+) (Fig. 12.41B). Bubbles or cracks in the tube indicate the production of CO_2 or H_2. Drawing a circle around the A for the acid butt; that is, Ⓐ, usually indicates this means the organism ferments glucose and sucrose; glucose and lactose; or glucose, sucrose, and lactose, with the production of gas.

Quality Control

Ⓐ, gas production: *Escherichia coli* (ATCC25922)

K/A,+/− gas production, H_2S+: *Salmonella enterica* subsp. *enterica* serovar Typhimurium (ATCC14028)

K/K: *Pseudomonas aeruginosa* (ATCC27853)

K/A, H_2S+: *Proteus mirabilis* (ATCC12453)

K/A: *Shigella flexneri* (ATCC12022)

Note: Gas production may also be indicated with a lower case (g) or upper case (G) as indicated:

Small amount of gas: g

Large amount of gas: G

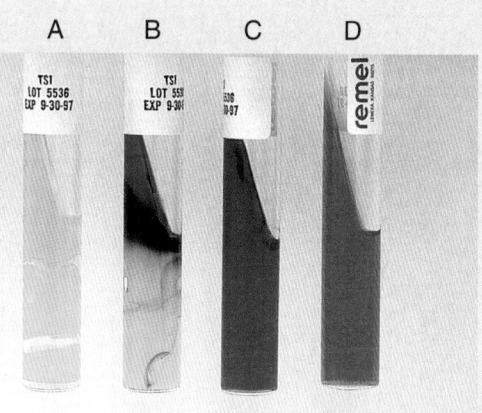

• **Fig. 12.41** Triple sugar iron agar. (A) Acid slant/acid butt with gas, no H_2S (A/A). (B) Alkaline slant/acid butt, no gas, H_2S-positive (K/A H_2S+). (C) Alkaline slant/alkaline butt, no gas, no H_2S (K/K). (D) Uninoculated tube.

PROCEDURE 12.42

Urease Test (Christensen's Method)

Purpose

This test is used to determine an organism's ability to produce the enzyme urease, which hydrolyzes urea. *Proteus* spp. may be presumptively identified by the ability to rapidly hydrolyze urea.

Principle

Urea is the product of decarboxylation of amino acids. Hydrolysis of urea produces ammonia and CO_2. The formation of ammonia alkalinizes the medium, and the pH shift is detected by the color change of phenol red from light orange at pH 6.8 to magenta (pink) at pH 8.1. Rapid urease-positive organisms turn the entire medium pink within 24 h. Weakly positive organisms may take several days, and negative organisms produce no color change or yellow because of acid production.

Media: Enzymatic digest of gelatin (1 g), dextrose (1 g), NaCl (5 g), KH_2PO_4 (2 g), urea (20 g), phenol red (0.012 g) per 1000 mL, pH 6.8.

Method

1. Streak the surface of a urea agar slant with a portion of a well-isolated colony or inoculate slant with one to two drops from an overnight brain-heart infusion broth culture.
2. Leave the cap on loosely and incubate the tube at 35°C–37°C in ambient air for 48 h to 7 days.

Expected Results

Positive: Change in color of slant from light orange to magenta (Fig. 12.42A).
Negative: No color change (agar slant and butt remain light orange) (Fig. 12.42B).

Limitations

Alkaline reactions may appear after prolonged incubation and may be the result of peptone or other protein utilization raising the pH. To eliminate false-positive reactions, perform a control test with the base medium without urea.

Quality Control

Positive: *Proteus vulgaris* (ATCC13315)
Weak positive: *Klebsiella pneumoniae* (ATCC13883)
Negative: *Escherichia coli* (ATCC25922)

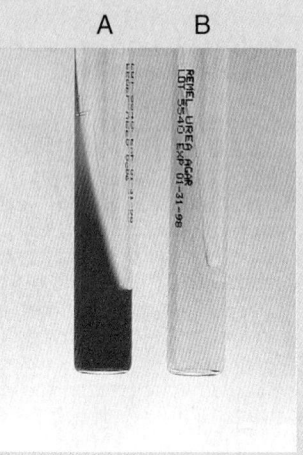

• **Fig. 12.42** Urea hydrolysis (Christensen's method). (A) Positive. (B) Negative.

PROCEDURE 12.43

X and V Factor Test

Purpose

The X and V factor test is used to differentiate *Haemophilus* spp. Members of the genus *Haemophilus* require accessory growth factors *in vitro*. Some *Haemophilus* spp. require X factor (hemin) alone, V factor (nicotinamide adenine dinucleotide [NAD]) alone, or a combination of the two.

Principle

A lawn of the test organism is streaked onto heart infusion agar, tryptic soy agar, *Haemophilus* agar, or nutrient agar. The impregnated disks or strips (X, V, or XV) are placed directly on the confluent inoculation, allowing diffusion of the accessory growth factor into the medium. The organisms will grow only around the disk that provides the appropriate factor for growth of the organism.

Method

1. Make a very light suspension (MacFarland 0.5) of the organism in sterile saline. *Note*: It is important not to carry over any X factor in the medium from which the organism is taken. Therefore, a loop, not a swab, should be used to make the suspension.
2. Dip a sterile swab into the organism suspension. Roll the swab over the entire surface of a trypticase soy agar plate.

3. Place the X, V, and XV factor disks on the agar surface. If using separate disks, place them at least 4–5 cm apart.
4. Incubate overnight at 35°C–37°C in ambient air.

Expected Results

Positive: Growth around the XV disk only shows a requirement for both factors (Fig. 12.43A). Growth around the V disk, no growth around the X disk, and light growth around the XV disk shows a V factor requirement (Fig. 12.43B).

Negative: Growth over the entire surface of the agar indicates no requirement for either X or V factor (Fig. 12.43C).

Quality Control

Positive:
Haemophilus influenzae (ATCC35056): Halo of growth around the XV disk, no growth on the rest of the agar surface
Haemophilus parainfluenzae (ATCC7901): Halo of growth around the XV and V disks
Haemophilus ducreyi (ATCC27722): Halo of growth around the XV and X disks

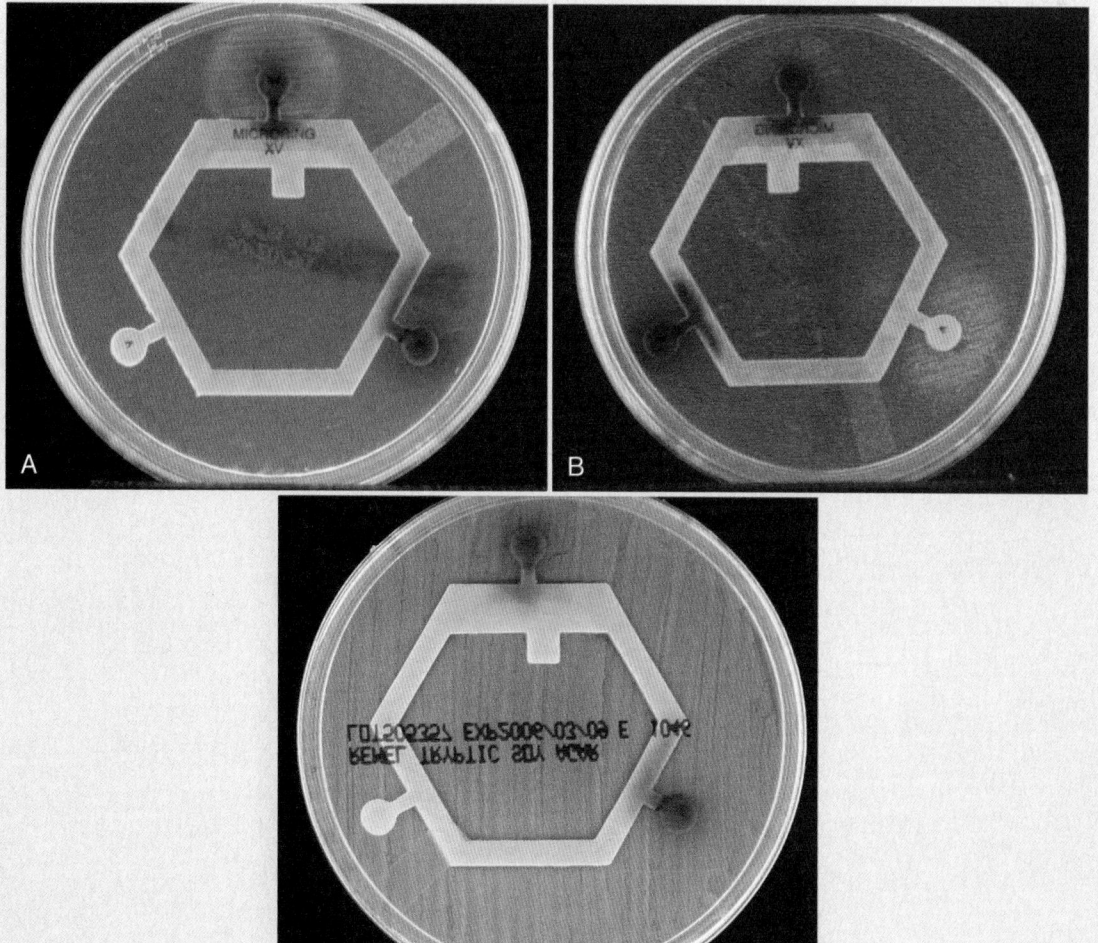

• **Fig. 12.43** X (hemin) and V (nicotinamide adenine dinucleotide [NAD]) factor test. (A) Positive: growth around XV disk only. (B) Positive: growth around V disk. (C) Negative: growth over entire plate.

Bibliography

Alatoom AA, Cunningham SA, Ihde SM, Mandrekar J, Patel R: Comparison of direct colony method versus extraction method for identification of gram-positive cocci by use of Bruker Biotyper matrix-assisted laser desorption ionization-time of flight mass spectrometry, *J Clin Microbiol* 49:2868–2873, 2011.

American Type Culture Collection, P.O. Box 1549, Manassas, Va 20108.

Baker JS, Hackett MF, Simard DJ: Variations in bacitracin susceptibility observed in *Staphylococcus* and *Micrococcus* species, *J Clin Microbiol* 23:963–964, 1986.

Becton, Dickinson & Co. *Quality Control Technical Bulletins.* Sparks, MD: BD Company.

Carroll KC, Pfaller MA, Landry ML, et al: *Manual of clinical microbiology,* ed 12, Washington, DC, ASM, 2019.

Chuard C, Reller LB: Bile-esculin test for presumptive identification of enterococci and streptococci: effects of bile concentration, inoculation technique, and incubation time, *J Clin Microbiol* 36:1135–1136, 1998.

Darling CL: Standardization and evaluation of the CAMP reaction for the prompt, presumptive identification of *Streptococcus agalactiae* (Lancefield group B) in clinical material, *J Clin Microbiol* 1:171–174, 1975.

Hawn CV, Beebe E: Rapid method for demonstrating bile solubility of *Diplococcus pneumoniae, J Bacteriol* 90:549, 1965.

Heimbrook ME, Wang WL, Campbell G: Staining bacterial flagella easily, *J Clin Microbiol* 26:2612–2615, 1989.

Technical data. Mumbai, India.

McDade JJ, Weaver RH: Rapid methods for the detection of gelatin hydrolysis, *J Bacteriol* 77:60–64, 1977.

Neogen Corp. Acumedia, 620 Lesher place, Lansing, Mich, 48912.

Oberhofer TR: Characteristics of human isolates of unidentified fluorescence pseudomonads capable of growth at 42°C, *J Clin Microbiol* 14:492–495, 1981.

Perez JL, Pulido A, Pantozzi F, Martin R: Butyrate esterase (4-methylumbelliferyl butyrate) spot test: a simple method for immediate identification of *Moraxella (Branhamella) catarrhalis, J Clin Microbiol* 28:2347–2348, 1990.

Pilsucki RW, Clayton NW, Cabelli VJ, Cohen PS: Limitations of the Moeller lysine and ornithine decarboxylase tests, *Appl Environ Microbiol* 37:254–260, 1979.

Qadri SM, DeSilva MI, Zubairi S: Rapid test for determination of esculin hydrolysis, *J Clin Microbiol* 12:472–474, 1980.

Scientific. *Technical Data.* Lenexa, KS.

Saffert RT, Cunningham SA, Ihde SM, Jobe KE, Mandrekar J, Patel R: Comparison of Bruker Biotyper matrix-assisted laser desorption ionization-time of flight mass spectrometer to BD Phoenix automated microbiology system for identification of gram-negative bacilli, *J Clin Microbiol* 49:887–892, 2011.

13

Staphylococcus, Micrococcus, and Similar Organisms

OBJECTIVES

1. Describe the general characteristics of *Staphylococcus* spp. and *Micrococcus* spp., including oxygenation, microscopic Gram staining characteristics, and macroscopic appearance on blood agar.
2. Correlate the culture and microscopic characteristics for the clinically relevant gram-positive coccus.
3. Describe the chemical principle and purpose of the primary plating media used for the isolation and differentiation of staphylococci, including 5% sheep blood agar, mannitol salt, phenylethyl alcohol, and colistin nalidixic acid agars.
4. Explain the principle of the coagulase test, including the different principles associated with the slide versus the tube test and the clinical significance.
5. List the various types of diseases and correlate patient populations specifically associated with *Micrococcus* spp., *Staphylococcus aureus, Staphylococcus saprophyticus,* and *Staphylococcus epidermidis.*
6. Outline the basic biochemical testing procedure to differentiate *Staphylococcus* spp. from *Micrococcus* spp., including coagulase-negative and coagulase-positive staphylococci.
7. Identify key biochemical reactions to identify the clinically significant *Staphylococcus* spp., and explain the chemical principle associated with each test.
8. Define methicillin-resistant *S. aureus* (MRSA) as it relates to antibiotic susceptibility.
9. Explain the D zone test principle and its clinical significance in the treatment of *S. aureus.*
10. Describe methods used to control the transmission of multiple drug-resistant organisms such as MRSA within the community and health care settings.
11. Define the following acronyms: MRSA, HA-MRSA, CA-MRSA, and LA-MRSA and understand their significance to antibiotic resistance in the population.

GENERA AND SPECIES TO BE CONSIDERED

Staphylococcus aureus subsp. *anaerobius*
Staphylococcus aureus subsp. *aureus*

Coagulase-negative staphylococci (most commonly encountered)
- *Staphylococcus epidermidis*
- *Staphylococcus haemolyticus*
- *Staphylococcus lugdunensis*
Staphylococcus saprophyticus subsp. *bovis*
Staphylococcus saprophyticus subsp. *saprophyticus*
Staphylococcus schleiferi subsp. *coagulans*
Staphylococcus schleiferi subsp. *schleiferi*
Coagulase variable
- *S. argenteus*
- *S. delphini*
- *S. intermedius*
- *S. pseudintermedius*
Coagulase-negative staphylococci
- *Staphylococcus auricularis*
  Staphylococcus capitis subsp. *capitis*
  Staphylococcus capitis subsp. *ureolyticus*
- *Staphylococcus caprae*
  Staphylococcus cohnii subsp. cohnii
- *Staphylococcus cohnii* subsp. *ureolyticus*
  Staphylococcus gallinarum
  Staphylococcus hominis subsp. *hominis*
  Staphylococcus hominis subsp. *novobiosepticus*
- *Staphylococcus massiliensis*
- *Staphylococcus massiliensis*
- *S. pasteurii*
- *Staphylococcus petrasii* subsp. *croceilyticus*
- *Staphylococcus petrasii* subsp. *jettensis*
- *Staphylococcus petrasii* subsp. *petrasii*
- *Staphylococcus pettenkoferi*
- *Staphylococcus rostra*
- *Staphylococcus saccharolyticus*
- *Staphylococcus sciuri*
- *Staphylococcus. simiae*
- *Staphylococcus simulans*
- Staphylococcus stepanovicii
- *Staphylococcus succinus* subsp. *casei*
- *Staphylococcus succinus* subsp. *succinus*
- *Staphylococcus vitulinus*
- *Staphylococcus warneri*
- *Staphylococcus xylosus*
Alloiococcus
Dermacoccus nishinomiyaensis
Kocuria spp.
Kytococcus spp.
Micrococcus spp.
Rothia mucilaginosa

TABLE 13.1	Epidemiology	
Organism	**Habitat (Reservoir)**	**Mode of Transmission**
Staphylococcus aureus	Normal microbiota: Anterior nares Nasopharynx Perineal area Skin Colonizer of mucosa	Endogenous strain: sterile site by traumatic introduction (e.g., surgical wound or microabrasions) Direct contact: person-to-person, fomites Indirect contact: aerosolized
Staphylococcus epidermidis	Normal microbiota: Skin Mucous membranes	Endogenous strain: sterile site, by implantation of medical devices (e.g., shunts, prosthetic devices) Direct contact: person-to-person
Staphylococcus haemolyticus *Staphylococcus lugdunensis*	Normal microbiota: Skin Mucous membranes (low numbers)	Same as previously indicated for *S. epidermidis*

Staphylococcus
  saprophyticus
	Normal microbiota:
	Skin
	Genitourinary tract
	Mucosa
		Endogenous strain: sterile urinary tract, notably in young,
		  sexually active females

Micrococcus spp. *Kocuria* spp. *Kytococcus* spp. *Rothia* spp. *Dermacoccus* spp. *Auritidibacter* spp. *Macrococcus* spp. *Planococcus* spp. *Aerococcus* spp. *Alloiococcus* spp.	Normal microbiota: Skin Mucosa Oropharynx	Endogenous strain: uncertain Rarely implicated in infections Immunocompromised hosts: brain abscess, meningitis, pneumonia, endocarditis

General Characteristics

The gram-positive cocci are a very heterogenous group with a high frequency of being isolated from patient specimens. Historically, the genus *Staphylococcus* was included with the genus *Micrococcus* in the family *Micrococcaceae*. However, molecular phylogenetic and chemical analysis indicates the two genera are not closely related and belong to different phyla, the Firmicutes and Actinobacteria, respectively. The *Staphylococcus* spp. are now combined with the *Bacillaceae*, *Planococcaceae*, and *Listeriaceae* into the order Bacillales. Forty-nine species, including 25 subspecies, are recognized in the genus *Staphylococcus*. Several of the *Micrococcus* species have been reclassified into the genera *Kocuria*, *Nesterenkonia*, *Kytococcus*, and *Dermacoccus*. These genera have been reorganized into two families, the *Micrococcaceae* and the *Dermacoccaceae*. The only other organism, *Alloiococcus otitidis*, that biochemically reacts similar to the families included in this chapter belongs to the family *Carnobacteriaceae*. The species described in this chapter are all catalase-positive, gram-positive cocci. The organisms are aerobic or facultative anaerobic with the exception of *Staphylococcus aureus* subsp. *anaerobius* and *Staphylococcus saccharolyticus*, which are obligate anaerobes, and may be catalase negative. However, only those belonging to the genus *Staphylococcus* are of primary clinical significance. *Staphylococcus* are non-motile and non–spore forming organisms. Several of the

coagulase-negative staphylococci (CoNS or non–*S. aureus*) species listed may be encountered in clinical specimens. The CoNS are subdivided into two groups based on their novobiocin susceptibility pattern. The CoNS group that demonstrates novobiocin susceptibility includes *Staphylococcus epidermidis*, *Staphylococcus capitis*, *Staphylococcus haemolyticus*, *Staphylococcus hominis* subsp. *hominis*, *Staphylococcus lugdunensis*, *S. saccharolyticus*, *Staphylococcus warneri*, and other species. The novobiocin-resistant group consists of *Staphylococcus cohnii*, *Staphylococcus kloosii*, *Staphylococcus saprophyticus*, and *Staphylococcus xylosus*. Three genera of skin-colonizing organisms, the *Micrococcus* spp., *Kocuria* spp., and *Kytococcus* spp., are easily confused with staphylococci. Occasionally, these genera will be associated with skin lesions and are more commonly isolated from immunocompromised patients.

Epidemiology

As outlined in Table 13.1, the staphylococci associated with infections in humans are colonizers (normal microbiota) of various skin and mucosal surfaces. There are three types of nasal carrier states associated with colonization of *S. aureus*: **persistent carriers** who harbor a single strain for an extended period, **intermittent carriers** who will harbor different strains over time, and **noncarriers,** individuals who do not harbor any organisms. Because the carrier state is common among the human population, infections are frequently acquired when colonizing strains gain access to a normally sterile site because of trauma or abrasion to the skin or mucosal surface. The traumatic event may be so minor that it goes unnoticed, which might impede a timely and accurate diagnosis. The prevalence of *S. aureus* carriers is high among health care providers (e.g., nurses, respiratory therapists), along with immunocompromised or immunosuppressed individuals. The healthcare environment, including all surfaces of health care settings and medical devices, are implicated in the transfer of pathogens. Vaginal carriage intermittently occurs in premenopausal women.

Staphylococci can be efficiently transmitted from person to person. Upon transmission, the organisms may become established as part of the recipient's normal microbiota and later introduced to sterile sites by trauma or invasive medical procedures, such as surgery. Person-to-person spread of staphylococci, particularly including antimicrobial-resistant strains, occurs in hospitals and presents a substantial infection-control concern. In addition, *S. aureus* infections cause outbreaks in prisons, dormitories, athletic environments, and educational settings throughout the community. The staphylococci can spread rapidly as a commensal organism in both humans and pets, and thus should be a consideration in the epidemiology of disease.

Pathogenesis and Spectrum of Disease

Without question, *S. aureus* is the most virulent species of staphylococci encountered. A wide spectrum of factors, not all of which are completely understood, contribute to this organism's ability to establish infections and cause several diseases. *S. aureus* and *S. epidermidis* produce a polysaccharide capsule that inhibits phagocytosis. The capsule, which is produced in various amounts by individual clinical isolates, may appear as a slime layer or biofilm and allows the organisms to adhere to inorganic surfaces and impairs or inhibits the penetration of antibiotics.

The chemical composition of the gram-positive cell affects the mediation of pathogenesis. The peptidoglycan resembles the endotoxin effect of gram negatives by activating complement, interleukin 1 (IL-1), and acting as a chemotactic factor for the recruitment of polymorphonuclear cells (PMNs). This cascade of events causes swelling and may lead to the exacerbation of tissue damage. *S. aureus* produces a surface protein, known as **protein A,** that is bound to the cytoplasmic membrane of the organism, and has a high affinity for the Fc receptor on IgG molecules as well as complement. This mechanism allows *S. aureus* to bind directly to immunoglobulins, thereby decreasing the immune-mediated clearance of organisms from the site of infection. Several toxins and enzymes mediate tissue invasion and survival at the infection site (Table 13.2). Staphylococcal species produce a variety of cytotoxins (alpha, beta, delta, and gamma toxins). Most strains of *S. aureus* produce **alpha toxin,** which disrupts smooth muscle in blood vessels and is toxic to erythrocytes, leukocytes, hepatocytes, and platelets. The

beta toxin, believed to work in conjunction with the alpha toxin, is a heat-labile sphingomyelinase, which catalyzes the hydrolysis of membrane phospholipids resulting in cell lysis. *S. aureus, S. epidermidis,* and *S. haemolyticus* are capable of producing **delta toxin,** which is cytolytic to erythrocytes and demonstrates nonspecific membrane toxicity to other mammalian cells. **Gamma toxin** is produced by all strains of *S. aureus* and may actually function in association with the **Panton-Valentine leukocidin (PVL).** Elaboration of these factors is chiefly responsible for the various skin, wound, and deep tissue infections commonly caused by *S. aureus.* Many of these infections can rapidly become life threatening if not treated and managed appropriately.

Thirty to fifty percent of all *S. aureus* strains are capable of producing one of eight distinct serologic types of a **heat-stable enterotoxin.** The enterotoxins are resistant to hydrolysis by the gastric and intestinal enzymes. The toxins, often found in milk products, are associated with pseudomembranous enterocolitis and toxic shock syndrome, and they may exacerbate the normal immune response, resulting in further tissue damage and systemic pathology.

Localized skin or soft tissue infections (SSTIs) may involve hair follicles (i.e., **folliculitis**) and spread into the tissue causing boils (i.e., **furuncles**). More serious, deeper infections result when the furuncles coalesce to form **carbuncles. Impetigo,** the *S. aureus* skin infection involving the epidermis, is characterized by the production of vesicles that rupture and crust over. Regardless of the initial site of infection, the invasive nature of this organism always presents a threat for deeper tissue invasion, bacteremia, and spread to one or more internal organs, including the respiratory tract. Furthermore, these serious infections have emerged more frequently among the general population and are associated with strains that produce the PVL toxin. PVL is toxic to white blood cells, preventing clearance of the organism by the immune system. These serious soft tissue "**community-associated**" infections are frequently mediated by methicillin-resistant *S. aureus* (community-acquired MRSA or CA-MRSA).

S. aureus also produces toxin-mediated diseases, such as **scalded skin syndrome** and **toxic shock syndrome.** In these cases, the organisms may remain relatively localized, but production of potent toxins causes systemic or widespread effects. With scalded skin syndrome (**Ritter disease**), which usually afflicts neonates, the **exfoliative toxin** is a serine protease that splits the intracellular bridges of the epidermidis, resulting in extensive sloughing of epidermis to produce a burnlike effect on the patient. The toxic shock syndrome toxin (TSST-1), also referred to as **pyrogenic exotoxin C,** has several systemic effects, including fever, desquamation, and hypotension potentially leading to shock and death.

Other coagulase-positive or variable staphylococci are normal microbiota of a variety of animal species, including dogs. These species include *Staphylococcus intermedius, Staphylococcus pseudintermedius,* and *Staphylococcus delphini.* These organisms may be associated with skin infections in

TABLE
13.2 **Pathogenesis and Spectrum of Diseases**

Organism	Virulence Factors	Spectrum of Diseases and Infections
Staphylococcus aureus	Polysaccharide capsule: inhibits phago-cytosis (slime layer or biofilm) Peptidoglycan: activates complement, IL-1, chemotactic to PMNs Teichoic acids: species specific, mediate binding to fibronectin Protein A: affinity for Fc receptor of IgG and complement. Exotoxins: cytotoxins (alpha, beta, delta, and gamma) Leukocidins, PVL Exfoliative toxins Enterotoxins: A-E, G-I heat stable Toxic shock syndrome toxin I (TSST-1); pyrogenic exotoxin C Enzymes: coagulase, clumping factor Catalase Hyaluronidase Fibrinolysin: staphylokinase Lipases Nucleases Penicillinase	Carriers: Persistent in older children and adults, nasophar-ynx Toxin mediated: Scalded skin syndrome: Ritter disease involves ≥90% of the body, pemphigus neonatorum is the localized form evident by a few blisters; both are exfoliative dermatitis caused by toxins A and B Toxic shock syndrome Food poisoning; preformed enterotoxins, resulting in gas-trointestinal symptoms within 2–6 h of consumption of contaminated food Localized skin infections: folliculitis Furuncles and carbuncles Impetigo Tissue and systemic: Wounds Bacteremia; any localized infection can become invasive and lead to bacteremia Endocarditis Osteomyelitis Cerebritis Pyelonephritis
Staphylococcus epider-midis	Exopolysaccharide "slime" or biofilm; antiphagocytic Exotoxins: delta toxin	Normal flora; nosocomial infections: bacteremia associated with indwelling vascular catheters; endocarditis involving prosthetic cardiac valves (rarely involves native valves); infection at intravascular catheter sites, commonly lead-ing to bacteremia; and other infections associated with CSF shunts, prosthetic joints, vascular grafts, postsurgi-cal ocular infections, and bacteremia in neonates under intensive care
Staphylococcus haemo-lyticus and *Staphylo-coccus lugdunensis*	Uncertain; probably similar to those described for *S. epidermidis*	*S. haemolyticus* Endocarditis Bacteremia Peritonitis Urinary tract Wound, bone, and joint infections *S. lugdunensis* Bacteremia Wound infections Endocarditis Endophthalmitis Septic arthritis Vascular catheter infections Urinary tract infections
Staphylococcus sapro-phyticus	Uncertain	Urinary tract infections in sexually active, young women; infections in sites outside urinary tract are not common
Staphylococcus schle-iferi	Uncertain	Endocarditis Septicemia Osteomyelitis Joint infections Wounds
Micrococcus spp. *Kocuria* spp. *Kytococcus* spp. *Rothia* spp. *Dermacoccus* spp. *Auritidibacter* spp. *Macrococcus* spp. *Planococcus* spp. *Aerococcus* spp. *Alloiococcus* spp.	Unknown; probably of extremely low virulence	Usually considered contaminants of clinical specimens; rarely implicated as cause of infections in humans Implicated in otitis externa Implicated in otitis media

CSF, Cerebrospinal fluid; *IL*, interleukin; *PMN*, polymorphonuclear cell; *PVL*, Panton-Valentine leukocidin.

dogs, as well as invasive infections in immunocompromised humans because of a bite or scratch wound.

The CoNS, among which *S. epidermidis* is the most commonly encountered, are substantially less virulent than *S. aureus* and are opportunistic pathogens. Their prevalence as health care–associated pathogens is as much, if not more, related to medical procedures and practices as to the organism's capacity to establish an infection. Infections with *S. epidermidis* and, less commonly, *S. haemolyticus* and *S. lugdunensis,* usually involve implantation of medical devices (Table 13.2). This kind of medical intervention improves the ability of these normally noninvasive organisms to cause infection. Two organism characteristics that enhance the likelihood of infection include production of a slime layer or biofilm, facilitating attachment to implanted medical devices, and the ability to acquire resistance to most of the antimicrobial agents used in health care environments. *S. lugdunensis* infections resemble *S. aureus* infections.

Although most coagulase-negative staphylococci are primarily associated with health care–associated infections (HAIs), urinary tract infections caused by *S. saprophyticus* are clear exceptions. This organism is most frequently associated with community-acquired urinary tract infections in young, sexually active females but is not commonly associated with HAIs or any infections at non–urinary tract sites. It is the second most common (after *Escherichia coli*) cause of urinary tract infections in young females.

Because coagulase-negative staphylococci are ubiquitous colonizers, they frequently act as contaminants in clinical specimens. This fact, coupled with the emergence of these organisms as health care–associated pathogens, complicates laboratory interpretation of their clinical significance. When these organisms are isolated from clinical specimens, every effort should be made to substantiate their clinical relevance in a particular patient.

The *Micrococcaceae* and *Dermacoccaceae* are generally normal microbiota of the skin and considered as harmless saprophytes; however, they can also act as opportunistic pathogens. Some of the genera including *Micrococcus, Kocuria,* and *Kytococcus* spp. have been associated with infections such as endocarditis, pneumonia, sepsis, FBRIs, and skin infections in immunocompromised patients. Foreign body–related infections (FBRIs), particularly catheter-related infections, significantly contribute to the increasing problem of nosocomial infections. However, recovery of the recently described environmental species of the *Micrococcaceae* and *Dermacoccaceae* should be assessed for clinical significance, as reported for *Kocuria rhizophila, Kocuria marina,* and *Dermacoccus barathri. Auritidibacter ignavus* has been cultivated from the ear swab of a patient with otitis externa; however, its role as a causative agent has not been clarified.

R. mucilaginosa has been implicated in cases of bacteremia, endocarditis, endophthalmitis, intravascular catheter-related and central nervous system infections, pneumonia, peritonitis, septicemia, and cervical necrotizing fasciitis. What, if any, virulence factors are produced by the remaining genera within this group is not known. Because these organisms are rarely associated with infections in healthy individuals, they are probably of low virulence and will not be discussed in detail in this chapter.

Alloiococcus otitis has been associated with infections of the middle ear; however, its role in the pathogenesis of otitis media remains a matter of debate. Some case reports have described other entities, such as endocarditis and endophthalmitis, some of which followed chronic otitis media.

Laboratory Diagnosis

Specimen Collection and Transport

No special considerations are required for specimen collection and transport of the organisms discussed in this chapter. Refer to Table 5.1 for general information on specimen collection and transport.

Specimen Processing

No special considerations are required for processing of the organisms discussed in this chapter. Refer to Table 5.1 for general information on specimen processing.

Direct Detection Methods

Microscopy

Most of the genera included within this chapter produce spherical, gram-positive cells. However, some of the species within the *Micrococcaceae* and *Dermacoccaceae* exhibit rod-shaped cells and are motile. During cell division, the organisms divide along both longitudinal and horizontal planes, forming pairs, tetrads, and, ultimately, irregular clusters (Fig. 13.1A). Gram stains should be performed on young cultures, because very old cells lose their ability to retain crystal violet and may appear gram variable or gram-negative. Micrococci typically appear as gram-positive cocci in tetrads, rather than large clusters (Fig. 13.1B). The additional related genera (i.e., *Kytococcus, Nesterenkonia, Dermacoccus, Arthrobacter,* and *Kocuria*) resemble the staphylococci microscopically.

Nucleic Acid Detection

Several nucleic acid amplification tests (NAAT) have been developed and approved by the US Food and Drug Administration (FDA) for the detection of staphylococci, most of which use single-locus polymerase chain reaction (PCR) amplification methods. Some of these tests are designed to detect MRSA and target *S. aureus* (specifically MRSA) from swab specimens or blood cultures. The assays detect the *mecA* gene (which encodes methicillin resistance) in conjunction with a species-specific target gene. Several of the most commonly used MRSA test systems include the BD GeneOhm MRSA ACP and StaphSR assays (BD, Franklin Lakes, NJ), the Xpert MRSA/SA tests for nasopharyngeal swabs and blood cultures (Cepheid, Sunnyvale, CA), and the Roche LightCycler MRSA Advanced Test (Roche Diagnostics, Indianapolis, IN). The rapid tests, such as the Cepheid Xpert MRSA/SA platform, offer turn-around times of approximately 1 hour

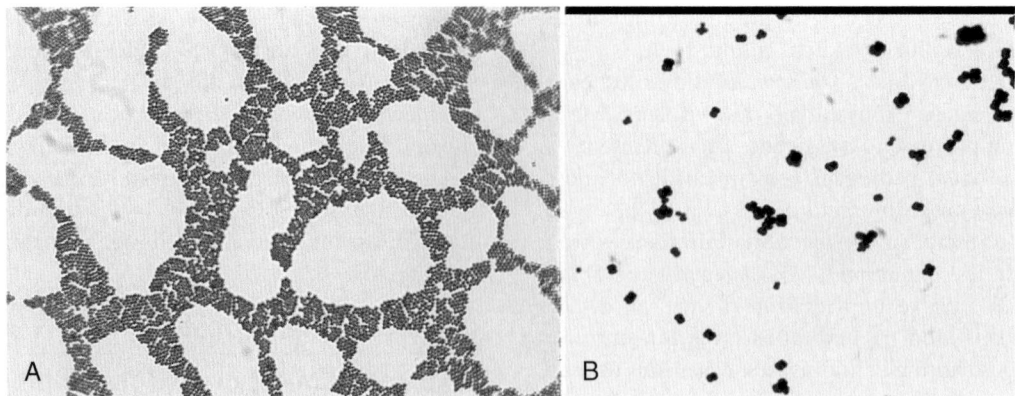

• **Fig. 13.1** (A) Indirect Gram stain of *Staphylococcus aureus* demonstrating characteristic clusters of gram-positive cocci. (B) Indirect Gram stain of *Micrococcus luteus* demonstrating characteristic tetrads or small clusters of gram-positive cocci.

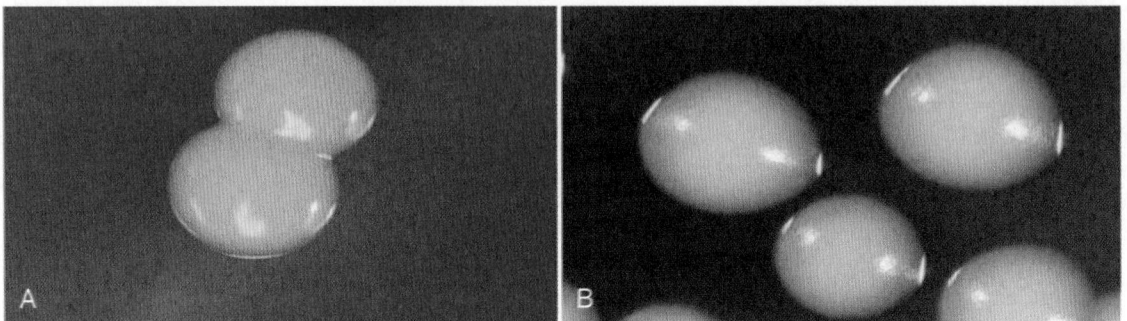

• **Fig. 13.2** (A) Yellow colonies of *Staphylococcus aureus* fermenting mannitol as evident by the yellow color of the agar. (Agar appears darkened due to laboratory bench under petri dish.) (B) White colonies of *Staphylococcus epidermidis*, no-mannitol fermenting, as evident by the original pink color of the agar. (Courtesy Malissa Tille, Sioux Falls, South Dakota.)

and facilitate systematic screening of hospital/clinic attendees. Such screening programs have proven to be cost-effective in many settings by reducing costs and unnecessary infection control measures to prevent HAIs.

Other molecular assays available include the Accuprobe, a commercially available DNA probe assay used for the confirmation of an identification of *S. aureus* (Hologic, Inc., San Diego, CA). *S. aureus* may also be identified by amplification of the *nuc* gene, which encodes a thermostable nuclease. The amplified DNA product is an approximately 270 bp fragment. The limit of detection for successful isolation and amplification is less than 10 colony-forming units or 0.69 pg of DNA and is highly specific. Additional amplification assays have been developed that detect species-specific genes or chromosomal sequences including 16S and 23S ribosomal ribonucleic acid (rRNA) genes and spacer regions, elongation factor (*tuf*), DNA gyrase (*gyrA*), superoxide dismutase (*sodA*), glyceraldehyde-3-phosphate dehydrogenase gene (*gap*), and a heat shock protein (*HSP60/GroE*). MRSA has been identified using the staphylococcal insertion sequence *IS431*.

A qualitative nucleic acid hybridization assay that targets rRNA sequences in *S. aureus* and CoNS has been developed by bioMérieux. The hybridization assay is based on the binding of a peptide nucleic acid (PNA) labeled with a fluorescent dye to *S. aureus* in a blood smear prepared from a positive blood culture bottle.

For first generation molecular tests, it has been historically recommended to perform a follow-up, culture-based confirmatory test. However, most modern FDA-approved MRSA/SA tests perform as stand-alone diagnostic tests and are characterized by very high sensitivity and specificity compared with culture.

Cultivation

Media of Choice

The organisms will grow on 5% sheep blood and chocolate agars. They also grow well in broth-blood culture systems and common nutrient broths, such as thioglycollate, dextrose, and brain-heart infusion broth.

Selective media can be used to isolate staphylococci from clinical material. Phenylethyl alcohol (PEA) or Columbia colistin-nalidixic acid (CNA) agars may be used to eliminate contamination by gram-negative organisms in heavily contaminated specimens such as feces. In addition, mannitol salt agar (MSA) may be used for this purpose. This agar contains a high concentration of salt (10%), the sugar mannitol, and phenol red as the pH indicator. *S. aureus* ferments mannitol and produces acid lowering the pH, which creates a yellow halo on this media (Fig. 13.2). Although MSA is not typically used in clinical identification, it may be useful to purify staphylococci from contaminating organisms for further characterization.

CHROMagar (originally invented by Alain Rambach) is a selective and differential media for the identification of MRSA. The medium is now available from a variety of manufacturers. These media are becoming more widely used for the direct detection of nasal colonization. The medium is selective because it contains cefoxitin, and MRSA is resistant to this antibiotic. The addition of chromogenic substrates hydrolyzed by the organisms produce a mauve-colored colony, allowing for the identification of the organisms. Other organisms will hydrolyze various chromogenic substances within the media, resulting in a variety of colored colonies from white to blue to green (Fig. 13.3).

Incubation Conditions and Duration

Visible growth on 5% sheep blood and chocolate agars incubated at 35°C in carbon dioxide (CO_2) or ambient air usually occurs within 24 hours of inoculation. MSA and other selective media may require incubation for at least 48 to 72 hours before growth is detected. CHRO-Magar requires storage and incubation in the dark for best results.

Colonial Appearance

Table 13.3 describes the colonial appearance and other distinguishing characteristics (e.g., hemolysis) of each genus and various staphylococcal species on 5% sheep blood agar. Growth on chocolate agar is similar. *Micrococcus* spp. are generally easily distinguishable from staphylococci species by the production of brightly colored yellow, orange, or

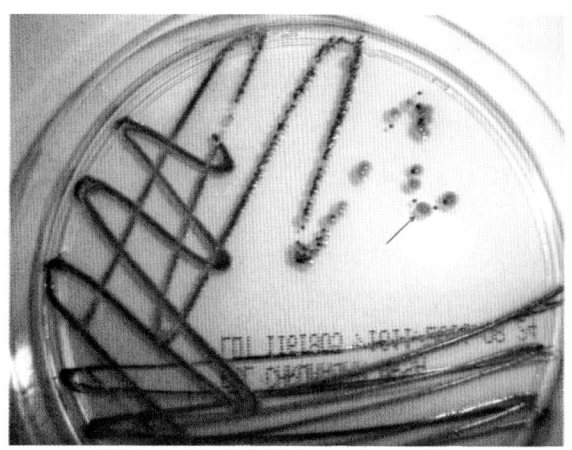

• **Fig. 13.3** CHROMagar for the identification of methicillin-resistant *Staphylococcus aureus* isolates through the selective and differential formation of mauve-colored colonies. (Courtesy Stacie Lansink, Sioux Falls, South Dakota.)

TABLE 13.3	Colonial Appearance and Characteristics on 5% Sheep Blood Agar
Organism	**Appearance**
Micrococcus spp. and related organisms[a]	Small to medium (1–2 µm); opaque, convex; nonhemolytic; wide variety of pigments (white, tan, yellow, orange, pink)
Staphylococcus aureus	Medium to large (0.5–1.5 µm); smooth, entire, slightly raised, low convex, opaque; most colonies pigmented creamy yellow; most colonies beta-hemolytic (Fig. 13.6)
Staphylococcus epidermidis	Small to medium; opaque, gray-white colonies; most colonies nonhemolytic; slime-producing strains are extremely sticky and adhere to the agar surface
Staphylococcus haemolyticus	Medium; smooth, butyrous, and opaque; beta-hemolytic (Fig. 13.7)
Staphylococcus hominis	Medium to large; smooth, butyrous, and opaque; may be unpigmented or cream-yellow-orange; nonhemolytic
Staphylococcus lugdunensis	Medium to large; smooth, glossy, entire edge with slightly domed center; unpigmented or cream to yellow-orange, may be beta-hemolytic
Staphylococcus warneri	Resembles *S. lugdunensis*
Staphylococcus saprophyticus	Large; entire, very glossy, smooth, opaque, butyrous, convex; usually white but colonies can be yellow or orange; nonhemolytic
Staphylococcus schleiferi	Medium to large; smooth, glossy, slightly convex with entire edges; unpigmented; may be hemolytic
Staphylococcus intermedius	Large; slightly convex, entire, smooth, glossy, translucent; usually nonpigmented; delayed to nonhemolytic
Staphylococcus hyicus	Large; slightly convex, entire, smooth, glossy, opaque; usually nonpigmented; nonhemolytic
Staphylococcus capitis	Small to medium; smooth, slightly convex, glistening, entire, opaque; *S. capitis* subsp. *ureolyticus* usually pigmented (yellow or yellow-orange); *S. capitis* subsp. *capitis* is nonpigmented; delayed to nonhemolytic

continued

TABLE 13.3 Colonial Appearance and Characteristics on 5% Sheep Blood Agar—cont'd

Organism	Appearance
Staphylococcus cohnii	Medium to large; convex, entire, circular, smooth, glistening, opaque; *S. cohnii* subsp. *urealyticum* usually pigmented (yellow or yellow-orange); *S. cohnii* subsp. *cohnii* is nonpigmented; delayed to nonhemolytic
Staphylococcus simulans	Large; raised, circular, nonpigmented, entire, smooth, slightly glistening; delayed to nonhemolytic
Staphylococcus auricularis	Small to medium; smooth, butyrous, convex, opaque, entire, slightly glistening; nonpigmented; nonhemolytic
Staphylococcus xylosus	Large; raised to slightly convex, circular, smooth to rough, opaque, dull to glistening; some colonies pigmented yellow or yellow-orange; nonhemolytic
Staphylococcus sciuri	Medium to large; raised, smooth, glistening, circular, opaque; most strains pigmented yellow in center of colonies; may be hemolytic
Staphylococcus caprae	Small to medium; circular, entire, convex, opaque, glistening; nonpigmented; delayed to nonhemolytic

aIncludes *Kytococcus, Nesterenkonia, Dermacoccus, Kocuria, Rothia* spp., *Auritidibacter* spp., *Macrococcus* spp., *Planococcus* spp., *Aerococcus* spp., *Alloiococcus* spp., and *Arthrobacter* spp.

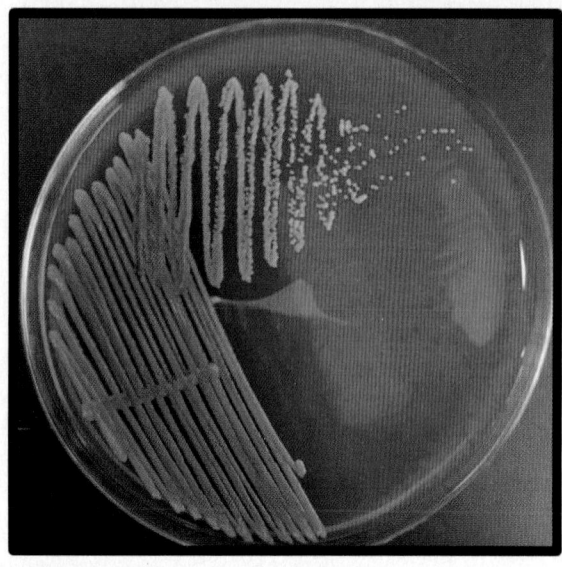

• **Fig. 13.4** *Micrococcus lylae* on TSA (tryptic soy agar) 5% sheep blood agar demonstrating a light pink pigmentation.)

light pink pigmentation (Fig. 13.4). *S. aureus* yields colonies surrounded by a yellow halo on MSA. In addition, small colony variants of *S. aureus* appear as small, pinpoint, nonhemolytic, and nonpigmented colonies on blood agar. **Small colony variants (SCVs)** may result from limited nutrients or other selective pressures and may revert to the normal *S. aureus* phenotype after subculture. However, other staphylococci (particularly *S. saprophyticus*) may also ferment mannitol and resemble *S. aureus* on this medium.

Approach to Identification

The commercial systems for identification of *Staphylococcus* spp. and *Micrococcus* spp. are discussed in Chapter 12 and are generally suitable for the identification of *S. aureus, S. epidermidis,* and *S. saprophyticus.* The identification of the other species varies from system to system. In addition, automated systems may not correctly identify nutritionally variant forms such as small colony variants and other unusual isolates, and therefore follow-up testing may be required for confirmatory identification of the isolates.

Gram stains are used in the clinical laboratory as the initial characterization method for all gram-positive cocci. Microscopic along with macroscopic colonial morphology (Table 13.3) provides a presumptive identification. The *Staphylococcus* spp. and *Micrococcus* spp. are distinguishable from the related family *Streptococcaceae* (Chapter 14) by the catalase test. However, some strains of catalase negative staphylococci have been identified. Table 13.4 shows how the catalase-positive, gram-positive cocci can be differentiated. Because they may show a pseudocatalase reaction—that is, they may appear to be catalase-positive—*Aerococcus* and *Enterococcus* are included in Table 13.4; *Rothia* (formerly *Stomatococcus*) is included for the same reason. Once an organism has been characterized as a gram-positive, catalase-positive, coccoid bacterium, complete identification may involve a series of tests, including (1) atmospheric requirements, (2) resistance to 0.04 U of bacitracin and furazolidone, and (3) possession of cytochrome C as determined by the microdase (modified oxidase) test. However, in the busy setting of many clinical and medical laboratories, microbiologists proceed immediately to a coagulase test based on recognition of a staphylococcal-like colony and a positive catalase test.

Microdase disks, a modified oxidase test, are available commercially (Remel, Inc., Lenexa, KS). This test is used for differentiating *Micrococcus* spp. from *Staphylococcus* spp. A visible amount of growth from an 18- to 24-hour-old culture is smeared on the disk; *Micrococcus* spp. turn blue

TABLE 13.4 **Differentiation Among Gram-Positive, Catalase-Positive Cocci**

Organism	Catalase	Microdase (Modified Oxidase)	Aerotolerance	Bacitracin (0.04 U)[a]	Resistance to:	
					Furazolidone (100 μg)[a]	Lysostaphin (≥200 g/L)
Staphylococcus	+[d]	−[c]	FA	R	S	S
Micrococcus	+	+	A[d]	S	R	R[e]
Macrococcus	+	+	A/FA[h]	R	S	S
Planococcus	+	ND	A	ND	R	S
Rothia	±	−	FA	R or S	R or S	R
Aerococcus	−[f]	−	FA[g]	S	S	R
Kocuria	+	+	A/FA[d]	R	S	S
Alloiococcus	±	−	A	ND	ND	ND
Enterococcus	−[f]	−	FA	R	S	R
Streptococcus	−	−	FA	R or S	S	R

[a]For bacitracin, susceptible ≥10 mm; for furazolidone, susceptible ≥15 mm.
[b]*S. aureus* subsp. *anaerobius* and *S. saccharolyticus* are catalase-negative and only grow anaerobically.
[c]*S. sciuri, Macrococcus caseolyticus, S. lentus,* and *S. vitulinus* are microdase-positive.
[d]*Kocuria (Micrococcus) kristinae* is facultatively anaerobic.
[e]Some strains of *Micrococcus, Arthrobacter (Micrococcus) agilis,* and *Kocuria* are susceptible to lysostaphin.
[f]Some strains may show a pseudocatalase reaction.
[g]Grows best at reduced oxygen tension and may not grow anaerobically.
[h]Organism is microaerophilic.
A, Strict aerobe; *FA,* facultative anaerobe or microaerophile; *ND,* no data available; *R,* resistant; *S,* sensitive; *+,* ≥90% of species or strains positive; *±,* ≥90% of species or strains weakly positive; *−,* ≥90% of species or strains negative.
Data compiled from Schumann P, Spröer C, Burghardt J, et al. Reclassification of the species *Kocuriaerythromyxa* (Brooks & Murray, 1981) as *Kocuriarosea* (Flügge, 1886). *Int J Syst Bacteriol.* 1999;49:393; Stackerbrandt E, Koch C, Gvozdiak O, et al. Taxonomic dissection of the genus *Micrococcus:* gen nov, *Nesterenkonia* gen nov, *Kytococcus* gen nov, *Dermacoccus* gen nov, and *Micrococcus* (Cohn, 1872) gen emend. *Int J Syst Bacteriol.* 1995;45:682; Caroll KC, Pfaller MA. *Manual of Clinical Microbiology.* 12th ed. Washington, DC: ASM Press; 2019.

within two minutes (Fig. 12.26). A variety of tests including the formation of acid from carbohydrates followed by tests for glycosidases, hydrolases, and peptidases are used for species identification and are included in a variety of identification panels.

Disk tests are used for the determination of bacitracin and furazolidone resistance (Fig. 13.5). A 0.04-U bacitracin-impregnated disk and a 100-μg furazolidone-impregnated disk are both available from Becton Dickinson. The disks are placed on the surface of a 5% sheep blood agar streaked in three directions with a cotton-tipped swab that has been dipped in a bacterial suspension prepared to match the turbidity of the 0.5 McFarland standard (i.e., the same as that used in preparing inoculum for disk diffusion susceptibility tests as described in Chapter 11). The tests are interpreted based on the inhibition or sensitivity of the bacteria by measuring the zone of inhibition present around the disk.

Additional rapid identification systems are available for presumptive screening for the detection of **clumping factor A,** a cell wall–associated adhesin for fibrinogen and protein A.

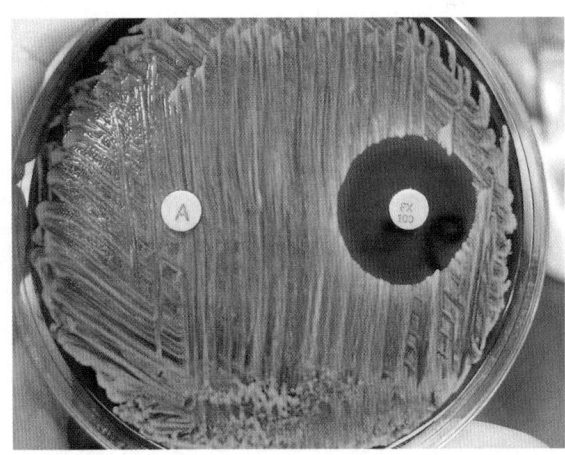

• **Fig. 13.5** *Staphylococcus epidermidis* screening plate showing resistance to bacitracin (Taxo A disk) and susceptibility to furazolidone (FX disk).

Comments Regarding Specific Organisms

Micrococcus spp. and related genera are (1) not lysed with lysostaphin, (2) resistant to the antibiotic furazolidone, (3) susceptible to 0.04 U of bacitracin, and (4) microdase-positive; they usually will only grow aerobically. In contrast, staphylococci are (1) lysed with lysostaphin, (2) resistant to 0.04 U of bacitracin, (3) susceptible to furazolidone, (4) microdase-negative, and (5) facultatively anaerobic.

Once an isolate is identified as, or strongly suspected to be, a species of staphylococci, a test for **coagulase** production is performed to separate *S. aureus* from the other species collectively referred to as coagulase-negative staphylococci.

The enzyme coagulase produced by *S. aureus* binds plasma fibrinogen and activates a cascade of reactions causing plasma to clot. An organism can produce two types of coagulase, referred to as bound and free (Procedure 12.12 includes information on coagulase tests). **Bound coagulase,** or clumping factor, is detected using a rapid slide test (i.e., the slide coagulase test), in which a positive test is indicated when the organisms agglutinate when mixed with plasma (Fig. 12.13A). Most, but not all, strains of *S. aureus* produce clumping factor and thus are readily detected by this test. Approximately 10% to 15% of strains may give a negative latex coagulase test as a result of the masking by capsular polysaccharides. In addition, false positives may occur because of auto agglutination from colonies grown on media with high salt concentrations.

Isolates suspected of being *S. aureus,* but failing to produce bound coagulase, must be tested for production of **extracellular** (i.e., **free**) **coagulase,** because *S. lugdunensis* and *S. schleiferi* may give a positive latex coagulase test. This extracellular coagulase test, referred to as the **tube coagulase** test, is performed by inoculation of a tube containing plasma and incubating at 35°C. Production of the enzyme results in a clot formation within 1 to 4 hours of inoculation (Fig. 12.12B). Some strains produce **fibrinolysin,** dissolve the clot after 4 hours of incubation at 35°C, and may appear to be negative if allowed to incubate longer than 4 hours. Because citrate-utilizing organisms may yield false-positive results, plasma containing ethylenediaminetetraacetic acid (EDTA) rather than citrate should be used. Differentiation of coagulase-positive staphylococci is included in Table 13.5.

Various commercial systems are available that substitute for the conventional coagulase tests previously described. Latex agglutination procedures that detect clumping factor and protein A and passive hemagglutination tests capable of detecting clumping factor are no longer used extensively because they often fail to detect MRSA strains, which are being isolated from an increasing number of community-acquired infections. In addition, the recent third-generation assays that include monoclonal antibodies to the capsular polysaccharide serotypes 5 and 8 or other molecules have a higher sensitivity but are less specific. False-positive reactions occur in the presence of some CoNS species, such as *S. haemolyticus, S. hominis,* and *S. saprophyticus.*

Table 13.5 lists the results for various tests used to differentiate the coagulase-positive staphylococci; *S. intermedius* is an important agent isolated from dog bite wound infections often misidentified as *S. aureus* if only coagulase testing is performed. Microbiologists should perform

additional confirmatory tests for cases in which coagulase-positive staphylococci are isolated from dog bite infections. Otherwise, catalase-positive, gram-positive cocci in clusters form a beta-hemolytic, white to yellow, creamy, opaque colony on blood agar (Fig. 13.6) that is latex coagulase-positive and tube coagulase-positive within 4 hours may be presumptively identified as *S. aureus.*

Many laboratories now speciate all staphylococci isolates due to the high degree of biochemical variability associated with clinical isolates. Definitive species identification should always include isolates from normally sterile sites (blood, joint fluid, or cerebrospinal fluid [CSF]); isolates from prosthetic devices, catheters, and shunts; and isolates from urinary tract infections that may be *S. saprophyticus.*

The coagulase-negative staphylococci may be identified based on the criteria shown in Tables 13.6 to 13.8. Isolates not identified to species are often reported as "coagulase-negative staphylococci" in some laboratories.

It is particularly important to differentiate *S. lugdunensis* from other coagulase-negative staphylococci from sterile sites because there are different interpretive criteria for susceptibility to oxacillin for this organism. *S. lugdunensis* is positive for both the 2-hour pyrrolidonyl aminopeptidase (PYR) and ornithine decarboxylase tests.

Serodiagnosis

Serologic testing for antibodies associated with infections from staphylococcal organisms is not clinically relevant because of low specificity and the presence of cross-reactive antibodies. Antibodies to teichoic acid, a major cell wall component of gram-positive bacteria, are usually produced in long-standing or deep-seated staphylococcal infections, such as osteomyelitis. This procedure is usually performed in reference laboratories. However, the clinical use of this assay is, at best, uncertain. The identification of protective antibodies in toxin-mediated syndromes such as toxic shock syndrome and staphylococcal scalded skin syndrome may be absent or present at very low levels. However, seroconversion after the onset of symptoms and during convalescence may be observed. Various kits are available for the detection of staphylococcal toxins in foods or patient specimens that may be helpful in clinical diagnosis. Additional assays for the detection of other staphylococcal proteins are being examined for their clinical use in identifying staphylococcal infections.

Matrix-Assisted Desorption Ionization Time of Flight

In recent years, alternative methods for identifying *S. aureus* and MRSA have been employed in the clinical laboratory, including matrix-assisted laser desorption ionization time-of-flight mass spectrometry (MALDI-TOF MS). MALDI-TOF MS (Chapter 7) follows culture-based assays in the diagnostic workflow. For example, this method can be used to discern between methicillin-sensitive *S. aureus* (MSSA) and MRSA and can provide information regarding strain

TABLE 13.5 Differentiation Among the Most Clinically Significant Clumping Factor or Tube Coagulase-Positive Staphylococci

Organism	Clumping Factor	Tube Coagulase	Heat Stable Nuclease	Alkaline Phosphatase	Ornithine Decarboxylase	Acetoin Production	Novobiocin Resistance	Polymyxin B Resistance	Beta-galactosidase	PYR[a]	D-Trehalose	D-Mannitol	Maltose	Sucrose	D-Mannose	Hemolysis
Staphylococcus aureus subsp. aureus	+	+	+	+	-	+	-	+	-	-	+	+	+	+	+	+
Staphylococcus aureus subsp. anaerobius	-	+	+	+	ND	-	-	ND	-	ND	-	-	-	+	-	-
Staphylococcus hyicus[bc]	-	V	+	+	-	-	-	+	-	-	+	-	-	+	+	-
Staphylococcus intermedius[b,d]	V	+	+	+	-	-	-	-	+	+	+	V	V	+	+	V
Staphylococcus delphini	-	+	-	+	ND	-	-	ND	ND	ND	+	+	+	+	+	+
Staphylococcus lugdunensis	+	-	-	-	+	+	-	V	-	+	+	-	+	+	+	+
Staphylococcus pseudintermedius[t]	-	+	ND	V	ND	+	-	+	+	+	+	V	+	+	+	+
Staphylococcus schleiferi subsp. coagulans	-	+	+	+	ND	+	-	ND	ND	ND	-	V	-	V	+	+
Staphylococcus schleiferi subsp. schleiferi	+	-	+	+	-	+	-	-	+	+	V	-	-	-	+	+
Staphylococcus sciuri subsp. rodentium	+	-	-	V	-	-	+	-	-	-	+	+	V	+	+	+

[a]Performed from disk (Becton Dickinson and Company, Sparks, MD) or tablet (KEY Scientific Products, Round Rock, Tex).

[b]Primarily isolated from animals.

[c]Rarely a cause of infections in humans.

[d]The hemolysis for S. intermedius is delayed.

ND, No data available; PYR, pyrrolidonyl aminopeptidase; V, variable; +, >90% of strains positive; -, >90% of strains negative.

Data compiled from Behme RJ, Shuttleworth R, McNabb A, et al. Identification of staphylococci with a self-educating system using fatty acid analysis and biochemical tests (published erratum appears in *J Clin Microbiol.* 1997;35:1043), *J Clin Microbiol.* 1996;34:2267; Hébert GA. Hemolysin and other characteristics that help differentiate and biotype *Staphylococcus lugdunensis* and *Staphylococcus schleiferi. J Clin Microbiol.* 1990;28:2425; Kloos WE, Wolfshohl JF. Identification of *Staphylococcus* species with API STAPH-IDENT System. *J Clin Microbiol.* 1982;16:509; Roberson JR, Fox LK, Hancock DD, et al. Evaluation of methods for differentiation of coagulase-positive staphylococci. *J Clin Microbiol.* 1992;30:3217; Caroll KC, Pfaller MA. *Manual of Clinical Microbiology.* 12th ed. Washington, DC: ASM Press; 2019.

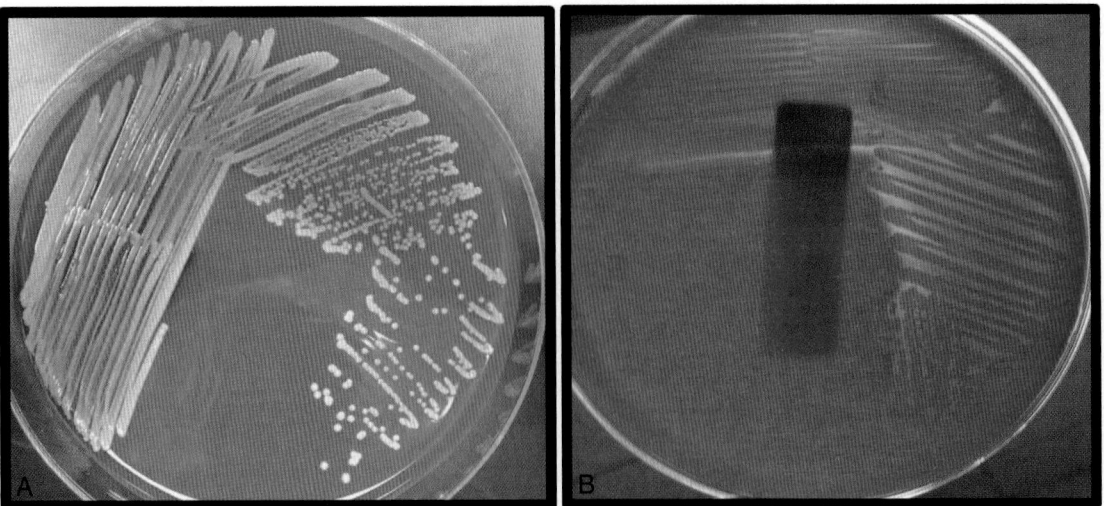

• **Fig. 13.6** (A) *Staphylococcus aureus* subsp. *aureus* demonstrating characteristic golden-yellow pigment on TSA 5% sheep blood agar. (B) Reverse demonstrating beta-hemolysis.

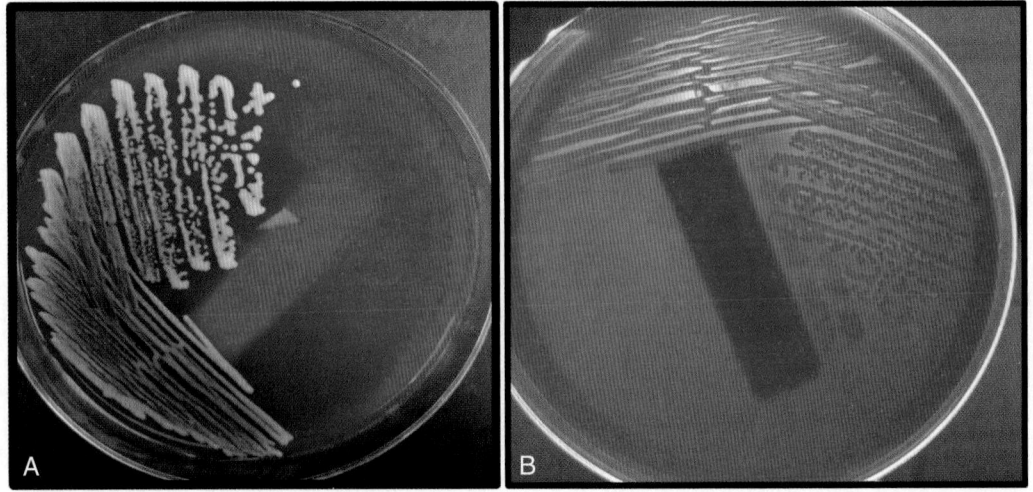

• **Fig. 13.7** (A) *Staphylococcus haemolyticus* demonstrating characteristic slightly mucoid colonies with white pigmentation on TSA 5% sheep blood agar; (B) reverse demonstrating weak beta-hemolysis.

virulence. Several studies have indicated that sampling directly from positive blood cultures for identification using MALDI-TOF MS has never misidentified a CoNS for a *S. aureus* or vice versa. In addition, it appears that CoNS are more often correctly speciated using this method. Identification of a pathogen directly from positive blood cultures may be possible within 20 minutes.

Antimicrobial Susceptibility Testing and Therapy

Identification of species using susceptibility testing is still useful in the differentiation of *S. saprophyticus* (novobiocin resistant) from other CoNS species (novobiocin sensitive).

In addition, polymyxin B resistance is common in clinical isolates of *S. aureus, S. epidermidis, S. hyicus, S. chromogenes,* and some strains of *S. lugdunensis.* Resistance is indicated by an inhibition zone diameter of <10 mm.

Antimicrobial therapy is vital to the management of patients suffering from staphylococcal infections (Table 13.8). Although a broad spectrum of agents may be used for therapy (Table 11.6 includes a detailed listing), most staphylococci are capable of acquiring and using one or more of the resistance mechanisms presented in Chapter 10. The unpredictable nature of any clinical isolate's antimicrobial susceptibility requires testing as a guide to therapy. As discussed in Chapter 11, several standard methods and commercial systems have been developed for testing staphylococci.

TABLE 13.6   Differentiation Among Coagulase-Negative, Pyrrolidonyl Aminopeptidase–Negative, Novobiocin-Resistant Staphylococci

Organism	Urease	Beta-Galactosidase	Alkaline Phosphatase	Acid From D-Trehalose	D-Mannitol	Maltose	Sucrose	D-Mannose
Staphylococcus cohnii subsp. *cohnii*	–	–	–	+	(d)	(d)	–	(d)
Staphylococcus cohnii subsp. *urealyticus*	+	–	+	+	+	(+)	–	+
Staphylococcus gallinarum	+	+	(+)	+	+	+	+	+
Staphylococcus hominis subsp. *novobiosepticus*	+	–	–	–	–	+	(+)	–
Staphylococcus lentus	-	+	>	+	+	(d)	+	(+)
Staphylococcus saprophyticus subsp. *saprophyticus*	+	(d)	–	+	(d)	+	+	–
Staphylococcus sciuri	–	+	+	+	+	(d)	+	(d)
Staphylococcus stepanovicii	+	ND	–	+	+	(+)	+	+
Staphylococcus Succinus subsp. *casei*	+	ND	+	+	+	+	+	+
Staphylococcus succinus subsp. *succinus*	+	ND	+	+	+	+	+	(d)
Staphylococcus vitulinus	-	(d)	-	(d)	-	–	+	–

(d), 11%–89% delayed positive; *PYR,* pyrrolidonyl aminopeptidase; *v,* variable; +, >90% of strains positive; –, >90% of strains negative; (+), delayed positive.
Data compiled from Caroll KC, Pfaller MA. *Manual of Clinical Microbiology.* 12th ed. Washington, DC: ASM Press; 2019.

TABLE 13.7 Differentiation Among Coagulase-Negative, Pyrrolidonyl Aminopeptidase–Negative, Novobiocin-Susceptible, Alkaline Phosphatase-Negative Staphylococci

Organism	Urease	Beta-Glucosidase	Acid from D-Trehalose	D-Mannitol	Maltose	Sucrose	D-Mannose
Staphylococcus auricularis	–	–	(+)	–	(+)	(d)	–
Staphylococcus capitis subsp. *capitis*	–	–	–	+	–	(+)	+
Staphylococcus capitis subsp. *ureolyticus*	+	–	–	+	+	+	+
Staphylococcus epidermidis	+	(d)	(d)	–	+	+	(+)
Staphylococcus hominis subsp. *hominis*	+	–	(d)	–	+	(+)	–
S. massiliensis	–	–	–	–	–	–	–
S. pasteuri	+	+	+	(d)	(d)	+	–
Staphylococcus warneri	+	+	+	(d)	(+)	+	–

(d), 11%–89% delayed positive; *PYR,* pyrrolidonyl aminopeptidase; *v,* variable results; +, >90% of strains positive; (+), >90% of strains delayed positive
–, >90% of strains negative; ±, 90% or more strains are weakly positive; ( ), reaction may be delayed.
Data compiled from Caroll KC, Pfaller MA. *Manual of Clinical Microbiology.* 12th ed. Washington, DC: ASM Press; 2019.

TABLE 13.8 Differentiation of Coagulase-Negative, Pyrrolidonyl Aminopeptidase–Positive, Novobiocin-Susceptible Staphylococci

Organism	Urease	Beta-Galactosidase	Alkaline-Phosphatase	Trehalose	Mannitol	Maltose	Sucrose	Mannose
Staphylococcus auricularis	-	(d)	-	(+)	-	(+)	(d)	-
Staphylococcus capitis subsp. *ureolyticus*	+	-	-	-	+	+	+	+
Staphylococcus caprae	+	-	(+)	(+)	(d)	(d)	-	+
Staphylococcus carnosus subsp. *carnosus*	-	-	+	(d)	+	-	-	+
Staphylococcus epidermidis	++	(d)	+	-	-	+	+	(+)
Staphylococcus equorum subsp. *equorum*	+	ND	(+)	+	+	(d)	+	+
Staphylococcus equorum subsp. *linens*	+	ND	(d)	-	ND	-	-	+
Staphylococcus haemolyticus	-	(d)	-	+	(d)	+	+	-
Staphylococcus petrasii subsp. *croceilyticus*	+	+	(d)	+	-	+	+	-
Staphylococcus petrasii subsp. *jettensis*	-	(d)	(d)	+	+	+	+	-
Staphylococcus petrasii subsp. *petrasii*	+	-	(d)	+	(d)	+	+	+
Staphylococcus petrasii subsp. *pragensis*	-	(d)	(d)	(d)	-	+	-	-
Staphylococcus pettenkoferi	+	ND	+	-	-	-	+	-
Staphylococcus rostri	-	ND	+	+	-	-	+	-
Staphylococcus schleiferi subsp. *schleiferi*	-	-	+	(d)	-	-	-	+
Staphylococcus simulans	+	-	(d)	(d)	+	+	+	(d)

(d), 11%–89% delayed positive; *PYR,* pyrrolidonyl aminopeptidase; *v,* variable; *ND,* not determined; +, >90% of strains positive; -, >90% of strains negative; (+), positive reactions may be delayed.
Data compiled from Caroll KC, Pfaller MA. *Manual of Clinical Microbiology.* 12th ed. Washington, DC: ASM Press; 2019.

Although penicillinase-resistant penicillins, such as methicillin, nafcillin, and oxacillin, are the mainstay of anti-staphylococcal therapy, resistance is common. The primary mechanism for this resistance is production of an altered penicillin-binding protein (i.e., PBP 2a), which renders all currently available beta-lactams essentially ineffective. Strains that carry the *mecA* gene, which encodes for PBP 2a, are referred to as MRSA. The *mecA* gene is carried on a mobile DNA element *(SSSmec)* that mediates wide dissemination of the antibiotic resistance. The prevalence of HA-MRSA has increased to >50% in some areas within the United States. In addition, an increasing prevalence of community-acquired (CA-MRSA) and **livestock-associated (LA-MRSA)** MRSA has been associated with clinical infections. In addition, beta-lactamase–producing strains should be considered resistant to all penicillins. Some strains have been identified that overproduce beta-lactamase and may appear resistant to oxacillin on routine disk diffusion sensitivity testing but do not possess the *mecA* gene. HA-MRSA are often resistant to aminoglycosides, fosfomycin, fusidic acid, glycopeptides, ketolides, lincosamides, macrolides, quinolones, rifampin, tetracyclines, and trimethoprim-sulfamethoxazole. Additional reports have identified isolates of *S. aureus* and CoNS resistant to linezolid, daptomycin, and tigecycline. CA-MRSA isolates are typically more susceptible to non–beta-lactam antibiotics.

MRSA isolates can also contain two subpopulations within a single culture, one that is oxacillin sensitive and one that is resistant. The resistant population grows much more slowly and is undetectable by routine susceptibility methods. **MRSA screen agar** may be used to clarify and interpret the oxacillin sensitivity pattern for such isolates. The MRSA screen agar uses oxacillin and promotes the growth of the resistant population by the addition of 2% to 4% NaCl. This medium is incubated at 35°C for a full 24 hours to determine the oxacillin-resistance pattern. Any growth on the MRSA screen agar indicates oxacillin resistance. Successful detection of mixed populations may be enhanced by incubation at a lower temperature, 30°C to 35°C for up to 48 hours. Alternatively, cefoxitin (30 µg) disk diffusion can be used to detect methicillin resistance in *S. aureus* and *S. lugdunensis*. An inhibition zone of ≤19 mm is reported as resistant and ≥20 mm is reported as sensitive. Other CoNS should be reported as resistant with a zone diameter of ≤24 mm. If microdilution testing is used to detect *mecA* resistance using either oxacillin or cefoxitin, *S. aureus* and *S. lugdunensis* should be reported as follows: resistant to cefoxitin (minimal inhibitory concentrations [MIC] ≥8µg/L) and oxacillin (MIC ≥4 µg/L) with CoNS resistant to oxacillin at an MIC ≥0.5 µg/L. Susceptibility testing with cefoxitin is the recommended method for the detection of penicillinase-resistant strains.

In addition to the increased penicillin resistance in *S. aureus,* many CoNS within the health care settings are now becoming resistant because of the production of beta-lactamase. Many isolates are resistant to methicillin and other antibiotics.

Interpretive guidelines for *S. aureus* with penicillin MICs of ≤12 µg/mL or zones of ≥29 mm using screen tests should be retested using disk diffusion. The same interpretive guidelines as indicated here for *S. aureus* are recommended for use with *S. lugdunensis*. However, it is important to use nitrocefin-based testing in place of penicillin for reliable results. Isolates that are beta-lactamase-positive should demonstrate a disk diffusion zone with a clear, sharp zone at the edge of the disk or "cliff." If the isolates demonstrate a fuzzy zone or "beach" edge, the isolate should be considered beta-lactamase-negative. In addition, any isolates that demonstrate a high level of mupirocin resistance should be retested using disk diffusion (200-µg mupirocin disk) or by broth microdilution using a single mupirocin 256 µg/mL well.

The increasing incidence of methicillin-resistant *Staphylococcus* spp. isolated from infections has resulted in an increase in the use of macrolide antibiotics for treatment. Lincomycin antibiotics such as clindamycin are hydrophobic and capable of diffusing into the tissues, providing a means for killing deep infections with *Staphylococcus* spp. However, macrolide resistance may be expressed as a **constitutive** (constant) **mechanism** or an **inducible** (expressed under specific conditions) **mechanism** that is activated by the presence of erythromycin. This is typically identified in erythromycin-resistant strains of *S. aureus*. Although erythromycin and clindamycin are different classes of antibiotics, their resistance mechanisms are similar. Resistance is mediated by either an efflux pump, *msrA,* resulting in macrolide resistance or the activity of a methylase enzyme that alters the ribosomal binding site, *erm,* which confers resistance to macrolides-lincosamide-streptogramin B and is referred to as **MLS$_B$** resistant. The MLS$_B$ resistance phenotype is the macrolide resistance that may be expressed as a constitutive or inducible mechanism. To determine the organism's susceptibility to clindamycin, a modified Kirby Bauer test, known as the **D zone,** has been used in microbiology laboratories. Two antibiotic disks are used: a clindamycin (2 µg) disk is placed 15 mm from an erythromycin disk (15 µg) on a Mueller Hinton agar plate streaked with confluent growth of the isolate. If the organism is able to express inducible clindamycin resistance in the presence of erythromycin, the cells will demonstrate a resistance in the zone of inhibition nearest the erythromycin disk demonstrating a characteristic D zone pattern. If this occurs, an alternate therapy is required for successful treatment of the infection.

Vancomycin is the most commonly used cell wall–active agent that retains activity and is an alternative drug of choice for the treatment of infections with resistant strains. High-level resistance to vancomycin (MIC >8 µg/mL) has been described in several clinical *S. aureus* isolates, and strains with MIC in the intermediate range have been encountered. These reduced **vancomycin-intermediate susceptible *S. aureus*** (VISAs, MIC 4 to 8 µg/mL) are believed to have structural alterations within the organism's cell wall. VISAs are also often resistant to teicoplanin. **Vancomycin-resistant *S. aureus* (VRSA)** are currently defined by the identification of an MIC ≥16 µg/mL and are readily detected using standard microdilution techniques. Intermediate vancomycin-resistant CoNS are currently defined as having an MIC 8 to 16 µg/mL. However, as resistance patterns increase, the detection of VISA has proved to be unreliable and probably underreported. Two relatively new agents available for use against such resistant strains are linezolid and daptomycin. Because of the substantial clinical and public health impact of vancomycin resistance emerging among staphylococci, laboratories should have a heightened awareness of this resistance pattern.

Staphylococcus spp. that demonstrate no intrinsic antibiotic resistance include *S. aureus, S. lugdunensis, S. epidermidis,* and *S. haemolyticus.* Intrinsic resistance has been reported in *S. saprophyticus* (novobiocin, fosfomycin, and fusidic acid), *S. capitis* (fosfomycin), *S. cohnii* (novobiocin), and *S. xylosus* (novobiocin). In addition, gram-positive bacteria are intrinsically resistant to polymyxin B/colistin, nalidixic acid, and aztreonam. Any clinical isolates that are identified as oxacillin-resistant *S. aureus* or coagulase-negative staphylococci should be considered resistant to all other beta-lactam antibiotics.

Because *Micrococcus* spp. are rarely encountered in clinically significant infections, therapeutic guidelines and standardized testing methods do not exist (Table 13.8). However, *in vitro* results indicate that these organisms generally appear to be susceptible to most beta-lactam antimicrobials.

Prevention

There are no approved antistaphylococcal vaccines. Health care workers identified as intranasal carriers of an epidemic strain of *S. aureus* are treated with topical mupirocin and, in some cases, with rifampin. Some physicians advocate the use of antibacterial substances such as gentian violet, acriflavine, chlorhexidine, or bacitracin to the umbilical cord stump to prevent staphylococcal disease in hospital nurseries. During epidemics, current recommendations require that all full-term infants be bathed with 3% hexachlorophene as soon after birth as possible and daily thereafter until discharge.

The Centers for Disease Control and Prevention recommend a concerted effort to battle multiple drug-resistant organisms identified in health care settings. Current recommended strategies for the control of spread and prevention of infection within health care settings include the screening of patients for MRSA before admission along with a variety of contact isolation procedures. Guidelines for the prevention and control of such organisms are included in the Campaign to Reduce Antimicrobial Resistance in Healthcare Settings (www.cdc.gov/drugresistance/healthcare/default.htm).

ⓔ Visit the Evolve site for a complete list of procedures, review questions, and case studies.

Bibliography

Barker KF, O'Driscoll JC, Bhargava A. *Staphylococcus lugdunensis, J Clin Pathol* 44:873–874, 1991.

Becker K, Rutsch F, Uekötter A, et al.: *Kocuriarhizophila* adds to the emerging spectrum of micrococcal species involved in human infections, *J Clin Microbiol* 46:3537–3539, 2008.

Behme RJ, Shuttleworth R, McNabb A, Colby WD: Identification of staphylococci with a self-educating system using fatty acid analysis and biochemical tests (published erratum appears in *J Clin Microbiol* 35:1043, 1997), *J Clin Microbiol* 34:2267, 1996.

Bosley GS, Whitney AM, Pruckler JM, et al.: Characterization of ear fluid isolates of *Alloiococcus otitidis* from patients with recurrent otitis media, *J Clin Microbiol* 33:2876–2880, 1995.

Brakstad OG, Aasbakk K, Maeland JA: Detection of *Staphylococcus aureus* by polymerase chain reaction amplification of the nuc gene. In *methods for dilution antimicrobial susceptibility testing for bacteria that grow aerobically; approved standard-eight ed. CLSI document M07-A8,* Wayne, PA, 2009, Clinical and Laboratory Science Institute.

Cakar M, Demirbas S, Yildizoglu U, et al.: First report of endocarditis by *Alloiococcus otitidis* spp. in a patient with a history of chronic otitis, *J Infect Public Health* 6:494–495, 2013.

Caroll KC, Pfaller MA: *Manual of clinical microbiology,* ed 12, Washington, DC, 2019, ASM Press.

Clinical and Laboratory Standards Institute: *Methods for dilution antimicrobial susceptibility tests for bacteria that grow aerobically; M07-A10,* Wayne, PA, 2015, CLSI.

Clinical and Laboratory Standards Institute: *Performance standards for antimicrobial disk susceptibility testing; M02-A12,* Wayne, PA, 2015, CLSI.

Clinical and Laboratory Standards Institute: *Performance standards for antimicrobial susceptibility testing; M100-S25,* Wayne, PA, 2015, CLSI.

Dhagat PV, Gibbs KA, Rohde RE: Prevalence of Staphylococcus, including Methicillin Resistant *Staphylococcus aureus* (MRSA), in a Physical Therapy Educational Facility, *J Allied Health* 44(4):215–218, 2015.

Felkner M, Rohde RE, Valle-Rivera AM, et al.: Methicillin-resistant *Staphylococcus aureus* nasal carriage rate in Texas county jail inmates, *J Correct Health Care* 13:289–295, 2007.

Gibbs KA, Rohde RE, Sanders B, et al.: *Staphylococcus* and MRSA prevalence in physical therapist education programs: are students at risk? *J Phys Ther Educ* 32(1):65–69, 2018.

Hébert GA: Hemolysins and other characteristics that help differentiate and biotype *Staphylococcus lugdunensis* and *Staphylococcus schleiferi, J Clin Microbiol* 28:2425–2431, 1990.

Hébert GA, Crowder CG, Hancock GA, Jarvis WR, Thornsberry C: Characteristics of coagulase-negative staphylococci that help differentiate these species and other members of the family *Micrococcaceae, J Clin Microbiol* 26:1939–1949, 1988.

Holt JG: *Bergey's manual of determinative bacteriology,* 9th ed., Baltimore, MD, 1994, Williams & Wilkins.

Isaac DW, Pearson TA, Hurwitz CA, Patrick CC: Clinical and microbiologic aspects of *Staphylococcus haemolyticus* infections, *Pediatr Infect Dis J* 12:1018–1021, 1993.

Kecojevic A, Ranken R, Ecker DJ, et al.: Rapid PCR/ESI-MS-based molecular genotyping of *Staphylococcus aureus* from nasal swabs of emergency department patients, *BMC Infect Dis* 14:16, 2014.

Kloos WE, Ballard DN, Webster JA, et al.: Ribotype delineation and description of *Staphylococcus sciuri* subspecies and their potential as reservoirs of methicillin resistance and staphylolytic enzyme genes, *Int J Syst Bacteriol* 47:313–323, 1997.

Kloos WE, Bannerman TL: Update on clinical significance of coagulase-negative staphylococci, *Clin Microbiol Rev* 7:117–140, 1994.

Kloos WE, George CG, Olgiate JS, et al.: *Staphylococcus hominis* subsp. *novobiosepticus* subsp. nov., a novel trehalose- and N-acetyl-D-glucosamine-negative, novobiocin- and multiple-antibiotic-resistant subspecies isolated from human blood cultures, *Int J Syst Bacteriol* 48:799–812, 1998.

Kloos WE, Schleifer KH: Simplified scheme for routine identification of human *Staphylococcus species*, *J Clin Microbiol* 1:82–88, 1975.

Koontz F: Is there a clinical necessity to identify coagulase-negative staphylococci to the species level? "Okay, so I was wrong!", *Clin Microbiol Newsl* 20:78, 1998.

LeLoir Y, Baron F, Gautier M: *Staphylococcus aureus* and food poisoning, *Genet Mol Res* 2:63–76, 2003.

Lee JY, Kim SH, Jeong HS, et al.: Two cases of peritonitis caused by *Kocuria marina* in patients undergoing continuous ambulatory peritoneal dialysis, *J Clin Microbiol* 47:3376–3378, 2009.

Loonen AJ, Jansz AR, Stalpers J, Wolffs PF, van den Brule AJ: An evaluation of three processing methods and the effect of reduced culture times for faster direct identification of pathogens from BacT/ALERT blood cultures by MALDI-TOF MS, *Eur J Clin Microbiol Infect Dis* 31:1575–1583, 2012.

Lyytikäinen O, Vaara M, Järviluoma E, Rosenqvist K, Tiittanen L, Valtonen V: Increased resistance among *Staphylococcus epidermidis* isolates in a large teaching hospital over a 12-year period, *Eur J Clin Microbiol Infect Dis* 15:133–138, 1996.

Maraki S, Papadakis IS: *Rothia mucilaginosa* pneumonia: a literature review, *Infect Dis(Lond).* 47:125–129, 2015.

McGowin CL, Rohde RE, Whitlock GC: Other pathogens of significant public health concern. In Hu P, Hedge M, Lennon PA, editors: *Modern clinical molecular techniques (New Edition)*, New York, NY, 2012, Springer Press.

McKenzie JF, Garcia SA, Patterson T, Rohde RE: Snapshot prevalence and characterization of staphylococcus species, including MRSA, in a student athletic facility: an undergraduate research project, *Clin Lab Sci* 25:156–164, 2012.

Mulligan ME, Murray-Leisure KA, Ribner BS, et al.: Methicillin-resistant *Staphylococcus aureus*: a consensus review of the microbiology, pathogenesis, and epidemiology with implications for prevention and management, *Am J Med* 94:313–328, 1993.

Patel R: MALDI-TOF MS for the diagnosis of infectious diseases, *Clin Chem* 61:100–111, 2015.

Roberson JR, Fox LK, Hancock DD, Besser TE: Evaluation of methods for differentiation of coagulase-positive staphylococci, *J Clin Microbiol* 30:3217–3219, 1992.

Rohde RE, Denham R, Brannon A: Methicillin resistant *Staphylococcus aureus*: carriage rates and characterization of students in a Texas University, *Clin Lab Sci* 22:176–184, 2009.

Rohde RE, Patterson T, Covington B, Vásquez BE, Redwine G, Carranco E: *Staphylococcus*, not MRSA? A final report of carriage and conversion rates in nursing students, *Clin Lab Sci* 27:21–31, 2014.

Savini V: *Pet-To-Man travelling staphylococci - A world in progress,* ed 1, Academic Press, Elsevier, 2018.

Shantala GB, Shetty AD, Rahul RK, et al.: Detection of inducible clindamycin clinical isolates of *Staphylococcus aureus* by the disc diffusion induction test, *J Clin Diagn Res* 5:35–37, 2011.

Stackebrandt E, Koch C, Gvozdiak O, Schumann P: Taxonomic dissection of the genus *Micrococcus: Kocuria* gen. nov., *Nesterenkonia* gen. nov., *Kytococcus* gen. nov., *Dermacoccus* gen. nov., and *Micrococcus* (Cohn, 1872) gen. emend, *Int J Syst Bacteriol* 45:682–692, 1995.

Takahashi N, Shinjoh M, Tomita H, et al.: Catheter-related blood stream infection caused by *Dermacoccus barathri*, representing the first case of *Dermacoccus* infection in humans, *J Infect Chemother* 21:613–616, 2015.

Tano K, von Essen R, Eriksson PO, Sjöstedt A: *Alloiococcus otitidis*—otitis media pathogen or normal bacterial flora? *APMIS* 116:785–790, 2008.

Vandenesch F, Etienne J, Reverdy ME, Eykyn SJ: Endocarditis due to *Staphylococcus lugdunensis*: report of 11 cases and review, *Clin Infect Dis* 17:871–876, 1993.

Woodford N, Johnson AP, Morrison D, Speller DC: Current perspectives on glycopeptide resistance, *Clin Microbiol Rev* 8:585–615, 1995.

Yassin AF, Hupfer H, Siering C, Klenk HP, Schumann P: *Auritidibacter gnavus* gen. nov., sp. nov., of the family *Micrococcaceae* isolated from an ear swab of a man with otitis externa, transfer of the members of the family *Yaniellaceae* Li et al. 2008 to the family *Micrococcaceae* and emended description of the suborder *Micrococcineae*, *Int J Syst Evol Microbiol* 61:223–230, 2011.

14

Streptococcus, Enterococcus, and Similar Organisms

OBJECTIVES

1. Describe the general characteristics of *Streptococcus* spp. and *Enterococcus* spp., including oxygenation, microscopic Gram-staining characteristics, and macroscopic appearance on blood agar.
2. Explain the Lancefield classification system for *Streptococcus* spp.
3. Identify the clinical infections associated with *Streptococcus* spp., *Enterococcus* spp., and related gram-positive cocci.
4. Describe the patterns of hemolysis for clinically significant species of streptococci and enterococci.
5. Explain the chemical principles for isolation of *Streptococcus* spp. and *Enterococcus* spp. on selective and differential media; include 5% sheep blood agar and Enterococcosel agar.
6. Compare and contrast streptolysin O and streptolysin S, including oxygen stability, immunogenicity, and appearance on blood agar.
7. Describe the major significance of serologic testing procedures for antistreptolysin O and antistreptolysin S, in combination with anti-DNase for diagnosis of poststreptococcal sequelae.
8. Explain the activity for the virulence factors of *Streptococcus pyogenes* and the pathogenic effects of each including M protein, hyaluronic acid capsule, streptokinase, F protein, hyaluronidase, and the streptococcal pyrogenic exotoxins.
9. Explain the significance of *Streptococcus agalactiae* (group B) in perinatal infections.
10. Identify the two major virulence factors associated with *Streptococcus pneumoniae,* and describe their effect on the pathogenesis of the infection.
11. List the appropriate clinical specimens for isolation of the individual *Streptococcus* spp., *Enterococcus,* and *Aerococcus viridans, Abiotrophia, Granulicatella, Gemella, Leuconostoc,* and *Pediococcus.*
12. Identify a clinical isolate based on the results from standard laboratory diagnostic procedures.

GENERA AND SPECIES TO BE CONSIDERED

Beta-hemolytic streptococci
- *Streptococcus pyogenes* (group A)
- *Streptococcus agalactiae* (group B)
- *Streptococcus dysgalactiae* subsp. *equisimilis* (group A, C, G, L)

Alpha-hemolytic streptococci
- *Streptococcus pneumoniae* (*S. mitis* group)
- *Streptococcus pseudopneumoniae* (*S. mitis* group)

Viridans streptococci (alpha-hemolytic)
- *Streptococcus mutans* group (*S. criceti, S. ratti, S. downei*)
- *Streptococcus salivarius* group (*S. salivarius* subsp. *salivarius, S. vestibularis*)
- *Streptococcus mitis* group (*S. australis, S. cristatus, S. gordonii, S. infantis, S. lactarius, S. massiliensis, S. mitis, S. oralis* subsp. *dentisani, S. oralis* subsp. *oralis, S. oralis* subsp. *tigurinus, S. parasanguinis, S. peroris, S. pneumoniae, S. pseudopneumoniae, S. rubneri, S. sanguinis, S. sinensis*)

Streptococcus bovis group (*S. equinus, S. gallolyticus, S. infantarius, S. alactolyticus*)
- Beta-, Alpha-, and Gamma-hemolytic
- *Streptococcus anginosus* group (*S. anginosus, S. constellatus, S. intermedius*)

Enterococci (recovered from human sources)
Group 1[a]
- *Enterococcus avium*
- *Enterococcus raffinosus*
- *Enterococcus gilvus*
- *Enterococcus pallens*
- *Enterococcus pseudoavium*
- *Enterococcus hawaiiensis*

Group 2
- *Enterococcus faecium*
- *Enterococcus casseliflavus*
- *Enterococcus gallinarum*
- *Enterococcus mundtii*
- *Enterococcus faecalis*
- *Enterococcus thailandicus*

General Characteristics

The organisms discussed in this chapter comprise several families of bacteria in the order Lactobacillales, including the two large families *Streptococcaceae* and *Enterococcaceae,* as well as the *Aerococcaceae, Lactobacillaceae, Carnobacteriaceae* and *Leuconostocaceae.* These organisms are all catalase-negative, gram-positive cocci 0.5 to 1.2 μm in diameter and arranged predominantly in pairs or chains, with some forming irregular clusters.

The *Streptococcaceae* consist of a large family of medically important species in the genus *Streptococcus.* Microscopically the gram-positive cells within the genus *Streptococcus* are generally arranged in chains or pairs. These organisms can be differentiated based on cell wall structure, hemolytic patterns on sheep blood agar (beta, alpha, or gamma), reaction of antibodies to specific bacterial antigen, the Lancefield Classification scheme, and biochemical identification relating to physiologic characteristics. This traditional system of classification is still useful within the clinical laboratory, although it differs in some cases with the molecular analysis of the 16S ribosomal ribonucleic acid (rRNA) sequences. Of the streptococci considered in this chapter, those that are most commonly encountered in infections in humans include *S. pyogenes, S. agalactiae, S. pneumoniae,* and the viridans streptococci group.

The genus *Enterococcus* includes organisms that were previously included in the *Streptococcaceae* family. However, due to the introduction of molecular methods, these organisms have been placed in a separate family, the *Enterococcaceae.* There are approximately 57 species included in the genus *Enterococcus,* 21 species that have been isolated from human sources. The members of this genus microscopically produce cocci arranged in pairs, short chains, or as small irregular clusters. Like the streptococci, organisms within this genus produce hemolysis on sheep blood agar (beta, alpha, or gamma); however, the hemolytic patterns vary within a single species and are therefore not as useful in the identification of specific species. Enterococci are commensal organisms of the human gastrointestinal (GI) tract that cause a variety of opportunistic infections. *E. faecalis* and *E. faecium* are the most common species encountered in human infections.

The remaining diverse group of organisms included in this chapter are considered contaminants and are infrequently isolated as opportunistic agents of infection. Many of these organisms are often confused and misidentified as streptococci or enterococci in the clinical laboratory. Microscopically, these gram-positive cocci may appear pleomorphic and arranged in pairs, chains, or clusters. The majority of these organisms are facultative anaerobes. Macroscopically, none of these organisms are beta-hemolytic on routine sheep blood agar.

Epidemiology

Many of these organisms are commonly found as part of the normal human microbiome of the pharynx, mouth, lower GI tract, and vagina. When other normal microbiota are depleted, when bacterial inoculum increases, when virulence factors are heightened, and/or when adaptive immunity is impaired, the bacteria can cause disease. However, some species are encountered in clinical specimens as contaminants or as components of mixed cultures with minimal or unknown clinical significance (Table 14.1). When these organisms gain access to normally sterile sites (blood, cerebrospinal fluid [CSF], pleural fluid, peritoneal fluid, pericardial fluid, bone, joint fluids, organs, vitreous fluid, and vascular tissue), they can cause life-threatening infections.

The upper respiratory tract and skin lesions serve as the primary sites of infection and transmissions of *S. pyogenes.* *S. pyogenes* can cause pharyngitis, scarlet fever, streptococcus toxic shock, puerperal fever, infection of skin, and poststreptococcal disease, and a severe invasive infection, necrotizing fasciitis.

S. pneumoniae, included in the *S. mitis* group, can be found as part of the normal upper respiratory microbiota in about half the population. Because the organism invades the lower respiratory tract, it can cause pneumonia; this is discussed separately in this chapter. *S. pneumoniae* causes 95% of all bacterial pneumonias. In addition, *S. pneumoniae* is the leading cause of acute otitis media in children up to the age of 3 and is a major cause of bacterial meningitis

TABLE 14.1 **Epidemiology, Pathogenesis, and Spectrum of Disease**

Organism	Habitat (Reservoir)	Mode of Transmission	Virulence Factors	Spectrum of Disease
Streptococcus pyogenes (group A)	Not considered normal microbiota Colonizes skin and upper respiratory tract of humans; carried on nasal, pharyngeal, and sometimes anal mucosa; presence in specimens is almost always considered clinically significant	Direct contact: person to person Indirect contact: aerosolized droplets from coughs or sneezes Upper respiratory tract and skin are reservoirs for transmission	Protein F mediates epithelial cell attachment (fibronectin binding); hyaluronic acid capsule inhibits phagocytosis; M protein is antiphagocytic (<100 serotypes); produces several enzymes and hemolysins that contribute to tissue invasion and destruction, including streptolysin O, streptolysin S, streptokinase, DNase, and hyaluronidase. Streptococcal pyrogenic exotoxins (SPEs) mediate production of rash (i.e., scarlet fever) or multisystem effects that may result in death; C5a peptidase-destroying complement chemotactic factors	Acute pharyngitis, impetigo, cellulitis, erysipelas, necrotizing fasciitis and myositis, bacteremia with potential for infection in any of several organs, pneumonia, scarlet fever, streptococcal toxic shock syndrome
			Cross-reactions of antibodies produced against streptococcal antigens and human heart tissue	Rheumatic fever
			Deposition of antibody-streptococcal antigen complexes in kidney results in damage to glomeruli	Acute poststreptococcal glomerulonephritis
Streptococcus agalactiae (group B)	Normal microbiota: female genital tract and lower gastrointestinal tract Occasional colonizer of upper respiratory tract	Endogenous strain: gaining access to sterile site(s) probable Direct contact: person to person from mother *in utero* or during delivery; or nosocomial transmission by unwashed hands of mother or health care personnel	Uncertain; capsular material interferes with phagocytic activity and complement cascade activation	Infections most commonly involve neonates and infants, often preceded by premature rupture of mother's membranes; transient vaginal carriage in 10%–30% of females; infections often present as multisystem problems, including sepsis, fever, meningitis, respiratory distress, lethargy, and hypotension; infections may be classified as early onset (occur within first 5 days of life) or late onset (occur 7 days to 3 months after birth) Invasive infections are often seen in elderly and immunocompromised patients with comorbidities; pneumonia, endocarditis, meningitis and urinary tract infections

Continued

TABLE 14.1 Epidemiology, Pathogenesis, and Spectrum of Disease—cont'd

Organism	Habitat (Reservoir)	Mode of Transmission	Virulence Factors	Spectrum of Disease
Streptococcus dysgalactiae subsp. *equisimilis* and other group A, C, G, and L beta-hemolytic streptococci	Normal microbiota: skin, nasopharynx, gastrointestinal tract, genital tract	Endogenous strain: gain access to sterile site Direct contact: person to person	None have been definitively identified, but likely include factors similar to those produced by *S. pyogenes* and *S. agalactiae*	Cause similar types of acute infections in adults as described for *S. pyogenes* and *S. agalactiae*; upper respiratory tract infections, skin and soft tissue infections, and invasive infections including necrotizing fasciitis, STSS, bacteremia, arthritis, osteomyelitis, and endocarditis. Cases of glomerulonephritis and acute rheumatic fever have been reported
Streptococcus pneumoniae	Colonizer of nasopharynx	Direct contact: person to person with contaminated respiratory secretions	Polysaccharide capsule that inhibits phagocytosis is primary virulence factor; pneumolysin has various effects on host cells, and several other factors are likely involved in eliciting a strong cellular response by the host; secretory IgA protease	A leading cause of meningitis and pneumonia with or without bacteremia; also causes sinusitis, peritonitis, endocarditis, and otitis media
Viridans streptococci	Normal microbiota: oral cavity, gastrointestinal tract, female genital tract	Endogenous strain: gain access to sterile site; most notably results from dental manipulations	Production of extracellular complex polysaccharides (e.g., glucans and dextrans) enhance attachment to host cell surfaces, such as cardiac endothelial cells or tooth surfaces in the case of dental caries	Slowly evolving (subacute) endocarditis, sepsis, pneumonia, urogenital tract infections, meningitis, dental carries
Enterococcus spp.	Normal microbiota: humans, animals, and birds Colonizers	Endogenous strain: gain access to sterile sites Direct contact: person to person Contaminated medical equipment; immunocompromised patients are at risk of developing infections with antibiotic-resistant strains	Little is known about virulence; adhesions, cytolysins, and other metabolic capabilities may allow these organisms to proliferate as nosocomial/health care–associated pathogens; multidrug resistance also contributes to proliferation	Most infections are health care–associated and include urinary tract infections, bacteremia, endocarditis, mixed infections of abdomen and pelvis, wound infections, and, occasionally, ocular infections; central nervous system and respiratory infections are rare
Abiotrophia spp.	Normal microbiota: oral cavity and upper respiratory tract	Endogenous strains: gain access to normally sterile sites	Unknown	Endocarditis; also isolated from ophthalmic, central nervous system, peritonitis, musculoskeletal infections, and septic arthritis
Leuconostoc spp.	Foods and vegetation; normal microbiota of the alimentary tract	Transiently colonize the gastrointestinal tract after ingestion; from that site the organism gains access to sterile sites	Unknown; probably of low virulence; opportunistic organisms that require impaired host defenses to establish infection; intrinsic resistance to certain antimicrobial agents (e.g., resistant to vancomycin) may enhance survival of some species in the hospital setting	Neonate bacteremia, wounds, gastrointestinal infections and isolated from sterile fluids in adults including blood

Organism	Habitat (Reservoir)	Mode of Transmission	Virulence Factors	Spectrum of Disease
Lactococcus spp. (group N)	Foods and vegetation; normal microbiota of the alimentary tract	Endogenous strains: gain access to normally sterile sites	Hemolysins, fibronectin-binding protein and potential antibiotic resistance genes to tetracycline and sulfonamides	Endocarditis, urinary tract infections, bacteremia and septicemia, osteomyelitis, peritonitis and other abscesses
Dolosicoccus pauciyorans	Unknown	Unknown	Unknown	Bacteremia
Dolosigranulum pigrum	Nasopharyngeal normal microbiota	Endogenous strains: gain access to normally sterile sites	Unknown	Health care–associated pneumonia, septicemia, synovitis, arthritis, and gastrointestinal infections
Globicatella sp.	Unknown	Unknown	Unknown	Bacteremia, urinary tract infections, meningitis
Granulicatella spp.	Normal microbiota: oral cavity and upper respiratory tract	Endogenous strains: gain access to normally sterile sites	Unknown	Endocarditis; also isolated from ophthalmic, central nervous system, peritonitis, musculoskeletal infections, and septic arthritis
Pediococcus spp.	Foods and vegetation; normal microbiota of the alimentary tract	Transiently colonize the gastrointestinal tract after ingestion; from that site they gain access to sterile sites	Unknown; probably of low virulence; opportunistic organisms that require impaired host defenses to establish infection; intrinsic resistance to certain antimicrobial agents (e.g., resistant to vancomycin) may enhance survival of some species in the hospital setting	Bacteremia and sepsis; hepatic abscess
Aerococcus spp.	Environmental; occasionally found on skin	Unknown	Bacterial adhesions and antiphagocytic polysaccharide capsule	Endocarditis, bacteremia, and urosepsis; *Aerococcus urinae* is notably associated with urinary tract infections
Facklamia spp.	Normal microbiota of the female genital tract	Unknown	Unknown	Bacteremia, wound, and genitourinary tract infections
Gemella spp.	Normal microbiota of human oral cavity and upper respiratory tract	Endogenous strains: gain access to normally sterile sites	Unknown	Endocarditis, meningitis, brain abscess, ocular infections, septic arthritis, osteomyelitis, peritonitis, and other wounds
Ignavigranum sp.	Unknown	Unknown	Unknown	Wound and abscesses
Helcococcus sp.	Normal microbiota of the skin	Endogenous strains: gain access to normally sterile sites	Unknown	Skin and soft tissue infections, most notably foot infections; bacteremia, pleural empyema and prosthetic joint infections
Vagococcus fluvialis	Uncertain; seen in domestic animals	Unknown	Unknown	Isolated from blood cultures and peritoneal fluid

STSS, Streptococcal toxic shock syndrome.

in infants, young children, and adults in the United States. Similarly, *S. pyogenes* may be carried in the upper respiratory tract of humans; it should be deemed clinically important whenever it is encountered. *S. agalactiae* (group B) is a common cause of pneumonia in 0- to 2-month-old patients following inhalation of organisms as neonates pass down the birth canal. It can also cause meningitis and sepsis in neonates. Prenatal transmission of the organism may also result in stillbirth.

Enterococci are predominantly inhabitants of the GI tract of humans and, less commonly, in other areas such as the oral cavity, genitourinary tract, skin, and perineal area. The GI tract is considered the main reservoir for disease associated with these organisms.

At the other extreme, the remaining organisms within this chapter are generally inhabitants of the human oral cavity, upper respiratory tract, skin, and genitourinary tract. Most of these organisms, such as *Leuconostoc* spp. and *Pediococcus* spp., are generally considered contaminants in the clinical laboratory, but are increasingly identified in association with a variety of infections.

Many of the organisms listed in Table 14.1 are spread person to person by various means and, subsequently, establish a state of colonization or carriage; infections may then develop when colonizing strains gain entrance to normally sterile sites. In some instances, this may involve trauma (medically or nonmedically induced) to skin or mucosal surfaces or, as in the case of *S. pneumoniae* pneumonia, may result from aspiration into the lungs of organisms colonizing the upper respiratory tract.

Pathogenesis and Spectrum of Disease

The capacity of the organisms listed in Table 14.1 to produce disease and the spectrum of infections they cause vary widely with the different genera and species.

Beta-Hemolytic Streptococci

Beta-hemolytic streptococci are characterized by Lancefield groups, based on carbohydrates in the cell wall. Beta-hemolytic streptococci are considered opportunistic bacteria. However, some Lancefield groups are clinically significant, such as *S. pyogenes* (group A) and *S. agalactiae* (group B). The beta-hemolytic group includes the large colony-forming pyogenic strains of streptococci with group A, C, G, or L antigens (*S. dysgalactiae* subsp. *equisimilis*) and strains with group B (*S. agalactiae*) antigen. Small colony-forming beta-hemolytic strains with group A, C, F, or G (*S. anginosus* group) are included in the viridans group.

Group A *S. pyogenes,* the most clinically important Lancefield group A, produces several factors that contribute to its virulence; it is one of the most aggressive pathogens encountered in clinical microbiology laboratories. Among these factors are streptolysin O and S, which contribute to virulence and are responsible for the beta-hemolytic pattern on blood agar plates used as a guide to identify this species. **Streptolysin S** is an oxygen-stable, nonimmunogenic hemolysin capable of lysing erythrocytes, leukocytes, and platelets in the presence of room air. **Streptolysin O** is immunogenic, capable of lysing the same cells and cultured cells, is inactivated by oxygen, and will produce hemolysis in the absence of room air. Streptolysin O is also inhibited by the cholesterol in skin lipids, resulting in the absence of the development of protective antibodies associated with skin infection. The infections caused by *S. pyogenes* may be localized or systemic; other problems may arise because of the host's antibody response to the infections caused by these organisms. Localized infections include acute pharyngitis, for which *S. pyogenes* is the most common bacterial cause, and skin infections, such as impetigo and erysipelas (see Chapter 75 for more information on skin and soft tissue infections).

S. pyogenes infections are prone to progression with involvement of deeper tissues and organs, a characteristic that has earned the designation in general publications as the "flesh-eating bacteria." Such systemic infections (necrotizing fasciitis) are life threatening. In addition, even when infections remain localized, **streptococcal pyrogenic exotoxins (SPEs)** may be released and produce scarlet fever, which occurs in association with streptococcal pharyngitis and is manifested by a rash of the face and upper trunk. The SPEs are erythrogenic toxins produced by lysogenic strains. They are heat labile and rarely found in group C and G streptococci. The SPEs act as superantigens, activating macrophages and T-helper cells and inducing the release of powerful immune mediators, including interleukin (IL)-1, IL-2, IL-6, tumor necrosis factor (TNF)-alpha, TNF-beta, interferons, and cytokines, which induce shock and organ failure. Streptococcal toxic shock syndrome, typified by multisystem involvement including renal and respiratory failure, rash, and diarrhea, is a serious disease mediated by production of potent SPE.

Other complications that result from *S. pyogenes* infections are the poststreptococcal diseases rheumatic fever and acute glomerulonephritis. The poststreptococcal diseases are mediated by the presence of the M protein, not present in any other Lancefield groups. The **M protein** consists of two alpha helical polypeptides anchored in the cytoplasmic membrane of the organism and extending through the cell wall to the outer surface. The outer amino terminus of the protein is highly variable, consisting of greater than 100 serotypes. Class 1M protein is associated with rheumatic fever, and class I or II is typically associated with glomerulonephritis. Rheumatic fever, which is manifested by fever, endocarditis (inflammation of heart muscle), subcutaneous nodules, and polyarthritis, usually follows respiratory tract infections and is believed to be mediated by antibodies produced against *S. pyogenes* M protein that cross-react with human heart tissue. Acute glomerulonephritis, characterized by edema, hypertension, hematuria, and proteinuria, can follow respiratory or cutaneous infections and is mediated by antigen-antibody complexes that deposit in glomeruli, where they initiate damage.

The organism adheres and invades the epithelial cells through the mediation of various proteins and enzymes. Internalization of the organism is believed to be important for persistent and deep tissue infections.

S. pyogenes is also a powerful modulator of the host immune system, preventing clearance of the infection. The M protein is able to bind beta globulin factor H, a regulatory protein of the alternate complement pathway involved in the degradation of C3b. The M protein also binds to fibrinogen-blocking complement alternate pathway activation. In addition, all strains produce a C5a peptidase, which is a serine protease capable of inactivating the chemotactic factor for neutrophils and monocytes (C5a).

Group B *S. agalactiae* (GBS) infections are usually associated with neonates and are acquired before or during the birthing process (Table 14.1). The organism is known to cause septicemia, pneumonia, and meningitis in newborns. Colonization of the maternal urogenital or GI tract occurs in 10% to 30% of pregnant women. The Centers for Disease Control and Prevention (CDC) recommends screening all pregnant women for GBS carriage between 35 and 37 weeks of gestation. All carriers should be treated with an intrapartum antibiotic prophylaxis.

S. dysgalactiae subsp *equisimilis* (Lancefield groups A, C, G, and L) clinically produces a similar spectrum of disease (i.e., pharyngitis, skin and soft tissue infections, and bacteremia) as *S. pyogenes* it is less commonly encountered. The organism harbors similar virulence factor genes and has been associated with poststreptococcal sequelae, including acute rheumatic fever and glomerulonephritis.

Streptococcus pneumoniae

S. pneumoniae contains the C polysaccharide unrelated to the Lancefield grouping and is still one of the leading causes of morbidity and mortality. The organism is the primary cause of community-associated bacterial pneumonia, meningitis, and otitis media. The antiphagocytic property of the polysaccharide capsule is associated with the organism's virulence. There are more than 90 different serotypes of encapsulated strains of *S. pneumoniae*. Nonencapsulated strains are avirulent. The organism may harmlessly inhabit the upper respiratory tract, with a 5% to 75% carriage rate in humans. *S. pneumoniae* is capable of spreading to the lungs, paranasal sinuses, and middle ear. In addition, this organism accesses the bloodstream and the meninges to cause acute, purulent, and often life-threatening infections. *S. pseudopneumoniae,* a closely related species that is nonencapsulated, insoluble in bile, and optochin susceptible, causes respiratory tract infections in patients with previous conditions such as chronic obstructive pulmonary disease.

S. pneumoniae is capable of mobilizing inflammatory cells mediated by its cell wall structure, including peptidoglycan, teichoic acids, and a pneumolysin. The **pneumolysin** activates the classic complement pathway. The pneumolysin mediates suppression of the oxidative burst in phagocytes, providing for effective evasion of immune clearance. In addition, the organism contains **phosphorylcholine** within the cell wall, which binds receptors for platelet-activating factor in endothelial cells, leukocytes, platelets, and tissue cells of the lungs and meninges, providing for entry and spread of the organism.

Infection with *S. pneumoniae* can be prevented through a series of vaccinations. There are two vaccines currently available, a 13-valent conjugate vaccine and a 23-valent capsular polysaccharide vaccine. Vaccine use has reduced the nasopharyngeal carrier rate and the number of invasive infections associated with the organism.

Viridans Streptococci

The viridans group includes a large and complex group of human streptococci that are not groupable by Lancefield serology. The viridans group of streptococci includes five groups, each containing several species. The groups include the *mutans* group, *salivarius* group, *bovis* group, *anginosus* group (previously *S. milleri* group), and *mitis* group. Organisms in the streptococcus viridans group typically demonstrate no hemolysis or alpha-hemolysis (greening) on sheep blood agar and smell like butterscotch, especially on chocolate agar. However, some viridan streptococci can produce beta-hemolysis, such as the S. *anginosus* group, which presents as small colony-forming beta-hemolytic strains with groups A, C, F, and G antigens.

S. salivarius group organisms are isolated primarily from the oropharynx and blood. *S. salivarius* has been reported in bacteremia, endocarditis, and meningitis. Several species of the *S. mutans* group have been isolated from the human oropharynx including *S. criceti, S. ratti,* and *S. downei. S. mutans* and *S. sobrinus* are the most commonly isolated species associated with dental carries. Species from the *S. bovis* group may be isolated in cases of bacteremia, septicemia, and endocarditis.

Organisms in the *S. anginosus* group are normal microbiota in the oropharynx, urogenital, and GI tract. Small-colony (<0.5 mm) beta-hemolytic group A, C, F, and G (or no group) organisms are considered normal microbiota of the throat and typically not reported when screening for beta-hemolytic streptococcus of the throat. However, they can cause bacteremia and disseminated deep-seated infections, especially in immunocompromised patients. Viridans streptococci are not highly invasive; however, they enter tissue during dental or surgical procedures, which could lead to tooth abscesses, abdominal infections, bacteremia, or valve endocarditis and late-onset prosthetic valve endocarditis. *S. anginosus* is frequently isolated from the urogenital tract, *S. constellatus* from the respiratory tract, and *S. intermedius* from liver and brain abscesses.

Similarly, to the *S. anginosus* group, organisms of the *S. mitis* group, other than *S. pneumoniae,* are also commensals of the oropharynx, urogenital, and GI tract. They may also be transient colonizers of the skin and identified as contaminants in blood cultures. These organisms may be isolated in cases of endocarditis. Immunocompromised patients may develop septicemia or pneumonia. Infections with organisms in the *S. mitis* group may be difficult to treat due to the presence of penicillin resistance.

Enterococcus spp.

Enterococcus microscopic morphology is similar to streptococci on Gram stain. *Enterococcus* species commonly colonize the GI tract; however, they can be isolated from the oropharynx, female genital tract, and skin. Everyone has *Enterococcus* in the digestive system, but few people get sick from the endogenous strains. Typically, *Enterococcus* isolates are not as virulent as other gram-positive cocci and are often seen in polymicrobial infections in immunosuppressed hosts. Clinical manifestations include urinary tract infections; bacteremia; endocarditis; and intraabdominal, pelvic, wound, and soft tissue infections. The increasing resistance to antibiotics has caused an increase in health care–associated infections.

More than 57 *Enterococcus* species exist, including commensals that lack potent toxins and other well-defined virulence factors. Virulence factors associated with enterococci continue to be a topic of increasing research interest because of an increasing likelihood to cause health care–associated infections, especially *E. faecium*. Enterococci are considered the second and third leading cause of urinary tract infections, wound infections, and bacteremia in the United States. Some of the virulence factors identified in *Enterococcus* species include aggregation substance, capsular polysaccharides, surface carbohydrates, ability to translocate across intact intestinal mucosa, hemolysin, lipoteichoic acid, gelatinase, superoxide production, peptide inhibitors, and the ability to adhere to extracellular matrix proteins. The ability of these organisms to form biofilms is implicated in endocarditis, endodontic, and urinary tract infections, as well as the ability to adhere to medical devices and implants, resulting in infection.

Compared with other clinically important gram-positive cocci, *Enterococcus* (especially *E. faecium* and *E. faecalis)* is intrinsically more resistant to the antimicrobial agents commonly used in acute and long-term health care settings. They are not known to secrete toxins; however, the resistance of enterococci to multiple antibiotics allows them to survive and proliferate, especially in patients receiving multiple antimicrobials, causing superinfection. Most enterococci are also intrinsically resistant to aminoglycosides and β-lactams. In addition, these organisms are capable of acquiring and exchanging genes encoding resistance to antimicrobial agents. This genus was the first clinically relevant group of gram-positive cocci to acquire and disseminate resistance to vancomycin; hence the name **vancomycin-resistant *Enterococcus*** (VRE). Vancomycin is an antibiotic used to treat infections caused by gram-positive bacteria that are resistant to antibiotics typically used for treatment. The spread of this troublesome resistance marker from enterococci to other clinically relevant organisms, such as *Staphylococcus aureus*, is a serious public health concern.

Recommended treatment includes a combination of a cell-wall active agent, either a β-lactam or vancomycin, and an aminoglycoside. Combination treatment is synergistic and, generally, is sufficient even in the presence of intrinsic resistance to one of the antibiotics.

A wide variety of enterococci species can be isolated from human infections. *E. faecalis* and *E. faecium* are the pathogenic species most commonly encountered. *E. faecalis* and *E. faecium* have been isolated from the respiratory tract and the myocardium. Between these two species, *E. faecalis* is the most commonly encountered, but the incidence of *E. faecium* infections is on the rise in many hospitals. Vancomycin resistance is seen more frequently with *E. faecium* than with *E. faecalis*.

Vagococcus fluvialis, Lactococcus garvieae, and *Lactococcus lactis* can be misidentified as enterococci. *Vagococcus* spp. are motile, differentiating them from the lactococci. Both lactococci and vagococci are susceptible to vancomycin and fail to form gas in Mann, Rogosa, and Sharpe (MRS) broth; are pyrrolidonyl arylamidase (PYR) and leucine aminopeptidase (LAP) positive; and grow in 6.5% NaCl broth.

Miscellaneous Other Gram-Positive Cocci

The other genera listed in Table 14.1 are of low virulence and are almost exclusively associated with infections involving compromised hosts. Certain intrinsic features, such as resistance to vancomycin among *Leuconostoc* spp. and *Pediococcus* spp., may contribute to the ability of these organisms to survive in the hospital environment. However, whenever they are encountered, strong consideration must be given to their clinical relevance and potential as contaminants. These organisms can also challenge many identification schemes used for gram-positive cocci, and they may be misidentified as viridans streptococci.

Laboratory Diagnosis

Specimen Collection and Transport

No special considerations are required for specimen collection and transport of the organisms discussed in this chapter. Refer to Table 5.1 for general information on specimen collection and transport.

Specimen Processing

No special considerations are required for processing of the organisms discussed in this chapter. Refer to Table 5.1 for general information on specimen processing.

Direct Detection Methods

Antigen Detection

Antigen detection screening methods are available for several streptococcal antigens. Detection of antigens is possible using latex agglutination or enzyme-linked immunosorbent assay (ELISA) technologies. These commercial kits are generally very specific, but false-negative results may occur if specimens contain low numbers of *S. pyogenes.* Sensitivity has ranged from approximately 60% to greater than 95% depending on the methodology and other variables; thus, many microbiologists recommend collecting two throat swabs from each patient. If the first swab yields a positive result by a direct antigen method, the second swab can be discarded. However, for those specimens in which the rapid antigen test yielded a negative result, a blood agar plate or selective streptococcal blood agar plate should be inoculated with the second swab. To increase recovery for diagnosing streptococcal pharyngitis, a two-plate culture method is recommended where both sheep blood agar and trimethoprim-sulfamethoxazole (SXT) blood agar is inoculated.

The urine antigen test for the *S. pneumoniae* C-polysaccharide has a demonstrated sensitivity between 50% and 80%. The method has proven to be effective in adult patients who received antimicrobial treatment prior to a primary culture for identification of the organism. However, the test is unable to distinguish between previous and current infections, as well as carrier status often seen in children. The test is not recommended for use with children under 6 years of age, and recommended in conjunction with other laboratory diagnostic methods in adults.

S. pneumoniae and *S. agalactiae* (group B) antigen detection kits are available for diagnosing meningitis using CSF; however, direct extraction and latex particle agglutination has demonstrated a low (<30%) sensitivity. These tests are not recommended for routine diagnostic use.

Latex agglutination test kits are available for rapid detection of beta-hemolytic streptococcus Lancefield groups A, B, C, F, and G from primary culture plates. In addition, the latex agglutination test provides a rapid and simple method for definitive identification.

Nucleic Acid Detection

Molecular methods, or nucleic acid–based testing, are available, making diagnosis more rapid and specific when compared with traditional identification schemes. There are numerous methods available for the direct detection of *S. pyogenes* and *S. agalactiae.* Methods for the detection of *S. pyogenes* from throat swabs exceed the sensitivity (90% to 100%) of direct antigen testing for group A. Some of these methods do not require culture as a back-up for negative specimens. In addition to the direct nucleic acid detection methods for *S. agalactiae,* some assays recommend culture enrichment in selective broth prior to detection. These methods can be used to screen pregnant women for group B streptococci colonization. These tests are not recommended for group B screening immediately prior to delivery. Once the pregnant female arrives at the hospital, delivery of the fetus is generally imminent and does not provide sufficient time to administer antibiotic treatment for colonization.

The literature indicates that nucleic acid-based testing for *S. pneumoniae* is available due to a large variety of nonstandardized laboratory developed tests (LDTs) for the detection of the pneumococcal surface antigen, the pneumolysin gene, and the autolysin gene. In addition, a Food and Drug Administration (FDA)-cleared multiplex assay (the FilmArray Meningitis/Encephalitis Panel [bioMerieux Inc., Durham, NC]) includes the detection of *S. pneumoniae* from CSF. False-positive results are reported to occur requiring careful interpretation and correlation with additional laboratory testing. An additional FDA-cleared FilmArray Pneumonia Panel launched that detects 33 infectious targets from lower respiratory specimens, including 8 bacteria, 8 viruses, and 7 antimicrobial resistance genes. A second FilmArray Panel—the Pneumonia Panel Plus—detects 18 bacteria, 7 antibiotic resistance markers, and 9 viruses from lower respiratory samples. Both panels include *S. pneumoniae, S. pyogenes,* and *S. agalactiae.* The overall reported sensitivity is 96.2% and 98.3% specificity. Additional nucleic acid tests are available for the indirect detection of streptococci from automated blood culture bottles. These assays accurately detect *S. pyogenes* and *S. agalactiae,* but have not demonstrated reliable identification of *S. pneumoniae* or other streptococci, such as the viridans group.

The direct detection of vancomycin-resistant *(van)* genes in enterococci from rectal swabs and fecal specimens has reportedly improved detection over conventional culture techniques. The nucleic acid targets used in these systems are proprietary, and therefore sensitivity and specificity vary. In addition, vancomycin-resistant determinants are not unique to enterococci and may be found in other GI bacteria. Despite the limitations, reports indicate that the use of the assay has improved patient treatment and reduced the spread of related health care–associated infections increasing the rapid diagnosis and implementation of isolation and infection control measures.

Gram Stain

All the genera described in this chapter are gram-positive cocci. Cellular division for the streptococci and enterococci occurs along a single axis; thus, they grow in chains or pairs. In contrast, some of the aerobic gram-positive organisms that are infrequently isolated, such as *Aerococcus, Pediococcus, Facklamia, Dolosigranulum,* and *Helcococcus,* divide along multiple axes, which results in a cluster or irregular grouping of cells. Microscopically, streptococci and enterococci are typically round or oval-shaped, occasionally forming elongated cells that resemble pleomorphic corynebacteria or lactobacilli. However, they can appear rodlike, especially if the patient has been on antibiotics or the culture is very young, making Gram stains difficult to interpret. The cells may also appear gram-negative if cultures are dying. The cell walls will be deteriorating, resulting in the failure of the primary stain, crystal violet, being retained in the cell wall. In addition, *Gemella* spp. are easily decolorized, and *S. pneumoniae* is typically lancet-shaped and occurs singly, in pairs, or in short chains (Fig. 14.1). Gram stains made from blood cultures or broth cultures will show more chaining than those made from agar plates.

Growth in broth should be used for determination of cellular morphology if there is a question regarding

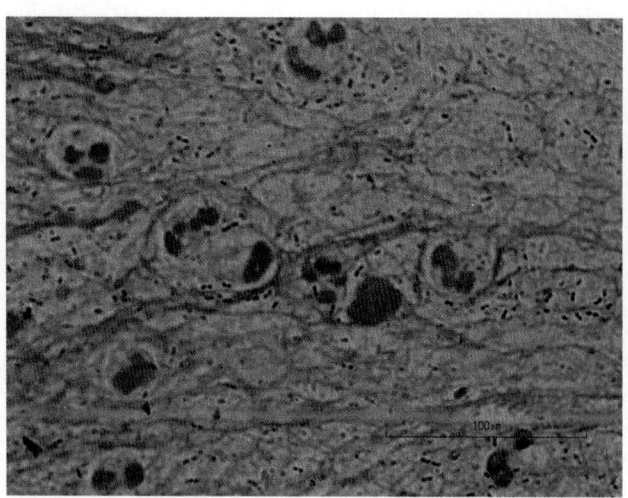

• **Fig. 14.1** *Streptococcus pneumoniae* lancet-shaped diplococci in Gram stain; note the encapsulated organisms, evident by the clear "halo."

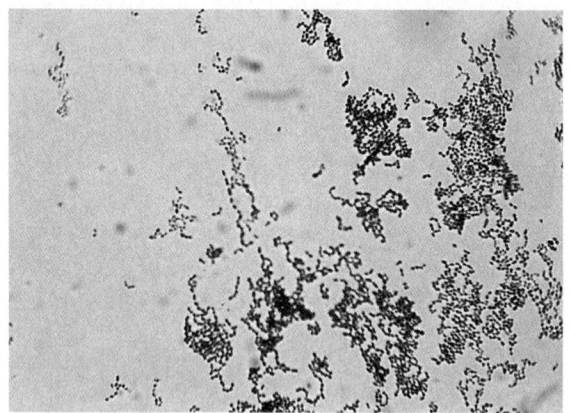

• **Fig. 14.2** Chains of streptococci seen in Gram stain prepared from broth culture.

staining characteristics from solid media. In fact, the genera described in this chapter are subdivided based on whether they have a "strep"-like Gram stain or a "staph"-like Gram stain. For example, *Streptococcus* and *Abiotrophia* growing in broth form long chains of cocci (Fig. 14.2), whereas *Aerococcus*, *Gemella*, and *Pediococcus* grow as large, spherical cocci arranged in small clusters (tetrads) or pairs, or as individual cells. *Leuconostoc* may elongate to form coccobacilli, although cocci are the primary morphology. The cellular arrangements of the genera in this chapter are noted by Tables 14.2 through 14.5.

Cultivation

Media of Choice

The organisms discussed in this chapter will grow on standard laboratory media, such as 5% sheep blood and chocolate agars. Some of the infrequently isolated genera, such as *Halococcus*, may require longer incubations of 48 to 72 hours on chocolate agar before visible growth is apparent. Streptococci will grow on gram-positive selective media such as **Columbia agar with colistin and nalidixic acid (CNA)** and **phenylethyl alcohol agar (PEA)**. CNA agar will inhibit

gram-negative organisms, staphylococci, *Bacillus* spp., and coryneforms, making it useful for specimens with mixed flora.

Abiotrophia and *Granulicatella* will not grow on blood and demonstrate reduced growth on chocolate agars unless **pyridoxal (vitamin B$_6$)** is supplied either by placement of a pyridoxal disk, by cross streaking with *Staphylococcus,* or by inoculation of vitamin B$_6$–supplemented culture media.

Blood culture media support the growth of all of these organisms, as do common nutrient broths, such as thioglycollate or brain-heart infusion. Blood cultures that appear positive and show chaining gram-positive cocci on Gram stain, but do not grow on subculture, should be subcultured again with a pyridoxal disk to consider the possibility of nutrient–variable pyridoxal–dependent organisms, such as *Abiotrophia* or *Granulicatella* bacteremia.

Other selective media are available for isolating certain species from clinical specimens. For isolating group A streptococci from throat swabs, the most common medium is 5% sheep blood agar supplemented with SXT to suppress the growth of normal microbiota. A bacitracin disc is placed on the initial inoculum, first quadrant, to aid in identification. However, this medium also inhibits growth of groups C, F, and G beta-hemolytic streptococci.

To detect genital carriage of group B streptococci during pregnancy, a vaginal or rectal swab is inoculated into Todd-Hewitt broth, such as LIM (Chapter 7). Todd-Hewitt broths contain antimicrobials (gentamicin, nalidixic acid, or CNA), which suppress the growth of normal vaginal microbiota and allow growth of GBS. After 24-hour incubation, the LIM broth is subcultured to 5% sheep blood agar. LIM broth can be subcultured to commercially available chromogenic agar, designed specifically for detection of GBS with sensitivity close to 100%. Latex agglutination confirmation test can be performed directly from the plates on suspected colonies. All plates negative for GBS should be incubated for an additional 24 hours.

Differentiation of enterococci, group D streptococci, and lactococci has been traditionally based on the ability of the organisms to hydrolyze esculin in the presence of 40% bile; other streptococci do not. The esculetin in bile esculin agar reacts with an iron salt to form a dark brown precipitate surrounding the colonies. **Enterococcosel agar** is a selective differential medium based on the esculin hydrolysis and is selective by incorporation of inhibitory oxgall (bile salts) to inhibit growth of other gram-positive organisms, with the exception of group D streptococci, and sodium azide to inhibit growth of gram-negative organisms. However, occasionally, other bacteria may display the dark brown precipitate. Bile esculin agar and enterococcosel agar with vancomycin is used for a primary screening to detect vancomycin-resistant enterococci.

Due to the increase in incidence of vancomycin resistance in clinical isolates of enterococci, numerous methods for the isolation and differentiation of these organisms are available that include agar and broth-based methods. No current consensus is available as to what media provides optimal recovery; however, broth selective-enrichment using BHI

TABLE 14.2 Differentiation of Clinically Relevant Beta-hemolytic *Streptococcus* Species (Catalase-Negative, Gram-Positive Cocci Primarily in Chains)

Species	Lancefield Group	PYR	VP	Hippurate	Bacitracin	Trehalose	Sorbitol	CAMP
S. agalactiae	B	–	–	+	R	V	–	+
S. dysgalactiae subsp. equisimilis	A, C, G, L	–	–	–	R	+	V	–
S. pyogenes	A	+	–	–	S	+	–	–
S. angino sus group[a]	A, C, G, F, Nontypeable	–	+	–	R	+	–	–

[a]*S. anginosus* group may demonstrate beta-, alpha- or gamma-hemolysis.
+, positive; –, negative; v, variable; R, resistant; S, susceptible.

(brain heart infusion), BE-azide (bile esculin), and Enterococcosel broth medias supplemented with vancomycin have been used to improve recovery of the organisms prior to plating to either routine or selective media such as chromogenic agar. A variety of commercially available chromogenic agars can be used for the detection of vancomycin-resistant enterococci. The various media also contain varying concentrations of vancomycin but are also useful in the identification of the two most common isolates, *E. faecium* and *E. faecalis.*

Incubation Conditions and Duration

Most of the organisms included in this chapter are facultative anaerobes, with some preferring a CO_2-enriched environment. Laboratories typically incubate blood or chocolate agar plates in 5% to 10% carbon dioxide, which is the preferred atmosphere for *S. pneumoniae* and is acceptable for all other genera discussed in this chapter. Visualization of beta-hemolysis is enhanced by anaerobic conditions in some organisms such as *S. pyogenes.* The blood agar plates should be inoculated by stabbing the inoculating loop into the agar several times (Fig. 14.3A). Colonies will grow throughout the depth of the agar, producing subsurface oxygen-sensitive hemolysins (i.e., streptolysin O) (Fig. 14.3B). Most organisms will grow on agar media within 48 hours of inoculation.

Colonial Appearance

Tables 14.2 through 14.5 either indicate or are separated by hemolysis on 5% sheep blood agar and other distinguishing characteristics. The beta-hemolytic streptococci may have a distinctive buttery odor. Viridans streptococci have a butterscotch odor, especially on chocolate agar.

Approach to Identification

None of the commercial identification systems accurately identify all species of viridans streptococci, enterococci, or the infrequently isolated genera. Polymerase chain reaction (PCR) is a rapid, reliable, reproducible technique for identification of *Streptococcus* spp. and *Enterococcus* spp. There are various PCRs for the different groups and their target genes.

Matrix-Assisted Laser Desorption Ionization Time-of-Flight Mass Spectrometry

Matrix-assisted laser desorption ionization time-of-flight mass spectrometry (MALDI-TOF MS) has been developed to determine species of *Streptococcus* and the commonly isolated *Enterococcus* species. However, limitations do occur. For example, correct identification of *S. dysgalactiae* to the subspecies level is not always reliable. Another limitation is that the MALDI-TOF MS cannot always distinguish between *S. pneumoniae* and members of the *S. mitis* group (*S. mitis* and *S. oralis*). Use of a P disk for optochin sensitivity or a bile solubility test will aid in differentiating these bacteria. Reliable identification of species within the *S. mitis* and *S. bovis* groups are also unreliable. MALDI-TOF MS methods are limited based on the size of the database. Several of the infrequently isolated organisms have, however, been successfully identified using this technique, including *Aerococcus, Lactococcus, Leuconostoc, Weisella,* and *Pediococcus.* It should be noted that the identification of gram-positive bacteria improves with the use of extraction procedures before application on the target because of the thickness of the peptidoglycan layer in the cell wall.

Comments Regarding Specific Organisms

Useful characteristics for differentiation among catalase-negative, gram-positive cocci are shown in Tables 14.2 through 14.5.

The cellular arrangement and the type of hemolysis are important considerations in identification. If the presence of hemolysis is uncertain, the colony should be moved aside with a loop, and the medium directly beneath the original colony should be examined by holding the plate in front of a light source.

A screening test for vancomycin susceptibility is often useful for differentiating among many alpha-hemolytic

TABLE 14.3 Differentiation of *Enterococcus* Species (Catalase-Negative, Alpha-, Beta-, or Gamma-hemolytic, PYR Positive, Gram-Positive Cocci Primarily in Pairs and Chains)

Species	ARA	ARG	GAL	LAC	MAN	MGP	PYU	RAF	SOR	SBL	SUC	TEL	TRE	XYL
E. avium	+	-	v	+	+	v	+	-	+	+	+	-	+	-
E. caccae	-	-	-	-	-	+	-	-	-	-	+	-	+	-
E. canintestini	-	+	-	+	-	+	+	+	-	-	+	-	+	-
E. casseliflavus	+	+	+	+	+	+	v	+	-	v	+	-	+	+
E. cecorum	-	-	+	+	-	-	+	+	+	-	+	-	+	-
E. dispar	-	+	+	+	-	+	+	+	-	-	-	-	+	-
E. durans	-	+	v	+	-	+	-	-	-	-	-	-	-	-
E. faecalis	-	+	-	+	+	-	+	-	-	-	+	+	+	-
E. faecium	+	+	v	+	+	-	-	v	-	v	+	-	+	-
E. gallinarum	+	+	+	+	+	+	+	+	-	-	+	-	+	+
E. gilvus	-	-	-	+	+	-	+	+	+	+	+	-	+	-
E. hawaiiensis	-	-	-	-	+	-	+	-	+	+	-	-	+	-
E. hirae	-	+	v	+	-	-	-	+	-	-	+	-	+	-
E. italicus	-	-	-	+	v	v	+	-	-	v	+	-	+	v
E. malodoratus	-	-	+	+	+	v	+	+	+	+	+	-	+	+
E. massiliensis	+	+	+	-	-	+	-	+	-	-	+	-	+	+
E. mundtii	+	+	v	+	+	-	-	+	-	v	+	-	+	+
E. pallens[a]	-	-	-	ND	+	-	+	+	+	+	+	-	+	+
E. pseudoavium	-	-	v	+	+	+	+	-	+	+	+	-	+	v
E. raffinosus	+	-	-	+	+	v	+	+	+	-	+	-	+	-
E. thailandicus	-	+	-	+	+	-	-	-	-	-	+	-	+	-

+, 90% or more of the strains are positive; −, 90% or more of the strains are negative; v, variable 11%–89% of the strains are positive; *ND*, no data.
ARA, Arabinose; *ARG*, arginine; *GAL*, 1-naphthyl-Beta-D-galactopyranoside; *LAC*, lactose; *MAN*, mannitol; *MGP*, methal-alpha-d-glucopyranoside; *PYU*, pyruvate; *RAF*, raffinose; *SOR*, sorbose; *SBL*, sorbitol; *SUC*, sucrose; *TEL*, tellurite; *TRE*, trehalose; *XYL*, xylose.
[a]PYR negative.

TABLE 14.4 Differentiation of Catalase-Negative, Gram-Positive Coccoid Organisms Primarily in Chains

Organisms	Gram Stain From Thio Broth	Hemolysis[a] (α, β, or γ)	Cytochrome[b]/Catalase	Van	LAP	PYR	Gas in MRS Broth	Motility	On BE	In 6.5% NaCl Broth	Growth At 10°C	Growth At 45°C	Comments
Leuconostoc	cb, pr, ch	α, γ	−/−	R	V	−	+	−	V	V	V	V	
Streptococcus gallolyticus subsp. *gallolyticus*	c, ch	α, γ	−/	S	+	−	−	−	+	−	−	+	
Viridans streptococci	c, ch	α, γ	−/−	S	+	−	−	−	−	−	−	V	
Abiotrophia	c, ch	α, γ	−/−	S	V	V	−	−	−	−	−	V	Satellitism around *Staphylococcus aureus*
Granulicatella	c, pr, ch	α	−/−	S	+	+	−	−	NT	−	−	V	Satellitism around *S. aureus*
Lactococcus	cb, ch	α, γ	−/−	S	+	V	−	−	+	V	+	V[c]	
Dolosicoccus	c, pr, ch	α	−/−	S	−	+	−	−	−	−	−	−	
Globicatella	c, ch, pr	α, γ	−/−	S	−	V	−	−	+	+	+	V	
Vagococcus	c, ch	α, γ	−/−	S	+	+	−	+	+	V	+	V	
Weissella confusa	Elongated bacilli[d]	α	−/−	R	−	NT	+	V	+	V	NT	+	Arginine positive

[a]Hemolysis tested on tryptic soy agar with 5% sheep blood.
[b]Cytochrome enzymes as detected by the porphyrin broth test.
[c]Majority of strains will not grow at 45°C in 48 hours or less.
[d]From blood agar, the organism resembles a gram-positive coccobacillus.

+, 90% or more of species or strains are positive; −, 90% or more of species or strains are negative; α, alpha-hemolytic; β, beta-hemolytic; γ, gamma-hemolytic; *BE*, bile esculin hydrolysis; c, cocci; cb, coccobacilli; ch, chaining; *LAP*, leucine aminopeptidase; *MRS*, gas from glucose in Mann, Rogosa, Sharp *Lactobacillus* broth; *NT*, not tested; pr, pairs; *PYR*, pyrrolidonyl arylamidase; *thio*, thioglycollate broth; V, variable reactions; *Van*, vancomycin (30 μg) susceptible (S) or resistant (R).

TABLE 14.5 Differentiation of Catalase-Negative, Gram-Positive, Coccoid Organisms Primarily in Clusters or Tetrads

Organisms	Gram Stain From Thio Broth	Hemolysis[a] α, β, or γ	Cytochrome[b]/ Catalase	Van	LAP	PYR	Gas in MRS Broth	Motility	On BE	In 6.5% NaCl Broth	Growth At 10°C	Growth At 45°C	Comments
Facklamia	c, pr, ch, cl	α, γ	−/−	S	+	+	−	−	NT	+[c]	−	−	
Dolosigranulum	c, cl	γ	−	S	+	+ wk	−	−	−	+	−	−	
Ignavigranum ruoffiae	c, pr, cl	α	−/−	S	+	+	−	−	−	+	−	−[d]	Enhanced growth around *Staphylococcus aureus*; sauerkraut odor on SBA
Gemella	c, pr, ch, cl, tet[e]	α, γ	−/−	S[f]	V[g]	V[h]	−	−	−	−	−	−	
Pediococcus[i]	c, pr, tet, cl	α, γ	−/−	R	+	−	−	−	+	V	−	V	
Aerococcus	c, pr, tet, cl	α	−/−	S	+	−	−	−	−	+	−	V¼[j]	
Aerococcus urinae													
A. viridans	c, pr, tet, cl	α	−/+[wk]	S	−	+	−	−	V	+	V	V	
Helcococcus[k]	c, pr, ch, cl	γ	−/−	S	−	+	−	−	−	+[l]	−	−	Lipophilic

[a]Hemolysis tested on tryptic soy agar with 5% sheep blood.

[b]Cytochrome enzymes as detected by the porphyrin broth test.

[c]*Facklamia hominis*, *F. ignava*, and *F. languida* are positive, and *F. sourekii* is negative.

[d]Positive after 7 days.

[e]*Gemella haemolysans* easily decolorizes when Gram stained. They resemble *Neisseria* with adjacent flattened sides of pairs of cells.

[f]There is one literature report of a vancomycin-resistant *G. haemolysans*.

[g]*G. haemolysans* and *G. sanguinis* are LAP negative, and *G. morbillorum* and *G. bergeri* are positive.

[h]Weakly positive. Use a large inoculum.

[i]The most commonly isolated pediococci are arginine deaminase positive.

[j]If inoculated too heavily, the organism will grow at 45°C.

[k]Lipophilic—growth stimulated on HIA (heart infusion agar) with 1% horse serum or 0.1% Tween.

[l]Owing to the fact that *Helcococcus* is lipophilic, the salt broth may appear to be negative unless supplemented with 1% horse serum or 0.1% Tween 80.

+, 90% or more of species or strains are positive; +[wk], strains or species may be weakly positive; −, 90% or more of species or strains negative; α, alpha-hemolytic; β, beta-hemolytic; γ, gamma-hemolytic; *BE*, bile esculin hydrolysis; *c*, cocci; *cb*, coccobacilli; *ch*, chaining; *cl*, clusters; *LAP*, leucine aminopeptidase; *MRS*, gas from glucose in Mann, Rogosa, Sharp *Lactobacillus* broth; *NT*, not tested; *pr*, pairs; *PYR*, pyrrolidonyl arylamidase; *SBA*, 5% sheep blood agar; *tet*, tetrads; *thio*, thioglycollate broth; *V*, variable; *Van*, vancomycin (30 μg) susceptible reactions, (S) or resistant (R).

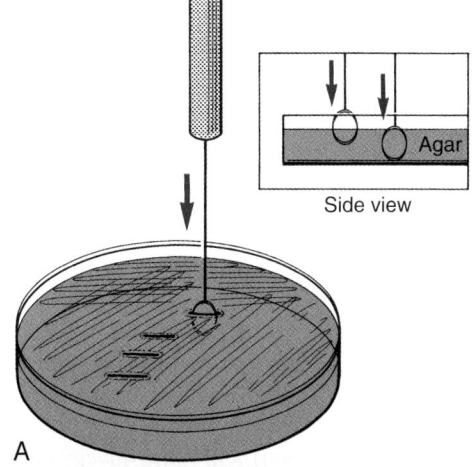

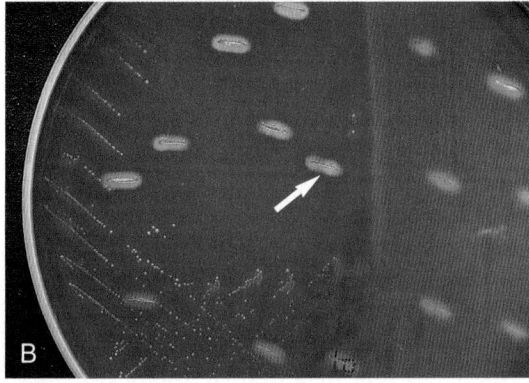

• **Fig. 14.3** Diagrammatical representation for stabbing the inoculating loop vertically into the agar after streaking the blood agar plate (A) allows subsurface colonies to display hemolysis caused by streptolysin O. (B) Sheep blood agar plate demonstrating enhanced beta-hemolysis surrounding a vertical stab.

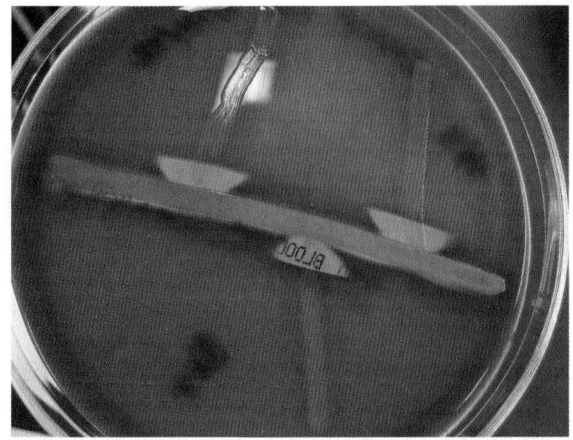

• **Fig. 14.4** Positive Christie, Atkins, Munch-Petersen reaction as indicated by enlarged zone of hemolysis shaped like the tip of an arrow; *Streptococcus agalactiae* intersecting with *Streptococcus aureus* streak line.

cocci. All streptococci, aerococci, gemellas, lactococci, and most enterococci are susceptible to vancomycin (any zone of inhibition), whereas pediococci, leuconostocs, and many lactobacilli are typically resistant (growth up to the disk).

Leuconostoc produces gas from glucose in MRS broth, which distinguishes it from all other genera, except the lactobacilli; however, unlike *Leuconostoc* spp., lactobacilli appear as elongated bacilli when Gram stained from thioglycollate broth. Several organisms (e.g., *Leuconostoc, Pediococcus, Lactococcus, Helcococcus, Globicatella, Tetragenococcus,* and *Aerococcus viridans*) will show growth on BE agar and in 6.5% salt broth; therefore, these two tests can no longer solely be used to identify enterococci.

Serologic grouping of cell wall carbohydrates (Lancefield classifications) is used to identify species of beta-hemolytic streptococci. The Lancefield Group carbohydrate latex agglutination procedures are available as commercial kits. Serologic tests have the advantage of being rapid, confirmatory, and easily performed on one or two colonies. However, they are more expensive than biochemical screening tests.

The PYR and hippurate or Christie, Atkins, Munch-Petersen (CAMP) tests can be used to identify groups A and B streptococci, respectively; however, use of the 0.04-U bacitracin disk is no longer recommended for *S. pyogenes,* because groups C and G streptococci are also susceptible to this agent. *S. pyogenes* is the only species of beta-hemolytic streptococci associated with human infections that will give a positive PYR reaction. A brown halo around colonies on bile esculin agar and a positive PYR reaction is generally indicative of *Enterococcus* sp.

S. agalactiae is able to hydrolyze hippurate and is positive in the CAMP test. The CAMP test detects production of a diffusible, extracellular protein that enhances the hemolysis of sheep erythrocytes by *Staphylococcus aureus.* A positive test is recognized by the appearance of an arrowhead shape at the juncture of the *S. agalactiae* and *S. aureus* streaks (Fig. 14.4). Occasionally, nonhemolytic strains of *S. agalactiae* may be encountered. Identification of such isolates can be accomplished using the serologic agglutination approach. Enterococci can also be hippurate hydrolysis positive.

Table 14.2 shows the differentiation of the clinically relevant beta-hemolytic streptococci. Minute beta-hemolytic streptococci are all likely to be of the *S. anginosus* group; a positive Voges-Proskauer test and negative PYR test identify a beta-hemolytic streptococcal isolate as such.

Colonies suspicious as *S. pneumoniae* (small, gray, moist, alpha-hemolytic; center may be depressed) must be tested for either bile solubility or susceptibility to optochin (ethylhydrocupreine hydrochloride). The bile solubility test is confirmatory and is based on the ability of bile salts to induce lysis of *S. pneumoniae. Streptococcus pseudopneumoniae* is generally insoluble, along with other alpha-hemolytic streptococci. In the optochin test, which is presumptive, a filter paper disk ("P" disk) impregnated with optochin is placed on a blood agar plate previously streaked with a lawn of the suspect organism. The plate is incubated at 35°C for 18 to 24 hours and examined for a zone of inhibition. *S. pneumoniae* produce a zone of inhibition, whereas viridans streptococci grow up to the disk and thus are resistant. Occasional strains of *S. oralis, S. mitis,* and *S. pseudopneumoniae* are optochin sensitive. Optochin disk tests should be incubated under 5% CO_2, and all tests should be confirmed by a bile solubility test.

Once *S. pneumoniae* has been ruled out as a possibility for an alpha-hemolytic isolate, viridans streptococci, and enterococci must be considered. Keep in mind that *Aerococcus, Abiotrophia, Granulicatella, Dolosicoccus, Dolosigranulum, Ignavigranum Facklamia, Gemella, Globicatella, Helcococcus, Lactococcus, Leuconostoc,* and *Pediococcus* can all resemble viridian streptococcus. In addition, *Pediococcus* can be confused with enterococci, because they are bile-esculin positive and cross-react with group D antisera. Carbohydrate fermentation tests are performed in heart infusion broth with bromocresol purple indicator. Although alpha-hemolytic streptococci are not often identified beyond the genus, there are cases (e.g., endocarditis, isolation from multiple blood cultures) in which full identification is indicated. This is particularly true for blood culture isolates from the *S. bovis* group that have been associated with GI malignancy and may be an early indicator of GI cancer. Organisms in the *S. bovis* group possess group D antigen that may be detected using commercially available typing sera. However, this is not a definitive test, because other organisms (e.g., *Leuconostoc*) may also produce a positive result.

Except for species infrequently isolated from humans (*E. bulliens, E. canintestini, E. cecorum, E. columbae, E. devriesei, E. moraviensis, E. pallens, E. saccharolytics, E. termitis,* and *E. viikkiensis*), all enterococci hydrolyze PYR and possess group D antigen. Identifying the species of enterococcal isolates is important for understanding the epidemiology of antimicrobial resistance among isolates of this genus and for managing patients with enterococcal infections. Most clinical laboratories identify *Enterococcus* spp. presumptively by demonstrating that the isolate is PYR and LAP (hydrolyze leucine-β-naphthylamide) positive and grows in 6.5% NaCl. However, *S. urinalis* and the commonly isolated *Enterococcus* spp. exhibit identical reactions in the tests listed here and only differ in the ability to grow at 10°C (*S. urinalis* cannot). Table 14.3 includes biochemical reactions that can be used to separate the species of enterococci isolated from human infections.

Serodiagnosis

Individuals with disease caused by *S. pyogenes* produce antibodies against various antigens. The most common are antistreptolysin O (ASO), anti-DNase B, antistreptokinase, and antihyaluronidase. Pharyngitis seems to be followed by rises in antibody titers against all antigens, whereas patients with pyoderma, an infection of the skin, only show a significant response to anti-DNase B. Use of serodiagnostic tests is most useful to demonstrate prior streptococcal infection in patients from whom *Streptococcus* spp. have not been cultured but who present with sequelae suggestive of rheumatic fever or acute glomerulonephritis. Serum obtained as long as 2 months after infection usually demonstrates increased antibodies. As with other serologic tests, an increasing titer over time is most useful for diagnosing previous streptococcal

infection. *S. dysgalactiae* subsp. *equisimilis* isolates can also produce streptolysin O following upper respiratory infection, and therefore elevated ASO titers are not specific to *S. pyogenes*.

There are no commercial systems available for detection of antibodies related to infection with enterococci.

Antimicrobial Susceptibility Testing and Therapy

For *S. pyogenes*, penicillin is the drug of choice; however, some strains of *S. agalactiae* demonstrate a decreased susceptibility to penicillin due to a mutation in the penicillin-binding protein. Macrolides and clindamycin are used in patients who are allergic to penicillin. However, if a macrolide such as erythromycin is being considered for use, testing is required to detect resistance that has emerged among some of these organisms. Susceptibility and resistance patterns to erythromycin can be used as a predictor for sensitivity patterns in streptococci to azithromycin, clarithromycin, and dirithromycin.

The emergence of resistance to a variety of different antimicrobial classes in *S. pneumoniae* and viridans streptococci dictates that clinically relevant isolates be tested using *in vitro* susceptibility. When testing is performed, methods that produce minimum inhibitory concentration (MIC) data for beta-lactams are preferred. The level of resistance (i.e., MIC in micrograms per milliliter) can provide important information regarding therapeutic management of the patient, particularly in cases of pneumococcal meningitis in which relatively slight increases in MIC can have substantial effects on the clinical efficacy of penicillins and cephalosporins. Vancomycin resistance has not been described in *S. pneumoniae* or viridans streptococci.

S. pneumoniae or other beta-hemolytic *Streptococcus* spp. that demonstrate resistance to erythromycin and are susceptible or intermediate to clindamycin should be examined for inducible clindamycin resistance, as previously described for *Staphylococcus* spp. in Chapter 13. Disk diffusion using Mueller Hinton or tryptic soy agar supplemented with 5% sheep blood may be used. Place a 14 μg erythromycin disk and a 2 μg disk 12 mm apart. If inducible resistance is present, the clindamycin zone adjacent to the erythromycin disk will demonstrate the classic flattening or D-zone appearance. Alternately, a broth microdilution using Mueller Hinton containing lysed horse blood (2.5% to 5%) may be used by adding 1 μg/mL erythromycin and 0.5 μg/mL clindamycin within a single well. Any visible growth within the well would indicate inducible clindamycin resistance. Automated analyzers have replaced the D-zone test by including the antibiotics and a combined test in the panels. Fluoroquinolone resistance among streptococci is also an increasing concern.

Enterococci are intrinsically resistant to a wide array of antimicrobial agents, and they are generally resistant to killing by any of the single agents (e.g., ampicillin or vancomycin) that are bactericidal for most other gram-positive cocci. Effective bactericidal activity can only be achieved with the combination of a cell wall–active agent, such as ampicillin or vancomycin, and an aminoglycoside, such as gentamicin or streptomycin. The performance of *in vitro* susceptibility testing with clinical isolates from systemic infections is critical for determining which combination of agents may still be effective therapeutic choices. Enterococci species identified in human infections that have had prolonged exposure to vancomycin have been identified that are no longer able to grow in the absence of the antibiotic. These organisms are now considered an unusual phenotype of vancomycin-dependent enterococci (VDE) and require D-alanyl-D-alanine production for cell wall synthesis.

For uncomplicated urinary tract infections, bactericidal activity is usually not required for clinical efficacy, so single agents such as ampicillin, nitrofurantoin, or a quinolone are often sufficient.

All gram-positive bacteria demonstrate intrinsic antibiotic resistance to polymyxin B/colistin, nalidixic acid, and aztreonam. In addition, several species of enterococci are intrinsically resistant to additional antibiotics. Careful consideration is required when reporting susceptibilities. Cephalosporins, aminoglycosides (except for high-level resistance screening), clindamycin, and trimethoprim-sulfamethoxazole may appear to be effective in the laboratory using *in vitro* methods, but they are not clinically effective and should not be reported as susceptible.

Prevention

A single-dose, 23-valent vaccine (Pneumovax, Merck & Co., Inc., West Point, PA) to prevent infection by the most common serotypes of *S. pneumoniae* is available in the United States. The CDC recommends pneumococcal conjugate vaccine (PCV13) for infants and young children, all adults younger than 65 years, and people 6 years or older with risk factors. Pneumococcal polysaccharide vaccine (PPSV23) is recommended for all adults 65 years or older and for children 2 years and older with medical conditions such as sickle cell disease, diabetes, cochlear implants, damaged spleen, CSF leaks, diseases that affect the immune system, or chronic heart or lung failure. The vaccine is not effective in children younger than 2 years of age. The serotypes included in this vaccine account for the majority of cases of bacteremia, meningitis, and otitis media in children younger than 6 years of age.

Ⓔ Visit the Evolve site for a complete list of procedures, review questions, and case studies.

Bibliography

Arbique JC, Poyart C, Trieu-Cuot P, et al.: Accuracy of phenotypic and genotypic testing for identification of *Streptococcus pneumoniae* and description of *Streptococcus pseudopneumoniae* sp. nov, *J Clin Microbiol* 42:4686–4696, 2004.

Berger S: *GIDEON guide to medically important bacteria*, Gideon Informatics, 2019.

Bhat DP, Nagaraju L, Asmar BI, Aggarwal S: *Abiotrophia* endocarditis in children with no underlying heart disease: a rare but a virulent organism, *Congenit Heart Dis* 9:E116–E120, 2014.

Binghuai L, Yanli S, Shuchen Z, Fengxia Z, Dong L, Yanchao C: Use of MALDI-TOF mass spectrometry for rapid identification of group B *Streptococcus* on chromID Strepto B agar, *Int J Infect Dis* 27:44–48, 2014.

Buchan BW, Windham S, Faron ML, et al.: *Clinical evaluation and potential impact of a semi-quantitative multiplex molecular assay for identification of pathogenic bacteria and viruses N Lower respiratory specimens, poster.* Available at: https://www.biomerieux.pt/sites/clinic/files/2018_ats_buchan_clinical_evalaution_and_potential_impact_of_semi-quant_mx_molec_assay_for_pneumonia.pdf. [Accessed 17 February 2019].

Camelo-Castillo A, Henares D, Brotons P, et al.: Nasopharyngeal microbiota in children with invasive pneumococcal disease: identification of bacteria with potential disease-promoting and protective effects, *Front Microbiol* 10:11, 2019.

Carkaci D, Højholt K, Nielsen XC, et al.: Genomic characterization, phylogenetic analysis, and identification of virulence factors in *Aerococcus sanguinicola* and *Aerococcus urinae* strains isolated from infection episodes, *Microb Pathog* 112:327–340, 2017.

Carroll KC, Pfaller MA, Landry ML, et al.: *Manual of clinical microbiology*, ed 12, Washington, DC, 2019, ASM Press.

Chapin KC, Blake P, Wilson CD: Performance characteristics and utilization of rapid antigen test, DNA probe, and culture for detection of group a streptococci in an acute care clinic, *J Clin Microbiol* 40:4207–4210, 2002.

Cherkaoui A, Emonet S, Fernandez J, Schorderet D, Schrenzel J: Evaluation of matrix-assisted laser desorption ionization-time of flight mass spectrometry for rapid identification of beta-hemolytic streptococci, *J Clin Microbiol* 49:3004–3005, 2011.

Collins MD, Hutson RA, Falsen E, Nikolaitchouk N, LaClaire L, Facklam RR: An unusual *Streptococcus* from human urine, *Streptococcus urinalis* sp. nov, *Int J Syst Evol Microbiol* 50:1173–1178, 2000.

Collins MD, Lawson PA: The genus *Abiotrophia* (Kawamura et al.) is not monophyletic: proposal of *Granulicatella* gen. nov., *Granulicatella adiacens* comb. nov., *Granulicatella elegans* comb. nov. and *Granulicatella balaenopterae* comb. nov, *Int J Syst Evol Microbiol* 50:365–369, 2000.

Corona PS, Haddad S, Andrés J, González-López JJ, Amat C, Flores X: Case report: first report of a prosthetic joint infection caused by *Facklamia hominis*, *Diagn Microbiol Infect Dis* 80:338–340, 2014.

De Paulis AN, Bertona E, Gutiérrez MA, Ramírez MS, Vay CA, Predari SC: *Ignavigranum ruoffiae*, a rare pathogen that caused a skin abscess, *JMM Case Rep* 5, 2018:e005137.

Dolka B, Chrobak-Chmiel D, Czopowicz M, Szeleszczuk P: Characterization of pathogenic Enterococcus cecorum from different poultry groups: Broiler chickens, layers, turkeys, and waterfowl, *PLoS One* :e0185199 12, 2017.

Eraclio G, Ricci G, Quattrini M, Moroni P, Fortina MG: Detection of virulence-related genes in *Lactococcus garvieae* and their expression in response to different conditions, *Folia Microbiol (Praha)* 63:291–298, 2018.

Facklam RR: Newly described, difficult-to-identify, catalase-negative, gram-positive cocci, *Clin Microbiol Newsl* 23:1–7, 2001.

Garcia-Granja PE, López J, Ladrón R, San Román JA: Infective endocarditis due to *Leuconostoc* species, *Rev Esp Cardiol (Engl ED)* 71:592–594, 2018.

Glazunova OO, Raoult D, Roux V: Streptococcus massiliensis sp. nov., isolated from a patient blood culture, *Int J Syst Evol Microbiol* 56:1127–1131, 2006.

Goh SH, Facklam RR, Chang M, et al.: Identification of *Enterococcus* species and phenotypically similar *Lactococcus* and *Vagococcus* species by reverse checkerboard hybridization to chaperon in 60 gene sequences, *J Clin Microbiol* 38:3953–3959, 2000.

Harimaya A, Takada R, Hendolin PH, Fujii N, Ylikoski J, Himi T: High incidence of *Alloiococcus otitidis* in children with otitis media, despite treatment with antibiotics, *J Clin Microbiol* 44:946–949, 2006.

Hassan AA, Abdulmawjood A, Yildirim AO, Fink K, Lämmler C, Schlenstedt R: Identification of streptococci isolated from various sources by determination of cfb gene and other CAMP-factor genes, *Can J Microbiol* 46:946–951, 2000.

LaClaire L, Facklam R: Antimicrobial susceptibility and clinical sources of *Dolosigranulum pigrum* cultures, *Antimicrob Agents Chemother* 44:2001–2003, 2000.

Leber AL: *Aerobic bacteriology, clinical microbiology procedures handbook*, ed 4, Washington, DC, 2016, ASM Press.

Lebreton F, Willems RJL, Gilmore MS: Enterococcus diversity, origins in nature, and gut colonization. In *Enterococci: From Commensals to Leading Causes of Drug Resistant Infection*, 2014. Available at: https://www.ncbi.nlm.nih.gov/books/NBK190427/. [Accessed 2 March 2019].

Lévesque S, Longtin Y, Domingo MC, et al.: Enterococcus pallens as a potential novel human pathogen: three cases of spontaneous bacterial peritonitis, *JMM Case Reports*, 2016. Available at: https://www.microbiologyresearch.org/docserver/fulltext/jmmcr/3/1/jmmcr005024.pdf?expires=1551577025&id=id&accname=guest&checksum=DCA3CB340F1A072DED6EEE7D570F8E25. [Accessed 2 March 2019].

Manero A, Blanch AR: Identification of Enterococcus spp. with a Biochemical Key, *Appl Environ Microbiol* 65:4425–4430, 1999.

Poisson DM, Evrard ML, Freneaux C, Vivès MI, Mesnard L: Evaluation of CHROMagar™ StrepB agar, an aerobic chromogenic medium for prepartum vaginal/rectal Group B *Streptococcus* screening, *J Microbiol Methods* 84:490–491, 2011.

Poyart C, Quesne G, Trieu-Cuot P: Taxonomic dissection of the *Streptococcus bovis* group by analysis of manganese-dependent superoxide dismutase gene (sodA) sequences: reclassification of "*Streptococcus infantarius* subsp. *coli*" as *Streptococcus lutetiensis* sp. nov. and of *Streptococcus bovis* biotype II.2 as *Streptococcus pasteurianus* sp. nov, *Int J Syst Evol Microbiol* 52:1247–1255, 2002.

Rallu F, Barriga P, Scrivo C, Martel-Laferrière V, Laferrière C: Sensitivities of antigen detection and PCR assays greatly increased compared to that of the standard culture method for screening for group B *Streptococcus* carriage in pregnant women, *J Clin Microbiol* 44:725–728, 2006.

Schlegel L, Grimont F, Ageron E, Grimont PA, Bouvet A: Reappraisal of the taxonomy of the *Streptococcus bovis/Streptococcus equinus* complex and related species: description of *Streptococcus gallolyticus* subsp. *gallolyticus* subsp. nov., *S. gallolyticus* subsp. *macedonicus* subsp. nov. and *S. gallolyticus* subsp. *pasteurianus* subsp. nov, *Int J Syst Evol Microbiol* 53:631–645, 2003.

Schlegel L, Grimont F, Collins MD, Régnault B, Grimont PA, Bouvet A: *Streptococcus infantarius* sp. nov., *Streptococcus infantarius* subsp. *infantarius* subsp. nov. and *Streptococcus infantarius* subsp. *coli* subsp. nov., isolated from humans and food, *Int J Syst Evol Microbiol* 50:1425–1434, 2000.

Tan JS, File TM: *Streptococcus species* (group G and group C streptococci, viridans group, nutritionally variant streptococci). *Antimicrobe: Infectious Disease Antimicrobial Agents*. Available at: http://www.antimicrobe.org/b241.asp. [Accessed 9 July 2016].

Tanasupawat S, Sukontasing S, Lee JS: *Enterococcus thailandicus* sp. nov., isolated from fermented sausage ('mum') in Thailand, *Int J Syst Evol Microbiol* 58:1630–1634, 2008.

Tyrrell GJ, Turnbull L, Teixeira LM, et al.: *Enterococcus gilvus* sp. nov. and *Enterococcus pallens* sp. nov. isolated from human clinical specimens, *J Clin Microbiol* 40:1140–1145, 2002.

15

Bacillus and Similar Organisms

OBJECTIVES

1. Describe the general characteristics of *Bacillus anthracis*, including colonial morphology and Gram stain appearance.
2. State the location of the organisms in the natural environment, and list the modes of transmission as they relate to human infections.
3. Describe the four forms of *B. anthracis* infection, including source, route of transmission, signs, and symptoms.
4. Summarize the types of infections associated with *Bacillus cereus* group organisms.
5. Outline the laboratory tests used to differentiate *B. anthracis* from other *Bacillus* species.
6. State the culture media used to differentiate *Bacillus* spp., and include the chemical principle and interpretation.
7. Describe the general approach (method and target sequences) and difficulties associated with the molecular identification of *B. anthracis*.
8. Summarize the approach to species differentiation within the genera *Bacillus, Brevibacillus,* and *Paenibacillus.*
9. Indicate the appropriate therapy for *B. anthracis* and other *Bacillus* spp. infections.

GENERA AND SPECIES TO BE CONSIDERED

Bacillus cereus Group
- *Bacillus anthracis*
- *Bacillus cereus* (type species)
- *Bacillus thuringiensis*
- *Bacillus mycoides*
- *Bacillus pseudomycoides*
- *Bacillus megaterium*
- *Bacillus cytotoxicus*
- *Bacillus toyonensis*
- *Bacillus weihenstephanensis*

Bacillus circulans Group
- *Bacillus circulans* (type species)
- *Bacillus firmus*
- *Bacillus coagulans*

Bacillus subtilis Group
- *Bacillus licheniformis*
- *Bacillus amyloliquefaciens*
- *Bacillus subtilis* (type species)
- *Bacillus pumilus*

Other Related Organisms
- *Brevibacillus* spp.
- *Lysinibacillus spp.*
- *Paenibacillus* spp.

General Characteristics

Bacillus species previously were phenotypically classified. With the development of whole genome sequencing the *Bacillus* spp. have been evaluated closely. Some phylogenetic classifications are inconsistent due to the presence of virulence or other accessory genes on mobile genetic elements such as plasmids. *Bacillus* spp. and related genera *Brevibacillus, Lysinibacillus,* and *Paenibacillus* are aerobic or facultatively anaerobic, mesophilic, gram-positive, spore-forming rods, although some asporogenous species exist in the environment. *Bacillus* remains the largest genus within the group, including more than 100 genera that are ubiquitous in the environment in both terrestrial and aquatic habitats. The majority of the aerobic, spore-forming species are nonpathogenic and commonly encountered in the diagnostic microbiology. However, only approximately 5% of the isolates are of clinical significance and are considered opportunistic pathogens.

Bacillus anthracis

Clinical microbiologists are sentinels for recognition of a bioterrorist event, especially involving microorganisms such as *B. anthracis.* Even though this organism is rarely found, sentinel laboratory protocols require ruling out the possibility of anthrax before reporting any blood, cerebrospinal fluid (CSF), or wound cultures in which a large gram-positive aerobic rod is isolated. *B. anthracis,* along with the other species within the genus, are capable of forming spores within the mother cell or **endospores.** The endospores are

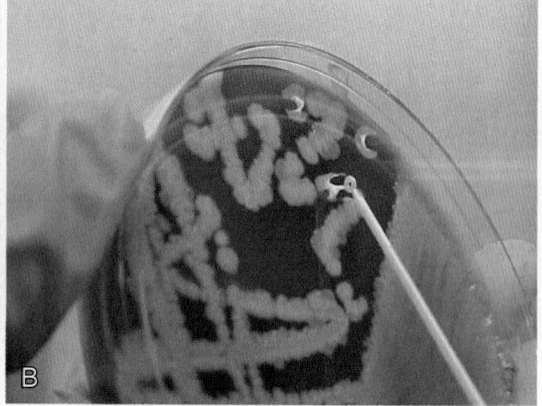

• **Fig. 15.1** Colonies of *B. anthracis* on sheep-blood agar demonstrating the characteristic comet tail or Medusa-head morphology. (Courtesy Robert Paolucci, National Naval Medical Center, Bethesda, MD.)

produced during conditions of environmental stress such as nutrient deprivation, temperature extremes, and drying or desiccation. The endospores are able to survive the harsh environmental conditions that also include resistance to radiation and disinfectants. The highly resistant nature of the endospore provides a mechanism for dissemination and survival of the organism in the environment.

Despite the widespread occurrence of bacilli in the environment, human cases of anthrax are rare in Europe and North America. *B. anthracis* should be suspected if typical nonhemolytic "comet tail or Medusa head" or ground-glass colonies are observed on 5% sheep-blood agar (Fig. 15.1). A rapid test, the Red Line Alert Test (Tetracore, Inc., Rockville, MD) is a Federal Food and Drug Administration (FDA)-cleared immunochromatographic test that presumptively identifies *B. anthracis* from blood agar within 15 minutes (Fig. 15.2). This test is a presumptive test and should not be used independently for the diagnosis of anthrax. The sentinel laboratory anthrax protocol to rule out nonhemolytic, nonmotile *Bacillus* spp. as potential isolates of *B. anthracis* is continually updated and is available from the American Society for Microbiology (ASCM) at https://asm.org/index.php/policy/sentinel-level-clinical-microbiology-guidelines.html.

Epidemiology

B. anthracis remains the most widely recognized bacillus in clinical microbiology laboratories. **Anthrax** is primarily a disease of wild and domestic animals including sheep, goats, horses, and cattle. The decline in animal and human infections is a result of the development of veterinary and human vaccines as well as improvements in industrial applications for handling and importing animal products.

The organism is normally found in the soil and primarily causes disease in herbivores. Humans acquire infections when inoculated with the endospores, by either traumatic introduction, injection, ingestion, or inhalation during exposure to contaminated animal products, such as hides (Table 15.1). Although rare, person-to-person transmission

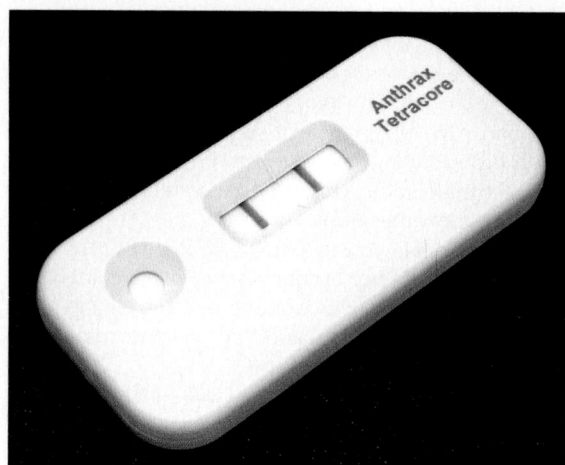

• **Fig. 15.2** Red line alert test. A red line appears on the cassette if the culture isolate is presumptive *Bacillus anthracis*. (Courtesy Tetracore, Inc., Rockville, MD.)

has been reported from mother to child, between siblings, and nosocomial spread from an infected umbilical lesion. *B. anthracis* produces endospores that may be effectively used as an agent of biologic warfare. Chapter 79 provides additional information).

Pathogenesis and Spectrum of Disease

B. anthracis is the most highly virulent species and is the causative agent of anthrax. The four forms of disease are cutaneous, gastrointestinal (ingestion), inhalation or woolsorters' disease, and injectional anthrax (Table 15.2). The **cutaneous anthrax** accounts for most human infections and is associated with contact with infected animal products. Infection results from close contact and inoculation of endospores through a break in the skin. After inoculation and an incubation period of approximately 2 to 6 days in most cases, a small papule appears that progresses to a ring of vesicles. The vesicles then develop into an ulceration. The typical presentation of the ulceration is a black, necrotic lesion known as an **eschar** (Fig. 15.3). The eschar

TABLE 15.1   Epidemiology

Species	Habitat (Reservoir)	Mode of Transmission
Bacillus anthracis	Soil: contracted by various herbivores	Direct contact: animal tissue or products such as wool or hair (infecting organisms) Trauma or insect bites: organisms or spores Inhalation: spores; woolsorters' disease Ingestion: contaminated meat Injection: contaminated drugs
Bacillus cereus group, *Bacillus cereus* type species, *Bacillus circulans, B. firmus, Bacillus licheniformis, Bacillus subtilis*, other *Bacillus* spp., *Brevibacillus* sp., and *Paenibacillus* spp.	Vegetative cells and spores ubiquitous in nature; may transiently colonize skin or the gastrointestinal or respiratory tracts	Trauma Associated with immunocompromised patients Predominantly ingestion of food (rice) contaminated with *B. cereus*–type species or toxins formed by this organism
Bacillus cytotoxicus	Vegetative cells and spores ubiquitous in nature	Predominantly ingestion of rehydrated foods contaminated with species or toxins formed by this organism

TABLE 15.2   Pathogenesis and Spectrum of Disease

Species	Virulence Factors	Spectrum of Diseases and Infections
Bacillus anthracis	Capsule exotoxins (edema toxin and lethal toxin) swelling and tissue death	Causative agent of anthrax, of which there are three forms: Cutaneous anthrax occurs at site of spore penetration 2–5 days after exposure and is manifested by progressive stages from an erythematous papule to ulceration and finally to formation of a black scar (i.e., eschar); may progress to toxemia and death Pulmonary anthrax, also known as woolsorters' disease, follows inhalation of spores and progresses from malaise with mild fever and nonproductive cough to respiratory distress, massive chest edema, cyanosis, and death Gastrointestinal anthrax may follow ingestion of spores and affects either the oropharyngeal or the abdominal area; most patients die of toxemia and overwhelming sepsis Injectional anthrax after the intravenous injection of contaminated drugs; soft tissue infections that lack the eschar associated with cutaneous anthrax. May result in death of shock, coma, organ failure, and necrotizing fasciitis.
Bacillus cereus	Enterotoxins and pyogenic toxin	Food poisoning of two types: diarrheal type, characterized by abdominal pain and watery diarrhea, and emetic type, which is manifested by profuse vomiting; *B. cereus*–type species is the most commonly encountered of *Bacillus* in opportunistic infections, including posttraumatic eye infections, endocarditis, and bacteremia; infections of other sites are rare and usually involve intravenous drug abusers or immunocompromised patients.
Bacillus circulans, B. firmus, Bacillus licheniformis, Bacillus subtilis, other Bacillus spp., *Brevibacillus* sp., and *Paenibacillus* spp.	Virulence factors unknown	Food poisoning has been associated with some species but is uncommon; these organisms may also be involved in opportunistic infections similar to those described for *B. cereus*.
Bacillus thuringiensis	Cereulide enterotoxin	Food poisoning and other infections such as wound, burn, pulmonary, and ocular infections.
Bacillus cytotoxicus	Cytotoxin K, enterotoxin	Severe food poisoning

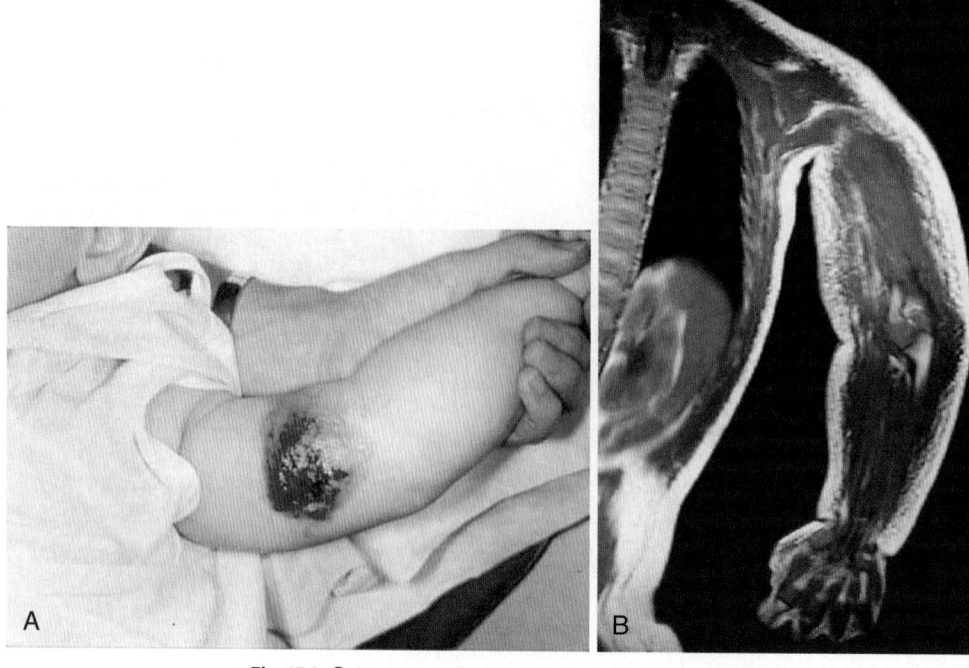

• **Fig. 15.3** Cutaneous anthrax eschar on a 7-month-old child.

may become thick and surrounded by edema. The lesion, however, is usually painless. The patient presents with no fever, and the lesion lacks purulence. If any of these symptoms are present, the patient may be experiencing a secondary bacterial infection. Cutaneous anthrax infections can be effectively treated with antibiotics. Fatalities may occur when the lesions form on the face or neck and cause an obstructed airway after edema or progression to systemic disease. The mortality rate for untreated cutaneous anthrax is low, at approximately 1%.

Gastrointestinal (ingestion) anthrax results from ingestion of endospores and presents in two forms: oral or oropharyngeal, with the lesion appearing in the buccal cavity or on the tongue, tonsils, or pharyngeal mucosa, and gastrointestinal anthrax, with the lesions developing typically in the mucosa of the terminal ileum or cecum. Oropharyngeal symptoms may include sore throat, lymphadenopathy, and edema of the throat (neck), and chest. The initial symptoms of gastrointestinal anthrax may be nonspecific with progression to abdominal pain, nausea, vomiting, anorexia, fever, bloody diarrhea, and hematemesis (vomiting of blood). The mortality rate of gastrointestinal anthrax is much higher than that of cutaneous anthrax and associated with toxemia and sepsis. This may be associated with the delayed treatment of the disease because of the nonspecific nature of the symptoms resulting in the failure of the patient to seek appropriate medical care.

Inhalation anthrax, previously referred to as pulmonary anthrax, is the result of the inhalation of endospores. The endospores are then ingested by macrophages in the lungs and transported to the lymph nodes, leading to the development of systemic infection. The disease appears flulike and includes symptoms such as fever, chills, fatigue, a nonproductive cough, and nausea or vomiting that then progresses to respiratory distress, edema, cyanosis, shock, and death. Patients typically demonstrate abnormal chest x-rays with pleural effusion, infiltrates, and mediastinal widening. **Woolsorters' disease** and **ragpickers' disease** are terms used to describe respiratory infections that result from exposure to endospores during the handling of animal hides, hair, fibers, and other animal products.

Injectional anthrax is associated with injection of contaminated drugs of abuse, frequently heroin. Animal skins are often used to move contraband, such as illegal drugs, to avoid detection by custom authorities. Although injectional anthrax is a skin infection, the symptoms significantly differ from a cutaneous infection. The skin around the injection site may appear bruised, but the characteristic lesion or eschar is absent. The infection typically presents as a severe soft tissue infection leading to rapid systemic dissemination and septic shock.

Although when properly identified anthrax is a treatable disease, complications may occur. Patients can develop meningitis within 6 days after exposure. Successful recovery, however, results in long-term immunity to subsequent infections.

Virulence in *B. anthracis* is attributed to the production of two plasmid-borne anthrax toxins referred to as **lethal toxin (LT)** and **edema toxin (ET)**. Each of these toxins consists of two proteins: the **protective antigen (PA)** and the functional enzyme, **lethal factor (LF)** and **edema factor (EF).** The PA facilitates the transport of the other protein into the cell. ET is responsible for edema, whereas LT is primarily responsible for death. Loss of the toxin-encoding plasmid from a *B. anthracis* strain appears to attenuate or reduce the pathogenesis of the organism. In addition, acquisition of the virulence plasmid also enhances the pathogenesis of other *Bacillus* spp. organisms.

B. cereus Group (not *B. anthracis*)

B. cereus, previously a single clinically relevant species, consists of a group of organisms that are classified as individual species. These include a variety of species: crystal-forming *B. thuringiensis;* a cold-tolerant *B. weihenstephanensis;* heat-tolerant *B. cytotoxicus;* a probiotic, *B. toyonensis;* and morphologic variants, *B. mycoides* and *B. pseudomycoides. B. anthracis* is actually included within the *Bacillus cereus* group but for medical reasons is presented independently in this text.

Epidemiology

B. cereus group is found within the soil and widely distributed in nature. The organisms are considered opportunistic pathogens and often associated with foodborne illness.

Pathogenesis and Spectrum of Disease

B. cereus organisms are often associated with infections in immunocompromised patients who have debilitating disease such as cancer or diabetes. The organisms may be associated with localized skin infections or systemic conditions such as bacteremia, endocarditis, and septicemia. Additional sites of infection include the urinary or respiratory tract. Health care–associated infections have also been identified and linked to contaminated material such as gowns, gloves, linens, and dressings, as well as medical devices including catheters, ventilators, and bronchoscopy equipment. As previously described for *B. anthracis*, infections with *B. cereus* group organisms have also been linked to contaminated drugs.

B. cereus group "food poisoning" is associated with the ingestion of a wide variety of foods including meats, vegetables, desserts, sauces, and milk. A higher incidence is seen after the ingestion of rice dishes. After ingestion, patients present with one of two types of symptoms: diarrhea and abdominal pain within 8 to 16 hours, or nausea and vomiting (emetic food poisoning) within 1 to 5 hours. *B. cereus* produces several toxins implicated in the diarrheal symptoms, including **hemolysin BL (HBL), nonhemolytic enterotoxin (Nhe),** and **cytotoxin K (CytK;** also referred to as hemolysin IV). The three toxins are believed to act synergistically, with Nhe responsible for the major symptoms in the diarrheal presentation of the infection. The emetic form of illness is associated with a heat-stable, proteolysis, and acid-resistant toxin, **cereulide** produced in food. The cereulide toxin is encoded on a plasmid-borne gene cluster and has been identified in a subset of *B. cereus* and *B. thuringiensis* isolates.

In addition to the food poisoning associated with *B. cereus,* the type-specific species is a serious pathogen of the eye, causing progressive endophthalmitis. Identification of

B. cereus from a patient's eye can cause permanent damage and should be reported to the primary care provider immediately.

B. thuringiensis

B. thuringiensis can also produce the cereulide enterotoxin. In addition, *B. thuringiensis* toxins have been commercialized for the control of insects that cause agricultural damage, such as moths, beetles, flies, and parasitic worms (nematodes). Occupational exposure to insecticides and pesticides containing the organism has resulted in the identification of the organism in feces without the presence of gastrointestinal symptoms. Additional rare cases of wound, burn, pulmonary, and ocular infections have been associated with the isolation of *B. thuringiensis.*
- *B. subtilis, Brevibacillus* spp., *Lysinibacillus* spp., and *Paenibacillus* spp.
- *B. subtilis* (type species) has been identified in clinical specimens in a variety of cases, including pneumonia, bacteremia, septicemia, surgical wounds, and meningitis after head trauma, and other surgical infections. Rare human infections have been associated with a variety of *Bacillus* spp., including *B. licheniformis, B. circulans, B. firmus, B. coagulans, B. megaterium, B. pumilus, Paenibacillus polymyxa, Brevibacillus* spp., *Lysinibacillus* spp., and others. In contrast to the type species of the genus *Bacillus*, the cell wall of *Lysinibacillus* spp. contains peptidoglycan with lysine, aspartic acid, alanine, and glutamic acid. Many of these organisms are common environmental contaminants, including *Bacillus amyloliquefaciens*. Identification of these organisms is not recommended unless isolated from a sterile site (e.g., blood) or found in large numbers in pure culture. Identification and interpretation should be closely evaluated in conjunction with the patient's signs and symptoms and consultation with the attending physician.

Epidemiology
- Most *Bacillus* spp., other than *B. anthracis, B. cereus,* and *B. thuringiensis,* are generally considered to be opportunistic pathogens of low virulence and are associated with immunocompromised patients after exposure to contaminated materials.

Pathogenesis and Spectrum of Disease

The endospores of *Bacillus* spp. are ubiquitous in nature, and contamination of various clinical specimens may occur. The clinical significance of the isolate should be carefully established during the identification of the microorganism.

Laboratory Diagnosis

Specimen Processing

With few exceptions, special processing considerations are not required. The organisms are capable of survival in fresh clinical specimens and standard transport medium. Refer to Table 5.1 for general information on specimen processing.

Specimens collected from patients suspected of having anthrax should be placed in leak-proof containers and placed in a secondary container. Cutaneous anthrax specimens should be collected from underneath the eschar. Two specimens of the vesicular fluid should be collected from underneath the lesion by rotating the swabs beneath the eschar. For histochemical testing, the physician may collect a punch biopsy that should be placed in 10% formalin. Inhalation anthrax specimens should include blood cultures, pleural fluid, and a serum specimen for serology. Again, the physician may collect a biopsy of bronchial or pleural tissue. Specimens required for gastrointestinal anthrax include blood cultures, ascites fluid, and material from any lesions as well as serum for serologic testing. The preferred specimens from patients suspected of infection with *B. anthracis* should be collected before antibiotic therapy. In addition, specimens should also be collected from the potential source of infection, such as the animal carcass.

Clinical specimens for the isolation of *Bacillus* species other than *B. anthracis* and *B. cereus* group organisms may be handled safely under normal standard laboratory practices. The exceptions are processing procedures that may produce aerosols or for foods implicated in *B. cereus* food poisoning outbreaks and animal hides or products and environmental samples for the isolation of *B. anthracis*. These specimens may contain endospores that pose an aerosolization and inhalation risk to the laboratory professional, requiring the use of personal protective equipment, including a proper respiratory mask.

Specimen processing may include heat or alcohol shock before plating on solid media. The pretreatment removes contaminating organisms, and only the spore-forming bacilli survive. This technique is considered an enrichment and selection procedure designed to increase the chance for laboratory isolation of the organisms.

Despite the publicity associated with *B. anthracis* as a potential agent of biologic warfare, the organism is not highly contagious. Disinfection with formaldehyde, glutaraldehyde, or hydrogen peroxide and peracetic acid should be performed before the disposal of specimens suspected of containing a large number of spores. *B. anthracis* is classified by the Department of Health and Human Services/Centers for Disease Control and Prevention (CDC) and the US Department of Agriculture/Animal and Plant Health Inspection Service (APHIS) as a select agent. Any laboratory in possession of the organism must register with one of these agencies and notify the organization within 7 days upon identification of the organism. If the organism is identified in an unregistered laboratory, the isolate must be shipped, using the request to transfer select agents and toxins approval from CDC or APHIS, to a registered laboratory for proper disposal.

Direct Detection Methods

Microscopically the organisms appear as large gram-positive rods in singles, pairs, or serpentine chains (Fig. 15.4A and

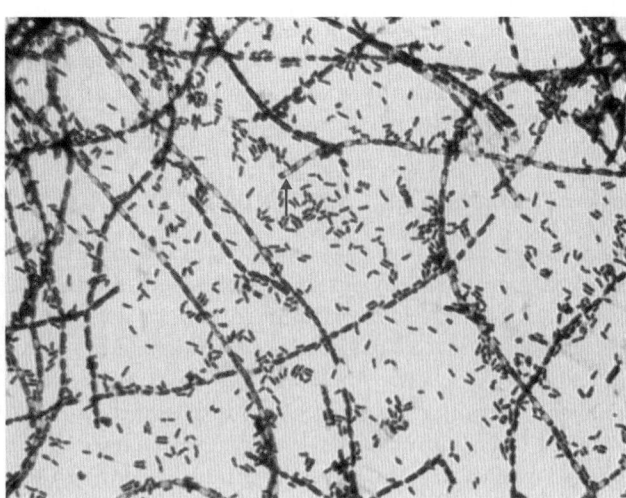

• **Fig. 15.4** *Bacillus anthracis* demonstrating serpentine form on a Gram stain when grown in culture. Note the endospore, as designated by the *arrow*.

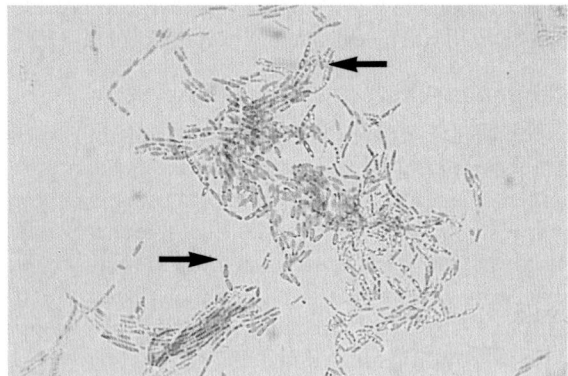

• **Fig. 15.5** Gram stain of *Bacillus cereus*. The *arrows* indicate endospores, the clear area inside the gram-positive vegetative cell.

B). Cells generally stain gram positive, but older cultures are more likely to appear gram variable or gram negative. In addition, because the organisms produce endospores that do not Gram stain, even young cultures may appear gram variable. The unstained areas within the cell may indicate sporulation or formation of endospores.

Bacillus spp. are the only clinically relevant aerobic organisms capable of producing endospores in the presence of oxygen. Sporulation is inhibited by high concentrations of CO_2. The production of spores may be induced by growth in triple sugar iron (TSI), urea, or nutrient agar containing 5 mg/L manganese sulfate. Endospores may appear as intracellular or extracellular clear oval structures upon Gram staining. Special staining is required to visualize endospores. The smear is covered with malachite green, and a piece of filter paper is placed over the stain. The microscope slide is heated for several minutes to force the dye into the cell walls of the endospore. During the heating process, it is important to keep the filter paper moist so that the stain is steamed rather than baked into the endospores. A safranin counterstain follows the primary stain. The endospores stain green, and the vegetative cells will appear pink from the secondary stain, safranin (Fig. 15.5).

The vegetative cell width of *B. anthracis, B. cereus, B. mycoides, B. thuringiensis,* and *B. megaterium* is usually greater than 1 μm, and the endospores do not cause swelling of the cell. The vegetative cell width of *B. subtilis, B. pumilus,* and *B. licheniformis* is less than 1 μm, and the endospores do not cause swelling of the cell. The cell width of *B. circulans, B. firmus, B. coagulans, B. sphaericus, B. brevis, Paenibacillus macerans, P. alvei,* and *P. polymyxa* is less than 1 μm, and the endospores cause the cell to swell. When determining cell width, only the cells that stain gram-positive should be measured. Organisms that fail to retain the crystal violet appear narrower.

Direct examination of blood smears may also reveal encapsulated rods or "ghost" capsules after antibiotic treatment when stained using polychrome methylene blue (M'Fadyean). The toxin-encoding virulence plasmid of *B. anthracis* also codes for the biosynthesis of the capsule. Therefore, strains that have lost the plasmid may be mistaken for nonencapsulated *B. cereus* organisms or, conversely, other species may acquire the plasmid and appear encapsulated. This may complicate the interpretation of molecular assays that identify *B. anthracis* based on the presence of the capsule gene (*capBCA*) as the nucleic acid target within the assay. A positive molecular amplification assay, polymerase chain reaction (PCR), from a normally sterile site is considered a presumptive diagnosis for anthrax infection.

Direct detection of *B. anthracis* in clinical and environmental samples is also available using antigen-based methods. The immunohistochemical method available from the CDC uses antibodies specific to the organism's cell wall antigen or capsule for the detection of *B. anthracis.*

Nucleic Acid Detection

The most rapid detection method and differentiation of *B. anthracis* in the United States public health system is completed using a PCR (amplification assay) for the detection of several targets located on the chromosome and virulence plasmids. The use of multiple nucleic acid targets improves the specificity of the assay as well as the identification of strains that have lost the virulence plasmid. A positive nucleic acid test from any clinical specimen collected from a sterile site is considered a presumptive diagnostic test for anthrax. However, additional confirmatory testing is recommended because of the potential for environmental contamination from a non–anthrax-associated lesion.

Various methods exist for the genetic analysis of *B. anthracis.* There are several sequence methods, including multilocus sequence typing (MLST) and multiple-locus variable-number tandem-repeat analysis. MLST has been used to discriminate different isolates of *B. cereus.* Each of these assays examines a variety of genes and compares the genetic pattern among isolates. Additional genotyping techniques that examine single nucleotide polymorphisms and DNA microarrays are available for strain typing.

In addition to identification of the organism, bioterrorist threats and hoaxes may require the analysis of other materials. The Norwegian Defense Research Establishment has developed a protocol for the examination of suspicious powders by matrix-assisted laser desorption ionization time-of-flight mass spectrometry (MALDI-TOF MS). This method is able to accurately distinguish *Bacillus* endospores from other materials and differentiate *B. anthracis* from other *Bacillus* spp.

Cultivation

Media of Choice

All *Bacillus* and related genera grow well on 5% sheep blood agar, chocolate agar, routine blood culture media, and nutrient broths. Isolates susceptible to nalidixic acid will not grow on Columbia agar with nalidixic acid and colistin (CNA), a selective and differential medium for gram-positive organisms. Phenylethyl alcohol agar (PEA), an additional selective agar for gram-positive organisms, is useful for the removal of contaminating organisms and the isolation of *Bacillus* spp. **Polymyxin-lysozyme-EDTA-thallous acetate (PLET)** can be used for selection and isolation from contaminated specimens. Colonies appear as creamy white, domed, circular colonies. In addition, bicarbonate agar is used to induce *B. anthracis* capsule formation, providing a means for presumptive morphologic identification.

B. cereus media referred to as mannitol, egg yolk, and polymyxin B agar (**MEYP or MYP**); polymyxin B, egg yolk, mannitol, bromothymol blue (**PEMBA**); and *B. cereus* medium (**BCM**) have been developed for the specific isolation and identification of the organism. These media take advantage of the phospholipase C–positive reaction on egg yolk agar, lack of production of acid from mannitol, and incorporation of pyruvate or polymyxin as the selective agents. More recently, chromogenic medium that uses chromogenic substrates in place of egg yolk for the identification of phospholipase C include *B. cereus/B. thuringiensis* media (R&F Laboratories, Downers Grove, IL) and *B. cereus* group medium (Biosynth Chemistry and Biology, Staad, Switzerland).

Heat shock treatment can be used for the growth and enhancement of endospores from clinical specimens. Heat treatment at 70°C for 30 minutes or 80°C for 10 minutes is effective for killing vegetative cells and retaining spores for most *Bacillus* spp. *B. anthracis* heat treatment is carried out at lower temperatures, 62°C to 65°C for 15 to 20 minutes. After heat treatment, samples are plated to culture medium along with a sample of untreated specimen to ensure maximal recovery of the isolate.

Incubation Conditions and Duration

Most species will produce detectable growth within 24 hours after incubation at 35°C, in ambient air, or in 5% carbon dioxide (CO_2). Bicarbonate agar requires incubation in CO_2.

Colonial Appearance

Table 15.3 describes the colonial appearance on blood agar and other distinguishing characteristics (e.g., hemolysis)

TABLE 15.3	Colonial Appearance and Other Characteristics
Organism	Appearance on 5% Sheep Blood Agar
Bacillus anthracis	Medium-large, gray, flat, irregular with swirling projections ("Medusa head" or "comet tail") or ground-glass appearance; nonhemolytic
Bacillus cereus, Bacillus cytotoxicus, and Bacillus thuringiensis	Large, feathery, spreading; beta-hemolytic
Bacillus mycoides	Rhizoid colony that resembles a fungus; weakly beta-hemolytic
Bacillus megaterium	Large, convex, entire, moist; nonhemolytic
Bacillus licheniformis	Large blister colony; becomes opaque with dull to rough surface with age; beta-hemolytic
Bacillus pumilus	Large, moist, blister colony; may be beta-hemolytic
Bacillus subtilis	Large, flat, dull, with ground-glass appearance; may be pigmented (pink, yellow, orange, or brown); may be beta-hemolytic
Bacillus circulans	Large, entire, convex, butyrous; smooth, translucent surface; may be beta-hemolytic
Bacillus firmus	Soft, smooth, and usually nonpigmented, but occasionally may be pigmented (yellow, pale orange, or salmon pink), may be beta-hemolytic
Bacillus coagulans	Medium-large, entire, raised, butyrous, creamy-buff; may be beta-hemolytic
Bacillus sphaericus	Large, convex, smooth, opaque, butyrous; nonhemolytic
Brevibacillus brevis	Medium-large, convex, circular, granular; may be beta-hemolytic
Paenibacillus macerans	Large, convex, fine granular surface; nonhemolytic
Paenibacillus alvei	Swarms over agar surface; discrete colonies are large, circular, convex, smooth, glistening, translucent or opaque; may be beta-hemolytic
Paenibacillus polymyxa	Large, moist blister colony with "amoeboid spreading" in young cultures; older colonies wrinkled; nonhemolytic

of each species of *Bacillus* or related genera. Colonies of *B. anthracis* growing on bicarbonate agar appear large and mucoid.

Approach to Identification

All *Bacillus* spp. isolates should be evaluated to rule out the presence of *B. anthracis* (Fig. 15.6). If *B. anthracis* cannot be ruled out, it must be sent to an appropriate laboratory for confirmation. Commercial biochemical identification systems or molecular techniques may be used in clinical laboratories for identification of *Bacillus* spp. Species differentiation within the genera *Bacillus, Brevibacillus,* and *Paenibacillus* is based on the size of the vegetative cell, sporulation resulting in swelling of the vegetative cell, and biochemical analysis (Table 15.4), including the production of the enzyme lecithinase (Fig. 15.7).

Serodiagnosis

Serologic methods are available for the detection of *B. cereus* toxin in food and feces: the Oxoid BCET-RPLA (Oxoid Ltd., Basingstoke, United Kingdom) and the TECRA VIA

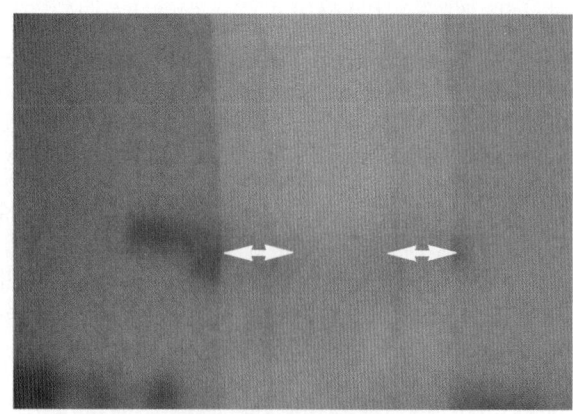

• **Fig. 15.6** Lecithinase production by *Bacillus cereus* on egg yolk agar. The organism has been streaked down the center of the plate. The positive test for lecithinase is indicated by the opaque zone of precipitation around the bacterial growth *(arrows).*

(TECRA Diagnostics, New South Wales, Australia). Indirect hemagglutination and enzyme-linked immunosorbent assays are available to detect antibodies to *B. anthracis.* Serodiagnostic methods are not used to diagnose infections caused by other opportunistic *Bacillus* spp. Serodiagnosis of *B. anthracis* is typically available for the detection of the

TABLE 15.4 Differentiation of Clinically Relevant *Bacillus* spp., *Brevibacillus* spp., and *Paenibacillus* spp

Organism	Bacillary Body Width >1 μm	Wide Zone Lecithinase	Spores Swell Sporangium	Voges-Proskauer	Glucose With Gas	Fermentation of: Mannitol	Fermentation of: Xylose	Anaerobic Growth	Citrate	Indole	Motility	Parasporal Crystals
Bacillus anthracis	+	+	−	+	−	−	−	+	V	−	−	−
Bacillus cereus	+	+	−	+	−	−	−	+	+	−	+	−
Bacillus thuringiensis	+	+	−	+	−	−	−	+	+	−	+	+
Bacillus cytotoxicus	+	+	−	w+	−	−	−	w+	−	−	+	−
Bacillus mycoides	+	+	−	+	−	−	−	+	+	−	−	−
Bacillus megaterium	+	−	−	−	−	+ or (+)	V	−	+	−	+	−
Bacillus licheniformis	−	−	−	+	−	+	+	+	+	−	+	−
Bacillus pumilus	−	−	−	+	−	+	+	−	+	−	+	−
Bacillus subtilis	−	−	−	+	−	+	+	−	+	−	+	−
Bacillus circulans	−	−	+	−	−	+	+	V	−	−	+	−
Bacillus firmus	−	−	−	−	−	+	+	−	−	−	+	−
Bacillus coagulans	−	−	V	V	−	−	V	+	V	−	+	−
Brevibacillus brevis	−	−	+	−	−	+	−	−	V	−	+	V
Paenibacillus macerans	−	−a	+	−	−	+	+	+	−	−	+	−
Paenibacillus alvei	−	−	+	+	−	−	−	+	−	+	+	−
Paenibacillus polymyxa	−	−a	+	+	−	V	+	+	−	−	+	−

aWeak lecithinase production only seen under the colonies.

+, 90% or more of species or strains are positive; −, 90% or more of species or strains are negative; V, variable reactions; ( ), reactions may be delayed; w, weak.

Compiled from Drobniewski FA. *Bacillus cereus* and related species. *Clin Microbiol Rev* 1993;6:324;Caroll KC, Pfaller MA. *Manual of Clinical Microbiology.* 12th ed. Washington, DC: ASM Press; 2019; and Parry JM, Turnbull PC, Gibson JR. *A Colour Atlas of Bacillus Species*, London: Wolf Medical Publications; 1983.

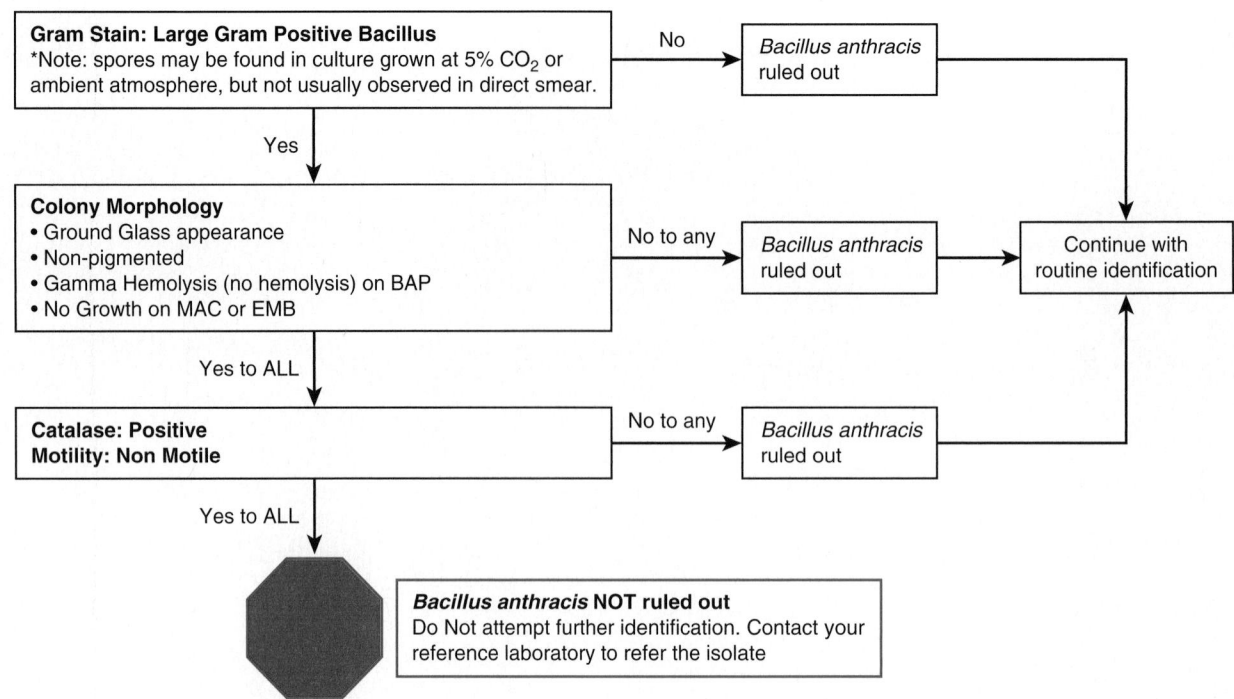

• **Fig. 15.7** Testing algorithm for *Bacillus* spp. for determination of possible *B. anthracis*. *BAP*, Blood agar plate; *EMB*, eosin methylene blue [agar]; *MAC*, *Mycobacterium avium* complex;

PA antigen or toxin protein, LF, and EF. However, in outbreak situations, serologic tests may be of limited clinical use because of the time required for an infected patient to seroconvert. Effective treatment of anthrax requires a rapid response and diagnostic testing.

Matrix-Assisted Laser Desorption Ionization Time-of-Flight Mass Spectrometry

MALDI-TOF MS has been used to identify many endospore-forming *Bacillus* species; however, endospores affect the identification accuracy when using MALDI-TOF MS because they change the protein composition of samples. Culture conditions directly influence endospore formation and *Bacillus* growth and therefore can influence the classification of *Bacillus* species using MALDI-TOF MS. Studies that are examining the identification and quantification of PA, LF, and EF are currently being developed that would provide for a rapid diagnosis of inhalation anthrax. Ultimately, the more rapid the diagnosis, the better the outcome and the reduction in anthrax-associated fatalities.

Antimicrobial Susceptibility Testing and Therapy

Although intravenous ciprofloxacin for 7 to 10 days with the addition of one (aminoglycoside) or two additional drugs has been established as the preferred therapy for severe cases of anthrax, the infrequent nature with which other species are encountered limits recommendations concerning therapy (Table 15.5). Most strains of *B. anthracis* are susceptible to penicillin; however, because of the presence of inducible beta-lactamases in some strains it is not the recommended treatment of choice without the administration of an additional antimicrobial agent. Treatment for cutaneous or uncomplicated anthrax typically consists of oral ciprofloxacin or doxycycline for 7 to 10 days. Nonetheless, the threat of bioterrorism has spawned interest in the development of *in vitro* testing of antimicrobial agents against *B. anthracis*. The Clinical and Laboratory Standards Institute (CLSI) has published technical guidelines and interpretive criteria required for antimicrobial susceptibility testing for *Bacillus* spp.

Unlike *B. anthracis*, *B. cereus* and *B. thuringiensis* are resistant to penicillin, cephalosporins, and beta-lactamase inhibitor combinations because of the production of penicillinases and a beta-lactamase. Most *Bacillus* spp. will grow on the media under the conditions recommended for testing the common organisms encountered in clinical specimens (see Chapter 11 for more information regarding validated testing methods). Technical information regarding the testing of the additional species is provided in CLSI document M45, "Methods for Antimicrobial Dilution and Disk Susceptibility Testing of Infrequently Isolated or Fastidious Bacteria." Careful evaluation of the organism's clinical significance must be established before extensive antimicrobial susceptibility testing efforts are undertaken. Recommended antimicrobial susceptibility testing for other nonanthrax

TABLE 15.5	Antimicrobial Therapy and Susceptibility Testing			
Species	Therapeutic Options	Resistance to Therapeutic Options	Validated Testing Methods[a]	Comments
Bacillus anthracis	Ciprofloxacin or doxycycline plus one or two other antibiotics; other agents that may demonstrate *in vitro* activity include rifampin, vancomycin, penicillin, ampicillin, chloramphenicol, imipenem, clindamycin, and clarithromycin	Beta-lactamases	See CLSI document M100: Performed in Approved Reference Laboratories Only	
Other *Bacillus* spp., *Brevibacillus* sp., *Paenibacillus* spp.	No definitive guidelines; vancomycin, ciprofloxacin, imipenem, and aminoglycosides may be effective	*B. cereus* frequently produces beta-lactamase	See CLSI document M45: Methods for Antimicrobial Dilution and Disk Susceptibility Testing of Infrequently Isolated or Fastidious Bacteria	Whenever isolated from clinical specimens, the potential for the isolate to be a contaminant must be strongly considered

[a]Validated testing methods include those standard methods recommended by the Clinical Laboratory Science Institute (CLSI) and those commercial methods approved by the US Federal Food and Drug Administration (FDA).

Bacillus spp. include clindamycin, vancomycin, and the fluoroquinolones. Cases associated with *Bacillus* spp. infections have been reported in which the *in vitro* susceptibility results did not directly correlate with effective treatment.

Prevention

A cell-free inactivated vaccine (BioThrax, Emergent Biodefense Operations, Lansing, MI) given in three primary doses followed by two boosters thereafter (0 weeks, 1 month, 6 months, 12 months, and 18 months) is available for immunizing high-risk adults (i.e., public health laboratory workers, workers handling potentially contaminated industrial raw materials, and military personnel) against anthrax. Chemoprophylaxis with ciprofloxacin (or doxycycline) is recommended after aerosol exposure to *B. anthracis*, such as in a bioterrorist event.

(e) Visit the Evolve site for a complete list of procedures, review questions, and case studies.

Bibliography

Ahmed I, Yokota A, Yamazoe A, Fujiwara T: Proposal of *Lysinibacillus boronitolerans* gen. nov. sp. nov., and transfer of *Bacillus fusiformis* to *Lysinibacillus fusiformis* comb. nov. and *Bacillus sphaericus* to *Lysinibacillus sphaericus* comb. nov, *Int J Syst Evol Microbiol* 57(Pt 5):1117–1125, 2007.

Ash C, Priest FG, Collins MD: Molecular identification of rRNA group 3 bacilli (Ash, Farrow, Wallbanks and Collins) using a PCR probe test, *Antonie Van Leeuwenhoek* 64:253, 1993.

Bennett J, Dolin R, Blaser M: *Principles and practice of infectious diseases,* ed 9, Philadelphia, 2020, Elsevier-Saunders.

Boyer AE, Gallegos-Candela M, Quinn CP, et al.: High-sensitivity MALDI-TOF MS quantification of anthrax lethal toxin for diagnostics and evaluation of medical countermeasures, *Anal Bioanal Chem* 407:2847–2858, 2015.

Caroll KC, Pfaller MA: *Manual of clinical microbiology,* ed 12, Washington, DC, 2019, ASM Press.

Claus D, Berkeley RC: Genus bacillus. In Vos P, Garrity G, Jones D, et al., editors: *Bergey's manual of systematic bacteriology* (vol 3). New York, NY, 2009, Springer.

Drobniewski FA: *Bacillus cereus* and related species, *Clin Microbiol Rev* 6:324–338, 1993.

Gordon RE, Hyde JL, Moore Jr JA, et al.: *Bacillus firmus-Bacillus lentus*: a series or one species? *Int J Syst Bacteriol* 27:256–262, 1977.

Guinebretière MH, Auger S, Galleron N, et al.: *Bacillus cytotoxicus* sp. nov. is a novel thermotolerant species of the *Bacillus cereus* Group occasionally associated with food poisoning, *Int J Syst Evol Microbiol* 63(Pt 1):31–40, 2013.

Hollis DG, Weaver RE: *Gram-positive organisms: a guide to identification,* Atlanta, 1981, Centers for Disease Control.

Shida O, Takagi H, Kadowaki K, Komagata K: Proposal for two new genera, *Brevibacillus* gen. nov. and *Aneurinibacillus* gen. nov, *Int J Syst Bacteriol* 46:939–946, 1996.

Shu LJ, Yang YL: *Bacillus* classification based on matrix-assisted laser desorption ionization time-of-flight mass spectrometry-effects of culture conditions, *Sci Rep* 7(1):15546, 2017.

Turnbull P, Böhm R, Cosivi O, et al.: *Guidelines for the surveillance and control of anthrax in humans and animals,* Geneva, Switzerland, 1998, World Health Organization.

16

Listeria, Corynebacterium, and Similar Organisms

OBJECTIVES

1. Describe the general characteristics of the *Corynebacterium* spp., including Gram stain morphology, culture media, and colonial appearance.
2. List two selective and differential media used to identify *Corynebacterium diphtheriae*, and describe the chemical principle for each.
3. Identify the clinically relevant indicators (e.g., signs, symptoms) associated with the need to identify *Corynebacterium* spp.
4. Describe four methods used to detect *C. diphtheriae* toxin, along with the chemical principle of each test.
5. Describe two methods used to observe motility in *Listeria monocytogenes.*
6. Explain how diphtheria is controlled by immunization, and describe the course of treatment for individuals exposed to the disease.
7. Define "cold enrichment," and explain how it enhances the isolation of *L. monocytogenes.*
8. List the foods pregnant women and immunocompromised patients should avoid to reduce the risk of infection with *L. monocytogenes.*
9. Describe the clinical significance of identification of *Corynebacterium pseudotuberculosis, Corynebacterium urealyticum, Corynebacterium glucuronolyticum,* and *Corynebacterium ulcerans.*

GENERA AND SPECIES TO BE CONSIDERED

- *Arcanobacterium haemolyticum*
- *Arthrobacter* spp.
- *Brevibacterium* spp.
- *Cellulomonas* spp.
- *Cellulosimicrobium* spp.
- *Corynebacterium amycolatum*
- *Corynebacterium aurimucosum*
- *Corynebacterium coyleae*
- *Corynebacterium diphtheriae* (toxigenic and nontoxigenic)
- *Corynebacterium glucuronolyticum*
- *Corynebacterium jeikeium*
- *Corynebacterium kroppenstedtii*
- *Corynebacterium macginleyi*
- *Corynebacterium propinquum*
- *Corynebacterium pseudodiphtheriticum*
- *Corynebacterium pseudotuberculosis* (toxigenic)

- *Corynebacterium resistens*
- *Corynebacterium simulans*
- *Corynebacterium striatum*
- *Corynebacterium tuberculostearicum*
- *Corynebacterium ulcerans* (toxigenic)
- *Corynebacterium urealyticum*
- *Dermabacter* spp.
- *Exiguobacterium* spp.
- *Leifsonia aquatica*
- *Listeria monocytogenes*
- *Microbacterium* spp.
- *Oerskovia* spp.
- Other *Corynebacterium* spp.
- *Rothia* spp.
- *Turicella otitidis*

General Characteristics

The genera of bacteria described in this chapter are catalase-positive, gram-positive rods. They are non–acid-fast, non–spore-forming, and mostly nonbranching rods. *Rothia* and *Oerskovia* spp. are included with the gram-positive rods because some species are rodlike. Furthermore, although *Oerskovia* spp. exhibit extensive branching and vegetative hyphae and penetrate into the agar surface, they do not display aerial hyphae, as do *Nocardia* spp. *Corynebacterium* spp. are aerobic or facultative anaerobic fastidious organisms that may demonstrate slow growth on an enriched medium. The additional genera, including *Arthrobacter, Brevibacterium, Cellulomonas, Cellulosimicrobium, Dermabacter, Exiguobacterium, Leifsonia, Microbacterium, Rothia,* and *Turicella,* are **coryneform bacteria**. These organisms demonstrate similar morphology to that of *Corynebacterium* spp. and may be isolated in medical device–associated infections. *Listeria monocytogenes* is a facultative anaerobic, catalase-positive, nonbranching, oxidase-negative, gram-positive rod. These organisms are commonly misidentified as diphtheroids, cocci, or diplococci in clinical specimens. The organisms are associated with infection in specific populations of immunocompromised patients as well as being associated with foodborne illness in healthy individuals.

Epidemiology

Most of the organisms listed in Table 16.1 are part of the normal human microbiome and colonize various parts of the

**TABLE
16.1**   **Epidemiology**

Organism	Habitat (Reservoir)	Mode of Transmission
Listeria monocytogenes	Colonizer: Animals, soil, and vegetable matter; widespread in these environments	Direct contact: Human gastrointestinal tract Ingestion of contaminated food, such as meat and dairy products Endogenous strain: Colonized mothers may pass organism to fetus. Portal of entry is probably from gastrointestinal tract to blood and in some instances from blood to meninges.
Corynebacterium diphtheriae	Colonizer: Human nasopharynx but only in carrier state; not considered part of normal microbiota Isolation from healthy humans is not common	Direct contact: Person to person by exposure to contaminated respiratory droplets Contact with exudate from cutaneous lesions Exposure to contaminated objects
Corynebacterium glucuronolyticum	Colonizer of the male genitourinary tract	Uncertain Endogenous strain: Access to normally sterile site
Corynebacterium jeikeium	Colonizer: Skin microbiota of hospitalized patients, most commonly in the inguinal, axillary, and rectal sites	Uncertain Direct contact: May be person to person Endogenous strain: Selection during antimicrobial therapy Introduction during placement or improper care of intravenous catheters
Corynebacterium ulcerans	Normal microbiota: Humans and cattle	Uncertain Zoonosis: Close animal contact, especially during summer
Corynebacterium pseudotuberculosis	Normal microbiota: Animals such as sheep, goats, and horses	Uncertain Zoonosis: Close animal contact, but infections in humans are rare
Corynebacterium pseudodiphtheriticum	Normal microbiota: Human pharyngeal and occasionally skin microbiota	Uncertain Endogenous strain: Access to normally sterile site
Corynebacterium urealyticum	Normal microbiota: Human skin	Uncertain Endogenous strain: Access to normally sterile site
Leifsonia aquatica	Environment: Fresh water	Uncertain
Corynebacterium striatum	Normal microbiota: Skin	Uncertain Endogenous strain: Access to normally sterile site
Corynebacterium amycolatum	Normal microbiota: Human conjunctiva Skin Nasopharynx	Uncertain Endogenous strain: Access to normally sterile site
Corynebacterium coyleae	Uncertain: Probably part of normal human microbiota	Uncertain Rarely implicated in human infections
Brevibacterium spp.	Normal microbiota: Human Various foods	Uncertain Rarely implicated in human infections
Dermabacter spp.	Normal microbiota: Human skin	Uncertain Rarely implicated in human infections

TABLE 16.1	Epidemiology—cont'd	
Organism	**Habitat (Reservoir)**	**Mode of Transmission**
Turicella otitidis	Uncertain: Probably part of normal human microbiota	Uncertain Rarely implicated in human infections
Arthrobacter spp., *Microbacterium* spp., *Cellulomonas* spp., and *Exiguobacterium* sp.	Uncertain: Probably environmental	Uncertain Rarely implicated in human infections

human body, found in the environment, or associated with various animals. The genus *Corynebacterium* includes approximately 105 species. More than 56 of the species cause human infection. These organisms are widely distributed throughout the mucous membranes and on the skin and are capable of causing opportunistic, localized, or systemic infection. The genus *Listeria* includes 17 species with only *L. monocytogenes* known to be pathogenic to humans. The two most notable pathogens discussed in this chapter are *L. monocytogenes* and *Corynebacterium diphtheriae*. However, these two species differ markedly in epidemiology. *L. monocytogenes* is widely distributed in nature and occasionally colonizes the human gastrointestinal tract. Many foods are contaminated with *L. monocytogenes,* including milk, raw vegetables, cheese, and meats. Humans only carry *C. diphtheriae*, and in rare cases, the bacterium is isolated from healthy individuals. Primary transmission for *C. diphtheriae* is through respiratory secretions or exudates from skin lesions.

In contrast to these two organisms, *C. jeikeium* is often encountered in clinical specimens, mostly because it tends to proliferate as skin microbiota of hospitalized individuals. However, *C. jeikeium* is not considered highly virulent. The penetration of the patient's skin by intravascular devices is usually required for this organism to cause infection. Additional common nosocomial pathogens include *C. urealyticum*, *C. amycolatum*, and *C. striatum*. The clinical significance of coryneform bacteria is often difficult to determine.

Many of the other organisms discussed in this chapter, *Exiguobacterium, Arthrobacter, Cellulomonas, Cellulosimicrobium, Leifsonia, Microbacterium,* and *Oerskovia,* are primarily opportunistic pathogens found in the environment. *Arcanobacterium* has been recovered from wounds and the human pharynx; however, the natural habitat is currently unknown. The remaining genera, *Dermabacter, Turicella, Rothia,* and *Brevibacterium,* include a variety of species that have been isolates from several clinical specimens.

Pathogenesis and Spectrum of Disease

Listeria monocytogenes, by virtue of its ability to survive within phagocytes, and *Corynebacterium diphtheriae* and *C. ulcerans,* by production of an extremely potent cytotoxic exotoxin, are the most virulent species listed in Table 16.2. Not all strains of *C. diphtheriae* are toxin-producing strains or considered

toxigenic. The toxin gene is present in strains that have acquired the gene *tox* by viral transduction. The result is the incorporation of the toxin gene into the organism's genome. The toxin gene blocks protein synthesis in human cells, causing the cell to die. The toxin is extremely lethal. Only toxin-producing strains of *C. diphtheriae* cause diphtheria. Diphtheria can be characterized as respiratory or cutaneous illness. Patients suffering from respiratory diphtheria present with symptoms of pharyngitis, dysphagia (difficulty swallowing), low-grade fever, cervical and submandibular lymphadenopathy, general malaise, and headache. A large pseudomembrane composed of cellular debris, caused by toxigenic cellular killing, may appear in the nasopharynx, resulting in obstruction of the patient's airway. In addition, the toxin spreads hematogenously and may induce systemic organ damage, leading to cardiac arrest. Cutaneous diphtheria, which may still be endemic in tropical countries, can be caused by either toxigenic or nontoxigenic strains *of C. diphtheriae*. Shallow, chronic skin lesions characterize the infection.

L. monocytogenes is primarily transmitted through the ingestion of contaminated food. In adults, the organism is often the cause of a variety of focal infections such as endocarditis, arthritis, osteomyelitis brain abscesses, and pulmonary, gastrointestinal, and cutaneous infections, to name a few. The organism is also capable of causing septicemia that may lead to meningitis or meningoencephalitis. Vertical transmission from mother to fetus occurs transplacentally or through an infected birth canal. Cross infection has been identified in neonatal nurseries and is associated with contaminated mineral oil used for bathing infants. Once the organism has been phagocytized by white blood cells, it produces **listeriolysin O**, the major virulence factor. Listeriolysin O is a pore-forming toxin that reduces T-cell responsiveness. This toxin-induced unresponsiveness, in combination with phospholipases, enables the organism to escape from the phagosome of white blood cells, avoid intracellular killing, and spread to the bloodstream. In addition to listeriolysin O, the organism produces a bacterial surface protein, **Act A** that induces host cell actin polymerization. Actin polymerization within the host cell moves the infecting organism toward the host cell membrane, forming pseudopod-like projections that are ingested by neighboring cells. This provides a means of cell-to-cell spread of the organism. The bacterium eventually reaches the central

TABLE 16.2 Pathogenesis and Spectrum of Diseases

Organism	Virulence Factors	Spectrum of Diseases and Infections
Listeria monocytogenes	Listeriolysin O: A hemolytic and cytotoxic toxin that allows for survival within phagocytes. Internalin: Cell surface protein that induces phagocytosis. Act A: Induces actin polymerization on the surface of host cells, producing cellular extensions and facilitating cell-to-cell spread. Siderophores: Organisms capable of scavenging iron from human transferrin and of enhanced growth	Systemic: Bacteremia, without any other known site of infection. CNS infections: Meningitis, encephalitis, brain abscess, spinal cord infections. Neonatal: Early onset: Granulomatosis infantisepticum—*in utero* infection disseminated systemically that causes stillbirth. Late onset: Bacterial meningitis. Immunosuppressed patients
Corynebacterium diphtheriae	Diphtheria toxin: A potent exotoxin that destroys host cells by inhibiting protein synthesis	Respiratory diphtheria is a pharyngitis characterized by the development of an exudative membrane that covers the tonsils, uvula, palate, and pharyngeal wall, if untreated, life-threatening cardiac toxicity, neurologic toxicity, and other complications occur. Respiratory obstruction develops, and release of toxin into the blood can damage various organs, including the heart.
	Nontoxigenic strains: Uncertain	Cutaneous diphtheria is characterized by nonhealing ulcers and membrane formation. Immunocompromised patients, drug addicts, and alcoholics Invasive endocarditis, mycotic aneurysms, osteomyelitis, and septic arthritis
Corynebacterium glucuronolyticum	Unknown	Prostatitis, nongonococcal urethritis
Corynebacterium jeikeium	Unknown: Multiple antibiotic resistance allows survival in hospital setting	Systemic: Septicemia Skin infections: Wounds, rashes, and nodules Immunocompromised: Malignancies, neutropenia, AIDS patients Associated with indwelling devices such as catheters, prosthetic valves, and CSF shunts
Corynebacterium ulcerans	Unknown	Zoonosis: Bovine mastitis Has been associated with diphtheria-like sore throat, indistinguishable from *C. diphtheriae* Skin infections Pneumonia
Corynebacterium pseudotuberculosis	Unknown	Zoonosis: Suppurative granulomatous lymphadenitis
Corynebacterium pseudodiphtheriticum	Unknown Some strains have been identified that are resistant to macrolides	Systemic: Septicemia Endocarditis Pneumonia and lung abscesses; primarily in immunocompromised patients
Corynebacterium urealyticum	Unknown Multiple antibiotic resistance allows survival in hospital setting	Immunocompromised and elderly: Urinary tract infections Wound infections Rarely: endocarditis, septicemia, osteomyelitis, and tissue infections

Continued

TABLE
16.2   **Pathogenesis and Spectrum of Diseases—cont'd**

Organism	Virulence Factors	Spectrum of Diseases and Infections
Leifsonia aquatica	Unknown	Immunocompromised: Bacteremia Septicemia
Corynebacterium striatum	Unknown	Immunocompromised: Bacteremia Pneumonia and lung abscesses Osteomyelitis Meningitis
Corynebacterium amycolatum	Unknown Multiple antibiotic resistance patterns	Immunocompromised: Endocarditis Septicemia Pneumonia Neonatal sepsis
Corynebacterium coyleae	Unknown Multiple antibiotic resistance patterns	Uncertain disease association but has been linked to otitis media
Brevibacterium and *Dermabacter* sp.	Unknown	Immunocompromised: Rarely causes infections in humans Bacteremia in association with indwelling catheters or penetrating injuries
Turicella otitidis	Unknown	Uncertain disease association but has been linked to otitis media
Arthrobacter spp., *Microbacterium* spp., *Aureobacterium* spp., *Cellulomonas* spp., and *Exiguobacterium* sp.	Unknown	Uncertain disease association

AIDS, Acquired immunodeficiency syndrome; *CSF,* cerebrospinal fluid; *CNS,* central nervous system.

nervous system and the placenta, resulting in disease (**listeriosis**). Systemic disease manifestations include stillbirth and neonatal death, meningitis, bacteremia, encephalitis, and endocarditis. Localized infections may occur and include conjunctivitis, skin infections, and lymphadenitis. Reports of febrile gastroenteritis have been documented and are associated with foodborne outbreaks of *L. monocytogenes.*

Most of the remaining organisms in Table 16.2 are opportunistic, and infections are associated with immunocompromised patients. When *Corynebacterium* spp., *Listeria* spp., or the other genera of gram-positive rods are encountered, careful consideration must be given to their role as infectious agents or contaminants. *C. urealyticum* is associated with cystitis in hospitalized patients, in those who have undergone urologic manipulation, and in the elderly.

Laboratory Diagnosis

Specimen Collection and Transport

No special considerations are required for specimen collection and transport of the organisms discussed in this chapter. Refer to Table 5.1 for general information on specimen collection and transport.

Specimen Processing

No special considerations are required for processing of most of the organisms discussed in this chapter. Refer to Table 5.1 for general information on specimen processing. One exception is the isolation of *L. monocytogenes* from placental and other tissue. Because isolating *Listeria* organisms from these sources may be difficult, **cold enrichment** may be used to enhance the recovery of the organism. The specimen is inoculated into a nutrient broth and incubated at 4°C for several weeks to months. The broth is subcultured at frequent intervals to enhance recovery. Stool samples are inoculated into selective broth such as polymyxin-acriflavine-lithium chloride-ceftazidime esculin-mannitol (PALCAM) or *Listeria* enrichment broth, transported overnight, and plated to appropriate isolation media in the laboratory.

Direct Detection Methods

Gram stain of clinical specimens is the only procedure used for the direct detection of these organisms. Most of the genera in this chapter (except *Listeria, Rothia,* and *Oerskovia* spp.) are considered coryneform bacteria; that is, they are gram-positive, short or slightly curved rods with rounded

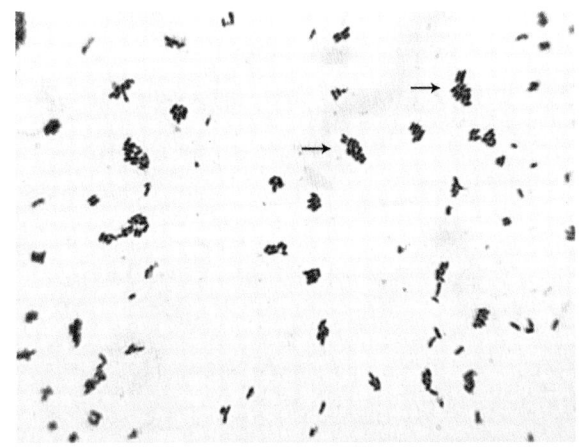

• **Fig. 16.1** Gram stain of *Corynebacterium diphtheriae.* Note palisading and arrangements of cells in formations that resemble Chinese letters *(arrows).*

ends; some have rudimentary branching. Cells are arranged singly, in "palisades" of parallel cells, or in pairs of cells connected after cell division to form **V** or **L** shapes. Groups of these morphologies seen together resemble and are often referred to as "Chinese letters" (Fig. 16.1). The Gram stain morphologies of clinically relevant species are described in Table 16.3. *L. monocytogenes* is a short, gram-positive rod that may occur singly or in short chains, resembling streptococci (Fig. 16.2).

Nucleic Acid Detection

Molecular methods to identify *C. diphtheriae,* including ribotyping, pulsed-field gel electrophoresis, and multilocus sequence typing, have demonstrated improved sensitivity and are effective for identification during an outbreak. Various polymerase chain reaction (PCR) techniques have been used for the quantitative detection of *L. monocytogenes* in food products. *L. monocytogenes* deoxyribonucleic acid (DNA), specifically the *hly* gene that encodes listeriolysin O, in cerebrospinal fluid (CSF) and tissue (fresh or paraffin blocks) can be detected by molecular assays. Two multiplex assays are currently commercially available for the direct detection of *Listeria* in clinical samples; the BioFire FilmArray Meningitis/Encephalitis (ME) Panel (BioFire Diagnostics, Salt Lake City, UT) and Verigene Gram-Positive Blood Culture (BC-GP) assay (Luminex Corporation, Austin, TX). The BioFire FilmArray ME Panel is a commercial multiplex test for *in vitro* diagnosis of infectious agents that cause meningitis and encephalitis, including *L. monocytogenes* in CSF specimens and five additional bacterial pathogens, seven viral pathogens, and *Cryptococcus neoformans/gattii.* The Verigene BC-GP assay is a microarray-based, multiplexed, molecular assay approved by the US Food and Drug Administration (FDA) for rapid detection and identification of 12 gram-positive targets, including *L. monocytogenes,* and has reported high sensitivity and specificity in BacT/Alert blood culture bottles. Diagnosis of listeriosis via traditional isolation and identification will still be available through standard culture and biochemical-based

microbiologic methods. However, implementation of nucleic acid detection methods has allowed for full integration into the workflow of the microbiology laboratory, contributing to significant reduction in turnaround time and identification.

Cultivation

Media of Choice

Corynebacterium spp. usually grow on 5% sheep blood and chocolate agars. Some coryneform bacteria do not grow on chocolate agar, and the lipophilic (lipid loving) species (e.g., *C. jeikeium, C. urealyticum, C. afermentans* subsp. *lipophilum, C. accolens,* and *C. macginleyi*) produce much larger colonies when cultured on 5% sheep blood agar supplemented with 1% Tween 80 (Fig. 16.4).

Selective and differential media for *C. diphtheriae* should be used for isolation of the organism if diphtheria is suspect. *C. diphtheriae* may be isolated from 5% sheep blood agar supplemented with 100 µg/mL of fosfomycin or by placing a 50-µg disk directly on the plate and examining the colonies that grow up to the disk. Nearly all other *Corynebacterium* species are susceptible to fosfomycin. Two media commonly used for the growth and isolation of *C. diphtheriae* are **cystine-tellurite blood agar** and **modified Tinsdale agar (TIN).** Tellurite blood agar may be used with or without cystine. Cystine enhances the growth of fastidious organisms, including *C. diphtheriae.* Both media contain a high concentration of potassium tellurite that is inhibitory to normal microbiota. Organisms capable of growing on Tinsdale agar are differentiated based on the conversion of the tellurite to tellurium. This conversion results in color variations of gray to black colonies on the two media. *C. diphtheriae* also produces a halo on both media. *C. diphtheriae* can be presumptively identified by observing brown-black colonies with a gray-brown halo on Tinsdale agar (Fig. 16.5). The brown halo is produced when the organism uses tellurite to produce hydrogen sulfide. The halo produced on cystine-tellurite blood agar appears brown because the organism is breaking down the cystine. In addition, **Loeffler medium,** which contains serum and egg, stimulates the growth of *C. diphtheriae* and the production of metachromatic granules in the cells. *C. diphtheriae* grows rapidly on the highly enriched agar and produces gray to white, translucent colonies within 12 to 18 hours. Primary inoculation of throat swabs to Loeffler serum slants is no longer recommended because of the inevitable overgrowth of normal oral microbiota.

Corynebacterium spp. are unable grow on MacConkey agar. They all are capable of growth in routine blood culture broth and nutrient broths, such as thioglycollate or brain-heart infusion. Lipophilic coryneform bacteria demonstrate better growth in broths supplemented with rabbit serum.

L. monocytogenes are auxotrophic for seven amino acids including leucine, isoleucine, valine, methionine, arginine, cysteine, and glutamine and require four additional vitamins including riboflavin, thiamine, biotin, and thioctic acid. Therefore, *L. monocytogenes* needs to be grown in a rich culture medium that provides all of the growth factors.

TABLE 16.3	Gram Stain Morphology, Colonial Appearance, and Other Distinguishing Characteristics	
Organism	**Gram Stain**	**Appearance on 5% Sheep Blood Agar**
Arthrobacter spp.	Typical coryneform gram-positive rods after 24 h, with "jointed ends" giving L and V forms, and coccoid cells after 72 h (i.e., rod-coccus cycle[a])	Large colony; resembles *Brevibacterium* spp.; nonhemolytic
Brevibacterium spp.	Gram-positive rods; produce typical coryneform arrangements in young cultures (<24 h) and coccoid-to-coccobacillary forms that decolorize easily in older cultures (i.e., rod-coccus cycle[a])	Medium to large; gray to white, convex, opaque, smooth, shiny; nonhemolytic; cheeselike odor
Cellulomonas spp.	Irregular, short, thin, branching, gram-positive rods	Small to medium; two colony types, one starts out white and turns yellow within 3 days and the other starts out yellow; nonhemolytic
C. amycolatum	Pleomorphic gram-positive rods with single cells, V forms, or Chinese letters	Small; white to gray, dry; nonhemolytic
C. aurimucosum	Typical coryneform gram-positive rods	Slightly yellowish sticky colonies; some strains black-pigmented; nonhemolytic
C. coyleae	Typical coryneform gram-positive rods	Small to medium; dry, slightly adherent, become yellowish with time; nonhemolytic
C. diphtheriae group[b]	Irregularly staining, pleomorphic gram-positive rods	Various biotypes of *C. diphtheriae* produce colonies ranging from small, gray, and translucent (biotype *intermedius*) to medium, white, and opaque (biotypes *mitis, belfanti*, and *gravis*); *C. diphtheriae* biotype *mitis* may be beta-hemolytic; *C. ulcerans* and *C. pseudotuberculosis* resemble *C. diphtheriae*
C. glucuronolyticum	Typical coryneform gram-positive rods	Small; white to yellow, convex; nonhemolytic
C. jeikeium	Pleomorphic; occasionally, club-shaped gram-positive rods arranged in V forms or palisades	Small; gray to white, entire, convex; nonhemolytic
C. pseudodiphtheriticum	Typical coryneform gram-positive rods	Small to medium; slightly dry; nonhemolytic
C. pseudotuberculosis	Typical coryneform gram-positive rods	Small, yellowish white, opaque, convex; matted surface; variable nonhemolytic and beta-hemolytic
C. striatum	Regular medium to large gram-positive rods; can show banding	Small to medium; white, moist and smooth (resembles colonies of coagulase-negative staphylococci); nonhemolytic
C. ulcerans	Typical coryneform gram-positive rods	Small, dry, waxy, gray to white; variable nonhemolytic and beta-hemolytic
C. urealyticum	Gram-positive coccobacilli arranged in V forms and palisades	Pinpoint (after 48 h); white, smooth, convex; nonhemolytic
Dermabacter spp.	Coccoid to short gram-positive rods	Small; gray to white, convex; distinctive pungent odor; nonhemolytic
Exiguobacterium acetylicum	Irregular, short, gram-positive rods arranged singly, in pairs, or short chains (i.e., rod-coccus cycle[a])	Golden yellow; nonhemolytic, and can be mucoid—needs to be differentiated from *B. anthracis*
Leifsonia aquatica	Irregular, slender, short gram-positive rods	Yellow; nonhemolytic to slightly alpha
Listeria monocytogenes	Regular, short, gram-positive rods or coccobacilli occurring in pairs (resembles streptococci)	Small; white, smooth, translucent, moist; beta-hemolytic
Microbacterium spp.	Irregular, short, thin, gram-positive rods	Small to medium; yellow; nonhemolytic to alpha-hemolytic

Organism	Gram Stain	Appearance on 5% Sheep Blood Agar
Oerskovia spp.	Extensive branching; hyphae break up into coccoid to rod-shaped elements	Yellow-pigmented; convex; creamy colony grows into the agar; dense centers; alpha- or beta-hemolytic
Rothia spp.	Extremely pleomorphic; predominately coccoid and bacillary (broth, Fig. 16.3A) to branched filaments (solid media, Fig. 16.3B)	Small, smooth to rough colonies; dry; whitish; raised; nonhemolytic
Turicella otitidis	Irregular, long, gram-positive rods	Small to medium; white to cream, circular, convex; nonhemlytic

aRod-coccus cycle means rods are apparent in young cultures; cocci are apparent in cultures older than 3 days.
bIncludes *C. diphtheriae, C. ulcerans,* and *C. pseudotuberculosis.*
Data from Mogrovejo DC, Perini L, Gostincar C, et al: Prevalence of antimicrobial resistance and hemolytic phenotypes in culturable arctic bacteria, *Front Microbiol* 11:570, 2020.

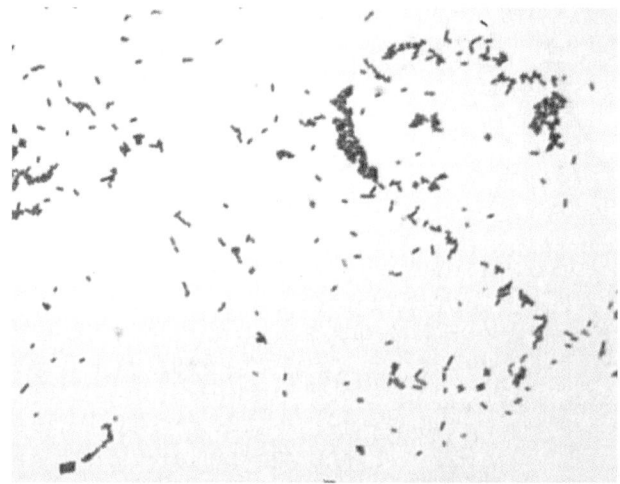

• **Fig. 16.2** Indirect (culture) Gram stain of *Listeria monocytogenes* (×1000).

Brain-heart infusion (BHI) is the most common nonselective media used for the cultivation of *Listeria* species. Some strains, such as *L. monocytogenes,* can also be cultivated in tryptic soy broth (TSB).

A wide variety of selective and differential media have been developed to aid in the identification of *L. monocytogenes* including modified Oxford agar (MOX) base and chromogenic media such as Brilliance *Listeria* Agar Base (Thermofisher Scientific, Waltham, MA) and CHROMagar *Listeria* (DRG International, Inc., Springfield, NJ). MOX medium comprises a Columbia agar base that provides the necessary amino acids, carbon, vitamins, and nitrogen for bacterial growth, supplemented with lithium chloride, esculin, ferric ammonium citrate, colistin, and moxalactam. Moxalactam inhibits staphylococci, bacilli, and *Proteus,* and colistin inhibits gram-negative bacilli to prevent the overgrowth of *L. monocytogenes* from contaminating mixed bacterial flora. The selectivity is enhanced by lithium chloride, which negatively affects the growth of enterococci. All species of *Listeria* are capable of hydrolyzing esculin in the media forming a black halo.

Chromogenic media, including Brilliance *Listeria* Agar and CHROMagar *Listeria,* can be used to differentiate *L. monocytogenes* from other *Listeria* spp. The detection of *L. monocytogenes* by chromogenic media usually involves cleavage of the substrate 5-bromo-4-chloro-3-indoxyl-beta-d-glucopyranoside by beta-d-glucosidase produced by *Listeria* spp., combined with l-alpha-phosphatidylinositol for the detection of phosphatidylinositol-specific phospholipase C (PI-PLC) and phosphatidylcholine-specific phospholipase C (PC-PLC). PI-PLC and PC-PLC, the major virulence factors, are only produced by pathogenic *L. monocytogenes* and *L. ivanovii.* Chromogenic media can be expensive and may not be suitable for routine laboratory use. In addition, some *Bacillus* spp., especially *Bacillus cereus,* and *Staphylococcus aureus* are beta-d-glucosidase, PI-PLC, and PC-PLC positive, and are capable of growth on chromogenic media resembling *L. monocytogenes.* Pathogenic *L. monocytogenes* will produce a blue-green colony surrounded by an opaque, white halo on CHROMagar Listeria. Other *Listeria* species will produce blue-green colonies without a halo. Gram-negative organisms are inhibited. Gram-positive organisms, other than *Listeria* species, will either be inhibited or produce white colonies.

Incubation Conditions and Duration

Detectable growth of *Corynebacterium* on 5% sheep blood and chocolate agars, incubated at 35°C in either ambient air or in 5% to 10% carbon dioxide, should occur within 48 to 72 hours after inoculation. The lipophilic organisms grow more slowly; it takes 3 days or longer to identify visible growth on routine media. For growth of *C. diphtheriae,* cystine-tellurite blood agar and modified Tinsdale agar should be incubated for at least 48 hours in ambient air. Five to ten percent of carbon dioxide (CO_2) retards the formation of halos on Tinsdale agar. The majority of the remaining corynebacteria will grow at 35°C to 37°C in CO_2. Some of the other genera, *Arthrobacter* and *Microbacterium* spp., have optimal growth temperatures between 30°C and 35°C. *L. monocytogenes* grows well on 5% sheep blood agar incubated at 35°C to 37°C in CO_2.

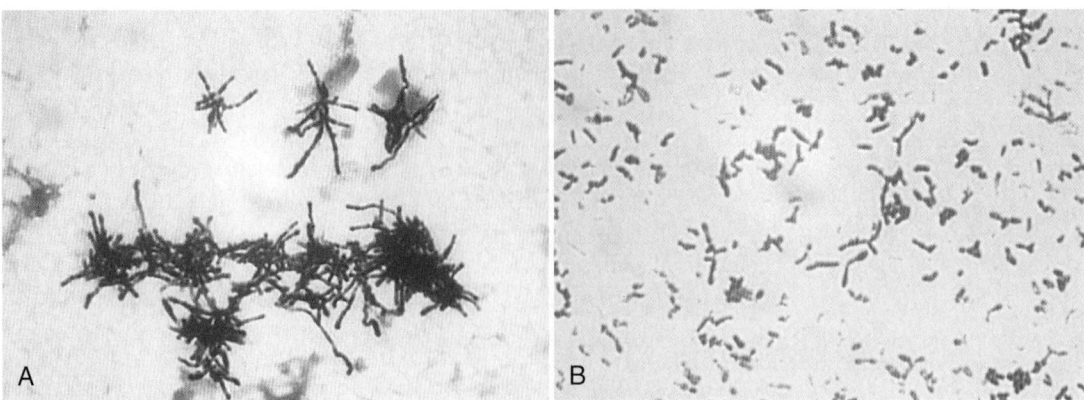

• **Fig. 16.3** (A) *Rothia dentocariosa* from broth. (B) *R. dentocariosa* from solid media. (Courtesy Deanna Kiska, SUNY Upstate Medical University, Syracuse, NY.)

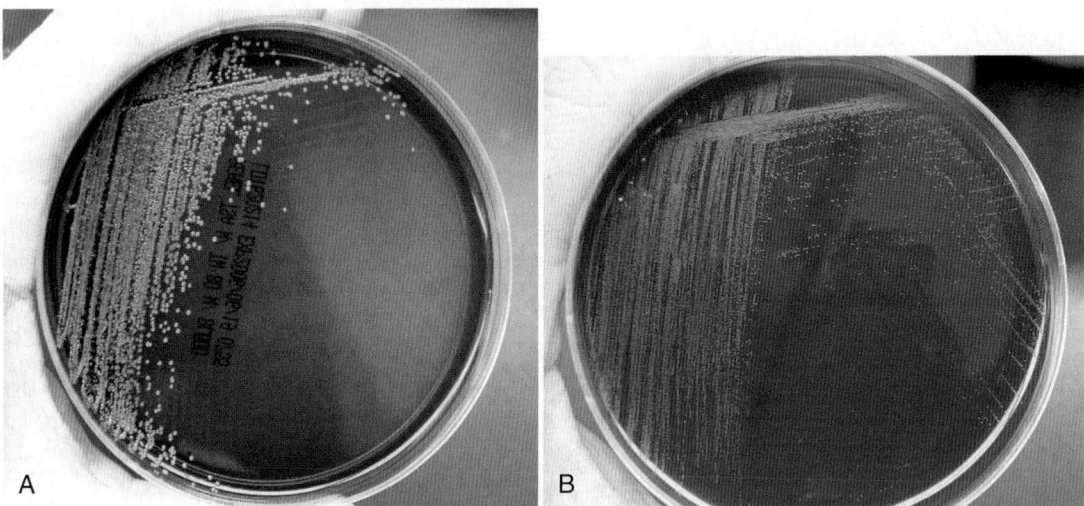

• **Fig. 16.4** *Corynebacterium urealyticum* on blood agar with Tween 80 (A) and blood agar (B) at 48 hours. This organism is lipophilic and grows much better on the lipid-containing medium.

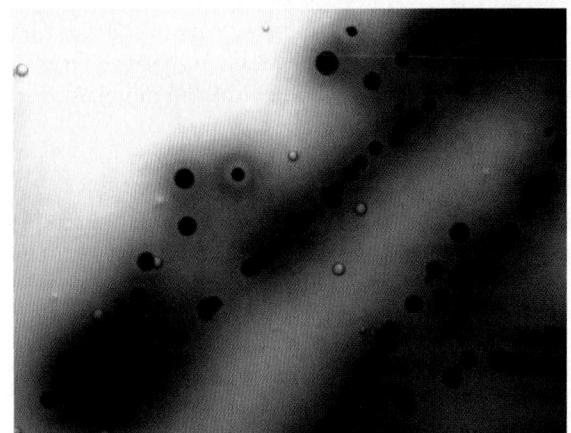

• **Fig. 16.5** Colony of *Corynebacterium diphtheriae* on Tinsdale agar. Note black colonies with brown halo.

Colonial Appearance

Table 16.3 describes the colonial appearance and other distinguishing characteristics (e.g., hemolysis and odor) of each clinically relevant genus or species of corynebacteria

on blood agar. Colonies of *C. diphtheriae* on cystine-tellurite blood agar appear black or gray, whereas those on modified Tinsdale agar are black with dark brown halos (Fig. 16.5).

Approach to Identification

Except for *L. monocytogenes* and a few *Corynebacterium* spp., identification of the organisms in this chapter generally is complex and problematic. A multiphasic approach is required for definitive identification. Phenotypic identification including biochemical testing may be sufficient to identify most organisms to the genus level and some of the more common species. However, definitive identification requires 16S ribosomal ribonucleic acid (rRNA) gene sequencing or the use of matrix-assisted desorption ionization time of flight (Chapter 7). Further complicating the situation is the fact that coryneformes are present as normal microbiota throughout the body. Thus only clinically relevant isolates should be identified fully. Indicators of clinical relevance include (1) isolation from normally sterile sites or multiple blood culture bottles, (2) isolation in pure culture or as the predominant organism from symptomatic patients who have not yielded any other known etiologic agent, and (3) isolation from urine if present as a pure culture at greater than 10,000 colony-forming units per milliliter (CFU/mL) or the predominant organism at greater than 100,000 CFU/mL. Coryneformes are more likely to be the cause of a urinary tract infection if the pH of the urine is alkaline or if **struvite crystals** composed of phosphate, magnesium, and ammonia are present in the sediment.

The API Coryne system (bioMérieux, St. Louis, MO), the RapID CB Plus (Thermo Fisher Scientific, Waltham, MA), and the BBL Crystal gram-positive identification system (Becton Dickinson, Franklin Lakes, NJ) are commercial products available for rapid identification of this group of organisms; however, the databases may not be current with recent taxonomic changes. Misidentifications can occur if the code generated using these kits is the exclusive criterion used for identification.

Table 16.4 shows the key tests needed to separate the genera discussed in this chapter. In addition to the features shown, the Gram stain and colonial morphology should be carefully noted.

Matrix-Assisted Laser Desorption Ionization Time-of-Flight Mass Spectrometry

Matrix-assisted laser desorption ionization time-of-flight mass spectroscopy (MALDI-TOF MS) has been used to reliably identify toxigenic strains of *Corynebacterium* spp. Currently, the existing identification capability of coryneform bacterial isolates by MALDI-TOF MS is limited. Some coryneform bacteria have been directly identified from the MALDI-TOF MS system using a lysis method (Sepsityper, bioMérieux, Durham, NC); however, caution should be used when interpreting due to inconsistencies in the spectra used for identification. MALDI-TOF MS has been used for rapid identification of *L. monocytogenes*; however, it is important to evaluate the results carefully, as the type of media used to grow the organism can alter the identification spectra. As the databases are improved, this technique will continue to provide a potential strategy for the improvement in identifying clinical isolates.

Serodiagnosis

Serodiagnostic techniques are not generally used for the laboratory diagnosis of infections caused by the organisms discussed in this chapter. Anti–listeriolysin O antibodies (IgG) can be detected in cases of listeriosis, although IgM antibodies are undetectable.

Comments on Specific Organisms

Two tests (halo on Tinsdale agar and urea hydrolysis) can be used to separate *C. diphtheriae* from other corynebacteria. Definitive identification of a *C. diphtheriae* as a true pathogen

requires demonstration of toxin production by the isolate in question. A patient may be infected with several strains at once; testing is performed using a pooled inoculum of at least 10 colonies. Several toxin detection methods are available:

- Guinea pig lethality test to ascertain whether diphtheria antitoxin (DAT) neutralizes the lethal effect of a cell-free suspension of the suspect organism
- Immunodiffusion test (Fig. 16.6)
- Tissue culture cell test to demonstrate toxicity of a cell-free suspension of the suspected organism in tissue culture cells and the neutralization of the cytopathic effect by DAT
- Enzyme immunoassays (EIAs)
- PCR to detect the toxin gene (*tox*)

Because the incidence of diphtheria in the United States is so low (fewer than five cases/year), it is not practical to perform these tests in routine clinical laboratories. Toxin testing is usually performed in reference laboratories.

Identification criteria for *Corynebacterium* spp. (including *C. diphtheriae*) are shown in Tables 16.5 through 16.9. Most clinically relevant strains are catalase positive, nonmotile, nonpigmented, and esculin and gelatin negative. Isolation of an organism failing to demonstrate any of these characteristics provides a significant clue that another genus shown in Table 16.4 should be considered. In addition, an irregular, gram-positive rod that is strictly aerobic, is nonlipophilic, and oxidizes or does not utilize glucose will likely be *Leifsonia aquatica* or *Arthrobacter, Brevibacterium,* or *Microbacterium* spp.

The enhancement of growth by lipids (e.g., Tween 80 or serum) of certain coryneform bacteria (e.g., *C. jeikeium* and *C. urealyticum*) is useful for preliminary identification. These two species are also resistant to several antibiotics commonly tested against gram-positive bacteria.

Listeria monocytogenes can be presumptively identified by observation of motility by direct wet mount. The organism exhibits characteristic end-over-end tumbling motility when incubated in nutrient broth at room temperature for 1 to 2 hours. Alternatively, characteristic motility can be seen by an umbrella-shaped pattern (Fig. 16.7) that develops after overnight incubation at room temperature of a culture stabbed into a tube of semisolid agar. *L. monocytogenes* ferments glucose and is Voges-Proskauer positive and esculin positive. Isolation of a small, gram-positive, catalase-positive rod with a narrow, soft zone of beta-hemolysis from blood or CSF should be considered strong presumptive evidence for listeriosis. *L. monocytogenes* can be differentiated from other *Listeria* spp. by a positive result on the Christie, Atkins, Munch-Petersen (CAMP) test, as described in Chapter 14 for the identification of *Streptococcus agalactiae*. A **reverse CAMP reaction** (i.e., an arrow of no hemolysis formed at the junction of the test organism with the staphylococci) is used to identify *C. pseudotuberculosis* and *C. ulcerans. C. urealyticum* is rapidly urease positive.

TABLE 16.4 Catalase-Positive, Non–Acid-Fast, Gram-Positive Rods

Organism	Metabolism[a]	Motility	Pigment[b]	Nitrate Reduction	Esculin	Glucose Fermentation	CAMP[c]	Mycolic Acid[d]	Cell Wall Diamino Acids[e]	Other Comments
Corynebacterium spp.	F/O	–	n, w, y, bl	v	–[f]	v	v	+[g]	meso-DAP	
Arthrobacter spp.	O	V[h]	w, g	v	v	–[i]	–	–	L-lys	Gelatin-positive
Brevibacterium spp.	O	–	w, g, sl y, t	v	–	–[i]	–	–	meso-DAP	Gelatin- and casein-positive; cheese odor
Microbacterium[j] spp.	F[k]/O[l]	V[m]	y, o, y-o	v	V[n]	v	–[o]	–	L-lys, D-orn	Gelatin and casein variable
Turicella spp.	O	–	w	–	–	–	+	–	meso-DAP	Isolated from ears
Dermabacter spp.	F	–	n, w	–	+	+	–	–	meso-DAP	Pungent odor; decarboxylates lysine and ornithine; gelatin positive
Cellulomonas spp.	F[k]	v	sl y, y	+	+	+	–	–	L-orn	Gelatin-positive; casein-negative
Leifsonia spp.	O	+	y	v	v	–[p]	–	–	DAB	Gelatin- and casein-negative
Cellulosimicrobium spp.	F	–	y	+	+	+	NT	–	L-lys	Hydrolyzes xanthine; colonies pit agar
Oerskovia spp.	F	v	y	+	+	+	NT	–	L-lys	Does not hydrolyze xanthine
Listeria monocytogenes	F	+[q]	w	–	+	+	+	–	meso-DAP	Narrow zone of beta-hemolysis on sheep blood agar; hippurate-positive
Exiguobacterium spp.	F	+	Golden	v	+	+	NT	–	L-lys	Most are oxidase positive; casein and gelatin positive
Rothia spp.	F	–	w	+	+	+	–	–	L-lys	If sticky, probably *R. mucilaginosa;* some strains are black pigmented

[a]*F,* Fermentative; *O,* oxidative.
[b]*bl,* Black; *c,* cream; *g,* gray; *n,* nonpigmented; *o,* orange; *sl,* slightly; *p,* pink; *t,* tan; *w,* white; *y,* yellow; *y-o,* yellowish-orange.
[c]CAMP test using a beta-lysin–producing strain of *Staphylococcus aureus.*
[d]Mycolic acids of various lengths are also present in the partially acid-fast *Nocardia, Gordonia,* and *Tsukamurella* and the completely acid-fast *Mycobacterium* genera.
[e]*DAB,* Diaminobutyric acid; *D-orn,* d-ornithine; *L-lys,* L-lysine; *L-orn,* L-ornithine; *meso-DAP,* meso-diaminopimelic acid.
[f]Of the significant clinical *Corynebacterium* isolates, only *C. matruchotii* and *C. glucuronolyticum* are esculin positive.
[g]Of the significant *Corynebacterium* isolates, *Corynebacterium amycolatum* does not have mycolic acid as a lipid in the cell wall, as determined by high-performance liquid chromatography (HPLC) profiling methods.
[h]Rod forms of some species are motile.
[i]Glucose may be variably oxidized, but it is not fermented.
[j]*Microbacterium* spp. now include the former *Aureobacterium* spp.
[k]Some grow poorly anaerobically.
[l]Slow and weak oxidative production of acid from some carbohydrates.
[m]Only the orange-pigmented species *M. imperiale* and *M. arborescens* are motile at 28°C.
[n]Positive reaction may be delayed.
[o]Some strains of *M. arborescens* are CAMP positive.
[p]Glucose is usually oxidized, but it is not fermented.
[q]Motile at 20°C–25°C.
NT, Not tested; *TSI,* triple sugar iron agar; *v,* variable reactions; *+,* ≥90% of species or strains positive; *–,* ≥90% of species or strains negative.

Antimicrobial Susceptibility Testing and Therapy

Definitive guidelines are established for antimicrobial therapy for *L. monocytogenes* against some antimicrobial agents. Because there is no resistance to the therapeutic agents of choice, antimicrobial susceptibility testing is not routinely necessary (Table 16.10).

As shown in Table 16.10, Clinical and Laboratory Standards Institute (CLSI) document M45 provides some guidelines for testing of *Corynebacterium* spp. Chapter 11 should be reviewed for strategies that can be used to provide susceptibility information and data when warranted.

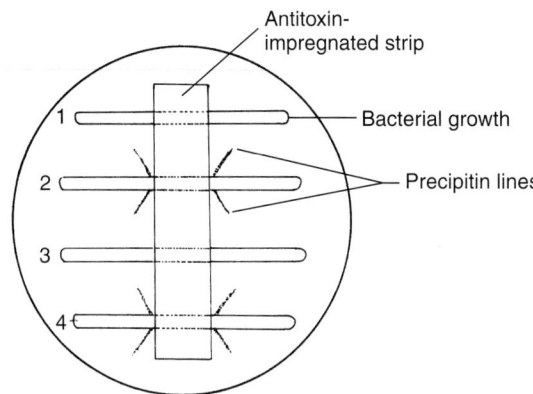

• **Fig. 16.6** Diagram of an Elek plate for demonstration of toxin production by *Corynebacterium diphtheriae.* A filter paper strip impregnated with diphtheria antitoxin is buried just beneath the surface of a special agar plate before the agar hardens. Strains to be tested, known positive and negative toxigenic strains are streaked on the agar's surface in a line across the plate and at a right angle to the antitoxin paper strip. After 24 hours of incubation at 37°C, the plates are examined with transmitted light for the presence of fine precipitin lines at a 45-degree angle to the streaks. The presence of precipitin lines indicates that the strain produced toxin that reacted with the homologous antitoxin. Line 1 is the negative control. *Line 2 is the positive control.* Line 3 is an unknown organism that is a nontoxigenic strain. Line 4 is an unknown organism that is a toxigenic strain.

It is important to note that some strains of *Corynebacterium* spp. may require 48 hours of incubation for growth. If growth is insufficient or if the isolate appears susceptible to beta-lactams at 24 hours, the medium should be incubated for a total of 48 hours before the result is reported.

Prevention

The only effective control of diphtheria is through immunization with a multidose diphtheria toxoid prepared by inactivation of the toxin with formaldehyde. There are currently four combination vaccines for the prevention of diphtheria, tetanus (Chapter 41), and pertussis (Chapter 36). Two of these are given to children younger than 7 years of age (DTap and DT), and two are given to older children and adults (Tdap and Td). Td boosters are recommended every 10 years to maintain active protection.

Treatment

Hyperimmune antiserum produced in horses, **DAT**, is a preparation of antibodies capable of toxin neutralization before its entry into the patient's cells. It is critical that DAT be administered as soon as a presumptive clinical diagnosis is completed. Because of hypersensitivity reactions to antibodies (proteins) produced in horses, it is recommended to question the patient regarding potential allergies and in some instances complete a skin scratch test to the forearm. DAT is no longer licensed in the United States, but a product is available from the Centers for Disease Control for use in other countries.

A single dose of intramuscular penicillin or a course of oral erythromycin is recommended for 14 days for all individuals that present with symptoms of diphtheria. In addition, prophylaxis may be indicated for individuals exposed to diphtheria. Immunized contacts should receive a booster dose of diphtheria toxoid; nonimmunized contacts should begin the primary series of immunizations.

TABLE 16.5	Fermentative, Nonlipophilic, Tinsdale-Positive *Corynebacterium* spp.[a]				
Organism	Urease[b]	Nitrate Reduction[b]	Esculin Hydrolysis[b]	Fermentation of Glycogen[b]	Lipophilic
C. diphtheriae	–	+	–	±	–
C. ulcerans[c,d]	+	–	–	+	–
C. pseudotuberculosis[c,d]	+	v	–	–	–

[a]Separation of lipophilic and nonlipophilic species can be determined by comparing growth on sheep blood agar and sheep blood agar with 1% Tween 80 or growth in brain-heart infusion broth with and without 1 drop of Tween 80 or rabbit serum.
[b]Reactions from API Coryne.
[c]Propionic acid produced as a product of glucose metabolism.
[d]Reverse CAMP positive.
v, Variable reactions; +, ≥90% of species or strains positive; –, ≥90% of species or strains are negative.
Data compiled from Coyle MB, Lipsky BA. Coryneform bacteria in infectious diseases: clinical and laboratory aspects. *Clin Microbiol Rev.* 1990;3:227; Funke G, Carlotti A. Differentiation of *Brevibacterium* spp. encountered in clinical specimens. *J Clin Microbiol.* 1994;32:1729; Gruner E, Steigerwalt AG, Hollis DG, et al. Human infections caused by *Brevibacterium casei,* formerly CDC groups B-1 and B-3. *J Clin Microbiol.* 1994;32:1511.

TABLE 16.6 Fermentative, Nonlipophilic, Tinsdale-Negative Clinically Relevant *Corynebacterium* spp.[a,b]

Organism	Urea[c]	Nitrate Reduction[c]	Propionic Acid[d]	Motility	Esculin Hydrolysis[c]	Fermentation of Glucose[c]	Maltose[c]	Sucrose[c]	Xylose[c]	CAMP[e]
C. amycolatum[f]	v	v	+	−	−	+	v	v	−	−
C. aurimucosum[g,h]	−	−	−	−	−	+	+	+	−	−
C. coyleae	−	−	ND	−	−	(+)	−	−	−	+
C. falsenii[i]	(+)	v	ND	−	v	(+)	v	−	−	−
C. freneyi[j]	−	v	−	−	−	+	+	+	−	ND
C. glucuronolyticum	v	v	+	−	v	+	v	+	v	+
C. imitans	−	v	ND	−	−	+	+	(+)	−	+
C. matruchotii	−	+	+	−	v +	+	+	+	−	−
C. riegelii	+	−	ND	−	−	−	(+)	−	−	−
C. simulans[k]	−	+	−	−	−	+	−	+	−	−
C. singulare	+	−	−	−	−	+	+	+	−	−
C. striatum	−	+	−	−	−	+	−	v	−	v
C. sundsvallense[g]	+	−	ND	−	−	(+)	+	+	−	−
C. thomsseniig	+	−	ND	−	−	(+)	+	+	−	−

[a]Consider also *Dermabacter, Cellulomonas, Exiguobacterium,* and *Microbacterium* spp. if the isolate is pigmented, motile, or esculin or gelatin positive (Table 16.4). The aerotolerant catalase-positive *Cutibacterium* spp. and *Actinomyces* spp. (Table 17.4) should also be considered in the differential with the organisms in this table.
[b]Separation of lipophilic and nonlipophilic species can be determined by comparing growth on sheep blood agar and sheep blood agar with 1% Tween 80 or growth in brain-heart infusion broth with and without 1 drop of Tween 80 or rabbit serum.
[c]Reactions from API Coryne.
[d]Propionic acid as an end-product of glucose metabolism.
[e]CAMP data using a beta-lysin–producing strain of *Staphylococcus aureus.*
[f]Most frequently encountered species in human clinical material; frequently misidentified as *C. xerosis.*
[g]Sticky colonies.
[h]Yellow or black-pigmented; black-pigmented strains have been previously listed as *C. nigricans;* may be pathogenic from female genital tract.
[i]Yellow after 72 hours.
[j]Grows at 42°C.
[k]Nitrite reduced.
ND, No data; *v,* variable reactions; +, ≥90% of species or strains are positive; +[W], (+), delayed positive reaction; −, ≥90% of species or strains are negative.

TABLE 16.7 Strictly Aerobic, Nonlipophilic, Nonfermentative, Clinically Relevant *Corynebacterium* spp.[a]

Organism	Oxidation of Glucose	Nitrate Reduction[b]	Urease[b]	Esculin Hydrolysis[b]	Gelatin[b]	CAMP[c]	Other Comments
C. afermentans subsp. afermentans	−	−	−	−	−	v	Isolated from blood; nonadherent colony
C. coyleae	−	−	−	−	−	+	Isolated from ears; dry, usually adherent colony
C. mucifaciens	+	−	−	−	NT	−	Slightly yellow, mucoid colonies
C. pseudodiphtheriticum	−	+	+	−	−	−	
C. propinquum	−	+	−	−	−	−	

[a]Separation of lipophilic and nonlipophilic species can be determined by comparing growth on sheep blood agar and sheep blood agar with 1% Tween 80 or growth in brain-heart infusion broth with and without 1 drop of Tween 80 or rabbit serum.
[b]Reactions from API Coryne.
[c]CAMP test using a beta-lysin–producing strain of *Staphylococcus aureus.*
NT, Not tested; *v,* variable reactions; +, ≥90% of species or strains are positive; −, ≥90% of species or strains are negative.

TABLE 16.8 Strictly Aerobic, Lipophilic, Nonfermentative, Clinically Relevant *Corynebacterium* spp.[a]

Organism	Nitrate Reduction[b]	Urease[b]	Esculin Hydrolysis[b]	Glucose	Maltose
			OXIDATION OF		
C. lipophiloflavum[c]	−	−	−	−	−
C. jeikeium[d]	−	−	−	+	v
C. afermentans subsp. *lipophilum*	−	−	−	−	−
C. urealyticum[d]	−	+	−	−	−

[a]Separation of lipophilic and nonlipophilic species can be determined by comparing growth on sheep blood agar and sheep blood agar with 1% Tween 80 or growth in brain-heart infusion broth with and without one drop of Tween 80 or rabbit serum.
[b]Reactions from API Coryne.
[c]Yellow.
[d]Isolates are usually multiply antimicrobial resistant.
v, Variable reactions; +, ≥90% of species or strains positive; −, ≥90% of species or strains negative.

TABLE 16.9 Lipophilic, Fermentative, Clinically Relevant *Corynebacterium* spp.[a]

Organism	Urease[b]	Esculin Hydrolysis[b]	Alkaline Phosphatase[b]	Pyrazinamidase[b]
C. kroppenstedtii[c]	−	+	−	+
C. bovis	−	−	+	−
C. accolens[d]	−	−	−	v
C. macginleyi[d]	−	−	+	−

[a]Separation of lipophilic and nonlipophilic species can be determined by comparing growth on sheep blood agar and sheep blood agar with 1% Tween 80 or growth in brain-heart infusion broth with and without one drop of Tween 80 or rabbit serum.
[b]Reactions from API Coryne.
[c]Propionic acid produced as a product of glucose metabolism.
[d]Nitrate reduced.
v, Variable reactions; +, ≥90% of species or strains positive; −, ≥90% of species or strains negative.

TABLE 16.10 Antimicrobial Therapy and Susceptibility Testing

Organism	Therapeutic Options	Resistance to Therapeutic Options	Validated Testing Methods[a]
Listeria monocytogenes	Ampicillin, or penicillin (MIC ≤2 μg/mL), with or without an aminoglycoside	Occasional resistance to tetracyclines	Yes, but testing is rarely needed to guide therapy; typically treated empirically
Corynebacterium diphtheriae	Antitoxin to neutralize diphtheria toxin plus penicillin or erythromycin to eradicate organism	Not to recommended agents; rare instances of penicillin or macrolide resistance	See CLSI document M45-A: Methods for Antimicrobial Dilution and Disk Susceptibility Testing of Infrequently Isolated or Fastidious Bacteria
Other *Corynebacterium* spp.	No definitive guidelines. All are susceptible to vancomycin and teicoplanin	Multiple resistance to penicillins, macrolides, aminoglycosides, fluoroquinolones, tetracyclines, clindamycin, and cephalosporins	See CLSI document M45-A: Methods for Antimicrobial Dilution and Disk Susceptibility Testing of Infrequently Isolated or Fastidious Bacteria
Brevibacterium spp., *Dermabacter* sp., *Arthrobacter* spp., *Microbacterium* spp., *Cellulomonas* spp., and *Exiguobacterium* sp.	No definitive guidelines	Unknown	Not available

[a]Validated testing methods include the standard methods recommended by CLSI and commercial methods approved by the US Food and Drug Administration (FDA). *CLSI,* Clinical and Laboratory Standards Institute; *MIC,* minimum inhibitory concentration.

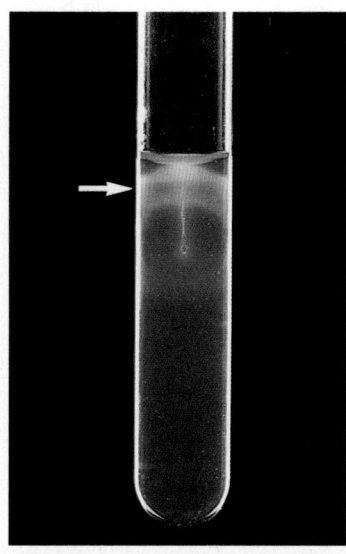

• **Fig. 16.7** Umbrella motility of *Listeria monocytogenes* grown at room temperature.

The general population should always properly wash raw vegetables and thoroughly cook vegetables and meat to prevent listeriosis. Patients who are immunocompromised and pregnant women should avoid eating soft cheeses (e.g., Mexican-style cheese, feta, brie, Camembert, and blue-veined cheese) to prevent food-borne listeriosis. In addition, leftover or ready-to-eat foods such as hot dogs or cold cuts (deli meats) should be thoroughly heated before consumption and only stored for a short period before disposal, because *L. monocytogenes* is able to replicate during refrigeration at 4°C.

ⓔ Visit the Evolve site for a complete list of procedures, review questions, and case studies.

Bibliography

Alibi S, Ferjani A, Gaillot O, Marzouk M, Courcol R, Boukadida J: Identification of clinically relevant *Corynebacterium* strains by Api Coryne, MALDI-TOF-mass spectrometry and molecular approaches, *Pathol Biol (Paris)* 63(4-5):153–157, 2015.

Barberis C, Almuzara M, Join-Lambert O, Ramírez MS, Famiglietti A, Vay C: Comparison of the Bruker MALDI-TOF mass spectrometry system and conventional phenotypic methods for identification of gram-positive rods, *PLoS One* 9(9):e106303, 2014.

Barreau C, Bimet F, Kiredjian M, Rouillon N, Bizet C: Comparative chemotaxonomic studies of mycolic acid-free coryneform bacteria of human origin, *J Clin Microbiol* 31:2085–2090, 1993.

Bennett J, Dolin R, Blaser M: *Principles and practice of infectious diseases,* ed 9, Philadelphia, 2020, Elsevier-Saunders.

Bernard K, Bellefeuille M, Hollis DG, Daneshvar MI, Moss CW: Cellular fatty acid composition and phenotypic and cultural characterization of CDC fermentative coryneform groups 3 and 5, *J Clin Microbiol* 32:1217–1222, 1994.

Caroll KC, Pfaller MA: *Manual of clinical microbiology,* ed 12, Washington, DC, 2019, ASM Press.

Centers for Disease Control and Prevention. *Diphtheria vaccination.* Available at: https://www.cdc.gov/vaccines/vpd/diphtheria/index.html. Accessed May 28, 2019.

Chen Y, Porter V, Mubareka S, Kotowich L, Simor AE: Rapid identification of bacteria directly from positive blood cultures by use of a serum separator tube, smudge plate preparation, and matrix-assisted laser desorption ionization-time of flight mass spectrometry, *J Clin Microbiol* 53:3349–3352, 2015.

Collins MD, Bernard KA, Hutson RA, Sjödén B, Nyberg A, Falsen E: Corynebacterium sundsvallense sp. nov., from human clinical specimens, *Int J Syst Bacteriol* 49:361–366, 1999.

Coyle MB, Lipsky BA: Coryneform bacteria in infectious diseases: clinical and laboratory aspects, *Clin Microbiol Rev* 3:227–246, 1990.

Daneshvar MI, Hollis DG, Weyant RS, et al.: Identification of some charcoal-black-pigmented CDC fermentative coryneform group 4 isolates as *Rothia dentocariosa* and some as *Corynebacterium aurimucosum*: proposal of *Rothia dentocariosa* (emend. Georg and Brown, 1967), *Corynebacterium aurimucosum* (emend. Yassin et al, 2002), and *Corynebacterium nigricans* (Shukla et al, 2003) pro synon. *Corynebacterium aurimucosum*, *J Clin Microbiol* 42:4189–4198, 2004.

De Benoist AC, White JM, Efstratiou A, et al.: Imported cutaneous diphtheria, United Kingdom, *Emerg Infect Dis* 10:511–513, 2004.

Evtushenko LI, Dorofeeva LV, Subbotin SA, Cole JR, Tiedje JM: *Leifsonia poae* gen. nov., sp. nov., isolated from nematode galls on *Poa annua*, and reclassification of "*Corynebacterium aquaticum*" (Leifson, 1962) as *Leifsonia aquatica* (ex Leifson, 1962) gen nov, nom rev, comb nov and *Clavibacter xyli* (Davis et al, 1984) with two subspecies as *Leifsonia xyli* (Davis et al, 1984) gen. nov., comb nov, *Int J Syst Evol Microbiol* 50:371–380, 2000.

Funke G, Carlotti A: Differentiation of *Brevibacterium* spp. encountered in clinical specimens, *J Clin Microbiol* 32:1729–1732, 1994.

Funke G, Efstratiou A, Kuklinska D, et al.: Corynebacterium imitans sp. nov. isolated from patients with suspected diphtheria, *J Clin Microbiol* 35:1978–1983, 1997.

Funke G, Falsen E, Barreau C: Primary identification of *Microbacterium* spp. encountered in clinical specimens as CDC coryneform group A-4 and A-5 bacteria, *J Clin Microbiol* 33:188–192, 1995.

Funke G, Hutson RA, Bernard KA, Pfyffer GE, Wauters G, Collins MD: Isolation of *Arthrobacter* spp. from clinical specimens and description of *Arthrobacter cumminsii* sp. nov. and *Arthrobacter woluwensis* sp. nov, *J Clin Microbiol* 34:2356–2363, 1996.

Funke G, Lawson PA, Bernard KA, Collins MD: Most *Corynebacterium xerosis* strains identified in the routine clinical laboratory correspond to *Corynebacterium amycolatum*, *J Clin Microbiol* 34:1124–1128, 1996.

Funke G, Lawson PA, Collins MD: *Corynebacterium mucifaciens* sp. nov., an unusual species from human clinical material, *Int J Syst Bacteriol* 47:952–957, 1997.

Funke G, Lawson PA, Collins MD: *Corynebacterium riegelii* sp. nov., an unusual species isolated from female patients with urinary tract infections, *J Clin Microbiol* 36:624–627, 1998.

Funke G, Lawson PA, Collins MD: Heterogeneity within human-derived Centers for Disease Control and Prevention coryneform group ANF-1-like bacteria and description of *Corynebacterium auris* sp. nov, *Int J Syst Bacteriol* 45:735–739, 1995.

Funke G, von Graevenitz A, Clarridge JE, Bernard KA: Clinical microbiology of coryneform bacteria, *Clin Microbiol Rev* 10:125–159, 1997.

Galan-Sanchez F, Aznar-Marin P, Marin-Casanova P, Garcia-Martos P, Rodriguez-Iglesias M: Urethritis due to *Corynebacterium glucuronolyticum*, *J Infect Chemother* 17:720–721, 2011.

Gruner E, Steigerwalt AG, Hollis DG, et al.: Human infections caused by *Brevibacterium casei*, formerly CDC groups B-1 and B-3, *J Clin Microbiol* 32:1511–1518, 1994.

Jadhav S, Gulati V, Fox EM, et al.: Rapid identification and source-tracking of *Listeria monocytogenes* using MALDI-TOF mass spectrometry, *Int J Food Microbiol* 202:1–9, 2015.

Jadhav S, Sevior D, Bhave M, Palombo EA: Detection of *Listeria monocytogenes* from selective enrichment broth using MALDI-TOF mass spectrometry, *J Proteomics* 97:100–106, 2014.

Jones GS, D'Orazio SE: Listeria monocytogenes: cultivation and laboratory maintenance, *Curr Protoc Microbiol* 31:9B.2.1–9B.2.7, 2013. https://doi.org/10.1002/9780471729259.mc09b02s31.

Leber AL, Everhart K, Balada-Llasat JM, et al.: Multicenter evaluation of BioFire FilmArray meningitis/encephalitis panel for detection of bacteria, viruses, and yeast in cerebrospinal fluid specimens, *J Clin Microbiol* 54(9):2251–2261, 2016.

McNeil MM, Brown JM: The medically important aerobic actinomycetes: epidemiology and microbiology, *Clin Microbiol Rev* 7:357–417, 1994.

Mestas J, Polanco CM, Felsenstein S, Dien Bard J: Performance of the Verigene gram-positive blood culture assay for direct detection of gram-positive organisms and resistance markers in a pediatric hospital, *J Clin Microbiol* 52(1):283–287, 2014.

Park SH, Chang PS, Ryu S, Kang DH: Development of a novel selective and differential medium for the isolation of *Listeria monocytogenes* [published correction appears in *Appl Environ Microbiol*.80(8):2645], *Appl Environ Microbiol* 80(3):1020–1025, 2014.

Riegel P, de Briel D, Prévost G, Jehl F, Monteil H: Genomic diversity among *Corynebacterium jeikeium* strains and comparison with biochemical characteristics and antimicrobial susceptibilities, *J Clin Microbiol* 32:1860–1865, 1994.

Riegel P, Ruimy R, de Briel D, et al.: Genomic diversity and phylogenetic relationships among lipid-requiring diphtheroids from humans and characterization of *Corynebacterium macginleyi* sp. nov, *Int J Syst Bacteriol* 45:128–133, 1995.

Shukla SK, Bernard KA, Harney M, Frank DN, Reed KD: Corynebacterium nigricans sp. nov.: proposed name for a black-pigmented *Corynebacterium* species recovered from the human female urogenital tract, *J Clin Microbiol* 41:4353–4358, 2003.

Zimmermann O, Spröer C, Kroppenstedt RM, Fuchs E, Köchel HG, Funke G: *Corynebacterium thomssenii* sp. nov., a *Corynebacterium* with N-acetyl-β-glucosaminidase activity from human clinical specimens, *Int J Syst Bacteriol* 48:489–494, 1998.

17

Erysipelothrix, Lactobacillus, and Similar Organisms

OBJECTIVES

1. Describe the Gram stain morphology of *Arcanobacterium, Lactobacillus, Erysipelothrix,* and *Gardnerella* spp.
2. Identify the media of choice and morphologic appearance of *Gardnerella* spp. and describe its incubation conditions, including time, oxygen requirements, and temperature.
3. List the disease states associated with *Erysipelothrix, Gardnerella,* and *Lactobacillus* spp.
4. Identify the correct specimens for the isolation of *Erysipelothrix, Gardnerella,* and *Lactobacillus* spp.
5. Explain why *in vitro* susceptibility testing is usually not necessary to guide therapy of *Erysipelothrix* or *Gardnerella* spp.

GENERA AND SPECIES TO BE CONSIDERED

- *Arcanobacterium haemolyticum*
- *Corynebacterium lipophiloflavum*
- *Erysipelothrix rhusiopathiae*
- *Gardnerella vaginalis*
- *Lactobacillus* spp.
- *Trueperella bernardiae*
- *Trueperella pyogenes*
- *Weissella confusa*

General Characteristics

The genera described in this chapter are all catalase-negative, non–spore-forming, gram-positive rods; some may exhibit rudimentary branching. *Erysipelothrix rhusiopathiae* is one of four species in the genus and is considered the only human pathogen. *E. rhusiopathiae* consists of several serovars based on peptidoglycan structure. The serovars most commonly associated with human infection include serovars 1 and 2. *Arcanobacterium* spp. consists of seven species; however, only *A. haemolyticum* has been recovered from clinical specimens. *Arcanobacterium* spp. demonstrate irregular, gram-positive rods on Gram stain. *Trueperella* spp. (*T. pyogenes* and *T. bernardiae*) demonstrate the same Gram stain morphology; however, they are Christie, Atkins, Munch-Petersen (CAMP) test negative, unlike

Arcanobacterium spp. *Gardnerella vaginalis* is the only species in the genus, and although it is a gram-positive bacterium, it has a much thinner layer of peptidoglycan than other organisms. As a result, the organism appears as a thin, gram-variable rod or coccobacilli. Although *Lactobacillus* spp. may be beneficial to the human host in immunocompetent individuals, numerous species have been isolated from serious infections in immunocompromised patients. The species most frequently isolated from invasive human infections include *L. acidophilus, L. casei, L. fermentum, L. plantarum, L. rhamnosus,* and *L. paracasei. Weissella confusa* is included in Tables 17.3 and 17.4 because it is easily confused on culture media with the organisms included in this chapter, and in rare cases, it has been isolated associated with bacteremia and endocarditis.

Epidemiology

Erysipelothrix spp. are found worldwide in a variety of vertebrate and invertebrate animals, including mammals, birds, and fish. Other domestic animals that may be infected include sheep, rabbits, cattle, and turkeys. The organism may be transmitted through direct contact or ingestion of contaminated water or meat. *Arcanobacterium haemolyticum* is a normal inhabitant of the mucosal membranes of cattle, sheep, dogs, cats, and pigs. *Trueperella bernardiae* has been identified in skin abscesses, but it is unclear whether the organism is normal microbiota of the skin or gastrointestinal tract in cows. *T. pyogenes* is found on the mucous membranes of cattle, sheep, and pigs. The organisms listed in Table 17.1 include those that are closely associated with animals and are contracted by humans through animal exposure (e.g., *E. rhusiopathiae* and *T. pyogenes*) and those that are normal human microbiota (e.g., *Lactobacillus* spp. and *Gardnerella vaginalis*).

Pathogenesis and Spectrum of Disease

G. vaginalis and *Lactobacillus* spp. (Table 17.2) are natural inhabitants of the human vagina. Vaginal infections with *G. vaginalis* are often found in association with a variety of

TABLE 17.1   Epidemiology

Species	Habitat (Reservoir)	Mode of Transmission
Erysipelothrix rhusiopathiae	Normal microbiota; carried by and causes disease in animals	Zoonosis; abrasion or puncture wound of skin with animal exposure
Arcanobacterium haemolyticum	Normal microbiota of human skin and pharynx	Uncertain; infections probably caused by person's endogenous strains
Gardnerella vaginalis	Normal microbiota: Human vaginal tissue Colonizers: Distal urethra of males	Endogenous strain
Lactobacillus spp.	Environmental: Widely distributed in foods and nature Normal microbiota: Human mouth, gastrointestinal tract, and female genital tract	Endogenous strain Infections rare
Trueperella spp.	Normal microbiota; carried by and causes disease in animals	Uncertain: Respiratory, abrasion, or undetected wound during exposure to animals

TABLE 17.2   Pathogenesis and Spectrum of Disease

Organisms	Virulence Factors	Spectrum of Diseases and Infections
Erysipelothrix rhusiopathiae	Capsule Neuraminidase Hyaluronidase Surface proteins	Localized: Erysipeloid, a skin infection that is painful and may spread slowly Systemic: Erysipeloid may cause diffuse skin infection with systemic symptoms Bacteremia Endocarditis is rare
Arcanobacterium haemolyticum	Unknown	Systemic: Pharyngitis Cellulitis and other skin infections
Gardnerella vaginalis	Uncertain Produces cell adherence factors and cytotoxin	Bacterial vaginosis; less commonly associated with urinary tract infections; bacteremia is extremely rare
Lactobacillus spp.	Uncertain	Most frequently encountered as a contaminant Immunocompromised: Bacteremia
Trueperella spp.	Unknown	When infections occur, they generally are cutaneous; pharyngitis is common and may be complicated by or lead to bacteremia (*T. pyogenes*)

mixed anaerobic flora. Extravaginal infections are uncommon but have been associated with postpartum endometritis, septic abortion, and cesarean birth.

Lactobacillus spp. are important for maintaining the proper pH balance in vaginal secretions. The organisms metabolize glucose to lactic acid, producing an acidic vaginal pH and resulting in an environment that is not conducive to the growth of pathogenic bacteria. Lactobacilli are frequently associated with dental caries. The organism enters the bloodstream during chewing, brushing teeth, and dental procedures, resulting in bacteremia and endocarditis. *W. confusa* is a *Lactobacillus*-like organism recovered in blood cultures from patients with clinical symptoms of endocarditis and is of particular concern because the organism is vancomycin resistant.

Erysipelothrix infections are associated with individuals employed in occupations such as fish handlers, farmers, slaughterhouse workers, food preparation workers, and veterinarians. Infections are typically a result of a puncture wound or skin abrasion. Three categories of human disease have been characterized, including localized skin lesions or cellulitis (**erysipeloid**), diffuse cutaneous infection with systemic symptoms, and bacteremia. Bacteremia results in dissemination of the organism and can manifest as endocarditis.

Arcanobacterium sp. and *Trueperella* spp. are primarily animal pathogens, but they have been associated with pharyngitis, septicemia, tissue abscesses, and ulcers in immunocompromised patients. *Arcanobacterium haemolyticum* is primarily associated with mild to severe pharyngitis.

T. bernardiae, in particular, can be recovered from the blood, abscesses, the urinary tract, joints, the eyes, and wounds. The organism has also been implicated in necrotizing fasciitis. *T. pyogenes* are typically isolated from infections in patients from rural environments and has been identified in abscesses, wounds, and blood infections.

Often the primary challenge is to determine the clinical relevance of these organisms when they are isolated in specimens from normally sterile sites.

Laboratory Diagnosis

Specimen Collection and Transport

Generally, no special considerations are required for specimen collection and transport of the organisms discussed in this chapter. Of note, skin lesions for *Erysipelothrix* should be collected by biopsy of the full thickness of skin at the leading edge of the discolored area. Refer to Table 5.1 for other general information on specimen collection and transport.

Specimen Processing

No special considerations are required for processing of the organisms discussed in this chapter. Refer to Table 5.1 for general information on specimen processing.

Direct Detection Methods

Gram staining of *Arcanobacterium* sp. demonstrates delicate, curved, gram-positive rods with pointed ends and occasional rudimentary branching. This branching is more pronounced after these organisms have been cultured anaerobically. The organisms may stain unevenly after 48 hours of growth on solid media and may exhibit coccal forms.

Lactobacillus is highly pleomorphic, occurring in long chaining rods and in coccobacilli and spiral forms (Fig. 17.1). *T. bernardiae* typically appears as short, gram-positive rods without branching.

E. rhusiopathiae stains as both short rods and long filaments. These morphologies correspond to two colonial types: (1) rough colonies that contain slender, filamentous, gram-positive rods with a tendency to over-decolorize and appear gram negative; and (2) smooth colonies that contain small, slender rods. This variability in staining and colonial morphology may be mistaken for a polymicrobial infection on both direct examination and culture.

Gardnerella organisms are small, pleomorphic, gram-variable or gram-negative coccobacilli and short rods. Wet mount and Gram staining of vaginal secretions are key tests for diagnosing bacterial vaginosis caused by *G. vaginalis.* A wet mount prepared in saline reveals the characteristic **"clue cells,"** which are large, squamous epithelial cells with numerous attached small rods. A

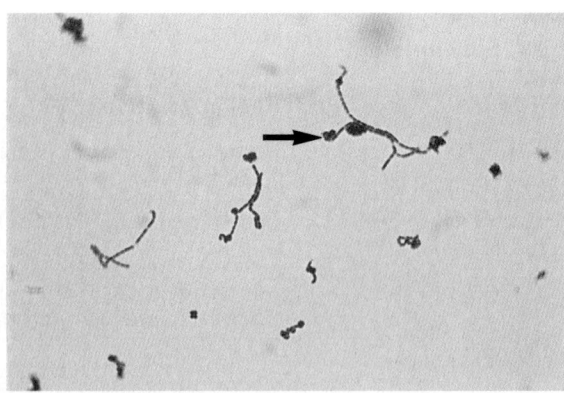

• **Fig. 17.1** Gram stain of *Lactobacillus* spp. Note spiral forms *(arrow).*

Gram-stained smear of the discharge shows the attached organisms to be gram-variable coccobacilli. In bacterial vaginosis, clue cells are typically present and large numbers of other gram-positive rods (i.e., lactobacilli), representing normal vaginal microbiota, are absent or few in number.

Nucleic Acid Detection

The direct detection of *Erysipelothrix* spp. by conventional and real-time PCR has been successful in animal tissue but has not been evaluated on human clinical samples. The BD Affirm vaginal deoxyribonucleic acid (DNA) probe (VDP) may be used for direct detection from genital specimens. Special vials containing transport reagent is used to stabilize the organism's nucleic acids before testing (Becton, Dickinson and Company, Franklin Lakes, NJ).

Large laboratories have also used 16S rRNA gene sequencing for the identification of organisms included in this chapter to the genus and species level.

Serodiagnosis

Serodiagnostic techniques are not generally used for the laboratory diagnosis of infections caused by the organisms discussed in this chapter.

Cultivation

Media of Choice

All the genera described in this chapter grow on 5% sheep blood and chocolate agars. They do not grow on MacConkey agar but do grow on Columbia colistin-nalidixic acid (CNA) agar. CNA agar is a nutritional base that may include 5% sheep blood to enhance the growth of fastidious organisms. The antibiotics colistin and nalidixic acid prevent the overgrowth of gram-negative organisms. All genera except *Gardnerella* spp. grow in commercially available blood culture broths. *Gardnerella* organisms are inhibited by sodium polyanethol sulfonate (SPS), which currently is used as an anticoagulant in most commercial blood culture media. An SPS-free medium or a medium with SPS that is

TABLE 17.3	Colonial Appearance on 5% Sheep Blood Agar and Other Characteristics
Organism	**Appearance**
Arcanobacterium haemolyticum	Small to large colonies with various appearances, including smooth, mucoid, white and dry, friable, and gray; may be surrounded by narrow zone of beta-hemolysis
Erysipelothrix rhusiopathiae	Two colony types: large and rough or small, smooth, and translucent; shows alpha-hemolysis after prolonged incubation
Gardnerella vaginalis	Pinpoint; nonhemolytic
Lactobacillus spp.	Multiple colonial morphologies, ranging from pinpoint, alpha-hemolytic colonies resembling streptococci to rough, gray colonies
Weissella confuse	Pinpoint; alpha-hemolytic and may be confused with organisms presented in this chapter

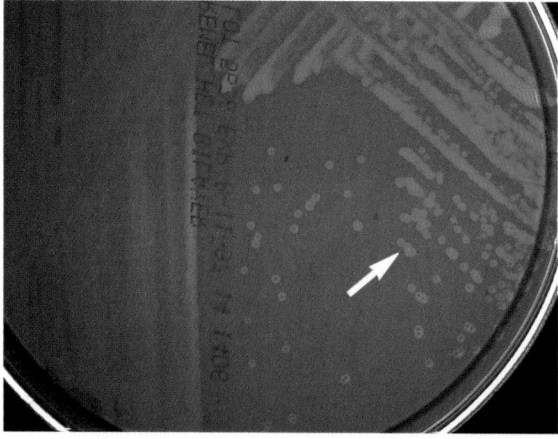

• **Fig. 17.2** *Gardnerella vaginalis* on human blood bilayer Tween (HBT) agar. Note small colonies with diffuse zone of beta-hemolysis *(arrow)*.

supplemented with gelatin should be used when *G. vaginalis* sepsis is suspected. A distinguishing biochemical characteristic of *E. rhusiopathiae* is the ability to produce H_2S.

Isolation of *G. vaginalis* from female genital tract specimens is best accomplished using the selective medium **human blood bilayer Tween (HBT) agar.** HBT is CNA agar with amphotericin B added to prevent the growth of yeasts and filamentous fungi. Human blood is layered over the top to enhance the beta-hemolytic pattern of *G. vaginalis*.

Incubation Conditions and Duration

Detectable growth of these organisms should occur on 5% sheep blood and chocolate agars, CNA, and HBT incubated at 35°C in 5% to 10% carbon dioxide (CO_2) within 48 hours of inoculation.

Colonial Appearance

Table 17.3 describes the colonial appearance and other distinguishing characteristics (e.g., hemolysis) of each genus on sheep blood agar. *G. vaginalis* produces small, gray, opaque colonies surrounded by a diffuse zone of beta-hemolysis on HBT agar (Fig. 17.2).

Approach to Identification

The identification of the four genera described in this chapter must be considered along with that of *Actinomyces, Bifidobacterium,* and *Cutibacterium* spp., which are discussed in Chapter 41. Although the latter genera are usually considered with the anaerobic bacteria, they grow on routine laboratory media in 5% to 10% CO_2. Some are catalase negative. Therefore as shown in Table 17.4, these

organisms must be considered together when a laboratory encounters catalase-negative, gram-positive, non–spore-forming rods.

Several commercial systems for fastidious gram-negative bacterial identifications will adequately identify *Gardnerella*. The HNID panel (*Haemophilus-Neisseria* identification panel, MicroScan, Beckman Coulter, Brea, California) works particularly well. However, rapid identification panels can be used for isolates from extragenital sources (e.g., blood).

Matrix-Assisted Laser Desorption Ionization Time-of-Flight Mass Spectrometry

Matrix-assisted laser desorption ionization time-of-flight mass spectroscopy (MALDI-TOF MS) has been effective in the identification of *E. rhusiopathiae* and *Lactobacillus* spp. Identification of *Weissella* using this technique is still in progress. MALDI-TOF MS represents a simple, reliable, and cost-saving tool with high discriminatory power and will undoubtedly provide an opportunity for improved identification of the species included in this chapter, with continued analysis of clinical isolates and incorporated into the database.

Comments Regarding Specific Organisms

A presumptive identification of *G. vaginalis* is sufficient for genital isolates, based on typical appearance on Gram stain, beta-hemolysis on HBT agar, and negative tests for oxidase and catalase. *Corynebacterium lipophiloflavum,* a bacterium isolated from females with bacterial vaginosis, is catalase positive and resembles *C. urealyticum*. Differentiation relies on *C. lipophiloflavum* producing a yellow pigment, weak urease activity, and slow acid production from glucose.

The beta-hemolytic *Arcanobacterium* sp. resembles the beta-hemolytic streptococci and can be differentiated by Gram stain morphology. *A. haemolyticum* and *Trueperella pyogenes* can be differentiated using liquefaction of gelatin;

TABLE 17.4 Biochemical and Physiologic Characteristics of Catalase-Negative, Gram-Positive, Aerotolerant, Non–Spore-Forming Rods

Organism	Urease	Nitrate Reduction	Beta-Hemolysis[b]	Fermentation[a] of:					CAMP[c]	GLC[d]	Other Comments
				Glucose	Maltose	Mannitol	Sucrose	Xylose			
Actinomyces israelii	−	v	−	+	+	vz	+	+	−	A, L, S	
Actinomyces odontolyticus	−	+	−[e]	+	v	−	+	v	−	A, S	Red pigment produced after 1 week on SBA
Actinomyces naeslundii	+	+	−	+	+	v	+	v	−	A, L, S	
Actinomyces radingae	−	−	−w	+	+	−	+	+	−	S?	Pyrazinamidase, beta-galactosidase–positive and esculin-positive
Actinomyces turicensis	−	−	−w	+	v	−	+	+	−	NT	Pyrazinamidase, beta-galactosidase–negative and esculin-negative
Actinomyces graevenitzii	−	−	−	+	+	−	+	−	ND	L > S	
Actinobaculum schaalii	−	−	−	+	+	−	v	+	+w	A, s	Beta-galactosidase–negative
Arcanobacterium haemolyticum	−	−	+	+	+	−	v	−	Reverse +[f]	A, L, S	Gelatin-negative at 48 h; beta-hemolysis is stronger on agar containing human or rabbit blood
Trueperella pyogenes	−	−	+[g]	+	v	v	v	+	−	A, L, S	Gelatin-positive at 48 h; casein-positive
Trueperella bernardiae	−	−	−	+	+	−	−	−	−	A, L, S	
Bifidobacterium adolescentis	−	−	−	+	+	−	+	+	ND	A > L (s)	
Erysipelothrix sp.	−	−	−	+[h]	−	−	−	−	−	A, L, S	H2S-positive in TSI butt; vancomycin-resistant; alpha-hemolytic
Lactobacillus spp.	−	−	−	+	+	v	+	ND	ND	L (a s)	Some strains vancomycin-resistant; alpha-hemolytic

TABLE 17.4   Biochemical and Physiologic Characteristics of Catalase-Negative, Gram-Positive, Aerotolerant, Non–Spore-Forming Rods—Cont'd

Organism	Urease	Nitrate Reduction	Beta-Hemolysis[b]	Fermentation[a] of: Glucose	Maltose	Mannitol	Sucrose	Xylose	CAMP[c]	GLC[d]	Other Comments
Cutibacterium acnes	–	+	–	+	–	–	–	–	+	A, P (iv L s)	Indole-positive; may show beta-hemolysis on rabbit blood agar
Gardnerella vaginalis	–	–	–	+	+	–	v	–[i]	ND	A (l s)	Beta-hemolysis on HBT; usually hydrolyzes hippurate
Weissella spp.	NT	–	–	+	+	–	+	v	NT	L (as)	Vancomycin-resistant, small, short rods; produces gas from MRS (Man, Rogosa and Sharpe) broth; alpha-hemolytic; esculin-positive; arginine-positive

HBT, Human blood bilayer Tween agar; *iv,* isovaleric acid; *ND,* not done; *NT,* not tested; *SBA,* 5% sheep blood agar; *TSI,* triple sugar iron agar; *v,* variable; *w,* weak; +, ≥90% of strains positive; –, ≥90% of strains negative.

[a]Fermentation is detected in peptone base with Andrade's indicator.

[b]On sheep blood agar.

[c]CAMP test using a beta-lysin–producing strain of *Staphylococcus aureus.*

[d]End products of glucose metabolism: *A,* Acetic acid; *L,* lactic acid; *P,* propionic acid; *S,* succinic acid; may or may not produce acid end product.

[e]May show hemolysis on brain-heart infusion agar with sheep or human blood.

[f]Reverse CAMP test; *Staphylococcus aureus* beta-lysins are inhibited by a diffusible substance produced by *A. haemolyticum* (Fig. 17.3).

[g]May also show beta-hemolysis on brain-heart infusion agar with human blood.

[h]Reaction may be weak or delayed.

[i]*Gardnerella vaginalis*–like organisms ferment xylose.

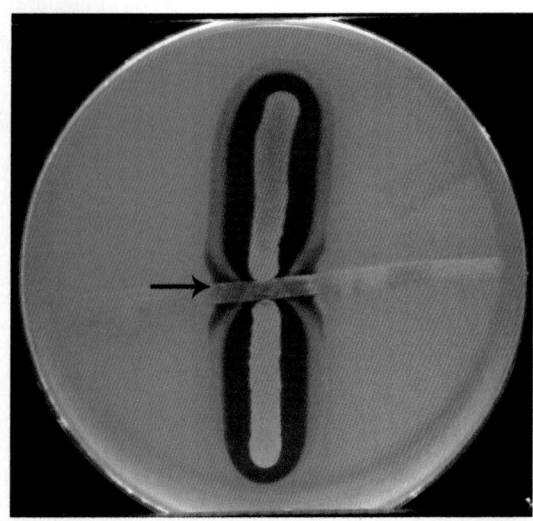

• **Fig. 17.3** Reverse Christie, Atkins, Munch-Petersen (CAMP) test. *Arcanobacterium haemolyticum* is streaked on a blood agar plate. *Staphylococcus aureus* is then streaked perpendicular to the *Arcanobacterium* path. A positive reverse CAMP test result is indicated (arrow).

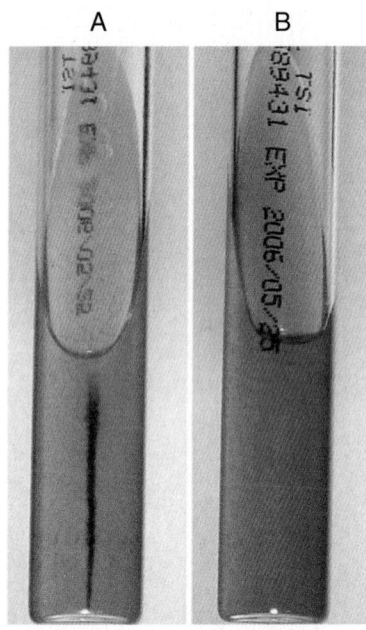

• **Fig. 17.4** H₂S production by *Erysipelothrix rhusiopathiae* in TSI (A). A negative TSI (B) is included for comparison. *TSI,* Triple Sugar Iron agar.

T. pyogenes is positive, and *A. haemolyticum* is negative. *Trueperella bernardiae* is nonhemolytic. *Arcanobacterium haemolyticum* is typically beta-hemolytic on human blood agar, although expression of hemolysis may vary by culture media and incubation conditions.

Erysipelothrix spp. is the only catalase-negative, gram-positive, non–spore-forming rod that produces hydrogen sulfide (H_2S) when inoculated into triple sugar iron (TSI) agar (Fig. 17.4). Some *Bacillus* spp. also blacken the butt of TSI, but they are catalase positive and produce spores. It is important to identify and report isolation of this organism in clinical samples, because intrinsic resistance to vancomycin has been identified.

Lactobacillus spp. are usually identified based on colony and Gram stain morphologies and catalase reaction (negative). Differentiation from viridans streptococci may be difficult, but the formation of rods in chains rather than cocci in thioglycollate broth is helpful. Alternatively, a Gram stain of growth just outside the zone of inhibition surrounding the 10-U penicillin disk placed on a blood agar plate and inoculated with a lawn of the organism should show long bacilli rather than coccoid forms if the organism is *Lactobacillus* spp.

Antimicrobial Susceptibility Testing and Therapy

The rarity with which most of these organisms are encountered as the cause of infection has made the development of validated *in vitro* susceptibility testing methods difficult (Table 17.5). However, most of the organisms are susceptible to the agents used to eradicate them; *in vitro* testing is not usually necessary to guide therapy. *Lactobacillus* spp. can be resistant to various antimicrobial agents. Fortunately, these organisms are rarely implicated in infections. When they are encountered in specimens from sterile sites, careful evaluation of their clinical significance is warranted before any attempt is made at performing a nonstandardized susceptibility test.

Susceptibility testing for *G. vaginalis* is not recommended. The organism is typically treated with metronidazole. Systemic infections have also been successfully treated with ampicillin or amoxicillin.

Although some of these organisms may grow on the media and under the conditions recommended for testing other bacteria (see Chapter 11 for more information regarding validated testing methods), this does not necessarily mean that interpretable and reliable results will be produced. Chapter 11 should be reviewed for preferable strategies that can be used to provide susceptibility information when validated testing methods do not exist for a clinically important bacterial isolate.

Prevention

Many of these organisms are ubiquitous in nature, and many are part of the normal human microbiome commonly encountered without deleterious effects on healthy human hosts. Currently there are no recommended vaccination or prophylaxis protocols for prevention and treatment of diseases caused by these organisms.

ⓔ Visit the Evolve site for a complete list of procedures, review questions, and case studies.

TABLE 17.5   Antimicrobial Therapy and Susceptibility Testing

Organism	Therapeutic Options	Resistance to Therapeutic Options	Validated Testing Methods[a]	Comments
Erysipelothrix rhusiopathiae	Susceptible to penicillins, cephalosporins, erythromycin, clindamycin, tetracycline, and ciprofloxacin	Not common; vancomycin resistance has been noted	See CLSI document M45 (Methods for Antimicrobial Dilution and Disk Susceptibility Testing of Infrequently Isolated or Fastidious Bacteria)	Susceptibility testing not needed to guide therapy
Arcanobacterium haemolyticum	No definitive guidelines; usually susceptible to penicillin, erythromycin, and clindamycin	Tetracycline and vancomycin resistance has been identified	Not available	Susceptibility testing not needed to guide therapy
Trueperella spp.	No definitive guidelines; usually susceptible to cephalosporins, penicillins, macrolides, tetracyclines, and aminoglycosides	Not known	Not available	Susceptibility testing not needed to guide therapy
Gardnerella vaginalis	Metronidazole is the drug of choice; also susceptible to ampicillin and amoxicillin	Not known	Not available	Susceptibility testing not needed to guide therapy
Lactobacillus spp.	No definitive guidelines; systemic infections may require the use of a penicillin with an aminoglycoside	Frequently resistant to cephalosporins; not killed by penicillin alone; frequently highly resistant to vancomycin	See CLSI document M45 (Methods for Antimicrobial Dilution and Disk Susceptibility Testing of Infrequently Isolated or Fastidious Bacteria)	Confirm that the isolate is clinically relevant and not a contaminant

[a]Validated testing methods include standard methods recommended by the Clinical and Laboratory Standards Institute (CLSI) and commercial methods approved by the US Food and Drug Administration (FDA).

Bibliography

Bennett J, Dolin R, Blaser M: *Principles and practice of infectious diseases,* ed 9, Philadelphia, 2020, Elsevier-Saunders.

Carlson P, Kontiainen S, Renkonen O: Antimicrobial susceptibility of *Arcanobacterium haemolyticum, Antimicrob Agents Chemother* 38:142–143, 1994.

Carroll KC, Pfaller MA, Landry ML, et al.: *Manual of clinical microbiology,* ed 12, Washington, DC, 2019, ASM.

Drancourt M, Oulès O, Bouche V, Peloux Y: Two cases of *Actinomyces pyogenes* infections in humans, *Eur J Clin Microbiol Infect Dis* 12:55–57, 1993.

Flaherty JD, Levett PN, Dewhirst FE, Troe TE, Warren JR, Johnson S: Fatal case of endocarditis due to *Weissella confusa, J Clin Microbiol* 41:2237–2239, 2003.

Foschi C, Laghi L, Parolin C, et al.: Novel approaches for the taxonomic and metabolic characterization of lactobacilli: integration of 16S rRNA gene sequencing with MALDI-TOF MS and1H-NMR, *PLoS One* 12(2):e0172483, 2017.

Funke G, Lucchini GM, Pfyffer GE, Marchiani M, von Graevenitz A: Characteristics of CDC group 1 and group 1-like coryneform bacteria isolated from clinical specimens, *J Clin Microbiol* 31:2907–2912, 1993.

Funke G, von Graevenitz A, Clarridge III JE, Bernard KA: Clinical microbiology of coryneform bacteria, *Clin Microbiol Rev* 10:125–159, 1997.

Lidbeck A, Nord CE: Lactobacilli and the normal human anaerobic microflora, *Clin Infect Dis* 16(Suppl 4):S181–S187, 1993.

Mackenzie A, Fuite LA, Chan TH, et al.: Incidence and pathogenicity of *Arcanobacterium haemolyticum* during a 2-year study in Ottawa, *Clin Infect Dis* 21:177–181, 1995.

Patel R, Cockerill FR, Porayko MK, Osmon DR, Ilstrup DM, Keating MR: Lactobacillemia in liver transplant patients, *Clin Infect Dis* 18:207–212, 1994.

Schuster MG, Brennan PJ, Edelstein P: Persistent bacteremia with *Erysipelothrix rhusiopathiae* in a hospitalized patient, *Clin Infect Dis* 17:783–784, 1993.

Spiegel CA: Bacterial vaginosis, *Clin Microbiol Rev* 4:485–502, 1991.

Vandamme P, Falsen E, Vancanneyt M, et al.: Characterization of *Actinomyces turicensis* and *Actinomyces radingae* strains from human clinical samples, *Int J Syst Bacteriol* 48:503–510, 1998.

18

Nocardia, Streptomyces, Rhodococcus, and Similar Organisms

OBJECTIVES

1. Describe the general characteristics of the aerobic actinomycetes, including their Gram stain morphology, microscopic morphology, colonial morphology, and biochemical reactions.
2. Describe the habitats of actinomycetes and the routes of transmission.
3. Describe the three types of skin infections caused by *Nocardia* spp. in immunocompromised individuals.
4. List the laboratory tests used to differentiate the clinically relevant aerobic actinomycetes.
5. List the laboratory tests used to differentiate the pathogenic *Nocardia* spp.
6. Describe the chemical structures required to classify an organism as acid-fast.
7. List the virulence factors associated with *Nocardia asteroides*.
8. Define the terms *mycetoma* and *actinomycetoma*.
9. List the various selective media used to isolate aerobic actinomycetes and describe their usefulness in achieving optimal recovery.

GENERA AND SPECIES TO BE CONSIDERED

Actinomadura spp.
Amycolatopsis congolensis
Dietzia spp.
Dermatophilus congolensis
Desmospora activa
Gordonia spp.
Kroppenstedtia spp.
Lawsonella spp.
Nocardia spp.
Nocardiopsis spp.
Pseudonocardia spp.
Rhodococcus spp.
Saccharomonospora spp.
Saccharopolyspora spp.
Segniliparus spp.
Streptomyces spp.
Thermoactinomyces spp.
Tsukamurella spp.
Williamsia spp.

The implementation of nucleic acid detection and sequencing technology has improved the identification and characterization of the organisms in the actinomycetes; as a result, there has been a significant increase in the number of species. It is important to emphasize that due to the change in the classification and identification of these organisms, the older literature containing clinical descriptions of organisms may not be reliable, making the assessment of the clinical significance of these isolates very difficult.

The actinomycetes are a large and diverse group of organisms that appear as gram-positive coccoid or rod-shaped cells. Many of the cells of all actinomycetes elongate to form branching, filamentous forms. Others will appear as beaded chains, may be coryneform, or fragment into various sized spores. The rate and extent of filament elongation with lateral branching and the formation of hyphae depend on the genus of actinomycetes, the growth medium, and the temperature of incubation. Some organisms form filaments, or hyphae, on the agar surface or into the agar, whereas others produce hyphae that extend into the air.

These organisms are aerobic, facultatively anaerobic, or obligately anaerobic. The actinomycetes belong to the order Actinomycetales. The medically relevant genus *Mycobacterium* (Chapter 42) and *Corynebacterium* spp. (Chapter 16) are also included in the order Actinomycetales, suborder Corynebacterium. Only the clinically relevant actinomycetes genera are considered in this chapter (Table 18.1). Another clinically significant aerobic actinomycete is *Tropheryma whipplei;* because this organism is extremely difficult to culture on artificial media, it is reviewed in Chapter 43. For purposes of discussion, the remaining genera of actinomycetes are divided into groups: those with cell walls that contain mycolic acid and are strongly acid fast, those that are partially or weakly acid fast, and those with cell walls that do not contain mycolic acid and therefore are not acid fast.

In general, the aerobic actinomycetes are not frequently isolated in the clinical laboratory; nevertheless, these organisms can cause serious human disease. Infections with these organisms

TABLE 18.1	Clinically Relevant Aerobic Actinomycetes[a]
Cell Wall Containing Mycolic Acid	**Genus**
Present	*Nocardia*
	Rhodococcus
	Gordonia
	Lawsonella
	Tsukamurella
	Corynebacterium
	Segniliparus
Absent	*Actinomadura*
	Amycolatopsis
	Desmospora
	Dermatophilus
	Dietzia
	Kroppenstedtia
	Nocardiopsis
	Pseudonocardia
	Saccharomonospora
	Saccharopolyspora
	Streptomyces
	Thermoactinomyces
	Williamsia

[a]Multiple genera classified as aerobic actinomycetes are associated with rare or occasional opportunistic infections. Clinical significance should be carefully evaluated.

are not only difficult to recognize in the clinical laboratory but the organisms are also difficult to isolate. Further complications include difficulty in classifying and identifying them as well as performing antibiotic susceptibilities on aerobic actinomycetes isolated from clinical specimens. The taxonomy of the aerobic actinomycetes is complex and continues to evolve. Only genomic sequencing is adequate to delineate species within this diverse phylogenetic group of organisms.

General Characteristics

The genera *Lawsonella* and *Segniliparus* are strongly acid-fast aerobic actinomyces and belong to the suborder *Corynebacterineae*, which includes the *Mycobacterium* and *Corynebacterium* spp. On the other hand, *Nocardia, Rhodococcus, Gordonia,* and *Tsukamurella* are partially acid-fast aerobic actinomycetes. *Nocardia, Gordonia,* and *Rhodococcus* belong to the family *Nocardiaceae,* and *Tsukamurella* is in the closely related *Tsukamurellaceae* family. However, the variability associated with the classification of an organism as partially acid fast depends on the particular strain and culture conditions. This characteristic should be interpreted with caution. The non–acid-fast genera include the *Actinomadura, Amycolatopsis, Dermatophilus congolensis, Dietzia, Nocardiopsis, Pseudonocardia, Saccharomonospora, Saccharopolyspora, Streptomyces,* and *Williamsia.* Finally, three genera—*Desmospora, Kroppenstedtia,* and *Thermoactinomyces*—are included in this section based on their chemotaxonomic and molecular features, which are related and typical of this group.

Acid-Fast Aerobic Actinomycetes

The newly identified genus *Lawsonella* contains a single species, *L. clevelandensis.* The organism is a significant inhabitant of the human microbiome residing in the nasal cavity. It has been isolated from only approximately seven clinical cases worldwide and is associated with abscesses and a respiratory illness that mimics *Nocardia* spp. infections. Microscopically the cells are filamentous pleomorphic gram-positive cocci to rods with prominent dark-staining round cells. Although the organism is aerobic, it is a fastidious, slow growing (5 to 10 days) bacterium. Growth can be enhanced in atmospheric conditions that contain greater than 1% O_2 tension. Macroscopically the organism appears as white, waxy, pinpoint nonhemolytic colonies on blood agar.

The second acid-fast genus, *Segniliparus,* includes two species, *S. rotundus* and *S. rugosus.* The bacterium, in particular *S. rugosus,* has been identified in respiratory illness and may be confused with fast-growing nonmycobacterium tuberculosis. The organisms are gram-positive nonbranching rods and may be isolated from respiratory infections in patients with cystic fibrosis as well as in cases of bronchiolitis and pneumonia in immunocompetent individuals. The organism grows well on media such as Löwenstein-Jensen (LJ) agar, used for the isolation of mycobacterium species, and appears as smooth, domed, wrinkled or rough colonies; it may produce soluble pigments. Although biochemical identification is possible using similar phenotypic diagnostic tests as those used for mycobacteria, identification is time consuming and expensive. Nucleic acid detection including 16S rRNA, polymerase chain reaction (PCR)-restriction fragment length polymorphism, and DNA-DNA hybridization; additional methods have been successfully used for identification at the species level. Identification and treatment of *Segniliparus* spp. is recommended. Successful antibiotic treatments include combinations of clarithromycin with amikacin, cefoxitin, or imipenem for 2 to 4 months.

Partially Acid-Fast Aerobic Actinomycetes
Nocardia spp.

The genus *Nocardia* consists of approximately 100 species. The organisms are gram positive (often with a beaded appearance), variably acid fast, catalase positive, and strictly aerobic. As they grow, *Nocardia* spp. form branched filaments that extend along the agar surface (**substrate hyphae**) and into the air (**aerial hyphae**). As the organisms age, Nocardiae fragment into pleomorphic rods or coccoid elements. Nocardiae are characterized by the presence of meso-diaminopimelic acid (DAP) and the sugars arabinose and galactose in the peptidoglycan of the cell wall.

Currently the taxonomy in the genus *Nocardia* is changing rapidly. Recognition and description of new species continue and remain controversial regarding the number of validly described species. *N. abscessus, N. cyriacigeorgica, N. nova complex, N. farcinica, N. asteroides, N. brasiliensis, N. otitidiscaviarum, N.*

pseudobrasiliensis, and *N. transvalensis* complex account for most of the disease in humans caused by *Nocardia* spp. The medically relevant species are summarized in Table 18.2.

Rhodococcus, Gordonia, and *Tsukamurella* spp.

Organisms belonging to the *Rhodococcus, Gordonia,* and *Tsukamurella* genera are similar to those of the *Nocardia* spp. in that they are gram-positive, aerobic, catalase-positive, partially acid-fast, branching, filamentous bacteria that can fragment into rods and cocci. The extent

of acid fastness depends on the amount and complexity of mycolic acids in the organism's cell wall and on culture conditions. The differentiation of these genera, as well as species identification, is difficult. In particular, the genus *Rhodococcus* consists of a very diverse group of organisms in terms of morphology, biochemical characteristics, and ability to cause disease. They may appear as coccoid to bacillary rods with some branching filaments that may appear beaded. All three genera are often dismissed as diphtheroids because of the Gram stain morphology. As

TABLE 18.2 Medically Relevant Species of *Nocardia*

Species	Skin and Soft Tissue		Ocular Infections	Respiratory	Disseminated
N. abscessus[a]	X		X	X	X
N. africana				X	
N. amikacin itolerans	X		X	X	
N. asiatica				X	
N. beijingensis	X		X	X	X
N. boionii	X				
N. brasiliensis[a]	X	X			
N. concava				X	X
N. cyriacigeorgica				X	X
N. elegans				X	X
N. farcinica[a]	X		X	X	X
N. kruczakiae	X		X	X	
N. mexicana	X			X	X
N. mikamii				X	X
N. niigatensis	X				
N. niwae	X				
N. nova[a]	X		X		
N. otitidiscaviarum	X			X	X
N. paucivorans					X
N. pseudobrasiliensis[a]				X	X
N. takedensis	X			X	
N. transvalensis				X	X
N. veteran[a]				X	
N. vinacea	X				
N. vulneris	X				
N. wallacei[a]					X

[a]Species most frequently isolated from human disease.

previously, mentioned, the taxonomy of these organisms continues to evolve; species included in these three genera are summarized in Table 18.3.

Non–Acid-Fast Aerobic Actinomycetes: *Streptomyces, Actinomadura, Amycolatopsis, Dermatophilus, Dietza, Nocardiopsis, Pseudonocarida, Saccharomonospora, Saccharopolyspora,* and *Williamsia* spp.

This is an extremely large and diverse group that as of this writing includes *Actinomadura, Amycolatopsis, D. congolensis, Dietzia, Nocardiopsis, Pseudonocardia* (54 species), *Saccharomonospora* (12 species), *Saccharopolyspora* (29 species and subspecies), *Streptomyces* (800 species and subspecies), and *Williamsia.* The non–acid-fast aerobic actinomycetes are gram-positive, rarely branching or branching filaments that do not contain mycolic acids in their cell walls; they are therefore non–acid fast. This group of actinomycetes

is heterogeneous and rarely encountered in the clinical laboratory. Only the non–acid-fast actinomycetes associated with human disease are addressed in this chapter (Table 18.4).

Thermophilic Actinomycetes

Another group of non–acid-fast actinomycetes, the thermophilic actinomycetes, is associated with infections in humans and includes the medically relevant genera *Desmospora* and *Kroppenstedtia.* These organisms are gram-positive filamentous bacteria that have been primarily associated with environmental sources. Although other non–acid-fast genera in the actinomyces are considered thermophilic—such as *Saccharomonospora* and *Saccharopolyspora*—at

TABLE 18.3 Species Included in the Genera *Rhodococcus, Gordonia,* and *Tsukamurella*

Genus	Species
Gordonia	G. amicalis
	G. araii
	G. bronchialis[a]
	G. efusa
	G. honkongensis
	G. otitidis
	G. polyisoprenivorans
	G. rubripertincta
	G. sputi
	G. terrae
	There are approximately 38 validly named species in this genus.
Rhodococcus	R. corybacteroides
	R. equi[a] (this has been proposed to be reclassified as R. hoagie.)
	R. fascians
	There are approximately 49 validly named species in this genus.
Tsukamurella	T. hongkongensis
	T. inchonensis
	T. paurometabola[a]
	T. pulmonis
	T. sinensis
	T. spunae
	T. strandjordii (previously Rhodococcus)
	T. tyrosinosolvens[a]
	There are approximately 14 validly named species in this genus.

[a]Species most frequently isolated from human disease.

TABLE 18.4 Non–Acid-Fast Aerobic Actinomycetes Associated With Human Disease

Genus	Number of Species	Species Associated With Human Disease
Actinomadura	60	A. chibensis, A. cremea, A. latina, A. madurae[a], A. nitrigenes, A. pelletieri[a], A. sputi
Amycolatopsis	70	A. benzoatilytica, A. orientalis, A. palatopharyngis
Dietzia	13	D. aurantiaca, D. cinnamea, D. maris, D. papillomatosis
Dermatophilus	1	D. congolensis[a]
Desmospora	2	D activa
Kroppenstedtia	4	K. eburnae, K. pulmonis, K. sanguinis
Nocardiopsis	46	N. dassonvillei[a]
Streptomyces	800	S. albus, S. bikiniensis, S. cacaoi subsp. cacaoi, S. somaliensis[a], S. thermocarboxyoydus, S. viridis. Note: Because of the large number of species, identification to the genus level is recommended.
Williamsia	10	W. deligens, W. muralis, W. serinedens

[a]Species most frequently isolated from human disease.

this time there is insufficient data to classify the two genera within the other groupings of clinically relevant actinomycetes.

Epidemiology and Pathogenesis

Acid-Fast Aerobic Actinomycetes

As previously described, *L. clevelandensis* has been identified as a constituent of the human microbiome, residing primarily in the nostrils. Infections most likely arise from opportunistic infections due to endogenous strains. *Segniliparus* spp. are considered emerging pathogens and generally associated with nonsterile human sources, including respiratory tract specimens. Studies to evaluate the pathogenicity of *Segniliparus* spp. have indicated that both species are capable of initiating multifocal granulomatous inflammatory conditions associated with cytokine activation and macrophage-induced tissue necrosis. Person-to-person transmission has not been identified with either genus.

Partially Acid-Fast Aerobic Actinomycetes
Nocardia spp.

Nocardia organisms are normal inhabitants of soil and water and are primarily responsible for the decomposition of plant material. Infections caused by *Nocardia* spp. are found worldwide. Because these organisms are ubiquitous, their isolation from clinical specimens does not always indicate infection. Rather, isolation may indicate colonization of the skin and upper respiratory tract or laboratory contamination, although the latter is rare. *Nocardia* infections can be acquired either by traumatic inoculation or by inhalation, particularly in immunocompromised patients. Hematogenous spread following a pulmonary infection may result in disease in a variety of body sites, with the brain being the most prominent secondary site of infection.

Nocardia spp., in particular *N. asteroides,* is the most commonly isolated human pathogen. It was previously designated *N. asteroides* complex. Molecular methods have been used to accurately differentiate the members of the complex. *N. asteroides* has been divided into six groupings, each with a different susceptibility pattern: *N. abscessus* (drug pattern I), *N. brevicatena/N. paucivorans* (drug pattern II), *N. nova* complex (drug pattern III), *N. transvalensis* complex (drug pattern IV), *N. farcinica* (drug pattern V), and *N. cyriacigeorgica* (drug pattern VI). It is currently believed that *N. asteroides sensu stricto* (type species) is rarely pathogenic. The mechanisms of pathogenesis are complex and not completely understood. However, the virulence of *Nocardia* spp. appears to be associated with several factors, such as stage of growth at the time of infection, resistance to intracellular killing, tropism for neuronal tissue, and ability to inhibit phagosome-lysosome fusion; other characteristics, such as production of large amounts of catalase and hemolysins, may also be associated with virulence.

Rhodococcus, Gordonia, and *Tsukamurella* spp.

Rhodococcus, Gordonia, and *Tsukamurella* spp. can be isolated from several environmental sources, especially soil and farm animals, as well as from fresh water and saltwater. Infection is primarily through the respiratory inhalation of the organisms. *Gordonia* spp. have been isolated from catheter-related or other medical device–associated infection.

Rhodococcus equi has been the organism most commonly associated with human disease, particularly in immunocompromised patients, such as those infected with the human immunodeficiency virus (HIV). Other species have also been implicated in human infections. *R. equi* is a facultative intracellular organism that can persist and replicate within macrophages. Virulence antigens A and B (VapA and VapB) have been associated with infection in animals. However, human isolates capable of causing infection may express one or none of the antigens, indicating that they are not directly involved in the pathogenesis of human infection. Transmission is likely through direct traumatic inoculation, inhalation, or ingestion of the organism from exposure to infected animal feces. Although *Gordonia* spp. and *Tsukamurella* are able to cause opportunistic infections in humans, little is known about their pathogenic mechanisms.

Non–Acid-Fast Aerobic Actinomycetes: *Streptomyces, Actinomadura, Amycolatopsis, Dermatophilus, Dietzia, Nocardiopsis, Pseudonocardia, Saccharomonospora, Saccharopolyspora, Williamsia* spp., and Thermophilic Actinomycetes

Aspects of the epidemiology of the non–acid-fast aerobic and thermophilic actinomycetes are not well understood. The organisms are generally associated with wounds and abrasions associated with contamination by environmental sources such as soil and water.

Acid-Fast Aerobic Actinomycetes

Abscesses and respiratory infections associated with *L. clevelandensis* are generally identified in immunocompromised individuals and likely associated with an endogenous strain of the organism. *Segniliparus* spp. have been predominantly isolated from respiratory illnesses including bronchiolitis and pneumonia; they have also been isolated from patients with cystic fibrosis.

Partially Acid-Fast Aerobic Actinomycetes

The partially acid-fast actinomycetes cause various infections in humans.

Nocardia spp.

Infections caused by *Nocardia* spp. can occur in immunocompetent and immunocompromised individuals.

Nocardia spp. cause a variety of skin infections in immunocompetent individuals; such infections are associated with contamination of existing wounds or traumatic inoculation.

- **Mycetoma,** a chronic, localized, painless, subcutaneous infection
- Lymphocutaneous infections
- Skin abscesses or cellulitis

In immunocompromised individuals, infection with *Nocardia* organisms can be contracted by inhalation and causes invasive pulmonary infections as well as disseminated infections. Patients receiving systemic immunosuppression—such as transplant recipients, individuals with impaired pulmonary immune defenses, and intravenous drug abusers—exemplify immunosuppressed patients at risk for these infections. Patients with pulmonary infections caused by *Nocardia* spp. can exhibit a wide range of symptoms, from an acute to a more chronic presentation. Unfortunately, no specific signs indicate pulmonary nocardiosis. Patients usually appear systemically ill, with fever, night sweats, weight loss, and a productive cough that may be bloody. Pulmonary infection can lead to complications such as pleural effusions, empyema, mediastinitis, and soft tissue infection. An acute inflammatory response follows infection, resulting in necrosis and abscess formation; granulomas are not usually formed.

Nocardia spp. can often spread hematogenously throughout the body from a primary pulmonary infection. Disseminated infection can result in lesions in the brain and skin; hematogenous dissemination involving the central nervous system is particularly common. Disseminated nocardiosis has a very poor prognosis.

Rhodococcus, Gordonia, and *Tsukamurella* spp.

The types of infections caused by *Rhodococcus, Gordonia,* and *Tsukamurella* spp. are listed in Table 18.5. For the most part, these organisms are considered opportunistic pathogens because most infections occur in immunocompromised individuals.

Non–Acid-Fast Aerobic Actinomycetes: *Streptomyces, Actinomadura, Amycolatopsis, Dermatophilus, Dietzia, Nocardiopsis, Pseudonocardia, Saccharomonospora, Saccharopolyspora, Williamsia* spp., and Thermophilic Actinomycetes

Infection caused by the non–acid-fast aerobic actinomycetes is usually associated with chronic, granulomatous lesions of the skin (mycetomas). Mycetoma is an infection of subcutaneous tissues that results in tissue swelling and drainage of the sinus tracts. Infections are acquired by traumatic inoculation of organisms (usually in the lower limbs) and are usually caused by fungi. A mycetoma caused by an actinomycete is an **actinomycetoma.**

Exudative lesions, cutaneous infections, pruritic skin rashes, and hairy leukoplakia of the tongue have been associated with *D. congolensis* infection. Wide varieties of infections have been identified in association with the non–acid-fast aerobic actinomycetes (Table 18.6).

The thermophilic actinomycetes—*Saccharopolyspora, Saccharomonospora,* and *Thermoactinomyces* spp.—are responsible for **hypersensitivity pneumonitis,** an allergic reaction to these agents. This occupational disease occurs in farmers, factory workers, and others who are repeatedly exposed to these agents. The disease has acute and chronic forms. Patients with acute hypersensitivity pneumonitis experience malaise, sweats, chills, loss of appetite, chest tightness, cough, and fever within 4 to 6 hours after exposure. Symptoms generally resolve within a day. Under some circumstances involving continued exposure to the organisms, patients suffer from a chronic form of disease, in which symptoms progressively worsen with subsequent development of irreversible lung fibrosis.

Laboratory Diagnosis

Specimen Collection, Transport, and Processing

Appropriate specimens should be collected aseptically from affected areas. For the most part, no special requirements are needed for specimen collection, transport, or processing of the organisms discussed in this chapter (refer to Table 5.1 for general information). When nocardiosis is clinically suspected, multiple early-morning pulmonary

TABLE 18.5	Infections Caused by *Rhodococcus, Gordonia,* and *Tsukamurella* spp.
Organism	**Clinical Manifestations**
Rhodococcus spp.	Pulmonary infections (pneumonia, lung abscess, pulmonary nodules) Bacteremia Skin, urinary tract, and wound infections Endophthalmitis Peritonitis Catheter-associated sepsis Abscesses: prostatic/splenic, thyroid, renal, brain, subcutaneous Osteomyelitis
Gordonia spp.	Skin infections Chronic pulmonary disease Catheter-associated sepsis Wound infection: sterna Bacteremia Central nervous system Associated with the use of medical devices
Tsukamurella spp.	Peritonitis Catheter-associated sepsis Skin infection Meningitis Bacteremia Pulmonary

specimens should be submitted for culture. Smears and cultures are simultaneously positive in only one-third of the cases. These organisms remain difficult to isolate because of low numbers of organisms present in the specimens and overgrowth by rapidly growing contaminating bacteria. The significance of random isolation of *Nocardia* spp. from the respiratory tract is questionable because these organisms are so widely distributed in nature. Some of the actinomycetes tend to grow as a microcolony in tissues, leading to the formation of granules. Most commonly,

these granules are formed in actinomycetomas, such as those caused by *Nocardia, Streptomyces, Nocardiopsis,* and *Actinomadura* spp. Therefore material from draining sinus tracts or a skin biopsy are excellent specimens for direct examination and culture. Aspirates of normally sterile fluids or biopsies may be necessary for diagnosis in immunocompromised patients. Commercial automated blood culture systems effectively support the growth of *Nocardia, Gordonia,* and *Tsukamurella* spp.

Direct Detection Methods

Direct microscopic examination of Gram-stained preparations of clinical specimens is of utmost importance in the diagnosis of infections caused by the aerobic actinomycetes. Often, the demonstration of gram-positive branching or partially branching beaded filaments provides the first clue to the presence of an aerobic actinomycete (Fig. 18.1). Unfortunately, the actinomycetes do not always exhibit such characteristic morphology. Often the organisms are not seen or appear as gram-positive cocci, rods, or short filaments. Nevertheless, if gram-positive, branching or partially branching organisms are observed, a modified acid-fast stain should be performed (i.e., using 1% sulfuric acid rather than 3% hydrochloric acid as the decolorizing agent) (Evolve Procedure 18.1). The modified acid-fast stain is positive in only about half of these smears, showing gram-positive beaded, branching filaments subsequently confirmed as *Nocardia* spp. Histopathologic examination of tissue specimens using various histologic stains, such as Gomori's methenamine-silver (GMS) stain, can also detect the presence of actinomycetes.

It is important to examine any biopsy or drainage material from actinomycetomas for the presence of granules. When observed, the granules are washed in saline, emulsified in 10% potassium hydroxide or crushed between two slides, Gram stained, and examined microscopically for the presence of filaments. Granules in *Nocardia* spp. infections are small yellow to orange and may be kidney shaped with clublike structures in the periphery. *Actinomadura* spp. granules are generally red to pink in color.

TABLE 18.6	Clinical Manifestations of Infections Caused by Non–Acid-Fast Aerobic Actinomycetes	
Organism	**Clinical Manifestations**
Streptomyces spp.	Actinomycetoma Other (rare): pericarditis, bacteremia, keratitis, pneumonia, and brain abscess
Actinomadura spp.	Actinomycetoma Other (rare): peritonitis, wound infection, pneumonia, and bacteremia
Amycolatopsis spp.	Pharyngeal mucosa
Dermatophilus congolensis	Exudative dermatitis with scab formation (dermatophilosis)
Dietzia spp.	Bacteremia Catheter-associated sepsis Prosthetics
Desmospora spp.	Respiratory
Kroppenstedtia spp.	Isolated from sterile body fluids including lung, blood, and cerebrospinal fluid. Clinical significance unknown.
Nocardiopsis spp.	Actinomycetoma and other skin infections Bacteremia Nasal abscesses

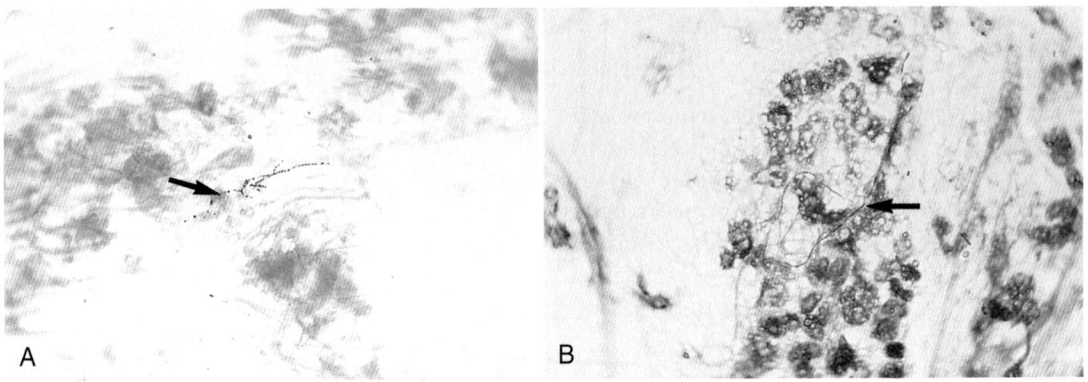

A   B

• **Fig. 18.1** (A) Gram stain of sputum obtained from a patient with pulmonary nocardiosis caused by *Nocardia asteroides*. (B) The same sputum stained with a modified acid-fast stain. The organism is indicated by the *arrow*.

Nucleic Acid Detection

Amplification techniques (i.e., polymerase chain reaction [PCR] involving the 16S ribosomal ribonucleic acid [rRNA] sequence) have been used to examine the relatedness among the genera and species within the non–acid-fast aerobic actinomycetes and thermophilic actinomycetes. When the MicroSeq System was used for identification, almost 15% of isolates were identified as *Nocardia* spp., but no definitive species were given. PCR paired with restriction endonuclease analysis can be used to identify commonly isolated *Nocardia* spp. Housekeeping heat-shock protein *(hsp65)* genes coupled with the 16S rRNA sequence are used in this assay. DNA sequencing of several genes including the 16S rRNA, a heat shock protein gene, and a housekeeping gene referred to as *secA1* (bacterial transport molecule) has been used for identification. Genus-level identification using the 16S rRNA sequence can also be used for *Nocardia, Pseudonocardia, Saccharopolyspora, Gordonia,* and *Nocardiopsis.* PCR of the 16S rRNA along with the *choE* gene can be used for the species level identification of *Rhodococcus.* Numerous other gene sequences have been examined to determine their value for organism characterization and identification. Gene sequencing of the 16S rRNA genes is the most reliable method for the differentiation of nearly all genera and species-level identification in the aerobic actinomycetes except *Tsukamurella* spp. Some species of *Nocardia* require additional discrimination. A 441-bp sequence of a heat-shock protein gene can be used for species that are very similar in the 16S rRNA sequence. The gyr B gene and secA1 gene sequences in *Gordonia* species provides greater species discrimination than the 16S rRNA. The *secA1* gene has also been used to identify species of *Tsukamurella.* However, many of these sequences are not currently available in public databases. These methods are also expensive and time-consuming and are not available in most clinical laboratories.

Matrix-Assisted Laser Desorption Ionization Time-of-Flight Mass Spectrometry

Numerous studies have examined the identification of the aerobic *Actinomycetes* for characterization and identification using matrix-assisted laser desorption ionization time-of-flight mass spectrometry (MALDI-TOF MS). Due to the limited growth of the isolates, it may be necessary to use the tube extraction method for proper identification. Limitations for the identification of the *Nocardia* and other aerobic actinomycetes is due to the lack of robustness in the available database libraries. Some libraries are able to discriminate some of the organisms discussed in this chapter to the genus level. As the databases expand, the use of MALDI TOF MS will continue to improve; however, direct sequencing is currently the method of choice and more accurate for specific species identification.

Cultivation

Many of the aerobic actinomycetes do not have complex growth requirements; they are able to grow on routine laboratory media such as sheep blood, chocolate, Sabouraud dextrose (SDA), LJ, and brain-heart infusion (BHI) agar. Buffered charcoal yeast extract (BCYE) agar has improved the recovery of *Nocardia* spp. Another actinomycete, *D. congolensis,* is unable to growth on SDA and LJ. However, because many of the aerobic actinomycetes grow slowly, they may be overgrown by other normal microbiota present in contaminated specimens. This is particularly true for the nocardiae that require a minimum of 48 to 72 hours of incubation before colonies become visible. Because of the slow growth and presence of contaminating microbiota, various selective media are used to recover nocardiae. Selective media formulated for the isolation of *Legionella* spp. from contaminated specimens, such as buffered charcoal yeast extract (BCYE) with polymyxin, anisomycin, and either vancomycin or cefamandole, have been successful in the recovery of nocardiae from contaminated specimens. Modified Thayer-Martin (MTM) medium has also been used. *Nocardia* spp. grow well on SDA agar; however, media containing chloramphenicol has shown to inhibit the growth of some species.

If other aerobic actinomycetes are considered, a selective medium, such as BHI with chloramphenicol and cycloheximide, is recommended in addition to routine agar to enhance isolation from contaminated specimens. Although most aerobic actinomycetes grow at 35°C, recovery is increased at 30°C. Selective and nonselective agars should be incubated at 35°C and 30°C; a total of four agar plates. Plates should be incubated for 2 to 3 weeks in ambient air. *D. congolensis* demonstrates enhanced growth in CO_2. *L. clevelandensis* requires incubation in atmospheres below 1% O_2. Plates should be examined daily for the first week and weekly thereafter using a dissecting microscope to identify tiny colonies. Aerobic actinomycetes have been recovered from a variety of blood culture media. However, growth times vary from collection to positivity from 3 to 19 days. It is recommended that if infection with aerobic actinomycetes is suspected, blood cultures should be incubated for a minimum of 3 weeks or terminal subcultures performed if the incubation period is not extended. The typical Gram-stain morphology and colonial appearance of the aerobic actinomycetes are summarized in Table 18.7. Examples of Gram stains and cultures of different aerobic actinomycetes are shown in Figs. 18.2 and 18.3.

Clinical laboratories are rarely asked to diagnose hypersensitivity pneumonitis caused by the thermophilic actinomycetes. These organisms grow rapidly on trypticase soy agar with 1% yeast extract. The ability to grow at temperatures of 50°C or greater is a characteristic of all thermophilic actinomycetes. Differentiation of the various infectious agents includes microscopic and macroscopic morphologies (Tables 18.7 and 18.8).

Approach to Identification

If Gram-stain morphology or colonial morphology suggests a possible actinomycete, an acid-fast stain should be performed first to rule out rapidly growing mycobacteria

| TABLE 18.7 | Typical Microscopic Morphology and Colonial Appearance | | |

Organism	Gram Stain[a]	Acid-Fast Stain	Colonial Appearance on Routine Agar
Actinomadura spp.	Moderate fine intertwining branches with short chains of spores; fragmentation	Negative	White to pink, cream to brown, yellow-gray, green or violet pigment, mucoid, molar tooth appearance after 2 weeks' incubation. Powdery aerial hyphae may be present; if no aerial hyphae are present, colonies may appear leathery.
Amycolatopsis spp.	Branching mycelium that fragments into rodlike cells	Negative	White to brown, yellow, or olive. May produce white aerial hyphae. May demonstrate a soluble brown pigment.
Dietzia spp.	Coccal and rod forms or coccobacilli; rarely branches	Negative	Nonhemolytic; round with red to salmon-pink pigment. Convex, entire, and glistening. May be indistinguishable from *Rhodococcus* spp.
Dermatophilus sp.	Branched filaments divided in transverse and longitudinal planes; fine tapered filaments	Negative	Round, adherent, gray-white colonies that later develop orange pigments; often beta-hemolytic.
Desmospora spp.	Branching filaments	Negative	Yellow with aerial hyphae, leathery colonies.
Gordonia spp.	Nonmotile short rods; may exhibit branching hyphae that fragment	Weak (modified acid fast)	Somewhat pigmented; *G. sputi:* smooth, mucoid, and adherent to media; *G. bronchialis:* dry and raised; other species smooth to wrinkled. Beige, orange, yellow, pink, or white to gray.
Kroppenstedtia spp.	Straight to curved rods, branching	Negative	Irregular, flat colonies, cream to beige. May appear dull and wrinkly. May have few aerial hyphae.
Lawsonella sp.	Irregular cocci to short rods, may have larger round dark-staining cells	Positive	Pinpoint, waxy.
Nocardia spp.	Branching fine, delicate filaments with fragmentation	Partially acid fast Weak (modified acid fast)	Extremely variable; adherent; some isolates are beta-hemolytic on sheep blood agar; wrinkled; often dry, chalky-white appearance to orange-tan pigment; crumbly.
Nocardiopsis spp.	Filamentous, branching, beaded rods	Partially acid fast Weak (modified acid fast)	White to cream, yellow to green, blue to gray. Colonies are wrinkled or folded and may have a yellow-green or brown soluble pigment present with few to abundant well-developed aerial hyphae.
Pseudonocardia spp.	Not well characterized	Negative	Yellow with white aerial hyphae, may appear fuzzy.
Rhodococcus spp.	Diphtheroid-like with minimal branching or coccobacillary; colonial growth appears as coccobacilli in zigzag configuration	Negative Weak (modified acid fast)	Nonhemolytic; round; often mucoid with orange to red, salmon-pink pigment developing within 4–7 days (pigment may vary widely),
Saccharomonospora spp.	Not well characterized	Negative	White aerial hyphae mature to gray or green to blue. May produce soluble pigments.
Saccharopolyspora spp.	Not well characterized	Negative	Slightly wrinkled or mucoid colonies that may be raised or convex. Few aerial hyphae.
Segniliparus spp.	Rod shaped	Positive	Smooth to wrinkled, convex. May be rough, nonpigmented but may produce a soluble pigment. Varies by species.
Streptomyces spp.	Extensive branching with chains and spores; does not fragment easily	Negative	Glabrous or waxy-heaped colonies; variable morphology including pigments, spore morphology and the presence of soluble pigment. Produces aerial hyphae.

TABLE 18.7	Typical Microscopic Morphology and Colonial Appearance—cont'd		
Organism	**Gram Stain[a]**	**Acid-Fast Stain**	**Colonial Appearance on Routine Agar**
Tsukamurella spp.	Mostly long rods that fragment; no spores or aerial hyphae	Negative Weak (modified acid fast)	May have rhizoid edges, dry, white to creamy to orange.
Williamsia spp.	Coccobacilli to short rods	Negative	Smooth yellow to orange or red colonies.

[a]Aerobic actinomycetes are gram-positive organisms that are often beaded in appearance.
Data compiled from McNeil MM, Brown JM. The medically important aerobic actinomycetes: epidemiology and microbiology. *Clin Microbiol Rev.* 1994;7:357; Hamid ME. *Dietzia* species as a cause of mastitis: isolation and identification of five cases from dairy cattle. *Afr J Microbiol Res.* 2013;7:3853–3857; Carroll KC, Pfaller MA, Landry ML, et al. *Manual of Clinical Microbiology.* 12th ed. Washington, DC: ASM; 2019; Souza WF, Silva RE, Goodfellow M, et al. *Amycolatopsis rhabdoformis* sp. nov., an actinomycete isolated from a tropical forest soil. *Int J System Evol Microbiol.* 2015;65:1786–1793.

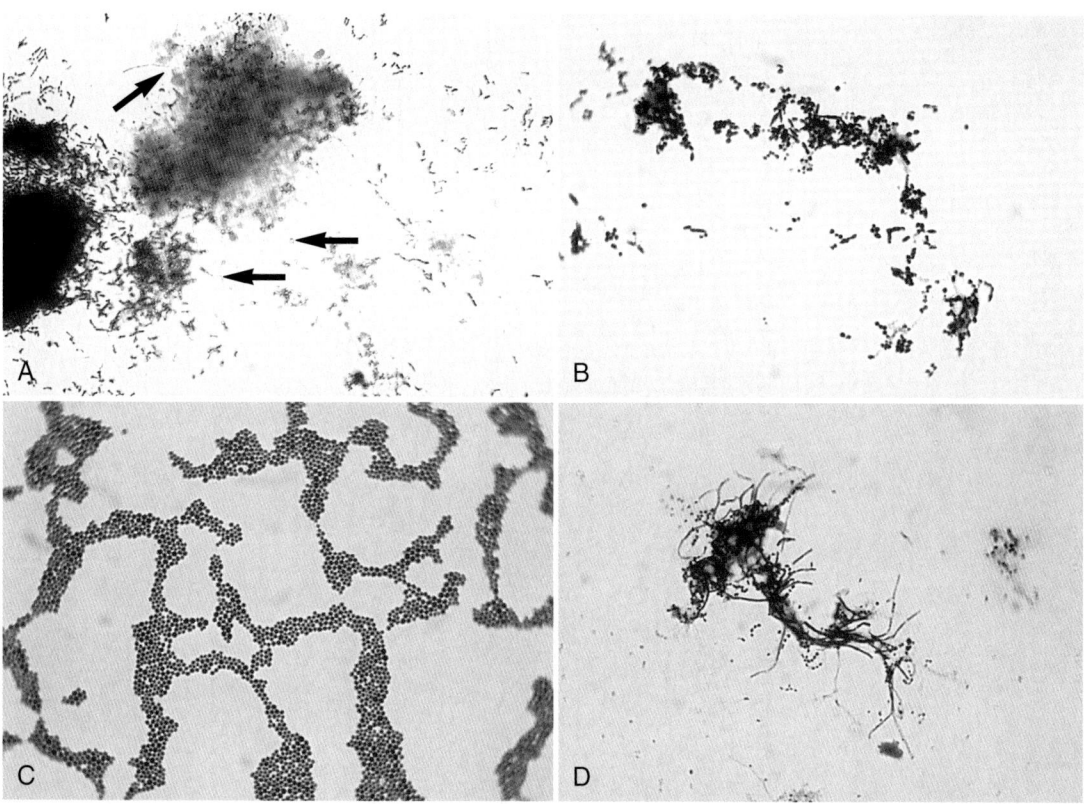

• **Fig. 18.2** Gram stains of different aerobic actinomycetes. (A) *Nocardia asteroides* grown on Löwenstein-Jensen medium. The *arrows* indicate branching rods. (B) *Rhodococcus equi* from broth. (C) *R. equi* grown on chocolate agar. (D) *Streptomyces* spp. grown on Sabouraud dextrose agar.

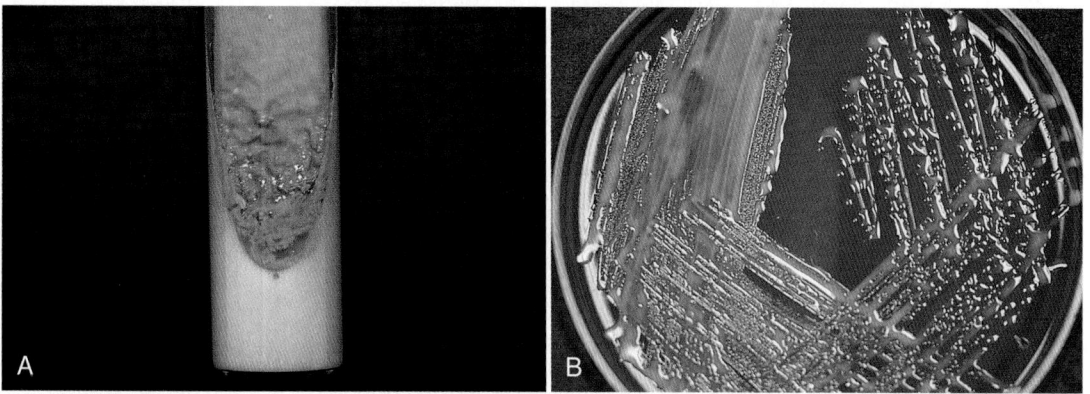

• **Fig. 18.3** Aerobic actinomycetes grown on solid media. (A) *Nocardia asteroides* grown on Löwenstein-Jensen medium. (B) *Rhodococcus equi* grown on chocolate agar.

TABLE 18.8 Preliminary Grouping of the More Commonly Isolated Clinically Relevant Aerobic Actinomycetes

Characteristics	Nocardia	Rhodococcus	Gordonia	Tsukamurella	Streptomyces	Actinomadura	Dermatophilus	Nocardiopsis
Partially acid fast	?	±	±	±	−	−	−	−
Lysozyme resistance	?	±	−	?	−	−	−	−
Urea hydrolysis	?	±	?	?	±	−	?	?
Nitrate reduction	±	±	?	−	±	?	−	?
Growth anaerobically	−	−	−	−	−	−	−	−

?, Predominantly positive; −, predominantly negative; ±, mostly positive with some negative isolates.

?, Predominantly positive; −, predominantly negative; ±, mostly positive with some negative isolates; −/?, mostly negative with some positive isolates; *NT*, not tested.

Note: Speciation is difficult; without verification with nucleic acid–based testing, biochemical identification may not be reliable.

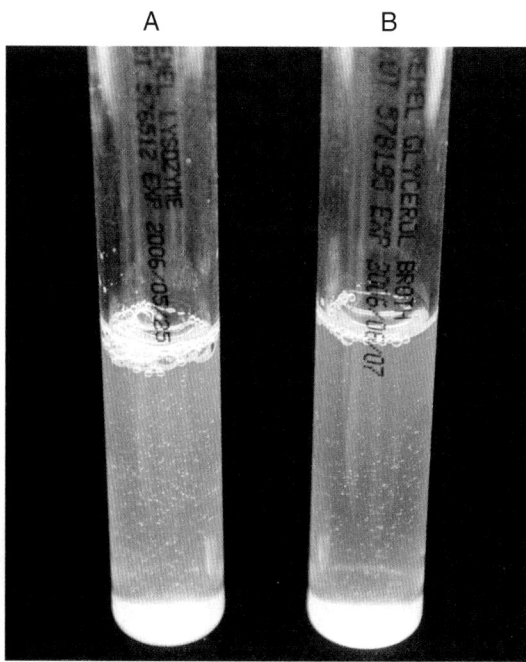

• **Fig. 18.4** Lysozyme (A) and glycerol (B) broths. The lysozyme broth demonstrates enhanced growth, which is typical of *Nocardia asteroides*.

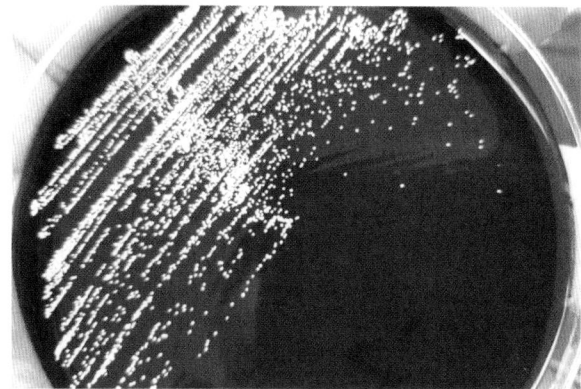

• **Fig. 18.5** *Nocardia asteroides* grown on chocolate agar. (Photo courtesy Brooks Kennedy, Houston, TX.)

(Chapter 42), followed by a modified acid-fast stain (Evolve Procedure 18.1). If the modified acid-fast stain results are positive, the isolate is a probable partially acid-fast aerobic actinomycete. If the acid-fast stain result is negative, these organisms are still not completely ruled out because of the variability of acid-fastness among isolates belonging to this group. Aerobic actinomycetes can be organized into major groupings by considering the following:

* Gram-stain morphology (Figs. 18.1 and 18.2)
* Modified acid-fast stain results
* Presence or absence of aerial hyphae and the presence of spores, their number and arrangement
* Growth or no growth in nutrient broth containing lysozyme (250 µg/mL (Fig. 18.4) (Evolve Procedure 18.2)
* Other tests: urea hydrolysis, nitrate reduction, and ability to grow anaerobically

Accurate identification of the pathogenic nocardiae to the species level can be problematic because no single method can identify all *Nocardia* isolates (Fig. 18.5). The methods used are time-consuming, often requiring 2 weeks. Useful phenotypic tests include the use of casein, xanthine, and tyrosine hydrolysis; growth at 45°C; acid production from rhamnose; gelatin hydrolysis; opacification of Middlebrook agar; and antimicrobial susceptibility patterns.

Many phenotypic tests are required to confirm the identification of the other actinomycetes at the level of speciation; these are beyond the capabilities of the routine clinical microbiology laboratory; such cases should be referred to a reference laboratory.

Serodiagnosis

No reliable serodiagnostic tests are available to help identify patients with active nocardiosis; such tests are used only to augment culture results. Infections caused by other aerobic actinomycetes currently cannot be diagnosed serologically.

Antimicrobial Susceptibility Testing and Therapy

A standard for susceptibility testing by broth microdilution and with cation-supplemented Mueller-Hinton broth has been approved by the Clinical and Laboratory Standards Institute (CLSI), along with interpretive guidelines. Break points and quality control guidelines are available and should be consulted for the most current information related to susceptibility treatment and therapeutic concerns.

Prevention

No vaccines are available for the prevention of infection with aerobic actinomycetes; some have been developed, but with little success. With respect to hypersensitivity pneumonitis caused by the thermophilic actinomycetes, patients must prevent the disease by avoiding exposure to these sensitizing microorganisms.

ⓔ Visit the Evolve site for a complete list of procedures, review questions, and case studies.

Bibliography

Bennett J, Dolin R, Blaser M: *Principles and practice of infectious diseases,* ed 9, Philadelphia, 2020, Elsevier-Saunders.

Buckwalter SP, Olson SL, Connelly BJ, et al.: Evaluation of matrix-assisted laser desorption ionization-time of flight mass spectrometry for identification of Mycobacterium species, *Nocardia* species, and other aerobic actinomycetes, *J Clin Microbiol* 54:376–384, 2016.

Carroll KC, Pfaller MA, Landry ML, et al.: *Manual of clinical microbiology*, ed 12, Washington, DC, 2019, ASM.

Chudy Onwugaje K, Vandermeer F, Quezada S: Mimicking abdominal tuberculosis: abdominal abscess caused by *Lawsonella clevelandensis* in inflammatory bowel disease, *Clin Gastroenterol Hepatol* 17:e92, 2019, https://doi.org/10.1016/j.cgh.2018.06.017.

Conville PS, Brown-Elliott BA, Smith T, Zelazny AM: The complexities of *Nocardia* taxonomy and identification, *J Clin Microbiol* 56(1), 2017https://doi.org/10.1128/JCM.01419-17.

Escapa IF, Chen T, Huang Y, Gajare P, Dewhirst FE, Lemon KP: New insights into human nostril microbiome from the expanded human oral microbiome database (eHOMD): a Resource for the Microbiome of the human aerodigestive tract, *mSystems* 3(6), 2018https://doi.org/10.1128/mSystems.00187-18.

Garrett MA, Holmes HT, Nolte FS: Selective buffered charcoal-yeast extract medium for isolation of nocardiae from mixed cultures, *J Clin Microbiol* 30:1891–1892, 1992.

Hamid ME: *Dietzia* species as a cause of mastitis: isolation and identification of five cases from dairy cattle, *Afr J Microbiol Res* 7: 3853–3857, 2013.

Kim JS, Kim WS, Lee K, et al.: Differential immune response to *Segniliparus rotundus* and *Segniliparus rugosus* infection and analysis of their comparative virulence profiles, *PLoS One* 8:e59646, 2013.

Kiska DL, Hicks K, Pettit DJ: Identification of medically relevant *Nocardia* species with an abbreviated battery of tests, *J Clin Microbiol* 40:1346–1351, 2002.

Kumaria A, Lucas EK, Crusz SA, Howarth SPS, Cartmill M: *Lawsonella clevelandensis* causing spinal subdural empyema, *Br J Neurosurg*1–3, 2018, https://doi.org/10.1080/02688697.2018.1540767.

Kumari R, Singh P, Lal R: Genetics and genomics of the genus *Amycolatopsis, Indian J Microbiol* 56:233–246, 2016.

Menezes MF, Sousa MJ, Paixão P, Atouguia J, Negreiros I, Simões MJ: *Lawsonella clevelandensis* as the causative agent of a breast abscess, *IDCases* 12:95–96, 2018, https://doi.org/10.1016/j.idcr.2018.03.014.

Perkin S, Wilson A, Walker D, McWilliams E: Dietzia species pacemaker pocket infection: an unusual organism in human infections, *BMJ Case Rep*, 2012, Available at: https://casereports.bmj.com/content/2012/bcr.10.2011.5011.

Roth A, Andrees S, Kroppenstedt RM, Harmsen D, Mauch H: Phylogeny of the genus *Nocardia* based on reassessed 16S rRNA gene sequences reveals underspeciation and division of strains classified as *Nocardia asteroides* into three established species and two unnamed taxons, *J Clin Microbiol* 41:851–856, 2003.

Saubolle MA, Sussland D: Nocardiosis: review of clinical laboratory experience, *J Clin Microbiol* 41:4497–4501, 2003.

Souza WF, Silva RE, Goodfellow M, et al.: *Amycolatopsis rhabdoformis* sp. nov., an actinomycete isolated from a tropical forest soil, *Int J Syst Evol Microbiol* 65:1786–1793, 2015.

Teng JLL, Tang Y, Wong SSY, et al.: MALDI-TOF MS for identification of *Tsukamurella* species: *Tsukamurella tyrosinosolvens* as the predominant species associated with ocular infections, *Emrg Microbes Infect* 7:80, 2018.

Weinstock DM, Brown AE: *Rhodococcus equi*: an emerging pathogen, *Clin Infect Dis* 34:1379–1385, 2002.

19

Enterobacterales

OBJECTIVES

1. Describe the general characteristics of the Enterobacterales, including oxygenation, microscopic Gram staining characteristics, and macroscopic appearance on blood and MacConkey agar (MAC).
2. Describe the chemical principle of the media used for the isolation and differentiation of Enterobacterales, including xylose-lysine-deoxycholate agar (XLD), *Salmonella-Shigella* agar (SS), Hektoen enteric agar (HE), MAC, eosin methylene blue agar (EMB), cefsulodin-irgasan-novobiocin agar (CIN), Simmons citrate agar (CIT), gram-negative broth (GN), Mac-Conkey agar with sorbitol (MAC-SOR), lysine iron agar (LIA), and triple sugar iron agar (TSI).
3. Describe the antigens used for serotyping in Enterobacterales, including bacterial location, chemical structure, heat stability, and nomenclature.
4. List the members of the Enterobacterales that are considered intestinal pathogens (and those that are extraintestinal pathogens).
5. Compare the interactions with the various pathotypes of *Escherichia coli* (i.e., uropathogenic *E. coli* [UPEC], meningitis/sepsis–associated *E. coli* [MNEC]; categories of diarrheagenic *E. coli* enterotoxigenic *E. coli* [ETEC], enteroinvasive *E. coli* [EIEC], enteroaggregative *E. coli* [EAEC], enteropathogenic *E. coli* [EPEC], and enterohemorrhagic *E. coli* [STEC]), including the route of transmission, types of infection, and pathogenesis.
6. Explain the clinical significance of *E. coli* O157:H7 and the recommended diagnostic testing for confirmation of infection.

7. Identify the serotype of *Shigella* spp. most often associated with shigellosis and hemolytic uremic syndrome.
8. Describe the difficulties associated with serotyping *Shigella* spp. and the process to resolve discrepancies in serotyping.
9. Explain the phenotypic and serologic identification of *Salmonella* serotype Typhi required for reporting a presumptive identification to the attending clinician.
10. Outline the basic biochemical testing procedure to differentiate Enterobacterales from other gram-negative rods.
11. Define the extended spectrum beta-lactamase (ESBL) test and describe the guidelines for interpretation, including the corrections required before reporting results.
12. Define multidrug-resistant typhoid fever (MDRTF) and the antibiotic susceptibility recommendations associated with identification of an MDRTF isolate.
13. Define an extended spectrum cephalosporin resistance and explain the clinical significance and identification in the clinical laboratory.
14. Describe the modified Hodge test (MHT) procedure, including the chemical principle and clinical significance of the test with regard to carbapenemase resistance.
15. Differentiate *Salmonella* spp. and *Shigella* spp. based on biochemical testing.
16. Differentiate *Yersinia* spp. from the major pathogens among the Enterobacterales.
17. Correlate signs and symptoms of infection with the results of laboratory diagnostic procedures for the identification of a clinical isolate in the Enterobacterale order.

GENERA AND SPECIES TO BE CONSIDERED

Opportunistic Pathogens

Citrobacter amalonaticus
Citrobacter braakii
Citrobacter farmeri
Citrobacter freundii
Citrobacter koseri
Citrobacter spp.
Cronobacter dubliniensis (previously *Enterobacter sakazakii*)
Cronobacter malonaticus (previously *Enterobacter sakazakii*)
Cronobacter muytjensii (previously *Enterobacter sakazakii*)
Cronobacter sakazakii (previously *Enterobacter sakazakii*)
Cronobacter turicensis (previously *Enterobacter sakazakii*)

Cronobacter universalis
Edwardsiella tarda
Enterobacter asburiae
Enterobacter bugandensis
Enterobacter cancerogenus
Enterobacter cloacae subsp. *cloacae*
Enterobacter hormaechei subsp. *hormaechei*
Enterobacter kobei
Enterobacter ludwigii
Enterobacter massiliensis
Other miscellaneous genera
Erwinia spp.
Escherichia coli (including extraintestinal)
Hafnia alvei

Hafnia paralvei
Klebsiella aerogenes
Klebsiella granulomatis (Chapter 43)
Klebsiella ozaenae
Klebsiella pneumoniae subsp. *pneumoniae*
Klebsiella pneumoniae subsp. *ozaenae*
Klebsiella pneumoniae subsp. *rhinoscleromatis*
Klebsiella oxytoca
Klebsiella quasipneumoniae
Klebsiella variicola
Kosakonia cowanii (previously *Enterobacter*)
Morganella morganii subsp. *morganii*
Morganella morganii subsp. *sibonii*
Pantoea agglomerans (previously *Enterobacter agglomerans*)
Pantoea ananatis
Pantoea spp.
Plesiomonas shigelloides
Pluralibacter gergoviae (previously *Enterobacter gergoviae* and *Enterobacter pyrinus*)
Proteus mirabilis
Proteus vulgaris
Proteus penneri
Providencia alcalifaciens
Providencia rettgeri

Providencia stuartii
Raoultella spp.
Serratia marcescens subsp. *marcescens*
Serratia marcescens subsp. *marcescens* biogroup 1
Serratia liquefaciens complex (*Serratia liquefaciens* sensu stricto, *Serratia proteamaculans,* and *Serratia grimesii*)
Serratia rubidaea
Serratia odorifera biogroups 1 and 2

Pathogenic Organisms
Primary Intestinal Pathogens
E. coli (diarrheagenic)
Escherichia spp.
P. shigelloides
Salmonella, all serotypes
Shigella dysenteriae (group A)
Shigella flexneri (group B)
Shigella boydii (group C)
Shigella sonnei (group D)

Pathogenic *Yersinia* spp.
Yersinia pestis
Yersinia enterocolitica subsp. *enterocolitica*
Yersinia pseudotuberculosis

The order Enterobacterales now includes seven families including *Enterobacteriaceae, Erwiniaceae, Pectobacteriaceae, Yersiniaceae, Hafniaceae, Morganellaceae,* and *Budvicaceae.* Although many members of the Enterobacterales cause severe disease, including opportunistic infections, there are a number of species whose clinical relevance is unknown or in question. It is helpful to consider the bacteria of this order as belonging to one of two major groups. The first group comprises species that either commonly colonize the human gastrointestinal tract or are most notably associated with human infections. Although many Enterobacterales that cause human infections are part of our normal gastrointestinal microbiota, there are exceptions, such as *Yersinia pestis, Yersinia enterocolitica,* and *Yersinia pseudotuberculosis.* The second group consists of genera capable of colonizing humans but are rarely associated with human infection and are recognized as environmental inhabitants or colonizers of other animals. For this reason, the discovery of these species in clinical specimens should alert laboratorians to possible identification errors. In some cases, careful confirmation of both the laboratory results and the clinical significance of the organism is warranted.

General Characteristics

Despite recent improvements in nucleic acid-based bacterial identification and the expanded use of techniques like whole genome multilocus sequencing typing (wgMLST), nucleic acid–based analysis has not proven definitive for identification of all organisms within Enterobacterales. While nucleic acid-based identification methods are redefining bacterial taxonomy and systematics, polyphasic classification is frequently used for the Enterobacterales. Molecular data in combination with phenotypic data such as Gram stain, bacterial morphology and arrangement, the absence of spore formation, oxidase, catalase, and other biochemical characteristics are often used for correct identification of Enterobacterales.

Epidemiology

Enterobacterales inhabit a wide variety of niches, including the human gastrointestinal tract, the gastrointestinal tract of other animals, and various environmental sites. Some are agents of zoonoses, causing infections in animal populations (Table 19.1). Just as the reservoirs for these organisms vary, so do their modes of transmission to humans.

For species capable of colonizing humans, infection may result when a patient's own bacterial strains (i.e., endogenous strains) establish infection in a normally sterile body site. The organisms can be passed from one patient to another. Such infections depend on the compromised state of a hospitalized patient and are acquired during the patient's hospitalization (nosocomial) or other health care–associated environment. However, this is not always the case. For example, although *Escherichia coli* is the most common cause of health care–associated infections, it is also the leading cause of community-acquired urinary tract infections.

Other species, such as *Salmonella* spp., *Shigella* spp., and *Y. enterocolitica,* inhabit the bowel and are acquired by ingestion of contaminated food or water. This is also the mode of transmission for the various types of *E. coli* known to cause gastrointestinal infections. In contrast, *Y. pestis* is unique among the Enterobacterales that infect humans. This is the only species transmitted from animals by an insect vector (i.e., flea bite).

Pathogenesis and Spectrum of Diseases

The clinically relevant members of the Enterobacterales can be separated into two groups: opportunistic pathogens and intestinal pathogens. *Salmonella* spp. and

TABLE 19.1   Epidemiology of Clinically Relevant Enterobacterales

Organism	Habitat (Reservoir)	Mode of Transmission
Escherichia coli and *Escherichia* spp.	Normal microbiota of the bowel of humans and other animals; may also inhabit female genital tract	Varies with the type of infection. For nongastrointestinal infections, organisms may be endogenous or spread person-to-person, especially in health care–associated environments. For gastrointestinal infections, the transmission mode varies with the strain of *E. coli* (Table 19.2); it may involve fecal-oral spread between humans in contaminated food or water or consumption of undercooked beef or unpasteurized milk from colonized cattle.
Shigella spp.	Only found in humans at times of infection; not part of normal microbiota	Person-to-person spread by fecal-oral route, especially in overcrowded areas, group settings (e.g., daycare), and areas with poor sanitary conditions.
Salmonella serotype Typhi *Salmonella* serotype Enteritidis	Only found in humans but not part of normal microbiota of the bowel	Person-to-person spread by fecal-oral route by ingestion of food or water contaminated with human excreta.
Other *Salmonella* spp.	Widely disseminated in nature and associated with various animals	Ingestion of contaminated food products processed from animals, frequently of poultry or dairy origin. Direct person-to-person transmission by fecal-oral route can occur in health care settings when handwashing guidelines are not followed.
Edwardsiella tarda	Gastrointestinal tract of fish, animals, and humans	Associated with the ingestion of contaminated water or close contact with a carrier animal. Carrier rate in humans in tropical regions that may result in endogenous spread of the organism.
Yersinia pestis	Carried by urban and domestic rats and wild rodents, such as the ground squirrel, rock squirrel, and prairie dog	From rodents to humans by the bite of flea vectors or by ingestion of contaminated animal tissues; during human epidemics of pneumonic (i.e., respiratory) disease, the organism can be spread directly from person-to-person by inhalation of contaminated airborne droplets; rarely transmitted by handling or inhalation of infected animal tissues or fluids.
Yersinia enterocolitica	Dogs, cats, rodents, rabbits, pigs, sheep, and cattle; not part of normal human microbiota	Consumption of incompletely cooked food products (especially pork), dairy products such as milk, and, less commonly, by ingestion of contaminated water or by contact with infected animals.
Yersinia pseudotuberculosis	Rodents, rabbits, deer, and birds; not part of normal human microbiota	Ingestion of organism during contact with infected animal or from contaminated food or water.
Citrobacter spp., *Enterobacter* spp., *Klebsiella* spp., *Morganella* spp., *Proteus* spp., *Providencia* spp., and *Serratia* spp.	Normal human gastrointestinal microbiota	Endogenous or person-to-person spread, especially in hospitalized patients.

Shigella spp. are among the latter group and are causative agents of typhoid fever and dysentery, respectively. *Y. pestis* is not an intestinal pathogen, but it is the causative agent of plague. Identification of these organisms in clinical material is serious and always significant. These organisms, in addition to others, produce various potent virulence factors and can cause life-threatening infections, especially when introduced to normally sterile sites (Table 19.2).

Opportunistic pathogens most commonly include *Citrobacter* spp., *Enterobacter* spp., *Klebsiella* spp., *Proteus* spp., *Serratia* spp., and a variety of other organisms. Although considered opportunistic pathogens, these organisms produce significant virulence factors, such as endotoxins capable of mediating fatal infections. However, because they generally do not initiate disease in healthy, uncompromised human hosts, they are considered opportunistic.

TABLE 19.2 Pathogenesis and Spectrum of Disease for Clinically Relevant Enterobacterales

Organism	Virulence Factors	Spectrum of Disease and Infections
Escherichia coli (as a cause of extraintestinal infections)	Several, including endotoxin, capsule production, and pili that mediate attachment to host cells.	Urinary tract infections, bacteremia, neonatal meningitis, and nosocomial infections of other various body sites. Most common cause of gram-negative health care–associated infections.
Enterotoxigenic *E. coli* (ETEC)	Pili that permit gastrointestinal colonization. Heat-labile (LT) and heat-stable (ST) enterotoxins that mediate secretion of water and electrolytes into the bowel lumen.	Travelers and childhood diarrhea, characterized by profuse, watery stools. Transmitted by contaminated food and water.
Enteroinvasive *E. coli* (EIEC)	Virulence factors uncertain, but organism invades enterocytes lining the large intestine in a manner nearly identical to *Shigella* spp.	Dysentery (i.e., necrosis, ulceration, and inflammation of the large bowel); usually seen in young children living in areas of poor sanitation.
Enteropathogenic *E. coli* (EPEC)	Bundle-forming pilus, intimin, and other factors that mediate organism attachment to mucosal cells of the small bowel, resulting in changes in cell surface (i.e., loss of microvilli).	Diarrhea in infants in developing, low-income nations; can cause a chronic diarrhea.
Enterohemorrhagic *E. coli* (STEC)	Toxin similar to Shiga toxin produced by *Shigella dysenteriae*. Most frequently associated with certain serotypes, such as *E. coli* O157:H7.	Inflammation and bleeding of the mucosa of the large intestine (i.e., hemorrhagic colitis); can also lead to hemolytic uremic syndrome, resulting from toxin-mediated damage to kidneys. Transmitted by ingestion of undercooked ground beef or raw milk.
Enteroaggregative *E. coli* (EAEC)	Probably involves binding by pili, ST-like, and hemolysin-like toxins; actual pathogenic mechanism is unknown.	Watery diarrhea that may be prolonged. Mode of transmission is not well understood.
Shigella spp.	Several factors involved to mediate adherence and invasion of mucosal cells, escape from phagocytic vesicles, intercellular spread, and inflammation. Shiga toxin role in disease is uncertain, but it does have various effects on host cells.	Dysentery defined as acute inflammatory colitis and bloody diarrhea characterized by cramps, tenesmus, and bloody, mucoid stools. Infections with *Shigella sonnei* may produce watery diarrhea.
Salmonella serotypes	Several factors help protect organisms from stomach acids, promote attachment and phagocytosis by intestinal mucosal cells, allow survival in and destruction of phagocytes, and facilitate dissemination to other tissues.	Three general categories of infection are seen: • Gastroenteritis and diarrhea caused by a wide variety of serotypes that produce infections limited to the mucosa and submucosa of the gastrointestinal tract. *Salmonella* serotype Typhi and *Salmonella* serotype Enteritidis are the serotypes most commonly associated with *Salmonella* gastroenteritis in the United States. • Bacteremia and extraintestinal infections occur by spread from the gastrointestinal tract. These infections usually involve *Salmonella* serotype Choleraesuis or *Salmonella* serotype Dublin, although any serotype may cause these infections. • Enteric fever (typhoid fever or typhoid) is characterized by prolonged fever and multisystem involvement, including blood, lymph nodes, liver, and spleen. This life-threatening infection is commonly caused by *Salmonella* serotype Typhi; *Salmonella* serotypes Paratyphi A, B, or C are rarely isolated in the United States.

<table>

TABLE 19.2 Pathogenesis and Spectrum of Disease for Clinically Relevant Enterobacterales—cont'd

Organism	Virulence Factors	Spectrum of Disease and Infections
Yersinia pestis	Multiple factors play a role in the pathogenesis of this highly virulent organism. These include the ability to adapt for intracellular survival and production of an antiphagocytic capsule, exotoxins, endotoxins, coagulase, and fibrinolysin.	Two major forms of infection are bubonic plague and pneumonic plague. Bubonic plague is characterized by high fever and painful inflammatory swelling of axilla and groin lymph nodes (i.e., the characteristic buboes); infection rapidly progresses to fulminant bacteremia that is typically fatal if untreated. Pneumonic plague involves the lungs and is characterized by malaise and pulmonary signs; the respiratory infection can occur as a consequence of bacteremic spread associated with bubonic plague or can be acquired by the airborne route during close contact with other individuals with pneumonic plague; this form of plague is also rapidly fatal.
Yersinia enterocolitica subsp. *enterocolitica*	Various factors encoded on a virulence plasmid allow the organism to attach to, invade the intestinal mucosa, and spread to lymphatic tissue.	Enterocolitis characterized by fever, diarrhea, and abdominal pain; also can cause acute mesenteric lymphadenitis, which may present clinically as appendicitis (i.e., pseudoappendicular syndrome). Bacteremia can occur with this organism but is uncommon.
Yersinia pseudotuberculosis	Similar to those of *Y. enterocolitica*.	Causes infections similar to those described for *Y. enterocolitica* but is much less common.
Citrobacter spp., *Enterobacter* spp., *Klebsiella* spp., *Morganella* spp., *Proteus* spp., *Providencia* spp., and *Serratia* spp.	Several factors, including endotoxins, capsules, adhesion proteins, and resistance to multiple antimicrobial agents.	Wide variety of health care–associated infections of the respiratory tract, urinary tract, blood, and several other normally sterile sites; most commonly infect hospitalized and seriously debilitated patients.

</table>

Although *E. coli* is a normal bowel inhabitant, its pathogenic classification is somewhere between that of the overt pathogens and the opportunistic organisms (Table 19.2). Diuretic strains of this species, such as **enterotoxigenic *E. coli* (ETEC), enteroinvasive *E. coli* (EIEC),** and **enteroaggregative *E. coli* (EAEC),** express potent toxins and cause serious gastrointestinal infections. In addition, in the case of **enterohemorrhagic *E. coli* (EHEC),** also referred to as **verocytotoxin producing *E. coli* (VTEC)** or **Shiga-like toxin–producing *E. coli* (STEC),** the organism may produce life-threatening systemic illness. Because the diarrheagenic *E. coli* capable of causing hemorrhagic colitis and hemolytic uremic syndrome (HUS) are not completely genetically defined, they will be collectively referred to as Shiga-toxin–producing *E. coli* or STEC throughout this text. Furthermore, as the leading cause of Enterobacterales infection, *E. coli* is likely to have greater virulence capabilities than the other species categorized as "opportunistic" Enterobacterales. Genetically, the four species of *Shigella* are technically non–gas producing biotypes of *E. coli*. However, the current nomenclature has not been changed primarily because of the disease presentation and differentiation in cases of shigellosis.

Specific Organisms

Opportunistic Human Pathogens
Citrobacter spp.

The genus *Citrobacter* now contains 13 species, with three species—*C. freundii*, *C. braakii*, and *C. koseri*—more commonly associated with human infection. *Citrobacter* organisms are inhabitants of the intestinal tract. Urinary tract infection is the most common clinical manifestation. However, additional infections, including wound infections, respiratory tract infections, bacteremia, endocarditis, septicemia, meningitis, brain abscess, and neurologic complications, have been associated with *Citrobacter* spp. These organisms are most often associated with infections in neonates or immunocompromised patients. Transmission is typically person-to-person. *C. freundii* may harbor inducible *AmpC* genes that encode resistance to ampicillin and first-generation cephalosporins. The primary human pathogens can be biochemically differentiated using indole; ornithine decarboxylase (ODC); malonate; and acid fermentation from adonitol, dulcitol, melibiose, and sucrose. *C. freundii* is indole-negative and sucrose-variable and positive for melibiose; *C. amalonaticus* is positive for indole and ODC; *C. braakii* is positive for ODC and variable for indole, dulcitol, and melibiose; *C. farmeri* is positive for indole, ODC, melibiose, and sucrose; *C. koseri* is variable for dulcitol and sucrose and negative for melibiose, and all other reactions are positive.

Cronobacter spp.

The *Cronobacter* genus is a group of opportunistic pathogens that includes 10 different species of which *Cronobacter malonaticus*, *Cronobacter muytjensii*, *Cronobacter sakazakii*, and *Cronobacter turicensis* are clinically relevant. Formerly considered a single species, *Enterobacter sakazakii*, nucleic acid-based testing revealed the true diversity of this group. *C. sakazakii* (neonatal infections) and *C. malonaticus* (adult infections) are the most commonly encountered isolates within the clinical environment. These organisms can cause bacteremia, meningitis, and necrotizing colitis in neonates. The association of *C. sakazakii* to neonatal infections may be correlated with the organism's ability to metabolize the sialic acid present in breast milk, infant formula, mucin, and gangliosides. The organism produces mucoid colonies on routine laboratory media resembling both *Enterobacter* and *Klebsiella* spp. when grown in culture (Fig. 19.1). The organism produces a yellow pigment that is enhanced by incubation at 25°C. *Cronobacter* spp. may be differentiated from *Enterobacter* spp. as Voges-Proskauer. In addition, the organism displays the following fermentation reactions: D-sorbitol–negative, raffinose-positive, L-rhamnose–positive, melibiose-positive, D-arabitol–positive, and sucrose-positive. Many commercial biochemical kits or systems are unable to differentiate the *Cronobacter* genus to the species level, resulting in erroneous identification of clinical isolates. *Cronobacter* is intrinsically resistant to ampicillin and first- and second-generation cephalosporins as a result of an inducible *AmpC* chromosomal beta-lactamase. Mutations to the *AmpC* gene may result in overproduction of

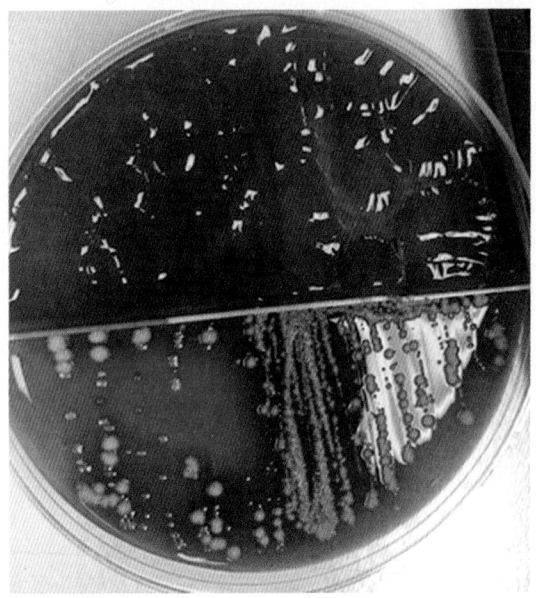

• **Fig. 19.1** Mucoid *Cronobacter sakazakii* on a sheep blood and eosin methylene blue (EMB) biplate isolated from a urinary tract specimen.

beta-lactamase, conferring resistance to third-generation cephalosporins.

Edwardsiella spp.

The genus *Edwardsiella* includes four species—*E. hoshinae*, *E. ictaluri*, *E. piscicida*, and *E. tarda*. *Edwardsiella tarda* is the most common isolated species in the clinical laboratory as a cause of gastroenteritis. The organism is typically associated with aquatic environments and is transmitted by contact with or consumption of infected fish. Immunocompromised individuals are particularly susceptible and may develop serious wound infections (myonecrosis); gastroenteritis; and occasionally septicemia, meningitis, and liver abscess. Systemic infections occur in patients with underlying liver disease or conditions resulting in iron overload.

Enterobacter spp.

Enterobacter spp. (*Enterobacter asburiae*, *Enterobacter bugandensis*, *Enterobacter cancerogenus*, *Enterobacter cloacae*, *Enterobacter hormaechei*, *Enterobacter kobei*, *Enterobacter ludwigii*, and *Enterobacter massiliensis*) are motile lactose fermenters that produce mucoid colonies. *Enterobacter* spp. are reported as one of the genera listed in the top 10 most commonly isolated health care–associated infections by the National Healthcare Safety Network. The infections are typically associated with contaminated medical devices, such as respirators and other medical instrumentation. The organisms can also be ingested from water, vegetables, and food products. The organism has a capsule that provides resistance to phagocytosis. *Enterobacter* spp. may harbor plasmids that encode multiple antibiotic resistance genes, requiring antibiotic susceptibility testing to identify appropriate therapeutic options. Notably, *Enterobacter aerogenes*, one of the most commonly encountered *Enterobacter* species second only to *E. cloacae* in many settings, was reclassified as *Klebsiella aerogenes*. Several of the *Enterobacter* species, including *E. cloacae*, *E. asburiae*, *E. hormaechei*, *E. kobei*, *E. ludwigii*, and *E. nimipressuralis*, have similar clinical presentations and biochemical reactions and therefore may be reported as *E. cloacae* complex.

Escherichia coli

Molecular analysis of *E. coli* (**uropathogenic *E. coli* [UPEC]**, **meningitis/sepsis–associated *E. coli* [MNEC]**, ETEC, EIEC, EAEC, enteropathogenic [EPEC], and STEC) continues to expand the classification of several pathotypes as well as commensal strains. However, the genetic diversity of this group continues to evolve with the implementation of polyphasic taxonomic studies. Recent reports indicate there are approximately 186 genomic types of *E. coli* and *Shigella* spp. that include pathogenic and commensal strains. The genomic variability is a result of overall plasmid (autonomous replicating extrachromosomal elements) diversity. These plasmids also harbor a large number of mobile genetic elements or transposons. The simple transposons referred to as insertion sequences are capable of flanking antibiotic resistance coding sequences or other virulence genes. The transposons are then able to excise from the plasmid or chromosome, carrying a cassette of genetic information capable of recombination into another bacterial strain. In addition to plasmids and transposons, bacteriophages are capable of promoting homologous recombination and horizontal gene transfer between organisms. One example is the pathogenic *E. coli* O157:H7. This particular strain contains 18 prophages (bacteriophages integrated into a chromosome or plasmid) and 6 prophagelike elements. Because these genetic elements are mobile and bacterial strains can readily gain or lose virulence genes, diagnosis of STEC strains becomes problematic in the diagnostic laboratory.

The genus consists of facultative anaerobic, glucose-fermenting, gram-negative, oxidase-negative rods capable of growth on MAC. In addition, the genus contains motile (peritrichous flagella) and nonmotile bacteria. Most *E. coli* strains are lactose fermenting, but this function may be delayed or absent in other *Escherichia* spp. (*Escherichia albertii*, *Escherichia blattae*, *Escherichia fergusonii*, and *Escherichia vulneris*). All species of *Escherichia*, except *E. blattae*, have been isolated from a variety of human clinical samples including stool, urine, sputum, blood, spinal fluid, peritoneal dialysate, and wounds (Table 19.3).

Pathogenic *E. coli* strains are grouped into diarrheagenic or intestinal and extraintestinal pathogens. Isolates of extraintestinal *E. coli* strains are separated into two categories: UPEC and MNEC. UPEC strains are the major cause of *E. coli*–associated community-acquired urinary tract infections. These strains contain a variety of pathogenicity islands that code for specific adhesions and toxins capable of causing disease, including cystitis and acute pyelonephritis that are not in the chromosomes of intestinal *E. coli* pathogens. MNEC causes neonatal meningitis resulting in high morbidity and mortality. Eighty percent of MNEC strains test positive for the K1 antigen. The organisms disseminate from the blood stream to the meninges and gain access to the central nervous system via membrane-bound vacuoles in microvascular endothelial cells. Once inside the cell, the organisms prevent lysosomal fusion and gain access to the central nervous system.

As mentioned, intestinal *E. coli* are classified as serotoxigenic (STEC), including strains that are considered enterohemorrhagic, or verotoxigenic, enterotoxigenic (ETEC), enteropathogenic (EPEC), enteroinvasive (EIEC), or enteroaggregative (EAEC) (Table 19.2). STEC causes hemorrhagic diarrhea, colitis, and **HUS.** HUS is characterized by a hemolytic anemia and low platelet count, and often results in kidney failure and death. Unlike dysentery, no white blood cells are found in the stool. Enterohemorrhagic (EHEC) strains may also carry the genes that code for the enterocyte effacement lesion found in EPEC strains. Although more than 150 non-O157 serotypes have been associated with diarrhea or HUS, the two most common are O157:H7 and O157: NM (nonmotile). The **O antigen** (156 serotypes) is a component of the lipopolysaccharide of the outer membrane, and the **H antigen** (56 serotypes) is the specific flagellin associated with the organism. ETEC produces a **heat-labile enterotoxin**

(LT) and a **heat-stable enterotoxin (ST)** capable of causing mild watery diarrhea. ETEC is uncommon in the United States but is an important pathogen in young children in developing countries and is associated with cases of traveler's diarrhea. ETEC typically produces mild, watery diarrhea and may be associated with abdominal cramps, nausea, and headache. Rarely does ETEC present with vomiting or fever. EIEC may produce a watery to bloody diarrhea as a result of direct invasion of the epithelial cells of the colon similar to *Shigella* spp. Cases are rare in the United States. EPEC typically does not produce exotoxins. The pathogenesis of these strains is associated with attachment and effacement of the intestinal cell wall through specialized adherence factors. Adherence of these organisms causes an **attachment and effacement lesion** in the colon. Symptoms of infection include prolonged, non-bloody diarrhea; vomiting; and fever, typically in infants or children. EAEC has been isolated from a variety of clinical cases of diarrhea. EAEC are often associated with pediatric diarrhea, foodborne outbreaks, and diarrhea in human immunodeficiency virus (HIV)–infected and acquired immune deficiency syndrome (AIDS) patients in the United States. The classification as aggregative results from the control of virulence genes associated with a global aggregative regulator gene, *AggR,* responsible for cellular adherence. EAEC-associated stool specimens typically are not bloody and do not contain white blood cells. Inflammation is accompanied by fever and abdominal pain.

Several new putative strains of *E. coli* have been isolated from patients presenting with watery diarrhea, enteritis, and extraintestinal infections. However, the roles of these strains in human disease are yet undefined and further studies are needed.

Erwinia spp.

The genus *Erwinia* includes organisms that were previously classified as *Pantoea* or *Enterobacter.* The organisms are typically plant pathogens but have been identified in human opportunistic infections. The use of newer technology, including matrix-assisted laser desorption ionization time-of-flight mass spectrometry (MALDI-TOF MS) and nucleic acid-based testing will improve the identification of this group of organisms.

Hafnia spp.

Two species, *Hafnia alvei* and *Hafnia paralvei,* are biochemically distinguishable and have been isolated from urine as well as respiratory and gastrointestinal infections. The organisms reside in the gastrointestinal tract of humans and many animals. *H. alvei* is more likely to be toxigenic than *H. paralvei.* Both organisms produce a verocytolytic toxin. In addition, infections are associated with consumption of contaminated food such as meat and dairy products. It is a motile non–lactose fermenter and is often isolated with other pathogens. Most infections with *Hafnia* spp. are identified in patients who are immunocompromised or have severe underlying disease (e.g., malignancies) or following surgery or trauma. The organism is often identified

TABLE 19.3 **Biochemical Differentiation of *Escherichia* species**

Species[a]	Acetate Utilization[a]	Growth in KCN[a]	Indole[a]	Gas from Glucose	Adonitol[a]	Arabinose[a]	Arabitol[a]	Cellobiose[a]	Dulcitol[a]	Lactose[a]	Sucrose[a]	Mannitol[a]	Raffinose[a]	Rhamnose[a]	Sorbitol[a]	Xylose[a]
E. albertii, biogroup 1	20	0	0	100	0	100	0	0	0	0	0	100	0	0	0	0
E. albertii, biogroup 2	0	0	100	40	0	100	0	0	0	0	0	100	0	0	100	0
E. blattae	0	0	0	100	0	100	0	0	0	0	0	0	0	100	0	100
E. coli	90	0	98	95	5	99	5	2	60	95	50	98	50	80	94	95
E. coli (inactive biotypes)	40	1	80	5	3	85	5	2	40	25	15	93	15	65	75	70
E. fergusonii	96	0	98	97	98	98	100	96	60	0	0	98	0	92	0	96
E. hermannii	78	94	99	97	0	100	8	97	19	45	45	100	40	97	0	100
E. vulneris	30	15	0	0	0	100	0	100	0	15	8	100	99	93	1	100

Numbers represent % of isolates that typically demonstrate the reaction.

Percent positives are based on 24 to 48 hours of incubation at 35°C to 37°C.

[a]Acid production.

Data obtained from Caroll KC, Pfaller MA. *Manual of Clinical Microbiology*. 12th ed. Washington, DC:ASM Press; 2019.

with other pathogens or opportunistic pathogens, making the clinical significance of isolation questionable. Successful treatment requires antibiotic susceptibility testing.

Klebsiella spp.

Klebsiella spp. (*Klebsiella pneumoniae* subsp. *pneumoniae*, *K. aerogenes*, *K. pneumoniae* subsp. *rhinoscleromatis*, *Klebsiella oxytoca*, *K. pneumoniae* subsp. *ozaenae*, *Klebsiella quasipneumoniae*, and *Klebsiella variicola*) are inhabitants of the nasopharynx and gastrointestinal tract. Isolates have been identified in association with a variety of infections, including liver abscesses, pneumonia, septicemia, and urinary tract infections. Some strains of *K. oxytoca* carry a heat-labile cytotoxin, which has been isolated from patients who have developed a self-limiting antibiotic-associated hemorrhagic colitis. K1 capsular clonal complex CC23^{K1}_ containing *K. pneumoniae* organisms are increasingly isolated from community-acquired pyogenic liver abscesses worldwide and demonstrate a hypervirulent (**hypermucoviscous**) phenotype (hvKP). A second K1 capsular clonal complex, CC82^{K1}, is associated with severe pneumonia and bloodstream infections. The hvKP clinical variants have the ability to spread in healthy patients because of an intrinsic resistance to serum complement and the bactericidal effects of neutrophils. *K. pneumoniae* subsp. *rhinoscleromatis* and *K. pneumoniae* subsp. *ozaenae* are agents of chronic infections, rhinoscleroma, and atrophic rhinitis (**ozena**). *K. pneumoniae* subsp. *ozaenae* has also been isolated in bloodstream, urinary tract, and respiratory tract infections. All of the *K. pneumoniae* subspecies are biochemically distinguishable; however, MALDI-TOF MS may not differentiate them. All strains of *K. pneumoniae* are resistant to ampicillin. In addition, they may demonstrate multiple antibiotic resistance patterns from the acquisition of multidrug-resistant plasmids with enzymes such as carbapenemase and cephalosporinases. Notably, *K. aerogenes* (formerly *E. aerogenes*) can also harbor mobile genetic elements that confer resistance to beta-lactam antimicrobials including carbapenems. Other mechanisms that confer resistance to carbapenems are known to occur in *K. aerogenes*.

Morganella spp.

Morganella spp. (*Morganella morganii* subsp. *morganii* and *M. morganii* subsp. *sibonii*) are ubiquitous throughout the environment and are normal microbiota of the gastrointestinal tract. They are often associated with stool specimens collected from patients with symptoms of diarrhea. *Morganella* spp. are emerging as opportunistic pathogens that cause skin and soft tissue and urinary tract infections. *Morganella* spp. are deaminase-positive and urease-positive and can express chromosomally encoded AmpC beta-lactamase leading to antimicrobial resistance.

Pantoea spp.

The genus *Pantoea* (*Pantoea agglomerans* and *Pantoea ananatis*) now includes more than 28 validly published species.

Pantoea spp. appear as a yellow-pigmented colony and are lysine-, arginine-, and ornithine-negative. In addition, the organism is indole-positive and mannitol-, raffinose-, salicin-, sucrose-, maltose-, and xylose-negative. *P. agglomerans* is the species most commonly isolated from human infections, however other species including *P. brenneri, P. conspicua, P. eucrina, P. ananatis,* and *P. septica* have been isolated from human infections. Sporadic infections with *P. agglomerans* and *P. ananatis* have been associated with traumatic injury from objects contaminated with soil (e.g., wound infections, septic arthritis, and osteomyelitis). Health care–associated infections with *P. agglomerans* have occurred from exposure to contaminated fluids (i.e., intravenous [IV] fluids, parenteral nutrition, and other administered fluids).

Plesiomonas shigelloides

Plesiomonas shigelloides is a freshwater inhabitant transmitted to humans by ingestion of contaminated water or exposure of disrupted skin and mucosal surfaces. *P. shigelloides* can cause gastroenteritis, most commonly in children. The organism is considered an emerging enteric pathogen associated with food- and water-borne illness. Disease presentation varies from acute watery to subacute chronic diarrhea and invasive, dysentery-like diarrhea. The organism has also been associated with extraintestinal infections, including meningitis in neonates, bacteremia, sepsis, and septic shock.

P. shigelloides is unusual in that it is among the few species of clinically relevant bacteria that decarboxylate lysine, ornithine, and arginine. It is important to distinguish *Aeromonas* spp. from *P. shigelloides,* because both are oxidase positive. This is accomplished by using the string test described in Chapter 25. The DNase test may also be used to differentiate these organisms. *Aeromonas* spp. are DNase-positive, and *Plesiomonas* organisms are DNase-negative. *P. shigelloides* can be detected by at least one commercially available nucleic acid amplification test.

Proteus spp. and *Providencia* spp.

The genera *Proteus* (*Proteus mirabilis, Proteus vulgaris, Proteus penneri, P. hauseri, P. terrae, P. cibarius*) and *Providencia* (*Providencia alcalifaciens, Providencia rettgeri,* and *Providencia stuartii*) are normal inhabitants of the gastrointestinal tract. They are motile, non–lactose fermenters capable of deaminating phenylalanine. *P. hauseri* can be differentiated from *P. vulgaris* by negative esculin and trehalose reactions. *Proteus* spp. are easily identified by their classic "swarming" appearance on culture media. However, some strains lack the swarming phenotype. *Proteus* has a distinct odor that is often referred to as a "chocolate cake" or "burnt chocolate" smell. However, for safety reasons, smelling plates is strongly discouraged in the clinical laboratory. Because of its motility, the organism is often associated with urinary tract infections; however, it also has been isolated from wounds and ears. The organism has also been associated with diarrhea and sepsis.

Providencia spp. are distributed worldwide and are common inhabitants in the environment and the gastrointestinal tracts of humans and animals. *Providencia* spp. are most commonly associated with urinary tract infections and isolated from the feces of children with diarrhea. These organisms may be associated with health care–associated outbreaks. These organisms are often misidentified as either *Proteus* or *Morganella* spp.

Raoultella spp.

The organisms in the genus *Raoultella* are very similar to *K. pneumoniae*. They can be differentiated by their ability to grow at 10°C and utilize sorbose. *R. ornithinolytica* has been identified in wound, urinary tract, and bloodstream infections. Both *R. planticola* and *R. terrigena* cause infections in all body sites with respiratory and urinary tract being the most common, very similar to *K. pneumoniae*. *Raoultella planticola* has been misidentified as *Klebsiella* using MALDI-TOF MS.

Serratia spp.

Serratia marcescens is known for colonization and the cause of pathogenic infections in health care settings. *Serratia* spp. (*S. marcescens* subsp. *marcescens*, *S. marcescens* subsp. *marcescens* biogroup 1, *Serratia liquefaciens*, *Serratia rubidaea*, and *Serratia odoriferous* biogroups 1 and 2) are motile, slow lactose fermenters and are DNase- and orthonitrophenyl galactoside (ONPG)–positive. *Serratia* spp. are ranked the twelfth most commonly isolated organism from pediatric patients in North America, Latin America, and Europe. Transmission may be person-to-person but is often associated with medical devices such as urinary catheters, respirators, IV fluids, and other medical solutions. *Serratia* spp. have also been isolated from the respiratory tract and wounds. The organism is capable of survival under very harsh environmental conditions and is resistant to many disinfectants. The red pigment (**prodigiosin** or 2-methyl-3-amyl-6-methoxyprodigiosene) produced by *S. marcescens* typically is the key to identification, although pigment-producing strains tend to be of lower virulence (Fig. 19.2). *S. liquefaciens*, *S. odoriferous*, and *S. rubidaea* have also been isolated from human infections. *Serratia* spp. are resistant to ampicillin and first-generation cephalosporins because of the presence of an inducible, chromosomal *AmpC* beta-lactamase. In addition, many strains have plasmid-encoded antimicrobial resistance to other cephalosporins, penicillins, carbapenems, and aminoglycosides.

Other Enterobacterales

Because of molecular methods, several organisms have been reclassified in Enterobacterales, creating new genera such as *Lelliottia*, *Pluralibacter*, and *Kosakonia* or moving them to other genera such as *Tatumella*, *Cedecea*, *Leminorella*, *Moellerella*, and *Kluyvera*. These organisms are either transient or commensal in the clinical setting or opportunistic pathogens in immunocompromised patients. *Kluyvera* has also been associated with infections in immunocompetent patients from a variety of clinical samples including blood, tissue, urine, cerebrospinal fluid (CSF), and peritoneal fluids. The organism is, however, more commonly associated with urinary and bloodstream infections. With the implementation

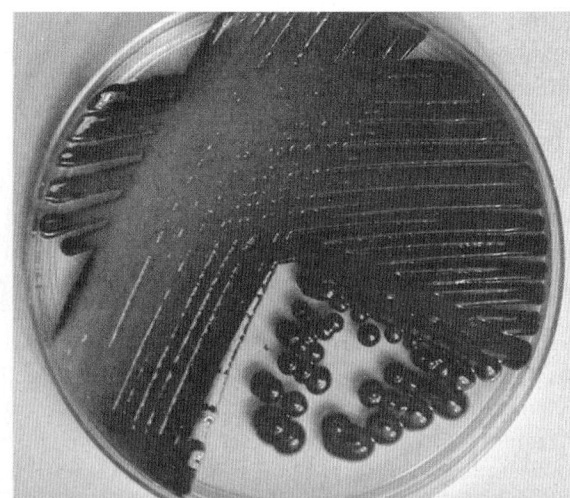

• **Fig. 19.2** Red-pigmented *Serratia marcescens* subsp. *marcescens* on MacConkey agar.

of advanced technology and methods including MALDI-TOF MS and nucleic acid-based methods, organisms that were rarely associated with human infection will likely be identified more frequently in the clinical laboratory.

Primary Intestinal Pathogens

Salmonella

Salmonella (all serotypes) are facultative anaerobic, motile, gram-negative rods commonly isolated from the intestines of humans and animals. Identification is primarily based on the ability of the organism to use citrate as the sole carbon source and lysine as a nitrogen source in combination with hydrogen sulfide (H_2S) production. The genus comprises two primary species, *Salmonella enterica* (human pathogen) and *Salmonella bongori* (animal pathogen). *S. enterica* is subdivided into six subspecies: subsp. *enterica* (group I), subsp. *salamae* (group II), subsp. *arizonae* (group IIIa), subsp. *diarizonae* (group IIIb), subsp. *houtenae* (group IV), and subsp. *indica* (group VI). *S. enterica* subsp. *enterica* can be further divided into serotypes with unique virulence properties. Serotypes are differentiated based on the characterization of the heat-stable O antigen, included in the LPS; the heat-labile H antigen flagellar protein; and the heat-labile **Vi antigen,** capsular polysaccharide. A DNA sequence–based method has been developed for molecular identification of DNA motifs in the flagella and O antigens. The primary identifiable *Salmonella* serotypes are *Salmonella* serotype Typhi associated with a severe disease called **typhoid fever.** Diarrhea and vomiting are not associated with typhoid fever. The symptoms are often headache, abdominal cramping, constipation, and high fever. The patient may present with a rash and appear confused. Human carriers have been identified. The disease is transmitted person-to-person or through contaminated food and water. A second serotype, *Salmonella* serotype Enteritidis, is associated with infections acquired from the ingestion of contaminated food or water. *Salmonella*-associated gastroenteritis is typically accompanied by diarrhea, fever, and abdominal cramps. Cases of gastroenteritis may cause extraintestinal infections such as bacteremia, urinary tract infection, or osteomyelitis. Transmission may be fecal-oral, person-to-person, or contact with infected animals.

Shigella spp.

Shigella spp. *(S. dysenteriae, Shigella flexneri, Shigella boydii, and Shigella sonnei)* are nonmotile; lysine decarboxylase–negative; citrate-, malonate-, and H$_2$S-negative; non–lactose fermenting; gram-negative rods that grow well on MAC. All strains ferment glucose without gas production, except a few strains (*S. flexneri* serotype 6 and *S. boydii* serotype 14). The four subgroups of *Shigella* spp. are *S. dysenteriae* (group A), *S. flexneri* (group B), *S. boydii* (group C), and *S. sonnei* (group D). Each subgroup has several serotypes. Serotyping is based on the somatic LPS O antigen. *Shigella* and inactive *E. coli* strains are often very difficult to distinguish. After presumptive identification of a suspected *Shigella* species based on traditional biochemical methods, serotyping should be completed, especially in the case of *S. dysenteriae*. Suspected strains of *Shigella* spp. that cannot be typed by serologic methods should be referred to a reference laboratory for further testing.

Shigellosis may begin as watery diarrhea, fever, and abdominal cramps. Progressive infection then leads to dysentery with stools that contain blood or mucus. Lesions in the intestinal tract typically remain confined to the large intestine. Bloodstream infections are rare. All *Shigella* are capable of causing dysentery. However, *S. dysenteriae* 1 produces the most severe forms of illness and may lead to HUS. *Shigella* spp. can generally be differentiated from *E. coli* based on its inability to ferment lactose, lack of motility, and negative indole reaction. However, nonreactive *E. coli* isolates cannot be differentiated from *Shigella* spp., requiring serological testing for further characterization.

Yersinia spp.

Yersinia spp. *(Y. pestis, Y. enterocolitica, and Y. pseudotuberculosis)* are gram-negative; catalase-, oxidase-, and indole-variable; non–lactose fermenting; facultative anaerobes capable of growth at temperatures ranging from 4°C to 43°C. The gram-negative rods exhibit an unusual bipolar or "safety pin" morphology that can be observed with **Wayson** stain. Based on the composition of the LPS in the outer membrane, colonies may present with either a rough form lacking the O-specific polysaccharide chain (*Y. pestis*) or a smooth form containing the lipid A-oligosaccharide core and the complete O-polysaccharide (*Y. pseudotuberculosis* and *Y. enterocolitica*). Complex typing systems exist to differentiate the various *Yersinia* spp., including standard biochemical methods coupled with biotyping (biochemical phenotypic methods), serotyping, bacteriophage typing, and antibiogram analysis. In addition, epidemiologic studies often include pulsed-field gel electrophoresis (PFGE) studies.

Y. pestis is most commonly transmitted by the bite of an infected flea resulting in **bubonic plague**. However, handling infected animals, inhaling infectious droplets, and ingestion of undercooked meat have also resulted in infections. Human-to-human transmission is possible with the **pneumonic** (respiratory) form of disease. *Y. enterocolitica* is found in the gastrointestinal tract of swine, rodents, and dogs. Transmission is primarily from the ingestion of contaminated food or water. Conversely, *Y. pseudotuberculosis* is found in a variety of wild and domesticated animals including rodents, birds, and rabbits. The mode of transmission is by contact with infected animals or the ingestion of contaminated food or water.

Laboratory Diagnosis

Specimen Collection and Transport

Enterobacterales are typically isolated from a variety of sources in combination with other more fastidious organisms. Fecal specimens should be collected from patients preferably within the first 4 days of illness and before administration of antimicrobials. In general, manufactured transport media such as Cary-Blair, Aimes, and Stuart transport media are satisfactory for isolation of *E. coli*, *Shigella*, and *Salmonella*. However, buffered glycerol saline should not be used for the recovery of *Campylobacter* or *Vibrio*. Table 5.1 includes general information on specimen collection and transport.

Specimen Processing

No special considerations are required for processing most of the organisms discussed in this chapter. Fecal specimens that are not processed within 1 to 2 hours of collection and all rectal swabs should be placed in cold transport medium and kept at 4°C. This is extremely important for the recovery of *Shigella* and *Campylobacter*. In addition, *Y. pestis* is considered a tier 1 Select Agent. Specimens suspected of containing *Y. pestis* should be moved to a biological safety cabinet immediately. Routine clinical diagnostic laboratories are strongly urged to work closely with a local or state public health laboratory if *Y. pestis* is suspected. Standard rule-out and refer methods are available for clinical laboratories that may encounter Select Agents during the course of clinical microbiology testing. Manipulation of specimens suspected of containing *Y. pestis* should be performed using Biosafety Level 3 (BSL-3) conditions by an approved Laboratory Response Network member laboratory. If samples for the identification of *Yersinia* spp. cannot be processed within 2 hours, the sample should be placed in Cary-Blair medium and transported at 2°C to 8°C. Refer to Table 5.1 for general information on specimen processing.

Direct Detection Methods

All Enterobacterales have similar microscopic morphology; therefore, Gram staining is not significant for the presumptive identification of Enterobacterales. Generally, isolation of gram-negative organisms from a sterile site, including CSF, blood, and other body fluids, is critical and may assist the physician in prescribing appropriate therapy.

Direct detection of Enterobacterales in stool by Gram staining is insignificant because of the abundance of gram-negative bacteria throughout the lower digestive tract. The presence of increased white blood cells may indicate an enteric infection. However, the absence of white blood cells in a stool sample is not sufficient to rule out a toxin-mediated enteric disease.

Other than Gram staining of patient specimens, specific procedures are required for direct detection of most Enterobacterales. Microscopically these organisms generally appear as coccobacilli or straight rods with rounded ends. *Yersinia* spp. demonstrate a bipolar staining that resembles a closed safety pin when stained with Wright-Giemsa or **Wayson stain;** this can be key characteristic for rapid diagnosis, although safety pin staining is not always visible.

Klebsiella granulomatis can be visualized in scrapings of lesions stained with Wright or Giemsa stain. Cultivation *in vitro* is very difficult, so direct examination is important diagnostically. Groups of organisms are seen in mononuclear endothelial cells. This pathognomonic entity or **Donovan body** is named after the physician who first visualized the organism in such a lesion. The organism stains as a blue rod with prominent polar granules, giving rise to the safety-pin appearance, surrounded by a large, pink capsule. Subsurface infected cells must be present; surface epithelium is not an adequate specimen. See Chapter 43 for additional information.

P. shigelloides tend to be pleomorphic gram-negative rods that occur singly; in pairs; in short chains; or even as long, filamentous forms.

Nucleic Acid Detection

Commercially available nucleic acid–based methods are available for the direct detection of the pathogens in Enterobacterales in both monoplex and multiplex platforms. The sensitivities and specificities vary among the assays but range from 83% to 100%.

In addition to nucleic acid–based methods for the detection of pathogenic Enterobacterales, polymerase chain reaction (PCR) amplification assays are used to distinguish multiple serotypes or pathotypes simultaneously. Both *E. coli* and *Shigella* produce verocytotoxins that have similar genetic structures and biologic activities. As the first Shiga-toxin identified, *Shigella dysenteriae* toxin is referred to as *Stx*. Because multiple subtypes have been identified using PCR, they are now classified according to the severity of disease associated with the presence of the specific toxin. Bloody diarrhea and HUS are primarily associated with Stx2d and severe disease with Stx2a and Stx2c.

Because of the variability associated with the pathogenicity of STEC strains, molecular probes for approximately 25 different genes have been used to characterize isolates. Some of these include the intimin adhesion and type II secretion system in the locus of enterocyte effacement (LEE) pathogenicity island, such as the *eae* gene and *hlyA* gene of the plasmid-encoded enterohemolysin. EPEC can be detected using a probe for the enteropathogenic adherence factor (EAF) plasmid and based on the absence of Stx. A specific probe (AA also known as CVD432) has been constructed from the pAA virulence plasmid to identify pathogenic strains of EAEC. *Shigella* and EIEC may be detectable using a molecular probe to the invasive plasmid-associated gene *ipaH*. As more and more isolates are characterized, nucleic acid–based testing will continue to provide a better method

for the detailed characterization of pathogenic *E. coli* strains and disease correlations to improve patient care.

It is important to note that there has been a significant increase in the identification of many Enterobacterales in human stool samples due to the high sensitivity of molecular platforms. The molecular diagnosis should not be used in cases of mild acute gastroenteritis or traveler's diarrhea lasting less than 14 days unless there are other risk factors associated with the patient's condition. The impact of molecular methods has markedly increased health care costs and has had a negative impact on public health and epidemiology efforts. Laboratories should continue to recover the isolates using culture-based methods for these reasons, as this information is critical for outbreak investigation and the identification of emerging serotypes and antibiotic resistance patterns.

Cultivation
Media of Choice

Most Enterobacterales grow well on routine laboratory media, such as 5% sheep blood, chocolate, and MACs. In addition to these media, selective agars, such as Hektoen enteric (HE) agar, xylose-lysine-deoxycholate (XLD) agar, and *Salmonella-Shigella* (SS) agar, are commonly used to cultivate enteric pathogens from gastrointestinal specimens (see Chapter 74 for more information about laboratory procedures for the diagnosis of bacterial gastrointestinal infections). The broths used in blood culture systems, as well as thioglycollate and brain-heart infusion broth, all support the growth of Enterobacterales. Gram-negative broth (GN) or Selenite broth (SEL) may be used as enrichment for the isolation of *Shigella* and other Enterobacterales. Media that are highly selective for the isolation of *Salmonella* spp. include CHROMagar *Salmonella*, brilliant green agar, and bismuth sulfite agar.

Cefsulodin-irgasan-novobiocin (CIN) agar is a selective medium specifically used for the isolation of *Y. enterocolitica* from gastrointestinal specimens. Similarly, MacConkey-sorbitol agar (MAC-SOR) is used to differentiate sorbitol-negative *E. coli* O157:H7 from other strains of *E. coli* that are capable of fermenting the sugar alcohol.

K. granulomatis (Chapter 43) will not grow on routine agar media. Recently the organism was cultured in human monocytes from biopsy specimens of genital ulcers of patients with **donovanosis**. Historically, the organism has also been cultivated on a special medium that contains growth factors found in egg yolk. In clinical practice, however, the diagnosis of **granuloma inguinale** is made solely on the basis of direct examination.

Table 19.4 presents a complete description of the laboratory media used to isolate Enterobacterales.

Incubation Conditions and Duration

Under normal circumstances, most Enterobacterales produce detectable growth in commonly used broth and agar media within 24 hours of inoculation. For isolation, 5% sheep blood and chocolate agars may be incubated at 35°C in carbon dioxide or ambient air. However, MAC and other selective agars (e.g., SS, HE, XLD) should be incubated only in ambient

TABLE 19.4   Biochemical Media Used in the Differentiation and Isolation of Enterobacterales

Media	Selective	Differential	Nutritional	Purpose
Blood agar (sheep) (BA)		Hemolysis of RBCs: Beta: complete lysis Alpha: partial, greening Gamma: nonhemolytic	Routinely used to cultivate moderately fastidious organisms; trypticase soy agar with 5%–10% defibrinated blood	Screening colonies for the oxidase enzyme
Bismuth sulfite agar	Selective inhibition of most gram-positive and gram-negative bacteria (bismuth sulfite and brilliant green)	Production of hydrogen sulfide (H_2S); ferrous sulfate. Positive reactions appear as brown to black precipitate.	Beef extract, peptones, and dextrose	Isolation of *Salmonella* spp.
Brilliant green agar	Selective; brilliant green is inhibitory to most gram-positive and gram-negative bacteria	Lactose and sucrose fermentation; positive (phenol red) fermenters appear as yellow to green colonies with bright yellow to green halos. *Salmonella* spp. appear as white to pink or red colonies surrounded by a bright halo.	Enzymatic digests of animal tissue, casein, lactose, and sucrose	Isolation of *Salmonella* spp.
Cefixime-tellurite-containing MacConkey (CT-SMAC)	Selective inhibition of most non-verocytotoxigenic *E. coli* and non–sorbitol fermenters (sorbitol, cefixime, and tellurite)	Fermentation of sorbitol in the presence of neutral red. Positive colonies appear pink and nonfermenters will appear colorless.	Pancreatic digests of gelatin, peptone, and sorbitol	Isolation and identification of *E. coli* O157-H7
Cefsulodin-irgasan-novobiocin agar (CIN)	Selective inhibition of gram-negative and gram-positive organisms	Fermentation of mannitol in the presence of neutral red. Macroscopic colonial appearance: colorless or pink colonies with red center.		Isolation of *Yersinia enterocolitica*
Citrate agar, Simmons (CIT)		Citrate as the sole carbon source, ammonium salt as nitrate. Ammonium salt alteration changes pH to alkaline, bromothymol blue shifts from green to blue.		Detect organisms capable of citrate utilization
Decarboxylases (ornithine, arginine, lysine)		Incorporate amino acid as differential media (e.g., lysine, arginine, or ornithine). Decarboxylation yields alkaline, pH-sensitive bromocresol purple dye. Basal medium serves as a control. Incubate for up to 4 days. Fermentative organisms turn media yellow, using glucose. (H+) increases, making optimal conditions for decarboxylation. Conversion of the amino acids to free amine groups raising the pH, reversing the yellow to purple. Nonfermenters turn the purple a deeper color.		Differentiate fermentative and nonfermentative gram-negative bacteria

Continued

TABLE 19.4				
Biochemical Media Used in the Differentiation and Isolation of Enterobacterales—cont'd				
Media	**Selective**	**Differential**	**Nutritional**	**Purpose**
Eosin/methylene blue agar (EMB)	Eosin Y and methylene blue dyes inhibit the growth of gram-positive bacteria.	Lactose and sucrose for differentiation based on fermentation. Sucrose is an alternate energy source for slow lactose fermenters, allowing quick differentiation from pathogens.		Identification of gram-negative bacteria. *Escherichia coli*: Lactose fermenter, forms blue-black with a metallic green sheen Other coliform fermenters: form pink colonies Nonfermenters: Translucent, either amber or colorless
Gram-negative broth (GN)	Deoxycholate and citrate salts inhibit gram-positive bacteria.		Increasing mannitol, which temporarily favors the growth of mannitol-fermenting, gram-negative rods (e.g., *Salmonella* and *Shigella* spp.)	Enhances the recovery of enteric pathogens from fecal specimens
Hektoen enteric agar (HE)	Bile salts inhibit gram-positive and many gram-negative normal intestinal flora.	Differential lactose, salicin, and sucrose with a pH indicator bromothymol blue and ferric salts to detect hydrogen sulfide (H_2S). Most pathogens ferment one or both sugars and appear bright orange to salmon pink because of the pH interaction with the dye. Nonfermenters appear green to blue green. H_2S production produces a black precipitate in the colonies.		Detection of enteric pathogens from feces or from selective enrichment broth
Lysine iron agar (LIA)		Contains lysine, glucose, and protein, bromocresol purple (pH indicator), and sodium thiosulfate/ferric ammonium citrate. Purple denotes alkaline (K), red color (R), acid (A). K/K: Organism decarboxylates but cannot deaminate, ferments glucose, first butt is yellow then turns back to purple. Decarboxylates lysine, producing alkaline; changes back to purple. K/A: Organism fermented glucose but was unable to deaminate or decarboxylate lysine. Bordeaux red and yellow butt. R/A: Organism deaminated lysine but could not decarboxylate it. The lysine deamination combines with the ferric ammonium citrate, forming a burgundy color. Blackening of the butt indicates production of H_2S.		Measures three parameters that are useful for identifying Enterobacterales (lysine decarboxylation, lysine deamination, and H_2S production)
MacConkey agar (MAC)	Bile salts and crystal violet inhibit most gram-positive organisms and permit growth of gram-negative rods.	Lactose serves as the sole carbohydrate. Lactose fermenters produce pink or red colonies; precipitated bile salts may surround colonies. Non–lactose fermenters appear colorless or transparent.		Selection for gram-negative organisms and differentiating Enterobacterales

TABLE 19.4   Biochemical Media Used in the Differentiation and Isolation of Enterobacterales—cont'd

Media	Selective	Differential	Nutritional	Purpose
MacConkey-sorbitol (MAC-SOR)		Same as regular MacConkey except D-sorbitol is substituted for lactose. Sorbitol-negative organisms are clear and may indicate *E. coli* O157:H7.		Used to isolate *Escherichia coli* O157:H7
Motility test medium		Nonmotile organisms grow clearly only on stab line, and the surrounding medium remains clear. Motile organisms move out of the stab line and make the medium appear diffusely cloudy.		Determine motility for an organism Identification and differentiation of Enterobacterales *Shigella* and *Klebsiella* spp.: nonmotile; *Yersinia* sp.: motile at room temperature *Listeria monocytogenes* (not an Enterobacterales): umbrella-shaped motility
Salmonella-Shigella agar (SS)	Bile salts, sodium citrate, and brilliant green, which inhibit gram-positive organisms and some lactose-fermenting, gram-negative rods normally found in the stool.	Lactose is the sole carbohydrate, and neutral red is the pH indicator. Fermenters produce acid and change the indicator to pink-red. Sodium thiosulfate is added as a source of sulfur for the production of hydrogen sulfide. Also includes ferric ammonium citrate to react with H_2S and produce a black precipitate in the center of the colony. *Shigella* spp. appear colorless. *Salmonella* spp. are colorless with a black center.		Select for *Salmonella* spp. and some strains of *Shigella* from stool specimens
Selenite broth	Selective inhibition of gram-positive and many gram-negative organisms.		Enzymatic digestion of casein and animal tissue and lactose.	Selective enrichment for the growth of *Salmonella* spp.
Triple sugar iron agar (TSI)		Contains glucose, sucrose, and lactose. Sucrose and lactose are present in 10 times the quantity of the glucose; phenol red is the pH indicator. Turns to yellow when sugars are fermented because of drop in pH. Sodium thiosulfate plus ferric ammonium sulfate as H_2S indicator. Acid/acid (A/A): Glucose and lactose or sucrose (or both) fermentation.		Differentiates glucose fermenters from non–glucose fermenters; also contains tests for sucrose and/or lactose fermentation, as well as gas production during glucose fermentation and H_2S production
		Gas bubbles: Production of gas. Visible air breaks or pockets in agar. Black precipitate: H_2S. Alkaline/acid (K/A): Glucose fermentation but not lactose or sucrose. Alkaline/alkaline (K/K): No fermentation of dextrose, lactose, or sucrose.		

Continued

TABLE 19.4	Biochemical Media Used in the Differentiation and Isolation of Enterobacterales—cont'd				
Media	**Selective**	**Differential**	**Nutritional**	**Purpose**	
Urea agar		Urea is hydrolyzed to form carbon dioxide, water, and ammonia. Ammonia reacts with components of the medium to form ammonium carbonate, raising the pH, which changes the pH indicator, phenol red, to pink. Limited protein in the medium prevents protein metabolism from causing a false-positive reaction.		Identification of Enterobacterales species capable of producing urease (*Citrobacter, Klebsiella, Proteus, Providencia,* and *Yersinia* spp.)	
Xylose-lysine-deoxycholate agar (XLD)	Sodium deoxycholate inhibits gram-positive cocci and some gram-negative rods. Contains less bile salts than other formulations of enteric media (e.g., SS, HE) and therefore permits better recovery.	Sucrose and lactose in excess concentrations and xylose in lower amounts. Phenol red is the pH indicator. Lysine is included to detect decarboxylation. Sodium thiosulfate/ferric ammonium citrate allows the production of H$_2$S. The following types of colonies may be seen: Yellow: Fermentation of the excess carbohydrates to produce acid; because of the carbohydrate use, the organisms do not decarboxylate lysine, even though they may have the enzyme. Colorless or red: Produced by organisms that do not ferment any of the sugars. Yellow to red: Fermentation of xylose (yellow), but because it is in small amounts, it is used up quickly, and the organisms switch to decarboxylation of lysine, turning the medium back to red. Black precipitate is formed from the production of H$_2$S.		Selective media used to isolate *Salmonella* and *Shigella* spp. from stool and other specimens containing mixed flora	

air. Unlike most other Enterobacterales, *Y. pestis* grows best at 25°C to 30°C. Colonies of *Y. pestis* are pinpoint at 24 hours but resemble those of other Enterobacterales after 48 hours. CIN agar, used for the isolation of *Y. enterocolitica*, should be incubated 48 hours at room temperature to allow for the development of the typical "bull's-eye" colonies (Fig. 19.3).

Colonial Appearance

Table 19.5 presents the colonial appearance and other distinguishing characteristics (pigment and odor) of the most commonly isolated Enterobacterales on MacConkey, HE, and XLD agars (Figs. 7.4, 7.6, and 7.8 for examples). All Enterobacterales produce similar growth on blood and chocolate agars; colonies are large, gray, and smooth. Colonies of *Klebsiella* or *Enterobacter* may be mucoid because of

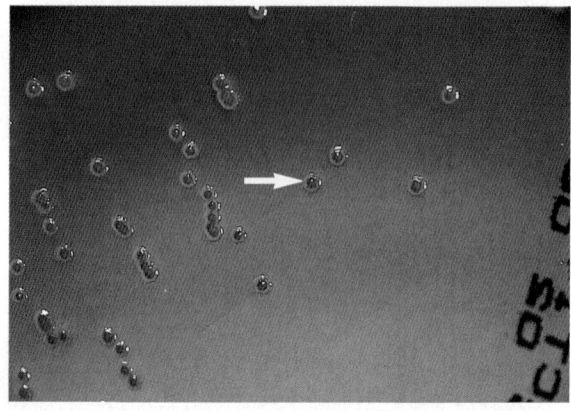

• **Fig. 19.3** Bull's-eye colony of *Yersinia enterocolitica (arrow)* on cefsulodin-irgasan-novobiocin (CIN) agar.

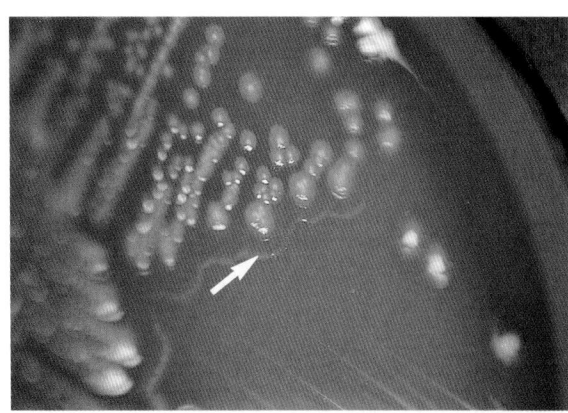

• **Fig. 19.4** *Proteus mirabilis* swarming on blood agar (*arrow* points to swarming edge).

their polysaccharide capsule. *E. coli* is often beta-hemolytic on blood agar, but most other genera are nonhemolytic. *P. mirabilis, P. penneri,* and *P. vulgaris* are motile and "swarm" on blood and chocolate agars. Swarming results in the production of a thin film of growth on the agar surface (Fig. 19.4) as the organisms spread from the original site of inoculation.

Colonies of *Y. pestis* on 5% sheep blood agar are pinpoint at 24 hours but exhibit a rough, cauliflower appearance at 48 hours. Broth cultures of *Y. pestis* exhibit a characteristic "stalactite pattern" in which clumps of cells adhere to one side of the tube.

Y. enterocolitica produces bull's-eye colonies (dark red or burgundy centers surrounded by a translucent border; Fig. 19.3) on CIN agar at 48 hours. However, because most *Aeromonas* spp. produce similar colonies on CIN agar, it is important to perform an oxidase test to verify that the organisms are *Yersinia* spp. (oxidase negative). The oxidase test should be performed on suspect colonies that have been subcultured to sheep blood agar (Table 19.4). Pigments present in the CIN agar will interfere with correct interpretation of the oxidase test results.

Approach to Identification

In the early decades of the twentieth century, Enterobacterales were identified using more than 50 biochemical tests in tubes. Many of these tests such as indole, methyl red, Voges-Proskauer, and citrate (known by the acronym **IMViC**) are still performed using conventional methods in some laboratories, principally reference and public health laboratories. Today, this type of conventional biochemical identification of enterics has become a historical footnote in most clinical and hospital laboratories in the United States.

In the latter part of the twentieth century, manufacturers began to produce panels of miniaturized tests for identification, first of enteric gram-negative rods and later of other groups of bacteria and yeast. Original panels were inoculated manually followed by incubation and manual interpretation of biochemical results. These panels ultimately gave way to semiautomated and automated systems, the most sophisticated of which inoculate, incubate, read, and discard the panels. Almost every commercial identification system can

be used to reliably identify commonly encountered Enterobacterales. Depending on the system, results are available within 4 hours or after overnight incubation. However, even the most sophisticated automated systems still struggle to provide high-confidence identification of some Enterobacterales, particularly organisms that require longer biochemical reaction times, are more biochemically inert, or are rarely encountered in the clinical laboratory. While the extensive computer databases used by these systems include information on unusual biotypes, rarely encountered species or newly discovered species may be underrepresented leading to misidentification or no identification at all.

Identification of enterics can be enhanced with nucleic acid–based methods such as gene sequencing (e.g., 16S ribosomal ribonucleic acid) or by newer methods such as whole genome or core genome multilocus sequence typing (wgMLST and cgMLST, respectively). Using nucleic acid–based methods, the genus *Plesiomonas,* composed of one species of oxidase-positive, gram-negative rods, is now included in Enterobacterales. *Plesiomonas* spp. cluster with the genus *Proteus* in the Enterobacterales by 16S rRNA sequencing. However, like all other Enterobacterales, *Proteus* organisms are oxidase-negative. The clustering together of an oxidase-positive genus and an oxidase-negative genus is a revolutionary concept in microbial taxonomy. Limitations of current commercial identification systems have been noted because of the genotypic classification of microorganisms. In addition, this technology has resulted in the need to combine genotypic and phenotypic traits in a polyphasic approach to resolve discrepancies as noted in the classification of *Cronobacter* spp. and *E. coli* pathotypes.

In the interests of cost containment, many clinical laboratories have traditionally used abbreviated schemes to identify commonly isolated enterics. *Escherichia* spp., for example, one of the most commonly isolated enteric genera, may be identified by a positive spot indole test (Procedure 12.40). This test, however, can no longer be used to presumptively identify *E. coli*. This is because of the isolation of other *Escherichia* spp. from clinical specimens. For identification of an organism such as *E. coli,* the characteristic colonial appearance on MAC, as described in Table 19.5, along with a positive spot indole must be verified with additional biochemical tests. A spot indole test can be used to separate swarming protease, such as *P. mirabilis* and *P. penneri,* which are negative, from the indole-positive *P. vulgaris*.

Table 19.6 provides an overview of common reactions for identifying biochemically unusual enteric pathogens. Fig. 19.5 depicts the biochemical reactions typically used to differentiate some of the representative enteric pathogens. Fig. 19.6 shows a urinary tract isolate of *E. coli* demonstrating strong lactose fermentation on EMB as indicated by the green metallic sheen.

Specific Considerations for Identifying Enteric Pathogens

Table 19.7 illustrates the use of biochemical profiles obtained with triple sugar iron (TSI) agar and lysine iron

TABLE 19.5 Colonial Appearance and Characteristics of the Most Commonly Isolated Enterobacterales[a]

Organism	Medium	Appearance
Citrobacter spp.	MAC	Late LF; therefore, NLF after 24 h; LF after 48 h; colonies are light pink after 48 h
	HE	Colorless
	XLD	Red, yellow, or colorless colonies, with or without black centers (H_2S)
Edwardsiella spp.	MAC	NLF
	HE	Colorless
	XLD	Red, yellow, or colorless colonies, with or without black centers (H_2S)
Enterobacter spp.	MAC	LF; may be mucoid
	HE	Yellow
	XLD	Yellow
Escherichia spp.	MAC	Most LF, some NLF (some isolates may demonstrate slow or late fermentation); generally flat, dry, pink colonies with a surrounding darker pink area of precipitated bile salts[b]
	HE	Yellow
	XLD	Yellow
Hafnia alvei	MAC	NLF
	HE	Colorless
	XLD	Red or yellow
Klebsiella spp.	MAC	LF; mucoid
	HE	Yellow
	XLD	Yellow
Morganella spp.	MAC	NLF
	HE	Colorless
	XLD	Red or colorless
Plesiomonas shigelloides	BAP	Shiny, opaque, smooth, nonhemolytic
	MAC	Can be NLF or LF
Proteus spp.	MAC	NLF; may swarm, depending on the amount of agar in the medium; characteristic foul smell
	HE	Colorless
	XLD	Yellow or colorless, with or without black centers
Providencia spp.	MAC	NLF
	HE	Colorless
	XLD	Yellow or colorless
Salmonella spp.	MAC	NLF
	HE	Green, black center as a result of H_2S production
	XLD	Red with black center
Serratia spp.	MAC	Late LF; *Serratia marcescens* may be red pigmented, especially if plate is left at 25°C (Fig. 19.2)
	HE	Colorless
	XLD	Yellow or colorless
Shigella spp.	MAC	NLF; *Shigella sonnei* produces flat colonies with jagged edges
	HE	Green
	XLD	Colorless

TABLE 19.5 **Colonial Appearance and Characteristics of the Most Commonly Isolated Enterobacterales^a—cont'd**

Organism	Medium	Appearance
Yersinia spp.	MAC	NLF; may be colorless to peach
	HE	Salmon
	XLD	Yellow or colorless

HE, Hektoen enteric agar; *LF*, lactose fermenter, pink colony; *MAC*, MacConkey agar; *NLF*, non–lactose fermenter, colorless colony; *XLD*, xylose-lysine-deoxycholate agar.

[a]Most Enterobacterales are indistinguishable on blood agar; see text for colonial description.

[b]Pink colonies on MacConkey agar with sorbitol are sorbitol fermenters; colorless colonies are non–sorbitol fermenters.

TABLE 19.6 **Biochemical Differentiation of Unusual LDC-, ODC-, and ADH-Negative Enterobacterales**

Genus	Gas from Glucose	Motility	KCN	VP	Acid Fermentation L-Arabitol	Sucrose	Trehalose
Budvicia			neg				
Leclercia	pos	pos	pos	neg	pos	pos	pos
Moellerella	pos	pos	V	neg	pos	neg	pos
Rahnella	pos	neg	neg	neg	neg	pos	pos
Tatumella	neg	neg	neg	neg	neg	pos	pos
Photorhabdus	neg	pos	neg	neg	neg	neg	neg

ADH, Arginine dihydrolase; *KCN*, potassium cyanide; *LDC*, lysine decarboxylase; *ODC*, ornithine decarboxylase; *neg*, negative 10%; *pos*, positive 90%; *V*, variable 11% to 89%; *VP*, Voges-Proskauer test.

agar (LIA) to presumptively identify enteric pathogens (see Chapter 12 for information on the principles, performance, and interpretation of these tests). Organisms that exhibit the profiles shown in Table 19.8 require further biochemical profiling and, in the case of *Salmonella* spp. and *Shigella* spp., serotyping to establish a definitive identification. Bacterial species not considered capable of causing gastrointestinal infections give profiles other than those shown, but further testing may be required.

In most clinical laboratories, serotyping of Enterobacterales is limited to the preliminary grouping of *Salmonella* spp., *Shigella* spp., and *E. coli* O157:H7. Typing should be performed from a non–sugar-containing medium, such as 5% sheep blood agar or LIA. Use of sugar-containing media, such as MacConkey or TSI agars, can cause the organisms to autoagglutinate.

Commercially available polyvalent antisera designated A, B, C₁, C₂, D, E, and Vi are used to preliminarily group *Salmonella* spp. Approximately 95% of the isolates belong to groups A through E. The antisera A through E contain antibodies against somatic ("O") antigens, and the Vi antiserum is prepared against the capsular ("K") antigen of *Salmonella* serotype Typhi. Typing is performed using a slide agglutination test. Complete typing of *Salmonella* spp., including the

use of antisera against the flagellar ("H") antigens, is performed at reference laboratories. Although rarely isolated in the United States, *Salmonella* serotypes Paratyphi A, B, and C can cause a disease similar to typhoid fever. *Salmonella* serotype Paratyphi B is associated with paratyphoid fever and gastroenteritis. Isolates associated with gastroenteritis are typically tartrate-positive, and those associated with paratyphoid fever are tartrate-negative.

Preliminary serologic grouping of *Shigella* spp. is also performed using commercially available polyvalent somatic ("O") antisera designated A (15 serotypes), B (8 serotypes), C (19 serotypes), and D (*S. sonnei*, single serotype). In some cases, slide agglutination testing with polyvalent antisera may be followed with monovalent testing for specific serotype identification. Monovalent antiserum for *S. dysenteriae* 1 is required but not widely available. As with *Salmonella* spp., *Shigella* spp. may produce a capsule, and therefore heating may be required before typing is successful. Isolates that produce a capsule will agglutinate poorly or not at all. These isolates should be suspended in saline and heated in a waterbath for 15 to 30 minutes at 100°C. After cooling, the organism should be tested for autoagglutination in normal saline. If the organism does not autoagglutinate, it can then be tested using antisera for subtyping. Subtyping of

Genus	Organism	Indole	VP	SC	H_2S	Urea	M 37°C	LDC	ADH	ODC	PDA	ONPG	LAC	SUC	ARA	MAN	ADO	SOR	RAF	RHA
	Escherichia coli	+	-	-	-	-	+	+	-v	+v	-	+	+	V	+	+	-	+	V	+
	Escherichia coli (inactive)	+	-	-	-	-	-	-v	-v	-	-	+	-v	-	+	+	-	+v	-	+v
	Edwardsiella tarda	+	-	-	+	-	+	+	-	+	-	-	-	-	-	-	-	-	-	-
	Ewingella americana	-	+	+	-	-	+v	-	-	-	-	+v	+v	-	-	+	-	-	-	-
Shigella	Shigella boydii	-v	-	-	-	-	-	-	-v	-	-	-	-	-	+	+	-	+v	-	-v
Shigella	Shigella dysenteriae	-v	-	-	-	-	-	-	-v	-	-	-v	-	-	-v	-	-	-v	-	-v
Shigella	Shigella flexneri	-v	-	-	-	-	-	-	-v	-	-	-	-	-	+v	+	-	-v	-v	-v
Shigella	Shigella sonnei	-	-	-	-	-	-	-	-	+	-	+	-	-	+	+	-	-v	-	+v
Salmonella	S. serotype Paratyphi A	-	-	-	+w	-	+	-	+v	+	-	-	-	-	+	+	-	+	-	+
Salmonella	S. serotype Typhi	-	-	-	+w	-	+	+	-	-	-	-	-	-	-	+	-	+	-	-
	Hafnia alvei	-	+	+	-	-	+	+	-	+	-	+	-	-	+	+	-	-	-v	-
Citrobacter	C. braakii	+v	-	+v	+v	-v	+	-	+	+	-	+	+	-	+	+	-	+	-	+
Citrobacter	C. freundii	-	-	+	+	-v	+	-	+v	-	-	+	+v	+v	+	+	-	+	-	+
Citrobacter	C. koseri	+	-	+	-	+v	+	-	+	+	-	+	-v	-v	+	+	+	+	+	+
	Pantoea agglomerans	-v	+v	V	-	-v	+	-	-	-	-v	+	-v	+v	+	+	-	-v	-v	-v
	Enterobacter cloacae	-	+	+	-	-v	+	-	+	+	-	+	+	+	+	+	+	-v	+	+
Klebsiella	K. aerogenes	-	+	+	-	-	+	+	-	+	-		+	+	+	+	+	+	+	+
Klebsiella	K. oxytoca	+	+	+	-	+	+	+	-	-	-	+	+	+	+	+	+	+	+	+
Klebsiella	K. pneumoniae	-	+	+	-	+	-	+	-	-	-	+	+	+	+	+	+	+	+	+
	Cronobacter sakazakii	-	+	+	-	-	+	-	+	+	+v	+	+	+	+	+	-	-	+	+
Serratia	S. marcescens biogroup 1	-	+v	-v	-	-	-v	+v	-v	+v	-	+v	-v	+	-	+	+v	+	-	-
Serratia	S. marcescens subsp. marcescens	-	+	+	-	-v	+	+	-	+	-	+	-	+	-	+	+v	+	-	-
Serratia	S. odorifera biogroup 1	+v	V	+	-	-v	+	+	-	+	-	+	+v	+	+	+	+v	+	-v	+v
Serratia	S. odorifera biogroup 2	V	+	+	-	-	+	+	-	-	-	+	+	-	+	+	+v	+	-	+
Proteus	P. mirabilis	-	V	+v	+	+	+	-	-	+	+	-	-	+	-	-	-	-	-	-
Proteus	P. penneri	-	-	-	-v	+	+	-	-	-	+v	-v	-	+	-	-	-	-v	-	-
Proteus	P. vulgaris	+	-	-v	+	+	+	-	-	-	+	-v	-	+	-	-	-	-	-	-
Providencia	P. alcalifaciens	+	-	+	-	-	+	-	-	-v	+	-v	-	-v	-v	-v	+	-v	-v	-v
Providencia	P. rettgeri	+	-	+	-	+	+	-	-	-	+	+v	-	+	-	+	+	-	-	+v
Providencia	P. stuartii	+	-	+	-	-v	+v	-	-	-	+	+v	-	V	-	-v	+	-	-	-
Morganella	M. morganii subsp. morganii	+	-	-	+v	+	+	V	-	+	+	+v	-	-	-	-	-	-	-	-
Morganella	M. morganii subsp. sibonii	V	-	-	+v	+	+v	-v	-	+v	+	-	-	+v	-	-	-	-	-	-
	Yersinia enterocolitica	V	-	-	-	+	-	-	-	+	-	+	-	+	+	+	-	+	-	-

• **Fig. 19.5** Biochemical differentiation of representative Enterobacterales. *ADH*, Arginine dihydrolase; *ADO*, adonitol; *ARA*, arabinose; *INO*, inositol; *LAC*, lactose; *LDC*, lysine decarboxylase; *M 37°C*, motility at 37°C; *MAN*, mannitol; *ODC*, ornithine decarboxylase; *ONPG*, o-nitrophenyl-B-D-galactopyranoside; *PDA*, phenylalanine deaminase; *RAF*, raffinose; *RHA*, rhamnose; *SC*, Simmons citrate; *SOR*, sorbitol; *SUC*, sucrose; *VP*, Voges Proskauer; +v, greater probability for a positive reaction ≥51%; -v, greater probability for negative reaction ≥51%; +, positive ≥80%; -, negative ≥80%; V, equal probability 50% as positive or negative; +w, weak reaction.

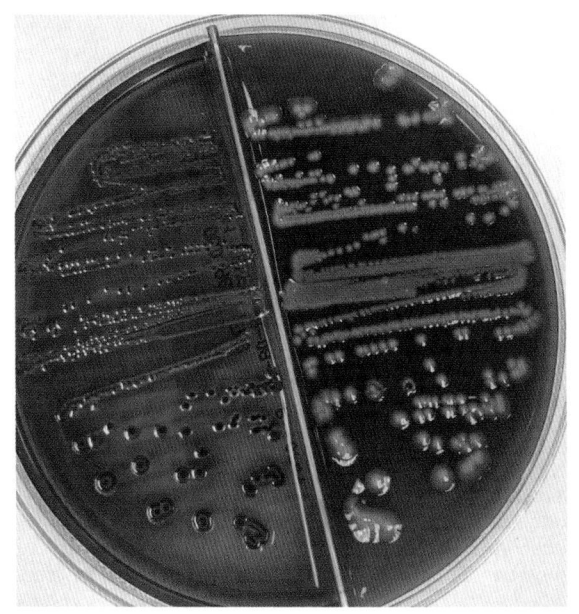

• **Fig. 19.6** *Escherichia coli* on a sheep blood agar, eosin methylene blue (EMB) biplate demonstrating strong lactose fermentation as evidenced by the extensive green metallic sheen on EMB.

Shigella spp. beyond the groups A, B, C, and D is typically performed in reference laboratories.

P. shigelloides, a new member of the Enterobacterales that can cause gastrointestinal infections (Chapter 25), might cross-react with *Shigella* grouping antisera, particularly group D, and lead to misidentification. This mistake can be prevented by performing an oxidase test.

Sorbitol-negative *E. coli* can be serotyped using commercially available antisera to determine whether the somatic "O" antigen 157 and the flagellar "H" antigen 7 are present. Latex reagents and antisera are now also available for detecting some non-O157, sorbitol-fermenting, Shiga-toxin–producing strains of *E. coli* (Meridian Diagnostics, Cincinnati, OH; Oxoid, Ogdensburg, NY). Some national reference laboratories therefore are simply performing tests for Shiga toxin rather than searching for O157 or non-O157 strains by culture. Laboratory tests to identify EPEC, ETEC, EIEC, and EAEC that cause gastrointestinal infections usually involve animal, tissue culture, or nucleic acid–based studies performed in reference laboratories. Nucleic acid amplification tests that detect and differentiate EPEC,

TABLE 19.7	TSI and LIA Reactions Used to Screen for Enteropathogenic Enterobacterales and *Aeromonas/Vibrio* spp.[a,b]	
TSI Reactions[c]	**LIA Reactions[c]**	**Possible Identification**
K/ⓐ or K/A H2S+	K/K or K/NC H2S+	*Salmonella* serotypes *Edwardsiella* spp.
K/A H2S+	K/K or K/NC H2S+	*Salmonella* serotypes (rare)
K/ⓐ	K/K or K/NC	*Salmonella* serotypes (rare)
K/A, H2S	K/K or K/NC H2S+	*Salmonella* serotype Typhi (rare)
K/ⓐ	K/A H2S+	*Salmonella* serotype Paratyphi A (usually H2S–)
K/ⓐ	K/A or A/A	*Escherichia* spp. *Salmonella* serotype Paratyphi A *Shigella flexneri* 6 (uncommon) *Aeromonas* spp. (oxidase positive)
K/A	K/K or K/NC	*Plesiomonas* sp. (oxidase positive) *Salmonella* serotype Typhi (rare) *Vibrio* spp. (oxidase positive)
K/A	K/A or A/A	*Escherichia* spp. *Shigella* groups A-D *Yersinia* spp.
A/ⓐ H2S+	K/K or K/NC H2S+	*Salmonella* serotypes (rare)
A/A	K/A or A/A	*Escherichia* spp. *Yersinia* spp. *Aeromonas* spp. (oxidase positive) *Vibrio cholerae* (rare, oxidase positive)
A/A	K/K or K/NC	*Vibrio* spp. (oxidase positive)

A, Acid; ⓐ, acid and gas production; H_2S, hydrogen sulfide; *K,* alkaline; *LIA,* lysine iron agar; *NC,* no change; *TSI,* triple sugar iron agar.
[a]*Vibrio* spp. and *Aeromonas* spp. are included in this table because they grow on the same media as the Enterobacterales and may be enteric pathogens; identification of these organisms is discussed in Chapter 26.
[b]TSI and LIA reactions described in this table are only screening tests. The identity of possible enteric pathogens must be confirmed by specific biochemical and serologic testing.
[c]Details regarding the TSI and LIA procedures can be found in Chapter 12.

TABLE 19.8 Therapy for Gastrointestinal Infections Caused by Enterobacterales

Organisms	Therapeutic Strategies
Enterotoxigenic *Escherichia coli* (ETEC), enteroinvasive *E. coli* (EIEC), enteropathogenic *E. coli* (EPEC), enterohemorrhagic *E. coli* (STEC), enteroaggregative *E. coli* (EAEC)	Supportive therapy, such as oral rehydration, is indicated in cases of severe diarrhea; for life-threatening infections, such as hemolytic uremic syndrome associated with STEC, transfusion and hemodialysis may be necessary. Antimicrobial therapy may shorten the duration of gastrointestinal illness, but many of these infections resolve without such therapy. Because these organisms may develop resistance, antimicrobial drug therapy for non–life-threatening infections may be contraindicated.
Shigella spp.	Oral rehydration; antimicrobial drug therapy may be used to shorten the period of fecal excretion and perhaps limit the clinical course of the infection. However, because of the risk of resistance, using antimicrobial drug therapy for less serious infections may be unwise.
Salmonella serotypes	For enteric fevers (e.g., typhoid fever) and extraintestinal infections (e.g., bacteremia), antimicrobial agents play an important role in therapy. Potentially effective agents for typhoid include quinolones, chloramphenicol, trimethoprim/sulfamethoxazole, and advanced-generation cephalosporins such as ceftriaxone; however, first- and second-generation cephalosporins and aminoglycosides are not effective. For nontyphoidal *Salmonella* bacteremia, a third-generation cephalosporin (e.g., ceftriaxone) is commonly used. For gastroenteritis, replacement of fluids is most important. Antimicrobial therapy generally is not recommended for treatment of the clinical infection or for shortening the amount of time a patient excretes the organism.
Yersinia enterocolitica and *Yersinia pseudotuberculosis*	The need for antimicrobial therapy for enterocolitis and mesenteric lymphadenitis is not clear. In cases of bacteremia, pseudotuberculosis piperacillin, third-generation cephalosporins, aminoglycosides, and trimethoprim/sulfamethoxazole are potentially effective agents. *Y. enterocolitica* is commonly resistant to ampicillin and first-generation cephalosporins, whereas *Y. pseudotuberculosis* isolates are generally susceptible.

ETEC, EHEC, EAEC, and STEC direct from a stool sample are also commercially available. Additionally, in 2019 the CDC officially migrated foodborne disease surveillance away from PFGE to wgMLST, which provides serotype information for foodborne pathogens.

The current recommendation for the diagnosis of Shiga toxin–producing *E. coli* includes testing all stools submitted from patients with acute community-acquired diarrhea to detect enteric pathogens (*Salmonella, Shigella,* and *Campylobacter* spp.). Stool samples should be cultured for O157 STEC on selective and differential agar and assayed for non-O157 STEC. Because it is impossible to distinguish O157 from other *E. coli* using routine media containing lactose, media containing D-sorbitol is used. Eighty percent of *E. coli* strains ferment sorbitol; however, O157 STEC is a nonsorbitol fermenter after 24 hours of incubation. In addition to MAC supplemented with sorbitol, additional media have been developed to assist in the identification of these organisms. CHROMagar O157 and cefixime-tellurite-containing MacConkey (CT-SMAC) demonstrate improved sensitivity for the isolation of O157 STEC. In addition, the stool samples should be tested using a Shiga-toxin detection assay or a nucleic acid–based assay to determine whether the sample contains a non-O157 STEC. To save media, some laboratories may elect to perform the assay first, and then attempt to grow organisms from broths with an assay-positive result on selective media. O157 STEC strains are beta-glucuronidase negative. In addition, O157 STEC strains and 60% to 80% of non-O157 STEC strains produce alpha-enterohemolysin (Ehly). A washed sheep blood agar supplemented with calcium (WSBA-CA) can be used to identify these isolates. Alpha-hemolytic *E. coli* strains are visible within 3 to 4 hours of incubation at 37°C, whereas enterohemolysins do not appear until 18 to 24 hours of incubation. In any case, any isolate or broth positive for O157 STEC, non-O157 STEC, or Shiga-toxin should be forwarded to the public health laboratory for confirmation and direct immunoassay testing. Identification of STEC is a reportable condition in many if not most public health jurisdictions. STEC isolates should be sent to the public health laboratory for additional epidemiologic analysis. Any specimens or enrichment broths that are positive for Shiga-toxin or STEC but negative for O157 STEC should also be sent to the public health laboratory for further testing. Isolation of ETEC, EPEC, EIEC, and EAEC are generally completed during major outbreaks at a public health or reference laboratory.

Most commercial systems can identify *Y. pestis* if a heavy inoculum is used. However, a suspected *Y. pestis* should never be identified using automated platforms. Instead, standard rule-out and refer methods should be used to presumptively identify *Y. pestis;* please contact your local or state public health laboratory for additional information regarding rule-out and refer procedures. Criteria used to presumptively identify *Y. pestis* include slow growing, gram-negative rods that are lactose non-fermenting on MAC. Additionally, *Y. pestis* is oxidase, indole, and urease negative, and catalase positive. Any isolate that meets these criteria should be tested by a Laboratory Response Network member-laboratory using LRN protocols in a BSL-3 facility. A variety of NAATs can be used for the detection of *Yersinia* spp. in patient specimens and a variety of platforms are available including multiplex assays.

Serodiagnosis

Serodiagnostic techniques are used for only two members of Enterobacterales: *Salmonella* serotype Typhi and *Y. pestis.* Agglutinating antibodies can be measured in the diagnosis of typhoid fever; a serologic test for *Salmonella* serotype Typhi A latex agglutination test for screening in SEL enrichment broth for *Salmonella,* Wellcolex Color *Salmonella* (Remel, Inc., Lenexa, KS), is available. The kit can be used to screen colonies isolated on primary culture media. The Vi antigen, as previously described, is not specific to *Salmonella* serotype Typhi. It has also been detected on *Salmonella* serotypes Dublin and Paratyphi C and some isolates of *Citrobacter* spp. The organism should be tested using O group D1 (O:9) antiserum and Vi antiserum. It is possible for the Vi capsular polysaccharide to mask the agglutination reaction of the O antigens and antiserum. If the Vi antiserum is positive and the O antiserum is negative, the isolate should be heated in boiling water for 15 minutes to remove the capsule. After it cools, the suspension should be retested for the O group D1 antiserum. A presumptive identification based on a positive Vi, O, urease negative, and typical reactions on TSI or Kilger Iron agar (KIA) may be reported.

Serologic diagnosis of plague is possible using enzyme-linked immunosorbent assay for the detection of *Y. pestis* F1 antigen in bubo aspirates and serum. This assay has been adapted to a lateral-flow immunochromatographic dipstick for field use. These tests are available commercially in the United States.

Matrix-Assisted Laser Desorption Ionization Time-of-Flight Mass Spectrometry

MALDI-TOF MS has become a very popular technique for identification of Enterobacterales. Based on the confidence level, the accuracy of the mass spectrometric identification was compared with 16S rRNA gene sequencing. Advances in microbial genomic research led to the recognition that many mass spectral peaks represent ribosomal proteins, and this proteomic technology can be used to identify clinically important bacteria such as Enterobacterales. Reference mass spectra libraries and software developed for data analysis are incorporated into commercial MALDI-TOF MS identification systems for use in clinical laboratories.

Antimicrobial Susceptibility Testing and Therapy

For many of the gastrointestinal infections caused by Enterobacterales, inclusion of antimicrobial agents as part of the therapeutic strategy is controversial or at least uncertain (Table 19.7).

For extraintestinal infections, antimicrobial therapy is a vital component of patient management (Table 19.8). Although a broad spectrum of agents may be used for therapy against Enterobacterales (see Table 11.6 for a detailed list), every clinically relevant species is capable of acquiring and using one or more of the resistance mechanisms discussed in Chapter 11. The unpredictable nature of any clinical isolate's antimicrobial susceptibility requires that testing be completed as a guide to therapy. Several standard methods and commercial systems have been developed for this purpose. Tables 19.9 and 19.10 present intrinsic patterns of resistance identified in Enterobacterales.

Extended Spectrum Beta-Lactamase–Producing Enterobacterales

Enterobacterales are capable of producing beta-lactamases that hydrolyze penicillins and cephalosporins, including the extended-spectrum cephalosporins (cefixime, ceftriaxone, ceftizoxime, and ceftazidime). These enzymes are referred to as extended spectrum beta-lactamases (**ESBLs**). A variety of chromogenic agars have been developed to identify ESBLs. One example, chromID ESBL (bioMérieux, Marcy l'Etoile, France), uses cefpodoxime as a substrate to increase the recovery and sensitivity of CTX-M type ESBL isolates. Some limitations must be considered when using this medium, including hyperproducing AmpC (*Enterobacter* and *Citrobacter* spp.) and hyperproducing penicillinase (*K. oxytoca*) false positives. Current automated susceptibility systems may not be able to accurately predict and detect ESBLs, AmpC, and *Klebsiella* carbapenemases (KPCs).

ESBLs can occur in bacteria other than *Klebsiella* spp., *E. coli,* and *P. mirabilis.* The Clinical and Laboratory Standards Institute (CLSI) has created guidelines (CLSI documents M-100 and M100-S25) for the minimum inhibitory concentration (MIC) and disk diffusion breakpoints for aztreonam, cefotaxime, cefpodoxime, ceftazidime, and ceftriaxone for *E. coli, Proteus* spp., and *Klebsiella* spp., as well as for cefpodoxime, ceftazidime, and cefotaxime for *P. mirabilis.* The sensitivity of the screening increases with the use of more than a single drug. ESBLs are inhibited by clavulanic acid and can be used as a confirmatory test in the identification process. Additionally, in cases where moxalactam, cefonicid, cefamandole, or cefoperazone is a treatment choice for infection caused by *E. coli, Klebsiella* spp., or *Proteus* spp., it is important to note that interpretive guidelines have not been evaluated, and ESBL testing should be performed.

TABLE 19.9	Antimicrobial Therapy and Susceptibility Testing of Clinically Relevant Enterobacterales			
Organism	Therapeutic Options	Potential Resistance to Therapeutic Options	Testing Methods[a]	Comments
Escherichia coli, Citrobacter spp., *Enterobacter* spp., *Morganella* spp., *Proteus* spp., *Providencia* spp., *Serratia* spp.	Several agents from each major class of antimicrobials, including aminoglycosides, beta-lactams, and quinolones, have activity. Table 11.7 includes a list of specific agents that should be selected for *in vitro* testing. For urinary tract infections, single agents may be used; for systemic infections, potent beta-lactams are used, typically in combination with an aminoglycoside.	Every species is capable of expressing resistance to one or more antimicrobials belonging to each drug class.	As documented in Chapter 11; disk diffusion agar dilution and commercial systems	*In vitro* susceptibility testing results are important for guiding broth dilution and therapy.
Yersinia pestis	Streptomycin is the therapy of choice; tetracycline and chloramphenicol are effective alternatives.	Yes, but rare.	See CLSI recommendations; testing must be performed only in a licensed reference laboratory.	Manipulation of cultures for susceptibility testing is dangerous for laboratory personnel and is not necessary.

[a]Validated testing methods include standard methods recommended by the Clinical and Laboratory Standards Institute (CLSI) and commercial methods approved by the US Food and Drug Administration (FDA).

If isolates test ESBL-positive, the results of the antibiotics listed should be reported as resistant.

The CLSI has revised the guidelines for susceptibility testing, lowering the breakpoints for cephalosporins and aztreonam. This eliminates the need for routine ESBL testing but requires an edit on reports to change cephalosporins, aztreonam, or penicillins that are indicated as susceptible to resistant. In addition, cefepime breakpoints have been reviewed and replaced the intermediate resistant category with what is referred to as "susceptible dose dependent," or SDD (Chapter 11). The treatment is based on higher doses, more frequent doses, or both.

Because of the problematic phenotypic detection for ESBLS, nucleic acid–based methods are becoming more widely used in the clinical microbiology laboratory. These tests detect the TEM and SHV beta-lactamase genes followed by nucleic acid sequencing. PCR amplification of the CTX-M beta-lactamase genes does not require sequencing, because amplification generally is sufficient evidence that the enzyme is responsible for the ESBL phenotype. It is highly recommended that laboratories institute screening primary clinical specimens using selective culture media such as MacConkey supplemented with cefotaxime and/or ceftazidime. These media are commercially available as BLSE agar (bioMérieux, Durham, NC) and EbSA ESBL agar (AlphaOmega B.V., The Netherlands). In addition to the chromogenic media, chromID ESBL (bioMérieux, Durham, NC) previously described, additional chromogenic media is available, including Brilliance ESBL (Oxoid Ltd., Basingstoke, United Kingdom) and CHROMagar ESBL CHROMagar, Paris, France).

Expanded-Spectrum Cephalosporin Resistance and Carbapenem Resistance

The explosion of molecular biology in the past two decades has provided molecular strategies to complement phenotypic identification of drug resistance. The bacterial chromosome represents the majority of the genetic make-up or genome within a single organism. However, many genes may be located on extrachromosomal elements such as transposons and plasmids, which are capable of independent replication and movement between organisms. Transposable elements are pieces of DNA that move from one genetic element to another, such as from the plasmid to the chromosome or vice versa (Chapter 2). In addition, these elements may have a complex structure, including the presence of integrins, which are genetic elements specifically designed to take up and incorporate or integrate genes such as those that encode antibiotic resistance. Multidrug resistant organisms are increasing in frequency on a worldwide basis because of these mobile genetic elements; a single bacterium can have numerous mobile elements that confer resistance as well as chromosomally encoded or intrinsic resistance.

AmpC beta-lactamases are clinically important cephalosporinases encoded on the chromosomes of many of the Enterobacterales and a few other organisms, where they mediate resistance to cephalothin, cefazolin, cefoxitin, most penicillins, and beta-lactamase inhibitor–beta-lactam combinations. In many bacteria, AmpC enzymes are inducible and can be expressed at high levels. Overexpression confers resistance to broad-spectrum cephalosporins including cefotaxime, ceftazidime, and ceftriaxone and is a problem especially in infections caused by *K. aerogenes* and *E. cloacae,* where an isolate initially susceptible to these agents may become resistant upon therapy. Transmissible plasmids have acquired genes for AmpC enzymes, which consequently can now appear in bacteria lacking or poorly expressing a chromosomal *blaAmpC* gene, such as *E. coli, K. pneumoniae,* and *P. mirabilis.* Resistance because of plasmid-mediated AmpC enzymes is less common than extended-spectrum beta-lactamase production in most parts of the world but may be both harder to detect and broader in spectrum. AmpC enzymes encoded by both chromosomal and plasmid genes are evolving to hydrolyze broad-spectrum cephalosporins more efficiently. Carbapenems, often considered a therapy of last resort for serious infections, can be a viable therapeutic option for infections caused by AmpC-producing bacteria. However, worldwide distribution of beta-lactamases known as carbapenemases, such as the *Klebsiella pneumoniae* carbapenemase (*kpc*), effectively neutralize carbapenems like meropenem, imipenem, ertapenem, and doripenem. These organisms are classified as carbapenem-resistant Enterobacterales (CRE) and are spreading at an alarming rate.

The spread of **carbapenem resistance in both healthcare and community settings is a serious concern worldwide.** Numerous **carbapenemases** exist and include KPC **(class A),** Verona integrin mediated carbapenemase (VIM), imipenemases (IMP), New Delhi metallo-beta-lactamases (NDM**; class B),** and oxacillinases (e.g., OXA-48; class D). Class A, C, and D beta-lactamases are the enzymes that contain serine at the active site. The **metallo-beta-lactamases** (class B) require a zinc ion for hydrolysis. Genes encoding the beta-lactamase enzymes can mutate in response to the heavy pressure exerted by antibiotic use. AmpC class **(class C)** genes that were originally carried on chromosomes can be found on plasmids. The last class of beta-lactamases is referred to as **oxacillinase (class D)** and contains a higher hydrolysis rate for oxacillin than penicillin.

Carbapenem resistance is most often mediated by mobile genetic elements that produce an enzyme capable of hydrolyzing almost all known beta-lactam antibiotics. These mobile genetic elements include the various classes of nontypeable plasmids (using current PCR-based replicon typing) and the IncHI family of plasmids. These plasmids demonstrate conjugative transfer (movement between individual bacterial cells) at a higher frequency at 30°C than at 37°C. The carbapenem resistance gene within these plasmids may also be included in a cassette of genes that are flanked by insertion sequences or small transposons that facilitate the movement of the gene between genetic elements. In addition, many of these genes, in particular the NDM (class B) are neither species- nor plasmid-specific, therefore indicating a limitless boundary for spread of this resistance. OXA-48 is carried on a composite transposon known as TN1999 or variants of the transposon known as TN1999.2 and TN1999.3. The metallo-beta-lactamases are also transferable via a plasmid, and in addition to beta-lactamase resistance, the strains are commonly resistant to aminoglycosides and fluoroquinolones while remaining susceptible to polymyxins.

These resistant determinants appear to be capable of existing in a very diverse genetic background and can move from one genetic element to another, one organism to another, and across genus and species lines in an unlimited capacity. It is therefore important for practitioners and laboratorians to not overlook or ignore any new emerging antibiotic patterns of resistance where they least expect them to occur.

Guidelines are currently available from the CDC to prevent CRE (e.g., contact precautions). Guidelines are available at http://www.cdc.gov/hai/organisms/cre/cre-toolkit/index.html.

Many of these organisms have been identified in patients in the United States after previous treatment outside of the United States. Techniques to identify AmpC beta-lactamase–producing isolates are available but are still evolving and are not optimized for the clinical laboratory. There are no published CLSI guidelines. Several laboratories have implemented an algorithm that includes screening for resistance to the cephamycins (i.e., cefoxitin and cefotetan), followed by an inhibitor-based confirmation test with boronic acid or cloxacillin. Some combination commercial E-tests or disks are also commercially available. The Modified Hodge Test (MHT) may be used as a screening test for carbapenemase resistance (Evolve Procedure 19.1). However, the MHT is notoriously nonspecific and a new test, the modified carbapenem inactivation method (mCIM), is now being used in many laboratories around the country as a replacement for the MHT. The mCIM uses a 10 μg meropenem disk incubated for 2 hours in an aqueous suspension of the carbapenemase producing organism. The carbapenem in the disk is degraded in a resistant organism. After incubation, the disk is removed from the suspension and placed on a Mueller-Hinton agar plate with a carbapenemase susceptible organism. Following overnight incubation, the zone of inhibition is measured to determine if the carbapenem was still active or had been inactivated by the test organism. In addition, there are PCR and DNA microarray methods available for the detection of the beta-lactamases and carbapenemases, such as the Check-MDR Arrays ESBL (the Netherlands) and the Cepheid GenXpert CARBA-R. Because of the rapidly changing resistance

TABLE 19.10 Intrinsic Antibiotic Resistance in Enterobacterales[a]

	Escherichia	Hafnia	Serratia	Yersinia	K.	Citrobacter		Enterobacter		Proteus			Providencia	
	hermannii	alvei	marcescens	enterocolitica	pneumoniae	C. freundii	C. koseri	E. cloacae	E. aerogenes	P. vulgaris	P. mirabilis	P. penneri	P. rettgeri	P. stuarti
Ampicillin	R	R	R	R	R	R	R	R	R	R		R	R	R
Amoxicillin/clavulanate	R	R	R	R		R		R	R	R		R	R	R
Ampicillin/sulbactam	R	R	R			R	R	R	R					
Piperacillin							R							
Ticarcillin	R			R	R		R							
Cephalosporins I: cefazolin and cephalothin	R	R	R	R		R		R	R	R		R	R	R
Cephamycins, cefoxitin, and cefotetan		R	R			R		R	R					
Cephalosporins II: cefuroxime			R			R		R	R	R			R	
Tetracyclines										R	R	R	R	R
Nitrofurantoin			R							R	R	R	R	R
Polymyxin B and colistin			R							R	R	R	R	R

[a]Cephalosporins III, cefepime, aztreonam, ticarcillin/clavulanate, piperacillin/tazobactam, and the carbapenems are not listed because the Enterobacterales have no intrinsic resistance to these antibiotics.
Modified from Clinical and Laboratory Standards Institute (CLSI). *Performance Standards for Antimicrobial Susceptibility Testing—Nineteenth Informational Supplement, M100-S25.* Wayne, PA: CLSI; 2015.

mechanisms present in Enterobacterales, it is important to consult the most recent guidelines for susceptibility testing and reporting criteria published annually by the CLSI.

Multidrug-Resistant Typhoid Fever

Multidrug-resistant typhoid fever (MDRTF) is caused by *Salmonella* serotype Typhi strains resistant to chloramphenicol, ampicillin, and cotrimoxazole. Isolates classified as MDRTF have been identified since the early 1990s in patients of all ages. The risk for the development of MDRTF is associated with the overuse, misuse, and inappropriate use of antibiotic therapy. Susceptibility tests should be performed using the typical first-line antibiotics, including chloramphenicol, ampicillin, and trimethoprim-sulfamethoxazole, along with a fluoroquinolone and a nalidixic acid (to detect reduced susceptibility to fluoroquinolones), a third-generation cephalosporin, and any other antibiotic currently used for treatment.

Prevention

Vaccines are available for typhoid fever and bubonic plague; however, neither is routinely recommended in the United States. An oral multiple-dose vaccine against *Salmonella* serotype Typhi strain Ty2la or a parenteral single-dose vaccine containing Vi antigen is available for people traveling to an endemic area or for household contacts of a documented *Salmonella* serotype Typhi carrier.

An inactivated multiple-dose, whole-cell bacterial vaccine is available for bubonic plague for people traveling to an endemic area. However, this vaccine does not provide protection against pneumonic plague. Individuals exposed to pneumonic plague should be given chemoprophylaxis with doxycycline (adults) or trimethoprim/sulfamethoxazole (children younger than 8 years of age).

ⓔ Visit the Evolve site for a complete list of procedures, review questions, and case studies.

Bibliography

Bear N, Klugman KP, Tobiansky L, Koornhof HJ: Wound colonization by *Ewingella americana*, *J Clin Microbiol* 23:650–651, 1986.

Caroll KC, Pfaller MA: *Manual of clinical microbiology*, ed 12, Washington, DC, 2019, ASM Press.

Clinical and Laboratory Standards Institute (CLSI): *Performance standards for antimicrobial susceptibility testing—nineteenth informational supplement, M100-S21*, Wayne, PA, 2011, CLSI.

Clinical and Laboratory Standards Institute (CLSI): *Performance standards for antimicrobial susceptibility testing; Twenty Third Informational Supplement, M100-S25*, Wayne, PA, 2015, CLSI.

Committee on Infectious Diseases: *2006 red book: report of the Committed on Infectious Diseases*, ed 27, Elk Grove Village, IL, 2006, American Academy of Pediatrics.

Laboratories Difco: *Differentiation of Enterobacteriaceae by biochemical tests*, Detroit, 1980, Difco Laboratories.

Dolejska M, Villa L, Poirel L, Nordmann P, Carattoli A: Complete sequencing of an IncHI1 plasmid encoding the carbapenemase NDM-1, the ARMA 16S RNA methylase and a resistance-nodulation-cell division/multidrug efflux pump, *J Antimicrob Chemother* 68:34–39, 2013.

Gould LH, Bopp C, Strockbine N, et al.: Recommendations for diagnosis of Shiga toxin-producing *Escherichia coli* infections by clinical laboratories, *MMWR Recomm Rep* 58:1–14, 2009.

Khan R, Rizvi M, Shukia I, Malik A: A novel approach for identification of members of *Enterobacteriaceae* isolated from clinical samples, *Biol Med* 3:313, 2011.

Mortimer CK, Peters TM, Gharbia SE, Logan JM, Arnold C: Towards the development of a DNA-sequence based approach to serotyping of *Salmonella enterica*, *BMC Microbiol* 4:31, 2004.

Noyal MJ, Menezes GA, Harish BN, Sujatha S, Parija SC: Simple screening tests for detection of carbapenemases in clinical isolates of nonfermentative Gram-negative bacteria, *Indian J Med Res* 129:707–712, 2009.

Oteo J, Hernandez JM, Espasa M, et al.: Emergence of OXA-48-producing *Klebsiella pneumoniae* and the novel carbapenemases OXA-244 and OXA-245 in Spain, *J Antimicrob Chemother* 68:317–321, 2013.

Passarelli-Araujo H, Palmeiro JK, Moharana K, et al.: Genomic analysis unveils important aspects of population structure, virulence, and antimicrobial resistance in *Klebsiella aerogenes*, *FEBS J* 286(19):3797–3810, 2019, https://doi.org/10.1111/febs.15005. Accessed 1 August 2019.

Pierce VM, Simner PJ, Lonsway DR, et al.: Modified carbapenem inactivation method for phenotypic detection of carbapenemase production among *Enterobacteriaceae*, *J Clin Microbiol* 55(8):2321–2333, 2017.

Rodriguez-Martinez JM, Fernandez-Echauri P, Fernandez-Cuenca F, Diaz de Alba P, Briales A, Pascual A: Genetic characterization of an extended-spectrum AmpC cephalosporinase with hydrolysing activity against fourth-generation cephalosporins in a clinical isolate of *Enterobacter aerogenes* selected *in vivo*, *J Antimicrob Chemother* 67:64–68, 2012.

Schultsz C, Geerlings S: Plasmid-mediated resistance in *Enterobacteriaceae*, changing landscape and implications for therapy, *Drugs* 72:1–16, 2012.

Willemsen I, Hille L, Vrolijk A, Bergmans A, Kluytmans J: Evaluation of a commercial real-time PCR for the detection of extended spectrum β-lactamase genes, *J Med Microbiol* 63:540–543, 2014.

Zaki S.A., Karande S.: Multidrug-resistant typhoid fever: a review, *J Infect Dev Ctries* 5:324–337, 2011.

20

Acinetobacter, Stenotrophomonas, and Other Organisms

OBJECTIVES

1. List the most common gram-negative organisms encountered in clinical specimens discussed in this chapter.
2. State the normal habitat for *Acinetobacter* spp. and the patients most at risk of infection.
3. Describe the Gram stain morphology of *Acinetobacter, Bordetella,* and *Stenotrophomonas* spp.
4. Describe the appearance and odor of *Stenotrophomonas maltophilia* when grown on blood agar.
5. Differentiate between the two groups of *Acinetobacter* organisms and identify the most dependable test to distinguish between the groups.

GENERA AND SPECIES TO BE CONSIDERED

Current Name

Acinetobacter baumannii
Acinetobacter calcoaceticus
Acinetobacter haemolyticus
Acinetobacter johnsonii
Acinetobacter junii
Acinetobacter lwoffii
Acinetobacter pittii
Acinetobacter radioresistens
Acinetobacter schindleri
Acinetobacter ursingii
Stenotrophomonas maltophilia
Bordetella holmesii
Bordetella parapertussis
Bordetella trematum
Burkholderia gladioli
Pseudomonas luteola
Pseudomonas oryzihabitans

General Characteristics

The organisms discussed in this chapter are a diverse group of nonfermenting gram-negative bacilli. These emerging pathogens are clinically important because they can cause a wide range of infections and are often multidrug resistant (MDR). Similar to the Enterobacterales, these organisms are oxidase negative and generally grow well on MacConkey agar. However, unlike the Enterobacterales, which ferment glucose, these organisms either oxidize glucose (i.e., they are saccharolytic) or do not utilize glucose (i.e., they are nonoxidizers, or asaccharolytic). Through the use of advanced molecular taxonomic techniques, 63 named species of *Acinetobacter* have been identified and reported as valid (http://www.bacterio.net/acinetobacter.html). The specific morphologic and physiologic features of the organisms are considered later in this chapter in the discussion of laboratory diagnosis. Of note, only *Acinetobacter* species and *Stenotrophomonas maltophilia* are routinely recovered from clinical specimens and discussed in depth; other less frequently encountered genera and species are mentioned briefly. According to DNA homology, the genus *Acinetobacter* is classified in the phylum Proteobacteria, class Gammaproteobacteria, order Pseudomonadales, family *Moraxellaceae.* The *Neisseriaceae* and the clinically relevant species *M. catarrhalis* are described in Chapters 27 and 39, respectively. The genus *Stenotrophomonas* is included in the same phylum Proteobacteria and class Gammaproteobacteria but classified in the order Xanthomonadales, family *Xanthomonadaceae. Acinetobacter baumannii* is one of the ESCAPE pathogens, a group of clinically significant health care–associated organisms that have a propensity for acquiring antimicrobial resistance determinants. Last, as some species of *Bordetella* have biochemical reactions that resemble those of *Acinetobacter* spp., they are briefly discussed in this chapter to help the reader distinguish them from other organisms but are discussed in detail in Chapter 36.

Epidemiology

The organisms discussed in this chapter most often inhabit environmental niches (e.g., water or soil) (Table 20.1). Species of *Acinetobacter* are distributed throughout the environment in soil and water. Clinical infections are more often identified in areas with temperate climates, and clinical

TABLE 20.1	Epidemiology	
Species	**Habitat (Reservoir)**	**Mode of Transmission**
Acinetobacter spp.	Widely distributed in nature, including the hospital environment; may become established as part of skin and respiratory microbiota of patients hospitalized for prolonged periods	Colonization of hospitalized patients from environmental factors; medical instrumentation (e.g., intravenous or urinary catheters) introduces organism to normally sterile sites
Stenotrophomonas maltophilia	Widely distributed in nature, including moist hospital environments; may become established as part of respiratory microbiota of patients hospitalized for prolonged periods	Colonization of hospitalized patients from environmental factors; medical instrumentation introduces organism to normally sterile sites (similar to transmission of *Acinetobacter* spp.)
Burkholderia gladioli	Environmental pathogen of plants; occasionally found in the respiratory tracts of patients with cystic fibrosis but not part of normal microbiota	Transmission to humans uncommon, mode of transmission not known
Pseudomonas luteola *Pseudomonas oryzihabitans*	Environmental, including moist hospital environments (e.g., respiratory therapy equipment); not part of normal human microbiota	Uncertain; probably involves exposure of debilitated hospital patients to contaminated fluids and medical equipment
Bordetella holmesii *Bordetella trematum*	Unknown or part of normal human microbiota	Unknown; rarely found in humans

infections with *Acinetobacter* seem to be higher in the summer months compared with other seasons. It is likely that the humid conditions are more favorable for growth. Some asaccharolytic *Acinetobacter* species are constituents of the human skin microbiota and contaminants when recovered from a positive blood culture. Carriage of *Acinetobacter* in the human gastrointestinal tract, respiratory tract, and on the skin is not uncommon.

S. maltophilia is ubiquitous in nature and is closely related to the genus *Pseudomonas*. It was first isolated from a human in 1943 and has undergone several taxonomic updates before finally being placed in a separate genus in 1993. These organisms are capable of survival on inanimate objects for extended periods (weeks to months). They are problematic in health care settings, where they frequently colonize the patients' environment and health care equipment. Both *Acinetobacter* spp. and *S. maltophilia* can contaminate potable or chlorinated water. The prevalence of these organisms is evidenced by the fact that, excluding the Enterobacterales and *Pseudomonas aeruginosa*, *Acinetobacter* spp. and *S. maltophilia* are the third and fourth most common gram-negative bacilli, respectively, encountered in clinical specimens.

Pathogenesis and Spectrum of Disease

All of the organisms listed in Table 20.2 are opportunistic pathogens. *Acinetobacter* spp. most often tend to infect intensive care unit (ICU) patients and patients residing in long-term care facilities. There are numerous risk factors related to colonization or infection with *Acinetobacter* among adult patients, including prior infection or colonization with methicillin-resistant *Staphylococcus aureus*, prior therapy with a beta-lactam antibiotic, prior

fluoroquinolone use, mechanical ventilation, tracheostomy, central venous catheterization, hemodialysis, malignancy, and enteral feeding. *Acinetobacter* spp. possess several key factors, including the ability to produce a lipopolysaccharide capsule, survival in dry environments, and adherence to mucosal epithelium via fimbriae; these contribute to the genus's virulence.

Infections with *S. maltophilia* in debilitated patients and those who are immunocompromised are often associated with high mortality rates. Infections caused by *S. maltophilia* are associated with the following risk factors: central venous catheterization, cystic fibrosis, ICU admission, malignancy, mechanical ventilation, neutropenia, previous broad-spectrum antibiotic therapy, recent surgery, and human immunodeficiency virus (HIV) infection. The rates of infection with *S. maltophilia* are increasing as the at-risk population increases. This is likely attributable to the increased utilization of medical devices and the use of broad-spectrum antimicrobial therapy to treat bacterial infections. *A. baumannii* has long been the species typically identified among nosocomial infections; however, other species are now being identified with increasing frequency due largely to the use of matrix-assisted laser desorption ionization time of flight (MALDI-TOF). Infections caused by *Acinetobacter* spp. and *S. maltophilia* usually involve the respiratory or genitourinary tract, bacteremia, and occasionally wound infections; however, infections including infective endocarditis, mastoiditis, peritonitis, and meningitis may also occur at several other body sites. Community-acquired infections with these organisms are less likely but can occur. The vast majority of infections are associated with health care. *Pseudomonas oryzihabitans* is rarely isolated in clinical specimens. Published case reports show that these bacteria have been isolated mainly from wounds but also occasionally from blood and dialysis fluid

TABLE 20.2	Pathogenesis and Spectrum of Diseases	
Species	**Virulence Factors**	**Spectrum of Disease and Infections**
Acinetobacter spp.	Unknown	Clinical isolates are often colonizers. True infections are usually noso-comial; occur during warm seasons; and most commonly involve the genitourinary tract, respiratory tract, wounds, soft tissues, and bacteremia.
Bordetella holmesii *Bordetella trematum*	Unknown	Bacteremia is the only type of infection described.
Burkholderia gladioli	Unknown	Role in human disease is uncertain; occasionally found in sputa of patients with cystic fibrosis, but clinical significance in this setting is uncertain.
Pseudomonas luteola *Pseudomonas oryzihabitans*	Unknown	Catheter-related infections, septicemia, and peritonitis, usually associ-ated with continuous ambulatory peritoneal dialysis, and miscella-neous mixed infections of other body sites.
Stenotrophomonas maltophilia	Unknown. Intrinsic resistance to almost every commonly used antibacterial agent supports the survival of this organism in the hospital environment.	Most infections are nosocomial and include catheter-related infections, bacteremia, wound infections, pneumonia, urinary tract infections, and miscellaneous infections of other body sites.

cultures. In contrast, *Pseudomonas luteola* is typically reported in skin infections, endocarditis, osteomyelitis, and meningitis after neurosurgical procedures. *Bordetella holmesii* is rare, but has been reported to cause severe systemic illness as well as pertussis-like symptoms and is commonly misidentified as *B. pertussis*, the causative agent of whooping cough (Chapter 36).

Laboratory Diagnosis

Specimen Collection and Transport

No special considerations are required for specimen collection and transport of the organisms discussed in this chapter. Refer to Table 5.1 for general information on specimen collection and transport.

Specimen Processing

No special considerations are required for processing of the organisms discussed in this chapter. Refer to Table 5.1 for general information on specimen processing.

Direct Detection Methods

Other than Gram staining patient specimens, there are no specific procedures for the direct detection of these organisms in clinical material. *Acinetobacter* spp. are plump coc-cobacilli that tend to resist alcohol decolorization, thus sometimes appearing gram positive. They also may be mis-taken for *Neisseria* spp. because of their similar microscopic appearance (i.e., shape and arrangement). The *Bordetella* spp. are coccobacilli or short rods. *S. maltophilia, P. oryzihabitans,* and *P. luteola* are short to medium-sized straight rods.

Cultivation

Media of Choice

All of the organisms discussed grow well on routine media such as Trypticase soy agar with 5% sheep blood and choco-late agars. Most of the organisms grow well on MacConkey agar, although *P. luteola* and *P. oryzihabitans* can sometimes be delayed or grow poorly on MacConkey agar. These organisms also grow well in the broth of blood culture sys-tems and in common nutrient broths, such as thioglycollate and brain-heart infusion.

Incubation Conditions and Duration

These organisms generally produce detectable growth on 5% sheep blood and chocolate agars when incubated at 35°C to 37°C in aerobic conditions or 5% carbon dioxide after 24 hours. MacConkey agar should be incubated only in ambient air.

Colonial Appearance

Table 20.3 describes the colonial appearance and other distinguishing characteristics (e.g., hemolysis and odor) of each genus when grown on Trypticase soy agar with 5% sheep blood and MacConkey agar.

Approach to Identification

Acinetobacter species and *S. maltophilia* are reliably identi-fied by most commercial identification systems including MicroScan (Beckman Coulter, Brea, CA) and Vitek 2 (bio-Mérieux, Marcy I'Etoile, France). These automated identi-fication systems can readily identify *A. baumannii* and *S. maltophilia*. Beyond these two primary pathogens, there

TABLE 20.3   Colonial Appearance and Characteristics

Organism	Medium	Appearance
Stenotrophomonas maltophilia	BA	Large, smooth, glistening colonies with uneven edges and lavender-green to light purple pigment; greenish discoloration underneath growth; ammonia smell; nonhemolytic (Fig. 20.1)
	Mac	NLF
Acinetobacter spp.	BA	Smooth, opaque, raised, creamy, and smaller than Enterobacterales; some genospecies are beta-hemolytic
	Mac	NLF, but colonies exhibit a purplish hue that may cause the organism to be mistaken for LF (Fig. 20.2)
Burkholderia gladioli	BA	Yellow; nonhemolytic
	Mac	NLF
Bordetella parapertussis	BA	Smooth, opaque, beta-hemolytic
	Mac	NLF, delayed growth
Bordetella holmesii	BA	Punctate, semiopaque, convex, round, with greening of blood usually accompanied by lysis
	Mac	NLF, delayed growth
Bordetella trematum	BA	Convex, circular, grayish cream to white; nonhemolytic
	Mac	NLF
Pseudomonas oryzihabitans	BA	Wrinkled, rough or smooth, transparent, yellow; nonhemolytic
	Mac	NLF
Pseudomonas luteola	BA	May be rough and smooth, opaque, yellow; nonhemolytic
	Mac	NLF

BA, Trypticase soy agar with 5% sheep blood; *LF,* lactose fermenter; *Mac,* MacConkey agar; *NLF,* non–lactose fermenter.

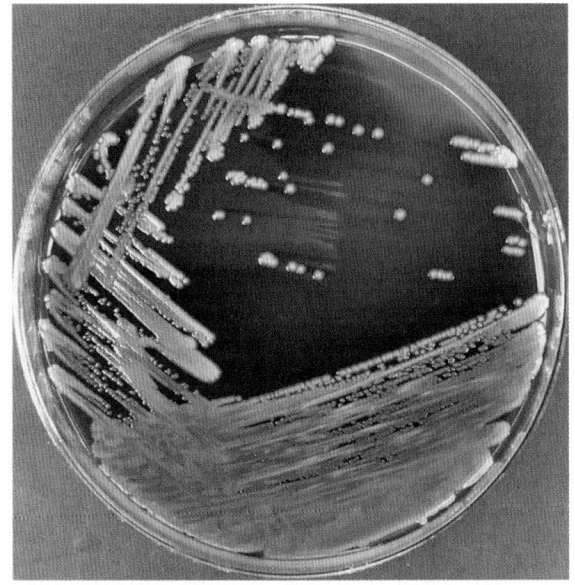

• **Fig. 20.1** Colony of *Stenotrophomonas maltophilia* on Trypticase soy agar with 5% sheep blood.

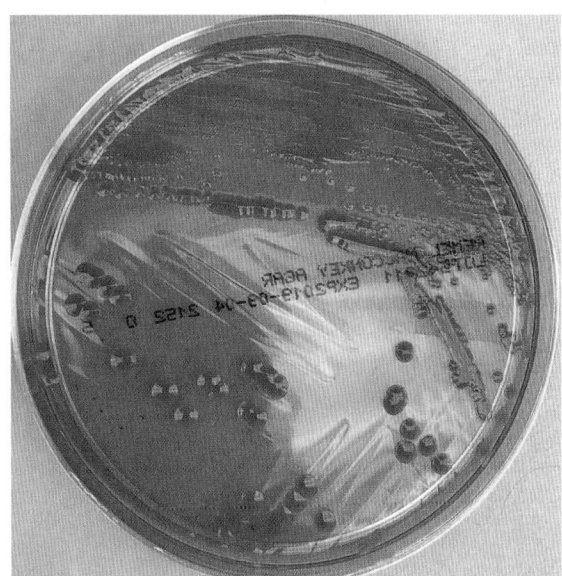

• **Fig. 20.2** Colony of *Acinetobacter* spp. on MacConkey agar. Note purple color.

TABLE 20.4   Key Biochemical and Physiologic Characteristics

Organism	Growth on Mac-Conkey	Motile	Oxi-dase	Oxidizes Glucose	Oxidizes Maltose	Esculin Hydrol-ysis	Lysine Decar-boxylase	Nitrate Reduc-tion	Urea Chris-tensen
Stenotropho-monas maltophilia	+	+	−	+	+	V	+	V	−
Saccharolytic Acineto-bacter	+	−	−	+	−	−	−	−	V
Asaccharolytic Acineto-bacter	+	−	−	−	V	−	−	−	V
Burkholderia gladioli[a]	+	+	V	+	−	−	−	V	V
Bordetella par-apertussis	+	−	−	−	−	−	ND	−	+
Bordetella holmesii[b]	+ or (+)	−	−	−	−	−	−	−	−
Bordetella trematum	+	+	−	−	−	−	−	V	−
Pseudomonas oryzihabitans	+	+ p, 1-2	−	+	+	−	−	−	V
Pseudomonas luteola	+	+ p, >2	−	+	+	+	−	V	V

[+], Greater than 90% of strains are positive; −, greater than 90% of strains are negative; (+), delayed; *ND,* no data; *p,* polar flagella; *V,* variable.
[a]*B. gladioli* is included with the oxidase-negative organisms because oxidase reactions are commonly weak and may be positive only with the Kovacs method.
[b]Brown soluble pigment.

is greater variability between the instruments in species-level identification with the other organisms included in this chapter. In those instances when a full identification is required (e.g., a sterile site), additional testing may be necessary using conventional biochemical and physiologic characteristics, such as those outlined in Table 20.4 or molecular techniques.

MALDI-TOF mass spectrometry has been shown to reliably and accurately identify *Acinetobacter* species where other conventional (i.e., biochemical) methods are unable to do so. This has led to the recognition of other species of *Acinetobacter* recovered from clinical specimens and is allowing microbiologists and infectious disease practitioners to learn more about the epidemiology of this ubiquitous genus. Nucleic acid–based methods, including amplification of the 16S ribosomal RNA (rRNA) gene, are routinely used to identify *Acinetobacter* spp. Both commercially available MALDI identification systems, the Biotyper CA System (Bruker Daltonics) and the Vitek MS (bioMérieux), can identify *S. maltophilia*. Other organisms in this chapter may be identified to the genus level by MALDI-TOF if the mass spectra for these organisms are included in the clinical or research databases and validated by the laboratory.

Comments Regarding Specific Organisms

The genus *Acinetobacter* has 63 named species that have been placed into homologous groups (**genomospecies**) based on deoxyribonucleic acid (DNA)–DNA hybridization studies. Genomospecies 1, 2, and 3 are often difficult to distinguish using phenotypic tests, and automated systems may result these as *Acinetobacter baumannii-calcoaceticus* complex. *Acinetobacter* species are oxidase negative, catalase positive, and nonmotile. The genus is divided into two groups: the saccharolytic (glucose oxidizing) species and the asaccharolytic (non–glucose-utilizing) species.

Most glucose-oxidizing nonhemolytic strains were previously identified as *A. baumannii,* and most non–glucose-utilizing, nonhemolytic strains were designated as *Acinetobacter lwoffi.* Other species that do not utilize glucose include *A. johnsonii, A. junii, A. radioresistens, A. schindleri, A. ursingii.* Some strains of *A. lwoffii* have been shown to oxidize glucose. Most beta-hemolytic strains are identified as *Acinetobacter haemolyticus.* Nitrate-reducing strains of asaccharolytic *Acinetobacter* spp. are difficult to differentiate from CDC group NO-1.

S. maltophilia is an oxidase-negative, nonfermentative, gram-negative bacillus that produces biochemical profiles similar to those of *Burkholderia cepacia.* A negative oxidase will rapidly rule out *B. cepacia. S. maltophilia* also oxidizes maltose faster than glucose (hence the species name, *maltophilia,* or "maltose loving"), and can produce a brown pigment on brain-heart infusion agar that contains tyrosine.

Pseudomonas spp. (previously *Chryseomonas* and *Flavimonas* spp.) are gram-negative, nonfermentative, oxidase-negative, catalase-positive bacilli. The organisms characteristically produce rough colonies that are often yellow pigmented on Trypticase soy agar with 5% sheep blood. *P. luteola* and *P. oryzihabitans* are oxidase negative, asaccharolytic, and nonmotile; they typically form small colonies on blood agar. Many of these species are nitrate reducers but fail to reduce nitrite.

Serodiagnosis

Serodiagnostic techniques are not generally used for the laboratory diagnosis of infections caused by the organisms discussed in this chapter.

Antimicrobial Resistance and Antimicrobial Susceptibility Testing

The gram-negative nonfermenting bacilli, including *Acinetobacter* spp. and *S. maltophilia,* are a significant health care concern because of their intrinsic mechanisms of antimicrobial resistance, which impart broad-spectrum antibiotic resistance, thereby making appropriate antimicrobial therapy selections difficult (Table 20.5). The World Health Organization has designated carbapenem-resistant *A. baumannii* (CRAB) as one of the critical priority pathogens for new antimicrobial drug development. *Acinetobacter* spp. are classified as MDR or extremely drug resistant (XDR) if they have chromosomally encoded AmpC beta-lactamases, mutations in porin channels, and overexpression of bacterial efflux pumps. *Acinetobacter* is notorious for its ability

TABLE 20.5 Antimicrobial Therapy and Susceptibility Testing

Species	Therapeutic Options	Potential Resistance to Therapeutic Options	Validated Testing Methods[a]	Comments
Acinetobacter baumannii	Beta-lactams: ampicillin-sulbactam, ceftazidime, cefepime, imipenem, meropenem. Aminoglycosides: gentamicin, amikacin. Other agents: fluoroquinolones, colistin, minocycline, tigecycline	Yes; resistance to beta-lactams, carbapenems, aminoglycosides, and quinolones	Disk diffusion or broth microdilution. See CLSI document M100, Performance Standards, for antimicrobial susceptibility testing.	*In vitro* susceptibility testing results are important for guiding therapy.
Bordetella holmesii	No definitive guidelines. Potentially active agents include penicillins, cephalosporins, and quinolones. Case report of 15 patients successfully treated with azithromycin.	Unknown	Not routinely performed.	See Chapter 36 for additional information.
Burkholderia gladioli	No definitive guidelines. Potentially active agents include imipenem, piperacillin-tazobactam, ciprofloxacin, tobramycin.	Yes	Extrapolated from *B. cepacia* complex. See CLSI document M100.	Rarely involved in human infections. Reliable therapeutic data are limited.
Pseudomonas luteola *Pseudomonas oryzihabitans*	No definitive guidelines. Potentially active agents include piperacillin/tazobactam, cefotaxime, ceftriaxone, ceftazidime, meropenem, fluoroquinolones, aminoglycosides, tetracyclines, trimethoprim-sulfamethoxazole.	Yes	See CLSI document M100, other non-Enterobacterales, MIC test methods only, no disk diffusion.	Rarely involved in human infection.
Stenotrophomonas maltophilia	Multiple resistance leaves few therapeutic choices; therapy of choice is trimethoprim-sulfamethoxazole. Potential alternatives include minocycline, ticarcillin/clavulanate, cefiderocol, levofloxacin, and chloramphenicol.	Yes; intrinsically resistant to most beta-lactams and aminoglycosides; frequently resistant to quinolones	Overnight minimal inhibitory concentration methods recommended. See CLSI document M100.	May be tested by various methods, but profiles obtained with beta-lactams can be seriously misleading.

[a]Validated testing methods include standard methods recommended by the Clinical and Laboratory Standards Institute (CLSI) and commercial methods approved by the US Food and Drug Administration (FDA).

to acquire beta-lactamase enzymes that reside in mobile genetic elements (i.e., plasmids), including serine and metallo-beta-lactamases (bla_{KPC} and bla_{IMP}, respectively), which, along with other beta-lactams, confer resistance to carbapenems. *Acinetobacter* species can encode resistance to fluoroquinolones through mutations in the *gyrA* and *parC* genes and become nonsusceptible to aminoglycosides by expressing aminoglycoside-modifying enzymes. A large survey of more than 39,000 unique isolates of *A. baumannii* was collected as part of a large surveillance study to evaluate trends in antimicrobial susceptibility testing. The study indicated that the prevalence of resistance to carbapenems and colistin had doubled, and MDR strains were more frequently identified in post–acute care facilities. The increase in carbapenem resistance may be due to the increased use of third-generation cephalosporins (e.g., ceftazidime and aztreonam) to treat *Acinetobacter* infections.

S. maltophilia exhibits resistance to a wide range of antibiotics, including beta-lactams, cephalosporins, aminoglycosides, tetracyclines, and polymyxins, through reduced membrane permeability, various enzymes, or efflux pumps. Susceptibility testing among this group of organisms can be challenging. Some automated methods for determining the minimal inhibitory concentration (MIC) for *Acinetobacter* spp. and other genera do not correlate well with disk diffusion methods. This underscores the importance of establishing the clinical significance of individual isolates before antimicrobial testing is performed (see Chapter 11 for a discussion of the criteria used to establish significance). Failure to do so could lead to inappropriate treatment of patients with expensive and potentially toxic agents. If susceptibility testing must be performed for these organisms, the use of an overnight MIC method is recommended.

Antimicrobial Therapy

For the treatment of infections caused by susceptible strains of *Acinetobacter* spp., many therapeutic options are available. Typical first-line agents include broad-spectrum cephalosporin (e.g., ceftazidime or cefepime), a beta-lactam/beta-lactamase inhibitor combination agent (e.g., ampicillin-sulbactam), or a carbapenem (e.g., imipenem, meropenem, or doripenem). *Acinetobacter* are intrinsically resistant to ertapenem making it an ineffective treatment. Resistance to beta-lactams or a carbapenem is a growing concern when used in monotherapy regimens. To prevent the development of resistance, a fluoroquinolone (e.g., levofloxacin) or an aminoglycoside (e.g., gentamicin or tobramycin) can be prescribed with a beta-lactam. For patients with a resistant *Acinetobacter* spp. infection, last-resort antibiotics like colistin and tigecycline have been used with some success, although resistance to each drug has been reported. In the setting of ventilator-associated infections, minocycline is another agent used for patients harboring resistant strains.

There are limited options for *S. maltophilia* infections because of the organism's high intrinsic resistance. Trimethoprim-sulfamethoxazole (TMP-SMX) is recommended as the primary drug of choice. For patients with hypersensitivity to TMP-SMX, other agents, including ticarcillin-clavulanic acid, fluoroquinolones, tigecycline, minocycline, rifampin, or moxifloxacin, should be considered if the organism tests susceptible *in vitro*. Resistance to TMP-SMX has been increasingly identified among *S. maltophilia* isolates, particularly in patients with cystic fibrosis.

Prevention

Because of their environmental niche and ability to survive in harsh conditions, these organisms can be difficult to control. Strategies for the prevention of infections should ensure that health care settings and patient environments are cleaned and sanitized regularly to prevent environmental contamination. Care should be taken to follow the proper aseptic techniques for the insertion of central venous catheters and other indwelling medical devices. All reusable medical equipment should be properly decontaminated or sterilized.

ⓔ Visit the Evolve site for a complete list of procedures, review questions, and case studies.

Bibliography

Caroll KC, Pfaller MA: *Manual of clinical microbiology,* ed 12, Washington, DC, 2019, ASM Press.

Clinical and Laboratory Standards Institute: *methods for dilution antimicrobial tests for bacteria that grow aerobically,* M7-A6, Villanova, PA, 2005, CLSI.

Clinical and Laboratory Standards Institute: *performance standards for antimicrobial disk susceptibility tests,* M2-A8, Villanova, PA, 2005, CLSI.

Clinical and Laboratory Standards Institute: *performance standards for antimicrobial susceptibility testing; m100-s29,* Wayne, PA, 2019, CLSI.

Denton M, Kerr KG: Microbiological and clinical aspects of infection associated with *Stenotrophomonas maltophilia, Clin Microbiol Rev* 11:57–80, 1998.

Esteban J, Valero-Moratalla ML, Alcazar R, Soriano F: Infections due to *Flavimonas oryzihabitans:* case report and literature review, *Eur J Clin Microbiol Infect Dis* 12:797–800, 1993.

Falagas ME, Kastoris AC, Vouloumanou EK, Rafailidis PI, Kapaskelis AM, Dimopoulos G: Attributable mortality of *Stenotrpohomonas maltophilia* infections: a systematic review of the literature, *Future Microbiol* 4:1103–1109, 2009.

Fournier PE, Richet H: The epidemiology and control of *Acinetobacter baumannii* in health care facilities, *Clin Infect Dis* 42:692–699, 2006.

Garrison MW, Anderson DE, Campbell DM, et al.: *Stenotrophomonas maltophilia:* emergence of multidrug-resistant strains during therapy and in an in vitro pharmacodynamic chamber model, *Antimicrob Agents Chemother* 40:2859–2864, 1996.

Lolans K, Rice TW, Munoz-Price LS, Quinn JP: Multicity outbreak of carbapenem-resistant *Acinetobacter baumannii* isolates producing the carbapenemase OXA-40, *Antimicrob Agents Chemother* 50:2941–2945, 2006.

Munoz-Price LS, Arheart K, Nordmann P, et al.: Eighteen years of experience with *Acinetobacter baumannii* in a tertiary care hospital, *Crit Care Med* 41:2733–2742, 2013.

Ottonello G, Dessi A, Pinna AP, et al.: *C. luteola* infection in pediatrics: description of a rare neonatal case and review of the literature, *J Chemother* 25:319–323, 2013.

Pittet LF, Emonet S, Schrenzel J, Siegrist CA, Posfay-Barbe KM: *Bordetella holmesii*: an under-recognized *Bordetella* species, *Lancet Infect Dis* 14:510–519, 2014.

Poirel L, Nordmann P: Carbapenem resistance in *Acinetobacter baumannii*: mechanisms and epidemiology, *Clin Microbiol Infect* 12:826–836, 2006.

Rahav G, Simhon A, Mattan Y, Moses AE, Sacks T: Infections with *Chryseomonas luteola* (CDC group Ve-1) and *Flavimonas oryzihabitans* (CDC group Ve-2), *Medicine* 74:83–88, 1995.

Reed RP: *Flavimonas oryzihabitans* sepsis in children, *Clin Infect Dis* 22:733–734, 1996.

Rice LB: Federal funding for the study of antimicrobial resistance in nosocomial pathogens: no ESKAPE, *J Infect Dis* 197:1079–1081, 2008.

Ritchie DJ, Garavaglia-Wilson A: A review of intravenous minocycline for treatment of multidrug-resistant *Acinetobacter* infections, *Clin Infect Dis* 59:S374–S380, 2014.

Seifert H, Strate A, Pulverer G: Nosocomial bacteremia due to *Acinetobacter baumannii*: clinical features, epidemiology, and predictors of mortality, *Medicine* 74:340–349, 1995.

Tacconelli E, Carrara E, Savoldi A, et al.: Discovery, research, and development of new antibiotics: the WHO priority list of antibiotic-resistant bacteria and tuberculosis, *Lancet Infect Dis* 18:318–327, 2018.

Tacconelli E, Cataldo MA, De Pascale G, et al.: Prediction models to identify hospitalized patients at risk of being colonized or infected with multidrug-resistant *Acinetobacter baumannii calcoaceticus* complex, *J Antimicrob Chemother* 62:1130–1137, 2008.

Wang CH, Lin JC, Lin HA, et al.: Comparisons between patients with trimethoprim-sulfamethoxazole-susceptible and trimethoprim-sulfamethoxazole-resistant *Stenotrophomonas maltophilia* monomicrobial bacteremia: a 10-year retrospective study, *J Microbiol Immunol Infect* 49:378–386, 2016.

Weyant RS, Hollis DG, Weaver RE, et al.: *Bordetella holmesii* sp nov: a new gram-negative species associated with septicemia, *J Clin Microbiol* 33:1–7, 1995.

Zilberberg MD, Kollef MH, Shorr AF: Secular trends in *Acinetobacter baumannii* resistance in respiratory and blood stream specimens in the United States, 2003 to 2012: a survey study, *J Hosp Med* 11:21–26, 2016.

21

Pseudomonas, Burkholderia, and Similar Organisms

OBJECTIVES

1. Describe normal sources (habitats) and routes of transmission for *Pseudomonas aeruginosa, Burkholderia cepacia, Burkholderia pseudomallei,* and *Burkholderia mallei.*
2. Identify factors that contribute to the pathogenicity of *P. aeruginosa* and explain the physiologic mechanism for each factor.
3. List common sites of infection and various disease states associated with *P. aeruginosa* and *Burkholderia* spp.
4. Compare and contrast the Gram stain appearance of the gram-negative bacilli discussed in this chapter.
5. Describe growth conditions, key biochemical tests, and antimicrobial susceptibility profiles used to identify *P. aeruginosa.*
6. Describe the media and chemical principles of each type, including differential and selective media that aid in the cultivation of the organisms included in this chapter.
7. Explain the difficulty with organism identification using phenotypic and physiological characteristics for the organisms included in this chapter.
8. List and briefly explain the efficacy of additional identification methods used.

GENERA AND SPECIES TO BE CONSIDERED

Current Name
Acidovorax delafieldii (*Pseudomonas delafieldii*)
Acidovorax facilis (*Pseudomonas facilis*)
Acidovorax temperans (*Pseudomonas* and *Alcaligenes* spp.)
Acidovorax wautersii
Brevundimonas diminuta (*Pseudomonas diminuta*)
Brevundimonas vesicularis (*Pseudomonas vesicularis*)
Burkholderia cepacia complex (*Pseudomonas cepacia*)
Burkholderia pseudomallei (*Pseudomonas pseudomallei*)
Burkholderia mallei (*Pseudomonas mallei*)
Cupriavidus spp. (*Ralstonia* spp.)
Pandoraea spp.
Pseudomonas aeruginosa

Current Name
Pseudomonas alcaligenes
Pseudomonas fluorescens
Pseudomonas mendocina
Pseudomonas monteilii
Pseudomonas pseudoalcaligenes
Pseudomonas putida
Pseudomonas stutzeri
Pseudomonas veronii
Ralstonia mannitolilytica (*Pseudomonas thomasii, Ralstonia pickettii* biovar 3)
Ralstonia insidiosa
Ralstonia pickettii (*Pseudomonas pickettii, Burkholderia pickettii*)

General Characteristics

At one time most of the species belonging to the genera *Brevundimonas, Burkholderia, Ralstonia,* and *Acidovorax* were members of the genus *Pseudomonas.* Organisms in these genera have many similar phenotypic characteristics but are genetically distinct. These organisms are organized into five unrelated rRNA homology groups using ribosomal ribonucleic acid (rRNA)–deoxyribonucleic acid (DNA) hybridization. *Pseudomonas* spp. belong to rRNA homology group I; *Burkholderia, Cupriavidus,* and *Ralstonia* spp. belong to rRNA homology group II; *Acidovorax* spp. belong to rRNA homology group III (along with genera *Comamonas* and *Delftia,* see Chapter 24); *Brevundimonas* spp. make up rRNA homology group IV (and for completeness, *Stenotrophomonas* spp. belong to group V). Phenotypically, they are aerobic, non–spore forming, straight or slightly curved, slender, gram-negative bacilli with cells that range from 1 to 5 μm long and 0.5 to 1 μm wide. All species except *Burkholderia mallei* are motile, having one or several polar flagella. Members of these genera use a variety of carbohydrate, alcohol, and amino acid substrates as carbon and energy sources. Although they can survive and possibly grow at relatively low temperatures (i.e., as low as 4°C), the optimal temperature range for growth of most species is 30°C to 37°C; that is, they are **mesophilic.**

Most of the organisms in this chapter are oxidase positive, grow on MacConkey agar, and oxidize glucose; *Pseudomonas* spp. are catalase positive. A few of the organisms are unable to utilize glucose, including *Pseudomonas alcaligenes, Ralstonia insidiosa,* and the *Cupriavidus* spp. These organisms are included here as they were previously included in the genus *Pseudomonas.*

Pseudomonas luteola and *Pseudomonas oryzihabitans* are oxidase negative and are discussed in Chapter 20. *Acidovorax facilis* is MacConkey negative.

Epidemiology

The genera included in this chapter are inhabitants of the environment and are not considered part of the normal human microbiota. These organisms have a worldwide distribution and are often associated with plant disease. They generally survive well in aqueous environments, making them potential opportunistic pathogens. Transmission usually involves human contact with heavily contaminated medical devices or solutions encountered in a health care setting.

Burkholderia, Cupriavidus, and *Ralstonia* spp.

Burkholderia cepacia complex, which is among the *Burkholderia* spp. found in the United States, is a complex of at least 20 distinct genomic species (**genomovars**) isolated from clinical specimens. Plants, soil, and water serve as reservoirs. These organisms are able to survive on or in medical devices and disinfectants. Intrinsic resistance to multiple antimicrobial agents and disinfectants contributes to the organism's survival in hospitals. Human colonization or infection with *B. cepacia* complex usually is a result of direct contact with contaminated foods, respiratory equipment and other devices, or medical solutions, including disinfectants. Interpatient transmission in patients with cystic fibrosis has been reported with strains of *B. cepacia.*

Burkholderia pseudomallei is another environmental inhabitant of niches similar to those of *B. cepacia* complex. Infections with *B. pseudomallei* were previously geographically restricted to tropical and subtropical areas of Australia and Southeast Asia. However, the distribution of the organism has now extended beyond these regions, with reports of infection in Africa, the Americas, China, other regions of Asia, India, Madagascar, and Mauritius. The organism is widely disseminated in soil, streams, ponds, and rice paddies. Human acquisition occurs through inhalation of contaminated debris or by direct inoculation through damaged skin or mucous membranes.

Although *Burkholderia mallei* mainly causes severe infections in horses and related animals, it has been identified in rare human localized suppurative or acute pulmonary infections. When transmission has occurred, it has been associated with close animal contact. *B. gladioli,* discussed in Chapter 20, is a plant pathogen rarely found in the sputa of patients with cystic fibrosis (CF); it is associated with chronic granulomatous disease (CGD) and other types of immunocompromise. The mode of transmission to humans is unknown.

Ralstonia pickettii, another environmental organism, is occasionally found in a variety of clinical specimens such as blood, the sputa of CF patients, and urine. The mode of transmission is uncertain, but normally sterile hospital fluids have been identified that are contaminated with this bacterial species as well as with *Ralstonia insidiosa* and *Ralstonia mannitolilytica.* *R. mannitolilytica* has been described in recurrent meningitis. Recent studies implicate this species as the causative agent for the majority of *Ralstonia* spp. infections in CF patients.

Cupriavidus spp. (*C. pauculus, C. gilardii, C. respiraculi,* and *C. taiwanensis*), were previously classified in the genera *Ralstonia.* These organisms have been recovered from patients with cystic fibrosis, bacteremia, peritonitis, and tenosynovitis. They have also been isolated from cerebrospinal fluid (CSF).

Acidovorax, Brevundimonas, and *Pandoraea* spp.

The genera *Acidovorax, Brevundimonas,* and *Pandoraea* comprise several environmental species that rarely inhabit human skin or mucosal surfaces. *Brevundimonas* spp. are environmental and encountered primarily in water, soil, and on plants, including fruits and vegetables. *Brevundimonas* spp. have been recovered from a variety of clinical specimens including blood, urine, and pleural fluid. *Acidovorax* spp. have been recovered from sputum in patients with CF; however, the organism's role in disease progression is unclear. *Pandoraea* spp. have been recovered from the blood and sputum of patients with chronic obstructive pulmonary disease, CGD, and other immunocompromised diseases. Because of the ubiquitous nature of these genera, their transmission to humans can occur in a variety of ways, and their clinical significance is unclear.

Pseudomonas spp.

In the clinical setting, *Pseudomonas aeruginosa* is the most commonly encountered gram-negative species that is not a member of Enterobacterales; it is an uncommon member of the normal human microbiota. The organism survives in various environments in nature. *P. aeruginosa* has been associated with colonization of immunocompromised patients who are neutropenic and have been previously treated for ventilator-associated pneumonia, in particular in patients with CF. Other *Pseudomonas* spp. are environmental inhabitants, but they are much less frequently found in clinical specimens than *P. aeruginosa*. Because they are rarely encountered in patient specimens, their mode of transmission to humans remains uncertain.

Pathogenesis and Spectrum of Disease

Burkholderia, Cupriavidus, and Ralstonia spp.

Because *Burkholderia, Cupriavidus, R. pickettii, R. insidiosa,* and *R. mannitolilytica* spp. are uncommon causes of infection in humans, very little is known about what, if any, virulence factors they exhibit.

The capacity of *B. cepacia* complex to survive in the hospital environment, which may be linked to the organism's intrinsic resistance to many antibiotics and disinfectants, provides the opportunity for this species to occasionally colonize and infect hospitalized patients. Person-to-person transmission has been described. In immunocompromised patients, especially those with CF or CGD, the organism can cause fulminant lung infections and bacteremia, resulting in death. Furthermore, CF patients infected with *B. cepacia* complex may be less likely to receive a lifesaving lung transplant because transplant success is compromised by the high risk of infection. In other patient populations, infections of the blood, urinary tract, and respiratory tract usually result from exposure to contaminated medical solutions or devices, but they are rarely fatal.

Infections or **melioidosis**, caused by *B. pseudomallei* (capable of survival in human macrophages) can range from being asymptomatic to severe. The disease has several forms, including the formation of skin abscesses as well as abscess formation in several internal organs, acute pulmonary disease, sepsis, and septic shock.

Except for *B. pseudomallei,* the additional *Burkholderia* spp. and organisms in the genera *Cupriavidus* and *Ralstonia* are generally considered nonpathogenic for healthy human hosts and are rarely encountered in human disease. The clinical significance of these organisms should be questioned when they are identified in clinical specimens.

Acidovorax, Brevundimonas, and Pandoraea spp.

Acidovorax and *Brevundimonas* spp. are rarely associated with human infections. *Acidovorax* spp. have been isolated from patients with CF, but the role of the organism in the disease is unclear. *Brevundimonas vesicularis* has

been isolated in clinical cases of bacteremia and from cervical specimens. *Brevundimonas diminuta* has been recovered from cancer patients in blood, urine, and pleural fluid, and *Brevundimonas vesicularis* has been identified in septicemia following open-heart surgery.

Pandoraea spp. have been increasingly identified in the sputum of patients with CF. In addition, patient-to-patient transmission has been reported in health care settings and attributed to poor infection control practices. The organisms have also been isolated from a variety of immunocompromised patients, as previously noted.

Pseudomonas spp.

Of the *Pseudomonas* spp., *P. aeruginosa* is the most thoroughly studied regarding infections in humans.

Although *P. aeruginosa* is an environmental inhabitant, it is also a successful opportunistic pathogen. Factors that contribute to the organism's pathogenicity include the production of exotoxin A, which kills host cells by inhibiting protein synthesis; exoenzymes S and T, which disrupt cytoskeleton organization; and the production of several proteolytic enzymes (e.g., elastases) and hemolysins (e.g., phospholipase C) capable of destroying cells and tissue. On the bacterial cell surface, pili and adhesions mediate and reinforce attachment to host cells. Some strains produce alginate, a polysaccharide polymer that inhibits phagocytosis, thus contributing to the infectious potential in CF patients (Fig. 21.1). This substance also protects the bacteria from dehydration and antibiotic activity. **Pyocyanin**, the blue phenazine pigment that contributes to the characteristic green color of *P. aeruginosa*, damages cells by producing reactive oxygen species. The latter are also bactericidal to the organism; to protect itself and prevent its destruction, the organism produces catalase enzymes.

P. aeruginosa also contains several genes involved in **quorum sensing**, a mechanism for detecting bacterial products

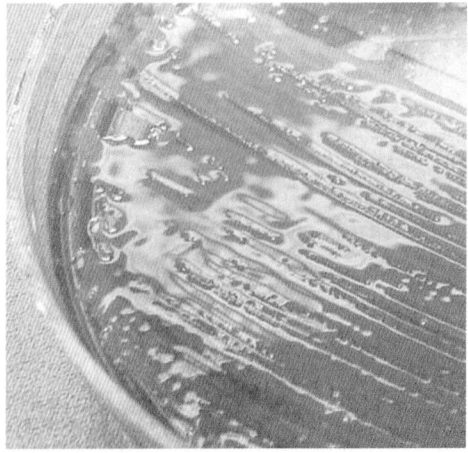

• **Fig. 21.1** Mucoid phenotype of *Pseudomonas aeruginosa* resulting from overproduction of alginate on dialyzed tryptic soy agar. The light blue pigment is caused by a low level of pyocyanin production. (Courtesy David Craft, PhD, D(ABMM), Penn State Hershey Medical Center.)

in the immediate environment. When the growth of the organism or neighboring bacteria reaches a critical mass, the concentration of these "inducing" molecules reaches a level that activates the transcription of virulence factors, including genes related to metabolic processes, enzyme production, and biofilm formation. It is also evident that *P. aeruginosa* does not form the same type of biofilm *in vivo* as is seen on artificial surfaces. Biofilm production related to the overproduction of alginate and the mucoid phenotype isolated from CF patients is associated with serious infections. *P. aeruginosa* forms microcolonies in tissue that are associated with quorum-sensing, biofilm-producing strains, which indicates that quorum sensing is also linked to the formation of microcolonies below the surface in severe wounds. These microcolonies contain DNA, mucus, actin, and other products from dying bacterial and host cells. In addition, *P. aeruginosa* can survive harsh environmental conditions and displays intrinsic resistance to a wide variety of antimicrobial agents, two factors that facilitate the organism's survival in the hospital setting. In addition, CF patients receive continuous antimicrobial therapy that naturally selects for the survival of highly drug-resistant strains of *P. aeruginosa*.

Even with the variety of potential virulence factors discussed, *P. aeruginosa* remains an opportunistic pathogen that requires compromised host defenses to establish infection. In normal, healthy hosts, either infection is in the outer ear or skin of swimmers or divers that spend significant amount of time in water, or it is associated with events that disrupt or bypass protection provided by the epidermis (e.g., burns, puncture wounds, use of contaminated needles by intravenous drug abusers, eye trauma with contaminated contact lenses). Deep wounds, severe burns, and the necrotic tissue found in diabetic foot infections and chronic ulcers are excellent environments for infection with *P. aeruginosa* and its growth. These infections, which may further spread to areas of the bone, heart, or eye, require a tissue biopsy to detect the organism within the biofilm.

In patients with CF, *P. aeruginosa* has a predilection for infecting the respiratory tract. Although organisms rarely invade through respiratory tissue and into the bloodstream of these patients, the consequences of respiratory involvement alone are serious and life threatening. In other patients, *P. aeruginosa* is a notable cause of health care–associated infections of the respiratory and urinary tracts, wounds, the bloodstream, and even the central nervous system. For immunocompromised patients, such infections are often severe and frequently life threatening. In some cases of bacteremia, the organism may invade and destroy the walls of subcutaneous blood vessels, resulting in the formation of cutaneous papules that become black and necrotic. This condition is known as **ecthyma gangrenosum.** Similarly, patients with diabetes may suffer a severe infection of the external ear canal (**malignant otitis externa**), which can progress to involve the underlying nerves and bones of the skull.

No known virulence factors have been identified in the numerous other *Pseudomonas* spp. However,

serious infections by most have occurred, including *P. fluorescens, P. putida, P. stutzeri, P. oryzihabitans, P. luteola* (Chapter 20), *P. alcaligenes, P. mendocina, P. pseudoalciagenes,* and *P. veronii.* When infections caused by these organisms occur, they usually involve a compromised patient exposed to contaminated medical materials. Such exposure may result in infections of the respiratory and urinary tracts and of wounds as well as bacteremia, osteomyelitis, endocarditis, and meningitis. Several of these species have been recovered from respiratory samples from patients with CF. However, because of their low virulence, their significance should be highly suspect.

Laboratory Diagnosis

Specimen Collection and Transport

No special considerations are required for collecting and transporting specimens of organisms discussed in this chapter. Table 5.1 provides general information regarding specimen collection and transport.

Specimen Processing

No special considerations are required for processing of the organisms discussed in this chapter. Table 5.1 provides general information regarding specimen processing.

Direct Detection Methods

Other than Gram staining, no specific procedures have been established for the direct detection from clinical samples of the organisms discussed in this chapter. These organisms usually appear as medium-size, straight rods on Gram staining (Fig. 21.2). Exceptions are *B. diminuta*, which is a long straight rod; *B. mallei*, which is a coccobacillus; and *B. pseudomallei*, which is a small gram-negative rod with bipolar staining.

Assays using real-time polymerase chain reaction (PCR) or culture-independent strategies, such as next-generation genome sequencing of bacterial isolates, are likely to provide alternative approaches for the direct detection of these

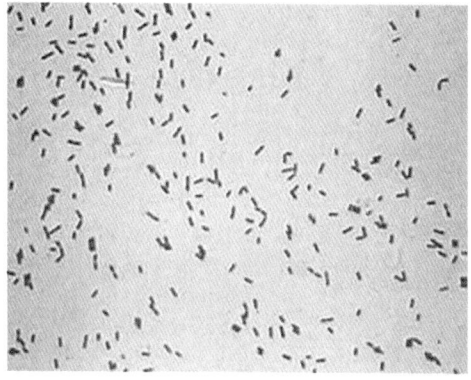

• **Fig. 21.2** Gram stain of *Pseudomonas aeruginosa.* (Courtesy David Craft, PhD, D[ABMM], Penn State Hershey Medical Center.)

organisms in clinical specimens. However, current molecular assays are not sensitive enough to replace conventional culture methods.

Nucleic Acid Detection

Although culture remains the standard approach for organism identification and antimicrobial susceptibility testing, screening by molecular methods may be useful when a large outbreak is being evaluated or in the course of environmental epidemiologic studies. PCR assays have been developed for various genes, including 16S rRNA, heat shock protein, pilin, and exotoxin A. Undoubtedly, with further development and expansion in molecular diagnostics, useful clinical assays related to rapid diagnosis for respiratory infections and other serious infections will continue to emerge.

Several genotyping methods have been developed to examine the heterogeneity and diversity of the pseudomonads, including restriction fragment length polymorphism (RFLP) by pulsed-field gel electrophoresis (PFGE); additional PCR-based typing methods, such as multiple locus variable-number tandem repeat (VNTR) of repetitive regions in the DNA; multilocus sequence typing (MLST) using several housekeeping genes; and single nucleotide polymorphisms (SNPs) typing using AT biochips (Clondiag Chip Technologies, Germany) directed against highly conserved genomic regions. Discriminatory techniques are typically limited to specialized reference laboratories and are not considered routine in laboratory testing; they include PCR ribotyping (i.e., fingerprinting of genomic DNA restriction fragments that contain all or part of the genes coding for the 16S and 23S rRNA), whole-genome sequencing (WGS), and multiplex species-specific PCR for species or strain identification. Real-time PCR targets that have been used to identify *B. pseudomallei* include 16S rRNA, flagellin (*fliC*), ribosomal protein subunit S21 (*rpsU*), and type III secretion system (TTS genes).

Similar nucleic acid detection and identification methods have been utilized to investigate the relationship and identification of the additional genera *Burkholderia, Ralstonia,* and *Pandoraea* included in this chapter. WGS of several strains of *Pseudomonas* spp. has been completed and is ongoing. Results are available at http://www.pseudomonas.com. WGS is becoming more affordable; however, international standards and criteria for species identification are yet to be determined prior to implementation in the routine clinical laboratory.

Cultivation

Media of Choice

Pseudomonas, Acidovorax, Brevundimonas, Burkholderia, Cupriavidus, and *Ralstonia* spp. grow well on routine laboratory media such as 5% sheep blood agar and chocolate agar (Figs. 21.3 and 21.4). Except for *B. vesicularis* and *Acidovorax facilis,* all usually grow on MacConkey agar. All genera also grow well in broth-blood culture systems and common nutrient broths, such as thioglycollate and brain-heart infusion.

Specific selective media, such as *Burkholderia cepacia* selective agar (BCSA), *Pseudomonas cepacia* (PC) agar, or **oxidative–fermentative base–polymyxin B–bacitracin–lactose (OFPBL) agar,** may be used to isolate *B. cepacia* complex and *Ralstonia* spp. from the respiratory secretions of CF patients (Table 21.1). BCSA contains peptones and sugars (i.e., sucrose and lactose) to supply nutrients for growth. Selective agents include crystal violet and vancomycin to inhibit gram-positive bacteria and gentamicin to inhibit a variety of gram-positive and gram-negative bacteria. Colonies of *B. cepacia* complex appear translucent, smooth to rough, and slightly raised; they cause the media to undergo a color change from red-orange to yellow. PC agar contains crystal violet, bile salts, polymyxin B, and ticarcillin to inhibit gram-positive and rapid-growing gram-negative organisms. Inorganic and organic components, including pyruvate and

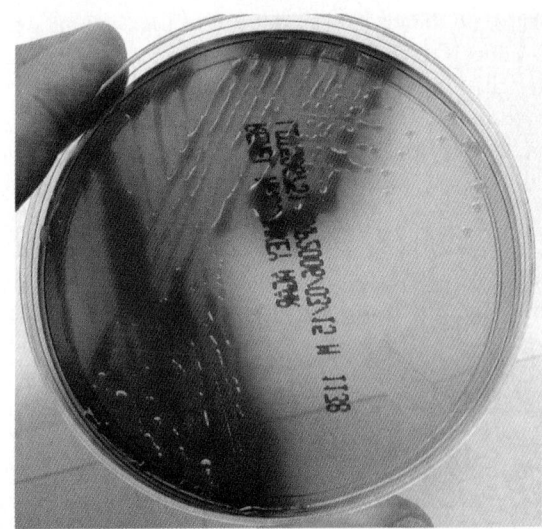

• **Fig. 21.3** *Pseudomonas stutzeri* on 5% sheep blood agar. Note the cream-colored colony and wrinkled colony topology. (Courtesy David Craft, PhD, D[ABMM], Penn State Hershey Medical Center.)

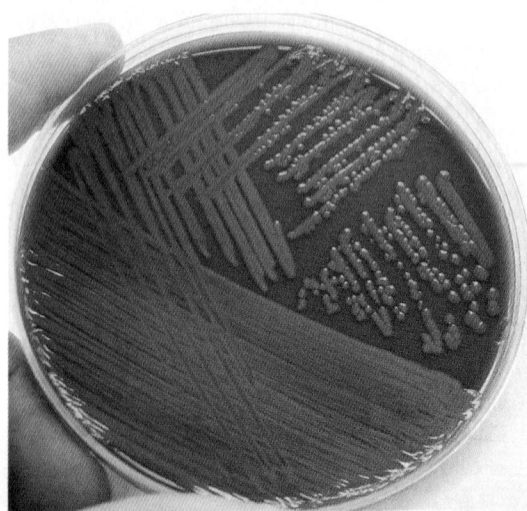

• **Fig. 21.4** *Burkholderia cepacia* on chocolate agar. Note the green pigment.

TABLE 21.1   Colonial Appearance and Other Characteristics of *Pseudomonas, Brevundimonas, Burkholderia, Ralstonia,* and Other Organisms

Organism	Medium	Appearance
Acidovorax spp. *(delafieldii, facilis, temperans)*	BA	No distinctive appearance; may have a yellow soluble pigment (except *A. facilis*), nonhemolytic
	Mac	NLF (*Acidovorax facilis* does not grow on Mac)
Brevundimonas diminuta	BA	Brown to tan pigment, nonhemolytic
	Mac	NLF
Brevundimonas vesicularis	BA	Yellow to orange pigment, nonhemolytic
	Mac	NLF; only 43% grow on Mac
Burkholderia cepacia complex	BA	Smooth and slightly raised; dirtlike odor, some species are beta-hemolytic May have a yellow or brown (*B. cenocepacia*) pigment
	Mac	NLF; colonies become dark pink to red because of oxidation of lactose after 4–7 days
	BCSA, PC, or OFPBL	Smooth
Burkholderia pseudomallei	BA	Cream to yellow-orange; smooth and mucoid (24–48 h) to dry and wrinkled (>3 days may resemble *Pseudomonas stutzeri*), generally nonhemolytic; putrid odor
	Mac	NLF, but appear as pink colonies (oxidize lactose)
	Ashdown	NLF
		Dry, wrinkled, violet-purple
Burkholderia mallei	BA	No distinctive appearance, may demonstrate a weak hemolysis
	Mac	NLF
Pandoraea spp.	BA	No distinctive appearance, nonhemolytic
	Mac	NLF
Pseudomonas aeruginosa	BA	Spreading and flat, serrated edges; confluent growth; often with metallic sheen; bluish green, red, or brown pigment; often beta-hemolytic; grapelike or corn tortilla–like odor; mucoid colonies seen in cystic fibrosis patients
	Mac	NFL
Pseudomonas fluorescens, Pseudomonas monteilii, Pseudomonas mosselii, Pseudomonas putida, and *Pseudomonas veronii, Pseudomonas alcaligenes, Pseudomonas pseudoalcaligenes*	BA	No distinctive appearance
	Mac	NLF
	Mac	NLF
Pseudomonas mendocina	BA	Smooth, nonwrinkled, flat, brownish-yellow pigment; nonhemlytic
	Mac	NLF
Pseudomonas stutzeri	BA	Dry, wrinkled, adherent, buff to brown; nonhemolytic
	Mac	NLF
	Mac	NLF
Ralstonia spp. *(insidiosa, mannitolilytica, pickettii)*	BA	No distinctive appearance; may take up to 72 h to produce visible colonies
	Mac	NLF

BA, 5% sheep blood agar; *BCSA, Burkholderia cepacia* selective agar; *Mac,* MacConkey agar; *NLF,* nonlactose fermenter; *OFPBL,* oxidative–fermentative base–polymyxin B–bacitracin–lactose; *PC, Pseudomonas cepacia* agar.

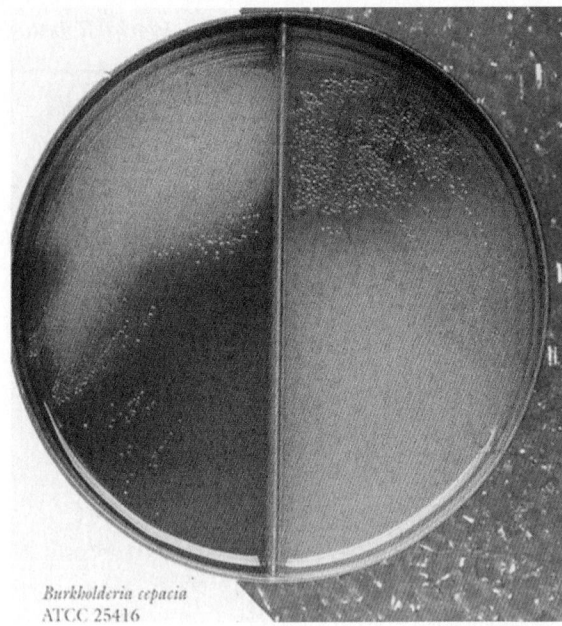

• **Fig. 21.5** *Burkholderia cepacia* complex colonies on (*left*) OFPBL agar, which change in color from green to yellow because of the acidic pH caused by the utilization of lactose; on (*right*) *Pseudomonas cepacia* (PC) agar, which change in color from yellow to pink because of the alkaline pH caused by the breakdown of pyruvate. (From Mahon C, Lehman D, Mansuelus G. *Textbook of Diagnostic Microbiology.* 5th ed. Philadelphia: Elsevier-Saunders; 2014.)

phenol red, are also added. *B. cepacia* complex species break down the pyruvate, creating an alkaline pH and resulting in a color change of the pH indicator (phenol red) from yellow to pink (Fig. 21.5). OFPBL incorporates bacitracin as an added selective agent and uses lactose fermentation to differentiate isolates. Most species of the *B. cepacia* complex ferment lactose and appear yellow, whereas nonfermenters appear green (Fig. 21.5). **Ashdown medium** is used to isolate *B. pseudomallei* when melioidosis is suspect. Preferred specimens include throat, rectal, or sputum samples. The medium contains crystal violet and gentamicin as selective agents to suppress the growth of contaminating organisms. Neutral red is incorporated into the medium and is taken up by the organism, making the dry, wrinkled colony appear violet-purple, which distinguishes it from other bacteria.

Incubation Conditions and Duration

Detectable growth on 5% sheep blood and chocolate agars, incubated at 35°C in carbon dioxide or ambient air, generally occurs 24 to 48 hours after inoculation. Growth on MacConkey agar incubated in ambient air at 35°C is detectable within this same period. Selective media used for patients with CF (e.g., BCSA, PC, or OFPBL) may require incubation at 35°C in ambient air for up to 72 hours before growth is detected. With Ashdown media, it may take up to 96 hours for growth to appear.

Colonial Appearance

Table 21.1 describes the colonial appearance and other distinguishing characteristics (e.g., hemolysis and odor) of

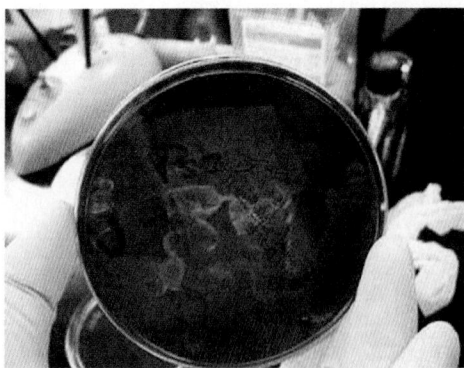

• **Fig. 21.6** *Pseudomonas aeruginosa* on 5% sheep blood agar. Note the beta-hemolysis; gray, gunmetal color and spreading flattened topology. (Courtesy David Craft, PhD, D[ABMM], Penn State Hershey Medical Center.)

each genus on common laboratory media (Fig. 21.6). Most species grow on MacConkey agar and appear as non–lactose fermenters at 24 hours.

Approach to Identification

Most manual and automated commercial systems available for phenotypic identification of these organisms reliably identify *Pseudomonas aeruginosa* and *Burkholderia cepacia* complex, but their reliability for the identification of other species is less certain. Examples of manual test systems include API 20NE (Biomerieux, Durham, NC), specifically for identification of most common nonfermenters within 24 to 48 hours, and rapid NF Plus (Remel, Lenexa, KS), which identifies bacteria by analysis of preformed enzymes within 4 hours. The Biolog Microbial ID System (Hayward, CA) can be used manually or in an automated format, and its database includes most of the clinically relevant nonfermenters. Automated systems include BD Phoenix (Franklin Lakes, NJ), Vitek-2 (Biomerieux, Durham, NC), and MicroScan (Beckman Coulter, Brea, CA), which provide identification (and susceptibility profiles) of many bacterial species, including most clinically relevant nonfermenters.

Tables 21.2–21.4 provide the key phenotypic characteristics for identifying the species discussed in this chapter. These tests provide useful information for presumptive organism identification, but definitive identification often requires the use of a more extensive battery of tests performed by reference laboratories.

Other Identification Methods

Cellular fatty acid analysis has been used to aid in the identification of clinical isolates for the nonfermenters discussed in this chapter. This method is very useful in differentiating *Cupriavidus* from other *Ralstonia* spp. Cellular fatty acid analysis is unable to differentiate *B. gladioli* (Chapter 20) from *B. cepacia* complex organisms. MALDI-TOF MS has been reported to be unreliable in the identification of many of the organisms included in this chapter.

TABLE 21.2 Biochemical and Physiologic Characteristics of *Acidovorax, Brevundimonas, Cupriavidus,* and *Ralstona* spp.

Organisms	Growth at 42°C	Nitrate Reduction	Gas From Nitrate	Gelatin Liquefied	Arginine Dihydrolase	Lysine Decarboxylase	Urea Hydrolysis	Oxidizes Glucose	Oxidizes Lactose	Oxidizes Mannitol	Oxidizes Xylose
Acidovorax delafieldii	50%	+	–	–	+	–	+	+	–	50%	85%
Acidovorax facilis	–	+	–	+	+	–	+	+	–	+	+
Acidovorax temperans	+	+	+	–	–	–	50%	+	–	50%	–
Brevundimonas diminuta	V38%	3%	–	68%	–	–	13%	21%	–	–	–
B. vesicularis	19%	5%	–	25%	–	–	2%	87%	–	–	27
Pandoraea (apista, pulmonicola, pnomenusa, sputorum, and *norimbergensis)* spp.	v	v	–	–	–	–	v	+w	–	–	–
Cupriavidus respiraculi	ND	v	v	ND	ND	–	–	–	–	ND	ND
C. gilardii	+	–	–	ND	ND	–	–	–	–	ND	–
C. pauculus	v	–	–	ND	ND	–	+	–	–	–	–
Ralstonia insidiosa	ND	+	ND	ND	–	–	v	–	v	ND	ND
Ralstonia mannitolilytica	+	–	–	v	–	–	+	+	+	+	+
Ralstonia pickettii	v	+	v	v	–	–	+	+	v	–	+

ND, No data; *v,* variable, %, percent of positive strains; +, >90% of strains are positive; –, >90% of strains are negative.
Updated from Carroll KC, Pfaller MA, Landry ML, et al. *Manual of Clinical Microbiology.* 12th ed. Washington, DC: ASM; 2019.

TABLE 21.3 Biochemical and Physiologic Characteristics Burkholderia cepacia Complex and Other Species

Organisms	Growth at 42°C	Nitrate Reduction	Gas From Nitrate	Gelatin Liquefied	Arginine Dihydrolase	Lysine Decarboxylase	Urea Hydrolysis	Oxidizes Glucose	Oxidizes Lactose	Oxidizes Mannitol	Oxidizes Xylose
Burkholderia cepacia complex	v	v	–	v	–	+/v	v	+	+/v	v	+/v
Burkholderia mallei	–	+	–	–	+	–	v	+	v	–	v
Burkholderia pseudomallei	+	+	+	v	+	–	v	+	+	+	+

ND, No data; v, variable; +, >90% of strains are positive; –, >90% of strains are negative.

TABLE 21.4   Biochemical and Physiologic Characteristics of *Pseudomonas* spp.

Organisms	Growth at 42°C	Nitrate Reduction	Gas From Nitrate	Gelatin Liquefied	Arginine Dihydrolase	Lysine Decarboxylase	Urea Hydrolysis	Oxidizes Glucose	Oxidizes Lactose	Oxidizes Mannitol	Oxidizes Xylose
Pseudomonas aeruginosa	+	+	+	v	+	–	v	+	–	v	+
Pseudomonas alcaligenes	v	54%	–	–	12%	–	–	–	–	–	–
Pseudomonas fluorescens	–	–	–	+	+	–	v	+	v	v	+
Pseudomonas mendocina	+	+	+	–	+	–	v	+	–	–	+
Pseudomonas monteilii	–	–	–	–	+	–	v	+	–	–	–
Pseudomonas mosselii	–	–	–	+	+	–	ND	+	–	v	–
Pseudomonas pseudoalcaligenes	94%	+	–	–	78%	–	3%	9%	–	–	18%
Pseudomonas putida	–	–	–	–	+	–	v	+	v	v	+
Pseudomonas stutzeri	v	+	+	–	–/+*	–	v	+	–	+	+
Pseudomonas veronii	–	+	+	v	+	ND	v	+	ND	+	+

ND, No data; v, variable; %, percent of positive strains; +, >90% of strains are positive; –, >90% of strains are negative.
Updated from: Carroll KC, Pfaller MA, Landry ML, et al. *Manual of Clinical Microbiology.* 12th ed. Washington, DC: ASM; 2019.

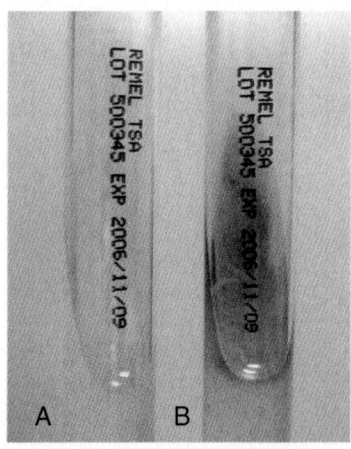

• **Fig. 21.7** An uninoculated tube (A) is shown for comparison. Note the blue-green color produced by pyocyanin and pyoverdine water-soluble pigments. *Pseudomonas aeruginosa* on tryptic soy agar (B).

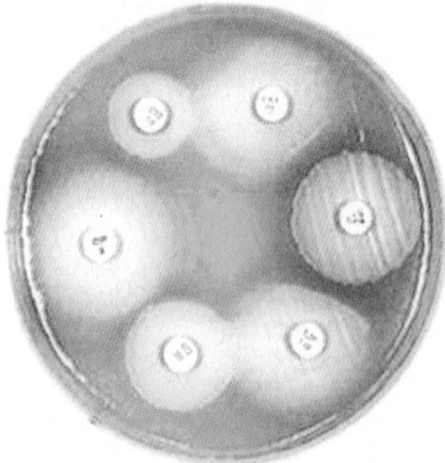

• **Fig. 21.8** Disk diffusion antimicrobial susceptibility test of *Pseudomonas aeruginosa* on Mueller Hinton agar. Note the blue-green pigment. (Courtesy David Craft, PhD, D[ABMM], Penn State Hershey Medical Center.)

Comments Regarding Specific Organisms

A convenient and reliable identification scheme for *P. aeruginosa* involves the following conventional tests and characteristics:

• Oxidase-positive
• Production of bright bluish (pyocyanin), green (**pyoverdin**), red (**pyrorubrin**), or brown (**pyomelanin**) diffusible pigment on Mueller-Hinton agar or trypticase soy agar (Figs. 21.7 and 21.8; Fig. 21.1)

P. aeruginosa, P. fluorescens, P. putida, P. veronii, P. monteilii, and *P. mosselii* comprise the group known as the fluorescent pseudomonads. These species all produce pyoverdine, a water-soluble yellow-green or yellow-brown pigment that fluoresces blue-green under ultraviolet (UV) illumination. *P. aeruginosa* can be distinguished from the others in this group by its ability to grow at 42°C and the production of pyocyanin. Mucoid strains of *P. aeruginosa* from CF patients may not exhibit the characteristic pigment and may react more slowly in biochemical tests than nonmucoid strains. The organisms may undergo

several phenotypic changes, including slow growth, changes in pigment production, and altered biochemical activity. Standard biochemical tests should be held for the complete 7 days before being recorded as negative for these strains. This slow biochemical activity often prevents identification of mucoid *P. aeruginosa* by commercial systems. *P. monteilii* can be distinguished from *P. putida* by its inability to oxidize xylose. Both can be distinguished from *P. fluorescens* by their inability to liquefy gelatin. *P. mosselii* liquefies gelatin but does not oxidize xylose, which separates it from *P. fluorescens.*

B. cepacia complex should be suspected whenever a nonfermentative organism that decarboxylates lysine is encountered. Lysine decarboxylation is positive in 80% of strains. Correct identification of the occasional lysine-negative (20%) or oxidase-negative (14%) strains requires full biochemical profiling. *Pandoraea* spp. may be differentiated from *B. cepacia* by the failure to decarboxylate lysine and the inability to liquefy gelatin.

The presumptive identification of other species in this chapter is at times difficult due to the variability in the phenotypic biochemical characteristics. However, it is important to provide some guidance in a few notable conditions. The initial identification of *B. cepacia* complex by a commercial system in a patient with CF requires confirmation by additional phenotypic and/or genotypic methods. The *B. cepacia* complex has 20 genomovars, and appropriate speciation is crucial. Likewise, if a rapid system identifies a clinical isolate as *B. gladioli* or *Acidovorax, Ralstonia, Cupriavidus,* or *Pandoraea* spp., confirmatory testing should be performed.

Serodiagnosis

Serodiagnostic techniques are not generally used for laboratory diagnosis of infections caused by the organisms discussed in this chapter. However, serologic tests may be performed as preliminary or adjunctive tests to culture-based diagnosis to improve the diagnosis of melioidosis. Many antibody detection formats are currently in use, but in general, they are not standardized and lack sensitivity. An indirect hemagglutination assay is available outside the United States to diagnose infections caused by *B. pseudomallei.* Acute and convalescent sera should be tested. However, single patient samples are frequently used, with a cut-off value based on a background seropositivity of the endemic population, making interpretation difficult. Furthermore, cross-reactions with antibodies produced against other organisms (e.g., *B. cepacia* complex and *P. aeruginosa*) can occur. A lateral flow immunoassay using monoclonal antibodies to the bacterial capsular polysaccharide specific for *B. pseudomallei* has been developed and demonstrated successful results when using sputum, urine, or purulent material. However, a significant decrease in sensitivity has been observed with blood specimens.

In addition, there are two approved commercial tests that detect IgG antibodies in serum or secretory IgA antibodies in saliva or mucosal secretions to *P. aeruginosa* antigens. Examining serum and mucosal secretions discriminates intermittent colonization and chronic infection, to monitor treatment, and to gauge the prognosis of CF patients.

Antimicrobial Susceptibility Testing and Therapy

Many of these organisms grow on the media and under the conditions recommended for testing of the more commonly encountered bacteria (see Chapter 11 for more information about validated testing methods); however, the ability to grow under test conditions does not guarantee reliable detection of important antimicrobial resistance. As such, even though testing can provide an answer, it poses a substantial risk of erroneous interpretations. Validated susceptibility testing method s (disk diffusion, broth dilution, agar dilution, and E-test) are available for a limited number of antibiotics.

Acidovorax, Brevundimonas, Cupriavidus, Pandoraea, and *Ralstonia* spp. are not typically encountered in human infections. Establishing the clinical significance of these species is important in the care of the patient because they may be present as colonizers and not pathogens. Antimicrobial treatment is not generally recommended for colonizing bacteria but would be warranted for an infecting pathogen. Potential therapies and susceptibility testing criteria are available for a limited number of antibiotics for *B. cepacia* complex. However, antimicrobial therapy rarely eradicates *B. cepacia* complex, as these organisms—especially those from the respiratory tracts of CF patients—are among the most resistant to antimicrobial therapy that have been identified in the clinical laboratory. At present optimal therapy for melioidosis remains controversial. *Burkholderia* spp. can express resistance to various antibiotics; therefore, it may be difficult to devise effective treatment options.

The Clinical Laboratory Standards Institute (CLSI) guidelines describe specific testing methods (e.g., disk diffusion and minimal inhibitory concentration) and provide interpretive standards for susceptibility reporting of *P. aeruginosa, B. cepacia,* and *Stenotrophomonas maltophilia* in the CLSI M100-S29 document. Guidelines for minimal inhibitory concentration assays for other non-Enterobacterales isolates, including *Pseudomonas* spp. other than *P. aeruginosa,* are included in the same document. Of the gram-negative nonfermenting bacilli, *P. aeruginosa* is the only species for which extensive *in vitro* susceptibility testing (Fig. 21.8) and therapeutic evidence exists (see Chapter 11 for a discussion of available testing methods).

Therapy usually involves the use of a beta-lactam developed for antipseudomonal activity and an aminoglycoside. The therapy used depends on several clinical factors and on the laboratory antimicrobial resistance profile for the *P. aeruginosa* isolate. *P. aeruginosa* isolated from patients with CF may require extended incubation for up to 24 hours before a reliable susceptibility pattern is evident. In addition, the organism may develop resistance during therapy with any antimicrobial agent within 3 to 4 days. Repeat susceptibility testing may be required to monitor the development of resistance.

P. aeruginosa is intrinsically resistant to various antimicrobial agents. However, *P. aeruginosa* also readily acquires resistance to the potentially active agents, necessitating susceptibility testing for each clinically relevant isolate.

Although antimicrobial resistance is also characteristic of the other *Pseudomonas* and *Brevundimonas* spp., the fact that these organisms are rarely clinically significant and the lack of validated testing methods prohibit the provision of specific guidelines. Antimicrobial agents used for *P. aeruginosa* infections are often considered for use against the other species. Before initiating treatment, it is critical to establish the clinical significance of the organism.

Prevention

Because these organisms are ubiquitous in nature and many are commonly encountered without deleterious effects on healthy human hosts, there are no recommended vaccination or prophylaxis protocols. Health care–associated infections can be minimized by ensuring that appropriate infection control guidelines are followed and protocols for the sterilization and decontamination of medical supplies are implemented.

Ⓔ Visit the Evolve site for a complete list of procedures, review questions, and case studies.

Bibliography

Abbott IJ, Peleg AY: *Stenotrophomonas, Achromobacter,* and nonmelioid *Burkholderia* species: antimicrobial resistance and therapeutic strategies, *Semin Respir Crit Care Med* 36:99–110, 2015.

Ambrose M, Malley RC, Warren SJ, et al.: *Pandoraea pnomenusa* Isolated from an Australian patient with cystic fibrosis, *Front Microbiol* 11:692, 2016, 7.

Bennett J, Dolin R, Blaser M: *Principles and practice of infectious diseases,* ed 9, Philadelphia, 2020, Elsevier-Saunders.

Bisharat N, Gorlachev T, Keness Y: 10 Years hospital experience in *Pseudomonas stutzeri* and literature review, *Open Infect Dis J* 6:21, 2012.

Cao H, Li M, Yang X, Zhang C: *Brevundimonas diminuta* bacteremia in a man with myelodysplastic syndrome, *Indian J Pathol Microbiol* 58:384–386, 2015.

Carroll KC, Pfaller MA, Landry ML, et al.: *Manual of clinical microbiology,* ed 12, Washington, DC, 2019, ASM.

Clinical Laboratory Standards Institute: *Performance standards for antimicrobial susceptibility testing: 29th informational supplement, M100-S29,* Wayne, PA, 2019, CLSI.

Davies JC, Rubin BK: Emerging and unusual gram-negative infections in cystic fibrosis, *Semin Resp Crit Care Med* 28:312–321, 2007.

De Baere T, Steyaert S, Wauters G, et al.: Classification of *Ralstonia pickettii* biovar 3/"thomasii" strains (Pickett 1994) and of new isolates related to nosocomial recurrent meningitis as *Ralstonia mannitolytica* spnov, *J Syst Evol Microbiol* 51(Pt 2):547–558, 2001.

Degand N, Lotte R, Segonds C, et al.: Epidemic spread of *Pandoraea pulmonicola* in a cystic fibrosis center, *BMC Infect Dis* 15:583, 2015, https://doi.org/10.1186/s12879-015-1327-8.

DeMarco ML, Ford BA: Beyond identification: emerging and future uses for MALDI-TOF mass spectrometry in the clinical microbiology laboratory, *Clin Lab Med* 33(3):611–628, 2013.

Houghton RL, Reed DE, Hubbard MA, et al.: Development of a prototype lateral flow immunoassay for the rapid diagnosis of melioidosis, *PLoS Negl Trop Dis* 8:e2727, 2014.

Lambiase Raia V, DelPezzo M, Sepe A, Carnovale V, Rossano F: Microbiology of airway disease in a cohort of patients with cystic fibrosis, *BMC Infect Dis* 6:4, 2006.

Lau SK, Sridhar S, Ho CC, et al.: Laboratory diagnosis of melioidosis: past, present and future, *Exp Biol Med* 240:742–751, 2015.

LiPuma JJ: The changing microbial epidemiology in cystic fibrosis, *Clin Microbiol Rev* 23:299–323, 2010.

Queenan AM, Bush K: Carbapenemases: the versatile β-lactamases, *Clin Microbiol Rev* 20:440–458, 2007.

Rebolledo PA, Vu CCI, Carlson RD, Kraft CS, Anderson EJ, Burd EM: Polymicrobial ventriculitis involving *Pseudomonas fulva*, *J Clin Microbiol* 52:2239–2241, 2014.

Regan KH, Bhatt J: Eradication therapy for *Burkholderia cepacia* complex in people with cystic fibrosis, *Cochrane Database Syst Rev*(10)CD009876, 2014.

Ryan MP, Adley CC: *Ralstonia* spp: emerging global opportunistic pathogens, *Eur J Clin Microbiol Infect Dis* 33:291–304, 2014.

Ryan MP, Pembroke JT, Adley CC: Genotypic and phenotypic diversity of *Ralstonia pickettii* and *Ralstonia insidiosa* isolates from clinical and environmental sources including high-purity water. Diversity in *Ralstonia pickettii*, *BMC Microbiol* 11:194, 2011.

Singh S, Bhatia BD: *Brevundimonas* septicemia: a rare infection with rare presentation, *Indian Pediatr* 52:901, 2015.

VanZandt KE, Greer MT, Gelhaus HC: Glanders: an overview of infection in humans, *Orphanet J Rare Dis* 8:131, 2013.

22

Achromobacter, Rhizobium, Ochrobactrum, and Similar Organisms

OBJECTIVES

1. Describe the general characteristics of the organisms discussed in this chapter, including their normal habitat, Gram stain characteristics, and morphology.
2. List the types of diseases associated with each organism.
3. Compare and contrast the Gram stain appearance of the various species.
4. Create an algorithm that outlines the major tests used to differentiate the genera included in this chapter.

GENERA AND SPECIES TO BE CONSIDERED

Current Name	Previous Name
Achromobacter denitrificans	*Alcaligenes dentrificans*
Achromobacter insuavis	
Achromobacter piechaudii	*Alcaligenes piechaudii*
Achromobacter pulmonis	
Achromobacter xylosoxidans	
Achromobacter spp.	
Haematobacter spp.	
Ochrobactrum anthropi	
Ochrobactrum haematophilum	CDC group Vd1-2 and *Achromobacter* groups A, C, and D
Ochrobactrum intermedium	
Ochrobactrum pseudogrignonense	
Orchobractrum pseudintermedium	
Oligellaurethralis	
Oligellauerolytica	
Pannonibacter phragmitetus	
Paracoccusyeei	CDC group EO-2
Paracoccus sanguinis	
Psychrobacter faecalis	Part of CDC group EO-2
Psychrobacter pulmonis	
Pseudochrobactrum asaccharolyticum	
Rhizobium pusense	
Rhizobium radiobacter	*Agrobacterium radiobacter*
Shewanella putrefaciens	*Alteromonas putrefaciens, Achromobacter putrefaciens,* CDC group Ib
Shewanella algae	
Wohlfahrtiimona schitiniclastica	

General Characteristics

Most of the organisms discussed in this chapter exist in the environment. However, several species have been isolated from clinical samples. *Achromobacter* species are gram-negative, nonsporulating, mostly motile rods with 1 to 20 peritrichous flagella. Motility in *A. pulmonis* is weak or absent and is strain-dependent in *A. insuavis*. They are strictly aerobic and nonfermentative. However, some strains are capable of anaerobic growth. Three *Haematobacter* species have been described: *H. massiliensis* (previously *Rhodobacter massiliensis*), *H. missouriensis* and *Hematobacter* genomic species 1. *Hematobacter* spp., *Paracoccus* spp., *Psychrobacter* spp., and *Wohlfahrtiimonas* spp. are oxidase-positive, indole-negative, trypsin-negative gram-negative rods. Three *Hematobacter* species have been described: *H. massiliensis* (previously *Rhodobacter massiliensis*), *H. missouriensis*, and *Hematobacter* genomic species 1 that have been isolated from the bloodstream of septic patients. The genus *Paracoccus* consists of approximately 48 species with two of clinical importance: *P. yeei* and *P. sanguinis*. The genus *Oligella* comprises two asaccharolytic small coccobacilli species, *O. ureolytica* and *O. urethralis*. *O. ureolytica* are motile by peritrichous flagella, and *O. urethralis* are nonmotile. *Psychrobacter* spp. includes 38 species but only *P. faecalis* and *P. pulmonis* are associated with human infection. *Wohlfahrtiimonas chitiniclastica* is a short coccoid rod that has been isolated from wounds, cellulitis, osteomyelitis, and bloodstream infections. In contrast to the previous group, *Ochrobactrum*, *Pannonibacter phragmitetus*, *Pseudochrobactrum*, *Rhizobium*, and *Shewanella* spp. are all oxidase-positive, indole-negative, trypsin-positive gram-negative rods that have been isolated from a variety of clinical specimens and infections. The specific morphologic and physiologic features are somewhat diverse. The organisms are considered later in this chapter in the laboratory diagnosis section.

Epidemiology

The habitats of the species listed in Table 22.1 vary from soil and water environments to the upper respiratory tract of various mammals. As predominantly environmental organisms, the diversity of the organisms' habitats is reflected in the various ways they are transmitted. For example, transmission of environmental isolates such as *Achromobacter denitrificans* typically involves exposure of debilitated patients to contaminated fluids or medical solutions. *A. xylosoxidans* is an opportunistic pathogen capable of causing a wide variety of infections and has been identified in health care–associated infections from contaminated disinfectants, dialysis fluids, saline solutions, and water. Some of the other bacteria have been discovered in clinical material, and several have been established as causes of human infections.

R. radiobacter inhabits the soil, and human infections occur by exposure to contaminated medical devices; it has been isolated from cystic fibrosis patients. *Psychrobacter* spp. are inhabitants of cold deep-sea environments and are rarely associated with human infection.

The specific environmental niche of *Ochrobactrum* is unknown, but this organism is capable of survival in water, including moist areas in the hospital environment. The organism may also be a transient colonizer of the human gastrointestinal tract. Similar to *R. radiobacter*, human infections caused by *Ochrobactrum* spp. are associated with implantation of intravenous catheters or other foreign bodies in patients with a debilitating illness. Acquisition by means of contaminated pharmaceuticals and through puncture wounds has also been documented. Because *O. intermedium* is phenotypically very similar to *O. anthropi*, it is possible that documented human infections may have been caused by *O. intermedium*. *O. haemophilum*, *O. pseudogrignonense* and *O. pseudintermedius* have been recovered from clinical samples; however, their significance is unclear.

Pathogenesis and Spectrum of Disease

Among the environmental organisms listed, *Achromobacter* spp. are most commonly associated with various infections, including bacteremia, meningitis, pneumonia, and peritonitis. They also have been implicated in outbreaks of health care–associated infections. *Achromobacter piechaudii* has been isolated from pharyngeal swabs, wounds, blood, and ear discharge. *Achromobacter xylosoxidans* increasingly has been recovered from patients with cystic fibrosis, along with *A. aegrifaciens*, *A. animicus*, *A. anxifer*, *A. dolens*, *A. insuavis*, *A. marplatenses*, *A. mucicolens*, *A. ruhlandi*, and *A. pulmonis*. It is unclear whether the organisms are implicated in causing clinical disease in patients with cystic fibrosis or whether they simply colonize the respiratory tract. *A. denitrificans* has been recovered from urine, prostate secretions, the buccal cavity, pleural fluid, and eye secretions. Because many of these organisms rarely cause human infections, little is known about what, if any, virulence factors they may produce to facilitate infectivity (Table 22.2). The fact that *R. radiobacter* and *Ochrobactrum* spp. infections commonly involve contaminated medical materials and immunocompromised patients and rarely, if ever, occur in healthy hosts, suggests that these bacteria have relatively low virulence. One report suggests that *R. radiobacter* is capable of capsule production. The ability of *Ochrobactrum* spp. to adhere to the silicone material of catheters may contribute to this organism's propensity to cause catheter-related infections.

For both *R. radiobacter* and *Ochrobactrum* spp., bacteremia is the most common type of infection (Table 22.2); peritonitis, endocarditis, meningitis, urinary tract, and pyogenic infections are much less commonly encountered. *R. radiobacter* is commonly isolated from blood, peritoneal dialysate, urine, and ascitic fluid. *Haematobacter* spp. have been identified on human skin and associated with bloodstream infections and endocarditis. *Shewanella* spp. have been isolated from skin, tissue, and ocular infections, as well as cases of osteomyelitis, otitis media, peritonitis, and blood infections. *S. algae* is the predominant species associated with clinical infection. *O. urethralis* and *O. ureolytica* have been isolated predominantly from the human urinary tract and associated with urosepsis. *Pannonibacter phragmitetus* has been identified in a liver abscess and in bloodstream infections. *Pseudochrobactrum asaccharolyticus* has been isolated from synovial fluid and wound infections.

Although other species listed in Table 22.2 may be encountered in clinical specimens, their clinical significance is uncertain, and such encounters should be carefully analyzed.

Laboratory Diagnosis

Specimen Collection and Transport

No special considerations are required for specimen collection and transport of the organisms discussed in this chapter. Refer to Table 5.1 for general information on specimen collection and transport.

Specimen Processing

No special considerations are required for processing the organisms discussed in this chapter. Refer to Table 5.1 for general information on specimen processing.

Direct Detection Methods

Other than Gram staining, no specific procedures are required for direct detection of these organisms in clinical material. *Achromobacter* spp. are medium to long straight rods. *Ochrobactrum* spp., are slender, short to long rods. *R. radiobacter* is a short, pleomorphic rod. *Psychrobacter* spp., *O. urethralis,* and *Paracoccus* spp. are coccobacilli. *P. yeei* has a characteristic O appearance on Gram staining (Fig. 22.1). *Shewanella* organisms are long, short, or filamentous rods. *O. ureolytica* is a short, straight rod.

TABLE 22.1	**Epidemiology**	
Species	**Habitat (Reservoir)**	**Mode of Transmission**
Achromobacter spp.	Environment, including moist areas of hospital Transient colonizer of human gastrointestinal or respiratory tract in patients with cystic fibrosis	Often not known Usually involves exposure to contaminated fluids (e.g., intravenous fluids, hemodialysis fluids, irrigation fluids), soaps, and disinfectants
Haematobacter spp.	Environment	Unknown; isolated from human skin
Ochrobactrum spp. CDC group OFBA-1	Uncertain, probably environmental; found in water and hospital environments; may also be part of human microbiota Uncertain, probably environmental; not part of human microbiota	Uncertain. Most likely involves contaminated medical devices, such as catheters or other foreign bodies, or contaminated pharmaceuticals Associated with puncture wounds Unknown; rarely found in humans
Pannonibacter phragmitetus	Environmental	Unknown
Paracoccus spp.	Environmental; not part of human microbiota	Identified in human peritonitis
Pseudochrobactrum assacharolyticus	Environmental	Unknown
Psychrobacter spp.	Environmental, particularly cold climates such as the Antarctic; not part of human microbiota	Unknown; rarely found in humans; has been found in fish, poultry, and meat products
Rhizobium radiobacter	Environmental, soil and plants; not part of human microbiota	Contaminated medical devices, such as intravenous and peritoneal catheters
Shewanella putrefaciens *Shewanella algae*	Environmental and foods; not part of human microbiota	Uncertain; infections associated with exposure to aquatic and marine habitats Isolated from abscesses, wounds, and ear infections and associated with cases of osteomyelitis, peritonitis, and septicemia
Wohlfahrtiimonas chitiniclastica	Environmental	Unknown

Cultivation

Media of Choice

The genera included in this chapter typically grow well on routine laboratory media such as 5% sheep blood, chocolate, and MacConkey agars. These organisms also grow well in the broth of blood culture systems and in common nutrient broths such as thioglycollate and brain-heart infusion.

Incubation Conditions and Duration

These organisms produce detectable growth on 5% sheep blood and chocolate agars in 5% carbon dioxide (CO_2) and on MacConkey agar in ambient air when incubated at 35°C for a minimum of 24 hours. *Psychrobacter* spp. are an exception in that they usually grow poorly or not at all on routine media such as TSA and grow best at 20°C to 25°C. *R. radiobacter* optimally grows at 25°C to 28°C but is also capable of growth at 35°C.

Colonial Appearance

Table 22.3 presents descriptions of the colonial appearance and other distinguishing characteristics (e.g., hemolysis and odor) of each genus when grown on 5% sheep blood or MacConkey agar.

Approach to Identification

The ability of most commercial identification systems to accurately identify the organisms discussed in this chapter is limited or uncertain. The key biochemical reactions used to presumptively differentiate among the genera discussed in this chapter are provided in Table 22.4. However, definitive identification of these organisms often requires performing an extensive battery of biochemical tests not commonly available in many clinical microbiology laboratories. MALDI-TOF MS has limited capabilities to identify the genera included in this chapter. Full identification of

TABLE 22.2	Pathogenesis and Spectrum of Disease	
Species	**Virulence Factors**	**Spectrum of Disease and Infections**
Achromobacter spp.	Unknown Survival in hospital the result of inherent resistance to disinfectants and antimicrobial agents	Infections usually involve compromised patients and include bacteremia, urinary tract infections, meningitis, wound infections, pneumonia, otitis media, peritonitis, and septicemia; occur in various body sites; can be involved in healthcare-associated outbreaks.
Ochrobactrum spp.	Unknown. Exhibits ability to adhere to silicone catheter material in a manner similar to staphylococci	Catheter- and foreign body–associated bacteremia. May also cause pyogenic infections, community-acquired wound infections, and meningitis in tissue graft recipients. Patients are usually immunocompromised or otherwise debilitated.
Oligella urethralis	Unknown	Urinary tract infections, particularly in females
Oligella ureolytica	Unknown	Also isolated from kidney, joint, and peritoneal fluid
Paracoccus yeei	Unknown	No infections described in humans. Rarely encountered in clinical specimens
Psychrobacter spp.	Unknown	Rare cause of infection in humans. Has been described in wound and catheter site infections, meningitis, and eye infections
Rhizobium radiobacter	Unknown. One blood isolate described as mucoid, suggestive of exopolysaccharide capsule production	Exposure of immunocompromised or debilitated patient to contaminated medical devices resulting in bacteremia and, less commonly, peritonitis, endocarditis, or urinary tract infection
Shewanella spp.	Unknown	Clinical significance uncertain; often found in mixed cultures. Implicated in cellulitis, otitis media, and septicemia; may be found in the respiratory tract, urine, feces, bile, cerebrospinal fluid, and pleural fluid

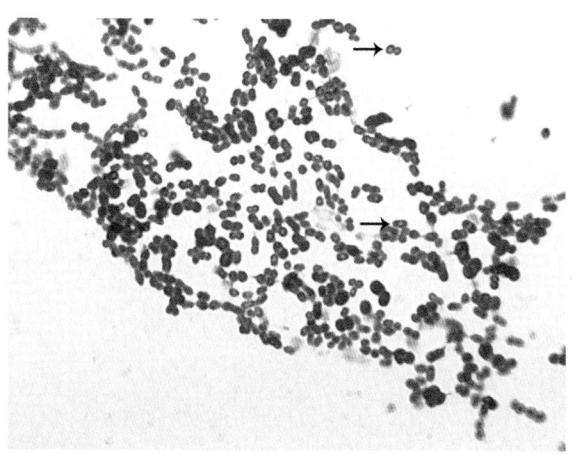

• **Fig. 22.1** *Paracoccus yeei*; note doughnut-shaped organism on Gram stain (arrows).

clinically relevant isolates may require identification by a reference laboratory and may include the use of 16S rRNA sequence analysis.

Comments Regarding Specific Organisms

The genus *Oligella* includes one nonmotile species (*O. urethralis*) and one motile species (*O. ureolytica*). Urea hydrolysis is a key test for differentiating between these species; *O. ureolytica* often turns positive within minutes. *O. urethralis* is urease and nitrate-reductase negative. *O. urethralis* may be easily confused with *Moraxella osloensis* (Chapter 27).

Achromobacter denitrificans reduces nitrate to nitrite and reduces nitrite to gas. *Achromobacter* species are oxidase and catalase positive and negative for urease, DNase, lysine decarboxylase, ornithine decarboxylase, arginine dihydrolase, and gelatinase. Overall, *Achromobacter* spp. show very limited to no saccharolytic reactions, making identification at the genus level difficult, and 16S rRNA may be required.

TABLE 22.3 Colonial Appearance and Characteristics

Organism	Medium	Appearance
Achromobacter denitrificans	BA	Small, convex, and glistening
	MAC	NLF
Achromobacter xylosoxidans	BA	Small, convex, and glistening
	MAC	NLF
Achromobacter piechaudii	BA	Nonpigmented, glistening, convex colonies surrounded by zone of greenish brown discoloration
	MAC	NLF
Ochrobactrum spp.	BA	Resembles colonies of Enterobacterales, only smaller
	MAC	NLF
Oligella spp.	BA	Small, opaque, whitish
	MAC	NLF
Paracoccus spp.	BA	Growth frequently mucoid
	MAC	NLF
Psychrobacter spp.	BA	No distinctive appearance but usually does not grow well at 35°C; grows best at 20°C; cultures (saccharolytic strains) smell like roses
	MAC	NLF
Rhizobium radiobacter	BA	No distinctive appearance
	MAC	NLF (mucoid pink after extended incubation [>48 h])
Shewanella spp.	BA	Convex, circular, smooth; occasionally mucoid; lavender greening of blood agar; soluble brown to tan pigment
	MAC	NLF
Wohlfahrtiimonas chitiniclastica	BA	Fast, slightly spreading colonies
	MAC	NLF

BA, 5% sheep blood agar; *MAC,* MacConkey agar; *NLF,* non–lactose fermenter.

TABLE 22.4 Key Biochemical and Physiologic Characteristics

Organism	Oxidizes Glucose	Oxidizes Xylose	Oxidizes Mannitol	Nitrate Reduction	Nitrite Reduction	Phenylalanine Deaminase	Esculin Hydrolyzed	Urease
Achromobacter denitrificans	−	−	−	+	+	ND	ND	−
Achromobacter xylosoxidans	−	−	−	+	+	ND	ND	−
Achromobacter piechaudii	−	−	−	+	−	ND	ND	−
Ochrobactrum anthropi	+	+	V	+	+	+	−	+
Ochrobactrum haematophilum	+	+	V	−	−	+	−	+
Orchrobactrum intermedium	+	+	V	+	+	+	−	V
Ochrobactrum pseudogrignonense	+	+	V	+	+	+	−	+
Paracoccus yeei	+	+	−	+	V	V	−	−
Pannonibacter phragmitetus	+	+	V	+	+	−	+	+
Psychrobacter faecalis	−	−	−	+	+	V	ND	−
Psychrobacter pulmonis	−	−	−	+	+	−	ND	−
Pseudochrobactrum asscharolyticus	+	+	−	−	−	+		−
Rhizobium radiobacter	+	+	+	V		−	+	−
Shewanella algae[ab]	−	−	−	+	ND	ND	−	ND
Shewanella putrefaciens[b]	V	−	−	+	−	−	−	−
Wohlfahrtiimona schitiniclastica	+1	+	−	−	−	+	ND	−

ND, No data available; V, variable; +, >90% of strains are positive; −, >90% of strains are negative; (+), delayed.
[a]Requires NaCl for growth.
[b]H$_2$S in butt of triple sugar iron (TSI) agar.
Data from Caroll KC, Pfaller MA. *Manual of Clinical Microbiology.* 12th ed. Washington, DC: ASM Press; 2019.

MALDI-TOF MS has been successfully used for the identification of *A. xylosoxidans, A. ruhlandi, A. insolitus,* and *A. spanius.*

P. yeei, formerly CDC group EO-2 (a **eugonic oxidizer**), has a biochemical profile very similar to that of the saccharolytic, nonhemolytic *Acinetobacter* spp., except that the latter are oxidase negative (see Chapter 20 for more information about this genus).

R. radiobacter produces acid from various carbohydrates. *R. radiobacter* may be differentiated from *Ochrobactrum* spp. by a positive beta-galactosidase test result. *Psychrobacter* spp. can be either saccharolytic or asaccharolytic, although all members of this genus have an optimal growth temperature of less than 35°C.

Pannonibacter phragmitetus can be differentiated from *Rhizobium, Ochrobactrum,* and *Pseudochrobactrum* by the inability to produce phenylalanine deaminase. In addition, *P. phragmitetus* is positive for the hydrolysis of tributyrin within 30 minutes. *Ochrobactrum* and *Pseudochrobactrum* do not hydrolyze tributyrin. *P. phragmitetus* is also capable of growth at 41°C.

Shewanella spp. are notable for the production of hydrogen sulfide (H_2S) in the butt of triple sugar iron (TSI) agar; this characteristic is rare among the nonfermentive gram-negative rods. *S. algae* is halophilic.

Serodiagnosis

Serodiagnostic techniques are not generally used in the laboratory diagnosis of infections caused by the organisms discussed in this chapter.

Antimicrobial Susceptibility Testing and Therapy

Although many of these organisms grow on the media and under the conditions recommended for testing of more commonly encountered bacteria, no standardized reference exists for antimicrobial resistance for these organisms. The lack of validated *in vitro* susceptibility testing methods does not allow definitive treatment and testing guidelines for the organisms listed in Table 22.5. Although susceptibility data for some of these bacteria are included in the literature, the lack of understanding of potential underlying resistance mechanisms prohibits the validation of the data.

Although standardized methods have not been established for the other species discussed in this chapter, *in vitro* susceptibility studies have been published, and

antimicrobial agents that have potential activity are noted. *A. xylosoxidans* demonstrates variable susceptibility to beta-lactams, ureidopenicillins, and carbapenems; the organism is resistant to narrow-spectrum penicillins and cephalosporins, including cefotaxime. Antimicrobial resistance patterns for additional species is rare; however, *A. spanius* and *A. insolitus* are resistant to most quinolones, macrolides, and cephalosporins.

Because *R. radiobacter* and *Ochrobactrum* infections are commonly associated with implanted medical devices, therapeutic management of the patient often involves removal of the contaminated material. Although definitive antimicrobial therapies for these infections have not been established, *in vitro* data suggest that certain agents could be more effective than others (Table 22.5). Most strains of *R. radiobacter* are susceptible to cephalosporins, carbapenems, tetracyclines, and gentamicin, but not tobramycin.

O. anthropi is commonly resistant to all currently available penicillins, cephalosporins, aztreonam, and amoxicillin-clavulanate but usually is susceptible to aminoglycosides, fluoroquinolones, imipenem, tetracycline, and trimethoprim-sulfamethoxazole. *O. anthropi* (colistin susceptible) may be differentiated from *O. intermedium* by colistin resistance. This resistance profile is sufficiently consistent with the species, making it potentially useful for confirming the organism's identification. The organism may also appear susceptible to trimethoprim-sulfamethoxazole and ciprofloxacin, but antimicrobial therapy without removal of the contaminated medical device may not successfully eradicate the organism.

Shewanella spp. are typically susceptible to most antimicrobial agents that are effective against gram-negative rods.

Review Chapter 11 for preferable strategies used to provide susceptibility information and data when validated testing methods do not exist for a clinically relevant bacterial isolate.

Prevention

Because these organisms are ubiquitous in nature and are not generally a threat to human health, no recommended vaccination or prophylaxis protocols have been established. Health care–associated infections are controlled by following appropriate sterile techniques and infection control guidelines and implementing effective protocols for the sterilization and decontamination of medical supplies.

ⓔ Visit the Evolve site for a complete list of procedures, review questions, and case studies.

TABLE 22.5	**Antimicrobial Therapy and Susceptibility Testing**			
Species	Therapeutic Options	Potential Resistance to Therapeutic Options	Validated Testing Methods[a]	Comments
Achromobacter denitrificans	No definitive guidelines. Potentially active agents include mezlocillin, piperacillin, ticarcillin/clavulanic acid, ceftazidime, imipenem, trimethoprim/sulfamethoxazole, and quinolones.	Capable of beta-lactamase production.	Not available.	
Achromobacter xylosoxidans	No definitive guidelines. Potentially active agents include imipenem, piperacillin, ticarcillin/clavulanic acid, ceftazidime, and trimethoprim-sulfamethoxazole.	Aminoglycosides, expanded spectrum cephalosporins other than ceftazidime, and quinolones demonstrated no activity. Resistant to tobramycin, azithromycin, and clarithromycin.	Not available.	
Achromobacter piechaudii	No definitive guidelines.	Resistant to ampicillin, cefpodoxime, and gentamicin.	Not available.	
Oligella urethralis *Oligella ureolytica*	No definitive guidelines. Potentially active agents include several penicillins, cephalosporins, and quinolones.	Produces beta-lactamases; may develop resistance to quinolones.	Not available.	
Ochrobactrum spp.	Optimal therapy uncertain. Treatment involves removal of foreign body. Potentially active agents include trimethoprim-sulfamethoxazole, ciprofloxacin, and imipenem; aminoglycoside activity variable.	Commonly resistant to all penicillins and cephalosporins.	Not available.	Grows on susceptibility testing media, but standards for interpretation of results do not exist.
Paracoccus yeei	No definitive guidelines.	Unknown.	Not available.	No clinical data.
Psychrobacter spp.	No definitive guidelines. Usually penicillin susceptible.	Unknown.	Not available.	Limited clinical data.
Rhizobium radiobacter	Optimal therapy uncertain. Treatment involves removal of foreign body. Potentially active agents include ceftriaxone, cefotaxime, imipenem, gentamicin, and ciprofloxacin.	Yes.	Not available.	Grows on susceptibility testing media, but standards for interpretation of results do not exist.
Shewanella spp.	No definitive guidelines. Generally susceptible to various antimicrobial agents.	Often resistant to ampicillin and cephalothin.	Not available.	

[a]Validated testing methods include standard methods recommended by the Clinical and Laboratory Standards Institute (CLSI) and commercial methods approved by the U.S. Food and Drug Administration (FDA).

Bibliography

Alnor D, Frimodt-MøllerN, Espersen F, Frederiksen W: Infections with the unusual human pathogens *Agrobacterium* species and *Ochrobactrum anthropi, Clin Infect Dis* 18:914–920, 1994.

Brugnaro P, Morelli E, Ebo F, et al.: The first Italian case report of leg ulcer and sepsis caused by *Shewanella algae* in a immunocompetent patient, *Infez Med* 27(2):179–182, 2019.

Caroll KC, Pfaller MA: *Manual of clinical microbiology,* ed 12, Washington, DC, 2019, ASM Press.

Chang HJ, Christenson JC, Pavia AT, et al.: *Ochrobactrum anthropi* meningitis in pediatric pericardial allograft transplant recipients, *J Infect Dis* 173:656–660, 1996.

Cheng JW, Wang P, Xiao M, et al.: First case report of endocarditis caused by *Haematobacter massiliensis* in China, *BMC Infect Dis* 17(1):709, 2017.

Cieslak TJ, Drabick CJ, Robb ML: Pyogenic infections due to *Ochrobactrum anthropi, Clin Infect Dis* 22:845–847, 1996.

Cieslak TJ, Robb ML, Drabick CJ, Fischer GW: Catheter-associated sepsis caused by *Ochrobactrum anthropi:* report of a case and review of related non-fermentative bacteria, *Clin Infect Dis* 14:902–907, 1992.

Dunne Jr WM, Tillman J, Murray JC: Recovery of a strain of *Agrobacterium radiobacter* with a mucoid phenotype from an immunocompromised child with bacteremia, *J Clin Microbiol* 31:2541–2543, 1993.

Khashe S, Janda JM: Biochemical and pathogenic properties of *Shewanella alga* and *Shewanella putrefaciens, J Clin Microbiol* 36:783–787, 1998.

Le Guern R, Wallet F, Vega E, Courcol RJ, Loïez C: *Psychrobacter sanguinis:* an unusual bacterium for nosocomial meningitis, *J Clin Microbiol* 52:3475–3477, 2014.

Lim JY, Ganzorig M, Huang SL, Lee K: First complete genome sequence of *Haematobacter massiliensis* OT1 (Chromosome and Multiple Plasmids) isolated from human skin, *Microbiol Resour Announc* 8(18), 2019. https://doi.org/10.1128/MRA.00292-19.

Lloyd-Puryear M, Wallace D, Baldwin T, Hollis DG: Meningitis caused by *Psychrobacter immobilis* in an infant, *J Clin Microbiol* 29:2041–2042, 1991.

Lozano F, Florez C, Recio FJ, Gamboa F, Gómez-Mateas JM, Martín E: Fatal *Psychrobacter immobilis* infection in a patient with AIDS, *AIDS* 8:1189–1190, 1994.

Nozue H, Hayashi T, Hashimoto Y, et al.: Isolation and characterization of *Shewanella algae* from human clinical specimens and emendation of the description of *S. algae (Simidu et al, 1990, 335), Int J Syst Bacteriol* 42:628–634, 1992.

Papalia M, Steffanowski C, Traglia G, et al.: Diversity of *Achromobacter* species recovered from patients with cystic fibrosis in Argentina, *Rev Argent Microbiol* S0325-7541(19):30048-3, 2019. https://doi.org/10.1016/j.ram.2019.03.004.

Pagotto A, Merluzzi S, Pillinini P, Valeri M: Bloodstream infection with *Oligellaureo lytica:* a case report and review of the literature, *Infez Med* 24(1):58–61, 2016.

Srinivas J, Pillai M, Vinod V, Dinesh RK: Skin and soft tissue infections due to *Shewanella algae*—an emerging pathogen, *J Clin Diagn Res* 9:DC16–DC20, 2015.

Validation of publication of new names and new combinations previously effectively published outside the IJSEM, *Int J Syst Evol Microbiol* 53:935–937, 2003.

Young JM, Kuykendall LD, Martínez-Romero E, et al.: A revision of *Rhizobium Frank,* 1889, with an emended description of the genus, and the inclusion of all species of *Agrobacterium conn,* 1942, and *Allorhizobium undicola de Lajudie et al, 1998,* as new combinations: *Rhizobium radiobacter, R. rhizogenes, R. rubi, R. undicola* and *R. vitis, Int J Syst Evol Microbiol* 51:89–103, 2001.

Zhou Y, Jiang T, Hu S, Wang M, Ming D, Chen S: Genomic insights of *Pannonibacter phragmitetus* 31801 isolated from a patient with a liver abscess, *Microbiologyopen* 6(6):e00515, 2017.

23

Chryseobacterium, Sphingobacterium, and Similar Organisms

OBJECTIVES

1. Describe the general characteristics of the organisms discussed in this chapter.
2. Identify the normal habitat and the routes of transmission for the organisms.
3. List the appropriate media for cultivation of the organisms listed, particularly *Elizabethkingia meningoseptica*.
4. Describe the colonial appearance of *E. meningoseptica*.
5. Outline the tests used to differentiate the major genera in this group, including *Elizabethkingia* spp., *Myroides* spp., *Sphingobacterium* spp., and *Bergeyella zoohelcum*.

GENERA AND SPECIES TO BE CONSIDERED

Current Name	Previous Name
Balneatrix alpica	
Bergeyella cardium	
Bergeyella zoohelcum	*Weeksella zoohelcum*, CDC group IIj
Chryseobacterium anthropi	CDC group IIe and IIc
Chryseobacterium gleum	CDC group IIb
Chryseobacterium hominis	CDC group IIc
Chryseobacterium indologenes	CDC group IIb
Chryseobacterium treverense	CDC group IIe
Elizabethkingia anophelis	
Elizabethkingia meningoseptica	*Flavobacterium meningosepticum*
Elizabethkingia miricola	
Empedobacter brevis	*Flavobacterium breve*
Myroides injenensi	
Myroides odoratus	*Flavobacterium odoratum*
Myroides odoratimimus	*Flavobacterium odoratum*
Sphingobacterium multivorum	*Flavobacterium multivorum* and CDC group IIK-2

Current Name	Previous Name
Sphingobacterium spiritivorum	*Flavobacterium spiritivorum* and CDC group IIK-3
Sphingobacterium thalpophilum	
Wautersiella falsenii	
Weeksella virosa	CDC group IIf

General Characteristics

The organisms discussed in this chapter belong to the family *Flavobacteriaceae* and are environmental inhabitants occasionally encountered in human specimens. All of the genera discussed are yellow-pigmented, oxidase-positive, indole-positive (except *Sphingobacterium* spp. and *Myroides* spp.), glucose oxidizers that generally grow well on Mac-Conkey agar. *Sphingobacterium* spp. have an unusually large amount of sphingophospholipid compounds in their cell membranes compared with other organisms discussed in this chapter. *Sphingobacterium mizutaii,* which does not grow on MacConkey agar, is discussed in further detail in Chapter 26.

Epidemiology

As environmental inhabitants, these organisms are found in various niches, most commonly soil and water reservoirs (Table 23.1). Most notable in terms of clinical relevance is their ability to persist in hospital environments, especially in moist areas. Although they are not considered part of the normal human microbiota, these species have been reported to colonize a patient's respiratory tract during hospitalization. Colonization often results from exposure to contaminated water or medical devices (e.g., respiratory equipment). Transmission also may occur directly from contaminated pharmaceutical solutions and, in the case of *Elizabethkingia* spp., from person to person.

TABLE 23.1 Epidemiology

Species	Habitat (Reservoir)	Mode of Transmission
Balneatrix alpica	Water, such as natural hot springs	Exposure to contaminated water
Bergeyella zoohelcum	Normal oral microbiota of dogs and other animals	Dog and cat bites
Chryseobacterium indologenes		Catheter-related infections
Elizabethkingia spp., *Chryseobacterium* spp., *Empedobacter brevis, Myroides* spp., *Sphingobacterium* spp.	Soil, plants, water, food, and hospital water sources, including incubators, sinks, faucets, tap water, hemodialysis systems, saline solutions, and other pharmaceuticals Not part of human microbiota	Exposure of patients to contaminated medical devices or solutions, but source is not always known

TABLE 23.2 Pathogenesis and Spectrum of Diseases

Species	Virulence Factors	Spectrum of Disease and Infections
Balneatrix alpaca	Unknown	Rarely isolated from clinical specimens. Associated with pneumonia and meningitis
Bergeyella cardium	Unknown	Endocarditis
Bergeyella zoohelcum	Unknown	Dog and cat bite wounds; can lead to bacteremia, septicemia, and meningitis
Chryseobacterium anthropic	Unknown	Wounds and bacteremia
Chryseobacterium indologenes	Unknown	Catheter-related bacteremia Bacteremia associated with malignancies and neutropenia
Elizabethkingia spp., *Chryseobacterium* spp., *Empedobacter brevis, Sphingobacterium* spp.	Specific virulence factors are unknown. Able to survive chlorinated tap water. *E. meningoseptica,* the species most often associated with human infections, can be encapsulated or produce proteases and gelatinases that destroy host cells and tissues.	Bacteremia (often associated with implanted devices, such as catheters, or contaminated medical solutions). *Elizabethkingia* spp. are particularly associated with meningitis in neonates and less commonly in children and adults. Other organisms are associated with pneumonia, mixed infections of wounds, ocular and urinary tract infections, and occasionally sinusitis, endocarditis, peritonitis, and fasciitis.
Myroides odoratus, Myroides odoratimimus	Pathogenesis unknown	Rarely isolated from humans Associated with urine, blood, wounds, and respiratory specimens
Weeksella virosa	Pathogenesis unknown	Genitourinary isolation most often. Has been isolated from postoperative wounds, peritonitis, and septicemia

Because of their ability to survive well in hospital environments, these organisms have the potential to contaminate laboratory culture media and blood culture systems. Whenever these species are encountered, their clinical significance and the potential for contamination should be carefully analyzed.

Pathogenesis and Spectrum of Disease

Because these are environmental organisms, no specific virulence factors have been identified. However, the ability to survive in chlorinated tap water may give these organisms an edge in their ability to thrive in potable water systems.

The development of infection requires exposure of debilitated patients to a contaminated source, often resulting in respiratory colonization. Subsequent infections, such as bacteremia or pneumonia, may develop. These infections are commonly caused by *E. anophelis, Chryseobacterium indologenes,* or *Myroides odoratus.* Infections of several other body sites, which may or may not be preceded by respiratory colonization, have been associated with the other species.

Meningitis caused by *E. meningoseptica* and *E. anophelis* is the most notable infection associated with the organisms listed in Table 23.2. This is a life-threatening infection, which may be accompanied by bacteremia and multiple

TABLE 23.3	Colonial Appearance and Characteristics	
Organism	Medium	Appearance
Balneatrix	BA	Pale yellow to brown, convex and smooth
Bergeyella zoohelcum	BA	Nonmucoid Sticky, nonpigmented
Chryseobacterium anthropi	BA	Sticky, nonpigmented to slightly salmon pink, rarely yellow
Chryseobacterium gleum	BA	Produces dark yellow flexirubin pigment, alpha-hemolytic
Chryseobacterium hominis	BA	Mucoid, slightly yellowish pigment
Chryseobacterium indologenes	BA	Circular, smooth, shiny with entire edge; dark yellow (flexirubin) to orange, beta-hemolytic
Elizabethkingia spp.	BA	Usually nonpigmented, although may exhibit a slight yellow or salmon-pink pigment; smooth, circular, large, shiny with entire edge
Empedobacter brevis	BA	Circular, smooth, shiny with entire edge; light yellow
Myroides spp.	BA	Yellow pigmented, fruity odor
Sphingobacterium spp.	BA	Small, circular, convex, smooth, opaque with light yellow pigment
Weeksella virosa	BA	Mucoid, slimy

BA, 5% sheep blood agar.

organ dysfunction. These organisms are both associated with moderate to large outbreaks in health care settings, which result in significant mortality. *Elizabethkingia* spp. meningitis can occur in infants, children, and compromised adults. *E. meningosepticum* strains have been identified that encode several cytolysin genes that contribute to the virulence of the organism. Historically, *E. meningosepticum* was considered the predominant human pathogen in this genus; however, more recently, *E. anopheles* has been associated with multiple outbreaks and appears to be a serious emerging human pathogen.

Infections caused by *C. indologenes* tend to occur more in immunocompromised individuals, such as those with leukemias or lymphomas, as well as preterm infants. *Sphingobacterium multivorum* and *S. spiritivorum* are the two most often clinically identified species of the genus. *S. multivorum* has been isolated from a variety of clinical specimens, whereas blood and urine isolates tend to be common for the detection of *S. spiritivorum*.

Laboratory Diagnosis

Specimen Collection and Transport

No special considerations are required for specimen collection and transport of the organisms discussed in this chapter. Refer to Table 5.1 for general information on specimen collection and transport.

Specimen Processing

No special considerations are required for processing the organisms discussed in this chapter. Refer to Table 5.1 for general specimen processing information.

Direct Detection Methods

Gram staining is used to detect these organisms in clinical material. The *Chryseobacterium* spp. and *Elizabethkingia* spp. are medium to long straight rods that often appear as "II-forms" (i.e., cells that appear thin in the center and thicker at the ends). *Empedobacter brevis* varies in being short to long rods. *Sphingobacterium* spp. are short straight rods; *S. thalpophilum* may exhibit II-forms. *Balneatrix alpaca* is a highly pleomorphic straight or curved gram-negative rod.

Cultivation
Media of Choice

All genera in this chapter grow well on routine laboratory media, such as trypticase soy agar with 5% sheep blood and chocolate agars. They also grow well in the broth of blood culture systems and in liquid media such as thioglycollate and brain-heart infusion broths. Some strains of the organisms in this chapter may have delayed growth or grow poorly on MacConkey agar.

Incubation Conditions and Duration

These organisms will produce detectable growth on blood and chocolate agars when incubated at 35°C to 37°C in either carbon dioxide or ambient air for a minimum of 24 hours. Growth on MacConkey agar is usually detectable within 24 hours of inoculation.

Colonial Appearance

Table 23.3 presents descriptions of the colonial appearance and other distinguishing characteristics of each genus on trypticase soy agar with 5% sheep blood, chocolate, and MacConkey agars.

Approach to Identification

Most commercial identification systems are limited or unreliable in the identification of the organisms discussed in this chapter. The key biochemical reactions used to presumptively differentiate the genera discussed in this chapter are included in Table 23.4. Matrix-assisted laser desorption/ionization time-of-flight mass spectrometry (MALDI-TOF MS) can be used to successfully identify some species of *Elizabethkingia, Chryseobacterium,* and *Sphingobacterium* spp. However, difficulties remain simply due to the missing spectra of described species within the databases. Definitive identification of these organisms may require a battery of biochemical tests not commonly available in many clinical microbiology laboratories. Full identification of clinically relevant isolates may require that they be sent to a reference laboratory.

Isolates of *E. meningoseptica* tend to have a more muddy colonial appearance, versus the yellow pigment of *C. indologenes.* Both are oxidase-positive, but *E. meningoseptica* is orthonitrophenyl galactoside (ONPG)-positive, whereas *C. indologenes* is ONPG-negative. They are oxidase-positive and grow poorly on MacConkey; they hydrolyze esculin but are otherwise biochemically non-reactive. *S. thalpophilum* can be differentiated from other clinically significant species by its ability to grow at 42°C and to reduce nitrate.

Comments Regarding Specific Organisms

The growth of *S. spiritivorum* and *Chryseobacterium* spp. is variable on MacConkey agar. Therefore, these organisms often need to be differentiated from the yellow-pigmented, MacConkey-negative, oxidase-positive genera considered in Chapters 26 and 30.

Serodiagnosis

Serodiagnostic techniques are not generally used for the laboratory diagnosis of infections caused by the organisms discussed in this chapter.

Antimicrobial Susceptibility Testing and Therapy

Validated susceptibility testing methods do not exist for these organisms. Although they grow on the media and under the conditions recommended for testing, the ability to grow and the ability to detect important antimicrobial resistances are not the same. The lack of validated *in vitro* susceptibility testing methods does not allow definitive treatment and testing guidelines to be given for any of the organisms listed in Table 23.5.

Although susceptibility data for some of these bacteria can be found in the literature, the lack of understanding of potential underlying resistance mechanisms prohibits the validation of such data. Review Chapter 11 for preferable strategies that can be used to provide susceptibility information and data when validated testing methods do not exist for a clinically important bacterial isolate.

In general, the species considered in this chapter are typically resistant to beta-lactams (including penicillins, cephalosporins, and carbapenems) and aminoglycosides commonly used to treat infections caused by other gram-negative bacilli. However, the susceptibility data can vary substantially with the type of testing method used. Many of these species often appear susceptible to, and may be treated with, antimicrobial agents that are considered effective against gram-positive bacteria; clindamycin, rifampin, and vancomycin are notable examples. Colistin has been successfully used to treat patients infected with *E. meningoseptica* and *C. indologenes.* Other studies have reported colistin resistance in these two organisms.

Prevention

Because these organisms are ubiquitous in nature and are not generally a threat to human health, no recommended vaccination or prophylaxis protocols have been established. Health care–associated infections are controlled using appropriate sterile technique, infection control, and implementation of effective protocols for sterilization and decontamination of medical supplies.

Visit the Evolve site for a complete list of procedures, review questions, and case studies.

TABLE 23.4 Key Biochemical and Physiologic Characteristics

Organism	Growth on MacConkey Agar	Mannitol	Arabinose	Esculin Hydrolysis	Gelatin	Urea	Nitrate Reduction	Nitrite Reduction	ONPG	PYR
Balneatrix alpica	–	+	–	–	–	–	+	–	–	–
Bergeyella zoohelcum	–	–	–	–	+	+	–	–	–	–
Chryseobacterium anthropi	–	–	–	–	+	–	–	–	–	+
Chryseobacterium gleam	+	–	+	+	+	73	73	54	–	+
Chryseobacterium hominis	–	–	–	+	+	–	65	65	–	+
Chryseobacterium indologenes	67	–	–	+	+	–	26	13	–	+
Chryseobacterium treverense	–	–	–	20	–	–	60	+	–	80
Elizabethkingia anophelis	+	+	–	+	–	–	ND	ND	+	ND
Elizabethkingia meningoseptica	83	+	–	+	+	–	–	88	+	+
Empedobacter brevis	+	–	–	–	+	–	–	–	–	+
Myroides injenensis	ND	–	ND	ND	+	+	–	ND	–	ND
Myroides odoratus	75	–	ND	–	+	+	–	+	+	+
Myroides odoratimimus	+	–	ND	–	+	+	–	+	–	+
Sphingobacterium multivorum	+	–	ND	+	–	+	–	–	+	+
Sphingobacterium spiritivorum	50	+	ND	+	–	+	–	–	75	+
Sphingobacterium thalpophilum	+	–	ND	+	–	+	+	–	+	+
Wautersiella falsenii	+	–	–	53	53	+	–	34	19	+
Weeksella virosa	–	–	–	–	+	–	–	–	–	+

Values are percentages; *ND*, no data; *ONPG*, beta-galactosidase; *PYR*, pyrrolindodyl aminopeptidase; −, >90% of strains are positive; −, >90% of strains are negative.
From Caroll KC, Pfaller MA. *Manual of Clinical Microbiology*. 12th ed. Washington, DC: ASM Press; 2019.

TABLE 23.5 **Antimicrobial Therapy and Susceptibility Testing**

Species	Therapeutic Options	Potential Resistance to Therapeutic Options	Validated Testing Methods[a]	Comments
Bergeyella zoohelcum	Susceptible to most antibiotics		Not available	
Chryseobacterium indologenes,[b] *Elizabethkingia* spp., *Empedobacter brevis, Sphingobacterium* spp.	No definitive guidelines. Potentially active agents include ciprofloxacin, rifampin, clindamycin, trimethoprim/ sulfamethoxazole, and vancomycin	Produce beta-lactamases and are frequently resistant to aminoglycosides, tetracyclines, and chloramphenicol	Not available	*In vitro* susceptibility results with disk diffusion may be seriously misleading.

[a]Validated testing methods include standard methods recommended by the Clinical and Laboratory Standards Institute (CLSI) and commercial methods approved by the US Food and Drug Administration (FDA).
[b]Multidrug-resistant strains have been isolated.

Bibliography

Arouna O, Deluca F, Camara M, et al.: *Chryseobacterium gleum* in a man with prostatectomy in Senegal: a case report and review of the literature, *J Med Case Rep* 11:118, 2017, https://doi.org/10.1186/s13256-017-1269-4.

Bennett J, Dolin R, Blaser M: *Principles and practice of infectious diseases*, ed 9, Philadelphia, 2020, Elsevier-Saunders.

Breurec S, Criscuolo A, Diancourt L, et al.: Genomic epidemiology and global diversity of the emerging bacterial pathogen *Elizabethkingia anopheles, Sci Rep* 6:30379, 2016.

Caroll KC, Pfaller MA: *Manual of clinical microbiology*, ed 12, Washington, DC, 2019, ASM Press.

Chen S, Soehnlen M, Downes FP, Walker ED: Insights from the draft genome into the pathogenicity of a clinical isolate of *Elizabethkingia meningoseptica* Em3, *Stand Genomic Sci* 12:56, 2017.

Choi MH, Kim M, Jeong SJ, et al.: Risk factors for *Elizabethkingia* acquisition and clinical characteristics of patients, South Korea, *Emerg Infect Dis* 25(1):42–51, 2019.

Giordano C, Falleni M, Capria AL, et al.: First report of *Wautersiella falsenii* genomovar 2 isolated from the respiratory tract of an immunosuppressed man, *IDCases* 4:27–29, 2016.

Gupta P, Zaman K, Mohan B, Taneja N: *Elizabethkingia miricola*: a rare non-fermenter causing urinary tract infection, *World J Clin Cases* 5(5):187–190, 2017.

Kim KK, Kim MK, Lim JH, et al.: Transfer of *Chryseobacterium meningosepticum* and *Chryseobacterium miricola* to *Elizabethkingia*

meningoseptica comb nov and *Elizabethkingia miricolacomb* nov, *Int J Syst Evol Microbiol* 55:1287–1293, 2005.

Lau SKP, Chow WN, Foo CH, et al.: *Elizabethkingia anopheles* bacteremia is associated with clinically significant infections and high mortality, *Sci Rep* 6:26045, 2016.

Mulliken JS, Langelier C, Budak JZ, et al.: *Bergeyella cardium*: clinical characteristics and draft genome of an emerging pathogen in native and prosthetic valve endocarditis, *Open Forum Infect Dis* 6(4):ofz134, 2019, https://doi.org/10.1093/ofid/ofz134.

Perrin A, Larsonneur E, Nicholson AC, et al.: Evolutionary dynamics and genomic features of *Elizabethkingia anophelis* 2015-2016 Wisconsin outbreak strain, *Nat Commun* 8:15483, 2017.

Reina J, Borrell N, Figuerola J: *Sphingobacterium multivorum* isolated from a patient with cystic fibrosis, *Eur J Clin Microbiol Infect Dis* 11:81–82, 1992.

Shailaja VV, Reddy AK, Ailmelu M, Sadanand LNR: Neonatal meningitis by multidrug resistant *Elizabethkingia meningosepticum* identified by 16S ribosomal RNA gene sequencing, *Int J Pediatr* 2014:918907, 2014.

Sharma D, Patel A, Soni P, et al.: *Empedobacter brevis* meningitis in a neonate: a very rare case of neonatal meningitis and literature review, *Case Rep Pediatr* 2016:7609602, 2016, https://doi.org/10.1155/2016/7609602.

Weaver KN, Jones RC, Albright R, et al.: Acute emergence of *Elizabethkingia meningoseptica* infection among mechanically ventilated patients in a long-term acute care facility, *Infect Control Hosp Epidemiol* 31:54–58, 2010.

24

Alcaligenes, Comamonas, and Similar Organisms

OBJECTIVES

1. Describe the normal habitat of the organisms discussed in this chapter and the means of transmission for human infection.
2. List the general characteristics of the bacteria discussed in this chapter.
3. Identify unusual biochemical reactions and incubation conditions required of organisms discussed in this chapter.
4. Outline the major tests used to identify the organisms in these groups.
5. Compare the appearance of the different genera in Gram stain preparations.
6. Describe the colonial appearance of the clinically significant species.

GENERA AND SPECIES TO BE CONSIDERED

Current Name	Previous Name
Advenella spp.	Alcaligenes spp.
Alcaligenes faecalis type species	Pseudomonas or Alcaligenes odorans
A. faecalis subsp. faecalis	
Comamonas spp.	
Delftia acidovorans	Comamonas acidovorans, Pseudomonas acidovorans
Kerstersia spp.	Alcaligenes sp.
Myroides spp.	Flavobacterium odoratum
Paenalcaligenes spp.	
Roseomonas spp.	

General Characteristics

The genera discussed in this chapter are considered together because most of them are usually oxidase-positive, non–glucose utilizers capable of growth on MacConkey agar. Many of the genera, *Alcaligenes, Kerstersia, Advenella* and *Paenalcaligenes,* belong to the family *Alcaligenaceae. Kerstersia* phenotypically resembles *Alcaligenes. Advenella* species are *Alcaligenes*-like. The organisms' specific morphologic and

physiologic features are presented later in this chapter in the discussion of laboratory diagnosis.

The genus *Alcaligenes* is limited to a single species, *A. faecalis,* with three subspecies: *A. faecalis* subsp. *faecalis, A. faecalis* subsp. *parafaecalis,* and *A. faecalis* subsp. *phenolicus. Alcaligenes* species are gram-negative, strict aerobic rods or coccobacilli that are oxidase and catalase positive. They are motile and have 1 to 12 peritrichous flagella. *Advenella* and *Kerstersia* are strictly aerobic, nonfermentative, gram-negative, rod-shaped or coccobacilli in pairs or short chains. Motility is strain-dependent. *Comamonas* spp. are typically environmental species that may be problematic opportunistic health care–associated pathogens. *Comamonas* and *Delftia* spp. are aerobic, non–spore-forming, and straight or slightly curved gram-negative rods with one or more polar flagella. *Paenalicaligenes* are small gram-negative rods. The genus *Myroides* contains two species: *M. odoratimimus* and *M. odoratus* (Chapter 23). The organisms are thin, nonmotile rods that develop a fruity smell similar to *A. faecalis. Roseomonas* spp. are coccoid, plump rods in pairs or short chains. They are typically motile by one or two polar flagella.

Epidemiology

The habitats of the species listed in Table 24.1 vary from soil and water environments to the upper respiratory tract of various mammals. Certain species have been exclusively found in humans, whereas the natural habitat for other organisms remains unknown. Some of these organisms have been known to colonize the upper respiratory tract. *Alcaligenes, Advenella*, and *Rosemonas* have been isolated from the respiratory tract of cystic fibrosis (CF) patients. In addition to environmental transmission, person-to-person transmission is believed to be involved in the spread of *Alcaligenes* among CF patients.

The diversity of the organisms' habitats is reflected in the various ways they are transmitted.

Pathogenesis and Spectrum of Disease

Identifiable virulence factors are not known for most of the organisms listed in Table 24.2. However, because infections usually involve exposure of compromised patients to contaminated materials, most of these species are probably of

TABLE 24.1 Epidemiology

Species	Habitat (Reservoir)	Mode of Transmission
Advenella	Environment	Unknown
Alcaligenes faecalis	Environment; soil and water, including moist hospital environments May transiently colonize the skin	Exposure to contaminated medical devices and solutions
Comamonas spp.	Environment, soil and water; can be found in the hospital environment Not part of human microbiota	Nosocomial opportunistic pathogens because of their ability to survive in aqueous environments
Delftia acidovorans	Environment, soil and water; can be found in the hospital environment Not part of human microbiota	Uncertain Rarely found in humans Probably involves exposure to contaminated solutions or devices
Kerstersia spp.	Environmental Colonizer of the upper respiratory tract	Uncertain
Myroides spp.	Unknown Probably environmental Not part of human microbiota	Unknown Rarely found in humans
Roseomonas spp.	Unknown	Unknown Rarely found in humans

TABLE 24.2 Pathogenesis and Spectrum of Disease

Species	Virulence Factors	Spectrum of Disease and Infections
Advenella spp.	Unknown	Recovered from the respiratory secretions of patients with cystic fibrosis
Alcaligenes faecalis	Unknown	Infections usually involve compromised patients. Often a contaminant; clinical significance of isolates should be interpreted with caution. Has been isolated from blood, respiratory specimens, and urine
Alcaligenes piechaudii	Unknown	Rare cause of human infection
Comamonas testosteroni *Comamonas* spp.	Unknown	Isolated from the respiratory tract, eye, and blood. Clinical significance is unclear
Delftia acidovorans	Unknown	Isolated from the respiratory tract, eye, and blood but rarely implicated as being clinically significant
Kerstersia spp.	Unknown	Associated with bacteremia; identified as a colonizer of the upper respiratory tract
Pseudomonas alcaligenes *P. pseudoalcaligenes*	Unknown; low virulence. Associated with administration of contaminated solutions and medicines	Recovered from the respiratory secretions of patients with cystic fibrosis
Roseomonas spp.	Unknown; uncommon isolates from humans	Clinical significance uncertain. Typically opportunistic infections. Most isolated from blood, wounds, exudates, abscesses, or genitourinary tract of immunocompromised or debilitated patients

low virulence. *A. faecalis* has been isolated from a wide range of clinical specimens and identified in bacteremia, ocular infections, pancreatic abscesses, bone infections, urine, and ear discharge. *Comamonas* spp. have been identified in cases of endocarditis, meningitis, and catheter-associated bacteremia. *C. testosteroni* has been the species most often associated with human infection. *Delftia acidovorans* has been associated with bacteremia, endocarditis, ocular infection, and otitis media. Both *C. testosteroni* and *D. acidovorans* have also been isolated from patients with CF. *M. odoratus* has been primarily isolated from the human urinary tract but has also been identified in wound, sputum, blood, and ear specimens. Other organisms, such *Advenella*, *Kerstersia*, and *Rosemonas* have been isolated from respiratory samples in CF patients. *Kerstersia gyiorum* has been isolated from wounds, chronic ear infections, bone, and sputum. *K. similis* has been isolated from leg wounds and other abscesses.

Laboratory Diagnosis

Specimen Collection and Transport

No special considerations are required for the collection and transport of the organisms discussed in this chapter. Refer to Table 5.1 for general information on specimen collection and transport.

Specimen Processing

No special considerations are required for processing of the organisms discussed in this chapter. Refer to Table 5.1 for general information on specimen processing.

Direct Detection Methods

Other than Gram staining of patient specimens, there are no specific procedures for the direct detection of these organisms in clinical material. *Roseomonas* spp. are coccobacilli.

Some *Roseomonas* spp. may appear as short, straight rods. *Myroides* spp. are pleomorphic rods and are either short or long and straight to slightly curved.

Alcaligenes, *Advenella*, and *Kerstersia* spp. are medium to long straight rods, as are *Cupriavidus pauculus* and *D. acidovorans*. The *Comamonas* spp. are pleomorphic and may appear as long paired curved rods or as filaments.

Cultivation
Media of Choice

All the genera included in this chapter grow well on 5% sheep blood, chocolate, and MacConkey agars. Most of these genera should also grow well in the broth of blood culture systems, as well as in common nutrient broths such as thioglycollate and brain-heart infusion.

Incubation Conditions and Duration

Most of the organisms produce detectable growth on media incubated at 35°C in ambient air or 5% carbon dioxide (CO_2).

Colonial Appearance

Table 24.3 describes the colonial appearance and other distinguishing characteristics (e.g., pigment and odor) of each genus on 5% sheep blood and MacConkey agars.

TABLE 24.3 Colonial Appearance and Characteristics

Organism	Medium	Appearance
Advenella spp.	BA MAC	Resembles *A. denitrificans* NLF
Alcaligenes faecalis	BA MAC	Feather-edged colonies usually surrounded by zone of green discoloration; produces a highly characteristic, fruity odor resembling apples or strawberries NLF
Alcaligenes piechaudii	BA MAC	Nonpigmented, glistening, convex colonies surrounded by zone of greenish brown discoloration NLF
Alcaligenes xylosoxidans	BA MAC	Small, convex, and glistening NLF
Comamonas spp.	BA MAC	No distinctive appearance NLF
Delftia acidovorans	BA MAC	No distinctive appearance NLF
Kerstersia spp.	BA MAC	Grey, flat colonies with spreading edges NLF
Myroides spp.	BA MAC	Most colonies are yellow, have a characteristic fruity odor, and tend to spread NLF
Roseomonas spp.	BA MAC	Pink-pigmented; some colonies may be mucoid NLF

BA, 5% sheep blood agar; *Mac*, MacConkey agar; *NLF*, non–lactose fermenter.

TABLE 24.4   Key Biochemical and Physiologic Characteristics for Rod-Shaped Motile Species With Polar Flagella

Organism	Number of Flagella	Oxidizes Mannitol	Insoluble Pigment	Growth at 42°C	Nitrate Reduction
Delftia acidovorans	>2	–	–	V	+
Comamonas spp.	>2	–	–	V	+
Roseomonas spp.[a]	1–2[b]	V	Pink	V	v

+, >90% of strains are positive; –, >90% of strains are negative; *V,* variable.
[a]Represents composite of several species and genomospecies.
[b]Genomospecies 5 is nonmotile.
Data compiled from Holt JG, Krieg NR, Sneath PH, et al, eds. *Bergey's Manual of Determinative Bacteriology.* 9th ed. Baltimore: Williams & Wilkins: 1994; and Carroll KC, Pfaller MA, Landry ML, et al. *Manual of Clinical Microbiology.* 12th ed. Washington, DC: ASM; 2019.

TABLE 24.5   Key Biochemical and Physiologic Characteristics for Rod-Shaped Motile Species With Peritrichous Flagella

Organism	Urea Hydrolysis	Nitrate Reduction	Gas from Nitrate	Growth on Cetrimide	Jordan's Tartrate[a]
Alcaligenes faecalis[b]	–	–	–	V	–
Alcaligenes piechaudii	–	+	–	+	+
Alcaligenes xylosoxidans		+	+	+	
Advenella	V	+	+	–	–

+, >90% of strains are positive; –, >90% of strains are negative; *V,* variable.
[a]Jordan's tartrate agar deep is a medium used to differentiate gram-negative enteric microorganisms based on the utilization of tartrate.
[b]Reduces nitrite.
Data compiled from Holt JG, Krieg NR, Sneath PH, et al, eds. *Bergey's Manual of Determinative Bacteriology.* 9th ed. Baltimore: Williams & Wilkins; 1994; and Carroll KC, Pfaller MA, Landry ML, et al. *Manual of Clinical Microbiology.* 12th ed. Washington, DC: ASM; 2019.

Approach to Identification

The ability of most commercial identification systems to accurately identify the organisms discussed in this chapter is limited or uncertain. Strategies for identification of these genera are based on the use of conventional biochemical tests and special staining for flagella. Although most clinical microbiology laboratories do not routinely perform flagella stains, motility and flagella placement are the easiest ways to differentiate among these organisms.

Many microbiologists groan at the mere mention of having to perform a flagella stain, but the method described in Procedure 12.17 is a wet mount that is easy to perform. At the very least, a simple wet mount to observe cells for motility helps distinguish between the motile and nonmotile genera. The motile organisms described in this chapter have peritrichous flagella (e.g., *Alcaligenes* spp.) or polar flagella (e.g., *Delftia, Comamonas* spp.).

Organisms are first categorized on the basis of Gram stain morphology and rod shape (Tables 24.4 and 24.5).

They are then further characterized based on whether the organisms have peritrichous flagella (Table 24.4), or flagellated by polar tufts (Table 24.5).

Comments Regarding Specific Organisms

In order to distinguish the genera included in this chapter, 16S rRNA sequence analysis is recommended. *Alcaligenes piechaudii* reduces nitrate to nitrite. *A. faecalis* has a fruity odor and reduces nitrite to gas. Urea hydrolysis is a key test for *Myroides* spp., which is also distinguished by production of a characteristic fruity odor.

D. acidovorans is unique in producing an orange color when Kovac's reagent is added to tryptone broth (indole test). *Advenella* can be separated from related species by the ability to assimilate phenyl acetate. *K. gyiorum* is positive for the oxidation of D-galacturonic acid and negative for D-serine, whereas *K. similis* is negative for the oxidation of D-galacturonic acid and positive for D-serine.

Roseomonas spp. must be separated from other pink-pigmented, gram-negative (e.g., *Methylobacterium* spp.) and gram-positive (e.g., certain *Rhodococcus* spp. or *Bacillus* spp.) organisms. *Roseomonas* spp. differ from *Rhodococcus* and *Bacillus* spp. by being resistant to vancomycin, as determined by using a 30-µg vancomycin disk on an inoculated 5% blood agar plate. Unlike *Methylobacterium* spp., *Roseomonas* spp. grow on MacConkey agar and at 42°C. All *Roseomonas* species strongly hydrolyze urea but not esculin and are beta-galactosidase negative.

Serodiagnosis

Serodiagnostic techniques are not generally used for the laboratory diagnosis of infections caused by the organisms discussed in this chapter.

Antimicrobial Susceptibility Testing and Therapy

Validated susceptibility testing methods do not exist for these organisms. Although they will grow on the media and under the conditions recommended for testing the more commonly encountered bacteria, this does not necessarily mean that interpretable and reliable results will be produced. Chapter 11 should be reviewed for preferable strategies that can be used to provide susceptibility information when validated testing methods do not exist for a clinically important bacterial isolate.

The lack of validated *in vitro* susceptibility testing methods does not allow definitive treatment and testing guidelines to be given for most organisms listed in Table 24.6. If antimicrobial sensitivity testing is required for *Alcaligenes*

TABLE 24.6   Antimicrobial Therapy and Susceptibility Testing

Species	Therapeutic Options	Potential Resistance to Therapeutic Options	Validated Testing Methods[a]	Comments
Advenella	No definitive guidelines	Unknown		
Alcaligenes faecalis	No definitive guidelines Potentially active agents include combinations of amoxicillin or ticarcillin with clavulanic acid, various cephalosporins, and ciprofloxacin	Capable of beta-lactamase production Commonly resistant to ampicillin, amoxicillin, ticarcillin, aztreonam, kanamycin, gentamicin, and nalidixic acid	Not available	Susceptible to combinations of amoxicillin or ticarcillin with clavulanic acid; cephalosporins and ciprofloxacin
Alcaligenes piechaudii	No definitive guidelines	Resistant to ampicillin, cefpodoxime, and gentamicin	Not available	
Alcaligenes xylosoxidans	No definitive guidelines Potentially active agents include imipenem, piperacillin, ticarcillin/clavulanic acid, ceftazidime, and trimethoprim-sulfamethoxazole	Aminoglycosides, expanded spectrum cephalosporins other than ceftazidime, and quinolones demonstrated no activity Resistant to tobramycin, azithromycin, and clarithromycin	Not available	
Comamonas acidovorans, Comamonas testosteroni, Comamonas spp.	No definitive guidelines Potentially active agents include extended- to broad-spectrum cephalosporins, carbapenems, quinolones, and trimethoprim-sulfamethoxazole	Unknown	Not available	*C. acidovorans* tends to be more resistant than the other two species, especially to aminoglycosides
Delftia acidovorans	No definitive guidelines	Frequently resistant to aminoglycosides	Not available	
Kerstersia spp.	No definitive guidelines	Unknown		Susceptible to ciprofloxacin and cefotaxime
Roseomonas spp.	No definitive guidelines Potentially active agents include aminoglycosides, imipenem, and quinolones	Generally resistant to cephalosporins and penicillins	Not available	

[a]Validated testing methods include standard methods recommended by the Clinical and Laboratory Standards Institute (CLSI) and commercial methods approved by the US Food and Drug Administration (FDA).

spp., methods include broth macrodilution and microdilution, agar dilution, breakpoint methods, and Etest.

Although standardized methods have not been established for the other species discussed in this chapter, *in vitro* susceptibility studies have been published, and antimicrobial agents that have potential activity are noted, where appropriate, in Table 24.6.

Prevention

Because the organisms may be encountered throughout nature and do not generally pose a threat to human health, there are no recommended vaccination or prophylaxis protocols. For those organisms occasionally identified in health care–associated infections, prevention of infection is best accomplished by following appropriate sterile techniques and infection control guidelines.

ⓔ Visit the Evolve site for a complete list of procedures, review questions, and case studies.

Bibliography

Balows A, Truper HG, Dworkin M, et al.: *The prokaryotes: a handbook on the biology of bacteria—ecophysiology, isolation, identification, applications,* ed 2, New York, NY, 1981, Springer-Verlag.

Carroll KC, Pfaller MA, Landry ML, et al.: *Manual of clinical microbiology,* ed 12, Washington, DC, 2019, ASM.

Castagnola E, Tasso L, Conte M, Nantron M, Barretta A, Giacchino R: Central venous catheter–related infection due to *Comamonas acidovorans* in a child with non-Hodgkin's lymphoma, *Clin Infect Dis* 19:559–560, 1994.

Deutscher M, Severing J, Balada-Llasat JM: *Kerstersia gyiorum* isolated from a bronchoalveolar lavage in a patient with a chronic tracheostomy, *Case Rep Infect Dis* 2014;2014:479581.

Doi Y, Poirel L, Paterson DL, Nordmann P: Characterization of a naturally occurring class D beta-lactamase from *Achromobacter xylosoxidans, Antimicrob Agents Chemother* 52:1952–1956, 2008.

Dunne Jr WM, Maisch S: Epidemiological investigation of infections due to *Alcaligenes* species in children and patients with cystic fibrosis: use of repetitive-element–sequence polymerase chain reaction, *Clin Infect Dis* 20:836–841, 1995.

Holt JG, Krieg NR, Sneath PH, et al.: *Bergey's manual of determinative bacteriology,* ed 9, Baltimore, MD, 1994, Williams & Wilkins.

Lan Y, Yan Q, Yan Y, Liu W: First case of *Kerstersia gyiorum* isolated from a patient with chronic osteomyelitis in China, *Front Lab Med* 1:141–143, 2017.

Rihs JD, Brenner DJ, Weaver RE, Steigerwalt AG, Hollis DG, Yu VL: *Roseomonas:* a new genus associated with bacteremia and other human infections, *J Clin Microbiol* 31:3275–3283, 1993.

Saiman L, Chen Y, Tabibi S, et al.: Identification and antimicrobial susceptibility of *Alcaligenes xylosoxidans* isolated from patients with cystic fibrosis, *J Clin Microbiol* 39:3942–3945, 2001.

Vancanneyt M, Segers P, Torck U, et al.: Reclassification of *Flavobacterium odoratum (Stutzer 1929)* strains to a new genus, *Myroides,* as *Myroidesodoratus* comb nov and *Myroidesodora timimus* spnov, *Int J Syst Bacteriol* 46:926, 1996.

Vandamme P, Heyndrickx M, Vancanneyt M, et al.: *Bordetella trematum* spnov, isolated from wounds and ear infections in humans, and reassessment of *Alcaligenes denitrificans (Rüger and Tan, 1983), Int J Syst Bacteriol* 46:849–858, 1996.

Wen A, Fegan M, Hayward C, Chakraborty S, Sly LI: Phylogenetic relationships among members of the *Comamonadaceae,* and description of *Delftia acidovorans* (den Dooren de Jong, 1926 and Tamaoka et al, 1987) gen nov, comb nov, *Int J Syst Bacteriol* 49:567–576, 1999.

Yabuuchi E, Kawamura Y, Kosako Y, Ezaki T: Emendation of the genus *Achromobacter* and *Achromobacter xylosoxidans* (Yabuuchi and Yano) and proposal of *Achromobacter ruhlandii* (Packer and Vishniac) comb nov, *Achromobacter piechaudii* (Kiredjian et al) comb nov, and *Achromobacter xylosoxidans* subsp *denitrificans* (Rüger and Tan) comb nov, *Microbiol Immunol* 42:429–438, 1998.

25

Vibrio, Aeromonas, Plesiomonas shigelloides, and Chromobacterium violaceum

OBJECTIVES

1. Describe the general characteristics of the organisms discussed in this chapter, including natural habitat, route of transmission, Gram stain reactions, and cellular morphology.
2. Describe the media used to isolate *Vibrio* spp. and the organisms' colonial appearance.
3. Explain the physiologic activity of the cholera toxin and its relationship to the pathogenesis of the organism.
4. Describe the clinical significance of *Aeromonas* spp., *Chromobacterium* spp., and *Vibrio* spp. other than *Vibrio cholerae*.
5. Correlate the patient's signs and symptoms and laboratory data to identify an infectious agent.

Current Name	Previous Name
Grimontia hollisae	CDC group EF-13, *Vibrio hollisae*
Vibrio alginolyticus	*Vibrio parahaemolyticus* biotype 2
Vibrio cholerae	
Vibrio cincinnatiensis	
Vibrio fluvialis	CDC group EF-6
Vibrio furnissii	
Vibrio harveyi	*Vibrio carchariae*
Vibrio metschnikovii	CDC enteric group 16
Vibrio mimicus	*Vibrio cholerae* (sucrose negative)
Vibrio parahaemolyticus	*Pasteurella parahaemolyticus*
Vibrio vulnificus	CDC group EF-3

General Characteristics

The organisms discussed in this chapter are considered together because they are all oxidase-positive, glucose-fermenting, gram-negative bacilli capable of growth on MacConkey agar. Their individual morphologic and physiologic features are presented later in this chapter in the discussion of laboratory diagnosis. Other halophilic (salt-loving) organisms, such as *Shewanella algae*, require salt but do not ferment glucose, as do the halophilic *Vibrio* spp.

Aeromonas spp. are gram-negative straight rods with rounded ends or coccobacillary facultative anaerobes that occur singly, in pairs, or in short chains. They are typically oxidase- and catalase-positive and produce acid from oxidative and fermentative metabolism. *Chromobacterium violaceum* is a facultative anaerobic, motile, gram-negative rod or cocci.

The family *Vibrionaceae* includes six genera, three of which are discussed in this chapter. The *Photobacterium* and *Grimontia* genera each include a single species. The genus *Vibrio* consists of 10 species of gram-negative, facultative anaerobic, curved or comma-shaped rods. Most *Vibrio* spp. require sodium for growth and glucose fermentation; with the exception of *Vibrio metschnikovii*, all species are motile and catalase- and oxidase-positive.

TABLE 25.1   Epidemiology

Species	Habitat (Reservoir)	Mode of Transmission
Vibrio cholerae	Niche outside of human gastrointestinal tract between occurrence of epidemics and pandemics is uncertain; may survive in a dormant state in brackish or saltwater; human carriers also are known, particularly in endemic regions	Fecal-oral route, by ingestion of contaminated washing, swimming, cooking, or drinking water; also by ingestion of contaminated shellfish or other seafood
Vibrio alginolyticus	Brackish or saltwater	Exposure to contaminated water
Vibrio cincinnatiensis	Unknown	Unknown
Photobacterium damsela	Brackish or saltwater	Exposure of wound to contaminated water
Vibrio fluvialis	Brackish or saltwater	Ingestion of contaminated water or seafood
Vibrio furnissii	Brackish or saltwater	Ingestion of contaminated water or seafood
Grimontia hollisae	Brackish or saltwater	Ingestion of contaminated water or seafood
Vibrio metschnikovii	Brackish, salt, and freshwater	Ingestion of contaminated water or seafood
Vibrio mimicus	Brackish or saltwater	Ingestion of contaminated water or seafood
Vibrio parahaemolyticus	Brackish or saltwater	Ingestion of contaminated water or seafood
Vibrio vulnificus	Brackish or saltwater	Ingestion of contaminated water or seafood
Aeromonas spp.	Aquatic environments around the world, including freshwater, polluted or chlorinated water, brackish water, and, occasionally, marine water; may transiently colonize gastrointestinal tract; often infect various warm- and cold-blooded animal species	Ingestion of contaminated food (e.g., dairy, meat, produce) or water; exposure of disrupted skin or mucosal surfaces to contaminated water or soil; traumatic inoculation of fish fins or fishing hooks
Chromobacterium violaceum	Environmental, soil and water of tropical and subtropical regions Not part of human microbiota	Exposure of disrupted skin to contaminated soil or water

Epidemiology

Many aspects of the epidemiology of *Vibrio* spp., *Aeromonas* spp., and *C. violaceum* are similar (Table 25.1). The primary habitat for most of these organisms is water; generally, brackish or marine water for *Vibrio* spp., freshwater for *Aeromonas* spp., and soil or water for *C. violaceum*. *Aeromonas* spp. may also be found in brackish water or marine water with a low salt content. None of these organisms are considered part of the normal human microbiota. Transmission to humans is by ingestion of contaminated water, fresh produce, meat, dairy products, or seafood or by exposure of disrupted skin and mucosal surfaces to contaminated water.

The epidemiology of the most notable human pathogen in this chapter, *Vibrio cholerae,* is far from being fully understood. This organism causes epidemics and pandemics (i.e., worldwide epidemics) of the diarrheal disease **cholera**. Since 1817, the world has witnessed seven cholera pandemics. In 2010, after a devastating earthquake in Haiti, more than 604,634 infections and 7436 deaths occurred as a result of *V. cholerae* O1 infections within a 24-month period. During these outbreaks the organism was spread among people by the fecal-oral route due to poor sanitation.

Most *V. cholerae* infections are asymptomatic, and therefore humans are likely the reservoir for infection in endemic regions. The form of the organism shed from infected humans is somewhat fragile and cannot survive long in the environment. However, evidence suggests that the bacillus has dormant stages that allow its long-term survival in brackish water or saltwater environments during interepidemic periods. These dormant stages are considered viable but nonculturable. Asymptomatic carriers of *V. cholerae* have been documented, but they are not thought to be a significant reservoir for maintaining the organism between outbreaks.

Pathogenesis and Spectrum of Disease

As a notorious pathogen, *V. cholerae* elaborates several toxins and factors that play important roles in the organism's virulence. **Cholera toxin (CT)** is primarily responsible for the key features of cholera (Table 25.2). Release of this toxin causes mucosal cells to hypersecrete water and electrolytes into the lumen of the gastrointestinal tract. The result is profuse, watery diarrhea, leading to dramatic fluid loss. The fluid loss results in severe dehydration and hypotension that, without medical intervention, frequently leads to death.

TABLE 25.2 Pathogenesis and Spectrum of Diseases

Species	Virulence Factors	Spectrum of Disease and Infections
Vibrio cholerae	Cholera toxin (CT); zonula occludens (Zot) toxin (enterotoxin); accessory cholera enterotoxin (Ace) toxin; O1 and O139 somatic antigens, hemolysin/cytotoxins, motility, chemotaxis, mucinase, and toxin coregulated (TCP) pili.	Cholera: profuse, watery diarrhea leading to dehydration, hypotension, and often death; occurs in epidemics and pandemics that span the globe. May also cause nonepidemic diarrhea and, occasionally, extra intestinal infections of wounds, respiratory tract, urinary tract, and central nervous system.
Vibrio alginolyticus	Specific virulence factors for the non–*V. cholerae* species uncertain.	Ear infections, wound infections; rare cause of septicemia; involvement in gastroenteritis is uncertain.
Vibrio cincinnatiensis		Rare cause of septicemia.
Photobacterium damsela		Wound infections and rare cause of septicemia.
Vibrio fluvialis		Gastroenteritis.
Vibrio furnissii		Rarely associated with human infections.
Grimontia hollisae		Gastroenteritis; rare cause of septicemia.
Vibrio metschnikovii		Rare cause of septicemia; involvement in gastroenteritis is uncertain.
Vibrio mimicus		Gastroenteritis; rare cause of ear infection.
Vibrio vulnificus		Wound infections and septicemia; involvement in gastroenteritis is uncertain.
Aeromonas spp.	Produces various toxins and factors, but their specific role in virulence is uncertain.	Gastroenteritis, wound infections, bacteremia, and miscellaneous other infections, including endocarditis, meningitis, pneumonia, conjunctivitis, and osteomyelitis.
Chromobacterium violaceum	Endotoxin, adhesins, invasins, and cytolytic proteins have been described.	Rare but dangerous infection. Begins with cellulitis or lymphadenitis and can rapidly progress to systemic infection with abscess formation in various organs and septic shock.

This toxin-mediated disease does not require the organism to penetrate the mucosal barrier. Therefore blood and the inflammatory cells typical of dysenteric stools are notably absent in cholera. Instead, "rice water stools," composed of fluids and mucous flecks, are the hallmark of CT activity.

V. cholerae is divided into three major subgroups: *V. cholerae* O1, *V. cholerae* O139, and *V. cholerae* non-O1/non-O139. The somatic antigens O1 and O139 associated with the *V. cholerae* cell envelope are positive markers for strains capable of epidemic and pandemic spread of the disease. Strains carrying these markers almost always produce CT, whereas non-O1/non-O139 strains do not produce the toxin and hence do not produce cholera. Therefore, although these somatic antigens are not virulence factors per se, they are important virulence and epidemiologic markers that provide important information about *V. cholerae* isolates. The non-O1/non-O139 strains are associated with nonepidemic diarrhea and extraintestinal infections.

V. cholerae produces several other toxins and factors that aid in the pathogen's ability to colonize, but the exact role of each in disease is still uncertain (Table 25.2). To effectively release toxin, the organism first must infiltrate and distribute itself along the cells lining the mucosal surface of the gastrointestinal tract. Motility and chemotaxis mediate the distribution of organisms, and mucinase production allows penetration of the mucous layer. **Toxin coregulated pili (TCP)** provide the means by which bacilli attach to mucosal cells for release of CT. The enterotoxin **zona occludens toxin (Zot)** has been shown to disrupt the tight junctions of the intestinal cells, effectively decreasing tissue resistance.

Depending on the species, other vibrios are variably involved in three types of infection: gastroenteritis, wound infections, and bacteremia. Although some of these organisms have not been definitively associated with human infections, others, such as *Vibrio vulnificus,* are known to cause fatal septicemia, especially in patients suffering from an underlying liver disease.

Aeromonas spp. are similar to *Vibrio* spp. in terms of the types of infections they cause. Although these organisms can cause gastroenteritis, especially in children, their role in intestinal infections is not always clear. Therefore, the significance of their isolation in stool specimens should be interpreted with caution. Severe watery diarrhea has been associated with *Aeromonas* strains that produce a heat-labile enterotoxin and a heat-stable enterotoxin. In addition to diarrhea, complications of infection with *Aeromonas* spp. include hemolytic-uremic syndrome (HUS) and kidney disease.

C. violaceum is not associated with gastrointestinal infections, but acquisition of this organism by contamination of wounds can lead to fulminant, life-threatening systemic infections.

Laboratory Diagnosis

Specimen Collection and Transport

Because no special considerations are required for isolation of these genera from extra intestinal sources, the general specimen collection and transport information provided in Table 5.1 is

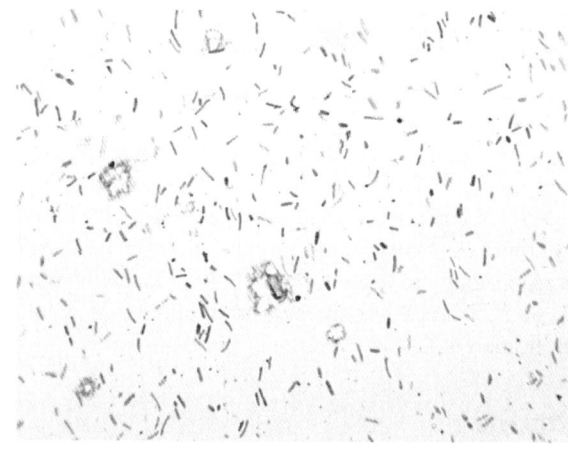

• **Fig. 25.1** Gram stain of *Vibrio parahaemolyticus.*

applicable. However, stool specimens suspected of containing *Vibrio* spp. should be collected and transported in Cary-Blair medium. Buffered glycerol saline is not acceptable, because glycerol is toxic to vibrios. Feces is preferable, but rectal swabs are acceptable during the acute phase of diarrheal illness.

Specimen Processing

No special considerations are required for processing of the organisms discussed in this chapter. Refer to Table 5.1 for general information on specimen processing.

Direct Detection Methods

V. cholerae toxin can be detected in stool using an enzyme-linked immunosorbent assay (ELISA) or a commercially available latex agglutination test (Oxoid, Inc., Odgensburg, NY), but these tests are not widely used in the United States.

A variety of rapid antigen tests are available worldwide, including the SMART II Cholera O1 and Bengal SMART O139 (investigational use only) (New Horizon Diagnostics Corporation, Columbia, MD) and immunochromatographic assays such as SD Bioline Cholera Ag O1/O139 (Standard Diagnostics, Gyeonggi-do, Republic of Korea) for the detection of *V. cholerae* in stool. The sensitivities and specificities vary for each assay.

Microscopically, vibrios are gram-negative, straight or slightly curved rods (Fig. 25.1). When stool specimens from patients with cholera are examined using dark-field microscopy, the bacilli exhibit characteristic rapid darting or shooting-star motility. However, direct microscopic examination of stools by any method is not commonly used for laboratory diagnosis of enteric bacterial infections.

A variety of multiplex nucleic acid–based testing methods have been developed for the detection of *V. cholerae.* The xTAG gastrointestinal panel (Luminex Corporation, Austin, TX) has been evaluated for the diagnosis of infectious disease for the isolation and differentiation of a variety of enteric pathogens including *Escherichia coli, Campylobacter, Yersinia,* and *V. cholerae.* In addition, the FilmArray (BioFire Diagnostics, Salt Lake City, UT) offers a multiplex polymerase chain reaction (PCR) system with an FDA-cleared gastrointestinal panel for *V.*

cholerae and *Vibrio* (*parahaemolyticus, vulnificus, and cholerae*). These assays are able to provide a quick diagnosis that appears sensitive and specific to pathogens capable of causing diarrhea.

Aeromonas spp. are gram-negative, straight rods with rounded ends or coccobacilli. Direct specimens may contain few or no white blood cells even though an infection is present. No molecular or serologic methods are available for direct detection of *Aeromonas* spp. Cells of *C. violaceum* are slightly curved, medium to long, gram-negative rods with rounded ends. A PCR amplification assay has been developed for the identification of *C. violaceum*.

Cultivation

Media of Choice

Stool cultures for *Vibrio* spp. are plated on the selective medium **thiosulfate citrate bile salts sucrose (TCBS) agar**. TCBS contains 1% sodium chloride, bile salts that inhibit the growth of Gram-positive organisms, and sucrose for the differentiation of the various *Vibrio* spp. Bromothymol blue and thymol blue pH indicators are added to the medium. The high pH of the medium (8.6) inhibits the growth of other intestinal microbiota. Although some *Vibrio* spp. grow very poorly on this medium, those that grow well produce either yellow or green colonies, depending on whether they are able to ferment sucrose (which produces yellow colonies). Alkaline peptone water (pH 8.4) may be used as an enrichment broth for obtaining growth of vibrios from stool. After inoculation, the broth is incubated for 5 to 8 hours at 35°C and then subcultured to TCBS. Oxidase testing is unreliable when performed on colonies grown on TCBS media.

The organisms will also grow on MacConkey or salmonella shigella (SS) agar. All species will appear as nonfermenters with the exception of *V. vulnificus*. Other species may be indistinguishable from other rapid sucrose-fermenting enterics when grown on Hektoen enteric (HE) or xylose-lysine-deoxycholate (XLD) media. Refer to Chapter 19 for a description of the enteric media included here.

Chromogenic *Vibrio* agar (CHROMagar Microbiology, Paris, France), which was developed for the recovery of *Vibrio parahaemolyticus* from seafood, supports the growth of other *Vibrio* spp. Colonies on this agar range from white to pale blue and violet.

Aeromonas spp. are indistinguishable from *Yersinia enterocolitica* on modified cefsulodin-irgasan-novobiocin (CIN) agar (4 μg/mL of cefsulodin); therefore, it is important to perform an oxidase test to differentiate the two genera; *Aeromonas* spp. are oxidase positive. Aeromonas agar is a relatively new alternative medium that uses D-xylose as a differential characteristic. These organisms typically grow on a variety of differential and selective agars used for the identification of enteric pathogens. They are also beta-hemolytic on blood agar.

C. violaceum grows on most routine laboratory media. The colonies may be beta-hemolytic and have an almond-like odor. Most strains produce **violacein,** an ethanol-soluble violet pigment.

All of the genera considered in this chapter grow well on 5% sheep blood, chocolate, and MacConkey agars. They

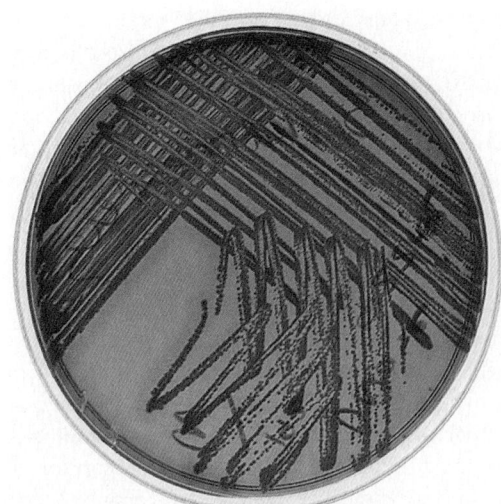

• **Fig. 25.2** Colonies of *Chromobacterium violaceum* on DNase agar. Note violet pigment.

also grow well in the broth of blood culture systems and in thioglycollate or brain-heart infusion broths.

Incubation Conditions and Duration

These organisms produce detectable growth on 5% sheep blood and chocolate agars when incubated at 35°C in carbon dioxide or ambient air for a minimum of 24 hours. MacConkey and TCBS agars should be incubated at 35°C in ambient air. The typical violet pigment of *C. violaceum* colonies (Fig. 25.2) is optimally produced when cultures are incubated at room temperature (22°C).

Colonial Appearance

Table 25.3 describes the colonial appearance and other distinguishing characteristics (e.g., hemolysis and odor) of each genus on 5% sheep blood and MacConkey agars. The appearance of *Vibrio* spp. on TCBS is described in Table 25.4 and shown in Fig. 25.3.

Approach to Identification

The colonies of these genera resemble those of the Enterobacterales but can be distinguished notably by their positive oxidase test result (except for *V. metschnikovii*, which is oxidase-negative). The oxidase test must be performed from 5% sheep blood or another medium without a fermentable sugar (e.g., lactose in MacConkey agar or sucrose in TCBS), because fermentation of a carbohydrate results in acidification of the medium, and a false-negative result may occur if the surrounding pH is below 5.1. Likewise, if the violet pigment of a suspected *C. violaceum* isolate interferes with performance of the oxidase test, the organism should be grown under anaerobic conditions (where it cannot produce pigment) and retested.

The reliability of commercial identification systems has not been widely validated for identification of these organisms, although most are listed in the databases of several systems. The API 20E system (bioMérieux, St. Louis, MO) is one of the best systems available for the identification of

TABLE 25.3 Colonial Appearance and Characteristics

Organism	Medium	Appearance
Aeromonas spp.	BA Mac	Large, round, raised, opaque; most pathogenic strains are beta-hemolytic except *Aeromonas caviae,* which is usually nonhemolytic Both NLF and LF
Chromobacterium violaceum	BA Mac	Round, smooth, convex; some strains are beta-hemolytic; most colonies appear black or very dark purple; cultures smell of ammonium cyanide (almondlike) NLF
Vibrio spp. and *Grimontia hollisae*	BA Mac	Medium to large, smooth, opaque, iridescent with a greenish hue; *V. cholerae, V. fluvialis,* and *V. mimicus* can be beta-hemolytic NLF except *V. vulnificus,* which may be LF
Photobacterium damsela	BA Mac	Medium to large, smooth, opaque, iridescent with a greenish hue; may be beta-hemolytic NLF

BA, 5% sheep blood agar; *LF,* lactose fermenter; *Mac,* MacConkey agar; *NLF,* non–lactose fermenter.

vibrios because the inoculum is prepared in 0.85% saline; the amount of salt is sufficient to allow growth of the halophilic organism.

Matrix-assisted laser desorption ionization time-of-flight mass spectrometry (MALDI-TOF MS) could provide a rapid identification method for the identification of vibrios isolated from clinical specimens. The VITEK MS (bioMérieux, St. Louis, MO) database includes *V. cholerae, V. parahaemolyticus, V. vulnificus,* as well as *V. alginolyticus, fluvialis, metschnikovii,* and *mimicus.* In a recent study, Cheng et al. (2015) evaluated the identification of *V. vulnificus, V. parahaemolyticus, V. fluvialis,* and 33 species of O1 and non-O139 *V. cholerae.* The system was not able to identify the serogroup types O1 and non-O139 to the species level.

Although MALDI-TOF MS does allow for the accurate identification of some species of *Aeromonas hydrophila/punctate, sobria,* and *jandaei,* it should be noted that the ability of most commercial identification systems to accurately identify *Aeromonas* organisms to the species level is limited and uncertain, and with some kits, difficulty arises in separating *Aeromonas* spp. from *Vibrio* spp. Identification of potential pathogens should be confirmed using conventional biochemical tests or serotyping. Tables 25.4 and 25.5 show several characteristics that can be used to presumptively group *Vibrio* spp., *Aeromonas* spp., and *C. violaceum.* New technologies such as nucleic acid–based testing and MALDI-TOF MS for additional isolates discussed in this chapter are typically not available because of clinical efficacy and database limitations.

Comments Regarding Specific Organisms

V. cholerae and *V. mimicus* are the only *Vibrio* spp. that do not require salt for growth. Therefore, a key test for distinguishing the halophilic species from *V. cholerae, V. mimicus,* and *Aeromonas* spp. is growth in nutrient broth with 6% salt. Furthermore, the addition of 1% NaCl to conventional biochemical tests is recommended to allow growth of halophilic species.

The **string test** can be used to differentiate *Vibrio* spp. from *Aeromonas* spp. In this test, organisms are emulsified in 0.5% sodium deoxycholate, which lyses *Vibrio* cells but not those of *Aeromonas* spp. Cell lysis releases deoxyribonucleic acid (DNA), which can be pulled up into a string with an inoculating loop (Fig. 25.4).

A **vibrostatic test** using 0129 (2,4-diamino-6,7-diisopropylpteridine)–impregnated disks also has been used to separate vibrios (susceptible) from other oxidase-positive glucose fermenters (resistant) and to differentiate *V. cholerae* O1 and non-O1 (susceptible) from other *Vibrio* spp. (resistant). However, recent strains of *V. cholerae* O139 and *V. cholera* O1 have demonstrated resistance; therefore, the dependability of this test is questionable.

Serotyping should be performed immediately to further characterize *V. cholerae* isolates. Toxigenic strains of serogroup O1 and O139 can be involved in cholera epidemics. Strains that do not type in either antiserum are identified as non-O1. Although typing sera are commercially available, isolates of *V. cholerae* are usually sent to a reference laboratory for serotyping.

Identification of *V. cholerae* or *V. vulnificus* should be reported immediately because of the life-threatening nature of these organisms.

Aeromonas spp. and *C. violaceum* can be identified using the characteristics shown in Table 25.5. *Aeromonas* spp. identified in clinical specimens should be identified as *A. hydrophilia, A. caviae* complex, or *A. veronii* complex.

Pigmented strains of *C. violaceum* are so distinctive that a presumptive identification can be made based on colonial appearance, oxidase, and Gram staining. Nonpigmented strains (approximately 9% of isolates) may be differentiated from *Pseudomonas, Burkholderia, Brevundimonas,* and *Ralstonia* organisms based on glucose fermentation and a positive test result for indole. Negative lysine and ornithine reactions are useful criteria for distinguishing *C. violaceum* from *Plesiomonas shigelloides.* In addition to the characteristics listed in

TABLE 25.4   Key Biochemical and Physiologic Characteristics of *Vibrio* spp. and *Grimontii hollisae*

Species	Oxidase	Indole	Gas From Glucose	Lactose	Sucrose	Lysine Decarboxylase[a]	Arginine Dihydrolase[a]	Ornithine Decarboxylase[a]	Growth in 0% NaCl[b]	Growth in 6% NaCl[b]	TCBS[c] Growth	Colony on TCBS[c]
Grimontii hollisae	+	+	−	−	−	−	−	−	−	+	Very poor	Green
Vibrio alginolyticus	+	V	−	−	+	+	−	V	−	+	Good	Yellow
Vibrio cholerae	+	+	−	V	+	+	−	+	+	V	Good	Yellow
Vibrio cincinnatiensis[d]	+	V	−	−	+	V	−	−	−	+	Very poor	Yellow
Photobacterium damsela	+	−	−	−	−	V	+	−	−	+	Reduced at 36°C	Green[e]
Vibrio fluvialis	+	V	−	−	+	−	+	−	−	+	Good	Yellow
Vibrio furnissii	+	V	+	−	+	−	+	−	−	+	Good	Yellow
Vibrio harveyi	+	+	−	−	V	+	−	−	−	+	Good	Yellow
Vibrio metschnikovii	−	V	−	V	+	V	V	−	−	V	May be reduced	Yellow
Vibrio mimicus	+	+	−	V	−	+	−	+	+	V	Good	Green
Vibrio parahaemolyticus	+	+	−	−	−	+	−	+	−	+	Good	Green[f]
Vibrio vulnificus	+	+	−	(+)	−	+	−	+	−	+	Good	Green[g]

[a]1% NaCl added to enhance growth.
[b]Nutrient broth with 0% or 6% NaCl added.
[c]Thiosulfate citrate bile salts sucrose agar.
[d]Ferments myoinositol.
[e]5% yellow.
[f]1% yellow.
[g]90% yellow.
+, >90% of strains are positive; −, >90% of strains are negative; (+), delayed; V, variable.

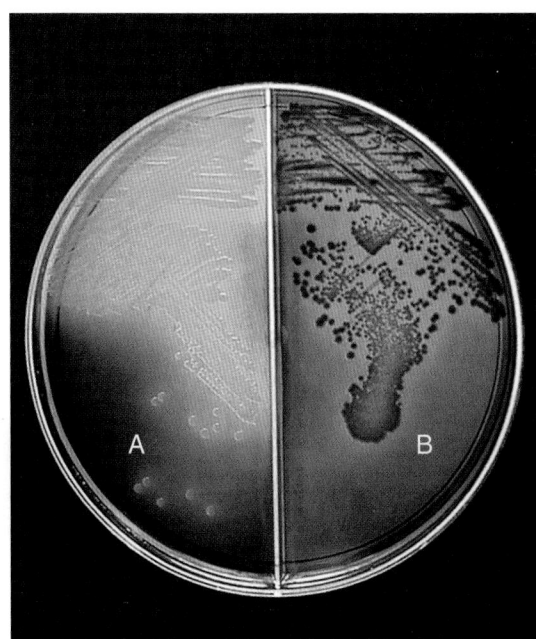

• **Fig. 25.3** Colonies of *Vibrio cholerae* (A) and *Vibrio parahaemolyticus* (B) on thiosulfate citrate bile salts sucrose agar.

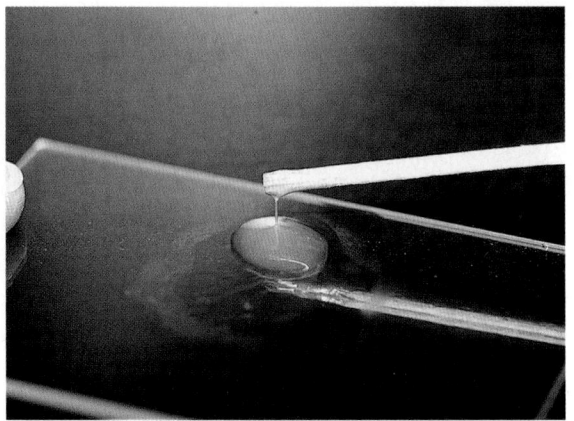

• **Fig. 25.4** String test used to differentiate *Vibrio* spp. (positive) from *Aeromonas* spp. and *Plesiomonas shigelloides* (negative).

Table 25.5, failure to ferment either maltose or mannitol also differentiates *C. violaceum* from *Aeromonas* spp.

Serodiagnosis

Agglutination, vibriocidal, or antitoxin tests are available for diagnosing cholera using acute and convalescent sera. However, these methods are most commonly used for epidemiologic purposes. Serodiagnostic techniques are not generally used for laboratory diagnosis of infections caused by the other organisms discussed in this chapter.

Antimicrobial Susceptibility Testing and Therapy

Two components of the management of patients with cholera are rehydration and antimicrobial therapy (Table 25.6).

Antimicrobials reduce the severity of the illness and shorten the duration of organism shedding. The Clinical and Laboratory Standards Institute (CLSI) has established methods for testing for *V. cholerae,* and the CLSI document should be consulted for this purpose.

The need for antimicrobial intervention for gastrointestinal infections caused by other *Vibrio* spp. and *Aeromonas* spp. is less clear. However, extraintestinal infections with these organisms and with *C. violaceum* can be life threatening, and directed therapy is required. *C. violaceum* is often resistant to beta-lactams and colistin.

Antimicrobial agents with potential activity are listed, where appropriate, in Table 25.6. It is important to note these organisms' ability to show resistance to therapeutic agents; especially noteworthy is the ability of *Aeromonas* spp. to produce various beta-lactamases.

Prevention

No cholera vaccine is available in the United States. However, the World Health Organization (WHO) now maintains a global stockpile of cholera vaccine to use in endemic hot spots and in emergency situations. Because of recent outbreaks, WHO developed a Global Task Force on Cholera Control. Information is available at http://www.who.int/cholera/task_force/en/. No approved vaccines or chemoprophylaxis exists for the other organisms discussed in this chapter.

ⓔ Visit the Evolve site for a complete list of procedures, review questions, and case studies.

Bibliography

Barzilay EJ, Schaad N, Magloire R, et al.: Cholera surveillance during the Haiti epidemic—the first 2 years, *N Engl J Med* 368:599–609, 2013.

Caroll KC, Pfaller MA: *Manual of clinical microbiology,* ed 12, Washington, DC, 2019, ASM Press.

Cheng WC, Jan IS, Chen JM, et al.: Evaluation of the Bruker Biotyper matrix-assisted laser desorption ionization-time of flight mass spectrometry system for the identification of blood isolates of *Vibrio* species, *J Clin Microbiol* 53:1741–1744, 2015.

Clark RB, Lister PD, Arneson-Rotert L, Janda JM: In vitro susceptibilities of *Plesiomonas shigelloides* to 24 antibiotics and antibiotic-beta-lactamase-inhibitor combinations, *Antimicrob Agents Chemother* 34:159–160, 1990.

Colwell RR: Global climate and infectious disease: the cholera paradigm, *Science* 274:2025–2031, 1996.

Committee on Infectious Diseases: *2006 red book: report of the Committee on Infectious Diseases,* ed 27, Elk Grove Village, IL, 2006, American Academy of Pediatrics.

Erler R, Wichels A, Heinemeyer EA, et al.: VibrioBase: a MALDI-TOF MS database for fast identification of *Vibrio* spp. that are potentially pathogenic in humans, *Syst Appl Microbiol* 38:16–25, 2015.

Feng W, Gu X, Sui W, et al.: The application and epidemiological research of xTAG GPP multiplex PCR in the diagnosis of infectious diarrhea, *Zhonghua Yi Xue Za Zhi* 95:435–439, 2015.

Jensen J, Jellinge ME: Severe septic shock and cardiac arrest in a patient with *Vibrio metschnikovii*: a case report, *J Med Case Rep* 8:348, 2014.

TABLE 25.5 Key Biochemical and Physiologic Characteristics of *Aeromonas* spp. and *Chromobacterium violaceum*

Species	Oxidase	Indole	Gas From Glucose	Esculin Hydrolysis	Fermentation of Sucrose	Lysine Decarboxylase	Arginine Dihydrolase	Ornithine Decarboxylase	Growth in 0% NaCl[a]	Growth in 6% NaCl[a]	TCBS[b] Growth
Aeromonas caviae complex	+	V	−	+	+	−	+	−	+	−	−
Aeromonas hydrophila complex	+	+	V	V	V	V	+	−	+	V	−
Aeromonas jandaei (*A. veronii* complex)	+	+	+	−	−	+	+	−	+	−	−
Aeromonas schubertii (*A. veronii* complex)	+	V	−	−	−	+	+	−	+	−	−
Aeromonas veronii biovar sobria	+	+	+	−	+	+	+	−	+	−	−
Aeromonas veronii biovar veronii	+	+	+	+	+	+	−	+	+	−	−
Chromobacterium violaceum[c]	V	V	−[d]	−	V	−	+	−	+	−	ND

+, >90% of strains are positive; −, >90% of strains are negative; ND, no data; V, variable.
[a] Nutrient agar with 0% or 6% NaCl added.
[b] Thiosulfate citrate bile salts sucrose agar.
[c] 91% produce an insoluble violet pigment; often, nonpigmented strains are indole-positive.
[d] Gas-producing strains have been described.

TABLE 25.6 Antimicrobial Therapy and Susceptibility Testing

Species	Therapeutic Options	Potential Resistance to Therapeutic Options	Validated Testing Methods[a]	Comments
Vibrio cholerae	Adequate rehydration plus antibiotics. *In vitro* susceptibility guidelines indicate susceptibilities to aminoglycosides, azithromycin, fluoroquinolones, extended-spectrum cephalosporins, carbapenems, and monobactams.	Known resistance to tetracycline, chloramphenicol, and trimethoprim-sulfamethoxazole	Refer to CLSI guidelines.	
Other *Vibrio* spp.	No definitive guidelines. For gastroenteritis, therapy may not be needed; for wound infections and septicemia; same as for *V. cholerae.*	Similar to resistance reported for *V. cholerae.*	Refer to CLSI guidelines.	
Aeromonas spp.	No definitive guidelines. For gastroenteritis, therapy may not be needed; for soft tissue infections and septicemia, potentially active agents include ceftriaxone, cefotaxime, ceftazidime, imipenem, aztreonam, amoxicillin-clavulanate, quinolones, and trimethoprim-sulfamethoxazole.	Capable of producing various beta-lactamases that mediate resistance to penicillins and certain cephalosporins.	Refer to CLSI guidelines.	
Chromobacterium violaceum	No definitive guidelines. Potentially active agents include cefotaxime, ceftazidime, imipenem, and aminoglycosides.	Variable activity of penicillins; poor activity of first- and second-generation cephalosporins.	Not available.	Grows on Mueller-Hinton agar, but interpretive standards do not exist.

[a]Validated testing methods include standard methods recommended by the Clinical and Laboratory Standards Institute (CLSI) and commercial methods approved by the US Food and Drug Administration (FDA).

Kimura B, Hokimoto S, Takahasi H: *Photobacterium histaminum* (Okuzumi et al, 1994) is a later subjective synonym for *Photobacterium damselae* subsp *damselae* (Love et al, 1981; Smith et al, 1991), *Int J Syst Evol Microbiol* 50:1339–1342, 2000.

Spina A, Kerr KG, Cormican M, et al.: Spectrum of enteropathogens detected by FilmArray GI Panel in a multicentre study of community-acquired gastroenteritis, *Clin Microbiol Infect* 21:719–728, 2015.

Thompson FL, Hoste B, Vandemeulebroecke K, Swings J: Reclassification of *Vibrio hollisae* as *Grimontia hollisae* gen nov, comb nov, *Int J Syst Evol Microbiol* 53:1615–1617, 2003.

Ti TY, Tan CW, Chong AP, Lee EH: Nonfatal and fatal infections caused by *Chromobacterium violaceum, Clin Infect Dis* 17:505–507, 1993.

Wei S, Zhao H, Xian Y, Hussain MA, Wu X: Multiplex PCR assays for the detection of *Vibrio alginolyticus, Vibrio parahaemolyticus, Vibrio vulnificus* and *Vibrio cholerae* with an internal amplification control, *Diagn Microbiol Infect Dis* 79:115–118, 2014.

26

Sphingomonas and Similar Organisms

OBJECTIVES

1. Identify cultivation methods and colonial characteristics for *Sphingomonas paucimobilis* and similar organisms.
2. State the initial clues that alert clinical laboratorians to the presence of this group of organisms in a patient specimen.
3. Explain the classification and identification algorithm for this group of organisms.
4. Describe the susceptibility testing methods appropriate for this group of organisms.
5. Explain the pathogenicity of organisms in this group.

ORGANISMS TO BE CONSIDERED

Current Name	Previous Name
Sphingobacterium mizutaii	
Sphingomonas parapaucimobilis	
Sphingomonas paucimobilis	*Pseudomonas paucimobilis,* CDC IIk-1

General Considerations

The organisms discussed in this chapter are considered together because they usually fail to grow on MacConkey agar, are oxidase-positive, and oxidatively utilize glucose.

Epidemiology, Spectrum of Disease, and Antimicrobial Therapy

As demonstrated in Table 26.1, these organisms are rarely or only occasionally isolated from human specimens and have limited roles as agents of infection. Because they are infrequently encountered in the clinical setting, little information is available on their epidemiology, ability to cause human infections, and potential for antimicrobial resistance. The genus *Sphingobacterium* is ubiquitous in nature in soil and aquatic environments. The only species discussed here, *Sphingobacterium mizutaii*, is the only species that is indole-positive and fails to grow on MacConkey agar. The remaining species are indole-negative and generally grow on MacConkey agar (Chapter 23). *Sphingomonas* spp. are associated with natural aquatic sources. *Sphingomonas* spp. have been isolated in cases of keratitis associated with contact lenses, bacteremia, and artificial medical device implants. These organisms are opportunistic pathogens, and when encountered in clinical specimens, their clinical significance and potential as contaminants should be carefully considered.

Laboratory Diagnosis

Specimen Collection and Transport

No special considerations are required for specimen collection and transport of the organisms discussed in this chapter. Refer to Table 5.1 for general information on specimen collection and transport.

Specimen Processing

No special considerations are required for processing of the organisms discussed in this chapter. Refer to Table 5.1 for general information on specimen processing.

Direct Detection Methods

No specific procedures other than microscopy are required for direct detection of these organisms in clinical material.

Serodiagnosis

Serodiagnostic techniques are not generally used for the laboratory diagnosis of infections caused by the organisms discussed in this chapter.

TABLE 26.1 Epidemiology, Spectrum of Disease, and Antimicrobial Therapy

Organism	Epidemiology	Disease Spectrum	Antimicrobial Therapy
Sphingobacterium mizutaii	Sphingobacteria are ubiquitous in nature.	Rarely involved in human infections; has been associated with blood, cerebrospinal fluid, and wound infections.	Erythromycin, trimethoprim-sulfamethoxazole, and pefloxacin.
Sphingomonas paucimobilis *Sphingomonas parapaucimobilis*	*S. paucimobilis* inhabits environmental niches and can exist in hospital water systems. Not part of human microbiota. Mode of transmission is uncertain but probably involves patient exposure to contaminated medical devices or solutions.	*S. paucimobilis* virulence factors are unknown. It has been implicated in community- and health care–associated infections, specifically in blood and urine infections.	No definitive guidelines; potentially active agents include trimethoprim-sulfamethoxazole, chloramphenicol, ciprofloxacin, and aminoglycosides; resistance to beta-lactams is known, but validated susceptibility testing methods do not exist.

TABLE 26.2 Colonial Appearance and Characteristics

Organism	Medium	Appearance
Sphingobacterium mizutaii	BA	Yellow pigmented colonies
Sphingomonas paucimobilis *Sphingomonas parapaucimobilis*	BA	Small, circular, smooth, convex; bright yellow growth pigment

BA, 5% sheep blood agar.

Cultivation

Media of Choice

Sphingomonas spp. and *S. mizutaii* grow well on routine laboratory media, such as 5% sheep blood and chocolate agars; however, they fail to grow on MacConkey agar. They usually grow well in thioglycollate and brain-heart infusion broths and in broths used in blood culture systems.

Incubation Conditions and Duration

Within 24 to 48 hours of inoculation and incubation, most of these organisms produce detectable growth on media incubated at 35°C to 37°C in 5% carbon dioxide (CO_2) or ambient air.

Colonial Appearance

Table 26.2 describes the colonial appearance and distinguishing characteristics (e.g., pigment) of each organism on 5% sheep blood agar.

Approach to Identification

The ability of many commercial identification systems, including matrix-assisted laser desorption ionization time-of-flight mass spectrometry (MALDI-TOF MS), to accurately identify the organisms discussed in this chapter may be limited or uncertain. Tables 26.3 and 26.4 show some biochemical tests that are helpful for presumptive differentiation among the various organisms in this group.

Comments Regarding Specific Organisms

Sphingobacterium mizutaii

S. mizutaii exhibits II-forms. It can produce a yellow pigment, and it does not grow on MacConkey agar. Frequently classified as nonmotile, the organism can be motile by gliding movement. It is able to grow in the presence of 40% bile, and it is oxidase-positive, catalase-positive, esculin-positive, indole-negative, and urease-negative (although a report exists that 20% are positive for Christensen urease). Key characteristics are shown in Table 26.3. Reported infections in humans have included septicemia (blood culture), meningitis (CSF specimen), and cellulitis (wound source). This bacterium has been reported to be susceptible to erythromycin, trimethoprim-sulfamethoxazole, and pefloxacin.

Sphingomonas paucimobilis

S. paucimobilis is a medium-size, straight, gram-negative rod with a single polar flagellum; growth requires at least 48 hours' incubation on sheep blood agar (Fig. 26.1). Optimal growth occurs at 30°C in 5% CO_2 or ambient air; it does grow at

TABLE 26.3 Key Biochemical and Physiologic Characteristics

Organism	Insoluble Pigment	Glucose Oxidized	Xylose Oxidized	Sucrose Oxidized	Esculin Hydrolysis	Motility
Sphingobacterium mizutaii	V[a]	+	(+)	+	+	nm
Sphingomonas spp.[b]	Yellow	+	+	+	+	+[c]

[a]Yellow pigment production may be enhanced by incubation at room temperature.
[b]Includes S. paucimobilis and S. parapaucimobilis.
[c]Usually nonmotile in motility medium, but motility is present on wet mount.
+, >90% strains positive; (+), delayed; nm, nonmotile; V, variable.
From Weyant RS, Moss CW, Weaver RE, et al, eds. *Identification of Unusual Pathogenic Gram-Negative Aerobic and Facultatively Anaerobic Bacteria*. 2nd ed. Baltimore: Williams & Wilkins; 1996.

TABLE 26.4 Specific Biochemical Characteristics for Differentiation of the *Sphingomonas* spp.

Biochemical Test	S. paucimobilis	S. parapaucimobilis
Oxidation of glucose	Positive	Positive
Oxidation of xylose	Positive	Positive
Oxidation of maltose	Positive	Positive
Esculin hydrolysis	Positive	Positive
Motility	Positive[a]	Positive
Indole	Negative	Negative
Susceptibility to polymyxin B	Susceptible	Variable
H$_2$S (lead acetate paper suspended over KIA)	Negative	Positive
Citrate	Negative	Positive
DNase	Positive	Negative

[a]Motility positive by wet mount or in motility medium incubated at 18°C to 22°C, but organism is nonmotile when incubated at 37°C.
H$_2$S, Hydrogen sulfide; KIA, Kligler iron agar.
Data compiled from Winn WC, Allen SD, Janda WM, et al. *Koneman's Color Atlas and Textbook of Diagnostic Microbiology*. 6th ed. Philadelphia: Lippincott Williams & Wilkins; 2006.

37°C but not at 42°C. It grows as a deep yellow colony on tryptic soy and blood agars. It is obligately aerobic, it grows in broth (e.g., brain-heart infusion, thioglycollate, blood culture media), and 90% of isolates do not grow on MacConkey agar (10% grow on MacConkey agar and appear as non–lactose fermenters). *S. paucimobilis* oxidatively utilizes glucose, xylose, and sucrose. Biochemical test results of interest include the following: esculin hydrolysis–positive, motile by wet mount or in motility medium when incubated at 18°C to 22°C (nonmotile when incubated at 37°C), oxidase-positive (90% to 94% positive), catalase-positive, urease-negative, and indole-negative. *S. paucimobilis* is susceptible to polymyxin B, a trait that distinguishes it from *Sphingobacterium* spp. Key characteristics are included in Table 26.4.

Antimicrobial susceptibility testing indicates that *S. paucimobilis* is susceptible to tetracycline, chloramphenicol, trimethoprim-sulfamethoxazole, and aminoglycosides.

Susceptibility to vancomycin has been noted when the organism is grown on sheep blood agar with a vancomycin disk (30 μg). *S. paucimobilis* is ubiquitous in soil and water and has been isolated environmentally from swimming pools, hospital equipment, and water and laboratory supplies. It has been associated with human infections and found in a variety of clinical specimens, specifically, peritonitis associated with wound infections (chronic ambulatory peritoneal dialysis, leg ulcer, empyema, splenic abscess, brain abscess); blood cultures; and CSF, urine, vaginal, and cervical samples. Recent literature indicates that *S. paucimobilis* is regarded as having minor clinical significance; however, community-acquired infection, diabetes mellitus, and alcoholism are significant risk factors for primary bacteremia. A retrospective study suggests that the prevalence of *S. paucimobilis* infection in humans seems to have increased in recent times, and although it

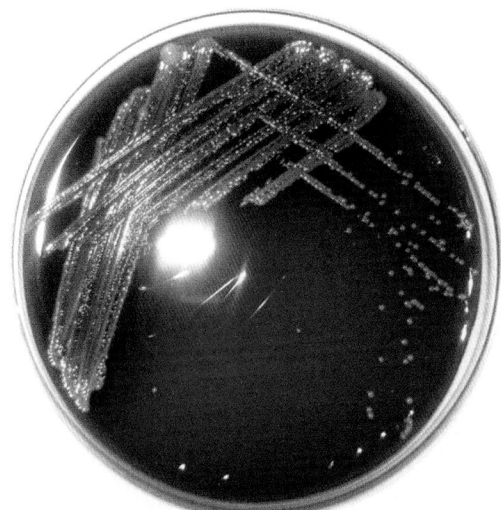

• **Fig. 26.1** *Sphingomonas paucimobilis* growth on blood agar. (From Seo SW, Chung IY, Kim E, et al. A case of postoperative *Sphingomonas paucimobilis* endophthalmitis after cataract extraction. *Kor J Ophthalmol.* 2008;22:63.)

has low virulence, infection can lead to septic shock, particularly in immunocompromised patients. Another report indicates that although this bacterium has low mortality associated with infection, it commonly causes complications in hospitalized patients.

Sphingomonas parapaucimobilis

S. parapaucimobilis is similar to *S. paucimobilis* in many ways. It is a medium-sized, straight, gram-negative rod that produces a deep yellow pigment. It is obligately aerobic, motile, and does not grow on MacConkey agar. *S. parapaucimobilis* can be distinguished from *S. paucimobilis* by several characteristics. *S. parapaucimobilis* is H₂S positive,

as indicated by blackening of lead acetate paper suspended over Kligler iron agar (KIA), it is Simmons citrate positive (*S. paucimobilis* is negative), and it is negative for extracellular DNAse (*S. paucimobilis* is positive). Like *S. paucimobilis*, *S. parapaucimobilis* is positive for OF glucose, OF xylose, and OF maltose but negative for OF mannitol. It has been distinguished from *Sphingobacterium* spp. by its susceptibility to polymyxin B; however, *S. parapaucimobilis* may demonstrate variable susceptibility to polymyxin B. Key characteristics are included in Table 26.4. Antimicrobial susceptibility testing indicates that *S. parapaucimobilis* displays variable resistance but is usually susceptible to tetracycline, chloramphenicol, sulfamethoxazole, aminoglycosides, third-generation cephalosporins, and fluoroquinolone. *S. parapaucimobilis* has been associated with human infections; specifically, it has been isolated from sputum, urine, and the vagina.

Antimicrobial Susceptibility

Antimicrobial susceptibility for this group of bacteria ranges from variable resistance to identifiable patterns of susceptibility. Standardized guidelines are not available. However, when clinically necessary, susceptibility testing should be completed using an overnight MIC or E-test method.

Prevention

Because these organisms are rarely implicated or identified in human infections, no vaccines or prophylactic measures are available.

Ⓔ Visit the Evolve site for a complete list of procedures, review questions, and case studies.

Bibliography

Boken DJ, Romero JR, Cavalieri SJ: Sphingomonas paucimobilis bacteremia: four cases and review of the literature, *Infect Dis Clin Pract* 7:286, 1998.

Caroll KC, Pfaller MA: *Manual of clinical microbiology*, ed 12, Washington, DC, 2019, ASM Press.

Charity RM, Foukas AF: Osteomyelitis and secondary septic arthritis caused by *Sphingomonas paucimobilis* infection, 33. 2005, pp 93–95.

Daneshvar MI, Hill B, Hollis DG, et al.: CDC group O-3: phenotypic characteristics, fatty acid composition, isoprenoid quinone content, and *in vitro* antimicrobic susceptibilities of an unusual gram-negative bacterium isolated from clinical specimens, *J Clin Microbiol* 36:1674–1678, 1998.

Freney J, Hansen W, Ploton C, et al.: Septicemia caused by *Sphingobacterium multivorum*, *J Clin Microbiol* 25:1126–1128, 1987.

Hollis DG, Moss CW, Daneshvar MI, Wallace-Shewmaker PL: CDC group IIc: phenotypic characteristics, fatty acid composition, and isoprenoid quinone content, *J Clin Microbiol* 34:2322–2324, 1996.

Lambiase A, Rossano F, Del Pezzo M, et al.: Sphingobacterium respiratory tract infection in patients with cystic fibrosis, *BMC Res Notes* 2:262, 2009.

Lemaitre D, Elaichouni A, Hundhausen M, et al.: Tracheal colonization with *Sphingomonas paucimobilis* in mechanically ventilated neonates due to contaminated ventilator temperature probes, *J Hosp Infect* 32:199–206, 1996.

Lin JN, Lai CH, Chen YH, et al.: *Sphingomonas paucimobilis* bacteremia in humans: 16 case reports and a literature review, *J Microbiol Immunol Infect* 43:35–42, 2010.

Refaat M, Zakka P, Khoury M, et al.: Cardiac implantable electronic device infections: observational data from a tertiary care center in Lebanon, *Medicine (Baltimore)* 98(16).e14906, 2019.

Reina J, Bassa A, Llompart I, Portela D, Borrell N: Infections with *Pseudomonas paucimobilis:* report of four cases and review, *Rev Infect Dis* 13:1072–1076, 1991.

Roca M, Garcia A, Peñas-Pardo L, Bosch-Aparicio N, Agustí J: *Sphingomonas paucimobilis* keratitis in a patient with neurotrophic keratopathy and severe neurosensory hypoacusis: treatment with penetrating keratoplasty and amniotic membrane grafting, *Oman J Ophthalmol* 11(3):291–293, 2018.

Saboor F, Amin F, Nadeem S: Community acquired *Sphingomonas paucimobilis* in a child - A rare case, *J Pak Med Assoc* 68(11):1714–1716, 2018.

Salazar R, Martino R, Sureda A, Brunet S, Subirá M, Domingo-Albós A: Catheter-related bacteremia due to *Pseudomonas paucimobilis* in neutropenic cancer patients: report of two cases, *Clin Infect Dis* 20:1573–1574, 1995.

Toh HS, Tay HT, Kuar WK, Weng TC, Tang HJ, Tan CK: Risk factors associated with *Sphingomonas paucimobilis* infection, *J Microbiol Immunol Infect* 44:289–295, 2011.

Weyant RS, Moss CW, Weaver RE, et al.: *Identification of unusual pathogenic gram-negative aerobic and facultatively anaerobic bacteria*, ed 2, Baltimore, 1996, Williams & Wilkins.

Willems A, Falsen E, Pot B, et al.: *Acidovorax, a new genus for Pseudomonas facilis, Pseudomonas delafieldii, E. Falsen (EF) group 13, EF group 16, and several clinical isolates, with the species Acidovorax facilis comb.nov., Acidovorax delafieldii comb.nov., and Acidovorax temperans sp.nov, Int J Syst Bacteriol* 40:384–398, 1990.

Winn WC, Allen SD, Janda WM, et al.: *Koneman's color atlas and textbook of diagnostic microbiology*, ed 6, Philadelphia, 2006, Lippincott Williams & Wilkins.

27

Moraxella and *Neisseria* spp.

GENERA AND SPECIES TO BE CONSIDERED

Current Name	Previous Name
Moraxella atlantae	
Moraxella canis	
Moraxella lacunata	
Moraxella lincolnii	
Moraxella nonliquefaciens	
Moraxella osloensis	
Neisseria animalis	
Neisseria animaloris	CDC EF-4a
Neisseria bacilliformis	
Neisseria elongata subspecies *elongata*	CDC group M6
Neisseria elongata subspecies *glycolytica*	
Neisseria elongata subspecies *nitroreducens*	
Neisseria oralis	
Neisseria weaverii	CDC group M5
Neisseria zoodegmatis	CDC EF-4b

General Characteristics

The organisms discussed in this chapter are either cocci, coccobacilli, or short- to medium-sized, gram-negative rods. This group of bacteria consists of several species within the genera *Moraxella* and *Neisseria*, other than the three frequently isolated pathogens, *Moraxella catarrhalis*, *Neisseria gonorrhoeae*, and *Neisseria meningitidis* (Chapter 39). Most of these organisms rarely cause opportunistic infection and should be considered as potential contaminants. The genus *Moraxella* includes approximately 20 species. *Moraxella osloensis*, *M. nonliquefaciens*, and *M. lincolnii* are considered normal human respiratory microbiota with low virulence. Many other *Moraxella* spp. are normal mucosal microbiota of a variety of animals including cattle, horses, goats, dogs, cats, camels, guinea pigs, rabbits, pigs, and sheep. *Neisseria weaveri*, *Neisseria animalis*, *N. bacilliformis*, *N. oralis*, *Neisseria animaloris*, *Neisseria zoodegmatis*, and *Moraxella canis*, are oropharyngeal flora in dogs and cats and are sometimes seen in humans following a bite wound. Subinhibitory concentrations of penicillin, such as occurs in the presence of a 10-unit penicillin disk, cause the coccoid forms of these bacteria to elongate to bacilli morphology. In contrast, true cocci, such as most *Neisseria* spp. and *M. catarrhalis*, with which these organisms may be confused, maintain their original cocci shape in the presence of penicillin. In addition, the organisms discussed in this chapter do not use glucose (except *N. animaloris*, *N. oralis*, *N. elongata* subsp. *glycolytica*, and some strains of *N. zoodegmatis*), do not ferment carbohydrates (i.e., are oxidizers or asaccharolytic), and most do not grow on MacConkey agar but will grow well on blood and chocolate agar, as well as in commercial blood culture systems. Specific morphologic and physiologic features are presented later in this chapter in the discussion of laboratory diagnosis.

Epidemiology, Spectrum of Disease, and Antimicrobial Therapy

Infections caused by *Moraxella* spp. and *Neisseria* spp. most likely result when a breakdown of the patient's mucosal or epidermal defensive barriers allows subsequent invasion of sterile sites by an organism that is part of the patient's normal microbiota (i.e., an endogenous

TABLE 27.1	**Epidemiology, Pathogenesis, and Spectrum of Disease**			
Organism	**Habitat (Reservoir)**	**Mode of Transmission**	**Virulence Factors**	**Spectrum of Disease and Infections**
Moraxella nonliquefaciens, Moraxella lacunata, Moraxella osloensis, Moraxella lincolnii, Moraxella canis, and Moraxella atlantae	Normal human microbiota that inhabit mucous membranes covering the nose, throat, other parts of the upper respiratory tract, conjunctiva, and, for some species (i.e., M. osloensis), the urogenital tract; may also colonize the skin	Infections are rare; when they occur, they are probably caused by the patient's endogenous strains; person-to-person transmission may be possible, but this has not been documented	Unknown; because they are rarely associated with infections, they are considered opportunistic organisms of low virulence	M. lacunata has historically been associated with eye infections, but these infections also may be caused by other Moraxella spp.; other infections include bacteremia, endocarditis and meningitis, septic arthritis, sinusitis, and respiratory infections
Neisseria elongata	Normal microbiota of upper respiratory tract	When infections occur, they are probably caused by the patient's endogenous strains	Unknown; this is considered an opportunistic organism of low virulence	Rarely implicated in infections; has been documented as a cause of bacteremia, endocarditis, and osteomyelitis
Neisseria animaloris, Neisseria weaveri, and Neisseria zoodegmatis	Oral microbiota of dogs	Dog bite	Unknown	Commonly found in infections of dog bite wounds

strain; Table 27.1). The fact that these organisms are rarely the cause of infection indicates that they have low virulence. No person-to-person transmission has been noted with the organisms included in this chapter. Whenever these organisms are encountered in clinical specimens, the possibility that they are contaminants should be seriously considered. This is especially the case when the specimen source may have been exposed to a mucosal surface.

Moraxella spp. have been isolated from cases of endocarditis, bacteremia, septic arthritis, and endophthalmitis. *M. catarrhalis* is the species most commonly associated with human infections, primarily of the respiratory tract. However, because the cellular morphology of this species is more similar to that of *Neisseria* spp. than that of the other *Moraxella* spp., details of this organism's characteristics are discussed in Chapter 39.

Data collected from the Centers for Disease Control and Prevention (CDC) show that these rare isolates may also be a cause of infection. In a study of the bacterium, *N. elongata* subsp. *nitroreducens,* one fourth of the isolates received at the CDC for analysis were from cases of bacterial endocarditis. Data collected during a 16-year period found that most of these isolates were from blood, but they were also recovered from wounds, respiratory secretions, and peritoneal fluid. Individuals at risk had preexisting heart damage or had undergone dental manipulations.

Laboratory Diagnosis

Specimen Collection and Transport

No special considerations are required for specimen collection and transport of the organisms discussed in this chapter. Refer to Table 5.1 for general information on specimen collection and transport.

Specimen Processing

No special considerations are required for processing of the organisms discussed in this chapter. Refer to Table 5.1 for general information on specimen processing.

Direct Detection Methods

Other than a Gram stain of patient specimens, there are no specific procedures for the direct detection of these organisms in clinical material. *Moraxella atlantae, Moraxella nonliquefaciens,* and *M. osloensis* may appear either as coccobacilli or as short, broad rods that tend to resist decolorization and may appear gram-variable. This is also true for *M. canis,* which appears as cocci in pairs or short chains. *Moraxella lacunata* is a coccobacilli or medium-sized rod, and *Moraxella lincolnii* is a coccobacilli that may appear in chains. *N. animaloris* and *N. zoodegmatis* are either coccobacilli or short, straight rods. *N. weaveri* and *N. bacilliforms* are medium-length, straight bacillus. All other species are cocci that appear in either singles or pairs.

Cultivation

Media of Choice

Moraxella spp. and the elongated *Neisseria* spp. grow well on 5% sheep blood and chocolate agars. Most strains grow slowly on MacConkey agar and resemble the non–lactose-fermenting Enterobacterales. Both genera also grow well in the broth of commercial blood culture systems and in common nutrient broths, such as thioglycollate and brain-heart infusion.

Incubation Conditions and Duration

Chocolate and 5% sheep blood agars should be incubated at 35°C in carbon dioxide or ambient air for a minimum of 48 hours. For those species that may grow on MacConkey agar, the medium should be incubated at 35°C in ambient air.

Colonial Appearance

Table 27.2 describes the colonial appearance and other distinguishing characteristics (e.g., pitting) of each species on 5% sheep blood and MacConkey agars. The ability of most commercial identification systems to accurately identify the organisms discussed in this chapter is limited or uncertain. Table 27.3 lists some conventional biochemical tests that can be used to presumptively differentiate the species in this chapter. This is a simplified scheme; clinically important

TABLE 27.2 Colonial Appearance and Characteristics

Organism	Medium	Appearance
Moraxella atlantae	BA	Small (<1 mm), pitting and spreading
	Mac	NLF
Moraxella lacunata	BA	Small gray to white colonies that pit the agar
	CHOC	Form dark halos
	Mac	No growth
Moraxella lincolnii	BA	Small (<1 mm), smooth, translucent to gray to white semiopaque; pitting is rare
	Mac	No growth
Moraxella nonliquefaciens	BA	Smooth, translucent to gray to white semiopaque; occasionally, colonies spread and rarely pit the agar; may appear mucoid
	Mac	NLF, if growth
Moraxella osloensis	BA	Smooth, translucent to gray to white semiopaque; rarely pit the agar
	Mac	NLF, if growth
Moraxella canis	BA	Large (>1 mm) and smooth grey to white; resemble colonies of Enterobacterales
	Mac	NLF
Neisseria elongata (all subspecies)	BA	Gray to white, semiopaque, smooth, glistening; may have dry, claylike consistency
	Mac	NLF, if growth
Neisseria animaloris	BA	Yellowish-white, convex, smooth hemolytic colonies
	Mac	NLF
Neisseria bacilliformis	BA	Grey to buff, smooth glistening
	Mac	No growth
Neisseria oralis	BA	Small, yellow, convex, glistening, α-hemolytic
	Mac	Not determined
Neisseria weaveri	BA	Small, smooth, semiopaque
	Mac	NLF, if growth
Neisseria zoodegmatis	BA	Yellowish-white convex, smooth hemolytic colonies
	Mac	No growth

BA, 5% Sheep blood agar; *Mac*, MacConkey agar; *ND*, not determined; *NLF*, non–lactose-fermenter.

TABLE 27.3　Key Biochemical and Physiologic Characteristics

Organism	Growth on MacConkey	Catalase	Nitrate Reduction	Nitrite Reduction	DNase	Digests Loeffler's Slant	Sodium Acetate Utilization	Growth in Nutrient Broth	Gelatinase	Tributyrin
Moraxella atlantae[b]	+	+	-	-	-		ND	-	-	-
Moraxella lacunata	-	+	+	-	-	+	-	-	+	+
Moraxella lincolnii	-	+	-	-[a]	-	-	-	-	-	-
Moraxella nonliquefaciens	-	+	+	-	-	-	-	V	-	+
Moraxella osloensis	V	+	V	-	-	-	+	+	-	+
Moraxella canis	+	+	+	V	+	-	+	+	-	+
Neisseria animaloris	ND	-	+	ND	ND	ND	ND	ND	ND	ND
Neisseria bacilliformis	-	V	+	ND	ND	ND	ND	ND	ND	ND
Neisseria elongata subsp. elongata	V	-	-	+	ND	ND	V	+	ND	ND
Neisseria elongata subsp. glycolytica	+	-	-	V	ND	ND	+	+	ND	ND
Neisseria elongata subsp. nitroreducens	V	+	+	+	ND	ND	V	V	ND	ND
Neisseria oralis	ND	-	+	ND	ND	ND	ND	ND	ND	ND
Neisseria weaverii	V	-	-	+	ND	ND	-	V	ND	ND
Neisseria zoodegmatis	-	-	V	ND	ND	ND	ND	ND	ND	ND

[a]Nitrite-positive strains have been reported.

[b]*M. atlantae* is positive for pyrrolidinyl aminopeptidase

+, Greater than 90% of strains positive; –, greater than 90% of strains negative; *ND*, no data; *V*, variable.

Note: Organisms listed are generally indole-negative.

isolates should be sent to a reference laboratory for definitive identification.

Approach to Identification

As previously mentioned, these organisms can be difficult to differentiate from gram-negative diplococci (see Chapter 39 for more information about gram-negative diplococci). In addition, these organisms are relatively biochemically inert. Elongation in the presence of penicillin is a useful criterion for differentiating them from true cocci. The effect of penicillin is determined by streaking a blood agar plate, placing a 10-unit penicillin disk in the first quadrant, and allowing overnight incubation at 35°C. A Gram stain of the growth taken from around the edge of the zone of inhibition readily demonstrates whether the isolate in question is a cocci or has elongated. *N. animators* and *N. zoodegmatis* are often misidentified as *Pasteurella* sp. or not identified at all because of slow growth. They are able to grow on sheep blood agar and chocolate agar in 48 hours. They are differentiated from *Pasteurella multocida* based on colonial morphology (yellow to white colonies) and indole negative. Matrix-assisted laser desorption ionization time-of-flight mass spectrometry (MALDI-TOF MS) may be a useful technique for identification of these organisms. Caution should be taken when identifying isolates of the *Neisseria* spp. from oropharyngeal clinical specimens to avoid misidentification. The lack of sufficient clinical isolates for comparison and the development of databases is problematic.

Comments Regarding Specific Organisms

M. nonliquefaciens and *M. osloensis*—the two most frequently isolated species—can be differentiated by the ability of *M. osloensis* to utilize acetate. *M. lacunata* is able to liquefy serum; growth of the organism results in the formation of depressions on the surface of Loeffler's serum agar slants. Most of the species considered in this chapter do not utilize glucose; *N. elongata* subsp. *glycolytica,* which produces acid from glucose in the rapid sugar test used for *Neisseria* spp., is the only exception. All *Neisseria* spp. are oxidase positive. *N. elongate* subsp. *nitroreducens* and some strains of *N. bacilliformis* are catalase positive, while all other species are catalase negative.

Serodiagnosis

Serodiagnostic techniques are not generally used for the laboratory diagnosis of infections caused by the organisms discussed in this chapter.

Antimicrobial Susceptibility

The rarity with which these organisms are encountered as the cause of infection and the lack of validated *in vitro* susceptibility testing methods does not allow definitive treatment guidelines. Although many of these organisms may grow on the media and under the conditions recommended for testing other bacteria, this does not necessarily mean that interpretable and reliable results will be produced. Chapter 11 provides preferable strategies that can be used to provide susceptibility information when validated testing methods do not exist for a clinically important bacterial isolate. In general, β-lactam antibiotics are considered to be effective against these species. However, some evidence suggests that β-lactamase–mediated resistance may be capable of spreading among *Moraxella* spp.

Prevention

Because these organisms do not generally pose a threat to human health, there are no recommended vaccination or prophylaxis protocols.

ⓔ Visit the Evolve site for a complete list of procedures, review questions, and case studies.

Bibliography

Alamri Y, Keene A, Pithie A: Acute cystitis caused by commensal *Neisseria oralis*: a case report and review of the literature, *Infect Disord Drug Targets* 17:64–66, 2017.

Carroll KC, Pfaller MA, Landry ML, et al.: *Manual of clinical microbiology*, ed 12, Washington, DC, 2019, ASM.

Fi A, Balada-Llasat JM, Pancholi P, et al.: A rare case of *Neisseria bacilliformis* native valve endocarditis, *Diagn Microbiol Infect Dis* 73:3788-379, 2012.

Gagnard JC, Hidri N, Grillon A, et al.: *Moraxella osloensis*, an emerging pathogen of endocarditis in immunocompromised patients? *Swiss Med Wkly* 145:w14185, 2015.

Grant PE, Brenner DJ, Steigerwalt AG, Hollis DG, Weaver RE: *Neisseria elongata* subsp. *nitroreducens* subsp. nov., formerly CDC group M-6, a gram-negative bacterium associated with endocarditis, *J Clin Microbiol* 28:2591–2596, 1990.

Heydecke A, Andersson B, Holmdahl T, Melhus A: Human wound infections caused by *Neisseria animaloris* and *Neisseria zoodegmatis,* former CDC Group EF-4a and EF 4b, *Infect Ecol Epidemiol* 3:3402, 2013.

Jannes G, Vaneechoutte M, Lannoo M, et al.: Polyphasic taxonomy leading to the proposal of *Moraxella canis* sp. nov. for *Moraxella catarrhalis*–like strains, *Int J Syst Bacteriol* 43:438–449, 1993.

Kodjo A, Richard Y, Tønjum T: *Moraxella boevrei* sp. nov., a new *Moraxella* species found in goats, *Int J Syst Bacteriol* 47:115–121, 1997.

Montejo M, Ruiz-Irastorza G, Aguirrebengoa K, et al.: Endocarditis due to *Neisseria elongata* subspecies *nitroreducens*, *Clin Infect Dis* 20:1431–1432, 1995.

Morel F, Jacquier H, Desroches M, et al.: Use of andromas and bruker MALDI-TOF MS in the identification of *Neisseria*, *Eur J Clin Microbiol Infect Dis* 37:2273–2277, 2018.

Meuleman P, Erard K, Herregods MC, Peetermans WE, Verhaegen J: Bioprosthetic valve endocarditis caused by *Neisseria elongata* subspecies *nitroreducens*, *Infection* 24:258–260, 1996.

Nagano N, Sato J, Cordevant C, Nagano Y, Taguchi F, Inoue M: Presumed endocarditis caused by BRO beta-lactamase-producing *Moraxella lacunata* in an infant with Fallot's tetrad, *J Clin Microbiol* 41:5310–5312, 2003.

Struillou L, Raffi F, Barrier JH: Endocarditis caused by *Neisseria elongata* subspecies *nitroreducens:* case report and literature review, *Eur J Clin Microbiol Infect Dis* 12:625–627, 1993.

Vandamme P, Gillis M, Vancanneyt M, Hoste B, Kersters K, Falsen E: *Moraxella lincolnii* sp. *nov.,* isolated from the human respiratory tract, and reevaluation of the taxonomic position of *Moraxella osloensis, Int J Syst Bacteriol* 43:474–481, 1993.

Wallace RJ, Steingrube VA, Nash DR, et al.: BRO β-lactamases of *Branhamella catarrhalis* and *Moraxella* subgenus *Moraxella,* including evidence for chromosomal β-lactamase transfer by conjugation in *B. catarrhalis, M. nonliquefaciens,* and *M. lacunata, Antimicrob Agents Chemother* 30:1845–1854, 1989.

Wong JD, Janda JM: Association of an important *Neisseria species, Neisseria elongata* subsp. *nitroreducens,* with bacteremia, endocarditis, and osteomyelitis, *J Clin Microbiol* 30:719–720, 1992.

28

Eikenella corrodens and Similar Organisms

OBJECTIVES

1. Identify and explain the key morphologic and biochemical characteristics for *Eikenella corrodens*.
2. Describe the normal habitat for *Eikenella* spp. and conditions that provide optimal conditions for the opportunistic bacteria to become a pathogen.
3. Define the acronym HACEK; what organisms does this acronym refer to, and what medical conditions are associated with these organisms?
4. Define the general characteristics for *Eikenella corrodens*, *Methylobacterium* spp., *Weeksella virosa*, and *Bergeyella zoohelcum*, and explain how the organisms are distinguished from one another.
5. Describe the Gram stain characteristics for each type of bacteria listed in Objective 4.
6. Identify the normal habitat for *Methylobacterium* and explain why the organism is commonly isolated from water distribution systems.
7. Explain how the pink colonies produced in culture by *Methylobacterium* spp. are differentiated from other species of bacteria capable of producing pink colonies.
8. Describe the culture techniques used to isolate *Eikenella corrodens* and *Methylobacterium* spp.
9. Correlate patient signs, symptoms, and laboratory results to identify the most probable etiologic agent associated with the data.

GENERA AND SPECIES TO BE CONSIDERED

Current Name

Asaia spp.
Eikenella corrodens
Methylobacterium spp.
Weeksella virosa
Bergeyella zoohelcum

General Characteristics

The organisms discussed in this chapter are considered together because they are predominantly asaccharolytic, oxidase-positive bacilli that fail to grow on MacConkey agar. Their individual morphologic and physiologic features are presented later in this chapter in the discussion of laboratory diagnosis.

Epidemiology, Spectrum of Disease, and Antimicrobial Therapy

The organisms listed in Table 28.1 are not commonly associated with human infections, but they are occasionally encountered in clinical specimens. *Eikenella corrodens* is normal microbiota of the human oral cavity and is often associated with periodontitis. The organism is a facultative anaerobe, nonmotile, gram-negative bacillus. Among the organisms considered in this chapter, *E. corrodens* is the organism most commonly isolated and is usually found in mixed infections resulting from human bites or clenched-fist wounds. The organism can be isolated from dental plaque and has been isolated in infections of the upper respiratory tract, osteomyelitis, bite wound infections, and endocarditis. It is an opportunistic pathogen predominantly in immunocompromised patients, causing abscesses and infections, and may lead to death. Patients with diabetes are often at risk for *Eikenella* infections because of the daily microtrauma to their skin via glucose monitoring and insulin injections. The organism is often the cause of soft tissue infections in intravenous drug abusers who lick the injection site or the needle.

This organism is also the "E," for *Eikenella*, in the HACEK group of bacteria known to cause subacute bacterial endocarditis (see Chapter 67 for more information regarding endocarditis and bloodstream infections). HACEK is an acronym used to represent the slow-growing gram-negative bacilli associated with endocarditis. The additional members of the HACEK group of bacteria include *Aggregatibacter aphrophilus*, *Aggregatibacter actinomycetemcomitans*, *Cardiobacterium hominis*, and *Kingella kingae*.

Methylobacterium spp. are gram-negative pleomorphic bacilli predominantly found in water and soil. The genus currently consists of over 50 recognized species. The three most common species isolated in clinical samples include *M. mesophilicum*, *M. extorquens*, and *M. zatmanii*.

TABLE 28.1 Epidemiology, Pathogenesis, and Spectrum of Disease

Organism	Habitat (Reservoir)	Mode of Transmission	Virulence Factors	Spectrum of Disease and Infections
Eikenella corrodens	Normal human microbiota of mouth and gastrointestinal tract	Person-to-person involving trauma associated with human teeth incurred during bites or clenched-fist wounds from facial punches; infection may be a result of the patient's endogenous strains (e.g., endocarditis)	Unknown; an opportunistic organism that usually requires trauma for introduction into normally sterile sites; also may enter bloodstream to cause transient bacteremia or be introduced by intravenous drug abuse	Human bite wound infections, head and neck infections, and aspiration pneumonias as part of a mixed infection; can also cause endocarditis that is slow to develop and indolent (i.e., subacute); less commonly associated with brain and intraabdominal abscesses
Methylobacterium spp.	Found on vegetation and occasionally in the hospital environment; not considered normal human microbiota	Uncertain; probably involves contaminated medical devices such as catheters	Unknown; an opportunistic organism probably of low virulence. Uncommon cause of infection	Bacteremia and peritonitis in patients undergoing chronic ambulatory peritoneal dialysis (CAPD)
Weeksella virosa	Uncertain; probably environmental; not considered normal human microbiota	Uncertain; rarely found in clinical material	Unknown; role in human disease is uncertain	Asymptomatic bacteriuria; also isolated from the female genital tract
Bergeyella zoohelcum	Normal oral microbiota of dogs and other animals; not considered normal human microbiota	Bite or scratch of dog or cat	Unknown; an opportunistic organism that requires traumatic introduction to normally sterile site	Dog and cat bite wound infections

The organisms have been isolated from numerous sterile body sites including blood, bone marrow, cerebrospinal fluid, synovial, ascites, and peritoneal fluids. The organisms are resistant to high temperatures, with drying and disinfectants contributing to the potential spread of these organisms in long-term health care facilities. They can be opportunistic pathogens of low virulence. Most human infections are associated with immunocompromised patients. *Asaia* spp. have been associated with infections in immunocompromised patients, including peritonitis and bacteremia. The colonies are pale pink on sheep blood agar and resemble *Methylobacterium*. Unlike the other organisms included in this chapter, *Asaia* spp. are oxidase negative and saccharolytic.

E. corrodens is usually susceptible to penicillin, cephalosporins, carbapenems, doxycycline, azithromycin, and fluoroquinolones. Beta-lactamase testing is recommended because penicillin-resistant, beta-lactamase–positive isolates have been described. Beta-lactamase–positive strains are susceptible to beta-lactam–beta-lactamase inhibitor combinations. *E. corrodens* is generally resistant to macrolides, clindamycin, and narrow-spectrum cephalosporins.

Methylobacterium are generally susceptible to aminoglycosides and trimethoprim-sulfamethoxazole.

Laboratory Diagnosis

Specimen Collection and Transport

No special considerations are required for specimen collection and transport for the organisms discussed in this chapter. Refer to Table 5.1 for general information on specimen collection and transport.

Specimen Processing

No special considerations are required for processing of the organisms discussed in this chapter. Refer to Table 5.1 for general information on specimen processing.

Direct Detection Methods

There are no specific procedures that are widely available for the direct detection of these organisms in clinical material. However, in the research setting, next-generation sequencing has shown success in the detection of pathogens directly from resected heart valves from patients with infective endocarditis. In the routine clinical laboratory, the Gram stain and microscopic observation remain readily available to rapidly provide critical information from a wide range of specimen types and facilitate appropriate therapy. *E. corrodens* is a slender, medium-length, gram-negative, straight bacillus with rounded ends. *Methylobacterium* is a vacuolated, pale-staining, short- to medium-length gram-negative bacillus that may resist decolorization. *Asaia* spp. are small to medium gram-negative bacilli. *Weeksella virosa* and *Bergeyella zoohelcum* are medium to long gram-negative bacilli with parallel sides and rounded ends that may form "II-forms" (parallel sides) similar to the *Sphingobacterium* (refer to Chapter 23 for more information regarding this genus).

Nucleic Acid Detection

E. corrodens is among a group of pathogens associated with dental plaque and the formation of polymicrobial biofilms associated with periodontal disease. Several studies have examined the three commercial nucleic acid–based identification systems for periodontopathogenic bacteria that are available in Europe. All three methods have been used to successfully identify *E. corrodens* from dental plaque, but are not currently available in the United States.

Cultivation

Media of Choice

E. corrodens grows slowly on blood and chocolate agar, with small colonies developing within 48 hours. The organism will not grow on MacConkey agar and displays limited growth in blood culture broth media, thioglycolate, and brain–heart infusion broth. The hallmark characteristics for the presence of *E. corrodens* in culture include the organism's tendency to pit or corrode the agar, to demonstrate a slightly yellow hue after several days, and to exude a chlorine bleach odor. Most strains require hemin for growth unless incubated in 5% to 10% CO_2. The organism grows well on Columbia-based blood agar.

Methylobacterium is difficult to grow on routine laboratory media, and it may take 4 to 5 days before identifiable colonies appear on sheep blood agar, modified Thayer-Martin, buffered charcoal-yeast extract (BCYE), and Middlebrook 7H11 agar. Reports have indicated that improved growth may be achieved using BCYE agar and Sabouraud agar. The organism is not capable of growth on MacConkey agar. In contrast to most other bacteria, optimal growth occurs at 25°C to 30°C. *Methylobacterium* produce small, dry, coral pink–pigmented colonies. *Roseomonas* also produce pink-pigmented colonies. The two genera can be differentiated by incubation at 42°C. *Roseomonas* is capable of growth at 42°C, whereas *Methylobacterium* is temperature sensitive and incapable of growth in increased temperatures.

TABLE 28.2	Colonial Appearance and Characteristics	
Organism	Medium[a]	Appearance
Asaia spp.	BA	Pale pink; do not appear darker when placed under UV light
Bergeyella zoohelcum	BA	Colonies may be sticky; tan to yellow
Eikenella corrodens	BA	Colonies are tiny at 24 h; mature colonies have moist, clear centers surrounded by flat, spreading growth; colonies may pit or corrode the agar surface; slight yellow pigmentation in older cultures; sharp odor of bleach
Methylobacterium spp.	BA	Pink to coral pigment, colonies appear darker pink under UV light; does not grow well on blood agar
Weeksella virosa	BA	Small colonies at 24 h; mature colonies mucoid and adherent with a tan to brown pigment

[a]These organisms usually do not grow on MacConkey agar; if breakthrough growth occurs, the organisms appear as non–lactose fermenters. *BA*, 5% Sheep blood agar; *UV*, ultraviolet.

In addition, *Methylobacterium* can metabolize acetate, but *Roseomonas* cannot.

Incubation Conditions and Duration

To detect growth on 5% sheep blood and chocolate agars, incubation at 35°C to 37°C in carbon dioxide for a minimum of 48 hours is required. In contrast to the other genera, *Methylobacterium* grows optimally at lower temperatures (25°C to 30°C).

Colonial Appearance

Table 28.2 describes the colonial appearance and other distinguishing characteristics (e.g., odor and pigment) of each genus on 5% sheep blood agar.

Approach to Identification

The ability of most commercial identification systems to accurately identify the organisms discussed in this chapter is limited or, at best, uncertain. Strategies for identification of these genera are based on conventional biochemical tests. A combination of phenotypic and genetic methods (16S ribosomal ribonucleic acid [rRNA] analysis) can be useful for the complete identification of the more unusual organisms. Matrix-assisted laser desorption ionization time-of-flight

TABLE 28.3	Key Biochemical and Physiologic Characteristics							
Organism	Catalase	Mannitol	Xylose	Urease	Nitrate Reduction	Indole	Arginine Dihydrolase
Asaia spp.[a]	+	+	+	−	−	ND	ND
Eikenella corrodens	−	−	−	−	+	−	−
Methylobacterium spp.[a]	+	−	+	+	−	−	ND
Weeksella virosa	+	−	−	−	−	+	−
Bergeyella zoohelcum	+	−	−	+	−	+	+

[a]Colonies are pigmented pink and must be differentiated from *Roseomonas* spp.; *Roseomonas* spp. usually grow on MacConkey agar and will grow at 42°C.
ND, No data; +, >90% of strains positive; −, >90% of strains negative.

mass spectrometry (MALDI-TOF MS) has also been successfully used to identify these organisms, and next-generation sequencing is available in research settings. Table 28.3 outlines basic criteria useful for differentiating the genera discussed in this chapter.

Comments Regarding Specific Organisms

Methylobacterium may be differentiated from other pink-pigmented, gram-negative bacilli (e.g., *Roseomonas* spp.) by the ability to utilize acetate and inability to grow at 42°C. Some strains of *Methylobacterium* weakly oxidize glucose.

The most recognizable feature of *E. corrodens* in culture is the distinctive bleachlike odor. The organism is asaccharolytic (does not utilize glucose or other carbohydrates). *E. corrodens* is oxidase positive, catalase negative, reduces nitrate to nitrite, and hydrolyzes both ornithine and lysine.

Weeksella and *Bergeyella* are oxidase and catalase positive. Both bacteria are indole positive, an unusual characteristic for most nonfermentative bacteria. *W. virosa* is urease negative and *B. zoohelcum* is urease positive, pyrrolidinyl aminopeptidase negative, and resistant to colistin. *W. virosa* will grow on selective media such as modified Thayer Martin (MTM) for *Neisseria gonorrhoeae* but can be differentiated from the gonococci using indole and Gram-stain morphology.

Serodiagnosis

Serodiagnostic techniques are not generally used for the laboratory diagnosis of infections caused by the organisms discussed in this chapter.

Prevention

Because these organisms do not generally pose a threat to human health, there are no recommended vaccination or prophylaxis protocols.

Visit the Evolve site for a complete list of procedures, review questions, and case studies.

Bibliography

Alotaibi F, Almusrea K: *Eikenella corrodens* skull osteomyelitis: case report and literature review, *Int J Neurol Neurosurg* 5:77–79, 2013.

Carroll KC, Pfaller MA, Landry ML, et al.: *Manual of clinical microbiology*, ed 12, Washington, DC, 2019, ASM.

Cercenado E, Cercenado S, Bouza E: In vitro activities of tigecycline (GAR-936) and 12 other antimicrobial agents against 90 *Eikenella corrodens* clinical isolates, *Antimicrob Agents Chemother* 47:2644–2645, 2003.

Cheng J, Hu H, Fang W, et al.: Detection of pathogens from resected heart valves of patients with infective endocarditis by next-generation sequencing, *Int J Infect Dis* 83:148–153, 2019.

Clinical Laboratory Standards Institute: *Methods for antimicrobial dilution and disk susceptibility testing of infrequently isolated or fastidious bacteria; Approved Guideline. CLSI Document M45*, Wayne, PA, 2016, Clinical Laboratory Standards Institute.

Couturier MR, Mehinovic E, Croft AC, Fisher MA: Identification of HACEK clinical isolates by matrix-assisted laser desorption ionization-time of flight mass spectrometry, *J Clin Microbiol* 49:1104–1106, 2011.

deMelo Oliveira MG, Abels S, Zbinden R, Bloemberg GV, Zbinden A: Accurate identification of fastidious gram-negative rods: integration of both conventional phenotypic methods and 16S rRNA gene analysis, *BMC Microbiol* 13:162, 2013.

Goncalves RJ, Murinello A, Gomes da Silva S, et al.: Hepatic abscess due to *Streptococcus anginosus* and *Eikenella corrodens*, secondary to gastric perforation by a fish bone, *GEPort J Gastroenterol* 26(4):414–419, 2019.

Lai CC, Cheng A, Liu WL, et al.: Infections caused by unusual *Methylobacterium* species, *J Clin Microbiol* 49:3329–3331, 2011.

Patas K, Douros K, Priftis KN, et al.: Isolation of *Aggregatibacter aphrophilus* from bronchoalveolar lavage in a paediatric patient presenting with haemoptysis, *New Microbes New Infect* 29:100509, 2019.

Powell EA, Blecker-Shelly D, Montgomery S, Mortensen JE: Application of matrix-assisted laser desorption ionization-time of flight mass spectrometry for identification of the fastidious pediatric pathogens *Aggregatibacter, Eikenella, Haemophilus,* and *Kingella*, *J Clin Microbiol* 51:3862–3864, 2013.

Prieto-Arevalo R, Muñoz P, Cuerpo G, et al.: Pulmonary infective endocarditis, *J Am Coll Cardiol* 73(21):2782–2783, 2019.

Saffert RT, Cunningham SA, Ihde SM, et al.: Comparison of bruker biotyper matrix-assisted laser desorption ionization-time of flight mass spectrometre to BD Phoenix automated microbiology system for identification of gram-negative bacilli, *J Clin Microbiol* 49:887–892, 2011.

Santigli E, Leitner E, Wimmer G, et al.: Accuracy of commercial kits and published primer pairs for the detection of periodontopathogens, *Clin Oral Investig* 20(9):2515–2528, 2016.

Shao S, Guo X, Guo P, Cui Y, Chen Y: *Roseomonas mucosa* infective endocarditis in patient with systemic lupus erythematosus: case report and review of literature, *BMC Infect Dis* 19:140, 2019.

Slenker AK, Hess BD, Jungkind DL, DeSimone JA: Fatal case of *Weeksella virosa* sepsis, *J Clin Microbiol* 50:4166–4167, 2012.

Tani A, Sahin N, Matsuyama Y, et al.: High-throughput identification and screening of novel *Methylobacterium* species using whole-cell MALDI-TOF/MS analysis, *PloS One* 7:e40784, 2012.

Teo WZW, Chung KC: Hand infections, *Clin Plast Surg* 46(3): 371–381, 2019.

Urban E, Terhes G, Radnai M, et al.: Detection of periodontopathogenic bacteria in pregnant women in traditional anaerobic culture method and by a commercial molecular genetic method, *Anaerobe* 16(3):283–288, 2010.

Weyant RS, Moss CW, Weaver RE, et al.: *Identification of unusual pathogenic gram-negative aerobic and facultatively anaerobic bacteria*, ed 2, Baltimore, 1997, Williams & Wilkins.

29

Pasteurella and Similar Organisms

OBJECTIVES

1. Describe the general characteristics of *Pasteurella* spp. and the additional organisms included in this chapter.
2. Describe the epidemiology associated with human infections caused by *Pasteurella* spp. and similar organisms, including the normal habitat and route of transmission.
3. Compare the Gram-stain appearance of the organisms included in this chapter.
4. Describe the antimicrobial therapy of choice for *Pasteurella* spp. and the appropriateness of antimicrobial susceptibility testing for these and similar organisms.
5. Identify limitations associated with the identification of *Pasteurella* spp. and similar organisms.

GENERA AND SPECIES TO BE CONSIDERED

Current Name	Previous Name
Mannheimia haemolytic	
[Pasteurella] aerogenes[a]	
[Pasteurella] bettyae[a]	
[Pasteurella] caballi[a]	
Pasteurella canis	
Pasteurella dagmatis	
Pasteurella multocida subsp. multocida	Pasteurella multocida
Pasteurella multocida subsp. gallicida	Pasteurella multocida
Pasteurella multocida subsp. septica	Pasteurella multocida
Pasteurella oralis	
Pasteurella stomatis	
Rodentibacter pneumotropicus	Pasteurella pneumotropica
Suttonella indologenes	Kingella indologenes

[a]*Pasteurella* incertae sedis (of uncertain placement).

General Characteristics and Taxonomy

The organisms discussed in this chapter are small, gram-negative, nonmotile, oxidase-positive bacilli that ferment glucose. Most of the organisms will not grow on MacConkey agar. The organisms included in this chapter are difficult to identify using conventional phenotypic methods and may require genomic sequencing including 16s rRNA analysis. The individual morphologic and physiologic features are presented later in this chapter in the discussion of laboratory diagnosis.

Taxonomy of *Pasteurella* spp. and similar organisms has significantly changed since the early 2000s and may be subject to additional revision. The family consists of over 90 named species in approximately 25 genera. The genus *Pasteurella* is included here and the remaining genera which include *Actinobacillus*, *Aggregatibacter* (aggregation of the former *Actinobacillus actinomycetemcomitans*, *Haemophilus aphrophilus*, *Haemophilus paraphrophilus*, and *Haemophilus segnis*), and *Haemophilus*, are included in Chapters 30 and 31. The only member of the family *Cardiobacteriaceae* that is associated with human infections is *Suttonella indologenes*.

Epidemiology, Spectrum of Disease, and Antimicrobial Therapy

Most of the organisms presented in this chapter constitute portions of both domestic and wild animal microbiota and are transmitted to humans during close animal contact, including bites. For most of these species, virulence factors are not recognized. As a result, the organisms may be considered opportunistic pathogens that require mechanical disruption of host anatomic barriers (i.e., bite wounds; Table 29.1). Of the organisms listed in Table 29.2, *Pasteurella multocida* subsp. *multocida* is most commonly encountered in clinical specimens. Reported virulence factors for this subspecies include lipopolysaccharide, cytotoxin, six serotypes of the antiphagocytic capsule, surface adhesins, and iron-acquisition proteins. Other manifestations of infection by *P. multocida* subsp. *multocida* can include respiratory disease and systemic disease such as endocarditis, septicemia, and rarely meningitis. Liver cirrhosis is viewed as a risk factor for systemic disease. Other organisms can be agents of systemic infection (*Rodentibacter pneumotropicus*) and genital tract–associated disease (*Pasteurella bettyae*).

TABLE 29.1 Epidemiology of Selected *Pasteurella* spp. and Similar Organisms

Organism	Habitat (Reservoir)	Mode of Transmission
Pasteurella multocida, other *Pasteurella* spp.	Commensal found in nasopharynx and gastrointestinal tract of wild and domestic animals; potential upper respiratory commensal in humans who have extensive occupational exposure to animals	Bite or scratch from a variety of veterinary hosts (usually feline or canine); infections may be associated with nonbite exposure to animals; less commonly, infections may occur without history of animal exposure
Suttonella indologenes	Unknown; rarely encountered in clinical specimens but may be part of the normal human microbiome	Unknown

TABLE 29.2 Pathogenesis and Spectrum of Disease of Selected *Pasteurella* spp. and Similar Organisms

Organism	Virulence Factors	Spectrum of Disease and Infections
Pasteurella bettyae	Unknown	Genital tract infection; neonatal infection
Pasteurella multocida subsp. *multocida*	Endotoxin, cytotoxin, surface adhesins, capsule associated with *P. multocida*	Focal soft tissue infection; chronic respiratory infection, usually in patients with preexisting chronic lung disease and heavy exposure to animals; systemic disease (hematogenous dissemination) such as meningitis, endocarditis, osteomyelitis, dialysis-associated peritonitis, septicemia
Pasteurella multocida subsp. *septica*	Unknown	Focal soft tissue infection
Rodentibacter pneumotropicus	Unknown	Rare systemic infection
Suttonella indologenes	Unknown	Rare ocular infection

TABLE 29.3 Antimicrobial Therapy and Susceptibility Testing for *Pasteurella* spp. and Similar Organisms

Organism	Therapeutic Options	Potential Resistance to Therapeutic Options	Validated Testing Methods
Pasteurella spp.	Penicillin, ampicillin, amoxicillin are recommended agents; doxycycline, amoxicillin-clavulanate are alternative agents; ceftriaxone, fluoroquinolones may be effective	Clindamycin, cephalexin, nafcillin, erythromycin (deduced from susceptibility testing)	CLSI document M45
Suttonella indologenes	Not well characterized; purported susceptibility to penicillins, chloramphenicol, tetracycline	Unknown	Not available

CLSI, Clinical and Laboratory Standards Institute.

An unusual feature of the organisms considered in this chapter is that most are susceptible to penicillin. Although most other clinically relevant gram-negative bacilli are intrinsically resistant to penicillin, it is the drug of choice for infections involving *P. multocida* and several other species listed in Table 29.3. The general therapeutic effectiveness of penicillin and the lack of resistance to this agent among *Pasteurella* spp. suggest that *in vitro* susceptibility testing is typically not indicated. This is especially true with isolates emanating from bite wounds. Moreover, bite wounds can be complicated by polymicrobial infection. In this case,

the empiric therapy directed toward multiple agents is generally also effective against *Pasteurella* spp. As a result, antimicrobial susceptibility testing for *Pasteurella* spp. may have greater utility for isolates recovered from sterile sources (blood, deep tissue) and from respiratory specimens obtained from immunocompromised patients. Clinical and Laboratory Standards Institute (CLSI) document M45-A2 does provide guidelines for broth microdilution (cation-adjusted Mueller Hinton broth medium supplemented with 2.5% to 5% lysed horse blood) and disk diffusion (Mueller Hinton agar medium supplemented with 5% sheep blood) antimicrobial susceptibility testing of *Pasteurella* spp. Both formats are incubated in 35°C ambient air. Interpretation of disk diffusion and broth microdilution formats occurs at 16 to 18 hours and 18 to 24 hours of incubation, respectively. Antimicrobial agents to consider for testing include penicillin, ampicillin, amoxicillin, amoxicillin-clavulanate, ceftriaxone, moxifloxacin, levofloxacin, tetracycline, doxycycline, erythromycin, azithromycin, chloramphenicol, and trimethoprim-sulfamethoxazole. Of these agents, breakpoints for categorical interpretation of resistance or intermediate susceptibility have only been established for erythromycin.

Laboratory Diagnosis

Specimen Collection and Transport

No special considerations are required for specimen collection and transport of the organisms discussed in this chapter. Refer to Table 5.1 for general information on specimen collection and transport.

Specimen Processing

No special considerations are required for processing of the organisms discussed in this chapter. Refer to Table 5.1 for general information on specimen processing.

Direct Detection Methods

Other than Gram staining, there are no commonly used procedures for the direct detection of these organisms from primary clinical material. *Pasteurella* spp. are typically short, straight bacilli, although *Pasteurella aerogenes* may also present as coccobacilli. Bipolar staining is frequent. The bacillus of *P. bettyae* is usually thinner than other species. *Mannheimia haemolytica* is a small bacillus or coccobacillus. *S. indologenes* is a broad, irregular staining gram-negative bacillus of variable length that may appear in pairs, chains, or rosettes.

Serodiagnosis

Serodiagnostic techniques are of little utility for the laboratory diagnosis of infections caused by the organisms discussed in this chapter.

Cultivation

Media of Choice

The bacteria described in this chapter grow well on routine laboratory media such as tryptic soy agar supplemented with 5% sheep blood (blood agar) and chocolate agar. With the exception of *P. aerogenes* and some strains of *P. bettyae* and *R. pneumotropicus,* most species do not grow on MacConkey agar. The presence of gram-negative bacilli in the direct Gram stain of a wound specimen followed by no growth on MacConkey agar provides a clue that *Pasteurella spp.* may be present in the culture, especially if the wound is

TABLE 29.4	Colonial Appearance and Characteristics of Selected *Pasteurella* spp. and Similar Organisms on Sheep Blood Agar
Organism	**Appearance**
Mannheimia haemolytica[a]	Convex, smooth, grayish, beta-hemolytic (feature may be lost on subculture)
Pasteurella aerogenes[a]	Convex, smooth, translucent, nonhemolytic[b]
Pasteurella bettyae,[c] *Pasteurella caballi, Pasteurella canis, Pasteurella, P. dagmatis*	Convex, smooth, nonhemolytic
Pasteurella multocida	Convex, smooth, gray, nonhemolytic; rough and mucoid variants can occur; may have a musty or mushroom odor
Pasteurella stomatis	Smooth, convex, nonhemolytic
Rodentibacter pneumotropicus	Smooth, convex, nonhemolytic
Suttonella indologenes	Resembles *Kingella* spp. (Chapter 30); may spread or pit the surface of blood agar

[a]Breakthrough growth may occur on MacConkey agar; will appear as a lactose fermenter.
[b]After 48 hours, colonies may be surrounded by a narrow green to brown halo or appear gamma-hemolytic.
[c]Breakthrough growth may occur on MacConkey agar; will appear as a nonlactose fermenter.

from a cat or dog bite. *M. haemolytica, Pasteurella* spp., and *S. indologenes* grow well in blood culture broth systems and common nutrient broths such as thioglycollate and brain-heart infusion. *Pasteurella* spp. may be differentiated from *Haemophilus* spp. via CO_2-independence and growth on media containing sheep blood.

Incubation Conditions and Duration

Inoculated blood and chocolate agar are incubated at 35°C in ambient air or an environment enriched with 5% CO_2 for a minimum of 24 hours. *S. indologenes* may grow especially slowly on primary media.

Colonial Appearance

Table 29.4 describes the colonial appearance and other distinguishing characteristics (e.g., hemolysis and odor) of these genera on blood agar.

Approach to Identification

Commercial biochemical identification systems will identify the most commonly isolated *Pasteurella* spp. but may not definitively identify the unusual *Pasteurella* spp. and

CHAPTER 29 *Pasteurella* and Similar Organisms 433

TABLE 29.5 Key Biochemical Characteristics of Selected *Pasteurella* spp. and Similar Organisms

Organism	Indole	Urea	Nitrate Reduction	Catalase	ODC[a]	Mannitol	Sucrose	Maltose
Mannheimia haemolytica	–	–	+	+	–	(+)	+	+
Pasteurella aerogenes	–	(+)	(+)	+	V	–	+	+
Pasteurella bettyae	(+)	–	(+)	–	–	–	–	–
Pasteurella caballi	–	–	(+)	–	(+)	(+)	(+)	(+)
Pasteurella canis	+	–	+	+	(+)	–	(+)	–
Pasteurella dagmatis	(+)	(+)	(+)	+	–	–	+	(+)
Pasteurella multocida	(+)	–	(+)	+	(+)	+	+	–
Pasteurella oralis	+	–	ND	+	+	–	+	+
Pasteurella stomatis	(+)	–	+	+	–	–	(+)	–
Rodentibacter pneumotropicus	(+)	(+)[b]	(+)	+	(+)	–	+	+
Suttonella indologenes	(+)	–	–	V	–	–	(+)	(+)

[a]Ornithine decarboxylase.
[b]May require a drop of rabbit serum on the slant or a heavy inoculum.
+, >90% of strains positive; (+), >90% of strains positive but reaction may be delayed (i.e., 2–7 days); –, >90% of strains negative; V, variable.
Data compiled from Angen O, Mutters R, Caugant DA, et al. Taxonomic relationships of the [*Pasteurella*] *haemolytica* complex as evaluated by DNA-DNA hybridization and 16S rRNA sequencing with proposal of *Mannheimia haemolytica* gen. nov., comb. nov., *Mannheimia granulomatis* comb. nov., *Mannheimia glucosida* sp. nov., *Mannheimia ruminalis* sp. nov. and *Mannheimia varigena* sp. nov. *Int J Syst Bacteriol.* 1999;49:67; Caroll KC, Pfaller MA. *Manual of Clinical Microbiology.* 12th ed. Washington, DC: ASM; 2019; and Weyant RS, Moss CW, Weaver RE, et al., eds. *Identification of Unusual Pathogenic Gram-negative Aerobic and Facultatively Anaerobic Bacteria.* 2nd ed. Baltimore: Williams & Wilkins; 1996.

similar organisms. Table 29.5 summarizes conventional biochemical tests that can assist in the presumptive differentiation or species confirmation of organisms discussed in this chapter. These organisms closely resemble those described in Chapter 30. Data discussed in both Chapters 29 and 30 can be considered when evaluating an isolate in the clinical laboratory. A more complete conventional biochemical battery, offered as part of a reference laboratory workup, may be required for definitive identification of the isolates. Historic methods used to definitively identify *Pasteurella* spp. and *Suttonella* sp. on the basis of cellular fatty acid analysis have been replaced with matrix-assisted laser desorption ionization time-of-flight mass spectrometry (MALDI-TOF MS) for the identification of the organisms more commonly isolated from clinical samples. In some cases, species identification may be unsatisfactory, requiring the use of 16s rRNA and *soda* gene sequencing.

Comments Regarding Specific Organisms

Pasteurella spp. typically yield a positive tetramethyl-p-phenylenediamine dihydrochloride-based oxidase result. With the exception of *P. bettyae* and *Pasteurella caballi*, these organisms are catalase positive; all *Pasteurella* spp. reduce nitrates to nitrites. *P. aerogenes* and some strains of *Pasteurella dagmatis* ferment glucose with the production of gas. *P. multocida* can be differentiated from other *Pasteurella* spp. based on positive reactions for ornithine decarboxylase and indole, with a negative reaction for urease. *P. multocida* subsp. *multocida* ferments sorbitol and fails to ferment dulcitol, *P. multocida* subsp. *gallicida* ferments dulcitol but not sorbitol, and *P. multocida* subsp. *septica* ferments neither carbohydrate.

M. haemolytica may be differentiated from members of the *Pasteurella* genus by its inability to produce indole or ferment mannose. *S. indologenes* can be separated from

Pasteurella spp. with a negative nitrate test and is delineated from *Kingella* spp. (Chapter 30) by indole production and sucrose fermentation.

Serodiagnosis

Serodiagnostic techniques are of little utility for the laboratory diagnosis of infections caused by the organisms discussed in this chapter.

Prevention

Because infections with these organisms are relatively rare and they do not pose a widespread threat to human health, there are no recommended vaccination or prophylaxis protocols.

ⓔ Visit the Evolve site for a complete list of procedures, review questions, and case studies.

Bibliography

Abrahamian FM, Goldstein EJ: Microbiology of animal bite wound infections, *Clin Microbiol Rev* 24:231–246, 2011.

Angen O, Mutters R, Caugant DA, Olsen JE, Bisgaard M: Taxonomic relationships of the [*Pasteurella*] *haemolytica* complex as evaluated by DNA-DNA hybridizations and 16S rRNA sequencing with proposal of *Mannheimia haemolytica* gen. nov., comb. nov., *Mannheimia granulomatis* comb. nov., *Mannheimia glucosida* sp. nov., *Mannheimia ruminalis* sp. nov. and *Mannheimia varigena* sp. nov, *Int J Syst Bacteriol* 49:67–86, 1999.

Bennett J, Dolin R, Blaser M: *Principles and practice of infectious diseases*, ed 9, Philadelphia, 2020, Elsevier-Saunders.

Caroll KC, Pfaller MA: *Manual of clinical microbiology*, ed 12, Washington, DC, 2019, ASM Press.

Clinical and Laboratory Standards Institute: *Methods for antimicrobial dilution and disk susceptibility testing of infrequently isolated or fastidious bacteria; M45*, ed 3, Wayne, PA, 2016, CLSI.

de Melo Oliveira MG, Abels S, Zbinden R, Bloemberg GV, Zbinden A: Accurate identification of fastidious gram-negative rods: integration of both conventional phenotypic methods and 16S rRNA gene analysis, *BMC Microbiol* 13:162, 2013.

Donnio PY, Lerestif-Gautier AL, Avril JL: Characterization of *Pasteurella* spp. strains isolated from human infections, *J Comp Pathol* 130:137–142, 2004.

Gregersen RH, Neubauer C, Christensen H, et al.: Characterization of *Pasteurellaceae*-like bacteria isolated from clinically affected psittacine birds, *J Appl Microbiol* 108:1235–1243, 2010.

Guillard T, Duval V, Jobart R, et al.: Dog bite wound infection by *Pasteurella dagmatis* misidentified as *Pasteurella pneumotropica* by automated system Vitek 2, *Diagn Microbiol Infect Dis* 65:347–348, 2009.

Harper M, Boyce JD, Adler B: *Pasteurella multocida* pathogenesis: 125 years after Pasteur, *FEMS Microbiol Lett* 265:1–10, 2006.

Janda WA: Update on family *Pasteurellaceae* and the status of genus *Pasteurella* and genus *Actinobacillus*, *Clin Microbiol Newsl* 33:135, 2011.

Nørskov-Lauritsen N, Kilian M: Reclassification of *Actinobacillus actinomycetemcomitans, Haemophilus aphrophilus, Haemophilus paraphrophilus,* and *Haemophilus segnis* as *Aggregatibacter actinomycetemcomitans* gen. nov., comb. nov., *Aggregatibacter aphrophilus,* comb. nov., and *Aggregatibacter segnis* comb. nov., and emended description of *Aggregatibacter aphrophilus* to include V factor-dependent and V factor-independent isolates, *Int J Syst Evol Microbiol* 56:2135–2146, 2006.

Ryan JM, Feder Jr HM: Dog licks baby. Baby gets *Pasteurella multocida* meningitis, *Lancet* 393(10186):E41, 2019.

Saffert RT, Cunningham SA, Ihde SM, Jobe KE, Mandrekar J, Patel R: Comparison of Bruker Biotyper matrix-assisted laser desorption ionization-time of flight mass spectrometre to BD Phoenix automated microbiology system for identification of gram-negative bacilli, *J Clin Microbiol* 49:887–892, 2011.

Teo WZW, Chung KC: Hand Infections, *Clin Plast Surg* 46(3):371–381, 2019.

Ujvari B, Makrai L, Magyar T: Virulence gene profiling and *ompA* sequence analysis of *Pasteurella multocida* and their correlation with host species, *Vet Microbiol* 233:190–195, 2019.

Weyant RS, Moss CW, Weaver RE, et al.: *Identification of unusual pathogenic gram-negative aerobic and facultatively anaerobic bacteria*, ed 2, Baltimore, 1996, Williams & Wilkins.

Wilkie IW, Harper M, Boyce JD, Adler B: *Pasteurella multocida:* diseases and pathogenesis, *Curr Top Microbiol Immunol* 36:1–22, 2012.

Wilson BA, Ho M: *Pasteurella multocida:* from zoonosis to cellular microbiology, *Clin Microbiol Rev* 26:631–655, 2013.

30

Actinobacillus, Kingella, Cardiobacterium, Capnocytophaga, and Similar Organisms

OBJECTIVES

1. Describe the general characteristics of the bacteria included in this chapter.
2. Describe the normal habitat and the routes of transmission for the organisms included in this chapter.
3. Identify the major clinical diseases associated with *Actinobacillus, Aggregatibacter, Kingella, Cardiobacterium,* and *Capnocytophaga* spp.
4. Explain the incubation conditions for these bacteria, including oxygenation, time, and temperature.
5. Define dysgonic.
6. List the media used to cultivate the organisms discussed in this chapter.
7. Discuss the unique colonial presentation of the various genera of the clinically significant species.

GENERA AND SPECIES TO BE CONSIDERED

Current Name	Previous Name
Actinobacillus spp.	
Actinobacillus equuli (horses and pigs)	
Actinobacillus hominis	
Actinobacillus lignieresii (sheep and cattle)	
Actinobacillus suis (pigs)	
Actinobacillus ureae	
Aggregatibacter spp.	
Aggregatibacter actinomycetemcomitans	*Actinobacillus actinomycetem-comitans*

Current Name	Previous Name
Aggregatibacter aphrophilus	*Haemophilus aphrophilus, Haemophilus paraphrophilus*
Aggregatibacter segnis	*Haemophilus segnis*
Capnocytophaga spp.	
Capnocytophaga canimorsus (dogs and cats)	CDC group DF-2
Capnocytophaga cynodegmi (dogs and cats)	CDC group DF-2
Capnocytophaga gingivalis	Formerly CDC group DF-1
Capnocytophaga granulosa	
Capnocytophaga haemolytica	
Capnocytophaga ochracea	Formerly CDC group DF-1
Capnocytophaga sputigena	Formerly CDC group DF-1
Cardiobacterium spp.	
Cardiobacterium hominis	
Cardiobacterium valvarum	
Dysgonomonas spp.	
Dysgonomonas capnocytophagoides	CDC group DF-3
Dysgonomonas gadei	
Dysgonomonas hofstadii	
Dysgonomonas mossii	
Kingella spp.	
Kingella denitrificans	
Kingella kingae	
Kingella oralis	
Kingella potus	
Leptotricha bucallis	

TABLE 30.1	Epidemiology		
Organism	**Habitat (Reservoir)**	**Mode of Transmission**	
Aggregatibacter actinomycetemcomitans	Normal microbiota of human oral cavity	Endogenous; enters deeper tissues by minor trauma to the mouth, such as during dental procedures	
Actinobacillus spp.	Normal oral microbiota of animals such as cows, sheep, and pigs; not part of the human microbiota	Rarely associated with human infection; transmitted by bite wounds or contamination of preexisting wounds during exposure to animals	
Kingella spp.	Normal microbiota of human upper respiratory and genitourinary tracts	Infections probably caused by patient's endogenous strains	
Cardiobacterium hominis and *Cardiobacterium valvarum*	Normal microbiota of the human upper respiratory tract	Infections probably caused by patient's endogenous strains	
Capnocytophaga gingivalis, Capnocytophaga ochracea, Capnocytophaga sputigena, and other species	Subgingival surfaces and other areas of the human oral cavity	Infections probably caused by patient's endogenous strains	
Capnocytophaga canimorsus and *Capnocytophaga cynodegmi*	Oral microbiota of dogs	Dog bite or wound (scratch), long exposure to dogs *Capnocytophaga cynodegmi*	
Dysgonomonas capnocytophagoides and other species	Uncertain; possibly part of human gastrointestinal microbiota	Uncertain; possibly endogenous	

General Characteristics

The organisms discussed in this chapter are **dysgonic**—that is, they grow slowly (48 hours at 35°C to 37°C) or poorly. Although they all ferment glucose, their fastidious nature requires that serum be added to the basal fermentation medium to enhance growth and detect fermentation byproducts. These bacteria are capnophiles—that is, they require additional carbon dioxide (5%–10% CO_2) for growth, and most species will not grow on MacConkey agar. *Actinobacillus actinomycetemcomitans* has been reclassified to be included in the *Aggregatibacter* genus based on 16S ribosomal ribonucleic acid (rRNA) sequencing. *Haemophilus aphrophilus* and *Haemophilus paraphrophilus* have been reclassified as a single species, *Aggregatibacter aphrophilus,* based on multilocus sequence analysis. *A. aphrophilus* now includes both the hemin-dependent and hemin-independent isolates. *Haemophilus segnis* has been reclassified as *Aggregatibacter segnis*. *A. segnis* requires V factor but does not require X factor.

Epidemiology, Pathogenesis, and Spectrum of Disease and Antimicrobial Therapy

The organisms listed in Table 30.1 are part of the normal microbiota of the nasopharynx or oral cavity of humans and other animals and are parasitic. Species associated with animals are indicated in the table at the beginning of the chapter. As such, the organisms generally are of low virulence and, except for those species associated with periodontal infections, usually cause infections in humans after introduction into sterile sites from trauma such as bites, droplet transmission from human to human, sharing paraphernalia, or manipulations in the oral cavity. Endogenous infections associated with normal microbiota are occasionally caused by *Aggregatibacter, Cardiobacterium,* and *Kingella* spp. *Cardiobacterium* spp. are not only associated with the human oropharynx and oral cavity, but they may also be identified in the gastrointestinal and urogenital tract. *Kingella* has also been isolated from the throat of children younger than 4 years of age. The natural habitat for *Dysgonomonas* is unknown. Rare isolates have been identified in the feces of immunocompromised patients.

The types of infections caused by these bacteria vary from periodontitis to endocarditis (Table 30.2). *Actinobacillus* spp. cause granulomatous disease in animals and have been associated with soft tissue infection in humans after animal bites. In addition, *Actinobacillus equuli* and *Actinobacillus suis* have been isolated from meningitis and the human respiratory tract in addition to animal bite wounds. Additional species (*Actinobacillus ureae* and *Actinobacillus hominis*) have been isolated from patients that have developed meningitis after trauma or surgery. *Actinobacillus* spp. may harbor a pore-forming protein toxin known as an **RTX leukotoxin,** which is cytotoxic and hemolytic. *A. actinomycetemcomitans* is often associated with periodontitis and may cause osteomyelitis and arthritis. Virulence factors include the RTX leukotoxin, **cytotoxic distending toxin (CDT),** and the **EmaA adhesin.** Several of these organisms, *Aggregatibacter actinomycetemcomitans, Aggregatibacter*

TABLE 30.2 Pathogenesis and Spectrum of Diseases

Organism	Virulence Factors	Spectrum of Diseases and Infections
Aggregatibacter spp.	Unknown; probably of low virulence; an opportunistic pathogen	*Aggregatibacter actinomycetemcomitans* has been associated with destructive periodontitis that may cause bone loss or endocarditis; endocarditis, often after dental manipulations; soft tissue and human bite infections, often mixed with anaerobic bacteria and *Actinomyces* spp.; *Aggregatibacter aphrophilus* is an uncommon cause of endocarditis and is the H member of the HACEK (AACEK) group of bacteria associated with slowly progressive (subacute) bacterial endocarditis
Actinobacillus spp.	Unknown for human disease; probably of low virulence	Rarely cause infection in humans but may be found in animal bite wounds, such as meningitis or bacteremia; association with other infections, such as meningitis or bacteremia, is extremely rare and involves compromised patients
Kingella spp.	Unknown; probably of low virulence; opportunistic pathogens	Endocarditis and infections in various other sites, especially in immunocompromised patients; *Kingella kingae* is associated with blood, bone, and joint infections of young children; periodontitis and wound infections
Cardiobacterium hominis	Unknown; probably of low virulence	Infections in humans are rare; most commonly associated with endocarditis, especially in persons with anatomic heart defects
Capnocytophaga gingivalis, Capnocytophaga ochracea, and *Capnocytophaga sputigena*	Unknown; produce a wide variety of enzymes that may mediate tissue destruction	Most commonly associated with periodontitis and other types of periodontal disease; less commonly associated with bacteremia in immunocompromised patients
Capnocytophaga canimorsus and *Capnocytophaga cynodegmi*	Unknown	Range from mild, local infection at the bite site to bacteremia culminating in shock and disseminated intravascular coagulation; most severe in splenectomized or otherwise debilitated (e.g., alcoholism) patients but can occur in healthy people; miscellaneous other infections such as pneumonia, endocarditis, and meningitis may also occur
Dysgonomonas capnocytophagoides and other species	Unknown; probably of low virulence	Role in disease is uncertain; may be associated with diarrheal disease in immunocompromised patients; rarely isolated from other clinical specimens, such as urine, blood, and wounds

aphrophilus, Aggregatibacter segnis, Cardiobacterium hominis, and *Kingella* spp., are the A, C, and K, respectively, of the HACEK group of organisms that cause slowly progressive (i.e., subacute) bacterial endocarditis, soft tissue infections, and other infections. *Capnocytophaga* are associated with septicemia and endogenous infections in immunocompetent and immunocompromised, often neutropenic patients. Infections with *C. canimorsus* and *C. cynodegmi* after a dog or cat bite can result in serious illness, including disseminated intravascular coagulation, renal failure, shock, and hemolytic-uremic syndrome. *Cardiobacterium* spp. are mainly isolated in cases of endocarditis associated with periodontal disease. *Kingella* spp. also can be involved in other serious infections involving children, typically those younger than 4 years, especially osteoarthritic infections. Systemic infections with *Kingella* spp., such as endocarditis, have been identified in immunocompromised adults. The pathogenic mechanisms are unknown, and disease associated with *Dysgonomonas* spp. is quite variable and includes diarrhea, bacteremia, blood, and wound infections.

Infections are commonly treated using beta-lactam antibiotics, occasionally in combination with an aminoglycoside (Table 30.3). Beta-lactamase production has been described in *Kingella* spp., but the impact of this resistance mechanism on the clinical efficacy of beta-lactams is uncertain. When *in vitro* susceptibility testing is required, Clinical and Laboratory Standards Institute (CLSI) document M45 provides guidelines for testing.

Laboratory Diagnosis

Specimen Collection and Transport

No special considerations are required for specimen collection and transport of the organisms discussed in this chapter. Refer to Table 5.1 for general information on specimen collection and transport. Transport media are recommended due to the slow growth and decreased viability of the genera included in this chapter.

TABLE 30.3	Antimicrobial Therapy and Susceptibility Testing		
Organism	Therapeutic Options	Potential Resistance to Therapeutic Options	Validated Testing Methods[a]
Aggregatibacter spp.	No definitive guidelines; for periodontitis, debridement of affected area; potential agents include ceftriaxone, ampicillin, amoxicillin-clavulanic acid, fluoroquinolone, or trimethoprim-sulfamethoxazole; for endocarditis, penicillin, ampicillin, or a cephalosporin (perhaps with an aminoglycoside) may be used	Some species appear resistant to penicillin and ampicillin, but clinical relevance of resistance is unclear	See CLSI document M45
Actinobacillus spp.	No guidelines (susceptible to extended-spectrum cephalosporins and fluoroquinolones)	Unknown (same as *Aggregatibacter*)	Not available
Kingella denitrificans, Kingella kingae	A beta-lactam with or without an aminoglycoside; other active agents include erythromycin, trimethoprim-sulfamethoxazole, and ciprofloxacin	Some strains produce beta-lactamase that mediates resistance to penicillin, ampicillin, ticarcillin, and cefazolin but have been reported susceptible to beta-lactam inhibitors	See CLSI document M45
Cardiobacterium hominis	For endocarditis, penicillin with or without an aminoglycoside; usually susceptible to other beta-lactams, chloramphenicol, and tetracycline	Beta-lactamase production is rare and may be neutralized with clavulanic acid	See CLSI document M45
Capnocytophaga gingivalis, Capnocytophaga ochracea, Capnocytophaga sputigena	No definitive guidelines; generally susceptible to clindamycin, erythromycin, tetracyclines, chloramphenicol, imipenem, and other beta-lactams; Multidrug-resistant strains have been identified	Beta-lactamase–mediated resistance to penicillin	Not available
Capnocytophaga canimorsus, Capnocytophaga cynodegmi	Penicillin is the drug of choice; also susceptible to penicillin derivatives, imipenem, and third-generation cephalosporins; Multidrug-resistant strains have been identified	Unknown	Not available
Dysgonomonas capnocytophagoides	Effective agents include tetracycline, macrolides, co-trimoxazole, and clindamycin	Variable resistance to beta-lactams and imipenem. Resistance has been identified to cephalosporins, aminoglycosides, and fluoroquinolones	Not available

[a]Validated testing methods include those standard methods recommended by the Clinical and Laboratory Standards Institute (CLSI) and those commercial methods approved by the US Food and Drug Administration (FDA).

Specimen Processing

No special considerations are required for processing of the organisms discussed in this chapter. Refer to Table 5.1 for general information on specimen processing.

Direct Detection Methods

Other than Gram stain of patient specimens, there are no specific procedures for the direct detection of these organisms in clinical material. *Actinobacillus* spp. are short to very short gram-negative bacilli. They occur singly, in pairs, and rarely in short chains and they tend to exhibit bipolar staining. This staining morphology gives the overall appearance of the dots and dashes of Morse code. *Aggregatibacter* spp. are very short bacilli but occasionally are seen as filamentous forms.

Kingella spp. stain as short, plump coccobacilli with squared-off ends that appear in pairs or clusters and may form short chains. The organisms may decolorize unevenly during the Gram stain and appear gram variable. *C. hominis* is a pleomorphic gram-negative rod with one rounded end and one tapered end, giving the cells a teardrop appearance. *C. hominis* tends to form pairs, short chains, clusters, or rosettes, when Gram stains are prepared from 5% sheep blood agar.

Capnocytophaga spp. are gram-negative, fusiform-shaped bacilli with one rounded end, one tapered end, and occasional filamentous forms; *C. cynodegmi* and *C. canimorsus* may be curved. *Dysgonomonas* spp. stain as short gram-negative rods or coccobacilli.

Nucleic Acid Detection

Amplification methods (such as polymerase chain reaction [PCR]) have been developed for the identification of some of the organisms discussed in this chapter. However, these tests are not routinely available in most clinical laboratories and are predominantly used in reference or research laboratories.

Serodiagnosis

Serodiagnostic techniques are not generally used for the laboratory diagnosis of infections caused by the organisms discussed in this chapter.

Cultivation
Media of Choice

All genera described in this chapter grow on 5% sheep blood and chocolate agars. Most are facultative anaerobes and will not grow on MacConkey agar. The use of selective media may enhance the recovery and identification of the organisms included in this chapter by suppressing normal microbiota. *Dysgonomonas capnocytophagoides* can be recovered from stool on CVA (cefoperazone-vancomycin-amphotericin B) agar. For recovery of *D. capnocytophagoides*, a *Campylobacter*-selective agar is incubated at 35°C instead of 42°C.

These genera grow in the broths of commercial blood culture systems and in common nutrient broths such as thioglycollate and brain–heart infusion. Growth of *Aggregatibacter* in broth media is often barely visible, with no turbidity produced. Microcolonies may be seen as tiny puffballs growing on the blood cell layer in blood culture bottles or as a film or tiny granules on the sides of a tube.

Incubation Conditions and Duration

The growth of all genera discussed in this chapter occurs best at 35°C and in the presence of increased CO_2. Sheep blood agar (5%) and chocolate agars should be incubated in a CO_2 incubator or candle jar. In addition, *Actinobacillus, Aggregatibacter,* and *Cardiobacterium* grow best in conditions of elevated moisture. *Capnocytophaga* requires CO_2 and enriched media. The organism is inhibited by sodium polyanethole sulfonate (SPS). Selective media containing bacitracin, polymyxin B, vancomycin, and trimethoprim, or Thayer-Martin and Martin Lewis agars have been used to isolate species of *Capnocytophaga*. Recovery of *Kingella kingae* from mixed cultures can be improved using media supplemented

with clindamycin or vancomycin. Thayer-Martin agar can be used to selectively isolate *Kingella* sp. Selective media containing cefoperazone, vancomycin, and amphotericin B can be used to isolate *Dysgonomonas* spp. from stool specimens.

Even when optimum growth conditions are met, the organisms discussed here are all slow growing; inoculated plates should be held 2–7 days for colonies to achieve maximal growth.

Colonial Appearance

Table 30.4 describes the colonial appearance and other distinguishing characteristics (e.g., hemolysis and pigment) of each genus on 5% sheep blood agar. Most species generally will not grow on MacConkey agar; exceptions are noted in Table 30.4.

Approach to Identification

Table 30.5 outlines some conventional biochemical tests that are useful for differentiating among *Actinobacillus, Aggregatibacter, Cardiobacterium,* and *Kingella,* four of the five HACEK bacteria that cause subacute bacterial endocarditis. *Haemophilus* spp. are included in Chapter 31. *A. aphrophilus* does not require either X or V factors for growth. However, it is catalase negative and ferments lactose or sucrose. *A. actinomycetemcomitans* yields the opposite reactions in these tests.

Table 30.6 shows key conventional biochemicals used to differentiate *Capnocytophaga* spp., *Dysgonomonas capnocytophagoides,* and aerotolerant *Leptotrichia buccalis*.

Comments Regarding Specific Organisms

Actinobacillus spp. are facultative anaerobic, nonmotile, gram-negative rods. The genus *Actinobacillus* is similar to *Aggregatibacter* and *Pasteurella* (Chapter 29), which must also be considered when a fastidious gram-negative rod requiring rabbit serum is isolated. *A. actinomycetemcomitans,* the most frequently isolated of the *Aggregatibacter* spp., can be distinguished from *A. aphrophilus* by a positive catalase test and negative lactose fermentation.

A. actinomycetemcomitans differs from *C. hominis* in being indole-negative and catalase positive; catalase is also an important test for differentiating *Kingella* spp., which are catalase negative, from *A. actinomycetemcomitans. C. hominis* is indole positive after extraction with xylene and the addition of Ehrlich's reagent; this is a key feature in differentiating it from *A. aphrophilus* and *A. actinomycetemcomitans. C. hominis* is similar to *Suttonella indologenes* (Chapter 29) but can be distinguished by its ability to ferment mannitol and sorbitol.

Kingella spp. are catalase negative, which helps to separate them from *Neisseria* spp. (Chapter 39), with which they are sometimes confused. *Kingella denitrificans* may be mistaken for *Neisseria gonorrhoeae* when isolated from modified Thayer-Martin agar. Nitrate reduction is a key test in differentiating *K. denitrificans* from *N. gonorrhoeae*, which is nitrate negative.

TABLE 30.4 Colonial Appearance and Characteristics on 5% Sheep Blood Agar

Organism	Appearance
Aggregatibacter actinomycetemcomitans	Pinpoint colonies after 24 h; rough, sticky, adherent colonies surrounded by a slight greenish tinge after 48 h; characteristic finding is presence of a 4- to 6-pointed-star–like configuration in the center of a mature colony growing on a clear medium (e.g., brain-heart infusion agar) resembling crossed cigars, which can be visualized by examining the colony under low power (10×) with a standard light microscope. Colonies may also pit the agar
Aggregatibacter aphrophilus	Round; convex with opaque zone near center on chocolate agar
Aggregatibacter segnis	Convex, grayish white, smooth or granular at 48 h on chocolate agar
Actinobacillus equuli[a]	Small colonies at 24 h that are sticky, adherent, smooth or rough, and nonhemolytic
Actinobacillus lignieresii[a]	Resembles *A. equuli*
Actinobacillus suis[a]	Beta-hemolytic but otherwise resembles *A. equuli* and *A. lignieresii*
Actinobacillus ureae	Resembles the pasteurellae (Chapter 31)
Cardiobacterium hominis	After 48 h, colonies are small, slightly alpha-hemolytic, smooth, round, glistening, and opaque; pitting may be produced
Capnocytophaga spp.	After 48–74 h, colonies are small- to medium-size, opaque, shiny, and nonhemolytic; pale beige or yellowish color may not be apparent unless growth is scraped from the surface with a cotton swab; gliding motility may be observed as outgrowths from the colonies or as a haze on the surface of the agar, similar to the swarming of *Proteus*
Dysgonomonas spp.	Pinpoint colonies after 24 h; small, wet, gray-white colonies at 48–72 h; usually nonhemolytic, although some strains may produce a small zone of beta-hemolysis; characteristic odor alternatively described as fruity strawberry-like odor or bitter
Kingella denitrificans	Small, nonhemolytic; frequently pits agar; can grow on *Neisseria gonorrhoeae* selective agar (e.g., Thayer-Martin agar)
Kingella kingae	Small, with a small zone of beta-hemolysis; may appear smooth with a central papilla or spread and pit agar

[a]May grow on MacConkey agar as tiny lactose fermenters.

TABLE 30.5 Biochemical and Physiologic Characteristics of *Actinobacillus* spp. and Related Organisms

Organism	Oxidase	Catalase	Nitrate Reduction	Indole	Urea	Esculin Hydrolysis	Fermentation of:[a] Xylose	Lactose	Trehalose
Aggregatibacter actinomycetemcomitans	V	+	+	–	–	–	V	–	–
Aggregatibacter aphrophilus	V	–	+	–	–	–	–	(+)	(+)
Aggregatibacter segnis	–	V	+	–	–	–	–	–	–
Actinobacillus equuli	+	V	+	–	(+)[b]	–	+	+	(+)
Actinobacillus hominis	+	+	+	–	+	V	+	+	+
Actinobacillus lignieresii	+	V	+	–	(+)[b]	–	+ or (+)	V	–
Actinobacillus suis	+	V	+	–	(+)[b]	+	+	+ or (+)	+

TABLE 30.5 **Biochemical and Physiologic Characteristics of *Actinobacillus* spp. and Related Organisms—Cont'd**

Organism	Oxidase	Catalase	Nitrate Reduction	Indole	Urea	Esculin Hydrolysis	Fermentation of:[a] Xylose	Lactose	Trehalose
Actinobacillus ureae	+	V	+	−	(+)[b]	−	−	−	−
Cardiobacterium hominis	+	−	−	+[c]	−	−	−	−	ND
Cardiobacterium valvarnum	+	−	−	V	−	−	−	−	ND
Kingella denitrificans	+	−	(+)[d]	−	−	−	−	−	ND
Kingella kingae[e]	+	−	−	−	−	−	−	−	ND
Kingella oralis[f]	+	−	−	−	−	−	−	−	ND
Kingella potus	+	−	−	−	−	−	−	−	ND

[a]May require the addition of 1–2 drops of rabbit serum per 3 mL of fermentation broth to stimulate growth.
[b]May require a drop of rabbit serum on the slant or a heavy inoculum.
[c]Weak reaction.
[d]Nitrate is usually reduced to gas.
[e]*K. kingea* maltose positive and can be differentiated from other *Kingella* spp., which are maltose negative.
[f]Alkaline phosphatase positive, which will differentiate the organism from *K. potus.*
ND, No data; *V,* variable; +, >90% of strains positive; (+), >90% of strains positive but reaction may be delayed (i.e., 2–7 days); −, >90% of strains negative.
Data compiled from Weyant RS, Moss CW, Weaver RE, et al, eds. *Identification of Unusual Pathogenic Gram-Negative Aerobic and Facultatively Anaerobic Bacteria.* 2nd ed. Baltimore: Williams & Wilkins; 1996; Caroll KC, Pfaller MA. *Manual of Clinical Microbiology.* 12th ed. Washington, DC: ASM Press; 2019.

TABLE 30.6 **Biochemical and Physiologic Characteristics of *Capnocytophaga* spp., *Dysgonomonas* spp., and Similar Organisms**

Organism	Oxidase	Catalase	Esculin Hydrolysis	Indole	Nitrate Reduction	Xylose Fermentation	Lactose Fermentation
C. granulosa	−	−	−	−	ND	−	+
C. gingivalis	−	−	−	−	−	−	V
C. canimorsus	(+)	(+)	V	−	−	−[b]	+
C. cynodegmi	(+)	(+)	+ or (+)	−	−	−	+
C. haemolytica	−	−	+	−	+	−	+
C. ochracea	−	−	V	−	V	−	+
C. sputigena	−	−	+	−	V	−	V
Leptotrichia buccalis[a]	−	−	V	−	−	−[c]	ND
Dysgonomonas capnocytophagoides/ D. gadei[a]	−	−	(+)	−	−	+ or (+)[c]	ND
D. hofstadii	−	−	−	+	ND	ND	ND
D. mossii	−	−	−	+	+	+	ND

[a]Lactic acid is the major fermentation product of glucose fermentation for *Leptotrichia buccalis,* and succinic acid and propionic is the major fermentation product of glucose fermentation for *Capnocytophaga* spp. and *Dysgonomonas capnocytophagoides.*
[b]*C. canimorsus* does not ferment the sugars inulin, sucrose, or raffinose; *C. cynodegmi* will usually ferment one or all of these sugars.
[c]May require the addition of 1–2 drops of rabbit serum per 3 mL of fermentation broth to stimulate growth.
ND, No data; *V,* variable; +, >90% of strains positive; (+), >90% of strains positive, but reaction may be delayed (i.e., 2–7 days); −, >90% of strains negative.
Data compiled from Jensen KT, Schonheyder H, Thomsen VF. In-vitro activity of β-lactam and other antimicrobial agents against *Kingella kingae. J Antimicrob Chemother* 1994;33:635; Weyant RS, Moss CW, Weaver RE, et al, eds. *Identification of Unusual Pathogenic Gram-Negative Aerobic and Facultatively Anaerobic Bacteria.* 2nd ed. Baltimore: Williams & Wilkins; 1996; Caroll KC, Pfaller MA. *Manual of Clinical Microbiology.* 12th ed. Washington, DC: ASM Press; 2019.

Capnocytophaga ochracea, Capnocytophaga sputigena, and *Capnocytophaga gingivalis* are catalase and oxidase negative. *Capnocytophaga canimorsus* and *Capnocytophaga cynodegmi* are catalase and oxidase positive; these species are also difficult to differentiate from each other. However, for most clinical purposes, a presumptive identification to genus, that is, *Capnocytophaga,* is sufficiently informative and precludes the need to identify an isolate to the species level. Presumptive identification of an organism, such as *Capnocytophaga* spp., can be made when a yellow-pigmented, thin, gram-negative rod with tapered ends that exhibits gliding motility (Table 30.4) and does not grow in ambient air, is isolated.

Dysgonomonas capnocytophagoides, although similar to the other organisms in this chapter, are oxidase negative. They are nonmotile, unlike the *Capnocytophaga,* which exhibit gliding motility. *D. capnocytophagoides* produces succinic and propionic acid, whereas *Capnocytophaga* produces only succinic acid. Cellular fatty acid analysis can provide information necessary to distinguish *Capnocytophaga, D. capnocytophagoides,* and the aerotolerant strains of *Leptotrichia buccalis.*

Matrix-assisted laser desorption ionization time-of-flight mass spectrometry (MALDI-TOF MS) have been used for the successful identification of the genera included in this chapter. Specific manufacturer's guidelines and databases should be consulted for identification.

Prevention

Because the organisms discussed in this chapter do not generally pose a threat to human health, there are no recommended vaccination or prophylaxis protocols.

ⓔ Visit the Evolve site for a complete list of procedures, review questions, and case studies.

Bibliography

Carbonnelle E, Grohs P, Jacquier H, et al.: Robustness of two MALDI-TOF mass spectrometry systems for bacterial identification, *J Microbiol Methods* 89:133–136, 2012.

Caroll KC, Pfaller MA: *Manual of clinical microbiology,* ed 12, Washington, DC, 2019, ASM Press.

Dingle TC, Butler-Wu SM: MALDI-TOF mass spectrometry for microorganism identification, *Clin Lab Med* 33:589–609, 2013.

Hassan IJ, Hayek L: Endocarditis caused by *Kingella denitrificans, J Infect* 27:291–295, 1993.

Hofstad T, Olsen I, Eribe ER: Dysgonomonas gen. nov. to accommodate *Dysgonomonas gadei* sp. nov., an organism isolated from a human gall bladder, and *Dysgonomonas capnocytophagoides* (formerly CDC group DF-3), *Int J Syst Evol Microbiol* 50:2189–2195, 2000.

Jensen KT, Schønheyder H, Thomsen VF: In-vitro activity of β-lactam and other antimicrobial agents against *Kingella kingae, J Antimicrob Chemother* 33:635–640, 1994.

Keys CJ, Dare DJ, Sutton H, et al.: Compilation of a MALDI-TOF mass spectral database for the rapid screening and characterisation of bacteria implicated in human infectious diseases, *Infect Genet Evol* 4:221–242, 2004.

Norskov-Lauritsen N, Kilian M: Reclassification of *Actinobacillus actinomycetemcomitans, Haemophilus aphrophilus, Haemophilus paraphrophilus* and *Haemophilus segnis* as *Aggregatibacter actinomycetemcomitans* gen. nov., comb. nov., *Aggregatibacter aphrophilus* comb. nov. and *Aggregatibacter segnis* comb. nov., and emended description of *Aggregatibacter aphrophilus* to include V factor-dependent and V factor-independent isolates, *Int J Syst Evol Microbiol* 56:2135–2146, 2006.

Pers C, Gahrn-Hansen B, Frederiksen W: *Capnocytophaga canimorsus* septicemia in Denmark, 1982-1995: review of 39 cases, *Clin Infect Dis* 23:71–75, 1996.

Sordillo EM, Rendel M, Sood R, Belinfanti J, Murray O, Brook D: Septicemia due to β-lactamase–*Kingella kingae, Clin Infect Dis* 17:818–819, 1993.

Weyant RS, Moss CW, Weaver RE, et al.: *Identification of unusual pathogenic gram-negative aerobic and facultatively anaerobic bacteria,* ed 2, Baltimore, 1996, Williams & Wilkins.

Yagupsky P, Dagan R: *Kingella kingae* bacteremia in children, *Pediatr Infect Dis J* 13:1148–1149, 1994.

31

Haemophilus

OBJECTIVES

1. List the general characteristics within the genus *Haemophilus,* including general habitat, atmosphere, and temperature requirements.
2. Describe the infections caused by *Haemophilus influenzae* and *Haemophilus ducreyi.*
3. Describe the difference in the typeable and nontypeable categories of *Haemophilus,* their virulence factors, and the disease they cause.
4. Describe the Gram stain and colonial morphology of the various *Haemophilus* spp.
5. Describe the isolation requirements necessary for optimal recovery of *Haemophilus,* including any special specimen processing or transport requirements.
6. Explain the satellite phenomenon and the chemical basis for the phenomenon.
7. List the X and V factor requirements for *H. influenzae, Haemophilus parainfluenzae,* and *H. ducreyi.*
8. Explain the principle of the porphyrin test.
9. Explain what routine susceptibility testing of clinical isolates for *H. influenzae* is necessary on strains of clinical significance (i.e., sterile sites).
10. Correlate patient signs, symptoms, and laboratory data to identify the most probable etiologic agent associated with an infection.

ORGANISMS TO BE CONSIDERED

Current Name

Haemophilus aegyptius
Haemophilus ducreyi
Haemophilus haemolyticus
Haemophilus influenzae
Haemophilus parainfluenzae
Haemophilus parahaemolyticus
Haemophilus paraphrohaemolyticus
Haemophilus pittmaniae
Haemophilus sputorum

General Characteristics

The genus *Haemophilus* contains significant genetic diversity. Members of the genus are small, nonmotile, pleomorphic gram-negative bacilli. The cells are typically coccobacillary or short rods. Species of the genus *Haemophilus* are fastidious organisms that require protoporphyrin IX (a metabolic intermediate of the hemin biosynthetic pathway), referred to as **X factor** and **V factor**, nicotine adenine dinucleotide (NAD), or nicotine adenine dinucleotide phosphate (NADP) for *in vitro* growth. These requirements vary by species. *Haemophilus* spp. are facultative anaerobes with optimal growth at 35°C to 37°C in a 5% to 7% CO_2-enriched atmosphere.

Epidemiology

As presented in Table 31.1, except for *Haemophilus ducreyi, Haemophilus* spp. normally inhabit the upper respiratory tract of humans. Asymptomatic colonization of the upper respiratory tract with *Haemophilus influenzae, Haemophilus parainfluenzae,* and Haemophilus *pittmaniae* is common. Colonization with *H. influenzae* type b, *H. parahaemolyticus,* and *H. haemolyticus* is rare. Although *H. ducreyi* is only found in humans, the organism is not part of our normal microbiota, and its presence in clinical specimens generally indicates infection. *H. ducreyi* colonization of the cervix has been noted following sexual intercourse.

Among *H. influenzae* strains, there are two broad categories: typeable and nontypeable *H. influenzae* (NTHi). Strains are typed based on capsular characteristics. The capsule is composed of a sugar-alcohol phosphate (i.e., polyribitol phosphate) complex. Differences in this complex are the basis for separating encapsulated strains into one of six groups: type a, b, c, d, e, or f. *H. influenzae* type b (Hib) was previously the most common type encountered in serious infections in humans. Nontypeable strains do not produce a capsule and are commonly encountered as normal inhabitants of the upper respiratory tract

Although person-to-person transmission plays a key role in infections caused by *H. influenzae* and *H. ducreyi,* infections caused by other *Haemophilus* strains and species likely arise endogenously as a person's own microbiota gains access to a normally sterile site (i.e., the colonizing organism invades the mucosa and enters the patient's bloodstream). As a result of widespread vaccination with the *H. influenzae* type b (Hib) vaccine, the distribution of capsular serotypes associated with invasive infections has shifted from predominantly type b, to 69.5% of nontypeable, 2.2% as type a, 3.6% as type b, 0.3% as type c, 0.3% as type d, 5.7% as type e, and 18.3% as type f. Encapsulated strains are protected from clearance from host phagocytes. Once in the circulation, the organism is able to spread to additional sites and tissues, including the lungs, pericardium, pleura, and meninges.

TABLE 31.1 *Haemophilus spp.* **Epidemiology, Pathogenesis, and Spectrum of Disease**

Organism	Habitat (Reservoir)	Mode of Transmission	Virulence Factors	Spectrum of Disease
H. aegyptius	Normal microbiota: upper respiratory tract	Endogenous strains	Uncertain	Purulent conjunctivitis, pinkeye
H. ducreyi	Not part of normal human microbiota; only found in humans during infection	Person-to-person: sexual contact	Uncertain, but capsular factors, pili, and certain toxins are probably involved in attachment and penetration of host epithelial cells	Chancroid; genital lesions progress from tender papules (i.e., small bumps) to painful ulcers with several satellite lesions; regional lymphadenitis is common
H. influenzae	Normal microbiota: upper respiratory tract	Person-to-person: respiratory droplets Endogenous strains	Capsule: Antiphagocytic types a–f Additional cell envelope factors mediate attachment to host cells Unencapsulated Nontypeable strains (NTHi): pili and other cell surface factors mediate attachment	Meningitis Epiglottitis Cellulitis with bacteremia Septic arthritis Pneumonia Localized infections Otitis media Sinusitis Conjunctivitis Immunocompromised patients: Chronic bronchitis Pneumonia Bacteremia
Haemophilus influenzae biotype *aegyptius*			Uncertain; probably similar to those of other *H. influenzae*	Purulent conjunctivitis single strain identified as the Brazilian purpuric fever, high mortality in children between ages 1 and 4; infection includes purulent meningitis, bacteremia, high fever, vomiting, purpura (i.e., rash), and vascular collapse
H. parainfluenzae	Normal microbiota: upper respiratory tract	Endogenous strains	Uncertain	Acute otitis media, sinusitis, bacteremia, and culture negative endocarditis
Other species: *H. haemolyticus* *H. parahaemolyticus* *H. paraphrohaemolyticus* *H. pittmaniae* *H. sputorum*	Normal microbiota: upper respiratory tract	Endogenous strains	Uncertain	May be implicated in lower respiratory tract infection, sinusitis, conjunctivitis, bacteremia, meningitis, wound infections, peritonitis, arthritis, or osteomyelitis

Pathogenesis and Spectrum of Disease

Production of a capsule and factors that mediate bacterial attachment to human epithelial cells are the primary virulence factors associated with *Haemophilus* spp. In general, infections caused by *H. influenzae* are often systemic and may be life-threatening (Table 31.1). Life-threatening illness associated with *Haemophilus* has become uncommon in the United States due widespread use of the Hib vaccine. Most serious infections caused by *H. influenzae* type b are biotypes I and II.

Many *H. influenzae* infections are caused by nontypeable strains (NTHi). Transmission is often via respiratory secretions. The organism is able to gain access to sterile sites from colonization in the upper respiratory tract. Clinical infections include otitis media (ear infection), sinusitis, bronchitis, pneumonia, and conjunctivitis. Immunodeficiencies and chronic respiratory problems such as chronic obstructive pulmonary disease may predispose an individual to infection with NTHi.

Chancroid is the sexually transmitted disease caused by *H. ducreyi* (Table 31.1). The initial symptom is the development of a painful genital ulcer and inguinal lymphadenopathy. Although small outbreaks of this disease have occurred in the United States, this disease is more common among socioeconomically disadvantaged populations inhabiting tropical environments. Epidemics of disease are associated with poor hygiene, prostitution, drug abuse, and poor socioeconomic conditions.

Other *Haemophilus* spp. have been associated with similar diseases as *H. influenzae* and are described in Table 31.1. *H. aegyptius* is an important cause of purulent conjunctivitis, commonly referred to as pinkeye. *H. haemolyticus* has been reported in cases of bacteremia, septic arthritis, and peritonitis.

Laboratory Diagnosis

Specimen Collection and Transport

Haemophilus spp. can be isolated from most clinical specimens. The collection and transport of these specimens are outlined in Table 5.1, with emphasis on the following points. First, *Haemophilus* spp. are susceptible to drying and temperature extremes. Specimens suspected of containing these organisms should be inoculated to the appropriate media immediately. Specimens susceptible to contamination with normal microbiota, such as a lower respiratory specimen, should be collected by bronchioalveolar lavage or bronchial washing. In cases of pneumonia or cerebrospinal fluid (CSF) infection or suspected infection of any other normally sterile body fluid, blood cultures also should be collected.

Second, the recovery of *H. ducreyi* from genital ulcers requires special processing. The ulcer should be cleaned with sterile gauze moistened with sterile saline. A cotton swab moistened with phosphate-buffered saline or broth is used to collect material from the base of the ulcer. To maximize the chance for recovering the organism, the swab is plated to special selective media within 10 minutes of collection. If there is a delay in processing, the swab may be placed in transport media such as Amies transport media or other transport media containing thioglycolate-hemin-based media containing albumin and glutamine. Specimens refrigerated at 4°C in Amies transport media have demonstrated the viability of *H. ducreyi* for up to 3 days. Additional specimens including lymph node aspirates, pus, and bubo aspirates have demonstrated a limited recovery of *H. ducreyi*.

Specimen Processing

Other than the precautions required for the collection of *H. ducreyi*, no special considerations are required for specimen processing. Collection of samples from genital specimens for direct nucleic acid detection of *H. ducreyi* should be processed according to the manufacturer's specifications. Refer to Table 5.1 for general information on specimen processing.

Direct Detection Methods
Direct Observation

Gram stain is generally used for the direct detection of *Haemophilus* in clinical material (Fig. 31.1). However, in some instances the acridine orange stain (see Chapter 6 for more information on this technique) is used to detect smaller numbers of organisms that may be undetectable by Gram staining.

To increase the sensitivity of direct Gram stain examination of body fluid specimens, especially CSF, specimens may be centrifuged (2000 rpm for 10 minutes), and the smear is prepared from the pellet deposited in the bottom of the tube. Most laboratories are now equipped with a cytocentrifuge (10,000 × *g* for 10 minutes) used for concentration of specimens. This is highly recommended over traditional centrifugation for nonturbid specimens. This concentration step can increase the sensitivity of direct microscopic examination from fivefold to tenfold. Cytocentrifugation of the specimen, in which clinical material is concentrated by

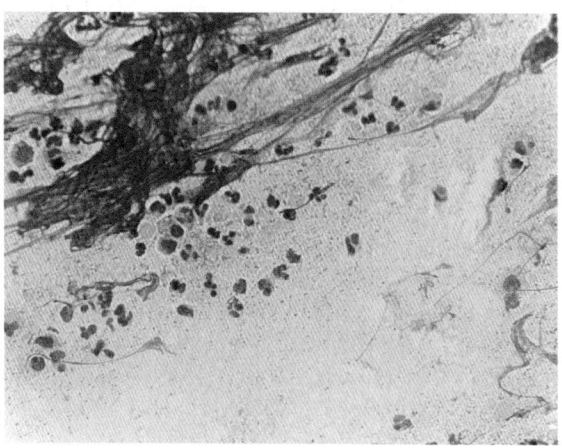

• **Fig. 31.1** Gram stain of *Haemophilus influenzae*.

centrifugation directly onto microscope slides, reportedly increases sensitivity of the Gram stain by as much as 100-fold (see Chapter 70 for information on infections of the central nervous system).

Gram stains of the smears from clinical specimens must be examined carefully to avoid confusion with the microscopic morphologies of *Brucella* spp., *Francisella* spp., or *Neisseria* spp. *Haemophilus* spp. stain a pale pink and may be difficult to detect in the pink background of proteinaceous material often found in clinical specimens. Under-decolorization may result in misidentification of *H. influenzae* as either *Streptococcus* spp. or *Listeria monocytogenes*.

Haemophilus species may appear as gram-negative coccobacilli with coccoid, coccobacillary, rod-shaped, or filamentous forms. *H. influenzae* appears as pleomorphic coccobacilli or small rods. *Haemophilus haemolyticus* are small coccobacilli or short rods with occasional cells appearing as tangled filaments.

H. parainfluenzae produce either small pleomorphic rods or long filamentous forms, whereas *Haemophilus parahaemolyticus* usually are short to medium-length bacilli. *A. aphrophilus* is short bacilli but occasionally is seen as filamentous forms. *Aggregatibacter segnis* (Chapter 30) may be difficult to distinguish from *H. parainfluenzae* biotype V unless molecular techniques are used. *H. ducreyi* may be either slender or coccobacillary. Traditionally, *H. ducreyi* cells are described as "railroad tracks" or "schools of fish." However, this morphology is rarely seen in clinical specimens.

Table 31.2 presents *H. influenzae* and *H. parainfluenzae* biotypes.

Antigen Detection

H. influenzae type b capsular polysaccharide in clinical specimens, such as CSF and urine, can be detected directly using commercially available particle agglutination assays (Chapter 9). Organisms in clinical infections are usually present at a sufficiently high concentration to be visualized by Gram stain. Latex tests lack sensitivity and specificity for detection of *H. influenzae* type b. False positives have been reported in CSF and urine of patients who have been recently immunized with the Hib vaccine. Most clinical laboratories no longer perform the latex test for the identification of *Haemophilus* spp.

Nucleic Acid Detection

Rapid screening procedures are very useful for patient therapy and evaluating outbreaks and have been developed for detection from CSF, plasma, serum, and whole blood. A polymerase chain reaction (PCR) for *H. influenzae* capsular types a and f has been developed. The PCR product is amplified for the specific capsular type for which the primer is designed. *H. influenzae* is also included in a variety of commercially available multiplex respiratory or meningitis/encephalitis panels. Detection from some clinical samples has been problematic based on the presence of small numbers of organisms in the sample, increasing the need for large samples and concentration procedures; however, specificity is high.

Diagnosis of chancroid and the identification of *H. ducreyi* have been successfully completed using a variety

TABLE 31.2	Differentiation of *Haemophilus influenzae* and *Haemophilus parainfluenzae* Biotypes		
Organism and Biotype	Indole	Ornithine Decarboxylase	Urease
H. influenzae			
I	pos	pos	pos
II	pos	neg	pos
III	neg	neg	pos
IV	neg	pos	pos
V	pos	pos	neg
VI	neg	pos	neg
VII	pos	neg	neg
VIII	neg	neg	neg
H. parainfluenzae			
I	neg	pos	neg
II	neg	pos	pos
III	neg	neg	pos
IV	pos	pos	pos
V	neg	neg	neg
VI	pos	pos	neg
VII	pos	neg	pos
VIII	pos	neg	neg

Modified from Carroll KC, Pfaller MA, Landry ML, et al. *Manual of Clinical Microbiology*. 12th ed. Washington, DC: ASM; 2019.

of molecular targets. Amplification of the 16S ribosomal ribonucleic acid (rRNA), the *rrs* (16S)-*rri* (23S) intergenic spacer region, or the heat shock protein gene *groEL* has been used in molecular assays. In addition, molecular detection has proven useful in the diagnosis of *H. parainfluenzae;* however, the detection of other *Haemophilus* spp. has not been successful. This has been particularly problematic in respiratory specimens in which the amplification of commensal *Haemophilus* spp. has made interpretations and positive results inconclusive for applications in diagnostic microbiology. It is not recommended that nucleic acid detection directly from clinical specimens be used as the sole determinant for the diagnosis of infection from respiratory specimens. Direct nucleic acid detection of *Haemophilus* spp. from blood cultures has significantly reduced turnaround time using the multiplex disease panels such as the FilmArray (BioFire Diagnostics, Salt Lake City, UT) or Verigene (Nanosphere, Inc., Northbrook, IL).

Cultivation
Media of Choice

Haemophilus spp. typically grow on chocolate agar as smooth, flat or convex, buff or slightly yellow colonies. Chocolate agar provides protoporphyrin IX (X factor) and NAD or NADP

(V factor), necessary for the growth of *Haemophilus* spp. X and V factor are both found in whole blood primarily inside the red blood cells or erythrocytes. Most strains will not grow on 5% sheep blood agar, which contains protoporphyrin IX but not NAD. X factor can be added to artificial bacteriologic media using crystalline hemin. In addition to X and V factors, fastidious species such as *H. ducreyi* and *H. aegyptius* require media supplemented with IsoVitale X (Becton-Dickinson) or Vitox (Thermofisher) for optimal growth. These formulas contain glucose, cysteine, glutamine, adenine, thiamine, vitamin B_{12}, guanine, iron, and aminobenzoic acid. Several bacterial species, including *Staphylococcus aureus, enterococci,* and *yeast,* lyse the red blood cells in the artificial media releasing X and V factors to supply growth requirements for *Haemophilus* spp. In addition, *S. aureus* also secretes NAD into the media as a metabolic byproduct. Tiny colonies of *Haemophilus* spp. may be seen growing on sheep blood agar very close to the colonies of bacteria that either lyse the red blood cells or are capable of producing V factor; this is known as the **satellite phenomenon** (Fig. 31.2). To examine an isolate for the satellite phenomenon, a single streak of a hemolysin-producing strain of *Staphylococcus* spp. is placed on a sheep blood agar plate that has been inoculated with a suspected *Haemophilus* spp. *Haemophilus* spp. will grow adjacent to the streak line where the nutrients are available.

Media used for the isolation of *Haemophilus* spp. include chocolate agar, enriched chocolate agar supplemented with 1% IsoVitale X or Vitox, or Levinthal medium. Levinthal medium is transparent and demonstrates iridescence of encapsulated strains of *Haemophilus*. A selective medium, such as horse blood–bacitracin agar or media containing a combination of bacitracin, vancomycin, and/or clindamycin may be used for isolation of *H. influenzae* from the respiratory secretions to avoid overgrowth by contaminating normal microbiota. The use of selective media is extremely important in patients with cystic fibrosis, patients with chronic bronchitis, conjunctivitis, or epiglottitis. Horse blood–bacitracin agar is designed to prevent overgrowth of *H. influenzae* by mucoid *Pseudomonas aeruginosa. Haemophilus* spp. are unable to grow on MacConkey agar.

H. ducreyi requires additional growth factors and special media for cultivation in the laboratory. Types of media used in the laboratory include (1) Mueller-Hinton–based chocolate agar supplemented with 1% IsoVitaleX and 3 μg/mL vancomycin; (2) GC agar base with 1% IsoVitaleX, 5% fetal bovine serum, 1% hemoglobin and 3 μg/mL vancomycin; (3) GC agar base with 5% Fildes enrichment (Becton-Dickenson), 5% horse blood, and 3 μg/mL vancomycin; or (4) 5% fresh rabbit blood agar with 3 μg/mL vancomycin. The vancomycin inhibits gram-positive colonizing organisms of the genital tract. Certain strains of *H. ducreyi* are sensitive to vancomycin; using more than one media type to optimize the recovery of *H. ducreyi* should be used to achieve optimal recovery.

Haemophilus spp. will grow in commercial blood culture broth systems, in common nutrient broths such as thioglycollate, and brain–heart infusion because the erythrocytes present in the sample lyse providing sufficient X and V factors

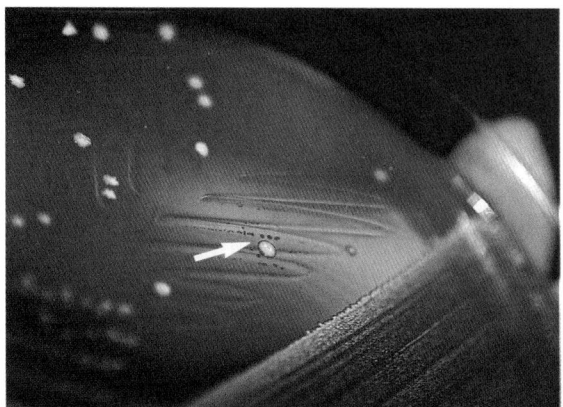

• **Fig. 31.2** *Haemophilus influenzae* satellite phenomenon *(arrow)* around colonies of *Staphylococcus aureus.*

for growth of the organisms. However, the growth is often slower, produces weakly turbid suspensions, and may not be readily visible. For this reason, blind subcultures to chocolate agar or examination of smears by AO or Gram stain have been used. Subcultures have not demonstrated a clinically significant effect on the isolation and detection of *Haemophilus* spp. from blood culture systems. Blood culture broth systems should not be used for the cultivation of other sterile body fluids such as synovial, pericardial, peritoneal, or pleural fluid due to the lack of red blood cells that provide X and V factors for growth. Blood culture bottles may be supplemented with 10 μg/mL of sterile hemin and NAD prior to inoculation with the clinical specimen to improve recovery.

Incubation Conditions and Duration

Most strains of *Haemophilus* spp. are able to grow aerobically and anaerobically (facultative anaerobes). Growth is stimulated by 5% to 7% carbon dioxide (CO_2). It is recommended that cultures be incubated in a CO_2 pouch or a CO_2 incubator. These organisms usually grow within 24 to 48 hours, but cultures are routinely held 72 hours before being discarded as negative. *H. ducreyi* and *H. aegyptius* may require as long as 5 days to grow.

Optimal growth of all *Haemophilus* spp., except *H. ducreyi*, occurs at 35°C to 37°C. Cultures for *H. ducreyi* should be incubated at 30°C to 33°C in 5% CO_2. In addition, *H. ducreyi* requires high humidity, which may be established by placing a sterile gauze pad moistened with sterile water inside the CO_2 pouch or vacuum atmospheric chamber.

Colonial Appearance

Table 31.3 describes the colonial appearance and other distinguishing characteristics (e.g., odor and hemolysis) of each species.

Approach to Identification

Commercial identification systems for *Haemophilus* spp. are available. All of the systems incorporate several rapid enzymatic tests and generally work well for identifying these organisms.

TABLE
31.3   **Colonial Appearance and Characteristics**

Organism	Medium	Appearance
Haemophilus aegyptius	CHOC	Small, flat, smooth, convex, and translucent. On semisolid media, agar content 0.4%, colonies may appear as "cometlike"
Haemophilus ducreyi	Selective medium	Small, flat, gray, smooth, and translucent to opaque at 48–72 h; may have slight beta-hemolysis on blood agar; colonies can be pushed intact across agar surface
Haemophilus haemolyticus	CHOC	Resembles *H. influenzae* except beta-hemolytic on rabbit or horse blood agar. May lose hemolytic ability on subsequent sub culturing
Haemophilus influenzae	CHOC	Unencapsulated strains are small, smooth, and translucent at 24 h; encapsulated strains form larger, more mucoid colonies; mouse nest odor; nonhemolytic on rabbit or horse blood agar. Colonies cultivated on Levinthal agar may demonstrate iridescence that may be yellow, red, green, or blue
Haemophilus influenzae biotype aegyptius	CHOC	Resembles *H. influenzae,* except colonies are smaller at 48 h
Haemophilus parahaemolyticus	CHOC	Resembles *H. parainfluenzae;* beta-hemolytic on rabbit or horse blood agar
Haemophilus parainfluenzae	CHOC	Medium to large off-white to yellow; general appearance is variable including smooth and translucent; granular with rough, serrated edges, or heaped and wrinkled; nonhemolytic on rabbit or horse blood agar; older colonies can be pushed intact across agar surface

CHOC, Chocolate agar.

Traditional identification criteria include hemolysis on horse or rabbit blood and the requirement for X and V factors for growth, carbohydrate fermentation pattern and additional biochemical tests (Table 31.4). Preliminary identification can be made for some *Haemophilus* spp. based on X and V factor requirements in conjunction with the porphyrin test. To establish X and V factor requirements, disks impregnated with each factor are placed on unsupplemented media, usually Mueller-Hinton agar or trypticase soy agar, inoculated with a 0.5 McFarland turbidity suspension of the organism (Fig. 12.42). After overnight incubation at 35°C in 5% to 7% CO_2, the plate is examined for growth around each disk. Many X factor–requiring organisms are able to carry over enough factor from the primary medium to give false-negative results (i.e., growth occurs at such a distance from the X disk as to falsely indicate that the organism does not require the X factor) and erroneous identification of *H. influenzae* as *H. parainfluenzae*. A specialized *Haemophilus* Tri (*Haemophilus* ID II, Thermofisher) or Quad (*Haemophilus* ID Quad, Thermofisher) plate may also be used to determine X and V factor requirements as well as hemolysis on horse blood agar. The *Haemophilus* quad plate is divided into four quadrants, each containing a different media and growth factors; quadrant 1—brain–heart infusion (BHI) agar supplemented with hemin (X factor), quadrant 2—BHI supplemented with IsoVitale X (V factor), quadrant 3—BHI supplemented with both X and V factors, and quadrant 4—horse blood agar (X factor) supplemented with V factor. The presence or absence of growth in each quadrant along with hemolytic properties in quadrant 4 are used to speciate *Haemophilus* isolates (Fig. 31.3).

The porphyrin test is another means for establishing an organism's X factor requirements and eliminates the potential problem of carryover. This test detects the presence of enzymes that convert D-aminolevulinic acid (ALA) into porphyrins or protoporphyrins. The porphyrin test may be performed in broth, in agar, or on a disk.

Isolates from CSF or respiratory tract specimens that (1) are gram-negative rods or gram-negative coccobacilli; (2) grow on chocolate agar in CO_2 but not blood agar or satellite around NAD-producing colonies on blood agar; and (3) are porphyrin negative and nonhemolytic on rabbit or horse blood may be identified as *H. influenzae*. More information on this topic is available online.

Matrix-assisted laser desorption ionization time-of-flight mass spectrometry (MALDI-TOF MS) has provided laboratories improved identification of the *Haemophilus* spp. in clinical specimens. *Haemophilus* species successfully identified using MALDI-TOF MS include *H. influenzae, H. parainfluenzae, H. haemolyticus,* and *H. parahaemolyticus.* In addition, sequencing and next generation sequencing of the 16S rRNA gene also provide definitive identification of these organisms. However, identification has been problematic for the discrimination of *H. influenzae* and *H. aegyptius,* due to high sequence homology in the 16S rRNA gene and the lack of biochemical diversity for phenotypic characterization. All indirect methods for identification of *Haemophilus* species including biochemical, MALDI-TOF, or sequencing require the cultivation and isolation of pure colonies for identification.

Whole genome sequencing for the detection and classification of antimicrobial resistance in a single assay is

TABLE 31.4 Key Biochemical and Physiologic Characteristics of *Haemophilus* spp.

Organism	X Facto	V Factor	Hemolysis	Catalase	Lactose	Glucose	Xylose	Sucrose	Mannose	Beta-galactosidase	Indole	Urease	ODC
Haemophilus influenzae	+	+	–	+	–	+	+	–	–	–	B	B	B
Haemophilus aegyptius	+	+	–	+	–	+[a]	–	–	–	–	–	+	–
Haemophilus haemolyticus	+	+	+	+	–	+	V	–	–	–	V	+	–
Haemophilus parahaemolyticus	–	+	+	V	–	+	–	+	–	V	–	+	–
Haemophilus parainfluenzae	–	+	–	V	–	+	–	+	+	V	B	B	B
Haemophilus pittmaniae	–	+	+	+W	–	+	–	+	+	+	ND	ND	ND
Haemophilus paraphrohaemolyticus	–	+	+	+	–	+	–	+	–	V	–	+	–
H. ducreyi	+	–	–[a]	–	–	V	–	–	–	–	–	–	+
H. sputorum	–	+	–[b]	ND	–	+	–	ND	–	+	+	+	–

[a]Delayed reactions in some strains.
[b]Produces hemolysis on horse and sheep blood.
+, >90% of strains positive; –, >90% of strains negative; V, indicates a variable reaction; W, indicates a weak reaction; B, reactions based on biotypes; see Table 31.2.
ND, Not determined; ODC, ornithine decarboxylase.

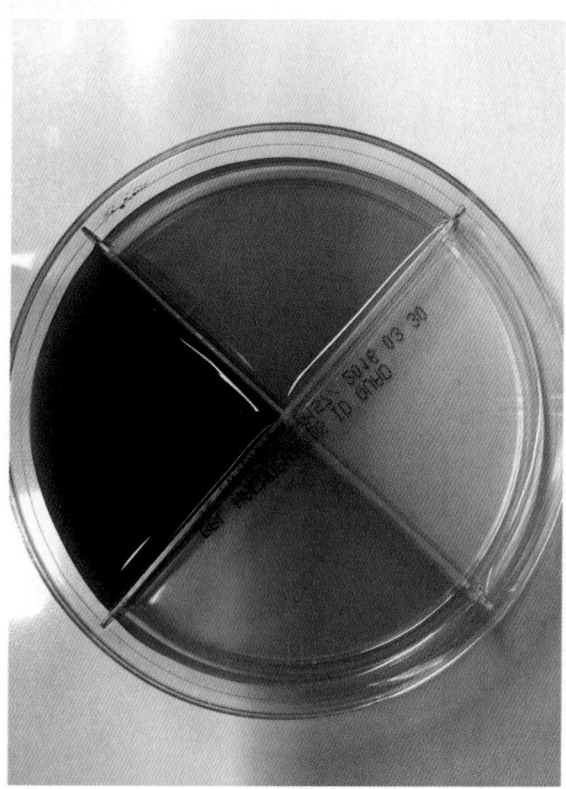

• **Fig. 31.3** *Haemophilus* Quad plate.

expected to become the future standard of care in the diagnostic microbiology laboratory. Turnaround time and annotation of the sequences can be completed in ≤24 hours, making outbreak investigations more effective for treatment and prevention of additional infections.

Serotyping

Serologic typing of *H. influenzae* may be used to establish an isolate as being any one of the six serotypes (i.e., a, b, c, d, e, and f) and should be completed as soon as possible after isolation and identification. The amount of capsular antigen produced by the organisms decreases over time, in particular on repeated subculturing in the laboratory. All *H. influenzae* from cases of invasive infections should be serotyped to determine what *H. influenzae* type is the cause of the infection. Testing can be performed using a slide agglutination test (Chapter 9); a saline control without the reagent antibodies should always be tested simultaneously alongside the patient's specimen to detect autoagglutination (i.e., the nonspecific agglutination of the test organism without homologous antiserum).

Molecular methods have also been used to type *H. influenzae*. The assays are based on the amplification of the outer membrane protein D gene *(glpQ)* from the capsule *(cap)* locus, the capsule producing gene *(bexA)*, the 16S rRNA, and the insertion-like sequence. PCR amplification has demonstrated an increased sensitivity compared with traditional serotyping.

Serodiagnosis

An enzyme-linked immunosorbent assay (ELISA) has been developed to detect antibodies to *H. ducreyi*. ELISA has been used to show seroconversion after Hib vaccination. None of the assays are commonly used for diagnostic purposes because of individual patient variability in the production of antibodies, antibody avidity, and persistence.

Antimicrobial Susceptibility Testing and Therapy

Standard methods have been established for performing *in vitro* susceptibility testing with clinically relevant isolates of *Haemophilus* spp. (see Chapter 11 for details on these methods). Although widespread *H. influenzae* is capable of producing beta-lactamase (penicillin resistance), cephalosporins and carbapenems as well as combination agents that contain a beta-lactamase inhibitor, such as clavulanate, sulbactam, or tazobactam combined with a beta-lactam, may be effective therapeutic agents. Other antimicrobials that remain useful for the treatment of *Haemophilus* infections include cephalosporins, macrolides, fluoroquinolones, and tetracyclines. Therefore, routine susceptibility testing of clinical isolates as a guide to therapy may not be necessary. Care should be taken when preparing inoculum concentrations (0.5 McFarland) for *Haemophilus* spp., in particular, beta-lactamase–producing strains of *H. influenzae,* because higher suspensions may lead to false-resistant results. In addition, beta-lactamase strains of *H. influenzae* that demonstrate elevated minimal inhibitory concentrations to ampicillin and amoxicillin have been identified. Cephalosporin activity is also decreased in these isolates. Rapid beta-lactamase testing using a chromogenic cephalosporin disk or spot test is sufficient for the majority of clinically significant isolates of *Haemophilus* spp. without further susceptibility testing.

Standardized and reliable susceptibility testing for *H. ducreyi* has not been developed and therefore should not be offered in a routine clinical microbiology laboratory. In addition, automated susceptibility testing for *H. influenzae* is unreliable and is not recommended.

Prevention

Several multiple-dose, protein-polysaccharide conjugate vaccines are licensed in the United States for *H. influenzae* type b. These vaccines have substantially reduced the incidence of severe invasive infections caused by type b organisms, and vaccination of children starting at 2 months of age is strongly recommended. The antibody to the Hib capsule and activation of the complement pathway within the host play a primary role in clearance and protection from infection. Newborns are protected for a short period after birth because of the presence of maternal antibodies.

ⓔ Visit the Evolve site for a complete list of procedures, review questions, and case studies.

Bibliography

Alfa M: The laboratory diagnosis of *H. ducreyi*, *Can J Infect Dis Med Microbiol* 16:31–34, 2005.

Carroll KC, Pfaller MA, Landry ML, et al.: *Manual of clinical microbiology*, ed 12, Washington, DC, 2019, ASM.

Committee on Infectious Diseases: *2006 Red book: report of the committee on infectious diseases*, ed 27, Elk Grove Village, IL, 2006, American Academy of Pediatrics.

Darville T, Jacobs RF, Lucas RA, Caldwell B: Detection of *Haemophilus influenzae* type b antigen in cerebrospinal fluid after immunization, *Pediatr Infect Dis J* 11:243–244, 1992.

Deshmukh D, Joseph J, Chakrabarti M, et al.: New insights into culture negative endophthalmitis by unbiased next generation sequencing, *Sci Rep* 9:844, 2019.

Falla TJ, Crook DW, Brophy LN, Maskell D, Kroll JS, Moxon ER: PCR for capsular typing of *Haemophilus influenzae*, *J Clin Microbiol* 32:2382–2386, 1994.

Lagergård T: *Haemophilus ducreyi*: pathogenesis and protective immunity, *Trends Microbiol* 3:87–92, 1995.

Leber AL: *Aerobic cultures, clinical microbiology procedures handbook*, ed 4, Washington, DC, 2016, ASM Press.

Leber AL, Everhart K, Balada-Llasat JM, et al.: Multicenter evaluation of BioFire filmarray meningitis/encephalitis panel for detection of bacteria, viruses, and yeast in cerebral spinal fluid specimens, *J Clin Microbiol* 54:2251–2261, 2016.

Nørskov-Lauritsen N: Classification, identification, and clinical significance of *Haemophilus* and *Aggregatibacter* species with host specificity for humans, *Clin Microbiol Rev* 29:214–240, 2014.

St Geme III JW: Nontypeable *Haemophilus influenzae* disease: epidemiology, pathogenesis, and prospects for prevention, *Infect Agents Dis* 2:1–16, 1993.

Van Dyck E, Bogaerts J, Smet H, Tello WM, Mukantabana V, Piot P: Emergence of *Haemophilus ducreyi* resistance to trimethoprim-sulfamethoxazole in rwanda, *Antimicrob Agents Chemother* 38:1647–1648, 1994.

32

Bartonella

OBJECTIVES

1. Explain the routes of transmission for *Bartonella* infections, and describe the organism's interaction with the host.
2. Discuss the clinical manifestations of trench fever, including signs, symptoms, and individuals at risk of acquiring the disease.
3. Explain the criteria used to diagnose *Bartonella henselae*.
4. Describe the methods for culturing *Bartonella*, including growth rates, media, incubation temperature, and other relevant conditions.
5. Describe the strategies to prevent exposure and infection by these organisms in immunocompromised individuals.

GENERA AND SPECIES TO BE CONSIDERED

Bartonella alsatica
Bartonella bacilliformis (type species)
Bartonella clarridgeiae
Bartonella elizabethae
Bartonella grahamii
Bartonella henselae
Bartonella koehlerae
Bartonella quintana
Bartonella rochalimae
Bartonella schoenbuchensis
Bartonella tribocorum
Bartonella vinsonii subsp. *arupensis*
Bartonella vinsonii subsp. *berkhoffii*

The *Bartonella* spp. are able to grow on chocolate agar and, albeit very slowly, on routine blood (trypticase soy agar with 5% sheep blood agar), typically appearing after 12 to 14 days and sometimes requiring as long as 45 days; neither organism grows on MacConkey agar. Presently, there is no optimal procedure for the isolation of these organisms from clinical specimens.

Bartonella

General Characteristics

The genus *Bartonella* spp. currently includes 35 named species. Fourteen species have been associated with human disease (Table 32.1) and four have been identified as presumptive human pathogens. Other members of the genus have been found in animal reservoirs such as rodents, ruminants, and moles. *Bartonella* spp. are most closely related to *Brucella abortus* and are short, gram-negative, pleomorphic coccobacillary or bacillary, facultative, intracellular bacteria that parasitize mammalian cells. They are fastidious organisms that are oxidase and catalase negative and grow best on blood-enriched media.

Epidemiology and Pathogenesis

Organisms belonging to the genus *Bartonella* cause numerous infections in humans; most of these infections are thought to be zoonoses. Interest in these organisms has increased because of their recognition as causes of an expanding array of clinical syndromes in immunocompromised and immunocompetent patients. For example, *Bartonella* species have been recognized with increasing frequency as a cause of culture-negative endocarditis. Humans acquire infection either naturally (infections caused by *Bartonella quintana* or *Bartonella bacilliformis*) or accidentally (other *Bartonella* species) via insect vectors or potentially by animal scratches or bites. Human infections can generally be divided into anthroponotic bartonellosis (humans as reservoirs) or zoonotic (animals as reservoirs) based on the normal host for the insect vector. Nevertheless, questions remain regarding the epidemiology of these infections; some epidemiologic information is summarized in Table 32.1.

Bartonella is a facultative intracellular bacterium that closely interacts with the host cells and has unique abilities to cause either acute or chronic infection as well as the proliferation of microvascular endothelial cells and angiogenesis (forming new capillaries from preexisting ones) or suppurative manifestations. Three *Bartonella* species (*Bartonella quintana, Bartonella*

TABLE 32.1	*Bartonella* spp. and Clinical Relevance in Human Accidental Hosts		
Organism	Habitat (Main Reservoir)	Mode of Transmission	Clinical Manifestation(s)
Bartonella alsatica	Rabbits	Fleas and ticks	Bacteremia and endocarditis
Bartonella bacilliformis	Humans	Sandflies	Carrión's disease[a] Chronic disease: Verruga peruana, bacteremia
Bartonella clarridgeiae	Cats	Fleas and ticks	Bacteremia Cat-scratch disease
B. elizabethae	Rats and gerbils	Fleas	Endocarditis
B. grahamii	Voles, mice, rats, and deer	Fleas, ticks, and leeches	Cat-scratch disease and neuroretinitis
B. henselae	Cats	Cats and dogs; bites or scratches, fleas, and ticks	Bacteremia Endocarditis Cat-scratch disease Bacillary angiomatosis Peliosis hepatitis or splenic peliosis Neuroretinitis
B. koehlerae	Cats	Fleas and ticks	Chronic bacteremia and endocarditis; implicated in arthritis peripheral neuropathies or tachyarrhythmias
B. quintana	Humans	Human body louse	Trench fever Chronic bacteremia Endocarditis Bacillary angiomatosis Chronic lymphadenopathy Pericarditis
B. rochalimae	Foxes, coyotes, dogs, rats, and skunks	Fleas and ticks	Fever and bacteremia
B. schoenbuchensis	Cattle, roe deer, and moose	Deer keds, biting flies, and ticks	Dermatitis
B. tribocorum	Rats and mice	Fleas and mites	Bacteremia
B. vinsonii subsp. *arupensis*	White-footed mice	Fleas and ticks	Bacteremia and endocarditis
B. vinsonii subsp. *berkhoffii*	Coyotes, dogs, and foxes	Ticks	Bacteremia, endocarditis, neurologic disorders, and rheumatic symptoms

[a]Disease confined to a small endemic area in South America; characterized by a septicemic phase with anemia, malaise, fever, and enlarged lymph nodes in the liver and spleen, followed by a cutaneous phase with bright red cutaneous nodules; usually self-limited.

bacilliformis, and *B. henselae*) are capable of causing angiogenic lesions. Research has demonstrated that some species are capable of interacting with host red blood cells, endothelial cells, and possibly bone marrow progenitor cells. Colonization of vascular endothelium is considered a crucial step in the establishment and maintenance of *Bartonella*-triggered angioproliferative lesions. Within several hours after infection of cultured human umbilical vein endothelial cells, *Bartonella* species adhere to and enter these cells by an actin-dependent process resembling other bacterial-directed phagocytosis or uptake into host cells. *B. henselae* possess nine outer membrane proteins (OMP), one of which is able to bind to endothelial cells.

Typically, *Bartonella* species multiply and persist in the red blood cells in the reservoir host and share common persistence and dissemination strategies. In addition to angioproliferation, bartonellae can inhibit endothelial cell apoptosis (programmed cell death); these organisms also activate monocyte and macrophage cells capable of producing potent angiogenic factors. Although more research is needed regarding the pathogenesis of infections caused by *Bartonella,* it is evident these organisms possess unique pathogenic strategies to expand their bacterial niche to sustain survival within the human host. It is evident that the pathologic response to these infections varies substantially with the status of the host immune system. For example, infection with the same *Bartonella* species, such as *B. henselae,* can cause a focal suppurative reaction (e.g., **cat-scratch disease [CSD]**) in immunocompetent patients or a multifocal angioproliferative lesion (e.g., **bacillary angiomatosis**) in immunocompromised patients. *B. quintana,* the causative agent for **trench fever,** also causes bacillary angiomatosis in immunocompromised patients.

Spectrum of Disease

The diseases caused by *Bartonella* species are listed in Table 32.1. Infection with *B. bacilliformis* presents as either an acute hemolytic bacteremia (**Oroya fever**) or a chronic vasoproliferative disease. The chronic form of infection is often referred to as **Carrion disease,** named after a medical student, Daniel Carrion, who died after self-inoculation with material from a wartlike lesion (**verruga**). The acute form of disease is a progressive, severe, febrile anemia. This is a result of intravascular hemolysis of erythrocytes infected with *B. bacilliformis.* Chronic bacteremia occurs in individuals who live in endemic areas. The chronic infection appears as cutaneous nodular angioproliferative lesions previously described as verruga. Depending on the status of the host and the disease presentation, mortality rates associated with *B. bacilliformis* range from 40% to 90% prior to the use of antibiotics.

Trench fever, caused by *B. quintana,* was largely considered a disease of the past. Clinical manifestations of trench fever range from a mild influenza-like headache and bone pain to splenomegaly (enlarged spleen) and a short-lived maculopapular rash. During the febrile stages of trench fever, infection may persist long after the disappearance of all clinical signs; some patients may have six or more recurrences. *B. quintana* has been reported in cases of bacteremia, blood-culture negative endocarditis, chronic lymphadenopathy, and bacillary angiomatosis. Bacillary angiomatosis is a vascular proliferative disease involving the skin (other organs such as the liver, spleen, and lymph nodes may also be involved). Prolonged bacteremia with *B. quintana* and *B. henselae* can cause epithelioid angiomatosis, a vasculoproliferative disease of the skin.

B. henselae is associated with bacteremia, endocarditis, and bacillary angiomatosis. Of note, observations indicate that *B. henselae* infections appear to be subclinical and are markedly underreported, because problems with current diagnostic approaches are recognized (see Laboratory Diagnosis). In addition, *B. henselae* is the primary cause of CSD with *B. grahamii* implicated in a few human cases. *B. henselae* also causes rheumatic manifestations and bacillary **peliosis hepatitis** or **splenic peliosis.** About 12,500 cases of CSD occur annually in the United States; about 33% of these occur in children ≤14 years of age. The infection begins as a papule or pustule at the primary inoculation site; regional tender lymphadenopathy develops in approximately 3 weeks. The spectrum of disease ranges from chronic, self-limited adenopathy to a severe systemic illness affecting multiple body organs in about 25% of CSD cases. Localized infections are common in immunocompetent patients, including ocular bartonellosis, but are rare in transplant patients. In addition, rare cases of optical neuropathy and unilateral loss of vision have been characterized in acute cases of CSD. Rheumatic manifestations may include myositis, arthritis with skin nodules in children, leukocytoclastic vasculitis,

erythema nodosum, or fever of unknown origin. Although complications such as a suppurative (draining) lymph nodes or encephalitis are reported, fatalities are rare. Zoonotic disease is caused by a variety of species and may be associated with blood culture–negative endocarditis or myocarditis. Diagnosis of CSD requires three of the following four criteria:

- History of animal contact plus site of primary inoculation (e.g., a scratch)
- Negative laboratory studies for other causes of lymphadenopathy
- Characteristic histopathology of the lesion
- A positive skin test using antigen prepared from heat-treated pus collected from another patient's lesion

Peliosis hepatitis caused by *B. henselae* may occur independently or in conjunction with cutaneous bacillary angiomatosis or bacteremia. Patients with bacillary peliosis hepatitis or splenic peliosis demonstrate gastrointestinal symptoms. Symptoms include fever, chills, and an enlarged liver and spleen that contain blood-filled cavities. This systemic disease primarily develops in patients infected with HIV and other immunocompromised individuals.

Laboratory Diagnosis

Specimen Collection, Transport, and Processing

Clinical specimens submitted to the laboratory for direct examination and culture include blood collected in a lysis-centrifugation blood culture tube (Isolator; Alere, Inc., Waltham, MA), sodium citrate or plastic EDTA tubes, aspirates, and tissue specimens (e.g., lymph node, spleen, or cutaneous biopsies). If a delay occurs when processing tissue specimens for culture of *Bartonella* spp., samples should be frozen at –20°C. Notably, attempts to culture *Bartonella* spp. in routine microbiology laboratories is not recommended due to low recovery rates. Fresh tissue samples and formalin-fixed, paraffin-embedded tissues from lymph nodes, lesions, infected organs and aspirated vitreous fluid, and cerebrospinal fluid can be processed for direct detection by nucleic acid testing. There are no special requirements for specimen collection, transport, or processing that enhances organism recovery. Refer to Table 5.1 for general information on specimen collection, transport, and processing.

Direct Detection Methods

Microscopy

Detection of *Bartonella* spp. during the histopathologic examination of tissue biopsies is enhanced using the Warthin-Starry silver stain or immunohistochemical techniques. Because of the fastidious nature of the organisms and slow growth associated with low levels of bacteremia in patients, these techniques lack sensitivity and specificity.

Nucleic Acid Detection

Tissue, body fluids, and blood can be successfully used for identification of *Bartonella* species from clinical samples by nucleic acid amplification detection. The 16S rRNA gene is extremely homologous within the genus and does not provide effective discrimination of *Bartonella* spp. Several other gene targets have been successfully used for identification, including citrate synthase (*gltA*), heat shock protein (*groEL*), riboflavin synthase (*ribC*), a cell division protein (*ftsZ*), and the 17-kDa antigen. In addition, the 16S–23S ribosomal ribonucleic acid (rRNA) gene intergenic transcribed spacer region has been used as a reliable method for the detection and the classification of *Bartonella* deoxyribonucleic acid (DNA) in clinical samples.

Cultivation

Bartonella spp. are slow-growing fastidious organisms that require heme for growth. Various agar bases such as Columbia agar, trypticase soy, brucella, or heart infusion agar supplemented with hemoglobin, 5% rabbit blood or hemin have been successfully used for the cultivation of the organisms. Lysed, centrifuged sediment of blood collected in an isolator tube or minced tissue is directly inoculated onto fresh chocolate and heart infusion agar plates containing 5% rabbit blood. Cultures should be incubated at 35°C to 37°C in 5% CO_2, except *B. bacilliformis* and *B. clarridgeiae*, which grow optimally at 25°C to 30°C in ambient air. Some species demonstrate improved growth on specific media: *B. henselae,* heart infusion agar; *B. quintana,* chocolate agar; *B. koehlerae* requires fresh chocolate agar. Due to the slow growth of these organisms, they should be incubated for at least 4 weeks in high humidity.

Biphasic or broth culture systems may be used for the isolation of *Bartonella* spp.; however, the organisms rarely reach a high level of turbidity or activate the CO_2 detector in automated systems. Subculturing and staining with acridine orange on negative cultures before discarding improves identification. Biopsy material is cultivated with an endothelial cell culture system; cultures are incubated at 35°C in 5% to 10% CO_2 for 15 to 20 days. Lymph node tissue, aspirates, or swabs can be inoculated onto laked horse blood agar slants supplemented with hemin; plates are sealed and incubated in 5% CO_2 up to 6 weeks at 37°C with 85% humidity. Heparinized plasma may also be cultured on T84 bladder carcinoma cells in a centrifugation shell-vial.

Approach to Identification

Bartonella spp. should be suspected when colonies of small, gram-negative bacilli are recovered after prolonged incubation (Fig. 32.1). Macroscopic colonial morphology is often variable. *B. henselae* may appear as irregular, dry, white "cauliflower-like" colonies that pit the agar or small, circular, tan, moist colonies. The majority of *Bartonella* spp. will appear tan and smooth on repeated subculture. The Gram-stain appearance of *Bartonella* as small, slightly curved gram-negative rods is similar to *Campylobacter, Helicobacter,* or *Haemophilus* spp. These organisms are all oxidase, urease, nitrate reductase, and catalase negative. Most of the *Bartonella* spp. are biochemically inert, making phenotypic methods for identification unreliable for identification from clinical specimens. Prolonged incubation requiring more than 7 days, microscopic and macroscopic morphologies in conjunction with negative oxidase, and catalase testing may be sufficient for preliminary identification. *Bartonella* spp. are not included in MALDI-TOF Reference databases. Nucleic acid amplification and sequencing is recommended for confirmation and identification of *Bartonella* species and strains.

Serodiagnosis

There are no US Food and Drug Administration-cleared serologic tests for the diagnosis of *Bartonella* infections.

Antimicrobial Susceptibility Testing and Therapy

Although there are no current standards or guidelines for antimicrobial susceptibility testing by the Clinical and Laboratory Standards Institute (CLSI) or the European Committee on Antimicrobial Susceptibility Testing (EUCAST), testing can be performed by agar dilution using blood or chocolate agar and microdilution methods with broth supplemented with blood.

Treatment recommendations for *Bartonella* diseases, including CSD, depend on the specific disease presentation and have demonstrated sensitivity to β-lactams, aminoglycosides, chloramphenicol, tetracyclines, macrolides,

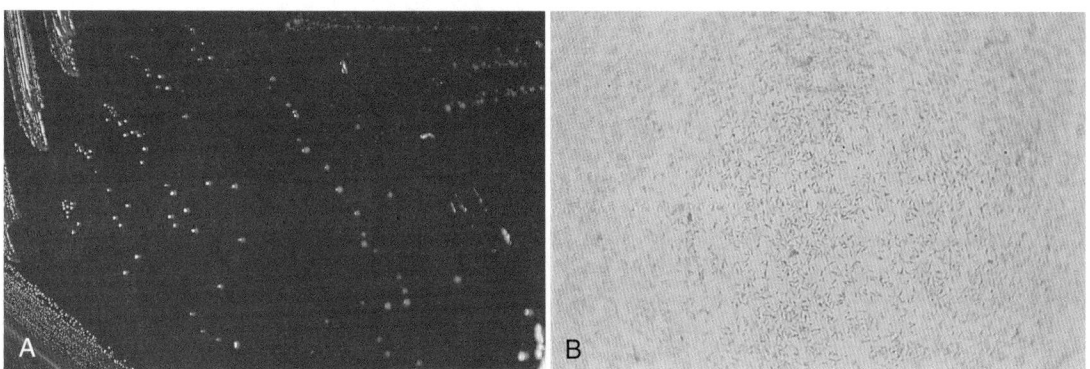

• **Fig. 32.1** (A) Colonies of *Bartonella henselae* on blood agar. (B) Gram stain of a colony of *B. henselae* from blood agar.

rifamycins, fluoroquinolones, and trimethoprim-sulfamethoxazole. The efficacy of various antibiotics for CSD is difficult to assess because of the self-limiting nature of the disease and the decrease in symptoms in the absence of therapy. In addition to the clinical presentation, the treatment must be specifically adapted to the correct *Bartonella* sp. Moreover, results of *in vitro* testing may not correlate with clinical efficacy; for example, the administration of penicillin is not effective therapy despite susceptibility *in vitro*. Suggested therapy for endocarditis, suspected or documented, is gentamicin with or without doxycycline, respectively. However, this treatment has been associated with kidney failure. Rifampin in combination with doxycycline is the current recommended treatment due to the intracellular penetration and bactericidal activity of rifampin.

Prevention

There are no vaccines available to prevent infections caused by *Bartonella* spp. Exposure to cats or cat fleas has been implicated in the transmission of *B. henselae* to humans. It is recommended that immunocompromised individuals avoid contact with cats, especially kittens, and control flea infestation.

ⓔ Visit the Evolve site for a complete list of procedures, review questions, and case studies.

Bibliography

Ak R, Doganay F, Akoglu EU, Ozturk TC: A challenging differential diagnosis of optic neuropathy in ED: CSD, *BMJ Case Rep* 2015; 2015:bcr2015210252.

Avidor B, Graidy M, Efrat G, et al.: *Bartonella koehlerae,* a new cat-associated agent of culture-negative human endocarditis, *J Clin Microbiol* 42:3462–3468, 2004.

Berger P, Papazian L, Drancourt M, La Scola B, Auffray JP, Raoult D: Ameba-associated microorganisms and diagnosis of nosocomial pneumonia, *Emerg Infect Dis* 12:248–255, 2006.

Breitschwerdt EB, Kordick DL: *Bartonella* infection in animals: carriership, reservoir potential, pathogenicity, and zoonotic potential for human infection, *Clin Microbiol Rev* 13:428–438, 2000.

Carroll KC, Pfaller MA, Landry ML, et al.: *Manual of clinical microbiology,* ed 12, Washington, DC, 2019, ASM.

Chan D, Geiger JA, Vasconcelos EJR, Oakley B, Diniz PPVP: *Bartonella rochalimae* detection by a sensitive and specific PCR platform, *Am J Trop Med Hyg* 99:840–843, 2018.

De Bruin A, Van Leeuwen AD, Jahfari S, et al.: Vertical transmission of *Bartonella schoenbuchensis* in *Lipoptena cervi, Parasit Vectors* 8:176, 2015.

Dehio C: Recent progress in understanding *Bartonella*-induced vascular proliferation, *Curr Opin Microbiol* 6:61–65, 2003.

Fournier PE, Robson J, Zeaiter Z, McDougall R, Byrne S, Raoult D: Improved culture from lymph nodes of patients with cat scratch disease and genotypic characterization of *Bartonella henselae* isolates in Australia, *J Clin Microbiol* 40:3620–3624, 2002.

Garcia-Caceres U, Garcia FU: Bartonellosis: an immunosuppressive disease and the life of Daniel Alcides Carrión, *Am J Clin Pathol* 95(Suppl 1):S58–S66, 1991.

Giladi M, Avidor B, Kletter Y, et al.: Cat scratch disease: the rare role of *Afipia felis, J Clin Microbiol* 36:2499–2502, 1998.

Greub G, Raoult D: *Bartonella:* new explanations for old diseases, *J Med Microbiol* 51:915–923, 2002.

Gutierrez R, Vayssier-Taussat M, Buffet JP, Harrus S: Guidelines for the isolation, molecular detection, and characterization of *Bartonella* species, *Vector Borne Zoonotic Dis* 17:42–50, 2017.

Jacomo V, Raoult D: Human infections caused by *Bartonella* spp. Parts 1 and 2, *Clin Microbiol Newsl* 22(1–5):9–13, 2000.

Jacomo V, Kelly PJ, Raoult D: Natural history of *Bartonella* infections (an exception to Koch's postulate), *Clin Diagn Lab Immunol* 9:8–18, 2002.

Kordick DL, Hilyard EJ, Hadfield TL, et al.: *Bartonella clarridgeiae:* a newly recognized zoonotic pathogen causing inoculation papules,

fever, and lymphadenopathy (cat scratch disease), *J Clin Microbiol* 35:1813–1818, 1997.

Kosoy M, McKee C, Albayrak L, Fofanov Y: Genotyping of *Bartonella* bacteria and their animal hosts: current status and perspectives, *Parasitology* 145:543–562, 2018.

LaScola B, Raoult D: Culture of *Bartonella quintana* and *Bartonella henselae* from human samples: a 5-year experience (1993-1998), *J Clin Microbiol* 37:1899, 1999.

Lawson PA, Collins MD: Description of *Bartonella clarridgeiae* sp nov isolated from the cat of a patient with *Bartonella henselae* septicemia, *Med Microbiol Lett* 5:640, 1996.

Lee RA, Ray M, Kasuga DT, et al.: Ocular bartonellosis in transplant recipients: two case reports and review of the literature, *Transpl Infect Dis* 17:723–727, 2015.

Maggi RG, Breitschwerdt EB: Potential limitations of the 16S-23S rRNA intergenic region for molecular detection of *Bartonella* species, *J Clin Microbiol* 43:1171–1176, 2005.

Manfredi R, Sabbatani S, Chiodo F: Bartonellosis: light and shadows in diagnostic and therapeutic issues, *Clin Microbiol Infect* 11:167–169, 2004.

Mazur-Melewska K, Mania A, Kemnitz P, Figlerowicz M, Służewski W: Cat-scratch disease: a wide spectrum of clinical pictures, *Postepy Dermatol Alergol* 32:216–220, 2015.

Mozayeni BR, Maggi RG, Bradley JM, Breitschwerdt EB: Rheumatological presentation of *Bartonella koehlerae* and *Bartonella henselae* bacteremias: a case report, *Medicine (Baltim)* 97(17).e0465, 2018, https://doi.org/10.1097/MD.0000000000010465.

Okaro U, Addisu A, Casanas B, Anderson B: *Bartonella* species, an emerging cause of blood-culture-negative endocarditis, *Clin Microbiol Rev* 30:709–746, 2017.

Oksi J, Rantala S, Kilpinen S, et al.: Cat scratch disease caused by *Bartonella grahamii* in an immunocompromised patient, *J Clin Microbiol* 51:2781–2784, 2013.

Oteo JA, Maggi R, Portillo A, et al.: Prevalence of *Bartonella* spp. by culture, PCR and serology, in veterinary personnel from Spain, *Parasit Vectors* 10:553–561, 2017.

Rolain JM, Brouqui P, Koehler JE, Maguina C, Dolan MJ, Raoult D: Recommendations for treatment of human infections caused by *Bartonella species, Antimicrob Agents Chemother* 48:1921–1933, 2004.

Silva BTGD, Souza AM, Campos SDE, et al.: *Bartonella henselae* and *Bartonella clarridgeiae* infection, hematological changes and associated factors in domestic cats and dogs from an Atlantic rain forest area, Brazil, *Acta Trop* 193:163–168, 2019.

33

Campylobacter, Arcobacter, and Helicobacter

OBJECTIVES

1. List the *Campylobacter* species most often associated with infections in humans, and explain how they are transmitted.
2. Identify the culture methods for optimum recovery of *Campylobacter* spp., including agar, temperatures, oxygenation, and length of incubation.
3. Describe how to isolate *Campylobacter* from blood, including special stains, atmospheric conditions, and length of incubation.
4. List the colonial morphology, microscopic characteristics, and biochemical reactions of *Campylobacter* and *Helicobacter*.
5. List the key biochemical test to identify *Helicobacter pylori* in specimens.
6. Describe how *H. pylori* colonize in the stomach and how motility plays an important role in the pathogenesis of the organism.
7. Differentiate the isolation and identification of *Campylobacter, Arcobacter,* and *Helicobacter* species, including *H. pylori* and enterohepatic helicobacters.
8. Describe why therapy is often problematic for *H. pylori*.

GENERA AND SPECIES TO BE CONSIDERED

Campylobacter coli
Campylobacter concisus
Campylobacter curvus
Campylobacter fetus subsp. *fetus*
Campylobacter fetus subsp. *venerealis*
Campylobacter gracilis
Campylobacter hominis
Campylobacter hyointestinalis subsp. *hyointestinalis*
Campylobacter jejuni subsp. *doylei*
Campylobacter jejuni subsp. *jejuni*
Campylobacter lari subsp. *lari*
Campylobacter pyloridis
Campylobacter rectus
Campylobacter showae
Campylobacter sputorum subsp. *sputorum*
Campylobacter upsaliensis
Campylobacter ureolyticus
Arcobacter cryaerophilus
Arcobacter butzleri
Arcobacter skirrowii
Helicobacter pylori

Helicobacter bizzozeronii
Helicobacter cinaedi
Helicobacter felis
Helicobacter fennelliae
Helicobacter heilmannii
Helicobacter suis
Helicobacter cinaedi
Helicobacter fennelliae
Helicobacter heilmannii
Helicobacter salomonis
Helicobacter suis
Helicobacter bilis
Helicobacter felis
Helicobacter canis
Helicobacter canadensis
Helicobacter pullorum

Because of their morphologic similarities and an inability to recover these organisms using routine laboratory media for primary isolation, the genera *Campylobacter, Arcobacter,* and *Helicobacter* are considered together in this chapter (Fig. 33.1). All organisms belonging to these genera are small, curved or straight, motile, gram-negative bacilli. When cultures are old or the organisms are exposed to air for long periods, they may form spherical or coccoid bodies. With few exceptions, most of these bacteria also have a requirement for a microaerobic (5% to 10% O_2) atmosphere with some species requiring the addition of 5% to 7% H_2.

Campylobacter and *Arcobacter*

General Characteristics

Campylobacter and *Arcobacter* spp. are relatively slow growing, fastidious, and, in general, asaccharolytic; organisms known to cause disease in humans are listed in Table 33.1.

Epidemiology and Pathogenesis

Most *Campylobacter* species are pathogenic and associated with a wide variety of diseases in humans and other animals. These organisms demonstrate considerable ecologic diversity. *Campylobacter* spp. are microaerobic (5% to 10% O_2) inhabitants of the gastrointestinal tracts of various animals,

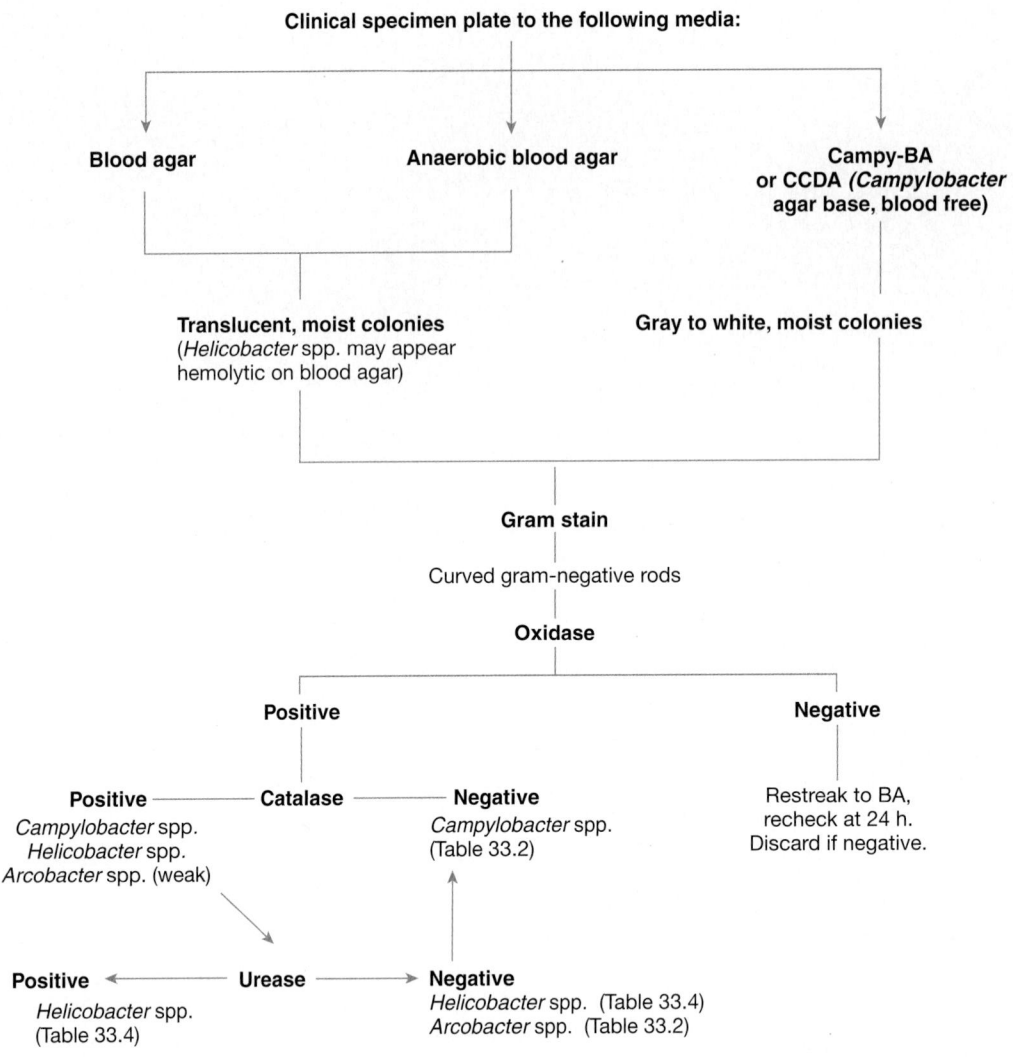

Clinical specimen plate to the following media:

Blood agar   Anaerobic blood agar   Campy-BA or CCDA *(Campylobacter* agar base, blood free)

Translucent, moist colonies
(Helicobacter spp. may appear hemolytic on blood agar)

Gray to white, moist colonies

Gram stain

Curved gram-negative rods

Oxidase

Positive   Negative

Positive —— Catalase —— Negative
Campylobacter spp.   *Campylobacter* spp.
Helicobacter spp.   (Table 33.2)
Arcobacter spp. (weak)

Restreak to BA, recheck at 24 h. Discard if negative.

Positive ◄—— Urease ——► Negative
Helicobacter spp.   *Helicobacter* spp. (Table 33.4)
(Table 33.4)   *Arcobacter* spp. (Table 33.2)

• **Fig. 33.1** Identification scheme for the differentiation of the genera *Helicobacter, Campylobacter,* and *Arcobacter. BAP,* Blood agar plate.

including poultry, dogs, cats, sheep, and cattle, as well as the reproductive organs of several species. In general, *Campylobacter* spp. produce three syndromes in humans: febrile systemic disease, periodontal disease, and, most commonly, gastroenteritis. Humans are the only recognized reservoir for *C. concisus, C. rectus, C. curvus,* and *C. showae* and implicated in periodontal disease.

Arcobacter spp. are aerotolerant and are also inhabitants of the gastrointestinal tracts of various animal species. Three of the eighteen species of *Arcobacter* have been identified in human infections. *Arcobacter* species appear to be associated with gastroenteritis. Studies have indicated that *Arcobacter butzleri,* one of the most common *Campylobacter*-like organisms isolated from stool, is often associated with persistent, watery diarrhea. The organism has also been isolated from patients with bacteremia, endocarditis, and peritonitis. The organism is found in the environment in untreated water. It is also prevalent in commercially prepared meats including chicken, beef, pork, lamb, and poultry. *Arcobacter cryaerophilus* has been isolated from patients with bacteremia

and diarrhea. *A. skirrowii* has been isolated from a patient with chronic diarrhea; however, the clinical significance of this isolate is unknown.

Within the genus *Campylobacter, Campylobacter jejuni* subsp. *jejuni* and *Campylobacter coli* are associated with clinically indistinguishable infections in humans and are transmitted via contaminated food, milk, or water. Outbreaks have been associated with contaminated drinking water and improperly pasteurized milk, among other sources. In contrast to other agents of foodborne gastroenteritis, including *Salmonella* and staphylococci, *Campylobacter* spp. does not multiply in food. Other *Campylobacter* spp. have been isolated from patients following consumption of untreated water as well as from immunocompromised patients or patients recently returned from international travel. In addition to food outbreaks, *Campylobacter* spp. may be present in poultry, cattle, sheep, pigs, and domestic pets. *C. lari* and *C. upsaliensis* have been identified in cases of gastrointestinal and urinary tract infections and bacteremia. *C. jejuni* subsp. *doylei* has been isolated from children with diarrhea and

TABLE 33.1   Source and Spectrum of Disease in Humans of Representative Species of *Campylobacter* and *Arcobacter*

Organism	Source	Spectrum of Disease in Humans
Campylobacter concisus, Campylobacter curvus, Campylobacter rectus, Campylobacter showae	Humans	Periodontal disease; gastroenteritis
Campylobacter gracilis	Humans	Deep-tissue infections: head, neck, and viscera; gingival crevices Peritonitis, bacteremia, and pulmonary infections
Campylobacter coli	Pigs, poultry, sheep, bulls, birds	Gastroenteritis[a] Septicemia
Campylobacter jejuni subsp. *jejuni*	Poultry, pigs, bulls, dogs, cats, birds, and other animals	Gastroenteritis[a] Septicemia Meningitis Proctitis
Campylobacter jejuni subsp. *doylei*	Humans	Gastroenteritis[a] Gastritis Septicemia
Campylobacter lari subsp. *concheus,* *Campylobacter lari* subsp. *lari*	Birds, poultry, other animals; river and seawater	Gastroenteritis[a] Septicemia Prosthetic joint infection Urinary tract infections
Campylobacter hyointestinalis subsp. *hyointestinalis*	Pigs, cattle, hamsters, deer	Gastroenteritis Proctitis
Campylobacter upsaliensis	Dogs, cats	Gastroenteritis Septicemia abscesses
Campylobacter fetus subsp. *fetus*	Cattle, sheep	Septicemia Gastroenteritis Abortion Meningitis
Campylobacter fetus subsp. *venerealis*	Cattle	Septicemia
Campylobacter pyloridis	Humans, shell fish	None reported
Campylobacter sputorum biovar *sputorum*	Humans, cattle, pigs	Abscesses Gastroenteritis
Campylobacter ureolyticus	Humans	Gastroenteritis
Arcobacter cryaerophilus	Pigs, bulls, and other animals	Gastroenteritis[a] Septicemia
Arcobacter butzleri	Pigs, bulls, humans, other animals; water	Gastroenteritis[a] Septicemia
Arcobacter skirrowii	Pigs, sheep, cattle, poultry, and humans	Gastroenteritis

[a]Most common clinical presentation.

from gastric biopsies in adults. In developed countries, most *C. jejuni* infections are transmitted by direct contact during the preparation and eating of chicken. Person-to-person transmission of *Campylobacter* infections plays only a minor role in the transmission of disease. There is a marked seasonality with the rates of *C. jejuni* infection in the United States; the highest rates of infection occur in late summer and early fall. *Campylobacter* spp. has been recognized as the most common causative agent of gastroenteritis in the United States.

Although infections with *C. jejuni* are evident in acute inflammatory enteritis of the small intestine and colon, the pathogenesis remains unclear. However, multiplication of organisms in the intestine leads to cell damage and an inflammatory response. Blood and polymorphonuclear neutrophils are often observed in stool specimens. Most strains of *C. jejuni* are susceptible to the nonspecific bactericidal activity of normal human serum; this susceptibility probably explains why *C. jejuni* bacteremia is uncommon.

Spectrum of Disease

As previously mentioned, *Campylobacter* spp. are the causative agent of gastrointestinal or extraintestinal infections. Extraintestinal infections including abscesses, bacteremia, cholecystitis, myocarditis, meningitis, abortion and neonatal sepsis, nephritis, pancreatitis, peritonitis, prostatitis, and septic arthritis have been reported following *Campylobacter* gastroenteritis.

The different campylobacters and their associated diseases are summarized in Table 33.1. Gastroenteritis associated with *Campylobacter* spp. is usually a self-limiting illness and does not require antibiotic therapy. Recently, postinfection complications with *C. jejuni* have been recognized and include reactive arthritis and **Guillain-Barré syndrome,** an acute demyelination (removal of the myelin sheath from a nerve) of the peripheral nerves. Studies indicate that 20% to 40% of patients with this syndrome were infected with *C. jejuni* 1 to 3 weeks before the onset of neurologic symptoms. Reactive arthritis, Reiter syndrome, and irritable bowel syndrome are also known to follow campylobacter infections.

Laboratory Diagnosis
Specimen Collection, Transport, and Processing

There are no special requirements for the collection, transport, and processing of clinical specimens for the detection of campylobacters; the two most common clinical specimens submitted to the laboratory are feces (rectal swabs are also acceptable for culture for infants and children) and blood. Specimens should be processed as soon as possible. Delays of more than 2 hours require the stool specimen to be placed either in Cary-Blair transport medium, modified Cary-Blair, Fecal Enteric Plus, or other equivalent transport medium. Cary-Blair or Fecal Enteric Plus transport medium is suitable for other enteric pathogens; specimens received in transport medium should be processed immediately or stored at 4°C until processed. *C. fetus, C. jejuni,* and *C. upsaliensis* have been successfully recovered from patient samples using automated blood culture systems.

Direct Detection

Upon Gram staining, *Campylobacter* spp. display a characteristic microscopic morphology as small, curved or seagull-winged, faintly staining, gram-negative rods (Fig. 33.2). *Campylobacter* spp. are difficult to visualize using the standard secondary safranin counterstain in the Gram stain procedure. Carbol-fuchsin or 0.1% aqueous basic fuchsin may be used to improve visualization from smears of stools or pure cultures. The presence of fecal white cells is not a recommended test for predicting bacterial infection with *Campylobacter;* the absence of fecal leukocytes does not rule out

infection. Other screening tests for inflammation, including fecal lactoferrin and calprotectin, lack sensitivity and specificity for the diagnosis of gastroenteritis.

Antigen Detection

The use of culture independent tests (CIDT) for the diagnosis of *Campylobacter* infections has increased. Several commercial antigen detection systems are available for the direct detection of *Campylobacter* in stool specimens. These enzyme immunoassays (EIAs) can be used to detect antigens in stool samples for several days if stored at 4°C. These include the Premiere *Campylobacter* assay and ImmunoCard Stat! (Meridian Bioscience, Cincinnati, OH) and the ProSpecT microplate assay (Thermo Fisher Scientific, Waltham, MA), which detect both *C. jejuni* and *C. coli* but are not able to differentiate them. In addition, some EIAs have been reported to cross-react with *Campylobacter upsaliensis.* Because of the poor specificity and positive predictive value of the antigen detection tests, it is recommended that these tests not be used independently to diagnose *Campylobacter* infections.

Nucleic Acid Detection

Nucleic acid amplification provides an alternative to culture methods for the detection of *Campylobacter* spp. from clinical specimens. The detection of *Campylobacter* deoxyribonucleic acid (DNA) in stools from a large number of patients with diarrhea suggests that *Campylobacter* spp. other than *C. jejuni* and *C. coli* may account for a proportion of cases of acute gastroenteritis in which no causative agent is identified. Five nucleic acid–based test methods are US Food and Drug Administration (FDA)–approved for use in the United States. These include the xTAG Gastrointestinal Pathogen Panel and the Verigene enteric pathogens test (Luminex Corporation, Toronto, CA), BioFire Film Array Gastrointestinal Panel (bioMérieux Co, Durham, NC), Verigene (Nanosphere Inc., Northbrook, IL), and Prodesse ProGastro SSCS (Hologic, Marlborough, MA). These assays are highly sensitive and often used as the primary diagnostic tool for the identification of *Campylobacter* infections.

Although CIDT are rapid and provide same-day diagnosis in patients with *Campylobacter* gastroenteritis, it is recommended that the laboratory continue to cultivate these organisms. Culturing is necessary for antimicrobial susceptibility and monitoring outbreaks and may be required by the manufacturer of the nucleic acid or other methods.

Media

Campy-BA is an enriched selective blood agar plate used to isolate *C. jejuni.* The medium is composed of a *Brucella* agar base; sheep red blood cells; and vancomycin, trimethoprim, polymyxin B, amphotericin B, and cephalothin. **Campy medium (CVA)** contains cefoperazone, vancomycin, and amphotericin B. The antibiotics in both media suppress the growth of normal fecal flora. *Campylobacter* **agar base**

Campylobacter, Arcobacter, and *Helicobacter* 461

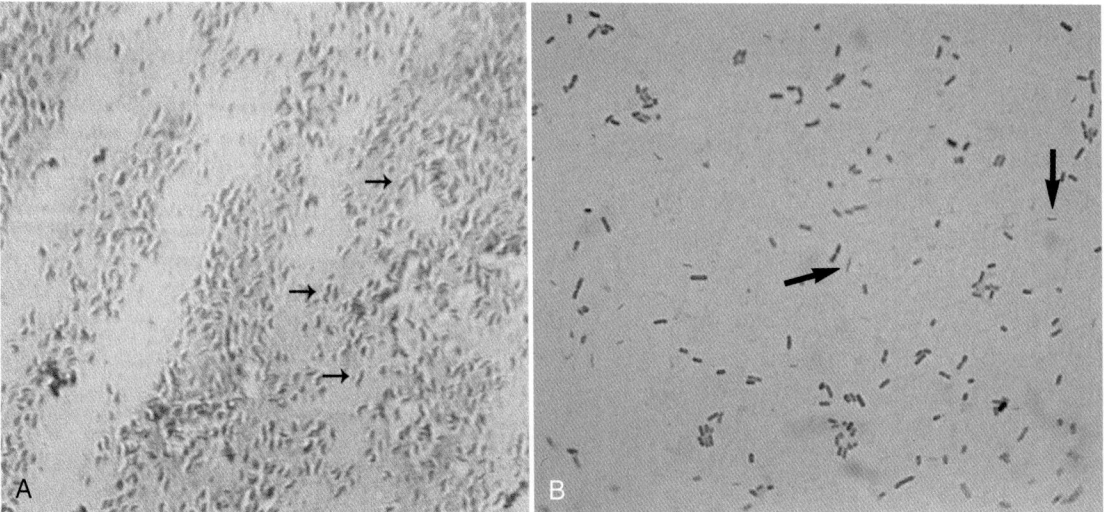

• **Fig. 33.2** (A) Gram stain appearance of *Campylobacter jejuni* subsp. *jejuni* from a colony on a primary isolation plate. Note seagull and curved forms *(arrows)*. (B) Appearance of *C. jejuni* subsp. *jejuni* in a direct Gram stain of stool obtained from a patient with campylobacteriosis. *Arrows* point to the seagull form.

blood free (CCDA) is a modified agar that does not include blood. The blood is replaced with charcoal, sodium pyruvate, and ferrous sulfate. The medium supports growth of most *Campylobacter* spp. An additional blood-free media is **charcoal-based selective medium (CSM).**

Cultivation

Stool

Successful isolation of *Campylobacter* spp. from stool requires selective media and optimal incubation conditions. Cultures should not be performed from formed stool for diagnostic purposes. Recommended inoculation of two selective agars is associated with increased recovery of the organisms. Reports indicate that CVA and CCDA demonstrate a higher recovery rate than blood-based media. Because *Campylobacter* and *Arcobacter* spp. have different optimum temperatures and atmospheric requirements, two sets of selective plates should be incubated, one at 42°C and one at 37°C with increased hydrogen. Extended incubation may be required (48 to 72 hours) before there is evidence of visible growth. In addition, *Campylobacter* spp. such as *C. concisus, C. upsaliensis, C. ureolyticus,* and *C. sputorum,* are not routinely isolated due to the nonthermophilic nature and/or inhibition by antibiotics included in the commonly used selective media.

A filtration method can also be used in conjunction with a nonselective medium to enhance recovery of *Campylobacter* and *Arcobacter* spp. A filter (0.45 to 0.65-μm pore-size polycarbonate or cellulose acetate) is placed on the agar surface, and a drop of stool is placed on the filter. The plate is incubated upright. After 60 minutes at 37°C, the filter is removed and the plates are reincubated in a microaerobic atmosphere. The organisms are motile and capable of migrating through the filter, producing isolated colonies on the agar surface and effectively removing contaminating stool microbiota. *C. concisus, A. butzleri, A.*

cryaerophilus, and *Helicobacter cinaedi* have been isolated after 5 to 6 days of incubation using the filter technique. An enrichment broth may be used for the recovery of *Arcobacter* or *Campylobacter* species from stool such as Preston enrichment, Campy-thio, and *Campylobacter* enrichment broth. The clinical advantage and cost-effectiveness of the use of enrichment broth has not been evaluated.

Blood

Campylobacter spp. are capable of growth in less than 5 days in most blood culture media, although they may require extended incubation periods of up to 2 weeks for detection. Subcultures should be incubated in 5% O_2, 10% CO_2, and 80% N_2 (microaerobic) environment. Turbidity may not be visible in blood culture media; therefore subcultures at 24 to 48 hours to a nonselective blood agar medium or microscopic examination using acridine orange stain may be necessary. The presence of *Campylobacter* spp. in blood cultures is effectively detected through carbon dioxide monitoring. Isolation from sources other than blood or feces is extremely rare. Recovery of the organisms is enhanced by inoculation (minced tissue, wound exudate) to a nonselective blood or chocolate agar plate and incubation at 37°C in a carbon dioxide–enriched, microaerobic atmosphere. Selective agars containing cephalosporin, rifampin, and polymyxin B may inhibit growth of some strains and should not be used for isolation from sterile sites.

Atmosphere

Campylobacter spp. require a microaerobic environment as previously indicated; however, not all species will grow in this environment. Some species, including *Campylobacter sputorum, C. concisus, C. mucosalis, C. curvus, C. rectus,* and *C. hyointestinalis* require increased hydrogen concentration for optimal growth. A gas mixture of 10% CO_2, 6% H_2, and 84% N_2 using an evacuation-replacement system such

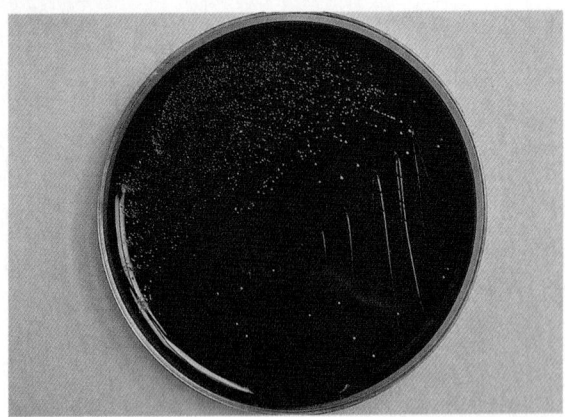

• **Fig. 33.3** Colonies of *Campylobacter jejuni* after 48 hours of incubation on a selective medium in a microaerobic atmosphere.

as the Anoxomat, Advanced Instruments, Norwood, MA (Chapter 40) is sufficient for growth of these organisms.

Approach to Identification

Plates should be examined for characteristic colonies, which are gray to pink or yellow gray and slightly mucoid; some colonies may exhibit a tailing effect along the streak line (Fig. 33.3). Colony morphology varies with the type of medium used for isolation. Suspicious-looking oxidase-positive colonies observed on selective media incubated at 42°C may be presumptively identified as *Campylobacter* spp., usually *C. jejuni* or *C. coli*. A wet preparation of the organism in broth can be examined for characteristic darting motility and curved morphology on Gram stain. Most isolates of *C. jejuni* subsp. *jejuni* can be distinguished from other *Campylobacter* species by the presence of sodium hippurate hydrolysis. *Campylobacter fetus* is incapable of growth at 42°C, and optimal growth is 37°C. Susceptibility or resistance to cephalothin and nalidixic-acid are no longer recommended for species identification due to the increasing fluoroquinolone resistance present in clinical isolates of *Campylobacter* spp. Table 33.2 provides characteristics for biochemical differentiation of the common clinically relevant organisms included in this chapter.

Almost all the pathogenic *Campylobacter* spp. are oxidase positive and catalase positive. Laboratories will commonly report stool isolates as "*Campylobacter* spp." Because *C. coli* and *C. jejuni* are similar, biochemically, molecular methods or MALDI-TOF is required to differentiate hippurate negative *C. jejuni*.

Most *Campylobacter* spp. are asaccharolytic, unable to grow in 3.5% NaCl, although strains of *Arcobacter* appear more resistant to salt and, except for *A. cryaerophilus*, unable to grow in ambient air requiring incubation in 10% O_2, 10% CO_2, and 80% N_2 at 37°C. Growth in 1% glycine is variable. Other tests useful for identifying these species are the rapid hippurate hydrolysis test, production of hydrogen sulfide (H_2S) in triple sugar iron agar slants, nitrate reduction, and hydrolysis of indoxyl acetate. Indoxyl acetate disks are available commercially. Cellular fatty acid analysis is useful for species identification. This method is not available in routine clinical microbiology laboratories.

Because *Campylobacter* and *Arcobacter* are difficult to identify using biochemical and phenotypic tests, nucleic acid (NAATS)–based amplification of the 16S and 23S ribosomal ribonucleic acid (rRNA) gene along with a variety of other targets and direct sequencing of the PCR products have successfully been used to identify most *Campylobacter* species. The assays accurately discriminate related taxa, including *Campylobacter*, *Arcobacter*, or *Helicobacter* species.

In addition to molecular methods, matrix-assisted laser desorption ionization time-of-flight mass spectrometry (MALDI-TOF MS) is increasingly being used to identify *Campylobacter* spp. Identification has been reported with 99% to 100% accuracy for *C. jejuni*, *C. coli*, *C. fetus* subsp. *fetus*, *Campylobacter lari*, and *A. butzleri*.

Serodiagnosis

Serodiagnosis is not widely applicable for the diagnosis of infections caused by these organisms.

Antimicrobial Susceptibility Testing and Therapy

C. jejuni and *C. coli* demonstrate variable susceptibility to many antimicrobial agents, including macrolides, tetracyclines, chloramphenicol, aminoglycosides, and quinolones. Erythromycin has been the drug of choice for patients with severe gastroenteritis (severe dehydration, bacteremia), with ciprofloxacin as an alternative therapeutic option. Ciprofloxacin resistance has been reported as high as 26.7% to 35.6% in *C. jejuni* and *C. coli*, with 25% to 50% resistance to erythromycin. Previously, fluoroquinolones were the antibiotic therapy most commonly prescribed for *Campylobacter* infection; however, a rapidly increasing proportion of *Campylobacter* strains worldwide have been identified as fluoroquinolone resistant. Parenteral therapy (not taken through the alimentary canal but by an alternate route, such as intravenously) is used to treat systemic *C. fetus* infections. *Arcobacter* spp. demonstrate variable resistance patterns to macrolides and fluoroquinolones.

The Clinical Laboratory Standards Institute (CLSI) recognizes broth microdilution and disk diffusion and ETEST (bioMérieux, Inc.) screening methods for susceptibility testing. Methodologies and breakpoints may vary; it is important to review the criteria used in the laboratory's region. Because of emerging resistance to fluoroquinolones, susceptibility testing is recommended for patients with *Campylobacter* spp. gastroenteritis. Susceptibility testing should be performed on all isolates from sterile fluids and body sites.

Prevention

No vaccines are available for *Campylobacter* spp. Infections caused by *Campylobacter* spp. are acquired by ingesting contaminated foodstuffs or water. Proper preparation and cooking of all foods derived from animal sources, particularly poultry, will decrease the risk of transmission. All milk

TABLE 33.2 Differential Characteristics of Clinically Relevant *Campylobacter* and *Arcobacter* spp.

Genus and Species	Growth at 25°C	H2 Required	Hippurate Hydrolysis	Catalase	H2S in Triple Sugar Iron Agar	Indoxyl Acetate Hydrolysis	Selenite Reduction	Urease
Campylobacter coli	-	-	-	+	-	+	+	-
Campylobacter concisus	-	+	-	-	+	-	V	-
Campylobacter curvus[a]	-	+	-	-	+	V	-	-
Campylobacter fetus subsp. *fetus*	+	-	-	+	-	-	V	+
Campylobacter fetus subsp. *venerealis*	+	-	-	V	-	-	V	-
Campylobacter gracilis	ND	ND	-	V	-	V	-	-
Campylobacter hominis[a]	-	+	-	-	-	-	-	ND
Campylobacter hyointestinalis subsp. *hycintestinalis*	V	V	-	+	+	-	+	-
Campylobacter jejuni subsp. *jejuni*	-	-	+	+	-	+	V	-
Campylobacter jejuni subsp. *doylei*	-	-	V	V	-	+	-	-
Campylobacter lari	-	-	-	+	-	-	V	V
Campylobacter pyloridis	ND	ND	-	+	ND	ND	ND	ND
Campylobacter rectus[a]	-	+	-	V	-	+	-	-
Campylobacter showae	-	+	-	+	-	V	-	-
Campylobacter sputorum bv. *sputorum*	-	+	-	-	+	-	V	-
Campylobacter upsaliensis	-	-	-	-	-	+	+	-
Campylobacter ureolyticus[a]	-	+	-	V	-	-	-	+
Arcobacter butzleri[b]	V	-	-	V	-	+	-	-
Arcobacter cryaerophilus[c]	+	-	-	V	-	+	-	-
Arcobacter skirrowii	+	-	-	+	-	+	ND	-

+, positive; –, negative; *ND,* test not determined; *V,* variable.
[a]Anaerobic, not microaerobic.
[b]Grows at 40°C.
[c]Aerotolerant, not microaerobic; except for a few strains, *A. cryaerophilus* cannot grow on MacConkey agar, but *A. butzleri* does.

should be pasteurized and drinking water chlorinated. Care must be taken during food preparation to prevent cross-contamination from raw poultry to other food items.

Helicobacter spp.

General Characteristics

Approximately 39 species are included in the genus *Helicobacter*, the majority of which colonize mammalian stomachs or enterohepatic regions (intestine, liver, and biliary tract). The genus *Helicobacter* consists of curved, helical or spiral, or fusiform microaerophilic, gram-negative rods with or without periplasmic fibers, with the majority of species exhibiting urease activity. The organisms may appear coccoid or spheroidal if cultivated for long periods or in suboptimal growth conditions.

Epidemiology and Pathogenesis

Helicobacter pylori's primary habitat is the human gastric mucosa. The organism is distributed worldwide and although acquired early in life in underdeveloped countries, the exact mode of transmission is unknown. An oral-oral, fecal-oral, and a common environmental source have been proposed as possible routes of transmission, with familial transmission associated with *H. pylori* infections. Research studies suggest mother-to-child transmission as well as among siblings and other household contacts as the most probable cause of intrafamilial spread. In industrialized nations, antibody surveys indicate that approximately 50% of adults older than 60 years are infected by *H. pylori*. Gastritis incidence increases with age. *H. pylori* has occasionally been cultured from feces and dental plaque, thereby suggesting a fecal-oral or oral-oral transmission.

The habitat for *H. heilmannii* and closely related species (*H. heilmannii*-like or HHLO) appears to be the human gastrointestinal tract with one or more species (*H salomonis, H. felis, H. suis*) of zoonotic origin. *H. heilmannii*, HHLO, and *H. pylori* may be normal microbiota of the human host. Additional enterohepatic species inhabit the intestinal and hepatobiliary tract of birds and mammals, such as *H. bilis, H. canadensis, H. canis, H. cinaedi, H. fennelliae,* and *H. pullorum.*

H. pylori is capable of colonizing the mucous layer of the antrum, cardia, and corpus of the stomach and areas of the gastric metaplasia of the proximal duodenum but fails to invade the epithelium. Motility allows *H. pylori* to escape the acidity of the stomach and burrow through and colonize the gastric mucosa in close association with the epithelium. In addition, the organism produces urease that hydrolyzes urea-forming ammonia (NH_3), significantly increasing the pH around the site of infection. The change in pH protects the organism from the acidic environment produced by gastric secretions. *H. pylori* also produces a protein called CagA and injects the protein into the gastric epithelial cells. The protein subsequently affects host cell gene expression, inducing cytokine release and altering cell structure, and interactions with

TABLE 33.3	Genes and Their Possible Role in Enhancing the Virulence of *Helicobacter pylori*
Gene	**Possible Role**
VacA	Exotoxin (VacA) Creates vacuoles in epithelial cells, decreases apoptosis, and loosens cell junctions
CagA	Pathogenicity island Encodes a type IV secretion system for transferring CagA proteins into host cells
BabA	Encodes outer membrane protein: mediates adherence to blood group antigens on the surface of gastric epithelial cells
IceA	Presence associated with peptic ulcer disease in some populations

neighboring cells, enabling *H. pylori* to successfully invade the gastric epithelium. Individuals who demonstrate positive antibody response to the CagA protein are at increased risk of developing both peptic ulcer disease and gastric carcinoma. Other possible virulence factors include adhesins for colonization of mucosal surfaces, mediators of inflammation, and a cytotoxin capable of causing damage to host cells (Table 33.3). Although *H. pylori* is noninvasive, untreated colonization persists despite the host's immune response.

Spectrum of Disease

H. pylori causes gastritis, peptic ulcer disease, and gastric cancer. However, most individuals tolerate the presence of *H. pylori* for decades with few, if any, symptoms. Infection with this organism is also a risk factor for the development of atrophic gastritis, gastric ulcer disease, gastric adenocarcinomas, and gastric mucosa–associated lymphoid tissue (MALT) lymphomas.

Enterohepatic helicobacters have been identified in association with human disease including *H. fennelliae, H. canis, H. cinaedi,* and *H. pullorum.* These isolates are transmitted from animals to humans and may be isolated from human blood or fecal samples. *H. cinaedi* and *H. fennelliae* have been isolated in cases of proctocolitis, gastroenteritis, neonatal meningitis, skin rashes, and bacteremia in immunocompromised patients. HHLO have been isolated in association with human cases of mild to moderate gastritis, peptic ulcer, and gastric MALT.

Laboratory Diagnosis
Specimen Collection, Transport, and Processing

Tissue biopsy material of the stomach for detection of *H. pylori* should be placed directly into transport media such as Stuart's transport medium, *Brucella* broth with 20% glycerol, or Portagerm pylori media (bioMérieux, Inc., Durham, NC) to prevent drying. Specimens for biopsy may be refrigerated up to 24 hours before processing; tissues should be minced and gently homogenized. If longer storage is required, samples should be frozen at –70°C in a 10% glycerol–containing medium.

Fecal specimens may be used for stool antigen tests but cannot be used for routine culture of gastric helicobacters. These samples should be tested immediately and stored at −20°C or according to the manufacturer's recommendations. Repeated freezing and thawing of specimens should be avoided. Enterohepatic helicobacters may be processed for culture using campylobacter protocols as previously described in this chapter.

Blood samples for serologic diagnosis of *Helicobacter* spp. infection may be collected, transported, and processed by standard methods. Gastric juice has been used for nucleic acid detection and culture of *H. pylori*.

Direct Detection

Gastric biopsy specimens that are preserved in 10% formaldehyde or paraffin-imbedded tissue are often used for the histopathologic diagnosis of *H. pylori* infection. Pathologists use the Warthin-Starry or other silver stains to examine biopsy specimens. Squash preparations of biopsy material can be performed and stained with rapid Giemsa stain, fluorescent acridine orange stain, or Gram stain. Gram stain using an alternate secondary stain, 0.5% carbolfuchsin or 0.1% basic fuchsin, enhances recognition of the bacteria's typical morphology. However, because of the presence of bacterial atypical morphologies, the results may not be interpreted correctly. Sampling error may occur during processing, resulting in no identification of the organisms.

Presumptive evidence of the presence of *H. pylori* in biopsy material may be obtained by placing a portion of crushed tissue biopsy material directly into urease broth, onto commercially available urease agar kits, or on a paper strip containing a pH indicator. These tests are collectively referred to as rapid urease tests (RUTs). A positive test is considered indicative of the organism's presence. The CLOtest (Kimberly-Clark, Neenah, Murray Hill, NG) is an example of an agar-gel based RUT (Fig. 33.4).

Another noninvasive indirect test to detect *H. pylori* is the urea breath test (UBT). This test relies on the presence of *H. pylori* urease. The patient ingests nonradioactively labeled natural isotope (^{13}C) urea, and if the organism is present, the urease produced by *H. pylori* hydrolyzes the urea to form ammonia and labeled bicarbonate that is exhaled as $^{13}CO_2$; the $^{13}CO_2$ is detected by a special spectrometer. This test has excellent sensitivity and specificity. EIA *H. pylori* stool antigen tests (Premier Platinum HpSA, Meridian Diagnostics, Inc., Cincinnati, OH, or IDEIA Hp StAR, Oxoid Ltd., Basingstoke, United Kingdom) and rapid immunochromatographic point of care assays using monoclonal antibodies (ImmunoCard STAT! HpSA, Meridian Bioscience, Cincinnati, OH, or *RAPID* Hp StAR, Oxoid Ltd., Basingstoke, United Kingdom) have been introduced to directly detect *H. pylori*.

Nucleic Acid Detection

A variety of nucleic acid–based methods have been developed to directly detect *H. pylori* and HHLO in clinical specimens and to identify bacterial strains and host genotype characteristics, bacterial density in the stomach, and antimicrobial

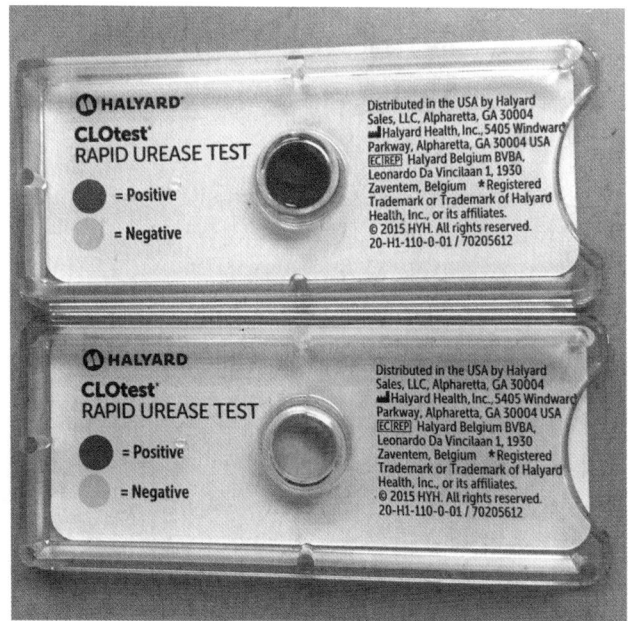

• **Fig. 33.4** CLOtest Rapid Urease Test indicating a positive reaction *(top test)* and a negative reaction *(bottom test)*.

resistance patterns. Polymerase chain amplification and fluorescence *in situ* hybridization using species-specific probes has enhanced the diagnosis and detection in gastric biopsy specimens. Amplification targets include the 16S RNA, 23S rRNA *ureA*, *glmM*, *vacA*, and *cagA* genes. Interpretation of nucleic acid–based methods should be used in conjunction with other diagnostics methods. There are no methods available for the detection of enterohepatic *Helicobacter* species of clinical relevance at the time of this writing.

Varieties of methods are under development for the direct detection of *H. pylori* nucleic acids in feces. These techniques are problematic in that DNA is often degraded when passing through the gastrointestinal tract as well as the presence of a variety of amplification enzyme inhibitors in feces. Potential new methods are expected to be placed in clinical trials and submitted for FDA approval that would not only detect the organism but also the presence of mutations that confer macrolide resistance.

Cultivation

Stool specimens submitted for culture of enterohepatic helicobacters such as *H. bilis*, *H. canadensis*, *H. canis*, *H. cinaedi*, *H. fennelliae*, and *H. pullorum* are inoculated onto selective media used for *Campylobacter* isolation but without cephalothin, such as Campy-CVA. *H. cinaedi*, *H. canis*, and *H. fennelliae* have been occasionally isolated from commercial blood culture systems in patients suspected of bacteremia. The recovery of *H. pylori* from tissue biopsy specimens, including gastric antral biopsies; nonselective agar media, including brain heart infusion agar, and *Brucella* agar with 5% sheep blood; **Wilkins Chalgren agar;** and trypticase soy agar have resulted in successful recovery of the organisms. The combination of a selective agar (Columbia agar with an egg yolk emulsion, supplements, and antibiotics) and a nonselective

TABLE 33.4 Differential Characteristics of *Helicobacter* Species

Species	Catalase	Urease	Indoxyl Acetate Hydrolysis	Nitrate	Alkaline Phosphatase	Gamma-glutamyl Transpeptidase
H. bilis	+	+	–	+	–	+
H. canis	–	–	+	–	+	+
H. canadensis	+	–	+	+	–	–
H. cinaedi	+	–	–	+	–	–
H. felis	+	+	–	+	+	+
H. fennelliae	+	–	+	–	+	–
H. heilmanni	ND	+	ND	ND	ND	ND
H. salomonis	+	+	+	+	+	+
H. suis	+	+	–		+	+
H. pullorum	+	–	–	+	–	ND

+, Positive; –, negative; *ND*, test not determined.

agar (modified chocolate agar with Columbia agar, 1% **Vitox**, and 5% sheep blood) was reported as the optimal combination for recovering *H. pylori* from antral biopsies. Incubation up to 1 week in a humidified, microaerobic environment (4% O_2, 5% CO_2, 5% H_2, and 86% N_2 atmosphere) at 35°C to 37°C may be required before growth is visible.

Approach to Identification

Colonies of *Helicobacter* spp. may require 4 to 7 days of incubation before growth is observed. Colonies may appear as small, translucent, circular colonies or swarming phenotypes from some gastric isolates. Culture plates should be reviewed daily for a minimum of 10 days before a negative culture is reported. Organisms are identified presumptively as *H. pylori* by the typical cellular morphology and positive results for oxidase, catalase, and RUT. *H. pylori* and some enterohepatic species may be definitively identified by using a similar approach to *Campylobacter* spp. However, on subculture these organisms may lose their classic morphology, making identification difficult. MALDI-TOF has been successfully used to identify *H. pylori* from cultures of gastric biopsy specimens (Table 33.4).

Serodiagnosis

Serologic diagnosis is also available for *H. pylori*. The immune response typically presents with a rise in immunoglobulin M (IgM), followed by immunoglobulin G (IgG) and immunoglobulin A (IgA), although 2% of patients fail to seroconvert. Numerous serologic EIAs designed to detect IgG and IgA antibodies to *H. pylori* are commercially available. Reported performance of these assays varies depending on the reference method used to confirm *H. pylori* infection, the antigen source for the assay, and the population studied. In addition to variability in assay performance, the clinical utility of IgA testing in these assays is controversial. In some cases, IgA has demonstrated a much lower sensitivity and specificity than IgG for the detection of *H. pylori* infections. These assays are incapable of differentiation of active versus past *H. pylori* infections. As of this writing, there are no serologic assays for the routine diagnosis of HHLO or enterohepatic *Helicobacter* spp.

Antimicrobial Susceptibility Testing and Therapy

Except for metronidazole and clarithromycin, most laboratory susceptibility assays are unsuccessful in predicting clinical outcome. Routine testing of *H. pylori* isolates' susceptibility to metronidazole is recommended using the ETEST and agar or broth dilution methods.

Therapy for *H. pylori* infection is problematic. *H. pylori* readily becomes resistant when metronidazole, clarithromycin, azithromycin, rifampin, or ciprofloxacin is prescribed as a single agent. Current regimens recommend triple-drug therapy including a proton pump inhibitor, clarithromycin, and either amoxicillin or metronidazole. An alternative treatment for *H. pylori* infection includes fluoroquinolone, levofloxacin, and a rifamycin (rifabutin). Similar treatments have demonstrated successful therapy in patients with gastritis and peptic ulcer disease associated with HHLO. No guidelines exist for the treatment of enterohepatic helicobacters.

Prevention

No vaccines are available for *H. pylori*.

ⓔ Visit the Evolve site for a complete list of procedures, review questions, and case studies.

Bibliography

Allos BM: *Campylobacter jejuni* infections: update on emerging issues and trends, *Clin Infect Dis* 32:1201–1206, 2001.

Blaser MJ: The biology of cag in the *Helicobacter pylori*-human interaction, *Gastroenterology* 128:1512–1515, 2005.

Bullman S, Lucid A, Corcoran D, Sleator RD, Lucey B: Genomic investigation into strain heterogeneity and pathogenic potential of the emerging gastrointestinal pathogen *Campylobacter ureolyticus, PloS One* 8:e71515, 2013.

Butzler JP: *Campylobacter,* from obscurity to celebrity, *Clin Microbiol Infect* 10:868–876, 2004.

Carroll KC, Pfaller MA, Landry ML, et al.: *Manual of clinical microbiology,* ed 12, Washington, DC, 2019, ASM Press.

Crowe SE: *Helicobacter* infection, chronic inflammation, and the development of malignancy, *Curr Opin Gastroenterol* 21:32–38, 2005.

Day AS, Jones NL, Lynetl JT, et al.: cagE is a virulence factor associated with *Helicobacter pylori*-induced duodenal ulceration in children, *J Infect Dis* 181:1370–1375, 2000.

Engberg J, On SL, Harrington CS, Gerner-Smidt P: Prevalence of *Campylobacter, Arcobacter, Helicobacter,* and *Sutterella* spp. in human fecal samples as estimated by a reevaluation of isolation methods for campylobacters, *J Clin Microbiol* 38:286–291, 2000.

Fitzgerald C, Patrick M, Gonzalez A, et al.: Multicenter evaluation of clinical diagnostic methods for detection and isolation of *Campylobacter* spp. from stool, *J Clin Microbiol* 54:1209–1215, 2016.

Gemmell MR, Berry S, Mukhopadhya I, et al.: Comparative genomics of *Campylobacter concisus*: analysis of clinical strains reveals genome diversity and pathogenic potential, *Emerg Microbes Infect* 7:116, 2018.

Gonzalez MD, Wilen CB, Burnham CA: Markers of intestinal inflammation for the diagnosis of infectious gastroenteritis, *Clin Lab Med* 35:333–344, 2015.

Gorkiewicz G, Feierl G, Schober C, et al.: Species-specific identification of campylobacters by partial 16S rRNA gene sequencing, *J Clin Microbiol* 41:2537–2546, 2003.

Hsieh YH, Wang YF, Moura H, et al.: Application of MALDI-TOF MS systems in the rapid identification of *Campylobacter* spp. of public health importance, *J AOAC Int* 101:761–768, 2018.

Han S, Zschausch H, Meyer HW, et al.: *Helicobacter pylori:* clonal population structure and restricted transmission within families revealed by molecular typing, *J Clin Microbiol* 38:3646–3651, 2000.

Konno M, Fujii N, Yakota S, et al.: Five-year follow-up study of mother-to-child transmission of *Helicobacter pylori* infection detected by a random amplified polymorphic DNA fingerprinting method, *J Clin Microbiol* 43:2246–2250, 2005.

Leber AL: Fecal and other gastrointestinal cultures and toxin assays; fecal cultures for campylobacter and related organisms and gastroenteritis panels. In *Clinical microbiology procedures handbook,* ed 4, Washington, DC, 2016, ASM Press.

Maher M, Finnegan C, Collins E, et al.: Evaluation of culture methods and a DNA probe-based PCR assay for detection of *Campylobacter* species in clinical specimens of feces, *J Clin Microbiol* 41:2980–2986, 2003.

Matsui H, Takahashi T, Murayama SY, et al.: Development of new PCR primers by comparative genomics for the detection of *Helicobacter suis* in gastric biopsy specimens, *Helicobacter* 19:260–271, 2014.

Nachamkin I, Nguyen P: Isolation of *Campylobacter* species from stool samples by use of a filtration method: assessment from a United States-based population, *J Clin Microbiol* 7:2204–2207, 2017.

O'Donovan D, Corcoran GD, Lucey B, Sleator RD: *Campylobacter ureolyticus:* a portrait of the pathogen, *Virulence* 5:498–506, 2014.

Pereira V, Abraham P, Nallapeta S, Shetty A: Gastric bacterial flora in patients harbouring *Helicobacter pylori* with or without chronic dyspepsia: analysis with matrix-assisted laser desorption ionization time-of-flight mass spectroscopy, *BMC Gastroenterol* 18:20, 2018.

Rieder G, Fischer W, Haas R: Interaction of *Helicobacter pylori* with host cells: function of secreted and translocated molecules, *Curr Opin Microbiol* 8:67–73, 2005.

Sakar SR, Hossain MA, Pual SK, Mahmud MC, Ray NC, Haque N: Use of modified blood agar plate for identification of pathogenic campylobacter species at Mymensingh Medical College, *Mymensingh Med J* 23:667–671, 2014.

Simala-Grant J, Taylor DE: Molecular biology methods for the characterization of *Helicobacter pylori* infections and their diagnosis, *APMIS* 112:886–897, 2004.

Vandenberg O, Dediste A, Houf K, et al.: *Arcobacter* species in humans, *Emerg Infect Dis* 10:1863–1867, 2004.

34

Legionella

GENUS AND SPECIES TO BE CONSIDERED

Legionella dumoffii
Legionella micdadei
Legionella longbeachae
Legionella pneumophila
   L. pneumophila subsp. *pneumophila*
   L. pneumophila subsp. *fraseri*
   L. pneumophila subsp. *pascullei*
Legionella spp.

Legionella belongs to the family *Legionellaceae,* which includes a single genus, *Legionella,* comprising approximately 59 species and 3 subspecies. *Legionella pneumophila* is the causative agent of **Legionnaires' disease,** a febrile and pneumonic illness with numerous clinical presentations. *Legionella* was discovered in 1976 by scientists at the Centers for Disease Control and Prevention (CDC) who were investigating an epidemic of pneumonia among Pennsylvania State American Legion members attending a convention in Philadelphia. There is retrospective serologic evidence of *Legionella* infection as far back as 1947. Bacteria resembling *Legionella* that are capable of living in amoebae have been designated as **Legionella-like amoebal pathogens (LLAPs).** *Legionella lytica,* one of the LLAPs, has been shown to cause human disease.

General Characteristics

All *Legionella* spp. are mesophilic (20°C to 42°C), obligately aerobic, faintly staining, thin, gram-negative, fastidious bacilli. *Legionella* do not grow on routine media and require a medium supplemented with iron, L-cysteine, branched-chain fatty acids, and ubiquinones and buffered to pH 6.9 for optimal growth. The organisms are asaccharolytic and utilize protein for energy generation. The overwhelming majority of *Legionella* spp. are motile. There are approximately 26 species of *Legionella* documented as human pathogens in addition to *L. pneumophila*. There have been more than 500 strains of *L. pneumophila* that have been completely sequenced, which indicates that the species is genetically diverse. The gene sequence for the lipopolysaccharide core and the O side chain for serogroup 1 demonstrates a predominance in clinical isolates of *L. pneumophila*. Box 34.1 is an abbreviated list of some of the species of *Legionella*.

Epidemiology

Legionellae are ubiquitous and widely distributed in the environment. As a result, most individuals are exposed to *Legionella* spp.; however, few develop symptoms. In nature, legionellae are found primarily in aquatic habitats and thrive at warmer temperatures; these bacteria can survive extreme ranges of environmental conditions for long periods; studies have shown that *Legionella* spp. are capable of survival for several months in free-flowing water. The organisms exist in microbial biofilms as intracellular parasites of free-living amoebae including *Acanthamoeba* and *Naegleria* spp. *Legionella* spp. have been isolated from most natural water sources investigated, including lakes, rivers, and marine waters, as well as moist soil. Organisms are also widely distributed in man-made facilities, including air-conditioning ducts and cooling towers; potable water; large, warm-water plumbing systems; humidifiers; whirlpools; and technical-medical equipment in hospitals. *L. longbeachae*, first isolated in Long Beach, California, is found predominantly in potting soil and compost.

Legionella infections are acquired exclusively from environmental sources; no person-to-person spread has been documented. Inhalation and aspiration of infectious aerosols (1–5 μm in diameter) are considered the primary means of transmission. Exposure to these aerosols can occur in the workplace or in industrial or health care settings; for example, nebulizers filled with tap water and showers have been implicated.

• BOX 34.1 *Legionella* spp. Isolated From Human Sources

Legionella pneumophila
Legionella anisa
Legionella birminghamensis
Legionella cardiaca
Legionella cincinnatiensis
Legionella micdadei
Legionella bozemanae
Legionella dumoffii
Legionella feeleii
Legionella gormanii
Legionella hackeliae
Legionella jordanis
Legionella lansingensis
Legionella londiniensis
Legionella lytica
Legionella maceachernii
Legionella nagasakiensis
Legionella norrlandica
Legionella longbeachae
Legionella oakridgensis
Legionella parisiensis
Legionella rubrilucens
Legionella sainthelensi
Legionella steelei
Legionella tucsonensis
Legionella wadsworthii

Pathogenesis and Spectrum of Disease

The virulence mechanisms of *Legionella* spp. are an important factor in the ability to infect and subsequently multiply within amoebae (*Acanthamoeba* and *Naegleria* spp.); *Tetrahymena* spp., a ciliated protozoan; and certain host cells. The organism can also multiply within biofilms, well-organized microcolonies of bacteria usually enclosed in polymer matrices that are separated by water channels that remove wastes and deliver nutrients. This contributes to the organism's survival in the environment. In addition, *L. pneumophila* exists in two well-defined, morphologically distinct forms in Hela cells: (1) a highly differentiated, cystlike form that is highly infectious, metabolically dormant, and resistant to antibiotics and detergent-mediated lysis and (2) a replicative intracellular form that is structurally similar to agar-grown bacteria. The existence of the cystlike form may account for the ability of *L. pneumophila* to survive for long periods between hosts (amoebae or humans).

L. pneumophila is considered a facultative intracellular pathogen. The organism causes disease by infecting human monocytes, predominantly alveolar macrophages. Once inside the macrophage, the organism is able to avoid destruction by the host's phagocytic cells and multiply. Molecular analysis of *L. pneumophila* has demonstrated that the organism's genome contains eukaryotic-like gene sequences that in effect subvert the normal eukaryotic cellular functions for intracellular survival. The pathogenesis of *L. pneumophila* has been extensively studied; however, little is known about the pathogenic mechanisms associated with other *Legionella* spp.

Legionella have a similar life cycle in both protozoa and human macrophages, as illustrated in Fig. 34.1:

- Binding of microorganisms to receptors on the surface of eukaryotic cells
- Penetration of microorganisms into phagocytes
- Escape from bactericidal attack
- Formation of a **replicative vacuole** (a compartment within the cell where bacterial replication occurs)

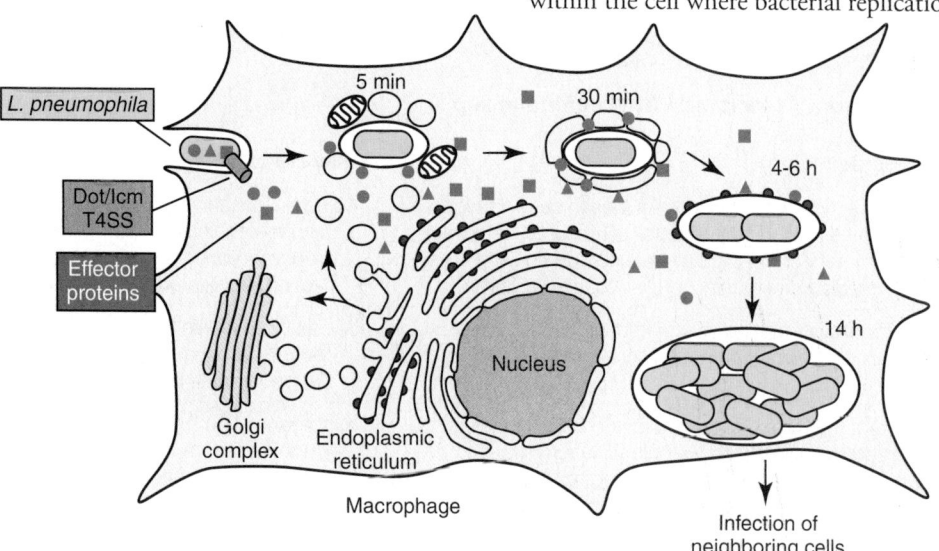

• Fig. 34.1 *Legionella pneumophila* cellular trafficking and growth mechanism inside a human macrophage. (Modified from 2009 annualreport.nichd.nih.gov/ump.html.)

- Intracellular multiplication and killing of the host cell

There are differences in the mechanisms used to enter and exit from the respective type of host cell. After infection, organisms are taken up by phagocytosis primarily in alveolar macrophages. Almost immediately following phagocytosis, *L. pneumophila* injects hundreds of pathogenicity effector molecules into the host macrophage using a type IVB secretion system (Dot or Icm). Strains that do not have the type IVB secretion system are avirulent. A type IVB secretion system has been identified in *Legionella dumoffii*. Once inside the host macrophage, the microorganism survives and replicates within a specialized, membrane-bound vacuole by resisting acidification and evading fusion with lysosomes. After replication, the organisms will kill the phagocytes, releasing them into the lungs. The organisms will again be phagocytized by a mononuclear cell, and multiplication of the organism will increase.

Many bacterial pathogens use secretion systems as a part of how they cause disease. *L. pneumophila* utilizes the type IVB secretion system, referred to as **defective organelle trafficking (Dot)** or **intracellular multiplication (Icm)**, to "trick" the eukaryotic macrophage into transporting the organism to the endoplasmic reticulum. In eukaryotic cells, most proteins secreted or transported inside vesicles to other cellular compartments are synthesized at the endoplasmic reticulum (ER) (Fig. 34.1). This Dot/Icm secretion system in *L. pneumophila* consists of 27 genes. Bacterial type IV secretion systems are bacterial devices that deliver macromolecules such as proteins across and into cells. After entry but before bacterial replication, *L. pneumophila*, residing in a membrane-bound vacuole, is surrounded by a ribosome-studded membrane derived from the host cell's ER and mitochondria. Thus, by exploiting host cell functions, *L. pneumophila* is able to gain access to the lumen of the ER, which supports its survival and replication where the environment is rich in peptides. A second type II secretion system has also been implicated in the virulence of some strains of *Legionella*. The **type II secretion system** carries numerous genes for enzymatic degradation, including lipases, proteinases, and a number of proinflammatory or tissue destructive proteins. The type II secretion system produces a number of novel proteins that permit growth of the organism in low temperatures, is required for biofilm establishment, sliding motility, and intracellular infection. Mutations within the type II secretion system result in decreased infectivity of the organism. *Legionella* is the only intracellular pathogen known to possess a functional type II secretion system. Several additional bacterial factors have also been identified as crucial for intracellular infection; some of these are listed in Box 34.2.

Finally, several cellular components and extracellular products of *L. pneumophila*, such as an extracellular cytotoxin that impairs the ability of phagocytic cells to use oxygen and various enzymes (e.g., phospholipase C), have been purified and proposed as virulence factors.

The sequestering of *Legionella* within macrophages also makes it difficult to treat the infection effectively with antimicrobial agents. Therefore, a competent cell-mediated immune response is also important for recovery from *Legionella* infections. Humoral immunity appears to play an insignificant role in the defense against this organism.

Legionellosis is a spectrum of clinical presentations, ranging from asymptomatic infection to severe, life-threatening diseases. Serologic evidence exists for the presence of asymptomatic disease, because many healthy people tested possess antibodies to *Legionella* spp. Table 34.1 provides a

---

• BOX 34.2   Examples of *Legionella pneumophila* Factors Crucial for Intracellular Infection

- Heat shock protein 60
- Outer membrane protein
- Macrophage infectivity potentiator
- Genes encoding for the type II secretion systems required for intracellular growth
- Type IV pili
- Flagella
- Dot/Icm type IVB secretion system

TABLE 34.1   Disease Spectrum Associated With *Legionella* spp.

	Epidemiology	Disease
Pneumonia (Legionnaires' disease)	Community and nosocomial, health care–associated transmission (inhalation of aerosolized particles); immunocompromised patients, particularly in cell-mediated immunity; rarely occurs in children	Acute pneumonia indistinguishable from other bacterial pneumonias; clinical syndrome may include nonproductive cough, myalgia, diarrhea, hyponatremia, hypophosphatemia, and elevated liver enzymes.
Pontiac fever	Community setting associated with employment (industrial or recreational) or other group	Self-limiting, febrile illness; symptoms may include cough, dyspnea, abdominal pain, fever, and myalgia; pneumonia does not occur.
Extrapulmonary	Rare, metastatic complications from underlying pneumonia; incidents of inoculation into sites via punctures have been identified; therapeutic bathing; highly associated with immunocompromised patients	Abscesses have been identified in the brain, spleen, lymph nodes, muscles, surgical wounds, and a variety of tissues and organs.

From Bennett J, Dolin R, Blaser M: *Principles and practice of infectious diseases*, ed 9, Philadelphia, 2020, Elsevier-Saunders.

more detailed description of the following three primary clinical manifestations:

- Legionnaires' disease is a severe pneumonia with a case fatality rate of 10% to 20%. It is a global public health issue. Legionnaires' disease occurs in sporadic, endemic, and epidemic forms. The incidence of the disease varies greatly and appears to depend on the geographic area, but it is estimated that *Legionella* spp. cause less than 1% to 5% of cases of pneumonia.
- A mild, self-limited, nonfatal, influenza-like (e.g., fever, headache, malaise) respiratory infection known as **Pontiac fever.**
- Other rare extrapulmonary sites, such as wound abscesses, encephalitis, or endocarditis.

The disease can affect anyone but principally affects those who are susceptible because of age, illness, immunosuppression, or other risk factors, such as heavy smoking. The clinical manifestations after infection with a particular species are primarily caused by differences in the host's immune response and perhaps by inoculum size; the same *Legionella* spp. gives rise to different expressions of disease in different individuals.

L. longbeachae is the second most common cause of legionellosis. Infections associated with *L. longbeachae* are particularly common in Australia, but cases have been documented in other countries including the United States. The infection is most likely due to inhalation or aspiration of contaminated dust compost or soil and can be very serious, often leading to hospitalization and sometimes death. *Legionella micdadei* is believed to be associated with approximately 60% of Legionnaire's disease not caused by *L. pneumophila* or *L. longbeachae*. This organism has been predominantly isolated from immunocompromised patients.

There are a few bacteria that grow within amoebae and are closely related phylogenetically based on 16S ribosomal ribonucleic acid (rRNA) gene sequencing to *Legionella* species: LLAPs. Several LLAPs have been assigned to the *Legionella* genus. One LLAP has been isolated from the sputum of a patient with pneumonia after the specimen was incubated with the amoeba *Acanthamoeba polyphaga*. Serologic surveys of patients with community-acquired pneumonia suggest LLAPs may be occasional human pathogens.

Laboratory Diagnosis

Although culture remains the gold standard for the diagnosis of Legionnaires' disease, it is currently diagnosed with a urinary antigen test that is highly accurate for *L. pneumophila* serogroup 1. The use of selective culture media yields a high sensitivity and specificity. Other diagnostic tests, including serotyping and nucleic acid sequencing are used to fully characterize clinical isolates of *Legionella* spp.

Specimen Collection and Transport

Specimens from which *Legionella* can be isolated include respiratory tract secretions of all types, including expectorated sputum, additional lower respiratory specimens including pleural fluid, bronchoscopy specimens, and lung biopsy specimens. Rare sources associated with infection include other sterile body fluids, such as pericardial fluid and specimens from kidney, liver, spleen, myocardium, respiratory sinuses, skin, soft tissues, wounds, peritoneal fluid, joint fluids, bone marrow, and intestine. Because sputum from patients with Legionnaires' disease is usually nonpurulent and may appear bloody or watery, the grading system used for screening sputum for routine cultures may not be applicable. Patients with Legionnaires' disease usually have detectable numbers of organisms in their respiratory secretions, even for some time after antibiotic therapy has been initiated. If the disease is present, the initial specimen is often likely to be positive. However, additional specimens should be processed if the first specimen is negative, and suspicion of the disease persists. Pleural fluid has not yielded many positive cultures in studies performed in several laboratories, but it may contain organisms and should be processed if available. Urine for antigen collection should be collected in a sterile container. The sample should be transported to the laboratory and refrigerated if a delay in processing occurs. Specimens should be transported without holding media, buffers, or saline, which may inhibit the growth of *Legionella*. The organisms are hardy and are best preserved by maintaining specimens in a small, tightly closed container to prevent desiccation and transporting them to the laboratory within 30 minutes of collection. If a longer delay is anticipated, specimens should be refrigerated. If moisture of the specimens cannot be ensured, 1 mL of sterile broth may be added. Samples collected for *Legionella* spp. nucleic acid testing do not require special collection or processing.

Specimen Processing

All specimens for *Legionella* culture should be handled and processed in a class II biologic safety cabinet (BSC). When specimens from nonsterile body sites are submitted for culture, selective media or treatment of the specimen to reduce the numbers of contaminating organisms is proposed. Brief treatment of sputum specimens with hydrochloric acid before culture has been shown to enhance the recovery of legionellae. However, this technique is time consuming and is recommended for specimens from patients with cystic fibrosis. Respiratory secretions may be held for up to 48 hours at 5°C before culture; if culturing is delayed longer, then the specimen may be frozen.

Tissues are homogenized before smears and cultures are performed, and clear, sterile body fluids are centrifuged for 30 minutes at 4000 × *g*. The sediment is then vortexed and used for culture and smear preparation. Blood for culture of *Legionella* may be processed with the lysis-centrifugation tube system (Isolator, Alere, Inc., Waltham, MA) and plated directly to **buffered charcoal–yeast extract (BCYE) agar.** Specimens collected by bronchoalveolar lavage are quite dilute and therefore should be concentrated at least tenfold by centrifugation before culturing.

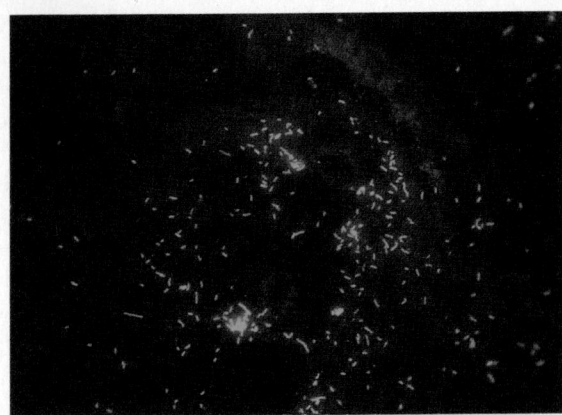

• **Fig. 34.2** Fluorescent antibody–stained *Legionella pneumophila*.

Direct Detection Methods

Several laboratory methods are used to detect *Legionella* spp. directly in clinical specimens.

Microscopy

Legionella spp. are small, gram-negative coccobacilli or short rods when directly observed in a clinical specimen. However, in indirect microscopy when examining an isolate from artificial culture media, the organism appears as long, filamentous bacilli. *Legionella* spp. have a thin cell wall and stain poorly in the Gram procedure if neutral red or safranin is used as the counterstain. This characteristic is related to the composition of the cell walls, which have large amounts of branched-chain cellular fatty acids. Because of their faint staining, intracellular form in human tissues and large amounts of proteinaceous material in clinical specimens, *Legionella* spp. are not usually detectable directly in clinical material by Gram stain. The use of 0.1% fuchsin substituted for safranin in the Gram-stain procedure may enhance the visibility of the organisms. Organisms can be observed on histologic examination of tissue sections using silver stains. However, these stains generally lack sensitivity and produce significant artifacts making interpretation highly complex. *L. micdadei* stains with acid-fast stain in fresh and formalin fixed tissue.

Direct immunofluorescent microscopy is the most sensitive and specific method for the detection of *L. pneumophila* in respiratory samples and tissue. The sensitivity of the DFA test ranges from 25% to 75%, and its specificity is greater than 95%. If positive, organisms appear as brightly fluorescent rods (Fig. 34.2). The high complexity of the test and lack of highly reproducible sensitivity discourage many laboratories from offering DFA testing, and it is rarely used except during autopsies.

Antigens

Microtube-based enzyme immunoassay (EIA) methods can be used to serologically diagnose *L. pneumophila* serogroup 1 in tissues. Several EIA serologic diagnostic kits are commercially available, with sensitivity ranging from 80% to 90% and a specificity of about 98%. The sensitivity of kits for testing antibody from other serotypes is still unknown.

Rapid detection of *Legionella* antigen in urine and other body fluids has been accomplished by commercially available EIA kits and by immunochromatography (ICT); however, the ICT have demonstrated up to a 40% decrease in sensitivity compared to the microtube-based immunoassays. Detecting the antigen in urine allows for early diagnosis of the infection. The antigen is detectable in most patients between 1 and 3 days after the onset of symptoms and may persist for some weeks or months. The urine antigen assays are 90% to 99.9% specific, which is similar to the traditional culture method, but may have greater sensitivity than culture. Compared with other diagnostic methods, the advantages of urinary antigen detection are striking. Specimens are easily obtained, the antigen is detectable very early in the course of disease, and the test is rapid and specific. A rapid immunochromatographic assay for detecting *L. pneumophila* serogroup 1 antigen in urine is also available. This assay detects urinary antigen within a very short time and does not require laboratory equipment. Concentration of urine improves the sensitivity of both the EIA and immunochromatographic assays without decreasing their specificity. A drawback of the immunochromatographic urine antigen assay is that it only detects the presence of antigen of *L. pneumophila* serogroup 1, which constitutes 80% to 90% of all *Legionella* infections. In addition, false positives may occur in urine in the presence of rheumatoid-like factors, urinary sediment, and freeze thawing of urine. All positive urine antigen tests should be confirmed. The urine sample should be clarified by brief centrifugation and boiled for 5 to 15 minutes (dependent on protocol) to remove rheumatoid-like factors.

Nucleic Acid Detection

Polymerase chain reaction (PCR) assays have been extensively used to detect deoxyribonucleic acid (DNA) from environmental and clinical samples, particularly those from the respiratory tract. Traditionally, the rRNA (16S and 23S) genes and the macrophage infectivity protein (*mip*) gene have been used for assays targeting the *Legionella* genus and the serogroup 1 target (*wzm*) gene for *L. pneumophila*–specific assays. Assays for *Legionella* and *L. pneumophila* using real-time PCR platforms have also been described. With respiratory samples, *Legionella* PCR has a reported specificity of more than 99% and sensitivity of 80% to 100%. An important feature of *Legionella* PCR is that the method can potentially detect all serogroups of *L. pneumophila* and other species and is therefore useful in the early diagnosis of infections, particularly in health care–associated cases and outbreak investigations.

Although no FDA-cleared nucleic acid–based tests are available in the United States, they are available in Europe. Nucleic acid amplification tests have demonstrated an 11% increase in positive yields over urine antigen testing. This may be a result of the predominance of serogroup I and the Pontiac subgroup in infections. NAAT may also demonstrate improved sensitivity in immunocompromised patients because of the low sensitivity of urine testing in these patients.

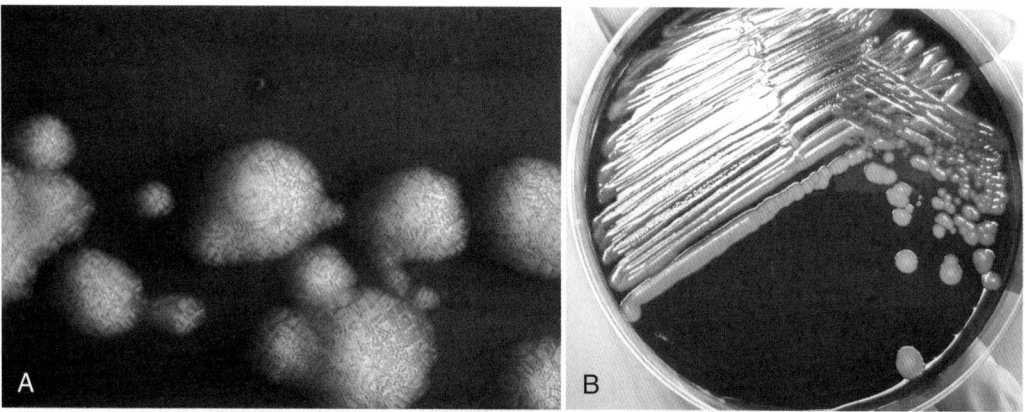

• **Fig. 34.3** (A) Colonies of *Legionella pneumophila* demonstrating the cut-glass internal granular speckling. (B) Colonies of *Legionella pneumophila* on buffered charcoal–yeast extract agar demonstrating blue-green glistening. (Photo courtesy Brooks Murillo-Kennedy, Houston, TX.)

Cultivation

The specimen should be processed for cultivation by diluting the specimen 1:10 in tryptic soy broth or distilled water to reduce inhibition by tissue and serum factors or decontamination for sputum and respiratory specimens to remove contaminating and inhibitory normal microbiota. Decontamination to reduce contaminating microbiota in sputum and respiratory samples should be completed using a 1:10 dilution of a low pH KCl-HCl buffer (pH 2.2) and incubating at room temperature for 4 minutes prior to plating. An alternative method for decontamination is heading at 50°C for 30 minutes. Primary isolation of *Legionella* spp. should be carried out by inoculating a nonselective media and two different selective media. Specimens for recovery of *Legionella* should be inoculated to at least one BCYEα agar plate containing L-cysteine and α-ketoglutarate without inhibitory agents. This medium contains charcoal to detoxify the medium, remove carbon dioxide (CO_2), and modify the surface tension to allow the organisms to proliferate more easily. BCYEα is also prepared with ACES buffer (N-[2-Acetoamido]-2-aminoethanesulfonic acid) and the growth supplements cysteine (required by *Legionella*), yeast extract, alpha-ketoglutarate, and iron. Additional selective media, such as the BCYEα with polymyxin B, anisomycin (to inhibit fungi), and cefamandole, is recommended for specimens, such as sputum, that are likely to be contaminated with other human microbiota. Less selective media containing polymyxin B, anisomycin, and vancomycin should be used to isolate *Legionella* spp. other than *L. pneumophila*. *L. micdadei* has been recovered from BCYEα supplemented with bovine serum albumin from a guinea pig spleen, but no data is available for direct culture from human specimens. BCYEα with natamycin, aztreonam, and vancomycin has been used to isolate *L. longbeachae* from environmental samples.

Culture plates are incubated at 35°C to 37°C in a humid atmosphere for up to 14 days and are examined every 3 or 4 days. Even the detection of one or a few colonies is sufficient to confirm the diagnosis. Some *Legionella* spp. may be stimulated by increased 2% to 5% concentration of CO_2,

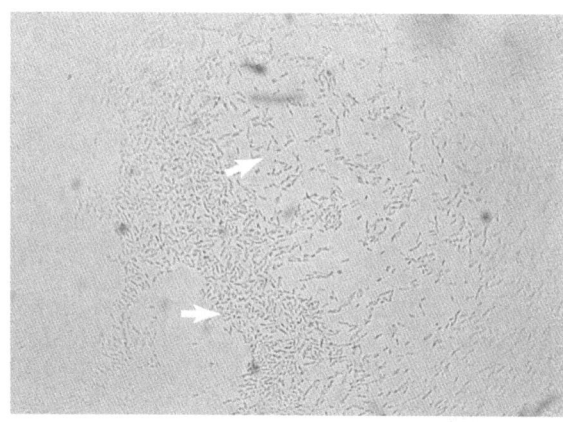

• **Fig. 34.4** Gram stain of a colony of *Legionella pneumophila* showing thin, gram-negative bacilli *(arrows)*.

including *Legionella sainthelensi* and *Legionella oakridgensis*. The low level of CO_2 will not prevent the growth of *L. pneumophila*. If this concentration is not possible, incubation in air is preferable to 5% to 10% CO_2, which may inhibit some legionellae, specifically *L. pneumophila*. At 5 days, colonies are 3 to 4 mm in diameter, gray-white to blue-green, glistening, convex, and circular and may exhibit a cut-glass type of internal granular speckling (Fig. 34.3). A Gram stain yields thin, gram-negative bacilli (Fig. 34.4).

Approach to Identification

Because *Legionella* spp. are biochemically inert, and many tests produce equivocal results, extensive biochemical testing is of little use. Definitive identification generally requires the facilities of a specialized reference laboratory. Using a long-wave UV light in a dark room, suspect colonies of *L. pneumophila* will appear pale yellow-green with diffusion of the pigment into the medium. It is important to note that some young colonies will not fluoresce. Other species of *Legionella* will fluoresce a brilliant bluish white or a brilliant red. *L. pneumophila* colonies should be Gram stained, using 0.1% fuchsin as the counterstain, to determine whether bacteria are small to filamentous, gram-negative rods. Colonies should be plated to two media, including a BYCEα plate

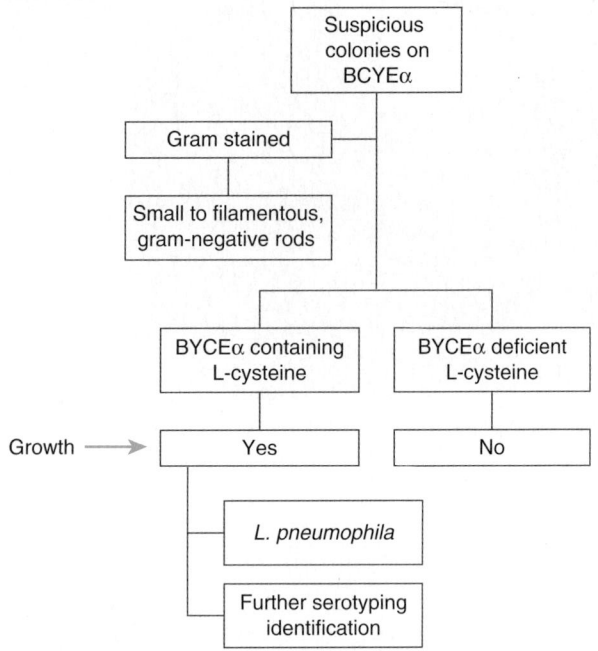

• **Fig. 34.5** Presumptive identification of *Legionella pneumophila* in culture.

containing L-cysteine and one made without. *L. pneumophila* will only grow on the BYCEα L-cysteine media, providing a more definitive identification. In addition, if only a small amount of growth is present on the primary medium, the growth may be emulsified in sterile water and used for subculturing, staining, and serologic identification. *F. tularensis* is the only other gram-negative bacterium that demonstrates L-cysteine growth dependence; however, the colonial morphology is opaque and homogenous. In addition, some serotyping reagents for *Legionella* spp. will cross-react with *F. tularensis*. Once the isolate has been determined to be L-cysteine dependent, further identification is completed using serotyping. Many different bacteria, including *Bordetella pertussis* have been reported to cross-react with serologic reagents used for the characterization and identification of *Legionella* spp. It is important to correlate all diagnostic testing with cellular and colonial morphology to avoid misidentification of other bacteria as *Legionella* spp. Gram-negative rods that demonstrate the colonial morphology and L-cysteine growth dependency may be presumptively reported as *Legionella* spp. If the organism is reactive in the serogroup 1 typing assay, the organism may be presumptively identified as *L. pneumophila* (Fig. 34.5).

Further identification of isolates can be completed using matrix-assisted laser desorption ionization time-of-flight mass spectrometry (MALDI-TOF MS) or DNA sequencing. MALDI-TOF MS databases include either no *Legionella* spp. or only *L. pneumophila*. This method is unable to distinguish serogroup designations. The research use only database in MALDI-TOF MS systems has been successfully used to identify 80% to 90% of isolates being tested in reference laboratories. Upon completion of sufficient data collection, the MALDI-TOF MS databases may be used to identify the organism upon FDA clearance.

Serodiagnosis

Most patients with legionellosis have been diagnosed retrospectively by detection of a fourfold rise in anti-*Legionella* antibody with an indirect fluorescent antibody (IFA) test. Serum specimens should be tested no closer than 2 weeks apart. Diagnostic efficacy associated with serologic testing increases with the collection and testing of acute and convalescent paired sera. Convalescent sera should be collected at 4, 6, and 12 weeks after the appearance of the disease. Disease is confirmed by a fourfold rise in titer to more than 128. A single serum with a titer of more than 256 and a characteristic clinical picture may be presumptive for legionellosis; however, because as many as 12% of healthy persons yield titers as high as 1:256, this practice is strongly discouraged. Unfortunately, individuals with Legionnaires' disease may not exhibit an increase in serologic titers until as long as 10 weeks after the primary illness, or they may never display significant antibody titer increases. It is essential to correlate serologic findings with the patient's clinical presentation because of the variation in antibody response associated with legionellosis. Most patients will develop a classic IgM, IgG, and IgA response. However, some patients may develop antibodies for a single class (in other words, IgG, IgM, or IgA only). Commercially prepared antigen-impregnated slides for IFA testing are available from numerous suppliers.

Antimicrobial Susceptibility Testing and Therapy

In vitro susceptibility studies are not predictive of clinical response and should not be performed for individual isolates of legionellae. Antimicrobial agents such as quinolones, tetracycline, and the macrolides (e.g., clarithromycin and azithromycin) are active against *L. pneumophila*. Penicillins, cephalosporins of all generations, and aminoglycosides are not effective and should not be used. Low-level resistance to ciprofloxacin was recently identified; however, the clinical significance is unclear. Macrolides and quinolones have also demonstrated effective treatment for infections with *L. micdadei, L. dumoffii,* and *L. longbeachae*.

Prevention

Although under development, a vaccine against *Legionella* infections is not currently available. The effectiveness of other approaches to the prevention of *Legionella* infections, such as the elimination of its presence from cooling towers and potable water, is uncertain.

Legionellosis is a notifiable disease in most industrialized countries. An important piece of information for surveillance of the disease is the history of exposure. The incubation period for legionellosis is normally between 2 and 10 days. Thus, during an outbreak, an exposure history for 2 weeks before the onset of illness should be obtained from the patient. In the presence of a pneumonic illness, a laboratory diagnosis will support clinical suspicion of the infection and help classify the case. Many countries have developed guidelines or regulations for the control of *Legionella* in water systems and for the prevention of legionellosis.

(e) Visit the Evolve site for a complete list of procedures, review questions, and case studies.

Bibliography

Amemura-Maekawa J, Kura F, Chida K, et al.: *Legionella pneumophila* and other *Legionella* species isolated from Legionellosis patients in Japan between 2008 and 2016, *Appl Environ Microbiol* 84(18):e00721-18, 2018.

Becton, Dickinson & Company: *BD ProbeTec ET legionella pneumophila (LP) amplified DNA assay, package insert,* Sparks, MD, 2006, Becton, Dickinson & Company.

Bennett J, Dolin R, Blaser M: *Principles and practice of infectious diseases,* ed 9, Philadelphia, 2020, Elsevier-Saunders.

Centers for Disease Control and Prevention. *Legionnaires' disease surveillance summary report, 2014–2015.* Published October 2018.

Garduño RA, Garduño E, Hiltz M, Hoffman PS: Intracellular growth of *Legionella pneumophila* gives rise to a differentiated form dissimilar to stationary-phase forms, *Infect Immun* 70:6273–6283, 2002.

Greenberg D, Chiou CC, Famigilleti R, Lee TC, Yu VL: Pediatric legionellosis: implications for underdiagnoses, *Lancet Infect Dis* 6:529–535, 2006.

Hlavsa MC, Cikesh BL, Roberts VA, et al.: Outbreaks associated with treated recreational water – United States, 2000–2014, *MMWR Morb Mortal Wkly Rep* 67(19):547–551, 2018.

Harb OS, Kwaik YA: Interaction of *Legionella pneumophila* with protozoa provides lessons, *ASM News* 66:609, 2000.

Helbig JH, Uldum SA, Bernander S, et al.: Clinical utility of urinary antigen detection for diagnosis of community-acquired, travel-associated, and nosocomial Legionnaires' disease, *J Clin Microbiol* 41:838–840, 2003.

Herpers BL, de Jongh BM, van der Zwaluw K, van Hannen EJ: Real-time PCR assay targets the 23S-5S spacer for direct detection and differentiation of *Legionella* spp. and *Legionella pneumophila*, *J Clin Microbiol* 41:4815–4816, 2003.

Jarraud S, Descours G, Ginevra C, et al.: Identification of *Legionella* in clinical samples, *Methods Mol Biol* 954:27–56, 2013.

Korevaar E, Khoo CA, Newton HJ: Genetic manipulation of non-pneumophila *Legionella*: protocols developed for *Legionella longbeachae, Methods Mol Biol* 1921:145–157, 2019.

Marrie TJ, Raoult D, LaScola B, et al.: *Legionella*-like and other amoebal pathogens as agents of community-acquired pneumonia, *Emerg Infect Dis* 7:1026, 2001.

McDade JE, Shepard CC, Fraser DW, Tsai TR, Redus MA, Dowdle WR: Legionnaires' disease: isolation of a bacterium and demonstration of its role in other respiratory disease, *N Engl J Med* 297(22):1197–1203, 1977.

Mercante JW, Winchell JM: Current and emerging *Legionella* diagnostics for laboratory and outbreak investigations, *Clin Microbiol Rev* 28:95–133, 2015.

Muder RR, Yu VL: Infection due to *Legionella* species other than *Legionella pneumophila, Clin Infect Dis* 35:990, 2002.

Murdock DR: Diagnosis of *Legionella* infection, *Clin Infect Dis* 36:64–69, 2003.

Osborne AJ, Jose BR, Perry J, et al.: Complete genome sequences of two geographically distinct *Legionella micdadei* clinical isolates, *Genome Announc* 5(22):1–2, 2017.

Pasculle W: Update on *Legionella, Clin Microbiol Newsl* 22:97, 2000.

Pedro-Botet L, Yu VL: *Legionella:* macrolides or quinolones, *Clin Microbiol Infect* 12(Suppl 3):25–30, 2006.

Qin T, Zhou H, Ren H, et al.: Distribution of secretion systems in the genus *Legionella* and its correlation with pathogenicity, *Front Microbiol* 8:388, 2017.

Qui J: Effector translocation by the *Legionella* Dot/Icm type IV secretion system, *Curr Top Microbiol Immunol* 376:103, 2013.

Roy CR, Tilney LG: The road less traveled: transport of *Legionella* to the endoplasmic reticulum, *J Cell Biol* 158:415, 2002.

Salcedo SP, Holden DW: Bacterial interactions with the eukaryotic secretory pathway, *Curr Opin Microbiol* 8:92, 2005.

Stout JE, Sens K, Mietzner S, et al.: Comparative activity of quinolones, macrolides and ketolides against *Legionella* species using in vitro broth dilution and intracellular susceptibility testing, *Int J Antimicrob Agents* 25:302–307, 2005.

Yu VL, Stout JE: Rapid diagnostic testing for community-acquired pneumonia: can innovative technology for clinical microbiology be exploited? *Chest* 136:1618–1621, 2009.

35

Brucella

GENERA AND SPECIES TO BE CONSIDERED

Classified as Select Agents

Brucella abortus
Brucella melitensis
Brucella suis

Other Species

Brucella canis
Brucella ceti
Brucella microti
Brucella neotomae
Brucella ovis
Brucella papionis
Brucella pinnipedialis

The family *Brucellaceae* comprises three genera: *Ochrobactrum* (Chapter 22), *Mycoplana,* and *Brucella. Brucella* spp. are discussed in this chapter. Brucellae are free-living organisms that are subcategorized into 10 recognized species. Eight of the species are terrestrial, and four of those have been associated with human disease: *Brucella abortus* (seven biovars), *Brucella melitensis* (three biovars), *Brucella suis* (five biovars), and *Brucella canis.* Two marine species, *B. ceti* and *B. pinnipedialis,* are also known to cause human disease. Of the four terrestrial species known to cause human infection, all but *B. canis* are considered Category B select agents. Brucellosis is a reportable disease in all 57 states and territories; it is mandatory that disease cases be reported to state and territorial

jurisdictions when identified by a health provider, hospital, or laboratory. Reporting requirements vary by jurisdiction. Brucellosis is also a nationally notifiable condition. Notification of brucellosis cases (without direct personal identifiers) to the Centers for Disease Control and Prevention (CDC) by state and territorial jurisdictions is voluntary for nationwide aggregation and monitoring of disease data. Clinical or diagnostic laboratories and other entities that have identified *B. suis, B. melitensis,* or *B. abortus* are required to immediately (within 24 hours) notify the CDC Division of Select Agents and Toxins (DSAT) (http://selectagents.gov).

General Characteristics

Brucellae are small, facultative, intracellular, nonmotile, aerobic, gram-negative coccobacilli or short bacilli that stain poorly by conventional Gram stain. Many isolates require supplementary carbon dioxide (CO_2) for growth, especially on primary isolation. *Brucella* spp. are closely related to *Bartonella, Rhizobium,* and *Agrobacterium* spp.

Epidemiology and Pathogenesis

The disease brucellosis occurs worldwide, especially in Mediterranean and Persian Gulf countries, India, and parts of Mexico and Central and South America. The organisms are capable of survival for extended periods (e.g., soil, 10 weeks; aborted fetuses, 11 weeks; bovine stool, 17 weeks; milk and ice cream, 3 weeks); they can survive in fresh cheese for several months. Animals are carriers and do not typically demonstrate symptoms of disease. The most prominent symptom in animals is the infectious abortion of the fetus. **Brucellosis** is a zoonosis and is recognized as a cause of devastating economic loss among domestic livestock.

Each of the *Brucella* spp. that are pathogenic for humans has a limited number of preferred animal hosts (Table 35.1). In the host, *Brucella* spp. tends to localize in tissues rich in erythritol (e.g., placental tissue), a four-carbon alcohol that enhances their growth. Humans become infected by four primary routes:

• Ingestion of infected unpasteurized animal milk products (most common means of transmission)
• Inhalation of infected aerosolized particles (laboratory-acquired infection is the most important source of transmission)

TABLE 35.1	*Brucella* spp. and Their Respective Natural Animal Hosts	
Organism	**Preferred Animal Host**
Brucella abortus	Cattle and buffalos
Brucella melitensis	Sheep, goats, or camels
Brucella suis	Swine and a variety of wild animals
Brucella canis	Dogs
Brucella ovis	Rams (not associated with human infection)
Brucella microti	Red foxes (not associated with human infection)
Brucella neotomae	Desert and wood rats (not associated with human infection)
Brucella papionis	Baboons and bull frogs (not associated with human infection)
Brucella pinnipedialis	Marine mammals, seals (rare human infection)
Brucella ceti	Dolphins, cetaceans (rare human infection)

- Direct contact with infected animal parts through ruptures of skin and mucous membranes
- Accidental inoculation of mucous membranes by aerosolization

Rare cases of transmission by blood and bone marrow transplantation and by sexual intercourse, in addition to neonatal brucellosis, have been reported. Individuals considered at risk for contracting brucellosis include dairy farmers, livestock handlers, slaughterhouse employees, veterinarians, and laboratory personnel (public health, medical, and research). The organism has a very low infectious dose (100 organisms or fewer). Mishandling and misidentification of the organism is often associated with laboratory transmission of the organism.

Brucella spp. are facultative, intracellular parasites that are able to exist in both intracellular and extracellular environments. After infecting a host, brucellae are ingested by neutrophils, within which they replicate, causing cell lysis. Neutrophils containing viable organisms circulate in the bloodstream and are subsequently phagocytized by mononuclear phagocytic cells in the spleen, liver, and bone marrow. If the infection goes untreated, granulomas develop in these organs, and the brucellae survive in monocytes and macrophages. Brucellae show a tendency to invade and persist in the human host by inhibiting apoptosis (programmed cell death). Resolution of the infection depends on the host's nutritional and immune status, the size of the inoculum and route of infection, and the *Brucella* species causing the infection; in general, *B. melitensis* and *B. abortus* are more virulent for humans.

Survival and multiplication of *Brucella* in phagocytic cells are features essential to the establishment, development, and chronicity of the disease. *Brucella* spp. can change from a smooth to a rough colonial morphology based on the composition of the cell wall lipopolysaccharide O-side chain (LPS); those with a smooth LPS are more resistant to intracellular killing by neutrophils than those with a rough LPS. The smooth phenotype has been identified in *B. abortus* and *B. melitensis*. Brucellae ensure intracellular survival by interfering with the phagosome-lysosome fusion in macrophages and epithelial cells. In addition, like *Legionella* spp. (Chapter 34), brucellae use a type IV secretion system, VirB, for intracellular survival and replication. Unlike *Legionella* spp., however, brucellae modulate phagosome transport to avoid being delivered to lysosomes. Essentially, VirB is involved in controlling the maturation of the *Brucella* vacuole into an organelle that allows replication. In the mouse model, if nucleic acid mutations occur in this region, *B. abortus* is unable to establish chronic infections. In addition, *Brucella* spp. produce urease, which provides protection during passage through the digestive system when the organism is ingested in food products. Urease breaks down urea, producing ammonia, and neutralizes the gastric pH. Despite our current knowledge, many questions remain about the pathogenesis of disease caused by *Brucella* spp.

Spectrum of Disease

The clinical manifestations of brucellosis vary greatly, ranging from asymptomatic infection to serious, debilitating disease. For the most part, brucellosis is a systemic infection that can involve any organ of the body. Symptoms, which are nonspecific, include fever, chills, weight loss, night sweats, headache, muscle aches, fatigue, and depression. Lymphadenopathy and splenomegaly are common physical findings. After an incubation period of about 2 to 4 weeks, the onset of disease is commonly insidious. Complications can occur, such as arthritis, spondylitis (inflammation of the vertebrae), genital, pulmonary, and renal complications, and endocarditis. Neurobrucellosis occurs in approximately 3% to 5% of infections and can result in mild symptoms such as fever and headache to meningitis, coma, and paralysis. Relapse is considered an important feature of brucellosis; it is associated with delayed initiation of treatment, ineffective antibiotic therapy, and positive blood culture findings during the initial presentation.

Laboratory Diagnosis

Specimen Collection, Transport, and Processing

Samples for the diagnosis and identification of infections associated with *Brucella* spp. may be used for culture, serology, or nucleic acid–based testing. The gold standard for the definitive diagnosis of brucellosis is isolation of the organisms in cultures of blood; bone marrow; cerebrospinal fluid

(CSF); pleural, abdominal, and synovial fluids; urine; spleen or liver abscesses; or other tissues. Bone marrow or blood are considered the best specimens for culture. If processing is delayed, the specimen may be held in the refrigerator. Some research laboratories offer nucleic acid–based testing on blood (serum or whole blood), CSF, and bone marrow specimens for the identification of the organism.

It is essential that the clinical microbiology laboratory be notified whenever brucellosis is suspected:

- To ensure that specimens are cultivated in an appropriate manner for optimal recovery from clinical specimens
- To prevent accidental exposure of laboratory personnel handling the specimens, because *Brucella* spp. are considered category B select agents (specimen labels should indicate that *Brucella* spp. are a potential pathogen). All specimens should be handled using a BS-3 or BSL-2 with BSL-3 precautions.

Blood for culture can be collected routinely (Chapter 67) into most commercially available blood culture bottles and the lysis-centrifugation system (Isolator, Alere, Waltham, MA). For other clinical specimens, no special requirements must be met for collection, transport, or processing.

Within 2 hours of obtaining a high-confidence presumptive or confirmatory result, a Laboratory Response Network (LRN) Laboratory Director or a designee must notify:

- the State Public Health Laboratory Director,
- the State Epidemiologist,
- the Health Officer for the State Public Health Department,
- the CDC Emergency Operations Center (EOC), and
- the FBI Weapons of Mass Destruction (WMD) POC.

For emergency and non-emergency situations, LRN laboratories will submit data for all samples, including positive and negative results related to the event, within 12 hours of obtaining each result. The LRN is a national network of local, state, federal, military, and international public health, food testing, veterinary diagnostic, and environmental testing laboratories that provides laboratory infrastructure and capacity to respond to biological and chemical public health emergencies. More information on the LRN is included in Chapter 79.

Direct Detection Methods

Direct stains of clinical specimens are not particularly useful for the diagnosis of brucellosis.

Nucleic Acid Detection

Conventional and real-time polymerase chain reaction (PCR) assays are reliable and specific means of directly detecting *Brucella* organisms in clinical specimens. Sensitivity varies among assays, ranging from 50% to 100%. This variation is related to the differences in nucleic acid extraction procedures, specimen type, and detection formats. Several gene targets have been used, including a cell surface protein (BCS P31), a periplasmic protein (BP26), 16S

ribosomal ribonucleic acid (rRNA), and transposon insertion sequence 711(IS711). Although nucleic acid–based testing can be used for rapid identification, standardization is needed to improve the use in routine laboratories.

Serodiagnosis

Because isolating brucellae is difficult, a serologic test is widely used (e.g., serum agglutination test [SAT] or microplate agglutination [MAT]). This technique detects antibodies to *B. abortus*, *B. melitensis*, and *B. suis;* however, the SAT does not detect *B. canis* antibodies. An indirect Coombs test is performed after the SAT. This test detects nonagglutinating or incomplete antibodies in complicated and chronic cases of brucellosis.

The serology associated with *Brucella* infection follows the classic antibody response: IgM appears initially, followed by IgG. A titer of 1:160 or greater in the SAT is considered diagnostic if this result fits the clinical and epidemiologic findings. The SAT can cross-react with class M immunoglobulins with a variety of bacteria, such as *Francisella tularensis* and *Vibrio cholerae*. Enzyme-linked immunosorbent assays (ELISAs) also have been developed. Purified LPS or protein extracts are primarily used in ELISAs. However, currently no reference antigen exists; therefore, it is important to identify the antigen used in the commercial system when evaluating test results. In patients with neurobrucellosis, ELISA offers significant diagnostic advantages over conventional agglutination methods.

Additional serologic assays are commercially available, including a lateral flow dipstick for screening outbreaks and an immunocapture agglutination method. The immunocapture assay demonstrates sensitivity and specificity similar to a Coombs test and is less cumbersome to perform. The dipstick test has a high degree of sensitivity (>90%). Microarrays that contain numerous antigens are being evaluated for their efficacy in elucidating differential antibody responses from patients during different stages of disease. Serologic testing should be interpreted with care, as methods lack standardization of antigen preparation, methodologies, and detection.

Cultivation

Cultivation and identification of *Brucella* spp. remain the primary method used for laboratory diagnosis of brucellosis. Although most isolates of *Brucella* spp. grow on blood and chocolate agars (some isolates are also able to grow on MacConkey agar), more enriched agars and special incubation conditions generally are needed to achieve optimal recovery of these fastidious organisms from clinical specimens. Brucella agar or infusion base is recommended for specimen types other than blood. The addition of 5% heated horse or rabbit serum enhances growth on all media. Thayer-Martin or Martin-Lewis medium may be used to isolate the organisms from mixed cultures or contaminated specimens. Cultures should be incubated in 5% to 10% CO_2 in

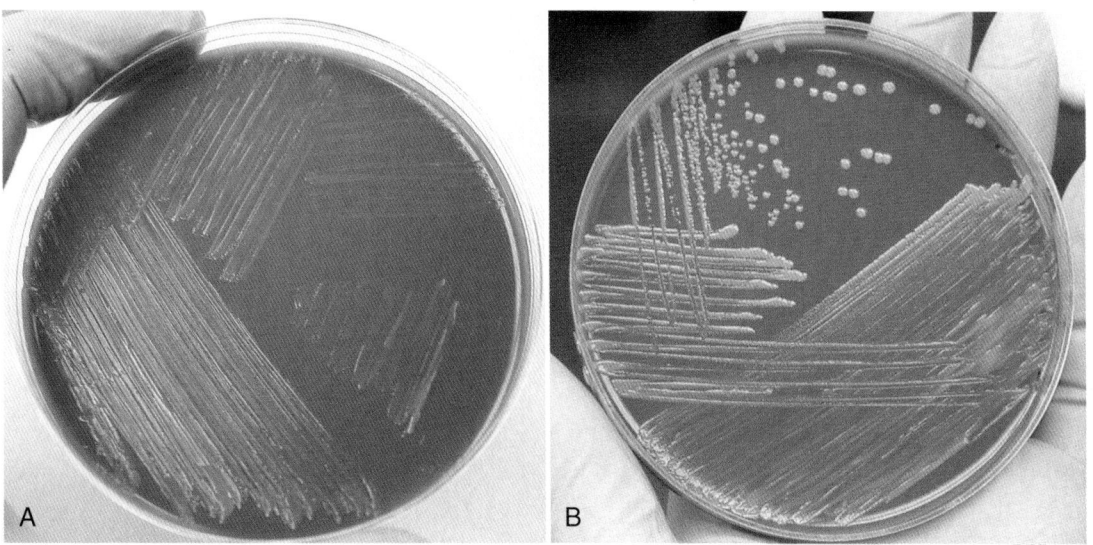

• **Fig. 35.1.** Growth of *Brucella* spp. on chocolate agar after incubation for 2 days (A) and 4 days (B).

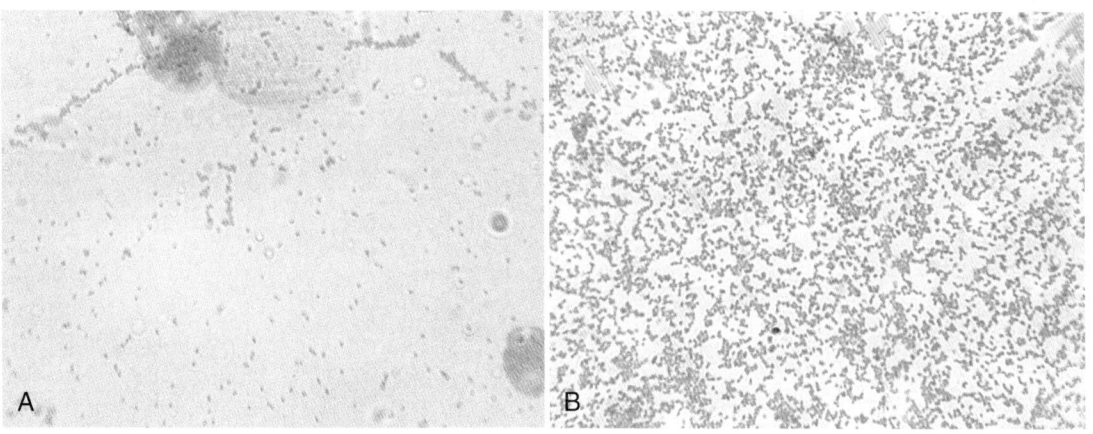

• **Fig. 35.2.** *Brucella melitensis* with traditional Gram stain (A) and Gram stain with 2-minute safranin counterstain (B) to allow easier visualization of the organism.

a humidified atmosphere; inoculated plates are incubated for up to 3 weeks before they are considered negative and discarded.

Commercial blood culture systems (e.g., BacT/Alert [bioMérieux, Durham NC], BACTEC [Becton Dickinson, Franklin Lakes, NJ], and lysis-centrifugation systems) all have successfully detected brucellae in blood. Other blood culture bottles, such as those with brain-heart infusion and trypticase soy broth support the growth of brucellae if the bottles are continuously vented and placed in a CO_2 incubator. Most isolates can be detected within 5 to 7 days using commercial systems. Bottles need not be incubated longer than 10 to 14 days. Culture bottles may not become turbid. All subculture plates should be held for a minimum of 10 days.

On culture, colonies appear small, convex, smooth, translucent, gamma-hemolytic, and slightly yellow and opalescent after at least 48 hours of incubation (Fig. 35.1). Rough variants may be seen with *B. canis.* The colonies may become brownish with age.

Approach to Identification

Brucellosis is the most commonly reported laboratory-acquired bacterial infection; therefore, all handling and manipulations of suspected *Brucella* spp. should be performed using BSL-3 precautions in a BSL-2 or higher biologic safety cabinet. Gram stain of the organisms reveals small coccobacilli that resemble fine grains of sand (Fig. 35.2). *Brucella* spp. are catalase and urease positive, and most strains are oxidase positive. *B. canis* may be oxidase variable. Other nonfermentative, urea-positive, oxidase- and catalase-positive, gram-negative coccobacilli that may be confused with brucellae are *Bordetella, Haemophilus, Psychrobacter, Paracoccus, Methylobacterium, Cupriavidus,* and *Oligella* spp. (Table 35.2).

Brucella spp. are differentiated by the rapidity with which the organism hydrolyzes urea, its relative ability to produce hydrogen sulfide (H_2S), its requirements for CO_2, and its susceptibility to the aniline dyes thionine and basic fuchsin (Table 35.3). For determination of the CO_2 requirement, identical plates of *Brucella* agar or brain-heart infusion agar

TABLE 35.2 Characteristics of Organisms That Resemble *Brucella* spp.

	Brucella spp.	*Bordetella* spp.	*Cupriavidus pauculus*	*Haemophilus* spp.[a]	*Methylobacterium* spp.[b]	*Oligella ureolyticus*[c]	*Paracoccus yeei*[d]	*Psychrobacter immobilis*	*Psychrobacter phenylpyruvicus*
Gram stain	Faintly staining, tiny coccobacilli	Bacilli	Bacilli	Tiny coccobacilli	Vacuolated bacilli	Tiny coccobacilli	cocci	Coccobacilli to short rods	Coccobacilli and bacilli; decolorize poorly
Motility	−	+	+	−	−	+	−	−	−
Urea	+	+	+	V	V	+	+	V	+

[a]Demonstrates no growth on blood agar; will satellite *Staphylococcus aureus.*
[b]Produces a pink pigment and appears mucoid on blood agar.
[c]Primarily a urinary tract pathogen.
[d]Mucoid on blood agar.
+, positive; −, negative; *V*, variable.
Modified from Leber, AL. *Aerobic Bacteriology, Clinical Microbiology Procedures Handbook.* 4th ed. Washington, DC: ASM Press; 2016.

TABLE 35.3 Characteristics of Human Pathogenic *Brucella* spp.

Species	CO_2 Required for Growth	H_2S Produced	Time to Positive Urease	Inhibition by Dye	
				Thionine[a]	Fuchsin[a]
Brucella abortus	±	+ (most strains)	2 h (rare 24 h)	+	−
Brucella melitensis	−	−	2 h (rare 24 h)	−	−
Brucella suis	−	±	15 min	−	+ (most)
Brucella canis	−	−	15 min	−	+

[a]Dye tablets (Key Scientific Products, Round Rock, TX).
+, >90% of strains positive; −, >90% of strains negative; ±, variable results.

should be given equal inocula (e.g., with a calibrated loop) of a broth suspension of the organism to be tested. One plate should be incubated in CO_2 and the other plate in ambient air. Most strains of *B. abortus* do not grow in ambient air but show growth in CO_2. Presumptive identification can be reported based on the colonial morphology and a positive catalase, oxidase, urease, and slide agglutination reaction with specific *B. abortus* or *B. melitensis* antisera. *Brucella* spp. isolates should be sent to state or other reference laboratories for confirmation or definitive identification because most clinical laboratories lack the necessary media and containment facilities required for further analysis.

Subtyping of biovars may be performed using a variety of molecular techniques, including pulsed-field electrophoresis, random amplification of polymorphic DNA, amplified fragment length polymorphism, various PCR techniques, and multilocus DNA target sequence typing.

MALDI-TOF MS is an important and increasingly available tool in clinical microbiology laboratories because it allows a rapid and accurate identification of bacteria. MALDI Biotyper software is a convenient molecular method that can be used for diagnosing brucellosis. This method requires strict culture conditions and sample preparation to ensure correct identification. Accurate identification of *Brucella* species using MALDI-TOF MS has been achieved by constructing a *Brucella* reference library based on multilocus variable-number tandem repeat analysis (MLVA) data. MLVA is a technique that utilizes multiple repeat nucleic acid sequences that are distributed in different variations across an organism's genome. Comparing MS-spectra from *Brucella* species against a custom-made MALDI-TOF MS reference library can be used as a rapid identification method for *Brucella* species. This method was able to identify 99.3% of 152 isolates tested to the species level, and *B. suis* biovar 1 and 2 were identified as the correct biovar. This demonstrates that for *Brucella*, even minimal genomic differences between the biovars translate to specific proteomic differences and clearly identifiable spectra using MALDI-TOF MS.

Antimicrobial Susceptibility Testing and Therapy

Because of the fastidious nature of the brucellae and their intracellular localization, *in vitro* susceptibility testing is not reliable. In addition, the organisms rarely develop antibiotic resistance, and laboratory safety is a consideration. To prevent relapse of infection, patients with brucellosis undergo prolonged treatment (6 weeks) with antimicrobials that can penetrate macrophages and act in the acidic intracellular environment. Clear guidelines for treatment and duration of therapy remain unclear. Combination therapy with two or more antimicrobials results in fewer relapses than using a single antimicrobial. Doxycycline, rifampin, streptomycin, gentamicin, aminoglycosides, or ceftriaxone are some of the antimicrobials that are used to treat brucellosis. In some instances, surgical drainage may also be required to treat the localized foci of infection and prevent the development of disseminated infection.

Prevention

Successful vaccines against *Brucella* infection have been developed for livestock. However, the development of human vaccines has met with serious medical contraindications and low efficacy. The prevention of brucellosis in humans depends on elimination of the disease in domestic livestock as well as heating dairy products and related food to reduce disease transmission.

ⓔ Visit the Evolve site for a complete list of procedures, review questions, and case studies.

Bibliography

Boschiroli ML, Ouahrani-Betlache S, Foulongne V, et al.: Type IV secretion and *Brucella* virulence, *Vet Microbiol* 90:341–348, 2002.

Caroll KC, Pfaller MA: *Manual of clinical microbiology*, ed 12, Washington, DC, 2019, ASM Press.

Centers for Disease Control and Prevention: *Brucellosis reference guide: exposures, testing and prevention*, 2017. Available at: https://www.cdc.gov/brucellosis/pdf/brucellosi-reference-guide.pdf.

Ferreira L, Vega Càstaño S, Sánchez-Juanes F, et al.: Identification of *Brucella* by MALDI-TOF mass spectrometry. Fast and reliable identification from agar plates and blood cultures, *PloS One* 5(12):e14235, 2010, https://doi.org/10.1371/journal.pone.0014235.

Guzmán-Verri C, González-Barrientos R, Hernández-Mora G, et al.: *Brucella ceti* and brucellosis in cetaceans, *Front Cell Infect Microbiol* 2:3, 2012.

Jimenez de Bagues MP, Dudal S, Dornand J, Gross A: Cellular bioterrorism: how *Brucella* corrupts macrophage physiology to promote invasion and proliferation, *Clin Immunol* 114:227–238, 2004.

Karger A, Melzer F, Timke M, et al.: Interlaboratory comparison of intact-cell matrix-assisted laser desorption ionization-time of flight mass spectrometry results for identification and differentiation of Brucella spp., *J Clin Microbiol* 51:3123–3126, 2013.

Leber AL: Aerobic bacteriology. In *Clinical microbiology procedures Handbook*, ed 4, Washington, DC, 2016, ASM Press.

Lista F, Reubsaet FA, De Santis R, et al.: Reliable identification at the species level of *Brucella* isolates with MALDI-TOF-MS, *BMC Microbiol* 11:267, 2011, https://doi.org/10.1186/1471-2180-11-267.

Pappas G, Akritidis N, Bosilkovski M, Tsianos E: *Brucellosis, N Engl J Med* 352:2325–2336, 2005.

Roy CR: Exploitation of the endoplasmic reticulum by bacterial pathogens, *Trends Microbiol* 10:418, 2002.

Scholz HC, Nockler K, Gollner C, et al.: *Brucella inopinata* sp. nov., isolated from a breast implant infection, *Int J Syst Evol Microbiol* 60:801–808, 2010.

Smith LD, Ficht TA: Pathogenesis of *Brucella*, *Crit Rev Microbiol* 17:209–230, 1990.

Yagupsky P: Detection of *Brucellae* in blood cultures, *J Clin Microbiol* 37:3437–3742, 1999.

36

Bordetella pertussis, Bordetella parapertussis, and Related Species

OBJECTIVES

1. Describe the general characteristics of the *Bordetella* spp.
2. State the normal habitat and routes of transmission for *Bordetella pertussis* and *Bordetella parapertussis*.
3. Describe the three stages of pertussis, including the duration and symptoms.
4. Describe the proper collection and transport of specimens for the detection of bordetellae.
5. Explain the limitations of nucleic acid-based methods for detecting *B. pertussis,* including assay specificity and sensitivity.
6. Describe the optimal conditions for culturing *B. pertussis,* including specimens of choice for optimal recovery.
7. Outline the major tests used to identify and differentiate *B. pertussis* and *B. parapertussis*.
8. Correlate the patient's signs, symptoms, and laboratory results to identify the etiologic agent associated with infection.

GENERA AND SPECIES TO BE CONSIDERED

Bordetella ansorpii (putative species)
Bordetella avium
Bordetella bronchialis
Bordetella bronchiseptica (Chapter 24)
Bordetella flabilis
Bordetella hinzii
Bordetella holmesii
Bordetella muralis
Bordetella pertussis
Bordetella parapertussis (Chapter 20)
Bordetella petrii
Bordetella pseudohinzii (considered a proposed species)
Bordetella sputigena
Bordetella trematum (Chapter 20)

The genus *Bordetella* includes four primary human pathogens: *B. bronchiseptica, B. holmesii, B. pertussis,* and *B. parapertussis.* Three new species have been identified from human respiratory specimens: *B. bronchialis, B. flabilis,* and *B. sputigena.* These organisms have been identified in patients with cystic fibrosis (CF). *B. bronchiseptica* is reviewed in Chapter 24 because it grows on MacConkey agar. Although *B. parapertussis* and *B. holmesii* can also grow on MacConkey agar, they are discussed here with *B. pertussis* because they are associated with human upper respiratory tract infections, with almost identical symptoms, epidemiology, and therapeutic management. Additional *Bordetella* species may cause rare asymptomatic infections in immunocompromised patients; these include *B. hinzii, B. holmesii, B. petrii, B. trematum,* and *B. ansorpii* (described species that remains putative, not validly named). (See the chapter cross-references in the preceding table for information on organisms not discussed in this chapter.)

General Characteristics

General features of *Bordetella* spp. other than *B. pertussis* and *B. parapertussis* are summarized in Chapter 24. In contrast to *B. bronchiseptica, B. pertussis* and *B. parapertussis* are nonmotile and infect only humans. In the evolutionary process, these exclusive human pathogens have a close genetic relationship. They remain separate species based on their chemotaxonomic differences, pathogenesis, and host range.

Epidemiology and Pathogenesis

Before the introduction of the vaccine (and currently in nonimmunized populations), pertussis (whooping cough) periodically appears as an epidemic disease that cycles approximately every 2 to 5 years. Transmission occurs person-to-person through inhalation of respiratory droplets. Humans are the only known reservoir.

Pertussis is a highly contagious, acute infection of the upper respiratory tract caused primarily by *B. pertussis* and less commonly by *B. parapertussis.* The latter agent generally has a less severe clinical presentation both in duration of symptoms and in the percentage of identified cases. *B. holmesii* causes a pertussis-like illness, but little is known about the biology, virulence mechanisms, and pathogenic significance. Additional species of bordetellae, *B. bronchiseptica, B. petrii, B. avium, B ansorpii,* and *B. hinzii* are rarely isolated from the respiratory secretions of patients with respiratory illness. Pertussis occurs worldwide, with millions of cases reported annually. Although the incidence has decreased significantly since vaccination became widespread, outbreaks of pertussis occur periodically. *B. pertussis* infections appear to be endemic in adults and adolescents because of a natural decrease in immune protection from natural infections and vaccine-induced immunity; these infections may serve as the source of the epidemic cycles involving unvaccinated or partially immunized infants and children. CF patients often present with polymicrobial respiratory infections and may serve as a source for periodic outbreaks. The microbiome of CF patients demonstrates a high degree of variability; however, only six genera, including *Bordetella* spp., are routinely identified from CF specimens.

Pathogenesis

B. pertussis, the primary pathogen of whooping cough, uses several mechanisms to overcome the immune defenses of healthy individuals. The mechanisms are complex and involve the interplay of several virulence factors (Table 36.1). Some factors help establish infection, others are toxigenic to the host, and still others override specific components of the host's mucosal defense system. For example, when *B. pertussis* reaches the host's respiratory tract, the surface adhesins attach to respiratory ciliated epithelial cells and paralyze the beating cilia by producing a tracheal cytotoxin. The organism produces a major virulence factor, pertussis toxin (PT). PT enters the bloodstream, subsequently binding to specific receptors on host cells. After binding, PT disrupts several host cell functions, such as initiation of host cell translation; the inability of host cells to receive signals from the environment causes a generalized toxicity. The center membrane of *B. pertussis* blocks access of the host's lysozyme to the bacterial cell wall via its outer membrane. *B. pertussis* and *B. parapertussis* share two nearly identical virulence control systems encoded by the *bags (Bordetella virulence gene)* and *plrSR* (persistence in the lower respiratory tract) loci that are responsive to variation in environmental conditions. Because of this very complex system, *Bordetella* organisms appear to be able to alter phenotypic expression, enhancing transmission, colonization, and survival.

Spectrum of Disease

Several factors influence the clinical manifestations of *B. pertussis* (Box 36.1). Classic pertussis is usually a disease of children and can be divided into three symptomatic stages: catarrhal, paroxysmal, and **convalescent.** During the **catarrhal stage,** symptoms are the same as for a mild cold with a runny nose and mild cough; this stage may last several weeks. Episodes of severe and violent coughing increase in number, marking the beginning of the **paroxysmal**

TABLE 36.1	Major Virulence Determinants of *Bordetella pertussis*
Function	**Factor/Structure**
Adhesion (auto transporters)	Fimbriae (FIM), types 2 and 3: Serotype-specific agglutinins for colonization of respiratory mucosa Filamentous hemagglutinin (FHA): Mediates adhesion to the ciliated upper respiratory tract Pertactin (PRN): Mediates eukaryotic cell binding and is highly immunogenic Tracheal colonization factor Brk A[a]
Toxicity	Pertussis toxin (encoded by the ptx gene, an A/B toxin related to cholera toxin): Induces lymphocytosis and suppresses chemotaxis and oxidative responses in neutrophils and macrophages Adenylate cyclase hemolysin: Hemolyzes red cells and activates cyclic adenosine monophosphate, thereby inactivating several types of host immune cells Dermonecrotic toxin (exact role unknown) Tracheal cytotoxin (ciliary dysfunction and damage) Endotoxin (lipopolysaccharide) Type III secretion[b] *Bordetella*-secreted protein regulator (BSPR)[c]
Overcome host defenses	Outer membrane: Inhibits host lysozyme Siderophore production: Prevents host lactoferrin and transferrin from limiting iron

[a]Plays a role in pathogenesis by conferring serum resistance.
[b]This type of secretion allows *Bordetella* organisms to transport proteins directly into host cells; it is required for persistent tracheal colonization.
[c]This transcriptional regulator is involved in mediation of the type III secretion system during iron-starved conditions.

> **• BOX 36.1   Factors Known to Affect the Clinical Manifestation of *Bordetella pertussis* Infection**

- Patient's age
- Previous immunization or infection
- Presence of passively acquired antibody
- Antibiotic treatment

stage. As many as 15 to 25 paroxysmal coughing episodes can occur in 24 hours; these are associated with vomiting and with "whooping," which is the result of air rapidly inspired into the lungs past the swollen glottis. Lymphocytosis occurs, although, typically, the patient has no fever and no signs and symptoms of systemic illness. This stage may last 1 to 6 weeks.

In addition to classic pertussis, *B. pertussis* can cause mild illness and asymptomatic infection, primarily in household contacts and in a number of unvaccinated and previously vaccinated children. Since the 1990s, a shift in the age distribution of pertussis cases to adolescence and adults has been observed in highly vaccinated populations. Adults and adolescents are now recognized as a reservoir for transmitting infection to vulnerable infants. Among these immunized individuals, a prolonged cough may be the only manifestation of pertussis; a scratchy throat, other pharyngeal symptoms, and episodes of sweating commonly occur in adults with pertussis. A number of studies have documented that 13% to 32% of adolescents and adults with an illness involving a cough of 6 days' duration or longer have serologic or culture evidence of *B. pertussis* infection. Organisms that may produce pertussis-like symptoms include adenoviruses, respiratory syncytial virus, human parainfluenza viruses, influenza viruses, and *Mycoplasma pneumoniae*.

Other *Bordetella* species have been associated with infection in immunocompromised patients. *B. bronchiseptica*, *B. holmesii*, and *B. hinzii* produce a pertussis-like respiratory illness. *B. trematum* has been isolated from individuals working with poultry, and *Bordetella ansorpii* has been associated with septicemia.

Laboratory Diagnosis

Specimen Collection, Transport, and Processing

Confirming the diagnosis of pertussis is challenging. Culture, which is most sensitive early in the illness, has been the traditional diagnostic standard for pertussis and shows nearly 100% specificity but varied sensitivity. Organisms may become undetectable by culture 2 weeks after the start of paroxysms. Nasopharyngeal aspirates (vacuum assisted), nasopharyngeal wash (syringe method), or a nasopharyngeal swab (calcium-alginate or Dacron on a wire handle) are acceptable specimens, because *B. pertussis* colonizes the ciliated epithelial cells of upper respiratory tract. Calcium-alginate swabs with aluminum shafts are not recommended for polymerase chain reaction (PCR) because they may inhibit the polymerase enzyme in PCR detection. Flocked swabs may be used but have not been validated for PCR or culture of *B. pertussis*. In addition, cotton swabs may be inhibitory to specimen growth and are not recommended. If possible, two nasopharyngeal swabs should be collected, one from each nostril. Specimens obtained from the throat, sputum, or anterior nose are unacceptable because these sites are not lined with ciliated epithelium. For collection, the swab is bent to conform to the nasal passage and held against the posterior aspect of the nasopharynx. If coughing does not occur, another swab is inserted into the other nostril to initiate the cough. The swab is left in place during the entire cough, removed, and immediately inoculated onto a selective medium at the bedside (Table 36.2) or placed in appropriate transport media. Samples should be collected before the administration of antibiotics.

Transport time is critical and should not exceed 48 hours. *B. pertussis* and *B. parapertussis* are highly sensitive to metabolites and other toxic substances present in microbiological

TABLE 36.2	Examples of Selective Media for Primary Isolation of *Bordetella pertussis* and *Bordetella parapertussis*
Agar Media	**Description**
Bordet-Gengou	Potato infusion agar with glycerol and sheep blood with methicillin or cephalexin[a] (short shelf-life)
Regan-Lowe[b]	Charcoal agar with 10% horse blood and cephalexin (4- to 8-week shelf-life)
Stainer-Scholte	Synthetic agar lacking blood products

[a]Cephalexin is superior to methicillin and penicillin for inhibiting normal respiratory flora.
[b]Regan-Lowe agar has been found to work best for recovery of *B. pertussis* from nasopharyngeal swabs.

media, requiring special fluid transport media. Half-strength Regan-Lowe agar enhances recovery when used as a transport and enrichment medium. Cold casein hydrolysate medium and casamino acid broth (available commercially) have proved to be effective transport media, particularly for the preparation of slides for direct fluorescent antibody staining. Dry swabs may be transported in ambient air for PCR testing.

Direct Detection Methods

Because of the limitations associated with culture and serologic diagnostic methods, significant effort has been put into developing nucleic acid amplification methods. Nucleic acid–based diagnostic tests for the direct detection of *B. pertussis* and *B. parapertussis* genes by various PCR procedures, including real-time PCR, have replaced DFA in the clinical laboratory. These assays have a diagnostic sensitivity at least comparable (and in most cases superior) to that of culture. Sensitivity of the assays appears to decrease with the duration of the cough, but they may be useful in diagnosis for up to 4 to 6 weeks. A word of caution: Positive results have been obtained with samples containing *B. holmesii* and *B. bronchiseptica* (Chapter 24) depending on the sequence targeted in conventional and real-time PCR assays. Most laboratories use transposon insertion sequence IS481 for *B. pertussis* and IS1001 for *B. parapertussis*; however, strains of *B. holmesii*, *B. parapertussis*, and *B. bronchiseptica* that carry IS481 have been identified, and thus, careful interpretation of results and correlation with the clinical presentation are required. The addition of transposon insertion sequence IS1002, which is closely related to IS481, and *recA* significantly improves the specificity of the nucleic acid amplification and species identification. (Table 36.3). Additional PCR assays are available for the detection of the PT promoter, PT, *recA*, filamentous hemagglutinin and the porin genes. However, because these are single-copy genes and not multicopy insertion sequences, assay sensitivity is reduced. Nasopharyngeal swabs (rayon or Dacron swabs on plastic shafts) and aspirates are the two types of samples primarily used for pertussis PCR; calcium-alginate swabs are unacceptable, as previously mentioned, because they inhibit PCR-based detection.

TABLE 36.3 Sequences Used to Differentiate *Bordetella* spp.

Organism	IS481	IS1001	IS1002	RecA
B. pertussis	+			
B. parapertussis		+	+	
B. bronchiseptica	+	+	+	
B. holmesii	+			+

From Martini H, Detemmerman, Soetens O, et al. Improving specificity of *Bordetella pertussis* detection using a four target real-time PCR. *PLoS One.* 2017;12:e0175587.

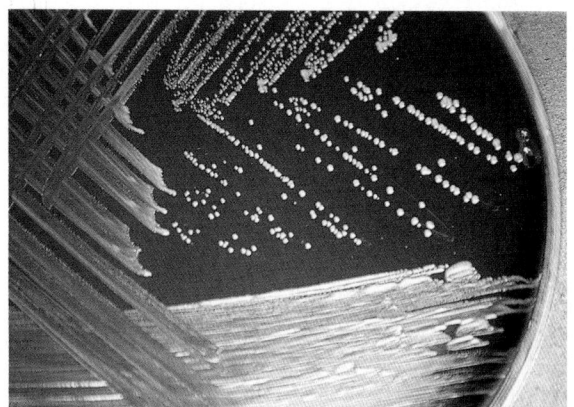

• **Fig. 36.1** Growth of *Bordetella pertussis* on Regan-Lowe agar.

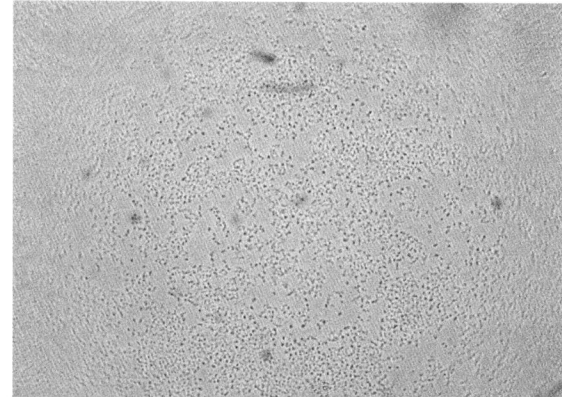

• **Fig. 36.2** Typical Gram stain appearance of *Bordetella pertussis.*

Cultivation

Cultivation is generally 100% specific; however, it has been replaced with PCR in most laboratories for routine diagnosis. Plates are incubated at 35°C in a humidified atmosphere without elevated carbon dioxide for up to 12 days. Most isolates are detected in 3 to 7 days; *B. parapertussis* appears in 2 to 3 days. Colony morphology is not distinct for the identification of other *Bordetella* spp.

Regan-Lowe agar, Bordet-Gengou agar, and Stainer-Scholte synthetic medium are suitable culture media. Regan-Lowe agar contains beef extract, starch, casein digest, and charcoal supplemented with horse blood. Bordet-Gengou agar is a potato fusion base containing glycerol and either sheep or horse blood. Most media contain cephalexin as an additive for suppression of contaminating organisms. Young colonies of *B. pertussis* and *B. parapertussis* are small and shiny, resembling mercury drops; colonies become whitish gray with age (Fig. 36.1).

Sensitivity of culture approaches 100% in the best of hands and depends on the stage of illness at the time of specimen collection, the technique used for specimen collection, specimen adequacy and transport, and culture conditions.

Approach to Identification

A Gram stain of the organism reveals minute, faintly staining coccobacilli singly or in pairs (Fig. 36.2). Use of a 2-minute safranin "O" counterstain or a 0.2% aqueous basic fuchsin counterstain enhances their visibility. *Bordetella* spp. characteristics are presented in Table 36.4. Whole-cell agglutination reactions in specific antiserum can be used for species identification. 16S rRNA gene sequencing or ribotyping and matrix-assisted laser desorption ionization time-of-flight mass spectrometry (MALDI-TOF MS) are often used to identify these organisms.

Serodiagnosis

Although several serologic tests are available for the diagnosis of pertussis, including agglutination and enzyme immunoassay, the enzyme-linked immunosorbent assay (ELISA) or bead-based assays are recommended for serologic diagnosis at this time.

The current most reliable serologic test available for diagnosis is an anti-PT (antibody to pertussis toxin) ELISA that has been used with acute and paired convalescent sera successfully in older children, adolescents, and adults. A titer greater than 100 to 125 IU/mL has been reported as a reliable indicator of exposure of patients to PT-producing bacteria. Serological assays cannot distinguish infection versus vaccine-induced immunity for *B. pertussis* and is unable to detect infection with *B. parapertussis.*

Antimicrobial Susceptibility Testing and Therapy

Laboratories currently do not perform routine susceptibility testing of *B. pertussis* and *B. parapertussis* because the organisms remain susceptible to some penicillins or the macrolides (clarithromycin, azithromycin), ketolides, quinolones, and other antibiotics, such as tetracyclines, chloramphenicol, and trimethoprim-sulfamethoxazole. Three erythromycin-resistant isolates of *B. pertussis* have been discovered; therefore, continued surveillance of *B. pertussis* is advised. Both *B. pertussis* and *B. parapertussis* are resistant to most oral cephalosporins and *B. bronchiseptica* is resistant to many penicillins, cephalosporins, and trimethoprim-sulfamethoxazole. Routine antimicrobial susceptibility testing for *Bordetella pertussis* and *B. parapertussis* is not recommended due to the lack of standardization; however, testing for other *Bordetella* isolates should be reported based on the laboratories' procedures for other fastidious gram-negative bacilli.

<table>
<tr><th>TABLE 36.4</th><th colspan="6">Characteristics That Differentiate the Major Isolates of Bordetella spp.</th></tr>
<tr><th>Characteristic</th><th>B. hinzii</th><th>B. holmesii</th><th>B. pertussis</th><th>B. parapertussis</th><th>B. bronchiseptica</th></tr>
<tr><td>Oxidase</td><td>+</td><td>(+)</td><td>+</td><td>−</td><td>+</td></tr>
<tr><td>Motility</td><td>+</td><td>−</td><td>−</td><td>−</td><td>+</td></tr>
<tr><td>Nitrate</td><td>−</td><td>−</td><td>−</td><td>−</td><td>+</td></tr>
<tr><td>Urease</td><td>−</td><td>−</td><td>−</td><td>+ (24 h)</td><td>+ (4 h)</td></tr>
<tr><td>Growth</td><td></td><td></td><td></td><td></td><td></td></tr>
<tr><td>Regan-Lowe agar</td><td>ND</td><td>2–3 days</td><td>3–4 days</td><td>2–3 days</td><td>1–2 days</td></tr>
<tr><td>Blood agar</td><td>−</td><td>+</td><td>−</td><td>+</td><td>+</td></tr>
<tr><td>MacConkey agar</td><td>+</td><td>(+)</td><td>−</td><td>−</td><td>+</td></tr>
</table>

ND, not determined; (+), <10% positive.

Prevention

Whole-cell vaccines to prevent pertussis, made from various *B. pertussis* preparations, are manufactured in many countries and are efficacious in controlling epidemic pertussis. As recommended by the Centers for Disease Control and Prevention (CDC), the United States uses three different formulas for diphtheria, tetanus, and pertussis vaccines. Children should receive five doses of DTaP vaccine before they are 6 years of age. Adolescents between 11 and 12 years of age, and adults, who have never received the vaccine, should receive a single dose of Tdap. Expectant mothers should receive a Tdap during pregnancy between 27 and 36 weeks. This should also be given to any children 7 to 10 years of age who are not fully immunized against pertussis. Capital letters in the vaccine indicate full strength doses of the vaccine components (D) diphtheria, (T) tetanus, and (P) pertussis. Lowercase letters indicate reduced doses that are used in adolescent and adult formulations. The lowercase *a* indicates that the pertussis component is acellular or simply a part of the organism. Td vaccine can be given as a booster for adults every 10 years. Prompt recognition of clinical cases and treatment of contacts and cases are also very important in preventing the transmission of *B. pertussis* and *B. parapertussis;* viable organisms can be recovered from untreated patients for 3 weeks after the onset of cough. To prevent nosocomial outbreaks, patients with suspected or confirmed pertussis should be placed on droplet precautions.

(e) Visit the Evolve site for a complete list of procedures, review questions, and case studies.

Bibliography

Abe A, Nishimura R, Tanaka N, et al.: The *Bordetella* secreted regulator Bsp I is translocated into the nucleus of host cells via its N-terminal moiety: evaluation of bacterial translocation by the *Escherichia coli* type III secretion system, *PLoS One* 10(8):e0135140, 2015.

Bone MA, Wilk AJ, Perault AI, et al.: *Bordetella* PLrSR regulatory system controls BvgAS activity and virulence in the lower respiratory tract, *Proc Natl Acad Sci U S A* 114:1519, 2017.

Carroll KC, Pfaller MA, Landry ML, et al.: *Manual of clinical microbiology,* ed 12, Washington, DC, 2019, ASM Press.

Coburn B, Wang PW, Diaz Caballero J, et al.: Lung microbiota across age and disease stage in cystic fibrosis, *Sci Rep* 5:10241, 2015.

Gordon KA, Fusco J, Biedenbach DJ, Pfaller MA, Jones RN: Antimicrobial susceptibility testing of clinical isolates of *Bordetella pertussis* from Northern California: report from the SENTRY antimicrobial surveillance program, *Antimicrob Agents Chemother* 45:3599–3600, 2001.

Hewlett EL, Edwards KM: Pertussis: not just for kids, *N Engl J Med* 352:1215, 2005.

Leber AL: *Bordetella* cultures. In *Clinical microbiology procedures handbook,* ed 4, Washington, DC, 2016, ASM Press.

Marko DC, Saffert RT, Cunningham SA, et al.: Evaluation of the Bruker Biotyper and Vitek MS matrix-assisted laser desorption ionization-time of flight mass spectrometry systems for identification of nonfermenting gram-negative bacilli isolated from cultures from cystic fibrosis patients, *J Clin Microbiol* 50:2034–2039, 2012.

Martini H, Detemmerman, Soetens O, et al.: Improving specificity of *Bordetella pertussis* detection using a four target real-time PCR, *PLoS One* 12. e0175587, 2017.

Mattoo S, Cherry JD: Molecular pathogenesis, epidemiology, and clinical manifestations of respiratory infections due to *Bordetella pertussis* and other *Bordetella* subspecies, *Clin Microbiol Rev* 18:326–382, 2005.

Spilker T, Barrah R, Lipuma JJ: Complete genome sequences of *Bordetella flabilis, Bordetella bronchialis,* and *Bordetella pseudohinzii, Genome Announc* 4(5). e01132, 2016.

Vandamme PA, Peeters C, Cnockaert M, et al.: *Bordetella bronchialis* sp. nov., *Bordetella flabilis* sp. nov., and *Bordetella sputigena* sp. nov. isolated from human respiratory specimens, and reclassification of *Achromobacter seiminum* as *Verticia sediminum* gen.nov.comb.nov, *Int J Syst Evol Microbiol* 65:3674, 2015.

37

Francisella

OBJECTIVES

1. List the media of choice for optimal recovery and cultivation of *Francisella tularensis*.
2. Describe the optimal incubation conditions for *F. tularensis*.
3. Describe the normal habitat and mode of transmission of *Francisella* spp.
4. Describe the symptoms of tularemia, and differentiate the various clinical presentations, including ulceroglandular, glandular, oculoglandular, oropharyngeal, systemic (typhoidal), and pneumonic tularemia.
5. Describe the clinical presentations that can be associated with non-*tularensis Francisellaceae*.
6. Differentiate *F. tularensis* from other potential biothreat agents with similar clinical findings.

GENERA AND SPECIES TO BE CONSIDERED

Francisella tularensis
   subsp. *tularensis* (type A)
   subsp. *holarctica* (type B)
   subsp. *mediasiatica*
Francisella halioticida
Francisella hispaniensis
Francisella noatunensis
Francisella novicida
Francisella persica
Francisella philomiragia

The family *Francisellaceae* includes two genera, *Francisella* and *Allofrancisella*. *Allofrancisella* spp. are environmental organisms that are not associated with disease. *Francisella tularensis* is the cause of tularemia, an acute fatal illness that affects animals and humans. Additional species of *Francisella* cause opportunistic infections in immunocompromised patients.

Tularemia is a reportable disease in all 57 states and territories; it is mandatory that disease cases be reported to state and territorial jurisdictions when identified by a health provider, hospital, or laboratory. Reporting requirements vary by jurisdiction. Tularemia is also a nationally notifiable condition. Notification of cases of tularemia (without direct personal identifiers) to the Centers for Disease Control and Prevention (CDC) by state and territorial jurisdictions is voluntary for nationwide aggregation and monitoring of disease data. Clinical or diagnostic laboratories and other entities that have identified *F. tularensis* are required to immediately (within 24 hours) notify the CDC

Division of Select Agents and Toxins (DSAT). http://selectagents.gov.

Francisella organisms are facultative, intracellular pathogens that require cysteine, cystine, or another sulfhydryl and a source of iron for enhanced growth. This indicates that the organisms require a complex medium for isolation and growth.

General Characteristics

Organisms belonging to the genus *Francisella* are faintly staining, tiny, gram-negative coccobacilli that are oxidase- and urease-negative, weakly catalase-positive, nonmotile, non–spore forming, strict aerobes (*F. philomiragia* and *F. hispaniensis* are oxidase-positive). Current members of the species *F. tularensis* share greater than 99% identity based on 16S ribosomal ribonucleic acid (rRNA) sequence analysis. However, the range of deoxyribonucleic acid (DNA) relatedness in the remaining species varies from 39% to 97%. The most current taxonomy and clinical spectrum of disease is summarized in Table 37.1. For the most part, different subspecies are associated with different geographic regions.

Epidemiology and Pathogenesis

Francisellaceae is widely distributed throughout the environment. *F. tularensis* is the agent of human and animal tularemia. Tularemia is caused by two subspecies, *F. tularensis* subsp. *tularensis* (type A) and *F. tularensis* subsp. *holarctica* (type B). *Francisella novicida* and *F. philomiragia* are present in the environment and are opportunistic human pathogens, with infection occurring in either immunocompromised or patients with a recent history of dry drowning or near drowning. *F. hispaniensis* has been identified associated with a bacteremia in a small number of cases. Worldwide in distribution, *F. tularensis* is carried by many species of wild rodents, rabbits, beavers, and muskrats in North America. Humans become infected by handling the carcasses or skin of infected animals, by inhaling infective aerosols or ingesting contaminated freshwater, through insect vectors (primarily deerflies and ticks in the United States), and by being bitten by carnivores that have themselves eaten infected animals. Some francisellae persist in waterways, and transmission of *F. novicida* and *F. philomiragia* is associated with contact or inhalation of saltwater or brackish water, including near drowning victims. Rare cases of infection in immunocompromised patients with *F. hispaniensis* have been associated with exposure to brackish or saltwater.

Most cases in the United States are sporadic, occurring during the summer months in the states of South Dakota, Arkansas, Missouri, and Oklahoma.

The capsule of *F. tularensis* appears to be a necessary component for expression of full virulence, allowing the organism to avoid immediate destruction by polymorphonuclear neutrophils (PMNS). In addition to being extremely invasive, *F. tularensis* is an intracellular parasite that can survive in the cells of the reticuloendothelial system, where it resides after a bacteremic phase. Granulomatous lesions may develop in various organs. The genome of *F. tularensis* includes a pathogenicity island that encodes 18 genes involved in the virulence of the organism including an atypical type VI secretion system (T6SS) that is required for intracellular growth. The T6SS attaches to the outer membrane of cells and is anchored to the cell with a baseplate attached to the membrane complex. The T6SS then ejects effector molecules into the target cell, which allows the organism to enter the cell, escape the phagosome, and replicate in the cell. Fewer than 50 organisms are required to infect humans through either aerosol or cutaneous routes. *F. tularensis* subsp. *tularensis* is the most virulent for humans, with an infectious dose of less than 10 colony-forming units. *F. philomiragia* has been isolated from several patients, many of whom were immunocompromised or victims of near-drowning incidents. The organism is present in animals and ground water.

Spectrum of Disease

The disease associated with *F. tularensis*, **tularemia,** is recognized worldwide. In the United States the clinical

TABLE 37.1   Most Recent Taxonomy of the Genus *Francisella* and Key Characteristics

Organism	Primary Region	Disease in Humans	Requires Cystine/Cysteine
Francisella tularensis subsp. *tularensis* (type A)	North America (United States and Canada)	Most severe: Tularemia (all forms, see Table 37.2)	+
Francisella tularensis subsp. *holarctica* (type B)	Europe, former Soviet Union, Japan, North America	Moderate to severe: Tularemia (all forms)	+
Francisella novicida	North America, Thailand, and Australia	Mild illness; virulent in immunocompromised patients	−
Francisella philomiragia	North America, Turkey, Switzerland, and Australia	Rare, mild illness; virulent in immunocompromised individuals	−
Francisella hispaniensis	United States and Spain	Rare disease in humans	+

TABLE 37.2   Clinical Manifestations of *Francisella tularensis* Infection

Types of Infection	Clinical Manifestations and Description	Recommended Specimen Type Based on Clinical Manifestation
Ulceroglandular	Common; ulcer and lymphadenopathy; rarely fatal	Whole blood; serum; swabs from visible lesions; aspirates from lymph nodes or lesions
Glandular	Common; lymphadenopathy; rarely fatal	Whole blood; serum; aspirates from lymph nodes or lesions
Oculoglandular	Conjunctivitis, lymphadenopathy	Whole blood; serum; swabs from visible lesions; aspirates from lymph nodes or lesions
Oropharyngeal	Ulceration in the oropharynx	Whole blood; serum; pharyngeal swabs, bronchial/tracheal washes or aspirates, sputum, transthoracic lung aspirates, and pleural fluid
Systemic (typhoidal) tularemia	Acute illness with septicemia; 30%–60% mortality rate; no ulcer or lymphadenopathy	Whole blood; serum; pharyngeal swabs, bronchial/tracheal washes or aspirates, sputum, transthoracic lung aspirates, and pleural fluid
Pneumonic tularemia	Acquired by inhalation of infectious aerosols or by dissemination from the bloodstream; pneumonia; most serious form of tularemia	Whole blood; serum; pharyngeal swabs, bronchial/tracheal washes or aspirates, sputum, transthoracic lung aspirates, and pleural fluid

manifestations have been referred to as **rabbit fever, deer fly fever**, glandular type of tick fever, Ohara's or yato-byo disease, water rat trappers' disease, and **market men's disease.** The clinical manifestation depends on the mode of transmission, the virulence of the infecting organism, the immune status of the host, and the length of time from infection to diagnosis and treatment. The typical clinical presentation after inoculation of *F. tularensis* through abrasions in the skin or by arthropod bites includes the development of a lesion at the site and progresses to an ulcer; lymph nodes adjacent to the site of inoculation become enlarged and often necrotic. Once the organism enters the bloodstream, patients become systemically ill with high temperature, chills, headache, and generalized aching. Clinical manifestations of infection with *F. tularensis* range from mild and self-limiting to fatal; they include glandular, ulceroglandular, oculoglandular, oropharyngeal, systemic, and pneumonic forms. These clinical presentations are summarized in Table 37.2.

Laboratory Diagnosis

The United States classifies *F. tularensis* as a Tier 1 select agent. Any laboratory receiving or maintaining the organism must register with the Federal Select Agent program (http://www.selectagents.gov). Diagnostic laboratories are exempt from registration under the condition that the organism and all infectious materials are properly disposed of or transferred within 7 days of identification. *F. tularensis* is a Biosafety Level 2 pathogen, a designation that requires technologists to wear gloves and to work in a biologic safety cabinet (BSC) when handling clinical material that potentially harbors this agent. The organism is designated Biosafety Level 3 when the laboratorian is working with cultures; therefore, a mask is recommended for the handling of all clinical specimens and is very important for preventing aerosol acquisition of *F. tularensis*. Because tularemia is one of the most common laboratory-acquired infections, most microbiologists do not attempt to work with infectious material from suspected patients. Specimens should be analyzed in reference laboratories, state, or other public health laboratories that are equipped to handle *Francisella* spp.

Specimen Collection, Transport, and Processing

The most common specimens submitted to the laboratory are scrapings from infected ulcers, lymph node biopsies, and respiratory samples, including sputum, pharyngeal swabs, bronchial or tracheal washes or aspirates, and pleural fluid. Whole blood is an acceptable specimen for all types of tularemia; however, false-negative results may occur during early stages of disease. Serum is generally collected from all patients early in disease and during convalescence. The blood should be separated from the serum as soon as possible, preferably within 24 hours. The serum may be stored at 2°C to 8°C for up to 10 days. If long-term storage is required, the serum may be frozen. To minimize the loss of viable organisms, samples should be transported to the laboratory within 24 hours. If specimens are held longer than 24 hours, they should be refrigerated in Amie's transport medium. *F. tularensis* should remain viable for up to 7 days stored at ambient temperature in Amie's medium. Swab specimens should be placed in Amie's transport media containing charcoal. Specimens for molecular testing may be placed in guanidine isothiocyanate buffer for up to 1 month.

Specimen collection for the identification of *F. tularensis* is highly dependent on the type of clinical manifestation. A detailed description of the recommended type of specimen associated with the patient's clinical presentation is included in Table 37.3. In light of concerns about bioterrorism, laboratories must keep in mind that isolation of *F. tularensis* from blood cultures might be considered a potential bioterrorist attack; *F. tularensis* is considered one of the Select Biological Agents of Human Disease (Chapter 79).

TABLE 37.3 Characteristics of Organisms That Resemble *Francisella* sp.

	Acinetobacter spp.	*Bartonella* spp.	*Brucella* spp.[a]	*Francisella* spp.	*Haemophilus* spp.[b]	*Pasteurella multocida*	*Yersinia pestis*
Gram-stain morphology	Broad coccobacilli	Thin bacilli	Tiny coccobacilli	Very tiny coccobacilli	Small coccobacilli	Small coccobacilli	Small bacilli
Oxidase	–	–	+	–	V	+	–
Urease			+		V		

+, ≥90% positive; –, less than or equal to 10% positive; *V*, variable (11%–89% positive).
[a]Growth of some strains is enhanced by the presence of hemin (X factor).
[b]Requires hemin (X factor) and NAD (V factor) or NAD only for growth.
Modified from Caroll KC, Pfaller MA. *Manual of Clinical Microbiology.* 12th ed. Washington, DC: ASM Press; 2019.

Direct Detection Methods

Gram staining of clinical material is of little use with primary specimens unless the concentration of organisms is high, as in swabs from wounds or ulcers, tissues, and respiratory aspirates. The organisms tend to counterstain poorly with safranin. Replacing safranin with basic fuchsin may enhance identification. The organisms appear as tiny, single, and pleomorphic gram-negative rods. Gram staining may be of little diagnostic use. Fluorescent antibody stains and immunohistochemical stains are commercially available for direct detection of the organism in lesion smears and tissues and are typically available in reference laboratories.

Nucleic Acid Detection

Conventional and real-time polymerase chain reaction (PCR) assays have been developed to detect *F. tularensis* directly in clinical specimens. Of significance, several patients with clinically suspected tularemia with negative serology and culture had detectable DNA by PCR. PCR or the *tul4* gene, which is unique to *Francisella* spp., demonstrates a sensitivity of approximately 75%. Real-time PCR assays are available in the Laboratory Response Network (LRN) throughout the United States. These assays target multiple genes from the organisms, including the *tul4*, *iglC*, *fopA*, and *ISFtu2* elements. PCR assays are limited by the inability to discriminate between *F. tularensis* and *F. novicida*. Gene sequencing of 16s rRNA does not sufficiently differentiate the two species but does identify the organism to the genus level.

A high-throughput nucleic acid based test Biothreat Panel (BT) has been FDA cleared using the BioFire FilmArray system (BioFire Diagnostics, Salt Lake City, UT) for the detection of potential biothreat agents in environmental samples, but has not been approved for clinical diagnostic use. The BT panel tests for 16 pathogens and 26 targets, including two targets for *F. tularensis*.

Serodiagnosis

Because of the risk of infection to laboratory personnel and other inherent difficulties with culture, diagnosis of tularemia is usually accomplished serologically by whole-cell agglutination (febrile agglutinins or newer enzyme-linked immunosorbent assay techniques). Serum antibody detection is useful for all forms of tularemia. After the initial specimen, a convalescent sample should be collected at 14 days and preferably up to 3 to 4 weeks after the appearance of symptoms. A fourfold difference in titers in acute versus convalescent phase serum samples, in conjunction with one additional positive diagnostic test, such as culture or molecular tests, is considered a presumptive diagnosis for tularemia. However, clinical management or monitoring treatment is of little use in cases of tularemia. Patients who present with acute illness may produce all three major diagnostic antibodies—IgM, IgA, and IgG—simultaneously. In addition, antibodies may persist for 10 years.

Cultivation

Isolation of *F. tularensis* is difficult. The organism is strictly aerobic and is enhanced by enriched media containing sulfhydryl compounds (cysteine, cystine, thiosulfate, or IsoVitaleX) for primary isolation. Two commercial media for cultivation of the organism are available: glucose cystine agar (BBL; Microbiology Systems, Sparks, Maryland) and cystine-heart agar (Beckton Dickinson, Franklin Lakes, New Jersey, BBL); both require the addition of 5% sheep or rabbit blood. *F. tularensis* may grow on chocolate agar supplemented with IsoVitaleX, the nonselective buffered charcoal-yeast extract agar (BCYE) used for isolation of legionellae, or in modified Mueller-Hinton broth and tryptic soy broth supplemented with 1% to 2% IsoVitaleX. Growth is not enhanced by carbon dioxide. All species grow at 35°C to 37°C, with the exception of *F. noatunensis*, which has an optimal growth temperature of 22°C and demonstrates no growth at 37°C.

These slow-growing organisms require 2 to 4 days for maximal colony formation; they are weakly catalase-positive and oxidase-negative. Some strains may require up to 2 weeks to develop visible colonies. *F. philomiragia* is less fastidious than *F. tularensis*. Although *F. philomiragia* does not require cysteine or cystine for isolation, it is similar to *F. tularensis* in that it is a small, coccobacillary rod that grows poorly or not at all on MacConkey agar. This organism grows well on heart infusion agar with 5% rabbit blood or BCYE agar with or without cysteine. *F. tularensis* can be detected in commercial blood culture systems in 2 to 5 days. Because the organisms Gram stain poorly, an acridine orange stain may be required to visualize the organisms in a positive blood culture bottle.

Approach to Identification

Colonies are transparent, mucoid, and easily emulsified. Although carbohydrates are fermented, isolates should be identified serologically (by agglutination) or by a fluorescent antibody stain. Ideally, isolates should be sent to a reference laboratory for characterization.

F. philomiragia differs from *F. tularensis* biochemically; *F. philomiragia* is oxidase-positive by Kovac's modification, and most strains produce hydrogen sulfide in triple sugar iron agar medium, hydrolyze gelatin, and grow in 6% sodium chloride (no strains of *F. tularensis* share these characteristics).

Laboratory exposures have occurred in association with the management of *Francisella* species isolated from clinical specimens. Twelve microbiology employees were exposed to *F. tularensis* even though bioterrorism procedures were in place; the organism had been isolated from blood, respiratory, and autopsy specimens and grew on chocolate agar. In this situation, multiple cultures were handled on open benches without any additional personal protective equipment for a culture that appeared consistent with a *Haemophilus* species. As a result of this report, microbiologists

• BOX 37.1 Indications of a Possible *Francisella* Sp.

- Unusual Gram stain: small, poorly staining gram-negative rods seen mostly as single cells or amorphous gram-negative mass without distinct cell forms *(Francisella philomiragia)*
- Subcultures yield primarily pinpoint colonies on chocolate agar
- Oxidase-negative; weak or negative catalase test
- Negative satellite on X and V tests
- Small, gram-negative coccobacillus observed in a Gram-stained smear of a positive blood culture in which time to detection is longer than 24 hours
- Organism requires prolonged incubation on chocolate agar

must be aware of not only the key characteristics of this group of organisms (Box 37.1), but also the possible pitfalls in their identification (e.g., some strains grow well on sheep blood agar; identification kits may incorrectly suggest an identification of *Actinobacillus actinomycetemcomitans*). See Table 37.3 for differentiation of *F. tularensis* and similar gram-negative bacteria. If *F. tularensis* is suspect, all culture petri dishes should be taped from the top to the bottom in two places to keep them together for safety purposes.

Matrix-assisted laser desorption ionization time-of-flight mass spectrometry (MALDI-TOF MS) has been used to differentiate the species and subspecies of *Francisella*. However, identification of the different species may be limited due to the lack of availability of spectra within the commercial databases. Safety considerations should be considered prior to using MALDI-TOF MS. Use of the ethanol-formic acid tube extraction process inactivates *F. tularensis*, whereas the direct colony and formic acid extraction on the target plate is not as reliable.

Antimicrobial Susceptibility Testing and Therapy

The organism is susceptible to aminoglycosides, and streptomycin is the drug of choice. Gentamicin is a possible alternative; doxycycline and chloramphenicol may be used, although these two agents have been associated with a higher rate of relapse after treatment. Fluoroquinolones appear promising for treatment of even severe tularemia. Tularemia is an end-stage disease and is not transmitted person-to-person. Many species carry genomic or plasmid-borne copies of several beta-lactamases, despite the fact that introduction into humans is always from a natural reservoir where there should be minimal exposure to beta-lactams to maintain selective pressure. However, the development of resistance to the recommended antibiotics by *Francisella* is rare.

Antimicrobial susceptibility testing for *F. tularensis* is not generally performed in routine laboratories for safety considerations and the rare occurrence of the development of antibiotic resistance in the organism. Interpretive criteria and quality control limits for broth microdilution have been published by the Clinical and Laboratory Standards Institute (CLSI).

Prevention

The primary means of preventing tularemia is to reduce the possibility of exposure to the etiologic agent in nature, such as by wearing protective clothing to prevent insect bites and by refraining from handling dead animals. An investigative live-attenuated vaccine is available.

ⓔ Visit the Evolve site for a complete list of procedures, review questions, and case studies.

Bibliography

Bennett J, Dolin R, Blaser M: *Principles and practice of infectious diseases*, ed 9, Philadelphia, 2020, Elsevier-Saunders.

Caroll KC, Pfaller MA: *Manual of clinical microbiology*, ed 12, Washington, DC, 2019, ASM Press.

Clemens DL, Lee BY, Horwitz MA: The *Francisella* type VI secretion system, *Front Cell Infect Microbiol* 8:121, 2018.

Clinical and Laboratory Standards Institute: *Performance standards for antimicrobial disk susceptibility testing; M02-A12*, Wayne, PA, 2015, CLSI.

Cunningham S, Patel R: Importance of using Bruker's security-relevant library for biotyper identification of *Burkholderia pseudomallei, Brucella* species, and *Francisella tularensis, J Clin Microbiol* 51:1639–1640, 2013.

Ellis J, Oyston PC, Green M, Titball RW: Tularemia, *Clin Microbiol Rev.* 15:631–646, 2002.

Friis-Møller A, Lemming LE, Valerius NH, Bruun B: Problems in identification of *Francisella philomiragia* associated with fatal bacteremia in a patient with chronic granulomatous disease, *J Clin Microbiol* 42:1840–1842, 2004.

Hollis DG, Weaver RE, Steigerwalt AG, et al.: *Francisella philomiragia* comb. nov. (formerly *Yersinia philomiragia*) and *Francisella tularensis* biogroup *novicida* (formerly *Francisella novicida*) associated with human disease, *J Clin Microbiol* 27:1601–1608, 1989.

Leber AL: Bioterrorism readiness plan. In *Clinical microbiology procedures handbook*, ed 4, Washington, DC, 2016, ASM Press.

Leski TA, Ansumana R, Taitt CR, et al.: Use of the FilmArray System for detection of *Zaire ebolavirus* in a small hospital in Bo Sierra Leone, *J Clin Microbiol* 53(7):2368–2370, 2015.

Limaye AP, Hooper CJ: Treatment of tularemia with fluoroquinolones: two cases and review, *Clin Infect Dis* 29:922–924, 1999.

Shapiro DS, Schwartz DR: Exposure of laboratory workers to *Francisella tularensis* despite a bioterrorism procedure, *J Clin Microbiol* 40:2278–2281, 2002.

Sjöstedt A: Virulence determinants and protective antigens of *Francisella tularensis, Curr Opin Microbiol* 6:66–71, 2003.

38

Streptobacillus spp. and *Spirillum minus*

OBJECTIVES

1. Describe the natural habitats of *Streptobacillus* spp. and *Spirillum minus.*
2. List the two ways in which *Streptobacillis* spp. are transmitted to humans.
3. Define Haverhill fever, rat-bite fever, and sodoku.
4. List the symptoms of rat-bite fever.
5. Describe the optimal conditions for culturing *S. moniliformis,* including media, supplements, atmospheric conditions, and length of incubation.
6. Describe the different appearances of *S. moniliformis* colonial morphology when grown on various media.
7. Describe how *S. minus* is detected in the laboratory.
8. Compare and contrast the microscopic appearance of *S. minus* and *S. moniliformis* in Gram-stained or other smears.

GENERA AND SPECIES TO BE CONSIDERED

Streptobacillus hongkongensis
Streptobacillus moniliformis
Streptobacillus notomysis
Spirillum minus

Streptobacillus are nonmotile, facultative anaerobic, filamentous gram-negative bacilli that require media containing blood, serum, or ascites fluid as well as incubation under carbon dioxide (CO_2) for isolation from clinical specimens. *S. moniliformis* and *S. notomysis* cause rat-bite fever or Haverhill fever in humans. *S. hongkongensis* has been isolated from patients with arthritis. *Spirillum minus* has never been grown in culture, but both are causative agents of rat-bite fever. Two additional species of *Streptobacillus* spp. have been identified in animals: *S. felis* was isolated from the lung of a cat and *S. ratti* from a black rat. Neither of these two species have been isolated from human infections.

Streptobacillus spp.

General Characteristics

The genus *Streptobacillus* is a member of the *Leptotrichiaceae* family. The *Streptobacillus* genus includes three species

that have been isolated from human infections, *S. moniliformis, S. hongkongensis,* and *S. notomytis.* The organisms are facultative, nonmotile anaerobes that tend to be highly pleomorphic.

Epidemiology and Pathogenesis

The natural habitat of *Streptobacillus* spp. is the upper respiratory tract (nasopharynx, larynx, upper trachea, and middle ear) of wild and laboratory rats (mice, gerbils, squirrels, ferrets, weasels) and other rodents such as ferrets, gerbils, mice, and squirrels; in addition, this organism occasionally has been isolated from other animals, such as cats and dogs that have fed on rodents. *Streptobacillus* spp. are pathogenic for humans and are transmitted by two routes:

- A bite from any of the organisms previously listed, or possibly through direct contact with rat feces or saliva.
- Ingestion of contaminated food, such as unpasteurized milk or milk products and, less frequently, water.

The incidence of *Streptobacillus* spp. infections is unknown, but human infections appear to occur worldwide.

The pathogenic mechanisms associated with *Streptobacillus* spp. are unknown. The organism is known to spontaneously develop L forms (bacteria without cell walls), which may allow its persistence.

Spectrum of Disease

Despite the different modes of transmission, the clinical manifestations of *Streptobacillus* spp. infection are similar. When *S. moniliformis* is acquired by ingestion, the disease is called **Haverhill fever.**

Patients with rat-bite or Haverhill fever develop acute onset of chills, fever, headache, vomiting, and often severe joint pains. Symptoms usually occur within 3 to 10 days after exposure to an infected animal. Febrile episodes may persist for weeks or months. In the first few days of illness, patients develop a rash on the palms, soles of the feet, and other extremities. Complications can occur, including endocarditis, bacteremia, septicemia, septic arthritis, pneumonia, pericarditis, brain abscess, amnionitis, prostatitis, and pancreatitis. Blood culture negative endocarditis has been reported with *S. moniliformis.*

Laboratory Diagnosis

Specimen Collection, Transport, and Processing

Unfortunately, the diagnosis of rat-bite fever caused by *Streptobacillus* spp. is often delayed because of lack of exposure history, an atypical clinical presentation, and the unusual microbiologic characteristics of the organism. Organisms may be cultured from blood or aspirates from infected joints, lymph nodes, or lesions. No special requirements have been established for the collection, transport, and processing of these specimens, except for blood. Because recovering *Streptobacillus* spp. from blood cultures are impeded by concentrations of sodium polyanethol sulfonate (SPS) used in blood culture bottles, an alternative to most commercially available bottles must be used. After collection by routine procedures (Chapter 67), blood and joint fluids are mixed with equal volumes of 2.5% citrate to prevent clotting and are then inoculated to brain-heart infusion cysteine broth supplemented with heated horse serum and yeast extract, commercially available fastidious anaerobe broth without SPS, or thiol broth.

Direct Detection Methods

Pus or exudates should be smeared, stained with Gram or Giemsa stain, and examined microscopically (Fig. 38.1). *Streptobacillus* spp. are pleomorphic, gram-negative rods. Cells may appear straight of variable size or as long, tangled chains and filaments with bulbar swellings. The cells may also appear spiral shaped and resemble a string of pearls. Direct detection of the 16S ribosomal ribonucleic acid (rRNA) gene sequence for *S. moniliformis* using polymerase chain reaction (PCR) analysis can be performed from the specimen or from the culture of the organism.

Cultivation

As previously mentioned, *S. moniliformis* requires the presence of blood, ascitic fluid, or serum for growth. Growth occurs on blood agar (15% sheep, horse, or rabbit); incubated in a very moist environment with 5% to 10% carbon dioxide (CO_2), usually after 48 hours of incubation at 37°C.

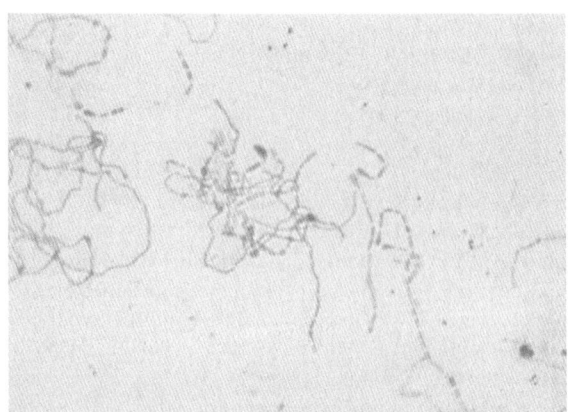

• **Fig. 38.1** Gram stain of *Streptobacillus moniliformis* from growth in thioglycollate broth with 20% serum. (Courtesy Robert E. Weaver, Centers for Disease Control and Prevention, Atlanta, GA.)

Colonies are nonhemolytic. The addition of 10% to 30% ascitic fluid (available commercially from some media suppliers) or 20% horse serum should facilitate recovery of the organism. *S. hongkongensis* has been successfully recovered from clinical specimens using Columbia agar base enriched with sheep blood either anaerobically or increased (5%) CO_2. In broth cultures, the organism grows as "fluff balls" or "bread crumbs" near the bottom of the tube or on the surface of the red blood cell layer in blood culture media. Colonies grown on brain-heart infusion agar supplemented with 20% horse serum are small, smooth, glistening, colorless or grayish, and have irregular edges.

Colonies are embedded in the agar and may have a "fried egg" appearance, with a dark center and a flattened, lacy edge. These colonies are also referred to as **L-phase** colonies because they have undergone spontaneous transformation to the L form. Staining of L-form colonies yields coccobacillary or bipolar-staining coccoid forms (usually a special stain, such as the Dienes stain performed by pathologists, is required). Acridine orange stain also reveals the bacteria when Gram stain fails because of a lack of cell wall constituents.

As previously stated, Gram-stained organisms from standard colonies show extreme pleomorphism, with long, looped, filamentous forms, chains, and swollen cells. The club-shaped cells can be two to five times the diameter of the filament. Carbolfuchsin counterstain or Giemsa stain may be necessary for visualization (Fig. 38.1).

Approach to Identification

S. moniliformis does not produce indole and is catalase-, oxidase-, and nitrate-negative, in contrast to organisms with which the *Streptobacillus* sp. may be confused, such as *Actinobacillus* spp., *Aggregatibacter aphrophilus,* and *Cardiobacterium* spp. In addition, *S. moniliformis* is nonmotile and urea- and lysine decarboxylase–negative; hydrogen sulfide (H_2S) is not produced in triple sugar iron agar but can be detected using lead acetate paper. MALDI-TOF MS has been used to identify *S. moniliformis* from pure culture. In addition, nucleic acid amplification and 16S rRNA sequencing has been used to identify *Streptobacillus* spp. from culture and culture-negative clinical samples.

Serodiagnosis

Serologic diagnosis of rat-bite fever is also useful; most patients develop agglutinating titers to the causative organism. The specialized serologic tests are performed at national reference laboratories because the disease is extremely rare in the United States. A titer of 1:80 is considered diagnostic unless a fourfold rise in titer is demonstrated.

Antimicrobial Susceptibility Testing and Therapy

No standardized methods have been established for determining *S. moniliformis* susceptibility to various antimicrobials. Different *in vitro* techniques, such as agar dilution and disk diffusion, have had similar results. Although *S. moniliformis* is susceptible to a broad spectrum of antibiotics, penicillin is regarded as the drug of choice for human rat-bite fever. Combination therapy with penicillin and an aminoglycoside is recommended for systemic infections such as endocarditis to enhance the elimination of the cell wall-deficient L forms.

Prevention

There are no vaccines available to prevent rat-bite fever. Disease is best prevented by avoiding contact with animals known to harbor the organism. Individuals with frequent animal contact should wear gloves, practice regular hand-washing, and avoid hand-to-mouth contact when handling rats or cleaning rat cages.

Spirillum minus

General Characteristics

Spirillum minus is a gram-negative, helical, strictly aerobic organism.

Epidemiology and Pathogenesis

Little information is available regarding the epidemiology or pathogenesis of *S. minus,* but it is supposed to be similar in some regard to that of *Streptobacillus* spp. The mode of transmission of infection is by a rat bite.

Spectrum of Disease

Spirillum minus also causes rat-bite fever but is primarily seen in Asia and is referred to as **sodoku** (*so,* rat; *doku,* poison). The clinical signs and symptoms are similar to those caused by *Streptobacillus,* except that arthritis is rarely seen in patients with sodoku, and swollen lymph nodes are prominent; febrile episodes are also more predictable in sodoku. The bite wound heals spontaneously, but 1 to 4 weeks later, it ulcerates to form a granulomatous lesion; at the same time, the patient develops symptoms of fever; headache; and a generalized, blotchy, purplish, maculopapular rash. Differentiation between rat-bite fever caused by *S. minus* and that caused by *Streptobacillus* is usually accomplished based on the clinical presentation of the two infections and isolation of the latter organism in culture. The incubation period for *S. minus* is much longer than that for streptobacillary rat-bite fever, which has occurred within 12 hours of the initial bite.

Laboratory Diagnosis
Specimen Collection, Transport, and Processing

Specimens commonly submitted for diagnosis of sodoku include blood, exudate, or lymph node tissues. There are no requirements for specimen collection, transport, or processing of the organisms discussed in this chapter. Refer to Table 5.1 for general information on this subject.

Direction Detection Methods

Because *S. minus* cannot be grown on synthetic media, diagnosis relies on direct visualization of characteristic spirochetes in clinical specimens using Giemsa or Wright stains or dark-field microscopy. *S. minus* appears as a thick, spiral, gram-negative organism with two or three coils and polytrichous polar flagella. Diagnosis is made by injection of lesion material or blood into experimental white mice or guinea pigs and subsequent recovery 1 to 3 weeks after inoculation.

Serodiagnosis

There is no specific serologic test available for *S. minus* infection.

Antimicrobial Susceptibility Testing and Therapy

Because this spirochete is nonculturable, routine antimicrobial susceptibility testing is not performed.

Prevention

No vaccines are available to prevent rat-bite fever. Disease is best prevented by avoiding contact with animals known to harbor the organism.

ⓔ Visit the Evolve site for a complete list of procedures, review questions, and case studies.

Bibliography

Buranakitjaroen P, Nilganuwong S, Gherunpong V: Rat-bite fever caused by *Streptobacillus moniliformis, Southeast Asian J Trop Med Public Health* 25:778–781, 1994.

Carroll KC, Pfaller MA, Landry ML, et al.: *Manual of clinical microbiology,* ed 12, Washington, DC, 2019, ASM.

Freundt EA: Experimental investigations into the pathogenicity of the L-phase variant of *Streptobacillus moniliformis, Acta Pathol Microbiol Scand* 38:246–258, 1956.

Lambe Jr DW, McPhedran AM, Mertz JA, Stewart P: *Streptobacillus moniliformis* isolated from a case of Haverhill fever: biochemical characterization and inhibitory effect of sodium polyanethol sulfonate, *Am J Clin Pathol* 60:854–860, 1973.

McEvoy MB, Noah ND, Pilsworth R: Outbreak of fever caused by *Streptobacillus moniliformis, Lancet* ii:1361, 1987.

Ogawa Y, Kasahara K, Lee ST, et al.: Rat-bite fever in human with *Streptobacillus notomytis* infection, Japan, *Emerg Infect Dis* 24(7):1377–1379, 2018.

Rupp ME: *Streptobacillus moniliformis* endocarditis: case report and review, *Clin Infect Dis* 14:769–772, 1992.

Shanson DC, Pratt J, Greene P: Comparison of media with and without "Panmede" for the isolation of *Streptobacillus moniliformis* from blood cultures and observations on the inhibitory effect of sodium polyanethol sulfonate, *J Med Microbiol* 19:181–186, 1985.

Torres-Miranda D, Moshgriz M, Siegle M: *Streptobacillus moniliformis* mitral valve endocarditis and septic arthritis: the challenges of diagnosing rat-bite fever endocarditis, *Infect Dis Rep* 10:39–41, 2018.

Wullenweber M: *Streptobacillus moniliformis:* a zoonotic pathogen— taxonomic considerations, host species, diagnosis, therapy, geographical distribution, *Lab Anim* 29:1–15, 1985.

39

Neisseria and *Moraxella catarrhalis*

OBJECTIVES

1. Identify the clinical specimens or sources for the isolation of pathogenic *Neisseria* spp.
2. List the *Neisseria* species considered normal microbiota and the sites where they colonize the human body.
3. Explain the routes of transmission for the organisms discussed in this chapter; include the clinical relevance of asymptomatic carriers.
4. Define and describe the diseases associated with *Moraxella catarrhalis* and the pathogenic *Neisseria* spp., *Neisseria gonorrhoeae* and *Neisseria meningitidis* (i.e., pelvic inflammatory disease, disseminated gonococcal infection, ophthalmia neonatorum, pharyngitis, meningitis, and septicemia); include the signs and symptoms, treatments, and prognosis.
5. Describe the method of transport that yields optimal recovery of *N. gonorrhoeae,* including transport media, growth temperatures, and atmospheric conditions.
6. Describe the benefits of amplified testing for *N. gonorrhoeae* as it relates to diagnostic and clinical efficacy.
7. Identify the optimal growth conditions for the *Neisseria* species.
8. Name the appropriate biochemical tests for differentiating the *Neisseria* species, and explain the chemical principle for each test.
9. Biochemically differentiate the organisms in this chapter using carbohydrate use (cysteine trypticase agar [CTA]) and orthonitrophenyl galactoside (ONPG).
10. Describe the appropriate therapeutic agents for *N. gonorrhoeae.*
11. Compare and contrast the laboratory identification of *M. catarrhalis* and *Neisseria* spp.
12. Analyze laboratory data and disease signs and symptoms for correlation and identification of the etiologic agents discussed in this chapter.

GENERA AND SPECIES TO BE CONSIDERED

Current Name	Previous Name
Moraxella catarrhalis	Branhamella catarrhalis, Neisseria catarrhalis
Neisseria gonorrhoeae	
Neisseria meningitidis	

Current Name	Previous Name
Other *Neisseria* spp.	
Neisseria cinerea	
Neisseria lactamica	
Neisseria polysaccharea	
Neisseria subflava	*Neisseria flava, Neisseria perflava*
Neisseria sicca	
Neisseria mucosa	
Neisseria flavescens	

General Characteristics

Species of the family *Neisseriaceae,* genus *Neisseria,* are discussed in this chapter, along with the family *Moraxellaceae,* species *Moraxella catarrhalis,* because of their biochemical and morphologic similarities. The organisms are all oxidase-positive, gram-negative diplococci that do not elongate when exposed to subinhibitory concentrations of penicillin. The rodlike *Neisseria* spp. and other *Moraxella* spp. are described in Chapter 27, and the genus *Acinetobacter,* an important clinical pathogen that is part of the family *Moraxellaceae,* is discussed in Chapter 20.

It is important to note that the implementation of next generation sequencing is beginning to identify inconsistencies in the differentiation of species among the current *Neisseria* taxonomy. Sequencing of the 16S rRNA gene generally provides sufficient interpretive criteria for identification within the genus *Neisseria.* However, lateral gene transfer can occur between species and as low as 1% diversity has been identified in the 16S rRNA sequence of *Neisseria* spp. Therefore, although the genus currently includes 30 described species, as additional target sequences are analyzed, species designations may change as more information becomes available.

Epidemiology

The *Neisseria* spp. are predominantly considered normal microbiota that reside on the mucous membranes of either humans or animals. Humans are the only natural host for

TABLE 39.1	Epidemiology	
Organism	Habitat (Reservoir)	Mode of Transmission
Moraxella catarrhalis	Normal microbiota of upper respiratory tract; occasionally colonizes female genital tract.	Spread of patient's endogenous strain to normally sterile sites. Person-to-person nosocomial spread by respiratory droplets may occur.
Neisseria gonorrhoeae	Not part of normal microbiota. Only found on mucous membranes of genitalia, anorectal area, oropharynx, or conjunctiva at time of infection.	Person-to-person spread by sexual contact, including rectal intercourse and orogenital sex. May be spread from the infected mother to newborn during birth. Asymptomatic carriers are a significant reservoir for increased disease transmission.
Neisseria meningitidis	Colonizes oropharyngeal and nasopharyngeal mucous membranes of humans. Humans commonly carry the organism without symptoms.	Person-to-person spread by respiratory droplets, usually in settings of close contact (e.g., dormitories, prisons, shelters).
Other *Neisseria* spp.	Normal microbiota of the upper respiratory tract.	Spread of patient's endogenous strain to normally sterile sites. Person-to-person spread may also be possible, but these species are not common causes of human infections.

N. gonorrhoeae, a clinically significant pathogen found in the urogenital tract, which is never considered normal microbiota. Asymptomatic carriers of *N. gonorrhoeae* are the primary reservoir for dissemination within the human population. The actual prevalence of cases of infection with *N. gonorrhoeae* is likely significantly higher than what is reported by the US Centers for Disease Control and Prevention (CDC) because of the number of unrecognized and underreported cases.

The two major pathogenic species of *Neisseria, N. gonorrhoeae* and *N. meningitidis,* are transmitted person to person. *N. gonorrhoeae* is sexually transmitted, and *N. meningitidis* is spread via respiratory droplets. Infections caused by *M. catarrhalis* and the other *Neisseria* spp. usually involve a patient's endogenous strain. Except for *Neisseria gonorrhoeae* and *Neisseria animaloris,* the organisms considered in Table 39.1 are normal commensal organisms present in the upper respiratory tract of humans.

Pathogenesis and Spectrum of Disease

As noted in Table 39.2, infections caused by *M. catarrhalis* are usually localized to the respiratory tract and rarely disseminate. Among young children, cases of acute otitis media caused by *M. catarrhalis* have been widely recognized. *M. catarrhalis* can also infect older adults but tends to cause chronic upper respiratory infections in this population.

According to the CDC, *N. gonorrhoeae* is the second most commonly reported sexually transmitted infection (STI) in the United States. In 2017, there were a total of 555,608 reported cases of gonorrhea infection, up from 333,004 reported cases in 2013. This equates to a rate of 171.9 cases/100,000 population, a 75.2% increase since the low in 2009. Infections usually remain localized to

the mucosal surfaces where the host is initially exposed to the organism (e.g., cervix, conjunctiva, oropharynx, anorectal area, or urethra of males). Localized infections may be asymptomatic or acute with a pronounced purulent response. The most common clinical presentation associated with *N. gonorrhoeae* is uncomplicated urethritis in men and genital infections in the endocervix in women. However, not all infections remain localized, and dissemination from the initial infection site can lead to severe disseminated disease (Table 39.2). Disseminated diseases with *N. gonorrhoeae* are uncommon but may result in serious morbidity and mortality, including gonococcal arthritis, endocarditis, and meningitis. Infants are at risk for acquiring infection in the eyes when passing through the birth canal. *N. gonorrhoeae* strains can also produce capsules, endotoxins, and adherence proteins to enhance protection from the host's immune responses (Table 39.2).

N. meningitidis, a leading cause of fatal bacterial meningitis in children and adults, exclusively infects humans and can be found colonizing the oropharynx and nasopharynx in approximately 10% of the population. Strains of *N. meningitidis* can be differentiated based on their distinct capsular polysaccharides. There are 12 serogroups, with eight commonly implicated in infections (A, B, C, X, Y, Z, W135, and L). The pathogenesis of the organism is related to nasopharyngeal colonization and the organism's virulence factors. The organism possesses pili that aid in organism attachment to the mucosal epithelium; opacity proteins that also play a role in host attachment; production of lipooligosaccharide, similar to lipopolysaccharide (endotoxin) of enteric gram-negative bacilli, which aids the organism in evading complement-mediated cell lysis; and the different capsular polysaccharides, which act as barriers to prevent phagocytosis.

N. meningitidis also causes a severe disseminated infection commonly referred to as invasive meningococcal

TABLE 39.2   Pathogenesis and Spectrum of Disease

Organism	Virulence Factors	Spectrum of Disease and Infections
Moraxella catarrhalis	Uncertain; factors associated with cell envelope probably facilitate attachment to respiratory epithelial cells.	Most infections are localized to sites associated with the respiratory tract and include otitis media, sinusitis, and pneumonia. Lower respiratory tract infections often target elderly patients and those with chronic obstructive pulmonary disease. Rarely causes disseminated infections such as bacteremia, meningitis, and endocarditis. Carried frequently in children and older adults; not typically isolated from the oropharynx of healthy adults.
Neisseria gonorrhoeae	Several surface factors, such as pili (types T1 and T2 virulent and T3–T5 avirulent), mediate the exchange of genetic material between strains and attachment to human mucosal cell surface, invasion of host cells, and survival through the inhibition of phagocytosis in the presence neutrophils. Genetic-phase variation of pilus structure between types T1 and T5 allows the organism to vary its antigenic structure, preventing recognition by host immune cells. Capsule, lipooligosaccharide (endotoxin), and outer cell membrane proteins I–III are important in antigenic variation and for eliciting an inflammatory response. Protein II (Opa) facilitates adherence to phagocytic and epithelial cells. Protein II (RMP) blocks the bactericidal effect of host immunoglobulin G (IgG). Outer membrane porin (PorB) provides protection from the host's immune response, including serum complement–mediated cell death.	A leading cause of sexually transmitted infections. Genital infections include acute purulent urethritis, prostatitis, and epididymitis in males and acute cervicitis in females. These infections also may be asymptomatic in females. Other localized infections include pharyngitis, anorectal infections, and conjunctivitis (e.g., ophthalmia neonatorum of newborns acquired during birth from an infected mother). Disseminated infections result when the organism spreads from a local infection to cause pelvic inflammatory disease or disseminated gonococcal infection that includes bacteremia, arthritis, and metastatic infection at other body sites. Pelvic inflammatory disease (PID) may cause sterility, ectopic pregnancy, or perihepatitis, also referred to as Fitz-Hugh–Curtis syndrome.
Neisseria meningitidis	Surface structures, perhaps pili, facilitate attachment to mucosal epithelial cells and invasion to the submucosa. Once in the blood, survival is mediated by production of a polysaccharide capsule. Endotoxin release mediates many of the systemic manifestations of infection, such as shock. Cellular proteins are similar to those described for *N. gonorrhoeae*, including Por and Opa. Two porin proteins are produced (PorA and PorB). IgA protease degrades membrane-associated IgA, increasing the host's susceptibility to invasion.	Life-threatening, acute, purulent meningitis. Meningitis may be accompanied by appearance of petechiae (i.e., rash) that is associated with meningococcal bacteremia (i.e., meningococcemia). Bacteremia leads to thrombocytopenia, disseminated intravascular coagulation, and shock. Disseminated disease is often fatal. Less common infections include conjunctivitis, pneumonia, and sinusitis.
Other *Neisseria* spp.	Unknown; probably of low virulence.	Rarely involved in human infections. When infections occur, they can include bacteremia, endocarditis, and meningitis.

disease (IMD). The clinical presentation of IMD includes symptoms of meningitis and septicemia. It is believed that IMD is transmitted by individuals who present as carriers of *N. meningitidis*. Although there is no standard for assessing carriage rates of meningococcal specific serogroups, it appears that some specific serogroups are prevalent in different age groups and demonstrate a regional distribution. Identifying the primary serogroups within a population can be used in conjunction with epidemiologic data and can provide valuable information for the prevention of transmission and disease with the appropriate vaccine.

The other *Neisseria* spp. are not considered pathogens and are often referred to as saprophytic *Neisseria*. They are often viewed as normal microbiota in respiratory culture specimens and not fully identified. Some species (e.g., *N. sicca, N. lactamica, N. bacilliformis, N. elongate,* and *N. subflava*) have been occasionally identified as the causative agent of infectious endocarditis or bacteremia. Additional species, discussed in Chapter 27, may cause soft tissue infections following an animal bite.

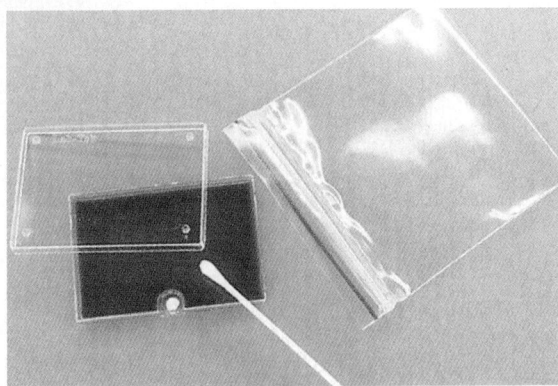

• **Fig. 39.1** JEMBEC system. Plate contains modified Thayer-Martin medium. The CO_2-generating tablet is composed of sodium bicarbonate and citric acid. After inoculation, the tablet is placed in the well, and the plate is closed and placed in the zippered plastic pouch. The moisture in the agar activates the tablet, generating a CO_2 atmosphere in the pouch.

Laboratory Diagnosis

Specimen Collection and Transport

The pathogenic *Neisseria* spp. described in this chapter are sensitive to drying and temperature extremes. In addition to general information on specimen collection and transport provided in Table 5.1, there are some special requirements for isolation of *N. gonorrhoeae* and *N. meningitidis*.

Swabs, although not optimal, are acceptable for the collection of culture-based samples for *N. gonorrhoeae* and should be plated as soon as possible. Reduced recovery of the organism may result as soon as 30 minutes after collection. Dacron-, polyurethane-, rayon-, or nylon-tipped swabs may be used for culture-based collection. Swabs should be placed in a suitable transport media such as Amie's charcoal to prevent dehydration and inhibit toxic fatty acids that may be present in the fibers. Cotton-tipped swabs and those with wooden shafts should be avoided because they can be inhibitory or toxic to *N. gonorrhoeae*. Calcium alginate swabs, oil-based lubricants, and cotton buds should not be used because they have been found to be inhibitory to organism recovery. Refrigeration of samples transported in liquid Amie's media has demonstrated sufficient recovery of *N. gonorrhoeae* in culture after 24 hours. *N. gonorrhoeae* should be inoculated to growth media immediately after specimen collection for optimal organism recovery. The sample should then be placed in a container able to sustain an atmosphere of increased carbon dioxide (CO_2) during transport. Specially packaged media consisting of selective agar in plastic trays that contain a CO_2-generating system are commercially available (JEMBEC plates). The JEMBEC system (Fig. 39.1) consists of a modified Thayer-Martin plate, CO_2-generating pill, and plastic bag. After collection, the specimen should be inoculated as soon as possible by cross-streaking the agar surface in a "Z" formation to obtain isolated colonies, activating the CO_2-generating pill, and placing the agar in the plastic bag. This system is then transported to the laboratory at room temperature. Upon receipt in the laboratory, the plate should be incubated at 37°C in 3% to 5% CO_2. Alternatively, the specimen may be sent and streaked in the laboratory and then properly incubated. Additional commercial transport systems may be useful when the collection site is separate from the diagnostic laboratory.

Molecular assays for the identification of *N. gonorrhoeae* generally provide specific specimen collection and transport systems that can be used for either urine, vaginal, or urethral specimens. In the absence of a specific collection device, Dacron- or rayon-tipped swabs are recommended with the use of Amie's transport media. Calcium alginate swabs reportedly inhibit nucleic acid amplification.

Recovery of *N. gonorrhoeae* or *N. meningitidis* from normally sterile body fluids requires no special methods, except for blood cultures. Both organisms are sensitive to sodium polyanethol sulfonate (SPS), the preservative typically found in blood culture broths. If a blood culture broth is inoculated, the SPS content should not exceed 0.025%. In addition, if blood is first collected in Vacutainer tubes containing SPS (Becton Dickinson, Sparks, MD), the specimen must be transferred to the broth culture system within 1 hour of collection.

Nasopharyngeal swabs collected to detect *N. meningitidis* carriers should be plated immediately to the JEMBEC system, or they should be submitted on swabs placed in charcoal transport media and plated within 5 hours of collection.

Specimen Processing

The JEMBEC system should be incubated at 35°C to 37°C as soon as the plate is received in the laboratory.

Any volume of clear fluid greater than 1 mL suspected of containing either of these pathogens should be centrifuged at room temperature at $1500 \times g$ for 15 minutes. The supernatant fluid should then be removed and saved, and the sediment should be vortexed and inoculated onto the appropriate media (see Cultivation section).

Any specimens or cultures in which *N. meningitidis* is a consideration should be handled in a biologic safety cabinet to prevent laboratory-acquired infections.

Direct Detection Methods
Gram Stain

The majority of the members of the genus *Neisseria* and *M. catarrhalis* appear as gram-negative diplococci (Fig. 39.2) with adjacent sides flattened. The cells are described as "kidney- or coffee bean–shaped" diplococci; other *Neisseria* spp. appear as gram-negative rods or elongated coccoid forms. Direct Gram staining of urethral discharge from symptomatic males with urethritis is an important test for gonococcal disease. The appearance of gram-negative diplococci inside polymorphonuclear leukocytes (PMNs) is diagnostic in this situation. However, because the normal vaginal and rectal microbiota are composed of gram-negative coccobacilli,

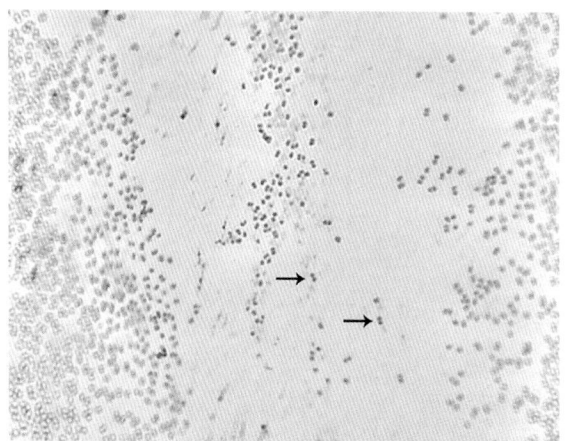

• **Fig. 39.2** Gram stain of *Neisseria gonorrhoeae* showing gram-negative diplococci *(arrows)*.

which can resemble *Neisseria* spp., direct examination of endocervical secretions in symptomatic females or rectal specimens is presumptive evidence of gonococcal infection, and the diagnosis must be confirmed by additional testing. In addition, avirulent strains may be present in specimens as extracellular diplococci; these are not pathogenic. Pharyngeal specimens should not be Gram stained, because nonpathogenic, commensal *Neisseria* spp. may be present, and the presence of these organisms is not diagnostic of infection.

The direct Gram stain of body fluids for either *N. gonorrhoeae* or *N. meningitidis* is best accomplished using a cytocentrifuge to concentrate small numbers of organisms 100-fold.

Nucleic Acid Detection

Nucleic acid–based methods have replaced old enzyme-linked immunosorbent assay systems for rapid diagnosis of *N. gonorrhoeae*. The US Food and Drug Administration (FDA) has approved a number of amplified tests for the *in vitro* detection of *N. gonorrhoeae* from clinical specimens. (For a discussion of nucleic acid–based methods, see Chapter 8.)

Amplified assays are commercially available from a variety of manufacturers. Nucleic acid amplification tests are superior to culture. The sensitivity, specificity, and positive predictive value (PPV) of the molecular assays for *N. gonorrhoeae* vary between manufacturers due to the use of different genomic target regions in the assays. A few of these tests are cartridge-based, point-of-care assays that require minimal training and rapid turnaround. Additional test systems are suitable for large-scale screening programs and can be fully integrated into automated molecular testing systems. However, the results obtained from the automated molecular test systems are not admissible as evidence in medicolegal cases or cleared for oropharyngeal, rectal, ocular, or pediatric specimens. An advantage of many of the FDA-approved nucleic acid–based tests for *N. gonorrhoeae* is the ability to detect *Chlamydia trachomatis* from the same specimen, because coinfections are common. For additional

information regarding *C. trachomatis,* refer to Chapter 43. *N. gonorrhoeae* DNA can be found in a specimen for up to 3 weeks after a successful treatment regimen; therefore, amplified nucleic acid–based methods should not be used to assess rates of cure.

Nucleic acid–based methods are also available for the detection of *N. meningitidis*. Sequence-based typing methods combined with serologic typing are currently recommended. Real-time assays are advantageous because they can quantify the amount of amplifiable template (DNA) in the sample. Molecular targets for identification include polymerase chain reaction (PCR) and sequencing of a variety of genes, including *porA, porB, fetA* (associated with *porA*), global housekeeping genes, *penA* (penicillin susceptibility), and factor H binding protein. The two genes recommended for species-specific identification by the CDC include the *ctrA* gene that is exclusive to *N. meningitidis* and is responsible for forming part of the capsule biosynthesis locus, and the copper-zinc superoxide dismutase gene, *sodC*, which has only been described in strains of *N. meningitidis*. The *sodC* gene is advantageous as a target for use in qPCR (quantitative PCR) assays because it can be used to detect nongroupable strains of *N. meningitidis* that do not contain *ctrA*. The polysialyltransferase genes *csb, csc, csw,* and *csy* can be used for serogrouping of B, C, W, and Y. At the time of this writing, the bioMerieux FilmArray meningitis/encephalitis panel is the only FDA-approved molecular assay available for the detection of *N. meningitidis*, along with 13 other viral and bacterial pathogens.

It is important to follow the manufacturer's recommendations when evaluating nucleic acid–based diagnostic tests for the identification of *Neisseria* spp. Some of the assays have limitations with regard to the type of specimen that may be used, cross reactivity with nonpathogenic species, and assay inhibition and false-negative results caused by substances present in patient samples.

Cultivation

Media of Choice

N. meningitidis, M. catarrhalis, and saprophytic *Neisseria* spp. grow well on trypticase soy agar with 5% sheep blood and enriched media, such as chocolate agar. *N. gonorrhoeae* is more fastidious and typically does not grow on blood agar but will grow on chocolate agar. Because gonococci and sometimes meningococci must be isolated from sites that contain large numbers of normal microbiota (e.g., genital tract or upper respiratory tract), selective media have been developed to facilitate their recovery. The first of these was Thayer-Martin medium, a chocolate agar with an enrichment supplement (IsoVitaleX), and the antimicrobials colistin (to inhibit gram-negative bacilli), nystatin (to inhibit yeast), and vancomycin (to inhibit gram-positive bacteria). This original medium was subsequently modified to include trimethoprim (to inhibit the swarming observed with *Proteus* spp.), and its name was changed to modified Thayer-Martin medium (MTM). Martin-Lewis (ML) medium is similar to MTM except that anisomycin, an antifungal agent, is substituted for nystatin and the concentration of vancomycin is increased. GC-LECT agar is a selective medium that contains additional antimicrobials to inhibit bacteria found in oropharyngeal specimens; it includes vancomycin and lincomycin (to inhibit gram-positive bacteria), colistin (to inhibit gram-negative bacteria), amphotericin B (to inhibit yeast), and trimethoprim (to inhibit swarming *Proteus* spp. and *Capnocytophaga* spp.).

New York City (NYC) medium, a transparent clear-to-yellow medium containing lysed horse blood, horse plasma, yeast dialysate, and the same antimicrobials as MTM, also has been used. The advantage of NYC medium is that genital mycoplasmas (*Mycoplasma hominis* and *Ureaplasma urealyticum;* refer to Chapter 44) also grow on this medium. Some strains of *N. gonorrhoeae* are inhibited by the concentration of vancomycin in the selective media. The addition of nonselective chocolate agar is recommended, especially in suspect cases that are culture-negative or for sterile specimens (e.g., joint fluid).

Unlike the pathogenic species, some of the saprophytic *Neisseria* spp. may grow on MacConkey agar, although poorly. *N. gonorrhoeae* and *N. meningitidis* will grow in most broth blood culture media but grow poorly in common nutrient broths such as thioglycollate and brain-heart infusion. *M. catarrhalis* and the other *Neisseria* spp. grow well in almost any broth medium.

Incubation Conditions and Duration

Agar plates should be incubated at 35°C to 37°C for 72 hours in a CO_2-enriched, humid atmosphere. *N. gonorrhoeae, N. meningitidis,* and *M. catarrhalis* grow best under conditions of increased CO_2 (3% to 7%). This atmosphere can be achieved using a candle jar, CO_2-generating pouch, atmospheric vacuum system, or CO_2 incubator. If incubating using a candle jar, only white, unscented candles should be used because other types may be toxic to *N. gonorrhoeae* and *N. meningitidis.*

Humidity can be provided by placing a pan with water in the bottom of a CO_2 incubator or by placing a sterile gauze pad soaked with sterile water in the bottom of a candle or vacuum jar.

All cultures should be held for 72 hours prior to resulting a negative culture for *N. gonorrhoeae* and *N. meningitidis.*

Colonial Appearance

Table 39.3 describes the colonial appearance and other distinguishing characteristics (e.g., pigment) of *M. catarrhalis* and the *Neisseria* spp. on chocolate agar.

Approach to Identification

Various commercial systems are available for the rapid identification of the coccoid *Neisseria* spp. and *M. catarrhalis.* These systems use biochemical or enzymatic substrates and work very well for the pathogenic species (*N. gonorrhoeae, N. meningitidis,* and *M. catarrhalis*). A heavy inoculum of the organism is required, but because these systems detect

TABLE 39.3	Colonial Appearance and Other Characteristics on Chocolate Agar[a]
Organism	**Appearance**
Moraxella catarrhalis	Large, pinkish to brown, opaque, smooth; friable "hockey puck" consistency: colony may be moved intact over the surface of the agar.
Neisseria gonorrhoeae	Small, grayish white, convex, translucent, shiny colonies with either smooth or irregular margins; may be up to five different colony types on primary plates.
Neisseria meningitidis	Medium, smooth, round, moist, gray to white; encapsulated strains are mucoid; may be greenish cast in agar underneath colonies.
Neisseria cinerea	Small, grayish white; translucent; slightly granular.
Neisseria elongata	Small, grayish white; translucent
Neisseria flavescens	Medium, yellow, opaque, smooth.
Neisseria lactamica	Small, nonpigmented or yellowish, smooth, transparent.
Neisseria mucosa	Large, grayish white to light yellow, translucent; mucoid because of capsule.
Neisseria polysaccharea	Small, grayish white to light yellow, translucent, raised.
Neisseria sicca	Large, nonpigmented, wrinkled, coarse and dry, adherent.
Neisseria subflava	Medium, greenish yellow to yellow, smooth, entire edge.

[a]Appearance on blood agar is the same as on chocolate agar except for pigmentation; colonies are less opaque on blood agar. Note: *N. gonorrhoeae* does not grow on classic sheep blood agars.

the activity of preformed enzymes, viability of the organisms in the inoculum is not essential. Manufacturers' instructions should be followed exactly; several systems have been developed for strains isolated on selective media and should not be used to test other gram-negative diplococci.

Biochemical Identification

Table 39.4 presents some conventional biochemical tests that traditionally have been used to identify these organisms. The extent to which identification of isolates is carried out depends on the source of the specimen and the suspected species of the organism involved.

An isolate from a child or a person involved in a case of sexual abuse must be identified unequivocally because of the medicolegal ramifications of the results. It is recommended that these organisms be identified using at least two different types of tests (i.e., biochemical, immunologic, enzymatic,

TABLE 39.4 Biochemical and Physiologic Characteristics of *Moraxella catarrhalis* and Coccoid *Neisseria* spp.

Organism	Growth On:			Rapid Fermentation Sugars								
	Modified Thayer-Martin[a]	Nutrient Agar at 35°C	Blood or Chocolate Agar at 25°C	Glucose	Maltose	Lactose	Sucrose	Fructose	Nitrate Reduction	Gas from Nitrate Reduction	0.1% Nitrite Reduction	Superoxol (30% H_2O_2)
Moraxella catarrhalis[b]	V	+	+	–	–	–	–	–	+	–	V	1 to 4+
Neisseria cinerea[c]	V	+	–	–[d]	–	–	–	–	–	–	+	Weak 2+
Neisseria elongata[e]	V	+	+	–	–	–	–	–	–	–	–	Neg
Neisseria flavescens	–	+	+	–	–	–	–	–	–	–	+[f]	2+
Neisseria gonorrhoeae[g]	+	–	–	+	–	–	–	–	–	–	–	Strong 4+
Neisseria lactamica	+	V	V	+	+	+	–	–	–	–	+	1 to 3+
Neisseria meningitidis	+	–	–	+	+	–	–	–	–	–	V	1 to 4+
Neisseria mucosa	–	+	+	+ or (+)	+	–	+	+	+	+	+	Weak 2+
Neisseria polysaccharea	–	–	–	+	+	–	–	–	–	–	–	Weak 1+ to 3+
Neisseria sicca[h]	–	+	+	+ or (+)	+	–	+	+	–	–	+	2+
Neisseria subflava[i]	–	+	+	V	+	–	–	–	–	–	+	2+

aGrowth defined as >10 colonies.
bButyrate and DNase positive.
cN. cinerea may be differentiated from N. flavescens by a positive reaction with the amylosucrase test.
dN. cinerea may appear glucose-positive in some rapid systems and be mistaken for N. gonorrhoeae. However, N. cinerea grows on nutrient agar at 35°C and reduces nitrite, unlike N. gonorrhoeae.
eN. elongata subsp. glycolytica is positive for acid production from glucose.
fN. subflava biovar flava is positive for acid production from fructose and N. subflava biovar perflava is positive for acid production from sucrose and fructose.
gKingella denitrificans may grow on modified Thayer-Martin agar and be mistaken for N. gonorrhoeae on microscopic examination. However, K. denitrificans can reduce nitrate and is catalase negative, unlike N. gonorrhoeae.
hOnly 2 of 10 strains were tested.
iNeisseria subflava produces a yellow pigment on Loeffler agar; N. sicca does not.
+, >90% of strains positive; (+), >90% of strains positive but reaction may be delayed (i.e., 2–7 days); –, >90% of strains negative; V, variable.
Data compiled from Centers for Disease Control; Carroll KC, Pfaller MA, Landry ML, et al. Manual of Clinical Microbiology. 12th ed. Washington, DC: ASM; 2019; and Weyant RS, Moss CW, Weaver RE, et al, editors. Identification of Unusual Pathogenic Gram-negative Aerobic and Facultatively Anaerobic Bacteria. 2nd ed. Baltimore: Williams & Wilkins; 1996.

amplified nucleic acid–based testing or by matrix-assisted laser desorption ionization time-of-flight mass spectroscopy (MALDI-TOF MS). Isolates from normally sterile body fluids should also be completely identified. However, isolates from genital sites in adults at risk of STI can be identified presumptively (i.e., oxidase-positive, gram-negative diplococci that grow on gonococcal selective agar). Likewise, an oxidase-positive, gram-negative diplococcus that hydrolyzes tributyrin using the enzyme butyrate esterase from an eye or ear culture can be identified as *M. catarrhalis* (Fig. 12.7).

Matrix-Assisted Laser Desorption Ionization Time-of-Flight Mass Spectrometry

MALDI-TOF MS is an automated mass spectrometry system that can identify organisms based on their protein structure (Chapter 7). Two major mass spectrometry systems are available for and have demonstrated the ability to identify *Neisseria* and *Moraxella* species. There have been reports of misidentification of commensal *Neisseria* species as *N. meningitidis*. Only organisms that are FDA-cleared for the specific MALDI-TOF MS system may be reported; however, other species may be validated by the individual laboratory.

Comments About Specific Organisms

Determination of carbohydrate utilization patterns historically has been performed in cysteine trypticase soy agar (CTA) with 1% glucose (dextrose), maltose, lactose, and sucrose (Evolve Procedure 39.1). This medium is no longer widely used because it does not work well for oxidative *Neisseria* spp., specifically *N. gonorrhoeae* and *N. meningitidis*. Carbohydrate utilization patterns are currently determined by inoculating an extremely heavy suspension of the organism to be tested in a small volume of buffered, low-peptone substrate with the appropriate carbohydrate. These methods do not require subculture or growth, and results are available in approximately 4 hours. Other rapid identification kits that are commercially available include the *Neisseria* Preformed Enzyme Test (PET) (BioConnections, Knypersley, United Kingdom), the RapID NH (Thermo-Fisher Scientific, Waltham, MA), or the API NH (bioMérieux, Marcy-l'Étoile, France). Each of these different kits has varying levels of sensitivity for correctly identifying *N. gonorrhoeae*, especially if the strain is proline iminopeptidase (Pip) negative.

Saprophytic *Neisseria* spp. are not routinely identified in the clinical laboratory. *Neisseria cinerea* may be misidentified as *N. gonorrhoeae* if the isolate produces a weak positive glucose (dextrose) reaction. However, it grows on nutrient agar at 35°C, whereas the gonococcus does not. Moreover, *N. cinerea* is inhibited by colistin, whereas *N. gonorrhoeae* is not.

M. catarrhalis can be differentiated from the gonococci and meningococci based on its growth on blood agar at 22°C and on nutrient agar at 35°C, the reduction of nitrate to nitrite, its inability to use carbohydrates, and its production of DNase. Severe *M. catarrhalis* is the only member of this group of organisms that hydrolyzes DNA.

Chromogenic substrate enzyme tests for beta-galactosidase, gamma-glutamyl aminopeptidase, and prolyl-hydroxyl prolyl aminopeptidase are available for the differentiation of *N. gonorrhoeae*, *N. meningitidis*, *N. lactamica*, and *M. catarrhalis*. *M. catarrhalis* lacks all three of these enzymes. The presence of prolyl-hydroxyl prolyl aminopeptidase alone identifies an organism as *N. gonorrhoeae*. The presence of beta-galactosidase and gamma-glutamyl aminopeptidase indicates *N. meningitidis*. Two commercial chromogenic substrate kits are the Gonocheck II (EY Laboratories, San Mateo, CA) and BactiCard *Neisseria* (Remel Laboratories, Lenexa, KS). A limitation of these methods is misidentification of various nonpathogenic strains of *Neisseria* spp. In addition, isolate colonies on selective media should be used to prevent misidentification of contaminants as a *Neisseria* spp. Modified chromogenic substrate kits, such as the Bacti-Card *Neisseria*, can be used to identify and speciate *Neisseria* and *Haemophilus* organisms from selective and nonselective media. These modified tests use a combination of enzyme substrate tests and additional biochemical tests.

N. lactamica may grow on selective media and may be confused with *N. meningitidis*. The ONPG test (Procedure 12.32) is used to determine an organism's ability to produce beta-galactosidase, which is an indicator of lactose utilization. *N. lactamica* is ONPG positive, and *N. meningitidis* is ONPG negative.

The eugonic fermenter *N. animaloris* propagates well on routine laboratory media and ferments glucose (dextrose); this distinguishes it from dysgonic fermenters that grow poorly on blood and chocolate agars (Chapter 27). *N. animaloris* ferments no carbohydrates other than glucose and is indole negative and arginine dihydrolase positive.

Immunoserologic Identification

A single particle agglutination method is available for immunoserologic identification of *N. gonorrhoeae* in the United States. The GonoGen II test (Becton Dickinson, Sparks, MD) can be performed from colonies growing on primary plates in which isolates are typed with specific monoclonal antibodies. The GonoGen II is a colorimetric test that uses antibodies adsorbed to metal sol particles. False-positives have occurred with *N. lactamica* and *N. meningitidis*, as well as false-negatives with other isolates. Extended protein extraction methods can be used to improve the sensitivity and specificity of the test.

Serotyping

Twelve different serogroups are distinguishable for *N. meningitidis*. Antisera are commercially available for identifying *N. meningitidis* serogroups A, B, C, H, I, K, L, W135, X, Y, and Z. Some manufacturers produce polyvalent antisera containing combinations of serogroups for identification. Serologic identification is usually performed by slide agglutination. A, B, C, W135, and Y are the serotypes that most commonly cause systemic disease in the United States. Serotyping is an important tool that reference or public health laboratories should possess to help aid in the identification of clusters of cases that may be related during outbreak investigations.

Nucleic acid amplification methods referred to as genogrouping are more reliable for the identification of commensal strains of *Neisseria* species. Whole genome sequencing is expected to replace serotyping.

Antimicrobial Susceptibility Testing and Therapy

Although beta-lactamase production is common among *M. catarrhalis* isolates, many beta-lactam antimicrobials maintain activity against these isolates. Because several other agents are also effective, susceptibility testing to guide therapy is not routinely required.

Standard methods have been established for performing *in vitro* susceptibility testing with *N. gonorrhoeae* and *N. meningitidis* (Chapter 11). The Clinical and Laboratory Standards Institute (CLSI) recommends the use of agar dilution for minimum inhibitory concentration (MIC) measurements and GC agar containing 1% growth supplement for *N. gonorrhoeae* disk diffusion methods.

In addition, various agents can be considered for testing and therapeutic use. Historically, fluoroquinolones were widely used to treat gonorrhea; however, resistance to these agents has emerged (i.e., fluoroquinolone-resistant *N. gonorrhoeae* [FRNG]), and they are no longer recommended for treatment of gonococcal infections.

The Gonococcal Isolate Surveillance Project (GISP) is a national collaborative surveillance project in the United States. The program was established in 1986 to analyze and monitor antimicrobial resistance trends among *N. gonorrhoeae*. Participating regional labs test isolates for resistance to antimicrobials that were commonly prescribed to treat gonococcal urethritis, including azithromycin, cefixime, ceftriaxone, ciprofloxacin, gentamicin, penicillin, and tetracycline.

Because of increasing resistance of fluoroquinolones reported in 2007, the CDC stopped recommending these agents (e.g., ciprofloxacin, levofloxacin) for treatment of gonococcal urethritis. This left cephalosporins as the only treatment option. In 2010, the CDC recommended dual therapy of a cephalosporin with azithromycin or tetracycline. Between 2006 and 2011, MICs to the oral cephalosporin cefixime have increased, and more treatment failures were reported throughout the world. As a result, in 2015 the CDC issued an update to their treatment guidelines that suggests a single-dose intramuscular injection of 250 mg of ceftriaxone taken along with either a 1-g oral dose of azithromycin or 100 mg oral doxycycline twice daily for 7 days. However, because many patients may be co-infected with *C. trachomatis*, dual therapy with azithromycin is recommended for eliminating both infections, as *C. trachomatis* is susceptible to a 1-g oral dose of azithromycin. Patients with severe penicillin

immunoglobulin E (IgE)-mediated allergies may warrant treatment with an alternative regimen; however, there are limited data on their utility. Alternative therapy includes a single-dose of 320 mg oral gemifloxacin with 2 g of oral azithromycin, or a single-dose intramuscular injection with 240 mg gentamicin and 2 g oral dose of azithromycin.

Although beta-lactamase production in *N. meningitidis* is rare, decreased susceptibility to penicillin, mediated by altered penicillin-binding proteins, is emerging. Resistance to sulfonamides is also quite common. The CLSI recommends that susceptibility testing be performed by disk diffusion on Mueller-Hinton agar or using cation-adjusted Mueller-Hinton broth in microdilution. All testing should occur within a biologic safety cabinet to minimize laboratory-acquired infections.

Prevention

The CDC recommends vaccination against *N. meningitidis* to prevent meningitis in adolescents and young adults. Currently, 11- to 12-year-olds should be vaccinated with a quadrivalent meningococcal conjugate vaccine. The two quadrivalent vaccines in the United States protect against serogroups A, C, W, and Y. The CDC recommends that a booster vaccine be given around age 16. If the initial vaccine is given to an adolescent between 13 and 15 years of age, the booster should be administered at age 18, when the patient enters a period of increased risk. Children with weakened immune systems (human immunodeficiency virus [HIV] positive, asplenia, complement deficiency, or some immunosuppressive drugs) should be given the quadrivalent vaccines earlier; depending on the age and disease, this may start as early as 8 weeks old and is given in multiple doses. There is also a vaccine available for serogroup B *N. meningitidis*. Historically, this vaccine was recommended only for people 10 years of age and older who had been identified as being at increased risk for exposure to serogroup B (e.g., community outbreak). However, the Advisory Committee on Immunization Practices has revised their position and allows individual clinical decision-making regarding the use of the serogroup B meningococcal vaccine. This is a multistep vaccination, and for each dose, the same manufacturer should be used because they are not interchangeable.

Ophthalmia neonatorum occurs when *N. gonorrhoeae* from an infected mother is transmitted to the newborn during vaginal delivery. Previously, this was a leading cause of neonatal blindness. Prophylactic administration of antimicrobials after birth has dramatically reduced the development of gonococcal conjunctivitis. The CDC recommends a single dose of 0.5% erythromycin ophthalmic ointment into each eye at birth. Silver nitrate is no longer manufactured in the United States, and povidone-iodine has not been adequately studied and is therefore not recommended.

ⓔ Visit the Evolve site for a complete list of procedures, review questions, and case studies.

Bibliography

Abadi FJ, Yakubu DE, Pennington TH: Antimicrobial susceptibility of penicillin-sensitive and penicillin-resistant meningococci, *J Antimicrob Chemother* 35: 687-190, 1995.

Bennett DE, Mulhall RM, Cafferkey MT: PCR-based assay for detection of *Neisseria meningitidis* capsular serogroups 29E, X, and Z, *J Clin Microbiol* 42:1764–1765, 2004.

Blondeau JM, Ashton FE, Isaacson M, et al.: *Neisseria meningitidis* with decreased susceptibility to penicillin in Saskatchewan, Canada, *J Clin Microbiol* 33:1784–1786, 1995.

Bratcher HB, Harrison OB, Maiden MCJ: Genome sequencing and interrogation of genome databases: a guide to *Neisseria meningitidis* genomics, *Methods Mol Biol* 1969:51–82, 2019.

Carroll KC, Pfaller MA, Landry ML, et al.: *Manual of clinical microbiology*, ed 12, Washington, DC, 2019, ASM.

Centers for Disease Control and Prevention (CDC): *Sexually transmitted disease surveillance 2017: gonorrhea*, 2018. Available at: https://www.cdc.gov/std/stats17/gonorrhea.htm.

Centers for Disease Control and Prevention (CDC): *Sexually transmitted disease treatment guidelines*, 2015. Available at: https://www.cdc.gov/std/tg2015/gonorrhea.htm.

Clinical and Laboratory Standards Institute (CLSI): 29th edition, *Performance standards for antimicrobial susceptibility testing*, M100, Wayne, PA, 2018, CLSI.

Committee on Infectious Diseases: *2006 red book: report of the Committee on Infectious Diseases*, ed 27, Elk Grove Village, IL, 2006, American Academy of Pediatrics.

Dolan Thomas J, Hatcher CP, Satterfield DA, et al.: sodC-based real-time PCR for detection of *Neisseria meningitidis*, *PloS One* 6:e19361, 2011.

Guldemir D, Turan M, Bakkaloglu Z, et al.: Optimization of real-time multiplex polymerase chain reaction for the diagnosis of acute bacterial meningitis and *Neisseria meningitidis* serogrouping, *Mikrobiyol Bul* 52:221–232, 2018.

Heiddal S, Sverrisson JT, Yngvason FE, et al.: Native valve endocarditis due to *Neisseria sicca*: case report and review, *Clin Infect Dis* 16:667, 1993.

Hong E, Bakhalek Y, Taha MK: Identification of *Neisseria meningitidis* by MALDI-TOF MS may not be reliable, *Clin Microbiol Infect* 25:717–722, 2019.

Kam KM, Wong PW, Cheung MM, Ho NK: Detection of quinolone-resistant *Neisseria gonorrhoeae*, *J Clin Microbiol* 34:1462–1464, 1996.

Meyer GA, Shope TR, Waecker Jr NJ, Lanningham FH: *Moraxella (Branhamella) catarrhalis* bacteremia in children, *Clin Pediatr (Phila)* 34:146–150, 1995.

Peterson ME, Li Y, Shanks H, et al.: Serogroup-specific meningococcal carriage by age group: a systemic review and meta-analysis, *BMJ Open* 9(4):e024343, 2019.

Rosenstein NE, Perkins BA, Stephens DS, et al.: Meningococcal disease, *N Engl J Med* 344:1378–1388, 2001.

Satterwhite CL, Torrone E, Meites E, et al.: Sexually transmitted infections among US women and men: prevalence and incidence estimates, 2008, *Sex Transm Dis* 40:187–193, 2013.

Tanaka M, Matsumoto T, Kobayashi I, Uchino U, Kumazawa J: Emergence of in vitro resistance to fluoroquinolones in *Neisseria gonorrhoeae* isolated in Japan, *Antimicrob Agents Chemother* 39:2367–2370, 1995.

Unemo M, Golparian D, Eyre DW: Antimicrobial resistance in *Neisseria gonorrhoeae* and treatment of gonorrhea, *Methods Mol Biol* 1997:37–58, 2019.

Vandamme P, Holmes B, Bercovier H, Coenye T: Classification of Centers for Disease Control group eugonic fermenter (EF)-4a and EF-4b as *Neisseria animaloris* sp. nov. and *Neisseria zoodegmatis* sp. nov., respectively, *Int J Syst Evol Microbiol* 56:1801–1805, 2006.

Verghese A, Berk SL: *Moraxella (Branhamella) catarrhalis*, *Infect Dis Clin North Am* 5:523–538, 1991.

Weyant RS, Moss CW, Weaver RE, et al.: *Identification of unusual pathogenic gram-negative aerobic and facultatively anaerobic bacteria*, ed 2, Baltimore, 1996, Williams & Wilkins.

Woods CR, Smith AL, Wasilauskas BL, Campos J, Givner LB: Invasive disease caused by *Neisseria meningitidis* relatively resistant to penicillin in North Carolina, *J Infect Dis* 170:453–456, 1994.

40

Overview and General Laboratory Considerations

OBJECTIVES

This chapter provides an overview of the methods used to identify anaerobic microorganisms. The detailed technical procedures discussed are designed for use in conjunction with specifics provided in Chapter 41 to develop a clear understanding of the full process, from specimen collection to identification. However, readers should consider the following general objectives for the information and methods provided.

1. State the specific diagnostic purpose for the test methodology.
2. Briefly describe the test principle associated with the test methodology.
3. Outline limitations and describe a process for troubleshooting or reporting results if a test result is equivocal or indistinguishable.
4. State the appropriate quality-control organisms and results used with each testing procedure.
5. Define and differentiate obligate (strict), moderate, facultative, and aerotolerant anaerobes.
6. List suitable specimens for isolation of anaerobic bacteria and characteristics of these specimens that might suggest the presence of an anaerobic infection.
7. Explain the proper techniques for collecting, transporting, and processing clinical specimens for anaerobic bacteriology.
8. Explain the use of antigen detection methodologies in the diagnosis of anaerobic infections.
9. List the media used for cultivation of anaerobic bacteria.
10. Describe the appropriate incubation conditions for cultivation of anaerobic bacteria.
11. Describe the procedures for the identification of and antibiotic susceptibility testing for anaerobic bacteria.

General Characteristics

The organisms described in this chapter and in Chapter 41 are common etiological agents of a variety of clinical conditions. The organisms included in this chapter are predominant in the human microbiome and are often opportunistic pathogens. These organisms do not grow in the presence of oxygen (O_2); they are **obligate** or **strict anaerobes** (0% O_2).

Obligate anaerobes are killed upon brief exposure (less than a few minutes) to atmospheric oxygen. Obligate anaerobes include *Prevotella* spp., *Fusobacterium* spp., and *Bacteroides* spp., which are included in these chapters. These chapters also include some **aerotolerant organisms** (5% O_2), such as *Actinomyces* spp., *Bifidobacterium* spp., and *Clostridium* spp., which are capable of growth in the presence of either reduced or atmospheric oxygen (microaerobic) but grow best under anaerobic conditions. Finally, **facultative anaerobes** do not require atmospheric oxygen but are capable of growth in oxygen and anaerobic environments.

Anaerobic organisms lack superoxide dismutase and catalase, the enzymes required to break down reactive oxygen species produced during respiration or aerobic metabolism. In addition, oxygen has a high affinity for organic compounds containing nitrogen, hydrogen, carbon, and sulfur, which interfere with normal biologic activity. Because they are unable to protect themselves against the action of oxygen, anaerobes require an environment free of oxygen to survive and grow.

Specimen Collection and Transport

The importance of proper collection and transport of specimens for anaerobic culture cannot be overemphasized. Because indigenous anaerobes are often present in large numbers as normal microbiota on mucosal surfaces, even minimal contamination of a specimen can produce misleading results. Box 40.1 shows the specimens acceptable for anaerobic culture; Box 40.2 presents specimens that are likely to be contaminated and therefore are unacceptable for anaerobic culture. In general, material for anaerobic culture is best collected by tissue biopsy or by aspiration using a needle and syringe to prevent contamination with normal microbiota. After collection, the air must be expelled from the device to prevent the reduction or loss of viable anaerobes in the sample. Because of the potential for contamination with normal microbiota, swabs are generally not recommended for the collection of anaerobes.

However, as previously described in Chapter 5, flocked swabs commercially available from numerous manufacturers have an improved design that enhances the recovery of both aerobes and anaerobes but are still prone to contamination and can be used when no other specimen type may be collected.

A crucial factor in obtaining valid results with anaerobic cultures is the transport of the specimen; the lethal effect of atmospheric oxygen must be nullified until the specimen can be processed in the laboratory. Recapping a syringe and transporting the needle and syringe to the laboratory is no longer acceptable because of safety concerns involving needle stick injuries. Even aspirates must be injected into an oxygen-free transport tube or vial. A large variety of transport devices that contain prereduced anaerobic media for the preservation of microorganisms are available commercially.

Macroscopic Examination of Specimens

Upon receipt in the laboratory, specimens should be inspected for characteristics that strongly indicate the presence of anaerobes: (1) foul odor; (2) sulfur granules (associated with *Actinomyces* spp., *Propionibacterium* spp., or *Eubacterium* sp.); and (3) brick red fluorescence under long wavelength ultraviolet (UV) light (associated with pigmented *Prevotella* or *Porphyromonas* spp.).

Direct Detection Methods

Gram Staining

The Gram stain is an important rapid tool for anaerobic bacteriology. Gram stain morphology from direct specimens should be carefully noted if an anaerobic infection is suspected, because organisms may no longer be viable and additional testing, such as anaerobic cultures, may demonstrate no growth. Not only does a properly performed Gram stain reveal the types and relative numbers of microorganisms and host cells present, it also serves as a quality control measure for the adequacy of anaerobic techniques. The absence of leukocytes does not rule out the presence of a serious anaerobic infection, however, because certain organisms, such as clostridia, produce necrotizing toxins that destroy white blood cells. A positive Gram stain with a negative culture may indicate (1) poor transport methods, (2) excessive exposure to air during specimen processing, (3) failure of the system (jar, pouch, or chamber) to achieve an anaerobic atmosphere, (4) inadequate types of media or old media, or (5) killing of microorganisms by antimicrobial therapy.

Standard Gram stain procedures and reagents are used, except that the safranin counterstain is left on for 3 to 5 minutes. Gram-negative anaerobes often stain poorly with safranin, resulting in failure to visualize pathogenic organisms. As an alternative, 0.5% aqueous basic fuchsin can be used as the counterstain to improve identification of gram-negative anaerobes. In addition, some gram-positive anaerobes (e.g., *Clostridium* spp.) stain pink. Enhanced Gram stain reagents are available that contain different concentrations in the reagents, in addition to a Gram enhancer, which is applied after decolorization to suppress the red color in the background, aiding the differentiation of gram-negative anaerobes.

Table 40.1 presents the cellular morphology seen with Gram staining of common anaerobes.

TABLE 40.1   Minimal Criteria Grouping Gram Stain Morphology, Aerotolerance, and Clinical Significance of Anaerobic Bacteria

Organism	Gram Stain[a]	Clinical Significance
Actinobaculum spp.	Gram-positive slightly curved rods; some species may branch	Urinary tract infections
Actinomyces spp.	Gram-positive, branching, beaded or banded, thin, filamentous rods	Actinomycosis; orocervicofacial, thoracic, and abdominopelvic forms
Actinotignum spp.	Gram-positive straight or slightly curved rods	Urinary tract infections
Alloscardovia spp.	Gram-positive short irregular shaped rods	Urinary tract infections
Alistipes spp.	Gram-negative rods	Appendicitis, intraabdominal fluids, abscesses, and urine
Anaerococcus spp.	Gram-positive cocci arranged in short chains or tetrads	Wound infections
Anaeroglobus sp.	Gram-negative cocci with cells approximately 0.5–1.1 µm in diameter	Postoperative wounds
Atopobium spp.	Elongated gram-positive cocci or coccobacilli; occur singly, in pairs, or in short chains	Bacterial vaginosis
Bacteroides spp.	Gram-negative, straight rods with rounded ends; occur singly or in pairs; cells may be described as resembling a safety pin (Fig. 41.4)	Bacteremia, ulcers, abscesses, bronchial secretions, bone, intraabdominal infections; body fluids
Bifidobacterium spp.	Gram-positive diphtheroid; coccoid or thin, pointed shape; or larger, highly irregular, curved rods with branching; rods terminate in clubs or thick, bifurcated (forked) ends ("dog bones")	Predominantly bacterium but may be isolated from a variety of sources
Bilophila wadsworthia	Gram-negative, pale-staining, delicate rods	Intraabdominal infections, abscesses, and bacteremia
Bulleidia spp.	Gram-positive short, straight, or slightly curved; singly or in pairs	Periodontitis and abscesses
Catabacter spp.	Gram-positive coccobacilli or short rods	Bacteremia
Clostridioides difficile	Gram-positive straight rods; may produce chains of up to six cells aligned end to end; spores oval and subterminal	Antibiotic associated disease, diarrhea, and colitis
Clostridium botulinum	Gram-positive, straight rods; occur singly or in pairs; spores usually subterminal and resemble a tennis racket	Food poisoning, botulism; wound botulism and infant botulism, a life-threatening neuromuscular disorder
Clostridium clostridioforme	Gram-positive rod that stains gram negative; long, thin rods; spores usually not seen; elongated football shape with cells often in pairs	Variety of human infections that may be serious and invasive
Clostridium histolyticum		Bacteremia; trauma associated gas gangrene; skin and other soft tissue infections
Clostridium novyi	Gram-positive rods with subterminal spores	Skin and other soft tissue infections; cutaneous gas gangrene
Clostridium perfringens	Gram-variable straight rods with blunt ends; occur singly or in pairs; spores seldom seen but if present are large and central to subterminal, oval, and swell cell; large boxcar shapes	Bacteremia; trauma-associated gas gangrene, skin and other soft tissue infections; enteric foodborne disease (food poisoning); enteritis necroticans and necrotizing enterocolitis; anaerobic cellulitis
Clostridium ramosum	Gram-variable straight or curved rods; spores rarely seen but are round and terminal; more slender and longer than *C. perfringens*	Abscesses, peritonitis, bacteremia, and chronic otitis media in children; bacteremia in adults

Continued

TABLE 40.1	Minimal Criteria Grouping Gram Stain Morphology, Aerotolerance, and Clinical Significance of Anaerobic Bacteria—cont'd	

Organism	Gram Stain[a]	Clinical Significance
Clostridium septicum	Gam positive in young cultures but becomes gram negative with age; stains unevenly; straight or curved rods; occur singly or in pairs; spores sub-terminal, oval, and swell cells	Bacteremia; trauma-associated gas gangrene; skin and other soft tissue infections; spontaneous nontraumatic gas gangrene
Clostridium sordellii	Gram-positive rods; subterminal spores	Skin and other soft tissue infections; cutaneous gas gangrene; gynecological infections; anaerobic cellulitis
Clostridium tertium	Gram-variable rods; terminal spores	Neutropenic enterocolitis and meningitis in immunocompromised patients
Clostridium tetani	Gram positive, becoming gram negative after 24-h incubation; occur singly or in pairs; spores oval and terminal or subterminal with drumstick or ten-nis racket appearance	Tetanus associated with puncture wounds
Cryptobacterium spp.	Gram-positive short rods in chains	Oral infections
Curtobacterium spp.	Pleomorphic gram-positive rods, may be branching	Associated with prosthetic infections such as joints and heart valves
Eggerthella spp.	Gram-positive, small, straight rod with rounded ends	Bacteremia
Eggerthii spp.	Gram-positive irregular rods in short chains	Dental abscess with bacteremia; empy-ema
Eisenbergiella spp.	Gram-positive medium to long, wavy filamentous rods with tapered ends	Bacteremia
Eubacterium spp.	Gram-positive pleomorphic rods or coccobacilli; occur in pairs or short chains; *Eubacterium alactolyticum* has a seagull-wing shape similar to *Campylobacter* spp.; *Eubacterium nodatum* is similar to *Actinomyces* spp. with beading, fila-ments, and branching	Oral and other various infections; abscesses, bacteremia, sinusitis, tonsil-litis
Filifactor spp.	Gram-positive short, regular bacilli	Oral infections
Finegoldia magna	Gram-positive cocci with cells >0.6 μm in diameter; in pairs and clusters; resemble staphylococci	Infections in various body sites including endocarditis, meningitis, pneumonia, skin, and soft tissue; bone and joint infections, chronic wounds and ulcers, septic arthritis, upper respiratory infec-tions; bacteremia
Fusobacterium spp.	Gram-negative, pale-staining, irregularly stained, highly pleomorphic rods with swollen areas, fila-ments, and large, bizarre, round bodies	Oral and other various infections; abscesses, bacteremia, sinusitis, tonsil-litis
Lactobacillus spp.	Gram-variable pleomorphic rods or coccobacilli; straight, uniform rods have rounded ends; short coccobacilli resemble streptococci	Bacteremia, endocarditis, intraabdominal abscesses; various other infections
Leptotrichia spp.	Gram-negative, large, fusiform rods with one pointed end and one blunt end	Bacteremia in immunocompromised patients; lesions in the oral and gastro-intestinal mucosa; endocarditis; bacte-rial vaginosis
Mobiluncus spp.	Gram-variable, small, thin, curved rods; the two spe-cies can be divided based on cell length	Vaginal tract; bacterial vaginosis
Mogibacterium spp.	Gram-positive short rods	Oral infections
Moryella spp.	Gram-positive elongated rods with pointed ends	Abscesses
Olsenella spp.	Short, elliptical gram-positive rods; occur singly, in pairs, or short chains	Dental caries

TABLE 40.1 Minimal Criteria Grouping Gram Stain Morphology, Aerotolerance, and Clinical Significance of Anaerobic Bacteria—cont'd

Organism	Gram Stain[a]	Clinical Significance
Parabacteroides spp.	Gram-negative rods	Intraabdominal infections, bacteremia
Paraeggerthella sp.	Gram-positive, coccobacilli in chains	Bacteremia
Parvimonas micros	Gram-positive cocci with cells <0.7 μm in diameter; occur in packets and short chains	Oral pathogen, periodontal infections, skin and wound infections, intraabdominal infections, septicemia, gynecological infections, otitis media, and sinus infection
Peptoniphilus spp.		Pressure ulcers and rhinosinusitis
Peptostreptococcus spp.	Gram-positive, large coccobacillus; often in chains	Polymicrobial infections in a variety of body sites; acute and chronic wound infections
Porphyromonas spp.	Gram-negative coccobacilli	Periodontal disease, necrotizing ulcerative gingivitis, abscesses, intraabdominal, bacterial vaginosis, synovial fluid (arthritis)
Prevotella spp.	Gram-negative rods or coccobacilli; occur in pairs or short chains	Oral infections, necrotizing ulcerative gingivitis, pericoronitis, abscesses; associated with respiratory infections in cystic fibrosis patients, ventilator-associated pneumonia
Propionibacterium spp.	Gram-positive, pleomorphic, diphtheroid-like rod; club-shaped to palisade arrangements; called *anaerobic diphtheroids*	Acne and superficial skin infections
Propionimicrobium spp.	Gram-positive diphtheroid or club-shaped rods	Urinary tract infections
Pseudoramibacter spp.	Gram-positive pleomorphic rods that occur in pairs	Oral infections
Scardovia spp.	Gram-positive small, coccoid rods	Dental caries
Slackia spp.	Gram-positive cocci, coccobacilli, rods; singly or in clumps	Oral infections or abscesses
Solobacterium spp.	Gram-positive short, straight, or slightly curved rods that occur in pairs or short chains	Bacteremia; various infections
Tannerella spp.	Gram-negative rods	Periodontal disease, bacterial vaginosis, synovial fluid (arthritis)
Veillonella spp.	Gram-negative, tiny diplococci in clusters, pairs, and short chains	Polymicrobial infections of various body sites; meningitis, osteomyelitis, prosthetic joint infections, pleuropulmonary infection, bacteremia, and endocarditis
Varibaculum spp.	Gram-positive short, straight, or curved rods, diphtheroid	IUD infections

Specimen Processing

Specimens for anaerobic culture may be processed in the biologic safety cabinet, after which they are incubated in anaerobic jars or pouches or in an anaerobic chamber.

Anaerobe Jars or Pouches

The most commonly used system for creating an anaerobic atmosphere is the **anaerobe jar.** Anaerobe jars are available commercially from several companies. For example, the GasPak (Fig. 40.1) is made by Becton Dickinson (Sparks, MD); other companies that produce these devices include EM Diagnostic Systems (Gibbstown, NJ) and Oxoid USA (Columbus, MD). All of these systems use a clear, heavy plastic jar with a lid clamped down to make it airtight. Anaerobic conditions can be set up by two methods. The first method uses a commercially available envelope containing a hydrogen and CO_2 generator activated either by adding water (GasPak) or by the moisture on the agar plates (EM Diagnostic Systems and Oxoid USA). The production of heat within a few minutes (detected by touching the top

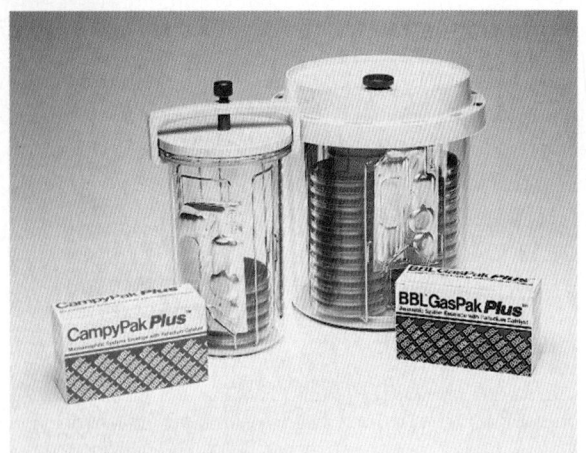

• **Fig. 40.1** GasPak anaerobe jar (BD Diagnostic Systems, Sparks, MD). Inside the jar are inoculated plates, an activated gas-generating envelope, and an indicator strip. A wire-mesh basket attached to the lid of the jar contains palladium-coated alumina pellets that catalyze the reaction to remove oxygen. Newer models of the GasPak jar use reagent packs that simply require the addition of water to catalyze a reaction (see text). (From Mahon CR. *Textbook of Diagnostic Microbiology.* 5th ed. St. Louis: Elsevier; 2015.)

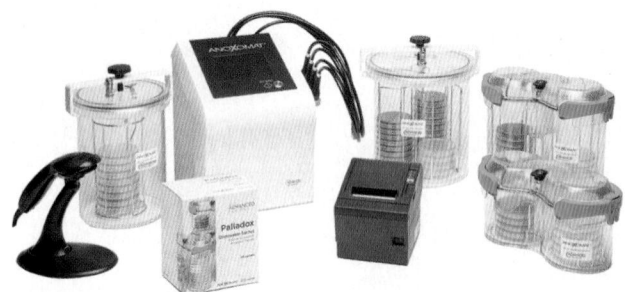

• **Fig. 40.2** Advanced Anoxomat System for the cultivation of anaerobic, microaerophilic, and capnophilic organisms. (Photos courtesy Advanced Instruments, Inc., Norwood, MA.)

of the jar) and subsequent development of moisture on the walls of the jar are indications that the catalyst and generator envelope are functioning properly. Reduced conditions are achieved in 1 to 2 hours, although the methylene blue or resazurin indicators take longer to decolorize.

Alternatively, the **evacuation-replacement** method can be used to create a specific environment in a short period. Air is removed from the sealed jar by drawing a vacuum and replaced with a combination of three different gases. The final fill of the jar is made with a gas mixture containing 80% to 90% nitrogen, 5% to 10% hydrogen, and 5% to 10% CO_2. Many anaerobes require CO_2 for maximal growth. The Anoxomat (Advanced Instruments, Inc., Norwood, MA; Fig. 40.2) is a complete system for the culturing of anaerobes, capnophiles, and microaerophilic organisms. The system provides the flexibility of creating optimal conditions in separate jars and may be adapted to the laboratory's needs. The atmosphere in the jars is monitored using an indicator to check anaerobiosis. The disadvantage is that plates must be removed from the jars to view bacterial growth on the plates.

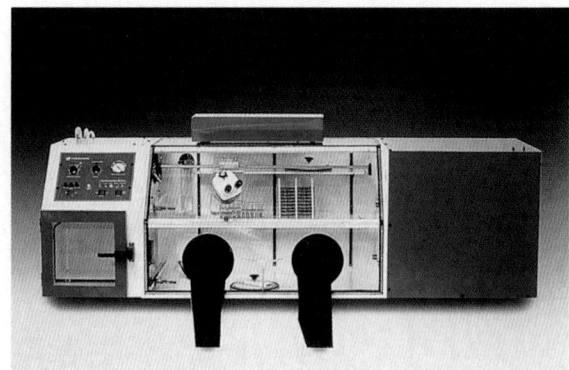

• **Fig. 40.3** Gloveless anaerobe chamber. Anaerobic chambers were developed more than 40 years ago, and a variety of new models are being used in cutting-edge research. (Courtesy Anaerobe Systems, Morgan Hill, CA.)

Anaerobe bags or **pouches** are useful for laboratories processing small numbers of anaerobic specimens. A widely used anaerobic pouch is the BD Biobag Type A (Becton Dickinson and Company, Franklin Lakes, NJ). Besides specimen transport, the pouch can be used to incubate one or two agar plates. If moisture or condensation has not accumulated on the inside of the bag or pouch, it is possible to view the plates without removing them from the bag.

Holding Jars

If anaerobic jars or pouches are used for incubation, holding jars should be used during specimen processing and examination of cultures. Holding jars are anaerobic jars with loosely fitted lids attached by rubber tubing to nitrogen gas. Uninoculated plates are kept in holding jars pending use for culture setup, and inoculated plates are kept in holding jars pending incubation or examination; this minimizes exposure to oxygen.

Anaerobe Chamber

Anaerobic chambers, or **glove boxes,** are made of molded or flexible clear plastic. The flexible clear plastic chambers are the most widely used type. Specimens and other materials are placed in the chamber through an air lock. The technologist uses gloves (Forma Scientific, Marietta, OH) or sleeves (Sheldon Manufacturing, Cornelius, OR) to form airtight seals around the arms (Fig. 40.3). Media stored in the chamber are kept oxygen-free, and all work on a specimen, from inoculation through workup, is performed under anaerobic conditions. A gas mixture of 5% CO_2, 10% hydrogen, and 85% nitrogen, plus a **palladium catalyst** (reacts with water to produce hydrogen and carbon dioxide), maintain the anaerobic environment inside the chamber.

Anaerobic Media

Initial processing of anaerobic specimens involves inoculation of appropriate media. Table 40.2 lists commonly used anaerobic media. Primary plates should be freshly prepared or used within 2 weeks of preparation. Plates stored for longer

TABLE 40.2 Common Anaerobic Media

Medium	Components/Comments	Primary Purpose
Anaerobic blood agar (Ana BA)	May be prepared with Columbia, Schaedler, CDC, *Brucella,* or brain-heart infusion base supplemented with 5% sheep blood, 0.5% yeast extract, hemin, L-cystine, and vitamin K_1.	Nonselective medium for isolation of anaerobes and facultative anaerobes
Bacteroides bile esculin agar (BBE)	Trypticase soy agar base with ferric ammonium citrate and hemin; bile salts and gentamicin act as inhibitors.	Selective and differential for *Bacteroides fragilis* group; good for presumptive identification
Laked kanamycin-vancomycin (LKV)	*Brucella* agar base with kanamycin (75 µg/ mL), vancomycin (7.5 µg/mL), vitamin K_1 (10 µg/mL), and 5% laked blood.	Selective for isolation of *Prevotella* and *Bacteroides* spp.
Anaerobic phenylethyl alcohol agar (PEA)	Nutrient agar base, 5% blood, phenylethyl alcohol.	Selective for inhibition of enteric gram-negative rods and swarming by some clostridia
Egg yolk agar (EYA)	Egg yolk base.	Nonselective for determination of lecithinase and lipase production by clostridia and fusobacteria
Cycloserine cefoxitin fructose agar (CCFA)	Egg yolk base with fructose, cycloserine (500 mg/L), and cefoxitin (16 mg/L); neutral red indicator.	Selective for *Clostridioides difficile*
Cooked meat (also called chopped meat) broth	Solid meat particles initiate growth of bacteria; reducing substances lower oxidation-reduction potential (Eh).	Nonselective for cultivation of anaerobic organisms; with addition of glucose, can be used for gas-liquid chromatography
Peptone–yeast extract–glucose broth (PYG)	Peptone base, yeast extract, glucose, cysteine (reducing agent), resazurin (oxygen tension indicator), salts.	Nonselective for cultivation of anaerobic bacteria for gas-liquid chromatography
Thioglycollate broth	Pancreatic digest of casein, soy broth, and glucose to enrich growth of most bacteria. Thioglycollate and agar reduce Eh. May be supplemented with hemin and vitamin K_1.	Nonselective for cultivation of anaerobes, facultative anaerobes, and aerobes

periods accumulate peroxides and become dehydrated; this results in growth inhibition. Reduction of media in an anaerobic environment eliminates dissolved oxygen but has no effect on the peroxides. Prereduced, anaerobically sterilized (PRAS) media are produced, packaged, shipped, and stored under anaerobic conditions. They are commercially available from a variety of manufacturers (Fig. 40.4) and have an extended shelf life of up to 6 months.

In general, anaerobic media should include a nonselective anaerobic blood agar (BA) (containing horse or sheep blood, additional hemin, and vitamin K) and all of the following selective media: *Bacteroides* **bile esculin agar (BBE), laked kanamycin-vancomycin BA (LKV), anaerobic phenylethyl alcohol agar (PEA), and an anaerobic broth.** In addition, aerobic 5% sheep BA, chocolate agar, and MacConkey agar are set up because most anaerobic infections are polymicrobic and may include aerobic or facultative anaerobic bacteria. A backup broth, usually thioglycollate, is inoculated to enrich small numbers of anaerobes in tissues and other sterile specimens and in some cases should be held for up to 14 days. Most anaerobes grow well on any of these media.

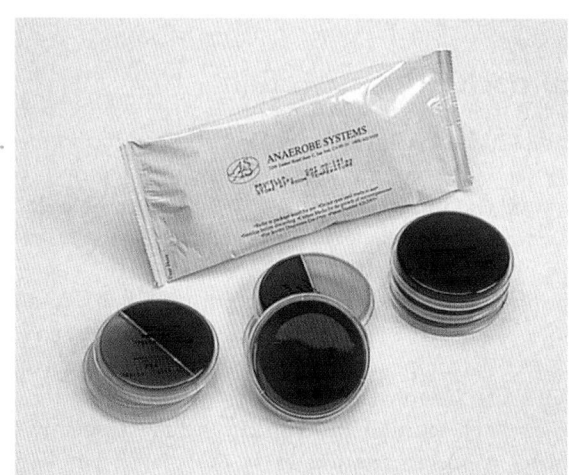

• **Fig. 40.4** Prereduced, anaerobically sterilized (PRAS) plated media. (Courtesy Anaerobe Systems, Morgan Hill, CA.)

Cultures for *Clostridioides difficile* are plated on a special selective medium, **cycloserine cefoxitin fructose agar (CCFA)** or **egg yolk agar (EYA).** There are also selective media for groups of anaerobes, such as *Actinomyces* spp., although they are rarely used in the clinical laboratory.

Special anaerobic blood culture systems containing various media, including thioglycollate broth, thiol broth, and Schaedler broth, are commercially available. Although many anaerobes will grow in the aerobic blood culture bottle, it is better to use an unvented anaerobic broth when attempting to isolate these organisms from blood or bone marrow.

Incubation Conditions and Duration

Inoculated plates should be immediately incubated under anaerobic conditions at 35°C to 37°C for 48 hours. In general, cultures should not be exposed to oxygen until after 48 hours' incubation, because anaerobes are most sensitive to oxygen during their log phase of growth. Plates may be removed from the anaerobic environment at 24 hours, briefly evaluated, and returned to the anaerobic environment. Plates incubated in an anaerobe chamber or bag can be examined at 24 hours without oxygen exposure for typical colonies of *B. fragilis* group or *Clostridium perfringens.* Plates that show no growth at 48 hours should be incubated for at least 5 days before being discarded. Thioglycollate broth can be incubated anaerobically with the cap loose or anaerobically with the cap tight. Broths should be inspected daily for 7 days.

In addition to the anaerobic media, a chocolate agar plate (CHOC) should be inoculated to determine whether the anaerobe is a facultative or strict obligate anaerobe. The CHOC should be placed in the CO_2 incubator. A 5% sheep BA plate is inoculated and placed in an anaerobic environment. The plates should be incubated at 35°C to 37°C for 48 hours. This test is referred to as an **aerotolerance test.** If an organism is a true strict anaerobe, there should be no visible growth on the chocolate plate after incubation. However, some anaerobes are aerotolerant and will be visible on the sheep BA plate, including *Propionibacterium* spp., *Clostridium* spp., *Lactobacillus* spp., *Actinomyces* spp., and other genera.

Approach to Identification

The direct Gram stain is essential in the identification of a potential anaerobic infection and may be the only procedure available in some laboratories. Table 40.1 provides an overview of many anaerobic bacteria including the expected Gram stain results and clinical significance. The complete identification of anaerobes can be costly, often requiring various biochemical tests. Most clinical laboratories no longer perform complete identification of anaerobes because presumptive identification is just as useful in assisting the physician in determining appropriate therapy. Therefore, the approach to identification taken in this chapter emphasizes simple, rapid methods to identify commonly isolated anaerobic bacteria. Identification should proceed in a stepwise fashion, beginning with examination of the primary plates.

Examination of Primary Plates

Anaerobes are usually present in mixed culture with other anaerobes and facultative bacteria. The combination of selective and differential agar plates yields information that suggests the presence and perhaps the types of one or more anaerobes. Primary anaerobic plates should be examined with a hand lens (8×) or, preferably, a stereoscopic microscope. Colonies should be described from the various media and semi-quantitated.

All colony morphotypes from the nonselective anaerobic BA should be characterized and subcultured to purity plates, because facultative and obligate anaerobic bacteria commonly have similar colonial appearances. Colonies on PEA are processed further if they are different from colonies growing on the anaerobic BA or if colonies on the anaerobic BA are impossible to subculture because of overgrowth by swarming clostridia, *Proteus,* or other organisms.

The backup broth (e.g., thioglycollate) should be Gram stained; if cellular types are seen that were not present on the primary plates, the broth should be subcultured. In addition, if no growth is seen on the primary plates, the backup broth should be subcultured to the battery of anaerobic media included in the primary plating setup. The broth should be subcultured even if it appears clear to ensure no anaerobic organisms are present.

Subculture of Isolates

A single colony of each distinct morphotype is examined microscopically using a Gram stain and is subcultured for aerotolerance testing. Fig. 40.5 presents a basic algorithm for processing isolated colonies. A sterile wooden stick or platinum loop should be used to subculture colonies to:
- A CHOC to be incubated in carbon dioxide (CO_2) for aerotolerance
- An anaerobic BA plate and a chocolate plate to be incubated anaerobically (purity plate)

The CHOC should be inoculated first, so that if only the anaerobic BA plate grows, there is no question of not having enough organisms to initiate growth. The following antibiotic identification disks are placed on the first quadrant of the purity plate (Evolve Procedure 40.1):
- Kanamycin, 1 mg
- Colistin, 10 µg
- Vancomycin, 5 µg

These disks aid preliminary grouping of anaerobes and verify the Gram stain results, but they do not imply susceptibility of an organism for antibiotic therapy.

Three other disks may be added to the anaerobic BA plate at this time. A nitrate disk may be placed on the second quadrant for subsequent determination of nitrate reduction; a sodium polyanethol sulfonate (SPS) disk can be placed near the colistin disk for rapid presumptive identification of *Peptostreptococcus anaerobius* if gram-positive cocci are seen on Gram staining; and a bile disk may be added to the second quadrant to detect bile inhibition if gram-negative rods are seen on Gram staining.

If processing is performed on the open bench, all plates should promptly be incubated anaerobically, because some

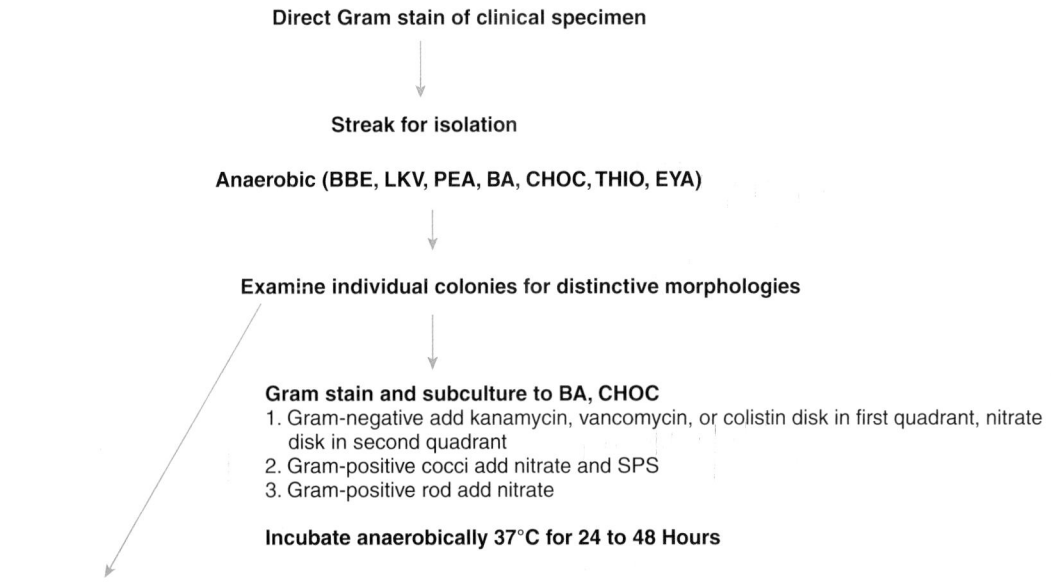

Direct Gram stain of clinical specimen

↓

Streak for isolation

Anaerobic (BBE, LKV, PEA, BA, CHOC, THIO, EYA)

↓

Examine individual colonies for distinctive morphologies

↓

Gram stain and subculture to BA, CHOC
1. Gram-negative add kanamycin, vancomycin, or colistin disk in first quadrant, nitrate disk in second quadrant
2. Gram-positive cocci add nitrate and SPS
3. Gram-positive rod add nitrate

Incubate anaerobically 37°C for 24 to 48 Hours

Aerotolerance Test: Subculture organisms to a CHOC plate, incubate 37°C for 24 to 48 hours in 5% CO_2 to detect slow growing aerobes such as *Capnocytophaga*, *Eikenella*, and *Actinobacillus* spp.

• **Fig. 40.5** Algorithm for isolation and identification of anaerobic bacteria. *BA*, Sheep blood agar; *BBE*, *Bacteroides* bile esculin agar; *CHOC*, chocolate agar; *EYA*, egg yolk agar (for suspected *Clostridium* spp.); *LKV*, laked kanamycin-vancomycin agar; *PEA*, phenylethyl agar; *SPS*, sodium polyanethol sulfonate; *THIO*, thioglycollate enrichment broth (should be examined daily and incubated for up to 7 days if no growth is identified on primary media; subculture to anaerobic media if growth is detected in broth culture).

clinical isolates (e.g., *Fusobacterium necrophorum* subsp. *necrophorum* and some *Prevotella* spp.) may die after relatively short exposure to oxygen. The primary plates are reincubated, along with the purity plates, for an additional 48 to 72 hours and are again inspected for slowly growing or pigmenting strains.

Presumptive Identification of Isolates

Information from the primary plates in conjunction with the atmospheric requirements, Gram stain results, and colony morphology of a pure isolate provides preliminary differentiation of many anaerobic organisms. Considering the specimen source and expected organisms from the site can be a useful aid in this process. Phenotypic characteristics for the identification of commonly isolated groups of anaerobic bacteria are included in Chapter 41.

Definitive Biochemical Identification

Various techniques can be used for definitive identification of anaerobic bacteria. Such methods may include the following:
• PRAS biochemicals
• Miniaturized biochemical systems (e.g., API 20A [bioMérieux, St. Louis, MO])
• Rapid, preformed enzyme detection panels (e.g., RapID-ANA II [Remel, Lenexa, KS]; BBL Brand Crystal Anaerobe ID [Becton Dickinson]; Rapid Anaerobe Identification Panel [MicroScan, Beckman Coulter, Brea, CA]; Vitek ANI card [bioMérieux]).

For commonly isolated anaerobic bacteria, the commercial identification systems and biochemical kits reliably identify the anaerobic bacteria. However, caution must be used in interpretation, and the results must be correlated with other clinical information, including the site of infection, Gram staining results, and colonial morphology. The high cost of some methods alone does not justify their use in most clinical laboratories.

Rapid Identification Methods

Nucleic acid–based testing has been used to identify anaerobic organisms. These methods include polymerase chain reaction (PCR), multiplex PCR, and oligonucleotide microarrays.

Matrix-assisted laser desorption ionization time-of-flight mass spectrometry (MALDI-TOF MS) has been used to identify anaerobes from clinical specimens (Chapter 7). MALDI-TOF MS is less expensive than traditional culture-based biochemical testing and nucleic acid–based testing. MALDI-TOF MS has also been used to detect the hydrolysate of meropenem and ertapenem identifying carbapenemase-producing anaerobic bacteria.

Antimicrobial Susceptibility Testing and Therapy

When mixed infections are encountered, definitive information about the identification of each species present usually does not affect therapeutic management. Because most clinically

TABLE 40.3 Summary of Antimicrobial Susceptibility Testing Methods for Anaerobic Bacteria

Test Conditions	Agar Dilution	Broth Microdilution	E-Test
		Test Methods	
Medium	*Brucella* agar supplemented with hemin (5 µg/mL), vitamin K (1 µg/mL), and 5% (V/V) laked sheep blood	*Brucella* broth supplemented with hemin (5 µg/mL), vitamin K (1 µg/mL), and lysed horse blood (5%)	*Brucella* blood agar
Inoculum size	1×10^5 CFU/spot	1×10^6 CFU/mL	0.1–1 McFarland standard, swab plate
Incubation conditions	Anaerobic, 35°C–37°C	Anaerobic, 35°C–37C	Anaerobic, 35°C–37°C
Incubation duration	48 h	48 h	24–48 h

CFU, Colony-forming units; *V/V,* volume/volume.

relevant anaerobes are susceptible to first-line antimicrobials, knowledge of their presence and Gram stain morphologies in mixed cultures is usually sufficient for guiding therapy. Therefore, definitive identification methods that follow the schemes outlined should be judiciously applied to clinical situations in which an anaerobic organism is isolated in pure culture from a normally sterile site (e.g., clostridial myonecrosis).

The therapeutic options for each of the major groups of anaerobic bacteria change rapidly; therefore, therapeutic use of the antimicrobial agents listed generally requires the performance of antimicrobial susceptibility testing with anaerobic isolates (Table 40.3). Although standard susceptibility testing methods have been established for testing anaerobic bacteria against various antimicrobial agents, the fastidious nature of many species and the labor intensity involved in using these methods indicate that testing should be done only under recommended circumstances (Box 40.3).

Although certain commercial methods (e.g., E-test, Spiral Gradient; Chapter 11) may facilitate anaerobic susceptibility testing in some way, the difficulty of assigning clinical significance to many anaerobic isolates and the availability of several highly effective empiric therapeutic choices significantly challenge a laboratory policy of routinely performing susceptibility testing with these organisms. Because of the difficulty associated with the growth, identification, and susceptibility testing of anaerobes, inclusion of these organisms in nucleic acid direct detection systems such as the Biofire blood culture identification system is important to initiate effective therapy in systemic disseminated infections.

ⓔ Visit the Evolve site for a complete list of procedures, review questions, and case studies.

Bibliography

Bennett J, Dolin R, Blaser M: *Principles and practice of infectious diseases*, ed 9, Philadelphia, 2020, Elsevier-Saunders.
Carroll KC, Pfaller MA, Landry ML, et al.: *Manual of clinical microbiology*, ed 12, Washington, DC, 2019, ASM Press.

BOX 40.3 Indications for Performing Antimicrobial Susceptibility Testing With Anaerobic Bacteria

- To establish patterns of susceptibility of anaerobes to new antimicrobial agents
- To periodically monitor susceptibility patterns of anaerobic bacteria collected in and among specific geographic areas or particular health care institutions
- To assist in the therapeutic management of patients, when such information may be critical because of the following:
  - Known resistance of a particular species to commonly used agents
  - Therapeutic failures and/or persistence of an organism at a site of infection
  - Lack of a precedence for therapeutic management of a particular infection
  - Severity of an infection (e.g., brain abscess, osteomyelitis, infections of prosthetic devices, and refractory or recurrent bacteremia)

Modified from Clinical and Laboratory Standards Institute (CLSI). Document M11-A8.

Committee on Infectious Diseases: *2006 red book: report of the Committee on Infectious Diseases*, ed 27, Elk Grove Village, IL, 2006, American Academy of Pediatrics.
Coy B: *The role of the anaerobic chamber in microbiology today*, American Laboratory, 2010.
Leber AL: *Anaerobes, clinical microbiology procedures handbook*, ed 4, Washington, DC, 2016, ASM Press.
Minutes Microlog: *Biolog, inc.: Gram-negative and gram-positive bacteria*, Volume 1. 2003, Issue 1. Hayward, CA.
Ny P, Ozaki A, Pallares J, et al.: Antimicrobial stewardship opportunities in patients with bacteremia not identified by BioFire FilmArray, *J Clin Microbiol*, 2019, https://doi.org/10.1128/JCM.01941-18.
Sawai T, Koga S, Ide S, et al.: An iliopsoas abscess caused by *Parvimonas micra*: a case report, *J Med Case Rep* 13:47, 2019.
Veloo ACM, Welling GW, Degener JE: Antimicrobial susceptibility of clinically relevant gram-positive anaerobic cocci collected over a three-year period in the Netherlands, *Antimicrob Agents Chemother* 55:1199–1203, 2011.

41

Overview of Anaerobic Organisms

OBJECTIVES

1. For each group of organisms listed, provide the general characteristics, including Gram stain reactions, colonial morphology, growth requirements (media, oxygen requirement, and temperature), laboratory identification, and clinical significance.
2. Differentiate normal anaerobic bacteria from pathogenic bacteria isolated from clinical specimens.
3. Describe the pathogenesis and virulence factors associated with the *Clostridium* species *Clostridium perfringens, Clostridium botulinum, Clostridioides difficile, Clostridium septicum,* and *Clostridium tetani.*
4. Define and discuss the pathogenesis for anaerobic cellulitis, gas gangrene, clostridial gastroenteritis, pseudomembranous enterocolitis, botulism, actinomycosis, bacterial vaginosis, and enteritis necroticans.
5. Differentiate the four forms of botulism (food poisoning, wound botulism, infant botulism, and botulism resulting from intestinal colonization).
6. Compare paralysis associated with botulism with tetanus.
7. Explain the procedure for spore isolation and growth using the ethyl alcohol shock procedure.
8. List the appropriate specimen collection, transport, and storage conditions for the recovery of anaerobic organisms.
9. Explain aerotolerance testing, including how to perform the test, what media are used, and the reason or reasons the media is important.
10. Identify the special potency antibiotics and explain the typical resistance patterns used to identify the various anaerobic groups (e.g., gram-positive cocci, gram-negative cocci).
11. Correlate disease signs and symptoms with laboratory data to identify the etiologic agent of infection.

GENERA AND SPECIES TO BE CONSIDERED

Current Name	Previous Name
Gram-Positive, Spore-Forming Bacilli	
Clostridioides difficile	
Clostridium argentinense	
Clostridium baratii	
Clostridium bartlettii	
Clostridium botulinum	
Clostridium butyricum	

Current Name	Previous Name
Clostridium histolyticum	
Clostridium novyi	
Clostridium perfringens	
Clostridium septicum	
Clostridium sordellii	
Clostridium tertium	
Clostridium tetani	
Clostridium clostridioforme group	*C. clostridioforme, C. hathewayi, C. bolteae*
Other *Clostridium* spp.	
Gram-Positive, Non–Spore-Forming Bacilli	
Actinobaculum massiliense	
Actinomyces gerencseriae	
Actinomyces graevenitzii	
Actinomyces israelii	
Actinomyces naeslundii	
Actinomyces neuii	
Actinomyces radingae	
Actinomyces turicensis	
Actinomyces odontolyticus	
Other *Actinomyces* spp.	
Actinotignum schaalii	*Actinobaculum schaalii*
Actinotignum urinale	*Actinobaculum urinale*
Atopobium minutum	*Lactobacillus minutum*
Atopobium parvulum	*Streptococcus parvulum*
Atopobium spp. *(A. deltae, A. fossor, A. rimae,* and *A. vaginae)*	
Bifidobacterium spp.	
Collinsella aerofaciens	*Eubacterium aerofaciens*
Cutibacterium acnes	*Propionibacterium acnes*
Cutibacterium avidum	
Cutibacterium granulosum	
Eggerthella lenta	*Eubacterium lentum*
Eggerthella sinensis	
Eubacterium spp.	
Lactobacillus spp.	
Mobiluncus curtisii	
Mobiluncus mulieris	

Continued

As previously described in Chapter 40, the organisms in this chapter predominantly do not grow in the presence of oxygen.

Epidemiology

Most of the anaerobic bacteria that cause infections in humans are also part of our normal microbiota. The ecology of these organisms is such that various species and genera exhibit preferences for the body sites they inhabit (**endogenous anaerobes**). The gram-positive cocci account for approximately one-third of the anaerobic organisms isolated from clinical samples. Other pathogenic anaerobes (e.g., *Clostridium botulinum* and *Clostridium tetani*) are soil and environmental inhabitants (**exogenous anaerobes**) and not considered part of the normal human microbiota.

The ways in which anaerobic infections are acquired are summarized in Table 41.1. Person-to-person, health care–associated transmission of *Clostridioides difficile* among hospitalized patients presents an enormous clinical and infection control dilemma. Most anaerobic infections occur when a patient's normal microbiota gains access to a sterile site as a result of disruption of some anatomic barrier.

Pathogenesis and Spectrum of Disease

The types of infections and diseases in humans caused by anaerobic bacteria span a wide spectrum. Certain species, such as *C. botulinum* and *C. tetani,* produce some of the most potent toxins known. In contrast, specific virulence factors for the organisms commonly encountered in infections (e.g., *Bacteroides fragilis* group, *C. difficile*) are not well understood (Table 41.2).

Most anaerobic infections involve a mixture of anaerobic and facultative anaerobic organisms (e.g., Enterobacterales), which creates problems in identification and diagnosis to establish the extent to which a particular anaerobic species contributes to infection. In addition, as ubiquitous members of the normal microbiota, anaerobic organisms commonly contaminate clinical materials. For these reasons, assigning clinical significance to anaerobic bacteria isolated in the laboratory is important, although often difficult.

Gram-Positive, Spore-Forming Bacilli

The clostridia are endospore forming, obligate anaerobic (or aerotolerant), catalase-negative, gram-positive bacilli (Fig. 41.1). Using chemotaxonomic and polyphasic characterization, *Clostridium difficile* has now been placed into a new genus, *Clostridioides*. The genus *Clostridium* contains more than 240 species and subspecies. *Clostridioides* and *Clostridium* will be included together throughout this chapter as clostridia. The clostridia microscopic morphology appear long, short, straight, or curved pleomorphic rods arranged in pairs or short chains. If spores are not present on Gram stain, the ethanol shock spore or heat shock spore test can separate this group from the non–spore-forming

TABLE 41.1 Acquisition of Anaerobic Infections and Diseases

Mode of Acquisition	Examples
Endogenous strains of normal microbiota gain access to normally sterile sites, usually as a result of one or more predisposing factors that compromise normal anatomic barriers (e.g., surgery or accidental trauma) or alter other host defense mechanisms (e.g., malignancy, diabetes, burns, immunosuppressive therapy, aspiration)	Wide variety of infections involving several anatomic locations, including bacteremia, head and neck infections, dental and orofacial infections, pneumonia and other infections of the thoracic cavity, intraabdominal and obstetric and gynecologic infections, bite wound and other soft tissue infections, and gangrene (i.e., clostridial myonecrosis). Organisms most commonly encountered in these infections include *Bacteroides fragilis* group, *Prevotella* spp., *Porphyromonas* spp., *Fusobacterium nucleatum*, *Peptostreptococcus* spp., and *Clostridium perfringens*.
Contamination of existing wound or puncture by objects contaminated with toxigenic *Clostridium* spp.	Tetanus (*Clostridium tetani*), gas gangrene (*Clostridium perfringens*, and, less commonly, *Clostridium septicum, Clostridium novyi*, and others).
Associated with medically induced abortions, normal vaginal delivery, and cesarean section delivery	*Clostridium sordellii* infections in young healthy women resulting in fatal postpartum infections.
Ingestion of preformed toxins in vegetable- or meat-based foods	Botulism (*Clostridium botulinum*) and other clostridial food poisonings (*C. perfringens*).
Colonization of gastrointestinal tract with a potent toxin-producing organism	Infant botulism (*C. botulinum, Clostridium butyricum*, and *Clostridium baratii*).
Person-to-person spread	Health care–associated spread of *Clostridioides difficile*–induced diarrhea and pseudomembranous colitis; bite wound infections caused by a variety of anaerobic species.

TABLE 41.2 Pathogenesis and Spectrum of Disease for Anaerobic Bacteria

Organism	Virulence Factors	Spectrum of Disease and Infections
Gram-Positive Bacilli, Spore-Forming		
Clostridium perfringens	Produces several exotoxins; alpha-toxin, the most important, mediates destruction of host cell membranes; enterotoxin inserts and disrupts membranes of mucosal cells; beta-toxin is a cytotoxin.	Gas gangrene (myonecrosis) and necrotizing fasciitis: Life-threatening, toxin-mediated destruction of muscle and other tissues after traumatic introduction of the organism. Food poisoning: Caused by release of the toxin after ingestion of large numbers of the organism. Usually self-limiting and benign; manifested by abdominal cramps, diarrhea, and vomiting. Enteritis necroticans (necrotizing enteritis; NEC): Life-threatening infection that causes ischemic necrosis of the jejunum. Often associated with immunocompromised patients (e.g., those with diabetes, alcohol-induced liver disease, or neutropenia). NEC, a gastrointestinal disease that causes bowel necrosis and inflammation, affects low-birth-weight, premature infants.
Clostridium sordellii	Produces a variety of bacterial proteases and phospholipases. Produces up to seven exotoxins, including lethal toxin (LT), hemorrhagic toxin (HT), and enterotoxins A, B, and C.	Gas gangrene of the uterus following abortion, normal delivery, or cesarean section. Patient presents with little or no fever, lack of purulent discharge, hypotension, peripheral edema, and an increased white blood cell (WBC) count. Infection is typically fatal, and death is rapid.
Clostridium tetani	Produces tetanospasmin (TeNT), a neurotoxic exotoxin that disrupts nerve impulses to muscles.	Tetanus (commonly known as lockjaw). Organism establishes a wound infection and elaborates TeNT, a potent toxin that mediates generalized muscle spasms. If the disease goes untreated, spasms continue to be triggered by even minor stimuli, leading to exhaustion and, eventually, respiratory failure.

Continued

TABLE 41.2	Pathogenesis and Spectrum of Disease for Anaerobic Bacteria—cont'd	
Organism	**Virulence Factors**	**Spectrum of Disease and Infections**
Clostridium botulinum	Produces an extremely potent neurotoxin (BoNT).	Foodborne botulism: Results from ingestion of pre-formed toxin in nonacidic vegetable or mushroom foodstuffs. Absorption of the toxin leads to nearly complete flaccid (rag doll) paralysis of respiratory and other essential muscle groups. Infant botulism: Occurs when the organism elaborates the toxin after it has colonized the gastrointestinal tract of infants (i.e., infant botulism). Wound botulism: Occurs when *C. botulinum* produces the toxin from an infected wound site. Intestinal botulism: Intestinal colonization has been associated with surgery and administration of antibiotics. Occurs in children and adults.
Clostridioides difficile	Produces toxin A (TcdA), an enterotoxin, and toxin B (TcdB), a cytotoxin. Both toxin A and toxin B are classified as large clostridial cytotoxins. The toxins glycosylate guanosine triphosphate (GTP) signaling proteins, leading to a breakdown of the cellular cytotoxin and cell death.	Organism requires diminution of normal gut microbiota by the activity of various antimicrobial agents to become established in the gut of hospitalized patients. Once established, elaboration of one or more toxins results in antibiotic-associated diarrhea or potentially life-threatening inflammation of the colon. When the surface of the inflamed bowel is overlaid with a "pseudomembrane" composed of necrotic debris, white blood cells, and fibrin, the disease is referred to as pseudomembranous colitis. Only strains producing toxin A or toxin B (or both) cause infections.
Gram-Positive Bacilli, Non–Spore-Forming		
Actinobaculum spp.	Unknown	Associated with urinary tract infections. Identified in a variety of severe infections including urosepsis, bacteremia, cellulitis, spondylodiscitis, and endocarditis.
Actinotignum schaalii	Unknown; often associated as a predominant member in polymicrobial biofilms in urinary tract infections.	Most commonly associated with urinary tract infections; has been isolated in endocarditis, abscesses, cellulitis, and bacteremia. There is an approximately 15% mortality rate in cases of bacteremia and severe sepsis.
Actinomyces spp.	No well-characterized virulence factors. Infections usually require disruption of the protective mucosal surface of the oral cavity, respiratory tract, gastrointestinal tract, and/or female genitourinary tract.	Usually involved in mixed oral or cervicofacial, thoracic, pelvic, and abdominal infections caused by the patient's endogenous strains. Also involved in periodontal disease and dental caries. Identified in a variety of soft tissue infections, including perianal, groin, ancillary, breast, and other abscesses.
Atopobium spp.	Atopobium vaginae is a predominant organism isolated concurrently as a constituent of *Gardnerella vaginalis* biofilm associated with bacterial vaginosis.	Identified in association with dental and respiratory infections and bacteremia. Isolated from various infections in the genital tract, including bacterial vaginosis.
Bifidobacterium spp.	Unknown, no differences have been identified in invasive versus noninvasive strains using whole genome sequencing (Esaiassen, 2017).	Commonly associated with dental infections, periodontal disease, peritonitis, pneumonia, abdominal abscesses, and bacteremia.
Cryptobacterium curtum	Overproduction of citrulline during bacterial metabolism in periodontal infections has been linked to the development of rheumatoid arthritis.	Associated with chronic periodontitis, endodontic infections, and dental abscesses. Translocation to other areas of the body have implicated the organism in the development of pelvic abscesses, gynecologic infections, and wounds.

TABLE 41.2   Pathogenesis and Spectrum of Disease for Anaerobic Bacteria—cont'd

Organism	Virulence Factors	Spectrum of Disease and Infections
Cutibacterium spp.	Different species produce factors that may be associated with virulence; *C. avidum* produces an extracellular polysaccharide-like structure that may be associated with biofilm formation and avoiding phagocytosis produces neuraminidase that may also be involved in pathogenicity; *C. granulosum* produces pililike structures involved in adherence; *C. acnes'* ability to produce biofilm and increase adherence is well documented: lipase is produced by most species resulting in the hydrolysis of triglycerides and sebum contributing to cutaneous skin lesions; all three species listed here produce hyaluronidase that may be involved in tissue damage.	Associated with inflammatory process in acne. Identified in systemic opportunistic infections, including endocarditis, central nervous system (CNS) infections, osteomyelitis, and arthritis. As part of normal skin flora, the organism is considered the most common anaerobic contaminant of blood cultures and is often ignored.
Eggerthella spp.	Some species are able to oxidase bile acids in the gastrointestinal tract. It is unknown if this is associated to the pathogenicity of the organism.	Recovered from a variety of infections including intraabdominal and periabdominal infections. Associated with meningitis, necrotizing pneumonia, osteomyelitis, and other disseminated infections. Mortality ranges from 20% to 40% in cases of human infections.
Eubacterium spp.	Unknown	Usually associated with mixed infections of the oral cavity, abdomen, pelvis, or genitourinary tract.
Lactobacillus spp.	Pili and adhesion proteins that make the organisms useful in probiotics, also enhances the organism's ability to cause infection in other areas of the body.	Associated with advanced dental caries. Organism has been identified in endocarditis, meningitis, intraabdominal infections, liver abscesses, septicemia, and bacteremia. Several species are commonly used in probiotics to maintain and restore normal intestinal bacterial microbiota. Severe infections do occur when these organisms translocate out of their normal environment, often in patients with underlying comorbidities.
Olsenella spp.	Unknown	Predominantly associated with dental infections and periodontitis, and bacteremia.
Propionimicrobium lymphophilum	Unknown	Predominantly associated with urinary tract infections.
Pseudopropionibacterium propionicum	Unknown	Known to cause actinomycosis as well as oral and eye infections.
Pseudoramibacter alactolyticus	Unknown	Primarily associated with dental infections including periodontitis, endodontic infections, dental caries, and oral abscesses.
Slackia spp.	Unknown	Predominantly associated with chronic periodontitis, polymicrobial abscesses in various body sites, and bacteremia.
Varibaculum spp.	Unknown	Associated with IUD, cerebral, post-auricular, submandibular, breast abscesses and other soft-tissue infections. Has been isolated from urine, sinus, and vaginal tract specimens.

Continued

TABLE 41.2	Pathogenesis and Spectrum of Disease for Anaerobic Bacteria—cont'd	
Organism	**Virulence Factors**	**Spectrum of Disease and Infections**
Other miscellaneous genera: *Anaerostipes, Bulleidia, Catonella, Eggerthia, Lachnoanaerobaculum, Moryella, Oribacterium, Robinsoniella, Filifactor*	*Filifactor alocis* is known to induce proinflammatory cytokine secretion in gingival epithelial cells inducing apoptosis contributing to tissue damage in periodontal disease.	Many of these genera are associated with similar infections as the other non–spore-forming gram-positive bacilli including dental infections, genitourinary, vaginal, abscesses, soft-tissue infections, and bacteremia.
Mobiluncus spp. (considered gram-variable)	Unknown	Organisms are found in the vagina and have been associated with bacterial vaginosis, but their precise role in gynecologic infections is unclear. Eighty-two percent of neovaginal samples from transgender patients are positive for *M. curtisii*. Organisms have been isolated from breast, hepatic, and intraabdominal abscesses, and bacteremia.
Gram-Negative Bacilli		
Bacteroides fragilis group, other *Bacteroides* spp., *Prevotella* spp., *Porphyromonas* spp. *Fusobacterium nucleatum* and other *Fusobacterium* spp.	Anaerobic, gram-negative bacilli that produce capsules, endotoxin, and succinic acid, which inhibit phagocytosis, and produce various enzymes that mediate tissue damage.	Most infections still require some breach of mucosal integrity that allows the organisms to gain access to deeper tissues. Organisms most commonly encountered in anaerobic infections. Infections are often mixed (polymicrobial) with infections caused by other anaerobic and facultative anaerobic organisms. Infections occur throughout the body, usually as localized or enclosed abscesses, and may involve the cranium, periodontium, thorax, peritoneum, liver, and female genital tract. May also cause bacteremia, aspiration pneumonia, septic arthritis, chronic sinusitis, decubitus ulcers, and other soft tissue infections. The hallmark of most but not all infections is the production of a foul odor. In general, infections caused by *B. fragilis* group occur below the diaphragm; pigmented *Prevotella* spp., *Porphyromonas* spp., and *F. nucleatum* generally are involved in head and neck and pleuropulmonary infections.
Bilophila wadsworthia	Unknown	Significant pathogen commonly isolated in intraabdominal polymicrobial abscesses.
Leptotrichia spp.	Unknown	Increasingly isolated from immunocompromised patients associated with oral or gastrointestinal lesions and bacteremia. Some isolates have been identified in infective endocarditis in immunocompetent patients.
Sutterella wadsworthensis	Unknown	Commonly isolated from a variety of infections including appendicitis, peritonitis, rectal, or perirectal abscesses.
Gram-Positive Cocci		
Anaerococcus lactolyticus	No definitive virulence factors known.	Diabetic and pressure ulcers.

TABLE 41.2	Pathogenesis and Spectrum of Disease for Anaerobic Bacteria—cont'd	
Organism	**Virulence Factors**	**Spectrum of Disease and Infections**
Anaerococcus prevotii	No definitive virulence factors known.	Predominantly isolated from vaginal discharges and ovarian, peritoneal, sacral, and lung abscesses; has been identified in blood cultures.
Anaerococcus vaginalis	No definitive virulence factors known.	Diabetic and pressure ulcers; has been identified in blood cultures.
Finegoldia magna	Demonstrated ability to form biofilm as well as several virulence factors including adhesion factors and extracellular transpeptidases that promote colonization.	Most often found in infections associated with skin and soft tissue, bone, and joint infections; chronic wounds such as diabetic and pressure ulcers. The organism has also been isolated from disseminated infections such as endocarditis, meningitis, pneumoniae, septic arthritis, and upper respiratory infections.
Murdochiella asaccharolyticus	No definitive virulence factors known.	Isolated from abdominal and sacral abscesses and polymicrobial bacterial vaginosis.
Parvimonas micra	*P. micra* has been shown to produce a variety of enzymes capable of tissue destruction, including collagenase, hemolysin, and elastase; induces production of **gingipain** (extracellular proteases) in polymicrobial infections with *Porphyromonas gingivalis,* causing biofilm formation and down regulation of inflammatory cytokines.	Normal oral microbiota; however often associated with periodontal, endodontic, and peritonsillar infections. It is also isolated in polymicrobial infections in various body sites including cutaneous, wound, otitis media, sinus, pleural empyema and septic-pulmonary embolism, intraabdominal, anorectal abscess, septicemia, gynecological, vertebral osteomyelitis, and prosthetic joint infections.
Peptoniphilus spp.	No definitive virulence factors known.	Most often associated with pressure ulcers and chronic rhinosinusitis; has been isolated from bone, joint, and bloodstream infections.
Peptostreptococcus anaerobius	No definitive virulence factors known.	Most often isolated from polymicrobic infections, including abscesses of the brain, ear, jaw, oral and pleural cavities, pelvis, urogenital tract, wound infections, and abdominal cavity.
Peptostreptococcus stomatis		Has been isolated in polymicrobial abscesses associated with colorectal cancer.
Gram-negative cocci		
Veillonella spp.	No definitive virulence factors known.	May be involved in mixed infections. Organisms have been isolated in increasingly serious infections, including meningitis, osteomyelitis, endocarditis, bacteremia, pleuropulmonary, and prosthetic infections.

anaerobic bacilli (Evolve Procedure 41.1). Some strains of *Clostridium perfringens, Clostridium ramosum,* and *Clostridium clostridioforme* may not produce spores or survive a spore test, so it is important to recognize these organisms using other characteristics. Some clostridia typically stain gram negative, although they are susceptible to vancomycin on the disk test. Several species of clostridia grow aerobically (*Clostridium tertium, Clostridium carnis, Clostridium histolyticum,* and occasional strains of *C. perfringens*), but they produce spores only under anaerobic conditions. *C. perfringens* may appear weakly catalase-positive.

Clostridia are widespread in nature because of their ability to form spores, referred to as endospores, in the mother cell (Table 41.3). In addition, they are present in large numbers as normal microbiota in the gastrointestinal tract of humans and animals, the female genital tract, and the oral mucosa.

C. botulinum is listed by the Centers for Disease Control and Prevention (CDC) as a potential agent of bioterrorism (Chapter 79). Spores of *C. botulinum* are widely distributed in soil and aquatic environments. Botulism is diagnosed by the demonstration of **botulinum neurotoxin (BoNT)** in serum, feces, gastric contents, vomitus, or a suspect food (food poisoning) or environmental specimen (potential bioterrorism incident). Aerosolized botulinum toxin is highly unstable, and the more likely route would be intentional food intoxication. This means that most hospital laboratories must know how to package and ship such a specimen to the state health department or CDC. *C. botulinum*

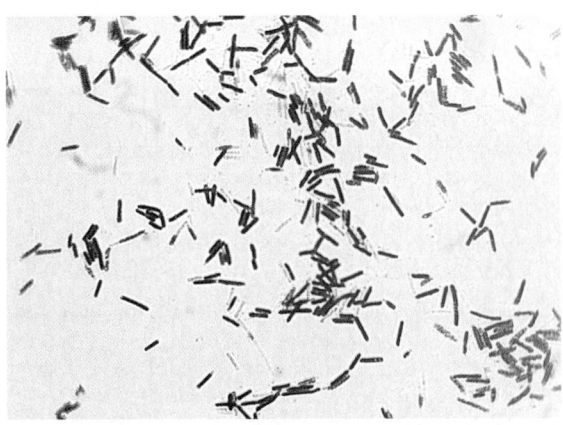

• **Fig. 41.1** Gram stain of *Clostridium perfringens*.

is rarely isolated in the clinical microbiology laboratory. In addition to *C. botulinum,* BoNT can be produced by *Clostridium butyricum, Clostridium baratii,* and *Clostridium argentinense.* Table 41.2 describes the pathogenesis of the commonly encountered *Clostridium* spp.

Laboratory Diagnosis and Specimen Collection

As stated in Chapter 40, the proper collection and transport of specimens for anaerobic culture cannot be overemphasized. General considerations are included in the discussion in Chapter 40. However, special collection instructions must be followed for some clostridial illnesses, specifically suspected gas gangrene or necrotizing fasciitis (*C. perfringens* and *C. ramosum*), foodborne *C. perfringens* and *C. botulinum,* *C. difficile* pseudomembranous enterocolitis, *Clostridium septicum* neutropenic enterocolitis (NEC), and enteritis necrotans (*C. perfringens*). Food and freshly passed fecal specimens must be sent to a public health laboratory for confirmation of *C. perfringens* food poisoning; these should be transported at 4°C. The specimens should be processed within 24 hours of collection. The clinical diagnosis of botulism is confirmed by demonstration of botulinum toxin in serum, feces, vomitus, or gastric contents, as well as by recovery of the organism from the stool of patients (Fig. 41.1). Several methods are available, including cell culture assays, enzyme-linked immunosorbent assay (ELISA), and reverse passive latex agglutination.

C. perfringens–associated enteritis necroticans infection requires the collection of three blood cultures from three different venipuncture sites, stool (25 g or 25 mL of liquid) and bowel contents, or bowel tissue. Specimens should be Gram stained, cultured, and isolated. Follow-up tests to identify the organism are determined by the interpretation of the initial Gram stain. The isolate should be serologically typed. If gas gangrene or necrotizing fasciitis is suspect, multiple tissue samples are collected from the site of infection, because organisms may not be uniformly distributed throughout the infection. As with enteritis necroticans, samples should be Gram stained for early presumptive diagnosis. It is important to note any gram-positive rods because sporulation is not always noted in tissue for *C. perfringens* and *C. ramosum.* If spores are noted, the location (terminal,

subterminal, or central) and the shape (spherical or oval) should be noted. In addition, polymerase chain reaction (PCR) testing is available for *C. perfringens.*

Suspected *C. difficile* infection (CDI) requires the collection of a freshly passed stool specimen (10 to 20 mL preferred; minimum 5 mL or 5 g) for culture, nucleic acid amplification, and toxin assays for both toxin A and toxin B. Nontoxigenic strains can colonize patients. Assays that detect the organism alone should be combined with an assay to determine toxin status. Only liquid or unformed stools should be processed for CDI to prevent unnecessary treatment of patients colonized with the bacterium. Formed stools or rectal swabs are adequate to detect carriers by culture or nucleic acid–based tests but are inadequate for toxin assays. Specimens should be cultured within 2 hours after collection. Figs. 41.2 and 41.3 demonstrate the isolation of *C. difficile* on **cycloserine cefoxitin fructose agar (CCFA)** and anaerobic blood agar. Specimens may be stored in anaerobic transport bags at 4°C for up to 48 hours; however, this reduces the recovery rate of viable organisms in culture. Specimens for toxin assays may be stored at 4°C for 72 hours or frozen at –70°C if a longer delay is expected.

Varieties of immunoassays are commercially available for the identification of *C. difficile* enterotoxin. In addition, a variety of nucleic acid–based platforms and assays have been developed for the amplification of the toxin A *(tcdA),* toxin B *(tcdB),* toxin C *(tcdC),* and binary toxin *(cdt)* genes. Stool samples may be submitted for nucleic acid–based testing. The assays include amplification of the glutamate dehydrogenase (GDH) gene or 16S ribosomal ribonucleic acid (rRNA) as internal control housekeeping genes. Detection of the GDH and 16S rRNA genes without the presence of a toxin gene would indicate a nonpathogenic strain or carrier state. Some studies indicate that nucleic acid–based testing without a confirmatory test leads to overdiagnosis of CDI, cannot differentiate a disease state from a carrier state, and should be limited to patients who present with diarrhea. Cell culture cultivation or toxin assays are still recommended.

The CDC maintains a 24-hours-a-day, 365-days-per-year hotline to provide emergency assistance in cases of botulism. Botulinum toxin is a potential bioweapon. Acceptable specimens for the diagnosis of *C. botulinum* or *C. tetani* infection include serum, feces, enema fluid, gastric aspirates, vomitus, tissue, exudates, or postmortem specimens. Specimens for infant botulism should include serum and stool; those for wound botulism should include serum, stool, and tissue biopsy. Serum specimens should be collected immediately after the onset of symptoms. All specimens should be stored and shipped at 4°C. Detection of the toxin BoNT is diagnostic for *C. botulinum* infection. The mouse bioassay remains the recommended method of analysis for the identification of BoNT. The bioassay requires splitting the specimen into two samples. One sample is boiled at 80°C for 10 minutes, inactivating the toxins. The two samples are independently injected intraperitoneal into two separate mice. One mouse serves as the negative control (inactivated specimen), and the other serves as the "test" sample. The

TABLE 41.3   Characteristics of Clinically Significant *Clostridium* Species and *Clostridioides difficile*

Species	Spore Location	Gelatin	Lecithinase	Lipase	Indole	Esculin	Nitrate
C. argentinense	ST	+	−	−	−	−	−
C. baratii	ST	−	+	−	−	+	V
C. bifermentans	ST	+	+	−	+	V	−
C. bolteae	ST	−	−	−	−	V	−
C. botulinum Types A, B, and F	ST	+	−	+	−	+	−
Types B, E, and F-nonproteolytic	ST	+	−	+	−	−	−
Types C and D	T	+	V	+	V	−	−
C. butyricum	ST	−	−	−	−	+	−
C. cadaveris	T	+	−	−	+	−	−
C. carnis	ST	−	−	−	−	+	−
C. clostridioforme	ST	−	−	−	−	+	−
Clostridioides difficile	ST(T)	+	−	−	−	+	−
C. glycolicum	ST	−	−	−	−	V	−
C. hastiforme	T	+	−	−	−	−	V
C. hathewayi	ST	−	−	−	−	+	−
C. histolyticum	ST	+	−	−	−	−	−
C. indolis	T	−	−	−	+	+	V
C. innocuum	T	−	−	−	−	+	−
C. limosum	ST	+	+	−	−	−	−
C. novyi	ST	+	+	+	−	−	−
C. paraputrificum	T(ST)	−	−	−	−	+	V
C. perfringens	ST	+	+	−	−	V	V
C. putrificum	T(ST)	+	−	−	−	V	−
C. ramosum	T	−	−	−	−	+	−
C. septicum	ST	+	−	−	−	+	V
C. sordellii	ST	+	+	−	+	V	−
C. sphenoides	ST(T)	−	−	−	+	+	V
C. sporogenes	ST	+	−	+	−	+	−
C. subterminale	ST	+	V	−	−	V	−
C. symbiosum	ST	−	−	−	−	−	−
C. tertium	T	−	−	−	−	+	V
C. tetani	T	+	−	−	V	−	−

+, Positive reaction; −, negative reaction; *V,* variable reaction; *ST,* subterminal; *T,* terminal; superscript indicates variability.
From Caroll KC, Pfaller MA. *Manual of Clinical Microbiology*. 12th ed. Washington, DC: ASM Press; 2019.

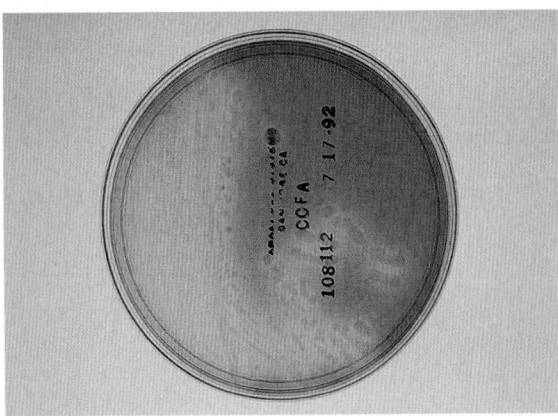

• **Fig. 41.2** *Clostridioides difficile* on cycloserine cefoxitin fructose agar (CCFA). (Courtesy Anaerobe Systems, Morgan Hill, CA.)

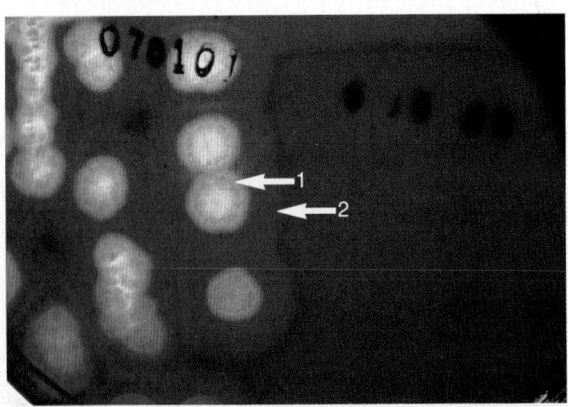

• **Fig. 41.3** *Clostridium perfringens* on anaerobic blood agar. Note double zone of beta-hemolysis. 1, First zone; 2, second zone. (Courtesy Anaerobe Systems, Morgan Hill, CA.)

mice are observed for neurologic symptoms. The presence of toxin is presumptively indicated with the development of symptoms and death in the test animal but not the control animal. The toxins associated with *C. botulinum*, *C. tetani*, and *C. perfringens* (BoNT, **tetanus neurotoxin [TeNT]**, and **iota toxin**) are considered extremely dangerous. The CDC recommends the use of Biosafety Level 3 practices and precautions, including immunization for the toxins; however, the vaccine is no longer available from the CDC.

The specimens of choice for *C. septicum* NEC include three different blood cultures from three different venipuncture sites, stool, and lumen contents or tissue from the involved ileocecal area; a muscle biopsy or aspirate of fluid from the sample should also be collected if myonecrosis (death of muscle tissue) is suspected. Table 41.4 provides an identification scheme for representative anaerobic organisms.

Nucleic Acid Detection and MALDI-TOF MS (Gram-Positive)

Nucleic acid detection using 16s rRNA gene sequencing may be useful for the identification of asaccharolytic species of clostridia. *C. tetani* can be directly detected by PCR. BoNT toxin and *C. difficile* toxin genes can be detected using real-time PCR assays; however, as previously indicated, toxin activity should be determined using an alternate method. Nontoxigenic strains may harbor the genes but do not produce the BoNT. Matrix-assisted laser desorption ionization time-of-flight mass spectrometry (MALDI-TOF MS) can be used to identify clostridia species more effectively than biochemical methods. Some clostridia may require pretreatment with formic acid for optimal extraction in MALDI-TOF MS.

Gram-Positive, Non–Spore-Forming Bacilli

Many genera of gram-positive, non–spore-forming bacilli are infrequently isolated as opportunistic infections. Some of the more commonly isolated genera include *Actinobaculum*, *Actinomyces*, *Actinotignum*, *Atopobium*, *Bifidobacterium*, *Eubacterium*, *Eggerthella*, *Collinsella*, *Cryptobacterium*, *Cutibacterium*, anaerobic *Lactobacillus*, *Mobiluncus*, *Olsenella*,

Paraeggerthella, *Atopobium*, *Propionimicrobium*, and *Varibaculum*. These organisms are typically normal microbiota on the mucosal surfaces of the human digestive tract and urogenital tract and on the skin. Many of the organisms are identified in polymicrobic infections of the mucosal surface, such as the oral or vaginal cavity or the urogenital tract.

The genera *Actinomyces* (anaerobic and aerotolerant) and *Mobiluncus* (strictly anaerobic) include species that show non–acid-fast, gram-positive, pleomorphic branching rods or coccobacilli. Direct examination and the macroscopic presence in purulent exudate of "sulfur granules," which reveal gram-positive filaments when crushed, is diagnostic for an infection with *Actinomyces* spp. *Mobiluncus* spp., a cause of bacterial vaginosis, usually is diagnosed on Gram staining of vaginal secretions by observation of gram-variable, curved rods with tapered ends. It is rarely isolated in the clinical laboratory because vaginal secretions are not acceptable specimens for anaerobic culture. *Actinobaculum* spp. are typically rod-shaped facultative anaerobes that are normal microbiota of the human genitourinary tract. *Propionibacterium* spp. are anaerobic and aerotolerant, pleomorphic, gram-positive rods. The bacterium produces propionic acid from glucose. *Bifidobacterium* spp. are strictly anaerobic or microaerophilic, gram-positive, pleomorphic rods that appear as rods or are branched or club-shaped. *Lactobacillus* spp. contain microaerophilic, catalase-negative, gram-positive rods capable of producing lactic acid from glucose fermentation. The genus *Eubacterium* remains poorly characterized, although its species are commonly isolated from oral infections. *Eggerthella* and *Paraeggerthella* are associated with intraabdominal and periabdominal infections, as well as bloodstream infections, which have a high mortality. The pathogenic mechanisms and the spectrum of diseases associated with these organisms are included in Table 41.2.

Laboratory Diagnosis

Differentiation of the gram-positive, non–spore-forming anaerobes can be determined using the characteristics that include hemolysis, fluorescence under long-wave UV illumination, and colony and Gram stain morphology. Follow-up tests to identify the organism is determined by the

TABLE 41.4	Differentiation of Representative Gram-Negative Bacilli and Gram-Positive Cocci			
	Gram-Negative Bacilli			
Test Method	Bacteroides fragilis	Bacteroides thetaiotaomicron	Bacteroides ovatus	Fusobacterium nucleatum
Arabinose	Neg	Pos	Pos	Neg
Bile 20%, growth	Pos	Pos	Pos	Neg
Catalase	Pos	Pos	Pos	Neg
Colistin (Col)	R	R	R	S
Esculin hydrolysis	Pos	Pos	Pos	Neg
Gelatinase	0	0	0	0
Indole	Neg	Pos	Pos	Pos
Kanamycin (Km)	R	R	R	S
Nitrate	Neg	Neg	Neg	Neg
Vancomycin (Van)	R	R	R	R

	Gram-Positive Bacilli		
Test Method	Peptostreptococcus anaerobius	Peptostreptococcus asaccharolyticus	Finegoldia magna
Indole	Neg	Pos	Neg
Nitrate	Neg	Neg	Neg
Sodium polyanethol sulfonate (SPS)	S	R	R

>10 mm = sensitive for Km, Van, Col; <12 mm = sensitive for SPS.
Neg, Negative reaction; *Pos,* positive reaction; *R,* resistant; *S,* sensitive.
From Caroll KC, Pfaller MA. *Manual of Clinical Microbiology.* 12th ed. Washington, DC: ASM Press; 2019.

interpretation of the initial Gram stain results. Additional tests include an aerotolerance test (Evolve Procedure 41.2) or growth in 5% CO_2, followed by routine screening of special-potency antibiotic susceptibility patterns. The gram-positive organisms typically are resistant to colistin (10 μg), susceptible to vancomycin (5 μg), and have variable sensitivity to kanamycin (1 mg). Additional rapid testing includes a 15% catalase test, production of indole, nitrate reduction, and motility. Many of these organisms are relatively biochemically inert, rendering phenotypic biochemical identification unreliable.

Nucleic Acid Detection and MALDI-TOF MS (Gram-Negative)

No rapid molecular amplification tests are available in the clinical laboratory at the time of this writing. Sequencing of the 16S rRNA is considered the gold standard for organism identification; however, not all organisms in this group can be characterized using this gene. Additional sequencing of housekeeping genes is required for some organisms. Whole genome sequencing (WGS) has the potential to replace 16S rRNA methods; however, sufficient WGS

databases are not currently available. MALDI-TOF MS has been successfully used to identify commonly isolated anaerobes; however, formic acid extraction is required to achieve optimal spectra and identification of the anaerobic gram-positive rods. In addition, due to the lack of information in available FDA-cleared databases, identification has relied on the research use only (RUO) databases in addition to other available testing methods. MALDI-TOF MS identification is expected to improve as the databases become optimized and approved for the detection of these organisms in the clinical laboratory. Table 41.4 provides an identification scheme for representative anaerobic organisms.

Gram-Negative Rods
Bacteroides fragilis Group

The anaerobic gram-negative rods typically are isolated from the mucosal surfaces of the human oral cavity and gastrointestinal tract (Fig. 41.4). (Table 41.2 presents an overview of the pathogenesis and infections associated with these organisms.) The *Bacteroidaceae* family consists of the saccharolytic, bile-resistant, nonpigmented *B. fragilis* group. The genus consists of approximately 50 species, more than

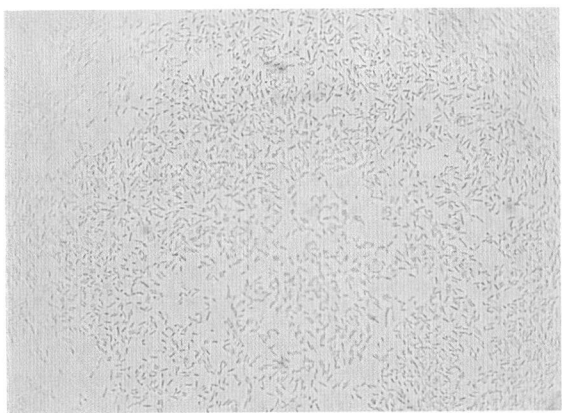

• **Fig. 41.4** Gram stain of *Bacteroides fragilis*.

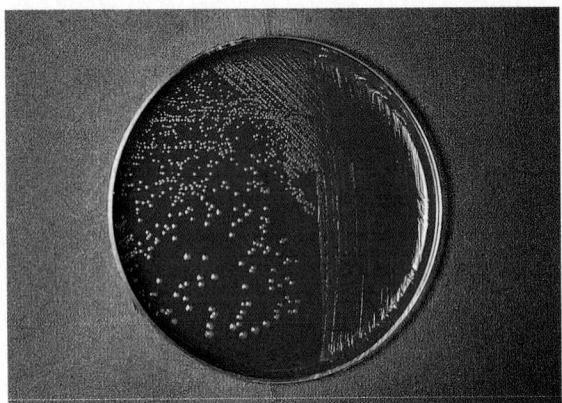

• **Fig. 41.5** *Bacteroides fragilis* on anaerobic blood agar.

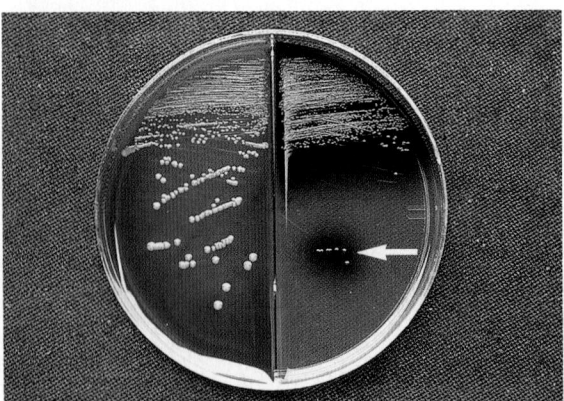

• **Fig. 41.6** *Bacteroides fragilis* on a biplate containing anaerobic blood agar and *Bacteroides* bile esculin agar (BBE) (*arrow*). (Courtesy Anaerobe Systems, Morgan Hill, CA.)

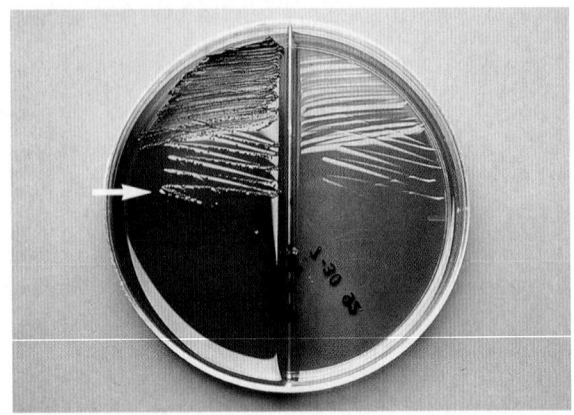

• **Fig. 41.7** *Prevotella disiens* on laked kanamycin-vancomycin blood agar. Note the black pigment (*arrow*).

25 of which have been isolated from human infection. *B. fragilis* is the most common organism isolated from clinical specimens, followed by *Bacteroides thetaiotaomicron* and *Bacteroides ovatus*. These organisms have been associated with a variety of infections.

The gram-negative *B. fragilis* group grows in 20% bile. These organisms are almost always resistant to all three special-potency antibiotic disks (Figs. 41.5 and 41.6). Rare strains of *B. fragilis* are susceptible to colistin.

Nonpigmented *Prevotella* spp.

Prevotella spp. are ubiquitous in the oral cavity and are an important component of dental biofilms. *Prevotella* organisms have been identified in the esophagus and stomach and isolated from human feces. Most are bile-sensitive, kanamycin-resistant, gram-negative rods. Colistin susceptibility is variable, and almost all strains are catalase- and indole-negative.

Pigmented *Porphyromonas* and *Prevotella* spp.

The *Porphyromonadaceae* family comprises seven genera, including *Butyricimonas, Coprobacter, Parabacteroides, Porphyromonas, Tannerella, Odoribacter,* and *Barnesiella*. *Porphyromonas* generally is considered the major pathogen in the *Porphyromonadaceae* family. There are approximately 19 species of *Porphyromonas* spp., 10 of which are commonly

isolated from humans (*P. asaccharolytica, P. bennonis, P. bronchialis, P. catoniae, P. endodontalis, P. gingivalis, P. pasteri, P. pogonae, P. somerae,* and *P. uenonis*). Most *Porphyromonas* spp. are asaccharolytic and pigmented. The *Prevotellaceae* includes saccharolytic organisms that have been isolated from a variety of body sites, including the oral cavity and feces. Colonies that fluoresce brick red or produce brown to black pigment are included in the pigmented *Prevotella* (Fig. 41.7) and *Porphyromonas* spp. (Fig. 41.8). Some species appear coccobacillary on Gram staining.

Fusobacteriaceae

The *Fusobacteriaceae* family includes the genera *Fusobacterium, Leptotrichia,* and *Sneathia*. These organisms are nonmotile, pleomorphic rods and typically are isolated from the oral cavity as integral components of dental biofilms or from the female genital tract (Fig. 41.9). The gram-negative *Fusobacterium* spp. (Fig. 41.10) are sensitive to kanamycin, and most strains fluoresce chartreuse. Different species have characteristic cell and colony morphologies.

The genus *Leptotrichia* includes seven validly described species. *Leptotrichia* spp. are saccharolytic, very large, fusiform rods with one pointed end and one blunt end that typically produce lactic acid. Colonies are large, gray, and

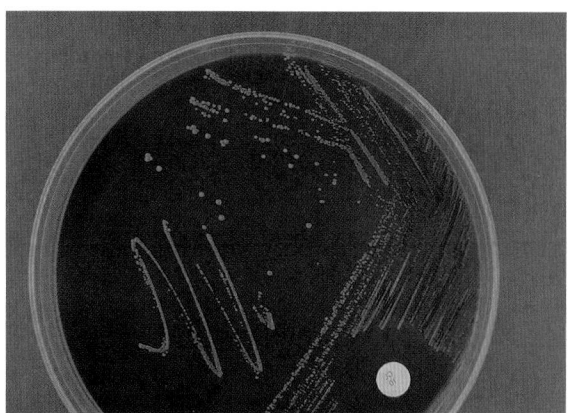

• **Fig. 41.8** *Porphyromonas* spp. on anaerobic blood agar. Red fluorescence is seen under ultraviolet light (365 nm). (Courtesy Anaerobe Systems, Morgan Hill, CA.)

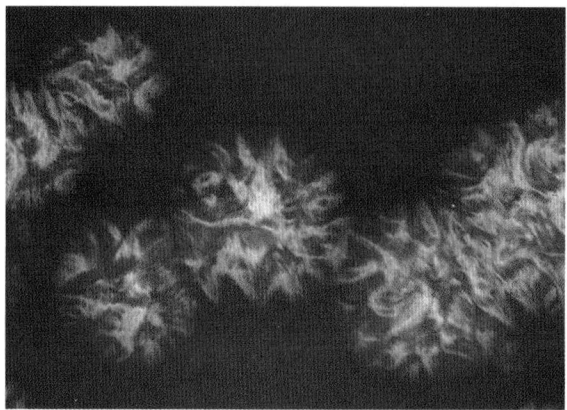

• **Fig. 41.9** *Fusobacterium nucleatum* subsp. *nucleatum* on anaerobic blood agar. Note the bread crumb–like colonies and greening of the agar.

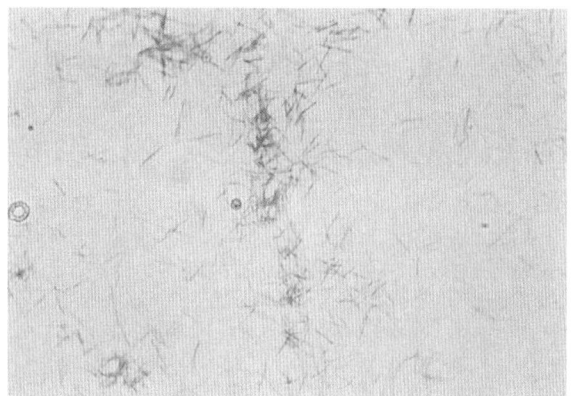

• **Fig. 41.10** Gram stain of *Fusobacterium nucleatum* subsp. *nucleatum.* Note the pointed ends.

convoluted. They are most often isolated from the oral cavity or urogenital tract.

Proteobacteria

The phylum Proteobacteria contains a variety of clinically significant organisms, including *Bilophila wadsworthia, Desulfovibrio, Desulfomicrobium,* and *Sutterella wadsworthensis. B.*

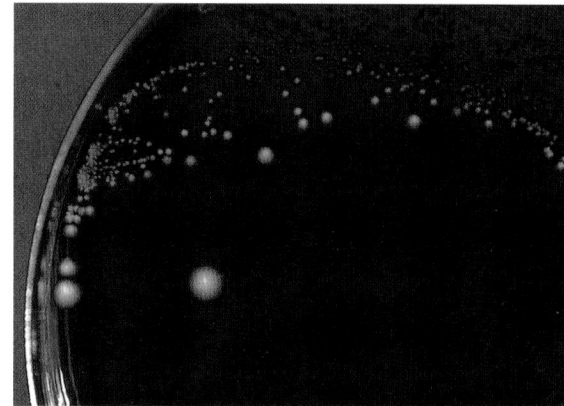

• **Fig. 41.11** *Peptostreptococcus anaerobius* on anaerobic blood agar.

wadsworthia is an anaerobic, asaccharolytic, bile-resistant, gram-negative rod. *S. wadsworthensis* is an asaccharolytic, bile-resistant, short, gram-negative rod. *B. wadsworthia* phenotypically resembles *Campylobacter ureolyticus* (Chapter 33) but is resistant to bile and is strongly catalase-positive. *Desulfomicrobium* spp. are motile, spiral-shaped organisms capable of reducing sulfate. *Desulfomicrobium orale* has been associated with periodontal disease. There are more than 70 species of *Desulfovibrio.* These organisms are rarely associated with human infections.

Anaerobic Gram-Positive and Gram-Negative Cocci

As stated earlier in this chapter and in Chapter 40, the proper collection and transport of specimens for anaerobic culture cannot be overemphasized. General considerations are included in the discussion in Chapter 40. The gram-positive anaerobic cocci typically are part of the normal microbiota of the oral cavity, upper respiratory tract, gastrointestinal tract, female genitourinary tract, and skin. The anaerobic cocci are non–spore forming and may appear slightly elongated. The cells vary in size and may be arranged in tetrads, chains, clusters, pairs, or clumps. Carbohydrate utilization varies among the genera. In addition, organisms typically classified as aerobic, such as *Staphylococcus epidermidis,* include strictly anaerobic strains. *Staphylococcus saccharolyticus* and *Staphylococcus aureus* subsp. *anaerobius* grow under anaerobic conditions, although after subculture they may develop aerotolerance. If a gram-positive coccus demonstrates resistance to metronidazole (5 μg) after 48 hours of incubation, it is likely a *Streptococcus* species. Among anaerobic gram-positive cocci, the genera of clinical importance are *Peptostreptococcus* (Fig. 41.11), *Finegoldia, Gallicola, Parvimonas, Peptoniphilus, Murdochiella, Peptococcus, Ezakiella, Staphylococcus,* and *Anaerococcus.*

The gram-negative anaerobic cocci are part of the normal microbiota of the oral cavity and the gastrointestinal, genitourinary, and respiratory tracts of humans. The category of anaerobic gram-negative cocci is based on Gram stain morphology. This category includes the genera *Veillonella, Megasphaera, Anaeroglobus, Negativicoccus,* and *Acidaminococcus.*

The genus *Veillonella* is ubiquitous as part of the normal microbiota of the human oral cavity and the genitourinary, respiratory, and gastrointestinal tracts. Human microbiome studies have begun to look at the balance of various anaerobic gram-negative cocci in normal and diseased tissue. In some instances, there are increased numbers of gram-negative cocci associated with abnormal clinical presentations such as *Megasphaera* in high-risk human papilloma viral infections and *Negativicoccus* in ground glass nodules associated with lung adenocarcinoma. When isolated from a clinical specimen, *Veillonella* are typically part of a mixed or polymicrobial culture.

Laboratory Diagnosis

Direct examination of clinical specimens reveals gram-positive or gram-negative cocci in chains, pairs, or singly. Some gram-positive cocci, in particular *Peptoniphilus asaccharolyticus*, are easily over-decolorized and can be misidentified as gram-negative. Follow-up tests to identify the organism are determined by the initial Gram stain. Organisms typically are isolated on anaerobic blood agar and can be differentiated using the special-potency antibiotic disks previously described in this chapter. Gram-positive cocci are sensitive to vancomycin and resistant to colistin. Gram-negative cocci typically are resistant to vancomycin. *Peptostreptococcus anaerobius* (≥12 mm) and *Parvimonas micra* (<12 mm) demonstrate sensitivity to sodium polyanethol sulfonate (SPS). *P. micra* also produces a milky halo around the colonies on blood agar. Interpretation and identification of either gram-positive or gram-negative cocci from a clinical specimen should be reported with caution and should correlate with the patient's signs and symptoms. Table 41.4 provides an identification scheme for representative anaerobic organisms.

Nucleic Acid Detection and MALDI-TOF MS

Nucleic acid–based methods have been developed to identify both anaerobic gram-positive and gram-negative cocci in the clinical laboratory. These methods include 16S rRNA sequencing, PCR, and oligonucleotide array assays. However, these methods are not without limitations. *Veillonella* demonstrates very low 16s rRNA variation making this method insufficient for species identification. Additional anaerobic cocci genera and species identifications are limited due to the lack of available reference sequence information in the databases. MALDI-TOF MS has been successfully used to identify many of the commonly isolated anaerobic gram-positive cocci. This method is also based on the spectra of 16s ribosomal proteins and housekeeping genes and may pose similar limitations on the identification of *Veillonella* spp. that are seen in nucleic acid–based methods.

Result Reporting

It is of primary importance to determine whether the clinical sample was properly collected when considering the isolation and identification of an anaerobic organism.

Interpretations should be carefully interpreted because of the potential for contamination of specimens with the patient's normal microbiota. In addition, recent or current antimicrobial therapy should be reviewed.

Isolation of anaerobes from normally sterile sites is considered clinically significant, and should be identified and reported to the clinician.

Prevention

A multiple-dose vaccine is available for the prevention of tetanus. The immunogen, which is adsorbed **tetanus toxoid** (inactivated toxin), is administered with diphtheria toxoid and pertussis vaccine as a triple antigen called Tdap. Single boosters of diphtheria and tetanus (Td or Tdap) or tetanus alone are recommended every 10 years. These vaccines can be used to catch up individuals who did not complete their full childhood vaccinations of DTap.

Immunoprophylaxis in wound management depends on the type of wound. Completely immunized individuals with minor or uncontaminated wounds do not require specific treatment. However, completely immunized individuals with major or contaminated wounds should get a booster of tetanus toxoid if they have not had one in the previous 5 years. Finally, a partially immunized individual or one who has never been immunized should receive a dose of tetanus toxoid immediately. In addition, passive immunization with human **tetanus immune globulin (TIG)** should be given if an individual has a major wound or a wound contaminated with soil that contains animal feces.

Individuals who have eaten food suspected of containing botulinum toxin should be purged with **cathartics** (laxatives), have their stomach pumped, and be given high enemas.

ⓔ Visit the Evolve site for a complete list of procedures, review questions, and case studies.

Bibliography

Ai D, Pan H, Han R, et al.: Using decision tree aggregation with random forest model to identify gut microbes associated with colorectal cancer, *Genes (Basel)* 10(2):E112, 2019.

Caroll KC, Pfaller MA: *Manual of clinical microbiology*, ed 12, Washington, DC, 2019, ASM Press.

Cattoir V: *Actinobaculum schaalii*: review of an emerging uropathogen, *J Infect* 64:260–267, 2012.

Chen Y, Hong Z, Wang W, et al.: Association between the vaginal microbiome and high-risk human papillomavirus infection in pregnant Chinese women, *BMC Infect Dis* 19(1):677, 2019, https://doi.org/10.1186/s12879-019-4279-6.

Corvec S: Clinical and biological features of *Cutibacterium* (formerly *Propionibacterium) avidum*, an underrecognized microorganism, *Clin Microbiol Rev* 31(3):e00064-17, 2018.

Diop K, Diop A, Khelaifia S, et al.: Characterization of a novel-Gram-stain-positive anaerobic coccus isolated from female genital tract: genome sequence and description of *Murdochiella vaginalis* sp. nov, *Microbiologyopen* 7(3):e00570, 2018.

Dowell VR, Hawkins TM: *Laboratory methods in anaerobic bacteriology: CDC laboratory manual.* Centers for Disease Control, DHHS Pub No (CDC) 81-8272, Atlanta, 1981, US Department of Health & Human Services.

Dzink JL, Sheenan MT, Socransky SS: Proposal of three subspecies of *Fusobacterium nucleatum* Knorr 1922: *Fusobacterium nucleatum* subsp. nucleatum subsp. nov., comb. nov.; *Fusobacterium nucleatum* subsp. *polymorphum* subsp. nov., nom. rev., comb. nov.; and *Fusobacterium nucleatum* subsp. *vincentii* subsp. nov., nom. rev., comb. nov, *Int J Syst Bacteriol* 40:74–78, 1990.

Esaiassen E, Hjerde E, Cavanagh JP, et al.: *Bifidobacterium* bacteremia: clinical characteristics and a genomic approach to assess pathogenicity, *J Clin Microbiol* 55(7):2234–2248, 2017.

Gardiner BJ, Korman TM, Junckerstorff RK: *Eggerthella lenta* bacteremia complicated by spondylodiscitis, psoas abscess and meningitis, *J Clin Microbiol* 52:1278–1280, 2014.

Hardy L, Jespers V, Dahchour N, et al.: Unraveling the bacterial vaginosis-associated biofilm: a multiplex *Gardnerella vaginalis* and *Atopobium vaginae* fluorescence in situ hybridization assay using peptide nucleic acid probes, *PLoS One* 10(8):e0136658, 2015.

Harris SC, Devendran S, Mendez-Garcia C, et al.: Bile oxidation by *Eggerthella lenta* strains C592 and DSM 2243, *Gut Microbes* 9(6):523–539, 2018.

Hiranmayi KV, Sirisha K, Ramaji Rao MV, et al.: Novel pathogens in periodontal microbiology, *J Pharm Bioallied Sci* 9(3):155–163, 2017.

Holdeman LV, Cato EP, Moore WEC, editors: *Anaerobic laboratory manual,* ed 4, Blacksburg, VA, 1977, Virginia Polytechnic Institute and State University.

Holdeman LV, Cato EP, Moore WEC, editors: *Anaerobic laboratory manual: update,* ed 4, Blacksburg, VA, 1987, Virginia Polytechnic Institute and State University.

Ikeda M, Kobayashi, Suzuki T, et al.: *Propionimicrobium lymphophilum* and *Actinotignum schaalii* bacteraemia: a case report, *New Microbes New Infect* 18:18–21, 2017.

Jousimies-Somer HR, Summanen P, Citron DM, et al.: *Wadsworth anaerobic bacteriology manual,* ed 6, Belmont, CA, 2002, Star.

Johnson CC: Susceptibility of anaerobic bacteria to β-lactam antibiotics in the United States, *Clin Infect Dis* 16(Suppl 4):S371, 1993.

Kageyama A, Benno Y, Nakase T: Phylogenetic and phenotypic evidence for the transfer of *Eubacterium aerofaciens* to the genus *Collinsella* as *Collinsella aerofaciens* gen. nov., comb. nov, *Int J Syst Bacteriol* 49:557–565, 1999.

Kageyama A, Benno Y, Nakase T: Phylogenetic evidence for the transfer of *Eubacterium lentum* to the genus *Eggerthella* as *Eggerthella lenta* gen. nov., comb. nov, *Int J Syst Bacteriol* 49:1725–1732, 1999.

Koransky JR, Allen SD, Dowell VR: Use of ethanol for selective isolation of spore forming microorganisms, *Appl Environ Microbiol* 35:762, 1978.

Kotaskova I, Obrucova H, Malisova B, et al.: Molecular techniques complement culture-based assessment of bacteria composition in mixed biofilms of urinary tract catheter-related samples, *Front Microbiol* 10:462, 2019.

Liderot K, Larsson M, Borang S, et al.: Polymicrobial bloodstream infection with *Eggerthella lenta* and *Desulfovibrio desulfuricans, J Clin Microbiol* 48:3810, 2010.

Lopez-Oliva I, Paropkari AD, Saraswat S, et al.: Dysbiotic subgingival microbial communities in periodontally healthy patients with rheumatoid arthritis, *Arthritis Rheumatol* 70(7):1008–1013, 2018.

Muller-Schulte E, Heimann KC, Treder W: *Peptoniphilus asaccharolyticus*-commensal, pathogen or synergist? Two case reports on invasive *Peptoniphilus asaccharolyticus* invasive infection, *Anaerobe* 59:159–162, 2019.

Neilands J, Davies JR, Bikker FJ, et al.: *Parvimonas micra* stimulates expression of ginigpains from *Porphyromonas gingivalis* in multispecies communities, *Anaerobe* 55:54–60, 2019.

Omar AB, Ahmadi N, Ombada M, et al.: Breaking bad: a case of *Lactobacillus* bacteremia and liver abscess, *J Community Hosp Intern Med Perspect* 9(3):235–239, 2019.

Ren Y, Su H, She Y, et al.: Whole genome sequencing revealed microbiome in lung adenocarcinomas presented as ground-glass nodules, *Transl Lung Cancer Res* 8(3):235–246, 2019.

Renz N, Mudrovcic S, Perka C, et al.: Orthopedic implant-associated infections caused by *Cutibacterium* spp.–a remaining diagnostic challenge, *One* 13(8):e0202639, 2018.

Rossi F, Amadoro C, Colavita G: Members of the *Lactobacillus* Genus Complex (LGC) as opportunistic pathoges: a review, *Microorganisms* 7(5):126, 2019.

Salameh A, Klotz SA, Zangeneh TT: Disseminated infection caused by *Eggerthella lenta* in a previously health young man: a case report, *Case Rep Infect Dis,* 2012, https://doi.org/10.1155/2012/517637.

Shinjo T, Fujisawa T, Mitsuoka T: Proposal of two subspecies of *Fusobacterium necrophorum* (Flügge) Moore and Holdeman: *Fusobacterium necrophorum* subsp. *necrophorum* subsp. nov., nom. rev. (ex Flügge 1886), and *Fusobacterium necrophorum* subsp. *funduliforme* subsp. nov., nom. rev. (ex Halle1898), *Int J Syst Bacteriol* 41:395–397, 1991.

Watanabe T, Yokoe M, Noguchi Y: Septic pulmonary embolism associated with periodontal disease: a case report and literature review, *BMC Infect Dis* 19(1):74, 2019.

42

Mycobacteria

OBJECTIVES

1. Describe the general characteristics of the *Mycobacterium* spp., including oxygen requirements, staining patterns and cellular morphology, artificial media required for cultivation and growth, and macroscopic colonial pigmentation.
2. Explain the chemical composition of the bacterial cell wall.
3. Explain the microscopic staining characteristics of *Mycobacterium* spp. using the Gram stain and acid-fast staining methods.
4. List the most common of the pathogenic *Mycobacterium* spp. and state for each the natural habitat, mode of transmission, and reservoir.
5. Differentiate *Mycobacterium tuberculosis* clinical infections based on the signs and symptoms of the following: primary infection, latent infection, disseminated infection, and reactivation.
6. Compare the current safety and containment methods recommended for handling mycobacterial infectious materials and routine bacteriology in a diagnostic laboratory.
7. Describe the purified protein derivative (PPD) test, also referred to as the tuberculin skin test. What is the significance of a positive result?
8. List the clinical specimens acceptable for recovery of mycobacteria and describe the limitations of recovery from each type of specimen.
9. Justify the use of deoxyribonucleic acid (DNA) probes and molecular sequencing or amplification methods and

matrix-assisted laser desorption ionization time-of-flight mass spectrometry (MALDI-TOF MS) to identify *Mycobacterium* spp.
10. Evaluate the effectiveness of the staining procedures—Kinyoun, Ziehl-Neelsen, and fluorescent staining (auramine-rhodamine or acridine orange)—for identifying mycobacteria.
11. Describe the requirements for using digestion and decontamination procedures to improve the recovery of *Mycobacterium* spp.
12. Explain the limitations of digestion and decontamination procedures.
13. Explain the methods commonly used for the biochemical identification of *Mycobacterium* spp. (i.e., niacin, nitrate, urease, modified catalase, Tween 80, tellurite, arylsulfatase, thiophene-2-carboxylic acid hydrazide [TCH], and 5% NaCl tests), including the purpose, principle, and control organisms used for each.
14. Describe the basic process and safety requirements associated with the extraction and processing of *Mycobacterium* spp. for MALDI-TOF MS TOF.
15. Describe the role of the human immunodeficiency virus (HIV) and acquired immunodeficiency syndrome (AIDS) in the dissemination and/or pathogenesis of infections with *Mycobacterium* spp.
16. Explain the recommended susceptibility testing methods and state when susceptibility testing is required or recommended for *Mycobacterium* spp.

MAJOR GENERA AND SPECIES TO BE CONSIDERED

Mycobacterium tuberculosis Complex

M. tuberculosis
M. bovis
M. bovis bacillus Calmette-Guérin (BCG)
M. africanum
M. caprae
M. canettii
M. microti
M. mungi
M. orygis
M. pinnipedii

Nontuberculous Mycobacteria

Slow-Growing Pathogens
M. avium complex (10 species, not listed here)
M. gordonae
M. haemophilum
M. kansasii

M. malmoense
M. marinum
M. ulcerans
M. xenopi

Rapid-Growing Opportunistic Pathogens
M. fortuitum group (10 species)
M. chelonae/abscessus group (6 species and 3 subspecies)
M. mucogenicum group (3 species)
M. smegmatis group (2 species)

Early Pigmented Rapid-Growing Opportunistic Pathogens
M. bacteremicum
M. canariasense
M. cosmeticum
M. mageritense/M. wolinskyi group (2 species)
M. monacense
M. neoaurum

Nonculturable Nontuberculosis Mycobacteria
M. leprae

Traditionally, *Mycobacterium* spp. have been classified according to phenotypic characteristics. However, since the late 1980s, molecular diagnostics have been used to shift the characterization of these organisms to genotypic studies. This chapter discusses both the phenotypic characterization and the new taxonomy based on molecular genetic data.

The organisms that belong to the genus *Mycobacterium* are aerobic (although *M. tuberculosis*, *M. bovis* BCG, and *M. avium* subsp. *paratuberculosis* demonstrate growth in reduced oxygen concentrations), non–spore-forming (except for *Mycobacterium marinum* and *M. avium* subsp. *paratuberculosis*), nonmotile, very thin, slightly curved or straight rods (0.2–0.6 × 1–10 μm). Some species may display a branching morphology. *Mycobacterium* is the only genus in the *Mycobacteriaceae* family (order Actinomycetales, class Actinomycetes). Genera that are closely related to *Mycobacterium* include *Corynebacterium*, *Nocardia*, *Rhodococcus*, *Segniliparus*, *Tsukamurella*, and *Gordonia*.

Mycobacterium spp. have an unusual cell wall; it contains N-glycolylmuramic acid instead of N-acetylmuramic acid and has a very high lipid content, which creates a hydrophobic permeability barrier. Because of this structure, mycobacteria are difficult to stain with commonly used basic aniline dyes such as those used in Gram staining. Although these organisms cannot be readily Gram stained, they are generally considered gram positive. However, they resist decolorization with acidified alcohol (3% hydrochloric acid) after prolonged application of a basic fuchsin dye or with heating of this dye after its application. This important property of mycobacteria, which derives from their cell wall structure, is referred to as **acid fastness;** this characteristic distinguishes mycobacteria from other genera. **Rapid-growing mycobacteria (RGM),** in which growth is apparent sooner than 7 days after subculture to Lowenstein-Jensen medium, may partially or completely lose this characteristic as a result of their growth characteristics.

Another important feature of many species is that they grow more slowly than most other human pathogenic bacteria because of their hydrophobic cell surface. Because of this hydrophobicity, organisms tend to clump, so that nutrients are not easily allowed into the cell. A single cell's generation time (the time required for a cell to divide into two independent cells) may range from approximately 20 to 36 hours for *Mycobacterium ulcerans*. **Slow-growing mycobacteria,** by definition, require more than 7 days to produce colonies on solid media. The variation in generation times among the mycobacteria results in the formation of visible colonies in 2 to 60 days at optimum temperature.

The genus *Mycobacterium* includes several highly pathogenic species included in the *M. tuberculosis* complex—*M. uclerans* and the nonculturable *M. leprae*. There are also more than 180 species of nonculturable **nontuberculosis mycobacteria (NTM),** many of which are increasingly found in opportunistic pathogens that are found throughout the environment.

The NTM slow-growing mycobacteria comprise more than 90 species, several of which are clinically significant.

These organisms produce a spectrum of infections in humans and animals ranging from localized lesions to disseminated disease. Some species cause only human infections and others have been isolated from a wide variety of animals. Many species are also found in water and soil.

For the most part, mycobacteria can be divided into two major groups based on fundamental differences in epidemiology and association with disease: those belonging to the *M. tuberculosis* complex and the others to the NTM group.

Mycobacterium tuberculosis Complex

Tuberculosis was endemic in animals in the Paleolithic period, long before it ever affected humans. This disease (also called **consumption**) has been recognized in all ages and climates. For example, tuberculosis was the subject of a hymn in a sacred text from India dating from 2500 BC, and deoxyribonucleic acid (DNA) unique to *M. tuberculosis* was identified in lesions from the lung of 1000-year-old human remains found in Peru.

General Characteristics

In the clinical microbiology laboratory, the term **complex** is commonly used to describe two or more species for which distinction is complicated and has little or no medical importance. The mycobacterial species that occur in humans and belong to the *M. tuberculosis* complex include *M. tuberculosis*, *Mycobacterium bovis*, *M. bovis* BCG, *Mycobacterium africanum*, *Mycobacterium caprae*, *Mycobacterium microti*, *Mycobacterium canettii*, *Mycobacterium mungi*, *Mycobacterium orygis*, and *Mycobacterium pinnipedii*. All these species are capable of causing tuberculosis. It should be noted that species identification might be required for epidemiologic and public health reasons. The organisms that belong to the *M. tuberculosis* complex are considered slow growers and their colonies are nonpigmented.

Epidemiology and Pathogenesis
Epidemiology

M. tuberculosis is the cause of most cases of human tuberculosis, particularly in developed countries. *M. tuberculosis* complex organisms are not able to replicate in the environment and are therefore isolated to growth in tissues of humans and other warm-blooded animals. An estimated 2.4 billion people, or one-third of the world's population, are infected with *M. tuberculosis*. This reservoir of infected individuals results in approximately 10 million new cases of tuberculosis and 2.9 million deaths annually. Tuberculosis continues to be a public health problem in the United States. An additional complicating factor in the management of tuberculosis is the increasing incidence of coinfection with HIV. HIV-associated tuberculosis remains a significant challenge to world health, with an estimated 1.1 million individuals living with HIV-associated tuberculosis. In the United States, tuberculosis is typically found among the poor, the homeless, intravenous drug users, alcoholics, the elderly—in general, medically underserved populations. Another area of concern is the increased identification of multidrug-resistant tuberculosis (MDR-TB) and extensively drug-resistant tuberculosis (XDR-TB). Although the organisms belonging to the *M. tuberculosis* complex have numerous characteristics in common, including extreme genetic homogeneity, they differ in certain epidemiologic aspects (Table 42.1).

TABLE 42.1	Epidemiology of Organisms Belonging to *Mycobacterium tuberculosis* Complex That Cause Human Infections		
Organism	**Habitat**	**Primary Route of Transmission**	**Distribution**
Mycobacterium tuberculosis	Patients with cavitary disease are primary reservoir.	Person-to-person by inhalation of droplet nuclei: droplet nuclei containing the organism (infectious aerosols, 1–5 μm) are produced when people with pulmonary tuberculosis cough, sneeze, speak, or sing; infectious aerosols may also be produced by manipulation of lesions or processing of clinical specimens in the laboratory. Droplets are so small that air currents keep them airborne for long periods; once inhaled, they are small enough to reach the lungs' alveoli.[a]	Worldwide
Mycobacterium bovis	Humans and a wide range of host animals, such as cattle, nonhuman primates, goats, cats, buffalo, badgers, possums, dogs, pigs, and deer.	Ingestion of contaminated milk from infected cows[b]; airborne transmission.[c]	Worldwide
Mycobacterium bovis BCG	Commercial vaccine strain that has been maintained by serial passage *in vitro*.	A heterogenous population of strains currently exist and are transmitted via immunization. They are attenuated strains that react similar to *M. bovis*.	Worldwide
Mycobacterium africanum	Humans.[d]	Inhalation of droplet nuclei.	East and West tropical Africa; some cases have been identified in the United States
Mycobacterium caprae	Predominately infects a wide range of animals: goats, cattle, sheep, pigs, wild boars, red deer, and foxes. Endemic in wild ruminants and dairy cattle in Australia.	Inhalation of droplet nuclei, leading to pulmonary manifestations.	Europe
Mycobacterium microti	Humans rarely; small animals (e.g., voles and other wild rodents); domestic cats, wild boars, badgers, and goats.	Inhalation of droplet nuclei; potentially transmitted by the ingestion of contaminated raw goat milk cheese or other animal products.	Europe; Great Britain, Netherlands
Mycobacterium mungi	Natural reservoir is the banded mongoose; rarely infects humans.	Unclear; likely inhalation of droplet nuclei.	Africa
Mycobacterium canettii	Natural reservoir has not been clearly defined. Rarely infects humans.	Unclear; inhalation of droplet nuclei most likely.	Africa
Mycobacterium orygis	Larger mammals; oryxes, gazelles, antelopes, and waterbucks.	Unclear; likely inhalation of droplet nuclei or direct contact; zoonotic.	Africa
Mycobacterium pinnipedii	Humans rarely; predominantly infects a wide range of animals (pigs, rabbits, camels, tapirs, and sea lions; possibly cattle).	Inhalation of droplet nuclei; however, transmission from sea lions to humans has been demonstrated in zoologic settings.	Europe

BCG, Bacillus Calmette-Guérin.
[a]Infection can occasionally occur through the gastrointestinal tract or skin.
[b]The incidence has decreased significantly in developed countries since the introduction of universal pasteurization of milk and milk products and the institution of effective control programs for cattle.
[c]Can be transmitted human to human, animal to human, and human to animal.
[d]Infections in animals have not been totally excluded.

Pathogenesis

The pathogenesis of tuberculosis caused by organisms of the *M. tuberculosis* complex is discussed in Chapter 68. Inhalation of a single viable organism has been shown to lead to infection, although close contact is usually necessary. Of those who become infected with *M. tuberculosis,* 15% to 20% develop disease. The disease usually occurs some years after the initial infection, when the patient's immune system breaks down for some reason other than the presence of tuberculosis bacilli in the lung. In a small percentage of infected hosts, the disease becomes systemic, affecting a variety of organs.

After the ingestion of unpasteurized dairy products from infected cows, *M. bovis* may penetrate the gastrointestinal mucosa or invade the lymphatic tissue of the oropharynx. The organism is also often transmitted by the inhalation of infectious droplets from infected cattle. An attenuated strain of *M. bovis,* **bacillus Calmette-Guérin (BCG),** has been used extensively in many parts of the world to immunize susceptible individuals against tuberculosis. Because mycobacteria are the classic examples of intracellular pathogens and the body's response to BCG hinges on cell-mediated immunoreactivity, immunized individuals are expected to react more aggressively against all antigens that elicit cell-mediated immunity. In rare cases, an individual's immune system is so compromised that it cannot handle the BCG, so that systemic BCG infection may develop.

M. africanum demonstrates physiologic and biochemical properties that place it intermediately between *M. tuberculosis* and *M. bovis.* This organism has been primarily identified as the cause of approximately half of the cases of tuberculosis in West Africa, but it has also been found in the United States in patients who previously resided in Africa. *M. caprae* can be identified by its susceptibility to pyrazinamide. This organism is associated with approximately 31% of the cases of human tuberculosis. Reservoir hosts for the organism include goats, cattle, sheep, pigs, wild boars, deer, and fox. *M. microti,* typically found in rodents, guinea pigs, rabbits, cats, llamas, and meerkats, usually fails to grow in culture. It has been identified in tuberculosis in both immunocompetent and immunosuppressed patients. *M. canettii* has been primarily identified in cases of lymphadenitis and generalized tuberculosis in immunocompromised individuals. This organism has also been primarily associated with infections in individuals who previously resided or currently reside in Africa. *M. pinnipedii* is transmitted from sea lions to humans and has been associated with granulomatous lesions in the lymph nodes, lungs, pleura, and spleen. It is also pathogenic in guinea pigs, rabbits, camels, and possibly cattle. The two additional species in the *M. tuberculosis* complex reservoir hosts include the banded mongoose *(M. mungi)* or large mammals such as gazelles, antelopes, waterbucks, and oryxes *(M. orygis).* The latter causes a disease in humans that is indistinguishable from tuberculosis.

Spectrum of Disease

Tuberculosis may mimic other diseases, such as pneumonia, neoplasm, or fungal infections. In addition, clinical manifestations in patients infected with *M. tuberculosis* complex may range from asymptomatic to acutely symptomatic. Patients who are symptomatic can have systemic symptoms, pulmonary signs and symptoms, signs and symptoms related to other organ involvement (e.g., the kidneys), or a combination of these features. Cases of pulmonary disease caused by *M. tuberculosis* complex organisms are clinically, radiologically, and pathologically indistinguishable.

Primary tuberculosis typically is considered a disease of the respiratory tract. Common presenting symptoms include low-grade fever, night sweats, fatigue, anorexia (loss of appetite), and weight loss. A patient who presents with pulmonary tuberculosis usually has a productive cough, along with low-grade fever, chills, myalgias (aches), and sweating; however, these signs and symptoms are similar for influenza, acute bronchitis, and pneumonia.

Upon respiratory infection with *M. tuberculosis* complex organisms, the cellular immune system's T cells and macrophages migrate to the lungs, where the organisms are phagocytized by the macrophages. However, these organisms are capable of intracellular multiplication in the macrophages. Often the host is unable to eliminate the organisms, and the result is a systemic hypersensitivity to *Mycobacterium* antigens. **Granulomas,** or hard tubercles, form in the lung from the lymphocytes, macrophages, and cellular pathology, including the formation of **giant cells** (cellular fusion displaying multiple nuclei). If the *Mycobacterium* antigen concentration is high, the hypersensitivity reaction may result in tissue necrosis caused by enzymes released from the macrophages. In this case no granuloma forms, and a solid or semisolid **caseous** material is left at the site of the primary lesion.

In some patients infected with primary active tuberculosis, the disease may spread via the lymph system or hematogenously, leading to **meningeal** or **miliary (disseminated) tuberculosis.** This most often occurs in patients with depressed or ineffective cellular immunity.

As previously mentioned, in a small percentage of patients, organs besides the lungs can become involved after infection with *M. tuberculosis* complex organisms. These organs include the following:

- Genitourinary tract
- Lymph nodes (cervical lymphadenitis)
- Central nervous system (meningitis)
- Bone and joint (arthritis and osteomyelitis)
- Peritoneum
- Pericardium
- Larynx
- Pleural lining (pleuritis)

Disseminated tuberculosis can be diagnosed by a positive tuberculin skin test (described later in the chapter).

Patients may also have **latent tuberculosis** (i.e., they have no apparent signs, symptoms, or pathologic condition).

A patient with latent tuberculosis is not infectious and does not have active disease, although the organism is present in granulomas. Patients with latent tuberculosis may progress to active disease (also referred to as **reactivation tuberculosis**) at any time. Reactivation tuberculosis typically occurs after an incident in which cellular immunity is suppressed or damaged as a result of a change in lifestyle or other health condition.

Individuals infected with HIV are particularly susceptible to developing active tuberculosis. These patients are likely to have rapidly progressive primary disease instead of a subclinical infection.

Diagnosing tuberculosis is more difficult in people infected with HIV because chest radiographs of the pulmonary disease often lack specificity, and patients frequently are **anergic** (lack a biologic response) to tuberculin skin testing, a primary means of identifying individuals infected with *M. tuberculosis*. The **tuberculin skin test,** or **purified protein derivative (PPD) test,** is based on the premise that after infection with *M. tuberculosis,* an individual develops a delayed hypersensitivity cell-mediated immunity to certain antigenic components of the organism. To determine whether a person has been infected with *M. tuberculosis,* a culture extract of *M. tuberculosis* (i.e., PPD of tuberculin) is injected intracutaneously. After 48 to 72 hours, an infected individual will show a delayed hypersensitivity reaction to the PPD, characterized by erythema (redness) and, most important, induration (firmness because of the influx of immune cells). The diameter of induration is measured and then interpreted as to whether the patient has been infected with *M. tuberculosis;* different interpretive criteria are used for different patient populations (e.g., immunosuppressed individuals, such as those infected with HIV). The PPD test is not 100% sensitive or specific, and a positive reaction to the skin test does not necessarily signify the presence of disease.

Immunodiagnostic methods that measure the release of interferon gamma by T cells following stimulation with MTBC antigens provide specific and rapid results that demonstrate equivalent and increased sensitivity compared to the PPD test. Two commercially available interferon gamma release assays (IGRAs) approved by the US Food and Drug Administration (FDA) are available in the United States. The T-Spot TB test (Oxford Immunotec, Oxford, UK) offers next-day results and does not require a follow-up visit with a physician. The assay measures T cells that have been activated by *M. tuberculosis* antigens. Peripheral blood mononuclear cells (PBMCs) are incubated with *M. tuberculosis*–specific antigens, thus stimulating any sensitized T cells in the patient sample. T-cell cytokines released in the sample are measured, using antibody to capture them, and then detected with a secondary antibody conjugated to alkaline phosphatase. This assay should be interpreted in correlation with the patient's signs and symptoms.

An enzyme-linked immunosorbent assay (ELISA) called QuantiFERON-TB Gold Plus (Qiagen, Germantown, MD) is also available. The assay measures a component of the cell-mediated immune response to *M. tuberculosis* to diagnose latent tuberculosis infection and is not generally used to identify active tuberculosis disease. It is based on the quantification of interferon-gamma released from sensitized lymphocytes in heparinized whole blood that has been incubated overnight with a mixture of synthetic peptides simulating two proteins in *M. tuberculosis.* The test assesses responses to multiple antigens, can be performed in a single patient visit, and is less subject to reader bias and error. An important feature is that the results of the assay are unaffected by previous BCG vaccination. Guidelines published by the Centers for Disease Control and Prevention (CDC) recommend the use of this assay in all circumstances in which the tuberculin skin test is currently used (e.g., contact investigations and the evaluation of recent immigrants). The guidelines also provide specific cautions for interpreting negative results in individuals from selected populations.

Nontuberculous Mycobacteria

The NTM include all mycobacterial species that do not belong to the *M. tuberculosis* complex. Currently approximately 180 species of NTM have been recognized, with about 90 species classified as slow growing. The members of this large group of mycobacteria are often opportunistic pathogens. Those most often isolated from clinical specimens are discussed in this chapter. Significant geographic variability is seen both in the prevalence of NTM disease and the species responsible. As previously mentioned, NTM are present everywhere in the environment and sometimes colonize the skin as well as the respiratory and gastrointestinal tracts of healthy individuals. Little is known about how infection is acquired, but some mechanisms appear to be trauma, inhalation of infectious aerosols, and ingestion; a few diseases are nosocomial or are acquired as an iatrogenic infection. In contrast to *M. tuberculosis* complex, NTM are not usually transmitted from person to person, nor does isolation of these organisms necessarily mean that they are associated with a disease process. Interpretation of a positive NTM culture is complicated because these organisms are widely distributed in nature, their pathogenic potential varies greatly from one species to another, and humans can be colonized by these mycobacteria without necessarily developing infection or disease. With few exceptions, little is known about the pathogenesis of infections caused by these bacterial agents.

In 1959, Runyon classified NTM into four groups (**Runyon groups I to IV**) based on the phenotypic characteristics of the various species, most notably their growth rates and colonial pigmentation (Table 42.2). Runyon's system first categorizes the slow-growing NTM (Runyon groups I to III) and then the rapid growers (Runyon group IV). One other NTM, *M. leprae,* which cannot be cultivated on artificial media, is also reviewed. As with many classification schemes, the Runyon classification does not always hold true. For example, some NTM can be either a photochromogen or a nonphotochromogen.

TABLE 42.2   Runyon Classification of Nontuberculous Mycobacteria

Runyon Group Number	Group Name	Description
I	Photochromogens	NTM colonies that develop pigment on exposure to light after being grown in the dark and take longer than 7 days to appear on solid media
II	Scotochromogens	NTM colonies that develop pigment in the dark or light and take longer than 7 days to appear on solid media
III	Nonphotochromogens	NTM colonies that are nonpigmented regardless of whether they are grown in the dark or light and take longer than 7 days to appear on solid media
IV	Rapid growers	NTM colonies that grow on solid media and take fewer than 7 days to appear

NTM, Nontuberculous mycobacteria.

Because it is difficult to determine the clinical significance of an NTM that has been isolated from a clinical sample, several clinical classification schemes have also been proposed. One such scheme classifies NTM recovered from humans into four major groups (pulmonary, lymphadenitic, cutaneous, or disseminated) based on the clinical disease they cause. Other NTM classifications are based on the pathogenic potential of a species.

Slow-Growing Nontuberculous Mycobacteria

The slow-growing NTM can be subdivided into three groups based on the phenotypic characteristics of the species. *Mycobacterium* spp. synthesize **carotenoids** (a group of yellow to red pigments) in varying amounts and thus can be categorized into three groups—photochromogens, scotochromogens, and nonphotochromogens—based on the production of those pigments Some of these NTM are considered potentially pathogenic for humans, whereas others are rarely associated with disease.

Photochromogens

The **photochromogens** (Table 42.3) are slow-growing NTM that produce colonies requiring light to form pigment.

Scotochromogens

The **scotochromogens** (Table 42.4) are slow-growing NTM that produce pigmented colonies whether grown in the dark or the light. The epidemiology of the potentially pathogenic scotochromogens has not been definitively described. In contrast to potentially pathogenic nonphotochromogens, these agents are rarely recovered in the clinical laboratory.

Nonphotochromogens

The **nonphotochromogens** (Table 42.5) are slow-growing NTM that produce unpigmented colonies whether grown in the dark or the light. Of the organisms in this group, *Mycobacterium terrae* complex (*M. terrae* and *M. nonchromogenicum*)

and *Mycobacterium gastri* are considered nonpathogenic for humans. *M. arupense, M. kumamotonense, M. heraklionense,* and *M. virginiense* are pathogenic when associated with tenosynovitis or osteomyelitis. The other nonphotochromogens are considered potentially pathogenic, and many are commonly recovered in the clinical laboratory. The nonphotochromogens belong to *M. avium* complex (MAC); they are commonly isolated in the clinical laboratory and able to cause infection in the human host.

Mycobacterium avium Complex

Largely because of the increasing populations of immunosuppressed patients, the incidence of infection caused by MAC—as well as these organisms' clinical significance—has changed significantly since they were first recognized as human pathogens in the 1950s. The introduction of **highly active antiretroviral therapy (HAART)** has dramatically reduced the infections caused by these organisms in patients with AIDS.

General Characteristics. Taxonomically, MAC comprises *M. avium, Mycobacterium intracellulare, M. avium* subsp. *avium, M. avium* subsp. *paratuberculosis, M. avium* subsp. *silvaticum* (wood pigeon bacillus), *M. avium* subsp. *hominissuis, M. arosiense, M. vulneris, M. marseillense, M. bouchedurhonense, M. chimaera, M. colombiense, M. yogonense,* and *M. timonense.* Although *M. avium* and *M. intracellulare* are clearly different organisms, they so closely resemble each other that the distinction cannot be made by routine laboratory determinations or on clinical grounds. As a result, these organisms are sometimes referred to as *M. avium-intracellulare.* Furthermore, because isolation of *M. avium* subsp. *paratuberculosis* in a routine laboratory setting is exceedingly rare, the term MAC is most commonly used to report the isolation of *M. avium-intracellulare.*

Epidemiology and Pathogenesis. MAC is an important pathogen in both immunocompromised and immunocompetent populations. These organisms are among the most commonly isolated NTM in the United States. MAC is particularly noteworthy for its potentially pathogenic role in pulmonary infections in patients with AIDS and in those who

TABLE 42.3	Characteristics of Representative Nontuberculous Mycobacteria—Photochromogens		
Organism	**Epidemiology**	**Pathogenicity**	**Type of Infection**
Mycobacterium kansasii	Infection more common in white males; natural reservoir is tap water; aerosols are involved in transmission.	Potentially pathogenic	Chronic pulmonary disease; extrapulmonary diseases, such as cervical lymphadenitis and cutaneous disease
Mycobacterium asiaticum	Not commonly encountered, tropical climates and commonly found in environmental water (primarily seen in Australia). No human-to-human transmission has been reported.	Frequent colonizer, potentially pathogenic	Pulmonary disease and extrapulmonary disease in a variety of organs and musculoskeletal system bursitis and tenosynovitis
Mycobacterium branderi	Unclear, environmental exposure suspected.	Potentially pathogenic	Ulcerative tenosynovitis, pulmonary disease, and wound infections
Mycobacterium marinum	Natural reservoirs are freshwater and saltwater as a result of contamination from infected fish and other marine life. Transmission is by contact with contaminated water and organism entry by means of trauma or small breaks in the skin; associated with aquatic activity usually involving fish.	Potentially pathogenic	Cutaneous disease; bacteremia
Mycobacterium intermedium	Environmental water sources.	Potentially pathogenic	Pulmonary disease (chronic bronchitis) and dermatitis
Mycobacterium nebraskense	Cutaneous infections have been identified in dogs and cats.	Potentially pathogenic	Pulmonary disease and cutaneous infections

are not infected with HIV. The organisms are ubiquitous in the environment and have been isolated from natural water, soil, dairy products, pigs, chickens, cats, and dogs. As a result of extensive studies, it is generally accepted that natural waters serve as the major reservoir for most human infections.

Infections caused by MAC are acquired by inhalation or ingestion. The pathogenesis of MAC infections is not clearly understood. The organisms are commonly associated with respiratory disease clinically similar to tuberculosis in adults, lymphadenitis in children, and disseminated infection in patients with HIV. However, these organisms and other environmental NTM have extraordinary starvation survival. They can persist well over a year in tap water, and MAC tolerates temperature extremes. In addition, similar to legionellae, *M. avium* can infect and replicate in protozoa. Amoeba-grown *M. avium* is more invasive toward human epithelial and macrophage cells.

MAC cultures can have an opaque glossy-white colony morphology or can produce a smaller translucent colony morphology. Studies suggest that transparent colonies are more virulent because they are more drug resistant, are isolated more commonly from the blood of patients with

AIDS and appear more virulent in macrophage and animal models. In addition, a third morphology appears as a dry flat colony that can be confused with *M. tuberculosis.* Some colonies may also produce a yellow pigment as they age.

M. avium subsp. *paratuberculosis* is known to cause an inflammatory bowel disease (known as **Johne disease**) in cattle, sheep, and goats. It has also been isolated from the bowel mucosa of patients with Crohn disease, a chronic inflammatory bowel disease of humans. The organism is extremely fastidious, seems to require a growth factor (mycobactin, produced by other species of mycobacteria), and may take as long as 6 to 18 months for primary isolation. Whether these and other mycobacteria contribute to the development of Crohn disease or are simply colonizing an environmental niche in the bowel of these patients remains to be elucidated.

Clinical Spectrum of Disease. The clinical manifestations of MAC infections are summarized in Table 42.5.

Other Nonphotochromogens

Several other mycobacterial species that are considered nonphotochromogens are potentially pathogenic in humans. The

TABLE 42.4 Characteristics of Representative Nontuberculous Mycobacteria—Scotochromogens

Organism	Epidemiology/Habitat	Pathogenicity	Type of Infection
Mycobacterium europaeum	May be a colonizer that leads to infection	Potentially pathogenic	Pulmonary disease and lymphadenitis; infections are most often associated with immunocompromised individuals with other respiratory diseases or comorbidities
Mycobacterium szulgai	Water and soil	Potentially pathogenic	Pulmonary disease, and extrapulmonary infections; cervical adenitis; bursitis
Mycobacterium scrofulaceum	Raw milk, soil, water, dairy products	Potentially pathogenic	Cervical adenitis in children, bacteremia, pulmonary disease, skin infections
Mycobacterium interjectum	Unknown; respiratory likely	Potentially pathogenic	Chronic lymphadenitis, pulmonary disease and polyangiitis; may lead to disseminated disease
Mycobacterium heckeshornense	Unknown; environmental	Potentially pathogenic	Pulmonary disease (cavitary and nodular), lymphadenitis, tenosynovitis and osteomyelitis
Mycobacterium lentiflavum	Environmental water	Potentially pathogenic	Pulmonary disease, lymphadenitis, spondylodiscitis, skin and disseminated disease. Frequently isolated from patients with cystic fibrosis.
Mycobacterium mantenii	Environmental water	Potentially pathogenic	Pulmonary disease and lymphadenitis
Mycobacterium palustre	Unknown	Potentially pathogenic	Lymphadenitis
Mycobacterium parmense	Unknown	Potentially pathogenic	Lymphadenitis
Mycobacterium tusciae	Unknown—isolated from tap water	Potentially pathogenic	Cervical lymphadenitis (rare)
Mycobacterium kubicae	Unknown	Potentially pathogenic	Pulmonary disease
Mycobacterium gordonae	Tap water (pipelines and laboratory faucets), fresh water, soil	Potentially pathogenic	Pulmonary pneumonitis and other hypersensitivity lung disease primarily in immunocompromised patients
Mycobacterium cookii	Sphagnum moss, surface waters in New Zealand	Nonpathogenic[a]	NA
Mycobacterium hiberniae	Sphagnum moss, soil in Ireland	Nonpathogenic[a]	NA

[a]Rarely if ever causes disease.
NA, Not applicable.

epidemiology and spectrum of disease for these organisms are summarized in Table 42.5. In addition to the species in this table, other more recently characterized species of mycobacteria that are nonphotochromogens have been described, such as *Mycobacterium celatum* and *Mycobacterium conspicuum.* These agents appear to be potentially pathogenic in humans.

Rapidly Growing Nontuberculous Mycobacteria

Mycobacteria that produce colonies on solid media in 7 days or earlier constitute the second major group of NTM,

or rapidly growing mycobacteria (RGM). Currently approximately 89 species have been classified into this group.

General Characteristics

The large group of organisms that constitute the RGM is divided into six major groups of potentially pathogenic species based on pigmentation and molecular studies. The common human pathogens in this group include *Mycobacterium abscessus* subsp. *abscessus, Mycobacterium chelonae,* and *Mycobacterium fortuitum.* Two new species—*M. celeriflabum* and *M saopaulense*—have been isolated from human samples. Unlike most other mycobacteria, most RGM can grow on

TABLE 42.5   Characteristics of the Representative Nontuberculous Mycobacteria—Nonphotochromogens and Species Considered Potential Pathogens

Organism	Epidemiology	Type of Infection
Mycobacterium avium complex	Environmental sources, including natural waters and soil	Patients without AIDS: pulmonary infections in patients with preexisting pulmonary disease; cervical lymphadenitis; and disseminated disease[a] in immunocompromised patients who are HIV negative Patients with AIDS: disseminated disease.
Mycobacterium celatum	Unknown	Immunocompetent patients: primarily children and the elderly. Immunocompromised: 32% of patients also infected with HIV; pulmonary disease and lymphadenitis.
Mycobacterium xenopi[b]	Water, especially hot water taps in hospitals; believed to be transmitted in aerosols	Primarily pulmonary infections in adults; less common, extrapulmonary infections (bone, lymph nodes, sinus tract) and disseminated disease
Mycobacterium ulcerans	Stagnant tropical waters; also harbored in an aquatic insect's salivary glands; infections occur in tropical or temperate climates. Third most common mycobacterial disease worldwide.	Indolent cutaneous and subcutaneous infections (African Buruli ulcer or Australian Bairnsdale ulcer); severe limb deformities with contractures and scarring are common
Mycobacterium lacus	Unknown; genetically related to M. malmoense and M. marinum	Bursitis with caseating granulomas after trauma
Mycobacterium malmoense	Most cases from England, Wales, and Sweden. Little is known about epidemiology; to date, isolated only from humans and captured armadillos.	Chronic pulmonary infections, primarily in patients with preexisting disease; cervical lymphadenitis in children; less common, infections of the skin or bursae
Mycobacterium genavense	Isolated from pet birds (parrots and parakeets), dogs, and tap water	Disseminated disease in patients with AIDS (wasting disease characterized by fever, weight loss, hepatosplenomegaly, anemia)
Mycobacterium haemophilum	Unknown; optimal growth temperature is 28°C–30°C and requires hemin or hemoglobin	Disseminated disease; cutaneous infections that appear as multiple skin lesions or ulcerations and associated with abscesses, fistulas, or osteomyelitis, cervical lymphadenitis, or pulmonary nodules
Mycobacterium heidelbergense	Unknown	Lymphadenitis in children; also isolated from sputum, urine, and gastric aspirate
Mycobacterium shimoidei	To date, has not been isolated from environmental sources; widespread geographically	Tuberculosis-like pulmonary infection; disseminated disease
Mycobacterium simiae	Tap water and hospital water tanks; rarely isolated	Tuberculosis-like pulmonary infection
Mycobacterium terrae complex	Trauma and respiratory routes; may be found in aquatic environments	Tenosynovitis and pulmonary disease

[a]Disseminated disease can involve multiple sites, such as bone marrow, lungs, liver, lymph nodes.
[b]Can be either nonphotochromogenic or scotochromogenic.
AIDS, Acquired immunodeficiency syndrome; *HIV*, human immunodeficiency virus.

routine bacteriologic media and on media specific for the cultivation of mycobacteria. On Gram staining, these organisms appear as weakly gram-positive rods resembling diphtheroids.

Epidemiology and Pathogenesis

The rapidly growing mycobacteria considered potentially pathogenic can cause disease in either healthy or immunocompromised patients. Like many other NTM, these organisms are ubiquitous in the environment and are present worldwide. They have been found in soil, marshes, rivers, and municipal water supplies (tap water) and in marine and terrestrial life forms. Infections caused by RGM can be acquired in the community from environmental sources. They can also be health care–associated infections resulting from medical interventions (including bone marrow transplantation), wound infections, and catheter sepsis. These organisms may be commensals on the skin. They gain entry into the host through inoculation into the skin and subcutaneous tissues as a result of trauma, injections, or surgery and may also be acquired through animal contact or from posttraumatic wound infections.

The RGM can also cause disseminated cutaneous infections. The description of chronic pulmonary infections caused by RGM suggests a possible respiratory route for the acquisition of organisms present in the environment. Of the potentially pathogenic rapidly growing NTM, *M. fortuitum* group, *M. chelonae,* and *M. abscessus* subsp. *abscessus* are commonly encountered; these three account for approximately 90% of clinical disease. Little is known about the pathogenesis of these organisms.

Spectrum of Disease

The spectrum of disease caused by the most commonly encountered rapid growers is summarized in Table 42.6. The most common infection associated with RGM is posttraumatic wound infection. An increase in wound infections has been associated with planktonic *M. abscessus* subsp. *abscessus,* which can be identified as a rough colonial phenotype on artificial media; these organisms are capable of infecting macrophages. The smooth colonial phenotype is typically identified in biofilms and lacks infectivity. Disseminated cutaneous infection due to *M. abscessus* and *M. chelonae* is common and presents as multiple chronic and painful red draining nodules often in the lower extremities. *M. abscessus* subsp. *abscessus* and *M. abscessus* subsp. *massiliense* are increasingly identified in the respiratory tracts of patients with cystic fibrosis.

Noncultivatable Nontuberculous Mycobacteria—*Mycobacterium leprae*

The nontuberculous mycobacterium *M. leprae* is a close relative of *M. tuberculosis.* This organism causes **leprosy** (also called **Hansen disease**)—a chronic disease of the skin, mucous membranes, and nerve tissue. Leprosy remains a worldwide public health concern owing to the development of drug-resistant isolates.

General Characteristics

M. leprae has not yet been cultivated *in vitro,* although it can be cultivated in the armadillo and in the footpads of mice. Molecular biologic techniques have provided most of the information about this organism's genomic structure and its various genes and their products. Polymerase chain reaction (PCR) assays have been used to detect and identify *M. leprae* in infected tissues, blood, and urine. A line probe assay, GenoType Leprae DR (Hain Lifescience, Nehren, Germany), has been developed that can detect the organism and resistance patterns to rifampicin, ofloxacin, and dapsone in clinical specimens. Paucibacillary patients require highly sensitive methods for the identification of organisms

and diagnosis. Droplet digital PCR (ddPCR) can detect infectious disease in samples that have very low copy numbers of nucleic acid. Routine diagnosis of leprosy is based on distinct clinical manifestations, such as hypopigmented skin lesions and peripheral nerve involvement, in conjunction with a skin smear that tests positive for acid-fast bacilli (AFB).

Epidemiology and Pathogenesis

Understanding of the epidemiology and pathogenesis of leprosy is hampered by the inability to grow the organism in culture. In tropical countries, where the disease is most prevalent, it may be acquired from infected humans; however, infectivity is very low. Prolonged close contact and the host's immunologic status play important roles in infectivity.

Epidemiology

The primary reservoir for *M. leprae* is infected humans. The disease is transmitted person to person through inhalation or contact with infected skin. The more important mode of transmission appears to be inhalation of *M. leprae* discharged in the nasal secretions of an infected individual.

Pathogenesis

Although the host's immune response to *M. leprae* plays a key role in the control of infection, the immune response is also responsible for the damage to skin and nerves; in other words, leprosy is both a bacterial and an immunologic disease. After acquisition of *M. leprae,* the infection passes through many stages characterized by their histopathologic and clinical features. Although the infection has many intermediate stages, the two primary phases are a **silent phase,** during which the leprosy bacilli multiply in the skin in macrophages, and an **intermediate phase,** in which the bacilli multiply in peripheral nerves and begin to cause sensory impairment. More severe disease states may follow. A patient may recover spontaneously at any stage.

Spectrum of Disease

Based on the host's response, the spectrum of disease caused by *M. leprae* ranges from subclinical infection to intermediate stages of disease to full-blown and serious clinical manifestations involving the skin, upper respiratory system, testes, and peripheral nerves. The two major forms of the disease are a localized form, called **tuberculoid leprosy,** and a more disseminated form, called **lepromatous leprosy.** Patients with lepromatous leprosy are anergic to *M. leprae* because of a defect in their cell-mediated immunity. Because the organisms' growth is unimpeded, these individuals develop extensive skin lesions containing numerous AFB; the organisms can spill over into the blood and disseminate. In contrast, individuals with tuberculoid leprosy do not have an immune defect; the disease is localized to the skin and nerves. In tuberculoid leprosy, a few organisms may be observed in the skin lesions. Most of the serious sequelae associated with leprosy are the result of this organism's tropism for peripheral nerves.

TABLE 42.6	**Common Types of Infections Caused by Rapidly Growing Mycobacteria**
Organism	**Common Types of Infection**
Mycobacterium abscessus subsp. *abscessus* Mycobacterium abscessus subsp. *bolletii* Mycobacterium abscessus subsp. *massiliense*	Disseminated disease, primarily in immunocompromised individuals; skin and soft tissue infections; pulmonary infections; postoperative infections; health care–associated infections
Mycobacterium fortuitum	Postoperative infections in breast augmentation and median sternotomy; skin and soft tissue infections; pulmonary infections, usually single, localized lesions Central nervous system (CNS) disease is rare but has high morbidity and mortality
Mycobacterium chelonae	Skin and soft tissue infections, postoperative wound infections, keratitis
Less Common Types of Infection (More Than 10 Cases)	
Mycobacterium bacteremicum	Skin and soft tissue infections, postoperative wound infections
Mycobacterium franklinii	Sinopulmonary disease and extrapulmonary sites
Mycobacterium mageritense	Pulmonary disease, endocarditis, and disseminated infection
Mycobacterium peregrinum	Skin and soft tissue infections; bacteremia
Mycobacterium mucogenicum	Posttraumatic wound infections, catheter-related sepsis, health care–associated infections
Mycobacterium smegmatis	Skin or soft tissue infections; less frequently, pulmonary infections
Mycobacterium boenickei	Bone and joint infections
Mycobacterium canariasense	Bacteremia
Mycobacterium cosmeticum	Pulmonary and urosepsis
Mycobacterium goodii	Bone and joint infections, osteomyelitis
Mycobacterium houstonense	Bone and joint infections
Mycobacterium immunogenum	Hypersensitivity pneumonitis
Mycobacterium neoaurum (closely related to M. lacticola)	Catheter-related sepsis
Mycobacterium phocaicum	Catheter-related sepsis
Mycobacterium porcinum	Surgical site infection
Mycobacterium senegalense	Catheter-related sepsis
Rare Infections (Fewer Than 10 Cases)	
Mycobacterium aubagnense	Various opportunistic health care–associated infections
Mycobacterium brisbanense	Various opportunistic health care–associated infections
Mycobacterium brumae	Various opportunistic health care–associated infections
Mycobacterium celeriflavum	Various opportunistic health care–associated infections
Mycobacterium elephantis	Various opportunistic health care–associated infections
Mycobacterium iranicum	Various opportunistic health care-associated infections
Mycobacterium monacense	Various opportunistic health care–associated infections
Mycobacterium moriokaense	Various opportunistic health care–associated infections
Mycobacterium neworleansense	Various opportunistic health care–associated infections
Mycobacterium novocastrense	Various types of opportunistic health care–associated infections
Mycobacterium saopaulense	Cervical abscess and various opportunistic health care–associated infections
Mycobacterium septicum	Various opportunistic health care–associated infections
Mycobacterium setense	Bone and joint infections
Mycobacterium wolinskyi	Skin and soft tissue infections, bone infection, osteomyelitis

Laboratory Diagnosis of Mycobacterial Infections

Specimens received by the laboratory for mycobacterial smear and culture must be handled in a safe manner. Tuberculosis ranks high among laboratory-acquired infections; therefore laboratory and hospital administrators must provide laboratory personnel with the facilities, equipment, and supplies needed to reduce this risk to a minimum. *M. tuberculosis* has a very low infective dose for humans (i.e., an infection rate of approximately 50% with exposure to fewer than 10 AFB). All tuberculin-negative personnel should have a skin test or one of the IGRAs at least annually and more frequently if any laboratory incidents have been identified within the facility. The CDC recommends Biosafety Level 2 practices, containment equipment, and facilities for preparing acid-fast smears and culture for nonaerosolizing manipulations. If *M. tuberculosis* is grown and then propagated and manipulated, biologic safety cabinet (BSC) class II safety precautions are required; however, Biosafety Level 3 practices are recommended. BSC Level 3 practices are recommended for opening centrifuge vials, adding reagents to biochemical testing media, setting up molecular tests, and sonication, these practices include restricted laboratory access, negative-pressure airflow, and special personal protective equipment (e.g., certified respirators). Respiratory devices should be certified through the National Institute for Occupational Safety and Health (NIOSH). All work surfaces should be disinfected before and after working with specimen samples. Effective disinfectants for *Mycobacterium* spp. include Amphyl (Reckitt Benckiser North America, Wayne, NJ), 0.05% to 0.5% sodium hypochlorite, and phenol-soap mixtures.

Specimen Collection and Transport

AFB can infect almost any tissue or organ of the body. Successful isolation of these organisms depends on the quality of the specimen obtained and the use of appropriate processing and culture techniques by the mycobacteriology laboratory. In suspected mycobacterial disease, as in all other infectious diseases, the diagnostic procedure begins at the patient's bedside. Collection of proper clinical specimens requires careful attention to detail by health care professionals. Most specimens are respiratory samples such as sputum, tracheal or bronchial aspirates, and specimens obtained by bronchial alveolar lavage. Other samples may include urine, gastric aspirates, tissue (biopsy) specimens, cerebrospinal fluid (CSF), and pleural and pericardial fluid. Blood or fecal specimens may be collected from immunocompromised patients. Specimens should be collected in sterile, leakproof, disposable, and appropriately labeled containers without fixatives and placed in bags to contain leakage. If transport and processing will be delayed longer than 1 hour, all specimens except blood should be refrigerated at 4°C until processed.

Pulmonary Specimens

Pulmonary secretions may be obtained by any of the following methods: spontaneously produced or induced sputum, gastric lavage, transtracheal aspiration, bronchoscopy, and laryngeal swabbing. Most specimens submitted for examination are sputum, aerosol-induced sputum, bronchoscopic aspirations, or gastric lavage samples. Spontaneously produced sputum is the specimen of choice. To raise sputum, patients must be instructed to take a deep breath, hold it momentarily, and then cough deeply and vigorously. Patients must also be instructed to cover their mouths carefully while coughing and to discard tissues in an appropriate receptacle. Saliva and nasal secretions should not be collected, nor should the patient use oral antiseptics during the collection period. Sputum specimens must be free of food particles, residues, and other extraneous matter.

The aerosol (saline) induction procedure can best be used on ambulatory patients who are able to follow instructions. Aerosol-induced sputum specimens have been collected from children as young as 5 years of age. This procedure should be performed in an enclosed area with appropriate airflow. Operators should wear particulate respirators and take appropriate safety measures to prevent exposure. The patient is told that the procedure is being performed to induce coughing and thus to raise sputum that the patient cannot raise spontaneously and that the salt solution is irritating. The patient is instructed to inhale slowly and deeply through the mouth and to cough at will, vigorously and deeply, coughing and expectorating into a collection tube. The procedure is discontinued if the patient fails to raise sputum after 10 minutes or feels discomfort. Ten milliliters of sputum should be collected; if the patient continues to raise sputum, a second specimen should be collected and submitted. Specimens should be delivered to the laboratory promptly and refrigerated if processing is to be delayed.

Sputum collection guidelines recommend the collection of three specimens at least 8 hours apart. One of the three specimens should be an early morning sample. In many cases, the third specimen demonstrates minimal recovery of organisms, and this collection may not be recommended in some laboratories. Pooled specimens are unacceptable because of the increased risk of contamination.

Gastric Lavage Specimens

Gastric lavage is used to collect sputum from patients who may have swallowed sputum during the night. The procedure is limited to senile, nonambulatory patients; children younger than 12 years of age (specimen of choice); and patients who fail to produce sputum by aerosol induction. The most desirable gastric lavage is collected at the patient's bedside before the patient arises and before exertion empties the stomach. Gastric lavage cannot be performed as an office or clinic procedure.

The collector should wear a cap, gown, and particulate respirator mask and should stand beside (not in front of) the patient, who should sit up on the edge of the bed or in a chair if possible. The Levine collection tube is inserted through a nostril, and the patient is instructed to swallow the tube. When the tube has been fully inserted, a syringe is attached to the end of the tube and filtered distilled water is injected into the tube. The syringe is then used to withdraw 5 to 10 mL of gastric secretions, which is expelled slowly down the sides of the 50-mL conical collecting tube. Samples should be adjusted to a neutral pH. The laboratory may choose to provide sterile receptacles containing 100 mg of sodium carbonate to reduce the acidity; this improves the recovery of organisms. The top of the collection tube is screwed on tightly, and the tube is held upright during prompt delivery to the laboratory. Three specimens should be collected over a period of consecutive days. Specimens should be processed within 4 hours.

Bronchial lavages, washings, and brushings are collected and submitted by medical personnel. These are the specimens of choice for detecting NTM and other opportunistic pathogens in patients with immune dysfunction.

Urine Specimens

The incidence of urogenital infections shows little sign of decreasing. About 2% to 3% of patients with pulmonary tuberculosis show urinary tract involvement, but 30% to 40% of patients with genitourinary disease have tuberculosis at some other site. The clinical manifestations of urinary tuberculosis, which are variable, include frequency of urination (most common), dysuria, hematuria, and flank pain. Definitive diagnosis requires recovery of AFB from the urine.

Early morning voided urine specimens (40 mL minimum) in sterile containers should be submitted daily for at least 3 consecutive days. The collection procedure is the same as for collecting a clean-catch midstream urine specimen (Chapter 72). The 24-hour urine specimen is undesirable because of excessive dilution, higher contamination, and difficulty in concentrating. Catheterization should be used only if a midstream voided specimen cannot be collected.

Fecal Specimens

Acid-fast staining or culture (or both) of stool from patients with AIDS or from other immunocompromised patients has been used to identify patients who may be at risk for developing disseminated MAC disease. The clinical utility of this practice remains controversial; however, if screening stains or cultures are positive, dissemination often follows. Feces should be submitted in a clean, dry, wax-free container without preservative or diluent. Contamination with urine should be avoided.

Tissue and Body Fluid Specimens

Tuberculous meningitis is uncommon but occurs in both immunocompetent and immunosuppressed patients. A sufficient quantity of specimen is crucial for the isolation of AFB from CSF. Very few organisms may be present in the spinal fluid, which makes their detection difficult. At least 10 mL of CSF is recommended for the recovery of

mycobacteria. Similarly, as much as possible of other body fluids (5 to 10 mL minimum)—such as pleural, peritoneal, and pericardial fluids—should be collected in a sterile container or syringe with a Luer-tip cap. Tissues must not be immersed in saline or wrapped in gauze. Swabs are discouraged because the recovery of organisms is decreased. Two cultures should be set up so that one set may be incubated at 30°C for *Mycobacterium* spp. that grow at lower temperatures (*Mycobacterium haemophilum, M. marinum, M. terrae* complex, *M. lentiflavum,* and *M. ulcerans*).

Blood Specimens

Immunocompromised patients, particularly those infected with HIV, can have disseminated mycobacterial infections; most of these are caused by MAC. A blood culture positive for MAC is always associated with clinical evidence of disease. Recovery of mycobacteria is improved with blood collection in either a broth or the Isolator lysis-centrifugation system (Chapter 67). Some studies have indicated that the lysis-centrifugation system is advantageous because quantitative data can be obtained with each blood culture; in patients with AIDS, quantitation of such organisms can be used to monitor therapy and determine prognosis. However, the necessity of quantitative blood cultures remains unclear.

Blood for culture of mycobacteria should be collected as for routine blood cultures. Blood collected in regular phlebotomy procedures in anticoagulants such as sodium polyanethol sulfonate (SPS), heparin, and citrate may be used to inoculate cultures for the recovery of *Mycobacterium* spp. Conventional blood culture collection systems are unacceptable for the isolation of *Mycobacterium* spp. However, specialized automated systems and culture media are available for growth of *Mycobacterium* spp., including the Myco/F Lytic Bottles (Becton-Dickinson, Franklin Lakes, NJ) and the BacT/ALERT MB Blood medium (bioMérieux, Durham, NC).

Wounds, Skin Lesions, and Aspirates

An aspirate is the best type of specimen for culturing a skin lesion or wound. The skin should be cleansed with alcohol before aspiration of the material into a syringe. If the volume is insufficient for aspiration, pus and exudates may be obtained on a swab and then placed in a transport medium, such as Amie or Stuart medium (dry swabs are unacceptable). However, a negative culture of a specimen obtained on a swab is not considered reliable, and this should be noted in the culture report.

Specimen Processing

Processing to recover AFB from clinical specimens involves several complex steps, each of which must be carried out with precision. Body fluid specimens from sterile sites can be inoculated directly to media (small volume) or concentrated ($\geq$3000 *g* for 15 minutes) to reduce volume. Sterile tissue samples may be ground in sterile 0.85% saline or 0.2%

bovine albumin and inoculated directly to media. Other specimens require decontamination and concentration. A processing scheme is shown in Fig. 42.1, and the procedures are explored in detail in the following discussions.

Contaminated Specimens

Most specimens submitted for mycobacterial culture consist of organic debris, such as mucin, tissue, serum, and other proteinaceous material contaminated with organisms. A typical example of such a specimen is sputum. Laboratories must process these specimens to kill or reduce contaminating bacteria that can rapidly outgrow mycobacteria, and mycobacteria are released from mucin and/or cells. After decontamination, mycobacteria are concentrated, usually by centrifugation, to enhance their detection by acid-fast stain and culture. Unfortunately, there is no single ideal method for decontaminating and digesting clinical specimens. Although they are continuously faced with the inherent limitations of various methods, laboratories must strive to maximize the survival and detection of mycobacteria while maximizing the elimination of contaminating organisms. RGM are especially susceptible to high or prolonged exposure to 2% or more of sodium hydroxide (NaOH). Digestion-decontamination procedures should be as gentle as possible.

Inadequate Specimens and Rejection Criteria

The identification and detection of *Mycobacterium* spp. is costly and time consuming. It is essential that the laboratory have a detailed policy regarding the rejection of inadequate specimens for the identification of these organisms. Specimens should be rejected according to the following guidelines: (1) insufficient volume, (2) contamination with saliva, (3) dried swabs, (4) pooled sputum or urine, (5) container has been compromised or is broken or leaking, and (6) length of time from collection to processing is too long.

Overview

Commonly used digestion-decontamination methods are the NaOH method, the Zephiran-trisodium phosphate method, and the *N*-acetyl-L-cysteine (NALC)–2% NaOH method. The NALC-NaOH method is presented in detail in Evolve Procedure 42.1. Another decontaminating procedure that uses oxalic acid is very useful for treating specimens known to harbor gram-negative rods, particularly *Pseudomonas* and *Proteus* spp., which are extremely troublesome contaminants. It is important to note that oxalic acid, NaOH, and mild hydrogen chloride (HCl) may reduce the recovery of *M. ulcerans.*

NaOH, a commonly used decontaminant that is also mucolytic, should be used with caution. It not only reduces contamination but also reduces recovery of *Mycobacterium* spp. as alkalinity increases, temperature rises, and exposure time increases. The sample should be homogenized by centrifugal swirling, minimizing physical agitation. The container should then be allowed to sit for 15 minutes so that aerosolized droplets can fall to the bottom, thus reducing the risk of infection for the laboratory professional.

Several agents can be used to liquefy a clinical specimen, including NALC, dithiothreitol (Sputolysin), and enzymes. None of these agents are inhibitory to bacterial cells. In most procedures, liquefaction (release of the organisms from mucin or cells) is enhanced by vigorous mixing with a vortex-type mixer in a closed container. After mixing as previously described, the container should be allowed to stand for 15 minutes before opening so as to prevent the dispersion of fine aerosols generated during mixing. Of utmost importance during processing is strict adherence to processing and laboratory safety protocols. All these procedures should be carried out in a BSC.

After digestion and decontamination, specimens are concentrated by centrifugation at greater than or equal to 3000 *g*. See Evolve Procedure 42.2 for specimen preparation considerations.

Special Considerations

Many specimen types besides respiratory samples contain normal microbiota and require decontamination and concentration.

Aerosol-induced sputum should be treated as sputum. Gastric lavages should be processed within 4 hours of collection or neutralized with 10% sodium carbonate (check with pH paper to make sure the specimen is at neutral pH) and refrigerated until processed, as for sputum. If more than 10 mL of watery-appearing aspirate was obtained, the specimen can be centrifuged at 3600× *g* for 30 minutes, the supernatant decanted, and the sediment processed as for sputum.

Urine specimens should be divided into a maximum of four 50-mL centrifuge tubes and centrifuged at 3600× *g* for 30 minutes. The supernatant should be decanted, leaving approximately 2 mL of sediment in each tube. The tubes are vortexed to suspend the sediments, and sediments are combined. If necessary, distilled water can be added to a total volume of 10 mL. This urine concentrate is treated as for sputum or with the Sputolysin–oxalic acid method.

For fecal specimens, approximately 0.2 g of stool (a portion about the size of a pea) is emulsified in 11 mL of sterile filtered distilled water. The suspension is vortexed thoroughly, and particulate matter is allowed to settle for 15 minutes. Ten milliliters of the supernatant is then transferred to a 50-mL conical centrifuge tube and decontaminated using the oxalic acid or the NALC-NaOH method.

Swabs and wound aspirates should be transferred to a sterile 50-mL conical centrifuge tube containing a liquid medium (Middlebrook 7H9, Dubos Tween albumin broth) at a ratio of 1 part specimen to 5 to 10 parts liquid media. The specimen is vortexed vigorously and allowed to stand for 20 minutes. The swab is removed, and the resulting suspension is processed as for sputum.

Large pieces of tissue should be finely minced with a sterile scalpel and scissors. This material is homogenized in a sterile tissue grinder with a small amount of sterile saline (0.85%) or sterile 0.2% bovine albumin; the suspension is then processed as for sputum. If the tissue is not known to be sterile, it is homogenized and half is directly inoculated

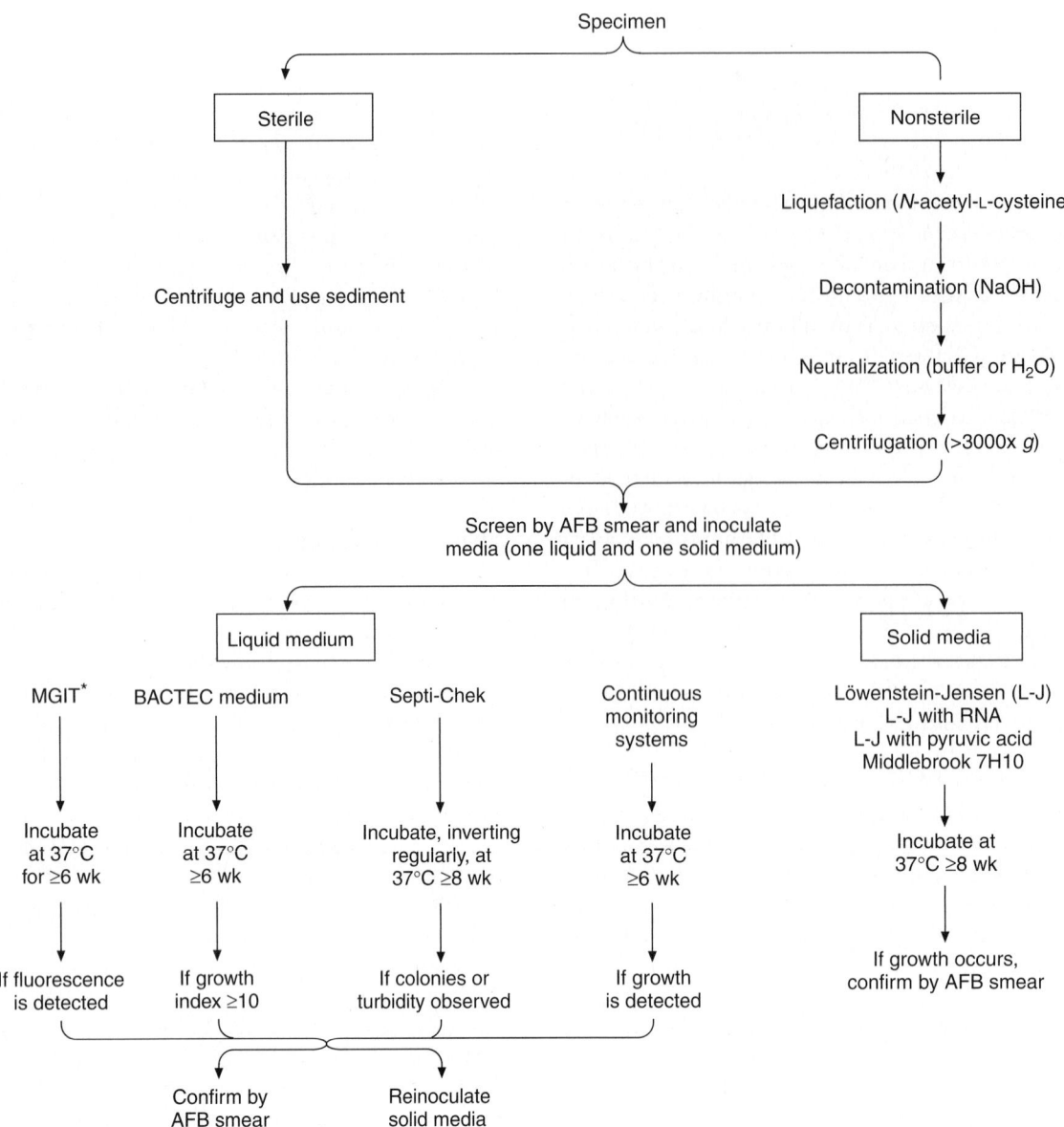

Specimen

Sterile → Centrifuge and use sediment

Nonsterile → Liquefaction (*N*-acetyl-ʟ-cysteine) → Decontamination (NaOH) → Neutralization (buffer or H$_2$O) → Centrifugation (>3000x *g*)

Screen by AFB smear and inoculate media (one liquid and one solid medium)

Liquid medium

MGIT* → Incubate at 37°C for ≥6 wk → If fluorescence is detected

BACTEC medium → Incubate at 37°C ≥6 wk → If growth index ≥10

Septi-Chek → Incubate, inverting regularly, at 37°C ≥8 wk → If colonies or turbidity observed

Continuous monitoring systems → Incubate at 37°C ≥6 wk → If growth is detected

Confirm by AFB smear

Reinoculate solid media

Solid media

Löwenstein-Jensen (L-J)
L-J with RNA
L-J with pyruvic acid
Middlebrook 7H10
→ Incubate at 37°C ≥8 wk → If growth occurs, confirm by AFB smear

*Mycobacterium Growth Indicator Tube.

• **Fig. 42.1** Flowchart for specimen processing to isolate mycobacteria. *AFB,* Acid-fast bacilli.

to solid and liquid media. The other half is processed as for sputum. If the tissue is collected aseptically (i.e., it is sterile), it may be processed without being treated with NALC-NaOH.

Specimens Not Requiring Decontamination

Tissues or body fluids collected aseptically usually do not require the digestion and decontamination methods used with contaminated specimens. The processing of clinical specimens that do not routinely require decontamination for acid-fast culture is described here. If such a specimen appears contaminated because of color, cloudiness, or foul odor, Gram staining is performed to detect bacteria other than AFB. Specimens found to be contaminated should be processed as described in the preceding section.

CSF should be handled aseptically and centrifuged for 30 minutes at 3600× *g* to concentrate the bacteria. The supernatant is decanted and the sediment is vortexed thoroughly before the smear is prepared and the media inoculated. If an insufficient quantity of CSF is received, the specimen should be used directly for smear and culture. Recovery of AFB from CSF is difficult; additional solid or liquid media should be inoculated if material is available.

Pleural fluid should be collected in sterile anticoagulant (1 mg/mL ethylenediaminetetraacetic acid [EDTA] or 0.1 mg/mL heparin). If the fluid becomes clotted, it should be liquefied with an equal volume of Sputolysin and vigorously mixed. To lower the specific gravity and density of pleural fluid, 20 mL is transferred to a sterile 50-mL centrifuge tube and the specimen is diluted by filling the tube with distilled water. The tube is inverted several times to mix the suspension and then centrifuged at 3600× *g* for 30 minutes. The supernatant should be removed and the sediment suspended for smear and culture.

Joint fluid and other sterile exudates can be handled aseptically and inoculated directly to media. Bone marrow aspirates may be injected into Pediatric Isolator tubes (Alere, Waltham, MA), which help to prevent clotting; the specimen can be removed with a needle and syringe for the preparation of smears and cultures. As an alternative, these specimens can either be inoculated directly to media or, if clotted, treated with Sputolysin or glass beads and distilled water before concentration.

Direct Detection Methods

Microscopy

Microscopy is considered a reasonably sensitive and rapid procedure for the presumptive identification of *Mycobacterium* spp. in clinical specimens. The preferred specimens are pretreated and/or concentrated before microscopy.

Acid-Fast Stains

The cell walls of mycobacteria contain long-chain multiple cross-linked fatty acids called **mycolic acids**. These contribute to the characteristic of acid-fastness that distinguishes mycobacteria from other bacteria. Mycobacteria are not the only group with this unique feature. Species of *Nocardia* and *Rhodococcus* are also partially acid fast; *Legionella micdadei*, a causative agent in pneumonia, is partially acid fast in tissue. Cysts of the genera *Cryptosporidium* and *Isospora* are distinctly acid fast. The mycolic acids and lipids in the mycobacterial cell wall account for the unusual resistance of these organisms to the effects of drying and harsh decontaminating agents in addition to the property of acid fastness.

When Gram stained, mycobacteria usually appear as slender, poorly stained and beaded gram-positive bacilli (Fig. 42.2); sometimes they appear as "gram neutral" or "gram ghosts" by failing to take up either crystal violet or safranin. Acid fastness is affected by the age of colonies, the medium on which growth occurs, and exposure to ultraviolet light. Rapidly growing species appear to be acid-fast variable.

Three types of staining procedures are used in the laboratory for the rapid detection and confirmation of AFB: fluorochrome, Ziehl-Neelsen, and Kinyoun. Smears for all methods are prepared in the same way. A modified Ziehl-Neelsen stain has improved the detection of organisms in CSF and of intracellular organisms in WBCs.

Visualization of AFB in sputum or other clinical material should be considered presumptive evidence of tuberculosis because staining does not specifically identify *M. tuberculosis*. The report form should indicate this. For example, *M. gordonae,* a nonpathogenic scotochromogen commonly found in tap water, has been identified when tap water or deionized water has been used in the preparation of smears or even when patients have rinsed their mouths with tap water before using an aerosolized saline solution to induce

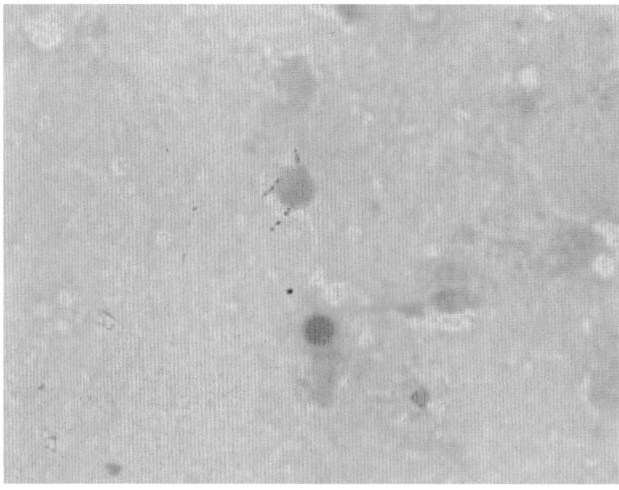

• **Fig. 42.2** Gram staining of *Mycobacterium marinum* demonstrates a beaded appearance. (Courtesy Stacie Lansink, Sioux Falls, SD.)

sputum. However, the incidence of false-positive smears is very low when good quality control is maintained. Conversely, acid fast–stained smears of clinical specimens require at least 10^4 AFB per milliliter for detection from concentrated specimens.

AFB direct detection is less expensive than nucleic acid detection (NAAT) methods and can enhance the NAAT interpretations. AFB microscopy remains useful in determining infectiousness, monitoring treatment, and arriving at decisions on when to release patients from respiratory isolation.

Methods

Fluorochrome Stain. Fluorochrome staining is the screening procedure recommended for laboratories that have a fluorescent (ultraviolet) microscope (Evolve Procedure 42.3). Fluorochrome stain is more sensitive than the conventional carbolfuchsin stains because the fluorescent bacilli stand out brightly against the background (Fig. 42.3). Because the smear can be examined initially at lower magnifications (250–400×), more fields can be visualized in a short period. In addition, a positive fluorescent smear may be restained using the conventional Ziehl-Neelsen or Kinyoun procedure, thereby saving the time needed to make a fresh smear. Screening of specimens with rhodamine or rhodamine-auramine B results in a higher yield of positive smears and substantially reduces the time needed to examine smears.

One drawback of the fluorochrome stains is that many rapid growers may not appear fluorescent with these reagents. All positive fluorescent smears should be confirmed with a Ziehl-Neelsen stain or by having them examined by another laboratory professional. It is important to wipe the immersion oil from the objective lens after examining a positive smear because stained bacilli can float off the slide into the oil, possibly contributing to a false-positive reading for the next smear examined.

Fuchsin Acid-Fast Stains. The classic carbolfuchsin stain (Ziehl-Neelsen) requires heating of the slide for

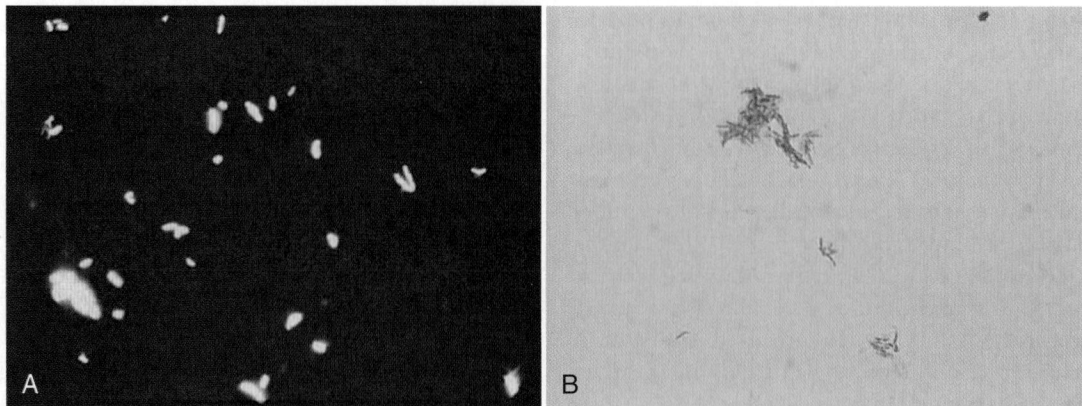

• **Fig. 42.3** *Mycobacterium tuberculosis* stained with (A) fluorochrome stain (×400) and (B) Kinyoun acid-fast stain (×1000).

better penetration of the stain into the mycobacterial cell wall; hence it is also known as the **hot stain procedure** (Evolve Procedure 6.3). With Ziehl-Neelsen staining, *Mycobacterium* spp. appear red or have a red-blue beaded appearance, whereas nonmycobacteria appear blue.

Evolve Procedure 6.4), describes the Kinyoun acid-fast stain. The method is similar to Ziehl-Neelsen staining but no heat is used (Fig. 42.3); this is known as the **cold stain procedure.** If present, typical AFB appear as purple to red, slightly curved, short or long rods (2 to 8 μm); they also may appear beaded or banded *(Mycobacterium kansasii)*. For some nontuberculous species, such as MAC, they appear pleomorphic and usually coccoid.

Examination, Interpretation, and Reporting of Smears

Before a smear is reported as negative, it should be examined carefully by scanning at least 300 oil immersion fields (magnification 1000×), equivalent to three full horizontal sweeps of a smear that is 2 cm long and 1 cm wide. Because the fluorescent stain can be examined using a lower magnification (250 or 450×) than that required for a fuchsin-stained smear, the equivalent number of fields (30) can be examined in less time, which makes the fluorochrome stain the preferred method.

When acid-fast organisms are observed on a smear, the report should include information about the type of staining method used and the quantity of organisms. The recommended interpretations and ways to report smear results are shown in Table 42.7.

The overall sensitivity of an acid-fast smear ranges from 20% to 80%. Factors such as specimen type, staining method, and culture method can influence the sensitivity of an acid-fast smear. In general, the specificity of an acid-fast smear examination is very high. However, cross-contamination of slides during the staining process and use of water contaminated with saprophytic mycobacteria can lead to false-positive results. Staining receptacles should not be used; AFB can also be transferred from one slide to another in immersion oil. For these reasons, the best course is to confirm a positive result.

Although not without some limitations because of its simplicity and speed, the stained smear is an important and useful test, particularly for the detection of smear-positive patients ("infectious reservoirs"), who pose the greatest risk to others in their environment.

Antigen-Protein Detection

The detection of microbial products or components has been used in recent years to diagnose infections caused by *M. tuberculosis*. For example, **lipoarabinomannan (LAM),** which is a major cell-wall component in *M. tuberculosis,* has been developed into an ELISA (Clearview TB ELISA, Alere Inc., Waltham, MA) and a point-of-care lateral flow assay (Determine TB; Alere). A point-of-care urine lipoarabinomannan assay has been successfully used to diagnose intrathoracic tuberculosis (ITTB) and latent tuberculosis. The test is approximately 73% to 76% sensitive but demonstrates a high specificity of approximately 93%.

Immunodiagnostic Testing

As previously discussed, interferon-gamma release assays have become more widely used for the diagnosis of tuberculosis. The available test systems, T-SPOT-TB (Oxford Immunotec, Oxford, UK and QuantiFERON Gold TB Plus (QFT-Plus; Qiagen, Germantown, MD), do not typically cross react with nontuberculous mycobacterium, are not affected by the BCG vaccine, and are not as variable as the historical serologic tuberculin skin tests. The T-SPOT-TB assay is an enzyme-linked immunospot assay that requires isolation and incubation of PBMCs. It takes approximately 2 days and is technically complicated. The QuantiFERON assay measure IFN-gamma by an ELISA. The QFT-Plus assay measures the stimulation of T-cell interferon-gamma in whole blood in a tube precoated with *M. tuberculosis* antigens. It yields results in approximately 8 hours. Neither assay distinguishes between latent and active infections, nor can they predict the likelihood that a patient will progress to active disease. In addition, specificity and sensitivity vary in the population tested, including immunocompromised patients and children. Variation is associated

TABLE 42.7 Acid-Fast Smear Reporting

Number of AFB Seen, Fuchsin Stain (1000× Magnification)	Number of AFB Seen, Fluorochrome Stain (450× Magnification)	Number of AFB Seen, Fluorochrome Stain (250× Magnification)	Report
0	0	0	No AFB seen
1–2/300 fields	1–2/70 fields	1–2/30 fields	Indeterminate; request another specimen for repeat testing
1–9/100 fields	2–18/50 fields	1–9/10 fields	1 +
1–9/10 fields	4–36/10 fields	1–9/field	2 +
1–9/field	4–36/field	10–90/field	3 +
> 9/field	>36/field	>90/field	4 +

AFB, Acid-fast bacilli.
Modified from Kent PT, Kubica GP. *Public Health Mycobacteriology: A Guide for the Level III Laboratory,* Washington, DC: Centers for Disease Control and Prevention; 1985; Carroll KC, Pfaller MA. *Manual of Clinical Microbiology.* 12th ed. Washington, DC: ASM Press; 2019.

with the patient's CD4 cell count; therefore, interpretations and results should be evaluated with caution.

Nucleic Acid Detection

Nucleic acid probes for the indirect detection and identification of *M. tuberculosis* complex and the *M. avium* complex from culture media are available (AccuProbe, Hologic, San Diego, CA). This technique can detect *M. avium, M. intracellulare, M. tuberculosis, M. africanum, M. microti, M. pinnipedii,* and *M. canettii,* but it cannot differentiate them at the species level. The assay also lacks enough sensitivity to be used for direct detection of the organisms in clinical samples.

Genetic Sequencing and Nucleic Acid Amplification

PCR-based sequencing for mycobacterial identification consists of PCR amplification of mycobacterial DNA with genus-specific primers and sequencing of the amplicons. The organism is identified by comparison of the nucleotide sequence with reference sequences. The most reliable sequence for identification of mycobacteria to the genus level is the approximately 1500 bp 16S ribosomal ribonucleic acid (rRNA) gene. However, only a 600-bp sequence at the 5′ end is required for identification. The sequence homogeneity in the *M. tuberculosis* complex prevents the use of this sequence to differentiate these species. This region contains both conserved and variable regions, which makes it an ideal target for identification purposes.

Despite the accuracy of PCR-based sequencing to identify mycobacteria, problems remain: the sequences in some databases are not accurate, no present consensus exists as to the quantitative definition of a genus or species based on 16S rRNA gene sequence data, and procedures are not standardized. In addition, the 16S rRNA 5′ region contains two hypervariable regions, A and B. The A region provides the signature sequences for species identification. However,

M. chelonae and *M. abscessus* both require additional sequencing, because the A and B regions are identical and the 3′ end of the 16S rRNA contains a 4-bp sequence difference.

Several other genes have also been used to identify mycobacterial species, including the 23S rRNA, ITS 1, *hsp65, rpoB,* and *gyrB* gene. The 23S rRNA sequence is 3100 bp in length, which limits accurate sequencing. ITS 1 is a spacer sequence located between the 16S and 23S rRNA genes. This sequence, which is 200 to 330 bp, is more easily analyzed. The limitation of this sequence is that it is not a genus-specific sequence; therefore results may be affected by contaminating bacteria. The 65-kDa heat shock protein, also referred to as the *groEL2* gene, is a 440-bp fragment that can be amplified and analyzed with restriction digestion followed by agarose electrophoresis. The *hsp65* is highly conserved but contains a greater variation in polymorphisms than the 16S rRNA, particularly in a 441-bp region referred to as the "Telanti fragment." This allows for the differentiation of *Mycobacterium* spp. based on the variation in restriction fragment length polymorphisms (RFLPs). Repetitive sequence–based PCR, Diversilab (bioMérieux, Durham, NC), demonstrates better species discrimination than RFLP.

Line probe assays (DNA strip assays) involve PCR amplification coupled with a reverse hybridization step. The target sequence is amplified using biotinylated primers. The amplicon is then hybridized to membrane-immobilized sequence-specific probes for each species. The membrane is developed using an enzyme-mediated reaction and color indicator to analyze the banding pattern. Banding patterns are species-specific based on the immobilized probe map on the membrane. A commercially available system in which the 16S-to-23S rRNA spacer region of mycobacterial species (INNO-LiPA v2 Mycobacteria; Innogenetics, Ghent, Belgium) has been successfully used to directly detect and identify several of the most clinically relevant mycobacterial species in aliquots of positive liquid culture. The assay can be used to identify the MTBC and 13 NTM species. However, the results should be interpreted cautiously because some cross-reactivity has occurred with closely related species.

Another commercial system, GenoType Mycobacterium (Hain Lifescience GmbH, Nehren, Germany), which uses a similar format, has additional probes for *M. celatum, Mycobacterium malmoense, Mycobacterium peregrinum, M. phlei,* and two subgroups of *M. fortuitum,* in addition to a supplemental kit that allows for the identification of 16 additional mycobacterial species.

The *rpoB* gene encodes the beta-subunit in the organism's RNA polymerase. Mutations in this gene confer rifampin resistance in *M. tuberculosis.* Different regions in this gene have been used to identify rapid-growing isolates, but little data are available for the slow-growing species. Finally, the *gyrB* gene encodes the beta-subunit in the organism's topoisomerase II. Several single nucleotide polymorphisms have been identified in this gene that are useful in distinguishing species in the *M. tuberculosis* complex. After amplification, identification and differentiation of species require restriction analysis and gel electrophoresis.

Additional molecular techniques, such as conventional and real-time PCR, have been used to detect *M. tuberculosis* directly in clinical specimens. The Xpert MTB/RIF (Cepheid, Sunnyvale, CA) is a real-time PCR, cartridge-based molecular beacon probe assay that also detects the mutations associated with rifampin resistance. The assay can detect the presence or absence of mutations and is unable to recognize silent mutations resulting in incorrect interpretations as rifampin resistance. The CDC recommends follow-up confirmation should be completed using sequencing technology. The Xpert MTB/Rif Ultra (Cepheid, Sunnyvale, CA), is capable of detecting some of the mutations that would previously go undetected. The Xpert MTB/RIF assay is approved on both smear-positive and smear-negative respiratory specimens only.

The Amplified *M. tuberculosis* Direct Test (AMTD; Gen-Probe Hologic, San Diego CA) uses rRNA released from the mycobacteria by means of a lysing agent, sonication, and heat. The specific DNA probe is allowed to react with the extracted rRNA to form a stable DNA-RNA hybrid. Any nonhybridized DNA acridinium ester probes are chemically degraded. When an alkaline hydrogen peroxide solution is added to activate the chemiluminescence, only the hybrid bound acridinium ester emits light. The amount of light emitted is directly proportional to the amount of hybridized probe. The light is measured using a chemiluminometer.

As previously indicated, the commercially available tests are limited in the number of species they can identify. Some clinical laboratories have developed their own PCR assays to detect *M. tuberculosis* directly in clinical specimens.

Due to the limitation associated with amplified probe assays, sequencing-based methods—including traditional Sanger sequencing, pyrosequencing, next-generation sequencing and whole genome sequencing—are being used to resolve discrepancies associated with detecting drug resistance in *Mycobacterium* spp. In addition, genome sequencing is important for epidemiologic students to resolve the transmission of clustered patients and identify false-positive cultures that cause patients to undergo unnecessary treatment. Genotyping and sequencing are essential for tuberculosis control programs. The CDC has established a national tuberculosis genotyping system and a National TB Molecular Surveillance Center that performs whole genome sequencing on all newly diagnosed patients in the United States. Details and updates are available at https://www.cdc.gov/tb/topic/laboratory/default.htm.

DNA Microarrays

DNA microarrays are also attractive for rapid examination of large numbers of DNA sequences by a single hybridization step. This approach has been used to simultaneously identify mycobacterial species and detect mutations that confer rifampin resistance in mycobacteria. Fluorescent-labeled PCR amplicons generated from bacterial colonies are hybridized to a DNA array containing nucleotide probes. The bound amplicons emit a fluorescent signal that is detected with a scanner. With this approach, 82 unique 16S rRNA sequences allow for the differentiation of 54 mycobacterial species and 51 sequences that contain unique *rpoB* gene mutations (rifampin resistance).

Matrix-Assisted Laser Desorption Ionization Time-of-Flight Mass Spectrometry

The current approaches for early identification of *Mycobacterium* spp. in culture include PCR and traditional phenotypic identification schemes. MALDI-TOF MS uses a proteomic-based technique to identify clinical mycobacterial isolates by protein profiling and can be used for accurate and rapid identification of various microorganisms. (See Chapter 7 for more information on MALDI-TOF MS.) Isolates of *M. tuberculosis* are consistently identified using MALDI-TOF MS; however, discrimination of the other species included in the *M. tuberculosis* complex is limited. Correct identification of clinically relevant strains of tuberculoid and NTM species has also been demonstrated; however, the capacity to identify all the species is limited to the information available in the current databases. In addition, identification is limited based on successful cultivation *in vitro.* Moderate growth in culture is required from a specimen to have sufficient sample size for the application to MALDI-TOF MS, whereas sequencing techniques require minimal or scant growth.

The application of MALDI-TOF MS to the identification of mycobacterial species requires an extraction process prior to placing the organism on the target plate. This involves chemical and physical disruption of the mycobacterial cell wall. See Fig. 42.4 for the processing of mycobacterial species and extraction required for identification using MALDI-TOF MS. Extraction should be completed in a BSL-3 or BSL-2 using BSL-3 practices.

Cultivation

A combination of different culture media is required to optimize recovery of mycobacteria from culture; at least one solid

Liquid sample processing method by protein extraction and inactivation for mycobacteria

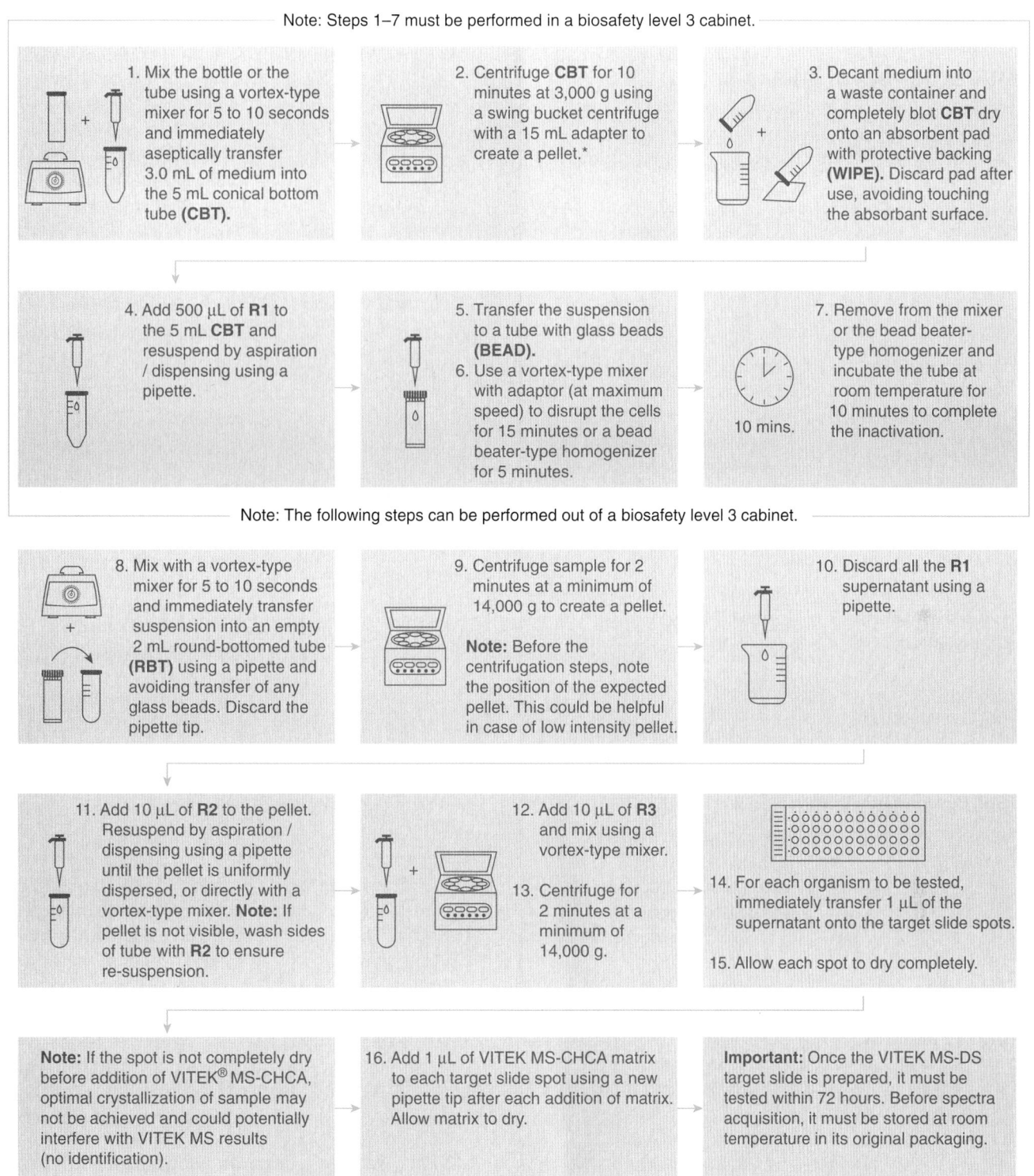

Note: Steps 1–7 must be performed in a biosafety level 3 cabinet.

1. Mix the bottle or the tube using a vortex-type mixer for 5 to 10 seconds and immediately aseptically transfer 3.0 mL of medium into the 5 mL conical bottom tube (CBT).

2. Centrifuge CBT for 10 minutes at 3,000 g using a swing bucket centrifuge with a 15 mL adapter to create a pellet.*

3. Decant medium into a waste container and completely blot CBT dry onto an absorbent pad with protective backing (WIPE). Discard pad after use, avoiding touching the absorbant surface.

4. Add 500 µL of R1 to the 5 mL CBT and resuspend by aspiration / dispensing using a pipette.

5. Transfer the suspension to a tube with glass beads (BEAD).
6. Use a vortex-type mixer with adaptor (at maximum speed) to disrupt the cells for 15 minutes or a bead beater-type homogenizer for 5 minutes.

10 mins.

7. Remove from the mixer or the bead beater-type homogenizer and incubate the tube at room temperature for 10 minutes to complete the inactivation.

Note: The following steps can be performed out of a biosafety level 3 cabinet.

8. Mix with a vortex-type mixer for 5 to 10 seconds and immediately transfer suspension into an empty 2 mL round-bottomed tube (RBT) using a pipette and avoiding transfer of any glass beads. Discard the pipette tip.

9. Centrifuge sample for 2 minutes at a minimum of 14,000 g to create a pellet.

Note: Before the centrifugation steps, note the position of the expected pellet. This could be helpful in case of low intensity pellet.

10. Discard all the R1 supernatant using a pipette.

11. Add 10 µL of R2 to the pellet. Resuspend by aspiration / dispensing using a pipette until the pellet is uniformly dispersed, or directly with a vortex-type mixer. Note: If pellet is not visible, wash sides of tube with R2 to ensure re-suspension.

12. Add 10 µL of R3 and mix using a vortex-type mixer.

13. Centrifuge for 2 minutes at a minimum of 14,000 g.

14. For each organism to be tested, immediately transfer 1 µL of the supernatant onto the target slide spots.

15. Allow each spot to dry completely.

Note: If the spot is not completely dry before addition of VITEK® MS-CHCA, optimal crystallization of sample may not be achieved and could potentially interfere with VITEK MS results (no identification).

16. Add 1 µL of VITEK MS-CHCA matrix to each target slide spot using a new pipette tip after each addition of matrix. Allow matrix to dry.

Important: Once the VITEK MS-DS target slide is prepared, it must be tested within 72 hours. Before spectra acquisition, it must be stored at room temperature in its original packaging.

• Fig. 42.4 Matrix-assisted desorption ionization time-of-flight workflow for extraction and processing *Mycobacterium* isolates. (Courtesy Biomerieux Inc., Durham, NC.)

medium in addition to a liquid medium should be used. The ideal media combination should be economical and should support the most rapid and abundant growth of mycobacteria, allow for the study of colony morphology and pigment production, and inhibit the growth of contaminants.

Solid Media

Solid media, such as those listed in Box 42.1, are recommended because of the development of characteristic reproducible colonial morphology, good growth from small inocula, and a low rate of contamination. Optimally, at

---

• BOX 42.1 **Suggested Media for Cultivation of Mycobacteria From Clinical Specimens[a]**

Media	Comments	Media	Comments
Solid		Petragnani medium	Contains twice the concentration of malachite than Löwenstein-Jensen green (an inhibitor of contaminating organisms); improves recovery from heavily contaminated specimens
Agar Based—Growth Within 10–12 Days			
Middlebrook	Contains 2% glycerol, which enhances the growth of *Mycobacterium avium* complex (MAC)		
Middlebrook 7H10	Supplemented with carbenicillin (for inhibition of pseudomonads), polymyxin B, trimethoprim lactate, and amphotericin B	Heme-supplemented media (egg or agar based)	Supplemented with hemin, hemoglobin, or ferric ammonium citrate; increases recovery of *Mycobacterium haemophilum*
Middlebrook 7H10 selective			
Middlebrook 7H11	Contains 0.1% enzymatic hydrolysate of casein, which improves recovery of isoniazid-resistant *Mycobacterium tuberculosis*	**Liquid[b]**	
Middlebrook 7H11 selective		BACTEC 12B medium	Used in the MGIT960 system; PANTA is added before incubation; ^{14}C-labeled palmitic acid is metabolized to produce $^{14}CO_2$, which is detected by the instrument
Middlebrook 7H11	Supplemented with mycobactin J, which provides for growth of *Mycobacterium genavense*		
Middlebrook 7H11 thin pour plates, 10 × 90 mm (Remel, Lenexa, KS)	Enhances visibility of colonies within 11 days	Middlebrook 7H9 broth	
		Dubos Tween albumin	
		Septi-Chek AFB	20 mL of Middlebrook 7H9 broth is incubated in 20% CO_2; solid phase contains three media: modified L-J, Middlebrook 7H11, and a chocolate agar slab
Middlebrook biplate (7H10/7H11S agar)			
Egg Based—Growth Within 18–24 Days		**Media Used in Commercially Supplied Growth and Semiautomated or Fully Automated Systems**	
Löwenstein-Jensen (L-J)	Commonly used medium; good recovery of *M. tuberculosis* but poor recovery of many other species; *M. genavense* fails to grow	Mycobacteria Growth Indicator Tube [MGIT] (Becton Dickinson Microbiology Systems, Cockeysville, MD)	MGIT 960 (fully automated system); MGIT is a modified Middlebrook 7H9 broth that incorporates a fluorescence-quenching–based oxygen sensor for detection
L-J Gruft	Supplemented with penicillin and nalidixic acid		
L-J Mycobactosel	Supplemented with cycloheximide, lincomycin, and nalidixic acid	Versa TREK Culture System (Trek Diagnostic Systems, Cleveland, OH)	Modified Middlebrook 7H9 broth
L-J with pyruvic acid	Enhances recovery of *Mycobacterium bovis*		
L-J with glycerol	Enhances recovery of *Mycobacterium ulcerans*	MB/BacT Alert 3D (bioMérieux, Durham, NC)	Uses Middlebrook 7H9 broth

[a]For optimal recovery of mycobacteria, a minimum combination of liquid medium and solid media is recommended.
[b]Tween 80 added to liquid media acts as a surfactant, breaking up clumps of organisms and increasing recovery rates.

---

least two solid media (a serum [albumin] agar base medium, [e.g., Middlebrook 7H10] and an egg-potato base medium [e.g., Löwenstein-Jensen, or L-J]) should be used for each specimen (these media are available from commercial sources). All specimens must be processed appropriately before inoculation. It is imperative to inoculate test organisms to commercially available products for quality control (Evolve Procedure 42.4). An example of interpreting

> ● BOX 42.2 **Example of Interpreting Quality Control Test Results of Decontamination and Concentration Procedure**

	SPUTUM SPECIMEN						
	Unprocessed Quantification of Growth			Processed Quantification of Growth			
Sputum Sample	10^4	10^3	10^2	10^4	10^3	10^2	Interpretation
1	3+	2+	50–100 colonies	2+	1+ or 2+	Approximately 10 colonies	Media and decontamination procedures acceptable
2	3+	2+	50–100 colonies	1+	0	0	Media acceptable; procedures too toxic
3	2+ or 1+	2+ or 1+	0	1+ or 0	1+ or 0	0	One or more of the media are not supporting growth of acid-fast bacilli (AFB) adequately

0, No growth; *1+*, scanty, barely discernible countable colonies; *2+*, dense, discrete growth, not countable; *3+*, confluent, abundant growth

quality-control test results of decontamination and concentration procedures associated with culture is provided in Box 42.2.

Cultures are incubated at 35°C in the dark in an atmosphere of 5% to 10% carbon dioxide (CO_2) and high humidity. Tube media are incubated in a slanted position with screw caps loose for at least 1 week to allow for the evaporation of excess fluid and the entry of CO_2; plated media are either placed in a CO_2-permeable plastic bag or wrapped with CO_2-permeable tape. If specimens obtained from the skin or superficial lesions are suspected to contain *M. marinum* or *M. ulcerans,* an additional set of solid media should be inoculated and incubated at 25°C to 30°C. In addition, a chocolate agar plate (or placement of an X-factor [hemin] disk on conventional media) and incubation at 25°C to 33°C is needed for recovery of *M. haemophilum* from these specimens. RGM optimally require incubation at 28°C to 30°C.

Cultures are examined weekly for growth. Contaminated cultures are discarded and reported as "contaminated, unable to detect presence of mycobacteria"; additional specimens are also requested. If available, sediment may be recultured after enhanced decontamination or by inoculating the sediment to a more selective medium. Most isolates appear between 3 and 6 weeks; a few isolates appear after 7 or 8 weeks of incubation. When growth appears, the rates of growth, pigmentation, and colonial morphology are recorded. The typical colonial appearance of *M. tuberculosis* and other mycobacteria is shown in Fig. 42.5. After 8 weeks of incubation, negative cultures (those showing no growth) are reported, and the cultures are discarded.

Liquid Media

In general, use of a liquid media system reduces the turnaround time for the isolation of AFB to approximately 10 days, compared with 17 days or longer for conventional solid media. Several different systems are available for culturing and detecting the growth of mycobacteria in liquid media. Growth of mycobacteria in liquid media, regardless of the type, requires 5% to 10% CO_2; CO_2 is either already provided in the culture vials or is added according to the manufacturer's instructions. When growth is detected in a liquid medium, acid-fast staining of a culture aliquot is performed to confirm the presence of AFB, and the material is subcultured to solid agar. Gram staining can also be performed if contamination is suspected.

Interpretation

Although isolation of MAC organisms indicates infection, the clinician must determine the clinical significance of isolating NTM in most cases; in other words, does the organism represent mere colonization or significant infection? Because these organisms vary greatly in their pathogenic potential, can colonize an individual without causing infection, and are ubiquitous in the environment, interpretation of a positive NTM culture is complicated; therefore the American Thoracic Society has recommended diagnostic criteria for NTM disease to help physicians interpret culture results.

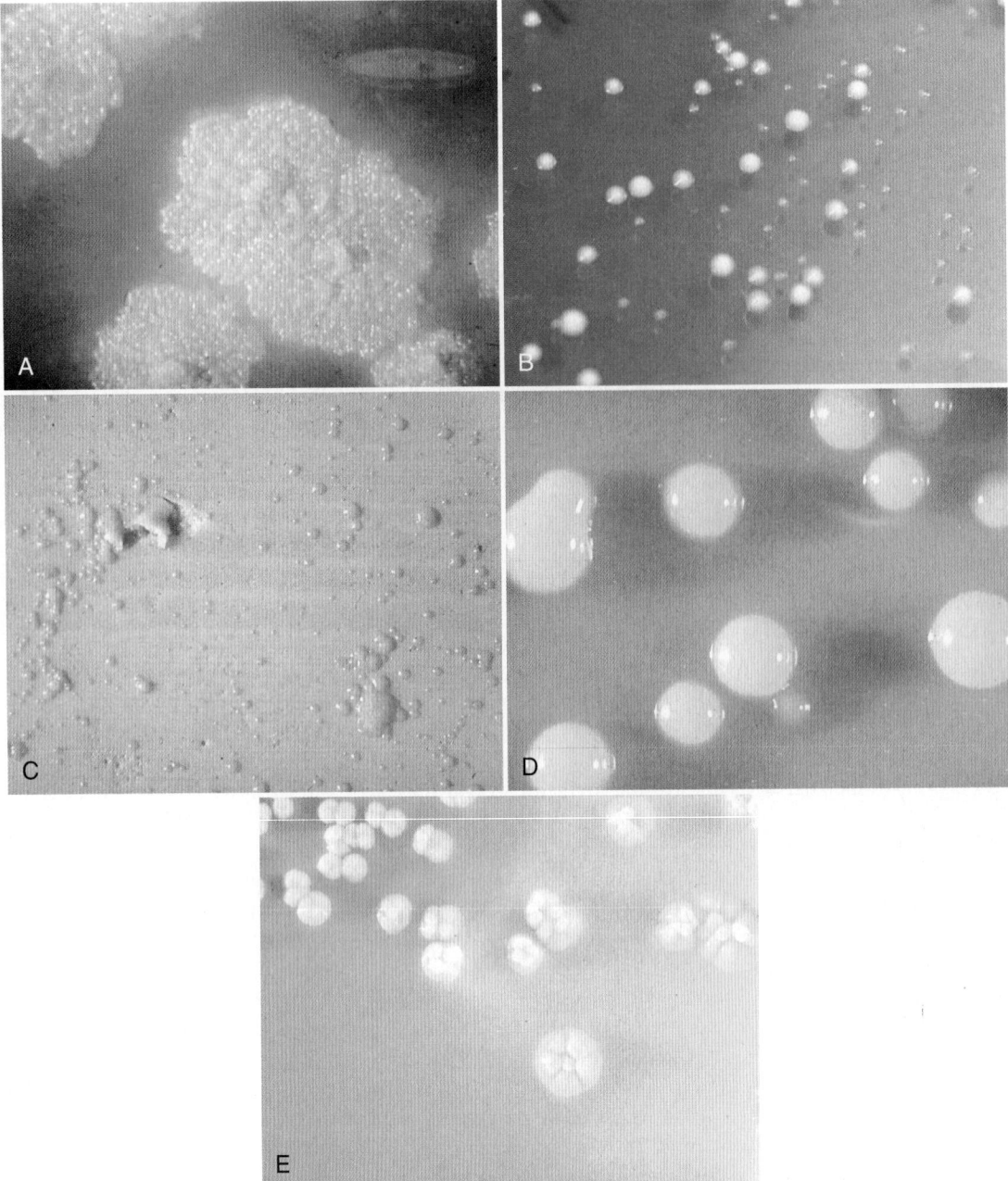

• **Fig. 42.5** Typical appearance of some mycobacteria on solid agar media. (A) *Mycobacterium tuberculosis* colonies on Löwenstein-Jensen agar after 8 weeks of incubation. (B) A different colonial morphology is seen on culture of one strain of *Mycobacterium avium* complex. (C) *Mycobacterium kansasii* colonies exposed to light. (D) Scotochromogen *Mycobacterium gordonae* showing yellow colonies. (E) Smooth, multilobate colonies of *Mycobacterium fortuitum* on Löwenstein-Jensen medium.

Approach to Identification

Regardless of the identification methods used, the first test always performed on organisms growing on solid or liquid mycobacterial media is acid-fast staining to confirm that the organisms are indeed mycobacteria. Identification of species other than MAC and the more commonly isolated NTM (MAC, *M. avium, M. intracellulare, M. gordonae,* and *M. kansasii*) has become challenging for routine clinical microbiology laboratories, particularly considering the ever-increasing number of new mycobacterial species.

Traditional methods (i.e., phenotypic methods) for identifying mycobacteria, particularly the NTM, are based on growth parameters, biochemical characteristics, and analysis of cell wall lipids, all of which are slow, cumbersome, and often inconclusive procedures. Over the past decade, the rate of non–AIDS-associated infections have been increasing, and many of the newly identified NTM species have been associated with various diseases. As a result, identification of species is vital to selecting effective antimicrobial therapy and to deciding whether to perform susceptibility testing on accurately speciated NTM. Newer species have been identified using nucleic acid sequencing with limited published phenotypic characteristics. Because of these issues and limitations with conventional phenotypic methods for identification, molecular and genetic investigations are becoming indispensable to identifying the NTM accurately. Therefore, for timely and accurate identification of mycobacteria, molecular approaches in conjunction with some phenotypic characteristics should be used.

Regardless of whether molecular or phenotypic methods are used, when growth is detected, broth subcultures of colonies growing in liquid media or on solid media (several colonies inoculated to Middlebrook 7H9 broth [5 mL] and incubated at 35°C for 5 to 7 days with daily agitation to enhance growth) are then used to determine pigmentation and growth rate and to inoculate all test media for biochemical tests if performed. Additional cultures may be inoculated and then incubated at different temperatures when more definitive identification is needed.

Conventional Phenotypic Tests

Growth Characteristics
Preliminary identification of mycobacterial isolates depends on the organisms' rate of growth, colonial morphology (Fig. 42.5), colonial texture, pigmentation, and, in some instances, the permissive incubation temperatures of mycobacteria. Despite the limitations of phenotypic tests, the mycobacterial growth characteristics are helpful for determining a preliminary identification (e.g., an isolate appears to represent RGM). To perform identification procedures, quality-control organisms should be tested along with unknowns (Table 42.8). The commonly used quality-control organisms can be maintained in broth at room temperature and transferred monthly. In this way they are always available for inoculation to test media along with suspensions of the unknown mycobacteria being tested.

Growth Rate. The rate of growth is an important criterion for determining the initial category of an isolate. Rapid growers usually produce colonies within 3 to 4 days after subculture. However, even a rapid grower may take longer than 7 days to initially produce colonies because of inhibition by a harsh decontaminating procedure; therefore the growth rate (and pigment production) must be determined by subculture (Evolve Procedure 42.5). The dilution of the organism used to assess the growth rate is critical. Even slow-growing mycobacteria appear to produce colonies in less than 7 days if the inoculum is too heavy. One organism particularly likely to exhibit false-positive rapid growth is *Mycobacterium flavescens*. It therefore serves as an excellent quality-control organism for this procedure.

Pigment Production. As previously discussed, mycobacteria can be categorized into three groups based on pigment production. Evolve Procedure 42.5 describes how to determine pigment production. To achieve optimum photochromogenicity, colonies should be young, actively metabolizing, isolated, and well aerated. Although some species (e.g., *M. kansasii*) turn yellow after a few hours of

light exposure, others (e.g., *Mycobacterium simiae*) may require prolonged exposure to light. Scotochromogens produce pigmented colonies even in the absence of light, and colonies often become darker with prolonged exposure to light (Fig. 42.6). One member of this group, *Mycobacterium szulgai*, is peculiar in that it is a scotochromogen at 35°C and nonpigmented when grown at 25°C to 30°C. For this reason, all pigmented colonies should be subcultured to test for photoactivated pigment at both 35°C and 25°C to 30°C. Nonchromogens are not affected by light.

Biochemical Testing
Once categorized into a preliminary subgroup based on its growth characteristics, an organism must be definitively identified to species or complex level. Although conventional biochemical tests can be used for this purpose, molecular methods have replaced biochemical tests for identifying mycobacterial species because of the previously discussed limitations of phenotypic testing. Although key biochemical tests are still discussed in this edition, the reader must be aware that this approach to identification will ultimately be replaced by molecular methods or at the very least be utilized to resolve unusual cases in the absence of availability of whole genome sequencing and/or database limitations. Table 42.9 summarizes distinctive properties of the more commonly cultivable mycobacteria isolated from clinical specimens; key biochemical tests for each of the major mycobacterial groupings, including *M. tuberculosis* complex, are listed in Table 42.10. The following sections address key biochemical tests.

Niacin. Niacin (nicotinic acid) plays an important role in the oxidation-reduction reactions that occur during mycobacterial metabolism. Although all species produce nicotinic acid, *M. tuberculosis* accumulates the largest amount. (*M. simiae* and some strains of *M. chelonae* also produce niacin.) Niacin therefore accumulates in the medium in which these organisms are growing. A positive niacin test (Evolve Procedure 42.6) is preliminary evidence that an organism that exhibits a buff-colored, slow-growing, rough colony may be *M. tuberculosis* (Fig. 42.7). However, this test is not sufficient to confirm identification. If sufficient growth is present on an initial L-J slant (the egg-base medium enhances accumulation of free niacin), a niacin test can be performed immediately. If growth on the initial culture is scant, the subculture used for growth rate determination can be used. If this culture yields rare colonies, the colonies should be spread around with a sterile cotton swab (after the growth rate has been determined) to distribute the inoculum over the entire slant. The slant then is incubated until light growth over the surface of the medium is visible. For reliable results, the niacin test should be performed from cultures on L-J medium that are at least 3 weeks old and show at least 50 colonies; otherwise, enough detectable niacin might not have been produced.

Nitrate Reduction. A nitrate reduction test is valuable for identifying *M. tuberculosis, M. kansasii, M. szulgai,* and

TABLE 42.8 Controls and Media Used for Biochemical Identification of Mycobacteria

Biochemical Test Tables Are Difficult to Review in This Format	Control Organisms		Result				Incubation
	Positive	Negative	Positive	Negative	Medium Used	Duration	Conditions
Niacin	Mycobacterium tuberculosis	Mycobacterium intracellulare	Yellow	No color change	0.5 mL DH₂O	15–30 min	Room temperature
Nitrate	Mycobacterium tuberculosis	Mycobacterium intracellulare	Pink or red	No color change	0.3 mL DH₂O	2 h	37°C bath
Urease	Mycobacterium fortuitum	Mycobacterium avium	Pink or red	No color change	Urea broth for AFB	1, 3, and 5 days	37°C incubator (without CO₂)
68°C Catalase	Mycobacterium fortuitum or Mycobacterium gordonae	Mycobacterium tuberculosis	Bubbles	No bubbles	0.5 mL phosphate buffer (pH, 7.0)	20 min	68°C bath
SQ Catalase	Mycobacterium kansasii or M. gordonae	Mycobacterium avium	>45 mm	<45 mm	Commercial medium	14 days	37°C incubator (with CO₂)
Tween 80	Mycobacterium kansasii	Mycobacterium intracellulare	Pink or red	No color change	1 mL DH₂O	5 or 10 days	37°C incubator (in the dark, without CO₂)
Tellurite	Mycobacterium avium	Mycobacterium tuberculosis	Smooth, fine, black precipitate (smoke-like action)	Gray clumps (no smokelike action)	Middlebrook 7H9 broth	7, then 3 additional days	37°C incubator (with CO₂)
Arylsulfatase	Mycobacterium fortuitum	Mycobacterium intracellulare	Pink or red	No color change	Wayne's arylsulfatase medium	3 days	37°C incubator (without CO₂)
5% NaCl	Mycobacterium fortuitum	Mycobacterium gordonae	Substantial growth	Little or no growth	Commercial slant with and without 5% NaCl	28 days	37°C incubator (with CO₂)
TCH	Mycobacterium bovis	Mycobacterium tuberculosis	No growth (i.e., susceptible)	Growth (i.e., resistant or ≥1% of colonies are resistant)	TCH slant	3 weeks	37°C incubator (with CO₂)

AFB, Acid-fast bacilli; *CO₂*, carbon dioxide; *DH₂O*, distilled water; *NaCl*, sodium chloride; *SQ*, semiquantitative; *TCH*, thiophene-2-carboxylic acid hydrazide.

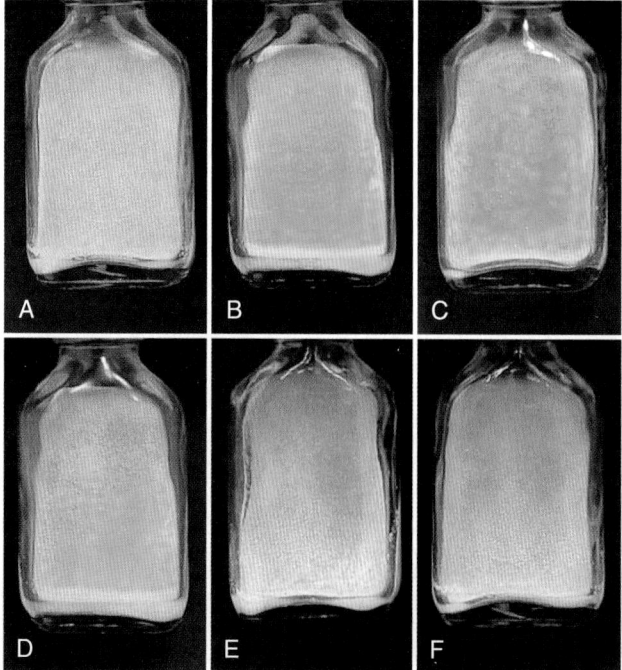

• **Fig. 42.6** Initial grouping of mycobacteria based on pigment production before and after exposure to light. In one test system, subcultures of each isolate are grown on two agar slants. One tube is wrapped in aluminum foil to prevent exposure of the organism to light, and the other tube is allowed light exposure. After sufficient growth has occurred, the wrapped tube is unwrapped, and the tubes are examined together. Photochromogens are nonpigmented when grown in the dark (A) and develop pigment after light exposure (B). Scotochromogens are pigmented in the dark (C); the color does not intensify after exposure to light (D). Nonphotochromogens are nonpigmented when grown in the dark (E) and remain so even after light exposure (F).

M. fortuitum. The ability of AFB to reduce nitrate is influenced by the age of the colonies, temperature, pH, and enzyme inhibitors. Although rapid growers can be tested within 2 weeks, slow growers should be tested after 3 to 4 weeks of luxuriant growth. Commercially available nitrate strips yield acceptable results with strongly nitrate-positive organisms, such as *M. tuberculosis.* This test may be tried first because of its ease of performance. The *M. tuberculosis*–positive control must be strongly positive in the strip test, or the test results are unreliable. If the paper strip test is negative or if the control test result is not strongly positive, the chemical procedure (Evolve Procedure 42.7) must be carried out using strongly and weakly positive controls.

Catalase. Most species of mycobacteria except for certain strains of *M. tuberculosis* complex (some isoniazid-resistant strains) and *M. gastri* produce the intracellular enzyme catalase, which splits hydrogen peroxide into water and oxygen. Catalase can be assessed by using the semiquantitative catalase test or the heat-stable catalase test.

• The semiquantitative catalase test is based on the relative activity of the enzyme, as determined by the height of a column of bubbles of oxygen (Fig. 42.8) formed by the action of untreated enzyme produced by the organism. Based on the semiquantitative catalase test, mycobacteria are divided into two groups: those that produce less than

45 mm of bubbles and those that produce more than 45 mm of bubbles.

• The heat-stable catalase test is based on the ability of the catalase enzyme to remain active after heating (i.e., it is a measure of the enzyme's heat stability). When heated to 68°C for 20 minutes, the catalase of *M. tuberculosis, M. bovis, M. gastri,* and *M. haemophilum* becomes inactivated.

Tween 80 Hydrolysis. The commonly nonpathogenic, slow-growing scotochromogens and nonphotochromogens produce a lipase that can hydrolyze Tween 80 (the detergent polyoxyethylene sorbitan monooleate) into oleic acid and polyoxyethylated sorbitol, whereas pathogenic species do not. Tween 80 hydrolysis is useful for differentiating species of photochromogens, nonchromogens, and scotochromogens. Because laboratory-prepared media have a very short shelf life, the CDC recommends use of a commercial Tween 80 hydrolysis substrate (Becton-Dickinson, Franklin Lakes, NJ, or Remel Laboratories, Lenexa, KS) that is stable for up to 1 year.

Tellurite Reduction. Some species of mycobacteria reduce potassium tellurite at variable rates. The ability to reduce tellurite in 3 to 4 days distinguishes members of MAC from most other nonchromogenic species. All rapid growers reduce tellurite in 3 days.

Arylsulfatase. The enzyme arylsulfatase is present in most mycobacteria. Test conditions can be varied to distinguish the different forms of the enzyme. The rate at which the enzyme breaks down phenolphthalein disulfate into phenolphthalein (which forms a red color in the presence of sodium bicarbonate) and other salts helps to differentiate certain strains of mycobacteria. The 3-day test is particularly useful for identifying the potentially pathogenic rapid growers *M. fortuitum* and *M. chelonae.* Slow-growing *M. marinum* and *M. szulgai* are positive in the 14-day test (Fig. 42.9).

Growth Inhibition by Thiophene-2-Carboxylic Acid Hydrazide. The thiophene-2-carboxylic acid hydrazide (TCH) growth-inhibition test is used to distinguish *M. bovis* from *M. tuberculosis* because only *M. bovis* is unable to grow in the presence of 10 mg/mL of TCH.

Other Tests. Other tests are often performed to make more subtle distinctions between species (Table 42.10). However, performing all the procedures necessary for definitive identification of mycobacteria is not cost-effective for routine clinical microbiology laboratories; therefore specimens that require further testing can be forwarded to regional laboratories.

Antimicrobial Susceptibility Testing and Therapy

Drug-resistant tuberculosis is a major health threat; more than 500,000 cases of multidrug-resistant (MDR) tuberculosis occur each year. MDR tuberculosis is resistant to rifampin and isoniazid, the two drugs most often used as

TABLE 42.9 Distinctive Properties of Commonly Cultivable Mycobacteria Encountered in Clinical Specimens

Group/Complex	Species	Optimal Temp (°C)	Usual Colonial Morphology[a]	Niacin	Growth on TCH (10 mg/mL)[b]	Nitrate Reduction	Semiquantitative Catalase (45 mm)	68°C Catalase	Tween Hydrolysis, 5 Days	Tellurite Reduction	Tolerance to 5% NaCl	Arylsulfatase, 3 Days	Iron Uptake	Growth on MacConkey Agar	Urease	Pyrazinamidase, 4 Days
Mycobacterium tuberculosis complex	M. tuberculosis	37	R	+	+	+	−	−	−[c]	∓	−	−	−	−	±	+
	Mycobacterium bovis	37	Rt	−	−	−	−	−	−	∓	−	−	−	−	±	−
	Mycobacterium africanum	37	R	V	V	V	−	−	−	−	−	−	−	−	+	−
Photochromogens	Mycobacterium marinum	30	S/SR	∓	+	−	−	−	+	∓	−	−	∓[d]	−	−/+	+
	Mycobacterium kansasii	35	SR/S	−	+	+	+	+	+	∓	−	−	−	−	+	−
	Mycobacterium simiae	37	S	±	+	−	+	+	+	−	−	−	−	N/A	±	+
	Mycobacterium asiaticum	37	S	−	+	−	+	+	+	−	−	−	−	N/A	−	−
Scotochromogens	Mycobacterium scrofulaceum	37	S	−	+	−	+	+	−	∓	−	−	V	−	V	±
	Mycobacterium szulgai	37	S or R	−	+	+	+	+	∓[c]	±	−	−	V	−	+	+
	Mycobacterium gordonae	37	S	−	+	−	+	+	+	−	−	−	V	−	V	±
Nonphotochromogens	Mycobacterium avium complex	35–37	St/R	−	+	−	+	±	−	+	−	−	−	∓	−	+
	Mycobacterium genavense[e]	37	St	−	+	−	−	+	+	N/A	N/A	−	−	N/A	+	+
	M. gastri	35	S/SR/R	−	+	−	+	−	+	∓	−	−	−	−	∓	−
	Mycobacterium malmoense	30	S	−	+	−	−	±	+	+	−	−	−	N/A	−	+
	Mycobacterium haemophilum[f]	30	R	−	+	−	−	−	−	−	−	−	−	−	−	+
	Mycobacterium shimoidei	37	R	−	+	−	−	−	+	N/A	−	−	−	−	−	+
	Mycobacterium ulcerans	30	R	−	+	−	−	+	−	N/A	−	N/A	−	N/A	−	−
	Mycobacterium flavescens[g]	37	S	−	+	+	+	+	+	∓	+	−	−	−	+	+
	Mycobacterium xenopi[h]	42	Sf	−	+	−	−	+	−	∓	−	−	±	−	−	V

TABLE 42.9 Distinctive Properties of Commonly Cultivable Mycobacteria Encountered in Clinical Specimens—cont'd

Group/Complex	Species	Optimal Temp (°C)	Usual Colonial Morphology[a]	Niacin	Growth on TCH (10 mg/mL)[b]	Nitrate Reduction	Semiquantitative Catalase (45 mm)	68°C Catalase	Tween Hydrolysis, 5 Days	Tellurite Reduction	Tolerance to 5% NaCl	Arylsulfatase, 3 Days	Iron Uptake	Growth on MacConkey Agar	Urease	Pyrazinamidase, 4 Days
	Mycobacterium terrae complex Mycobacterium terrae Mycobacterium triviale[i] Mycobacterium nonchromogenicum	35	SR	–	–	+	+	+	+	–	–	–		–	V	–	V
Rapidly growing	Mycobacterium fortuitum group	28–30	Sf/Rf	–	+	+	+	+	V	+	+	+	+	+	+	+
	Mycobacterium chelonae	28–30	S/R	–/+	+	–	+	V	V	+	–	–	+	+	+	+
	Mycobacterium abscessus	28–30	S/R	–	N/A	–	+	V	V	+	+	–	+	+	+	N/A
	Mycobacterium smegmatis	28–30	R/S	–	+	+	+	+	+	+	+	+	–	–	N/A	N/A

[a]R, Rough; S, smooth; SR, intermediate in roughness; t, thin or transparent; f, filamentous extensions.
[b]TCH, Thiophene-2-carboxylic acid hydrazide.
[c]Tween hydrolysis may be positive at 10 days.
[d]Arylsulfatase, 14 days, is positive.
[e]Requires mycobactin for growth on solid media.
[f]Requires hemin as a growth factor.
[g]Young cultures may be nonchromogenic or have only pale pigment that may intensify with age.
[h]Strains of M. xenopi can be nonphotochromogenic or scotochromogenic.
[i]M. triviale is tolerant to 5% NaCl, and a rare isolate may grow on MacConkey agar.
Data from Carroll KC, Pfaller MA. Manual of Clinical Microbiology. 12th ed. Washington, DC: ASM Press; 2019.
+, Present; –, absent; ±, usually present; ∓, usually absent; N/A, the information is not currently available or the property is unimportant; V, variable.

TABLE 42.10 Key Biochemical Reactions to Help Differentiate Organisms Belonging to the Same Mycobacterial Group

Mycobacterial Group	Key Biochemical Tests
Mycobacterium tuberculosis complex	Niacin, nitrate reduction; susceptibility to thiophene-2-carboxylic acid hydrazide (TCH) if Mycobacterium bovis is suspected
Photochromogens	Tween 80 hydrolysis, nitrate reduction, pyrazinamidase, 14-day arylsulfatase, urease, niacin
Scotochromogens	Permissive growth temperature, Tween 80 hydrolysis, nitrate reduction, semiquantitative catalase, urease, 14-day arylsulfatase
Nonphotochromogens	Heat-resistant and semiquantitative catalase activity, nitrate reduction, Tween 80 hydrolysis, urease, 14-day arylsulfatase, tellurite reduction, acid phosphatase activity
Rapidly growing	Growth on MacConkey agar, nitrate reduction, Tween 80 hydrolysis, 3-day arylsulfatase, iron uptake

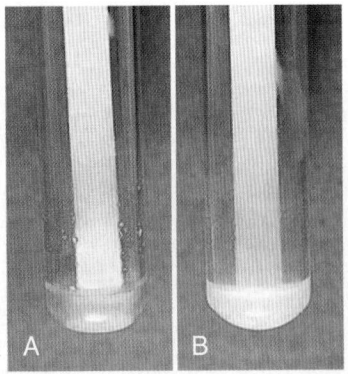

• **Fig. 42.7** Niacin test performed with filter paper strips. (A) With a positive test result, the liquid turns yellow. (B) With a negative result, the liquid remains milky white or clear.

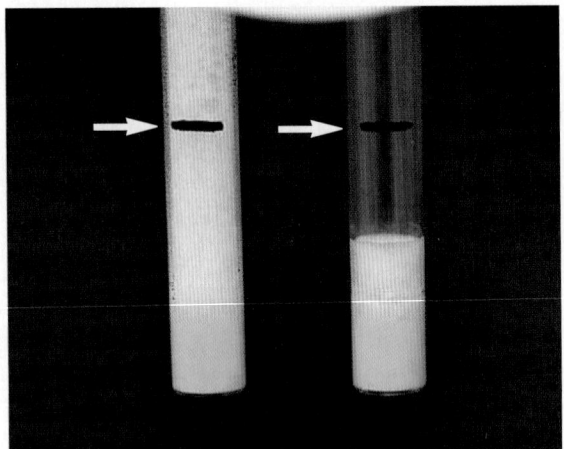

• **Fig. 42.8** Semiquantitative catalase test. The tube on the *left* contains a column of bubbles that has risen past the line *(arrow)*, indicating 45-mm height (a positive test result). The tube on the *right* is the negative control.

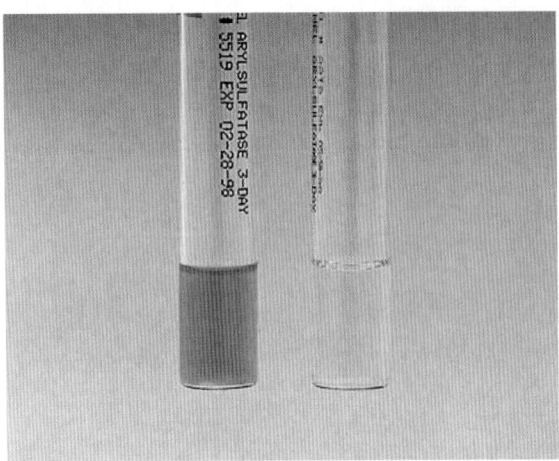

• **Fig. 42.9** A positive arylsulfatase test result is shown on the *left;* the tube containing the negative control is on the *right.*

effective treatment against tuberculosis. In addition, strains of XDR TB are emerging that are resistant not only to rifampin and isoniazid, but also to quinolones and other drugs, such as aminoglycosides and capreomycin.

Standardized methods for susceptibility testing, including direct and indirect testing and new molecular tools, currently are available for susceptibility testing.

M. tuberculosis Complex

In vitro drug susceptibility testing should be performed on the first isolate of *M. tuberculosis* from all patients. Susceptibility testing of *M. tuberculosis* requires meticulous care in the preparation of the medium, selection of adequate samples of colonies, standardization of the inoculum, use of appropriate controls, and interpretation of results. Laboratories that see very few positive cultures should consider sending isolates to a reference laboratory for testing. Isolates must be saved in sterile 10% skim milk in distilled water at −70°C for possible future additional studies (e.g., susceptibilities if the patient does not respond well to treatment).

Direct Versus Indirect Susceptibility Testing

Susceptibility tests may be performed by either the direct or indirect method. The direct method uses the smear-positive concentrate containing more than 50 AFB per 100 oil immersion fields as the inoculum; the indirect method uses a culture as the inoculum source. Although direct testing provides more rapid results, it is less standardized and contamination may occur.

Conventional Methods

The development of primary drug resistance in tuberculosis represents an increase in the proportion of resistant organisms. The increase in resistant organisms results from a spontaneous mutation and subsequent selection to predominance of the drug-resistant mutants by the action of a single or ineffective drug therapy. A poor clinical outcome is predicted with an agent when more than 1% of bacilli in the test population are resistant. If an isolate is reported as resistant to a drug, treatment failure is likely if this drug is used for therapy.

Drug resistance is defined for *M. tuberculosis* complex in terms of the critical concentration of the drug. The **critical concentration** of a drug is the amount of drug required to prevent growth above the 1% threshold of the test population of tubercle bacilli. Initial isolates of *M. tuberculosis* are tested against five antimicrobials, which are referred to as **primary drugs** (Box 42.3). If resistance to any of the primary drugs is detected, a second battery of agents is tested (Box 42.3).

Molecular Methods for the Determination of Susceptibility

Several technologies show promise of being faster, more reliable, and/or easier to perform than most conventional methods of susceptibility testing. As previously indicated,

Primary Drugs
Isoniazid
Rifampin
Ethambutol
Pyrazinamide

Secondary Drugs
Amikacin
Amithiozones
Bedaquiline
Ethionamide
Capreomycin

Secondary Drugs—cont'd
Clofazimine
Doxycycline or minocycline
Linezolid
Levofloxacin
Moxifloxacin
Kanamycin
Cycloserine
p-Aminosalicylic acid
Rifabutin
Streptomycin

the Cepheid Xpert is FDA approved in the United States for the detection of rifampicin mutations in *M. tuberculosis*. Another molecular method as previously discussed, the line probe assay (INNO-LiPA Rif TB; Innogenetics, Ghent, Belgium), is a commercially available reverse hybridization–based probe assay for rapid detection of rifampin mutations leading to rifampin resistance in *M. tuberculosis*. Many different genotypic assays are currently available for drug susceptibility testing. Most are based on PCR amplification of a specific region of an *M. tuberculosis* gene, followed by analysis of the amplicon for specific mutations associated with resistance to a drug. The presence or absence of mutations can then be detected by several methods, such as automated sequencing.

As previously mentioned, high-density DNA probe assays (Chapter 8) have been used to detect rifampin resistance and to identify mycobacterial species identification.

The CDC currently offers a molecular drug resistance sequencing method for culture isolates or nucleic acid test sediments positive for *M. tuberculosis* complex organisms. Susceptibility testing should be repeated if the patient remains culture positive after 3 months following appropriate therapy or fails to respond clinically to therapy.

Therapy

Therapy directed against *M. tuberculosis* depends on the susceptibility of the isolate to various antimicrobial agents. To prevent the selection of resistant mutants, treatment of tuberculosis requires four drugs: isoniazid, rifampin, ethambutol, and pyrazinamide. Initial therapy includes all four drugs for 8 weeks. However, if drug susceptibility is determined for isoniazid, rifampin, and pyrazinamide, ethambutol may be discontinued. This is the preferred therapy for initial treatment, followed by isoniazid and rifampin for an additional 18 weeks. The most common two-drug regimen is isoniazid (INH, also known as **isonicotinoylhydrazine**) and rifampin. The combination is administered for 9 months in cases of uncomplicated tuberculosis; if pyrazinamide is added to this regimen during the first 2 months, the total duration of therapy can be shortened to 6 months.

Ethambutol may also be added to the regimen. INH prophylaxis is recommended for individuals with a recent skin test conversion who are disease free.

Nontuberculous Mycobacteria

In general, the treatment of patients infected with NTM requires more individualized therapy than does the treatment of patients with tuberculosis. This individualization is based on the species of mycobacteria recovered, the site and severity of infection, antimicrobial drug susceptibility results, concurrent diseases, and the patient's general condition.

Susceptibility testing should be performed on clinically significant, rapidly growing mycobacteria. Skin and soft tissue infections, if susceptible, are treated with clarithromycin and at least one additional drug based on susceptibility testing. Pulmonary infections with *M. abscessus* should also be treated with a multidrug regimen that includes clarithromycin, if susceptible, and then additional drugs based on susceptibility testing.

Prevention

As previously mentioned, prophylactic chemotherapy with INH is used when known or suspected primary tuberculous infection poses a risk of clinical disease. At present, the BCG vaccine is the only vaccine available against tuberculosis. The effectiveness of this live vaccine is controversial, because studies have demonstrated ineffectiveness to 80% protection. The greatest potential value for this vaccine is in developing countries with high prevalence rates for tuberculosis. At least four types of antituberculosis vaccines are currently being evaluated in experimental studies in animals.

ⓔ Visit the Evolve site for a complete list of procedures, review questions, and case studies.

Bibliography

Al-Rubaye DS, Henihan G, Al-Abasly AK, et al.: Genotypic assessment of drug-resistant tuberculosis in Baghdad and other Iraqi provinces using low-cost and density (LCD) DNA microarrays, *J Med Microbiol* 65:114–122, 2015.

Arttawejkul P, Kongpolprom N: A case of pulmonary infection caused by *Mycobacterium asiaticum*: difficulties on diagnostic and therapeutic approaches, *Respir Med Case Rep* 24:150–152, 2018.

Badak FZ, Kiska DL, Setterquist S, Hartley C, O'Connell MA, Hopfer RL: Comparison of mycobacteria growth indicator tube with BACTEC 460 for detection and recovery of mycobacteria from clinical specimens, *J Clin Microbiol* 34:2236–2239, 1996.

Banales JL, Pineda PR, Fitzgerald JM, Rubio H, Selman M, Salazar-Lezama M: Adenosine deaminase in the diagnosis of tuberculous pleural effusions: a report of 218 patients and review of the literature, *Chest* 99:355–357, 1991.

Biswal M, Singh G, Jain V, et al.: P201: first report in the world of *Mycobacterium bacteremicum* causing a cluster of postlaparotomy surgical wound infections, *Antimicrob Resist Infect Control* 2(Suppl 1):201, 2013.

Brown-Elliott BA, Griffith DE, Wallace RJ: Newly described or emerging human species of nontuberculous mycobacteria, *Infect Dis Clin North Am* 16:187–200, 2002.

Brown-Elliott BA, Griffith DE, Wallace RJ: Diagnosis of nontuberculous mycobacterial infections, *Clin Lab Med* 22:911–925, 2002.

Carroll KC, Pfaller MA: *Manual of clinical microbiology*, ed 12, Washington, DC, 2019, ASM Press.

Carpenter RJ, Graf PC: Pott's disease? AIDS-associated *Mycobacterium heckeshornense* spinal osteomyelitis and diskitis, *J Clin Microbiol* 53(2):716–718, 2015.

Chen P, Shi M, Feng GD, et al.: A highly efficient Ziehl-Neelsen stain: identifying de novo intracellular *Mycobacterium tuberculosis* and improving detection of extracellular *M. tuberculosis* in cerebrospinal fluid, *J Clin Microbiol* 50:1166–1170, 2012.

Cheng X, Sun L, Zhao Q, et al.: Development and evaluation of a droplet digital PCR assay for the diagnosis of paucibacillary leprosy in skin biopsy specimens, *PLoS Negl Trop Dis* 13(3):e0007284, 2019.

Colston MJ: The microbiology of *Mycobacterium leprae:* progress in the last 30 years, *Trans R Soc Trop Med Hyg* 87:504–507, 1993.

Forbes BA, Hall GS, Miller MB, et al.: Practice guidelines for clinical microbiology laboratories: mycobacteria, *Clin Microbiol Rev* 31(2):e00038-17, 2018.

Ghielmetti G, Scherrer S, Friedel U, et al.: Epidemiological tracing of bovine tuberculosis in Switzerland, multilocus variable number of tandem repeat analysis of *Mycobacterium bovis* and *Mycobacterium caprae*, *PLoS One* 12(2):e0172474, 2017.

Greendyke R, Byrd TF: Differential antibiotic susceptibility of *Mycobacterium abscessus* variants in biofilms and macrophages compared to that of planktonic bacteria, *Antimicrob Agents Chemother* 52:2019–2026, 2008.

Griffith DE, Girard WM, Wallace RJ: Clinical features of pulmonary disease caused by rapidly growing mycobacteria, *Am Rev Respir Dis* 147:1271–1278, 1993.

Gautam H, Singla M, Jain R, et al.: Point-of-care urine lipoarabinomannan antigen detection for diagnosis of tuberculosis in children, *Int J Tuberc Lung Dis* 23(6):714–719, 2019.

Harries AD, Lawn SD, Getahun H, Zachariah R, Havlir DV: HIV and tuberculosis–science and implementation to turn the tide and reduce deaths, *J Int AIDS Soc* 15:17396, 2012.

Havlik Jr JA, Metchock B, Thompson III SE, Barrett K, Rimland D, Horsburgh CR: A prospective evaluation of *Mycobacterium avium* complex colonization of the respiratory and gastrointestinal tracts of persons with human immunodeficiency virus infection, *J Infect Dis* 168:1045–1048, 1993.

Heifets L: Mycobacterial infections caused by nontuberculous mycobacteria, *Semin Respir Crit Care Med* 25:283–295, 2004.

Horsburgh Jr C, Metchock BG, McGowan Jr JE, Thompson SE: Clinical implications of recovery of *Mycobacterium avium* complex from the stool or respiratory tract of HIV-infected individuals, *AIDS* 6:512–514, 1992.

Jacobs Jr WR, Barletta RG, Udani R, et al.: Rapid assessment of drug susceptibilities of *Mycobacterium tuberculosis* by means of luciferase reporter phages, *Science* 260:819–822, 1993.

Kent PT, Kubica GP: *Public health mycobacteriology: a guide for the level III laboratory*, Atlanta, 1985, US Department of Health and Human Services, Public Health Service, Centers for Disease Control and Prevention.

Lapierre SG, Fellag M, Magan C, Drancourt M: *Mycobacterium malmoense* pulmonary infection in France, a case report, *BMC Res Notes* 10:436, 2017.

Lipsky BA, Gates J, Tenover FC, Plorde JJ: Factors affecting the clinical value of microscopy for acid-fast bacilli, *Rev Infect Dis* 6:214–222, 1984.

Marjani M, Farshidpour M, Tabarsi P, Sheikholslami FM, Farnia P: Isolation of *Mycobacterium branderi*, an unusual species from an acute myelogenous leukemia patient, *Avicenna J Med* 4(1):17–19, 2014.

Mazurek GH, Jereb J, LoBue P, et al.: Guidelines for using the QuantiFERON-TB Gold test for detecting *Mycobacterium tuberculosis* infection, United States, *MMWR Recomm Rep* 54(RR-15):49–55, 2005.

McMullen AR, Mattar C, Kirmani N, et al.: Brown-pigmented *Mycobacterium mageritense* as a cause of prosthetic valve endocarditis and bloodstream infection, *J Clin Microbiol* 53(8):2777–2780, 2015.

Mediavilla-Gradolph MC, De Toro-Peinado I, Bermúdez-Ruiz MP, et al.: Use of MALDI-TOF MS for identification of nontuberculous mycobacterium species isolated from clinical specimens, *BioMed Res Int* 2015:854078, 2015.

Michelet L, de Cruz, Krystel, Phalente Y, et al.: *Mycobacterium microti* infection in dairy goats, France, *Emerg Infect Dis* 22(3):569–570, 2016.

Mijs W, de Haas P, Rossau R, et al.: Molecular evidence to support a proposal to reserve the designation *Mycobacterium avium* subsp. *avium* for bird-type isolates and *M. avium* subsp. *hominissuis* for the human/porcine type of *M. avium*, *Int J Syst Evol Microbiol* 52:1505–1518, 2002.

Morris A, Reller LB, Salfinger M, Jackson K, Sievers A, Dwyer B: Mycobacteria in stool specimens: the nonvalue of smears for predicting culture results, *J Clin Microbiol* 31:1385–1387, 1993.

Moschella SL: An update on the diagnosis and treatment of leprosy, *J Am Acad Dermatol* 51:417–426, 2004.

Nagano N: *Mycobacterium shimoidei,* a rare non-tuberculosis mycobacteria pathogen identified by matrix-assisted laser desorption ionization time-of-flight mass spectrometry, *Respirol Case Rep* 7(5):e00428, 2019.

Nebreda Mayoral T, Andrés Andres AG, Fuentes Carretero S, et al.: Cervicofacial lymphadenitis due to *Mycobacterium mantenii*: rapid and reliable identification by MALDI-TOF MS, *New Microbes New Infect* 22:1–3, 2017.

Nogueira CL, Whipps CM, Matsumoto CK, et al.: *Mycobacterium saopaulense* sp. nov., a rapidly growing mycobacterium closely related to members of the *Mycobacterium chelonae-Mycobacterium abscessus* group, *Int J Syst Evol Microbiol* 65(Pt 12):4403–4409, 2015.

Oliveira FM, Da Costa AC, Procopio VO, et al.: *Mycobacterium abscessus* subsp. *massiliense myca_0076* and *mycma_0077* Genes code for ferritins that are modulated by iron concentration, *Front Microbiol* 9:1072, 2018.

O'Reilly LM, Daborn CJ: The epidemiology of *Mycobacterium bovis* infections in animals and man: a review, *Tuber Lung Dis* 76(Suppl 1):1–46, 1995.

Oxford Immunotec, Ltd: *T-spot TB, package insert*, Oxfordshire, England, 2012, An Aid in the Diagnosis of Tuberculosis Infection.

Pfaller MA: Application of new technology to the detection, identification, and antimicrobial susceptibility testing of mycobacteria, *Am J Clin Pathol* 101:329–337, 1994.

Phelippeau M, Delord M, Drancourt M, Brouqui P: Respiratory tract isolation of *Mycobacterium europaeum* following influenza infection in an immunocompromised patient: a case report, *J Med Case Rep* 8:463, 2014.

Phelippeau M, Dubus JC, Reynaud-Gaubert M, et al.: Prevalence of *Mycobacterium lentiflavum* in cystic fibrosis patients, France, *BMC Pulm Med* 15:131, 2015.

Primm TP, Lucero CA, Falkinham JO: Health impacts of environmental mycobacteria, *Clin Microbiol Rev* 17:98–106, 2004.

Runyon EH: Anonymous mycobacteria in pulmonary disease, *Med Clin North Am* 43:273–290, 1959.

Santos M, Gil-Brusola A, Escandell A, Blanes M, Gobernado M: *Mycobacterium genavense* infections in a tertiary hospital and reviewed cases in non-HIV patients, *Patholog Res Int* 2014:371370, 2014.

Shinnick TM, Good RC: Mycobacterial taxonomy, *Eur J Clin Microbiol Infect Dis* 13:884–901, 1994.

Singh AK, Marak RS, Maurya AK, et al.: Mixed cutaneous infection caused by *Mycobacterium szulgai* and *Mycobacterium intermedium* in a healthy adult female: a rare case report, *Case Rep Dermatol Med* 2015:607519, 2015.

Sotello D, Hata DJ, Reza M, et al.: Disseminated *Mycobacterium interjectum* infection with bacteremia, hepatic and pulmonary involvement associated with a long-term catheter infection, *Case Rep Infect Dis* 2017:6958204, 2017.

Springer B, Tortoli E, Richter I, et al.: *Mycobacterium conspicuum* sp. nov., a new species isolated from patients with disseminated infections, *J Clin Microbiol* 33:2805–2811, 1995.

Steele JH, Ranney AF: Animal tuberculosis, *Am Rev Tuber* 77:908–922, 1958.

Taylor Z, Nolan CM, Blumberg HM: Controlling tuberculosis in the United States: recommendations from the American Thoracic Society, CDC, and the Infectious Diseases Society of America, *MMWR Recomm Rep* 54:1–81, 2005.

Timm K, Welle M, Friedel U, et al.: *Mycobacterium nebraskense* infection in a dog in Switzerland with disseminated skin lesions, *Vet Dermatol* 30(3):262-e80, 2019.

Tortoli E: Impact of genotypic studies on mycobacterial taxonomy: the new mycobacteria of the 1990s, *Clin Microbiol Rev* 16:319–354, 2003.

Utsugi H, Usui Y, Nishihara F, et al.: *Mycobacterium gordonae*-induced humidifier lung, *BMC Pulm Med* 15:108, 2015.

Vernet G, Jay C, Rodrigue M, Troesch A: Species differentiation and antibiotic susceptibility testing with DNA microarrays, *J Appl Microbiol* 96:59–68, 2004.

Welch DF, Guruswamy AP, Sides SJ, Shaw CH, Gilchrist MJ: Timely culture for mycobacteria which utilizes a microcolony method, *J Clin Microbiol* 31:2178–2184, 1993.

Wolinsky E: Mycobacterial diseases other than tuberculosis, *Clin Infect Dis* 15:1–10, 1992.

Woods GL: Mycobacterial susceptibility testing and reporting: when, how, and what to test, *Clin Microbiol Newsl* 27:67, 2005.

Yajko DM, Nassos PS, Sanders CA, et al.: Comparison of four decontamination methods for recovery of *Mycobacterium avium* complex from stools, *J Clin Microbiol* 31:302–306, 1993.

43

Obligate Intracellular and Nonculturable Bacterial Agents

OBJECTIVES

1. Define the following: bubo, proctitis, bartholinitis, salpingitis, elementary body, reticulate body, Whipple disease, morulae, and Donovan body.
2. Describe the general characteristics for the organisms included in this chapter, including Gram stain characteristics, cultivation methods (media and growth conditions), transmission, and clinical significance.
3. Explain the mechanism and location for the replication of *Chlamydia* spp.
4. Compare the clinical manifestations and diagnosis of trachoma and other oculogenital infections associated with *Chlamydia* spp.
5. List the appropriate specimens used for the isolation of the organisms included in this chapter.
6. Describe the correct collection method for a specimen submitted for *Chlamydia trachomatis* screening from the female genital tract.
7. Explain the three stages associated with lymphogranuloma venereum, and compare the disease with other genital infections.
8. Describe the laboratory methods used for the diagnosis of *Chlamydia* infections, including sensitivity, limitations, and appropriate use for culture, cytology, antigen (direct fluorescent antibody), and nucleic acid amplification testing (NAAT).
9. Compare hybridization and amplification nucleic acid–based testing for chlamydia.
10. Describe the triad of symptoms associated with *Rickettsia* spp.
11. Compare human monocytic ehrlichiosis (HME) and granulocytic anaplasmosis (HGA).
12. Distinguish and describe the three groups of *Rickettsia* based on mode of transmission, clinical manifestations, and intracellular growth characteristics.
13. Describe the Weil-Felix reaction, including chemical principle and limitations.
14. Describe the clinical significance for *Coxiella burnetii* phase I and phase II forms, including laboratory diagnosis.
15. Explain the limitations of the laboratory tests used to diagnose disease caused by the obligate intracellular and nonculturable bacteria.
16. Correlate signs, symptoms, laboratory data, and antimicrobial susceptibility results for identification of organisms included in this chapter.

GENERA AND SPECIES TO BE CONSIDERED

Current Name	Previous Name
Chlamydia abortus	
Chlamydia trachomatis	
Chlamydia psittaci	*Chlamydophila psittaci*
Chlamydia pneumoniae	*Chlamydophila pneumoniae*
Rickettsia rickettsii	
Rickettsia parkeri	
Rickettsia prowazekii	
Rickettsia typhi	
Rickettsia spp.	
Orientia tsutsugamushi	
Ehrlichia chaffeensis	
Anaplasma phagocytophilum	*Ehrlichia phagocytophila, Ehrlichia equi*, and human granulocytic ehrlichiosis agent
"*Candidatus neoehrlichia mikurensis*"	Newly proposed genus and species
Neorickettsia sennetsu	*Ehrlichia sennetsu*
Coxiella burnetii	
Tropheryma whipplei	
Klebsiella granulomatis	*Calymmatobacterium granulomatis*

Organisms addressed in this chapter are obligate intracellular bacteria and considered either extremely difficult to culture or unable to be cultured. Organisms of the genera *Chlamydia, Rickettsia, Orientia, Anaplasma,* and *Ehrlichia* are prokaryotes that differ from most other bacteria with respect to their very small size and obligate intracellular development cycles. Three other organisms, *Coxiella, Klebsiella granulomatis,* and *Tropheryma whipplei,* are discussed in this chapter because they are difficult to cultivate or are nonculturable.

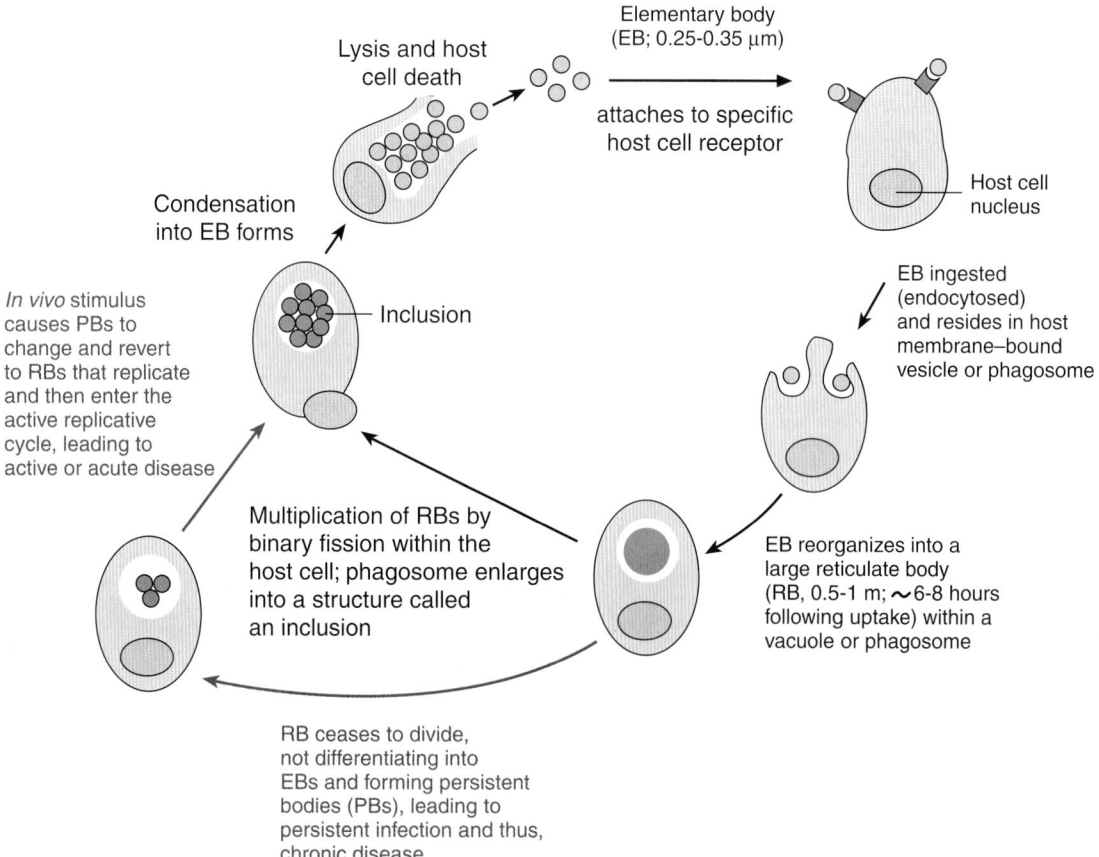

• **Fig. 43.1** The life cycle of chlamydiae. The entire cycle takes approximately 48 to 72 hours.

Chlamydia

The *Chlamydia* spp. are members of the order Chlamydiales and the family *Chlamydiaceae.* Members of the order Chlamydiales are obligate intracellular bacteria once regarded as viruses because, like viruses, the chlamydiae require biochemical resources of eukaryotic host cells such as adenosine triphosphate to fuel intracellular growth and replication. *Chlamydia* spp. are similar to gram-negative bacilli in that they have lipopolysaccharide (LPS) as a component of the cell wall. However, the chlamydial LPS has little endotoxic activity. Chlamydiae have a major outer membrane protein (MOMP) that is antigenically diverse in *Chlamydia trachomatis* yet highly conserved in *Chlamydia pneumoniae.* MOMP variation in *C. trachomatis* is used to separate the species into 15 antigenically distinct serovars, designated A through L.

Chlamydiae have a unique developmental cycle characterized by an intracellular, replicative form, known as the **reticulate body (RB),** and a metabolically inert, infective form, known as the **elementary body (EB).** Upon infection of a host cell, the EB differentiates into an RB. The RB divides by binary fission within a vacuole. As the number of RBs increase, the vacuole expands, forming an intracytoplasmic inclusion. The RBs differentiate into EBs, and 48 to 72 hours postinfection, the EBs are released from the host cell (Fig. 43.1). In addition to the replicative cycle associated with acute chlamydial infections, there is evidence that *Chlamydia* can persist in an aberrant form *in vitro,* depending on the amount of interferon-gamma (IFN-γ) and tryptophan in the host cell, as well as function of the tryptophan synthase encoded by the organism. Removal of IFN-γ or increase in tryptophan will result in differentiation of chlamydiae into an active EB infection. Therapeutic implications of this persistence *in vivo* have not yet been completely defined. Evidence suggests that activity of the tryptophan synthase gene in *C. trachomatis* differs between isolates recovered from the eye versus the genital tract.

C. trachomatis, C. pneumoniae, and *Chlamydia psittaci* are important causes of human infection; *C. psittaci* and *Chlamydia pecorum* are common pathogens among animals. *Chlamydia abortus* is associated with spontaneous abortion and fetal loss in sheep and calves. There are reports of pregnant women who have experienced spontaneous abortions after exposure to animals infected with *C. abortus.* The three major species that infect humans differ with respect to their antigens, host cell preference, antibiotic susceptibility, EB morphology, and inclusion morphology (Table 43.1).

Chlamydia trachomatis

Over the past few decades, the importance of both acute and chronic infections caused by *C. trachomatis* has been recognized. *C. trachomatis* infections are often associated

TABLE 43.1 Differential Characteristics Among Chlamydiae That Cause Human Disease

Property	Chlamydia trachomatis	Chlamydia psittaci	Chlamydia pneumoniae
Host range	Humans (except one biovar that causes mouse pneumonitis)	Birds, lower mammals, humans (rare)	Humans
Elementary body morphology	Round	Round	Pear-shaped
Inclusion morphology	Round, vacuolar	Variable, dense	Round, dense
Glycogen-containing inclusions	Yes	No	No
Plasmid DNA	Yes	Yes	No
Susceptibility to sulfonamides	Yes	No	No

DNA, Deoxyribonucleic acid.

TABLE 43.2 Primary Syndromes Caused by *Chlamydia trachomatis*

Serovars	Clinical Syndrome	Route(s) of Transmission
A, B, Ba, C	Endemic trachoma (multiple or persistent infections that ultimately lead to blindness)	Hand to eye from fomites, flies
L1, L2, L3	Lymphogranuloma venereum	Sexual
D–K	Urethritis, cervicitis, pelvic inflammatory disease, epididymitis, infant pneumonia, and conjunctivitis (does not lead to blindness)	Sexual, hand to eye by autoinoculation of genital secretions; eye to eye by infected secretions; neonatal

with infertility and ectopic pregnancy, and frequently these infections are asymptomatic, which facilitates transmission and contributes to increased prevalence.

General Characteristics

C. trachomatis infects humans almost exclusively and is responsible for various clinical syndromes. Based on MOMP antigenic differences, *C. trachomatis* is divided into 15 different serovars associated with different primary clinical syndromes (Table 43.2).

Epidemiology and Pathogenesis

C. trachomatis causes significant infection and disease worldwide. In the United States, *C. trachomatis* is the most common sexually transmitted bacterial pathogen and a major cause of pelvic inflammatory disease (PID), ectopic pregnancy, and infertility (see Chapters 39 and 73 for more information on PID). An estimated 3 million cases of *C. trachomatis* infection occur annually in the United States. In 2017, more than 1.7 million cases of *C. trachomatis* infection were reported to the Centers for Disease Control and Prevention (CDC) from 50 states and the District of Columbia. However, the CDC estimates as many as 2.86 million cases of chlamydia occur annually. Genital tract infections caused by *C. trachomatis* were identified more frequently in females 14 and 24 years of age; the CDC estimates that 1 in 20 sexually active women in this age group have chlamydia.

However, it is important to note that data reported to the CDC, especially with regard to *Chlamydia,* come as a result of screening programs that primarily target females between the ages of 15 and 24 years. In addition to young women, the CDC notes disparity in chlamydia infection according to race and ethnicity. Non-Hispanic blacks are 5.6 times more likely to be infected with chlamydia compared with non-Hispanic whites. Rectal and pharyngeal chlamydial infections disproportionately impact men who have sex with men (MSM).

Ocular trachoma is the leading infectious cause of blindness worldwide, with an estimated 84 million cases resulting in blindness for 7 to 9 million. Remote rural areas of Africa, Asia, Central and South America, Australia, and the Middle East are hyperendemic for trachoma, where the prevalence rate of *C. trachomatis* is 60% to 90% in preschool children. Trachoma causes 3% of the cases of blindness in individuals around the world, with females more likely to be affected as a result of their exposure to children, who serve as the major reservoir of the organism.

C. trachomatis infections are primarily transmitted from human to human by direct contact with infected secretions. Some infections, such as neonatal pneumonia or **inclusion conjunctivitis,** are transmitted from mother to infant during birth. The various routes of transmission for *C. trachomatis* infection are summarized in Table 43.2. The natural habitat of *C. trachomatis* is humans. The mechanisms by which

C. trachomatis causes inflammation and tissue destruction is not completely understood. The chlamydiae can infect a variety of different cells, including epithelial cells of the mucosa and blood vessels, smooth muscle cells, and monocytes. The chlamydial EB is phagocytosed into a host cell and resides in a vacuole that fails to fuse with a lysosome. This leads to the intracellular persistence of the organism and escape from the host immune response. Chlamydiae are able to either turn on or turn off apoptosis (programmed cell death pathways) in infected host cells. By inducing host cell death, the organism facilitates its transmission to neighboring host cells and downregulating inflammation in the acute disease process, whereas, by inhibiting apoptosis, the organism keeps the host cell alive, allowing for sustained survival in chronic infections.

The host's immune response accounts for the majority of the tissue destruction after infection with *C. trachomatis.* Infected epithelial cells secrete proinflammatory cytokines including interleukin (IL)-1α, tumor necrosis factor (TNF), and IL-6. Quickly upon infection, neutrophils and monocytes migrate to the mucosa and eliminate exposed EBs. Later, CD4 T helper cells migrate to the site of infection. Responding neutrophils and T helper cells release cytokines, resulting in the influx of additional immune cells. The importance of multiple, recurrent infections with *C. trachomatis* are associated with the development of ocular trachoma. Immunity provides little protection from reinfection and appears to be short lived after infection with *C. trachomatis.*

Spectrum of Disease

As previously mentioned, infection with different *C. trachomatis* serovars can lead to several clinical diseases. The diseases are summarized in Table 43.2.

Trachoma

Trachoma results from chronic inflammation of the conjunctiva and remains a major cause of preventable blindness worldwide. The organism is acquired through contact with infected secretions on towels or fingers or by flies. Early symptoms of infection include mild irritation and itching of the eyes and eyelids. There may also be some discharge from the infected eye. The infection progresses slowly with increasing eye pain, blurred vision, and photophobia. Repeated infections result in scarring of the inner eyelid that may then turn the eyelid in toward the eye (**entropion**). As the inner eyelid continues to turn in, the eyelashes follow (**trichiasis**), resulting in rubbing and scratching of the cornea. The combined effects of the mechanical damage to the cornea and inflammation result in ulceration, scarring, and loss of vision.

Lymphogranuloma Venereum

Lymphogranuloma venereum (LGV) is a sexually transmitted disease rarely identified in North America but is relatively frequent in Africa, Asia, and South America. It is reemerging in Europe, especially in homosexual males.

In contrast to serovars A through K, which also cause sexually transmitted infections, *C. trachomatis* serovars L1, L2, L2b, and L3 are invasive, leading to regional lymphadenopathy. The disease is characterized by a brief appearance of a primary genital lesion at the initial infection site. This lesion is often small and may be unrecognized, especially by female patients. The second stage, acute lymphadenitis, often involves the inguinal lymph nodes, causing them to enlarge and become matted together, forming a large area of groin swelling, or **bubo.** During this stage, infection may become systemic and cause fever or may spread locally, causing granulomatous proctitis. Advanced disease, which is more common in females than males, can result in genital hyperplasia, rectal fistulas, rectal stricture, draining sinuses, and other manifestations.

Oculogenital Infections

C. trachomatis can cause acute inclusion conjunctivitis in adults and newborns. The organism is acquired when contaminated genital secretions get into the eyes such as during passage of the neonate through the birth canal. Autoinfection rarely occurs. The organism can be acquired from swimming pools and poorly chlorinated hot tubs or by sharing eye makeup. Inclusion conjunctivitis is associated with swollen eyes and a purulent discharge. In contrast to trachoma, inclusion conjunctivitis does not lead to blindness in adults (or newborns).

Genital tract infections caused by *C. trachomatis* have surpassed gonococcal *(Neisseria gonorrhoeae)* infections as a top cause of sexually transmitted disease in the United States. Similar to gonococci, *C. trachomatis* causes urethritis, cervicitis, bartholinitis (Bartholin glands or greater vestibular glands), proctitis, salpingitis (infection of the fallopian tubes), epididymitis, and acute urethral syndrome in females. In the United States, 60% of cases of nongonococcal urethritis are caused by chlamydiae. Both chlamydiae and gonococci are major causes of PID, contributing significantly to the rising rate of infertility and ectopic pregnancies in young women. After a single episode of PID, as many as 10% of women may become infertile because of tubal occlusion. The risk increases dramatically with each additional episode.

Many genital chlamydial infections in both sexes are asymptomatic or not easily recognized by clinical criteria; asymptomatic carriage in both males and females may persist, often for months. As many as 50% of males and 70% to 80% of females identified as having chlamydial genital tract infections have no symptoms. Of significance, these asymptomatic infected individuals serve as a large reservoir to sustain transmission of the organism within a community.

When symptomatic, patients with a genital chlamydial infection will have an unusual discharge and pain or a burning sensation, symptoms similar to those for gonorrhea.

Perinatal Infections

Approximately one-fourth to one-half of infants born to females infected with *C. trachomatis* develop inclusion conjunctivitis. Usually, the incubation period is 5 to 12 days after birth, but it may be as long as 6 weeks. Although most develop inclusion conjunctivitis, approximately 10% to 20% of infants develop pneumonia. Perinatal-acquired *C. trachomatis* infection may persist in the nasopharynx, urogenital tract, or rectum for more than 2 years.

Laboratory Diagnosis

C. trachomatis is commonly diagnosed by nucleic acid amplification tests (NAATs). Additional diagnostic methods for *C. trachomatis* infection include cytology, culture, direct detection of antigen, and serologic testing.

Specimen Collection and Transport

The organism can be recovered or detected in infected cells of the urethra, cervix, conjunctiva, nasopharynx, rectum, and material aspirated from the fallopian tubes and epididymis. The endocervix is the preferred anatomic site to collect screening specimens from female patients. The specimen for *C. trachomatis* culture should be collected after all other specimens (e.g., those for Gram-stained smear, *N. gonorrhoeae* culture, or Papanicolaou [Pap] smear). A large swab should be used to remove all secretions from the cervix. The swab supplied or specified by the manufacturer should be used for nonculture tests. The swab or endocervical brush is inserted 1 to 2 cm into the endocervical canal, rotated against the wall for 10 to 30 seconds, withdrawn without touching any vaginal surfaces, and placed in the appropriate transport medium or applied to a slide prepared for direct fluorescent antibody (DFA) testing.

Urethral specimens should not be collected until 2 hours after the patient has voided. A urogenital swab is gently inserted into the urethra (females, 1 to 2 cm; males, 2 to 4 cm), rotated at least once for 5 seconds, and then withdrawn. Swabs should be placed into the appropriate transport medium or onto a slide prepared for DFA testing. Screening of rectal or pharyngeal specimens for *C. trachomatis* by nucleic acid tests has proven useful in homosexual male patients. Urine specimens in appropriate transport media provided by manufacturers of nucleic acid testing methodologies are also available for both male and female patients. Because chlamydiae are relatively labile, viability can be maintained by keeping specimens cold and minimizing transport time to the laboratory. Specimens should be submitted in a chlamydial transport medium such as 2SP (0.2 M sucrose-phosphate transport medium with antibiotics); a number of commercial transport media are available. Specimens should be refrigerated upon receipt, and if the specimen cannot be processed for culture within 24 hours, they should be frozen at −70°C.

Direct Detection Methods

Cytologic Examination. Cytologic examination of cell scrapings from the conjunctiva of newborns or persons with ocular trachoma can be used to detect *C. trachomatis* inclusions, usually after Giemsa staining. Cytology has been used to evaluate endocervical and urethral scrapings, including those obtained for Pap smears. However, this method is insensitive

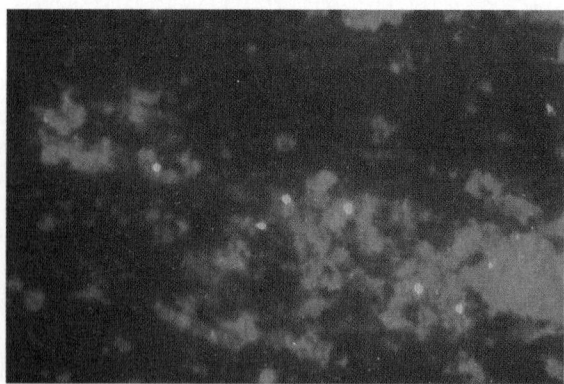

• **Fig. 43.2** Appearance of fluorescein-conjugated, monoclonal antibody–stained elementary bodies in direct smear of urethral cell scraping from a patient with chlamydial urethritis. (Courtesy Syva Co, San Jose, CA.)

compared with culture or other methods discussed in the following sections.

Antigen Detection. Fluorescent monoclonal specific antibody antigen detection of *C. trachomatis* species-specific outer membrane proteins makes it possible to detect the organism within 30 minutes. These methods can be used to identify the organism in inclusion conjunctivitis in infants. DFA staining methods use fluorescein-isothiocyanate–conjugated monoclonal antibodies to either MOMP or LPS of *C. trachomatis* to detect EBs in smears of clinical material (Fig. 43.2). The sensitivity and specificity of DFA are similar to those of culture. Chlamydial antigen can be detected by enzyme immunoassays (EIAs). Numerous US Food and Drug Administration (FDA)-approved kits are commercially available. These assays use polyclonal or monoclonal antibodies that detect chlamydial LPS. These tests are not species-specific for *C. trachomatis* and may cross-react with LPS of other bacterial species present in the vagina or urinary tract and thereby produce a false-positive result.

Nucleic Acid Detection. FDA-approved NAATs for the laboratory diagnosis of *C. trachomatis* infection use three different formats: polymerase chain reaction (PCR), strand displacement amplification (SDA), and transcription-mediated amplification (TMA). The first two assay formats amplify DNA sequences present in the cryptic plasmid that is present in 7 to 10 copies in the chlamydial EB, whereas the last format amplifies 23s ribosomal RNA (rRNA) sequences. Studies clearly indicate that NAATs are more sensitive than culture and other non–nucleic acid amplification assays. Because of the increased sensitivity of detection, first-voided urine specimens from symptomatic and asymptomatic males and females are acceptable specimens to detect *C. trachomatis,* thereby affording a noninvasive means of chlamydia testing. NAATs are the preferred methodology for detecting *C. trachomatis* in most clinical situations because of increased sensitivity, ease of specimen collection, and the availability of automated high-volume methods. Table 43.3 summarizes the possible uses of the different methodologies available for the detection of *C. trachomatis;* however,

NAATs are used almost exclusively for the laboratory detection of *C. trachomatis.*

Serodiagnosis

Serologic testing has limited value for diagnosis of urogenital infections in adults. Serology can be used to diagnose LGV. Antibodies to a genus-specific antigen can be detected by complement fixation (CF), and a single-point titer greater than 1:64 is indicative of LGV. This test is not useful in diagnosing trachoma, inclusion conjunctivitis, or neonatal infections. The microimmunofluorescence assay (micro-IF), a tedious and difficult test, is used for type-specific antibodies of *C. trachomatis* and can be used to diagnose LGV. A high titer of immunoglobulin M (IgM) (1:32) suggests a recent infection; however, not all patients produce IgM. In contrast to CF, micro-IF may be used to diagnose trachoma and inclusion conjunctivitis using acute and convalescent phase sera. Detection of *C. trachomatis*–specific IgM is useful in the diagnosis of neonatal infections. Negative serology can reliably exclude chlamydial infection.

Based on numerous studies, these culture-independent tests are more reliable for the detection of infection in patients who are symptomatic and shedding large numbers of organisms than in those who are asymptomatic and most likely shedding fewer organisms. For the most part, these assays have sensitivities of greater than 70% and specificities of 97% to 99% in populations with a prevalence of *C. trachomatis* infection of 5% or more. In a low-prevalence population (i.e., less than 5%), a significant proportion of positive tests will be falsely positive. A positive result in a low-prevalence population should be handled with care, and a positive result should be verified. Positive results can be validated by the following methods:

- Culture
- Performing a second culture-independent test that identifies a *C. trachomatis* antigen or nucleic acid sequence that is different from that used in the screening test
- Using a blocking antibody or competitive probe that verifies a positive test result by preventing attachment of a labeled antibody or probe used in the standard assay

Cultivation

Culture-independent methods for the diagnosis of *C. trachomatis* are frequently compared with culture. However, culture is not performed as frequently, with NAAT used almost exclusively for genital tract infections.

Several eukaryotic cell lines can be used to culture *C. trachomatis,* including cycloheximide-treated McCoy, HeLa, and monkey kidney cells. After shaking the clinical specimens with 5-mm glass beads, centrifugation of the specimen onto the cell monolayer (usually growing on a coverslip in the bottom of a vial, commonly called a **"shell vial"**) facilitates adherence of EBs. After 48 to 72 hours of incubation, monolayers are stained with a fluorescein-labeled monoclonal antibody that is either species specific, targeting the MOMP of *C. trachomatis,* or genus specific, targeting the LPS. The monolayers are examined microscopically for inclusion formation.

TABLE 43.3	Use of Different Laboratory Tests to Diagnose *Chlamydia trachomatis* Infections	
Patient Population	**Specimen Type**	**Acceptable Diagnostic Test**
Prepubertal girls	Vaginal	NAAT, culture
Neonates and infants	Nasopharyngeal	NAAT, culture, DFA
	Rectal	Culture
	Conjunctiva	Culture, DFA, EIA, NAAT
Women	Cervical	NAAT,[a] culture, DFA, EIA, NAH, NAAT
	Vaginal	NAAT[a]
	Urethral	NAAT, culture, DFA, EIA
	Urine	NAAT[a]
Children, women, and men	Rectal	Culture, DFA, NAAT[a]
Men	Urethral	NAAT[a] (DFA, EIA)
	Urine[b]	NAAT[a]

DFA, Direct fluorescent antibody staining; *EIA,* enzyme immunoassay; *NAAT,* nucleic acid amplification test; *NAH,* nucleic acid hybridization.
[a]Must be confirmed in a population with a low prevalence (<5%) of *C. trachomatis* infection.
[b]EIA can be used on urine from symptomatic men but not on urine from older men. A positive result must be confirmed in a population with a low prevalence of *C. trachomatis* infection.

Iodine can be used to detect inclusions but is less specific and not recommended.

Although culture specificity approaches 100%, the sensitivity of culture is estimated at between 70% and 90% in experienced laboratories. Limitations of *Chlamydia* culture contributing to the lack of sensitivity include prerequisites to maintain viability of patient specimens by either rapid or frozen transport and to ensure the quality of the specimen submitted for testing (i.e., endocervical specimens devoid of mucus and containing endocervical epithelial or metaplastic cells or urethral epithelial cells). In addition, successful culture requires a sensitive cell culture system and a minimum of at least 2 days turnaround time between specimen receipt and the availability of results. Despite these limitations, culture is still recommended as the method of choice in some situations (Table 43.3). As of this writing, only chlamydia cultures should be used in situations with legal implications (e.g., sexual abuse), when the possibility of a false-positive test is unacceptable. However, local and state requirements may vary.

Antibiotic Susceptibility Testing and Therapy

Because *C. trachomatis* is an obligate intracellular bacterium, susceptibility testing is not practical in the routine clinical microbiology laboratory setting and is performed in only a few laboratories. In addition, no standardized *in vitro* assay or an understanding of the relationship between *in vitro* test results and clinical outcome after treatment exist. Antibiotics typically used in infections with *C. trachomatis* include azithromycin, doxycycline, erythromycin and other macrolide antibiotics, tetracyclines, and fluoroquinolones.

Prevention

Because no effective vaccines are available, strategies to prevent chlamydial urogenital infections focus on trying to manifest behavioral changes. By identifying and treating individuals with genital chlamydia before infection is transmitted to sexual partners or from pregnant females to babies, the risk of acquiring or transmitting infection may be significantly decreased.

Chlamydia psittaci

Although members of this chlamydial species are common in birds and domestic animals, infections in humans are relatively uncommon.

General Characteristics

C. psittaci differs from *C. trachomatis* in that it is sulfonamide resistant and in the morphology of its EBs and inclusion bodies (Table 43.1).

Epidemiology and Pathogenesis

C. psittaci is an endemic pathogen of all bird species. Psittacine birds (e.g., parrots, parakeets) are a major reservoir for human disease, but outbreaks have occurred among turkey-processing workers and pigeon aficionados. The birds may show diarrheal illness or may be asymptomatic. Humans acquire the disease by inhalation of aerosols. The organisms are deposited in the alveoli; some are ingested by alveolar macrophages and carried to regional lymph nodes. From there they are disseminated systemically, growing within cells of the reticuloendothelial system. Human-to-human transmission is rare, thus obviating the need for isolating patients if admitted to the hospital.

Spectrum of Disease

Disease usually begins after an incubation period of 5 to 15 days. Onset may be insidious or abrupt. Clinical findings associated with this infection are diverse and include pneumonia, severe headache, mental status changes, and hepatosplenomegaly. The severity of infection ranges from unapparent or mild disease to a life-threatening systemic illness with significant respiratory problems.

Laboratory Diagnosis

Diagnosis of **psittacosis** is typically by serologic means. Because of hazards associated with working with the agent, only laboratories with Biosafety Level 3 biohazard containment facilities can culture *C. psittaci* safely. State health departments take an active role in consulting with clinicians about possible cases. CF and indirect immunofluorescence have been used to detect anti–*C. psittaci*

antibodies in patients with suspected psittacosis. Either a fourfold rise in titer between acute and convalescent serum samples or a single IgM titer of 1:32 or greater in a patient with an appropriate illness is considered diagnostic of an infection.

Finally, amplification of rRNA sequences using a PCR assay followed by restriction fragment length polymorphism (RFLP) is able to identify and distinguish all nine chlamydial species, including *C. psittaci*. There are no current commercially available nucleic acid–based tests for the diagnosis of *C. psittaci*.

Antibiotic Susceptibility Testing and Therapy

Because *C. psittaci* is an obligate intracellular pathogen and its incidence of infection is rare, susceptibility testing is not practical in the routine clinical microbiology laboratory. Tetracycline is the drug of choice for psittacosis. If left untreated, the fatality rate is approximately 20%.

Prevention

Disease is prevented by treating infected birds or by quarantining imported birds for a month.

Chlamydia pneumoniae

The TWAR strain of *C. pneumoniae* was first isolated from the conjunctiva of a child in Taiwan in 1965. It was initially considered a psittacosis strain because the inclusions produced in cell culture resembled those of *C. psittaci*. The Taiwan isolate (TW-183) is serologically related to a pharyngeal isolate (AR-39) isolated from a college student in the United States, and thus the new strain was called "TWAR," an acronym for TW and AR (acute respiratory). Only one serotype of *C. pneumoniae* has been identified.

General Characteristics

C. pneumoniae does not exhibit the antigenic diversity characteristic of *C. trachomatis* or *C. psittaci*; all *C. pneumoniae* isolates tested to date are immunologically similar based on MOMP homogeneity. One significant difference between *C. pneumoniae* and the other chlamydiae is the pear-shaped appearance of its EBs (Fig. 43.3).

Epidemiology and Pathogenesis

C. pneumoniae appears to be a strict human pathogen; there are no documented bird or animal reservoirs. The pathogen is transmitted from person to person by aerosolized droplets via the respiratory route. Although the spread of infection is low, antibody prevalence starts to rise in school-aged children and reaches 30% to 45% in adolescents. By adulthood, more than half of adults in the United States are seropositive for *C. pneumoniae* antibodies. Of interest, *C. pneumoniae* infections are both endemic and epidemic. Unfortunately, little is known about the pathogenesis of *C. pneumoniae* infections. However, *C. pneumoniae* infection is similar to *C. trachomatis* in that both infections elicit an inflammatory response that contributes to tissue damage.

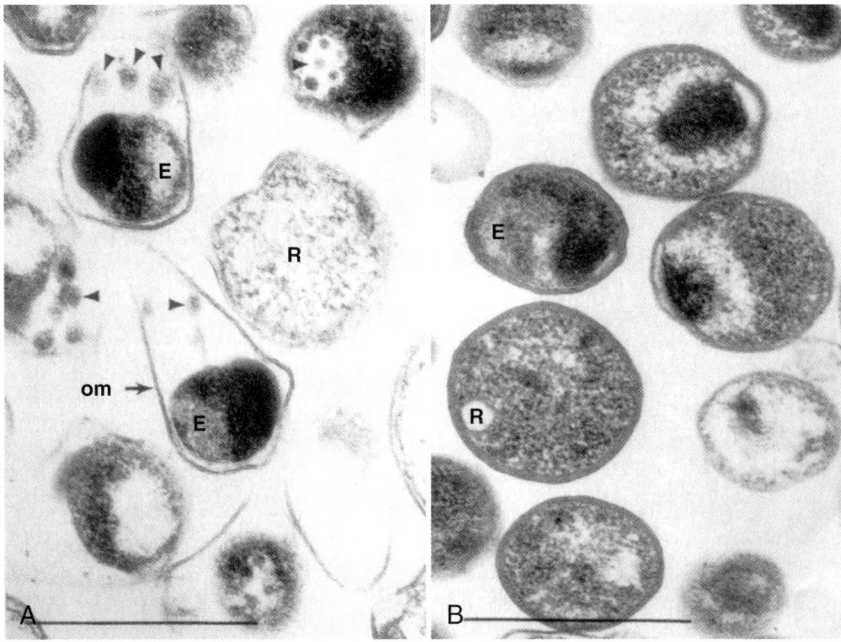

• **Fig. 43.3** Electron micrograph of *Chlamydia pneumoniae* (A) and *Chlamydia trachomatis* (B) (bar = 50.5 μm), *E*, Elementary body; *om*, outer membrane; *R*, reticulate body; *arrowhead*, small electron-dense bodies of undetermined function. (From Grayston JT, Kuo C-C, Campbell La, Wang S-P. *Chlamydia pneumoniae* sp. nov. for *Chlamydia* sp. strain TWAR. *Int J Syst Bacteriol.* 1989;39:88.)

Spectrum of Disease

C. pneumoniae has been associated with pneumonia, bronchitis, pharyngitis, sinusitis, and a flulike illness. It causes 5% to 10% of cases of community-acquired pneumonia. Infection in young adults is usually mild to moderate. The primary differential diagnosis of infectious origin is *Mycoplasma pneumoniae*. Severe pneumonia may occur in older or respiratory-compromised patients. Of note, asymptomatic infection or unrecognized, mild symptomatic illnesses caused by *C. pneumoniae* are common. In addition, an association exists between *C. pneumoniae* infection and the development of asthmatic symptoms. Finally, an association between coronary artery disease and other atherosclerotic syndromes and *C. pneumoniae* infection has been suggested by seroepidemiologic studies. The organism has been identified in atheromatous plaques, yellow deposits within arteries containing cholesterol and other lipid material. This etiologic role by this organism has been questioned and is still under intense scrutiny. An excellent and comprehensive review of the literature related to whether *C. pneumoniae* is a cause of atherosclerosis was published in 2008 by Watson and Alp. Their research indicated, "it is difficult to attribute causality to a common infectious agent in a highly prevalent multifactorial disease." They also stated that "*C. pneumoniae* is neither alone sufficient nor is it necessary to cause atherosclerosis or its clinical consequences in humans," but they allowed for the possibility that treatment of *C. pneumoniae* may reduce the risk of atherosclerosis development.

Laboratory Diagnosis

In the laboratory, *C. pneumoniae* infections are diagnosed using cell culture, serology, or NAAT methods.

Direct Detection Methods

Assays that directly detect *C. pneumoniae* antigens have poor sensitivity. A variety of NAATs, including conventional and real-time PCR assays, have been developed to detect *C. pneumoniae* in clinical specimens. Several of these amplification assays are commercially available, including at least on nested multiplex PCR test. NAATs have been used to detect *C. pneumoniae* in throat swabs and other specimens, such as nasopharyngeal, bronchoalveolar lavage fluids, and sputum.

Serodiagnosis

C. pneumoniae infection can also be diagnosed using serology. However, serologic testing has had variable success and questionable validity. CF using a genus-specific antigen is not specific for *C. pneumoniae*. A micro-IF test using *C. pneumoniae* EBs as antigen is more reliable. However, availability is limited to specialized laboratories. A four-fold rise in either IgG or IgM is diagnostic, and a single IgM titer of 16 or greater or an IgG titer of 512 or greater suggests recent infection

Cultivation

Specimens for isolation are usually swabs of the oropharynx; techniques for isolation of the organism from sputum are unsatisfactory. Swabs should be placed into chlamydial transport media, transported on ice, and stored at 4°C. Organisms are rapidly inactivated at room temperature or by rapid freezing or thawing. A cell culture procedure similar to *C. trachomatis* is available, but more sensitive HL or Hep-2 cell lines are often substituted for McCoy cells. Multiple blind passages might be necessary to improve recovery rates. *C. pneumoniae* species-specific monoclonal antibodies can detect the organism in cell culture.

Antibiotic Susceptibility Testing and Therapy

Methods for susceptibility testing of *C. pneumoniae* have been largely adapted from those used for *C. trachomatis.* Similar to *C. trachomatis,* susceptibility testing is not practical for the clinical microbiology laboratory, and the methods are not standardized. Treatment with tetracycline, doxycycline, macrolides, fluoroquinolones, and erythromycin has been successful.

Prevention

Little is known regarding effective ways to prevent *C. pneumoniae* infections beyond standard respiratory precautions.

Rickettsia, Orientia, Anaplasma, and Ehrlichia

The rickettsias and rickettsia-like organisms are members of two families: the *Rickettsiaceae* (*Rickettsia* and *Orientia tsutsugamushi*) and the *Anaplasmataceae* (*Ehrlichia, Anaplasma,* and *Neorickettsia*). *O. tsutsugamushi* (formerly called *Rickettsia tsutsugamushi*) was placed into its own genus primarily based on the lack of LPS, the presence of a 54- to 58-kDa major surface protein, and the lack of a 17-kDa lipoprotein, all of which make it different from the other species of *Rickettsia*. "*Candidatus neoehrlichia mikurensis*" is a new bacterium that is present in *Ixodes* ticks and has been documented in human infections.

Coxiella and *Bartonella,* two other genera of intracellular bacteria that cause human disease, were at one time included in the *Rickettsiaceae* family. However, based on phylogenetic differences, these two genera were removed from the *Rickettsiaceae* family and separated into two families, *Coxiellaceae* and *Bartonellaceae*. *Bartonella* spp. can be cultured on standard bacteriologic media; this group of organisms is discussed in Chapter 32. Because *Coxiella burnetii* can survive extracellularly, unlike the rickettsiae, yet requires cultivation in cell culture similar to the rickettsiae, this organism is discussed separately in this chapter.

General Characteristics

Rickettsiaceae and *Anaplasmataceae* are obligate, intracellular parasites. These bacterial agents survive briefly outside of a host (reservoir or vector) and multiply only intracellularly. Organisms are small (0.3 μm × 1 to 2 μm), pleomorphic, gram-negative bacilli that multiply by binary fission in the cytoplasm of host cells; the release of bacteria results in the lysis of the host cell.

Epidemiology and Pathogenesis

Rickettsiaceae and *Anaplasmataceae* are arthropod-borne pathogens typically spread by ticks, fleas, or lice. These pathogens principally infect animals, but humans can become accidental hosts if bitten by an infected arthropod. Human infection can also occur by inhalation of infectious aerosols. Characteristics, including the respective arthropod vector of the prominent species of *Rickettsia, Orientia, Anaplasma,* and *Ehrlichia,* are summarized in Table 43.4.

Members of the genus *Rickettsia* share genetic and antigenic properties that result in similar mechanisms of host cell infection and pathogenesis. The infection process typically begins with the introduction of rickettsiae into the host bloodstream following a bite by an arthropod vector. Rickettsiae then bind to endothelial cells lining the blood vessel wall. Endothelial cells engulf the bacteria, which results in the formation of a protective vacuolar niche in the host cell cytoplasm. The bacterium then escapes the vacuole and enters the host cell cytoplasm, where the bacterium multiplies, ultimately leading to cell injury and death. Subsequent vascular lesions caused by *Rickettsia*-induced damage to endothelial cells account for the changes that occur throughout the body, particularly in the skin, heart, brain, lung, and muscle. Rickettsiae also have numerous ways to evade human host defenses such as cell-to-cell spread, escaping from the phagosome, and entering into a latent state (primarily *Rickettsia prowazekii*).

Members of the family Anaplasmataceae, principally *Ehrlichia* and *Anaplasma,* are also obligate intracellular parasites. Similar to other obligate intracellular parasites, these pathogens have reduced viability outside host cells and, once released, must rapidly induce signals for their own uptake into another host cell that is unique to each genus. *Ehrlichia chaffeensis* primarily infects monocytes and causes **human monocytic ehrlichiosis (HME),** whereas *A. phagocytophilum* infects bone marrow–derived cells, primarily infecting neutrophils, causing **human granulocytic anaplasmosis (HGA).**

Candidatus neoehrlichiamikurensis is transmitted by ticks. The reservoir appears to be small mammals such as field mice and voles found in Europe and Asia. Cases have been reported predominantly in immunocompromised patients in Europe and immunocompetent patients in China.

Spectrum of Disease

Rickettsiaceae are divided into three groups: the spotted fever group, the typhus group, and the scrub typhus group (*O. tsutsugamushi),* based on the arthropod mode of transmission, clinical manifestations, rate of intracellular growth,

TABLE 43.4   Characteristics of *Rickettsia, Orientia, Anaplasma,* and *Ehrlichia* spp.

Agent	Disease	Vector	Distribution	Diagnostic Tests
Spotted Fever Group				
Rickettsia africae	African tick bite fever	Ticks	Sub-Saharan Africa, Caribbean	NAAT
Rickettsia conorii	Mediterranean and Israeli spotted fevers; Indian tick typhus; Kenya tick typhus	Ticks	Southern Europe, Middle East, Africa	Serology, immunohistology, NAAT
Rickettsia heilongjiangensis	Far Eastern tick-borne rickettsiosis	Ticks	Russia	NAAT
Rickettsia honei	Flinders Island spotted fever	Ticks	Australia and Thailand	NAAT and serology
Rickettsia japonica	Japanese spotted fever	Ticks	Japan and Korea	NAAT
Rickettsia rickettsii	Rocky Mountain spotted fever	Ticks (*Dermacentor* spp.)	North and South America; particularly in southeastern states and Oklahoma in the United States	Serology, immunohistology, NAAT
Rickettsia parkeri	Mild illness with no reported fatalities	Ticks	North and South America	Serology, immunohistochemical, NAAT
Rickettsia sibirica	North Asian tick typhus, lymphangitis-associated rickettsiosis	Ticks	Asia, Europe, and Africa	NAAT
Rickettsia slovaca	Tick-borne lymphadenopathy	Ticks	Eurasia	NAAT, serologic, and culture
Typhus Group				
Rickettsia prowazekii	Epidemic typhus	Lice	Worldwide	Serology, PCR, or RFLP
	Brill-Zinsser disease	None; recrudescent disease	Worldwide	Serology, PCR, or RFLP
Rickettsia typhi	Murine typhus	Fleas	Worldwide	Serology, PCR, or RFLP
Scrub Typhus Group				
Orientia tsutsugamushi	Scrub typhus	Chiggers	South and Southeast Asia, South Pacific	Serology, conventional or nested PCR
Ehrlichia/Anaplasma/Neorickettsia				
Ehrlichia chaffeensis	Human monocytic ehrlichiosis	Ticks (*Amblyomma americanum*—Lone Star tick)	Southeast, South Central, and mid-Atlantic United States	Serology, PCR, immunohistology, immunocytology
Ehrlichia ewingii		Ticks (*Amblyomma americanum*—Lone Star tick)	United States (overlapping with *E. chaffeensis*)	PCR with species-specific primers
Anaplasma	Human granulocytic anaplasmosis	Ticks (*Ixodes* spp.)	United States, Europe	Serology, PCR, immunohistology, phagocytophilum peripheral blood smear, immunocytology
Neorickettsia sennetsu	Sennetsu fever	Ticks	Southeast Asia (primarily Japan)	Serology

NAAT, Nucleic acid amplification tests; *PCR,* polymerase chain reaction; *RFLP,* restriction fragment length polymorphism.

rate of intracellular burden, and extent of intracellular growth (Table 43.4). *Rickettsiaceae* are often suspected when the triad of fever, headache, and rash is the primary clinical manifestation in patients with an exposure to insect vectors. Infections caused by these organisms may be severe and are sometimes fatal.

Although HME and HGA cause distinct infections, their clinical findings are similar. In general, patients with ehrlichial infections present with nonspecific symptoms such as fever, headache, and myalgias; rashes occur only rarely. The illness can range from asymptomatic to mild to severe.

Laboratory Diagnosis

Because rickettsial and ehrlichial infections can be severe or even fatal, a timely diagnosis is essential.

Direct Detection Methods

Immunohistology and conventional and real-time PCR have been used to diagnose rickettsial and ehrlichial infections. Biopsy of skin tissue from the rash caused by the spotted fever group rickettsiae is the preferred specimen. Organisms are detected using polyclonal fluorescein-labeled antibodies or enzyme-labeled antibodies using indirect procedures. The sensitivity of these techniques is approximately 70% and depends on correct tissue sampling, examination of multiple tissue levels, and biopsy before or during the first 24 hours of therapy (Table 43.4).

Direct detection of *Ehrlichia* and *Anaplasma* from peripheral blood or cerebrospinal fluid (CSF) includes PCR amplification, direct microscopic examination of Giemsa-stained or Wright-stained specimens, or immunocytologic or immunohistologic stains with *E. chaffeensis* or *Anaplasma* species-specific antibodies. Direct microscopic examination of Giemsa-stained or Diff-Quik–stained peripheral blood buffy-coat smears can detect **morulae** (cytoplasmic vacuoles containing enriched organisms) during the febrile stage of infection in ehrlichiosis. Morulae-like structures also can be observed in CSF cells and tissues. Finally, recent reports have described the development of rapid, species-specific real-time PCR assays to detect single or coinfections with *Anaplasma* spp. or *Ehrlichia* spp. in peripheral blood specimens.

Serodiagnosis

Serodiagnosis is the primary method used for the identification of rickettsial disease and ehrlichiosis. Serologic assays for the diagnosis of rickettsial infections include the indirect immunofluorescence assay (IFA), EIA, *Proteus vulgaris* OX-19 and OX-2 and *Proteus mirabilis* OX-K strain agglutination (**Weil-Felix reaction**), line blot, and Western immunoblotting. The Weil-Felix

reaction (Evolve Procedure 43.1), the fortuitous agglutination of certain strains of *P. vulgaris* by serum from patients with rickettsial disease, may still be performed in developing countries, but because false-positive and false-negative tests are a continuing problem, these tests have been replaced by more accurate serologic methods such as IFA.

Except for latex agglutination, IFA, and DFA testing for diagnosing Rocky Mountain spotted fever (RMSF), no serologic test is useful for diagnosis of RMSF in time to influence therapy. Serologic diagnosis provides little clinical utility in the early stage of infection because antibodies to rickettsiae, other than *R. rickettsia,* cannot be reliably detected until at least 2 weeks following onset of symptoms. However, with new tests under development, the potential exists for improved serologic diagnosis of rickettsial diseases.

The sensitivity and specificity of serologic assays for ehrlichiosis remains unknown but are presumed to be relatively high; indirect immunofluorescent antibody testing is available for *E. chaffeensis* or *A. phagocytophilum.* A four-fold or greater rise in antibody titer during the course of disease is considered clinically significant.

Cultivation

Although the rickettsiae can be cultured in cell culture and embryonated eggs, the risk of laboratory-acquired infection is extremely high, limiting the availability of culture to a few specialized laboratories. Blood should be collected in a sterile, heparin-containing vial as early as possible following symptom onset. Similarly, punch biopsies of skin or eschars (slough or dead skin) are also acceptable but must be collected early in the course of disease. The same specimens are also acceptable for PCR.

Ehrlichia and *Anaplasma* cell culture conditions are not standardized and are not widely available. The preferred specimen for culture is peripheral blood obtained in a sterile, ethylenediaminetetraacetic acid (EDTA) or acid-citrate-dextrose (ACD) tube. If processing of specimens is delayed, they should be transported overnight at 4°C.

Antibiotic Susceptibility Testing and Therapy

Tetracyclines, especially doxycycline, are the primary drugs of choice for treatment of most infections caused by *Rickettsia, Ehrlichia,* or *Anaplasma* species. Depending on the specific species of *Rickettsia,* some fluoroquinolones or chloramphenicol have been used for successful treatment.

Prevention

The best means of preventing rickettsial and ehrlichial infection is to avoid contact with arthropod vectors.

Coxiella

C. burnetii is the causative agent of **Q fever,** an acute systemic infection that primarily affects the lungs.

General Characteristics

C. burnetii is smaller than *Rickettsia* spp. and is more resistant to various chemical and physical agents. Phylogenetic studies of this gram-negative coccobacillus have demonstrated that it is far removed from the rickettsiae and most closely related to *Legionella.* In contrast to the rickettsiae, *C. burnetii* can survive extracellularly and can only be cultured in lung cells. The organism has a sporelike life cycle and can exist in two antigenic states. When isolated from animals, *C. burnetii* is in phase I (**large-cell variant form**) and is highly infectious. In its phase II form (**small-cell variant**) the organism acts like a spore assisting in the extracellular survival of the organism. *C. burnetii* has been cultivated in cell lines and is not considered infectious in culture.

Epidemiology and Pathogenesis

The most common animal reservoirs for the zoonotic disease caused by *C. burnetii* are cattle, sheep, and goats. Organisms are shed in the urine, feces, milk, and birth products of infected animals. Usually, the infected animals are asymptomatic. Humans are infected through the inhalation of contaminated aerosols. Of significance, because of the resistance of the small-cell variant to desiccation and sunlight, *C. burnetii* is able to withstand harsh environmental conditions. Q fever is endemic worldwide except in New Zealand.

After infection, *C. burnetii* is phagocytized by host cells and multiplies within vacuoles. The incubation period is typically 2 to 4 weeks. After infection and proliferation in the lungs, organisms ingested by macrophages are carried to the lymph nodes and subsequently can disseminate hematogenously.

Spectrum of Disease

After the incubation period, initial clinical manifestations of *C. burnetii* infections are systemic and nonspecific: headache, fever, chills, and myalgias. In contrast to rickettsial infections, a rash does not develop. Both acute and chronic forms of the disease are recognized. The clinical manifestations are listed in Box 43.1.

Laboratory Diagnosis

Cultivation of *C. burnetii* must be performed in a Biosafety Level 3 containment facility to avoid laboratory-acquired infections. No laboratory-acquired infections have been documented with the use of a shell vial cultures. Shell vial cultures containing human lung fibroblasts can be inoculated with buffy coat or biopsy specimens for the isolation of *C. burnetii.* Once inoculated, cultures are incubated for 6 to 14 days at 37°C in carbon dioxide. The organism is

> **• BOX 43.1 Clinical Manifestations of *Coxiella burnetii* Infection**
>
> Febrile, self-limited illness
> Atypical pneumonia
> Granulomatous hepatitis
> Endocarditis
> Neurologic manifestations (e.g., encephalitis, meningoencephalitis)
> Osteomyelitis

detected using a direct immunofluorescent assay. Immunohistochemistry detection is useful for identification in cardiac valve tissues during chronic Q fever.

Nucleic acid amplification, PCR, is a useful technique for the diagnosis of Q fever. However, it is important that testing be performed within 4 weeks of symptom onset. Serology has been the most commonly used diagnostic tool. Three serologic techniques are available: IFA, CF, and EIA. IFA is considered the reference method for both acute and chronic Q fever. IFA is highly specific and sensitive and is recommended for its reliability, cost effectiveness, and ease of performance. Many reference and state health laboratories perform phase I and phase II IgG and IgM serologic assays. However, reports indicate that if completed early in the disease process, PCR provides a more sensitive diagnosis than serology.

Antibiotic Susceptibility Testing and Therapy

Because *C. burnetii* does not multiply in bacteriologic culture media, susceptibility testing is performed in a limited number of laboratories. Tetracyclines are recommended for the treatment of acute and chronic Q fever.

Prevention

The best way to prevent infection with *C. burnetii* is to avoid contact with infected animals. A vaccine is commercially available in Australia and Eastern European countries and under development in the United States.

Tropheryma whipplei

Although observed in diseased tissue, some organisms are nonculturable yet associated with specific disease processes, making the development of "traditional" diagnostic assays difficult (e.g., serology or antigen detection). With the ability to detect and classify bacteria using molecular techniques such as PCR to amplify ribosomal DNA sequences followed by sequencing and phylogenetic analysis, *T. whipplei* was identified as the causative agent of **Whipple disease.**

General Characteristics

Phylogenetic analysis shows that this organism is a gram-positive actinomycete not closely related to any other genus known to cause infection. The organism stains poorly with conventional Gram stain and is acid-fast negative.

Epidemiology, Pathogenesis, and Spectrum of Disease

Whipple disease, found primarily in middle-aged male patients, is characterized by the presence of periodic acid-Schiff (PAS)-staining macrophages (indicating mucopolysaccharide or glycoprotein) in almost every organ system. The bacillus is observed in macrophages and affected tissues, but it has never been cultured. Patients develop diarrhea, weight loss, arthralgia, lymphadenopathy, hyperpigmentation, often a long history of joint pain, and a distended and tender abdomen. Neurologic and sensory changes often occur. Although less common than intestinal or articular involvement, cardiac manifestations can also occur, including endocarditis. It has been suggested that a cellular immune defect is involved in the pathogenesis of this disease.

Colonization of healthy adults is well established by identification of the organism in stool and saliva of asymptomatic individuals. Additional specimens that may harbor the organism include dental plaque, intestinal biopsy tissue, and gastric juice.

Laboratory Diagnosis

Detection of *T. whipplei* is limited to a few laboratories using conventional and real-time PCR from any infected tissue or organ. Stool and saliva is used to screen and identify carriers. However, PCR should not be considered a definitive diagnosis because of the prevalence of carriage in otherwise healthy individuals.

Antibiotic Susceptibility Testing and Therapy

The organism is nonculturable, resulting in the inability to perform susceptibility testing. Patients usually respond well to long-term therapy with antibacterial agents, including trimethoprim-sulfamethoxazole, macrolides, aminoglycosides, tetracycline, and penicillin; however, tetracycline has been associated with serious relapses. Colchicine therapy appears to control symptoms. Without treatment, the disease is uniformly fatal.

Prevention

Little is known about the prevention of this disease.

Klebsiella granulomatis

K. granulomatis is the etiologic agent of **granuloma inguinale,** or **donovanosis,** a sexually transmitted disease.

General Characteristics

K. granulomatis is an encapsulated, pleomorphic, gram-negative bacillus that is usually observed in vacuoles in the cells of large mononuclear cells.

Epidemiology and Pathogenesis

Granuloma inguinale is uncommon in the United States but is recognized as a major cause of genital ulcers in India, Papua New Guinea, the Caribbean, Australia, and parts of South America. The causative agent is sexually transmitted, although there is a possibility that other modes of transmission may exist. Infectivity of this bacillus is presumed to be low, because sexual partners of infected patients often do not become infected or require repeated exposures to become infected.

Spectrum of Disease

Granuloma inguinale is characterized by the presence of enlarged subcutaneous nodules that evolve to form beefy, erythematous, granulomatous, painless lesions that bleed easily. The lesions, which usually occur on the genitalia, have been mistaken for neoplasms. Patients often have inguinal lymphadenopathy.

Laboratory Diagnosis

The organism can be visualized in scrapings of lesions stained with Wrights or Giemsa stain. Subsurface infected cells must be present; surface epithelium is not an adequate specimen. Groups of organisms can be seen within mononuclear endothelial cells and is referred to as a Donovan body. This pathognomonic characteristic of *K. granulomatis* is named after the physician who first visualized the organism in a lesion. The organism stains as a blue rod with prominent polar granules, giving rise to a "safety pin" appearance, surrounded by a large, pink capsule.

Cultivation *in vitro* is difficult, but it can be completed using media containing some of the growth factors found in egg yolk. More recently, this agent was cultured in human monocytes from biopsies of genital ulcers of patients with donovanosis.

Antibiotic Susceptibility Testing and Therapy

No antibiotic susceptibility testing is performed. Trimethoprim-sulfamethoxazole and doxycycline are the most effective drugs for the therapy of granuloma inguinale. Ciprofloxacin, azithromycin, or erythromycin (in pregnancy) also provide effective treatment for granuloma inguinale.

Ⓔ Visit the Evolve site for a complete list of procedures, review questions, and case studies.

Bibliography

Bastian I, Bowden FJ: Amplification of *Klebsiella*-like sequences from biopsy samples from patients with donovanosis, *Clin Infect Dis* 23:1328–1330, 1996.

Bristow CC, Morris SR, Little SJ, Mehta SR, Klausner JD: Meta-analysis of the Cepheid Xpert® CT/NG assay for extragenital detection of *Chlamydia trachomatis* (CT) and *Neisseria gonorrhoeae* (NG) infections, *Sex Health* 16(4):314–319, 2019. https://doi.org/10.1071/SH18079.

Carroll KC, Pfaller MA, Landry ML, et al.: *Manual of clinical microbiology*, ed 12, Washington, DC, 2019, ASM.

Centers for Disease Control and Prevention: Sexually transmitted diseases treatment guidelines, 2010, *MMWR Recomm Rep* 59(RR-12):1–110, 2010.

Chapman AS, Bakken JS, Folk SM, et al.: Diagnosis and management of tickborne rickettsial diseases: Rocky Mountain spotted fever, ehrlichioses, and anaplasmosis–United States, *MMWR Recomm Rep* 55(RR-4):1–27, 2006.

Cook RL, Hutchison SL, Østergaard L, Braithwaite RS, Ness RB: Systematic review: noninvasive testing for *Chlamydia trachomatis* and *Neisseria gonorrhoeae*, *Ann Intern Med* 142:914–925, 2005.

Darville T, Hiltke TJ: Pathogenesis of genital tract disease due to *Chlamydia trachomatis*, *J Infect Dis* 201(Suppl 2):S114–S125, 2010.

De Sousa R, Pereira BI, Nazareth C, et al.: *Rickettsia slovaca* infection in humans, Portugal, *Emerg Infect Dis* 19(10):1627–1629, 2013.

De Vries HJC, Morre SA, White JA: International union against sexually transmitted infections (IUSTI): 2010 European guideline on the management of lymphogranuloma venereum, *Int J STD AIDS* 21:533, 2010.

Doyle CK, Labruna MB, Breitschwerdt EB, et al.: Detection of medically important *Ehrlichia* by quantitative multicolor TaqMan real-time polymerase chain reaction of the dsb gene, *J Mol Diagn* 7:504–510, 2005.

Everett KD, Andersen AA: Identification of nine species of the *Chlamydiaceae* using PCR-RFLP, *Int J Syst Bacteriol* 49:803–813, 1999.

Everett KD, Bush RM, Andersen AA: Emended description of the order Chlamydiales, proposal of *Parachlamydiaceae* fam.nov. and *Simkaniaceae* fam.nov., each containing one monotypic genus, revised taxonomy of the family *Chlamydiaceae*, including a new genus and five new species, and standards for the identification of organisms, *Int J Syst Bacteriol* 49:415–440, 1999.

Gaydos CA, Quinn TC: Urine nucleic acid amplification tests for the diagnosis of sexually transmitted infections in clinical practice, *Curr Opin Infect Dis* 18:55–60, 2005.

Hogan RJ, Mathews SA, Mukhopadhyay S, Summersgill JT, Timms P: Chlamydial persistence: beyond the biphasic paradigm, *Infect Immun* 72:1843–1855, 2004.

Jensenius M, Fournier PE, Raoult D: Rickettsioses and the international traveler, *Clin Infect Dis* 39:1493–1499, 2004.

Johnson RE, Green TA, Schachter J, et al.: Evaluation of nucleic acid amplification tests as reference tests for *Chlamydia trachomatis* infections in asymptomatic men, *J Clin Microbiol* 38:4382–4386, 2000.

Jouglet M, Wuillaume I, Buchs C, Reix P, Schweitzer C, Coutier L: Neonatal low respiratory tract *Chlamydia trachomatis* infection: diagnostic and treatment management, *Respir Med Case Rep* 28:100852, 2019. https://doi.org/10.1016/j.rmcr.2019.100852.

Kellogg JA: Impact of variation in endocervical specimen collection and testing techniques on frequency of false-positive and false-negative chlamydia detection results, *Am J Clin Pathol* 104:554–559, 1995.

Kularatne SA, Gawarammana IB: Validity of the Weil-Felix test in the diagnosis of acute rickettsial infections in Sri Lanka, *Trans R Soc Trop Med Hyg* 103:423–424, 2009.

Lepidi H, Fenollar F, Dumler JS, et al.: Cardiac valves in patients with Whipple endocarditis: microbiological, molecular, quantitative histologic, and immunohistochemical studies of 5 patients, *J Infect Dis* 190:935–945, 2004.

Mahajan SK, Kashyap R, Kanga A, Sharma V, Prasher BS, Pal LS: Relevance of Weil-Felix test in diagnosis of scrub typhus in India, *J Assoc Physicians India* 54:619–621, 2006.

McMenemy A: Whipple's disease, familial Mediterranean fever, adult-onset Still's disease, and enteropathic arthritis, *Curr Opin Rheumatol* 4:479–483, 1992.

Musso D, Raoult D: *Coxiella burnetii* blood cultures from acute and chronic Q-fever patients, *J Clin Microbiol* 33:3129–3132, 1995.

O'Connell CM, Ferone ME: *Chlamydia trachomatis* genital infections, *Microb Cell* 3(9):390–403, 2016.

Paddock CD, Childs JE: *Ehrlichia chaffeensis*: a prototypical emerging pathogen, *Clin Microbiol Rev* 16:37–64, 2003.

Parola P, Paddock CD, Raoult D: Tick-borne rickettsioses around the world: emerging diseases challenging old concepts, *Clin Microbiol Rev* 18:719–756, 2005.

Raby E, Pearn T, Marangou AG, et al.: New foci of spotted fever group Rickettsiae including *Rickettsia honei* in Western Australia, *Trop Med Infect Dis* 1(1):E5, 2016.

Raoult D, Marrie T: Q fever, *Clin Infect Dis* 20:489–495, 1995.

Relman DA, Schmidt TM, MacDermott RP, Falkow S: Identification of the uncultured bacillus of Whipple's disease, *N Engl J Med* 327:293–301, 1992.

Sachse K, Bavoil PM, Kaltenboeck B, et al.: Emendation of the family *Chlamydiaceae*: proposal of a single genus, *Chlamydia*, to include all currently recognized species, *Syst Appl Microbiol* 38:99–103, 2015.

Sirigireddy KR, Ganta RR: Multiplex detection of *Ehrlichia* and *Anaplasma* species pathogens in peripheral blood by real-time reverse transcriptase-polymerase chain reaction, *J Mol Diagn* 7:308–316, 2005.

Walker DH, Valbuena GA, Olano JP: Pathogenic mechanisms of diseases caused by *Rickettsia*, *Ann N Y Acad Sci* 990:1–11, 2003.

Watson C, Alp NJ: Role of *Chlamydia pneumoniae* in atherosclerosis, *Clin Sci (Lond)* 114:509–531, 2008.

Wyrick PB: *Chlamydia trachomatis* persistence *in vitro*: an overview, *J Infect Dis* 201(Suppl 2):S88–S95, 2010.

44

Cell Wall–Deficient Bacteria: *Mycoplasma* and *Ureaplasma*

This chapter addresses a group of bacteria, the mycoplasmas, which are the smallest known free-living forms; unlike all other bacteria, these prokaryotes do not have a cell wall. Although mycoplasmas are ubiquitous in the plant and animal kingdoms (more than 200 different species exist within this class), this chapter addresses the most prominent of the *Mycoplasma* spp. and *Ureaplasma* spp. that colonize or infect humans that are not of animal origin.

General Characteristics

Organisms in this chapter belong to the class Mollicutes (Latin, meaning "soft skin"). This class comprises four orders, which, in turn, contain five families and eight genera (Fig. 44.1). The mycoplasmas that colonize or infect humans belong to the family *Mycoplasmataceae*; this family comprises two genera, *Mycoplasma* and *Ureaplasma*. These organisms are highly fastidious and slow growing, and most are facultative anaerobes that require nucleic acid precursor molecules, fatty acids, and sterols such as cholesterol for growth. Morphologically, these bacteria have a very small cell size (approximately 0.3 to 1.0 μm in diameter). In addition, these organisms represent bacterial species that are highly reduced genetically; the *Mycoplasma* genus includes species with the smallest genomes

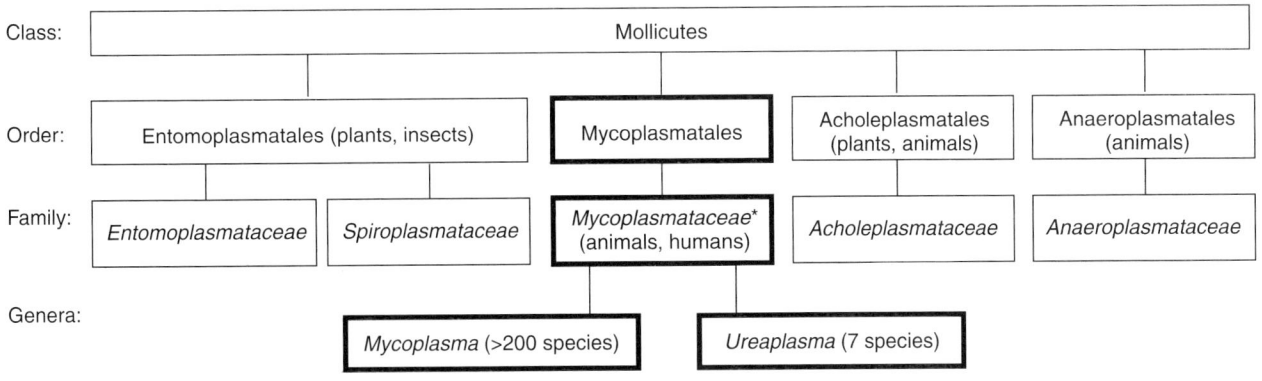

• **Fig. 44.1** Taxonomy of the class Mollicutes.

of all free-living bacteria. Mollicutes are descended from low G+C gram-positive bacteria (i.e., the *Firmicutes*), and their closest living relatives include bacilli, streptococci, and lactobacteria.

Epidemiology and Pathogenesis

Mycoplasmas are part of the human microbiota of the oropharynx and upper respiratory tract and can be part of the microbiota of the genitourinary tract. Besides those that are considered commensals, considerable evidence indicates the pathogenicity of some mycoplasmas; for others, a role in human disease is unclear.

Epidemiology

The mycoplasmas usually considered as commensals are listed in Table 44.1, along with their respective sites of colonization. These organisms are transmitted by direct sexual contact, by transplanted tissue from donor to recipient, or from mother to fetus during childbirth or *in utero*. *Mycoplasma pneumoniae* are transmitted by respiratory secretions. One species of *Acholeplasma* (organisms that are widely disseminated in animals), *Acholeplasma laidlawii*, has been isolated from the oral cavity of humans; however, the significance of these mycoplasmas and their colonization of humans remains uncertain.

Of the other mycoplasmas isolated from humans, the possible role that *Mycoplasma pirum, Mycoplasma amphoriforme, Mycoplasma fermentans,* and *Mycoplasma penetrans* might play in human disease is uncertain at this time. *M. pirum, M. fermentans,* and *M. penetrans* have been isolated from patients infected with human immunodeficiency virus (HIV); however, no clear link exists between acquisition or shedding of HIV and infections with these mycoplasmas. The potential for *M. penetrans* to play a role in the transition from HIV-positive patients

to clinical acquired immune deficiency syndrome (AIDS) has been examined but no connection has been fully demonstrated. In contrast, the ability of *M. genitalium* to facilitate both the shedding and the acquisition of HIV following exposure has been determined. *M. fermentans* has been isolated from specimens such as bronchoalveolar lavage, bone marrow, peripheral blood, and the throats of children with pneumonia. *M. fermentans* has also been associated with infection in children and immunocompromised individuals. *M. amphoriforme* has been detected in the lower respiratory tract in patients with chronic respiratory disease and antibody deficiencies, and isolation from healthy asymptomatic carriers has never been reported. However, until recent advances in molecular diagnostic offering for *M. pneumoniae*, the serologic cross reactivity between *M. pneumoniae* and *M. amphoriforme* may have masked primary respiratory tract infections with *M. amphoriforme* in previously healthy patients by miscategorizing them as *M. pneumoniae* infections. Prospective studies evaluating culture-positive, *M. pneumoniae* DNA-negative respiratory specimens can be evaluated to determine the role of *M. amphoriforme* as a primary or opportunistic pathogen. The presence of various *Mycoplasma* spp. infections in immunocompromised patients has been demonstrated by genital or respiratory tract colonization associated with medical procedures such as renal transplantation or genitourinary manipulations or following trauma resulting in wound infections.

Finally, the remaining species that have been isolated from humans—*M. pneumoniae, M. genitalium, M. phocicerebrale, Ureaplasma urealyticum, Ureaplasma parvum,* and *Mycoplasma hominis*—have well-established roles in human infections. *M. genitalium, U. urealyticum, U. parvum,* and *M. hominis* have been isolated from the genitourinary tract of humans, and *M. pneumoniae* has been isolated from the respiratory tract. *M. genitalium* accounts for approximately 15% to 20% of nongonococcal urethritis (NGU), which

TABLE 44.1 Mycoplasmas Isolated From Humans

Organism	Source of Isolation	Clinical Presentations
Mycoplasma amphoriforme	Respiratory tract	• Chronic bronchopneumonia and relapsing airway infection in immunocompromised patients • Primary atypical pneumonia or secondary pneumonia (proposed/suspected)
Mycoplasma buccale	Oropharynx	• Oral microbiome
Mycoplasma orale	Oropharynx	• Oral microbiome • Opportunistic pneumonia, infectious synovitis, osteomyelitis, or abscess in immunocompromised patients
Mycoplasma salivarium	Oropharynx, gingiva	• Oral microbiome • Opportunistic arthritis, submasseteric abscess,[a] gingivitis, or periodontitis in immunocompromised patients
Mycoplasma hominis	Genital tract, joints, respiratory tract (neonates), central nervous system (neonates)	• Vaginal microbiome • Bacterial vaginosis • Pelvic inflammatory disease • Pyelonephritis • Chorioamnionitis • Bronchopulmonary dysplasia (neonates) • Meningitis/meningoencephalitis (neonates) • Septic arthritis • Abscess (pelvic, brain, aortal) • Meningitis[a] • Osteomyelitis[a]
Mycoplasma pneumoniae		• Primary atypical pneumonia • Bronchitis • Pharyngitis • Meningoencephalitis • Pericarditis • Arthritis • Hemolytic anemia • Nephritis • Bell palsy • Stevens-Johnson syndrome
Mycoplasma faucium	Oropharynx	• Oral microbiome • Cerebral abscess[a]
Mycoplasma fermentans	Oropharynx, peripheral blood, respiratory tract, bone marrow, urine, genital tract	• Lipshütz ulcer[a] • Infectious rheumatoid arthritis • Malignant transformation (proposed) • Opportunistic pneumonia (proposed)
Mycoplasma lipophilum	Respiratory tract	• Pneumonia[a]
Mycoplasma penetrans	Urine, genital tract, blood, respiratory tract	• HIV disease progression (proposed) • Idiopathic nongonococcal urethritis
Mycoplasma phocicerebrale	Cutaneous lesions	• "Seal finger" (ulcerative keratitis secondary to seal bite)
Mycoplasma pirum	Rectum, peripheral blood, urine	• Gastrointestinal microbiome

TABLE 44.1	Mycoplasmas Isolated From Humans—cont'd	
Organism	**Source of Isolation**	**Clinical Presentations**
Mycoplasma genitalium	Genital tract, urine	• Nongonococcal urethritis • Prostatitis • Pelvic inflammatory disease • Infertility • Cervicitis • Sexually acquired reactive arthritis • Enhanced HIV transmission
Mycoplasma primatum	Genital tract, oropharynx	• Oral microbiome • Opportunistic keratitis[a]
Mycoplasma spermatophilum	Genital tract, semen	• Impaired fertility (proposed)
Acholeplasma laidlawii	Cutaneous burns	• Complex burn infections[a,b]
Ureaplasma parvum	Genital tract, urine, semen, blood, neonatal respiratory tract, neonatal central nervous system	• Urogenital microbiome • Chorioamnionitis • Preterm labor • Bronchopulmonary dysplasia (neonates) • Meningitis/meningoencephalitis (neonates) • Nongonococcal urethritis
Ureaplasma urealyticum	Genital tract, urine, semen, blood, neonatal respiratory tract, neonatal central nervous system	• Urogenital microbiome • Chorioamnionitis • Fatal hyperammonemia syndrome in immunocompromised patients • Preterm labor • Bronchopulmonary dysplasia (neonates) • Meningitis/meningoencephalitis (neonates) • Nongonococcal urethritis

HIV, Human immunodeficiency virus.

[a]This presentation has been reported less than 5 times.

[b]This presentation is described in a single report, and all *Acholeplasma*-positive lesions were coinfected with Gram-positive bacilli. Evidence for an association between *A. laidlawii* and burn infections or carriage in humans is minimal.

is urethritis not attributable to *Neisseria gonorrhoeae,* the most common cause of urethritis in males. *M. genitalium* is not associated with the presence of other mycoplasmas or ureaplasmas in the urogenital tract. In females, this organism can cause cervicitis, pelvic inflammatory disease (PID), and postinfectious tubal factor infertility. Both *Ureaplasma* and *Mycoplasma* species have been isolated from the internal organs of stillborn, premature, and spontaneously aborted fetuses. Although *M. genitalium* and, to a lesser extent, *M. hominis* are associated but not yet definitely implicated in pregnancy-related complications, *U. urealyticum* and *U. parvum* are recognized as causes of chorioamnionitis, preterm labor, and premature rupture of the membranes both in clinical studies and prospective studies using animal (sheep) models. In addition, delivery following invasion of the chorioamnion and amniotic fluid by ureaplasmas is strongly associated with risk for bronchopulmonary dysplasia and meningitis/meningoencephalitis in preterm infants. Recently, *Ureaplasma* sp. and *M. hominis* have been identified as a cause of hyperammonemia in immunocompromised patients.

Risks associated with prenatal ureaplasmosis are highly strain dependent. Infants are commonly colonized with benign strains of *U. urealyticum* and *M. hominis*. Once an individual reaches puberty, colonization with these organisms occurs primarily as a result of sexual contact. *M. hominis* is associated with bacterial vaginosis (BV) and should be considered in clinical BV when other agents have been ruled out. The organism also has a commensal relationship with the protozoal parasite *Trichomonas vaginalis*, wherein it invades *T. vaginalis* cells and lives intracellularly. This relationship may play a role in elevated pathogenicity for *T. vaginalis* in the form of enhanced cytopathology and metronidazole resistance. The role of *T. vaginalis* in the improved survival and enhanced transmission for *M. hominis* has been confirmed during antibiotic treatment. *M. hominis* is rarely associated with infection at distal body sites, most notably cerebral abscess.

M. pneumoniae is a cause of community-acquired atypical pneumonia, often referred to as walking pneumonia (Chapter 68). The organism causes infections worldwide, with an estimated 2 million cases per year in the United States. *M. pneumoniae* infection may also result in bronchitis or pharyngitis. *M. pneumoniae* may be transmitted person to person by respiratory secretions or indirectly via inanimate objects contaminated with respiratory secretions (fomites). Infections can occur singly or as outbreaks in closed populations such as families and military recruit camps. Pneumonia caused by *M. pneumoniae* may present as asymptomatic to mild disease, with early nonspecific symptoms including malaise, fever, headache, sore throat, earache, and nonproductive cough. This differs significantly from the classic symptoms associated with pneumonia associated with a *Streptococcus pneumoniae* infection (Chapters 14 and 68). *M. pneumoniae* strongly attaches to the mucosal cells and may reside intracellularly within host cells, resulting in a chronic persistent infection that may last for months to years. The infections do not follow seasonal patterns as seen with influenza and other respiratory pathogens. Besides respiratory infection, *M. pneumoniae* can cause extrapulmonary manifestations such as pericarditis, hemolytic anemia, arthritis, nephritis, Bell palsy, and meningoencephalitis. Finally, *M. phocicerebrale*, an oropharyngeal commensal and occasional cause of wound infections of seals, is the only confirmed mycoplasmal zoonosis described to date. This organism is associated with ulcerative keratitis secondary to marine mammal contact colloquially known as "seal finger."

Pathogenesis

In general, mycoplasmas colonize mucosal surfaces of the respiratory and urogenital tracts. Except for those mycoplasmas noted, most rarely produce invasive disease except in immunocompromised hosts or infections associated with medical device implants. Of the mycoplasmas that are established as causes of human infections, these agents predominantly reside extracellularly, attaching with great affinity to the surfaces of ciliated and nonciliated epithelial cells. Recently *M. fermentans*, *M. penetrans*, *M. genitalium*, *M. hominis*, and *M. pneumoniae* have been identified intracellularly. Intracellular invasion in bacterial infections is generally considered a means for immune evasion and may contribute to the persistent nature of infections, capacity for recrudescence after cessation of treatment, and difficulties in cultivation or isolation of *Mycoplasma* spp. *M. pneumoniae* has a complex and specialized attachment organelle that includes a P1 adhesin protein that primarily interacts with host cells. Similarly, *M. genitalium* uses a tip organelle to attach to host cells using the MgPa adhesion, which is homologous to the P1 adhesin of *M. pneumoniae*. With respect to the mycoplasmas that are clearly able to cause disease, many of the disease processes include a strong competent host immune response (inflammation), which leads

to long-term inflammatory syndromes because of the chronic nature of these infections. In addition to adherence properties and host immune responses to infection, the ability to directly cause cell death may also contribute to their pathogenicity. *M. pneumoniae* produces a potent ADP-ribosylating toxin ("community-acquired respiratory distress syndrome" [CARDS] toxin) that is strongly associated with disease capacity.

Of interest, the mycoplasmas associated with HIV patients (*M. fermentans*, *M. penetrans*, and *M. pirum*) are all capable of invading human cells and modulating the immune system. Based on these findings, some investigators have proposed that these mycoplasmas might play a role in certain disease processes in these patients.

Spectrum of Disease

The clinical manifestations of mycoplasmosis in humans are summarized in Table 44.1.

Laboratory Diagnosis

The laboratory diagnosis of mycoplasma infections can be extremely challenging because of complex and time-consuming culture requirements; however, the recent availability of rapid, molecular diagnostic tests represents a major step forward in the diagnosis of mycoplasmosis and ureaplasmosis. Accurate, rapid diagnosis for *M. pneumoniae* and *M. genitalium* is highly desired because penicillin and other beta-lactam agents are ineffective treatments. The laboratory diagnosis of the cell wall deficient organisms implicated in human diseases (i.e., *M. pneumoniae*, *U. urealyticum*, *U. parvum*, *M. hominis*, and *M. genitalium*) is addressed.

Specimen Collection, Transport, and Processing

Consistent with the diverse spectrum of diseases, various specimens are appropriate for the diagnosis of mycoplasma infections by culture or other means of detection. Acceptable specimens include body fluids (e.g., blood, joint fluid, amniotic fluid, urine, prostatic secretions, semen, pleural secretions, sputum, and bronchoalveolar lavage specimens); tissues; wound aspirates; and swabs of wounds, the throat, nasopharynx, urethra, cervix, or vagina. Blood for culture of genital mycoplasmas should be collected without anticoagulants and immediately inoculated into an appropriate broth culture medium. Mycoplasmas are inhibited by sodium polyethyl sulfonate (SPS), the anticoagulant typically found in commercial blood culture media. This may be overcome by the addition of 1% wt/vol of gelatin. However, commercial blood culture media and automated instruments are not adequate for the detection of *Mycoplasma* spp. Swab specimens should be obtained without the application of any disinfectants, analgesics, or lubricant. Dacron or polyester swabs on aluminum or plastic shafts should be used. Care must be taken when collecting urine samples to prevent contamination with lubricants or antiseptics used during gynecologic examination.

Because mycoplasmas have no cell wall, they are highly susceptible to drying; therefore, transport media is necessary, particularly when specimens are collected on swabs. Liquid specimens such as body fluids do not require transport media if inoculated to appropriate media within 1 hour of collection. Tissues should be kept moist; if a delay in processing is anticipated, they should also be placed in transport media. Specific media for the isolation of *Mycoplasma* spp. include those containing 10% heat-inactivated calf serum containing 0.2 M sucrose in a 0.02 M phosphate buffer, pH 7.2, such as SP4 glucose broth, or Shepard 10B broth. Additional commercial media available for cultivation of these organisms include Stuart medium, trypticase soy broth supplemented with 0.5% bovine serum albumin, Mycotrans (Irvine Scientific, Irvine, CA), and A3B broth (Remel, Inc., Lenexa, KS). Excessive delays in processing can result in decreased viability and recovery of organisms from clinical specimens. If the storage time is expected to exceed 24 hours before cultivation, the samples should be placed in transport media and frozen at –80°C. Frozen samples should be thawed in a hot water bath at 37°C. Transport and storage conditions of various types of specimens are summarized in Table 44.2.

Direct Detection Methods

No direct methods for identifying *M. pneumoniae, Ureaplasma* spp., or other *Mycoplasma* spp. in clinical samples are recommended, although some methods have been described, such as immunoblotting and indirect immunofluorescence. Direct detection by Gram staining may rule out the presence of other infectious organisms, but does not informatively stain cell wall–deficient mycoplasmas and ureaplasmas. Acridine orange or a fluorochrome stain may be useful to visualize organisms. However, these are nonspecific stains that will stain nucleic acids in bacteria as well as human cells.

Nucleic Acid Detection

Several amplification methods, such as polymerase chain reaction (PCR), have been developed for the detection of the clinically relevant *Mycoplasma* and *Ureaplasma* species, including US Food and Drug Administration (FDA)-cleared or approved tests to detect *M. pneumoniae* and *M. genitalium*. Various targets including 16S ribosomal ribonucleic acid (rRNA) sequences, insertion sequences, and organism-specific genes have been used in the development of these assays. As a result of the fast turnaround time, specificity, and lack of need to cultivate fastidious organisms, PCR amplification for the diagnosis of these organisms is currently the "gold standard." The Illumigene (Meridian Biosciences, Inc., Cincinnati, OH) ab FDA cleared assay, is a single-target isothermal loop-mediated PCR test that may be used for detection. When considering the use of

molecular amplification methods for the detection of infectious diseases, it is important to note that, although an organism is detectable, the patient's signs and symptoms must be correlated with the identified agent. It is possible to detect an organism by one method but not another—in other words, a patient may be PCR positive but culture negative or serologically negative for a *Mycoplasma* based on the patient's response to infection and current state of disease manifestation. Chapter 8 provides a more detailed description of the advantages, limitations, and methods used in the development of amplification assays. Multiplex real-time PCR assays that detect *M. pneumoniae* as well as other atypical respiratory tract pathogens such as *Chlamydia pneumoniae* and *Legionella pneumophila* are widely available in routine clinical laboratories. *M. genitalium* has been detected directly in urine and urethral swabs in males, using PCR methods targeting several unique genomic loci. In females, similar methods are used for detection from vaginal or cervical swabs. After successful implementation of commercial PCR-based diagnostics in Europe and Australia, a similar test for *M. genitalium* is also FDA cleared and available for use in the United States (Aptiva *M. genitalium* Assay by Hologic [Marlborough, MA]). Because macrolide resistance is increasing in *M. genitalium* at an alarming rate, the Australian company SpeeDx (Eveleigh, NSW, Australia) has developed ResistancePlus MG that detects the organism and the five distinct genotypes associated with macrolide resistance.

Cultivation

In general, the medium for mycoplasma isolation contains a beef or soybean protein with serum, fresh yeast extract, and other specific growth factors. As a result of the slow growth of these organisms, the medium must be highly selective to prevent overgrowth of faster-growing organisms that may be present in a clinical sample. Culture media and incubation conditions for these organisms are summarized in Table 44.3. Culture methods for *M. pneumoniae, U. urealyticum,* and *M. hominis* are provided in Evolve Procedures 44.1, 44.2, and 44.3, respectively. The quality control of the growth media with a fastidious isolate is of great importance.

For the most part, the different metabolic activity of the mycoplasmas for different substrates is used to detect their growth. Glucose (dextrose) is incorporated into media selective for *M. pneumoniae,* because this mycoplasma ferments glucose to lactic acid; the resulting pH change is then detected by a color change in a dye indicator. Similarly, urea or arginine can be incorporated into media to detect *U. urealyticum, U. parvum,* and *M. hominis,* respectively (Table 44.4). If a color change is observed (i.e., a change in pH detected by a chemical indicator added to the culture medium), a 0.1- to 0.2-mL aliquot is immediately subcultured to fresh broth and/or agar medium.

In some clinical situations, it may be necessary to provide quantitative information regarding the burden of

TABLE
44.2

Transport and Storage Conditions for *Mycoplasma* and Related Organisms

Specimen Type	Transport Conditions	Transport Media (Examples)[a]	Storage	Processing
Body fluid or liquid specimens[b]	Within 1 h of collection on ice or at 4°C	Not required	4°C up to 24 h[c]	Concentrate by high-speed centrifugation and dilute (1:10–1:1000) in broth culture media to remove inhibitory substances and contaminating bacteria; urine should be filtered through a 0.45-μm pore size filter
Swabs	Place immediately into transport media	0.5% albumin in trypticase soy broth modified Stuart 2SP (sugar-phosphate medium with 10% heat-inactivated fetal calf serum) Shepard 10B broth for ureaplasmas SP4 broth for other mycoplasmas and *M. pneumoniae*[d] *Mycoplasma* transport medium (trypticase phosphate broth, 10% bovine serum albumin, 100,000 U of penicillin/milliliter and universal transport media [Copan, Murrieta, CA])	4°C up to 24 h[c]	None
Tissue	Within 1 h of collection on ice or at 4°C	Not required as long as prevented from drying out	4°C up to 24 h[c]	Mince (not grind) and dilute (1:10 and 1:100) in transport media

[a]Not a complete list. A variety of commercial media is available.
[b]Except blood (see text).
[c]Can be stored indefinitely at −80°C if diluted in transport media after centrifugation.
[d]SP4 broth: sucrose phosphate buffer, 20% horse serum, *Mycoplasma* base, and neutral red.

TABLE
44.3

Cultivation of *Mycoplasma pneumoniae*, *Ureaplasma* spp., and *Mycoplasma hominis*

Organism	Media (Examples)	Incubation Conditions
M. pneumoniae	Biphasic SP4 (pH 7.4) Triphasic system (Mycotrim RS, Irvine Scientific, Irvine, CA) PPLO[a] broth or agar with yeast extract and horse serum Modified New York City medium	Broths: 37°C, ambient air for up to 4 weeks Agars: 37°C, ambient air supplemented with 5%–10% CO_2 or anaerobically in 95% N_2 plus 5% CO_2 All cultures should be retained for 4 weeks before reporting as negative
U. urealyticum/U. parvum[b]/*M. hominis*[c]	A7 or A8 agar medium (Remel, Lenexa, KS); penicillin should be included to minimize bacterial overgrowth[a] New York City medium Modified New York City medium SP4 glucose broth with arginine[d] SP4 glucose broth with urea[e] Triphasic system (Mycotrim GU, Irvine Scientific) Shepard 10B broth (or *Ureaplasma* 10C broth)[e]	Broths: 37°C, ambient air for up to 7 days Agars: 37°C in 5%–10% CO_2 or anaerobically in 95% N_2 plus 5% CO_2 for 2–5 days Genital cultures should be retained for 7 days before reporting as negative

PPLO, pleuropneumonia-like organisms.
[a]Commercially available.
[b]Uses urea and requires acidic medium.
[c]Converts arginine to ornithine and grows over a broad pH range.
[d]For *M. hominis* isolation.
[e]For *U. urealyticum* isolation.

Organism	Glucose Metabolism	Arginine Metabolism	Urease
M. fermentans	Positive	Positive	Negative
M. genitalium	Positive	Negative	Negative
M. hominis	Negative	Positive	Negative
M. pneumoniae	Positive	Negative	Negative
U. parvum	Negative	Negative	Positive
U. urealyticum	Negative	Negative	Positive

TABLE 44.4 Basic Biochemical Differentiation of the Major *Mycoplasma* and *Ureaplasma* spp.

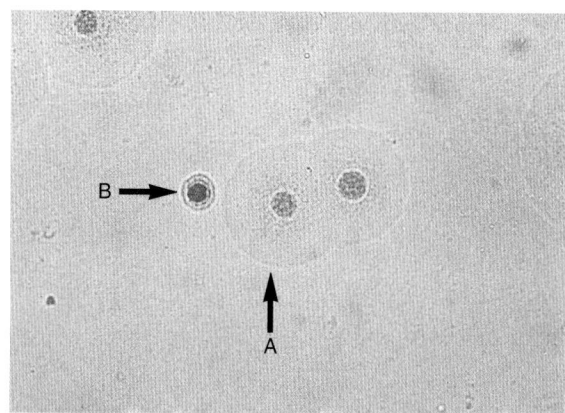

• **Fig. 44.3** Isolation of *Mycoplasma hominis* and *Ureaplasma urealyticum* (100× magnification). Note the "fried egg" appearance of the large *M. hominis* colony *(arrow A)* and the relatively small size of the *U. urealyticum* colony *(arrow B)*. (Courtesy Clinical Microbiology Laboratory, SUNY Upstate Medical University, Syracuse, NY.)

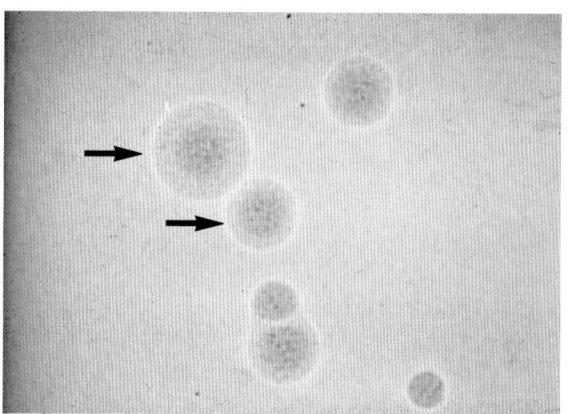

• **Fig. 44.2** Colonies of *Mycoplasma pneumoniae* visualized under 100× magnification. Note the variation in the size of the colonies *(arrows)*. (Courtesy Clinical Microbiology Laboratory, SUNY Upstate Medical University, Syracuse, NY.)

mycoplasmas in a clinical specimen. For example, quantitation of specimens taken at different stages during urination or after prostatic massage can help to determine the location of mycoplasmal infection in the genitourinary tract.

Approach to Identification

On agar, *M. pneumoniae* will appear as spherical, grainy, yellowish forms that are embedded in the agar, with a thin outer layer similar to those shown in Fig. 44.2. The agar surface is examined under 20× to 60× magnification using a stereomicroscope daily for *Ureaplasma* spp., at 24 to 72 hours for *M. hominis*, and every 3 to 5 days for *M. pneumoniae* and other slow-growing species. Because only *M. pneumoniae* and one serovar of *U. urealyticum* hemadsorb, *M. pneumoniae* is definitively identified by overlaying suspicious colonies with 0.5% guinea pig erythrocytes in phosphate-buffered saline. After 20 to 30 minutes at room temperature, colonies are observed for adherence of red blood cells.

Cultures for the genital mycoplasmas are handled in a similar fashion, including culture examination and the requirement for subculturing. Colonies may be definitively identified on A8 agar (Hardy Diagnostics, Santa Maria CA.) as *U. urealyticum* by urease production in the presence of a calcium chloride indicator. *U. urealyticum* colonies (15 to 60 μm in diameter) will appear as dark brownish clumps. Colonies that are typical in appearance for *U. urealyticum* are shown in Fig. 44.3. *M. hominis* colonies are large (approximately 20 to 300 μm in diameter) and are urease negative (Fig. 44.3), with a characteristic "fried egg" appearance (Fig. 44.4). Similar fried egg colonies are produced by *M. genitalium* but typically take several weeks to develop and thus are not useful for diagnostic purposes. On conventional blood agar, strains of *M. hominis*, but not of *U. urealyticum*, produce nonhemolytic, pinpoint colonies that do not Gram stain. These colonies can be stained with the Dienes or acridine orange stains. Numerous transport and growth media systems for the detection, quantitation, identification, and antimicrobial susceptibility testing of the genital mycoplasmas are commercially available in the United States and Europe.

Serodiagnosis

Laboratory diagnosis of *M. pneumoniae* is usually made serologically. Nonspecific production of cold agglutinins occurs in approximately half of patients with atypical pneumonia caused by this organism. Antibodies to *M. pneumoniae* are typically detectable after approximately 1 week of illness, peaking between 3 to 6 weeks, followed by a gradual decline. The antibody response to *M. pneumoniae* varies greatly from patient to patient. Some patients fail to produce a detectable immunoglobulin M (IgM) level, whereas in others the IgM level will persist

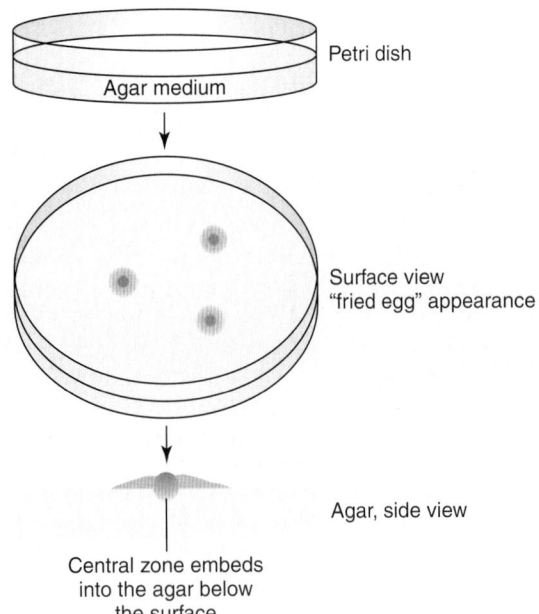

Petri dish
Agar medium

Surface view "fried egg" appearance

Agar, side view

Central zone embeds into the agar below the surface

• **Fig. 44.4** Colonial growth characteristics of *Mycoplasma* in agar medium.

for months. The variability associated with the antibody response necessitates the comparison of paired sera for proper diagnosis. In addition, cold agglutinins form in association with *M. pneumoniae* infection. The most widely used serologic tests are enzyme-linked immunosorbent assay (ELISA) tests, although indirect fluorescent antibody tests have been used with some success. IgM-specific tests such as the Immuno Card (Meridian Diagnostics, Cincinnati, OH) are commercially available, and a single positive result in children, adolescents, and young adults may be considered diagnostic in some cases. In addition, commercially available, membrane-based assay that simultaneously detects IgM and IgG against *M. pneumoniae* (Remel EIA, Lenexa, KS) has demonstrated good sensitivity and specificity compared with other tests. Several additional commercial assays are available that include enzyme immunoassay (EIA) microtiter assays.

Although serologic tests such as indirect hemagglutination and metabolism inhibition for genital mycoplasmas are available, they are rarely used. Because of the antigenic complexity of the mycoplasmas, and serologic cross reactivity among the outer membrane antigens, the development of a specific and useful serologic assay is a challenge.

Susceptibility Testing and Therapy

Although agar and broth dilution methods may be used to determine antibiotic susceptibilities, the complex growth requirements of mycoplasmas have restricted their performance to a few laboratories. The Human Mycoplasma Susceptibility Testing Subcommittee of the Clinical and Laboratory Standards Institute has formulated agar and broth dilution methods. Most mycoplasmal infections are treated empirically.

Most *M. pneumoniae* infections are self-limited and usually do not require treatment, but antibiotic treatment can markedly reduce or shorten the disease process. Because of the lack of a cell wall, *M. pneumoniae* and the other *Mollicutes* are innately resistant to all beta-lactam antibiotics, because this class of drugs interferes with cell wall synthesis. In addition, they are resistant to sulfonamides, trimethoprim, and rifampin. Susceptibility patterns vary by species to macrolides and lincosamides. *M. pneumoniae* and *M. genitalium* have historically been susceptible to the macrolides, tetracycline, ketolides, and fluoroquinolones. Although macrolides are still an appropriate first-line therapy for *M. pneumoniae*, they are rapidly becoming ineffective against predominant strains of *M. genitalium*. Single-dose macrolides (i.e., azithromycin) are beneficial for treating gonococcal and nongonococcal urethritis in sexually transmitted disease clinics, because the success of extended dosing regimens relies on patient compliance, which is often unreliable in high-risk clinical settings. Although this was initially a successful intervention against *M. genitalium* infection, the organism's facultative intracellular location affords it protection against macrolides during high-dose treatment, resulting in incomplete clearance, disease recrudescence, and increasing rates of macrolide resistance. Given the factors that single-dose macrolide treatment successfully addressed, it is predictable that outpatient treatment of *M. genitalium* will pose a unique challenge. Unfortunately, the susceptibility of *M. hominis* and *U. urealyticum* to various agents is not as predictable. For the most part, the tetracyclines are the drugs of choice for these agents, although resistance has been reported.

Multidrug-resistant mycoplasmas and ureaplasmas have been identified in genital and extragenital infections in immunocompromised patients. Treatment and clearance of these infections is extremely difficult and limited by the bacteriostatic concentrations of antimicrobials, as well as the slow growth and immune modulation associated with infections with these agents.

Prevention

No vaccines are available for the human mycoplasmas. Early studies both in human subjects and animal models have proven either ineffective or deleterious upon challenge, likely due to the inflammatory, immunomodulatory nature of the organisms. Urogenital transmission of mycoplasmas and ureaplasmas can be prevented through barrier protection, such as with the use of male condoms.

ⓔ Visit the Evolve site for a complete list of procedures, review questions, and case studies.

Bibliography

Ainsworth JG, Katseni V, Hourshid S, et al.: *Mycoplasma fermentans* and HIV-associated nephropathy, *J Infect* 29:323–326, 1994.

Bauer FA, Wear DJ, Angritt P, Lo SC: *Mycoplasma fermentans* (incognitus strain) infection in the kidneys of patients with acquired immunodeficiency syndrome and associated nephropathy: a light microscopic, immunohistochemical, and ultrastructural study, *Hum Pathol* 22:63–69, 1991.

Bennett J, Dolin R, Blaser M: *Principles and practice of infectious diseases*, ed 9, Philadelphia, 2020, Elsevier-Saunders.

Bharat A, Cunningham SA, Scott Budinger GR, et al.: Disseminated *Ureaplasma* infection as a cause of fatal hyperammonemia in humans, *Sci Transl Med* 7(284):284re3, 2015. https://doi.org/10.1126/scitranslmed.aaa8419.

Blanchard A: Mycoplasmas and HIV infection, a possible interaction through immune activation, *Wien Klin Wochenschr* 109(14–15):590–593, 1997.

Browning GF, Whithear KG, Geary SJ: Vaccines to control mycoplasmosis. In *Mycoplasmas: molecular biology, pathogenicity, and strategies for control*, Norfolk, NR, United Kingdom, 2005, Horizon Bioscience.

Caroll KC, Pfaller MA: *Manual of clinical microbiology*, ed 12, Washington, DC, 2019, ASM Press.

Dessì D, Delogu G, Emonte E, Catania MR, Fiori PL, Rappelli P: Long-term survival and intracellular replication of *Mycoplasma hominis* in *Trichomonas vaginalis* cells: potential role of the protozoon in transmitting bacterial infection, *Infect Immun* 73(2):1180–1186, 2005.

Gaydos CA: *Mycoplasma genitalium*: accurate diagnosis is necessary for adequate treatment, *J Infect Dis* 216(Suppl 2):S406–S411, 2017.

Goldenberg RL, Thompson C: The infectious origins of stillbirth, *Am J Obstet Gynecol* 189:861–873, 2003.

Loens K, Ursi D, Goossens H, Ieven M: Molecular diagnosis of *Mycoplasma pneumoniae* respiratory tract infections, *J Clin Microbiol* 4:4915–4923, 2003.

May M, Balish MF, Blanchard A: *The order Mycoplasmatales in the prokaryotes*, New York, NY, 2014, Springer Inc.

Mena L, Wang X, Mroczkowski TF, Martin DH: *Mycoplasma genitalium* infections in asymptomatic men and men with urethritis attending a sexually transmitted diseases clinic in New Orleans, *Clin Infect Dis* 35:1167–1173, 2001.

Montagnier L, Blanchard A: Mycoplasmas as cofactors in infection due to the human immunodeficiency virus, *Clin Infect Dis* 17(Suppl 1):S309–S315, 1993.

Razin S, Yogev D, Naot Y: Molecular biology and pathogenicity of mycoplasmas, *Microbiol Mol Biol Rev* 62:1094–1156, 1998.

Rittenschober-Böhm J, Waldhoer T, Schulz SM, et al.: Vaginal *Ureaplasma parvum* serovars and spontaneous preterm birth, *Am J Obstet Gynecol* 220(6):594.e1–594.e9, 2019. https://doi.org/10.1016/j.ajog.2019.01.237.

Sanchez PJ: Perinatal transmission of *Ureaplasma urealyticum*: current concepts based on review of the literature, *Clin Infect Dis* 17(Suppl 1):S107–S111, 1993.

Silwedel C, Speer CP, Glaser K: *Ureaplasma*-associated prenatal, perinatal, and neonatal morbidities, *Expert Rev Clin Immunol* 13(11):1073–1087, 2017.

Totten PA, Schwartz MA, Sjöström KE, et al.: Association of *Mycoplasma genitalium* with nongonococcal urethritis in heterosexual men, *J Infect Dis* 183:269–276, 2001.

Waites KB, Bebear CM, Robertson JA, et al.: *Cumitech 34, laboratory diagnosis of mycoplasmal infections*, Washington, DC, 2001, American Society for Microbiology.

Waites KB, Talkington DF: *Mycoplasma pneumoniae* and its role as a human pathogen, *Clin Microbiol Rev* 17:697–728, 2004.

Wang PJ, Xie CB: *Mycoplasma hominis* symbiosis and *Trichomonas vaginalis* metronidazole resistance, *Zhongguo Ji Sheng Chong Xue Yu Ji Sheng Chong Bing Za Zhi* 30(3):210–213, 2012.

45

The Spirochetes

GENERA AND SPECIES TO BE CONSIDERED

Treponema pallidum subsp. *pallidum*
Treponema pallidum subsp. *pertenue*
Treponema pallidum subsp. *endemicum*
Treponema carateum
Treponema denticola

Lyme Borreliosis

Borrelia afzelii
Borrelia bavariensis
Borrelia bissettiae
Borrelia burgdorferi sensu stricto
Borrelia garinii
Borrelia lusitaniae
Borrelia mayonii
Borrelia spielmanii
Borrelia valaisiana

Relapsing Fever

Borrelia caucasica
Borrelia crocidurae
Borrelia duttonii
Borrelia hermsii
Borrelia hispanica
Borrelia mazzottii
Borrelia miyamotoi (hard tick-borne relapsing fever)
Borrelia parkeri
Borrelia persica
Borrelia recurrentis
Borrelia turicatae
Borrelia venezuelensis
Brachyspira aalborgi
Brachyspira hominis (provisionally named)
Brachyspira pilosicoli

Pathogenic Species

Leptospira alexanderi
Leptospira alstonii
Leptospira borgpetersenii
Leptospira interrogans
Leptospira kirschneri
Leptospira mayottensis
Leptospira noguchii
Leptospira santarosai
Leptospira weilii

Intermediate Species

Leptospira broomii
Leptospira fainei
Leptospira inadai
Leptospira licerasiae
Leptospira venezuelensis
Leptospira wolffii

Saprophytic Species

Leptospira biflexa
Leptospira idonii
Leptospira meyeri
Leptospira terpstrae
Leptospira vanthielii
Leptospira wolbachii
Leptospira yanagawae

This chapter discusses the bacteria that belong to the phylum Spirochaetes. The phylum includes three orders, which include four medically relevant genera: the order Brachyspirales (*Brachyspira* spp.), the order Leptospirales (*Leptospira* spp.), and the order Spirochaetales. Within the order Spirochaetales, there are two families: *Borreliaceae* (*Borrelia* spp.) and *Spirochaetaceae* (*Treponema* spp.).

The spirochetes are all long, slender, helically curved organisms, with the unusual morphologic features of **axial fibrils** and an outer sheath. These fibrils, or **axial filaments,** are flagella-like organelles that wrap around the bacteria's cell walls, are enclosed within the outer sheath, and facilitate motility of the organisms. The fibrils are attached in the cell wall by platelike structures, called **insertion disks,** located near the ends of the cells. The protoplasmic cylinder gyrates around the fibrils, causing bacterial movement to appear as a corkscrewlike winding. Differentiation of genera *(Treponema)* within the family *Spirochaetaceae* is based on the number of axial fibrils **(endoflagella)**, the number of insertion disks present (Table 45.1), and biochemical and metabolic features. The spirochetes also fall into genera based loosely on their morphology (Fig. 45.1): *Treponema* appear as slender with tight coils; *Borrelia* (family *Borreliaceae*) are somewhat thicker with fewer and looser coils; and *Leptospira* (family *Leptospiraceae*) resemble *Borrelia*, except for their hooked ends. *Brachyspira* (family *Brachyspiraceae*) are comma-shaped or helical, with tapered ends with four flagella at each end.

Treponema
General Characteristics

The major pathogens in the genus *Treponema*—*Treponema pallidum* subsp. *pallidum*, *Treponema pallidum* subsp. *pertenue*, *Treponema pallidum* subsp. *endemicum*, and *Treponema carateum*—infect humans and have not been cultivated for more than one passage *in vitro*. Most species stain poorly with Gram staining or Giemsa methods and are best observed with the use of dark-field or phase-contrast microscopy. The organisms are microaerophilic.

Other treponemes such as *Treponema vincentii, T. denticola, T. refringens, T. socranskii, T. parvum, T. pectinovorum, T. putidum, T. lecithinolyticum, T. amylovorum, T. medium,* and *T. maltophilum* are normal microbiota of the oral cavity or the human genital tract. These organisms are cultivable anaerobically on artificial media. Acute necrotizing ulcerative gingivitis, also known as **Vincent disease,** is a

destructive lesion of the gums. Methylene blue–stained material from the lesions of patients with Vincent disease shows certain morphologic types of bacteria. Observed morphologies include spirochetes and fusiform; oral spirochetes, particularly unusually large ones, may be important in this disease, along with other anaerobes.

Epidemiology and Pathogenesis

Key features of the epidemiology of diseases caused by the pathogenic treponemes are summarized in Table 45.2. In general, these organisms enter the host by either penetrating intact mucous membranes (as is the case for *T. pallidum* subsp. *pallidum*—hereafter referred to as *T. pallidum*) or entering through breaks in the skin. *T. pallidum* is transmitted by sexual contact and vertically from mother to the unborn fetus. Neonates can also become infected from contact with contaminated lesions or infected maternal blood during the birthing process. Although rare in the United States, the transmission of *T. pallidum* in blood products still occurs in underdeveloped countries that do not have routine donor screening and processing facilities. After *T. pallidum* penetrates the host, the organism subsequently invades the bloodstream and spreads to other body sites. The mechanisms associated with disease pathology to the host are unclear. Molecular studies have not identified a *T. pallidum* protein that binds to host fibronectin and laminin receptors on various human cells. Binding to different host cells is apparent in cells that produce fibronectin. The organism has an inherent ability to cross the endothelial, blood-brain, and placental barriers. *T. pallidum* has been shown to activate platelets to aid in movement and dissemination throughout the host. As a result, *T. pallidum* has a remarkable **tropism** (attraction) to arterioles; infection ultimately leads to **endarteritis** (inflammation of the lining of arteries) and subsequent progressive tissue destruction.

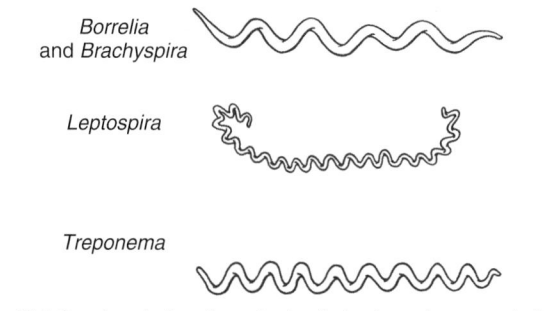

• **Fig. 45.1** Species designation of spirochetes based on morphology.

TABLE 45.1	Spirochetes Pathogenic for Humans		
Genus	Axial Filaments		Insertion Disks
Treponema	6–10		1
Borrelia	30–40		2
Leptospira	2		3–5

		Geographic		Clinical	
Agent	**Transmission**	**Location**	**Disease**	**Manifestations**[a]	**Age Group**
Treponema pallidum subsp. *pallidum*	Sexual contact or congenital (mother to fetus).	Worldwide	Venereal syphilis[b]	Refer to text in this chapter	All ages
Treponema pallidum subsp. *pertenue*	Traumatized skin contact with an infected lesion (person-to-person contact).	Humid, warm climates: Africa, South and Central America, Pacific Islands	Yaws	Skin—papules,[b] nodules, ulcers Primary lesion (mother yaw), disseminated lesions (frambesia) May progress to a latent stage and late infection involving destructive lesions to bone and cartilage	Children
Treponema pallidum subsp. *endemicum*	Mouth to mouth by utensils (person-to-person contact).	Arid, warm climates: North Africa, Southeast Asia, Middle East	Endemic nonvenereal syphilis	Skin/mucous membrane patches, papules, macules, ulcers, scars[b] May progress to disseminated oropharyngeal with generalized lymphadenopathy May demonstrate a latent stage, and late syphilis destructive to skin, bone, and cartilage	Children or adults; rarely congenital
Treponema carateum	Traumatized skin contact with an infected lesion (person-to-person contact).	Semiarid, warm climates: Central and South America, Mexico	Pinta	Skin papules, macules. Hyperkeratotic pigmented may lead to disseminated skin lesions and lymphadenopathy; late stage may result in pigmentary changes in skin (hyper- or hypopigmentation)	All ages but primarily children and adolescents

TABLE 45.2 Epidemiology and Spectrum of Disease of the Treponemes Pathogenic for Humans

[a]All diseases have a relapsing clinical course and prominent cutaneous manifestations.
[b]If untreated, organisms can disseminate to other parts of the body, such as bone.

Spectrum of Disease

In recent years, there has been a resurgence of primary and secondary syphilis cases in the United States, with a 10.5% increase in the number of reported cases between 2016 and 2017.

T. pallidum causes **venereal** (transmitted through sexual contact) **syphilis.** The clinical presentation of venereal syphilis is varied and complex, often mimicking many other diseases. The disease is divided into stages: incubating, primary, secondary, early nonprimary nonsecondary syphilis, unknown duration or late syphilis, and tertiary.

Primary syphilis is characterized by the appearance of one or more hard **chancres** (painless ulcers) that develop(s) at the site of inoculation, most commonly the genitalia. The primary stage is extremely infectious because the lesion contains a large number of organisms. Disease at this stage may be undetectable in the vagina or rectum. Within 3 to 6 weeks, the chancre heals spontaneously (without treatment). Dissemination of the organism occurs during this primary stage; once the organism has reached a sufficient number (usually within 4 to 10 weeks), clinical manifestations of **secondary syphilis** become apparent.

During secondary syphilis, the patient usually seeks medical attention. Systemic symptoms such as fever, weight loss, malaise, and loss of appetite are present in about half of patients. Common symptoms are flulike (fever, sore throat, and lymphadenopathy). The skin is the organ most commonly affected in secondary syphilis, with patients having a widespread rash (generally on the face, scalp, palms of hands, and soles of the feet) and generalized lymphadenopathy. Patchy hair loss may occur, such as a loss of eyebrows ("moth-eaten" area). This stage is a highly infectious state, again because large numbers of spirochetes are present. Aseptic meningitis may also occur. This stage may be mild and go unnoticed by the patient, or symptoms may disappear without treatment. This is when the disease becomes **subclinical** (asymptomatic) but not necessarily dormant (inactive). During this period, diagnosis can be made using serologic methods. Relapses are common during **early, nonprimary, nonsecondary** (≤1 year) **syphilis**. **Unknown duration or late latent syphilis** (≥1 year) is usually asymptomatic and noninfectious. Many untreated cases develop into tertiary syphilis.

Tertiary syphilis is the tissue-destructive phase that appears 10 to 25 years after the initial infection in up to 35% of untreated patients. Complications of syphilis at this stage include central nervous system disease (**neurosyphilis**) and cardiovascular abnormalities (**cardiovascular syphilis**), such as aortic valve insufficiency associated with the presence of cardiovascular lesions, eye disease (**ocular syphilis**), and granuloma-like lesions (**gummas**) that are soft, painless, and noninfectious, and found on the skin or in the bones or visceral organs. Neurosyphilis has been categorized into five major clinical presentations: asymptomatic, meningeal, meningovascular, parenchymatous, and gummatous.

As seen with primary and secondary syphilis, there has also been an increase in the number of reported congenital syphilis cases in recent years; cases of congenital syphilis have increased every year in the United States since 2013. **Congenital syphilis** is transmitted from a mother to an unborn fetus during any stage of infection but is most often associated with early syphilis. The unborn fetus may develop an asymptomatic infection or symptomatic infection. Clinical signs known as **Hutchinson's triad** (deafness, blindness, notched peg-shaped teeth) may occur. Additionally, poor bone formation may result, such as "saber shin" bowing of the tibia and the "bulldog" appearance of a deformed maxilla. Finally, neurosyphilis or neonatal death can occur.

The additional pathogenic treponemes are major health concerns in developing countries. Although morphologically and antigenically similar, these agents differ epidemiologically and with respect to their clinical presentation from *T. pallidum*. The diseases caused by these treponemes are summarized in Table 45.2.

Laboratory Diagnosis
Specimen Collection
Samples collected from ulcers and lesions should not be contaminated with blood, microorganisms, or tissue debris.

The site should be cleansed with sterile gauze moistened with saline. The sample should be placed on a clean glass slide and cover slipped. Polymerase chain reaction (PCR) samples should be collected on a sterile Dacron or cotton swab and placed in a cryotube containing nucleic acid transport medium or universal transport medium. Tissue or needle aspirates of lymph nodes should be placed in 10% buffered formalin at room temperature. To test for congenital syphilis, a small section of the umbilical cord is collected and fixed in 10% buffered formalin at room temperature until processed. A 3 to 4 cm section of umbilical cord distal from the placenta for the detection of congenital syphilis should be collected immediately following delivery and processed as a tissue. Serum is the specimen of choice for serology; however, plasma may be used in some assays. Plasma should be tested within 24 hours to avoid false-positive results. Capillary draws of whole blood, serum, or plasma may be used for rapid syphilis tests. Maternal serum may also be used to screen for congenital syphilis. Infants' serum should be used for immunoglobulin (Ig)M specific tests because cord blood specimens may be contaminated with maternal blood.

Serum, plasma, and cerebrospinal fluid (CSF) should be stored at 4°C if testing is delayed more than 4 hours and at –20°C if delayed more than 5 days. Samples collected for PCR, such as unfixed tissue, ulcer exudate, mucosal and skin lesions, CSF or amniotic fluid, and whole blood in EDTA, should be stored at –80°C if testing is delayed.

Direct Detection
Treponemes can be detected in material taken from skin lesions by dark-field examination or fluorescent antibody staining and microscopic examination. Material for microscopic examination is collected from suspicious lesions. The area around the lesion must first be cleansed with a sterile gauze pad moistened in saline. The surface of the ulcer is then abraded until some blood is expressed. After blotting the lesion until there is no further bleeding, the area is squeezed until serous fluid is expressed. Dark-field microscopy should be completed within 20 minutes of collection in order to identify motile treponemes. For other microscopic techniques, the surface of a clean glass slide is touched to the exudate, allowed to air dry, and transported in a dust-free container for fluorescent antibody staining. A *T. pallidum* fluorescein-labeled antibody is commercially available for staining. For dark-field examination, the expressed fluid is aspirated using a sterile pipette, dropped onto a clean glass slide, and cover slipped. The slide containing material for dark-field examination must be transported to the laboratory immediately. Because positive lesions may be teeming with viable spirochetes that are highly infectious, all supplies and patient specimens must be handled with extreme caution and carefully discarded as required for contaminated materials. Gloves should always be worn.

Material for dark-field examination is examined under 400× high-dry magnification for the presence of motile spirochetes. Treponemes are long (8 to 10 µm, slightly larger than a red blood cell) and consist of 8 to 14 tightly coiled, even spirals (Fig. 45.2). Once seen, characteristic forms should be verified by examination under oil immersion magnification (1000×). Although the dark-field examination depends greatly on technical expertise and the numbers of organisms in the lesion, it can be highly specific when performed on genital lesions. Dark-field methods cannot be used to evaluate oral or rectal lesions.

Lesion exudates or tissue samples may be used for direct fluorescent antibody detection for *T. pallidum* (DFA-TP). DFA-TP visualizes specimens on slides with fluorescein isothiocyanate (FITC) labeled antibodies. Polyclonal and monoclonal antibodies may be used; however, the US Food and Drug Administration (FDA) has not approved this test. Dark-field microscopy and fluorescent antibody methods are insensitive. Dark-field microscopy is no longer performed in most clinical laboratories.

Nucleic Acid Detection

Although nucleic acid–based assays are not currently available within many clinical laboratories, several methods have been developed using PCR for the detection of *T. pallidum*. These methods are primarily useful in the identification of organisms within exudate or lesions, and are sensitive and specific when used to analyze genital lesions. Commercially available extraction kits can be used, such as the QIAamp DNA mini kit (Qiagen, Inc., Valencia, CA).

Although there are currently no FDA-approved nucleic acid tests available for the detection of *T. pallidum*, the Center for Disease Control Laboratory Reference and Research Branch, Division of Sexually Transmitted Disease Prevention, has developed a multiplex PCR assay. The TaqMan-based assay simultaneously detects *T. pallidum, Haemophilus ducreyi,* and herpes simplex viruses (HSV1 and HSV2). In addition, laboratory-developed tests have been shown to detect atypical cases of syphilis in tonsillar, vertebral, and ocular syphilis. However, a major limitation of PCR is that the sensitivity of the test begins to decrease during secondary syphilis.

Serodiagnosis

Serologic tests for treponematosis measure the presence of two types of antibodies: treponemal and nontreponemal. Treponemal antibodies are produced against antigens of the organisms themselves, whereas nontreponemal antibodies, often referred to as **reagin antibodies,** are produced in infected patients against components of mammalian cells. Reaginic antibodies, although almost always produced in patients with syphilis, are also produced in patients with other infectious diseases such as leprosy, tuberculosis, chancroid, leptospirosis, malaria, rickettsial disease, trypanosomiasis, lymphogranuloma venereum (LGV), measles, chickenpox, hepatitis, and infectious mononucleosis; noninfectious conditions such as drug addiction; autoimmune disorders, including rheumatoid disease and systemic lupus erythematosus; and in conjunction with increasing age, pregnancy, and recent immunization. Nontreponemal serologic tests are useful in monitoring treatment, whereas treponemal tests are not, as titers tend to remain elevated, even after successful treatment. Serologic testing may be negative during the early course of infection.

Rapid Syphilis Tests

Rapid point-of-care immunochromatographic strip assays have been developed that detect treponemal antibodies from whole blood, serum, or plasma. These rapid tests are capable of detecting IgM and IgG antibodies with antigens bound to a solid phase membrane. The tests provide results within 20 to 25 minutes and are useful for screening in the clinical setting. Although the rapid tests demonstrate similar sensitivities and specificities in comparison to laboratory-based methods, follow-up nontreponemal antibody titers are required for further evaluation.

The Chembio DPP Syphilis Screen & Confirm Assay (Chembio Diagnostic Systems, Inc., Medford, NY) utilizes an immunochromatographic test strip and is able to detect both treponemal and nontreponemal antibodies by utilizing two test lines on the same strip. There are other rapid

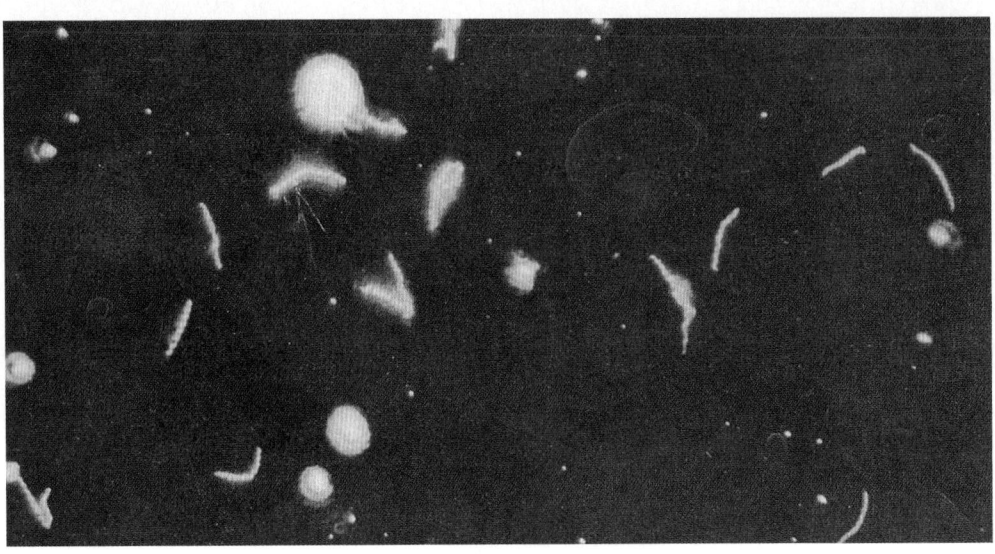

• **Fig. 45.2** Appearance of *Treponema pallidum* in dark-field preparation.

point-of-care immunochromatographic strip assays that qualitatively detect antibodies to both *T. pallidum* and HIV-1/2 (SD Bioline HIV/Syphilis Duo, Abbott, Lake Forest, IL; Chembio DPP HIV-Syphilis Assay, Chembio Diagnostic Systems, Inc., Medford, NY).

Nontreponemal Antibody Tests

The three nontreponemal serologic tests are the Venereal Disease Research Laboratory (VDRL), the TRUST assay, and the rapid plasma reagin (RPR) tests, which measure IgM and IgG antibodies. Each of these tests is a flocculation (or agglutination) test, in which soluble antigen particles are coalesced to form larger particles that are visible as clumps when they are aggregated in the presence of an antibody. The VDRL is used as a quantitative test and may be performed on serum or CSF in suspected cases of neurosyphilis. The RPR uses charcoal particles to detect antibodies in serum or plasma. There are numerous RPR kits commercially available that vary in methodology and procedures. Automated RPR tests use latex agglutination or immunoassay methods to increase the ability to screen multiple samples simultaneously. The TRUST assay is similar to the RPR but utilizes toluidine red in place of charcoal particles and is considered a macroflocculation. See Evolve Procedures 45.1 and 45.2 for details and limitations for the VDRL and RPR. Nontreponemal serologic tests for syphilis can be used to determine antibody quantitative titers, which are useful to follow the patient's response to therapy. The relative sensitivity of each test is shown in Table 45.3 to confirm that a positive nontreponemal test result is from syphilis rather than from one of the other infections or biologic false-positive conditions noted previously. For syphilis, traditional diagnosis is useful in active infections. However,

early or treated infections may be incorrectly diagnosed. In addition, primary testing using RPR or VDRL may result in a high rate of false positives. The CDC has recommended a **reverse algorithm** to detect early primary or treated infections that may be missed using traditional nonspecific screening methods. Reverse testing suggests the use of specific antibody testing for syphilis, using EIA for IgM and IgG or a similar technique. *T. pallidum* antibodies persist for many years after infection. Specific tests may then be followed by nonspecific screening tests, which become less reactive over time. However, reverse testing is not currently widely accepted, and more data are needed to resolve clinical diagnostic discrepancies (Fig. 45.3).

Treponemal Serologic Tests

Specific treponemal serologic tests are typically positive within 1 to 2 weeks after the appearance of the primary lesion and include automated enzyme immunoassays (EIAs) and agglutination tests, such as the *T. pallidum* particle agglutination (TP-PA) test, the microhemagglutination assay (MHA-TP), *T. pallidum* indirect hemagglutination (TPHA), particle gel immunoassay (PaGIA), the fluorescent treponemal antibody absorption (FTA-ABS) test, chemiluminescence immunoassays (CIAs), and microbead immunoassays (MBIA). Once positive, their usefulness is limited because these tests tend to yield positive results throughout the patient's life. The specificity of these tests is around 99%.

The FTA-ABS test is performed by overlaying whole treponemes fixed to a slide with serum from patients suspected of having syphilis. This test is typically performed after a positive VDRL or RPR screening test. The patient's serum is first absorbed with non–*T. pallidum* treponemal antigens (sorbent) to reduce nonspecific cross-reactivity.

TABLE 45.3	Sensitivity of Commonly Used Serologic Tests for Syphilis		
Method	**Primary**	**Secondary**	**Late**
Nontreponemal (Reaginic Tests)—Screening			
Venereal Disease Research Laboratory (reaginic) test (VDRL)	78%	100%	96%
Rapid plasma-reagin (RPR) card test and automated reagin test (ART)	86%	100%	98%
Specific Treponemal Tests—Confirmatory			
FTA-ABS	78%	93%	93%
TP-PA	95%	100%	87%
Trep-Sure EIA	95%	100%	99%
Centaur CIA	95%	100%	94%
Liason CIA	96%	100%	93%
Bioplex MBIA	96%	100%	94%

FTA-ABS, Fluorescent treponemal antibody absorption; *TP-PA, Treponema pallidum* particle agglutination; *EIA,* enzyme immunoassay; *CIA,* chemiluminescence immunoassay; *MBIA,* microbead immunoassay.

Fluorescein-conjugated antihuman antibody reagent is applied as a marker for specific antitreponemal antibodies in the patient's serum. This test should not be used as a primary screening procedure. It has been demonstrated that FTA-ABS is less sensitive than TP-PA and other immunoassays (CIA, EIA, MBIA) at all stages of syphilis, especially primary syphilis.

TP-PA (Fujirebio America, Fairfield, NJ) tests use gelatin particles sensitized with *T. pallidum* subsp. *pallidum* antigens. Serum samples are diluted in a microtiter plate, and sensitized gelatin particles are added. The presence of specific antibodies causes the gelatin particles to agglutinate and form a flat mat across the bottom of the microdilution well in which the test is performed. The MHA-TP is a passive hemagglutination assay of sensitized erythrocytes that are tested against the patient's serum. Agglutination indicates the presence of IgG or IgM antitreponemal antibodies in the patient's serum. TPHA is an indirect hemagglutination assay that uses sensitized red blood cells, which aggregate when exposed to positive patient serum. This test is similar to the MHA-TP. The PaGIA test, which uses gel immunoassay technology, is an established method in blood group serology. The assay contains recombinant antigens for the detection of *T. pallidum* antibodies in the patient's serum or plasma. The results are available in approximately 15 minutes.

Several EIAs are available that use direct, antibody class capture, indirect sandwich or competitive assay methodology. EIAs use recombinant antigens to detect IgM, IgG, or both. Trep-Sure EIA (Phoenix Biotech, Mississauga, Ontario, Canada) is a qualitative EIA that measures IgG and IgM treponemal antibodies. It utilizes microplates that are coated with treponemal antigens. Patient antibodies bind to these antigens, and horseradish peroxidase conjugated to treponemal antigens is added, which binds to the antigen-antibody complexes. A chromogenic reaction occurs when the substrate for horseradish peroxidase, tetramethylbenzidine is added. The reaction is detected with a spectrophotometer at 450 nm.

Several automated multiplex flow or MBIA systems exist that use bead-capture technology. These assays use a capture antibody attached to a suspension of small micropolystyrene beads. The beads are tagged with fluorophores of differing intensity, giving each a unique fingerprint. The sandwich immunoassay uses a flow cytometry dual-laser system for detection. There are currently three Luminex commercial platforms that use this technology: Abbott Architect (Abbott Laboratories, Abbott Park, IL), Bio-Rad Bioplex (Bio-Rad Laboratories, Hercules, CA), and Zeus AtheNA (Zeus Scientific, Branchburg, NJ).

CIA also utilize bead technology and are automated. This type of assay utilizes a luminescent molecule as the antigen conjugate. The Liaison Treponema screen (DiaSorin, Stillwater, MN) uses magnetic beads to capture patient antibodies with an isoluminol-antigen conjugate. Positive samples are detected using a flash-chemiluminescent signal. The ADVIA Centaur syphilis assay (Siemens Healthcare Diagnostics, Inc., Newark, DE) is a direct sandwich immunoassay utilizing acridinium ester-labeled *T. pallidum* recombinant antigens, which bind to patient antibodies present in the specimen. Streptavidin-coated magnetic latex particles with biotinylated *T. pallidum* antigens bind to the antigen-antibody complexes. A light signal is produced during the reaction.

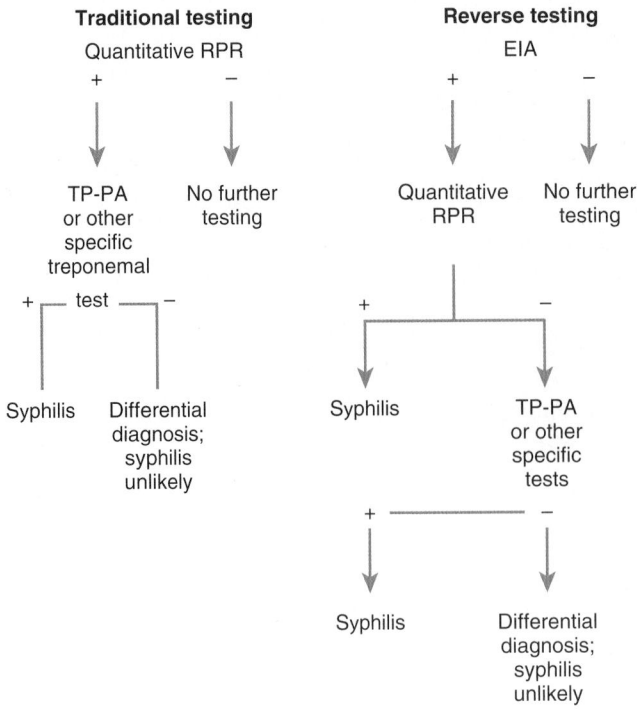

• **Fig. 45.3** Traditional testing versus reverse testing. *EIA,* Enzyme immunoassays; *RPR,* rapid plasma reagin; *TP-PA,* T. pallidum particle agglutination.

Antimicrobial Susceptibility Testing and Therapy

Because the treponemes cannot be cultivated, susceptibility testing is not performed. For all treponemal infections, penicillin G is the drug of choice. Ceftriaxone is also highly effective in most cases of syphilis, other than early syphilis. Tetracycline or doxycycline is often the treatment of choice when patients are allergic to penicillin. Treatment varies depending on the stage of disease and the host (e.g., children or adults, HIV-infected, or infected with congenital syphilis).

Prevention

No vaccines are available for the treponematoses. Prevention begins with early and appropriate treatment, thereby preventing person-to-person spread.

Borrelia

General Characteristics

Borreliosis is considered a **relapsing fever** transmitted by a human-specific body louse or the soft-body tick of the genus *Ornithodoros*. Organisms belonging to the genus

Borrelia are helical shaped and composed of 3 to 10 loose coils (Fig. 45.1) without hooked ends. They contain endoflagella located beneath the outer membrane that enables the organism to actively demonstrate a characteristic corkscrew motility. The cells contain a protoplasmic cylinder that is composed of a peptidoglycan layer and an inner membrane. In contrast to the treponemes, *Borrelia* spp. stain well with a Giemsa stain. Species that have been grown *in vitro* are microaerophilic or anaerobic.

Epidemiology and Pathogenesis

Although pathogens for mammals and birds, *Borrelia* are the causative agents of tick-borne and louse-borne relapsing fever and tick-borne Lyme disease in humans (Table 45.4).

Relapsing Fever

Human relapsing fever is caused by more than 20 species of *Borrelia* and is transmitted to humans by the bite of a louse or tick. *Borrelia recurrentis* is responsible for louse-borne or epidemic relapsing fever. This spirochete is transmitted from the louse *Pediculus humanus* subsp. *humanus*, and disease is found worldwide; humans are the only reservoir for *B. recurrentis*. All other borreliae that cause disease in the United States are transmitted via tick bites and are named after the species of tick, usually of

TABLE 45.4 Epidemiology and Spectrum of Disease of *Borrelia* spp. Pathogenic for Humans

Disease	Agent	Primary Arthropod Vector	Geographic Location	Clinical Manifestations
Lyme disease (Lyme borreliosis)	*Borrelia burgdorferi sensu lato* (*B. burgdorferi sensu stricto, B. mayonii, B. afzelii,*[a] *B. garinii,*[b] *B. valaisiana, B. lusitaniae, B. bavariensis, B. spielmanii, B. finlandensis, B. bissettiae, B. carolinensis*)	*Ixodes scapularis* and *I. pacificus* in the United States, *I. ricinus* in Europe, and *I. persulcatus* in Asia	Northeast, Mid-Atlantic, Upper Midwest, West Coast United States, Europe, and Asia	Refer to text in this chapter
Tick-borne relapsing fever (TBRF)	*Borrelia hermsii, B. turcatae,*[c] *B. parkeri, B. mazzottii, B. caucasica, B. crocidurae,*[c] *B. duttonii,*[c] *B. hispanica,*[c] *B. persica, B. venezuelensis*	*Ornithodoros* spp.	North America, South America, Europe, Asia, Africa	Refer to text in this chapter
Louse-borne relapsing fever (LBRF)	*Borrelia recurrentis*	*Pediculus humanus* subsp. *humanus*	Worldwide	Refer to text in this chapter
Hard tick-borne relapsing fever (HTBRF) or *Borrelia miyamotoi* disease (BMD)	*Borrelia miyamotoi*	*Ixodes scapularis* and *I. pacificus* in the United States, *I. ricinus* in Europe, and *I. persulcatus* in Asia	Northeast, Mid-Atlantic, Upper Midwest, West Coast United States, Europe, and Asia	Fever, chills, headache, myalgia, arthralgia, and fatigue. Neurologic involvement in immunocompromised. Skin lesions are rare.

[a]Acrodermatitis chronica atrophicans.
[b]Neuroborreliosis is strongly associated.
[c]Neurological involvement is common.

the genus *Ornithodoros* (soft tick), from which they are recovered. Common species in the United States include *Borrelia hermsii*, *Borrelia turicatae*, *Borrelia parkeri*, and *Borrelia mazzottii*. Depending on the organisms and the disease, their reservoir is either humans or rodents, in most cases. Although their pathogenic mechanisms are unclear, these spirochetes exhibit antigenic variability that may account for the cyclic fever patterns associated with this disease.

Lyme Disease

Although there are currently more than 20 different *Borrelia* genospecies within the *B. burgdorferi sensu lato* complex, only *Borrelia burgdorferi sensu stricto* (strict sense of *B. burgdorferi*), as well as *Borrelia garinii*, *Borrelia afzelii*, *Borrelia spielmanii*, *Borrelia lusitaniae*, and *Borrelia valaisiana*, and the recently discovered *Borrelia mayonii*, are agents of Lyme disease and are transmitted by the bite of *Ixodes* ticks. *B. burgdorferi* and *B. mayonii* (less commonly) cause Lyme disease in North America. Currently, *B. mayonii* has been detected in ticks in the Upper Midwest. **Lyme disease** is the most common vector-borne disease in North America and Europe and is an emerging problem in northern Asia. Hard ticks, belonging primarily to the genus *Ixodes*, act as vectors in the United States, including *Ixodes pacificus* in California and *Ixodes scapularis* in other areas. The ticks' natural hosts are deer and rodents. However, the adult ticks feed on a variety of mammals, including raccoons, domestic and wild carnivores, and birds. The ticks will attach to pets as well as to humans; all stages of ticks—larva, nymph, and adult—can harbor the spirochete and transmit disease. The nymphal form of the tick is most likely to transmit disease because it is active in the spring and summer, when people are dressed lightly and participate in outdoor activities in wooded areas. At this stage, the tick is the size of a pinhead and the initial tick bite may be overlooked. Ticks generally require a period of attachment of at least 24 hours before they transmit disease; however, other common diseases associated with *Ixodes* ticks, such as **anaplasmosis**, may be transmitted earlier on in the attachment period. Endemic areas of disease have been identified in many states, including Massachusetts, Connecticut, Maryland, Minnesota, Oregon, and California, as well as in Europe, Russia, Japan, and Australia. Direct invasion of tissues by the organism is responsible for the clinical manifestations. However, IgM antibodies are produced continually months to years after initial infection as the spirochete changes its antigens. *B. burgdorferi*'s potential ability to induce an autoimmune process in the host because of cross-reactive antigens may contribute to the pathology associated with Lyme disease. Moreover, by virtue of its ability to vary its surface antigens (e.g., outer surface protein [Osp] A to G), as well as avoid complement, *B. burgdorferi* is able to avoid the human host response. The pathologic findings associated with Lyme disease are also believed to result from the release of host cytokines initiated by the presence of the organism.

Spectrum of Disease

Relapsing Fever

Between 2 and 15 days after infection, patients have an abrupt onset of fever, headache, and myalgia that lasts for 4 to 10 days. Physical findings often include petechiae, diffuse abdominal tenderness, and conjunctival effusion. As the host produces specific antibodies in response to the agent, organisms disappear from the bloodstream, becoming sequestered (hidden) in different organs during the afebrile period. Subsequently, organisms reemerge with newly modified antigens and multiply, resulting in another febrile period. Subsequent relapses are usually milder and of shorter duration. In general, more relapses are associated with cases of untreated tick-borne relapsing fever, but louse-borne relapsing fevers tend to be more severe. *B. miyamotoi* can manifest as meningoencephalitis in immunocompromised patients.

Treatment of relapsing fever with antibiotics may result in the formation of the **Jarisch-Herxheimer reaction.** This reaction is associated with the clearance of the organisms from the bloodstream and the release of cytokines within hours of antibiotic treatment. The patient experiences tachycardia, chills, rigors, hypotension, fever, and diaphoresis. Death may be associated with the reaction. An acute respiratory distress syndrome has also been recognized in cases associated with tick-borne relapsing fever.

Lyme Disease

Lyme disease is characterized by three stages, not all of which occur in any given patient. The first stage, **early localized,** is characterized by **erythema migrans (EM),** a red, ring-shaped skin lesion sometimes with a central clearing ("bull's-eye" appearance) that first appears at the site of the tick bite but may develop at distant sites as well (Fig. 45.4). Patients may experience headache, fever, muscle and joint pain, and malaise during this stage. The **second stage, early disseminated,** beginning weeks to months after infection, may include arthritis, but the most important features are neurologic disorders (i.e., meningitis, neurologic deficits) and carditis. This is a result of the hematogenous spread of

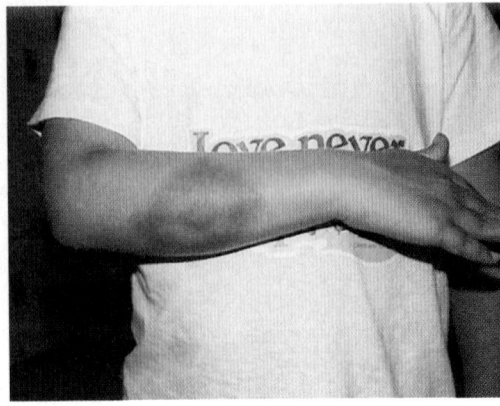

• **Fig. 45.4** Appearance of the classic erythema migrans lesion of acute Lyme disease.

spirochetes to organs and tissues. In addition, neurologic symptoms and infection may occur in the meninges, spinal cord, peripheral nerves, and brain (neuroborreliosis). The **third stage, late disseminated,** is usually characterized by chronic arthritis or **acrodermatitis chronica atrophicans (ACA),** a diffuse skin rash, and may continue for years. There is an association between *Borrelia* species and distinct clinical manifestations. For example, *B. garinii* has been associated with up to 72% of European cases of neuroborreliosis. Infection with *B. mayonii* has been associated with nausea and vomiting, as well as the presence of a diffuse skin rash and higher levels of spirochetemia, distinguishing it from *B. burgdorferi*.

Laboratory Diagnosis

Specimen Collection, Transport, and Processing

Peripheral blood in EDTA is the specimen of choice for direct detection of borreliae that cause relapsing fever. *B. burgdorferi* can be visualized, cultured, and identified using PCR; CSF samples may be used for nucleic acid detection in the diagnosis of *B. miyamotoi*–associated meningoencephalitis or in patients with neurological symptoms associated with *B. burgdorferi*. Serum should be collected for serology during acute and convalescent phases, separated by at least 2 weeks. Specimens submitted for stain or culture include blood, biopsy specimens, and body fluids, including joint and CSFs. Body fluids should be transported without any preservatives. Tissue biopsy specimens should be placed in sterile saline to prevent drying. Skin biopsies of the EM lesion can be used for culture and nucleic acid detection. Whole blood in EDTA can also be used for culture or nucleic acid detection during early disseminated infection. Synovial fluid and tissue may also be tested using nucleic acid tests to monitor treatment in Lyme arthritis.

Direct Detection Methods

Relapsing Fever

Clinical laboratories rely on direct observation of the organism in peripheral blood from patients for diagnosis. Organisms can be found in 70% of cases when blood specimens from febrile patients are examined. The organisms can be seen directly in wet preparations of peripheral blood (mixed with equal parts of sterile, nonbacteriostatic saline) under dark- or bright-field illumination, in which the spirochetes move rapidly, often pushing the red blood cells around. The organisms may be visualized by staining thick and thin films with Wright or Giemsa stains or the quantitative buffy coat (QBC) method, using procedures similar to those used to detect malaria. *B. miyamotoi* may be detected microscopically in CSF in patients experiencing meningoencephalitis. *B. burgdorferi* may be visualized in tissue sections stained with Warthin-Starry silver stain. In general, the number of spirochetes in the blood of patients with Lyme borreliosis is below the lower limits of microscopic detection, although *B. mayonii* may be seen on a blood smear due to high spirochetemia.

Nucleic Acid Detection

PCR has become important in diagnosing Lyme disease. PCR has detected *B. burgdorferi* DNA in clinical specimens from patients with early and late clinical manifestations; optimal specimens include synovial tissue, CSF, synovial fluid, and skin biopsies from patients with EM. PCR amplification of *B. burgdorferi* nucleic acid sequences has been successful from urine but is not recommended. Laboratories have used a variety of nucleic acid–based methods to increase sensitivity and specificity and decrease turnaround time for diagnosing Lyme borreliosis. PCR has confirmed EM with an overall sensitivity and specificity of 68% and 100%, respectively. The ability to detect spirochetes in blood or plasma by PCR is dependent on the stage of illness (from 40% of patients with secondary EM to only 9.5% of patients with primary EM); PCR also does relatively well in detecting *B. burgdorferi sensu lato* in synovial fluids. In contrast, variable results using PCR occur in CSF specimens obtained from patients with peripheral or central nervous system involvement with Lyme borreliosis. PCR testing can be used to diagnose Lyme borreliosis caused by *B. mayonii*. PCR has also been used for the detection of organisms within the relapsing fever *Borrelia* group. However, 16SrRNA gene sequences do not provide good discrimination between species. Other sequences have been used for speciation, including the chromosomally encoded flagellin sequence (*flaB*), the 16-23S ribosomal RNA intergenic spacer gene, and the glycerophosphodiester (*glpQ*) gene unique to relapsing fever *Borrelia* species.

Serodiagnosis

Relapsing Fever

Serologic tests for relapsing fever have not demonstrated reproducible or reliable data for diagnosis because of the many antigenic shifts *Borrelia* organisms undergo during the course of disease. Protein heterogeneity in strains of different species is quite variable. For example, the OspC protein has 21 major recognized antigenic types. In addition, patients may exhibit increased titers to *Proteus* OX K antigens (up to 1:80), but other cross-reacting antibodies are rare. EIA using recombinant GlpQ antigen has been successful in the relapsing fever *Borrelia* group. Patients infected with relapsing fever *Borrelia* can demonstrate reactivity in *B. burgdorferi* EIA antibody assays, including the C6 antibody assay. References laboratories and the CDC perform Western blot testing for relapsing fever. Infection is confirmed by Western blot when the organisms GlpQ and 22-kDa antigens are positive with IgG and IgM.

Lyme Disease

Despite its inadequacies, serology continues to be the standard for the diagnosis of Lyme disease. *B. burgdorferi* has numerous immunogenic lipids, proteins, lipoproteins, and carbohydrate antigens on its surface and outer membrane. The earliest antibody response and development of IgM are in response to the OspC membrane protein, the flagellar antigens (FlaA and FlaB), or the fibronectin-binding protein (BBK32). The IgM levels peak within several weeks but may be detectable for several months. The IgG response develops slowly during the first several weeks of disease and increases with antibody responses to Osp17 (decorin-binding protein) and additional proteins, including p39 (BmpA) and p58. The late-stage infection demonstrates IgG antibodies to numerous antigens.

Numerous serologic tests are commercially available. These include indirect immunofluorescence assays (IFA), which are being used less frequently, EIA, CIA, Immunoblots, and Western blots. The CDC recommends using validated and FDA approved IFA, CIA, or EIA as a first step, followed by an immunoblot, when performing serologic testing using the STTT. Measuring antibody by EIA or CIA are the most common screening methods used because they are quick, reproducible, and relatively inexpensive. However, false-positive rates are high, mainly as a result of cross-reactivity. In addition, there is a lack of standardization between assays regarding the antigenic composition and antibodies detected from different manufacturers. The specificity of IFA may be improved by the adsorption of serum with the Reiter *Treponema*, *Treponema phagedenis* sonicate, or egg yolk (IFA-ABS). Patients with syphilis, HIV infection, leptospirosis, mononucleosis, parvovirus infection,

rheumatoid arthritis, and other autoimmune diseases commonly show positive results. Capture EIAs have been developed to prevent false-positive reactions with rheumatoid factor. In addition, this may be overcome by pretreatment of the patient's sera with anti-IgG.

For the United States, the CDC recommends a two-step approach to the serologic diagnosis of Lyme disease. In the STTT, the first step is a sensitive screening test such as an EIA, IFA, or CIA; if this test is positive for IgM or IgG or equivocal, the result must be confirmed by separate IgM and IgG immunoblotting (Fig. 45.5). Western blots should not be performed without a previously positive CIA, IFA, or EIA result, as this decreases the specificity of the test and can lead to false-positive results. IgM immunoblot requires reactivity in at least two of the three antigens tested: 23 kDaOspC, 39, and 41 kDa antigens. An IgM immunoblot requires reactivity in at least 5 of 10 antigens included in the assay: 18, 23, 28, 30, 39, 41, 45, 58, 66, and 93 kDa. IgM should only be used during the first 30 days of the infection, whereas IgG may be used at any stage during the disease process. As with *B. burgdorferi*, Lyme borreliosis caused by *B. mayonii* can also be detected with two-tier serologic testing.

Recently, the CDC changed its recommendations for Lyme disease testing to include an MTTT. In this algorithm,

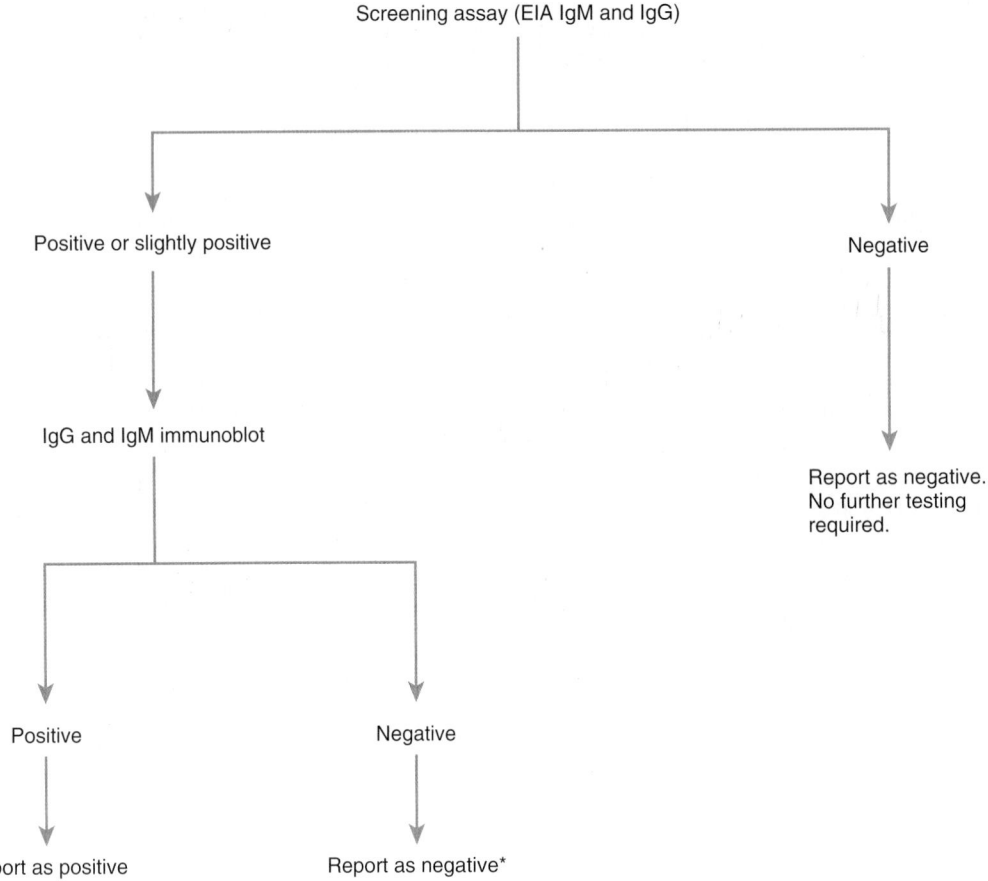

• **Fig. 45.5** Two-step serodiagnostic procedure. *Note: If neuroborreliosis is suspected, a paired sera and cerebrospinal fluid (CSF) specimen is recommended for testing. Any disease of short duration. For Lyme disease, it is recommended that a follow-up serologic test be performed at a later date. *EIA*, Enzyme immunoassays.

two EIAs are used: one as the primary screening test and the other as the second confirmatory test, which is performed if the first EIA is positive or equivocal. The FDA cleared ZEUS Scientific's EIAs (ZEUS ELISA) for use in the MTTT. The first-tier test, ZEUS ELISA *Borrelia* VlsE1/pepC10 IgG/IgM Test System, measures IgM and IgG antibodies to the *Borrelia burgdorferi* antigens VlsE1 and pepC10. Positive or equivocal results are followed by the second-tier test, either the ZEUS ELISA *Borrelia burgdorferi* IgG/IgM Test System, ZEUS ELISA *Borrelia burgdorferi* IgM Test System, or ZEUS ELISA *Borrelia burgdorferi* IgG Test System, which measure antibodies to *Borrelia burgdorferi* whole-cell antigen. All of the assays are horseradish peroxidase based. The MTTT allows for a greater ease of performance and interpretation as compared with the STTT by eliminating the need to perform a Western blot and decreases turnaround time.

In certain clinical situations, results of serologic tests must be interpreted with caution. For example, patients with Lyme arthritis commonly remain antibody-positive despite treatment but do not necessarily have a persistent infection. Conversely, patients with a localized EM may be seronegative. Because of these limitations and others, the FDA and the American College of Physicians have published guidelines regarding the use of laboratory tests for Lyme disease diagnosis. Of paramount importance is the clinician's determination before ordering serologic tests of the pretest probability of Lyme disease based on clinical symptoms and the incidence of Lyme disease in the population represented by the patient.

Cultivation

Although the organisms that cause relapsing fever can be cultured in nutritionally rich media under microaerobic conditions, the procedures are cumbersome and unreliable and are used primarily as research tools. Similarly, the culture of *B. burgdorferi* may be attempted, although the yield is low. The best specimens for culture in untreated patients include the peripheral area of the EM ring lesion or synovial tissue. CSF and blood or plasma (greater than 9 mL), in general, are of low diagnostic yield by culture. This seems to correlate with the duration of the neurologic disease—in other words, positive results decrease as the duration of the disease increases. To cultivate the organism, the plasma, spinal fluid sediment, or macerated tissue biopsy is inoculated into a tube of modified Kelly's medium (BSK II, BSK-H, or Preac-Mursic) and incubated at 30°C to 34°C for up to 12 weeks under microaerophilic conditions. Likewise, *B. mayonii* can be cultivated under these conditions in BSK II medium. Blind subcultures (0.1 mL) are performed weekly from the lower portion of the broth to fresh media, and the cultures are examined by dark-field microscopy or by fluorescence microscopy after staining with acridine orange for the presence of spirochetes. Because of the long incubation time and low sensitivity associated with cultivation, cultivation is often confined to reference or research laboratories.

Antimicrobial Susceptibility Testing and Therapy

Currently there are no standardized methods, and borreliae are difficult to culture; therefore, antimicrobial susceptibility testing is not routinely performed.

Several antibiotics, including tetracycline, are effective in treating relapsing fever, although it is associated with a higher rate of **Jarisch-Herxheimer reaction,** which can be life threatening. Doxycycline, amoxicillin, or cefuroxime and parenteral cephalosporins are drugs of choice during the first stage of Lyme disease. Broad-spectrum cephalosporins, particularly ceftriaxone or cefotaxime, have been used successfully with patients who either fail initial treatment or present in later stages of the disease, such as neuroborreliosis. Oral regimens are typically successful; however, patients with atrioventricular block may require intravenous (IV) therapy. Symptomatic treatment failures have been reported.

Prevention

Avoiding tick-infested areas; wearing protective clothing; checking the clothing, body, and pets for ticks; and removing them promptly also assist in the prevention of infection. There are no vaccines against infections caused by other *Borrelia* spp.

Brachyspira

General Characteristics

Brachyspira spp. are comma or helical shaped, with tapered ends containing four flagella. *Brachyspira aalborgi* requires anaerobic incubation and has not been isolated from animals, whereas *Brachyspira pilosicoli* colonizes the intestine of a variety of animal species. The organisms reside in the brush border within the intestine and appear as a basophilic fringe, referred to as a "false brush border," upon histologic staining with hematoxylin and eosin.

Epidemiology and Pathogenesis

B. aalborgi is most likely transmitted via fecal-oral contamination. *B. pilosicoli* infection results from ingesting water contaminated with feces from infected animals. *Brachyspira* spp. cause intestinal spirochetosis, which may manifest as chronic diarrhea. The organisms have been associated with crypt abscesses, ulceration, necrosis, and multiple organ failure. Pathogenic mechanisms are not well understood. Clinical significance must be carefully correlated with patient signs and symptoms.

Laboratory Diagnosis
Specimen Collection and Direct Detection

Fresh stool or rectal swabs may be collected and examined by dark-field microscopy. In addition, tissue biopsy specimens may be submitted for culture, PCR and histologic examination using periodic acid-Schiff (PAS) or hematoxylin and eosin staining. PCR amplification methods have been developed but are not available within the clinical laboratory.

Cultivation

Brachyspira spp. can be grown in the laboratory on brain-heart infusion (BHI) or tryptic soy agar containing 10% fetal bovine blood, 400 μg/mL of spectinomycin, and 5 μg/mL polymyxin in anaerobic conditions at 37°C. Increased growth can be seen at 41°C. Confluent growth patterns typically occur. *B. aalborgi* is weakly beta-hemolytic on BHI containing 10% fetal bovine blood.

Approach to Identification

B. aalborgi can be differentiated from *B. pilosicoli* by a strong positive hippurate hydrolysis reaction and a weak indole reaction. *B. pilosicoli* is indole-negative and has a weak hippurate hydrolysis reaction. Matrix-assisted laser desorption ionization and time-of-flight mass spectrometry have been successfully used for the identification of *Brachyspira* species.

Antimicrobial Susceptibility Testing and Therapy

Isolates of *B. pilosicoli* have demonstrated susceptibility to Augmentin (amoxicillin-clavulanic acid), ceftriaxone, chloramphenicol, meropenem, tetracycline, and metronidazole.

Leptospira

General Characteristics

The leptospires include both free-living and parasitic forms. The organisms are spiral-shaped, right-handed helices with hooked ends. The organisms contain two axial filaments and exhibit either a spinning motility or a rapid back-and-forth movement. *Leptospira* spp. are typically classified into three major groups, with *Leptospira interrogans sensu stricto* being the main species associated with human leptospirosis; in France, this organism is responsible for about 60% of human cases.

Molecular classification using 16S ribosomal ribonucleic acid (rRNA) sequencing currently separates the genus into three distinct groups of pathogens, intermediate pathogens, and environmental saprophytes.

The pathogens include more than 200 serologically defined types that were formerly designated as species and are now referred to as serovars, or serotypes, of *L. interrogans sensu stricto* and more than 60 serovars of *L. biflexa sensu lato*. Each serovar is usually associated with a particular animal host, and therefore serovar identification is important for epidemiology studies and prevention strategies. The genotypic classification scheme now includes approximately 23 genomospecies, which incorporates all current serovars of *Leptospira*. Serovars cross species lines as a result of the horizontal transfer of genetic elements, making it difficult to fully classify species phenotypically.

Epidemiology and Pathogenesis

Leptospirosis, a zoonosis, has a worldwide distribution but is most common in developing countries and warm climates via contact with infected animals or contaminated water. *L. interrogans* can infect most mammals throughout the world, as well as reptiles, amphibians, fish, birds, and invertebrates. The organism is maintained in nature by virtue of persistent colonization of renal tubules of carrier animals. Humans become infected through direct or indirect contact with the urine of infected animals. Humans and animals can be classified as a maintenance (infection is endemic) host or accidental host for leptospires. Leptospires enter the human host through breaks in the skin, mucous membranes, or conjunctivae. Infection can be acquired in home and recreational settings (e.g., swimming, hunting, canoeing) or in people who work in certain occupational settings (e.g., farmers, ranchers, abattoir workers, trappers, veterinarians).

Pathogenic leptospires rapidly invade the bloodstream after entry, and spread throughout all sites in the body, such as the central nervous system and kidneys. Virulent strains show chemotaxis toward hemoglobin as well, as the ability to migrate through host tissues. A number of potential virulence factors that might facilitate this process are shown in Box 45.1. How *L. interrogans* causes disease is not completely understood, but it appears that the presence of endotoxin and other toxins may play a role in activation of the hemostasis pathways as an autoimmune response in the human host.

Spectrum of Disease

Symptoms begin abruptly 2 to 30 days after infection and include fever, headache, and myalgia. The most common clinical syndrome is **anicteric leptospirosis,** which is a self-limiting illness consisting of a septicemic stage, with high fever and severe headache that lasts 3 to 7 days, followed by the immune stage. Symptoms associated with the immune stage (onset coincides with the appearance of IgM) are varied but are generally milder than those associated with the septicemic stage. The hallmark of the immune stage is aseptic meningitis. **Weil disease,** or **icteric leptospirosis,** is generally the most severe illness, with symptoms caused by liver, kidney, or vascular dysfunction with lethal pulmonary hemorrhage; death can occur in up to 10% of cases.

• BOX 45.1 Potential Virulence Factors of *Leptospira*

Hemolysins
Sphingomyelinases C and H
Proteolytic enzymes (thermolysin, collagenase)
Catalase
Cobalamin biosynthesis
Sialic acids
Fibronectin-binding protein for adhesion and invasion
Lipopolysaccharide and outer membrane proteins

Unfortunately, the clinical presentations of leptospirosis mimic those of many other diseases.

Laboratory Diagnosis

Specimen Collection, Transport, and Processing

During the first 10 days of illness, leptospires are present in the blood, CSF, and peritoneal dialysate. Urine specimens can be collected beginning in the second week of illness and up to 30 days after the onset of symptoms. Specimens may be collected in citrate, heparin, or oxalate anticoagulants. There are no other special requirements for specimen collection, transport, or processing. Citrate or ethylenediaminetetraacetic acid (EDTA) is the preferred anticoagulant for nucleic acid–based testing. Urine specimens should not be placed in preservatives and should be processed within 1 hour for optimal results. Urine specimens collected for nucleic acid testing can be placed in several commercial products and transported over long periods. Specimens should be transported at room temperature and inoculated for culture within 24 hours.

Direct Detection

Blood, CSF, and urine may be examined directly by dark-field microscopy. The detection of motile leptospires in these specimens is optimized after centrifuging at $1500\times g$ for 30 minutes; sodium oxalate or heparin-treated blood is initially spun at $500\times g$ for 15 minutes to remove blood cells. Other techniques, such as fluorescent antibody staining and hybridization techniques using leptospira-specific DNA probes, have also detected leptospires in clinical specimens.

Nucleic Acid Detection

Conventional and real-time PCR assays have been used to detect leptospires in blood, plasma, serum, urine, aqueous humor, CSF, autopsy tissue, and environmental samples. Nucleic acid detection is at least comparable to culture and useful in confirming diagnosis during the acute stages of the infection.

Cultivation

Albeit insensitive, the definitive method for laboratory diagnosis of leptospirosis is to culture the organisms from blood, CSF, or urine. A few drops of heparinized or sodium oxalate–anticoagulated blood are inoculated into tubes of semisolid media enriched with rabbit serum (Fletcher's or Stuart's) or bovine serum albumin. Urine should be inoculated soon after collection, because acidity (diluted out in the broth medium) may harm the spirochetes. One or two drops of undiluted urine and a 1:10 dilution of urine are added to 5 mL of medium. The addition of 200 μg/mL of 5-fluorouracil (an anticancer drug) may prevent contamination by other bacteria without harming the leptospires. Commercial media such as the Ellinghausen-McCullough-Johnson-Harris (EMJH) or Fletcher's medium (Difco EMJH or Difco Fletcher's medium; BD Diagnostic Systems, Sparks, MD) are available, which contain 5-fluorouracil for use at the patient's bedside. Tissue specimens, especially from the liver and kidney, may be aseptically macerated and inoculated in dilutions of 1:1, 1:10, and 1:100 as for urine cultures.

All cultures are incubated at room temperature or 30°C in the dark for up to 6 to 8 weeks. Because organisms grow below the surface, material collected from a few centimeters below the surface of broth cultures should be examined weekly for the presence of growth, using a direct wet preparation under dark-field illumination. Leptospires exhibit corkscrewlike motility.

Approach to Identification

Based on the number of coils and hooked ends, leptospires can be distinguished from other spirochetes. Physiologically, the saprophytes can be differentiated from pathogens by their ability to grow at 10°C and lower, or at least 5°C lower than the growth temperature of pathogenic leptospires. Leptospires may also be visualized using dark-field microscopy or immunofluorescence.

Serodiagnosis

Serodiagnosis of leptospirosis requires a fourfold or greater rise in titer of agglutinating antibodies. The microscopic agglutination test (MAT) using live cells is the standard serologic procedure. Serologic diagnosis of leptospirosis is performed using pools of bacterial antigens containing many serotypes in each pool. Positive results are indicated by the presence of agglutination using dark-field microscopy. However, a macroscopic agglutination procedure is more readily accessible to routine clinical laboratories. Reagents are available commercially. Indirect hemagglutination and an ELISA test for IgM antibody are also available; IgM-detection assays are primarily used because IgM antibodies become detectable during the first week of illness. Rapid immunochromatographic assays are now available for the detection of IgM and/or IgG antibodies to *Leptospira interrogans* (Abbott, Chicago, IL).

Molecular Typing Methods

Several nucleic acid–based amplification methods have been developed. However, PCR methodologies are not useful for the differentiation of serovars and therefore are of limited use in epidemiologic studies. Highly complex and labor-intensive techniques such as pulsed-field gel electrophoresis (PFGE) and restriction-fragment-length polymorphism (RFLP) and ribotyping are more useful for the identification of serovars. Nucleic acid sequencing has been used to successfully identify *Leptospira* directly in clinical specimens when the bacterial load was high.

Antimicrobial Susceptibility Testing and Therapy

Treatment of leptospirosis is supportive management and the use of appropriate antibiotics. Ceftriaxone, penicillin, amoxicillin, doxycycline, and tetracycline are recommended for the treatment of leptospirosis. Standardized procedures for antibiotic susceptibility are limited by the slow growth of the organisms and the need for serum during cultivation.

Prevention

General preventive measures include the vaccination of domestic livestock and pet dogs. In addition, protective clothing, rodent control measures, and preventing recreational exposures, such as avoiding freshwater ponds, are indicated in preventing leptospirosis.

ⓔ Visit the Evolve site for a complete list of procedures, review questions, and case studies.

Bibliography

Aguero-Rosenfeld ME, Wang G, Schwartz I, Wormser GP: Diagnosis of Lyme borreliosis, *Clin Microbiol Rev* 18:484–509, 2005.

Caroll KC, Pfaller MA: *Manual of clinical microbiology*, ed 12, Washington, DC, 2019, ASM Press.

Centers for Disease Control and Prevention: Discordant results from reverse sequence syphilis screening—five laboratories, United States, 2006-2010, *MMWR Morb Mortal Wkly Rep* 60:133–137, 2011.

Centers for Disease Control and Prevention: *Sexually transmitted disease surveillance 2017*, Atlanta, 2018, U.S. Department of Health and Human Services.

Church B, Wall E, Webb JR, Cameron CE: Interaction of *Treponema pallidum*, the syphilis spirochete, with human platelets, *PloS One* 14(1):e0210902, 2019.

Cutler S, Vayssier-Taussat M, Estrada-Peña A, Potkonjak A, Mihalca AD, Zeller H: A new *Borrelia* on the block: *Borrelia miyamotoi* – a human health risk? *Euro Surveill* 24(18), 2019. https://doi.org/10.2807/1560-7917.ES.2019.24.18.1800170.

Djokic V, Giacani L, Parveen N: Analysis of host cell binding specificity mediated by the Tp0136 adhesin of the syphilis agent *T. pallidum* subsp. *pallidum*, *PLoS Negl Trop Dis* 13(5):e0007401, 2019.

Erlandson KM, Klingler ET: Intestinal spirochetosis: epidemiology, microbiology and clinical significance, *Clin Microbiol Newsl* 27:91, 2005.

Fakile YF, Jost H, Hoover KW, et al.: Correlation of treponemal immunoassay signal strength values with reactivity of confirmatory treponemal testing, *J Clin Microbiol* 56(1):e01165-e01117, 26, 2017. https://doi.org/10.1128/JCM.01165-17.

Food and Drug Administration: *FDA clears new indications for existing Lyme disease tests that may help streamline diagnoses. [News release]*, Silver Spring, MD, 2019, US Department of Health and Human Services, Food and Drug Administration, Available at: https://www.fda.gov/news-events/press-announcements/fda-clears-new-indications-existing-lyme-disease-tests-may-help-streamline-diagnosesexternal.

Fouts DE, Matthias MA, Adhikarla H, et al.: What makes a bacterial species pathogenic? comparative genomic analysis of the genus *Leptospira*, *PLoS Negl Trop Dis* 10(2):e0004403, 2016. https://doi.org/10.1371/journal.pntd.0004403.

Hampson DJ: The spirochete *Brachyspirapilosicoli*, enteric pathogen of animals and humans, *Clin Microbiol Rev* 31(1):e00087-17, 2017. https://doi.org/10.1128/CMR.00087-17.

Johnson TL, Graham CB, Maes SE, et al.: Prevalence and distribution of seven human pathogens in host-seeking *Ixodes scapularis* (Acari: Ixodidae) nymphs in Minnesota, USA, *Ticks Tick Borne Dis* 9(6): 1499–1507, 2018. https://doi.org/10.1016/j.ttbdis.2018.07.009.

Li SJ, Zhang CC, Li XW, et al.: Molecular typing of *Leptospira interrogans* strains isolated from *Rattus tanezumi* in Guizhou province, southwest of China, *Biomed Environ Sci* 25:542–548, 2012.

Malincarne L, Schiaroli E, Ciervo A, et al.: Meningitis with cranial polyneuritis and cavernous sinus thrombosis by *Borrelia crocidurae*: first autochthonous case in Europe, *Int J Infect Dis* 82:30–32, 2019. https://doi.org/10.1016/j.ijid.2019.02.028.

Mead P, Petersen J, Hinckley A: Updated CDC recommendation for serologic diagnosis of Lyme disease, *MMWR Morb Mortal Wkly Rep* 68:703, 2019. https://doi.org/10.15585/mmwr.mm6832a4.

Package Insert: *ZEUS ELISA Borrelia VlsE1/pepC10 IgG/IgM test System*, Branchburg, NJ 08876, USA, ZEUS Scientific, Inc.

Package Insert: *ZEUS ELISA Borrelia burgdorferi IgG/IgM test System*, Branchburg, NJ 08876, USA, ZEUS Scientific, Inc.

Park IU, Fakile YF, Chow JM, et al.: Performance of treponemal tests for the diagnosis of syphilis, *Clin Infect Dis* 68(6):913–918, 2019. https://doi.org/10.1093/cid/ciy558.

Peeling RW, Mabey D, Kamb ML, Chen XS, Radolf JD, Benzaken AS: Syphilis, *Nat Rev Dis Primers* 3:17073, 2017. https://doi.org/10.1038/nrdp.2017.73.

Phillips ND, La T, Hampson DJ: *Brachyspira catarrhinii* sp. nov., an anaerobic intestinal spirochaete isolated from Vervet monkeys may have been misidentified as *Brachyspira aalborgi* in previous studies, *Anaerobe* 59:8–13, 2019. https://doi.org/10.1016/j.anaerobe.2019.05.004.

Pritt BS, Respicio-Kingry LB, Sloan LM, et al.: *Borrelia mayonii* sp. nov., a member of the *Borrelia burgdorferi* sensu lato complex, detected in patients and ticks in the upper Midwestern United States, *Int J Syst Evol Microbiol* 66(11):4878–4880, 2016.

Ratnam S: The laboratory diagnosis of syphilis, *Can J Infect Dis Med Microbiol* 16(1):45–51, 2005.

Shen AK, Mead PS, Beard CB: The Lyme disease vaccine—a public health perspective, *Clin Infect Dis* 52(Suppl 3):s247–s252, 2011. Available at: https://doi.org/10.1093/cid/ciq115.

Strnad M, Hönig V, Růžek D, Grubhoffer L, Rego ROM: Europe-wide meta-analysis of *Borrelia burgdorferi* sensu lato prevalence in questing *Ixodes ricinus* ticks, *Appl Environ Microbiol* 83(15):e00609–e00617, 2017. https://doi.org/10.1128/AEM.00609-17.

Spirochaetes. *National Center for Biotechnology Information (NCBI) taxonomy database*. Accessed May 15,2019. Available at: https://www.ncbi.nlm.nih.gov/Taxonomy/Browser/wwwtax.cgi?mode=Undef&id=203691&lvl=6&lin.

Talagrand-Reboul E, Boyer PH, Bergström S, Vial L, Boulanger N: Relapsing fevers: neglected tick-borne diseases, *Front Cell Infect Microbiol* 8:98, 2018. https://doi.org/10.3389/fcimb.2018.00098.

Wang Y, Li S, Wang Z, Zhang L, Cai Y, Liu Q: Prevalence and identification of *Borrelia burgdorferi* sensu lato genospecies in ticks from Northeastern China, *Vector Borne Zoonotic Dis* 19(5):309–315, 2019. https://doi.org/10.1089/vbz.2018.2316.

Wilske B: Diagnosis of Lyme borreliosis in Europe, *Vector Borne Zoonotic Dis* 3:215–227, 2003.

You M, Mo S, Leung WK, Watt RM: Comparative analysis of oral treponemes associated with periodontal health and disease, *BMC Infect Dis* 13:174, 2013. https://doi.org/10.1186/1471-2334-13-174.

Zhou C, Zhang X, Zhang W, Duan J, Zhao F: PCR detection for syphilis diagnosis: status and prospects, *J Clin Lab Anal* 33(5):e22890, 2019. https://doi.org/10.1002/jcla.22890.

46

Overview of the Methods and Strategies in Parasitology

OBJECTIVES

This chapter provides an overview of the general epidemiology, pathogenesis, spectrum of disease, and approach to the identification of parasites. The detailed technical procedures should be used in conjunction with additional organism-specific chapters in this section to provide a clear description of the process, from specimen collection to identification. However, students should consider the following general objectives for the methods provided:

1. State the specific diagnostic purpose for each test methodology as well as its advantages and disadvantages.
2. Briefly describe the principle associated with the test method.
3. Determine specimen acceptability for parasite identification, including collection method, collection time/receipt time, number or quantity of specimen, and presence of interfering and contaminating substances.
4. Select appropriate preservatives for parasite specimens and explain the chemical principle and rationale for the preservative, including polyvinyl alcohol (PVA), universal fixative, formalin, and sodium acetate acetic acid formalin (SAF).
5. Select the appropriate method of detection and identification of parasites based on the type of specimen.
6. Discuss the effectiveness of antibody serology, antigen detection, molecular methods, and the traditional processing of ova and parasites (O&Ps) for the diagnosis of various parasite infections.

P arasitic diseases are often associated with the earth's tropical zones; however, many parasitic organisms that infect humans are worldwide in distribution and occur with some frequency in the temperate zones. In addition, people who travel to and from areas where parasites are endemic may contract one of these infections and then seek medical attention in their home country, far distant from the expected geographic area. An increase in the number

of compromised patients, particularly those who are immunodeficient or immunosuppressed, has also led to increased interest in the field of parasitology. These individuals are greatly at risk for certain parasitic infections. Parasites that infect humans are classified into six major divisions:

- Protozoa (amebae, flagellates, ciliates, sporozoans, coccidia, microsporidia)
- Nematoda, or roundworms
- Platyhelminthes, or flatworms (cestodes, trematodes)
- Pentastomids, or tongue worms
- Acanthocephala, or thorny-headed worms
- Arthropoda (e.g., insects, spiders, mites, ticks)

The identification of parasitic organisms traditionally depends on the observation of characteristic morphologic criteria; accurate depiction of these criteria, in turn, depends on correct specimen collection, processing, and adequate fixation. Improperly submitted specimens may result in failure to detect the organisms or their misidentification. Tables 46.1 to 46.3 present information on the various groups of parasites, those that may be recovered from various body sites, the most frequently used specimen collection approaches, and appropriate processing methods.

Epidemiology

Parasites are usually restricted to specialized environments inside and outside of their hosts. The **host specificity** of any individual parasite greatly influences factors associated with transmission and control. A disease of wild or domestic animals, **zoonotic disease,** also occurs in humans. Animals that are potential sources of a parasitic infection for humans are **reservoir hosts.** Some parasitic organisms are free living during specific stages of their life cycles and do not depend on human or other living hosts for survival. In some cases, humans become an **accidental** or unintended **host.** When humans are the only host for a parasite or a stage of its development, control and prevention options are relatively easy to define. However, if an infection is zoonotic or has an

TABLE 46.1   Description of the More Common Groups of Human Parasites

Parasite Group	Description
Protozoa, Intestinal	
Amebae	Single-celled organisms; pseudopodia (motility), trophozoite, and cyst stages in the life cycle. Exceptions: Some have no identified cyst. Fecal-oral transmission of the infective cyst. *Entamoeba histolytica* causes amebiasis and is the most significant organism in this group.
Flagellates	Protozoa with characteristic flagella. Fecal-oral transmission. Exceptions: *Trichomonas* has a trophozoite and no cyst stage. Reproduction by longitudinal binary fission. Examples: *Giardia duodenalis* and *Dientamoeba fragilis*.
Ciliates	Single-celled protozoa; cilia (motility), which beat in a coordinated, rhythmic pattern, moving the trophozoite in a spiral path. Trophozoite and cyst stages in the life cycle; both stages show a large macronucleus and a micronucleus. Fecal-oral transmission. *Neobalantidium coli* is the single human pathogen in the group.
Coccidia	Protozoa; asexual and sexual life cycles. Fecal-oral transmission via contaminated food and/or water. Infective stage (oocyst) containing sporocysts and/or sporozoites. Examples: *Cryptosporidium* spp., *Cyclospora cayetanensis*, *Cystoisospora belli*, and *Sarcocystis* spp.
Microsporidia	Small (1–2.5 µm) intestinal protozoa. Transmission by ingestion, inhalation, or direct inoculation of spores. Nine genera cause disease in humans; the two most important are *Encephalitozoon* and *Enterocytozoon*.
Protozoa, Other Sites	
Amebae	Pathogenic free-living organisms associated with warm freshwater environments. Except for *Entamoeba gingivalis* (found in the mouth), they have been isolated from the central nervous system (CNS), eye, and other body sites. Examples: *Naegleria fowleri*—acute CNS infection and death. Chronic CNS disease (*Acanthamoeba* spp., *Balamuthia mandrillaris*), and *Acanthamoeba* spp. can also cause keratitis.
Flagellates	Have flagella (long, proteinaceous organelles used for motility). Sexual transmission. Examples: *Trichomonas vaginalis* is located in the genitourinary system. *Trichomonas tenax* can be identified in the mouth and is considered nonpathogenic.
Coccidia	Obligate intracellular, spore forming. Transmission is typically fecal-oral through ingestion of contaminated materials or food. Examples: *Cryptosporidium* spp. and *Toxoplasma gondii*.
Microsporidia	Small (1–2.5 µm) spore-forming protozoa. Transmission is typically by ingestion of spores. Life cycles vary considerably; some have an asexual life cycle, whereas others are complex and have both asexual and sexual life cycles and multiple hosts. Examples: *Encephalitozoon, Pleistophora, Trachipleistophora,* and *Anncaliia* spp.
Protozoa, Blood and Tissue	
Malaria, babesiosis	Arthropod vector–borne protozoa. Transmission via insect bite. Examples: *Plasmodium* spp. includes parasites that undergo exoerythrocytic and pigment-producing erythrocytic schizogony in vertebrates and a sexual stage followed by sporogony in mosquitoes. *Babesia* spp. are tick-borne and can cause severe disease in patients who have been splenectomized or otherwise immunologically compromised.
Flagellates (leishmaniae)	Trypanosomatid protozoa; two morphologic forms—promastigotes (anterior flagellum) in the insect host and amastigote (no flagella) in the vertebrate host. Transmission is through an insect vector. Recovery and identification of the organisms are related to body site. Recovery of leishmanial amastigotes is limited to the site of the lesion in infections other than those caused by the *Leishmania donovani* complex (visceral leishmaniasis).

TABLE 46.1   Description of the More Common Groups of Human Parasites—cont'd

Parasite Group	Description
Flagellates (trypanosomes)	Trypanosomatid protozoa; morphologic forms are identified based on the position, length, and attachment site of the flagella. At some time in their life cycle, these protozoa have the trypomastigote form with the typical undulating membrane and free flagellum at the anterior end. Transmission is typically through an insect vector. Some organisms cause African sleeping sickness (e.g., *Trypanosoma brucei gambiense, T. brucei rhodesiense*). The etiologic agent of American trypanosomiasis is *Trypanosoma cruzi,* which has amastigote and trypomastigote stages in the mammalian host and an epimastigote form in the arthropod host.
Nematodes, intestinal	Helminthic parasites; roundworms. Nematodes have separate sexes, are elongate-cylindrical and bilaterally symmetric with a triradiate symmetry at the anterior end. Nematodes have an outer cuticle layer, no circular muscles, and a pseudocele that contains all systems (digestive, excretory, nervous, and reproductive). Transmission is by ingestion of eggs or by skin penetration of larval forms from the soil. Examples: *Ascaris, Enterobius, Trichuris,* and *Strongyloides* spp. and hookworm.
Nematodes, tissue	Helminthic parasites; roundworms. Many of these organisms are rarely seen in the United States; however, some are important and are found worldwide. Diagnosis may be difficult if the only specimens are biopsy and/or autopsy, and interpretation must be based on examination of histologic preparations. Examples: *Trichinella* spp., visceral larva migrans (VLM), ocular larva migrans (OLM), cutaneous larva migrans (CLM).
Nematodes, filarial	Helminthic parasites; roundworms. Transmission is via arthropods. Adult worms tend to live in the tissues or lymphatics of the vertebrate host. The diagnosis is made based on recovery and identification of the larval worms (microfilariae) in the blood, other body fluids, or skin. Examples: *Wuchereria, Brugia, Loa,* and *Onchocerca* spp.
Cestodes, intestinal	Helminthic parasites; tapeworms. Adult tapeworm consists of a chain of egg-producing units called proglottids, which develop from the neck region of the attachment organ (scolex). Food is absorbed through the worm's integument. The intermediate host contains the larval forms acquired through ingestion of the adult tapeworm eggs. Transmission is through the ingestion of larval forms in poorly cooked or raw meat or freshwater fish. Examples: *Dipylidium caninum* (infection is acquired by accidental ingestion of dog fleas). *Hymenolepis nana* and *Hymenolepis diminuta* are transmitted via ingestion of certain arthropods (fleas, beetles). In addition, *H. nana* can be transmitted through egg ingestion (life cycle can bypass the intermediate beetle host). Humans can serve as both the intermediate and definitive hosts in *H. nana* and *Taenia solium* infections.
Cestodes, tissue	Tissue tapeworms. Transmission is through ingestion of certain tapeworm eggs or accidental contact with certain larval forms, leading to tissue infection. Humans serve as the accidental intermediate host. Examples: *T. solium, Echinococcus granulosus,* and several other species.
Trematodes, intestinal	Flatworms that are exclusively parasitic. Except for the schistosomes (blood flukes), flukes are hermaphroditic. They may be flattened; most have oral and ventral suckers. Transmission: Intestinal trematodes require a freshwater snail to serve as an intermediate host; these infections are food-borne (freshwater fish, mollusks, or plants). Example: *Fasciolopsis buski,* the giant intestinal fluke.
Trematodes, liver, lung	Transmission: Liver and lung trematodes require a freshwater snail to serve as an intermediate host; these infections are food-borne (freshwater fish, crayfish or crabs, or plants). Examples: Public health concerns include cholangiocarcinoma associated with *Clonorchis* and *Opisthorchis* infections, severe liver disease associated with *Fasciola* infections, and misdiagnosis of tuberculosis in individuals infected with *Paragonimus* spp.
Trematodes, blood	Schistosomes; sexes are separate. Males are characterized by an infolded body that forms the gynecophoral canal in which the female worm is held during copulation and oviposition. Transmission: Infection is acquired by skin penetration by the cercarial forms that are released from freshwater snails. The adult worms reside in the blood vessels over the small intestine, large intestine, or bladder. Examples: *Schistosoma mansoni, Schistosoma haematobium,* and *Schistosoma japonicum.*

TABLE 46.2 Body Sites and Parasite Recovery (Trophozoites, Cysts, Oocysts, Spores, Adults, Larvae, Eggs, Amastigotes, Trypomastigotes)

Site	Parasites	Site	Parasites
Blood		Liver, spleen	Capillaria hepatica
Red cells	Plasmodium spp.		Clonorchis/Opisthorchis
	Babesia spp.		Echinococcus spp.
			Entamoeba histolytica
White cells	Leishmania spp.		Fasciola hepatica
	Toxoplasma gondii		Leishmania donovani
			Toxocara spp.
Whole blood/plasma	Trypanosoma spp.		Microsporidia
	Microfilariae	Lung	Cryptosporidium spp.[a]
Bone marrow	Leishmania spp.		Dirofilaria immitis
	Trypanosoma cruzi		Echinococcus spp.
	Plasmodium spp.		Hookworm larvae
			Paragonimus spp.
Central Nervous System			Microsporidia
Cutaneous ulcers	Taenia solium (cysticerci)	Muscle	Gnathostoma spinigerum
	Echinococcus spp.		Taenia solium (cysticerci)
	Naegleria fowleri		Taenia/Multiceps spp.
	Acanthamoeba spp.		Trichinella spp.
	Balamuthia mandrillaris		Onchocerca volvulus (nodules)
	Sappinia diploidea		Spirometra/Diphyllobothrium spp.
	Toxoplasma gondii		Trypanosoma cruzi
	Microsporidia		Microsporidia
	Trypanosoma spp.	Skin	Ancylostoma spp.
	Leishmania spp.		Dracunculus medinensis
Intestinal tract	Entamoeba bangladeshi		Gnathostoma spinigerum
	Entamoeba histolytica		Leishmania spp.
	Entamoeba dispar		Onchocerca spp.
	Entamoeba coli		Microfilariae
	Entamoeba hartmanni		Taenia spp.
	Entamoeba polecki		Demodex spp.
	Endolimax nana		Sarcoptes scabiei
	Iodamoeba bütschlii		
	Blastocystis hominis	Urogenital system	Trichomonas vaginalis
	Giardia duodenalis		Schistosoma spp.
	Chilomastix mesnili		Baylisascaris procyonis
	Dientamoeba fragilis		Microsporidia
	Pentatrichomonas hominis		Microfilariae
	Neobalantidium coli		
	Cryptosporidium spp.	Eye	Acanthamoeba spp.
	Cyclospora cayetanensis		Dirofilaria spp.
	Cystoisospora belli		Toxoplasma gondii
	Sarcocystis spp.		Toxocara spp.
	Microsporidia		Loa loa
	Ascaris lumbricoides		Microsporidia
	Anisakis spp.		
	Enterobius vermicularis		
	Hookworm		
	Strongyloides stercoralis		
	Angiostrongylus spp.		
	Trichostrongylus spp.		
	Trichuris trichiura		
	Hymenolepis nana		
	Hymenolepis diminuta		
	Taenia saginata		
	Taenia solium		
	Diphyllobothrium latum		
	Clonorchis sinensis (Opisthorchis)		
	Paragonimus spp.		
	Schistosoma spp.		
	Fasciolopsis buski		
	Fasciola hepatica		
	Metagonimus yokogawai		
	Heterophyes heterophyes		

Note: This table does not include every possible parasite that can be identified in each body site; the most likely organisms have been listed.
[a]Disseminated in severely immunosuppressed individuals.

TABLE 46.3 Specimens and Body Site: Specimen Options, Collection and Transport Methods, and Processing

Specimens and/or Body Site	Specimen Options	Collection and Transport Methods	Specimen Processing	Comments
Stool for ova and parasites (O&Ps) examination	Fresh stool	½ pint waxed container; 30 min if liquid, 60 min if semiformed, 24 h if formed; delivery to laboratory	Direct wet smear (not on formed specimen), concentration, permanent stained smear	Stool specimens containing barium are unacceptable; intestinal protozoa may be undetectable for 5–10 days after barium use. Certain substances and medications also impede detection of intestinal protozoa: mineral oil, bismuth, antibiotics, antimalarial agents, and nonabsorbable antidiarrheal preparations. After administration of any of these compounds, parasitic organisms may not be recovered for a week to several weeks. Specimen collection should be delayed after barium or antibiotics are administered for 5–10 days or at least 2 weeks, respectively.
	Preserved stool[a]	5% or 10% formalin, MIF, SAF, Schaudinn's, PVA, modified PVA, single vial systems, universal fixative	Concentration, permanent stained smear. Depending on specimen (fresh or preserved) and patient's clinical history, immunoassays may also be performed.	
Stool for culture of nematodes	Fresh stool, entire stool specimen	½ pint waxed container; immediate delivery to laboratory	Filter paper strip, Petri dish, and agar plate, charcoal cultures are all available.	Fresh stool (do not refrigerate) is required for these procedures.
Stool for recovery of tapeworm scolex	Preserved stool, entire stool specimen	5% or 10% formalin (10% recommended)	The stool is filtered with a series of mesh screens and examined for the very small tapeworm scolex (proof of therapy efficacy) and/or proglottids.	After treatment for tapeworm removal, the patient should be instructed to take a saline cathartic and to collect all stool material passed for the next 24 h. The stool should be immediately placed in 10% formalin and thoroughly broken up and mixed with the preservative (1-gallon [3.8-L] plastic jars are recommended, half-full of 10% formalin).
	Adult worms, worm segments	Saline, 70% alcohol		
Cellophane tape preparation for pinworms	Surface sample from perianal skin; anal impression smear	Cellophane (Scotch) tape preparation or commercial sampling paddle or swab	Tape is lifted from a slide, a drop of xylene substitute is added, the tape is replaced, and the specimen is ready for examination under the microscope.	Specimens should be collected late at night after the person has been asleep for several hours or first thing in the morning before going to the bathroom or taking a shower. At least 4–6 consecutive negative tapes are required to rule out the infection.
Sigmoid colon	Sigmoidoscopy material, prepared as smears	Fresh or PVA or Schaudinn's smears; specimen is taken with a spatula rather than cotton-tipped swabs; transported as smears in preservative	Direct wet smear, permanent stained smears	Material from the mucosal surface should be aspirated or scraped; it should not be collected with cotton-tipped swabs. At least 6 representative areas of the mucosa should be sampled and examined (6 samples, 6 slides). A parasitology specimen tray (containing Schaudinn's fixative, PVA, and 5% or 10% formalin) should be provided, or a trained technologist should be available at the time of sigmoidoscopy to prepare the slides. Examination of sigmoidoscopy specimens does not take the place of routine O&Ps examinations. If the amount of material is limited, use of a fixative containing PVA is highly recommended.

Continued

TABLE 46.3   Specimens and Body Site: Specimen Options, Collection and Transport Methods, and Processing—cont'd

Specimens and/or Body Site	Specimen Options	Collection and Transport Methods	Specimen Processing	Comments
Duodenum	Duodenal contents	Entero-Test or aspirates; string in Petri dish or tube; immediate transport to laboratory	The specimen may be centrifuged (10 min at 500×) and should be examined immediately as a wet mount for motile organisms. Iodine also can be used. Direct wet smear of mucus; permanent stained smears can also be prepared.	A fresh specimen is required; the amount may vary from <0.5 mL to several milliliters of fluid. If the specimen cannot be completely examined within 2 h after collection, any remaining material should be preserved in 5%–10% formalin.
Entero-Test capsule (string)	Duodenal contents	Entero-Test (string test) in Petri dish (fresh) or preserved in PVA	Bile-stained mucus clinging to the yarn should be scraped off (mucus can also be removed by pulling the yarn between the thumb and finger) and collected in a small Petri dish; disposable gloves are recommended. Usually 4 or 5 drops of material are collected. The specimen should be examined immediately as a wet mount for motile organisms (iodine may be added later to facilitate identification of any organisms present). The pH of the terminal end of the yarn should be checked to ensure adequate passage into the duodenum (a very low pH means that it never left the stomach). The terminal end of the yarn should be yellow-green, indicating that it was in the duodenum (the bile duct drains into the intestine at this point). Permanent stained smears can also be prepared.	If the specimen cannot be completely examined within 1 h after removal of the yarn, the material should be preserved in 5%–10% formalin, or PVA-mucus smears should be prepared.
Urogenital tract	Vaginal discharge Urethral discharge Prostatic secretions	Saline swab, transport swab (no charcoal), culture medium, plastic envelope culture, air-dried smear for FA	Direct wet smear; fluorescence; urine must be centrifuged before examination.	Fresh specimens are required; an air-dried smear may be an option for fluorescence. Do not refrigerate swabs and/or culture containers at any time, because motility and/or ability to grow will probably be lost.
	Urine	Single unpreserved specimen, 24-h unpreserved specimen, early morning specimen Nucleic acid–based testing media according to manufacturer's instructions	Examination of urinary sediment may be indicated in certain filarial infections. Administration of the drug diethylcarbamazine (Hetrazan) has been reported to enhance the recovery of microfilariae from the urine. The triple-concentration technique is recommended for the recovery of microfilariae. The membrane filtration technique can be used with urine for the recovery of microfilariae. A membrane filter technique for the recovery of Schistosoma haematobium eggs has also been useful.	

TABLE 46.3 Specimens and Body Site: Specimen Options, Collection and Transport Methods, and Processing—cont'd

Specimens and/or Body Site	Specimen Options	Collection and Transport Methods	Specimen Processing	Comments
Sputum	Sputum	True sputum (not saliva)	Direct wet smear; permanent stained smears; fluorescence also available (Calcofluor for microsporidia). Sputum is usually examined as a wet mount (saline or iodine), using low and high dry power (10× and 400×). The specimen is not concentrated before preparation of the wet mount. If the sputum is thick, an equal amount of 3% sodium hydroxide (NaOH) (or undiluted chlorine bleach) can be added; the specimen is thoroughly mixed and then centrifuged. NaOH should not be used if the examiner is looking for *Entamoeba* spp. or *Trichomonas tenax*.	True sputum is required; all specimens, especially induced specimens and BAL, should be delivered immediately to the laboratory (do not refrigerate).
	Induced sputum	No preservative (10% formalin if time delay)		
	Bronchoalveolar lavage (BAL)	Sterile; immediate delivery to laboratory	After centrifugation, the supernatant is discarded, and the sediment can be examined as a wet mount with saline or iodine. If examination is delayed, the sputum should be fixed in 5% or 10% formalin to preserve helminth eggs or larvae or in PVA.	
Aspirates	Bone marrow	Sterile; immediate delivery to laboratory	Permanent stained smears; cultures can also be set (specifically designed for the recovery of blood parasites).	All aspirates for culture must be collected using sterile conditions and containers; this is mandatory for culture isolation of leishmania and trypanosomes.
	Cutaneous ulcers	Sterile plus air-dried smears		
	Liver, spleen	Sterile, collected in 4 separate aliquots (liver)		
	Lung			
	Transbronchial aspirate	Air-dried smears		
	Tracheobronchial aspirate	Air-dried smears		
Central nervous system	Cerebrospinal fluid (CSF)	Sterile	Direct wet smear, permanent stained smears; culture for free-living amebae (*Naegleria, Acanthamoeba* spp.).	All specimens must be transported immediately to the laboratory (STAT procedure).

Continued

TABLE 46.3 Specimens and Body Site: Specimen Options, Collection and Transport Methods, and Processing—cont'd

Specimens and/or Body Site	Specimen Options	Collection and Transport Methods	Specimen Processing	Comments
Biopsy	Intestinal tract	Routine histology	Direct wet smears, permanent stained smears; specimens to histology for routine processing.	The more material that is collected and tested, the more likely the organism is to be isolated and subsequently identified. Sterile collection is required for all specimens that will be cultured; bacterial and/or fungal contamination prevents isolation of parasites in culture.
	Cutaneous ulcers	Sterile, nonsterile to histopathology (formalin acceptable)		
	Eye	Sterile (in saline), nonsterile to histopathology		
	Scrapings	Sterile (in saline)		
	Cornea (scrapings)	Collected by physician, placed directly on microscope slide	Fixed using methyl alcohol and stained using Calcofluor white.	Helpful in diagnosis of *Acanthamoeba* keratitis.
	Liver, spleen	Sterile, nonsterile to histopathology		
	Lung			
	Brush biopsy	Air-dried smears		
	Open lung biopsy	Air-dried smears		
	Muscle	Fresh, squash preparation, nonsterile to histopathology		
	Skin biopsy	Nonsterile to histopathology (formalin acceptable)		
	Scrapings	Sterile (in saline), nonsterile to histopathology		
	Skin snip	Aseptic, smear or vial No preservative		
Blood	Smears of whole blood	Fresh (first choice) Thick and thin films; immediate delivery to laboratory	Thick and thin films, specialized concentrations and/or screening methods	Examination of blood films (particularly for malaria) is considered a STAT procedure; immediate delivery to the laboratory is mandatory.
	Anticoagulated blood	Anticoagulant (second choice) EDTA (first choice) Heparin (second choice)	Thick and thin films, specialized concentrations and/or rapid methods Quantitative Buffy Coat (QBC) Microhematocrit Centrifugation Method (Becton Dickinson, Tropical Disease Diagnostics, Sparks, MD)	Delivery to the laboratory within 30 min or less. If delayed, typical parasite morphology may not be seen in blood collected using anticoagulants. Knott concentration procedure: Used primarily to detect microfilariae in the blood, especially when a light infection is suspected. The disadvantage of the procedure is that the microfilariae are killed by the formalin and are no longer motile. Membrane filtration technique: This technique, using Nuclepore filters, has proved highly efficient in demonstrating filarial infections when microfilaria are of low density. It has also been successfully used in field surveys.

EDTA, Ethylenediaminetetraacetic acid; *FA,* fluorescent antibody; *MIF,* merthiolate-iodine-formalin; *PVA,* polyvinyl alcohol; *SAF,* sodium acetate–acetic acid–formalin.

[a]A number of new stool fixatives are available; some use a zinc sulfate base rather than mercuric chloride. Some collection vials can be used as a single-vial system; both the concentration and permanent stained smear can be performed from the preserved stool. However, not all single-vial systems (proprietary formulas) provide material that can be used for fecal immunoassay procedures. A universal fixative is now available (TOTAL-FIX) that contains no formalin, mercury, or PVA.

Modified from Garcia LS. *Diagnostic Medical Parasitology.* 6th ed. Washington, DC: ASM Press; 2016.

environmental phase, these measures can be complex, especially if more than one reservoir species or environmental resource is involved.

A human parasitic infection can be initiated through a variety of mechanisms and pathways depending on the species of microorganism. Many parasites of the intestinal tract are transmitted through ingestion of the infective form of the parasite in contaminated food or water (e.g., *Giardia duodenalis, Cryptosporidium* spp., *Ascaris lumbricoides*). Other parasites can be transmitted from host to host through sexual means (venereal transmission) (e.g., *Trichomonas vaginalis*), through skin penetration of infective larvae (e.g., *Strongyloides stercoralis,* hookworm), or through the bites of various arthropods (e.g., *Plasmodium, Trypanosoma, Leishmania*) (Table 46.4).

Pathogenesis and Spectrum of Disease

Although a number of parasites can cause serious and life-threatening disease, particularly in compromised patients, many organisms reach a "status quo" with the host and cause no significant damage. Obvious disease symptoms may not be the ultimate outcome of infection. Depending on the parasite, one or multiple body sites may be infected. Some parasitic infections can result in few or no symptoms, whereas infection with other parasites can result in devastating permanent damage and eventual death of the host. Some parasites multiply in the human body, whereas others mature but do not increase in number inside the body. These life-cycle differences play important roles in pathogenicity and disease outcome. It is also important to remember that a patient who is debilitated or immunocompromised (including the very young and the very old) may react differently to a parasitic infection than a healthy adult.

Certainly, it is not to the parasite's advantage to damage the host to the extent that severe illness or death results; this makes survival of the parasite difficult at best. When this occurs, long-term survival of the parasite may depend on rapid and efficient transmission from host to host or the parasite's ability to survive within the environment without a live host.

It is important to understand the life cycle of parasites in terms of potential prevention and control as well as mechanisms of infectivity and disease outcome (Table 46.5). Table 46.6 lists mechanisms of pathogenesis and the spectrum of parasitic diseases. Specific guidelines for physician requests are presented in Table 46.7.

Laboratory Diagnosis

As with all laboratory testing, the ability to detect and correctly identify human parasites is directly linked to the quality of the clinical specimen, submission of the appropriate specimen or specimens, appropriate processing and handling before analysis, relevant diagnostic test orders, and the experience and training of laboratory personnel (Table 46.8). A summary of human parasites and applicable collection fixatives, clinical specimens, diagnostic tests, the elements of a positive finding, and comments are presented in Tables 46.9 and 46.10.

Specimen Collection and Transport

Depending on its stage of development in the clinical specimen (adult, larvae, eggs, trophozoites, cysts, oocysts, spores), a particular parasite may not be able to survive outside the host. For this reason, clinical specimens should be transported to the laboratory immediately to increase the likelihood of finding intact organisms. Because a lag time often occurs between collection of the specimen and its arrival in the laboratory, most facilities routinely use preservatives for collection and transport (Fig. 46.1). This approach ensures that any parasites present maintain their morphology and can be identified after processing.

Correct processing depends on the use of appropriate fixatives, immediate fixation upon collection of the specimen, and adequate mixing between the fixative and specimen (Table 46.9). It is mandatory that specimen collection guidelines be available in plain and direct language for health care personnel or patients performing specimen collection and that all clients recognize the importance of following such guidelines. In areas with non-native English speakers, alternate language versions should be readily available to provide clear directions for specimen collection. Specimen rejection criteria must be included as a part of the guidelines; guidelines must be followed and enforced to limit the possibility of reporting misleading or incorrect results. Detailed specimen descriptions and body sites, in addition to collection and transport information, are included in Table 46.3.

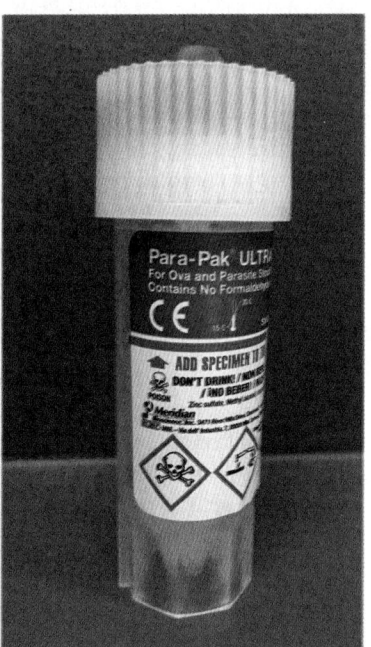

• **Fig. 46.1** Stool collection vial. Most laboratories recommend immediate placement of stool samples into a preservative such as this to preserve morphology.

TABLE 46.4 **Epidemiology of the More Common Groups of Human Parasites**

Parasite Group	Habitat (Reservoir)	Mode of Transmission	Prevention
Protozoa, Intestinal			
Amebae	Single-celled organisms generally found in humans. Although certain animals harbor some of these organisms, they are not considered important reservoir hosts.	Humans acquire infections by ingesting food and water contaminated with fecal material containing the resistant infective cyst stage of the protozoa. Various sexual practices have been documented in transmission.	Preventive measures include increased attention to personal hygiene, sanitation measures, and elimination of sexual activities that may involve fecal-oral contact.
Flagellates	The flagellates are generally found in humans. Although certain animals harbor some of these organisms, they are not considered important reservoir hosts; one exception may be animals such as the beaver that harbor *Giardia duodenalis*. Contaminated water supplies are also a source.	Humans acquire infections by ingesting food and water contaminated with fecal material containing the resistant infective cyst stage of the protozoa; the trophozoite forms may be transmitted from person to person in helminth eggs.	Preventive measures include increased attention to personal hygiene and sanitation measures, elimination of sexual activities that may involve fecal-oral contact, adequate water treatment (including filtration), and awareness of environmental sources of infection.
Ciliates	*Neobalantidium coli* is generally found in humans and pigs. In some areas of the world, pigs are considered important reservoir hosts.	Humans acquire infections by ingesting food and water contaminated with fecal material containing the resistant infective cyst stage of the protozoa.	Preventive measures include increased attention to personal hygiene and sanitation measures as well as the elimination of sexual activities that may involve fecal-oral contact.
Coccidia	Coccidia are found in humans. In some cases (e.g., cryptosporidiosis) animal reservoirs (cattle) can serve as important hosts. The muscle of various animals may contain sarcocysts that are infective for humans through the consumption of raw or poorly cooked meat. Numerous water-borne outbreaks with *Cryptosporidium* spp. have been reported throughout the world. Coccidian oocysts are extremely resistant to environmental conditions, particularly if kept moist.	These protozoa are acquired through ingestion of various meats or by fecal-oral transmission through contaminated food and/or water. The infective forms are called oocysts (*Cryptosporidium* spp., *Cystoisospora belli*, *Cyclospora cayetanensis*) or sarcocysts (*Sarcocystis* spp.), which are contained in infected meat. Cryptosporidia have also been implicated in nosocomial infections.	Preventive measures include increased attention to personal hygiene and sanitation measures and elimination of sexual activities that may involve fecal-oral contact. Adequate water treatment (including filtration) is mandatory; awareness of environmental sources of infection is also important.
Microsporidia	Microsporidia can infect every living animal, some of which probably serve as reservoir hosts for human infection. However, host specificity has not been well defined. The spores are environmentally resistant and can survive for years if kept moist.	Infection with microsporidial spores usually occurs through ingestion; however, inhalation of spores and direct inoculation from the environment almost certainly occur.	Preventive measures include increased attention to personal hygiene and sanitation measures, increased awareness of environmental exposure possibilities, and adequate water treatment.
Protozoa, Other Sites			
Amebae	Free-living amebae are associated with warm, freshwater environments; they are also found in soil. Although humans can harbor these organisms, person-to-person transfer is rare. Environmental sources are the primary link to human infection. Contaminated eye care solutions have been linked to organisms that cause keratitis.	Infection occurs through contact with contaminated water; organisms enter through the nasal mucosa and may travel via the olfactory nerve to the brain. Disease can be very severe and life-threatening; keratitis is also caused by these organisms, and infection can be linked to blindness or severe corneal damage. Eye infections can be linked to contaminated lens solutions or direct accidental inoculation of the eye from environmental water and/or soil sources.	Prevention includes avoidance of contaminated environmental water and soil sources and adequate care of contact lens systems.

TABLE 46.4   **Epidemiology of the More Common Groups of Human Parasites—cont'd**

Parasite Group	Habitat (Reservoir)	Mode of Transmission	Prevention
Flagellates	*Trichomonas vaginalis* infection is found in a large percentage of humans; humans may present as symptomatic or asymptomatic. Person-to-person transfer is very common; reinfection is also common, particularly if sexual partners are not treated.	*T. vaginalis* is found in the genitourinary system and is usually acquired by sexual transmission.	Prevention involves awareness of sexual transmission; treatment of all partners is necessary when infection is diagnosed in an individual patient.
Protozoa, Blood and Tissue			
Malaria, babesiosis	Humans harbor the five species of malaria (*Plasmodium vivax, P. ovale, P. malariae, P. knowlesi,* and *P. falciparum*). Other animals can carry *Babesia* spp., and animal reservoir hosts play a large role in human transmission.	These organisms are borne by arthropods, *Plasmodium* spp. by the female anopheline mosquito and *Babesia* spp. by one or more genera of ticks. Infections can be transmitted transplacentally, via shared needles, through blood transfusions, and from organ transplants.	Prevention involves vector control and awareness of transmission through blood transfusions, shared drug needles, congenital infections, and organ transplants. Careful monitoring of the blood supply is necessary. Malaria prophylaxis is recommended for persons traveling to endemic areas.
Flagellates (leishmaniae)	Some strains of leishmaniae have reservoir hosts (e.g., dogs for the Mediterranean strain of *Leishmania donovani* and wild rodents for the African strains of *L. donovani*). *Leishmania tropica* has been linked to the same animal reservoirs.	Transmission is through the bite of infected sandflies. Infection can be spread person-to-person contact (cutaneous lesions), blood transfusions, shared needles, and organ transplants.	Prevention includes vector control, avoiding environmental sources (e.g., dogs, wild rodents), and careful handling of all clinical specimens from infected patients.
Flagellates (trypanosomes)	Humans are the only known hosts for *Trypanosoma brucei gambiense* (West African trypanosomiasis); *Trypanosoma brucei rhodesiense* (East African trypanosomiasis) infections are found in a number of antelope and other ungulates that act as reservoir hosts. Rodents and some mammals are reservoir hosts for *Trypanosoma cruzi*.	Transmission is through the bite of the infected tsetse fly and through blood transfusion, shared needles, and organ transplants. Transmission of *T. cruzi* is through the infected feces of the triatomid bug; the bug takes a blood meal, immediately defecates, and the human host scratches the infected feces into the bite site; bug saliva contains an irritant that stimulates scratching.	Prevention relies on vector control and awareness of potential exposure/infection from blood sources (transfusions, shared needles, organ transplants). Laboratory accidents while handling infected blood have been reported.
Nematodes, intestinal	These roundworms generally do not have animal reservoirs relevant to human infection. One exception is the pig ascarid; human infections have been reported. These worms are found worldwide; *Ascaris lumbricoides* is probably the most common parasite in humans. *Strongyloides stercoralis* is particularly important as the causative agent of severe disease in the compromised host.	*A. lumbricoides* and *Trichuris trichiura* eggs must undergo development in the soil before they are infective; thus, children who play in the dirt are a particularly high-risk group. Ingestion of food and water contaminated with infective eggs is the primary route of infection. Hookworm and *S. stercoralis* infections are initiated by larval penetration of the skin from contaminated soil. Pinworm infection (*E. vermicularis*) is acquired through ingestion of infective eggs from the environment (hand-to-mouth).	Prevention includes avoiding ingestion of contaminated soil and/or avoiding frequenting soil contaminated with hookworm eggs (pets, soil, water, warmth, warm weather); treatment for pinworm is recommended, but reinfection is common.

Continued

TABLE 46.4 Epidemiology of the More Common Groups of Human Parasites—cont'd

Parasite Group	Habitat (Reservoir)	Mode of Transmission	Prevention
Nematodes, tissue	*Trichinella* spp. have a number of animal reservoir hosts, including bears, walruses, pigs, rodents, and other animals. Dog and cat hookworms cause cutaneous larva migrans (CLM), and the dog and cat ascarid, *Toxocara* spp., causes visceral and ocular larva migrans (VLM, OLM). These infections can be serious and cause severe disease if not treated.	*Trichinella* organisms are acquired by ingestion of raw or poorly cooked infected meat. CLM is caused by skin penetration of infective larvae from the soil; children should avoid sandboxes where dogs and cats are known to defecate. Larval migration is limited to the skin. VLM and OLM are caused by accidental ingestion of *Toxocara* spp. eggs from contaminated soil; larval migration occurs throughout the body, including the eyes.	Preventive measures include adequate cooking of infected meat; awareness of possibility of contaminated soils for dog and cat hookworms and/or ascarids; and covering of all sandboxes where pets have access to defecate and children play.
Nematodes, filarial	*Wuchereria bancrofti, Loa loa*, and *Onchocerca volvulus* have no animal reservoirs and are found only in humans, whereas *Brugia* spp. can be found in cats and monkeys. *Dracunculus medinensis* can infect dogs, cats, monkeys, and humans.	Filarial nematodes are transmitted through the bite of a blood-sucking arthropod (midges, mosquitoes, and flies). *Dracunculus* infections are acquired through ingestion of water contaminated with small crustaceans, *Cyclops* spp., which contain infective larvae.	Prevention involves vector control and protection of well-water sources.
Cestodes, intestinal	The human serves as the definitive host for beef (*Taenia saginata)* and pork (*Taenia solium)* tapeworms; cows/camels and pigs serve as intermediate hosts, respectively. Humans also serve as the intermediate host for *T. solium* (cysticercosis). *Diphyllobothrium latum* adult tapeworms can be found in a number of wild animals, the most important being dogs, bears, seals, and walruses, which serve as reservoir hosts; humans are the definitive host. *Hymenolepis nana* (dwarf tapeworm) can occur in rodents; humans can serve as both intermediate and definitive hosts, with development from the egg to adult worm occurring in the human intestine.	Human infection with the adult worm occurs through ingestion of raw or poorly cooked meat (beef, camel, pork) containing the intermediate forms, the cysticerci. Humans become the accidental intermediate host when eggs from an adult *T. solium* tapeworm are ingested. The cysticerci develop in the muscle and tissues of the human rather than the pig. Infection with the adult *D. latum* tapeworm occurs through ingestion of poorly cooked freshwater fish containing the sparganum or plerocercoid larval form. Infection with *H. nana* is primarily acquired through accidental ingestion of eggs from an adult tapeworm.	Preventive measures involve adequate cooking of infected meat and treatment of patients harboring adult tapeworms (accidental ingestion of eggs can lead to infection).
Cestodes, tissue	Adult worms are found in a variety of animals; the human becomes the accidental intermediate host after ingestion of eggs from the adult worms. Reservoir hosts include dogs, cats, and rodents.	Ingestion of certain tapeworm eggs or accidental contact with certain larval forms can lead to tissue infection with *Taenia solium, Echinococcus* spp., and several others.	Preventive measures involve increased attention to personal hygiene and sanitation measures.
Trematodes, intestinal	Fish-eating wild and domestic animals serve as reservoir hosts. The definitive host of *Fasciolopsis buski* is the pig.	Ingestion of water chestnut and caltrop (raw, peeled with the teeth) is the source of infection; metacercariae are encysted on the plant material. Pig feces are used to fertilize various water plant crops.	Preventive measures include avoiding eating raw water plants that may contain encysted larval forms of the flukes and adequate waste disposal of farm animal feces (pigs).

TABLE 46.4   Epidemiology of the More Common Groups of Human Parasites—cont'd

Parasite Group	Habitat (Reservoir)	Mode of Transmission	Prevention
Trematodes, liver, lung	Cats, dogs, and wild fish-eating mammals can serve as reservoir hosts for *Opisthorchis* spp., *Clonorchis sinensis*, and *Paragonimus* spp. *Fasciola hepatica* is normally a parasite of sheep, and *Fasciola gigantica* is a parasite of cattle; humans are accidental hosts.	Infection occurs through ingestion of encysted metacercariae in raw or poorly cooked fish, crabs, crayfish, and on plants. Infection with *Fasciola* spp. is not easily acquired (the parasite is not that well adapted to the human host).	Prevention requires thorough cooking of potentially infected fish, crabs, crayfish and avoiding eating raw water plants that may contain encysted metacercariae.
Trematodes, blood	*Schistosoma mansoni* and *S. haematobium* appear to be restricted to the human host; *S. japonicum* can be found in cattle, deer, dogs, and rodents; *S. mekongi* is found in dogs and rodents. The worms mature in the blood vessels, and eggs make their way outside the body in stool and/or urine. The freshwater snail is a mandatory part of the life cycle (contains developmental forms of schistosome).	Infection occurs through skin penetration by infected cercariae released from a freshwater snail containing the intermediate stages of the schistosome life cycle. Cercariae can be released from the snail intermediate host singly or in groups.	Prevention involves protection from potentially contaminated water sources; awareness of mode of transmission; and proper handling of human waste containing eggs (continued infection of snail intermediate hosts).

TABLE 46.5   Parasitic Infections: Clinical Findings in Normal and Compromised Hosts

Organism	Normal Host	Compromised Host
Entamoeba histolytica	Asymptomatic to chronic-acute colitis, extraintestinal disease may also occur (primary site: right upper lobe of liver).	Diminished immune capacity may lead to extraintestinal disease.
Free-living amebae *Naegleria fowleri* *Acanthamoeba* spp. *Balamuthia mandrillaris* *Sappinia* spp.	Patients tend to have eye infections with *Acanthamoeba* spp. linked to poor lens care.	Primary amoebic meningoencephalitis (PAM); granulomatous amebic encephalitis (GAE).
Giardia duodenalis	Asymptomatic to malabsorption syndrome.	Certain immunodeficiencies tend to predispose an individual to infection.
Toxoplasma gondii	Approximately 50% of individuals have antibody and organisms in tissue but are asymptomatic. It is important to note that a developing fetus may be severally affected if the mother is infected; this is highly dependent on the time (trimester) when the infection occurs.	Disease in compromised hosts tends to involve the central nervous system (CNS), with various neurologic symptoms; it can mimic neurologic symptoms of infection with the human immunodeficiency virus (HIV).
Cryptosporidium spp. *Cryptosporidium hominis* (humans) *Cryptosporidium parvum* (humans and animals)	Self-limiting infection with diarrhea and abdominal pain.	Because of the autoinfective nature of the life cycle, infection is not self-limiting and may produce fluid loss of more than 10 L/day; multisystem involvement may occur. No effective therapy is available.
Cyclospora cayetanensis	Self-limiting infection with diarrhea (3–4 days); relapses common.	Diarrhea may persist for 12 weeks or longer; biliary disease has also been reported in this group, particularly those with acquired immunodeficiency syndrome (AIDS).

Continued

TABLE 46.5 **Parasitic Infections: Clinical Findings in Normal and Compromised Host—cont'd**

Organism	Normal Host	Compromised Host
Cystoisospora belli	Self-limiting infection with mild diarrhea or no symptoms.	May lead to severe diarrhea, abdominal pain, and possibly death (rare case reports); diagnosis occasionally may be missed because of failure to recognize the oocyst stage; is not seen when concentrated from polyvinyl alcohol (PVA) fixative.
Sarcocystis spp.	Self-limiting infection with diarrhea or mild symptoms.	Symptoms may be more severe and last for a longer period.
Microsporidia *Anncaliia Nosema Vittaforma Encephalitozoon Enterocytozoon Pleistophora Trachipleistophora* "*Microsporidium*"	Little is known about these infections in the normal host. Most infections have been identified as causing intestinal symptoms *(Enterocytozoon, Encephalitozoon)* or eye infections *(Vittaforma, Encephalitozoon)*.	Organisms infect various parts of the body; diagnosis often depends on histologic examination of tissues; routine examination of clinical specimens (e.g., stool, urine) is becoming more common; infection can probably cause death.
Leishmania spp.	Asymptomatic to mild disease. Depending on species, infection can result in cutaneous, diffuse cutaneous, or mucocutaneous disease.	More serious manifestations of visceral leishmaniasis; some cutaneous species manifest visceral disease; infection is difficult to treat and manage; definite coinfection with AIDS.
Strongyloides stercoralis	Asymptomatic to mild abdominal complaints; can remain latent for many years because of low-level infection maintained by internal autoinfective life cycle.	Can result in disseminated disease (hyperinfection syndrome resulting from autoinfective nature of life cycle); abdominal pain, pneumonitis, sepsis-meningitis with gram-negative bacilli, eosinophilia; distinct link to certain leukemias or lymphomas; can be fatal.
Crusted (Norwegian) scabies	Infections can range from asymptomatic to moderate itching.	Severe infection with reduced itching response; hundreds of thousands of mites on the body; infection is very easily transferred to others; secondary infection is common.

TABLE 46.6 **Pathogenesis and Spectrum of Parasitic Diseases**

Parasite Group	Pathogenesis	Spectrum of Disease
Protozoa, Intestinal		
Amebae	Pathogens can cause severe disease; however, exposure does not always lead to disease; infection may be self-limiting; disease more likely in the compromised host.	Nonpathogens cause no disease, patients are asymptomatic; *Entamoeba histolytica* causes intestinal symptoms (bloody diarrhea) and the potential for amoebic liver abscess; other tissues may be involved, especially in the immunocompromised patient. "*Blastocystis hominis*" comprises a number of strains, some considered pathogenic; patients' conditions range from asymptomatic to severe diarrhea.
Flagellates	Not all patients are infected upon exposure; disease spectrum varies; some patients may remain asymptomatic; if nonexposed patients become infected, symptoms are much more likely to occur.	Nonpathogens cause no disease, patients are asymptomatic; *Giardia duodenalis* (malabsorption syndrome) and *Dientamoeba fragilis* cause intestinal symptoms ranging from "indigestion" to nonbloody diarrhea, cramping, gas, and so on.
Ciliates	*Neobalantidium coli* infection is rare in the United States; people who have regular contact with pigs are much more likely to become infected; wide range of symptoms.	*N. coli* causes intestinal symptoms, including severe watery diarrhea, similar to coccidial and microsporidial infections.

TABLE 46.6   Pathogenesis and Spectrum of Parasitic Diseases—cont'd

Parasite Group	Pathogenesis	Spectrum of Disease
Coccidia	All coccidia infective to humans can cause severe disease, particularly in the immunocompromised patient; infections in the immunocompetent patient tend to be self-limiting; *Cryptosporidium* spp. can maintain the infective cycle in the patient as a result of the autoinfective portion of the life cycle (the immunocompromised patient cannot produce antibody to limit this autoinfective cycle); huge water-borne outbreaks have been documented for *Cryptosporidium* spp.; infecting dose is low for *Cryptosporidium* spp.	*Cryptosporidium* spp., *Cyclospora cayetanensis,* and *Cystoisospora belli* cause intestinal symptoms, including severe watery diarrhea; infections are more severe in immunocompromised patients. Life-threatening infections can be seen with *Cryptosporidium* spp.; the organisms can disseminate to other tissues, primarily the lung. *Sarcocystis* can cause intestinal symptoms and/or muscle pain, depending on the mode of infection (ingestion of oocysts or infected meat).
Microsporidia	A number of genera are pathogenic for humans and for animals; wide range of body sites; disease varies, depending on patient's immune status; disease outcome is complicated by lack of treatment for some genera; albendazole is effective for *Encephalitozoon* spp.	Every human tissue may be infected; *Enterocytozoon bieneusi* and *Encephalitozoon intestinalis* are the most common and are found in the intestinal tract; the latter can also disseminate to other tissues, including the kidneys. Eye infections have been seen in both healthy and compromised patients; severe corneal infections seen.

Protozoa, Other Sites

Parasite Group	Pathogenesis	Spectrum of Disease
Amebae	Pathogenic for humans; disease ranging from acute meningoencephalitis to chronic encephalitis, cutaneous infections to keratitis, and the potential for other body sites; disease spectrum depends on patient's immune capacity and the organism involved; disease can be mild (*Acanthamoeba* spp.) to fatal *(Naegleria fowleri)*.	Infection occurs through contact with contaminated water; organisms enter through the nasal mucosa and may travel via the olfactory nerve to the brain. Disease caused by *N. fowleri* can be severe and life-threatening (primary amoebic meningoencephalitis [PAM]); chronic granulomatous amoebic encephalitis (GAE) can be caused by *Acanthamoeba* spp. and *Balamuthia mandrillaris;* keratitis is also caused by these organisms, and infection can be linked to blindness or severe corneal damage. Eye infections can be linked to contaminated lens solutions or to direct, accidental inoculation of the eye from environmental water and/or soil sources.
Flagellates	*Trichomonas vaginalis* causes genitourinary disease, depending on vaginal pH, presence or absence of other organisms, sexual practices, and other factors. Disease can vary from mild to severe.	*T. vaginalis* is found in the genitourinary system and is usually acquired by sexual transmission. Disease can be asymptomatic in the male but can cause pain, itching, and discharge in females; some strains of drug-resistant *Trichomonas* have been documented.

Protozoa, Blood and Tissue

Parasite Group	Pathogenesis	Spectrum of Disease
Malaria, babesiosis	*Plasmodium vivax, Plasmodium falciparum, Plasmodium ovale, Plasmodium knowlesi,* and *Plasmodium malariae* are pathogenic for humans; *P. falciparum* malaria is the leading cause of death in endemic areas; although the host can develop antibody, protection is strain specific and short-lived.	Malaria can cause a range of symptoms, with life-threatening illness caused by *P. falciparum/P. knowlesi;* symptoms include fever, chills, nausea, and central nervous system (CNS) symptoms; *Babesia* infections often mimic those seen with malaria but without the fever periodicity.
Flagellates (leishmaniae)	*Leishmania donovani* invades the spleen, liver, and bone marrow and can cause serious disease, particularly in compromised hosts.	Leishmaniasis can infect the skin and mucous membranes and the organs of the reticuloendothelial system; symptoms can be mild to life threatening.
Flagellates (trypanosomes)	Humans are the only known hosts for *Trypanosoma brucei gambiense* (West African trypanosomiasis); *Trypanosoma brucei rhodesiense* (East African trypanosomiasis) infections are found in a number of antelope and other hoofed mammals that serve as reservoir hosts. *Trypanosoma cruzi* (American trypanosomiasis) can be found in rodents and chickens.	*T. brucei gambiense* and *T. brucei rhodesiense* cause African sleeping sickness, with eventual invasion of the CNS, leading to coma and death; Chagas disease (*T. cruzi*) causes acute to chronic problems, primarily linked to cardiac disease and diminished cardiac capacity; the muscles of the gastrointestinal (GI) tract are also infected, leading to loss of function in terms of movement of food through the GI tract.

Continued

TABLE 46.6	Pathogenesis and Spectrum of Parasitic Diseases—cont'd	
Parasite Group	**Pathogenesis**	**Spectrum of Disease**
Nematodes, intestinal	These worms can cause mild to severe disease, depending on the worm burden (original number of eggs ingested or infective larvae penetrating the skin); young children and debilitated patients are more likely to be symptomatic; severe infections are seen in hyperinfections caused by *Strongyloides stercoralis* (autoinfective life cycle and immunocompromised patients); outcome varies tremendously from patient to patient and depends on the original infective dose.	*Ascaris lumbricoides, Trichuris trichiura*, and hookworm symptoms range from none to diarrhea, pain, and so on, depending on the worm burden; anemia may be seen with severe hookworm infection; *S. stercoralis* infections can involve many body tissues (disseminated disease) in the immunocompromised patient and can cause death; pinworm infection (*Enterobius vermicularis*) symptoms range from none to anal itching, irritability, loss of sleep, and so on.
Nematodes, tissue	Depending on the infective dose, *Trichinella* spp. can cause mild to severe disease; both cutaneous larva migrans (CLM) (dog/cat hookworm larvae) and toxocariasis (visceral larva migrans [VLM], ocular larva migrans [OLM]) through ingestion of dog/cat ascarid eggs cause serious disease if not treated; CLM, VLM, and OLM are seen in children more than adults.	*Trichinella* spp. can cause eosinophilia, muscle aches and pains, and death, depending on the worm burden; CLM can cause severe itching and eosinophilia as a result of larval migration in the skin; VLM and OLM are caused by larval migration throughout the body, including the eyes (mimics retinoblastoma).
Nematodes, filarial	*Wuchereria bancrofti, Loa loa*, and *Onchocerca volvulus* cause human disease; however, some filarial infections are not well adapted to humans and require many years of exposure before disease is evident; some infections are not evident, some cause multiple disease manifestations.	Symptoms range from asymptomatic to elephantiasis, blindness, skin changes, lymphadenitis, and lymphangitis; in some cases, Loeffler syndrome may also be seen.
Cestodes, intestinal	The beef (*Taenia saginata*), pork (*Taenia solium*), and freshwater fish (*Diphyllobothrium latum*) tapeworms infect humans and are generally found in the intestine as a single worm. In the case of cysticercosis, ingestion of *T. solium* eggs can cause mild to severe disease, depending on the infecting dose and body site (muscle, CNS). *Hymenolepis nana* (dwarf tapeworm) infection can lead to many worms in the intestinal tract (autoinfective cycle; the organism can go from egg to larval form to adult in the human host).	Human infection with the adult tapeworm can cause no symptoms, or mild intestinal symptoms may occur. When the human becomes the accidental intermediate host for *T. solium*, CNS symptoms may occur, including epileptic seizures. Infection with the adult *D. latum* tapeworm can cause intestinal symptoms, such as pain, diarrhea, and so on, but the patient may also be asymptomatic; a vitamin B_{12} deficiency may be seen. Infection with *H. nana* is primarily acquired from accidental ingestion of eggs from an adult tapeworm; symptoms may be absent, or diarrhea may be present.
Cestodes, tissue	*Echinococcus* spp. can cause severe disease, depending on the original infecting dose of tapeworm eggs; multiple organs can be involved, including brain, liver, lung, and bone; some cysts grow like a metastatic tumor; surgical removal can be very difficult if not impossible.	Depending on the body site, hydatid cysts can cause pain, anaphylactic shock (fluid leakage), or CNS symptoms. The patient may be unaware of infection until a cyst begins to press on other body organs or a large fluid leak occurs.
Trematodes, intestinal	Many genera and species are pathogenic for humans; disease severity depends on the infective dose of metacercariae; some patients may be unaware of the infection.	Intestinal trematodes can cause pain and diarrhea; intestinal toxicity can sometimes be seen in heavy infections with *Fasciolopsis buski*.
Trematodes, liver and lung	Many genera and species are pathogenic for humans; disease severity depends on the infective dose of metacercariae; some patients may be unaware of the infection.	*Paragonimus* spp. infection in the lungs can be severe, resulting in coughing, shortness of breath, and other symptoms; liver fluke infection can involve the bile ducts and gallbladder; symptoms depend on worm burden.
Trematodes, blood	Schistosomes are pathogenic for humans; however, the loading dose of cercariae from infected water sources determines the outcome of disease; very light infections may not produce symptoms; heavy infections can lead to death.	Symptoms may range from asymptomatic in light infections to severe organ failure resulting from deposition of eggs and subsequent granuloma formation in the tissues; "pipe-stem" fibrosis is seen in blood vessels; collateral circulation may develop; severe disease can cause death.

TABLE 46.7 Recommendations for Stool Testing

Patient and/or Situation	Test Ordered[a]	Follow-Up Test
Patient with diarrhea and acquired immuno-deficiency syndrome (AIDS) or other cause of immune deficiency. Potential water-borne outbreak (municipal/city water supply).	*Cryptosporidium* or *Giardia/Cryptosporidium* immunoassay.	If immunoassays are negative and symptoms continue, special tests for microsporidia (modified trichrome stain) and other coccidia (modified acid-fast stain), in addition to ova and parasites (O&Ps) examination, should be performed.
Patient with diarrhea (nursery school, day care center, camper, backpacker). Patient with diarrhea and potential water-borne outbreak (resort setting). Patient with diarrhea from areas where *Giardia* sp. is the most common parasite found.	*Giardia* or *Giardia/Cryptosporidium* immunoassay (perform testing on two stools before reporting as negative). Particularly relevant for areas of the United States where *Giardia* sp. is the most common organism found.	If immunoassays are negative and symptoms continue, special tests for microsporidia and other coccidia (see previous entry) and O&P examination should be performed.
Patient with diarrhea and relevant travel history. Patient with diarrhea who is a past or present resident of a developing country. Patient in an area of the United States where parasites other than *Giardia* sp. are found.	O&P examination, *Entamoeba histolytica* immunoassay; various tests for *Strongyloides* spp. may be relevant (even in the absence of eosinophilia).	If examinations are negative and symptoms continue, special tests for coccidia and microsporidia should be performed.
Patient with unexplained eosinophilia and possible diarrhea; if chronic, patient may also have history of respiratory problems (larval migration) and/or sepsis or meningitis (hyperinfection).	Although the O&P examination is a possibility, the agar plate culture for *Strongyloides stercoralis* is recommended (it is more sensitive than the O&P examination).	If tests are negative and symptoms continue, additional O&P examinations and special tests for microsporidia and other coccidia should be performed.
Patient with diarrhea (suspected food-borne outbreak).	Test for *Cyclospora cayetanensis* (modified acid-fast stain, autofluorescence).	If tests are negative and symptoms continue, special procedures for microsporidia and other coccidia and O&P examination should be performed.

[a]Depending on the particular immunoassay kit used, various single or multiple organisms may be included. Selection of a particular kit depends on many variables, such as clinical relevance, cost, ease of performance, training, personnel availability, number of test orders, training of physician clients, sensitivity, specificity, equipment, and time to result. Very few laboratories handle this type of testing in exactly the same way. Many options are clinically relevant and acceptable for good patient care. It is critical that the laboratory report indicate specifically which organisms could be identified using the kit; a negative report should list the organisms relevant to that particular kit.

Note: Two ordering/collection/processing/examination situations are considered STAT orders (i.e., they require immediate attention for potentially life-threatening situations): central nervous system (CNS) specimens to be examined for free-living amebae and blood films in potential malaria or other cases involving blood parasites.

Specimen Processing

Diagnostic parasitology procedures designed to detect organisms in clinical specimens typically depend on morphologic criteria and visual identification (Evolve Procedures 46.1 to 46.10). Many clinical specimens, such as those from the intestinal tract, contain numerous artifacts that complicate the differentiation of parasites from surrounding debris. Specimen preparation may require concentration methods designed to increase the chance of finding the organism(s) by removing some fecal debris. Microscopic examination requires review of the prepared clinical specimen using multiple magnifications; organism identification also depends on the skill of the microbiologist. Final identification is based on microscopic examination of stained preparations to identify key characteristics of the parasite form. (Table 46.3 includes specific details on specimen processing.)

Approach to Identification

Protozoa are small, ranging from 1.5 μm (microsporidia) to approximately 80 μm (*Neobalantidium coli*, a ciliate) in size. Some are intracellular and require multiple detection and staining methods for identification. Helminth infections are usually diagnosed by finding eggs, larvae, and/or adult worms in various clinical specimens, primarily from the intestinal tract (Fig. 46.2). Identification to the species level may require microscopic examination of the specimen. Recovery and identification of blood parasites can require concentration, culture, and microscopy. Confirmation of suspected parasitic infections depends on the proper collection, processing, and examination of clinical specimens; often multiple specimens may be necessary to find and confirm the existence of a parasitic infection and the identity of the suspected organism or organisms (Table 46.10).

TABLE 46.8	Stool Specimen Collection and Testing Options		
Option	**Pros**	**Cons**	
Rejection of stools from inpatients who have been in house for longer than 3 days.	Data suggest that patients who begin to have diarrhea after they have been inpatients for a few days are not symptomatic from parasitic infections but generally from other causes.	The chance always exists that the problem is related to a health care–associated (nosocomial) parasitic infection (rare); *Cryptosporidium* spp. and microsporidia may be possible considerations.	
Examination of a single stool (ova and parasites [O&Ps]). Data suggest that 40%–50% of organisms present are found with only a single stool examination. Two O&Ps examinations (concentration, permanent stained smear) are acceptable but not always as good as three specimens (may be a relatively cost-effective approach); any patient remaining symptomatic requires additional testing.	Some believe that most intestinal parasitic infections can be diagnosed from examination of a single stool. If the patient becomes asymptomatic after collection of the first stool, subsequent specimens may not be necessary.	Diagnosis from a single stool examination depends on the experience of the laboratory scientist, proper collection, and the parasite load in the specimen. In a series of three stool specimens, commonly all three specimens are not positive and/or may be positive for different organisms.	
Examine a second stool only after the first is negative and the patient is still symptomatic.	With additional examinations, yield of protozoa increases (*Entamoeba histolytica,* 22.7%; *Giardia lamblia,* 11.3%; and *Dientamoeba fragilis,* 31.1%).	Assumes the second (or third) stool is collected within the recommended 10-day period for a series of stools; protozoa are shed periodically. May be inconvenient for patient.	
Examination of a single stool and an immunoassay (enzyme immunoassay [EIA], fluorescent antibody [FA], lateral or vertical flow cartridge). This approach is a mix: one immunoassay may be acceptable; however, immunoassay testing of two separate specimens may be required to confirm the presence of *Giardia* antigen. One O&P examination is generally insufficient.	If the examinations are negative and the patient's symptoms subside, probably no further testing is required.	Patients may show symptoms (off and on), so ruling out parasitic infections with only a single stool and one fecal immunoassay may be difficult. If the patient remains symptomatic, then even if two *Giardia* immunoassays are negative, other protozoa may be missed (*Entamoeba histolytica/Entamoeba dispar* group, *Dientamoeba fragilis, Cryptosporidium* spp., microsporidia). It is not recommended to perform both the O&P and fecal immunoassay automatically as a stool examination for parasites.	
Pool three specimens for examination; perform one concentration and one permanent stain (the laboratory pools the specimens).	Three specimens are collected by the patient (three separate collection vials) over 7–10 days; pooling by the laboratory may save time and expense.	Organisms present in low numbers may be missed because of the dilution factor once the specimens have been pooled.	

Microscopic Examination

High-quality clinical-grade binocular compound brightfield microscopes, kept in good working condition, are essential for examining specimens for parasites. Organism identification depends on morphologic differences found after careful examination using a regular brightfield microscope at low (100×), high dry (400×), and oil immersion (1000×) magnifications. The use of a 50× or 60× oil-immersion objective for scanning can be very helpful, particularly when the 50× oil and 100× oil-immersion objectives are side by side. The microscope should be set up using Köhler illumination, which maximizes the brightness and uniformity of the light that contacts the specimen, providing optimal viewing conditions.

A stereoscopic microscope is recommended for larger specimens (e.g., arthropods, tapeworm proglottids,

various artifacts). The total magnification usually varies from approximately 10× to 45×, either with a zoom capacity or with fixed objectives (0.66×, 1.3×, 3×) used with 5× or 10× oculars. Depending on the density of the specimen or object to be examined, the light source must be directed from under the stage or onto the top of the stage.

Because size is an essential factor for the accurate description and identification of parasites, especially for the characterization of fecal protozoa, a stage micrometer and calibrated ocular must be used for final identification. The stage micrometer typically has a 0.1-mm line with increments every 0.01 mm. This stage micrometer line is then viewed using the ocular at each objective magnification on the microscope to calibrate the ocular's scaled line. This allows the microbiologist to determine the exact size of the parasitic element using the ocular (Fig. 46.3).

TABLE 46.9   Fecal Fixatives Used in Diagnostic Parasitology (Intestinal Tract Specimens)

Fixative	Concentration	Permanent Stained Smear Trichrome, Iron-Hematoxylin, Special Stains/*Coccidia* and *Microsporidia*	Immunoassays: *Giardia lamblia* *Cryptosporidium* spp.	Comments
5% or 10% formalin	Yes	No	Yes	Concentrations and IAs (EIA, FA, Rapids)
5% or 10% buffered formalin	Yes	No	Yes	Concentrations and IAs (EIA, FA, Rapids)
MIF	Yes	Polychrome IV stain	ND	No published data
SAF	Yes	Iron-hematoxylin best	Yes	Concentrations, permanent stains, and IAs (EIA, FA, Rapids)
Schaudinn's (Hg base) no PVA[a]	Rare	Yes	No	Permanent stains; Hg interferes with IAs; primarily used with fresh stool specimens (no fixative collection vials)
Schaudinn's (Hg base) with PVA[a]	Rare	Yes	No	Permanent stains; Hg and PVA interfere with IAs; considered gold standard fixative for permanent stains
Schaudinn's (Cu base) with PVA[b]	Rare	Yes	No	Permanent stains; PVA interferes with IAs; stains not as good as with Schaudinn's fixative using Hg or Zn
Schaudinn's (Zn base) with PVA[c]	Rare	Yes	No	Permanent stains; PVA interferes with IAs; the same fixative as TOTAL-FIX without PVA (see Commentary)
Ecofriendly ECOFIX (PVA)[d]	Rare	Yes	No	Permanent stains; PVA interferes with IAs; works best with ECOSTAIN; Wheatley's trichrome second best
Universal fixative,[e] ecofriendly TOTAL-FIX	Yes	Yes	Yes	No formalin, no mercury, no PVA; concentrations, permanent stains, special stains, fecal IAs

Commentary

The most common collection option (original public health approach) is a two-vial system: one vial of 5% or 10% formalin or buffered formalin and one vial of fixative containing the plastic adhesive polyvinyl alcohol (PVA). The formalin vial is used for concentration and fecal immunoassays, and the PVA vial is used for the permanent stained smear. Regulations for formalin originally were developed for industry, not the clinical laboratory, where amounts of formalin tend to be quite low. However, a laboratory using any amount of formalin must be monitored.

SEMIUNIVERSAL FIXATIVES

Examples of a semiuniversal fixative include sodium acetate–acetic acid–formalin (SAF) (no mercury or PVA; *contains formalin*) and ECOFIX (no mercury or formalin; *contains PVA*).

UNIVERSAL FIXATIVE

Currently, TOTAL-FIX is the only fixative that contains *no* formalin, *no* PVA, and *no* mercury. TOTAL-FIX can be used without adding PVA to the fixative; adequate drying time for smears before staining is the most important step (minimum of 1 hour in 37°C incubator; more time is required for thicker fecal smears). This fixative can be used for concentration, permanent stained smear, special stains for coccidia or microsporidia, and fecal immunoassays for *Giardia* and *Cryptosporidium* spp.

FORMALIN FIXATIVE

Formalin has been used for many years as an all-purpose fixative that is appropriate for helminth eggs and larvae and for protozoan cysts, oocysts, and spores. Two concentrations are commonly used: 5%, which is recommended for preservation of protozoan cysts, and 10%, which is recommended for helminth eggs

Continued

TABLE 46.9 Fecal Fixatives Used in Diagnostic Parasitology (Intestinal Tract Specimens)—cont'd

and larvae. Although 5% is often recommended for all-purpose use, most commercial manufacturers provide 10%, which is more likely to kill all helminth eggs. To help maintain organism morphology, the formalin can be buffered with sodium phosphate buffers (i.e., neutral formalin). Selection of specific formalin formulations is at the user's discretion. *Aqueous formalin permits examination of the specimen as a wet mount only, a much less accurate technique than a permanent stained smear for identifying intestinal protozoa.* However, the fecal immunoassays for *Giardia duodenalis* and *Cryptosporidium* spp. can be performed from the aqueous formalin vial. Fecal immunoassays for the *Entamoeba histolytica/E. dispar* group are limited to fresh or frozen fecal specimens or Cary-Blair transport medium. After centrifugation, special stains for the coccidia (modified acid-fast stains) and microsporidia (modified trichrome stains) can be performed from the concentrate sediment obtained from formalin-preserved stool material. Use of the sediment provides a more sensitive test.

OCCUPATIONAL SAFETY AND HEALTH ADMINISTRATION REGULATIONS ON THE USE OF FORMALDEHYDE

Formaldehyde has been in use for more than a century as a disinfectant and preservative, and it is found in a number of industrial products. Disagreement exists about the carcinogenic potential of lower levels of exposure, and epidemiologic studies of the effects of formaldehyde exposure among humans have given inconsistent results. Studies of industry workers with known exposure to formaldehyde report little evidence of increased cancer risk. In addition, people with asthma appear to respond no differently than healthy individuals after exposure to concentrations of formaldehyde up to 3 ppm. The federal Occupational Safety and Health Administration (OSHA) requires all workers to be protected from dangerous levels of vapors and dust. Formaldehyde vapor is the most likely air contaminant to exceed the regulatory threshold in a laboratory, particularly in anatomic pathology. Current OSHA regulations require vapor levels not to exceed 0.75 ppm (measured as a time-weighted average [TWA]) and 2 ppm (measured as a 15-minute short-term exposure). OSHA requires monitoring for formaldehyde vapor wherever formaldehyde is used in the work place. The laboratory must have evidence at the time of inspection that formaldehyde vapor levels have been measured. Both 8-hour and 15-minute exposures must have been determined.

If each measurement is below the permissible exposure limit and the 8-hour measurement is below 0.5 ppm, no further monitoring is required as long as laboratory procedures remain constant. If the 0.5-ppm, 8-hour TWA or the 2-ppm, 15-minute level is exceeded, monitoring must be repeated semiannually. If either the 0.75-ppm, 8-hour TWA or the 2-ppm, 15-minute level is exceeded (very unlikely in a routine microbiology laboratory setting), employees must be required to wear respirators. Accidental skin contact with aqueous formalin must be prevented with the use of proper clothing and equipment (gloves, laboratory coats). The amendments of 1992 add medical removal protection provisions to supplement the existing medical surveillance requirements for employees suffering significant eye, nose, or throat irritation and for those experiencing dermal irritation or sensitization from occupational exposure to formaldehyde. In addition, these amendments establish specific hazard-labeling requirements for all forms of formaldehyde, including mixtures and solutions composed of at least 0.1% formaldehyde in excess of 0.1 ppm. Additional hazard labeling, including a warning label that formaldehyde presents a potential cancer hazard, is required where formaldehyde levels, under reasonably foreseeable conditions of use, may potentially exceed 0.5 ppm. The final amendments also provide for annual training of all employees exposed to formaldehyde at levels of 0.1 ppm or higher.

Note: The use of monitoring badges may not be a sensitive enough method to correctly measure the 15-minute exposure level. Contact the OSHA office in your institution for monitoring options. Usually, the accepted method involves monitoring airflow in the specific area or areas in the laboratory where formaldehyde vapors are found.

POLYVINYL ALCOHOL ADHESIVE (NOT A FIXATIVE)

PVA is a water-soluble, synthetic polymer used as a viscosity-increasing agent in pharmaceuticals, as an adhesive in parasitology fecal fixatives, and as a lubricant and protectant in ophthalmic preparations. PVA is defined as a water-soluble polymer made by hydrolysis of a polyvinyl ester (e.g., polyvinyl acetate). It is used in adhesives, as a textile and paper sizer, and for emulsifying, suspending, and thickening solutions. PVA is not a fixative, but rather an adhesive to help glue stool material onto the slide; this is the only purpose of PVA as an additive to parasitology fecal fixative formulations.

PVA is a plastic resin that is incorporated into Schaudinn's fixative. Although some laboratories may perform a fecal concentration from a PVA-preserved specimen, some parasites do not concentrate well, and some do not exhibit the typical morphology that would be seen in concentration sediment from a formalin-based fixative. PVA fixative solution is highly recommended as a means of preserving cysts and trophozoites for later examination. Use of PVA fixative also allows specimens to be shipped (by regular mail service) from any location in the world to a laboratory for examination. PVA fixative is particularly useful for liquid specimens and should be used in the ratio of three parts PVA to one part fecal specimen.

Note: Very detailed information on all fixative options can be found in Garcia LS. *Diagnostic Medical Parasitology*. 6th ed. Washington, DC: ASM Press; 2016.

Cu, Copper; *EIA*, enzyme immunoassay; *FA*, fluorescent antibody; *Hg*, mercury; *IA*, immunoassay; *MIF*, merthiolate-iodine-formalin fixative; *ND*, no data; *PVA*, polyvinyl alcohol; *Rapids*, cartridge-format, membrane-flow IAs; *SAF*, sodium acetate–acetic acid–formalin; *Zn*, zinc.

[a]These two fixatives use the mercuric chloride base in the Schaudinn's fixative; this formulation is still considered the gold standard against which all other fixatives are evaluated (organism morphology after permanent staining).

[b]This modification uses a copper sulfate base rather than mercuric chloride; the morphology of stained organisms is not as good as with Hg or Zn.

[c]This modification (proprietary formula) uses a zinc base rather than mercuric chloride and works well with both trichrome and iron-hematoxylin.

[d]This fixative uses a combination of ingredients but is prepared from a proprietary formula (contains PVA).

[e]This modification uses a combination of ingredients, including zinc, but is prepared from a proprietary formula. The aim is to provide a universal fixative that can be used for the fecal concentration, permanent stained smear, and available immunoassays for *Giardia duodenalis*, *Cryptosporidium* spp., and *Entamoeba histolytica*. However, currently, fecal immunoassays for the *E. histolytica* require fresh or frozen specimens; testing can also be performed from stool submitted in Cary-Blair transport medium.

Microscopy for parasitology is labor intensive and requires significant knowledge and skills for the identification of the organisms. Techcyte Inc. (Lindon, Utah), has developed a digital artificial intelligence system for identifying O&Ps from stool samples. The system preclassifies the slides by screening out negative samples before the technologist reviews the positive slides for organism identification. The system is designed to reduce technologist time and cost.

Intestinal Tract

Stool specimens are the most common specimen submitted to the diagnostic laboratory for parasite identification. As a result, the most commonly performed procedure in parasitology is the traditional examination for O&Ps, although the use of rapid fecal immunoassays and molecular techniques has greatly increased over the past 10 years. Several other diagnostic techniques are available for the recovery and identification of parasitic organisms from the intestinal tract. Although many laboratories do not routinely offer all these relatively simple and inexpensive techniques, the clinician should be familiar with the relevance of information obtained from them. It is rarely necessary to examine stool specimens for scolices and proglottids of cestodes and adult nematodes and trematodes in order to

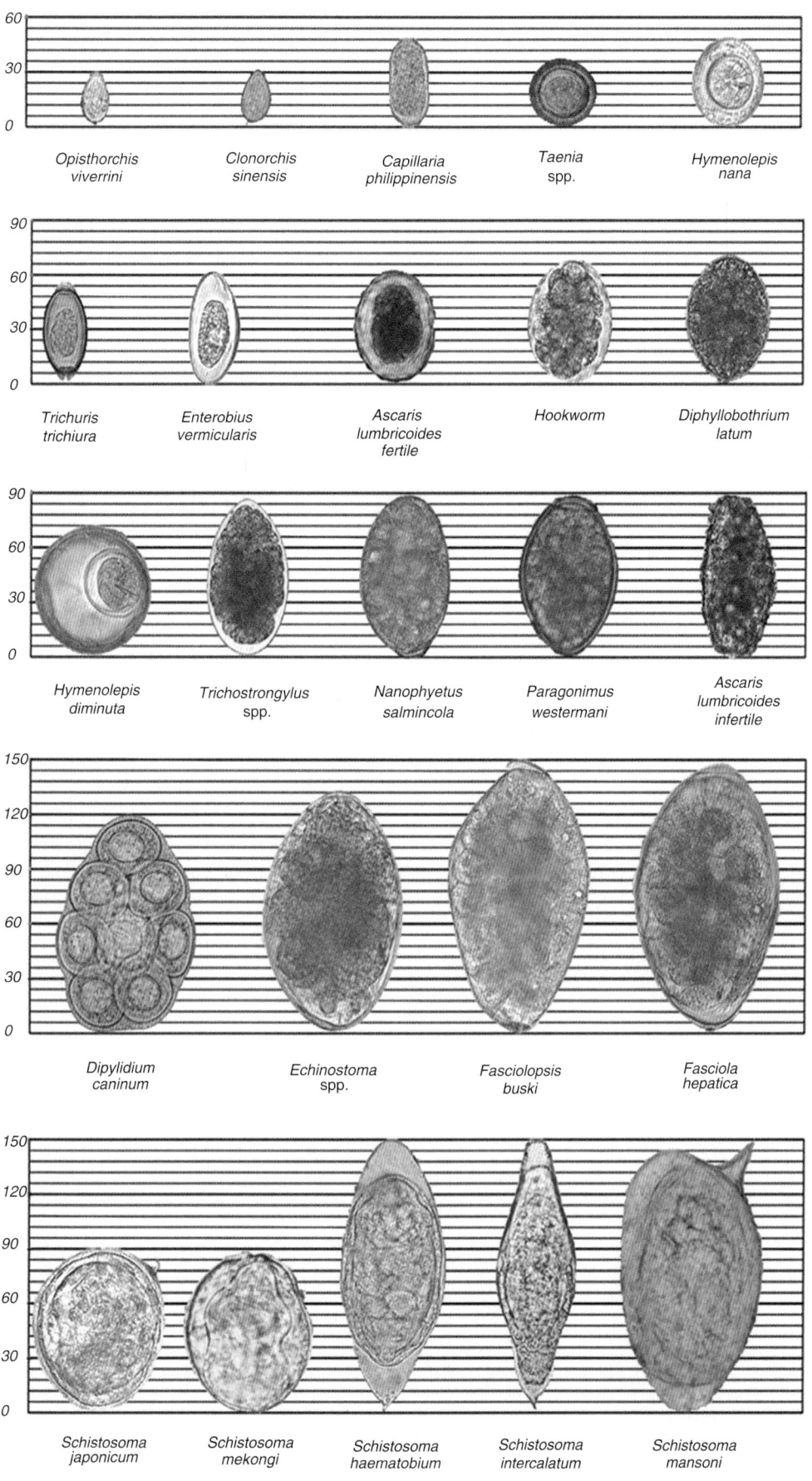

• **Fig. 46.2** Relative egg size of helminths that infect humans. Measurements are in micrometers (μm). (From Centers for Disease Control and Prevention. *Intestinal Parasites: Comparative Morphology Figures. Figure 6: Relative Sizes of Helminth Eggs.* https://www.cdc.gov/dpdx/diagnosticprocedures/stool /morphcomp.html. Accessed October 26, 2020.)

TABLE 46.10 Common Human Parasites: Diagnostic Specimens, Tests, and Positive Findings

Organism	Infection Acquired	Location in Host	Diagnostic Specimen	Diagnostic Test[a]	Positive Specimen	Comments
Intestinal Amebae *Entamoeba histolytica* *Entamoeba bangladeshi* *Entamoeba dispar* *Entamoeba hartmanni* *Entamoeba coli* *Entamoeba moshkovskii* *Entamoeba polecki* *Endolimax nana* *Iodamoeba bütschlii* *Blastocystis hominis*	Ingestion of food or water contaminated with infective cysts; fecal-oral transmission.	Intestinal tract; *E. histolytica* infection may disseminate to the liver (extraintestinal amebiasis); *Blastocystis* strains are pathogenic or nonpathogenic; cannot differentiate on morphology.	Stool; sigmoidoscopy specimens.	O&Ps examination; stained sigmoidoscopy slides; stool immunoassays.	Trophozoites and/or cysts.	Many of the protozoa can look very much alike; see diagnostic tables for details; immunoassays for *E. histolytica/E. dispar* group and *E. histolytica* (fresh, frozen stool, Cary Blair required).
Free-Living Amebae *Naegleria fowleri* *Acanthamoeba* spp. *Balamuthia mandrillaris* *Sappinia* spp.	Contaminated water or soil; dust, contaminated eye solutions; organisms may enter through nasal mucosa, travel to brain via olfactory nerve.	CNS; eye.	CSF, corneal scrapings, biopsy, eye care solutions; CSF examination STAT request.	Stains, culture, FA, biopsy; *B. mandrillaris* cannot be grown on agar culture, whereas *N. fowleri* and *Acanthamoeba* species can.	Trophozoites or cysts.	CNS disease life threatening with *N. fowleri* (PAM); other CNS infections more chronic (GAE); keratitis can lead to blindness.
Intestinal Flagellates *Giardia duodenalis* *Dientamoeba fragilis* *Chilomastix mesnili* *Pentatrichomonas hominis*	Ingestion of food or water contaminated with infective cysts or trophozoites (*D. fragilis*, *T. hominis*); fecal-oral transmission.	Intestinal tract.	Stool; duodenal specimens or Entero-Test capsule (string test) for *Giardia duodenalis*.	O&P examination; wet preparations or stains of duodenal material; stool immunoassays (can use fresh or formalin fixed specimens; no PVA); need two specimens for IA for *G. duodenalis*.	Trophozoites or cysts	*G. duodenalis* is very difficult to recover; stool immunoassays are more sensitive than routine O&Ps examinations; *D. fragilis* requires permanent stain for identification.
Urogenital Flagellates *Trichomonas vaginalis*	Sexually transmitted; wet towels less likely but possible.	Urinary tract; genital system; males may be asymptomatic.	Vaginal secretions, prostatic fluid, often recovered in urine sediment	Wet preparations, culture, immunoassays; molecular testing.	Trophozoites	Often diagnosed by motility in urine sediment or wet preparations.
Intestinal Ciliate *Neobalantidium coli*	Ingestion of food or water contaminated with infective cysts; fecal-oral transmission.	Intestinal tract.	Stool.	O&Ps examination; wet preparations better than permanent stained smear.	Trophozoites and/or cysts	Not common in the United States; associated with pigs; seen in proficiency testing specimens.

TABLE 46.10 Common Human Parasites: Diagnostic Specimens, Tests, and Positive Findings—cont'd

Organism	Infection Acquired	Location in Host	Diagnostic Specimen	Diagnostic Test[a]	Positive Specimen	Comments
Intestinal Coccidia *Cryptosporidium* spp. *Cyclospora cayetanensis* *Cystoisospora belli*	Ingestion of food or water contaminated with infective oocysts; fecal-oral transmission.	Intestinal tract; *Cryptosporidium* spp. can disseminate to other tissues in compromised host (lung, gallbladder).	Stool; biopsy; duodenal specimen; sputum.	Modified acid-fast stains; stool immunoassays; concentration, wet prep for *C. belli.*	Oocysts in stool or scrapings; other developmental stages in tissues.	*Cryptosporidium* spp. cause severe diarrhea in compromised patient; nosocomial transmission.
Intestinal Microsporidia[b] *Enterocytozoon bieneusi* *Encephalitozoon intestinalis*	Ingestion of food or water contaminated with infective spores; fecal-oral transmission.	Intestinal tract; organisms can disseminate to other body sites (kidney).	Stool; biopsy.	Modified trichrome stains; optical brightening agents; experimental immunoassays; biopsy and histology (tissue Gram stains).	Spores in stool; other developmental stages in tissues.	Can cause serious diarrhea in compromised host.
Microsporidia; Other Body Sites *Encephalitozoon* spp. *Anncaliia vesicularum* *Microsporidium* *Pleistophora* *Trachipleistophora* *Vittaforma* *Tubulinosema*	Ingestion of food or water contaminated with infective spores; fecal-oral transmission; inhalation; direct environmental contact to eyes; probably hands to eyes.	All tissues.	All body fluids and/or tissues relevant, depending on *body* site.	Modified trichrome stains; optical brightening agents; experimental immunoassays; biopsy and histology (tissue Gram stains).	Spores in stool, urine, other body fluids; developmental stages in tissues.	Can cause serious diarrhea in compromised host; a number of eye infections documented in immunocompetent patients.
Tissue Protozoa *Toxoplasma gondii*	Ingestion of raw meat; oocysts from cat feces.	Eye, CNS in compromised patient.	Biopsies (any tissue), CSF.	Serology, tissue culture; recovery from CSF.	Positive serology; recovery of trophozoites in CSF.	Many people have positive serologies for *T. gondii*; infections are serious in immunocompromised patients.
Intestinal Nematodes *Enterobius vermicularis* *Trichuris trichiura* *Ascaris lumbricoides* Hookworm *Strongyloides stercoralis*	Ingestion of food or water contaminated with infective eggs; penetration of skin by infective larvae in soil.	Intestine; *S. stercoralis* may disseminate (hyperinfection), primarily in immunocompromised patients.	Stool; duodenal contents (*S. stercoralis*); cellophane tape preps or paddles for *E. vermicularis.*	O&Ps examination; special concentrates and cultures; examination of tapes for *E. vermicularis.*	Adult worms, eggs and/or larvae, depending on the roundworm involved.	Review direct and indirect life cycles (migration through heart, lung, trachea to intestine), 4–6 consecutive tapes required to rule out *Enterobius* infection.

Continued

TABLE 46.10 Common Human Parasites: Diagnostic Specimens, Tests, and Positive Findings—cont'd

Organism	Infection Acquired	Location in Host	Diagnostic Specimen	Diagnostic Test[a]	Positive Specimen	Comments
Tissue Nematodes						
VLM, OLM (*Toxocara* spp.)	Ingestion of infective eggs.	Migration through tissues.	Serum.	Serology.	Positive serology.	Human is accidental host for VLM, OLM, and CLM.
CLM (dog/cat hookworm)	Skin penetration of larvae.	Skin tracks, migration.	Visual inspection.	Presence of tracks/skin.	Eosinophilia, visual tracks.	Outbreaks still occur.
Trichinella spp.	Ingestion of raw pork.	Muscle.	Serum, muscle biopsy.	Serology, squash prep.	Positive serology, larvae.	
Anisakis, others	Ingestion of raw marine fish.	Intestine.	Submission of larvae.	ID of larvae.	Positive larval ID.	Sometimes identified only after surgical removal.
Intestinal Cestodes	Ingestion of:	Intestine.				Eggs for the two *Taenia* spp. look alike; gravid proglottid or scolex is needed for identification.
Taenia saginata (beef)	Raw beef.		Stool and/or proglottids.	O&Ps, India ink proglottids.	Eggs, proglottid branches.	
Taenia solium (pork)	Raw pork.		Stool and/or proglottids.	O&P, India ink proglottids.	Eggs, proglottid branches.	
Diphyllobothrium latum	Raw freshwater fish.		Stool and/or proglottids.	O&P.	Eggs, proglottid shape.	
Hymenolepis nana	Tapeworm eggs.		Stool.	O&Ps.	Eggs.	
Hymenolepis diminuta	Grain beetles.		Stool.	O&Ps.	Eggs.	
Dipylidium caninum	Fleas from dogs/cats.		Stool and/or proglottids.	O&Ps.	Eggs, proglottid shape.	
Tissue Cestodes	Ingestion of:					
Echinococcus granulosus	Eggs from dog tapeworm.	Liver, lung, and so on.	Serum, hydatid cyst aspirate; biopsy.	Serology, centrifugation of fluid; histology.	Positive serology; hydatid sand, tapeworm. Tissue.	*E. granulosus* (enclosed cyst).
Echinococcus multilocularis	Eggs from fox tapeworm.					*E. multilocularis* (cyst wanders through tissue).
Taenia solium (pork)	Eggs from human tapeworm.	CNS, subcutaneous tissues.	Serum, scans, biopsy.	Serology, films, histology.	Positive serology, positive scans, tapeworm tissue.	Small, enclosed cysticerci (cysticercosis).

TABLE 46.10 Common Human Parasites: Diagnostic Specimens, Tests, and Positive Findings—cont'd

Organism	Infection Acquired	Location in Host	Diagnostic Specimen	Diagnostic Test[a]	Positive Specimen	Comments
Intestinal Trematodes	Ingestion of metacercariae:					
Fasciolopsis buski	On water chestnuts.	Intestine.	Stool.	O&Ps examination; M. yokogawai, H. heterophyes eggs very small; use high dry power.	Eggs in stool.	Eggs of F. buski look identical to those of the liver fluke, Fasciola hepatica.
Metagonimus yokogawai	In raw fish.					
Heterophyes heterophyes						
Liver and Lung Trematodes	Ingestion of metacercariae.					
Fasciola hepatica	On watercress.	Liver.	Stool.	O&Ps.	Eggs in stool.	Eggs of F. hepatica look almost identical to those of F. buski; lung fluke eggs in sputum resemble brown metal filings.
Clonorchis sinensis	In raw fish.	Liver, bile ducts.	Stool, duodenal drainage.	O&Ps.	Eggs in stool, and so on.	
Paragonimus spp.	In raw crabs.	Lung.	Stool, sputum.	O&Ps.	Eggs in stool. and/or sputum.	
Blood Trematodes						
Schistosoma mansoni	Skin penetration of cercariae released from the freshwater snail intermediate host.	Veins over the large intestine.	Because the adult worms may become located in the "incorrect" veins, both urine and stool (unpreserved) should be examined.	O&Ps; hatching test for egg viability (all specimens collected with no preservatives); concentrates performed with saline, not water.	Eggs in stool and/or urine.	When schistosomiasis is suspected, stool, random urine, and 24-h urine specimen (collected with no preservatives).
Schistosoma haematobium		Bladder.				
Schistosoma japonicum; Schistosoma mekongi		Small intestine.				
Malaria		Preerythrocytic				
Plasmodium vivax	Infection through mosquito bite, blood transfusion, shared drug needles; transplacental.	Liver.	Drawn immediately: STAT request. Blood draw every 6 h until confirmed as positive or negative.	Thick, thin blood films; rapid immunoassay methods (not yet FDA approved in United States); concentration methods.	Parasites present.	P. falciparum and P. knowlesi infections are medical emergencies; complete patient history mandatory (travel, prophylaxis, prior history); Giemsa or other bloodstain recommended.
Plasmodium ovale		Blood.				
Plasmodium malariae		Blood.				
Plasmodium knowlesi		Blood.				
Plasmodium falciparum		Blood. Blood plus capillaries of deep tissues (spleen, liver, bone marrow).				
Babesiosis						
Babesia spp.	Tick borne; transfusion; organ transplants.	Blood.	Blood.	Thick, thin blood films.	Parasites present.	Can mimic ring forms of P. falciparum; patient will have no travel history outside of United States.

Continued

TABLE 46.10 Common Human Parasites: Diagnostic Specimens, Tests, and Positive Findings—cont'd

Organism	Infection Acquired	Location in Host	Diagnostic Specimen	Diagnostic Test[a]	Positive Specimen	Comments
Trypanosomes						
Trypanosoma brucei gambiense	Bite of tsetse fly.	Blood, lymph nodes, CNS.	Blood, node aspirate, CSF.	Thick, thin films.	Trypomastigotes.	African sleeping sickness more common with *T. brucei gambiense.*
Trypanosoma brucei rhodesiense	Bite of tsetse fly.	Blood, lymph nodes, CNS.		Thick, thin films.	Trypomastigotes.	Chagas disease
Trypanosoma cruzi	Feces of triatomid bug (kissing bug) (bug feces scratched into bite site).	Blood, striated muscle (e.g., heart, GI tract).	Blood, cardiac changes, muscle biopsy.	Thick, thin films, histology; culture.	Trypomastigotes in blood, amastigotes in tissue.	(American trypanosomiasis) (xenodiagnosis an option).
Leishmaniae						
Leishmania tropica complex (cutaneous)	Bite of sand fly.	Macrophages of skin.	Skin biopsy.	Stained smears, cultures.	Amastigotes in clinical specimens indicated.	Animal inoculation rarely used; some research labs now using PCR.
Leishmania braziliensis complex (mucocutaneous)	Bite of sand fly.	Skin, mucous membranes.	Skin, membrane biopsy.	Stained smears, cultures.		
Leishmania donovani complex (visceral)		Spleen, liver, bone marrow (RE system).	Blood, bone marrow, liver/spleen biopsy.	Thick, thin blood films; stained smears, cultures.		
Filarial Nematodes						
Wuchereria bancrofti (S)	Bite of mosquito.	Lymphatics (adults), blood (microfilariae).	Blood.	Thick and thin films; various concentrations.	Microfilariae.	Elephantiasis possible; periodicity a factor in finding microfilariae; some microfilariae sheathed (S), some not (NS)
Onchocerca volvulus (NS)	Black fly.	Skin, nodules (adults), blood, eye (microfilariae).	Skin snips, blood; biopsy nodule.	Biopsy, tease skin apart in water; thick and thin films.	Microfilariae; adult in tissue nodules.	
Less Common						
Loa loa (S)	Black gnat.	Eye (adults), lymphatics (adults), blood (microfilariae) for all three.	Blood.	Thick, thin films; various concentrations.	Microfilariae, adult worm.	"African eye worm."
Brugia malayi (S)	Mosquito.				Microfilariae.	
Mansonella spp. (NS)	Mosquito.					

CLM, Cutaneous larva migrans; *CNS,* central nervous system; *CSF,* cerebrospinal fluid; *FA,* fluorescent antibody; *FDA,* Food and Drug Administration; *GAE,* granulomatous amoebic encephalitis; *IA,* immunoassay; *ID,* identification; *NS,* not sheathed; *OLM,* ocular larva migrans; *O&P,* ova and parasite; *PAM,* primary amoebic meningoencephalitis; *PCR,* polymerase chain reaction; *RE,* reticuloendothelium system; *S,* sheathed; *VLM,* visceral larva migrans

[a]Although serologic tests are not always mentioned, they are available for a number of parasitic infections. Unfortunately, most are not routinely available. Contact your state Public Health Laboratory or the Centers for Disease Control and Prevention (CDC) in Atlanta, Georgia.

[b]The microsporidia are classified with the fungi.

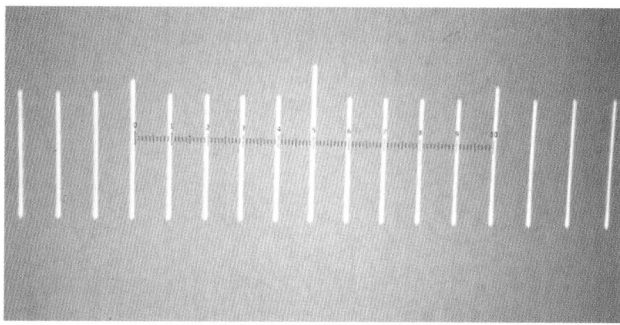

• **Fig. 46.3** Stage and ocular micrometer.

confirm the diagnosis or to identify the organism to the species level.

Other specimens from the intestinal tract—such as duodenal aspirates or drainage, mucus from the Entero-Test Capsule technique, and sigmoidoscopy material—can also be examined as wet preparations and as permanent stained smears after processing with trichrome or iron-hematoxylin staining.

Ova and Parasite Examination

The traditional O&Ps examination comprises three separate protocols: the direct wet mount, the concentration technique and indirect wet mount examination, and the permanently stained smear.

The **direct wet mount,** which requires fresh stool, is designed to enable the detection of motile protozoan trophozoites. The specimen is examined microscopically at low and high dry magnifications (100×, entire 22- by 22-mm cover slip; 400×, one-third to one-half of a 22- by 22-mm cover slip) (Box 46.1). However, because of potential problems resulting from the lag time between specimen passage and receipt in the laboratory, the direct wet examination has been eliminated from the routine O&Ps examination in many laboratories in the United States in favor of specimens collected in stool preservatives. The direct wet preparation is not performed for specimens received in the laboratory in preservatives. The various fixatives available are included in Table 46.9. Each preservative or combination of preservatives has advantages and disadvantages for different types of parasites and for different laboratory methods. Each laboratory should consider the types of parasites most commonly seen in their location and population and should select the preservatives that maximize the detection of such parasites.

The second part of the O&Ps is the **indirect** examination after specimen concentration, which is designed to facilitate recovery of protozoan cysts, coccidian oocysts, microsporidial spores, and helminth eggs and larvae (Box 46.2). Both flotation and sedimentation methods are available; the most common procedure is the formalin–ethyl acetate sedimentation method (previously the formalin-ether method) (Fig. 46.4). The concentrated specimen sediment can be examined as a wet preparation with or without iodine using low and high dry magnifications (100×, 400×) as indicated for the direct wet smear examination.

• BOX 46.1 Direct Smear: Review

Principle

To detect the presence of motile forms of parasites (primarily protozoan trophozoites or larvae); to diagnose organisms that cannot be identified from the permanent stain methods; to allow quick diagnosis of heavily infected patients; to estimate the worm burden of a patient.

Specimen

Any fresh liquid or soft stool specimen that has not been refrigerated or frozen.

Reagents

0.85% NaCl; Lugol's or D'Antoni's iodine.

Examination

Low-power examination (100×) of entire 22- by 22-mm cover slip preparation (both saline and iodine); high dry power examination (400×) of at least one-third of the cover slip area (both saline and iodine).

Results

Results from the direct smear examination should be considered presumptive. However, some organisms can be identified definitively (*Giardia duodenalis* cysts and *Entamoeba coli* cysts, helminth eggs and larvae, *Cystoisospora belli* oocysts). The report should be considered "preliminary"; the final report includes the results of the concentration and permanent stained smear.

Notes and Limitations

When iodine is added to the preparation, the organisms are killed and motility is lost. Specimens submitted in stool preservatives and fresh, formed specimens should not be examined using this procedure; the concentration and permanent stained smear techniques should be performed instead. Oil immersion examination (1000×) is not recommended (the organism morphology is not that clear).

The third part of the O&Ps examination is the permanently stained smear, which is designed to facilitate the identification of intestinal protozoa (Box 46.3). The permanently stained smear is the most important procedure performed to confirm the diagnosis of intestinal protozoan infections.

Several staining methods are available; the two most commonly used are the Wheatley modification of the Gomori tissue trichrome stain and the iron-hematoxylin stain (Fig. 46.5). This part of the O&PS examination is critical for confirmation of suspicious objects seen in the wet examination and for identification of protozoa that may not have been visible in the wet preparation. Permanently stained smears are examined using oil immersion objectives (600× or 800× for screening and 1000× for final review of 300 or more oil-immersion fields). The permanently stained smears also provide a permanent record for reexamination or confirmation.

Modified acid-fast stains are necessary for the identification of intestinal coccidia (Box 46.4), and modified trichrome stains are recommended for identification of

• BOX 46.2 Concentration: Review

Principle
To concentrate the parasites present, either through sedimentation or by flotation. The concentration is specifically designed to allow recovery of protozoan cysts, coccidian oocysts, microsporidian spores, and helminth eggs and larvae.

Specimen
Any stool specimen that is fresh or preserved in formalin (most common), polyvinyl alcohol (PVA; mercury based or non–mercury based), sodium acetate–acetic acid–formalin (SAF), merthiolate-iodine-formalin (MIF), or the newer fixatives for the single-vial system—universal fixatives containing no mercury, formalin, or PVA.

Reagents
Formalin, ethyl acetate, zinc sulfate 5% or 10% (specific gravity, 1.18 for fresh stool and 1.20 for preserved stool); 0.85% sodium chloride (NaCl); Lugol's or D'Antoni's iodine.

Examination
Low-power examination (100×) of entire 22- by 22-mm cover slip preparation (iodine recommended but optional); high dry power examination 400×) of at least one-third of the cover slip area (both saline and iodine).

Results
Results from the concentration examination should be considered presumptive. However, some organisms can be identified definitively (*Giardia duodenalis* cysts and *Entamoeba coli* cysts, helminth eggs and larvae, *Cystoisospora belli* oocysts). The report should be considered "preliminary" and should be coordinated with the findings from the permanent smear.

Notes and Limitations
Formalin–ethyl acetate sedimentation concentration is most commonly used. Zinc sulfate flotation may not detect operculated or heavy eggs (*Clonorchis* eggs, unfertilized *Ascaris* eggs). For the flotation technique, both the surface film and sediment must be examined before a negative result is reported. Smears prepared from concentrated stool are normally examined at low power (100×) and high dry power (400×). Oil-immersion examination (1000×) may be used with caution because the morphology of some organisms may not be clear. The addition of too much iodine may obscure helminth eggs (i.e., it produces an effect that mimics debris).

intestinal microsporidia (Box 46.5). These stains are specifically designed to enable the identification of coccidian oocysts and microsporidian spores, respectively.

Fig. 46.6 provides a diagrammatic overview of the processing of fecal specimens for parasite identification.

Recovery of the Tapeworm Scolex
The procedure for the recovery of the tapeworm scolex is rarely requested in the United States and is no longer clinically relevant because of the effective use of medication to treat tapeworm infections. However, stool specimens may be examined for scolices and gravid proglottids of cestodes for species identification. This procedure requires mixing a small amount of feces with water and straining the mixture

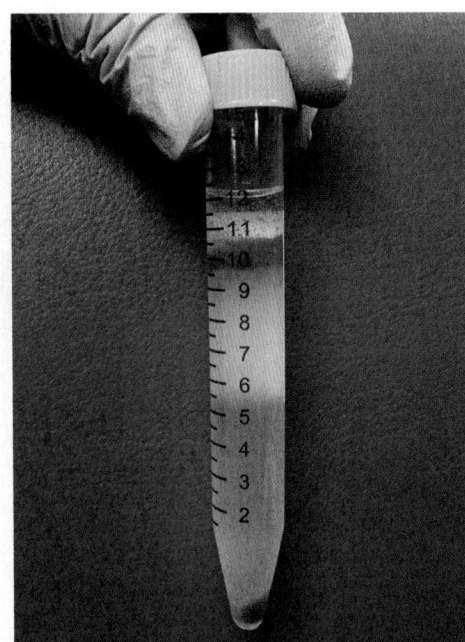

• **Fig. 46.4** Formalin–ethyl acetate concentration test tube after centrifugation showing four layers; from the bottom: sediment, formalin layer, debris plug, and ethyl acetate layer.

through a series of wire screens (graduated from coarse to fine mesh) to look for scolices and proglottids. The appearance of scolices after therapy is an indication of successful treatment. If the scolex has not been passed, it may still be attached to the mucosa. Because the scolex can continue to produce new proglottids, the infection will continue. If this occurs, the patient must be retreated to eradicate the infection completely.

Examination for Pinworm
Enterobius vermicularis, **pinworm** or **seatworm,** a roundworm parasite commonly found in children worldwide. The adult female worm migrates out of the anus, usually at night, and deposits her eggs in the perianal area. The adult female (8 to 13 mm long) may occasionally be found on the surface of a stool specimen or on the perianal skin. Because the eggs are usually deposited around the anus, they are not commonly found in feces and must be detected by other diagnostic means. Diagnosis of pinworm infection is usually based on the recovery of eggs, which are described as thick-shelled, football-shaped eggs with one slightly flattened side. Often, each egg contains a fully developed embryo and is infective within a few hours after being deposited (Fig. 46.7).

Sigmoidoscopy Material
Material obtained from sigmoidoscopy can be helpful in the diagnosis of amebiasis that has gone undetected by routine fecal examination. However, a series of at least three routine stool examinations for parasites should be completed before a sigmoidoscopy examination is performed. A sigmoidoscopy specimen should be processed immediately. All three methods of examination are recommended (direct,

• BOX 46.3 Permanent Stained Smear: Review

Principle

To allow the examination and recognition of detailed organism morphology under oil-immersion examination (100× objective for a total magnification of 1000×), primarily enabling the recovery and identification of intestinal protozoa.

Specimen

Any stool specimen that is fresh or preserved in polyvinyl alcohol (PVA; mercury based or non–mercury based), sodium acetate–acetic acid–formalin (SAF), merthiolate-iodine-formalin (MIF), or the newer single vial–system fixatives (universal fixatives).

Reagents

Trichrome, iron-hematoxylin, modified iron-hematoxylin, polychrome IV, or chlorazol black E stains and their associated solutions; dehydrating solutions (alcohols and xylenes or xylene substitutes); mounting fluid (optional). The use of true absolute alcohol (100% ethanol) is preferred over the use of 95%/5% alcohol.

Examination

The entire smear should be examined on low power (100×) for the presence of large parasite forms such as larvae or helminth eggs. Oil-immersion examination (1000×) should include at least 300 fields; additional fields may be required if suspect organisms have been seen in the wet preparations from the concentrated specimen.

Results

Most suspected protozoa and/or human cells can be confirmed by examination of the permanently stained smear. These reports should be categorized as "final" and are reported as such (the direct wet smear and the concentration examination provide "preliminary" results).

Notes and Limitations

The most commonly used stains are trichrome and iron-hematoxylin. Unfortunately, helminth eggs and larvae may take up the stain inconsistently and are not easily identified from the permanent stained smear. Coccidian oocysts and microsporidian spores also require other staining methods for identification.

Permanent stained smears are examined under oil-immersion examination (1000×). The slide may be screened using the 50× or 60× oil-immersion objectives, but the results should not be reported until the examination has been completed using the 100× oil-immersion lens. Confirmation of intestinal protozoa (both trophozoites and cysts) is the primary purpose of this technique.

Important Reminder

When nonmercury fixatives or one of the single-vial options (usually a zinc-based proprietary formula or one of the universal fixatives) is used, the iodine-alcohol step can be eliminated. After drying, the slides can be placed directly into the stain (trichrome or hematoxylin). However, if fecal specimens have been preserved with mercury-based fixatives, the iodine-alcohol step must be included in the routine staining protocol as well as subsequent rinse steps to remove the mercury and iodine. Some laboratories leave the staining protocol as is, including the iodine-alcohol step, which does not harm smears preserved with non–mercury based fixatives.

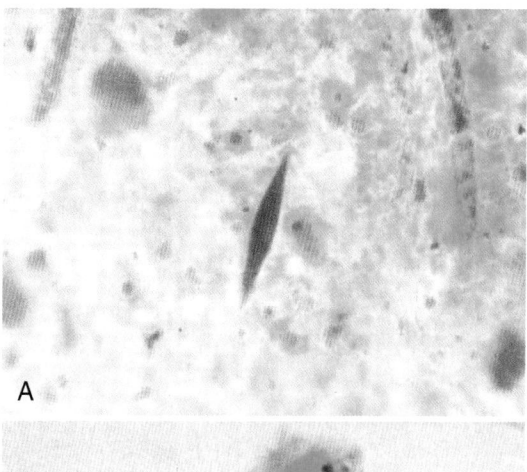

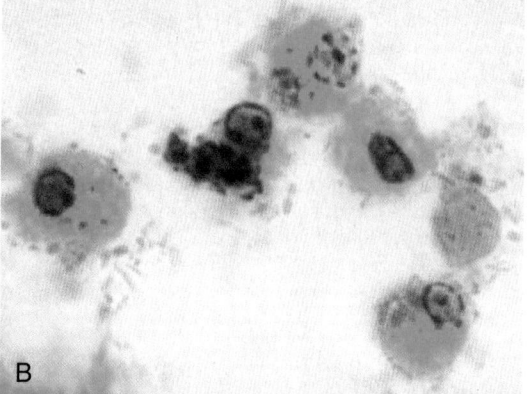

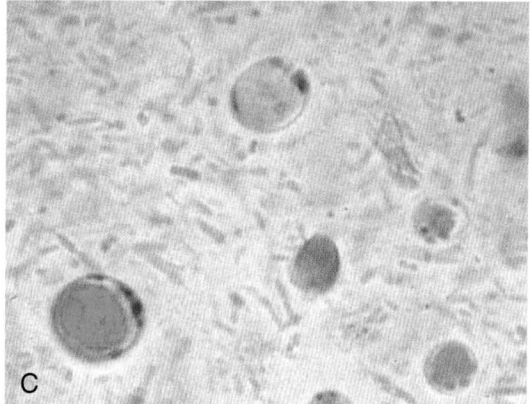

• **Fig. 46.5** Stool material stained with Wheatley's trichrome stain. (A) Charcot-Leyden crystals. (B) Polymorphonuclear leukocytes. (C) *Blastocystis hominis* central body forms (larger objects) and yeast cells (smaller, more homogeneous objects).

concentration, permanent smear). However, depending on the availability of trained personnel, proper fixatives, or the amount of specimen obtained, one or two procedures may be used. It is important to note that even the most thorough examination will be meaningless if the specimen has been improperly collected, fixed, and transported.

Duodenal Drainage

In patients infected with *G. duodenalis* or *S. stercoralis*, routine stool examinations may not be sufficient to identify the infecting organisms. Duodenal drainage material may increase the likelihood of identifying the parasites. However, the "falling leaf" motility often described for *Giardia*

• BOX 46.4 Modified Acid-Fast Permanent Stained Smear: Review

Principle

To provide contrasting colors for background debris and parasites. This technique is designed to allow examination and recognition of acid-fast characteristics of organisms under high dry power (40× objective, for a total magnification of 400×), primarily allowing recovery and identification of intestinal coccidian oocysts. The internal morphology of sporozoites can be seen within some *Cryptosporidium* oocysts under oil immersion (1000×); *Cyclospora* oocysts do not have a specific internal morphology.

Specimen

Any stool specimen that is fresh or preserved in formalin, sodium acetate–acetic acid–formalin (SAF), or the newer fixatives for the single-vial system (universal fixatives).

Reagents

Kinyoun's acid-fast stain, modified Ziehl-Neelsen stain, and their associated solutions; dehydrating solutions (alcohols and xylenes or xylene substitutes); mounting fluid (optional). The decolorizing agents are less intense than the acid alcohol used in routine acid-fast staining (this is what makes these "modified" acid-fast procedures). The recommended decolorizer is 1%–3% sulfuric acid. Many laboratories use 1% so that the *Cyclospora* oocysts retain more color.

Examination

High dry examination (400×) of at least 300 fields; additional fields may be required if suspicious organisms have been seen but are not clearly acid-fast stained.

Results

Identification of *Cryptosporidium* and *Cystoisospora* oocysts should be possible. *Cyclospora* oocysts, which are twice the size of *Cryptosporidium* oocysts, should be visible but tend to be more acid-fast variable. Although microsporidia are acid-fast, their small size makes recognition very difficult. Final laboratory results depend heavily on the appearance of the quality control (QC) slides and comparison with positive patient specimens.

Notes and Limitations

Both the cold and hot modified acid-fast methods are excellent for staining coccidian oocysts. Some clinicians believe that the hot method may result in better stain penetration, but the differences are probably minimal. Procedure limitations are related to specimen handling (proper centrifugation speeds and time, use of no more than two layers of wet gauze for filtration, and complete understanding of the difficulties in recognizing microsporidial spores). In addition, some controversy exists over whether the organisms lose the ability to take up acid-fast stains after long-term storage in 10% formalin. The organisms are more difficult to find in specimens from patients who do not have the typical watery diarrhea (more formed stool contains more artifact material).

• BOX 46.5 Modified Trichrome Permanent Stained Smear: Review

Principle

This technique is designed to allow examination and recognition of organism morphology under oil immersion examination (100× objective, for a total magnification of 1000×), primarily allowing recovery and identification of intestinal microsporidial spores. The internal morphology (horizontal or diagonal "stripes") may be seen in some spores under oil immersion.

Specimen

Any stool specimen that is fresh or preserved in formalin, sodium acetate–acetic acid–formalin (SAF), or the newer fixatives for the single-vial system (universal fixatives).

Reagents

Modified trichrome stain (using high dye–content chromotrope 2R) and associated solutions; dehydrating solutions (alcohols, xylenes, or xylene substitutes); mounting fluid (optional).

Examination

Oil immersion examination (1000×) of at least 300 fields; additional fields may be required if suspect organisms have been seen but are not clearly identified.

Results

Identification of microsporidial spores may be possible; however, their small size makes recognition difficult. Final laboratory results depend heavily on the appearance of the quality control (QC) slides and comparison with positive patient specimens.

Notes and Limitations

Because of the difficulty in getting dye to penetrate the microsporidial spore wall, this staining approach can be helpful. Procedure limitations are related to specimen handling (proper centrifugation speeds and time, use of no more than two layers of wet gauze for filtration, and complete understanding of the difficulties in recognizing microsporidial spores because of their small size [1–3 μm]).

Commercial Suppliers

Suppliers must be asked about specific fixatives and whether the fecal material can be stained with the modified trichrome stains and modified acid-fast stains. They should also be asked whether the fixatives prevent the use of any of the newer fecal immunoassay methods available for several of the intestinal amebae, flagellates, coccidia, and microsporidia.

---

trophozoites in fresh stool samples is rarely seen in these preparations. The organisms may be caught in mucus strands, and the movement of the flagella on the *Giardia* trophozoites may be the only subtle motility visible. *Strongyloides* larvae are usually very motile. It is important to keep the light intensity low for visualization of the moving parasites.

The duodenal fluid typically contains mucus, and the organisms tend to be located in the mucus threads. Therefore, centrifugation of the specimen before examination is important. Fluorescent antibody or immunoassay detection kits (*Cryptosporidium* or *Giardia*) can also be used with fresh or formalinized material. It is important to check the package insert of each kit to see which specimen types are acceptable.

If a presumptive diagnosis of giardiasis is reached as a result of a wet prep examination, the cover slip can be

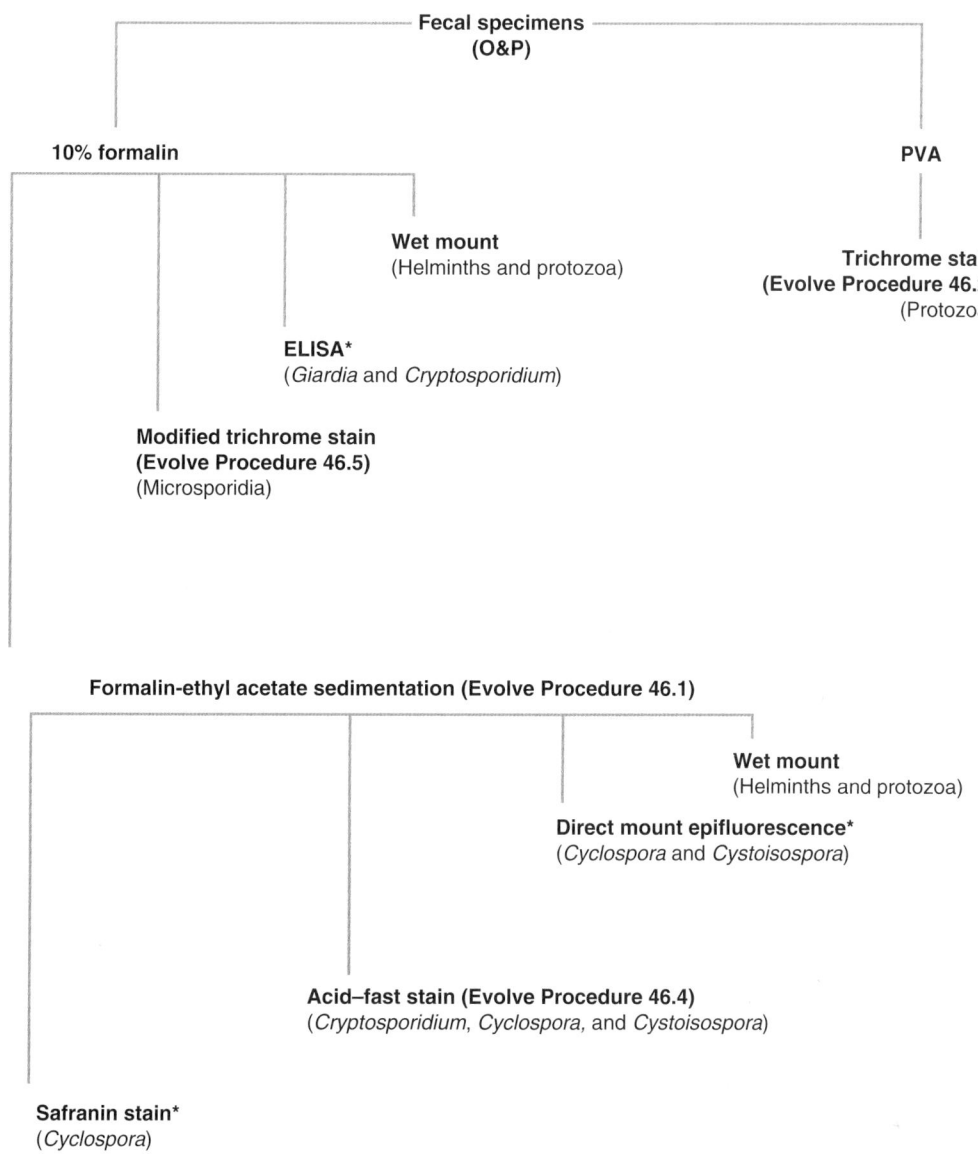

Fecal specimens (O&P)

10% formalin

PVA

Wet mount
(Helminths and protozoa)

Trichrome stain (Evolve Procedure 46.2)
(Protozoa)

ELISA*
(*Giardia* and *Cryptosporidium*)

Modified trichrome stain (Evolve Procedure 46.5)
(Microsporidia)

Formalin-ethyl acetate sedimentation (Evolve Procedure 46.1)

Wet mount
(Helminths and protozoa)

Direct mount epifluorescence*
(*Cyclospora* and *Cystoisospora*)

Acid–fast stain (Evolve Procedure 46.4)
(*Cryptosporidium*, *Cyclospora*, and *Cystoisospora*)

Safranin stain*
(*Cyclospora*)

• **Fig. 46.6** Processing of fecal specimens for ova and parasites (modified according to diagnostic guidelines established by the Centers for Disease Control and Prevention). *Indicates a special test procedure.

removed and the specimen fixed with Schaudinn's fluid, other fixatives containing polyvinyl alcohol (PVA), or a "universal fixative" (i.e., no formalin, mercury, or PVA) for subsequent staining with trichrome or iron-hematoxylin. If the amount of duodenal material submitted is very small, permanent stains can be prepared in lieu of using a portion of the specimen for a wet prep. This approach provides a permanent record; it may also improve the visualization of parasites using an oil-immersion examination of the stained specimen at 1000× compared with the examination of unstained organisms with minimal motility at a lower magnification.

Duodenal Capsule Technique (Entero-Test)

The duodenal capsule technique is a simple, convenient method for collecting duodenal contents, thus eliminating the need for intestinal intubation. The technique involves the use of a length of nylon cord coiled inside a gelatin capsule. The cord protrudes through one end of the capsule and is taped to the side of the patient's face. The capsule is swallowed. The gelatin dissolves in the stomach, and the weighted cord is carried by peristalsis into the duodenum. The cord is attached to the weight by a slipping mechanism; the weight is released and passes out in the stool when the cord is retrieved after 4 hours. The mucus collected on the cord is examined using the direct wet mount method for parasites, including *S. stercoralis, G. duodenalis, Cryptosporidium* spp., microsporidia, and the eggs of *Clonorchis sinensis*.

Urogenital Tract Specimens

T. vaginalis is typically identified by the examination of wet preparations of vaginal or urethral discharges, prostatic secretions, or urine sediment. Multiple specimens may be needed to detect the organisms. The specimens should be diluted with a drop of saline and examined for motile

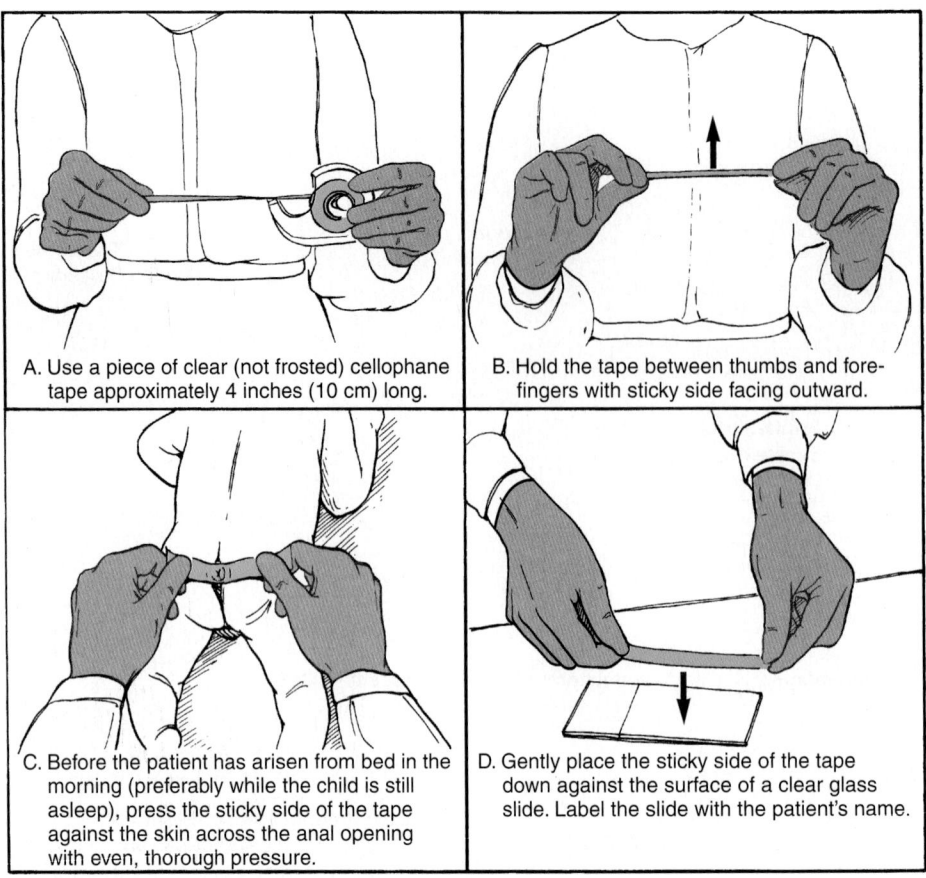

A. Use a piece of clear (not frosted) cellophane tape approximately 4 inches (10 cm) long.

B. Hold the tape between thumbs and fore-fingers with sticky side facing outward.

C. Before the patient has arisen from bed in the morning (preferably while the child is still asleep), press the sticky side of the tape against the skin across the anal opening with even, thorough pressure.

D. Gently place the sticky side of the tape down against the surface of a clear glass slide. Label the slide with the patient's name.

• **Fig. 46.7** Method of collecting a cellophane (Scotch) tape preparation for pinworm diagnosis. This method dispenses with the tongue depressor, requiring only tape and a glass microscope slide. The tape must be pressed deep into the anal folds.

organisms under low power (100×) with reduced illumination. As the jerky motility begins to diminish, the undulating membrane may often be observed under high dry power (400×). Unfortunately, the overall sensitivity of wet mount examinations is limited compared with culture and/ or molecular testing, such as polymerase chain reaction (PCR) analysis. Stained smears are usually not necessary for the identification of *T. vaginalis*. The number of false-positive and false-negative results reported from stained smears supports the value of confirmation by observation of motile organisms from the direct mount, culture media, or more sensitive direct antigen detection methods.

Sputum

Although not a common specimen, expectorated sputum may be submitted for parasitic examination. Organisms found in sputum that may cause pneumonia, pneumonitis, or Loeffler syndrome include the migrating larval stages of *A. lumbricoides*, *S. stercoralis*, and hookworm; the eggs of *Paragonimus* spp.; *Echinococcus granulosus* hooklets (Fig. 46.8); and the protozoa *Entamoeba histolytica*, *Entamoeba gingivalis*, *Trichomonas tenax*, *Cryptosporidium* spp., and possibly the microsporidia. Some of the smaller organisms must be differentiated from fungi such as

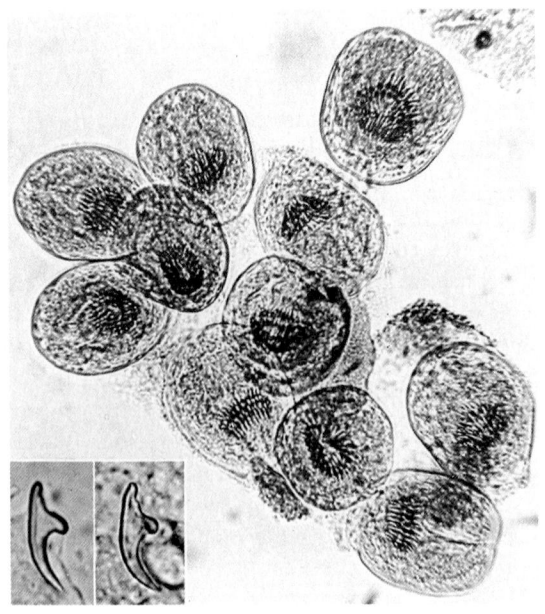

• **Fig. 46.8** *Echinococcus granulosus*, cyst. (Enlarged for detail, 500×).

Candida spp., *Pneumocystis jiroveci*, and *Histoplasma capsulatum*. In a *Paragonimus* infection, the sputum may be viscous, streaked with blood, and tinged with brownish flecks, which are clusters of eggs ("iron filings").

Induced sputa are collected after patients have used appropriate cleansing procedures to reduce oral contamination. The induction protocol is critical for the success of the procedure, and well-trained individuals such as respiratory therapists are needed to recover the organisms.

Aspirates

Examination of aspirated material for the diagnosis of parasitic infections may be extremely valuable, particularly when routine testing methods have failed to demonstrate the presence of the organisms. These specimens should be transported to the laboratory immediately after collection and processed as quickly as possible. Aspirates include liquid specimens collected from a variety of body sites. Aspirates most commonly processed in the parasitology laboratory include fine-needle aspirates and duodenal aspirates. Fluid specimens collected by bronchoscopy include bronchoalveolar lavages and bronchial washings.

Fine-needle aspirates may be submitted for slide preparation, culture, or both. Aspirates of cysts and abscesses for amebae may require concentration by centrifugation, digestion, microscopic examination for motile organisms in direct preparations, cultures, and microscopic evaluation of stained preparations. Aspiration of cyst material (usually liver or lung) for diagnosis of hydatid disease usually is performed when surgical techniques are used for cyst removal. The aspirated fluid is submitted to the laboratory and examined for hydatid sand (scolices) or hooklets; absence of this material does not rule out the possibility of hydatid disease because some cysts are sterile.

Bone marrow aspirates for *Leishmania* and *Trypanosoma cruzi* amastigotes or *Plasmodium* spp. require staining with any of the blood stains (Giemsa, Wright's, Wright-Giemsa combination, rapid stains, or Field's stain). Giemsa stain is the preferred stain for blood parasites because it provides better visibility of intracellular details for optimal morphology. Examination of specimens may confirm an infection previously missed by examination of routine blood films.

Cases of primary amoebic meningoencephalitis (PAM) are rare, but examination of spinal fluid may reveal the causative agent, *Naegleria fowleri,* one of the free-living amebae (Fig. 46.9). Although rare, this disease has a very high mortality rate. For this reason, a cerebrospinal fluid (CSF) sample with a request for examination for parasites is always considered a STAT procedure.

Biopsy Specimens

Biopsy specimens are recommended for diagnosis of tissue parasite infections. Impression smears, teased, and squash preparations of biopsy tissue from skin, muscle, cornea, intestine, liver, lung, and brain can be used for this purpose, in addition to standard histologic preparations. An impression smear is a collection of cells, microorganisms, or fluids produced by pressing the surface of the tissue specimen against a slide for review. Squash preparations are described

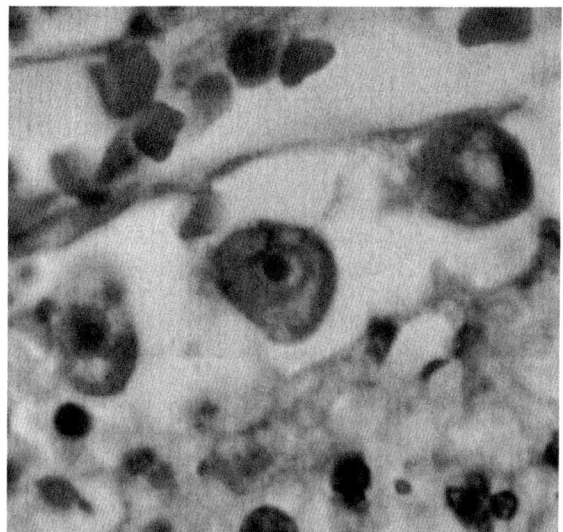

• **Fig. 46.9** *Naegleria fowleri* in brain tissue (hematoxylin and eosin stain).

in Chapter 6. Tissue for examination using permanent sections or electron microscopy should be fixed as specified by the processing laboratory. In certain cases, a biopsy may be the only means of confirming a suspected parasitic problem. Specimens examined as fresh material rather than as tissue sections should be kept moist in saline and submitted to the laboratory immediately.

Detection of parasites in tissue depends in part on specimen collection and adequate material to perform the recommended diagnostic procedures. Biopsy specimens are usually small and may not be representative of the diseased tissue. Multiple tissue samples often improve diagnostic results. To optimize the yield from any tissue specimen, all areas should be examined by as many procedures as possible. Tissues are collected using invasive procedures, many of which are very expensive and lengthy; consequently, these specimens deserve the most comprehensive procedures possible. A muscle biopsy for diagnosis of infection with *Trichinella* spp. can be processed as a routine histology slide or can be examined as a squash preparation (Fig. 46.10).

Tissue submitted in a sterile container on a sterile sponge dampened with saline may be used for cultures of protozoa after mounts for direct examination or impression smears for staining have been prepared. If cultures will be processed for parasites, sterile slides should be used for smear and mount preparation. Examination of tissue impression smears is detailed in Table 46.11.

Blood

Depending on the life cycle, a number of parasites may be recovered from blood specimens. Although organisms may be motile in fresh whole blood, species identification is typically accomplished from examination of permanently stained thick and thin blood films (Fig. 46.11). Blood films can be prepared from fresh, whole blood containing no anticoagulants, anticoagulated blood, or sediment from the various concentration procedures. The two most

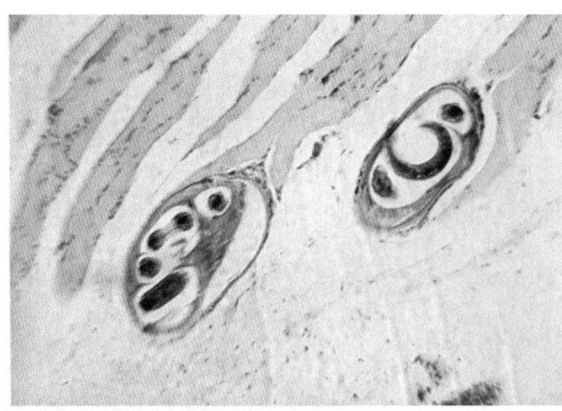

• **Fig. 46.10** *Trichinella* spp. larvae encysted in muscle.

commonly used hematology stains are Wright's and Giemsa stains. Many clinical laboratories use a commercial stain for hematology that is a combination of Wright's and Giemsa. The stain of choice is Giemsa stain because it provides optimal detail of intracellular malarial and other blood-borne parasites. However, blood parasites can also be seen on blood films stained using Wright's or other stains, including rapid staining options. Delafield's hematoxylin stain is often used to improve visibility of the microfilarial sheath. Multiple smears should be made as soon as the specimen is received in the laboratory, but initially only one should be stained and observed for parasites. The remaining slides can be stained with routine or specialized stains depending on what is observed on the first slide.

A request for examination of blood films for parasites is always a STAT request. Examination of any blood smear for parasitology should be performed by a highly experienced laboratory scientist.

Thin Blood Films

In any examination of thin blood films for parasitic organisms, the initial screening should be completed using the low-power microscope objective (10×).

Depending on the training and experience of the laboratory scientist, examination of a thin film for parasites usually takes 15 to 20 min (300 or more oil immersion fields at a magnification of 1000×). Some use a 50× or 60× oil-immersion objective to screen stained blood films; however, the chance is greater that small parasites (e.g., *Plasmodium* spp., *Babesia* spp., *Leishmania donovani*) will be missed at the lower total magnification (500× or 600×) compared with the 1000× total magnification achieved using the 100× oil-immersion objective.

Microfilarial organisms are rarely present in large numbers. Frequently only a few organisms are identified in each thin film preparation. Because microfilariae are carried with the smear during preparation and typically located at the edges or feathered end of the thin film, the entire film should be scanned to ensure that no microfilariae are missed. The feathered end of the film should be examined for intracellular and extracellular parasites. Because the cells

in the feathered end are spread further apart, the morphology and size of the infected red blood cells (RBCs) may be more clearly visible (Box 46.6).

Before a smear is reported as negative for the presence of parasites, a minimum of 300 fields should be examined. The request for blood film examination should be considered a STAT procedure, and all results (negative and positive) should be reported by telephone to the physician as soon as possible. If a result is positive, the appropriate government agencies (local, state, and federal) should be notified within a reasonable time, in accordance with guidelines and laws. It is important to note that one negative set of blood films is not sufficient to rule out blood parasites.

Both malaria and *Babesia* infections have been missed with automated differential instruments, delaying treatment. Although these instruments are not designed to detect intracellular blood parasites, the inability of the automated systems to distinguish between uninfected RBCs and those infected with parasites may pose diagnostic problems. Because automated systems may not be able to detect intracellular parasites, a manual differential should always be performed whenever a blood sample is submitted for parasitology.

Thick Blood Films

In the preparation of a thick blood film, the greatest concentration of blood cells is in the center of the film. The examination should be performed at low magnification to detect microfilariae. Examination of a thick film usually requires 5 to 10 min (approximately 100 oil-immersion fields). A search for malarial organisms and trypanosomes should be completed using oil immersion (total magnification of 1000×). Intact RBCs are commonly seen at the very periphery of the thick film; if infected, such cells may prove useful in the diagnosis of malaria (Box 46.7). However, a thin film preparation should always be used to confirm speciation of malarial and other blood parasite organisms.

Buffy Coat Films

L. donovani, trypanosomes, and *H. capsulatum* (a fungus with intracellular elements resembling those of *L. donovani*) may be detected in the peripheral blood. The parasite or fungus is detected in the neutrophils and large mononuclear cells found in the buffy coat (a layer of white blood cells seen just above the red cell layer after centrifugation of whole citrated blood). With *L. donovani*, the nuclear material stains dark red-purple, and the cytoplasm is light blue. In contrast, *H. capsulatum* is visible as a large dot of nuclear material (dark red-purple) surrounded by a clear halo. Trypanosomes and microfilariae may also concentrate with the buffy coat cells due to their size.

Direct Detection Methods

Significant progress has been made in the development and application of molecular methods for the diagnosis of parasitic infections, including the use of purified or

TABLE 46.11 Examination of Impression Smears

Tissue	Possible Parasite	Stain[a]
Lung	Microsporidia	Modified trichrome, acid-fast stain, Giemsa, tissue Gram stain, optical brightening agent (calcofluor), methenamine silver, electron microscopy (EM)
	Toxoplasma gondii	Giemsa, immune-specific reagent
	Cryptosporidium spp.	Modified acid-fast stain, immune-specific reagent
	Entamoeba histolytica	Giemsa, trichrome
Liver	*Toxoplasma gondii*	Giemsa
	Leishmania donovani	Giemsa
	Cryptosporidium spp.	Modified acid-fast stain, immune-specific reagent
	Entamoeba histolytica	Giemsa, trichrome
Brain	*Naegleria fowleri*	Giemsa, trichrome
	Acanthamoeba spp.	Giemsa, trichrome
	Balamuthia mandrillaris	Giemsa, trichrome
	Sappinia spp.	Giemsa, trichrome
	Entamoeba histolytica	Giemsa, trichrome
	Toxoplasma gondii	Giemsa, immune-specific reagent
	Microsporidia	Modified trichrome, acid-fast stain, Giemsa, tissue Gram stain, optical brightening agent (calcofluor), methenamine silver, EM
	Encephalitozoon spp.	Modified trichrome, acid-fast stain, Giemsa, optical brightening agent (calcofluor), methenamine silver, EM
Skin	*Leishmania* spp.	Giemsa
	Onchocerca volvulus	Giemsa
	Mansonella streptocerca	Giemsa
	Acanthamoeba spp.	Giemsa, trichrome
Nasopharynx, sinus cavities	Microsporidia	Modified trichrome, acid-fast stain, Giemsa, optical brightening agent (calcofluor), methenamine silver, EM
	Acanthamoeba spp.	Giemsa, trichrome
	Naegleria fowleri	Giemsa, trichrome
Intestine		
Small intestine	*Cryptosporidium parvum* (both small and large intestine)	Modified acid fast, immune-specific reagent
Jejunum	*Cyclospora cayetanensis*	Modified acid-fast
	Microsporidia *Enterocytozoon bieneusi* *Encephalitozoon intestinalis*	Modified trichrome, acid-fast stain, Giemsa, optical brightening agent (calcofluor), methenamine silver, EM
Duodenum	*Giardia duodenalis*	Giemsa, trichrome
Colon	*Entamoeba histolytica*	Giemsa, trichrome
Cornea, conjunctiva	Various genera of microsporidia *Acanthamoeba* spp.	Acid-fast stain, Giemsa, modified trichrome, methenamine silver, optical brightening agent (calcofluor), EM Giemsa, trichrome, calcofluor (cysts)
Muscle	*Trichinella spiralis*	Wet examination, squash preparation
	Microsporidia *Pleistophora* sp., *Anncaliia* sp., *Trachipleistophora* sp.	Modified trichrome, acid-fast stain, Giemsa, optical brightening agent (calcofluor), methenamine silver, EM

[a]Whenever Giemsa stain is mentioned in the table, any bloodstain is acceptable: Giemsa, Wright's, Wright-Giemsa combination, rapid blood stains.

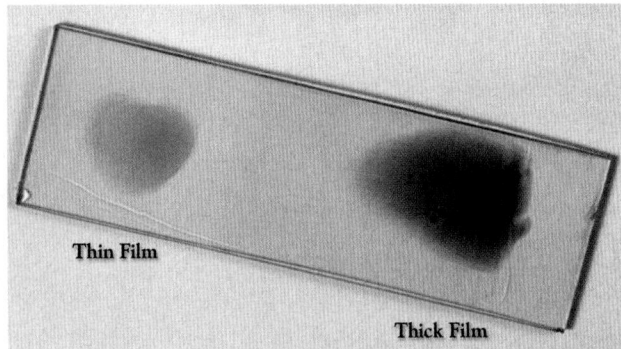

• **Fig. 46.11** Thin and thick blood smear for the identification of blood parasites. Most commonly used for identifying *Plasmodium* or *Trypanosoma* spp.

recombinant antigens and nucleic acid probes. The presence of parasite-specific antigen indicates current disease. Nucleic acid–based parasitic diagnostic tests are primarily available in specialized research or reference centers. PCR and other nucleic acid probe tests have been reported for almost all species of parasites. The demand for implementation of direct detection using molecular methods will continue to increase as the cost of these tests decreases and automation increases.

Intestinal Parasites

Immunoassays are generally simple and enable the simultaneous performance of many tests, thereby reducing overall costs. Antigen detection in stool specimens is often limited to the detection of one or two pathogens simultaneously. A routine O&P examination should also be performed to detect other parasitic pathogens. The current commercially available antigen tests (direct fluorescent antibody [DFA], enzyme immunoassay [EIA], indirect fluorescent antibody [IFA], and the cartridge formats) have excellent sensitivity and specificity compared with routine microscopy. Available antigen detection tests are listed in Table 46.12. The most common immunoassays are designed to confirm infection with *E. histolytica, G. duodenalis,* and *Cryptosporidium* spp.

Blood Parasites

Several new blood parasite antigen detection systems are available and have been effectively tested in field trials. Several quick screening tests are available for malaria using an immunochromogenic or antigen-capture EIA system (Table 46.12). Although these simple rapid methods are appropriate for population screening, a blood film from a positive patient must be examined to confirm the diagnosis and properly identify the species. Commercial PCR testing kits are currently available for *Plasmodium* spp. and *Wuchereria bancrofti.* Some of the rapid test kits for *Plasmodium* can detect all of the species that commonly infect humans but may not be able to differentiate the individual species. Other PCR kits are designed to specifically identify *P. falciparum.* Because PCR techniques

Principle

This technique is designed to allow examination and recognition of detailed organism morphology under oil-immersion examination (100× objective, for a total magnification of 1000×), primarily allowing recovery and identification of *Plasmodium* spp., *Babesia* spp., *Trypanosoma* spp., *Leishmania donovani,* and filarial blood parasites. The thin blood film is routinely used for specific parasite identification, although the number of organisms per field is significantly reduced compared with the thick blood film. The primary purpose is to allow malarial parasites to be visualized in the RBCs and to assess the size of infected RBCs compared with that of uninfected RBCs. RBC morphology is preserved using this method.

Specimen

Finger-stick blood, whole blood, or anticoagulated blood (ethylenediaminetetraacetic acid [EDTA] recommended). Multiple smears should be made within 1 h of collection, but initially only one smear should be stained. Additional smears can be stained if needed by different methods to enhance identification.

Reagents

Giemsa stain (films must be prefixed with absolute methanol before staining), Wright's stain (the stain contains the fixative), or Wright-Giemsa stains and their associated solutions; mounting fluid (optional).

Examination

Oil-immersion examination (1000×) of at least 300 fields; additional fields may be required if suspect organisms have been seen in the thick blood film. The slide may be screened using the newer 50× or 60× oil-immersion objectives, but the results should not be reported until the examination has been completed using the 100× oil-immersion lens. A blood film must be examined totally at a lower power to rule out the presence of microfilariae, which tend to be found near the edges of the smear.

Results

The thin blood film is routinely used for parasite identification to the species level (*Plasmodium* spp.). Both the thick and thin films should be examined before the final result is reported.

Notes and Limitations

The thin blood film is prepared exactly as one used for a differential count. A well-prepared film is thick at one end and thin at the other. The use of clean, grease-free slides is mandatory; long streamers of blood indicate that the slide used as a spreader was dirty or chipped. Streaks in the film usually are caused by dirt; holes in the film indicate grease on the slide. Although Giemsa stain is the stain of choice, blood parasites can be seen using other stains; however, the parasite morphology and color may not be consistent with that described for Giemsa-stained organisms. Giemsa stain does not stain the sheath of *Wuchereria bancrofti;* hematoxylin-based stains (e.g., Delafield's hematoxylin) are recommended for these organisms. The WBCs on the stained blood film serve as the quality control; if the WBC morphology and color are acceptable, then any parasites present will also appear normal and will be acceptable. Alternately, previously positive patient smears (if available) can be fixed with methanol and air dried, then stored in a sealed container at −70°C. These QC slides should be brought to room temperature before staining.

Thick Blood Films: Review

Principle

This technique is designed to allow examination and recognition of detailed organism morphology under oil-immersion examination (100× objective, for a total magnification of 1000×), primarily allowing recovery and identification of *Plasmodium* spp., *Babesia* spp., *Trypanosoma* spp., *Leishmania donovani,* and filarial blood parasites. The thick blood film is routinely used for detection of parasites, because the number of organisms per field is much greater than with the thin blood film. The primary purpose is to allow examination of a larger volume of blood than is seen with the thin blood film. RBC morphology is not preserved using this method.

Specimen

Finger-stick blood, whole blood, or anticoagulated blood (ethylenediaminetetraacetic acid [EDTA] recommended).

Reagents

Giemsa stain, Wright's stain, or Wright-Giemsa stains and their associated solutions; mounting fluid (optional).

Examination

Oil-immersion examination (1000×) of at least 300 fields; additional fields may be required if suspect organisms have been seen in the thin blood film. The slide may be screened using the newer 50× or 60× oil-immersion objectives, but the results should not be reported until the examination has been completed using the 100× oil-immersion lens. A blood film must be examined at a lower power to rule out the presence of microfilariae.

Results

The thick blood film is used to detect the presence of parasites; final identification may require examination of the thin blood film. Both should be examined before the final result is reported.

Notes and Limitations

The thick blood film is prepared by spreading a few drops of blood (using a circular motion) over an area approximately 2 cm in diameter. If whole blood is used, the examiner should continue stirring about 30 s to prevent the formation of fibrin strands. The use of clean, grease-free slides is mandatory. The film is allowed to air-dry at room temperature (heat is never applied to these films). Although Giemsa stain is the stain of choice, blood parasites can be seen using other stains; however, the parasite morphology and color may not be consistent with that described for Giemsa-stained organisms. Giemsa stain does not stain the sheath of *Wuchereria bancrofti*; hematoxylin-based stains (e.g., Delafield's hematoxylin) are recommended for these organisms. The WBCs on the stained blood film serve as the quality control; if the WBC morphology and color are acceptable, then any parasites present will also appear normal and will be acceptable. Alternately, previously positive patient smears (if available) can be held fixed with methanol and air-dried, then stored in a sealed container at −70°C. The QC slides should be brought to room temperature before staining.

can amplify the parasite's DNA, it can detect infection even when the number of parasites is low. It can also be used to confirm species identification when the morphology is unclear.

Cultivation

Parasite culture techniques are not routinely used to detect parasite infections in the United States. Any laboratory providing these types of cultures must maintain stock quality control (QC) cultures of specific organisms, often obtained from the American Type Culture Collection (ATCC). The relevant QC organisms are cultured simultaneously with the patient specimen, thus providing some assurance that the culture system functioned properly. The methods for *in vitro* culture are often complex, and QC is difficult and not feasible in the routine diagnostic laboratory. Some techniques may be available in certain institutions, particularly those in which research and consulting services are available. The cultivation of parasites is an essential technique for laboratories developing diagnostic testing methods, for epidemiologic analysis of outbreaks, for testing for drug resistance, or for the analysis of parasite life cycles.

Although *T. vaginalis* can be easily detected in vaginal or urethral secretions as well as urine sediment, accurate identification may require an experienced laboratory scientist. Several test kits are commercially available that allow quick culture confirmation of *Trichomonas* infection. OSOM *Trichomonas* and InPouch TV are two of the methods commonly used in physicians' offices or clinics. *Trichomonas* culture is very sensitive and specific, but it may take up to 7 days for growth. Physicians may request cultures when a patient is suspected to have a *Trichomonas* infection but is negative by microscopic examination. This is an example of an **axenic** culture method, in which the parasites are grown in pure culture without augmentation with bacteria.

Keratitis caused by *Acanthamoeba* may be confirmed by microscopic observation but also by culture of the parasite. Corneal scrapings or contact lenses are inoculated onto nutrient agar that has an overlay of *Escherichia coli* or *Enterobacter* spp., which serves as a food source for the ameba. The plate is observed for up to 7 days to detect the organism's growth on the agar surface. Identification of the organism is confirmed by microscopic morphology or PCR. This culture technique is called **monoxenic** because a single known bacterial species is used to help cultivate the organism. This same culture technique is used to recover and confirm granulomatous amebic encephalitis (GAE) caused by *Acanthamoeba* or PAM caused by another free-living amebic parasite, *N. fowleri*. In both cases, because of the critical nature of the infection, the organism identification must be confirmed by PCR or other antigen confirmation methods.

Larval-Stage Nematodes

The use of certain fecal culture methods (sometimes referred to as **coproculture**) is especially helpful for detecting light infections of hookworm, *S. stercoralis,* and *Trichostrongylus* spp. The rearing of infective-stage nematode larvae improves the diagnosis of hookworm and trichostrongyle infections, because the eggs of these species are identical and differentiation is based on larval morphology. These techniques are also useful for obtaining infective-stage larvae for research

TABLE 46.12 Example Antigen Detection Kits for Stool or Vaginal Discharge Specimens[a]

Organism/Kit Name	Manufacturer or Distributor[b]	Test Format/ Methodology
Cryptosporidium spp.		
PARA-TECT *Cryptosporidium* Antigen 96	Medical Chemical Corporation	EIA
ProSpecT Rapid (*Cryptosporidium*)	Remel	EIA
Xpect *Crypto*	Remel	RAPID
Cryptosporidium	TechLab	EIA
Crypto CELISA	Cellabs	EIA
Crypto CEL	Cellabs	IFA
Cryptosporidium spp. and *Giardia* sp.		
ColorPAC *Giardia/Cryptosporidium* RAPID	Becton Dickinson	RAPID
PARA-TECT *Cryptosporidium/Giardia*	Medical Chemical	DFA
Merifluor	Meridian Bioscience	DFA
ImmunoCard STAT *Cryptosporidium/Giardia*	Meridian Bioscience	RAPID
ProSpecT *Giardia/Cryptosporidium*	Remel	EIA
Xpect *Giardia/Cryptosporidium* RAPID	Remel	RAPID
Crypto/*Giardia* CEL	Cellabs	IFA
Cryptosporidium spp., *Giardia* sp., and *Entamoeba histolytica*		
Triage (fresh, frozen)	BioSite/Alere	RAPID
Entamoeba histolytica		
Entamoeba histolytica II	TechnLab	EIA
Entamoeba CELISA	Cellabs	EIA
E. histolytica	Wampole	EIA
Entamoeba histolytica/E. dispar		
ProSpecT	Remel	EIA
Giardia duodenalis		
Giardia CELISA	Cellabs	EIA
PARA-TECT *Giardia* Antigen 96	Medical Chemical Corporation	EIA
ProSpecT *Giardia*	Remel	EIA or RAPID
Giardia	Wampole	EIA
Giardia II	TechLab	EIA
Giardia EIA	Antibodies, Inc.	EIA
Giardia CEL	Cellabs	IFA
Simple-Read *Giardia*	Medical Chemical Corporation	Rapid
Trichomonas vaginalis		
Affirm VPIII	Becton Dickinson	Probe
T. vaginalis	Chemicon	DFA
OSOM *Trichomonas*	Sekisui Diagnostics	Rapid
Quik-Trich	PanBio	LA

DFA, Direct fluorescent antibody; *EIA,* enzyme immunoassay; *IFA,* indirect fluorescent antibody; *RAPID,* rapid immunochromatographic assay.
[a]The kits are available commercially in the United States for immunodetection of parasitic organisms or antigens in stool or vaginal discharge. This is a representative list; not every available kit is listed.

TABLE 46.12 **Example Antigen Detection Kits for Stool or Vaginal Discharge—cont'd**

bAntibodies, Inc., P O Box 1560, Davis, CA 95617-1560; Becton Dickinson, 1 Becton Dr., Franklin Lakes, NJ 07417; BioSite, 11030 Roselle St., San Diego, CA 92121; Cellabs, P O Box 421, Brookvale, NSW 2100, Australia; Chemicon, 28835 Single Oak Dr., Temecula, CA 92590; PanBio InDx, 1756 Sulfur Spring Rd., Baltimore, MD 21227; Genzyme Virotech, Gmbh, Lowenplatz 5, 66248, Russelheim, Germany; Medical Chemical Corporation, 19430 Van Ness Avenue, Torrance, CA 90501; Meridian Bioscience, Inc., 3471 River Hills Dr., Cincinnati, OH 45244; Novocastra, 30 Ingold Rd., Burlingame, CA 94010; Panbio Inc, 9075 Guilford Rd, Columbia, MD, 21046 Remel, 12076 Santa Fe Drive, Lenexa, KS 66215; Sekisui Diagnostics, LLC, One Wall Street, Burlington, MA 01803; TechLab, VPI Research Park, 1861 Pratt Dr., Blacksburg, VA 24060; Wampole Laboratories, P O Box 1001, Cranbury, NJ 08512;
Adapted from the Centers for Disease Control and Prevention. *Laboratory Identifications of Parasitic Diseases of public Health Concerns* (website). www.cdc.gov/dpdx/diagnosticprocedures/stool/antigendetection.html. https://www.cdc.gov/dpdx/diagnosticprocedures/other/vaginalswabs.html. Accessed June 29, 2019.

purposes. Diagnostic methods available include the **Harada-Mori** filter paper strip culture, the Petri dish/slant filter paper culture, the agar plate method, and the charcoal culture.

Blood Protozoa

Leishmaniasis is often diagnosed by observation of the non-motile **amastigote** stage of the parasite on blood smears, particularly as intracellular forms within monocytes and macrophages. The extracellular motile form, or **promastigote** stage found in tissue specimens, can also be cultured in specialized media (Novy-MacNeal-Nicolle [NNN] medium). This method is not part of a routine analysis in the clinical laboratory.

Recent breakthroughs have allowed scientists to cultivate the malarial parasites that infect humans and a number of other animal species. Although not used for diagnosis of malaria in the clinical laboratory, the ability to cultivate *Plasmodium* species has led to a number of significant developments, including a better understanding of the life cycle, development of analytical testing methods such as PCR, and research leading to the development of protective vaccines.

A unique cultivation method involves the use of intermediate hosts to isolate a parasitic organism from a human host. This technique is called **xenodiagnosis.** It was primarily used for the detection of chronic Chagas disease caused by *T. cruzi.* The insect vector Triatomid bug was allowed to take a blood meal from the patient and was examined for the presence of the trypanosomes in its gut. In addition to the detection of Chagas disease, other now archaic xenodiagnostic methods have been used to detect leishmaniasis and onchocerciasis.

Serodiagnosis

Serodiagnosis, or testing patient serum for the presence of antibodies, has been available for many years. However, serologic methods for the detection and identification of parasitic infections are not routinely offered by most clinical laboratories because of their high cost, difficulty of interpretation, low test volume, and limited sensitivity and specificity. Direct parasite detection and/or detection of parasite antigens are the methods of choice in all but a few situations. In parasitic infections where the organism reproduces in the host tissues, continuous antigenic stimulation of the host's immune system occurs as the infection progresses. In these cases, there is a positive correlation between clinical symptoms and serologic test results. Serodiagnosis

is recommended when the collection of a direct specimen may cause significant risk to the patient, as with echinococcosis or cysticercosis. Serodiagnosis is also recommended when the infection may be widespread, making specimen collection difficult, as with infections caused by *Toxoplasma* or *Toxocara* spp. Standard serologic techniques used in the laboratory for parasitic diagnostics include latex agglutination, enzyme-linked immunosorbent assay (ELISA)/EIA, IFA, and immunoblot techniques.

The Centers for Disease Control and Prevention (CDC) offers a number of serologic procedures for diagnostic purposes, some of which are not available elsewhere. Regulations for submitting specimens to the CDC may vary from state to state. Each laboratory should check with the appropriate county or state department of public health for specific instructions. Additional information on procedures and the interpretation of test results may be obtained directly from the CDC: http://www.cdc.gov/parasites/.

Prevention

The prevention of human parasitic infections is directly linked to understanding the life cycles of the various organisms and their modes of infection (Table 46.4). Preventive measures include avoiding direct exposure, as by improving personal hygiene, ensuring proper sanitation, and eliminating sexual activities that may involve fecal-oral contact. Adequate water treatment (including filtration) may be required, in addition to overall awareness of environmental sources of infection. In some cases, avoiding contaminated environmental water and soil sources may be important; for example, this is mandatory in dealing with systems of contact lens care, methods of sinus irrigation methods, potential infection with free-living amebae from municipal water supplies.

Chemoprophylactic agents to prevent clinical symptoms are given to individuals traveling to areas where malaria is endemic. These medications are effective against the erythrocytic forms but do not actually prevent infection with malaria; that is, the drugs do not prevent sporozoites from entering the host, traveling to the liver, and beginning the preerythrocytic developmental cycle. In general, chloroquine is the drug of choice, although different regimens may be used for chloroquine-resistant strains of malaria and for different species of malaria.

Vector control and awareness of transmission through blood transfusions, shared drug needles, congenital infections, and organ transplants are also important considerations in preventing human parasitic disease. Careful monitoring of the blood supply is required to prevent the transmission of parasites. This is particularly important in areas of the world where blood-borne parasites play a large role in human disease or in the case of blood donors who have recently traveled to endemic areas.

Adequate cooking of meat that may be infected is also important; cultural habits may influence the handling and eating of raw or poorly cooked foods. Prevention depends on a thorough understanding of the life cycle and epidemiology of all parasites that cause human disease. This information is critical to the prevention of human disease caused either by parasites limited to the human host or by parasites that can cause disease in humans and other animal hosts.

An example of a global initiative to eliminate parasitic infection can be seen in the management of Guinea worm disease, caused by the parasite *Dracunculus medinensis*. Individuals become infected with the worms by drinking contaminated water. In 1980, the CDC, World Health Organization (WHO), and other partners began a campaign to provide access to clean drinking water as well as identifying sources of potential infection. In 1986, there were 3.5 million cases of Guinea worm disease, primarily in Africa. Thanks to the efforts of the global Guinea Worm Eradication Program, only

25 human cases from Chad, Ethiopia, and South Sudan were reported worldwide in 2016. The ultimate goal is complete elimination of the parasite.

(WHO Collaborating Center for Research Training and Eradication of Dracunculiasis. Guinea Worm Wrap Up #245Cdc-pdf External, 2017, Centers for Disease Control and Prevention [CDC]: Atlanta, Georgia.)

Ectoparasites

Ectoparasites, member of the phylum Arthropoda, can affect human health in several ways. Arthropods can act as biologic vectors of disease, as when mosquitoes transmit malaria or when ticks transmit Lyme disease during a blood meal. They can also act as mechanical vectors—for example, when flies or cockroaches help transmit bacteria to food or water, causing enteric diseases. Mites and lice can act as biologic vectors of disease, but they can also cause disease directly by their presence (lice infestation) and the body's reaction to them (scabies). Although not true parasites, members of the Arthropoda can also affect humans through venomous bites (spiders) or stings (scorpions). Any arthropod that breaks the skin can also cause a secondary bacterial infection at the injury site (Table 46.13).

TABLE 46.13	Arthropods (Ectoparasites)		
Arthropods	**Organisms Transmitted**	**Other Impacts**	
Arachnida			
Ticks (Four pairs of legs; two pairs of mouth parts; no antennae; larval, nymph, and adult stages; separate sexes)	*Anaplasma* *Arboviruses* *Babesia* spp. *Borrelia burgdorferi* (Lyme disease) *Borrelia* sp. (relapsing fever) *Ehrlichia* spp. *Francisella* sp. *Rickettsia* spp. *Flavivirus* (tick-borne encephalitis)	Secondary bite wound infections Tick paralysis (toxin)	
Mites, infestation	St. Louis encephalitis western equine encephalitis *Rickettsia* sp.	Scabies (infestation) pruritus	
Spiders		Venom reaction to bite (e.g., brown recluse, black widow)	
Scorpions		Venom reaction to sting (e.g., bark scorpion)	
Insecta			
Fleas (three pairs of legs; rear legs much larger)	*Dipylidium caninum* *Hymenolepis nana* *Hymenolepis diminuta* *Yersinia pestis* *Rickettsia typhi* (murine typhus) *Francisella* sp.	Pruritus, site of bite	
Flies 1–2 pairs of wings; separate head, thorax, and abdomen)	*Trypanosoma rhodesiense* *Trypanosoma gambiense* *Leishmania* spp. *Onchocerca volvulus* *Loa loa* *Bartonella* (Oroya fever)	Mechanical transfer of disease; poor sanitation (dysentery, cholera)	

TABLE 46.13	Arthropods (Ectoparasites)—cont'd		
Arthropods	**Organisms Transmitted**	**Other Impacts**
Bugs (three pairs of legs; some have wings)	*Trypanosoma cruzi* (Triatomids including bed bugs)	Bite wound reactions; pruritus Mechanical transfer of disease; poor sanitation (dysentery, cholera, e.g., cockroaches)
Lice (wingless; three segments)	*Borrelia* (relapsing fever) *Bartonella* (trench fever) *Rickettsia prowazeki* (typhus)	Pruritus reaction to infestation; waste products
Mosquitoes (three pairs of legs, three segments; long abdomen; 3000+ species)	*Plasmodium* spp. *Wuchereria bancrofti* *Brugia malayi* Arboviruses *Flaviviruses* (dengue, yellow fever) *Togaviruses* (encephalitis)	Bite reaction—pruritus

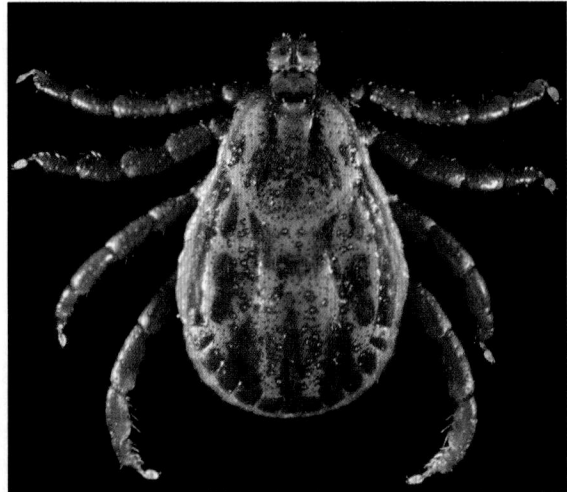

• **Fig. 46.12** Dorsal view of a male Rocky Mountain wood tick, *Dermacentor andersoni*. This tick species is a known North American vector of *Rickettsia rickettsii*, which is the etiologic agent of Rocky Mountain spotted fever (RMSF). (Courtesy the Division of Parasitic Diseases/Centers for Disease Control and Prevention.)

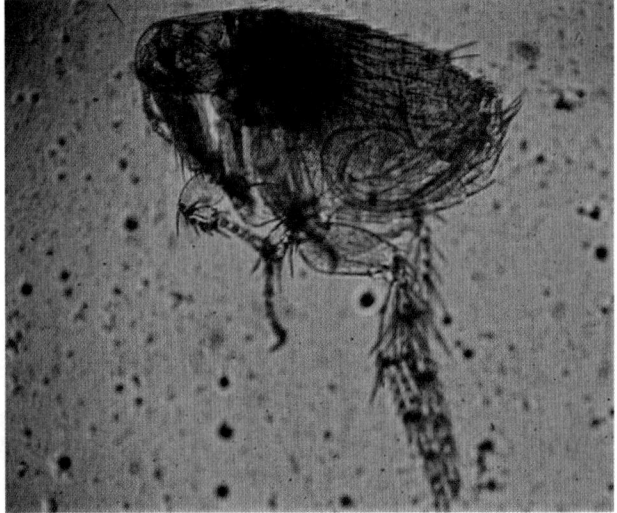

• **Fig. 46.13** *Xenopsylla cheopis,* the Oriental rat flea, the primary vector of bubonic plague and murine typhus. (400×)

Ectoparasites can be directly observed without a microscope, but it is better to place them in 70% to 95% ethanol to maintain their morphology and color and examine them using a stereomicroscope or low power on a light microscope. Permanent fixation can be obtained using Permount (Fisher Scientific, Pittsburgh, PA). Arthropods have four characteristics: a chitinized exoskeleton, pairs of jointed legs or appendages, bilateral symmetry, and a hemocele. Members of the Arachnida (ticks, mites, spiders, and scorpions) have four pairs of appendages (legs) (Fig. 46.12), whereas members of the Insecta (flies, lice, fleas, bugs, and mosquitoes) have three pairs of appendages (legs and wings) (Figs. 46.13 and 46.14). Identification is based on recognizing the morphologic characteristics of the arthropod and carefully describing the head, thorax, and abdomen as well as noting the number of legs or other appendages and the presence of antennae.

Ⓔ Visit the Evolve site for a complete list of procedures, review questions, and case studies.

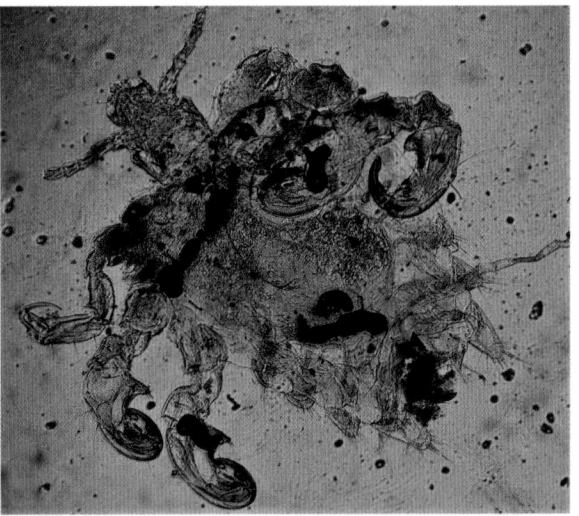

• **Fig. 46.14** *Pediculus* sp., louse that infests humans and transmits a variety of diseases including endemic typhus, trench fever, and relapsing fever.

47

Intestinal Protozoa

OBJECTIVES

1. Describe the basic life cycle, distinguishing morphologic characteristics, clinical disease (if pathogenic), laboratory diagnosis, and prevention for the organisms discussed in this chapter.
2. Define and identify the following parasitic structures: trophozoite, cyst, oocyst, spore, pseudopodia, flagella, cilia, chromatoidal bars, karyosome, central vacuole, cyst form, axoneme, cytostome, spiral groove, undulating membrane, ventral disc, shepherd's crook, axostyle, macronucleus, micronucleus, apical complex, sporocyst, sporozoite, spore, sarcocyst, and polar tubule.
3. Define life cycle processes, including merogony, gametogony, sporogony, schizogony, and the associated organism(s) and stages.
4. Correlate the parasitic life cycles with the specific diagnostic stages for the organisms listed.
5. Distinguish pathogenic from nonpathogenic protozoa.

PARASITES TO BE CONSIDERED

Protozoa

Amoebae (intestinal)
  Entamoeba bangladeshi
  Entamoeba histolytica
  *Entamoeba dispar**
  Entamoeba coli
  Entamoeba gingivalis
  Entamoeba hartmanni
  Entamoeba moshkovskii
  Entamoeba polecki
  Endolimax nana
  Iodamoeba bütschlii (buetschlii)
  Blastocystis spp.
Flagellates (intestinal)
  Giardia duodenalis
  Chilomastix mesnili
  Pentatrichomonas hominis
  Retortamonas hominis
Amoeba flagellate
  Dientamoeba fragilis
Ciliates (intestinal)
  Neoblantidium coli

*E*ntamoeba histolytica is considered a true pathogen, and *Entamoeba dispar* is used to designate nonpathogens. Additional morphologically identical species, *Entamoeba moshkovskii* and *Entamoeba bangladeshi*, have

been identified which are associated with noninvasive diarrhea. Although it was previously reported that 16% of identified *E. dispar* trophozoites contain ingested red blood cells, nucleic acid–based methods have been used to resolve this morphological discrepancy. All trophozoites containing red blood cells can be distinctly identified as *E. histolytica* using nucleic acid–based methods. Immunoassay kits and molecular assays are available for identifying the *E. histolytica/E. dispar* group and for differentiating *E. histolytica, E. dispar,* and *E. moshkovskii. E. bangladeshi* is a species that is indistinguishable from *E. histolytica* both physically and pathologically; little more is known regarding this species.

The protozoa are unicellular eukaryotic organisms, most of which are microscopic. They have a number of specialized organelles that are responsible for life functions and that allow further division of the group into classes. Most protozoa multiply by binary fission and are ubiquitous worldwide.

The important characteristics of the intestinal protozoa are presented in Tables 47.1–47.7. The clinically relevant intestinal protozoa are generally considered to be *Entamoeba histolytica, Entamoeba moshkovskii, Blastocystis hominis, Giardia duodenalis, Dientamoeba fragilis, Neobalantidium coli, Cystoisospora belli, Cryptosporidium* spp., *Cyclospora cayetanensis,* and the microsporidia. Nonpathogenic intestinal protozoa are listed in various figures and tables but are not discussed in detail.

Amoebae

The class Sarcodina, or Amoebae, includes the organisms capable of movement by means of cytoplasmic protrusions called **pseudopodia.** This group includes free-living organisms, in addition to nonpathogenic and pathogenic organisms found in the intestinal tract and other areas of the body (Tables 47.1 and 47.2). Occasionally, when fresh stool material is examined as a direct wet mount, motile trophozoites may be seen, as well as other, nonparasitic structures (Fig. 47.1).

Entamoeba histolytica
General Characteristics

Living **trophozoites** (motile feeding stage) of *E. histolytica* vary in size from about 12 to 60 μm in diameter. Organisms recovered from diarrheic or dysenteric stools generally are larger than those in formed stool from an asymptomatic individual. The motility has been described as rapid

TABLE 47.1 Intestinal Protozoa: Trophozoites of Common Amoebae

Characteristic	Entamoeba histolytica	Entamoeba dispar/moshkovskii/bangladeshi	Entamoeba hartmanni	Entamoeba coli	Endolimax nana	Iodamoeba bütschlii
Size[a] (diameter or length)	12–60 μm (usual range, 15–20 μm); invasive forms may be >20 μm	Same size range as E. histolytica	5–12 μm (usual range, 8–10 μm)	15–50 μm (usual range, 20–25 μm)	6–12 μm (usual range, 8–10 μm)	8–20 μm (usual range, 12–15 μm)
Motility	Progressive, with hyaline, fingerlike pseudopodia; motility may be rapid	Same motility as E. histolytica	Usually nonprogressive	Sluggish, nondirectional; blunt, granular pseudopodia	Sluggish, usually nonprogressive	Sluggish, usually nonprogressive
Nucleus (single) and visibility	Difficult to see in unstained preparations	Difficult to see in unstained preparations	Usually not seen in unstained preparations	Often visible in unstained preparation	Occasionally visible in unstained preparations	Usually not visible in unstained preparations
Peripheral chromatin (stained)	Fine granules, uniform in size and usually evenly distributed; may have beaded appearance.	Fine granules, uniform in size and usually evenly distributed; may have beaded appearance.	Nucleus may stain more darkly than in E. histolytica, although morphology is similar; chromatin may appear as solid ring rather than beaded (trichrome).	May be clumped and unevenly arranged on the membrane; may also appear as solid, dark ring with no beads or clumps.	Usually no peripheral chromatin; nuclear chromatin may be quite variable.	Usually no peripheral chromatin.
Karyosome (stained)	Small, usually compact; centrally located but may also be eccentric	Small, usually compact; centrally located but may also be eccentric	Usually small and compact; may be centrally located or eccentric	Large, not compact; may or may not be eccentric; may be diffuse and darkly stained	Large, irregularly shaped; may appear blotlike; many nuclear variations are common; may mimic E. hartmanni or Dientamoeba fragilis	Large, may be surrounded by refractile granules that are difficult to see ("basket nucleus")
Cytoplasm appearance (stained)	Finely granular, "ground glass" appearance; clear differentiation of ectoplasm and endoplasm; if present, vacuoles are usually small.	Finely granular, "ground glass" appearance; clear differentiation of ectoplasm and endoplasm; if present, vacuoles are usually small.	Finely granular.	Granular, with little differentiation into ectoplasm and endoplasm; usually vacuolated.	Granular, vacuolated.	Granular, may be heavily vacuolated.
Inclusions (stained)	Noninvasive organism may contain bacteria or red blood cells.	Organisms usually contain bacteria; in cytoplasm.	May contain bacteria; no RBCs.	Bacteria, yeast, other debris.	Bacteria.	Bacteria.

[a]These sizes refer to wet preparation measurements. Organisms on a permanent stained smear may be 1 to 1.5 μm smaller as a result of artificial shrinkage.
RBC, Red blood cell.

TABLE 47.2 Intestinal Protozoa—Cysts of Common Amoebae

Characteristic	Entamoeba histolytica/dispar/moshkovskii/bangladeshi	Entamoeba hartmanni	Entamoeba coli	Endolimax nana	Iodamoeba bütschlii
Size[a] (diameter or length)	10–20 μm (usual range, 12–15 μm)	5–10 μm (usual range, 6–8 μm)	10–35 μm (usual range, 15–25 μm)	5–10 μm (usual range, 6–8 μm)	5–20 μm (usual range, 10–12 μm)
Shape	Usually spherical	Usually spherical	Usually spherical; may be oval, triangular, or other shapes; may be distorted on permanent stained slide because of inadequate fixative penetration	Usually oval, may be round	May vary from oval to round; cyst may collapse because of large glycogen vacuole space
Nucleus (number and visibility)	Mature cyst: 4 nuclei; Immature cyst: 1–2 nuclei; nuclear characteristics difficult to see on wet preparation	Mature cyst: 4 nuclei; Immature cyst: 1–2 nuclei (2-nucleated cysts very common)	Mature cyst: 8 (occasionally 16 or more nuclei may be seen). Immature cysts with 2 or more nuclei are occasionally seen	Mature cyst: 4 Immature cysts: 2 very rarely seen and may resemble cysts of Enteromonas hominis	Mature cyst: 1
Peripheral chromatin (stained)	Peripheral chromatin present; fine, uniform granules, evenly distributed; nuclear characteristics may not be as clearly visible as in trophozoite.	Fine granules evenly distributed on the membrane; nuclear characteristics may be difficult to see.	Coarsely granular; may be clumped and unevenly arranged on membrane; nuclear characteristics not as clearly defined as in trophozoite; may resemble E. histolytica.	No peripheral chromatin.	No peripheral chromatin.
Karyosome (stained)	Small, compact, usually centrally located but occasionally may be eccentric	Small, compact, usually centrally located	Large, may or may not be compact and/or eccentric; occasionally may be centrally located	Smaller than karyosome seen in trophozoites but generally larger than those of genus Entamoeba	Larger, usually eccentric refractile granules may be on one side of karyosome ("basket nucleus")
Cytoplasm, chromatoidal bodies (stained)	May be present; bodies usually elongate, with blunt, rounded, smooth edges; may be round or oval	Usually present; bodies usually elongate with blunt, rounded, smooth edges; may be round or oval	May be present (less frequently than in E. histolytica); splinter shaped with rough, pointed ends	Rare chromatoidal bodies present; occasionally small granules or inclusions seen; fine linear chromatoidals may be faintly visible on well-stained smears	No chromatoidal bodies present; occasionally small granules may be present
Glycogen (stained with iodine)	May be diffuse or absent in mature cyst; clumped chromatin mass may be present in early cysts (stains reddish brown with iodine)	May or may not be present, as in E. histolytica	May be diffuse or absent in mature cyst; clumped mass occasionally seen in mature cysts (stains reddish brown with iodine)	Usually diffuse if present (stains reddish brown with iodine)	Large, compact, well-defined mass (stains reddish brown with iodine)

[a]Wet preparation measurements; in permanent stains, organisms usually are 1–2 μm smaller.

TABLE 47.3 Intestinal Protozoa—Trophozoites of Flagellates

Protozoa	Shape and Size	Motility	Number of Nuclei and Visibility	Number of Flagella (Usually Difficult to See)	Other Features
Dientamoeba fragilis	Shaped like amebae; 5–15 μm (usual range, 9–12 μm)	Usually nonprogressive; pseudopodia are angular, serrated, or broad lobed and almost transparent.	Percentage may vary, but 40% of organisms have 1 nucleus and 60% have 2 nuclei; not visible in unstained preparations; no peripheral chromatin; karyosome is composed of a cluster of 4–8 granules.	Internal flagella; not visible	Cytoplasm is finely granular and may be vacuolated with ingested bacteria, yeasts, and other debris; may be great variation in size and shape on a single smear.
Giardia duodenalis	Pear-shaped; length 10–20 μm; width, 5–15 μm	"Falling leaf" motility may be difficult to see if organism is in mucus; slight flutter of flagella may be visible using low light (duodenal aspirate or mucus from Entero-Test capsule).	2; not visible in unstained mounts.	4 lateral; 2 ventral, 2 caudal	Sucking disk occupies one half to three fourths of ventral surface; pear-shaped front view, spoon-shaped side view.
Chilomastix mesnili	Pear-shaped; length 6–24 μm (usual range, 10–15 μm); width, 4–8 μm	Stiff, rotary.	1; not visible in unstained mounts.	3 anterior, 1 in cytostome	Prominent cytostome extending one-third to one-half the length of the body; spiral groove across ventral surface.
Pentatrichomonas hominis	Pear-shaped; length 5–15 μm (usual range, 7–9 μm); width 7–10 μm	Jerky, rapid.	1; not visible in unstained mounts.	3–5 anterior, 1 posterior	Undulating membrane extends the length of the body; posterior flagellum extends free beyond end of body.
Trichomonas tenax	Pear-shaped; length 5–12 μm; average of 6.5–7.5 μm; width, 7–9 μm	Jerky, rapid.	1; not visible in unstained mounts.	4 anterior, 1 posterior	Seen only in preparations from mouth; axostyle (slender rod) protrudes beyond the posterior end and may be visible; posterior flagellum extends only halfway down the body; no free end.
Enteromonas hominis	Oval; 4–10 μm (usual range, 8–9 μm); width, 5–6 μm	Jerky.	1; not visible in unstained mounts.	3 anterior, 1 posterior	One side of the body is flattened; posterior flagellum extends free posteriorly or laterally.
Retortamonas intestinalis	Pear-shaped or oval; 4–9 μm (usual range, 6–7 μm); width, 3–4 μm	Jerky.	1; not visible in unstained mount.	1 anterior, 1 posterior	Prominent cytostome extends approximately one half the length of the body.

TABLE
47.4 **Intestinal Protozoa—Cysts of Flagellates**

Protozoa	Size	Shape	Number of Nuclei	Other Features
Dientamoeba fragilis	5–8 um	Oval to round	1–2	Distinct cyst wall with inner irregular cyst wall. Clear space apparent between outer and inner cyst wall.
Pentatrichomonas hominis, Trichomonas tenax	No cyst stage			
Giardia duodenalis	8–19 μm (usual range, 11–14 μm); width, 7–10 μm	Oval, ellipsoidal, or may appear round	4; not distinct in unstained preparations; usually located at one end	Longitudinal fibers in cysts may be visible in unstained preparations; deep-staining median bodies usually lie across the longitudinal fibers. Shrinkage is common, with the cytoplasm pulling away from the cyst wall; "halo" effect may be seen around the outside of the cyst wall because of shrinkage caused by dehydrating reagents.
Chilomastix mesnili	6–10 μm (usual range, 7–9 μm); width, 4–6 μm	Lemon or pear-shaped with anterior hyaline knob	1; not distinct in unstained preparations	Cytostome with supporting fibrils, usually visible in stained preparation; curved fibril alongside of cytostome, usually referred to as a "shepherd's crook."
Enteromonas hominis	4–10 μm (usual range, 6–8 μm); width, 4–6 μm	Elongate or oval	1–4; usually 2 lying at opposite ends of cyst; not visible in unstained mounts	Resembles *Endolimax nana* cyst; fibrils or flagella usually not seen.
Retortamonas intestinalis	4–9 μm (usual range, 4–7 μm); width, 5 μm	Pear-shaped or slightly lemon-shaped	1; not visible in unstained mounts	Resembles *Chilomastix* cyst; shadow outline of cytostome with supporting fibrils extends above nucleus; "bird beak" fibril arrangement.

TABLE
47.5 **Intestinal Protozoa—Ciliates**

Protozoa	Shape and Size	Motility	Number of Nuclei	Other Features
Neobalantidium coli trophozoite	Ovoid with tapering anterior end; 50–100 μm long, 40–70 μm wide (usual range, 40–50 μm)	Ciliates: rotary, boring; may be rapid	1 large kidney-shaped macronucleus; 1 small round micronucleus, which is difficult to see even in stained smear; macronucleus may be visible in unstained preparation.	Body covered with cilia, which tend to be longer near cytostome; cytoplasm may be vacuolated.
Cyst	Spherical or oval; 50–70 μm (usual range, 50–55 μm)		1 large macronucleus visible in unstained preparation; micronucleus difficult to see.	Macronucleus and contractile vacuole are visible in young cysts; in older cysts, internal structure appears granular; cilia difficult to see in cyst wall.

TABLE 47.6   Morphologic Criteria Used to Identify Intestinal Protozoa (Coccidia, *Blastocystis* spp.)

Protozoa	Shape and Size	Other Features
Cryptosporidium spp. *Cryptosporidium parvum* (humans and animals) *Cryptosporidium hominis* (humans)	Oocyst generally round, 4–6 μm; each mature oocyst contains four sporozoites.	Oocyst, diagnostic stage in stool, sporozoites occasionally visible within oocyst wall; acid-fast positive using modified acid-fast stains; various other stages in life cycle can be seen in biopsy specimens taken from gastrointestinal tract (brush border of epithelial cells) and other tissues; disseminated infection well documented in compromised host; oocysts immediately infective (in both formed and/or watery specimens); nosocomial infections documented; use enteric precautions for inpatients.
Cyclospora cayetanensis	Oocyst generally round, 8–10 μm; oocysts are not mature, no visible internal structure; oocysts may appear wrinkled.	Oocyst, diagnostic stage in stool; acid-fast variable using modified acid-fast stains; color range from clear to deep purple (tremendous variation); best results obtained with decolorizing solution consisting of 1% acid, 3% maximum; oocysts may appear wrinkled (like crumpled cellophane); mimic *Cryptosporidium* oocysts but are twice as large.
Cystoisospora belli	Ellipsoidal oocyst; range 20–30 μm long, 10–19 μm wide; sporocysts rarely seen broken out of oocysts but measure 9–11μm.	Mature oocyst contains two sporocysts with four sporozoites each; usual diagnostic stage in feces is immature oocyst containing spherical mass of protoplasm (intestinal tract). Oocysts are modified acid-fast positive. Whole oocyst may stain pink, but just the internal sporocysts stain if the oocyst is mature.
Sarcocystis hominis *Sarcocystis suihominis*	Oocyst thin-walled and contains two mature sporocysts, each containing four sporozoites; commonly thin oocyst wall ruptures; ovoid sporocysts each measure 10–16 μm long and 7.5–12 μm wide.	Thin-walled oocyst or ovoid sporocysts occur in stool (intestinal tract).
Blastocystis spp.	Organisms are generally round, measure approximately 6–40 μm, and are usually characterized by a large, central body (looks like a large vacuole); this stage has been called the *central body form*.	The more amebic form can be seen in diarrheal fluid but is difficult to identify. The central body forms vary tremendously in size, even on a single fecal smear; this is the most common form seen. Routine fecal examinations may indicate a positive rate much higher than other protozoa; some laboratories report figures of 20% and higher.

and unidirectional. Although this characteristic motility is described, **amebiasis** rarely is diagnosed based on motility seen in a direct wet mount. The cytoplasm is differentiated into a clear outer ectoplasm and a more granular inner endoplasm.

E. histolytica has directional and progressive motility, whereas the other amebae tend to move more slowly and at random. Motility is rarely seen even in a fresh direct wet mount from a patient with diarrhea or dysentery. The cytoplasm is generally more finely granular, and the presence of red blood cells (RBCs) in the cytoplasm is considered diagnostic for *E. histolytica* (Fig. 47.2); however, most patient samples do not demonstrate trophozoites with ingested red blood cells.

Permanent stained smears demonstrate accurate morphology compared with other techniques.

When the organism is examined on a permanent stained smear (trichrome or iron-hematoxylin stain), the morphologic characteristics of *E. histolytica*, *E. dispar*,

E. moshkovskii, and *E. bangladeshi* are readily seen. The nucleus is characterized by evenly arranged chromatin on the nuclear membrane and a small, compact, centrally located **karyosome** (condensed chromatin). As mentioned, the cytoplasm usually is described as finely granular, with few ingested bacteria and scant debris in vacuoles. In organisms isolated from a patient with dysentery, RBCs may be visible in the cytoplasm (Fig. 47.3), and such organisms should be identified as *E. histolytica*. Most often, infection with *E. histolytica/dispar* group is diagnosed on the basis of the organism's morphology, without the presence of RBCs. Newer techniques, including nucleic acid–based testing, are now available that provide a more specific identification and differentiation of *Entamoeba* spp. and are discussed later in this chapter.

As part of the life cycle, the trophozoites may condense into a round mass (**precyst**), and a thin wall is secreted around the immature cyst (Fig. 47.4). Two types of inclusions may be found in this immature cyst: a **glycogen mass**

TABLE 47.7 Microsporidia That Cause Human Infection

Microsporidia	Immunocompromised Patient	Immunocompetent Patient	Comments
Common			
Enterocytozoon bieneusi	Chronic diarrhea; wasting syndrome, cholangitis, acalculous cholecystitis, chronic sinusitis, chronic cough, pneumonitis; cause of diarrhea in organ transplant recipients	Self-limiting diarrhea in adults and children; traveler's diarrhea; asymptomatic carriers.	Short-term culture only; three strains identified but not named; AIDS patients with chronic diarrhea (present in 5%–30% of patients when CD4 lymphocyte counts are very low); pigs, nonhuman primates
Encephalitozoon hellem	Disseminated infection; keratoconjunctivitis; sinusitis, bronchitis, pneumonia, nephritis, uretertitis, cystitis, prostatitis, urethritis	Possibly diarrhea.	Cultured *in vitro*; detected in people with traveler's diarrhea and coinfection with *E. bieneusi*; pathogenicity unclear; spores not reported yet from stool; psittacine birds
Encephalitozoon intestinalis	Chronic diarrhea, cholangiopathy; sinusitis, bronchitis, pneumonitis; nephritis, bone infection, nodular cutaneous lesions	Self-limiting diarrhea; asymptomatic carriers.	Cultured *in vitro*; formerly *Septata intestinalis*; AIDS patients with chronic diarrhea; dogs, donkeys, pigs, cows, goats
Encephalitozoon cuniculi	Disseminated infection; keratoconjunctivitis, sinusitis, bronchitis, pneumonia; nephritis; hepatitis, peritonitis, symptomatic and asymptomatic intestinal infection; encephalitis	Not described; two HIV–serologically negative children with seizure disorder (suspect *E. cuniculi* infection) presumably were immunocompromised.	Cultured *in vitro*; wide mammalian host range
Uncommon			
Pleistophora sp.	Myositis (skeletal muscle)	Not described.	Tend to infect fish
Pleistophora ronneafiei	Myositis	Not described.	
Trachipleistophora hominis	Myositis; myocarditis keratoconjunctivitis; sinusitis	Keratitis.	Cultured *in vitro*; AIDS patients
Trachipleistophora anthropophthera	Disseminated infection; keratitis	Not described.	AIDS patients
Anncalia connori	Disseminated infection	Not described.	Formerly *Nosema connori*; often infects insects; disseminated in infant with SCID
Anncalia vesicularum	Myositis	Not described.	Formerly *Brachiola vesicularum*
Anncalia algerae	Myositis; nodular cutaneous lesions	Keratitis.	Formerly *Nosema algerae* or *Brachiola algerae*; cultured *in vitro*; skin nodules in boy with acute lymphocytic leukemia; found in arthropods
Nosema ocularum	Not described	Keratitis.	HIV–serologically negative individual
Vittaforma corneae	Disseminated infection; urinary tract infection	Keratitis.	Formerly *Nosema corneum*; cultured *in vitro*; non-HIV patient
Microsporidium ceylonensis[a]	Not described	Corneal ulcer, keratitis.	HIV–serologically negative individual, autopsy
Microsporidium africanum[a]	Not described	Corneal ulcer, keratitis.	HIV–serologically negative individual, autopsy
Microsporidia (not classified)		Keratoconjunctivitis in a contact lens wearer.	

[a]*Microsporidium* is a collective generic name for microsporidia that cannot be classified. *AIDS,* Acquired immunodeficiency syndrome; *HIV,* human immunodeficiency virus; *SCID,* severe combined immunodeficiency.

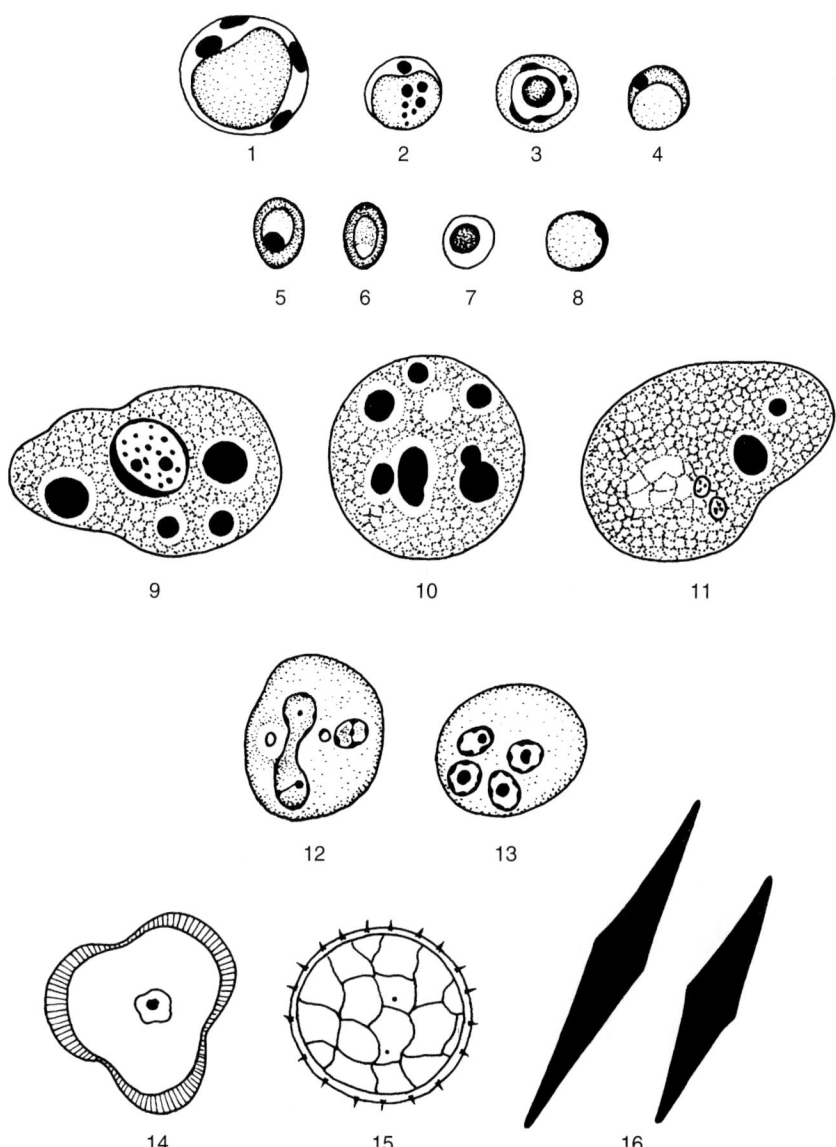

• Fig. 47.1 Various structures that may be seen in stool preparations. (1, 2, and 4) *Blastocystis* spp. (3 and 5–8) Various yeast cells. (9) Macrophage with nucleus. (10 and 11) Deteriorated macrophage without nucleus. (12 and 13) Polymorphonuclear leukocytes. (14 and 15) Pollen grains. (16) Charcot-Leyden crystals. (Modified from Markell EK, Voge M. *Medical Parasitology*. 5th ed. Philadelphia: WB Saunders; 1981.)

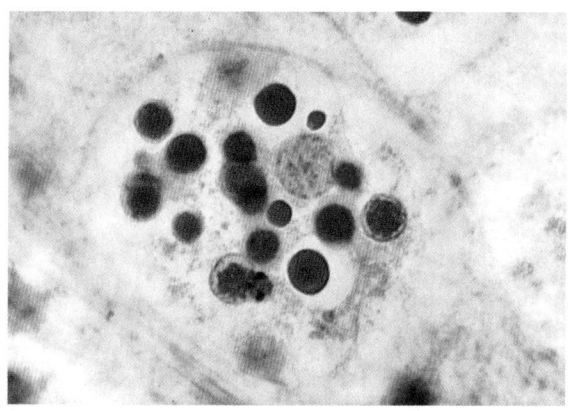

• Fig. 47.2 *Entamoeba histolytica* trophozoite containing ingested red blood cells.

and highly refractile **chromatoidal bars** (refractile chromatin structure) with smooth, rounded edges. As the cyst matures (**metacyst**) (Fig. 47.5 and Fig. 47.3), nuclear division occurs, with the production of four nuclei. Often chromatoidals may be absent in the mature cyst. Cyst morphology does not differentiate *E. histolytica, E. dispar, E. moshkovskii,* and *E. bangladeshi*; it may also resemble *Entamoeba coli.* Cyst formation occurs only in the intestinal tract; once the stool has left the body, cyst formation does not occur. The one-, two-, and four-nucleated cysts are infective and represent the mode of transmission from one host to another.

Epidemiology

Amebiasis is caused by infection with the true pathogen, *E. histolytica.* Evidence from molecular studies confirms the differentiation of pathogenic *E. histolytica* and non-pathogenic *E. dispar* (Fig. 47.6) as two distinct species. *E. histolytica* is considered the etiologic agent of **amebic colitis** (Fig. 47.7A) and **extraintestinal abscesses** (amebic liver abscess; Fig. 47.7B), whereas nonpathogenic *E. dispar* produces no intestinal symptoms and is not invasive in humans. Trophozoites found in tissue are diagnostic of extraintestinal *E. histolytica* infection. *E. moshkovskii* has been shown to cause diarrhea in school-age children and immunocompromised individuals. *E. bangladeshi* has been recovered from the feces of symptomatic and asymptomatic children.

Infection is acquired through the fecal-oral route from infective cysts contained in the feces. The cysts can be ingested in contaminated food or drink or contracted from fomites or various sexual practices that include accidental ingestion of fecal organisms. Flies and cockroaches have been implicated as mechanical vectors of contaminated fecal material.

The infection with all *Entamoeba* spp. occurs worldwide, particularly in areas with poor sanitation. It is estimated that *E. histolytica* infection kills more than 100,000 people each year.

Pathogenesis and Spectrum of Disease

The pathogenesis of *E. histolytica* is related to the organism's ability to directly lyse host cells and cause tissue destruction. Amebic lesions show evidence of cell lysis, tissue necrosis, and damage to the extracellular matrix. Evidence indicates that *E. histolytica* trophozoites interact with the host through a series of steps: adhesion to the target cell, phagocytosis, and cytopathic effect. Numerous other parasite factors also play a role. From the perspective of the host, *E. histolytica* induces both humoral and cellular immune responses; cell-mediated immunity is the major human host defense against this complement-resistant cytolytic protozoan.

The presentations of disease are seen with invasion of the intestinal mucosa or dissemination to other organs (most often the liver) or both. However, it is estimated that a small proportion (2% to 8%) of infected individuals have invasive disease beyond the lumen of the bowel. In addition, organisms may be spontaneously eliminated with no disease symptoms.

Asymptomatic Infection

Individuals harboring *E. histolytica* may have either a negative or a weak antibody titer and negative stools for occult

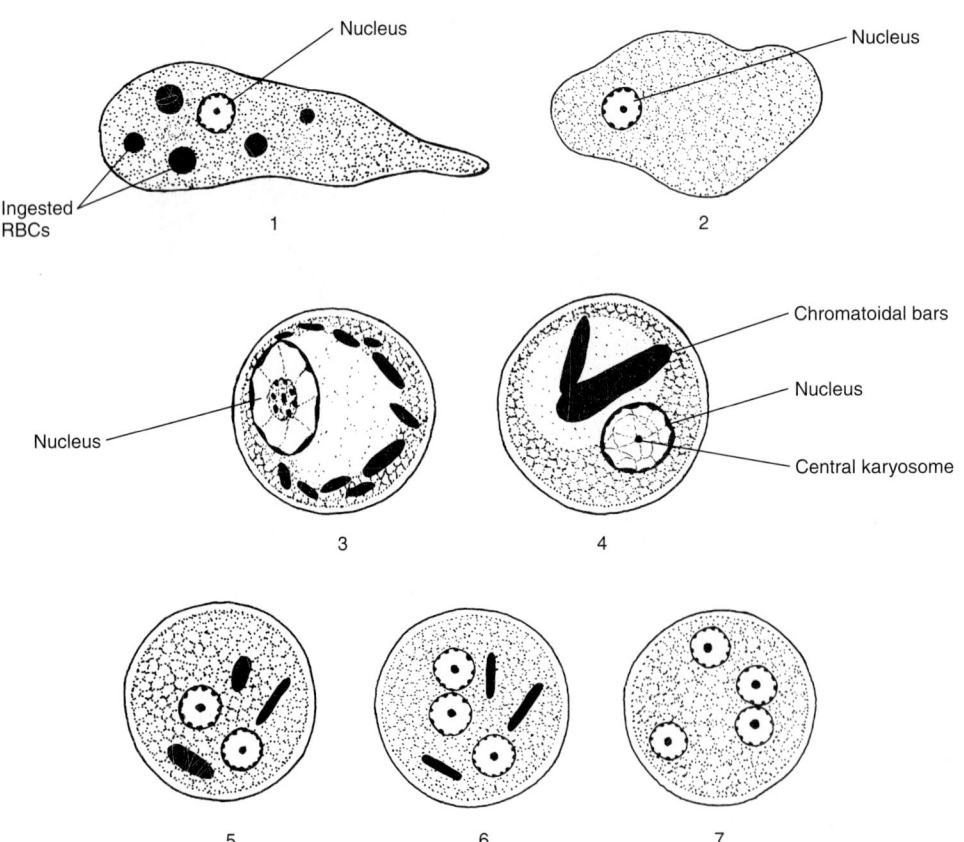

• **Fig. 47.3** (1) Trophozoite of *Entamoeba histolytica* (note ingested red blood cells *[RBCs]*). (2) Trophozoite of *Entamoeba histolytica/Entamoeba dispar* group (morphology does not allow differentiation between the *Entamoeba* species). (3 and 4) Early cysts of *E. histolytica/E. dispar* group. (5–7) Cysts of *E. histolytica/E. dispar* group. (8 and 9) Trophozoites of *Entamoeba coli*. (10 and 11) Early cysts of *E. coli*. (12–14) Cysts of *E. coli*. (15 and 16) Trophozoites of *Entamoeba hartmanni*. (17 and 18) Cysts of *E. hartmanni*. (From Garcia LS. *Diagnostic Medical Parasitology*. 4th ed. Washington, DC: ASM Press; 2001. Illustrations 4 and 11 by Nobuko Kitamura.)

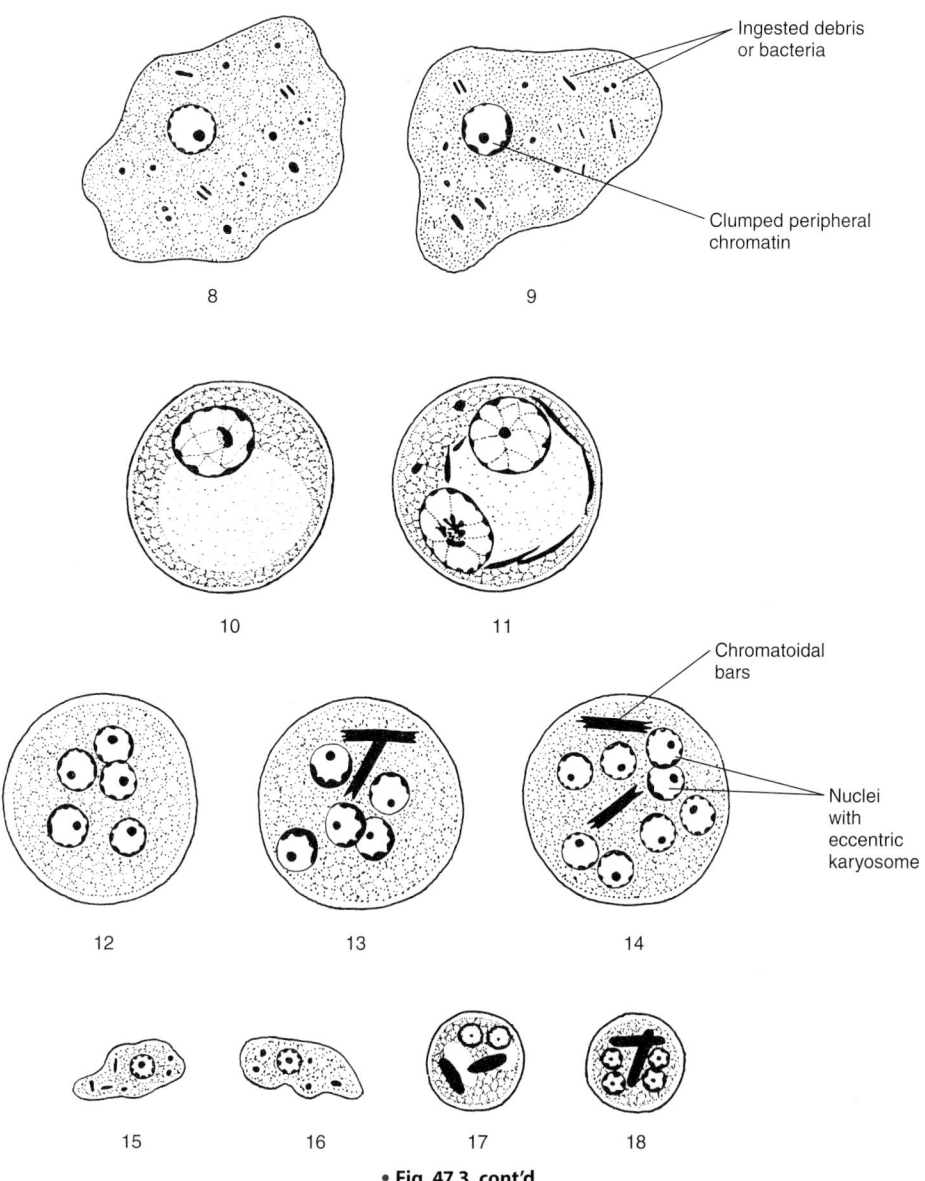

Ingested debris
or bacteria

Clumped peripheral
chromatin

8   9

10   11

Chromatoidal
bars

Nuclei
with
eccentric
karyosome

12   13   14

15   16   17   18

• **Fig. 47.3, cont'd**

blood. They also may be passing cysts detectable by a routine ova and parasite (O&P) examination. However, these cysts cannot be morphologically differentiated from those of the nonpathogenic species, most of the asymptomatic infections are actually due to *E. dispar.* Although trophozoites may be identified, they will not contain any phagocytized RBCs and cannot be differentiated from the nonpathogenic species. Molecular analyses of organisms isolated from asymptomatic individuals have indicated that the isolates typically identified are *E. dispar* or *E. moshkovskii,* and up to 80% belong to *E. histolytica.* Generally, asymptomatic patients never become symptomatic and may excrete cysts for a short period. Asymptomatic patients identified with *E. histolytica* are at risk for the development of invasive amebiasis.

Intestinal Disease

The incubation period varies from a few days to a much longer time; in an area where *E. histolytica* is endemic, it is impossible to determine exactly when exposure to the organism occurred. Normally, the incubation time ranges from 1 to 4 weeks. Tissue invasion by *E. histolytica* requires a contact-dependent process that involves colonic mucins and amebic lectins in the plasma membrane that mediate adherence to the host mucosa. After adherence, destruction of the host cells involves a process referred to as trogocytosis-like, in which the amebae essentially take bites out of the host cellular membrane. This process is enhanced by *E. histolytica* adherence that induces membrane blebbing that facilitates the **trogocytosis.** *E. histolytica* produces cysteine proteinases utilized in the degradation of colonic mucin glycoproteins, digestion of hemoglobin and villin, inactivation of immune modulators such as interleukin (IL)-18, and the digestion of the host's extracellular matrix. The digestive action of these proteases contributes to the development of amebic ulcers and tissue damage in the intestinal tract. Amebic ulcers often develop in the cecum, appendix, or adjacent portion of the ascending colon; however, they can also be found

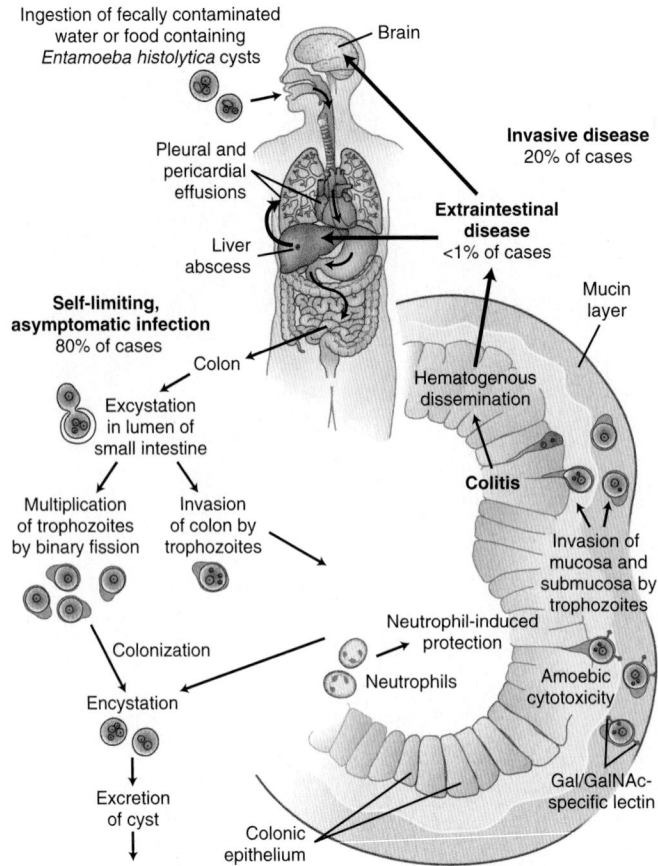

• **Fig. 47.4** Life cycle of *Entamoeba histolytica*.

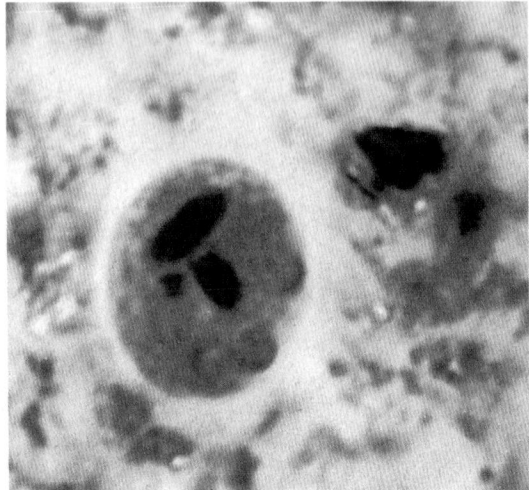

• **Fig. 47.5** *Entamoeba histolytica/Entamoeba dispar* group cyst.

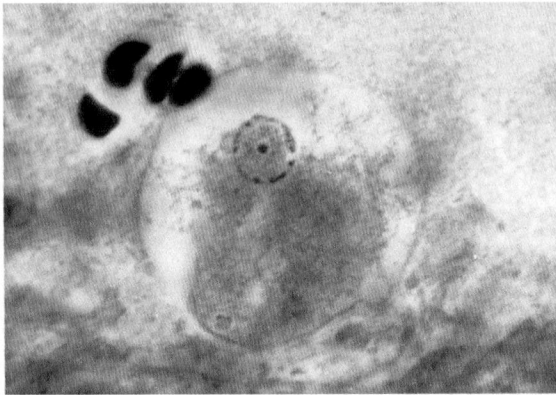

• **Fig. 47.6** *Entamoeba histolytica/Entamoeba dispar* group trophozoite; no ingested red blood cells are present.

in the sigmoidorectal area. Other lesions may occur from these primary sites. Ulcers usually are raised, with a small opening on the mucosal surface and a larger area of destruction below the surface (i.e., flask-shaped). The mucosal lining may appear normal between ulcers.

Invasive intestinal amebiasis has various clinical forms, all of which are generally acute: amebic diarrhea without dysentery, **dysentery** (bloody diarrhea), or **colitis, ameboma,** and **amebic liver abscess.** Dysentery and diarrhea account for 90% of cases of invasive intestinal amebiasis. The severity of symptoms can range from asymptomatic to severe symptoms that mimic ulcerative colitis. Ameboma, a granulomatous, localized lesion, can occur in patients with chronic ulcerative colitis and may be confused with colon cancer. Patients with colicky abdominal pain, frequent bowel movements, and **tenesmus** (a persistent feeling of needing to pass stool) may present with a gradual onset of disease. With the onset of dysentery, bowel movements are frequent (up to 10 per day). Fever is typically absent, and abdominal distention (swelling) or dehydration

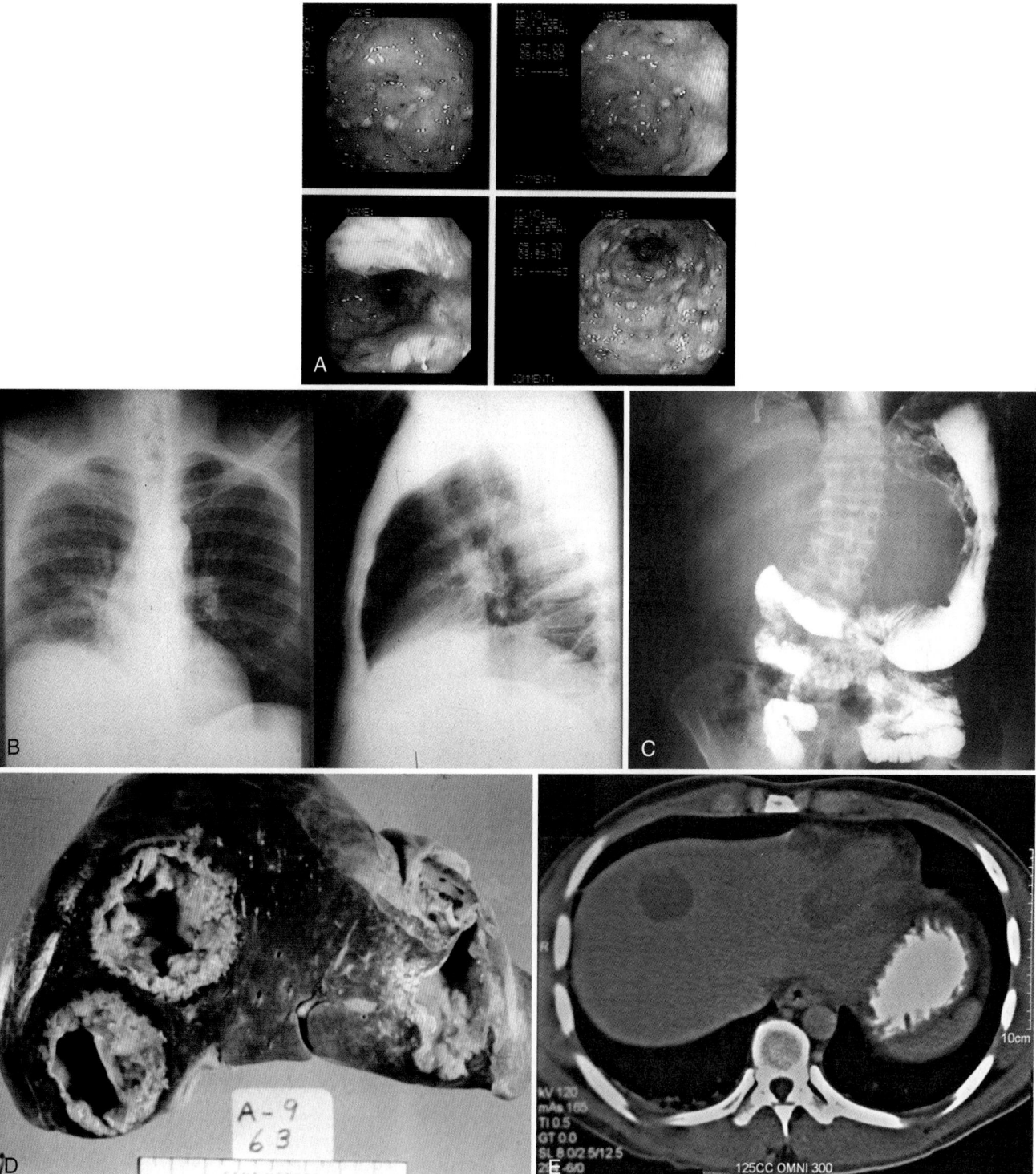

• **Fig. 47.7** Endoscopic and pathologic features of intestinal and extraintestinal amebiasis. (A) Colonoscopic appearance of intestinal amebiasis. (B) Left posteroanterior and right lateral chest radiographs in a patient with amebic liver abscess. (C) Luminal narrowing revealed by a barium-enema examination in a patient with ameboma. (D) Two abscesses in the right lobe and one abscess in the left lobe of a patient with an amebic liver abscess. (E) One abscess in the right lobe and one abscess in the left lobe of a patient with amebic liver abscess, shown on an abdominal computed tomography scan (CT scan).

is uncommon. Although dysentery may last for months, it varies from severe to mild and may lead to weight loss and prostration. In rare severe cases, symptoms may begin very suddenly and include profuse diarrhea, fever, and dehydration with electrolyte imbalances.

Hepatic Disease

Blood flow from the mesenteric veins surrounding the intestine returns blood, via the portal vein, to the liver, most commonly the upper right lobe. Amebae in the submucosa can be carried by the bloodstream to the liver. The onset of symptoms may be gradual or sudden; upper right abdominal pain and fever (38°C to 39°C) are the most consistent findings. Although the liver may be enlarged and tender, liver function tests may be normal or slightly abnormal (jaundice is rare). The abscess can be visualized radiologically, sonically, or by radionuclear scan; most patients have a single abscess in the right lobe of the liver. The most common complication is rupture of the abscess into the pleural space. An abscess also can extend into the peritoneum and through the skin. Hematogenous spread to the brain, lung, pericardium, and other sites is possible.

Pyogenic and amebic liver abscesses are the two most common hepatic abscesses. The severity of a **pyogenic abscess** depends on the bacterial source and the patient's underlying condition. An amebic abscess tends to be more prevalent in those with suppressed cell-mediated immunity, males, and younger individuals. *E. histolytica* cysts and trophozoites can be found in the stools of patients with liver abscess. About 60% of these patients have no intestinal symptoms or any history of dysentery. In addition, the patient's condition should be differentiated from hepatocellular carcinoma and echinococcal cysts (*Echinococcus granulosus,* or hydatid sand; see Chapter 54).

Metastatic Amebiasis

In addition to extraintestinal amebiasis, extraabdominal amebiasis may occur after liver involvement. Thoracic amebiasis is the most common extraabdominal manifestation that presents with empyema, bronchohepatic fistulas, and pericardial abscesses. Pericardial involvement is the second most common extraabdominal presentation resulting in pericarditis. Cerebral amebiasis has been noted after liver abscesses and other rare infections such as in the pharynx, heart, aorta, and scapula.

Laboratory Diagnosis

Routine Methods

The standard O&P examination is the recommended procedure for recovery and identification of *E. histolytica* in stool specimens. Microscopic examination of a direct saline wet mount may reveal motile trophozoites, which may contain RBCs. However, trophozoites with RBCs are identified in a limited number of cases. In many patients who do not present with acute dysentery, trophozoites may be present but do not contain RBCs, and the organisms may be pathogenic *E. histolytica*, or one of the other species: *E. dispar, E. moshkovskii,* or *E. bangladeshi.* An asymptomatic individual may have few trophozoites and possibly only cysts in the stool. Although the concentration technique is helpful for demonstrating cysts, the most important technique for the recovery and identification of protozoan organisms is the permanent stained smear (normally stained with trichrome or iron-hematoxylin). A minimum of three specimens collected over a period of not more than 10 days may be required for identification.

Sigmoidoscopy specimens may be very helpful for identifying organisms. At least six areas of the mucosa should be sampled. Smears from these areas should be examined after permanent staining. However, these specimens are not considered a substitute for the recommended minimum of three stool specimens submitted for O&P examination (direct wet mount, concentration, and permanent stained smear). Colonoscopy and biopsy material may also be helpful; however, amebae may be difficult to identify within the biopsy material. Periodic acid-Schiff (PAS) stains or immunoperoxidase with anti–*E. histolytica* antibodies may improve identification and diagnosis.

Liver aspirate material is rarely examined, and often the specimen is not collected properly. Aspirated material must be aliquoted into several different containers as it is removed from the abscess; amebae may be found only in the last portion of the aspirated material, theoretically material from the abscess wall, not necrotic debris from the abscess center.

Antigen Detection

A number of enzyme immunoassay (EIA) reagents are commercially available, and their specificity and sensitivity provide excellent options for the clinical laboratory. Some fecal antigen tests can differentiate the *E. histolytica*/*E. dispar* group from the rest of the *Entamoeba* spp., such as nonpathogenic *E. coli* or *E. hartmanni* (*E. histolytica* II test, TechLab, Blacksburg, VA). These kits require fresh or fresh frozen stool; fecal preservatives have been found to interfere with the *Entamoeba* spp. reagents. Other kits, such as the *E. histolytica* II test, TechLab, Blacksburg, can differentiate *E. histolytica* from *E. dispar.* Because of the specificity of the immunoassay reagents, the laboratory can inform the physician whether the *E. histolytica*/*E. dispar* group or organisms seen in the stool specimen are pathogenic *E. histolytica.*

If the laboratory does not use these reagents, the presence of *E. histolytica*/*E. dispar* group should be reported to the physician, accompanied by commentary related to the newer information on pathogenicity.

Additional antigen screening test kits are available but are unable to determine the species of amebae. Two examples of these tests include the RIDASCREEN *Entamoeba* (R-Biopharm, Darmstadt, Germany) and the Triage Micro Parasite Panel (Biosite Diagnostics Inc., San Diego, CA). However, the Triage Micro Parasite Panel has the distinct advantage of screening for the major intestinal parasites found in the United States including *G. duodenalis, Cryptosporidium parvum,* and *E. histolytica*/*E. dispar.*

Depending on each state's requirements, pathogenic *E. histolytica* generally is reported to the public health facility (county).

Histology

A histologic diagnosis of amebiasis can be made when the trophozoites in the tissue are identified. Organisms must be differentiated from host cells, particularly histiocytes and ganglion cells. PAS staining, as previously noted, can be used to help locate the organisms, which appear bright pink with a green-blue background (depending on the counterstain used). Hematoxylin and eosin staining also allows visualization of the typical morphology, thus allowing accurate identification. As a result of sectioning, some organisms exhibit the evenly arranged nuclear chromatin with the central karyosome, and some no longer contain the nucleus.

Nucleic Acid Detection

Nucleic acid–based amplification methods, including polymerase chain reaction (real-time and multiplex assays), have been developed for the identification of *E. histolytica* and *E. dispar*. The polymerase chain reaction assays (PCR) identify unique ribosomal ribonucleic acid (rRNA) or specific episomal (small circular nucleic acid) sequences to differentiate the organisms. Suitable samples for real-time PCR (Chapter 8) detection of *E. histolytica* or *E. dispar* include stool, liver or brain aspirates, cerebrospinal fluid, blood, saliva, and urine samples. Multiplex assays that are capable of detecting multiple types of organisms including viral, bacterial, and parasitic organisms capable of causing gastroenteritis would significantly improve diagnostic testing and enhance patient care. Several multiplex panels are available for the identification of *E. histolytica* including the xTAG Gastrointestinal Panel (Luminex Molecular Diagnostics, Austin, TX) for the detection of *E. histolytica*, *G. duodenalis*, and *Cryptosporidium* along with 13 bacterial species or pathogenic forms, 2 bacterial toxins, and 3 viral agents that cause gastroenteritis; the RIDAGENE Stool PCR panel (R. Biopharm AG, Darmstadt, Germany) differentiates *Giardia*, *Cryptosporidium*, *E. histolytica*, and *Dientamoeba*; the BD MAX Enteric Parasite Panel (Becton, Dickinson and Company, Sparks MD) differentiates *Giardia*, *Cryptosporidium*, and *E. histolytica*; and the BioFire FilmArray Gastrointestinal Panel that differentiates 13 bacterial, 5 viral, and parasitic pathogens *Cryptosporidium*, *Cyclospora*, *E. histolytica*, and *Giardia*. Stool specimens, however, may contain inhibitors that would prevent accurate detection using amplification methods; therefore, it is necessary that all assays include an amplification control. These tests are becoming more widely used and have proven to be more sensitive than microscopy and as sensitive as antigen-based immunoassays.

Antibody (Serologic) Detection

Serologic testing for intestinal disease is rarely recommended unless the patient has true dysentery; even in these cases, the titer (e.g., indirect hemagglutination) may be low and thus difficult to interpret. A definitive diagnosis of intestinal amebiasis should not be made without demonstrating the presence of the organisms and is not useful in the diagnosis of asymptomatic patients. In patients suspected of having extraintestinal disease, serologic tests are diagnostically more effective and a valuable tool in conjunction with either antigen or nucleic acid–based testing. Indirect hemagglutination and indirect fluorescent antibody tests have been reported positive with titers greater than or equal to 1:256 and greater than or equal to 1:200, respectively, in almost 100% of cases of amebic liver abscess. In the absence of STAT serologic tests for amebiasis, the decision on diagnosis must be made on clinical grounds and based on results of other diagnostic tests, such as scans. In addition, antibodies may persist for up to 10 years in patients who have had previous incidences of invasive amebiasis, making diagnosis complicated in subsequent infections.

Reporting of Results

It is important to note, when possible, the full taxonomic name of the infecting organism, including genus and species as well as the life cycle stage or form present, trophozoite or cyst. The laboratory should report *E. histolytica/dispar* group and provide a comment relative to other potentially pathogenic or nonpathogenic species. If full species identification is not available, the physician will be responsible to determine whether treatment is warranted based on the patient's condition and additional clinical information. Quantitation of organisms is not warranted.

Therapy

Two classes of drugs are used in the treatment of amebic infections: luminal amebicides, such as paromomycin, iodoquinol, or diloxanide furoate, and tissue amebicides, such as metronidazole, tinidazole, or dehydroemetine. Because of the differences in drug efficacy, it is important that the laboratory report indicate whether cysts, trophozoites, or both are present in the stool specimen.

Asymptomatic Infection

Patients found to have true *E. histolytica* in the intestinal tract, even if asymptomatic, should be treated to eliminate the organisms. Both diloxanide furoate and iodoquinol or paromomycin can be used to treat cysts in the lumen of the gut. In general, these treatments are ineffective against extraintestinal disease. If the patient is passing trophozoites and cysts, the recommended treatment is a tissue amebicide followed by a luminal amebicide.

The importance of using both luminal and tissue amebicides is emphasized in patients with amebic liver abscesses. Asymptomatic colonization may be present with the true pathogen, *E. histolytica*. In patients treated with a tissue amebicide, generally, a 100% clinical response to the hepatic lesions is seen; however, failure to eliminate the organism from the bowel can lead to secondary bouts with invasive disease and intestinal colonization. In addition, these carriers constitute a public health hazard because of continued shedding of infective cysts. Chemoprophylaxis is not recommended because of the potential for the development of drug resistance in the organisms.

Prevention

Humans are the reservoir host for *E. histolytica*, and infection can be transmitted to other humans, primates, dogs, cats, and possibly pigs. Accidental consumption of sewage-contaminated water provides another route of infection. Amebiasis is considered a zoonotic waterborne infection. The cyst stages are resistant to environmental conditions and can remain viable in the soil for 8 days at 28°C to 34°C, for 40 days at 2°C to 6°C, and for 60 days at 0°C. Cysts normally are removed by sand filtration or destroyed by 200 ppm of iodine, 5% to 10% acetic acid, or boiling. However, an asymptomatic carrier who is a food handler generally is believed to play the most important role in transmission. Proper disposal of contaminated feces is considered the most important preventive measure. Although vaccines have been discussed as a possibility for eliminating human disease, no vaccine is currently available.

Entamoeba coli
General Characteristics

The life cycle of *E. coli* is identical to that of *E. dispar*. After digestion of infective cysts, the organisms exist in the intestinal tract and produce trophozoites. Cyst formation occurs as the gut contents move through the intestinal tract; the excreted cysts are the infective form transmitted to humans and some animals.

E. coli trophozoites may appear larger than those of the other *Entamoeba* spp. and range from 15 to 50 μm in diameter (Figs. 47.3, 47.8, 47.9, and Table 47.1). Motility is sluggish with broad, short pseudopods. In wet preparations, differentiating nonpathogenic *E. coli* from pathogenic *E. histolytica* is almost impossible. On a permanent stained smear viewed at a higher magnification, the cytoplasm is granular with vacuoles containing bacteria, yeasts, and other food materials. The nucleus has a large, blotlike karyosome that may be eccentric rather than centrally located. The chromatin on the nuclear membrane tends to be clumped and irregular.

Early cysts often contain chromatoidal bars, which tend to be splinter-shaped and irregular. Eventually, the nuclei divide until the mature cyst, containing eight nuclei, is formed (Table 47.2 and Figs. 47.3 and 47.8). In rare cases, the number of nuclei reaches 16. The cysts measure 10 to 35 μm in diameter, and as they mature, the chromatoidal bars disappear. When the cyst of *E. coli* matures, it becomes more refractive to fixation; therefore, the cyst may be seen on the wet preparation but not on the permanent stained

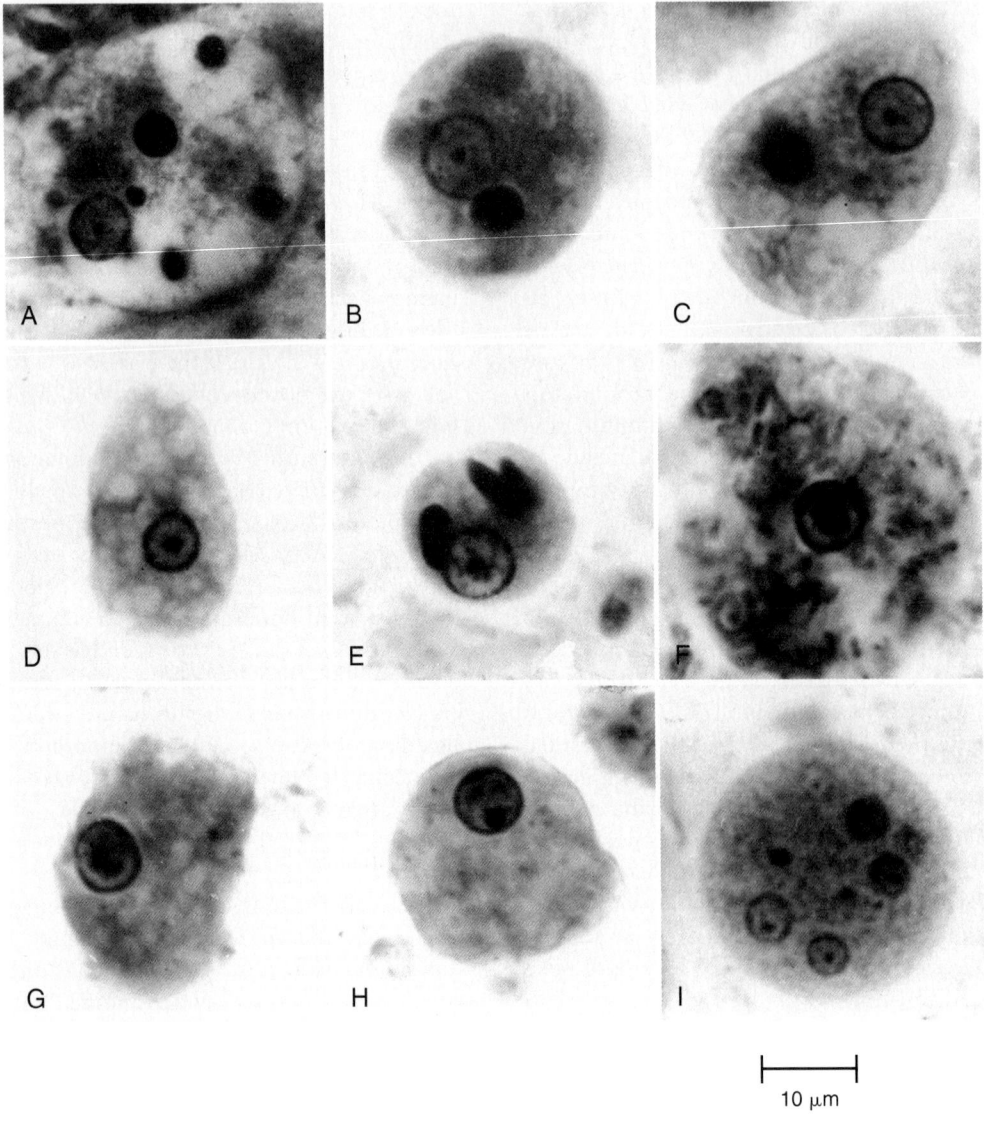

10 μm

• **Fig. 47.8** (A–C) Trophozoites of *Entamoeba histolytica* (note ingested red blood cells). (D) Trophozoite of *E. histolytica*/*Entamoeba dispar* group. (E) Early cyst of *E. histolytica*/*E. dispar* group. (F–H) Trophozoites of *Entamoeba coli*. (I) Cyst of *E. coli*.

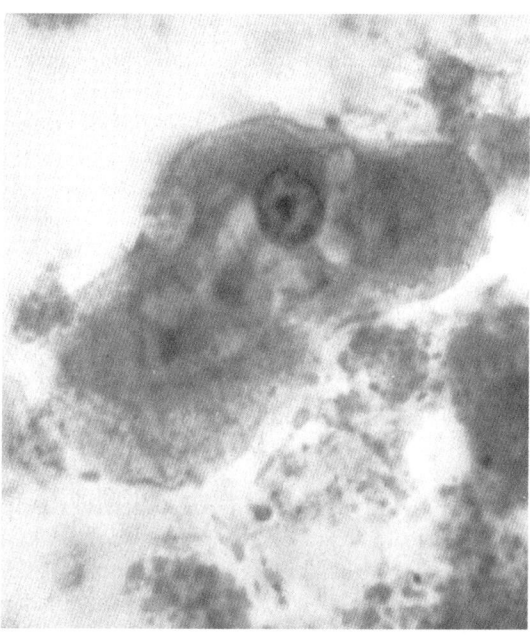

• **Fig. 47.9** *Entamoeba coli* trophozoite.

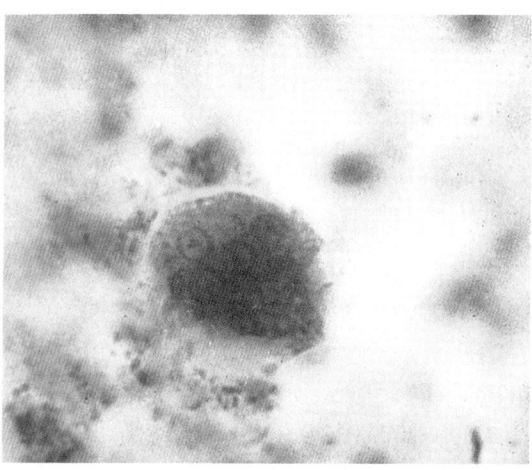

• **Fig. 47.10** *Entamoeba coli* cyst (trichrome stain) (poor preservation; typical appearance of some *E. coli* cysts).

smear. Occasionally, on trichrome smears, the cysts appear distorted and somewhat pink (Fig. 47.10).

Epidemiology

Transmission occurs through the ingestion of mature cysts from contaminated food or water. The organism is readily acquired. In some warmer climates or areas with poor sanitation and inadequate disposal of human excreta, the colonization rate with *E. coli* can be high.

Pathogenesis and Spectrum of Disease

E. coli are typically considered nonpathogenic and do not cause disease. However, it is important for the physician to correlate patient signs and symptoms with disease presentation. In addition, a patient that presents with a potential nonpathogenic protozoan may simultaneously be infected with a pathogenic species.

Laboratory Diagnosis

Unless the mature cyst with eight nuclei is seen, the morphologies of the other *Entamoeba* spp. and *E. coli* are similar in the trophozoite and immature cyst stages. Definitive identification may not be possible from examining permanent stained smears. Species specific immunoassay or nucleic acid based testing may be necessary to correctly identify the organism.

Therapy

Specific treatment is not recommended for nonpathogenic *E. coli*. Correct differentiation among the species is critical to good patient care. Because the amebae are acquired through fecal-oral contamination, pathogens and nonpathogens can be found in the same patient. Treatment is not recommended for infection with *E. coli*.

Prevention

Prevention depends on adequate disposal of human excreta and improved personal hygiene, preventive measures that apply to most of the intestinal protozoa.

Entamoeba hartmanni
General Characteristics

The life cycle of *E. hartmanni* is similar to that of *E. dispar*, with differences in size as the key characteristic for proper identification (Figs. 47.11 and 47.12). In wet preparations, *E. hartmanni* trophozoites range in size from 4 to 12 μm in diameter, and cysts range in size from 5 to 10 μm in diameter. On the permanent stained smear, the cysts tend to shrink because of dehydration. Therefore, the sizes of the organisms may be smaller (1 to 1.5 μm) than determined in the wet preparation measurements.

Trophozoites do not ingest RBCs, and their motility is slower (Table 48.1 and Figs. 47.3, 47.11, and 47.12). The morphologic characteristics of *E. hartmanni* are very similar to those of *E. histolytica*, with two exceptions. Commonly, *E. hartmanni* cysts may contain one or two nuclei and the mature cyst contains four nuclei. Mature cysts of *E. hartmanni* may retain their chromatoidal bars, a characteristic not seen in *E. histolytica* or *E. dispar*. *E. hartmanni*'s chromatoidal bars are similar to those of *E. histolytica* and *E. dispar* but smaller and more numerous (Table 47.2 and Figs. 47.11 and 47.12). At the species level, differentiation between *E. hartmanni* and the other *Entamoeba* spp. depends on size; therefore laboratories are required to use calibrated microscopes that are checked periodically for accuracy.

Epidemiology

Transmission occurs through the ingestion of mature cysts from contaminated food or water. If accurate identifications have been recorded, the colonization rate tends to match that of *E. histolytica*.

Pathogenesis and Spectrum of Disease

E. hartmanni is considered nonpathogenic and does not cause disease.

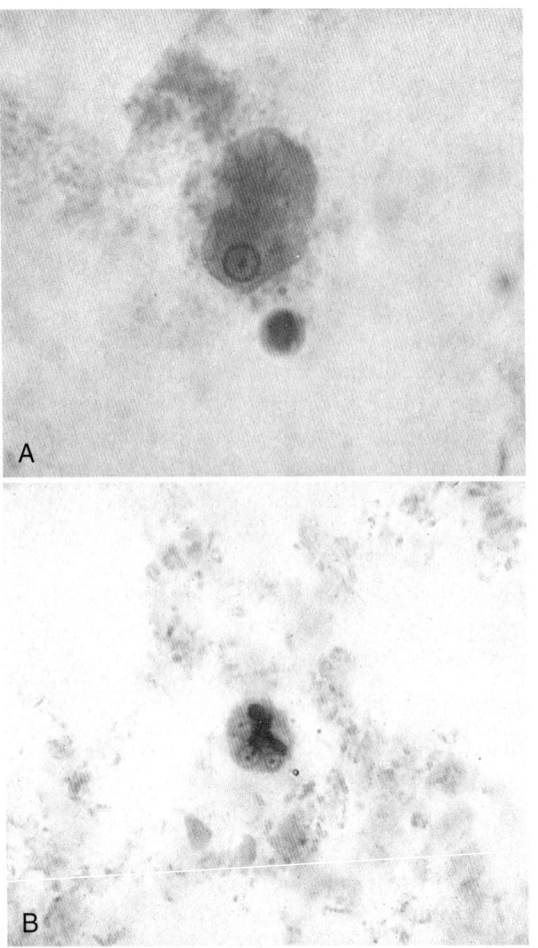

• **Fig. 47.11** (A) *Entamoeba hartmanni* trophozoite. (B) *E. hartmanni* cyst.

Laboratory Diagnosis

Unless the trophozoites and cysts match the size requirements, they are unlikely to be *E. hartmanni*. Definitive identification relies on examination of permanent stained smears and measurements made with the calibrated microscope, specific immunoassay, or nucleic acid–based testing.

Entamoeba polecki and Entamoeba gingivalis

Entamoeba polecki has been identified in human clinical samples but is not believed to be pathogenic. The organism is associated with pigs. The organism resembles the other *Entamoeba* spp., with the exception of containing a sharply defined round or oval mass that may be present on a permanent stained smear. *Entamoeba gingivalis* does not include a cyst stage and is considered nonpathogenic. The organism also ingests white blood cells and fragments may be visualized within vacuoles differentiating *E. gingivalis* from the other *Entamoeba* spp. A few cases of *E. gingivalis* being isolated from clinical specimens have been identified in vaginal, oral, tissue, and pulmonary infections.

Endolimax nana
General Characteristics

Endolimax nana, one of the smaller nonpathogenic amebae, has a worldwide distribution and occurs as commonly as *E. coli.*

E. nana has the same life cycle stages as *E. dispar* and the other nonpathogenic amebae. The trophozoite usually measures 6 to 12 μm in diameter (normal range, 8 to 10 μm) (Figs. 47.13–47.15, and Table 47.1). Although rarely seen, motility is sluggish and nonprogressive with blunt, hyaline pseudopods. In the permanent stained smear, normally no peripheral chromatin is seen on the nuclear membrane, and the karyosome is large, with either a central or an eccentric location in the nucleus (Figs. 47.14 and 47.15). *E. nana* shows more nuclear variation than any of the other amebae and can mimic *D. fragilis* or *E. hartmanni.* The cytoplasm may have small vacuoles containing ingested debris or bacteria, but it also may appear relatively clean.

Cysts usually measure 5 to 10 μm in diameter (normal range, 6 to 8 μm) (Table 47.2). Cysts as large as 14 μm have been seen. The cyst is usually oval to round, with the mature cyst containing four nuclei. The nuclei typically have no peripheral chromatin and are evenly distributed in the cyst. Occasionally, very small, slightly curved chromatoidal bars are present. The two-nucleated stage is not commonly seen, and frequently both trophozoites and cysts are present in clinical specimens.

Epidemiology

Transmission occurs through the ingestion of mature cysts from contaminated food or water. The cysts of *E. nana* are less resistant to desiccation *E. coli. E. nana* is also found in warm, moist climates and in other areas with poor sanitary conditions.

Pathogenesis and Spectrum of Disease

E. nana is considered nonpathogenic and does not cause disease.

Laboratory Diagnosis

Although cysts sometimes can be seen in a wet preparation, definitive identification of *E. nana* relies on examination of permanent stained smears.

Iodamoeba bütschlii (buetschlii)
General Characteristics

Iodamoeba bütschlii, one of the nonpathogenic amebae, has a worldwide distribution. Generally, the acquisition rate for this organism is not as high as that for *E. coli* and *E. nana.*

The life cycle stages of *I. bütschlii* are the same as those of *E. nana.* The trophozoite varies from 8 to 20 μm in diameter and demonstrates active motility in a fresh stool preparation (Table 47.1). The cytoplasm is granular, containing numerous vacuoles with ingested debris and bacteria. The cytoplasm is more vacuolated than in *E. nana* trophozoites. The nucleus has a large karyosome, which can be either centrally located or eccentric (Figs 47.16 and 47.17). On the permanent stained smear, the nucleus may appear to have a halo, and chromatin granules fan out around the karyosome. If the granules are on one side, the nucleus may appear to have a "basket nucleus" arrangement of chromatin, more commonly seen in the cyst. The trophozoites of *I. bütschlii* and

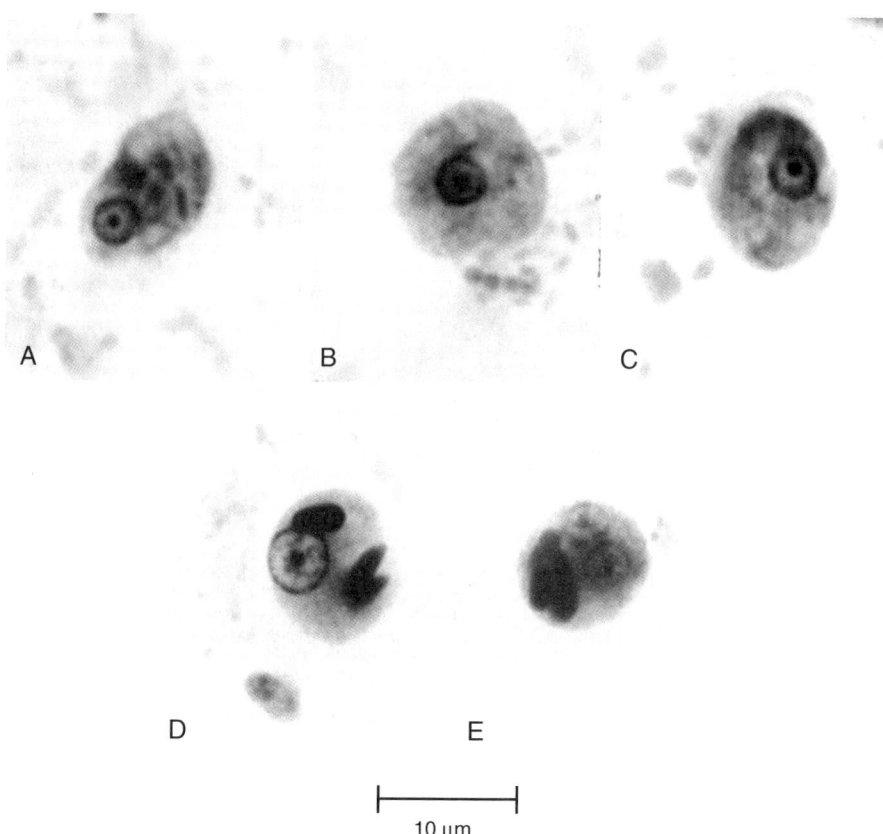

10 μm

• **Fig. 47.12** (A–C) Trophozoites of *Entamoeba hartmanni*. (D and E) Cysts of *E. hartmanni*.

E. nana may appear similar and are difficult to differentiate at the species level, even on the permanent stained smear. Both organisms are considered nonpathogenic. *E. nana* is recovered in clinical specimens much more commonly than is *I. bütschlii.*

I. bütschlii cysts are round to oval (Table 47.2). The glycogen vacuole is so large that occasionally the cyst collapses on itself. Because nuclear multiplication does not occur in the cyst form, the mature cyst contains a single nucleus. The cysts measure approximately 5 to 20 μm in diameter and are rarely confused with those of other amebae (Figs. 47.16 and 47.17).

Epidemiology

Transmission of *I. bütschlii* occurs through the ingestion of mature cysts from contaminated food or water. This organism is found in warm, moist climates and in other areas with a low standard of personal hygiene and poor sanitary conditions.

Pathogenesis and Spectrum of Disease

I. bütschlii is considered nonpathogenic and does not cause disease.

Laboratory Diagnosis

Although *I. bütschlii* cysts sometimes can be seen in a wet preparation, definitive identification relies on the examination of permanent stained smears.

Therapy

Specific treatment is not recommended for *I. bütschlii.* Because these nonpathogenic amebae are acquired through fecal-oral contamination, both pathogens and nonpathogens can be identified in the same patient. If few organisms are present, extended microscopic examination and multiple organism measurements are required for definitive identification. It is always important to report pathogens and nonpathogens, because they are acquired in similar ways.

Prevention (Nonpathogenic *Entamoeba*, *Endolimax*, and *Iodamoeba* spp.)

Prevention depends on adequate disposal of human excreta and improved personal hygiene, preventive measures that apply to most of the intestinal protozoa.

Blastocystis spp.
General Characteristics

Blastocystis (Fig. 47.1 and Table 47.6) consists of a number of different subtypes and subspecies that are indistinguishable morphologically, some of which are pathogenic and some of which are nonpathogenic. Although usually listed with the amebae, the organism's classification is still under review; different subtypes eventually may be classified as different species. In addition, based on molecular sequencing of the *SSU* rRNA gene, *Blastocystis* has been placed within a heterogenous group referred to as the **stramenopiles**. This group contains brown algae, slime molds, diatoms, and

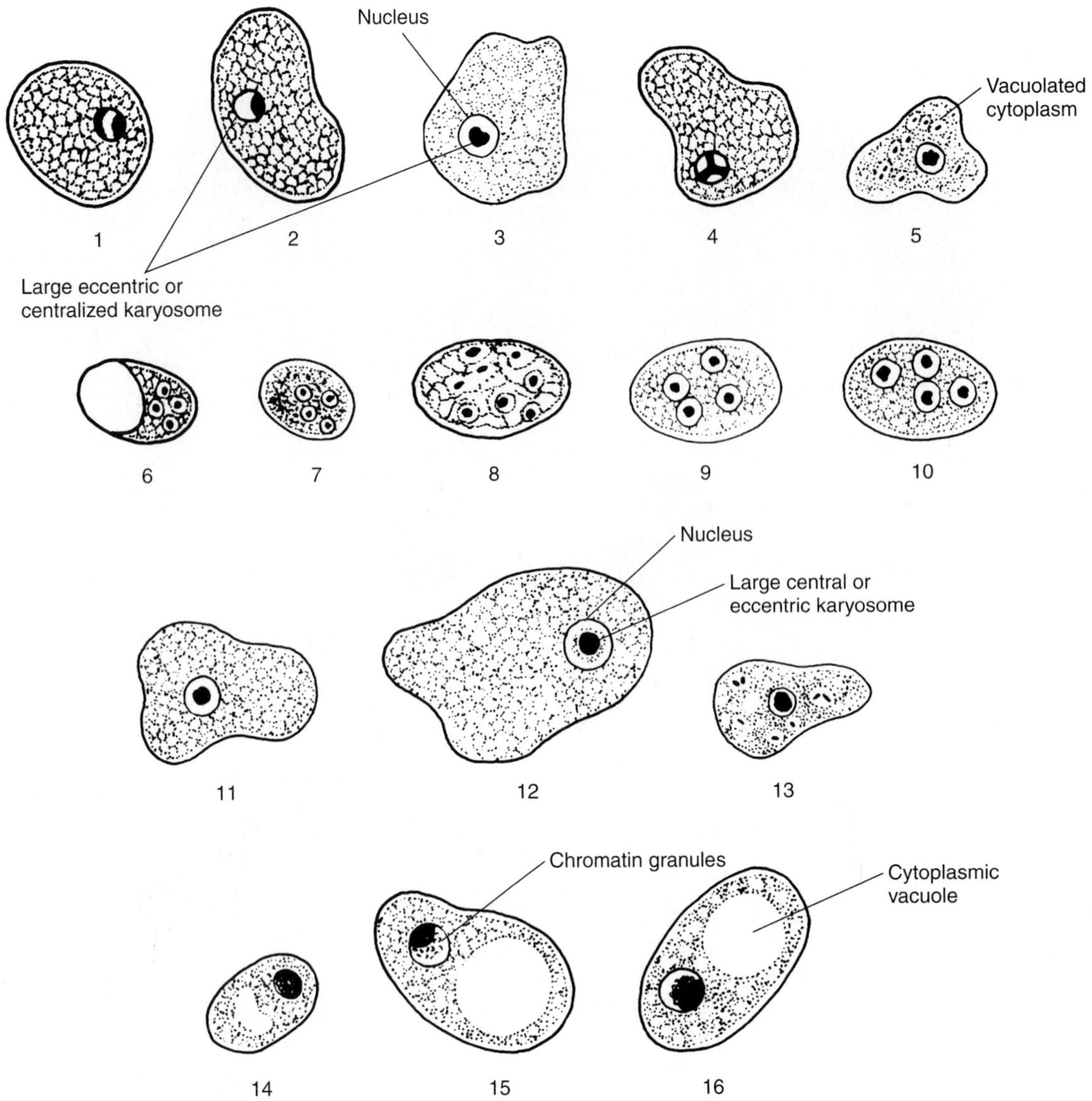

Nucleus

Large eccentric or
centralized karyosome

Vacuolated
cytoplasm

1   2   3   4   5

6   7   8   9   10

Nucleus

Large central or
eccentric karyosome

11   12   13

Chromatin granules

Cytoplasmic
vacuole

14   15   16

• **Fig. 47.13** (1–5) Trophozoites of *Endolimax nana*. (6–10) Cysts of *E. nana*. (11–13) Trophozoites of *Iodamoeba bütschlii*. (14–16) Cysts of *I. bütschlii*. (From Garcia LS. *Diagnostic Medical Parasitology*. 4th ed. Washington, DC: ASM Press; 2001.)

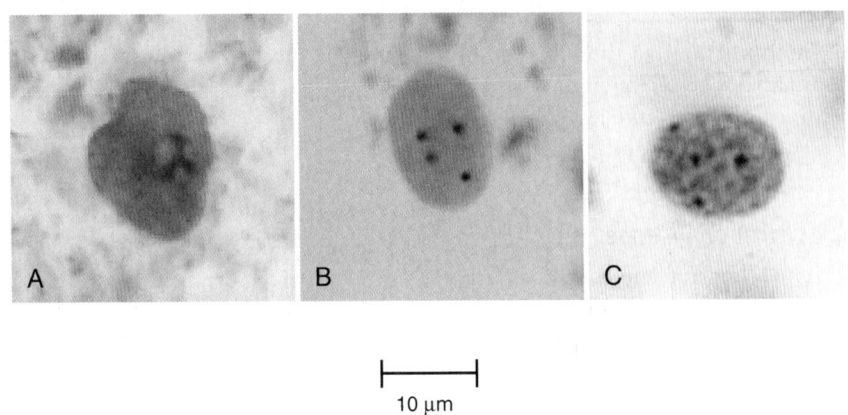

A   B   C

├─────── 10 µm ───────┤

• **Fig. 47.14** (A) Trophozoite of *Endolimax nana*. (B–C) Cysts of *E. nana*. (Courtesy Lynne Garcia, Santa Monica, CA.)

chrysophytes. Although the true role of this organism in terms of disease has been controversial, it is generally considered a causative agent of intestinal disease. The current recommendation is to report the presence of *Blastocystis* spp. and quantitate from the permanent stained smear (i.e., rare, few, moderate, many, packed); this information may be valuable in helping to assess the pathogenicity of the organism in the individual patient.

Blastocystis spp. consists of four major forms. The **cyst form** is the most recently described form of the life cycle stages. Thick-walled cysts are believed to be responsible for external transmission through the fecal-oral route; thin-walled cysts are believed to cause autoinfection. Cysts can vary in shape but are mostly ovoid or spherical. Cyst forms have also been identified that contain multiple vacuoles. The **central vacuole form** (also referred to as the **central body form**) is the most common form found in clinical stool samples. The large central vacuole can occupy most of the cellular volume. The **amoeboid form** is rarely seen but has been identified in stool specimens of patients with diarrhea. The **granular form** can be seen in cultures of *Blastocystis* spp. and is characterized by intracytoplasmic or intravacuolar granules.

Epidemiology

Transmission of *Blastocystis* is by the fecal-oral route from infective forms contained in the feces. The organisms can be ingested in contaminated food and drink or acquired from fomites or through various sexual practices that may include accidental ingestion of fecal organisms. As with *E. histolytica*, flies and cockroaches can be responsible for mechanical transmission. Human-to-human and animal-to-human transmission is probably more common than suspected.

Blastocystis is a common intestinal parasite of humans and animals, with a worldwide distribution. Depending on the geographic location, it may be detected in 1% to 40% of fecal specimens. *Blastocystis* may be the most common parasite found in the intestinal tract.

Pathogenesis and Spectrum of Disease

Blastocystis spp. can cause diarrhea, cramps, nausea, fever, vomiting, abdominal pain, and urticaria and may require therapy. A possible relationship between *Blastocystis* and intestinal obstruction and perhaps even infective arthritis has been suggested. In patients with other underlying conditions, the symptoms may be more pronounced. The incidence of this organism appears to be higher than suspected in stools submitted for parasite examination. In symptomatic patients in whom no other etiologic agent has been identified, *Blastocystis* should certainly be considered the possible pathogen. It has been suggested that proteases of genetic subtype 3 could be considered a virulence factor responsible for protein degradation and subsequent pathogenesis.

Laboratory Diagnosis
Routine Methods
Routine stool examinations are very effective in recovering and identifying *Blastocystis* spp.; the permanent stained

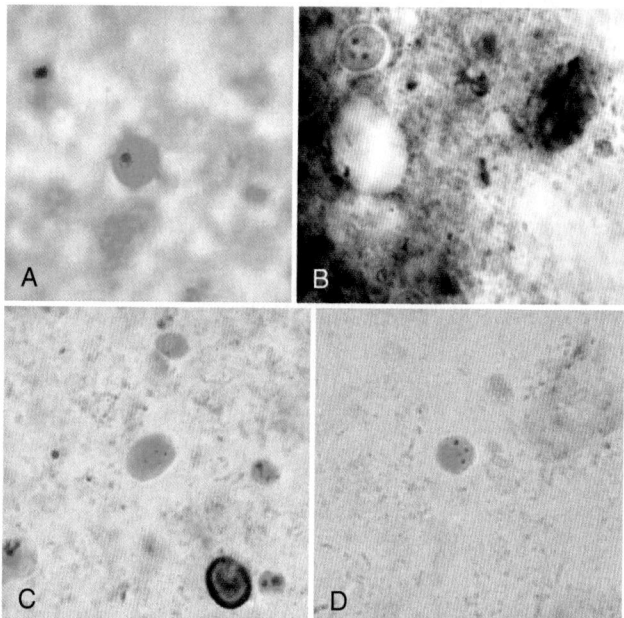

• **Fig. 47.15** (A) *Endolimax nana* trophozoite. (B) *E. nana* cyst, iodine stain. (C and D) *E. nana* cyst. (B, Courtesy Dr. Henry Travers, Sioux Falls, SD.)

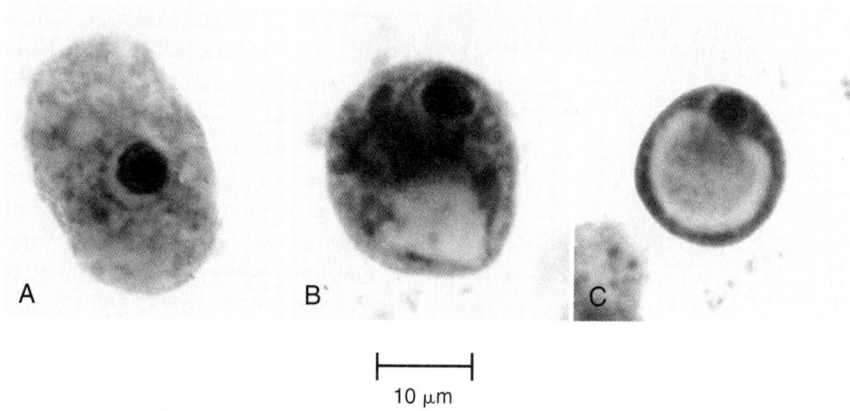

10 µm

• **Fig. 47.16** (A) Trophozoites of *Iodamoeba bütschlii*. (B and C) Cysts of *I. bütschlii*.

smear is the procedure of choice, because examination of wet preparations may not easily reveal the organism. If the fresh stool is rinsed in water before fixation (for the concentration method), *Blastocystis* organisms, other than the cysts, are destroyed, and a false-negative report may result.

Antigen Detection

Fecal immunoassays to detect *Blastocystis* antigen have been developed but are of little clinical use. The technique currently used is the enzyme-linked immunosorbent assay (ELISA).

Antibody (Serologic) Detection

ELISA and fluorescent antibody tests have been developed to detect serum antibody to *Blastocystis* spp. infections. A strong antibody response is consistent with the ability of this organism to cause symptoms. In addition, demonstration of serum antibody production both during and after *Blastocystis* symptomatic disease may provide immunologic evidence for the pathogenic role for this protozoan, although it may take 2 years or longer with chronic infections to develop a serologic response.

Reporting of Results

Unlike *E. histolytica,* the presence of *Blastocystis* spp. should be quantitated in the report (i.e., rare, few, moderate, or many). This may provide the clinician with some indication as to whether to consider the infection pathogenic. However, it is not important to state the life cycle stage or form of the organism present, because the central body form is the most common (90%) identified in clinical specimens. It is also important to remember that other possible pathogens should be adequately ruled out before a patient is treated for *Blastocystis* spp. infection.

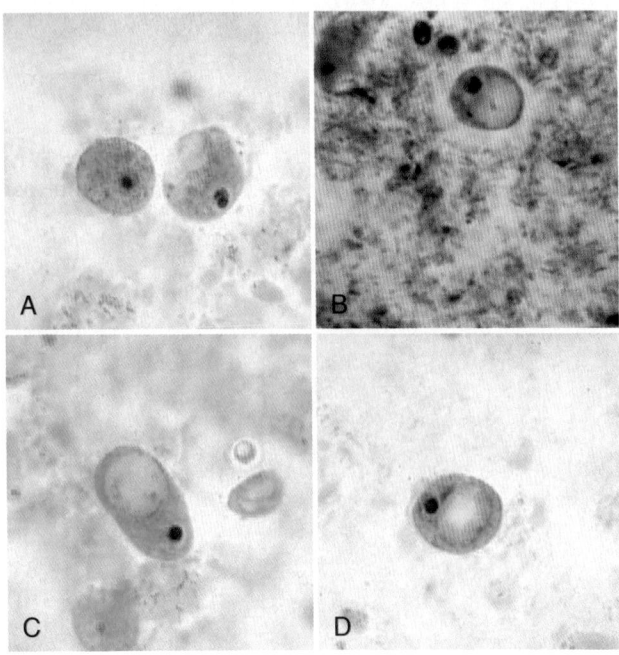

• **Fig. 47.17** (A) *Iodamoeba bütschlii* trophozoites. (B–D) *I. bütschlii* cyst. (B, Courtesy Dr. Henry Travers, Sioux Falls, SD.)

Therapy

Although clinical evidence is limited, *in vitro* susceptibility studies for numerous drugs have been completed for *Blastocystis* spp. Currently, metronidazole (Flagyl) appears to be the most appropriate drug. TMP-SMX (trimethoprim-sulfamethoxazole) and iodoquinol are also recommended with variable success. *Blastocystis* resistance to metronidazole has been reported.

Prevention

Prevention requires improved personal hygiene and sanitary conditions, in addition to proper disposal of fecal material.

Flagellates

The Mastigophora, or flagellates, have specialized locomotor organelles called flagella; these are long, thin, cytoplasmic extensions that may vary in number and position, depending on the species. Different genera of flagellates may live in the intestinal tract, the bloodstream, or various tissues.

Four common species of flagellates are found in the intestinal tract: *Giardia duodenalis, D. fragilis, Chilomastix mesnili,* and *Pentatrichomonas hominis* (Figs. 47.18–47.25, Tables 47.3 and 47.4). Several other smaller, nonpathogenic flagellates, such as *E. hominis* and *Retortamonas intestinalis* (Fig. 47.18), are rarely seen, and none are identified in the intestinal tract. The **sucking disk** and **axonemes** of *G. duodenalis,* the **cytostome** and **spiral groove** of *C. mesnili,* and the **undulating membrane** of *Trichomonas* spp. are all distinctive criteria for identification (Figs. 47.18–47.25).

G. duodenalis and *D. fragilis* are the flagellates considered pathogenic. *D. fragilis* has been associated with diarrhea, nausea, vomiting, and other nonspecific intestinal complaints. *Trichomonas vaginalis* is pathogenic but occurs in the urogenital tract. *Trichomonas tenax* is occasionally found in the mouth and may be associated with poor oral hygiene.

Giardia duodenalis
General Characteristics

G. duodenalis is the most common cause of intestinal infection worldwide. As a result of molecular techniques, *G. duodenalis* is the accepted species nomenclature for organisms isolated from human clinical specimens. However, significant genetic diversity does exist and has been subdivided into subgenotypes designated as A and B. Subgenotype B is only isolated from human specimens, whereas A has been identified in both animal and human samples. Other than *Blastocystis* spp., *G. duodenalis* is probably the most common protozoan organism identified in individuals in the United States. It causes symptoms ranging from mild diarrhea, flatulence, and vague abdominal pains to acute, severe diarrhea, to **steatorrhea** and a typical malabsorption syndrome. Various documented waterborne and foodborne outbreaks have occurred during the past several years. A number of animals may serve as reservoir hosts for *G. duodenalis.* Differentiation of flagellates is based on overall shape, numbers, and arrangements of flagella.

Both the trophozoite and cyst stages are included in the life cycle of *G. duodenalis.* Trophozoites divide by means of

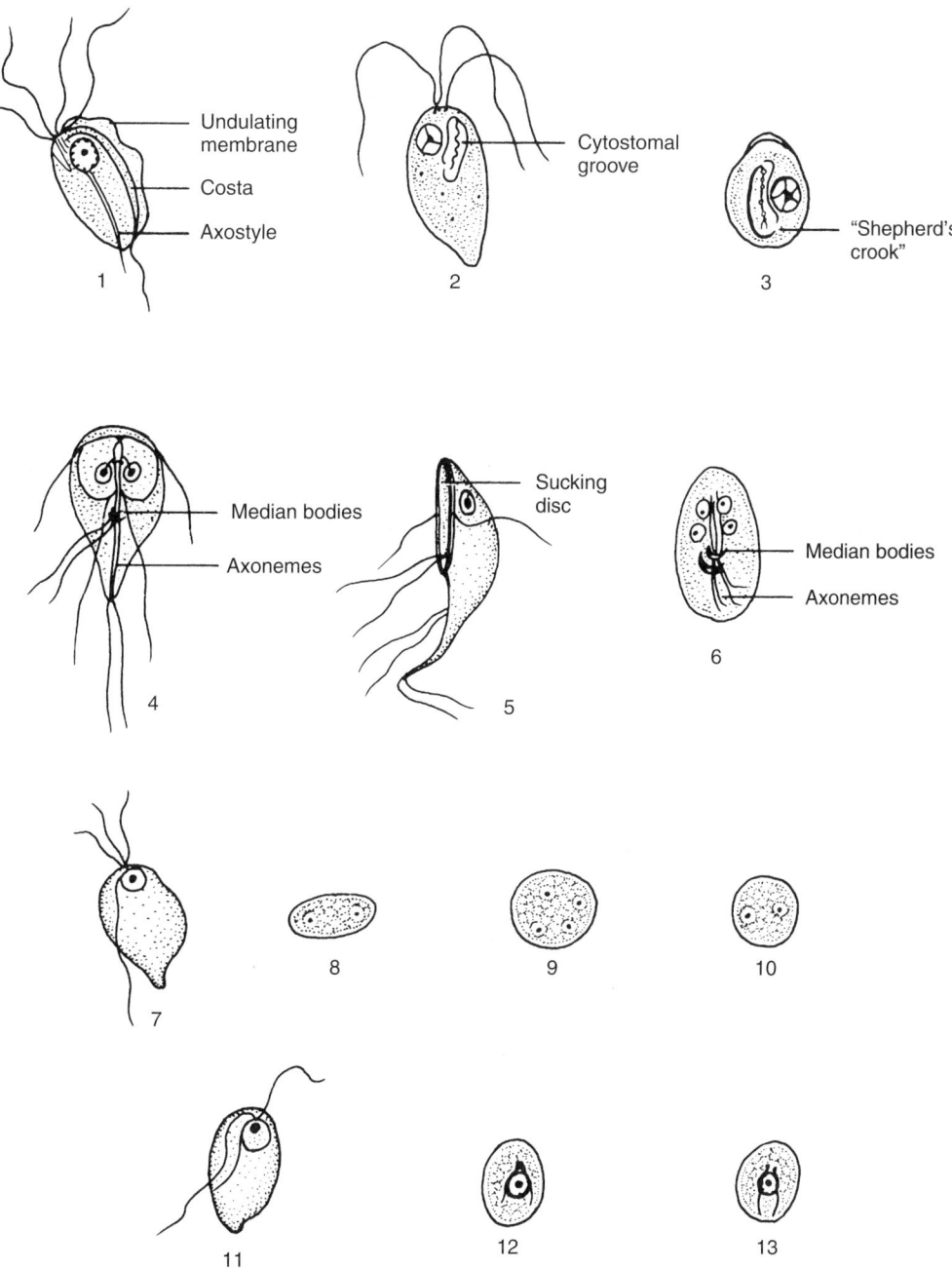

• **Fig. 47.18** (1) Trophozoite of *Pentatrichomonas hominis*. (2) Trophozoite of *Chilomastix mesnili*. (3) Cyst of *C. mesnili*. (4) Trophozoite of *Giardia duodenalis* (front view). (5) Trophozoite of *G. duodenalis* (side view). (6) Cyst of *G. duodenalis*. (7) Trophozoite of *Enteromonas hominis*. (8–10) Cysts of *E. hominis*. (11) Trophozoite of *Retortamonas intestinalis*. (12–13) Cysts of *R. intestinalis*. (From Garcia LS, Bruckner DA. *Diagnostic Medical Parasitology*. Washington, DC: ASM Press; 1993. Illustration 5 by Nobuko Kitamura. Illustrations 7-13 modified from Markell EK, Voge M. *Medical Parasitology*. 5th ed. Philadelphia: WB Saunders; 1981.)

longitudinal binary fission, producing two daughter trophozoites. The organism is found in the crypts in the duodenum. Trophozoites are the intestinal dwelling stage and attach to the epithelium of the host villi by means of the **ventral disk.** The attachment is substantial and results in disk "impression prints" when the organism detaches from the surface of the epithelium. Trophozoites may remain attached to or may detach from the mucosal surface. Because the epithelial surface sloughs off the tip of the villus every 72 hours, the trophozoites apparently detach at that time. *G. duodenalis* trophozoites are teardrop-shaped and have been described as "someone looking at you" (Figs. 47.18–47.20).

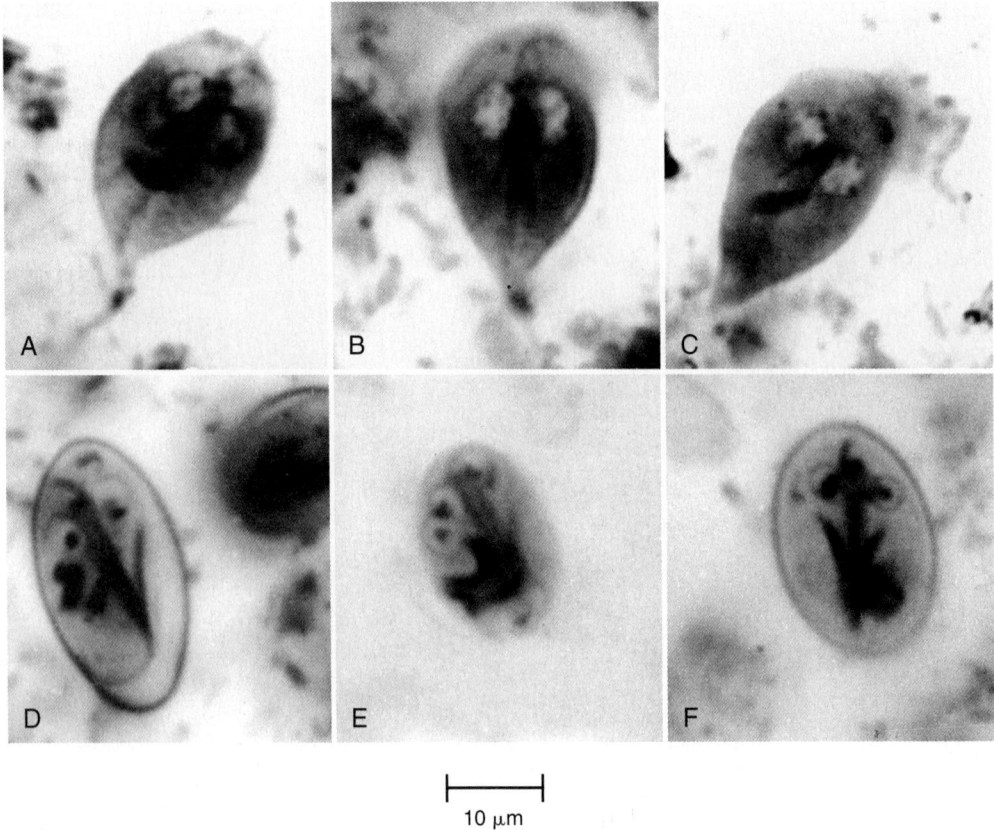

10 μm

• **Fig. 47.19** (A–C) Trophozoites of *Giardia duodenalis*. (D–F) Cysts of *G. duodenalis*.

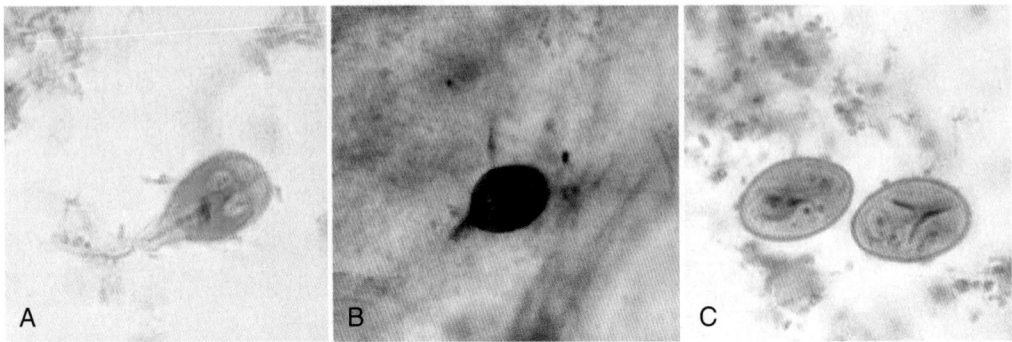

• **Fig. 47.20** (A) *Giardia duodenalis* trophozoite. (B) *G. duodenalis* trophozoite, iodine stain. (C) *G. duodenalis* cysts. (B, Courtesy Dr. Henry Travers, Sioux Falls, SD.)

Cyst formation takes place as the organisms move down through the jejunum after exposure to biliary secretions. The trophozoites retract the flagella into the axonemes, the cytoplasm becomes condensed, and the cyst wall is secreted (Figs. 47.18–47.20). As the cyst matures, the internal structures are doubled, so that when excystation occurs, the cytoplasm divides, producing two trophozoites. Excystation occurs in the duodenum or appropriate culture medium.

Epidemiology

Transmission of *G. duodenalis* occurs by ingestion of viable cysts. Although contaminated food or drink may be the source, intimate contact with an infected individual may also result in transmission of the organism. This organism is found more frequently in children or in groups living in close quarters. Outbreaks have been associated with poor sanitation facilities or sanitation breakdowns, as evidenced by infections of travelers and campers. Limited information is available on seasonal variations in giardiasis. Some data suggest an association with the cooler, wetter months of the year, which may implicate environmental conditions as advantageous to cyst survival. Certain occupations may place an individual at risk for infection, such as sewage and irrigation workers, who may be exposed to infective cysts. In situations in which young children are grouped together, such as in nursery schools, an increased incidence of exposure and subsequent infection of both children and staff members may be seen. A high incidence

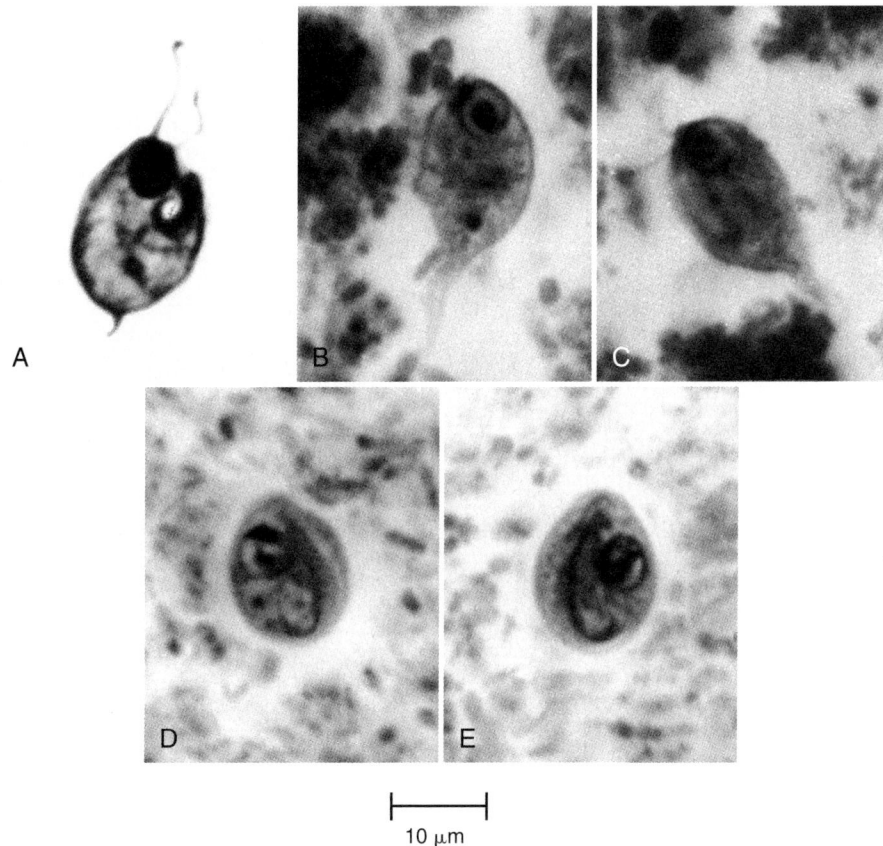

• **Fig. 47.21** (A–C) Trophozoites of *Chilomastix mesnili* (A, silver stain). (D and E) Cysts of *C. mesnili*.

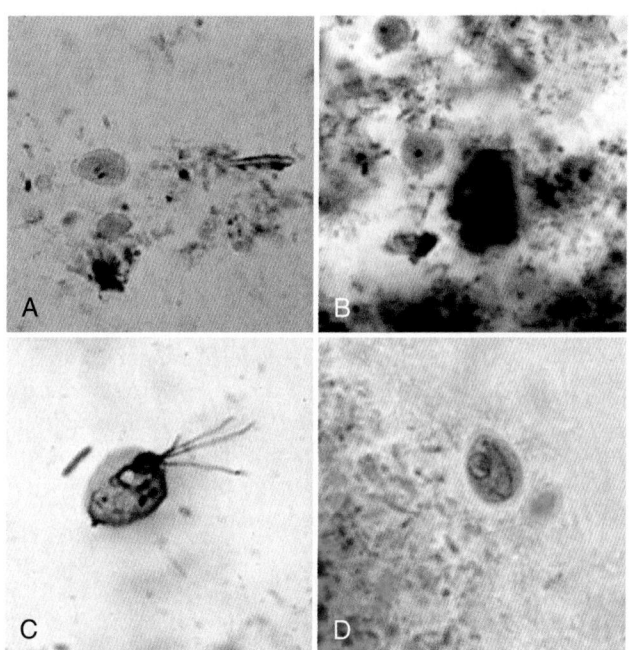

• **Fig. 47.22** (A) *Chilomastix mesnili* trophozoite (iodine stain). (B) *C. mesnili* cyst (iodine stain). (C) *C. mesnili* trophozoite (silver stain). (D) *C. mesnili* cyst. (A and B, Courtesy Dr. Henry Travers, Sioux Falls, SD.)

of giardiasis occurs in patients with immunodeficiency syndromes, particularly in those with common variable hypogammaglobulinemia. Giardiasis is the most common cause of diarrhea in these patients and may be associated with mild to severe villus atrophy.

Pathogenesis and Spectrum of Disease

The incubation period for giardiasis ranges from approximately 12 to 20 days. Giardiasis may not be recognized as the cause, because the infection mimics acute viral enteritis, bacillary dysentery, bacterial or other food poisonings, acute intestinal amebiasis, or "traveler's diarrhea" (toxigenic *Escherichia coli*). However, the type of diarrhea plus the lack of blood, mucus, and cellular exudate is consistent with giardiasis.

Asymptomatic Infection

Although the parasites in the crypts of the duodenal mucosa may reach very high numbers, they may not cause a pathologic condition. The organisms feed on the mucous secretions and do not penetrate the mucosa. Although organisms have been seen in biopsy material obtained from inside the intestinal mucosa, others have been seen attached to the epithelium.

Intestinal Disease

For unknown reasons, symptomatic patients may have irritation of the mucosal lining, increased mucus secretion, and dehydration. The onset of disease may be accompanied by nausea, anorexia, malaise, low-grade fever, and chills, in addition to a sudden onset of explosive, watery, foul-smelling diarrhea. Other symptoms include epigastric pain, flatulence, and diarrhea with increased amounts of fat and mucus in the stool but no blood. Weight loss often

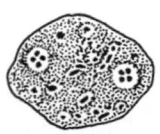 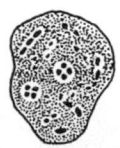 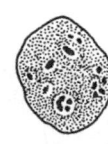

• **Fig. 47.23** Trophozoites of *Dientamoeba fragilis*.

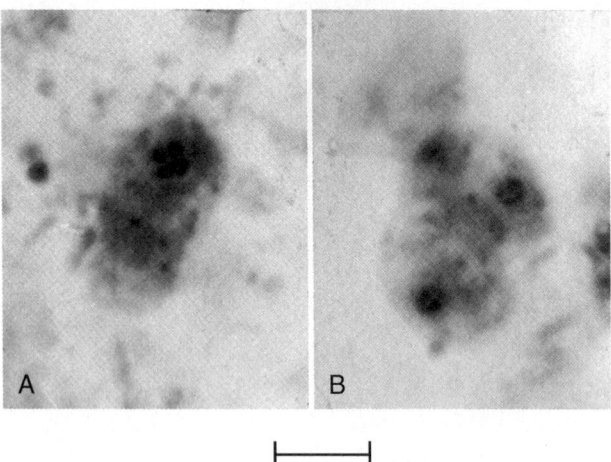

10 μm

• **Fig. 47.24** (A and B) Trophozoites of *Dientamoeba fragilis*.

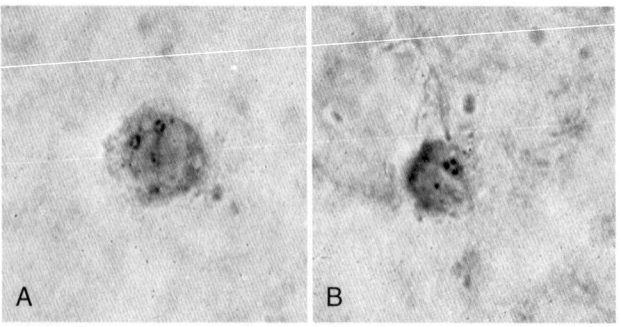

• **Fig. 47.25** (A) *Dientamoeba fragilis*, two nuclei. (B) *D. fragilis*, one nucleus.

accompanies these symptoms. Although some speculate that the organisms coating the mucosal lining may act to prevent fat absorption, this does not completely explain the prevention of the uptake of other substances normally absorbed at other intestinal levels. Severe malabsorption has been linked with isolated levothyroxine malabsorption, leading to severe hypothyroidism and secondary impairment of pancreatic function. In both cases, treatment with metronidazole led to complete remission of symptoms. Occasionally the gallbladder is involved, resulting in gallbladder colic and jaundice. *G. duodenalis* has been identified in bronchoalveolar lavage fluid.

Chronic Disease

The acute phase of infection is often followed by a subacute or chronic phase. Symptoms include recurrent, brief episodes of loose, foul-smelling stools and possibly increased distention and foul flatus. Between episodes of mushy stools, the patient may have normal stools or may be constipated.

Abdominal discomfort includes marked distention and belching with a rotten-egg taste. Chronic disease must be differentiated from amebiasis; disease caused by other intestinal parasites (e.g., *D. fragilis*, *Cryptosporidium* spp., *Cyclospora cayetanensis*, *Cystoisospora belli*, *Strongyloides stercoralis*); inflammatory bowel disease; and irritable colon. Based on symptoms such as upper intestinal discomfort, heartburn, and belching, giardiasis must be differentiated from duodenal ulcer, hiatal hernia, and gallbladder and pancreatic disease.

Antigenic Variation

Variation of the surface antigen during human infections with *G. duodenalis* has been documented. This capability suggests that variation may provide a mechanism for the organism to escape the host's immune response. The **variant-specific surface proteins (VSPs)** are a family of related, highly unusual proteins covering the surface of the organism. VSPs are resistant to the effects of intestinal proteases, which allows the parasites to survive in the protease-rich small intestine. Antigenic variation at the surface membrane of trophozoites is common; seemingly, the higher the rate of change, the more likely it is that a chronic infection would persist.

Laboratory Diagnosis

Routine Methods

Routine stool examinations are normally recommended for the recovery and identification of intestinal protozoa. However, in the case of *G. duodenalis*, because the organisms are attached securely to the mucosa by means of the sucking disk, a series of five or six stool samples may be examined without recovering the organism. The organisms also tend to be passed in the stool on a cyclic basis. The Entero-Test capsule can be helpful for recovering the organisms, as can the duodenal aspirate. Although cysts often can be identified on the wet stool preparation, many infections may be missed without examination of a permanent stained smear. If material from the string test (Entero-Test, HDC Corp., San Jose, CA) or mucus from a duodenal aspirate is submitted, it should be examined as a direct wet preparation for motility; however, motility may be represented by nothing more than a slight flutter of the flagella, because the organism is caught up in the mucus. After diagnosis, the positive specimen can be preserved as a permanent stain.

Antigen Detection

The development of fecal immunoassays to detect *Giardia* antigen in stool has dramatically improved the sensitivity seen with the routine O&P examination. The ELISA has been used to detect *Giardia* antigen in feces. Fluorescent methods with monoclonal antibodies have also proven extremely sensitive and specific in detecting *G. duodenalis* in fecal specimens. Other products are available as a cartridge format that uses an immunochromatographic strip–based detection system for *G. duodenalis* and/or *Cryptosporidium* spp. Any antigen detection system should always be reviewed for compatibility with stools submitted in preservatives rather than fresh specimens. Some limitations exist on the use of kits for organisms in the genus *Entamoeba.* However, commercial reagent kits for detecting *Giardia* and *Cryptosporidium* spp. can be used with formalin-based stool preservatives or with fresh or frozen specimens. Many of these cartridge format tests provide an answer within 10 minutes and are equal to or better than other immunoassays with regard to sensitivity and specificity. Many of the methods are being used to test patients suspected of having giardiasis or those who may be involved in an outbreak.

The detection of antigen in stool or visual identification of organisms by using monoclonal antibody reagents indicates current infection. The value of these detection assays as rapid, reliable immunodiagnostic procedures has been emphasized by the increase in *Giardia* infections and the greater awareness of particular incidences (e.g., nursery school settings). Because the organisms are shed so sporadically, use of a fecal immunoassay does not eliminate the need to analyze multiple stool specimens for sensitive detection of *G. duodenalis;* a minimum of two stools should be tested. If the first specimen is negative, it may represent a false negative.

Antibody Detection

Unfortunately, serodiagnostic procedures for antibody detection do not fulfill the criteria necessary for wide clinical use, particularly because they may indicate either past or present infection.

Histology

Trophozoites are detectable in the duodenum and proximal jejunum; however, mucosal invasion generally has been found in areas in which necrosis or mechanical trauma was present. Changes range from normal to almost complete villus atrophy, with a greater density of inflammatory infiltrate in the lamina propria when villus atrophy is present. The amount of villus damage seems to correlate with the degree of malabsorption. Apparently, patients with giardiasis also have reduced mucosal surface areas compared with control patients.

Histologic changes in the mucosal architecture in immunodeficient patients with giardiasis also range from mild to severe villus atrophy. It appears that giardiasis produces a more severe degree of villus damage in patients with hypogammaglobulinemia. In patients with acquired immunodeficiency syndrome (AIDS), giardiasis does not appear to be an important pathogen, although the infection has been identified in this group and in homosexual males.

Nucleic Acid Detection

There are three multiplex assays available in the United States to detect *G. duodenalis,* as previously discussed in this chapter.

Results and Reporting

It may be necessary to examine up to six stool specimens to rule out an infection with *Giardia* sp. This is because the organism remains securely attached to the intestinal mucosa, resulting in poor shedding or visibility in a stool specimen.

Organisms may also be passed intermittently or in cycles. A positive stool specimen does not require quantitation.

Prevention

The most effective practice for preventing the spread of infection in a childcare setting is thorough hand washing by the children, staff members, and visitors. Rubbing the hands together under running water is the most important part of washing away infectious organisms. Premoistened towelettes or wipes and waterless hand cleaners should not be used as substitutes for washing the hands with soap and running water. These guidelines are not limited to giardiasis but include all potentially infectious organisms.

Because wild animals and possibly domestic animals serve as reservoir hosts, personal hygiene, improved sanitary measures, and safe drinking water are considerations. Iodine has been recommended as an effective disinfectant for drinking water. Filtration systems have been recommended, although they have certain drawbacks, such as clogging.

Treatment

In most cases, treatment is not necessary, because infections are self-limiting; however, treatment will decrease the duration and prevent transmission to others. The treatments of choice include metronidazole, nitazoxanide, or tinidazole.

Chilomastix mesnili
General Characteristics

C. mesnili has both trophozoite and cyst stages and is somewhat more easily identified than are some of the smaller flagellates, such as *E. hominis* and *R. intestinalis* (Tables 47.3, 47.4 and Figs. 47.18 and 47.21). The *C. mesnili* trophozoite is pear-shaped, measuring 6 to 24 μm long and 4 to 8 μm wide. It has a single nucleus and a distinct oral groove, or **cytostome** (mouth), close to the nucleus. Flagella are difficult to see without obvious motility in a direct wet preparation. The morphology can be seen on the permanent stained smear; the cytostome may be visible in some trophozoites. The cysts are pear- or lemon-shaped and range from 6 to 10 μm long and 4 to 6 μm wide (Figs. 47.21 and 47.22). They have a single nucleus and a typical curved cytostomal fibril, called the **shepherd's crook.** The cyst's definitive morphology can be seen on a permanent stain.

Epidemiology

C. mesnili tends to have a cosmopolitan distribution, although it is found more commonly in warm climates. Transmission occurs through ingestion of infective cysts.

Pathogenesis and Spectrum of Disease

C. mesnili is considered nonpathogenic and does not cause disease.

Laboratory Diagnosis

Although cysts sometimes can be seen in a wet preparation, definitive identification of *C. mesnili* relies on examination of permanent stained smears.

Therapy

Specific treatment is not recommended for *C. mesnili*. Because these nonpathogenic organisms are acquired through fecal-oral contamination, both pathogens and nonpathogens can be found in the same patient. If few organisms are present, extended microscopic examination and multiple organism measurements are required for definitive identification. It is always important to report pathogens and nonpathogens, because they are acquired the same way.

Prevention

Prevention depends on adequate disposal of human excreta and improved personal hygiene, preventive measures that apply to most of the intestinal protozoa.

Dientamoeba fragilis
General Characteristics

D. fragilis has a worldwide distribution, and surveys report incidence rates of 1.4% to 19%. Much higher incidence figures have been reported for patients in mental institutions, missionaries, and Native Americans in Arizona. *D. fragilis* tends to be common in some pediatric populations, and the incidence is higher for patients younger than 20 years in some studies. Some speculate that *D. fragilis* may be infrequently recovered and identified; a low incidence or absence from survey studies may be a result of poor laboratory techniques and a general lack of knowledge about the organism.

The *D. fragilis* trophozoite is characterized as having one nucleus (20% to 40%) or two nuclei (60% to 80%). The nuclear chromatin usually is fragmented into three to five granules, and normally no peripheral chromatin is seen on the nuclear membrane. In some organisms, the nuclear chromatin tends to mimic that of *E. nana, E. hartmanni,* or even *C. mesnili,* particularly if the organisms are overstained with trichrome or iron-hematoxylin stain. The cytoplasm is usually vacuolated and may contain ingested debris and some large, uniform granules. The cytoplasm can also appear uniform and clean with few inclusions. Size and shape vary considerably among organisms, even on a single smear. The cyst has a distinct cell wall with a clear zone around the cyst that includes an axostyle, flagellar axonemes, and a costa. Cysts generally contain two nucleic with a large central karyosome. A precystic stage exists that is a compact spherical structure about half the size of a trophozoite. The cysts are rarely found in clinical samples.

Epidemiology

The transmission of *D. fragilis* has been postulated as associated with helminth eggs (e.g., *Ascaris* and *Enterobius* spp.) (Figs. 47.23–47.25). A cyst stage has been identified, although rarely present in clinical samples, and indicates that fecal-oral transmission occurs (Tables 47.3 and 47.4).

Pathogenesis and Spectrum of Disease

D. fragilis has been associated with a wide range of symptoms. Case reports of children infected with *D. fragilis* reveal a number of symptoms, including intermittent diarrhea, abdominal pain, nausea, anorexia, malaise, fatigue, poor weight gain, and unexplained eosinophilia. The most common symptoms in patients infected with this parasite appear to be intermittent diarrhea and fatigue. In some patients, both the organism and the symptoms persist or reappear until appropriate treatment is initiated.

Laboratory Diagnosis
Routine Methods

Diagnosis of *D. fragilis* infections depends on proper collection and processing techniques (a minimum of three fecal specimens). Although the survival time for this parasite has been reported as 24 to 48 hours in the trophozoite form, the survival time in terms of morphology is limited, and stool specimens must be examined immediately or preserved in a suitable fixative soon after defecation. It is particularly important to examine permanent stained smears of stool with an oil immersion objective (×100). The trophozoites have been recovered in formed stool; therefore, a permanent stained smear must be prepared for every stool sample submitted for examination. Organisms seen in direct wet mounts may appear as refractile, round forms that may actually represent the cysts or precystic forms; the nuclear structure cannot be seen without examination of the permanent stained smear.

Antigen Detection

Although fecal immunoassays for antigen detection are not yet available commercially, they have been developed using several test formats. Detection of deoxyribonucleic acid (DNA) from feces is being used in some laboratories.

Antibody Detection

On indirect immunofluorescence assay, serum samples from patients with confirmed *D. fragilis* infections showed positive titers, and all matched controls had positive titers ranging from 20 to 160. However, these tests are not routinely used, nor are the reagents commercially available.

Therapy

Although treatment is not generally recommended for infections with nonpathogenic flagellates, clinical improvement has been seen in adults receiving tetracycline, and symptomatic relief has been observed in children receiving diiodohydroxyquin, metronidazole, or tetracycline. Current recommendations include iodoquinol, paromomycin, or tetracycline. Although limited studies have been undertaken on the efficacy of various therapies, information continues to support the finding that elimination of this organism from symptomatic patients leads to clinical improvement. Treatment of *D. fragilis* infection with iodoquinol, paromomycin, or combination therapy results in eradication of the parasite and complete resolution of symptoms.

Prevention

Fecal-oral transmission has been documented. Therefore, transmission from ingestion of certain helminth eggs, or the fecal-oral route, indicate that the appropriate hygiene and sanitary measures to prevent contamination with fecal material are useful for the prevention of infection with *D. fragilis*, as with other intestinal parasites.

Pentatrichomonas hominis

P. hominis is probably the most commonly identified flagellate, other than *G. duodenalis* and *D. fragilis*. *P. hominis* has been recovered from all parts of the world, in both warm and temperate climates, and is considered nonpathogenic and noninvasive. It is not known to have a cyst stage (Fig. 47.18). *P. hominis* trophozoites live in the cecum and feed on bacteria. The trophozoite measures 5 to 15 μm long and 7 to 10 μm wide. It has a pyriform shape and has both an **axostyle** and an undulating membrane, which aid identification of the organism. The undulating membrane extends the entire length of the body, in contrast to that seen in the pathogen *T. vaginalis* (on which the membrane extends halfway down the body).

Epidemiology

Because *P. hominis* is not known to have a cyst stage, transmission probably occurs in the trophic form. If ingested in a substance such as milk, these organisms apparently can survive passage through the stomach and small intestine in patients with achlorhydria. *P. hominis* cannot be transplanted into the vagina, the natural habitat of *T. vaginalis*. The incidence of this organism is relatively low, but it tends to be recovered more often than *E. hominis* or *R. intestinalis*, two small nonpathogenic flagellates that are rarely seen and extremely difficult to identify (Fig. 47.18).

Pathogenesis and Spectrum of Disease

P. hominis is considered nonpathogenic and does not cause disease.

Laboratory Diagnosis

P. hominis trophozoites can sometimes be seen on a permanent stained smear, but definitive identification can be difficult. However, it is important to report the presence of the organism if seen.

Therapy

Specific treatment is not recommended for this nonpathogen.

Prevention

Prevention depends on adequate disposal of human excreta and improved personal hygiene, preventive measures that apply to most of the intestinal protozoa.

Retortamonas intestinalis

Retortamonas intestinalis is a small oval to elongated pyriform trophozoite. The trophozoite has a cystome that may not be evident, and the cyst stage is pear shaped. Both life cycle stages have a single nucleus. The organism is transmitted by the fecal-oral route; however, it is considered nonpathogenic, and therefore treatment is not warranted.

Ciliates

The class Ciliata, or ciliates, include species that move by means of **cilia,** or short extensions of cytoplasm that cover the surface of the organism. The ciliates also have two different types of nuclei, one **macronucleus** and one or more **micronuclei.** This group includes only one organism that infects humans, *Neobalantidium coli,* which infects the intestinal tract and may produce severe symptoms. Using current molecular techniques, the classification of this organism has been revised, although there seems to be discrepancy in the literature listing the organism as *Balantidium, Neobalantidium,* or *Balanitides coli.* An extensive molecular analysis was completed by Pomajbíková et al. (2013) which supports the new taxonomic designation of *Neobalantidium coli* (previously *Balantidium coli*).

Neobalantidium coli
General Characteristics

The life cycle of *N. coli* includes both the trophozoite and cyst stages (Fig. 47.26). The cyst form is the infective stage. After ingestion of the cysts and excystation, trophozoites secrete hyaluronidase, which aids the invasion of the colonic tissue.

The trophozoite is quite large, oval, and covered with short cilia. It measures approximately 50 to 150 μm long and 40 to 70 μm wide. The organism can be seen in a wet preparation on lower power. The anterior end is somewhat pointed and has a cytostome (primitive mouth opening); in contrast, the posterior end is broadly rounded. The cytoplasm contains many vacuoles with ingested bacteria and debris. The trophozoite has two nuclei: one very large, bean-shaped macronucleus and a smaller, round micronucleus. The organisms live in the large intestine. The trophozoites have a rapid, rotatory, boring motion because of the movement of the cilia. The cyst is formed as the trophozoite moves down the intestine. Nuclear division does not occur in the cyst; therefore, only two nuclei are present, the macronucleus and the micronucleus. The cysts measure 50 to 70 μm in diameter (Table 47.5).

Epidemiology

N. coli is widely distributed in hogs, particularly in warm and temperate climates, and in monkeys in the tropics. Human infection is found in warmer climates, sporadically in cooler areas, and in institutionalized groups with low levels of personal hygiene.

Pathogenesis and Spectrum of Disease

Some individuals with *N. coli* infection are asymptomatic, whereas others have severe dysentery, similar to that seen in patients with amebiasis. Symptoms include diarrhea or dysentery, tenesmus, nausea, vomiting, anorexia, and headache. Insomnia, muscular weakness, and weight loss have been reported. Diarrhea may persist for weeks to months, with or without subsequent development of dysentery. Tremendous fluid loss may occur, with diarrhea similar to that seen in cholera or in some coccidial or microsporidial infections.

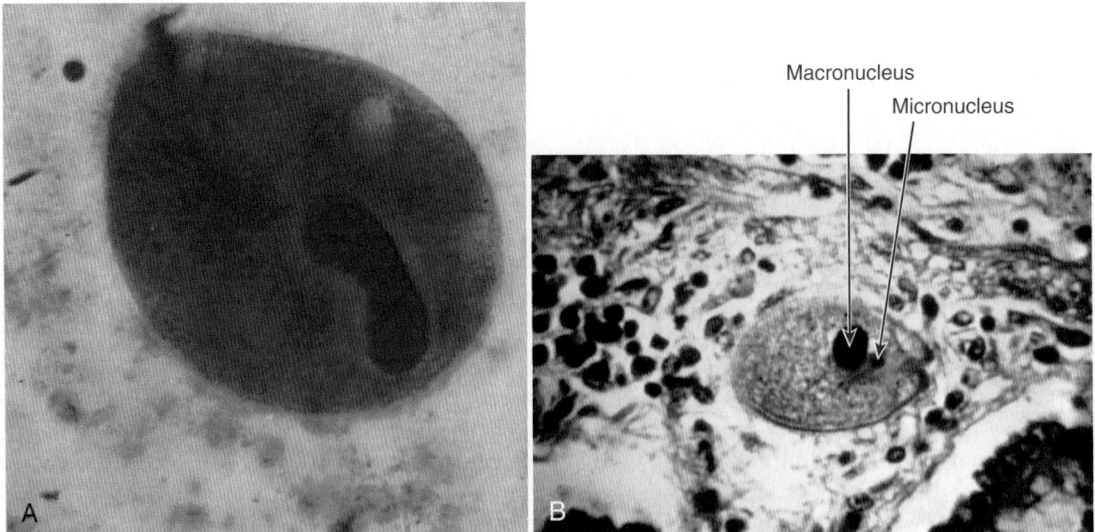

• **Fig. 47.26** (A) *Neobalantidium coli* trophozoite. (B) *N. coli* trophozoite. (B, Courtesy Dr. Henry Travers, Sioux Falls, SD.)

N. coli can invade tissue. It may penetrate the mucosa on contact, with cellular infiltration in the area of the developing ulcer. Some of the abscess formations may extend to the muscular layer. The ulcers may vary in shape, and the ulcer bed may be full of pus and necrotic debris. The organism has been reported to migrate from the intestine to the lungs causing a pneumonia-like illness in immunocompromised patients. Although the number of cases is small, extraintestinal disease (peritonitis, urinary tract infection, and inflammatory vaginitis) has been reported.

Laboratory Diagnosis

Routine stool examinations, particularly direct wet preparation examinations of fresh and concentrated material, demonstrate the presence of organisms. Organism recognition and identification on a permanent stained smear is usually difficult. These protozoa are large and stain very darkly, which obscures any internal morphology. *N. coli* organisms may be confused with helminth eggs or debris because of their size, particularly when the cilia are not visible. Recovery of *N. coli* from specimens in the United States is rare. However, laboratories should be able to identify these organisms in proficiency testing specimens.

Results Reporting

As previously noted, the organism is rarely identified, and care should be taken to not confuse the parasite with contaminating debris.

Therapy

Tetracycline is the drug of choice for treating *N. coli* infection, although it is considered investigational for this infection. Iodoquinol or metronidazole may be used as an alternative. Nitazoxanide, a broad-spectrum antiparasitic drug, may be another alternative.

Prevention

In areas where pigs are raised, the incidence of human infection can be quite high in pig farmers and slaughterhouse workers. Human infection is fairly rare in temperate areas, although infections can develop into an epidemic, particularly in areas of poor environmental sanitation and personal hygiene. This situation has been seen in mental hospitals in the United States. Preventive measures involve increased attention to personal hygiene and sanitation measures, because the mode of transmission is ingestion of infective cysts through contaminated food or water.

Sporozoa (Apicomplexa)

All the Apicomplexa are unicellular and have an **apical complex.** These structures can be seen in electron microscopy (EM) studies and are used to help classify the various organisms. Genera that develop in the gastrointestinal tract of vertebrates throughout their entire life cycle include *Cystoisospora, Cyclospora,* and *Cryptosporidium.* Genera capable of or requiring extraintestinal development are referred to as **cyst-forming coccidia;** they include *Sarcocystis* and *Toxoplasma* spp. The genera that cause disease in humans include *Cryptosporidium, Cyclospora, Cystoisospora, Sarcocystis,* and *Toxoplasma* (see Chapter 49 for a discussion of *Toxoplasma*).

Cryptosporidium spp.
General Characteristics

Cryptosporidium spp. are intracellular parasites that primarily infect epithelial cells of the stomach, intestine, and biliary ducts. The organism previously called *Cryptosporidium parvum,* thought to be the primary *Cryptosporidium* species infecting humans, now is classified as two species, *C. parvum* (mammals, including humans) and *Cryptosporidium hominis* (primarily humans) (Figs. 47.27 and 47.28, and

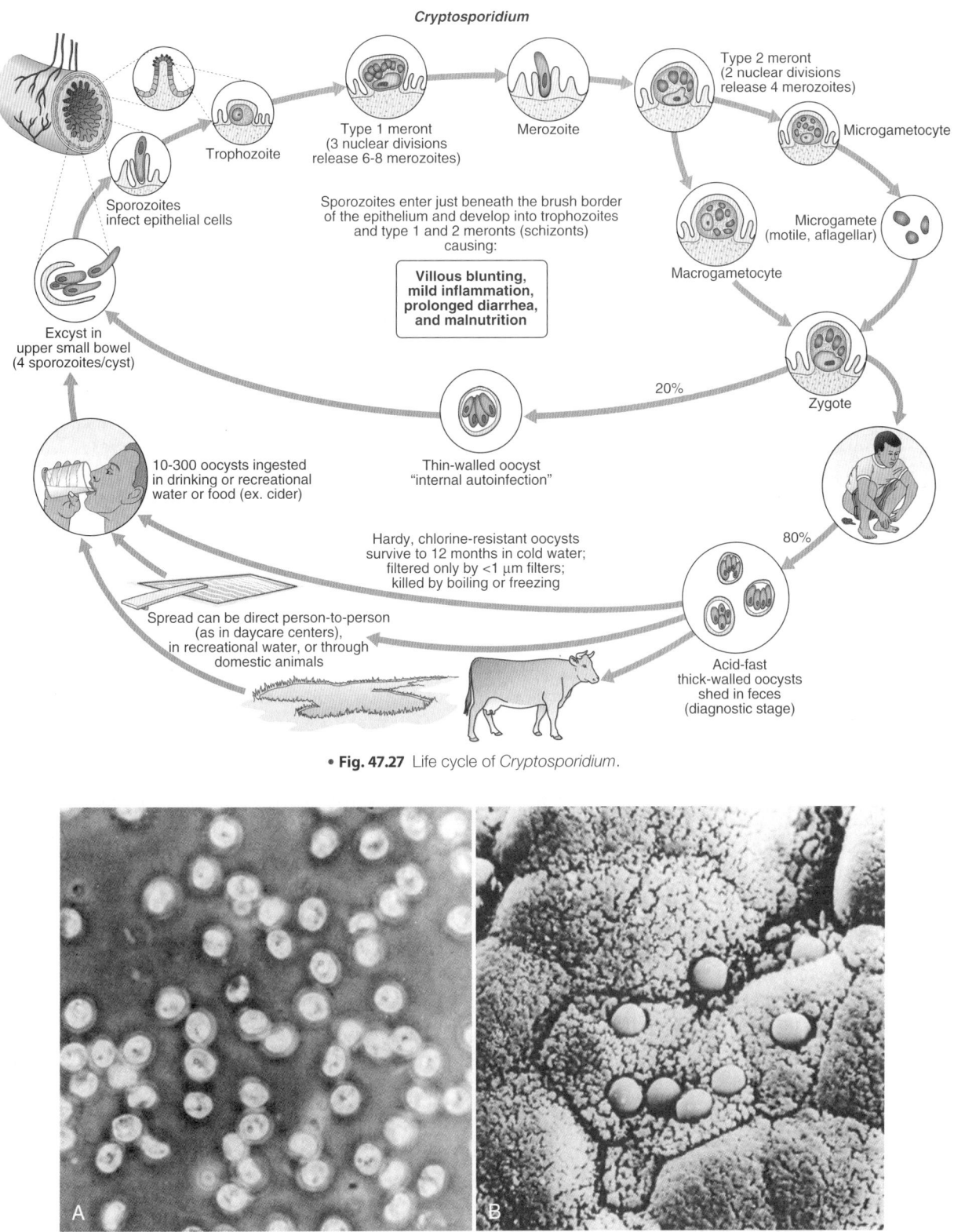

Cryptosporidium

Trophozoite

Sporozoites
infect epithelial cells

Type 1 meront
(3 nuclear divisions
release 6-8 merozoites)

Merozoite

Type 2 meront
(2 nuclear divisions
release 4 merozoites)

Microgametocyte

Sporozoites enter just beneath the brush border
of the epithelium and develop into trophozoites
and type 1 and 2 meronts (schizonts)
causing:

**Villous blunting,
mild inflammation,
prolonged diarrhea,
and malnutrition**

Microgamete
(motile, aflagellar)

Macrogametocyte

Excyst in
upper small bowel
(4 sporozoites/cyst)

20%

Zygote

Thin-walled oocyst
"internal autoinfection"

80%

10-300 oocysts ingested
in drinking or recreational
water or food (ex. cider)

Hardy, chlorine-resistant oocysts
survive to 12 months in cold water;
filtered only by <1 μm filters;
killed by boiling or freezing

Acid-fast
thick-walled oocysts
shed in feces
(diagnostic stage)

Spread can be direct person-to-person
(as in daycare centers),
in recreational water, or through
domestic animals

• **Fig. 47.27** Life cycle of *Cryptosporidium*.

• **Fig. 47.28** *Cryptosporidium*. (A) Oocysts recovered from a Sheather's sugar flotation; organisms measure 4 to 6 μm. (B) Scanning electron microscopy view of organisms at brush border of epithelial cells. (From Garcia LS, Bruckner DA. *Diagnostic Medical Parasitology*. Washington, DC: ASM Press; 1993.)

Table 47.6). Differentiation of these two species based on oocyst morphology is not possible. Currently, more than 20 established *Cryptosporidium* spp. have been reported in humans in immunocompetent and immunocompromised individuals.

Cryptosporidium infections begin with ingestion of viable oocysts (Fig. 47.27). Upon contact with gastric and duodenal fluid, each **oocyst** releases four **sporozoites,** which invade the epithelial cells and develop into trophozoites surrounded by a **parasitophorous vacuole** (layers of endoplasmic reticulum around an intracellular parasite). In the epithelial cells, trophozoites undergo two or three generations of asexual amplification, called **merogony,** leading to the formation of different types of **meronts** containing four to eight **merozoites.** The merozoites differentiate into sexually distinct stages in a process called **gametogony.** New oocysts are formed in the epithelial cells in a process called **sporogony.** About 20% of the oocysts are thin-walled and may excyst in the digestive tract of the host, leading to the infection of new cells (**autoinfection**). The remaining 80% of the oocysts are excreted into the environment; are resistant to low temperature, high salinity, and most disinfectants; and can initiate infection in a new host. *Cryptosporidium* oocysts in humans measure 4 to 6 μm in diameter.

Epidemiology

Humans can acquire cryptosporidiosis through several transmission routes, such as direct contact with infected people or animals or consumption of contaminated water (drinking or recreational) or food. The interval between ingestion of infective oocysts to completion of the life cycle and excretion of new oocysts usually is 4 to 10 days. The only extracellular stage in the *Cryptosporidium* life cycle is the oocysts; these are the environmental stage of the parasite and are immediately infectious when passed in the stool (Fig. 47.28).

Cryptosporidium spp. have a worldwide distribution, and the oocysts are ubiquitous in the environment. In developing countries, human *Cryptosporidium* infection occurs mostly in children younger than 5 years, with peak occurrence of infections and diarrhea in children younger than 2 years. In developed countries, pediatric cryptosporidiosis occurs in older children, probably because, due to better hygiene, exposure to contaminated environments occurs later. Cryptosporidiosis is also common in the elderly in nursing homes, where person-to-person transmission occurs. In the general population, sporadic infections occur in all age groups in the United States and the United Kingdom, and traveling to developing countries and consumption of contaminated food and water can lead to infection. Cryptosporidiosis is common in immunocompromised individuals, such as those with AIDS or primary immunodeficiency and cancer and transplant patients undergoing immunosuppressive therapy.

Calves and perhaps other animals serve as potential sources of human infection. Contact with these animals may be an unrecognized cause of gastroenteritis in humans in both rural and urban settings. Direct person-to-person transmission is also likely and may occur through direct or indirect contact with stool material. Direct transmission may occur during sexual practices involving oral-anal contact. Nucleic acid sequence analyses of the *gp60* (glycoprotein) gene for epidemiologic determination has indicated that human infections of *C. parvum* are not zoonotic. There are two major subtypes, IIa and IIc. The first subtype has been identified in humans and ruminants, therefore suggesting potential zoonotic transmission. The latter, IIc, has only been identified in humans and is therefore limited as a human (**anthroponotic**) pathogen. Subtype infection rates in humans varies geographically. Both IIa and IIc have been identified in human cases in developing countries; a third subtype, IId, has been identified in humans in the Middle Eastern countries. Indirect transmission may occur through exposure to positive specimens in a laboratory setting or from contaminated surfaces, food, or water.

Pathogenesis and Spectrum of Disease
Immunocompetent Individuals

In immunocompetent people with sporadic cryptosporidiosis in industrialized nations, the most common symptom is diarrhea. Clinical symptoms include nausea; low-grade fever; abdominal cramps; anorexia; and 5 to 10 watery, frothy bowel movements per day, which may be followed by constipation. Some patients may have diarrhea, and others may have few symptoms, particularly later in the course of the infection. In patients with the typical watery diarrhea, the stool contains mainly water and mucus. Often the organisms are entrapped in the mucus, and diagnostic procedures are performed accordingly. Generally, a patient with a normal immune system has a self-limited infection; however, patients who are immunocompromised may have a chronic infection with a wide range of symptoms. The illness usually lasts 9 to 21 days and may require hospitalization in up to 20% of those infected. Patients infected with *C. hominis* are more likely to have joint pain, eye pain, recurrent headache, dizziness, and fatigue than those infected with *C. parvum*.

Immunocompromised Individuals

Hemodialysis patients with chronic renal failure and renal transplant patients with cryptosporidiosis can have chronic, life-threatening diarrhea. In individuals infected with the human immunodeficiency virus (HIV), cryptosporidiosis increases as the CD4+ lymphocyte count falls, especially below 200 cells/μL. Sclerosing cholangitis and other biliary involvement are also seen in AIDS patients with cryptosporidiosis. The combination of AIDS and cryptosporidiosis often leads to increased mortality. In these patients, *Cryptosporidium* infections are not always confined to the gastrointestinal tract; additional symptoms (respiratory problems, cholecystitis, hepatitis, and pancreatitis) have been associated with extraintestinal infections. Although the clinical features of sclerosing cholangitis secondary to opportunistic infections of the biliary tree in patients with AIDS are well known, the mechanisms by which pathogens such as *Cryptosporidium* spp. cause disease are unclear.

Laboratory Diagnosis
Routine Methods

Oocysts in clinical specimens are difficult to see without special staining techniques, such as the modified acid-fast, Ziehl-Neelsen or Kinyoun's, or Giemsa method, or the newer immunoassay methods. Oocysts appear bright red to purple against a blue or green background when stained using a modified acid-fast stain. The four sporozoites may be seen in the oocyst in some of the organisms, although they are not always visible in freshly passed specimens.

Antigen Detection

Immunoassays are very helpful, because they are a more sensitive method of detecting organisms in stool specimens. A direct fluorescent antigen (FA) procedure with excellent specificity and sensitivity has been developed and results in a significantly increased detection rate over conventional staining and microscopy methods. Some of these reagents, particularly the combination direct FA product used to identify both *Giardia* spp. cysts and *Cryptosporidium* spp. oocysts, are being widely used in water testing and outbreak situations (Fig. 47.29). Most antibodies in commercial direct fluorescent antibody (DFA) kits react with oocysts of almost all *Cryptosporidium* species, making identification to the species level impossible. EIA tests also provide excellent specificity and sensitivity for laboratories using this approach, as do the immunochromatographic cartridge rapid test formats. However, high false-positive rates have been reported in rapid diagnostic tests. It is important to remember that if a patient is in the carrier state or undergoing self-cure, the number of oocysts may drop below the sensitivity levels of these kits. The inability to detect other *Cryptosporidium* spp. other than *C. hominis* and *C. parvum* may thus produce a false-negative result. Positive rapid diagnostic tests should be confirmed with additional testing and negative tests should be interpreted with caution and correlated with the patient's clinical presentation.

Nucleic Acid Detection

Molecular techniques, especially PCR and PCR-related methods, have been used to detect and differentiate *Cryptosporidium* spp., and a few of the PCR assays are commercially available. Several genus-specific PCR-restriction fragment length polymorphism–based genotyping tools have been developed for detecting and differentiating *Cryptosporidium* organisms at the species level. Other genotyping techniques are designed mostly for differentiation of *C. parvum* and *C. hominis* and cannot detect and differentiate other *Cryptosporidium* spp. or genotypes. Currently, three FDA-approved assays are available for the detection of *Cryptosporidium* in the United States: the xTAG Gastrointestinal Pathogen Panel, the FilmArray System GI Panel (BioFire Diagnostics, Salt Lake City, UT) and the BD MAX enteric parasite panel (Becton Dickinson Company, Sparks, MD) as previously noted.

Antibody Detection

In the United States, drinking untreated surface water has been identified as a risk factor for cryptosporidiosis; residents living in cities with surface-derived drinking water generally have higher antibody levels against *Cryptosporidium* spp. in their blood than those living in cities with ground water as drinking water. However, antibody detection is not available on a routine basis and currently is not used in the diagnosis of cryptosporidiosis.

Histology

In the examination of histologic preparations, developmental stages (sporozoites, trophozoites, merozoites, and oocysts) in the life cycle of *Cryptosporidium* spp. can be found at all levels of the intestinal tract, with the jejunum being the most heavily infected site. Routine hematoxylin and eosin staining is sufficient to demonstrate these parasites. Under regular light microscopy, the organisms are visible as small, round structures (about 1 to 3 µm in diameter) aligned along the brush border. They are intracellular but extracytoplasmic and are found in parasitophorous vacuoles. Developmental stages are more difficult to identify without a transmission electron microscope. It also is important to remember that in severely compromised patients, *Cryptosporidium* spp. have been found in other body sites, primarily the lungs, as a disseminated infection.

Results Reporting

Cryptosporidiosis is a reportable disease in the United States. An increase in reported cases may indicate an outbreak. Identification of oocysts in a patient's stool should be reported as *Cryptosporidium* positive. A positive antigen test should be reported as *Cryptosporidium*-presumptive with additional follow-up testing. Positive diagnosis should be referred to the appropriate public health laboratory for confirmation.

Therapy

Oral or intravenous rehydration and antimotility drugs are used whenever severe diarrhea is associated with cryptosporidiosis. Nitazoxanide is the only drug approved by the FDA for the treatment of cryptosporidiosis in immunocompetent individuals. This drug can shorten the clinical disease and reduce the number of parasites present. However, nitazoxanide is not effective in treating cryptosporidiosis in immunodeficient patients; paromomycin and spiramycin have been used in these individuals.

In industrialized nations, the most effective prophylaxis and treatment for cryptosporidiosis in patients with AIDS is

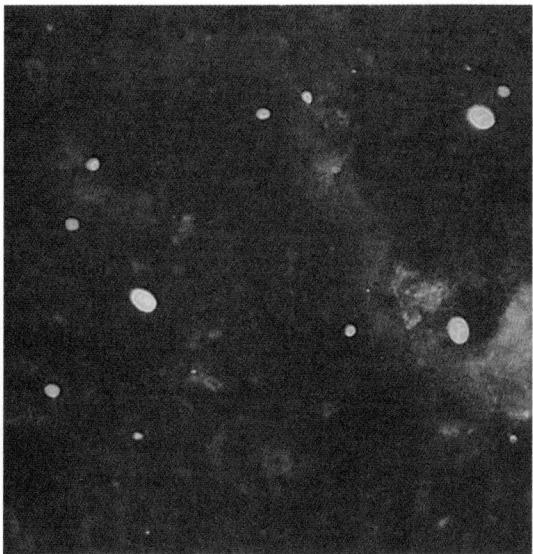

• **Fig. 47.29** *Cryptosporidium* oocysts and *Giardia* cysts stained with monoclonal antibody–conjugated fluorescent reagent. (Courtesy Merifluor, Meridian Diagnostics, Cincinnati, OH.)

highly active antiretroviral therapy (HAART). Eradication and prevention of the infection are related to replenishment of CD4+ cells in treated individuals and the antiparasitic activities of the protease inhibitors used in HAART. Relapse of cryptosporidiosis is common in patients with AIDS who have stopped HAART.

Prevention

Effective concentrations of most substances used for disinfection are not practical outside the laboratory, and high concentrations that significantly reduce oocyst infectivity are either very expensive or quite toxic. *Cryptosporidium* oocysts are highly resistant to most commercial disinfectants, including iodine water purification tablets. Although chlorine and related compounds can dramatically reduce the ability of oocysts to excyst or infect, high concentrations and long exposure times are required, making this approach impractical.

Cyclospora cayetanensis
General Characteristics

During the past few years, a number of outbreaks of diarrhea associated with *Cyclospora cayetanensis* have occurred;

the distribution is worldwide (United States, Caribbean, Central and South America, Southeast Asia, Eastern Europe, Australia, Nepal). These organisms are acid-fast variable and have been found in the feces of immunocompetent travelers to developing countries, immunocompetent individuals with no travel history, and patients with AIDS.

The life cycle of *C. cayetanensis* involves only humans as hosts. Oocysts are passed in the feces unsporulated (Fig. 47.30A). At room temperature (23°C to 25°C), small numbers of oocysts may sporulate within 10 to 12 days.

In clean wet mounts, *Cyclospora* organisms are seen as nonrefractile spheres, which are difficult to recognize as parasites. Unless a high number of oocysts are present, they may easily be mistaken for artifacts. They are acid-fast variable with the modified acid-fast stain; those that are unstained appear as glassy, wrinkled spheres (wrinkled cellophane). The oocysts are twice the size of those of *Cryptosporidium* spp. and measure 8 to 10 μm in diameter. Because it takes 10 days to 2 weeks for the oocysts to sporulate, no internal structures are visible (sporozoites), as can be seen in *Cryptosporidium* organisms.

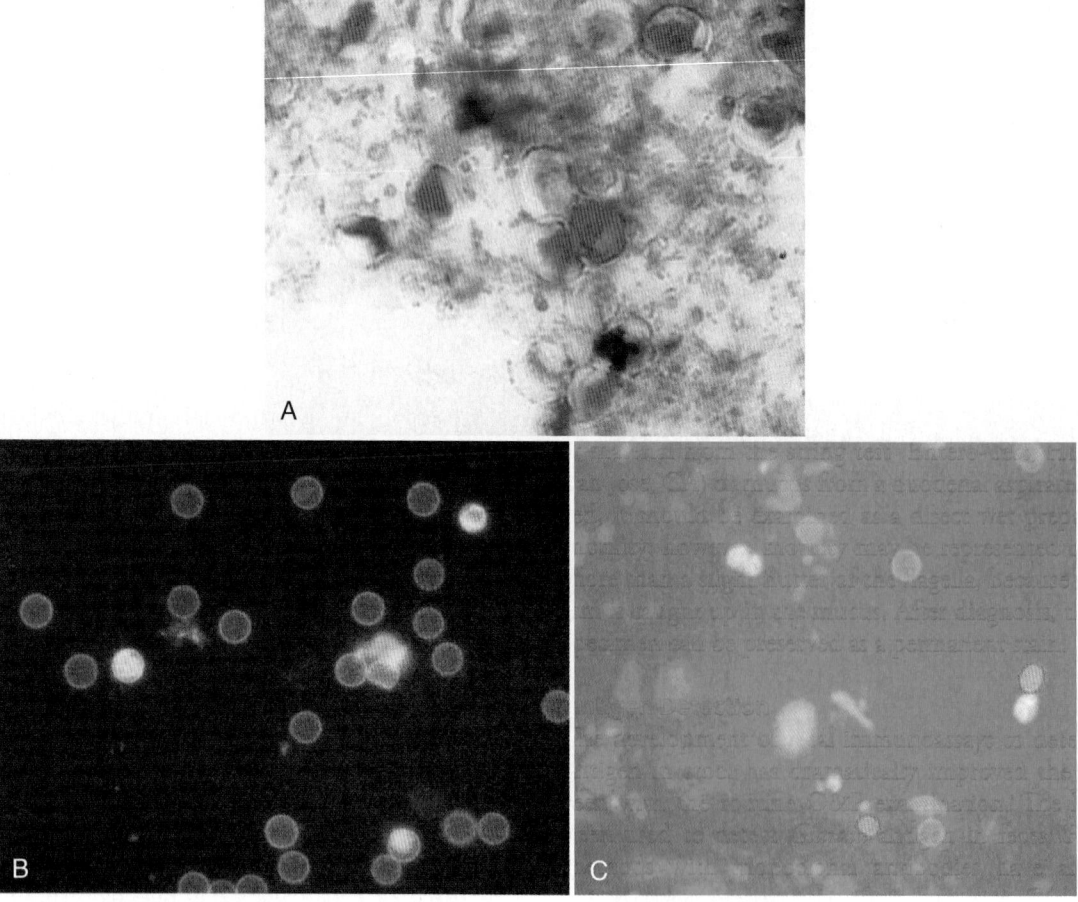

• **Fig. 47.30** (A) *Cyclospora cayetanensis* oocysts after modified acid-fast staining. Note the variability in the intensity of the stain. These oocysts measure 8 to 10 μm, twice the size of *Cryptosporidium* spp. (oil immersion, ×1000). (B and C) *Cyclospora cayetanensis* oocysts exhibiting autofluorescence (high dry power, ×400). (A and B, Courtesy Charles R. Sterling, University of Arizona. C, Courtesy E. Long, Centers for Disease Control and Prevention, Atlanta, GA.)

Epidemiology

Transmission of *C. cayetanensis* is by the fecal-oral route and often correlated with the ingestion of contaminated fruits and vegetables. However, direct person-to-person transmission has not been well documented and may not be a factor, because sporulation takes a number of days. Information on reservoir hosts is not well defined; however, in some areas humans appear to be the only host.

C. cayetanensis is endemic in Central and South America, the Caribbean, Mexico, Indonesia, Asia, Nepal, Africa, India, Southern Europe, and the Middle East. In endemic areas, contact with soil and water increases the risk of *Cyclospora* infection. Infections in most temperate areas correlate with the consumption of imported contaminated fruits and vegetables.

Pathogenesis and Spectrum of Disease

Although some patients are asymptomatic, others report a flulike illness, marked by nausea, vomiting, anorexia, weight loss, and explosive diarrhea lasting 1 to 3 weeks. The incubation period is not yet known. However, the onset of symptoms after infection generally averages 7 to 8 days, and the symptoms last 2 to 3 weeks. Oocyst shedding in the feces is highly variable and may range from 7 days to several months. Indigenous infections are confined primarily to tropical, subtropical, or warm temperate regions of the world. Outbreaks occur in other areas of the world as a result of contaminated foodstuffs.

In immunocompromised and immunocompetent patients, *C. cayetanensis* infection can be associated with biliary disease. With light and transmission EM, developmental stages have been seen in the gallbladder epithelium of AIDS patients with acalculous cholecystitis. In addition, oocysts have been seen in the bile of patients with active biliary disease.

Laboratory Diagnosis

C. cayetanensis oocysts do not routinely stain with the trichrome fecal stain; special methods are required for identification. The oocysts can be concentrated using routine methods; special stains can then be used to enhance morphology. A single negative stool specimen is not conclusive in the examination of stools for coccidia; three stool specimens collected on subsequent days must be examined before infection can be ruled out.

Special Stains

With modified acid-fast stains, the oocysts appear light pink to deep red, and some contain granules or have a bubbly appearance (described as wrinkled cellophane). It is very important to be aware of these organisms when the modified acid-fast stain is used, because *Cryptosporidium* spp. and other similar but larger structures (approximately twice the size of *Cryptosporidium* oocysts [8 to 10 μm]) are seen in the stained smear. Laboratories need to measure all acid-fast oocysts, particularly if they appear to be somewhat larger than *Cryptosporidium* spp. Variations on the safranin

staining technique stain *C. cayetanensis* oocysts orange or pinkish orange. Heating and other treatments have been used to increase the staining frequency of oocysts. The oocysts autofluoresce green (450 to 490 DM excitation filter) or blue (365 DM excitation filter) under ultraviolet (UV) epifluorescence (Fig. 47.30B and C). It is strongly recommended that during concentration (formalin ethyl acetate) of stool specimens, centrifugation be carried out for 10 minutes at 500× *g*. The concentration sediment can then be stained, enhancing the sensitivity of the microscopy examinations.

Nucleic Acid Detection and Serologic Tests

Several nucleic acid–based tests have been developed in research laboratories that detect a variety of organism-specific genes, including the 18S rRNA, 28S rRNA, and the cytochrome oxidase 1 sequence. Commercially available multiplex panels are also available for the detection of *C. cayetanensis* including the BioFire FilmArray Gastrointestinal panel, previously described. No antibody or antigen tests are available for the diagnosis of *C. cayetanensis* infection.

Results and Reporting

C. cayetanensis is reportable to both the local public health authorities and the Centers for Disease Control and Prevention. The organism has been associated with human outbreaks and contamination of food sources. Quantitation is not required. If a negative result is indicated, it is important to note that three samples have been examined before a negative is reported.

Therapy

Patients have been treated symptomatically with antidiarrheal preparations and have obtained some relief; however, the disease appears to be self-limiting within a few weeks. TMP-SMX, currently the drug of choice, is given orally twice daily for 7 days. Elimination of parasites, a decrease in diarrhea, and diminished abdominal pain occur within 2 to 3 days after treatment. Patients with AIDS may need higher doses and long-term maintenance treatment. However, more than 40% of patients have a recurrence of symptoms in 1 to 3 months after treatment. Patients who are allergic to sulfonamides have been effectively treated with ciprofloxacin.

Prevention

Individuals in endemic areas should wear gloves when gardening to prevent exposure to oocysts of *C. cayetanensis*. Thorough washing of produce may help remove oocysts. Most of the produce items implicated in the transmission of *C. cayetanensis* are consumed raw; thus cooking as a means of prevention is not relevant.

Cystoisospora belli
General Characteristics

Although *Cystoisospora belli* is found worldwide, certain tropical areas in the Western Hemisphere have specific locations where endemic infections occur. These organisms infect both adults and children, and intestinal involvement and symptoms are generally transient unless the patient is immunocompromised. *C. belli* has also been implicated in traveler's diarrhea. However, unlike with *Cryptosporidium* spp. and *C. cayetanensis,* large outbreaks have not been reported (Table 47.6).

C. belli oocysts are passed in the stool. They are long and oval, measuring 20 to 33 μm long by 10 to 19 μm wide. Usually the oocyst contains one immature **sporont,** but two may be present. Continued development occurs outside the body, with the development of two mature **sporocysts,** each containing four sporozoites, which can be recovered from the fecal specimen. The sporulated oocyst is the infective stage that excysts in the small intestine, releasing the sporozoites, which penetrate the mucosal cells and initiate the life cycle.

Epidemiology

C. belli oocysts are passed in the feces unsporulated or partially sporulated (Fig. 47.31). Oocysts complete sporulation within 72 hours, although it may take longer, depending on the temperature. The time required for unsporulated oocysts to appear in the feces after ingestion of sporulated oocysts is 9 to 17 days. Oocyst shedding is variable and depends on the immune status of the infected individual. Oocysts can be found for 30 to 50 days in immunocompetent patients, and immunosuppressed patients may continue to shed oocysts for 6 months or longer. Chronic infections can occur, and oocysts can be shed for months to years. In one particular case, an immunocompetent individual had symptoms for 26 years, and *C. belli* was recovered in stool a number of times over 10 years.

C. belli is thought to be the only species of *Cystoisospora* that infects humans, and no other reservoir hosts are recognized for this infection. However, *C. belli* sporozoites can become dormant as a single-organism-containing tissue cyst in the lymph nodes, liver, or spleen. The existence of these monozoic tissue cysts indicates there may be an unknown transport (paratenic) host in the life cycle of the organism. Transmission occurs through ingestion of water or food contaminated with mature, sporulated oocysts and possibly from the ingestion of tissue from the unknown paratenic host. Sexual transmission by direct oral contact with the anus or perineum also occurs, although this mode of transmission is probably much less common. The oocysts are very resistant to environmental conditions and may remain viable for months if kept cool and moist; oocysts usually mature within 48 hours after stool passage and are then infectious.

Pathogenesis and Spectrum of Disease

Symptoms include diarrhea (most common), weight loss, abdominal colic, and fever. Stools (usually 6 to 10 per day) are watery to soft, foamy, and offensive smelling, suggesting a malabsorption process. Many patients have eosinophilia, recurrences are quite common, and the disease is more severe in infants and young children.

Patients who are immunosuppressed, particularly those with AIDS, often present with profuse diarrhea associated with weakness, anorexia, and weight loss. Biopsies reveal an abnormal mucosa with short villi, hypertrophied crypts, and infiltration of the lamina propria with eosinophils, neutrophils, and round cells. Physicians should consider *C. belli* in AIDS patients with diarrhea who have immigrated from or traveled to Latin America, are Hispanics born in the United States, are young adults, or who have not received prophylaxis with TMP-SMX for *Pneumocystis* infection. It has also been recommended that patients with AIDS traveling to Latin America and other developing countries be advised of the waterborne and foodborne transmission of *C. belli* and that chemoprophylaxis should be considered.

Extraintestinal infections in immunocompromised patients have been reported. At autopsy, microscopic findings associated with *C. belli* infection were seen in the lymph nodes and walls of the small and large intestines, mesenteric and mediastinal lymph nodes, lymphatic channels, liver, and spleen. *C. belli* infections in the gallbladder epithelium and endometrial epithelium have also been reported, and oocysts have been recovered in bile specimens.

Laboratory Diagnosis

Examination of fresh material, either as a direct wet prep or as concentrated material, is recommended, rather than a permanent stained smear. The oocysts are very pale and transparent and can easily be overlooked. The light level of the microscope should be reduced, and additional contrast through staining may be required for optimal visualization. On the permanent stained smear, the organisms may take up excess stain and resemble helminth eggs or artifacts.

It is possible to have a positive biopsy specimen but not recover the oocysts in the stool because of the small numbers of organisms present. The oocysts are acid-fast and can also be demonstrated by using auramine rhodamine stains. Organisms tentatively identified using auramine rhodamine stains should be confirmed by wet prep examination or acid-fast stains, particularly if the stool contains other cells or excess artifact material (more normal stool consistency).

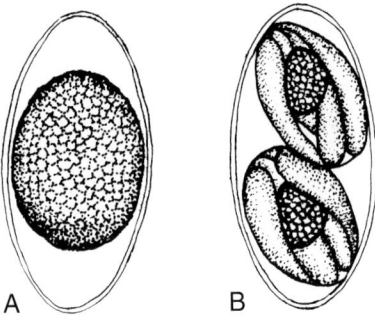

• **Fig. 47.31** (A) Immature oocyst of *Cystoisospora belli.* (B) Mature oocyst of *C. belli.* (Illustration by Nobuko Kitamura.)

Nucleic Acid Detection

Currently, there are no commercially available nucleic acid–based methods for the detection of *C. belli*. However, PCR assays have been developed for the detection of the organism in stool samples.

Histology

Developmental stages of *C. belli* have been reported for intestinal biopsy specimens of the duodenum, jejunum, and occasionally ileum. Intestinal development tends to occur in epithelial cells, although developing stages are occasionally reported from the lamina propria or submucosa. Extraintestinal infections in immunocompromised patients have been reported; the organisms become dormant as cysts in a variety of tissues, including the intestine, mesenteric lymph nodes, liver, and spleen; these cysts are called monozoic tissue **cysts**. In histologic sections, these cysts are thick-walled and measure 12 to 22 μm × 8 to 10 μm, and each contains a single dormant sporozoite or merozoite of about 8 to 10 μm × 5 μm. As immunity declines, these cysts can reactivate patient infections.

Results and Reporting

C. belli is typically easily identified in human stool specimens. Quantitation is not required. If a negative result is indicated, it is important to note that three samples have been examined before a negative is reported.

Therapy

The drug of choice to treat *C. belli* infection is TMP-SMX, which is given two to four times a day for 10 to 14 days. With this approach, the parasites are eliminated, the diarrhea stops, and the abdominal pain decreases within a few days. There is no standardized treatment for patients who are allergic or cannot tolerate sulfonamides. Pyrimethamine has been used as an effective alternate treatment.

Prevention

Because transmission occurs through the infective oocysts, prevention includes improved personal hygiene measures and sanitary conditions to eliminate possible fecal-oral transmission from contaminated food, water, and possibly environmental surfaces.

Sarcocystis spp.
General Characteristics

Two well-described *Sarcocystis* spp. include *Sarcocystis hominis* and *Sarcocystis suihominis*. Humans are the definitive host for both species, and the intermediate hosts are either cattle (*S. hominis*) or pigs (*S. suihominis*). When uncooked meat from these infected animals is ingested by humans, **gamogony** (fission resulting in the production of sporozoan gametes) can occur in the intestinal cells, with eventual production of the sporocysts in stool.

Sarcocystis spp. have an obligatory two-host life cycle. Intermediate hosts (herbivores and omnivores) become infected through ingestion of sporocysts excreted in the feces of the definitive hosts (carnivores and omnivores). The definitive hosts become infected through ingestion of mature cysts found in the muscles of the intermediate hosts. In some intermediate hosts, such as cattle and sheep, all adult animals may be infected. Extraintestinal human sarcocystosis is rare, with a much lower incidence than is seen with the intestinal infection. Humans who have ingested meat containing the mature sarcocysts serve as the definitive hosts. Fever, severe diarrhea, abdominal pain, and weight loss have been reported in immunocompromised hosts, although the number of patients with these symptoms has been quite small.

The sporocysts found in the stool are broadly oval and slightly tapered at the ends. They measure 9 to 16 μm long and contain four mature sporozoites and the **residual body** (Table 47.6). Normally, the oocyst contains two sporocysts (similar to *C. belli*); however, in *Sarcocystis* infections, the sporocysts are released from the oocyst and normally are seen singly. These sporocysts tend to be larger than *Cryptosporidium* oocysts that contain four sporozoites. The oocysts are fully sporulated when passed in the stool.

Pathogenesis and Spectrum of Disease

When humans (intermediate host) ingest oocysts from other animal stool sources, the **sarcocysts** that develop in human muscle are 7 to 16 μm long and cause few, if any, problems. No inflammatory response to these organisms occurs in the muscle, and no evidence of pathogenicity is seen. Patients demonstrate symptoms related to the disintegration of the sarcocysts and death of **intracystic bradyzoites**. Painful muscle swellings measuring 1 to 3 cm in diameter are associated with erythema of the overlying skin; these occur periodically and last 2 days to 2 weeks. Symptoms also include fever, diffuse myalgia, muscle tenderness, weakness, eosinophilia, and bronchospasm. Different types of skeletal and cardiac muscle sarcocysts have been found in humans. No specific therapy is required for this type of infection. Corticosteroids can reduce allergic inflammatory reactions.

Infections in humans can manifest primarily as intestinal disease if infected meat is ingested or as muscular disease if sporocysts are ingested. Intestinal disease occurs within a few hours after consumption of infected meat and is characterized by nausea, abdominal pain, and diarrhea. However, in both situations patients may be infected and asymptomatic.

Laboratory Diagnosis

A presumptive diagnosis of intestinal disease may be based on the patient's symptoms, particularly with documented ingestion of raw or poorly cooked meat. Confirmation of the diagnosis may depend on finding human fecal specimens containing sporocysts, which are passed in the stool 11 to 18 days after ingestion of beef or pork. Sporocysts of the two *Sarcocystis* spp. are very difficult to differentiate.

A muscle biopsy is appropriate for suspected symptomatic intramuscular infection in a patient with a history of travel to or residence in a tropical location. Sarcocysts in biopsy specimens can be identified by microscopy on routine histologic sections stained with hematoxylin and eosin. Most sarcocysts in humans have been found in skeletal and cardiac muscle; however, muscles in the larynx, pharynx, and upper esophagus have also been involved.

Nucleic Acid Detection

No molecular assays are currently available for the detection of sarcocystis in humans. Laboratory developed tests have used PCR to detect *Sarcocystis* spp. DNA in human stool and muscle biopsy tissue.

Results and Reporting

Identification of *Sarcocystis* spp. is very rare. However, it is not possible to differentiate the two species based on morphologic characteristics of the sporocysts. It is recommended that potential identification be confirmed by a reference laboratory and should be included in the final patient report.

Therapy

No known treatment or prophylaxis is available for intestinal infection, myositis, vasculitis, or related lesions caused by human sarcocystosis. Supportive therapy for patients with severe diarrhea is indicated. It is also unclear whether immunosuppressives are effective at reducing the inflammatory reactions seen in vasculitis or myositis. Without more definitive data, no course of therapy can be recommended.

Prevention

Cooking meat to an internal temperature higher than 67°C kills *Toxoplasma gondii* tissue cysts in meat; this temperature should also kill *Sarcocystis* tissue cysts in meat. Preventing cattle, buffalo, and swine from consuming human feces shedding infective oocysts also prevents animal infection. Most cases of human muscular *Sarcocystis* infection have been reported from the Far East. When humans are intermediate hosts, preventive measures involve careful disposal of animal feces that may contain the infective sporocysts. This may be impossible in wilderness areas, where wild animals may serve as reservoir hosts for many *Sarcocystis* spp.

Microsporidia

Microsporidia are obligate intracellular, spore-forming parasites. More than 200 microsporidial genera and 1500 species have been identified. Nine genera (*Anncaliia, Encephalitozoon, Endoreticulatus, Enterocytozoon, Nosema, Pleistophora, Vittaforma, Tubulinosema,* and *Trachipleistophora*) and unclassified microsporidia *(Microsporidium)* have been identified as causing human infections.

Although the microsporidia are true eukaryotes, they also have molecular and cytologic characteristics of prokaryotes. Microsporidia evolved from the fungi. Features shared with fungi include the presence of chitin and trehalose, similarities in cell cycles, and certain gene organizations. Microsporidia are considered highly derived fungi that underwent genetic and functional losses, resulting in one of the smallest eukaryotic genomes known. However, the life cycle of microsporidia is unique and unlike that of any fungal species. At this point, clinical and diagnostic issues and responsibilities often remain with the parasitologists.

General Characteristics

Human microsporidial infections have been documented worldwide. The spore, the only life cycle stage able to survive outside the host cell, is the infective stage (Fig. 47.32 and Table 47.7). Infection occurs with ingestion or inhalation of the infective spores, from which the infective **sporoplasm** (spore protoplasm) enters the host cell through the **polar tubule** (Fig. 47.33). The microsporidia multiply extensively in the host cell cytoplasm; the life cycle includes repeated divisions by binary fission (merogony) or multiple fission (schizogony) and spore production (sporogony). Both merogony and sporogony can occur in the same cell at the same time. During sporogony, a thick spore wall is formed, providing environmental protection for the spore.

Microsporidial spores measure 0.7 to about 4 μm in diameter. Mature spores contain a tubular extrusion apparatus (polar tube or tubule) for injecting infective spore contents (sporoplasm) into the host cell.

Epidemiology

Transmission possibilities include human-to-human and animal-to-human routes. Many questions relating to reservoir hosts and possible congenital infections are still unanswered. Primary infection occurs through inhalation or ingestion of spores from environmental sources or by zoonotic transmission. The presence of *Encephalitozoon intestinalis* has been confirmed in tertiary sewage effluent, surface water, and groundwater; *Enterocytozoon bieneusi* has been confirmed in surface water; and *Vittaforma corneae* has been confirmed in tertiary effluent. Ingestion or inhalation of the environmentally highly resistant spores is probably the normal mode of transmission. Direct contact with contaminated water or other infected animals including humans may also serve as a route of transmission.

E. bieneusi, an intestinal pathogen, serves as an example of infection potential. The spores are released into the intestinal lumen and are passed in the stool (Fig. 47.34). These spores are environmentally resistant and can be ingested by other hosts. Zoonotic transmission of microsporidia infecting humans has not been verified.

Microsporidiosis

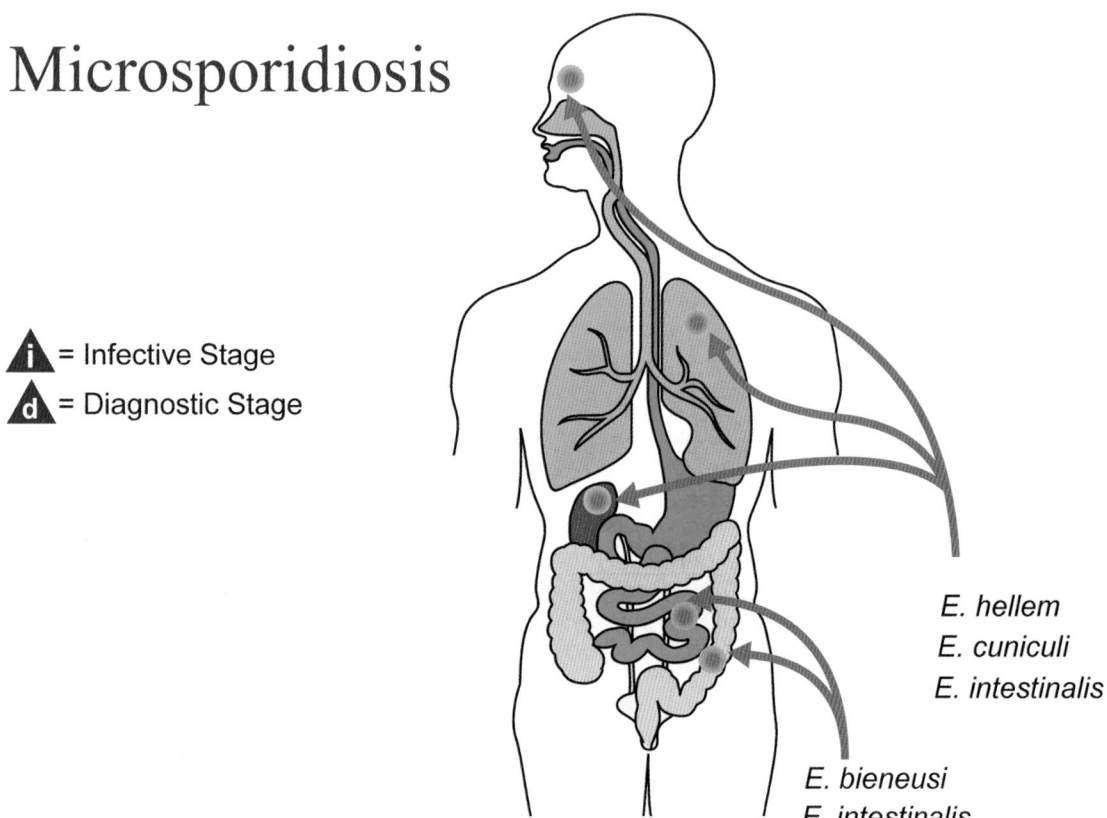

i = Infective Stage

d = Diagnostic Stage

E. hellem
E. cuniculi
E. intestinalis

E. bieneusi
E. intestinalis

Intracellular development of *E. bieneusi* and *E. intestinalis* spores.

Enterocytozoon bieneusi

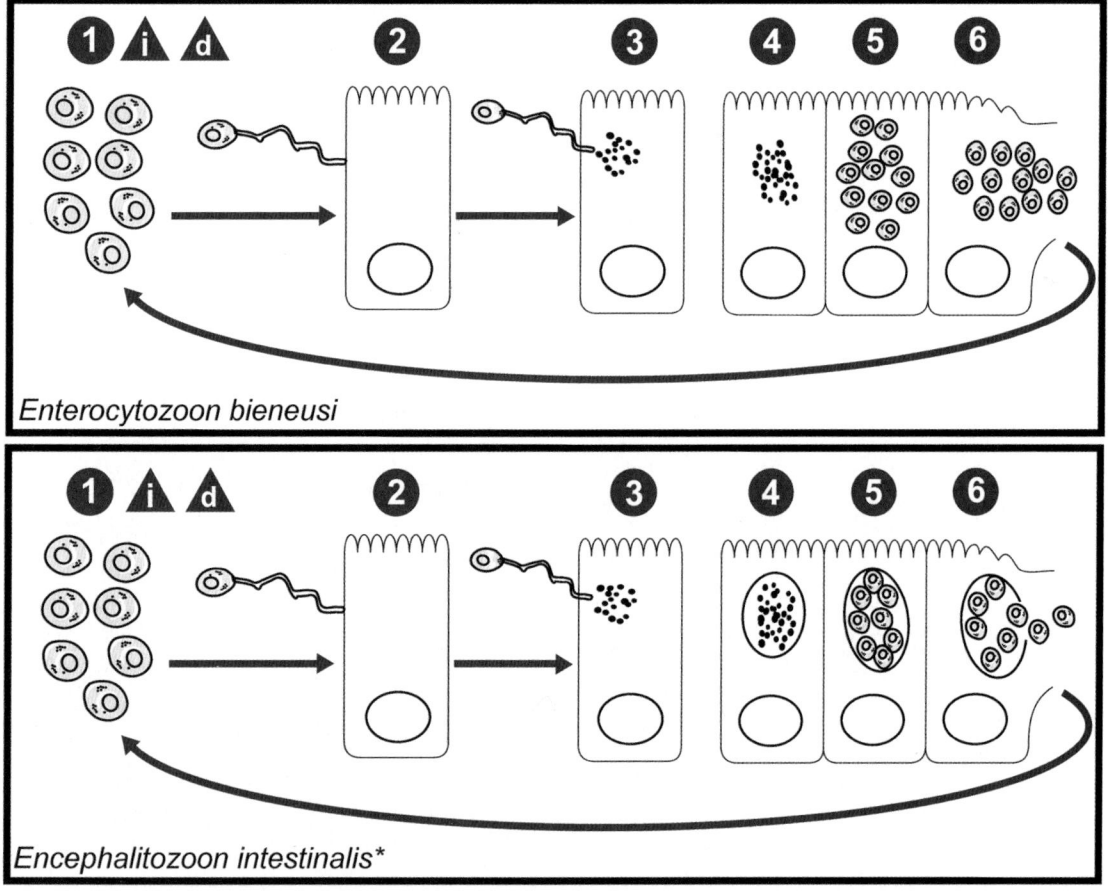

*Encephalitozoon intestinalis**

*Development inside parasitophorous vacuole also occurs in *E. hellem* and *E. cuniculi*.

• **Fig. 47.32** This is an illustration of the life cycle of the different species of microsporidia responsible for causing the diarrheal illness known as microsporidiosis. (Courtesy of the Division of Parasitic Diseases/ Centers for Disease Control and Prevention.)

Pathogenesis and Spectrum of Disease

Microsporidia were recognized as causing disease in animals as early as the 1920s but were not recognized as agents of human disease until the AIDS pandemic began in the mid-1980s.

Enterocytozoon bieneusi

A number of cases of *E. bieneusi* infection have been reported in patients with AIDS. Chronic intractable diarrhea, fever, malaise, and weight loss are symptoms of *E. bieneusi* infections, and these symptoms mimic those seen with cryptosporidiosis or isosporiasis. Often these patients have four to eight watery, nonbloody stools each day, accompanied by nausea and anorexia. Dehydration and D-xylose and fat malabsorption also may develop. These patients tend to be severely immunodeficient, with a CD4+ count usually below 200 cells/mm^3 and often below 100 cells/mm^3. Mixed infections with *E. bieneusi* and *E. intestinalis* have been reported. *E. bieneusi*

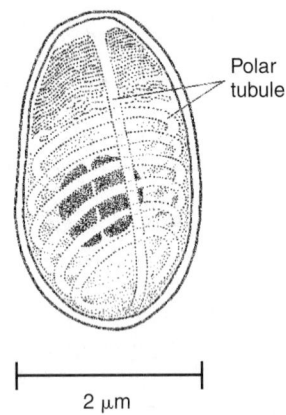

• **Fig. 47.33** Diagram illustrating the polar tubule in a microsporidian spore.

infection has been implicated in AIDS-related sclerosing cholangitis. However, demonstration of *E. bieneusi* spores in extraepithelial tissues does not always appear to be associated with subsequent development of systemic infection.

E. bieneusi spores have been identified in sputum and bronchoalveolar lavage fluid in addition to stool specimens. *E. bieneusi* can colonize the respiratory tract, and clinical specimens from these sources may reveal the presence of spores. Multiorgan microsporidiosis caused by *E. bieneusi* has been diagnosed in patients infected with HIV; organisms have been recovered in stools, duodenal biopsy specimens, nasal discharge, and sputum.

Infection with *E. bieneusi* has been reported in immunocompetent individuals; symptoms were self-limited, and diarrheal disease resolved within 2 weeks. *E. bieneusi* may be more commonly associated with sporadic diarrheal disease than was previously suspected, and the immune system may play a role in the control of this intestinal infection. It is possible that *E. bieneusi* may persist as an asymptomatic infection in immunocompetent individuals.

Encephalitozoon spp.

Both *Encephalitozoon cuniculi* and *Encephalitozoon hellem* have been isolated from human infections. The spectrum of disease in patients with AIDS, organ transplant recipients, and otherwise immunocompromised patients includes keratoconjunctivitis, intraocular infection, sinusitis, bronchiolitis, pneumonitis, nephritis, ureteritis, cystitis, prostatitis, urethritis, hepatitis, sclerosing cholangitis, peritonitis, diarrhea, and encephalitis. Clinical manifestations may vary, ranging from an asymptomatic carrier state to organ failure.

Encephalitozoon intestinalis

Encephalitozoon intestinalis infects primarily small intestinal enterocytes, but infection does not remain

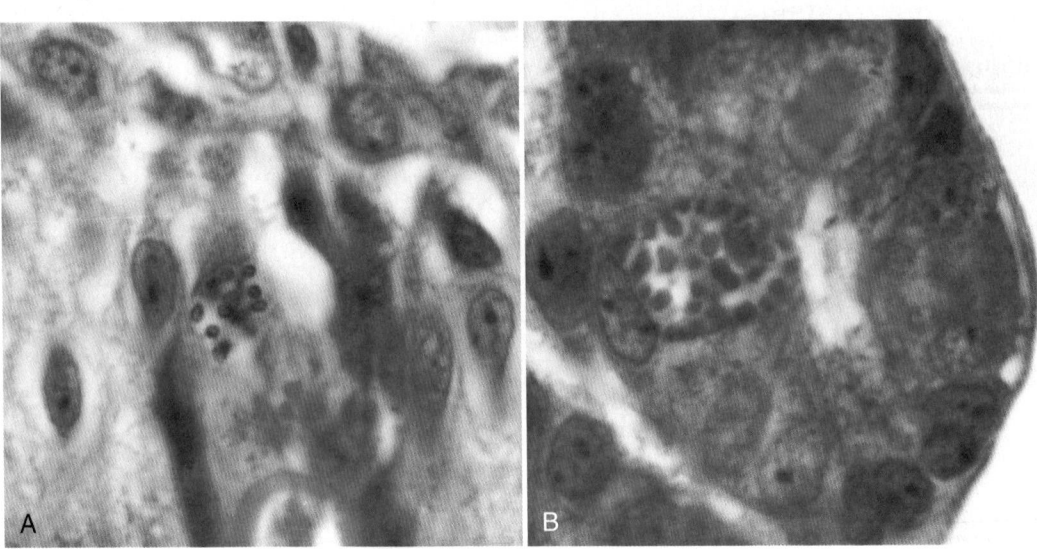

• **Fig. 47.34** Routine histology micrograph of microsporidian spores in enterocytes (Giemsa stain). (A) Note the fully formed spores. (B) These spores are not fully mature.

confined to epithelial cells. *E. intestinalis* is also found in lamina propria macrophages, fibroblasts, and endothelial cells. Dissemination to the kidneys, lower airways, and biliary tract appears to occur through infected macrophages. Fortunately, these infections tend to respond to therapy with albendazole, unlike infections caused by *E. bieneusi*.

Other Microsporidia

Different microsporidial species have been isolated from immunocompetent individuals who presented with keratoconjunctivitis, severe keratitis, or corneal ulcers. In addition, keratoconjunctivitis has been found in an immunocompetent contact lens wearer.

In immunocompromised patients, myositis has been seen in infections caused by *Pleistophora* spp., *Pleistophora ronneafiei*, *Trichomonas hominis*, *Anncaliia vesicularum*, and *Anncaliia algerae*. *Trachipleistophora anthropophthera* has been identified in cerebral, cardiac, renal, pancreatic, thyroid, hepatic, splenic, lymphoid, and bone marrow tissue. Disseminated infection caused by *Anncaliia connori* has also been identified.

Laboratory Diagnosis

The most commonly used stains are chromotrope-based stains (modified trichrome) and chemofluorescent optical brightening agents, including calcofluor white and other chemofluorescent stains. Regardless of the staining technique selected, the use of positive control material is highly recommended. Detection of the small microsporidial spores requires adequate illumination and magnification (i.e., magnification using the oil immersion objective [×100] for a total magnification of ×1000). Microsporidial spores may be identified in a variety of specimens including unconcentrated stool, body fluids (duodenal aspirates, bile, biliary aspirates, urine, bronchoalveolar lavage, cerebral spinal fluid, sputum, and nasal discharge), conjunctival specimens, and corneal scrapings.

Antigen Detection

Antigen detection tests have been developed, but the reagents are not widely available commercially.

Antibody Detection

Although the detection of antibody using a number of methods has been documented, cross-reactivity among the genera may occur. Currently, this approach is not commonly used.

Nucleic Acid Detection

Molecular techniques have been quite successful in identifying a number of the microsporidia; however, this approach is not yet widely used in clinical laboratories.

These laboratory-developed tests include PCR, real-time PCR, loop-mediated isothermal amplification technique (LAMP), and *in situ* hybridization for tissue biopsies. These tests can be universal panmicrosporidian or genus and species–specific assays.

Histology

Microsporidia do not tend to stain predictably, if at all, in tissues. However, spores occasionally can be seen very well with use of the PAS stain, silver stains, or acid-fast stains. Modified Gram stains also have proved sensitive. The spore has a small, PAS-positive posterior body; the spore coat stains with silver, and the spores are acid-fast variable. Tissue examination by EM techniques is still considered the best approach for differentiation of genera; however, this option is not available to all laboratories, and the sensitivity of EM may not be equal to that of other methods when examining stool or urine.

Results and Reporting

Immunocompetent patients may not produce significant numbers of microsporidia for identification. However, as a predominantly opportunistic pathogen in immunocompromised patients, stool examination along with additional body fluid or tissue specimens should be performed to properly assess the patient's condition if a microsporidia infection is suspected.

Therapy

Albendazole therapy can result in clinical cure of HIV-associated infection with *Encephalitozoon* spp., along with elimination of spore shedding. Albendazole is not effective for *Enterocytozoon* infections, although clinical improvement occurs in some patients. Oral purified fumagillin, nikkomycin Z, and fluoroquinolones have been shown to inhibit sporulation and eradicate *E. bieneusi* and *Vittaforma*. Antiretroviral combination therapy results in complete clinical response with elimination of intestinal microsporidia.

Prevention

The presence of infective spores in human clinical specimens suggests that taking precautions when handling body fluids and following personal hygiene measures, such as hand washing, may be important in preventing primary infections in the health care setting. However, the establishment of comprehensive guidelines for disease prevention requires more definitive information about sources of infection and modes of transmission.

ⓔ Visit the Evolve site for a complete list of procedures, review questions, and case studies.

Bibliography

Barbosa ADS, Barbosa HS, Souza SMO, et al.: *Balantioides coli*: morphological and ultrastructural characteristics of pig and non-human primate isolates, *Acta Parasitol* 63(2):287–298, 2018.

Bennett J, Dolin R, Blaser M: *Principles and practice of infectious diseases*, ed 9, Philadelphia, 2020, Elsevier-Saunders.

Carroll KC, Pfaller MA, Landry ML, et al.: *Manual of clinical microbiology*, ed 12, Washington, DC, 2019, ASM.

Clark DP: New insights into human cryptosporidiosis, *Clin Microbiol Rev* 12:554–563, 1999.

Espinosa-Cantellano M, Martinez-Paloma A: Pathogenesis of intestinal amebiasis: from molecules to disease, *Clin Microbiol Rev* 13:318–331, 2000.

Fayer R: *Cryptosporidium*: a water-borne zoonotic parasite, *Vet Parasitol* 126:37–56, 2004.

Fayer R: *Sarcocystis* spp. in human infections, *Clin Microbiol Rev* 17:894–902, 2004.

Feng Y, Xiao L: Zoonotic potential and molecular epidemiology of *Giardia* species and giardiasis, *Clin Microbiol Rev* 24:110–140, 2011.

Fotedar R, Stark D, Beebe N, et al.: Laboratory diagnostic techniques for *Entamoeba* species, *Clin Microbiol Rev* 20:511–532, 2007.

Garcia LS: *Diagnostic medical parasitology*, ed 6, Washington, DC, 2016, ASM Press.

Garcia LS: *Practical guide to diagnostic parasitology,* ed 2, Washington, DC, 2008, ASM Press.

Garcia LS, Shimizu RY: Detection of *Giardia lamblia* and *Cryptosporidium parvum* antigens in human fecal specimens using the ColorPAC combination rapid solid-phase qualitative immunochromatographic assay, *J Clin Microbiol* 38:1267–1268, 2000.

Garcia LS, Shimizu RY, Bernard CN: Detection of *Giardia lamblia, Entamoeba histolytica/E. dispar*, and *Cryptosporidium parvum* antigens in human fecal specimens using the EIA Triage Parasite Panel, *J Clin Microbiol* 38:3337–3340, 2000.

Haque R, Neveille LM, Hahn P, Petri Jr WA: Rapid diagnosis of *Entamoeba* infection by using *Entamoeba* and *Entamoeba histolytica* stool antigen detection ids, *J Clin Microbiol* 33:2558–2561, 1995.

Johnson EH, Windsor JJ, Clark CG: Emerging from obscurity: biological, clinical, and diagnostic aspects of *Dientamoeba fragilis*, *Clin Microbiol Rev* 17:553–570, 2004.

Lindsay DS, Dubey JP, Blagburn BL: Biology of *Isospora* spp. from humans, nonhuman primates, and domestic animals, *Clin Microbiol Rev* 10:19–34, 1997.

Mathis A, Weber R, Deplazes P: Zoonotic potential of the microsporidia, *Clin Microbiol Rev* 18:423–455, 2005.

Ortega YR, Sanchez R: Update on *Cyclospora cayetanensis*, a food-borne and waterborne parasite, *Clin Microbiol Rev* 23:218–234, 2010.

Pomajbikova K, Obornik M, Horak A, et al.: Novel insights into the genetic diversity of *Balantidium* and *Balantidium*-like cyst-forming ciliates, *PLoS Negl Trop Dis* 7(3):e2140, 2013.

Royer TL, Gilchrist C, Kabir MD, et al.: *Entamoeba bangladeshi* nov. sp., Bangladesh, *Emerg Infect Dis* 18:1543–1545, 2012.

Santi-Rocca J, Rigothier MC, Guillen N: Host-microbe interactions and defense mechanisms in the development of amoebic liver abscesses, *Clin Microbiol Rev* 22:65–75, 2009.

Schuster FL, Ramirez-Avila L: Current world status of *Balantidium coli*, *Clin Microbiol Rev* 21:626–638, 2008.

Sekar U, Shanthi M: Blastocystis: consensus of treatment and controversies, *Trop Parasitol* 3:35–39, 2013.

Shields JM, Olson BH: *Cyclospora cayetanensis*: a review of an emerging parasitic coccidian, *Int J Parasitol* 33:371–391, 2003.

Siberman JD, Sogin ML, Leipe DD, et al.: Human parasite finds taxonomic home, *Nature* 380:398, 1996.

Soleimanpour S, Babaei A, Roudi AM, et al.: Urinary infection due to *Balantioides coli*: a rare accidental zoonotic disease in an addicted and diabetic young female in Iran, *JMM Case Rep* 3(1):e000102, 2016.

Stark D, Garcia LS, Barratt JLN, et al.: Description of *Dientamoeba fragilis* cyst and precystic forms in human samples, *J Clin Microbiol* 52(7):2680–2683, 2014.

Tan KS: New insights on classification, identification, and clinical relevance of *Blastocystis* spp, *Clin Microbiol Rev* 21:639–665, 2008.

Tanyuksel M, Petri Jr WA: Laboratory diagnosis of amebiasis, *Clin Microbiol Rev* 16:713–729, 2003.

ten Hove RJ, van Lieshout L, Brienen EA, et al.: Real-time polymerase chain reaction for detection of *Isospora belli* in stool samples, *Diagn Microbiol Infect Dis* 61:280–283, 2008.

Thompson RC, Monis PT: Variation in *Giardia:* implications for taxonomy and epidemiology, *Adv Parasitol* 58:69–137, 2004.

Wilson M, Schantz PM: Parasitic immunodiagnosis. In Strickland GT, editor: *Hunter's tropical medicine and emerging infectious diseases*, ed 8, Philadelphia, 2000, WB Saunders.

Xiao L, Ryan UM: Cryptosporidiosis: an update in molecular epidemiology, *Curr Opin Infect Dis* 17:483–490, 2004.

48

Blood and Tissue Protozoa

OBJECTIVES

1. Explain the general life cycle of *Plasmodium* spp., including both asexual and sexual stages, exoerythrocytic and erythrocytic cycle trophozoites, schizonts, hypnozoites, merozoites, gametocytes, and sporozoites.
2. Describe the distinguishing morphologic characteristics, clinical disease, vectors, stages of infectivity, and laboratory diagnosis for *Plasmodium* spp., *Babesia* spp., and *Trypanosoma* and *Leishmania* spp.
3. Define paroxysm in malarial periodicity.
4. Compare and contrast recrudescence and relapse, including the physiologic basis for each during infection with malaria.
5. Compare and contrast the pathogenesis of infections with *Plasmodium falciparum, Plasmodium malariae, Plasmodium ovale, Plasmodium vivax,* and *Plasmodium knowlesi,* including variation in signs and symptoms.
6. Differentiate intracellular forms of *Babesia* spp. from *Plasmodium* spp.
7. Define and describe the life cycle stages of *Trypanosoma* and *Leishmania* spp., including amastigotes, promastigotes, trypomastigotes, epimastigotes, and metacyclic trypanosome forms when appropriate.
8. Compare and contrast the efficacy of various detection and diagnostic methods for blood and tissue parasites.

PARASITES TO BE CONSIDERED

Protozoa

Sporozoa, Flagellates (Blood, Tissue)
Sporozoa (Malaria and Babesiosis)
  Plasmodium vivax
  Plasmodium ovale
  Plasmodium malariae
  Plasmodium falciparum
  Plasmodium knowlesi
  Babesia spp.
Flagellates (Leishmaniae, Trypanosomes)
  Leishmania tropica complex
  Leishmania major complex
  Leishmania mexicana complex
  Leishmania braziliensis complex
  Leishmania donovani complex
  Leishmania enrietti complex
  Leishmania guyanensis complex
  Leishmania peruviana
  Trypanosoma brucei gambiense
  Trypanosoma brucei rhodesiense
  Trypanosoma cruzi
  Trypanosoma rangeli

Plasmodium spp.

Malaria has been well documented as an ancient disease in Egyptian and Chinese writing beginning in 2700 BCE. By 200 BCE, malaria was identified in Rome; it spread throughout Europe during the 12th century and arrived in England by the 14th century. By the early 1800s, malaria was found worldwide.

Malaria has played a tremendous role in world history, influencing the outcome of wars, the movement of populations, and the development and decline of various nations. Before the American Civil War, malaria was found as far north as southern Canada, but it was no longer endemic within the United States by the 1950s.

In 2018, the World Health Organization (WHO) estimated that 228 million individuals worldwide were infected with *Plasmodium* spp. As many as 405,000 people die each year of malaria, more than 67% (272,000) of whom are children. This is a significant decrease from previous years in part due to better access to testing and treatment, as well as improvements in prevention and surveillance, but we still have a long way to go. Approximately 1700 cases of malaria are diagnosed in the United States each year, primarily from individuals who traveled to endemic areas. Malaria is endemic in more than 90 countries, impacting a population of 2400 million people, representing 40% of the world's population. More than 90% of deaths caused by malaria occur in Africa, and another 5% occur in Southeast Asia. *Plasmodium falciparum* is the major species associated with deadly infections throughout the world. Unfortunately, prevention remains a complex problem, and no drug is universally effective for all *Plasmodium* species.

There are approximately 250 species of *Plasmodium*. However, only five species infect humans. Of the species that cause human disease, *Plasmodium vivax* and *P. falciparum* cause 95% of infections. *P. vivax* may be responsible for 80% of the remaining infections, because this species has the widest distribution in the tropics, subtropics, and temperate zones. *P. falciparum* is generally confined to the tropics, *Plasmodium malariae* is sporadically distributed, and *Plasmodium ovale* is confined mainly to central West Africa and some South Pacific islands. The fifth human malaria, *Plasmodium knowlesi,* a malaria parasite of long-tailed macaque monkeys, has been confirmed in human cases from Malaysian Borneo, Thailand, Myanmar, and the Philippines.

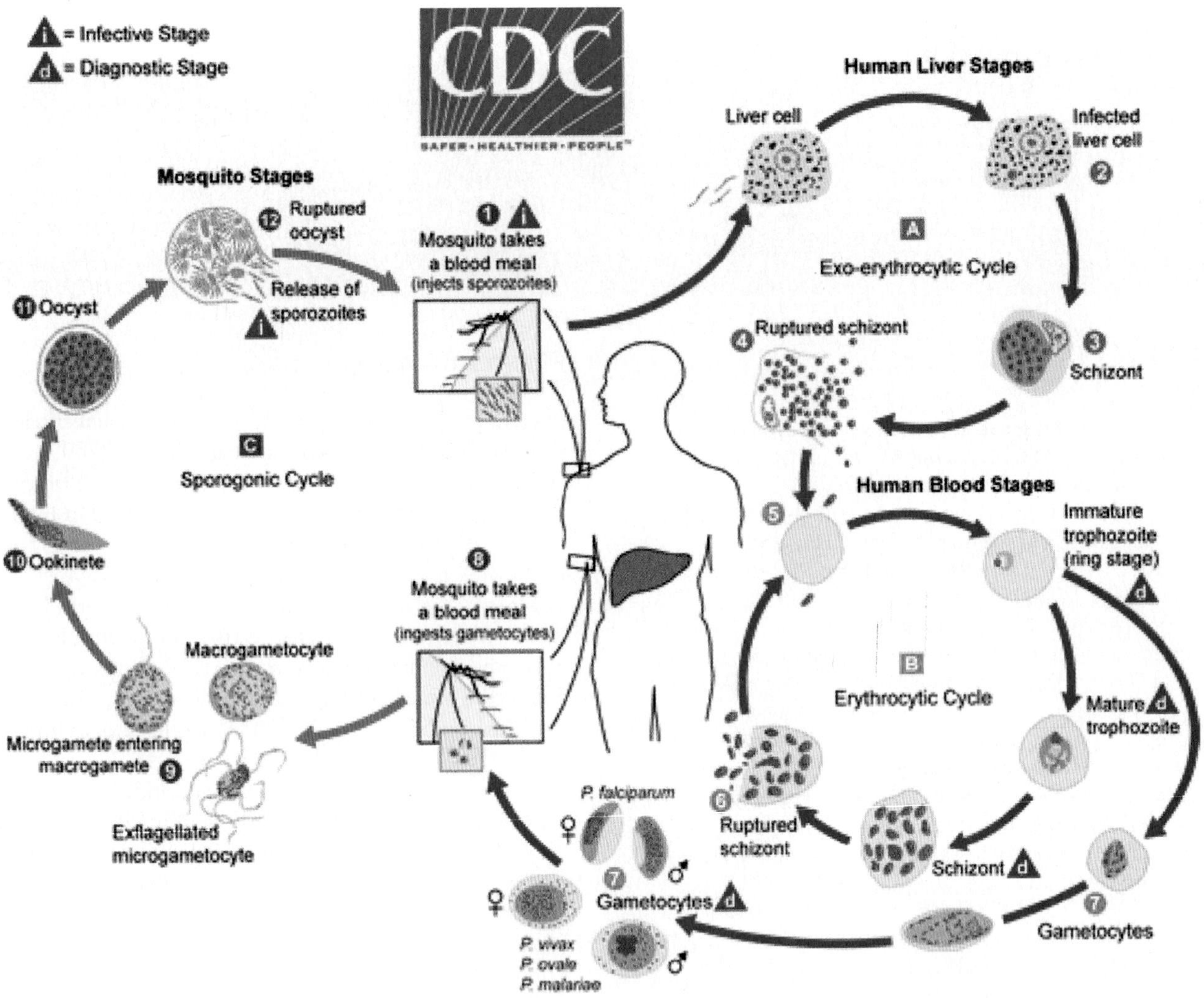

• **Fig. 48.1** Life cycle of *Plasmodium*. (Courtesy Division of Parasitic Diseases/Centers for Disease Control and Prevention.)

The vector for malaria is the female *Anopheles* mosquito. When the vector takes a blood meal, **sporozoites** contained in the salivary glands of the mosquito are discharged into the puncture wound (Fig. 48.1). Within an hour, these infective sporozoites are carried via the blood to the liver, where they penetrate hepatocytes and begin to grow, initiating the **preerythrocytic** or **primary exoerythrocytic** cycle. The sporozoites become round or oval and begin dividing repeatedly. **Schizogony** results in large numbers of exoerythrocytic **merozoites.** Once these merozoites leave the liver, they invade the red blood cells (RBCs), initiating the **erythrocytic cycle.** A dormant schizogony may occur in *P. vivax* and *P. ovale* organisms, which remain quiescent in the liver. These resting stages are known as **hypnozoites** and lead to a true relapse, often within 1 year or up to more than 5 years later. Delayed schizogony does not occur in *P. falciparum*, *P. malariae*, or *P. knowlesi.*

Once the RBCs and reticulocytes have been invaded, the parasites grow and feed on hemoglobin and other proteins inside the cells. Within the RBC, the merozoite (or young trophozoite) is vacuolated, ring-shaped, more or less amoeboid, and uninucleate. The excess protein and hematin present from the metabolism of hemoglobin combine to form malarial pigment. Once the nucleus begins to divide, the trophozoite is called a developing **schizont.** The mature schizont contains merozoites (the number depends on the species), which are released into the bloodstream. Many of the merozoites are destroyed by the immune system, but others invade RBCs and initiate a new cycle of **erythrocytic schizogony.** After several erythrocytic generations, some of the merozoites begin to undergo development into the male and female **gametocytes.**

Although malaria is often associated with travelers to endemic areas, other situations resulting in infection include blood transfusions, use of contaminated hypodermic needles, bone marrow transplantation, congenital infection, and transmission within the United States by indigenous mosquitoes that acquired the parasites from imported infections.

Plasmodium vivax (Benign Tertian Malaria)
General Characteristics

P. vivax infects only the reticulocytes; thus the parasitemia is limited to approximately 2% to 5% of the available RBCs in an otherwise healthy host (Tables 48.1–48.3 and Figs. 48.2–48.4 during the first few weeks of infection. The spleen will

TABLE 48.1   *Plasmodium* **spp.: Clinical Characteristics of the Five Human Infections**

Infection	Incubation Period	Prodromal Symptoms Severity / Initial Fever Pattern	Symptom Periodicity	Initial Paroxysm Severity / Mean Duration	Duration of Untreated Primary Attack	Duration of Untreated Infection	Parasitemia Limitations	Anemia	CNS Involvement	Nephrotic Syndrome
Plasmodium vivax	8–17 days	Mild to moderate / Irregular (48 h)	48 h	Moderate to severe / 10 h	3–8+ weeks	5–7 years	Young RBCs	Mild to moderate	Rare	Possible
Plasmodium ovale	10–17 days	Mild / Irregular (48 h)	48 h	Mild / 10 h	2–3 weeks	12 months	Young RBCs	Mild	Possible	Rare
Plasmodium malariae	18–40 days	Mild to moderate / Regular (72 h)	72 h	Moderate to severe / 11 h	3–24 weeks	20+ years	Old RBCs	Mild to moderate	Rare	Very common
Plasmodium falciparum	8–11 days	Mild / Continuous remittent	36–48 h	Severe / 16–36 h	2–3 weeks	6–17 months	All RBCs	Severe	Very common	Rare
Plasmodium knowlesi	9–12 days	Mild to moderate / Regular (24 h)	24–27 h	Moderate to severe / Not available	Not available	Not available	All RBCs	Moderate to severe	Possible	Probably common
Comments	All may be extended for months to years.	All may mimic influenza symptoms. Early symptoms may reflect lack of regular periodicity.		*P. knowlesi* can be as dangerous as *P. falciparum.*						*P. knowlesi* can be as dangerous as *P. falciparum.*

CNS, Central nervous system; *RBC,* red blood cell.

TABLE
48.2 **Plasmodia in Giemsa-Stained Thin Blood Smears**

	Persistence of Exoerythrocytic Cycle	Relapses	Time of Cycle	Appearance of Parasitized RBCs; Size and Shape	Schüffner Dots (Eosinophilic Stippling)	Color of Cytoplasm	Multiple Rings/Cell	All Developmental Stages Present in Peripheral Blood	Appearance of Parasite; Young Trophozoite (Early Ring Form)
Plasmodium vivax	Yes	Yes	44–48 h	1.5–2 times larger than normal; oval to normal; may be normal size until ring fills half of cell.	Usually present in all cells except early ring forms.	Decolorized, pale	Occasional	All stages present	Ring is ⅓ diameter of cell, cytoplasmic circle around vacuole; heavy chromatin dot.
Plasmodium malariae	No	No, but long-term recrudescence is recognized	72 h	Normal shape; size may be normal or slightly smaller.	None	Normal	Rare	Few ring forms, because ring stage is brief; mostly growing and mature trophozoites and schizonts	Ring often small than in *P. viva* occupying ⅛ of cell; heavy chromatin do vacuole at times "filled i pigment form early.
Plasmodium falciparum	No	No long-term relapses	36–48 h	Both normal.	None; occasionally comma-like red dots are present (Maurer dots).	Normal, bluish tinge at times	Common	Young ring forms and no older stages; few gametocytes	Delicate, small r with small ch matin dot (oft 2); scanty cyt plasm around small vacuole sometimes a edge of red c (appliqué form or filamentou slender form; may have multiple rings per cell.
Plasmodium ovale	Yes	Possible, but usually spontaneous recovery	48 h	60% of cells larger than normal and oval; 20% have irregular, frayed edges.	Present in all stages including early ring forms; dots may be larger and darker than in *P. vivax*.	Decolorized, pale	Occasional	All stages present	Ring is larger and more amoeboid than in *P. vivax*; otherwise similar *P. vivax*.
Plasmodium knowlesi	No	No	24 h	Normal shape, size.	No true stippling; occasional faint dots.	Normal	Common	All stages present	Rings ⅓ to ½ diameter of RBC; double chromatin dots; appliqué forms rare; multiple ring per RBC.

RBC, Red blood cell.

Growing Trophozoite	Mature Trophozoite	Schizont (Presegmenter)	Mature Schizont	Macrogametocyte	Microgametocyte	Main Criteria
Multishaped irregular amoeboid parasite; streamers of cytoplasm close to large chromatin dot; vacuole retained until close to maturity; increasing amounts of brown pigment.	Irregular amoeboid mass; 1 or more small vacuoles retained until schizont stage; fills almost entire cell; fine brown pigment.	Progressive chromatin division; cytoplasmic bands containing clumps of brown pigment.	16 (12–24) merozoites, each with chromatin and cytoplasm, filling entire red cell, which can hardly be seen	Rounded or oval homogeneous cytoplasm; diffuse delicate light brown pigment throughout parasite; eccentric compact chromatin	Large pink to purple chromatin mass surrounded by pale or colorless halo; evenly distributed pigment	Large pale red cell; trophozoite irregular; pigment usually present; Schüffner dots not always present; several phases of growth seen in one smear; gametocytes appear as early as third day.
Nonamoeboid rounded or band-shaped solid forms; chromatin may be hidden by coarse dark brown pigment.	Vacuoles disappear early; cytoplasm compact, oval, band shaped, or nearly round and almost filling cell; chromatin may be hidden by peripheral coarse dark brown pigment.	Similar to P. vivax except smaller; darker; larger pigment granules, peripheral or central.	8 (6–12) merozoites in rosettes or irregular clusters filling normal-sized cells, which can hardly be seen; central arrangement of brown-green pigment	Similar to P. vivax, but fewer in number; pigment darker and more coarse	Similar to P. vivax, but fewer in number; pigment darker and more coarse	Red cell normal in size and color; trophozoites compact, stain usually intense, band forms not always seen; coarse pigment; no stippling of red cells; gametocytes appear after a few weeks.
Heavy ring forms; fine pigment grains.	Not seen in peripheral blood (except in severe infections); development of all phases after ring form occurs in capillaries of viscera.	Not seen in peripheral blood (see previous entries).	Not seen in peripheral blood	Gender differentiation difficult; "crescent" or "sausage" shapes characteristic; may appear in "showers" with black pigment near chromatin dot, which is often central	Same as macrogametocyte (described in previous entries)	Development after ring stage takes place in blood vessels of internal organs; delicate ring forms and crescent-shaped gametocytes are only forms normally seen in peripheral blood; gametocytes appear after 7–10 days.
Ring shape maintained until late in development; nonamoeboid compared with P. vivax.	Compact; vacuoles disappear; pigment dark brown, less than in P. malariae.	Smaller and more compact than P. vivax.	¾ of cells occupied by 8 (8–12) merozoites in rosettes or irregular clusters	Smaller than P. vivax	Smaller than P. vivax	Red cell enlarged, oval, with fimbriated edges; Schüffner dots seen in all stages; gametocytes appear after 4 days or as late as 18 days.
Slightly amoeboid and irregular; band forms seen; very little pigment.	Denser cytoplasm (slightly amoeboid) band forms seen; little to no malaria pigment (scattered, fine brown grains).	Between 2 and 5 divided nuclear chromatin masses; abundant pigment granules occupy ⅔ of RBCs.	RBCs normal size; distorted/fimbriated RBCs very rare; occupy whole RBC; maximum of 16 merozoites; no rosettes; grapelike clusters	Occupy most of RBC; bluish cytoplasm; dense pink chromatin at periphery of parasite	Occupy most of RBC; cytoplasm pinkish purple; early forms similar to mature trophozoite	Ring forms compact; single/double chromatin dots, appliqué forms, multiple rings/RBC (mimic P. falciparum); overall RBCs not enlarged; developing stages mimic P. malariae (band forms, 16 merozoites in mature schizont, but no rosettes).

TABLE 48.3	Malaria Characteristics With Fresh Blood or Blood Collected Using EDTA With No Extended Lag Time	
Type of Malaria	**Characteristics**	
Plasmodium vivax (benign tertian malaria)	1 48-h cycle 2 Tends to infect young cells 3 Enlarged RBCs 4 Schüffner dots (true stippling) after 8–10 h 5 Delicate ring 6 Very amoeboid trophozoite 7 Mature schizont contains 12–24 merozoites	
Plasmodium malariae (quartan malaria)	1 72-h cycle (long incubation period) 2 Tends to infect old cells 3 Normal size RBCs 4 No stippling 5 Thick ring, large nucleus 6 Trophozoite tends to form "bands" across the cell 7 Mature schizont contains 6–12 merozoites	
Plasmodium ovale	1 48-h cycle 2 Tends to infect young cells 3 Enlarged RBCs with fimbriated edges (oval) 4 Schüffner dots appear in the beginning (in RBCs with very young ring forms, in contrast to *P. vivax*) 5 Smaller ring than *P. vivax* 6 Trophozoite less amoeboid than that of *P. vivax* 7 Mature schizont contains an average of 8 merozoites	
Plasmodium falciparum (malignant tertian malaria)	1 36–48–h cycle 2 Tends to infect any cell regardless of age, thus very heavy infection may result 3 All sizes of RBCs 4 No Schüffner dots (Maurer dots: may be larger, single dots, bluish) 5 Multiple rings/cell (only young rings, gametocytes, and occasional mature schizonts are seen in peripheral blood) 6 Delicate rings, may have two dots of chromatin/ring, appliqué or accolé forms 7 Crescent-shaped gametocytes	
Plasmodium knowlesi (simian malaria)[a]	1 24-h cycle 2 Tends to infect any cell regardless of age; thus very heavy infection may result 3 All sizes of RBCs, but most tend to be normal size 4 No Schüffner dots (faint, clumpy dots later in cycle) 5 Multiple rings/cell (may have 2–3) 6 Delicate rings, may have 2 or 3 dots of chromatin/ring, appliqué forms 7 Band form trophozoites commonly seen 8 Mature schizont contains 16 merozoites, no rosettes 9 Gametocytes round, tend to fill the cell 10 Early stages mimic *P. falciparum*; later stages mimic *P. malariae*	

EDTA, Ethylenediaminetetraacetic acid; *RBC*, red blood cell.
[a]Preparation of thick and thin blood films within 60 min of collection.

progress from being soft and palpable to hard, with continued enlargement during a chronic infection. If the infection is treated during the early phases, the spleen will return to its normal size. A secondary or dormant schizogony occurs in *P. vivax* and *P. ovale,* which remain quiescent in the liver as hypnozoites.

After a few days of irregular periodicity, a regular 48-hour cycle is established. An untreated primary attack may last from 3 weeks to 2 months or longer. Over time, the **paroxysms** (symptomatic period) become less severe and more irregular in frequency and then cease altogether. In approximately 50% of patients infected with *P. vivax,* relapses occur after weeks, months, or even after 5 years or more. The RBCs tend to be enlarged (young RBCs), there

may be **Schüffner dots,** which are small, round, red granulations (exclusively found in *P. vivax* and *P. ovale*) after 8 to 10 hours, and the developing rings are amoeboid and very actively (Fig. 48.5B) motile; hence the name vivax or lively. The mature schizont contains 12 to 24 merozoites, a key identification factor (Fig. 48.5A).

Pathogenesis and Spectrum of Disease

In patients who have never been exposed to malaria, symptoms such as headache, photophobia, muscle aches, anorexia, nausea, and sometimes vomiting may occur before organisms can be detected in the bloodstream. In other patients with prior exposure to the malaria, the parasites can be found in the bloodstream several days before symptoms appear.

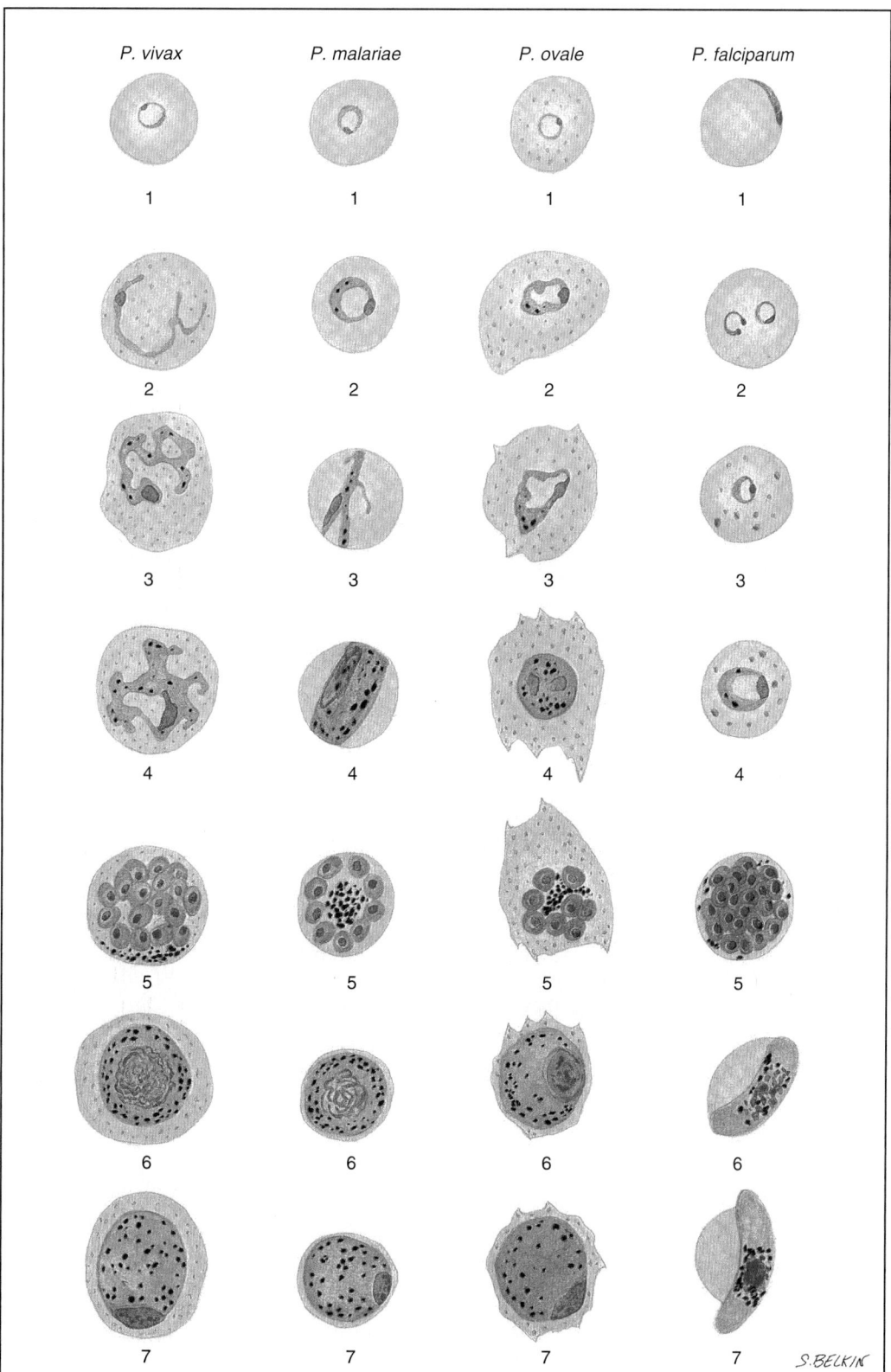

• **Fig. 48.2** Morphology of malaria parasites. *Plasmodium vivax: 1*, Early trophozoite (ring form). *2*, Late trophozoite with Schüffner dots (note enlarged red blood cell). *3*, Late trophozoite with amoeboid cytoplasm (very typical of *P. vivax*). *4*, Late trophozoite with amoeboid cytoplasm. *5*, Mature schizont with merozoites (18) and clumped pigment. *6*, Microgametocyte with dispersed chromatin. *7*, Macrogametocyte with compact chromatin. *Plasmodium malariae: 1*, Early trophozoite (ring form). *2*, Early trophozoite with thick cytoplasm. *3*, Early trophozoite (band form). *4*, Late trophozoite (band form) with heavy pigment. *5*, Mature schizont with merozoites (9) arranged in rosette. *6*, Microgametocyte with dispersed chromatin. *7*, Macrogametocyte with compact chromatin. *Plasmodium ovale: 1*, Early trophozoite (ring form) with Schüffner dots. *2*, Early trophozoite (note enlarged red blood cell). *3*, Late trophozoite in red blood cell with fimbriated edges. *4*, Developing schizont with irregularly shaped red blood cell. *5*, Mature schizont with merozoites (8) arranged irregularly. *6*, Microgametocyte with dispersed chromatin. *7*, Macrogametocyte with compact chromatin. *Plasmodium falciparum: 1*, Early trophozoite (accolé or appliqué form). *2*, Early trophozoite (one ring is in headphone configuration/double chromatin dots). *3*, Early trophozoite with Maurer dots. *4*, Late trophozoite with larger ring and Maurer dots. *5*, Mature schizont with merozoites (24). *6*, Microgametocyte with dispersed chromatin. *7*, Macrogametocyte with compact chromatin. Note: Without the appliqué form, Schüffner dots, multiple rings/cell, and other developing stages, differentiation among the species can be difficult. It is obvious that the early rings of all four species can mimic one another very easily. *One set of negative blood films cannot rule out a malarial infection.* (Reprinted by permission of the publisher from Garcia LS. *Diagnostic Medical Parasitology.* 5th ed. Washington, DC: ASM; 2007. Copyright by American Society for Microbiology.)

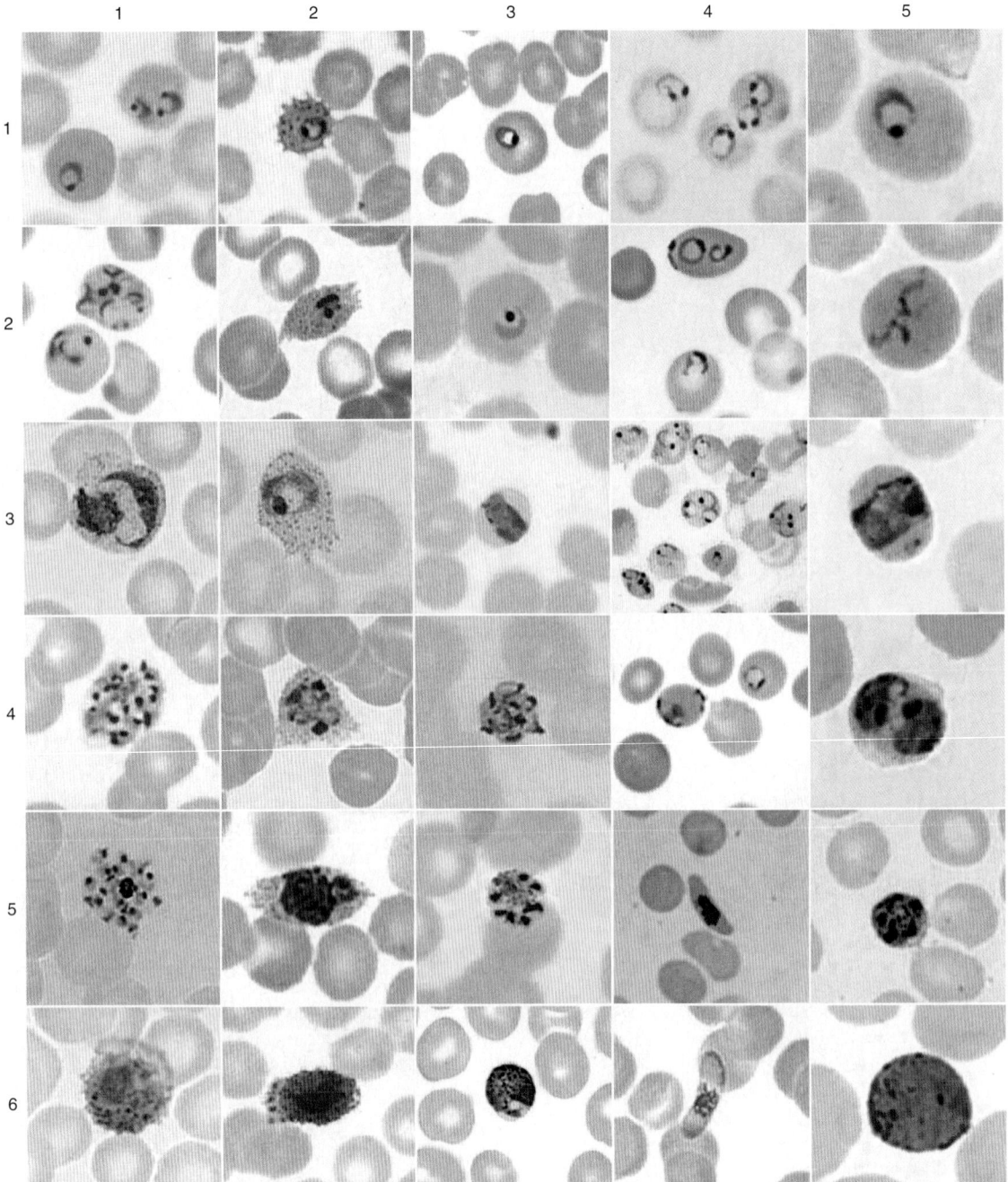

• **Fig. 48.3** Morphology of malaria parasites. *Column 1: Plasmodium vivax* (note enlarged infected red blood cells [RBCs]). (1) Early trophozoite (ring form) (note one RBC contains two rings—not that uncommon); (2) older ring, note ameboid nature of rings; (3) late trophozoite with Schüffner dots (note enlarged RBC); (4) developing schizont; (5) mature schizont with 18 merozoites and clumped pigment; (6) microgametocyte with dispersed chromatin. *Column 2: Plasmodium ovale* (note enlarged infected RBCs). (1) Early trophozoite (ring form) with Schüffner dots (RBC has fimbriated edges); (2) early trophozoite (note enlarged RBC, Schüffner dots, and RBC oval in shape); (3) late trophozoite in RBC with fimbriated edges; (4) developing schizont with irregular-shaped RBC; (5) mature schizont with eight merozoites arranged irregularly; (6) microgametocyte with dispersed chromatin. *Column 3: Plasmodium malariae* (note normal or smaller than normal infected RBCs). (1) Early trophozoite (ring form); (2) early trophozoite with thick cytoplasm; (3) late trophozoite (band form); (4) developing schizont; (5) mature schizont with nine merozoites arranged in a rosette; (6) microgametocyte with compact chromatin. *Column 4: Plasmodium falciparum.* (1) Early trophozoites (the rings are in the headphone configuration with double chromatin dots); (2) early trophozoite (accolé or appliqué form); (3) early trophozoites (note the multiple rings/cell); (4) late trophozoite with larger ring (accolé or appliqué form); (5) crescent-shaped gametocyte; (6) crescent-shaped gametocyte. *Column 5: Plasmodium knowlesi*—with the exception of image 5, these were photographed at a higher magnification (note normal or smaller than normal infected RBCs). (1) Early trophozoite (ring form); (2) early trophozoite with slim band form; (3) late trophozoite (band form); (4) developing schizont; (5) mature schizont with merozoites arranged in a rosette; (6) microgametocyte with dispersed chromatin. **Note:** Without the appliqué form, Schüffner dots, multiple rings per cell, and other developing stages, differentiation among the species can be very difficult. It is obvious that the early rings of all five species can mimic one another very easily. *Remember: One set of negative blood films cannot rule out a malaria infection.* (From Garcia LS. *Malaria Clin Lab Med* 30:93–129, 2010, with permission. Column 5 courtesy Centers for Disease Control and Prevention.)

Malaria Identification Rubric

1. How many ring forms are seen per cell?

    a. More than 1 ring form per cell → ***Plasmodium falciparum***

        i. Look for applique ring forms

        ii. Banana-shaped gametocytes

        iii. Typically only ring forms and gametocytes seen in peripheral blood

        iv. Schizonts have up to 24 merozoites (nuclei)

        v. Black Water Fever – Heme pigments in urine

    b. Only 1 ring form per cell → Go to next question

2. Are the infected RBCs larger than the noninfected RBC?

    a. Infected RBCs not enlarged → probably ***Plasmodium malariae*** or ***P. knowlesi***

        i. Difficult to distinguish without PCR

        ii. RBC may look smaller due to rounding

        iii. Look for band form trophozoites

        iv. Compact ring with large chromatin dot

        v. ***P. malariae***

            1. Every 3rd day paroxysm (quartan)

            2. Schizonts have 6 – 12 merozoites (nuclei) – may rosette

        vi. ***P. knowlesi***

            1. Every day paroxysm (quotidian)

            2. Schizonts have 8 – 10 merozoites (nuclei) – may rosette

    b. Infected RBCs larger than noninfected → Go to next question

3. Are the infected cells oval in shape?

    a. Yes, some cells oval → most likely ***Plasmodium ovale***

        i. No Schüffner's dots

        ii. RBCs may have rough edge – "comet cells"

        iii. Schizonts have 4 – 12 merozoites (nuclei)

    b. Not oval → ***Plasmodium vivax***

        i. Schüffner's dots (best seen with Giemsa stain)

        ii. Large spread-out or small ring forms

        iii. May see full array of stages

        iv. Schizonts have 12 – 24 merozoites (nuclei)

• **Fig. 48.4** Malaria identification rubric: This rubric is used for the identification and characterization of *Plasmodium* spp. from Giemsa-stained peripheral blood thin smears. All laboratory reports should include the body form of the parasite present in the smear, along with the genus and species when possible. (Developed by Janice Conway-Klaassen, University of Minnesota.)

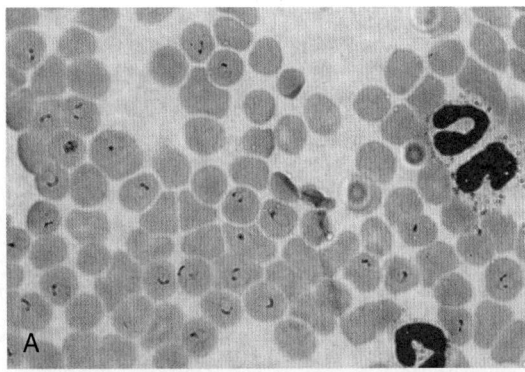
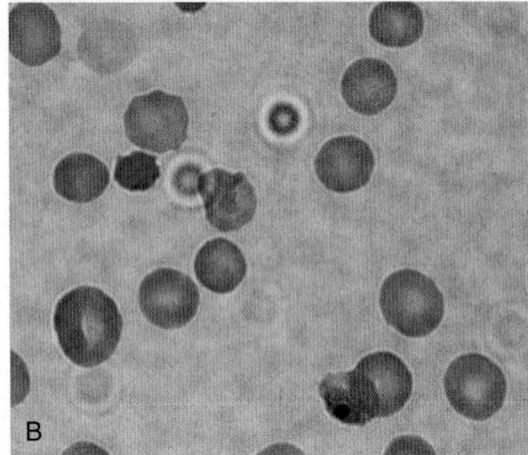

• **Fig. 48.5** (A) *Plasmodium falciparum.* Ring forms (trophozoites) (100× oil immersion). (B) *P. falciparum* microgametocyte appliqué form (100× oil immersion).

Severe complications are uncommon in *P. vivax* infections, although coma and sudden death or other symptoms of cerebral involvement have been reported, particularly in patients whose disease is caused by primaquine-resistant organisms. These patients can exhibit cerebral malaria, renal failure, circulatory collapse, severe anemia, hemoglobinuria, abnormal bleeding, acute respiratory distress syndrome, and jaundice. Acute cerebral malaria involves changes in mental status and if untreated may result in fatality within 3 days.

Plasmodium ovale

General Characteristics

P. ovale was first described in 1922 where the distinctive oval-shaped cells with ragged edges distinguish it from *P. vivax.* Although *P. ovale* and *P. vivax* infections are clinically similar, *P. ovale* malaria is usually less severe, tends to relapse less frequently, and usually ends with spontaneous recovery, often after no more than 6 to 10 paroxysms (Tables 48.1–48.3 and Figs. 48.2 and 48.3). Like *P. vivax, P. ovale* infects only the reticulocytes, so the parasitemia is limited to approximately 2% to 5% of the available RBCs in otherwise healthy individuals. For many years, the literature has stated that, as with *P. vivax,* a secondary or dormant schizogony occurs in *P. ovale,* which remain quiescent in the liver. However, newer findings indicate that hypnozoites have never been demonstrated in naturally occurring cases.

After a few days of irregular periodicity, a regular 48-hour cycle is established. Over time, the paroxysms become less severe and more irregular in frequency and then stop altogether. In some patients infected with *P. ovale,* relapses occur after weeks, months, or up to 1 year or more. The RBCs tend to be enlarged (young RBCs), Schüffner dots (also known as **James stippling**) are present from the beginning of the cycle, the developing rings are less amoeboid than those of *P. vivax,* and the mature schizont contains an average of eight merozoites.

Pathogenesis and Spectrum of Disease

The incubation period is similar to that for *P. vivax* malaria, but the frequency and severity of the symptoms are much less, with a lower fever and a lack of typical rigors. The geographic range is usually described as being limited to tropical Africa, the Middle East, Papua New Guinea, and Irian Jaya in Indonesia. However, *P. ovale* infections in Southeast Asia may cause benign and relapsing malaria in this area. Sequences of small subunit ribosomal RNA have identified two subtypes, *P. ovale curtisi* (classic type) and *P. ovale wallikeri* (variant type) which are morphologically indistinguishable. Human infections with variant-type *P. ovale* are associated with a higher level of parasitemia.

Plasmodium malariae (Quartan Malaria)

General Characteristics

P. malariae invades primarily the older RBCs, limiting the number of infected cells (Tables 48.1–48.3 and Figs. 48.2 and 48.3). The incubation period between infection and symptoms may be much longer than that for *P. vivax* or *P. ovale* malaria, ranging from approximately 27 to 40 days. A regular periodicity is seen from the beginning, with a more severe paroxysm, including a longer cold stage and more severe symptoms during the hot stage. Collapse during the sweating phase is not uncommon.

A regular periodicity of 72 hours is seen from the beginning of the erythrocytic cycle. The infection may end with spontaneous recovery, or there may be a **recrudescence** (recurrence of symptoms) or series of recrudescence over many years. These patients are left with a latent infection and persisting low-grade parasitemia for many, many years. The RBCs tend to be normal to small (old RBCs), there is no true stippling, the RBCs may have fimbriated edges, the developing rings tend to demonstrate "band" forms, and the mature schizont contains an average of 6 to 12 merozoites (Fig. 48.6).

Pathogenesis and Spectrum of Disease

Proteinuria is common in *P. malariae* infections and may be associated with clinical signs of nephrotic syndrome. With a chronic infection, kidney problems result from deposition within the glomeruli of circulating antigen-antibody complexes. A membrane proliferative type of glomerulonephritis is the most common lesion seen in quartan malaria. Because chronic glomerular disease associated with *P. malariae* infections is usually not reversible with therapy, genetic

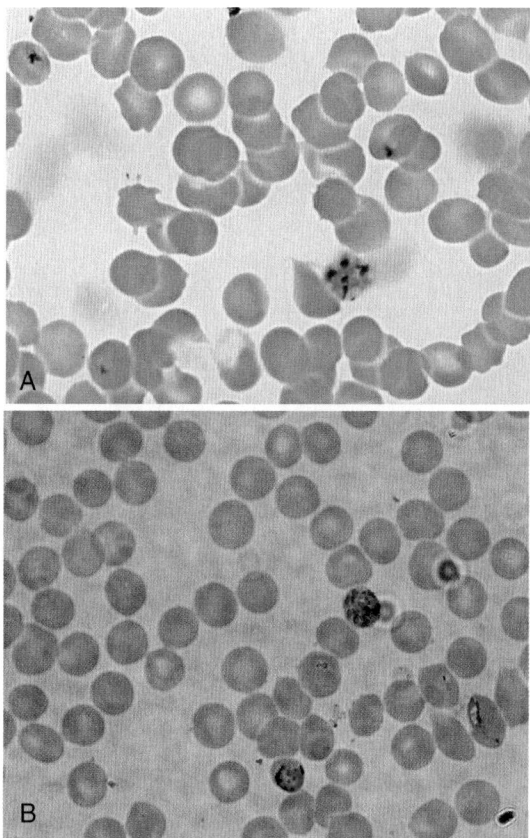

• **Fig. 48.6** (A) *Plasmodium malariae* schizont (100× oil immersion). (B) *P. malariae* schizont and developing trophozoite (100× oil immersion).

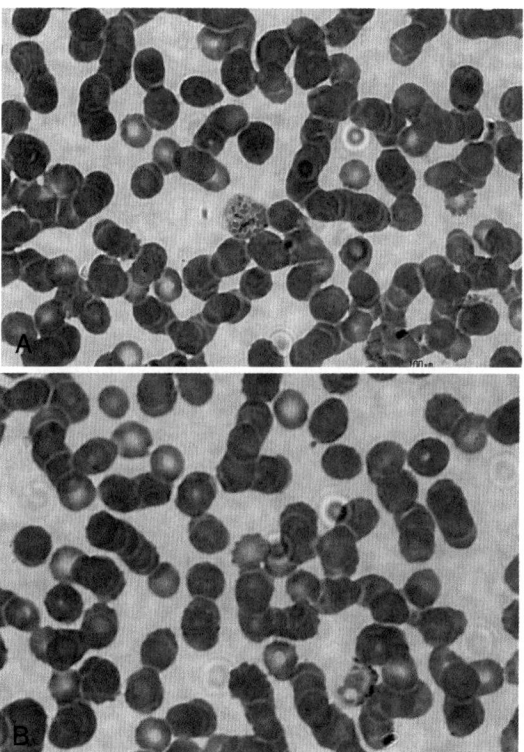

• **Fig. 48.7** (A) *Plasmodium vivax* schizont with late trophozoite and Schüffner dots. (B) *P. vivax* late trophozoite (100× oil immersion).

and environmental factors may play a role in the disease, as well. The patient may have a spontaneous recovery, or there may be a recrudescence or series of recrudescence over many years (>50 years). In these cases, patients are left with a latent infection and persisting low-grade parasitemia.

Plasmodium falciparum (Malignant Tertian Malaria)

General Characteristics

P. falciparum invades all ages of RBCs, and the number of infected cells may exceed 50% (Fig. 48.7; Tables 48.1–48.3 and Figs. 48.2 and 48.3). Schizogony occurs in the spleen, liver, and bone marrow rather than in the circulating blood. Ischemia caused by the obstruction of vessels within these organs by parasitized RBCs will produce various symptoms, depending on the organ involved. A decrease in the ability of the RBCs to change shape when passing through capillaries or the splenic filter may lead to plugging of the vessels. In addition, *P. falciparum* causes **cytoadherence,** allowing the parasites to bind to the surface of RBC and to vascular endothelial cells, a feature that is associated with severe malaria.

The asexual and sexual forms circulate in the bloodstream during infections by four of the *Plasmodium* species. However, as the parasite matures in *P. falciparum* infections, the RBC membrane becomes sticky and the cells adhere to the

endothelial lining of the capillaries of the internal organs. Thus, only the ring forms and the gametocytes (occasionally mature schizonts) normally appear in the peripheral blood. Periodicity of the cycle will not be established during the early stages, and the presumptive diagnosis may be totally unrelated to a possible malaria infection. If the fever demonstrates a synchronous cycle, it is usually a cycle of 36 to 48 hours. Because *P. falciparum* infects young and old RBCs, very heavy parasitemia can occur. The RBCs are all sizes; there is no true stippling, but **Maurer dots** (coarse granulation in the cytoplasm of RBCs) are sometimes present. A unique characteristic of *P. falciparum* is multiple parasite infections per cells, and therefore multiple rings may be seen. The rings are delicate and often have two dots of chromatin. Infected RBCs may show **appliqué** or **accolé** forms—ring forms located on the surface or marginal regions of the erythrocytes (Fig. 48.5B). The gametocytes of *P. falciparum* are crescent shaped, whereas other species are round.

Pathogenesis and Spectrum of Disease

The onset of a *P. falciparum* malaria attack occurs 8 to 12 days after infection and is characterized by 3 to 4 days of vague symptoms such as aches, pains, headache, fatigue, anorexia, or nausea. This stage is followed by fever, a more severe headache, and nausea and vomiting, with occasional severe epigastric pain. At the onset of fever, there may be a feeling of chilliness. As with the other *Plasmodium* spp., periodicity of the cycle will not be established during the early stages.

Severe or fatal complications can occur at any time and are related to the obstruction of vessels in the internal organs (liver, intestinal tract, adrenal glands, intravascular hemolysis/blackwater fever, and kidneys). **Blackwater fever** is a complication of malaria that is a result of RBC lysis, releasing hemoglobin into the bloodstream and urine, causing discoloration. The severity of the complications may not correlate with the peripheral blood parasitemia, particularly in *P. falciparum* infections in a patient who has never been exposed to malaria before (immunologically naïve).

Disseminated intravascular coagulation (DIC) is a rare complication and is seen with a high parasitemia, pulmonary edema, anemia, and cerebral and renal complications. Vascular endothelial damage from endotoxins and bound parasitized blood cells may lead to clot formation in small vessels. Cerebral malaria is more common in *P. falciparum* infections but can also occur in the other species. If the onset is gradual, the patient becomes disoriented or violent or may develop severe headaches and pass into coma. However, some patients, including those with no prior symptoms, may suddenly become comatose. Physical signs of central nervous system (CNS) involvement vary, and there is no correlation between the severity of the symptoms and the level of parasitemia.

Extreme fevers, 41.7°C (107°F) or higher, may occur in an uncomplicated malaria attack or in cases of cerebral malaria. Without vigorous therapy, the patient usually dies. Cerebral malaria is considered the most serious complication and the major cause of death with *P. falciparum;* it occurs in up to 10% of all *P. falciparum* patients admitted to the hospital and is responsible for 80% of fatal cases.

Plasmodium knowlesi (Simian Malaria, The Fifth Human Malaria)
General Characteristics

P. knowlesi invades all ages of RBCs, and the number of infected cells can be significantly more than are seen in *P. vivax, P. ovale,* and *P. malariae. P. knowlesi* infection should be considered in patients with a travel history to forested areas of Southeast Asia, especially if *P. malariae* is diagnosed, unusual forms are seen with microscopy, or if a mixed infection with *P. falciparum* and *P. malariae* is diagnosed. Because the disease is potentially fatal, proper identification to the species level is critical.

The early blood stages of *P. knowlesi* resemble those of *P. falciparum;* whereas the mature blood stages and gametocytes resemble those of *P. malariae* (Tables 48.1–48.3 and Figs. 48.2–48.4). Unfortunately, these infections are often misdiagnosed as the relatively benign *P. malariae;* however, infections with *P. knowlesi* can be fatal. The RBCs are all sizes, there is no true stippling (fine, granular, blue stippling in RBCs stained with Wright's stain or red when using eosin hematoxylin (Fig. 48.8), often there are multiple rings per RBC (there may be two to three rings), the rings are delicate and often have two to three dots of chromatin, band forms are typically seen with the developing trophozoites,

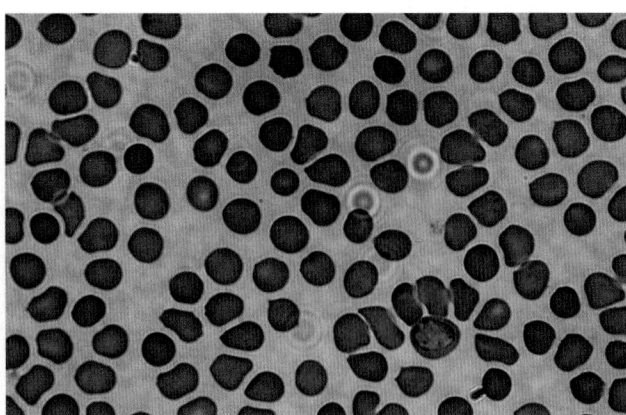

• **Fig. 48.8** *Plasmodium knowlesi* microgametocyte (100× oil immersion).

and the mature schizont contains 16 merozoites. The early stages mimic *P. falciparum,* whereas the later stages mimic *P. malariae.*

Because of different levels of parasitemia, low organism densities, and confusion among various morphologic criteria for identification, detection of mixed infections can be quite difficult. Even if a mixed infection is suspected, identification to the species level may not be possible using routine microscopy methods. However, using polymerase chain reaction (PCR) methods, it is likely that higher detection and identification rates of chronic and mixed malarial infections will be possible.

Pathogenesis and Spectrum of Disease

Patients exhibit chills, minor headaches, and daily low-grade fever. Patients who have been diagnosed with high numbers of *P. malariae* organisms by microscopy should receive intensive management as appropriate for severe *P. falciparum* malaria, assuming the infection is actually caused by *P. knowlesi.* Overall, these infections can be as severe as those caused by *P. falciparum,* with fatal outcomes.

Laboratory Diagnosis (All Species)
Routine Methods

Malaria is considered to be immediately life threatening, and a patient with the diagnosis of *P. falciparum* or *P. knowlesi* malaria should be considered a medical emergency because the disease can be rapidly fatal. This approach to the patient is recommended in situations in which *P. falciparum* or *P. knowlesi* cannot be ruled out as a possible diagnosis. Any laboratory providing the expertise to identify malarial parasites should do so on a 24-hour basis, 7 days a week.

Examination of a single blood specimen is not sufficient to exclude the diagnosis of malaria, especially when the patient has received partial prophylaxis or therapy and has a low number of organisms in the blood. Patients with a relapse case or an early primary case may also have few organisms in the blood smear. Regardless of the presence or absence of any fever periodicity, both thick and thin blood films should be prepared immediately, and at least 200 to 300 oil immersion fields should be examined on both films before a negative report is issued. If the initial specimen is negative, additional blood specimens should be examined over a 36-hour time frame. Although Giemsa stain is recommended for all parasitic blood work, the organisms can be seen with other bloodstains, such as Wright's stain, Wright-Giemsa, or the rapid Field's stain. Using any of the bloodstains, the white blood cells (WBCs) serve as the built-in quality control; if the WBCs look good, any parasites present will be more easily visualized. Fig. 48.7 compares the multinucleated stages (schizont) of *P. malariae* and *P. vivax*. Fluorescent nucleic acid stains, such as acridine orange, may also be used to identify organisms in infected RBCs. However, this may be more difficult to interpret because of the presence of WBC nuclei or RBC **Howell-Jolly bodies**. Acridine orange may be used in the **quantitative buffy coat (QBC)** (QBC Diagnostics, Becton Dickinson, Port Matilda, PA) method. The method provides a rapid screening tool (results are available in 15 minutes) that is technically simple. The test uses a 50-μL tube that contains all the reagents (anticoagulant) and stain (acridine orange) needed for completion of the assay. The microhematocrit tube can be used to collect either capillary or venous blood. The tube also contains a plastic float that is inserted in the tube after phlebotomy. The float is designed to separate specific layers of blood during centrifugation that allows a clear separation of RBCs, WBCs, and what is termed the **malaria detection zone**. Once the tube is centrifuged, it is examined under a fluorescent microscope, permitting rapid detection of stained malaria organisms.

For thin- and thick-smear microscopic films, blood collected using ethylenediaminetetraacetic acid (EDTA) anticoagulant is preferred; however, if the blood remains in the tube for any length of time before blood film preparation, Schüffner dots may not be visible after staining (e.g., *P. vivax*), and other morphologic changes in the parasites will be seen. In addition, the proper ratio between blood and anticoagulant is required to maintain organism morphology, so each collection tube should be filled to the top. Finger-stick blood is recommended, particularly when the volume of blood required is minimal (i.e., when no other hematologic procedures have been ordered). The blood should be free flowing when taken for smear preparation and should not be contaminated with alcohol used to clean the finger before the stick. However, the use of finger-stick blood is currently much less common, and venipuncture blood is the normal specimen collected for the laboratory. Identification to the species level is highly desirable because this information determines the recommended drug therapy. Patients with early *P. falciparum* infections may not have the crescent-shaped gametocytes in the blood. In addition, low parasitemia with the delicate ring forms may be missed; consequently, oil immersion examination at 1000× is mandatory.

Antigen-Based Tests

Several rapid diagnostic tests (RDTs) for malaria are now commercially available, some of which use monoclonal antibodies against the histidine-rich protein 2 (HRP2) or *Plasmodium* aldolase, whereas others detect species-specific parasite lactate dehydrogenase (pLDH). These procedures are based on an antigen capture approach in dipstick or cartridge formats of immuno-chromatographic antigen-detection tests. The BinaxNOW rapid malaria test (Alere, Waltham, MA) is US Food and Drug Administration (FDA) approved for use within the United States. The kit is designed to detect primarily *P. falciparum* and a panmalarial antigen common to the four primary malaria species that infect humans. However, because of sensitivity limitations in patients with a low parasitemia, the "gold standard" is still considered the examination of thick and thin blood films. Given the limitations associated with the rapid tests, it is recommended that results be confirmed using the standard thick and thin blood films. If the rapid test is negative, the thick and thin blood films must be examined on a STAT basis.

Nucleic Acid Detection

Other methods include direct detection of the five species by using a specific DNA probe after PCR amplification of target DNA sequences. Some laboratories are now using PCR for detection of malaria; the high sensitivity, rapidity, and simplicity of some of the methods are becoming much more relevant for diagnosis. Detection is possible for as few as 5 or 10 parasites per microliter of blood; thus, PCR detects many more cases of low-level parasitemia than do thick blood films. This approach is also valuable when the determination of species is questionable by microscopy or when mixed infections are suspected. Although these tests are more sensitive than the traditional blood films, they are primarily available as laboratory-developed tests and are not FDA approved. When a positive result is obtained using a nucleic acid–based test, it is still recommended that a thin and thick blood smear be completed to quantitate the level of parasitemia. Nucleic acid–based quantitation does not correlate with manual quantitation, because the assays are unable to differentiate the reproductive and extracellular forms from the organisms infecting the RBCs.

Automated Instruments

Using automated flow cytometry hematology instruments, there are potential limitations related to the diagnosis of blood parasite infections. *Plasmodium* spp. and *Babesia* spp. infections have been completely missed using such instrumentation. Failure to detect a light parasitemia is highly likely. Unfortunately, failure to make the diagnosis in many of these patients has resulted in delayed therapy. Although most of these instruments are not designed to detect intracellular blood parasites, the inability of the automated systems to discriminate between uninfected RBCs and those infected with parasites may pose serious diagnostic problems in situations in which the parasitemia is 0.5% or less.

Serologic Tests

Serologic tests have little to no clinical utility. This is primarily because of their inability to detect antibodies at the presentation of symptoms. It is also extremely difficult to differentiate a previous from an acute malaria infection. Serology is primarily used to screen donor blood units and for epidemiologic studies.

Results Reporting

In addition to reporting the species of *Plasmodium* identified, it is also important to quantify the level of parasitemia. This will help to guide and monitor the patient's treatment and potentially provide prognostic information to the clinician. Quantitation in the thick film may be reported based on the number of WBCs per microliter of blood in comparison to the number of organisms. If quantitation is completed on the thin smear, the parasitemia is reported as the percentage of infected RBCs in total erythrocytes; extracellular parasites are not included in the count. In addition, *Plasmodium* spp. gametocytes should not be included in the quantitation because they are not considered infectious and are not affected by antimalarial medications. Failure to exclude the reproductive forms of the parasite may result in erroneous changes in treatment due to either falsely elevated or depressed results.

Therapy

Malaria is serious health problem, both in residents of endemic areas and in travelers returning to nonendemic areas. Therapy has become more complex as a result of increased resistance of *P. falciparum* to a variety of drugs, resistance problems with *P. vivax*, and the need to treat severe disease complications. Antimalarial drugs are classified according to the stage of malaria against which they are targeted. These drugs are referred to as **tissue schizonticides** (which kill tissue schizonts), **blood schizonticides** (which kill blood schizonts), **gametocytocides** (which kill gametocytes), and **sporonticides** (which prevent formation of sporozoites within the mosquito). It is important for the clinician to know the species of *Plasmodium* involved in the infection, the estimated parasitemia, and the patient's travel history to assess the possibility of drug resistance related to the organism and geographic area.

Chloroquine-resistant *P. falciparum* is present in almost all endemic areas other than Central America and the Caribbean. Increasing resistance to sulfadoxine-pyrimethamine and mefloquine has been identified in *P. falciparum*. Therefore treatment with **artemisinin combination therapy (ACT)**—including artesunate-mefloquine, artemether-lumefantrine (Coartem), and artesunate-amodiaquine—has been instituted against *P. falciparum*. However, resistance to artesunate-mefloquine has already appeared in Southeast Asia. Current information on the distribution of drug-resistant *P. falciparum* is available from the Centers for Disease Control and Prevention (CDC) malaria hotline in Atlanta, Georgia (phone: 770-488-7788). Therapy for chloroquine-resistant *P. falciparum* remains very complex with continual changes; thus, consultation with an infectious disease specialist is highly recommended. Chloroquine resistance

continues to evolve and spread. Primaquine tolerance has been documented. Current CDC treatment guidelines are available at https://www.cdc.gov/malaria/diagnosis_treatment/index.html.

Molecular detection of specific single nucleotide polymorphisms associated with antimalarial resistance has been used successfully to identify resistance to sulfadoxine-pyrimethamine, chloroquine, mefloquine, quinine, and artemisinin. Methods are available that use PCR and DNA microarray formats, but they are primarily for reference and research laboratory use.

Babesia spp.

The genus *Babesia* includes approximately 100 species transmitted by ticks of the genus *Ixodes*. In addition to humans, these blood parasites infect a variety of wild and domestic animals. Cases of babesiosis have been documented worldwide, and several outbreaks in humans have occurred in the northeastern United States, particularly in Long Island, Cape Cod, and the islands off the East Coast (Homer). Although there are many species of *Babesia*, *Babesia microti* is the cause of most human infections in the United States. *Babesia duncani* and *B. duncani*–like organisms have also been reported associated with infections across Canada and in Washington, Oregon, and California. *Babesia divergens* tends to be more common in Europe, is often found in splenectomized patients, and causes a more serious form of the disease.

General Characteristics
Organism

Although the life cycle of *Babesia* spp. is similar to that of *Plasmodium* spp., no exoerythrocytic stage has been described; in addition, sporozoites injected by the bite of an infected tick (*Ixodes scapularis*–*B. microti* and *Ixodes ricinus*–*B. divergens*) invade erythrocytes directly. The specific vector for the transmission of *B. duncani* and *B. duncani*–like organisms has not been identified. Once inside the erythrocytes, the trophozoites reproduce by binary fission rather than schizogony. Once the tick begins to take a blood meal, the sporozoites are injected into the host with the tick's saliva.

The trophozoites of *Babesia* can mimic *P. falciparum* rings; however, there are differences that can help to differentiate the two organisms (Fig. 48.9). *Babesia* trophozoites vary in size from 1 to 5 μm; the smallest are smaller than *P. falciparum* rings. In addition, ring forms outside of the RBCs and two to three rings per RBC are much more common in *Babesia*. The ring forms of *Babesia* tend to be very pleomorphic and range in size, even within a single RBC. The diagnostic tetrads, the Maltese cross, although not seen in every specimen or species, may be present (Fig. 48.6).

Pathogenesis and Spectrum of Disease

Babesiosis caused by *B. microti* and *B. duncani* or *B. duncani*–like parasites may be mild to severe. Mild disease

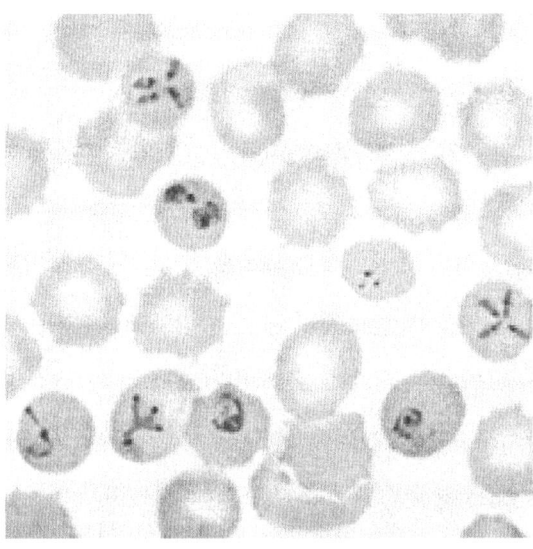

• **Fig. 48.9** *Babesia* in red blood cells.

resembles influenza-like illness, whereas severe disease is clinically similar to malaria, and symptoms include high fever, myalgias, malaise, fatigue, hepatosplenomegaly, and anemia. Usually, *B. microti* infections in the United States occur in nonsplenectomized individuals and are relatively mild. Infections with some of the other *Babesia* spp. from the United States and with *B. divergens* in Europe occur in splenectomized or immunocompromised individuals and are clinically more serious. A recent study found infections with *B. duncani* across Canada, not just in the Pacific Northwest region. Mortality among symptomatic cases of *B. microti* infection in the United States is 5%, whereas that in *B. divergens* infection in Europe is approximately 40%. In both areas, risk factors for severe disease include increasing age, splenectomy, and a compromised immune system. Infections with *Babesia* species from California, Washington, and other Western states tend to be more serious and can mimic the symptoms seen in *B. divergens*.

Laboratory Diagnosis
Routine Methods
The diagnosis of babesiosis should be considered for a patient with typical symptoms and a travel history including endemic areas, exposure to ticks, or recent blood transfusion. Examination of thick- and thin-stained blood films is the most direct approach to diagnosis. It is important to remember that the parasitemia may be low, and these organisms tend to be routinely missed using automated hematology instruments. Similar to malaria infections, the level of parasitemia should be reported to assist in the therapy and patient management in splenectomized or immunocompromised individuals.

Nucleic Acid Detection
Molecular methods such as PCR are available in some laboratories. Nucleic acid amplification acids have demonstrated increased sensitivity in cases of low parasitemia

in comparison to identification on blood films. Assays are available for *B. microti* and *B. divergens*; however, none are FDA approved/cleared.

Serologic Tests
Serologic testing has little use in the diagnosis of acute infections. Antibodies to *B. microti* typically appear within 2 weeks after the development of symptoms and persist for many years after infection. An indirect immunofluorescent test is available in the United States for the detection of antibodies in response to infection with *B. microti* (Imugen, Norwood, MA). Seroconversion in a paired acute versus convalescent or a fourfold rise in titer is indicative of a recent infection.

Results Reporting
Identification of *B. microti* organisms in the thin or thick smear should be immediately reported to the clinician. Quantitation is recommended. Serial smears should be completed if the initial smears are negative, because a negative single smear does not rule out a diagnosis of babesiosis.

Therapy
Mild cases caused by *B. microti* usually resolve spontaneously, and in more serious cases, treatment with clindamycin and quinine or atovaquone and azithromycin is used. In very severe cases of *B. microti* infection and in splenectomized or immunosuppressed patients with *B. divergens*, exchange transfusion can be used in addition to antimicrobials.

Prevention
Personal protective measures, such as long pants, long-sleeved shirts, and insect repellant, may reduce the risk of infection when outdoors in endemic areas for the tick vectors.

Trypanosoma spp.
Trypanosoma spp. are hemoflagellate protozoa that live in the blood and tissue of the human host belonging to the Class Kinetoplastea and Family Trypanosomatidae (Tables 48.4 and 48.5 and Fig. 48.10). African trypanosomiasis (sleeping sickness) is caused by *Trypanosoma brucei gambiense* and *T. brucei rhodesiense* species and is confined to the central belt of Africa. American trypanosomiasis (Chagas disease) is produced by *Trypanosoma cruzi* (Fig. 48.11A) and is confined to the Americas. *Trypanosoma rangeli* infects a wide range of mammals in South and Central America and produces an asymptomatic infection in humans. African trypanosomes and *T. rangeli* are transmitted directly into the bite wound by salivary secretions from the insect vector, whereas *T. cruzi* is transmitted through contamination of the bite wound with the feces from the reduviid bug.

<table>
<tr><td colspan="3">**TABLE 48.4**   **Characteristics of American Trypanosomiasis**</td></tr>
</table>

	Causative Organism	
Characteristic	***Trypanosoma cruzi***	***Trypanosoma rangeli***
Vector	Reduviid bug	Reduviid bug
Primary reservoirs	Opossums, dogs, cats, wild rodents	Wild rodents
Illness	Symptomatic (acute, chronic)	Asymptomatic
Diagnostic stage Blood Tissue	Trypomastigote Amastigote	Trypomastigote None
Recommended specimens	Blood, lymph node aspirate, chagoma	Blood

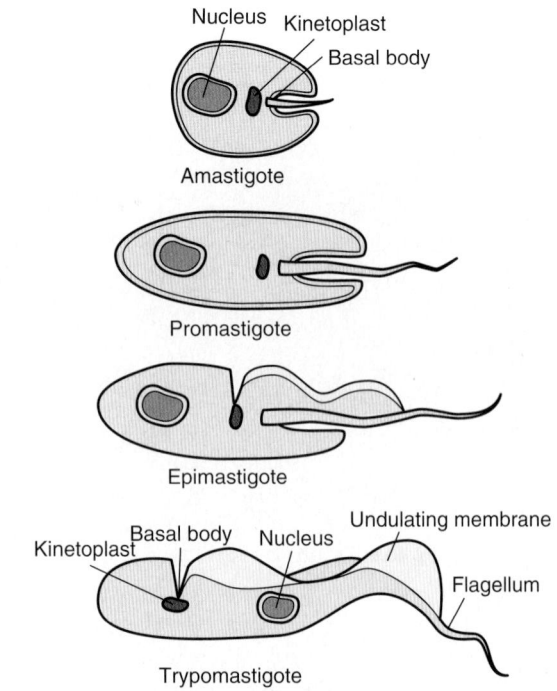

• **Fig. 48.10** Characteristic stages of species of *Leishmania* and *Trypanosoma* in human and insect hosts.

<table>
<tr><td colspan="3">**TABLE 48.5**   **Characteristics of East and West African Trypanosomiasis**</td></tr>
</table>

Characteristic	East African	West African
Organism	*Trypanosoma brucei rhodesiense*	*Trypanosoma brucei gambiense*
Vector	Tsetse fly, *Glossina morsitans* group	Tsetse fly, *Glossina palpalis* group
Primary reservoirs	Animals	Humans
Illness	Acute (early CNS invasion), <9 months	Chronic (late CNS invasion), months to years
Lymphadenopathy	Minimal	Prominent
Parasitemia	High	Low
Epidemiology	Anthropozoonosis, game parks	Anthroponosis, rural populations
Diagnostic stage	Trypomastigote	Trypomastigote
Recommended specimens	Chancre aspirate, lymph node aspirate, blood, CSF	Chancre aspirate, lymph node aspirate, blood, CSF

CNS, Central nervous system; *CSF*, cerebrospinal fluid.

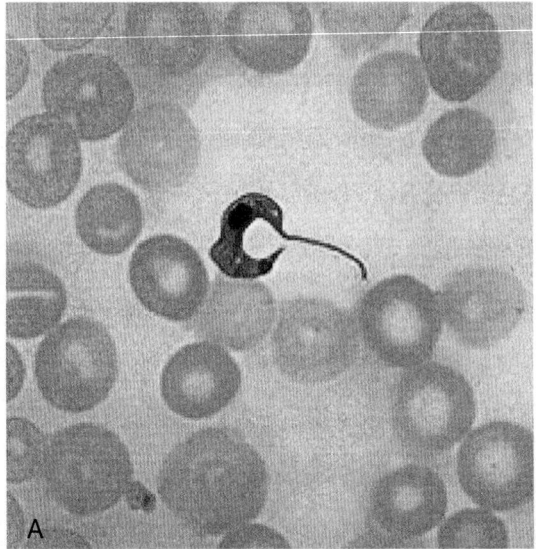

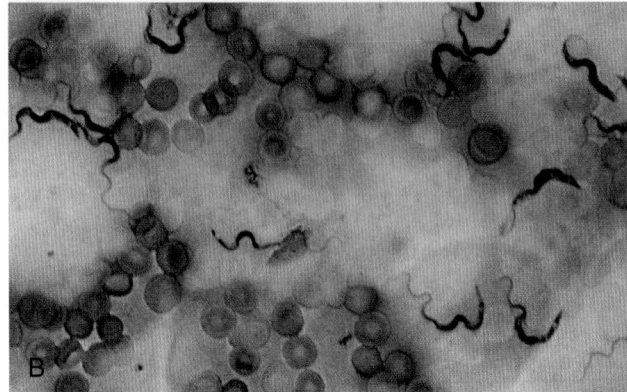

• **Fig. 48.11** (A) *Trypanosoma cruzi* trypomastigote. (B) *Trypanosoma brucei gambiense* trypomastigotes in a peripheral blood smear.

African Trypanosomiasis

The primary area of endemic infection with *T. brucei gambiense* (West African trypanosomiasis) coincides with the vector tsetse fly belt through the heart of Africa, where 300,000 to 500,000 people may be infected in Western and Central Africa. *T. brucei rhodesiense* (which causes Rhodesian trypanosomiasis or East African sleeping sickness) is more limited in distribution than *T. brucei gambiense,* found only in central East Africa, where the disease has been responsible for some of the most serious obstacles to economic and social development of Africa. Within this area, the tsetse flies prefer animal blood, which therefore limits the raising of livestock. The infection in humans has a greater morbidity and mortality than does *T. brucei gambiense* infection, and game animals, such as the bushbuck, and cattle are the natural reservoir hosts.

A unique feature of African trypanosomes is their ability to change the antigenic surface coat of the outer membrane of the **trypomastigote,** helping to evade the host immune response. The trypomastigote surface is covered with a dense coat of **variant surface glycoprotein (VSG).** There are approximately 100 to 1000 genes in the genome, responsible for encoding as many as 1000 different VSGs. More than 100 serotypes have been detected in a single infection. It is postulated that the trypomastigote changes its antigenic coat approximately every 5 to 7 days (antigenic variation). This change is responsible for successive waves of parasitemia every 7 to 14 days and allows the parasite to evade the host humoral immune response. Each time the antigenic coat changes, the host does not recognize the organism and must mount a new immunologic response. The sustained high immunoglobulin M (IgM) levels are a result of the parasite producing variable antigen types, and in an immunocompetent host, the absence of elevated IgM levels in serum rules out trypanosomiasis.

General Characteristics

Trypanosomal forms are ingested by the tsetse fly (*Glossina* spp.) when a blood meal is taken. The organisms multiply in the lumen of the midgut and hindgut of the fly. After approximately 2 weeks, the organisms migrate back to salivary glands where the organisms attach to the epithelial cells of the salivary ducts and then transform to their **epimastigote** forms. Multiplication continues within the salivary gland, and **metacyclic** (infective) **forms** develop from the epimastigotes in 2 to 5 days. While feeding, the fly introduces the metacyclic trypanosomal forms into the next victim in saliva injected into the puncture wound. The entire developmental cycle in the fly takes approximately 3 weeks, and once infected, the tsetse fly remains infected for life.

In fresh blood, the trypanosomes move rapidly among the RBCs. An undulating membrane and flagellum may be seen with slower-moving organisms. The trypomastigote forms are 14 to 33 µm long and 1.5 to 3.5 µm wide (Table 48.5, and Fig. 48.11B). With a bloodstain, the granular cytoplasm stains pale blue. The centrally located nucleus

stains reddish. At the posterior end of the organism is the **kinetoplast,** which also stains reddish, and the remaining intracytoplasmic flagellum (axoneme), which may not be noticeable. The flagellum arises from the kinetoplast, as does the undulating membrane. The flagellum runs along the edge of the undulating membrane until the undulating membrane merges with the trypanosome body at the anterior end of the organism. At this point, the flagellum becomes free to extend beyond the body.

Pathogenesis and Spectrum of Disease
Trypanosoma brucei gambiense

African trypanosomiasis caused by *T. brucei gambiense* (West African sleeping sickness) has a long, mild, chronic course that ends in death with CNS involvement after several years. This is unlike the disease caused by *T. brucei rhodesiense* (East African sleeping sickness), which has an acute, short course and ends fatally within 1 year.

After the host is bitten by an infected tsetse fly, a nodule or chancre at the site may develop after a few days. Usually, this primary lesion will resolve spontaneously within 1 to 2 weeks, and is rarely seen in patients living in an endemic area. Trypomastigotes may be detected in fluid aspirated from the ulcer. The trypomastigotes enter the bloodstream, causing a low-grade parasitemia that may continue for months with the patient remaining asymptomatic. This is considered **stage I disease,** where the patient can have systemic trypanosomiasis without CNS involvement. During this time, the parasites may be difficult to detect, even by thick blood film examinations. The infection may self-cure during this period without development of symptoms or lymph node invasion.

Symptoms may occur months to years after infection. When the lymph nodes are invaded, the first symptoms appear and include remittent, irregular fevers with night sweats. Headaches, malaise, and anorexia may also be present. The febrile periods of up to 1 week alternate with afebrile periods of variable duration. Many trypomastigotes may be found in the circulating blood during fevers, but few are seen during afebrile periods. Lymphadenopathy is a consistent feature of Gambian trypanosomiasis, and the enlarged lymph nodes are soft and painless. In addition to lymph node involvement, the spleen and liver become enlarged. With Gambian trypanosomiasis, the blood lymphatic stage may last for years before the sleeping sickness syndrome occurs.

When the organisms finally invade the CNS, the sleeping sickness stage of the infection is initiated (**stage II disease**). Behavioral and personality changes are seen during CNS invasion. This stage of the disease is characterized by steady progressive meningoencephalitis, apathy, confusion, fatigue, loss of coordination, and **somnolence** (state of drowsiness). In the terminal phase of the disease, the patient becomes emaciated and progresses to profound coma and death, usually from secondary infection. The typical signs of true sleeping sickness are seen in patients with Gambian disease.

Trypanosoma brucei rhodesiense

T. brucei rhodesiense produces a more rapid, fulminating disease than does *T. brucei gambiense*. Fever, severe headaches, irritability, extreme fatigue, swollen lymph nodes, and aching muscles and joints are typical symptoms. Progressive confusion, personality changes, slurred speech, seizures, and difficulty in walking and talking occur as the organisms invade the CNS. The early stages of the infection are like those of *T. brucei gambiense* infections. However, CNS invasion occurs early, the disease progresses more rapidly, and death may occur before there is extensive CNS involvement. The incubation period is short, often within 1 to 4 weeks, with trypomastigotes being more numerous and appearing earlier in the blood. Lymph node involvement is less pronounced. Febrile episodes are more common, and the patients are more anemic and more likely to develop myocarditis or jaundice. Some patients may develop persistent tachycardia, and death may result from arrhythmia and congestive heart failure. Myocarditis may develop in patients with Gambian trypanosomiasis but is more common and severe with the Rhodesian form.

Laboratory Diagnosis (All Species)

Routine Methods

Blood can be collected from either finger stick or venipuncture (use EDTA anticoagulant). Multiple thick and thin blood films should be made for examination, and multiple blood examinations should be completed before trypanosomiasis is ruled out. Parasites will be found in large numbers in the blood during the febrile period and in small numbers when the patient is afebrile. In addition to thin and thick blood films, a QBC concentration method is recommended to detect the parasites. Parasites can be detected on thin blood films with a detection limit at approximately 1 parasite/200 microscopic fields (high dry power magnification, ×400) and thick blood smears when the numbers are greater than 2000/mL, and when they are greater than 100/mL with hematocrit capillary tube concentration

Nucleic Acid Detection

Reference laboratories have used nucleic acid–based tests to detect infections and differentiate species, but these methods are not routinely used in the field. The PCR-based methods have not been standardized, and validation studies have not been performed. Few studies have compared the various PCR methods used for diagnostic purposes. In general, these tests are not available in the routine laboratory.

Antigen Detection

A simple and rapid test, the card indirect agglutination trypanosomiasis test (CATT), and LATEX/*T.b. gambiense* are available, primarily in areas of endemic infection, for the detection of circulating antigens in persons with African trypanosomiasis. These tests are not available for use in the United States. The sensitivity of the test (95.8% for *T. brucei gambiense* and 97.7% for *T. brucei rhodesiense*) is significantly higher than those for lymph node puncture,

microhematocrit centrifugation, and cerebrospinal fluid (CSF) examination after single and double centrifugation. Its specificity is excellent, and it has a high positive predictive value.

Antibody Detection

Serologic techniques that have been widely used for epidemiologic screening include indirect fluorescent antibody assays (IFA), enzyme-linked immunosorbent assays (ELISAs), the indirect hemagglutination test, and the card agglutination trypanosomiasis test. A major problem in endemic areas is that individuals have elevated antibody levels attributable to exposure to animal trypanosomes that are noninfectious to humans. Serum and CSF IgM concentrations are of diagnostic value. CSF antibody titers should be interpreted with caution because of the lack of reference values and the possibility that the CSF will contain serum as the result of a traumatic tap. In addition, antibodies to galactocerebrosides and neurofilaments along with elevated interleukin-10 may also indicate CNS involvement if present in the CSF.

Therapy

All drugs used in the therapy of African trypanosomiasis are toxic and require prolonged administration. Treatment should be started as soon as possible, and the antiparasitic drug selected depends on whether the CNS is involved. Suramin or pentamidine isethionate can be used when the CNS is not involved. Melarsoprol, a toxic trivalent arsenic derivative, is effective for both blood and CNS stages but is recommended for treatment of late-stage sleeping sickness. Eflornithine (DL-alpha-difluoromethylornithine; DFMO) has been used for more than 10 years for melarsoprol-resistant *T. brucei gambiense* infection with or without CNS involvement. Any individual treated for African trypanosomiasis should be monitored for 2 years after completion of therapy.

American Trypanosomiasis

American trypanosomiasis (Chagas disease) is a zoonosis occurring throughout the American continent and involves reduviid bugs/kissing bugs (vectors) living in close association with human reservoirs (dogs, cats, armadillos, opossums, raccoons, and rodents). Sylvatic cycles of *T. cruzi* transmission extend from southern Argentina and Chile to northern California. Transmission to humans depends on the defecation habits of the insect vector. In areas where the local species of reduviid bug does not ordinarily defecate while feeding, there are no human infections. This may explain why there are few human infections in the United States, even though sylvatic infections are known to occur in the southern states. A number of **autochthonous** (indigenous) cases have been reported in the United States, in both Texas and California. The reduviid species involved in transmitting the infection to humans vary with the geographic area. A very serious problem is disease acquisition through blood transfusion and organ transplantation.

A large number of patients with positive serologic results can remain asymptomatic. Patients can present with either acute or chronic disease.

Trypanosoma cruzi

General Characteristics

Trypomastigotes (Table 48.4) are ingested by the reduviid bug (triatomids, kissing bugs, or conenose bugs) as it obtains a blood meal. The trypomastigotes transform into epimastigotes (Fig. 48.10) that multiply in the posterior portion of the bug's midgut. After 8 to 10 days, trypomastigotes develop from the epimastigotes. Humans contract Chagas disease when the reduviid bug defecates while taking a blood meal and the parasites in the feces are rubbed or scratched into the bite wound or onto mucosal surfaces.

In humans, *T. cruzi* is found in two forms: **amastigotes** and trypomastigotes (Fig. 48.10). The trypomastigote form is present in the blood and infects the host cells. The amastigote form multiplies within the cell, eventually destroying the cell, and both amastigotes and trypomastigotes are released into the blood.

The trypomastigote (Fig. 48.11A) is approximately 20 μm long, and it usually assumes a C or U shape in stained blood films. Trypomastigotes occur in the blood in two forms: a long slender form and a short stubby one. The nucleus is situated in the center of the body, with a large oval kinetoplast located at the posterior extremity. A flagellum arises from the kinetoplast and extends along the outer edge of an undulating membrane until it reaches the anterior end of the body, where it projects as a free flagellum. When the trypomastigotes are stained with any of the blood stains, the cytoplasm stains blue and the nucleus, kinetoplast, and flagellum stain red or violet.

When the trypomastigote penetrates a cell, it loses its flagellum and undulating membrane and divides by binary fission to form an amastigote (Fig. 48.9). The amastigote continues to divide and eventually fills and destroys the infected cell. Both amastigote and trypomastigote forms are released from the cell. The amastigote is indistinguishable from those found in leishmanial infections. It is 2 to 6 μm in diameter and contains a large nucleus and rod-shaped kinetoplast that stains red or violet with bloodstains. The cytoplasm stains blue. Only the trypomastigotes are found free in the peripheral blood.

Pathogenesis and Spectrum of Disease

The clinical stages associated with Chagas disease are categorized as acute, indeterminate, and chronic. The acute stage represents the initial encounter of the patient with the parasite, whereas the chronic phase is the result of late sequelae. In children younger than the age of 5 years, the disease is seen in its acute form, whereas in older children and adults, the disease is milder and is commonly diagnosed in the subacute or chronic form. The incubation period in humans is approximately 7 to 14 days but is somewhat longer in some patients.

Acute symptoms occur 2 to 3 weeks after infection and include high fevers, enlarged spleen and liver, myalgia, erythematous rash, acute myocarditis, lymphadenopathy, keratitis, and subcutaneous edema of the face, legs, and feet. There may be symptoms of CNS involvement, which carry a very poor prognosis. Myocarditis is confirmed by electrocardiographic changes, tachycardia, chest pain, and weakness. Amastigotes proliferate within the cardiac muscle cells and destroy them, leading to conduction defects and a loss of heart contractility (Fig. 48.9). Death may result from myocardial insufficiency or cardiac arrest. In infants and very young children, fatal swelling of the brain can develop.

The chronic stage may be initially asymptomatic (indeterminate stage), and even though parasites are rarely seen in blood films, transmission by blood transfusion is a serious problem in endemic areas.

Chronic Chagas disease may develop years after undetected infection or after the diagnosis of acute disease. Approximately 30% of patients may develop chronic Chagas disease, including cardiac changes and enlargement of the colon and esophagus. Megacolon results in constipation, abdominal pain, and the inability to discharge feces. There may be acute obstruction leading to perforation, septicemia, and death. However, the most common clinical signs of chronic Chagas disease involve the heart, where enlargement of the heart and conduction changes are commonly seen.

Laboratory Diagnosis

Routine Methods. Trypomastigotes may be detected in blood by using thick and thin blood films or the buffy coat concentration technique (QBC). Any of the blood stains can be used for both amastigote and trypomastigote stages.

Nucleic Acid Detection. Referral laboratories have used molecular methods to detect infections with as few as one trypomastigote in 20 mL of blood, but these methods are not routinely used in the field. The PCR-based methods have not been standardized, and validation studies have not been performed. PCR-based methods have been used to monitor parasite load and therapy. As with African trypanosomiasis, there have been few studies that have compared the various PCR methods used for diagnostic purposes. In general, these tests are not available in the routine laboratory.

Xenodiagnosis. In endemic areas where reduviid bugs are readily available, xenodiagnosis can be used to detect light infections; this technique is helpful in the diagnosis of chronic infections when there are few trypomastigotes in the blood. Trypanosome-free bugs are allowed to feed on individuals suspected of having Chagas disease. If organisms are ingested in the blood meal, the parasites will multiply and be detected in the bug's intestinal contents, which should be examined monthly for flagellated forms over a period of 3 months.

Antigen Detection. Immunoassays have been used to detect antigens in urine and sera in patients with congenital infections and those with chronic Chagas disease. Antigen detection can also be valuable for early diagnosis and for diagnosis of chronic cases in patients with conflicting serologic test results.

Serologic Tests. Serologic tests for antibody detection include complement fixation, IFA, indirect hemagglutination tests, and ELISA. The use of synthetic peptides and recombinant antigens has improved the sensitivity and specificity of these tests. However, depending on the antigens used, cross-reactions have been noted to occur in patients with *T. rangeli* infection, leishmaniasis, toxoplasmosis, and hepatitis. The sensitivity and specificity of serologic tests for screening blood donors has improved; single-assay screening may be acceptable rather than the two-assay screening methods previously recommended.

Histology. In tissue, amastigotes can be differentiated from fungal organisms because they will not stain positive with periodic acid-Schiff (PAS), mucicarmine, or silver stains. Although the amastigotes of *T. cruzi* look like those in leishmaniasis, patient history, including geographic and/or travel history, and confirmation of organisms in striated muscle rather than reticuloendothelial tissues are very strong evidence for *T. cruzi* rather than *Leishmania donovani* as the causative agent.

Therapy

Nifurtimox (Lampit) and benznidazole (Radamil) reduce the severity of acute Chagas disease. Other drugs, allopurinol, fluconazole, itraconazole, and ketoconazole, have been used to treat a limited number of patients. However, drug therapy has little effect on reducing the progression of chronic Chagas disease. In some cases, surgery has been successfully used to treat cases of chagasic heart disease, megaesophagus, and megacolon.

Leishmania spp.

Leishmaniasis is caused by more than 20 species of the protozoan genus *Leishmania*. Although most laboratories rely on geographic distribution and clinical presentation for the identification of isolates, species differentiation is now based on molecular techniques. Depending on the species involved, infection with *Leishmania* spp. can result in cutaneous, diffuse cutaneous, diffuse, mucocutaneous, or visceral disease. Published disease burden estimates place leishmaniasis second in mortality and fourth in morbidity among all tropical diseases. Leishmaniasis is classified as one of the "most neglected diseases," based on its association with poverty and on the limited resources invested in diagnosis, treatment, and control. The WHO estimates that up to 1 million cases of cutaneous leishmaniasis (CL) and 50,000 to 90,000 cases of visceral leishmaniasis (VL) occur every year in 88 countries. Estimates indicate that approximately 350 million people are at risk for acquiring leishmaniasis, with 12 million currently infected.

Cases of leishmaniasis are seen each year in the United States and can be attributed to immigrants from countries with endemic infection, military personnel, and American travelers. Another concern is the potential for more infections occurring in areas of endemic infection in Texas and Arizona.

General Characteristics

The parasite has two distinct phases in its life cycle: **amastigote** and **promastigote** (Table 48.6, Fig. 48.12). The amastigote form is an intracellular parasite in the cells of the reticuloendothelial system and is oval shaped, measures 1.5 to 5 μm, and contains a nucleus and kinetoplast. *Leishmania* spp. exist as the amastigote in humans and as the promastigote in the insect host. The vector for all forms of human disease is the female phlebotomine sandfly. As the infected sandfly takes a blood meal, promastigotes are introduced into the human host. Depending on the species, the parasites then move from the bite site to the organs within the **reticuloendothelial system** (bone marrow, spleen, liver) or to the macrophages of the skin or mucous membranes.

More than 90% of **cutaneous leishmaniasis** cases occur in Afghanistan, Algeria, Iran, Iraq, Saudi Arabia, Syria, Brazil, and Peru. There has been an increase in the number of cases among military personnel deployed in Afghanistan, Iraq, and Kuwait. Autochthonous (native to origin) human infections have been described in Texas. Most of the cases of **mucocutaneous leishmaniasis** occur in Bolivia, Brazil, and Peru. More than 90% of the cases of **visceral leishmaniasis** are found in Brazil, East Africa, and South-East Asia.

In endemic areas with leishmaniasis, coinfection with human immunodeficiency virus (HIV)-positive patients is common. If coinfected patients are severely immunocompromised, up to 25% will die shortly after being diagnosed.

Pathogenesis and Spectrum of Disease

The first sign of cutaneous disease is a lesion (generally a firm, painless papule) at the bite site. Although a single lesion may appear insignificant, multiple lesions or disfiguring facial lesions may be devastating for the patient. Usually, the secondary lesions will have a similar appearance and will progress at the same speed. The original lesion may remain as a flattened plaque or may progress to a shallow ulcer. As the ulcer enlarges, it produces exudate and often becomes secondarily infected with bacteria or other organisms.

In mucocutaneous leishmaniasis, the primary lesions are similar to those found in CL. Untreated primary cutaneous lesions may develop into the mucocutaneous form in up to 80% of the cases. Dissemination to the nasal or oral mucosa may occur from the active primary lesion or may occur years later after the original lesion has healed. These mucosal lesions do not heal spontaneously, and secondary bacterial infections are common and may be fatal. The mucocutaneous form of leishmaniasis is primarily found in Brazil, Bolivia, and Peru.

Diffuse leishmaniasis, including diffuse CL, is characterized as a nodular disease that results in high parasitemia due to an inappropriate antibody response of the infected patient. This is significantly different than disseminated

TABLE 48.6   **Features of Human Leishmanial Infections[a]**

Species	Disease Type	Humoral Antibodies	Delayed Hypersensitivity	Parasite Quantity	Recommended Specimen
Leishmania donovani complex	VL	Abundant	Absent	Absent	Bone marrow, spleen, tissue
	CL, MCL	Variable	Present	Present	Skin or mucosal biopsy
	DL	Variable	Variable	Variable	Skin or tissue biopsy
Leishmania tropica complex	CL, DCL, MCL	Variable	Present	Present	Skin or mucosal biopsy, tissue
Leishmania major complex	CL	Present	Present	Present	Skin biopsy
Leishmania mexicana complex	CL, MCL	Variable	Present	Present	Skin or mucosal biopsy
	DCL	Variable	Absent	Abundant	Skin or mucosal biopsy
Leishmania braziliensis complex	CL	Present	Present	Present	Skin biopsy
	MCL	Present	Present	Scant	Skin or mucosal biopsy
Leishmania guyanensis complex	CL, MCL	Present	Present	Present	Skin or mucosal biopsy
Leishmania enrietti complex	CL, DL, VL	ND	ND	ND	Skin or tissue biopsy

CL, Cutaneous leishmaniasis; DCL, diffuse cutaneous leishmaniasis; DL, diffuse leishmaniasis; MCL, mucocutaneous leishmaniasis; VL, visceral leishmaniasis; ND, no data available.
[a]For culture, specimens must be collected aseptically; in older lesions, the number of parasites may be scant and difficult to recover.

leishmaniasis that demonstrates a very low parasitemia and an inappropriate cell-mediated response by the patient's immune system.

VL, also known as **kala azar**, has an incubation period that ranges from 10 days to 2 years but typically is 2 to 4 months. Common symptoms include fever, anorexia, malaise, weight loss, and, frequently, diarrhea. Clinical signs include nontender enlarged liver and spleen, swollen lymph nodes, and occasional acute abdominal pain. Darkening of facial, hand, foot, and abdominal skin is often seen in light-skinned persons in India. Death may occur after a few weeks or after 2 to 3 years in chronic cases. Most infected individuals will be asymptomatic or have very few or minor symptoms that will resolve without therapy. Since 1990, an increase in leishmaniasis in organ transplant recipients has been documented. Most of these cases have been VL.

Laboratory Diagnosis

After the cutaneous lesion exudate is removed, these lesions should be thoroughly cleaned with 70% alcohol. Specimens can be collected from the margin of the lesion by aspiration, scraping, or punch biopsy or by making a slit with a scalpel blade. Smears can be prepared from the material obtained and stained with any of the bloodstains; biopsy specimens should also be submitted for routine histologic examination. Specimens for visceral disease include lymph node aspirates, liver biopsy specimens, bone marrow specimens, and buffy coat preparations of venous blood. Amastigotes within reticuloendothelial cells have been detected in a number of different specimen types from HIV-positive patients. Stained smears can be examined for the presence of the amastigotes. Although the specimens can be cultured using special techniques, these procedures are not routinely available.

Nucleic Acid Detection

A single FDA-approved test for the detection of CL, SMART Leish PCR (Cepheid, Sunnyvale, CA) is available in the United States. Often the level of parasitemia in CL or mucocutaneous leishmaniasis is quite low, making identification difficult microscopically. PCR methods have excellent sensitivity and specificity for direct detection, for identification of causative species, and for assessment of treatment efficacy, although they are not routinely available in most laboratories.

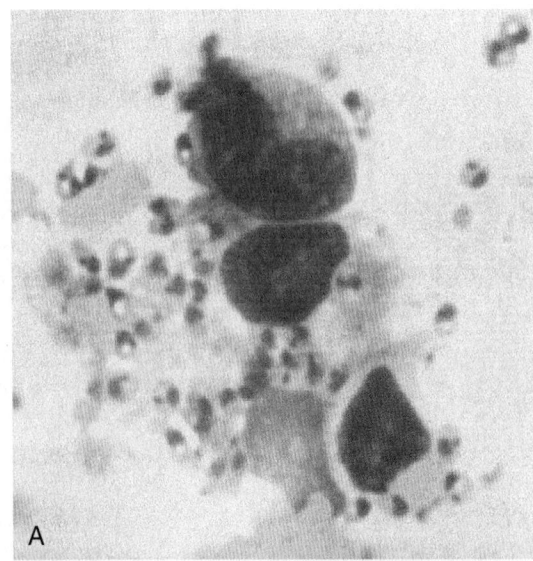

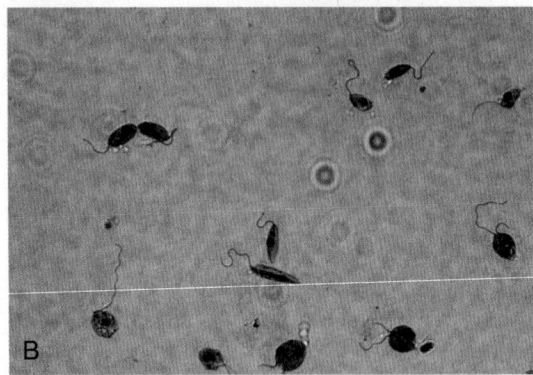

• **Fig. 48.12** (A) *Leishmania donovani*. (B) *L. donovani* amastigotes and promastigotes.

Serologic Tests

A rapid immunochromatographic dipstick test using the recombinant K39 antigen has become available for the qualitative detection of total anti–*Leishmania* immunoglobulins.

In patients with severe VL (kala-azar), there is a characteristic hypergammaglobulinemia, including both IgG and IgM. In highly suspect patients for the diagnosis of VL (assuming they are immunocompetent), if hypergammaglobulinemia is not present, this may be used to rule out the original diagnosis. Although serologic testing is available from some reference centers such as the CDC, serologic assays are not very useful for the diagnosis of mucocutaneous and VL.

Therapy

In simple CL, lesions usually heal spontaneously, although treatment options include cryotherapy, heat, photodynamic therapy, surgical excision of lesions, and chemotherapy. Standard therapy consists of injections of antimonial compounds; however, relapse is quite common, and the patient response varies depending on the infecting *Leishmania* species and type of disease.

Patients clinically cured of mucocutaneous infection continue to be PCR positive for many years after therapy; this disease is characterized by chronicity, latency, and metastasis with mucosal membrane involvement.

For many years, pentavalent antimony compounds have been the drugs of choice for the treatment of VL. However, with the first reports of primary treatment failures in the mid-1990s, additional drugs have been used and include lipid-associated amphotericin B for Mediterranean and Indian disease.

ⓔ Visit the Evolve site for a complete list of procedures, review questions, and case studies.

Bibliography

Alvar J, Aparicio P, Aseffa A, et al.: The relationship between leishmaniasis and AIDS: the second 10 years, *Clin Microbiol Rev* 21:334–359, 2008.

Atroosh WM, AL-Mekhlafi HM, Mahdy MA, et al.: The detection of pfcrt and pfmdr1 point mutations as molecular markers of chloroquine drug resistance, *Pahang, Malaysia, Malaria J.* 11:251–257, 2012.

Baird JK: Resistance to therapies for infection by *Plasmodium vivax*, *Clin Microbiol Rev* 22:508–534, 2009.

Bennett J, Dolin R, Blaser M: *Principles and practice of infectious diseases*, ed 9, Philadelphia, 2020, Elsevier-Saunders.

Carroll KC, Pfaller MA, Landry ML, et al.: *Manual of clinical microbiology*, ed 12, Washington, DC, 2019, ASM.

Chin-Hong PV, Schwartz BS, Bern C, et al.: Screening and treatment of Chagas disease in organ transplant recipients in the United States: recommendations from the Chagas in Transplant Working Group, *Am J Transplant* 11:672–680, 2011.

Cogswell FB, Collins WE, Krotoski WA, et al.: Hypnozoites of *Plasmodium simiovale*, *Am J Trop Med Hyg* 45:211–213, 1991.

Craig AG, Khairul MFM, Patil PR: Cytoadherence and severe malaria, *Malays J Med Sci* 19(2):5–18, 2012.

Eliades MJ, Shah S, Nguyen-Dinh P, et al.: Malaria surveillance—United States, 2003, *MMWR Surveill Summ* 54:25–40, 2005.

Freites CO, Gundacker ND, Pascale JM, et al.: First case of diffuse leishmaniasis associated with *Leishmania panamensis*, *Open Forum Infect Dis* 5(11):281, 2018, https://doi.org/10.1093/ofid/ofy281.

Garcia LS: *Diagnostic medical parasitology*, ed 6, Washington, DC, 2016, ASM Press.

Garcia LS: Malaria, *Clin Lab Med* 10:405–416, 2010.

Garcia LS: *Practical guide to diagnostic parasitology*, ed 2, Washington, DC, 2009, ASM Press.

Gemma S, Travagli V, Savini L, et al.: Malaria chemotherapy: recent advances in drug development, *Recent Pat Antiinfect Drug Discov* 5:195–225, 2010.

Hidron A, Vogenthaler N, Santos-Preciago JI, et al.: Cardiac involvement with parasitic infections, *Clin Microbiol Rev* 23:324–349, 2010.

Jongwutiwes S, Putaporntip C, Iwasaki T, et al.: Naturally acquired *Plasmodium knowlesi* malaria in human, Thailand, *Emerg Infect Dis* 10:2211–2213, 2004.

Koenderink JB, Kavishe RA, Rijpma SR, et al.: The ABCs of multidrug resistance in malaria, *Trends Parasitol* 26:440–446, 2010.

Kribs-Zaleta C: Estimating contact process saturation in sylvatic transmission of *Trypanosoma cruzi* in the United States, *PLoSNegl Trop Dis* 4:e656, 2010.

Lescure FX, Le Loup G, Freilij H, et al.: Chagas disease: changes in knowledge and management, *Lancet Infect Dis* 10:556–570, 2010.

Lou J, Lucas R, Grau GE: Pathogenesis of cerebral malaria: recent experimental data and possible applications for humans, *Clin Microbiol Rev* 14:810–820, 2001.

Murray CK, Gasser Jr RA, Magill AJ, et al.: Update on rapid diagnostic testing for malaria, *Clin Microbiol Rev* 21:L466–472, 2008.

Paranaiba LF, Pinheiro LJ, Torrecilhas AC, et al.: *Leishmania enrietti* (Muniz & Medina, 1948): a highly diverse parasite is here to stay, *PLos Pathog* 13(5):e1006303, 2017, https://doi.org/10.1371/journal.ppat.1006303.

QBC Malaria Test 4277-112-350, Phillipsburg, PA:QBC Diagnostics. Accessed August 09, 2016.

Richter J, Franken G, Mehlhorn H, et al.: What is the evidence for the existence of *Plasmodium ovale* hypnozoites? *Parasitol Res* 107:1285–1290, 2010.

Rodgers J: Human African trypanosomiasis, chemotherapy and CNS disease, *J Neuroimmunol* 211:16–22, 2009.

Scott JD, Scott CM: Human babesiosis caused by *Babesia duncani* has widespread distribution across Canada, *Healthcare* 6:49, 2018, https://doi.org/10.3390/healthcare6020049.

Singh B, Kim Sung L, Matusop A, et al.: A large focus of naturally acquired *Plasmodium knowlesi* infections in human beings, *Lancet* 363:1017–1024, 2004.

Spinello A, Galimberti L, Milazzo L, Corbellino M: Biology of human malaria plasmodia including *Plasmodium knowlesi*, *Mediterr J Hematol Infect Dis* 4:e2012013, 2012.

Vaidya Kuladeepa AS: Quantitative buffy coat (QBC) test and other diagnostic techniques for diagnosing malaria: review of literature, *Nat J Med Res* 2:386–388, 2012.

49

Protozoa From Other Body Sites

OBJECTIVES

1. Describe the distinguishing morphologic characteristics, clinical disease, basics of life cycle (source, stages of infectivity), and laboratory diagnosis for amoebae, flagellates, and coccidia.
2. Compare and contrast the morphologic forms of the *Naegleria* trophozoites, including specimens used for identification.
3. Compare and contrast *Naegleria fowleri, Balamuthia mandrillaris,* and *Acanthamoeba* spp., including routes of transmission, specimens, risk factors, and disease presentation.
4. Compare and contrast the specimen requirements and morphologic characteristics of *Trichomonas vaginalis* and *Trichomonas tenax.*
5. Identify the various morphologic forms of *Toxoplasma gondii* and correlate those with the clinical presentation of the infection (acute, chronic, and congenital).
6. Describe the various individual populations at risk for infection with *Toxoplasma* spp. and the disease symptoms and pathogenesis for each.
7. Define the following terms in relation to the appropriate parasite discussed in this chapter: axostyle, bradyzoite, tachyzoite, ectocyst, mesocyst, endocyst, and oocyst.

PARASITES TO BE CONSIDERED

Amoebae, flagellates (other body sites)
Amoebae
    Naegleria fowleri
    Acanthamoeba spp.
    Balamuthia mandrillaris
    Paravahlkampfia francinae
    Sappinia pedata
Flagellates
    Trichomonas vagina lis, Trichomonas tenax
Coccidia (other body sites)
Coccidia
    Toxoplasma gondii

Free-Living Amoebae

Infections caused by small, free-living amoebae belonging to the genera *Naegleria, Acanthamoeba,* and *Balamuthia* are generally not very well-known or recognized clinically but are often fatal in both immunocompetent and immunocompromised patients. In addition, methods for laboratory diagnosis are not routinely offered by most laboratories. However, hundreds of cases of **primary amoebic meningoencephalitis (PAM)** caused by *Naegleria fowleri* and **granulomatous amoebic encephalitis (GAE)** caused by *Acanthamoeba* spp. and *Balamuthia mandrillaris* (including several cases in patients with acquired immunodeficiency syndrome [AIDS]) have been documented. Other infections caused by these organisms result in *Acanthamoeba* keratitis, related primarily to poor lens care in contact lens wearers. Additionally, both *Acanthamoeba* spp. and *B. mandrillaris* can cause cutaneous infections in humans. *Sappinia pedata,* a free-living amoeba normally found in soil contaminated with the feces of elk and buffalo, was identified in an excised brain lesion from a 38-year-old immunocompetent man who developed a frontal headache, blurry vision, and loss of consciousness after a sinus infection. Additionally, *Paravahlkampfia francinae,* a species of the free-living amoeba genus *Paravahlkampfia,* was isolated from the cerebrospinal fluid (CSF) of a patient with a headache, sore throat, and vomiting, symptoms typical of PAM caused by *N. fowleri* from the environment.

Naegleria fowleri

General Characteristics

Although 30 species of *Naegleria* have been recognized based on sequencing data, *N. fowleri* is the only one that has been isolated in cases of amebic meningoencephalitis. There are both trophozoite and cyst stages in the life cycle of *N. fowleri,* with the stage present primarily dependent on environmental conditions. Trophozoites can be found in water or moist soil and can be maintained in tissue culture or other artificial media. The amoebae may enter the nasal cavity by inhalation or aspiration of water, dust, or aerosols containing the trophozoites or cysts. *N. fowleri* is incapable of survival in clean, chlorinated water. After inhalation or aspiration, the organisms then penetrate the nasal mucosa, probably through phagocytosis of the olfactory epithelial cells, and migrate via the olfactory nerves to the brain (Fig. 49.1).

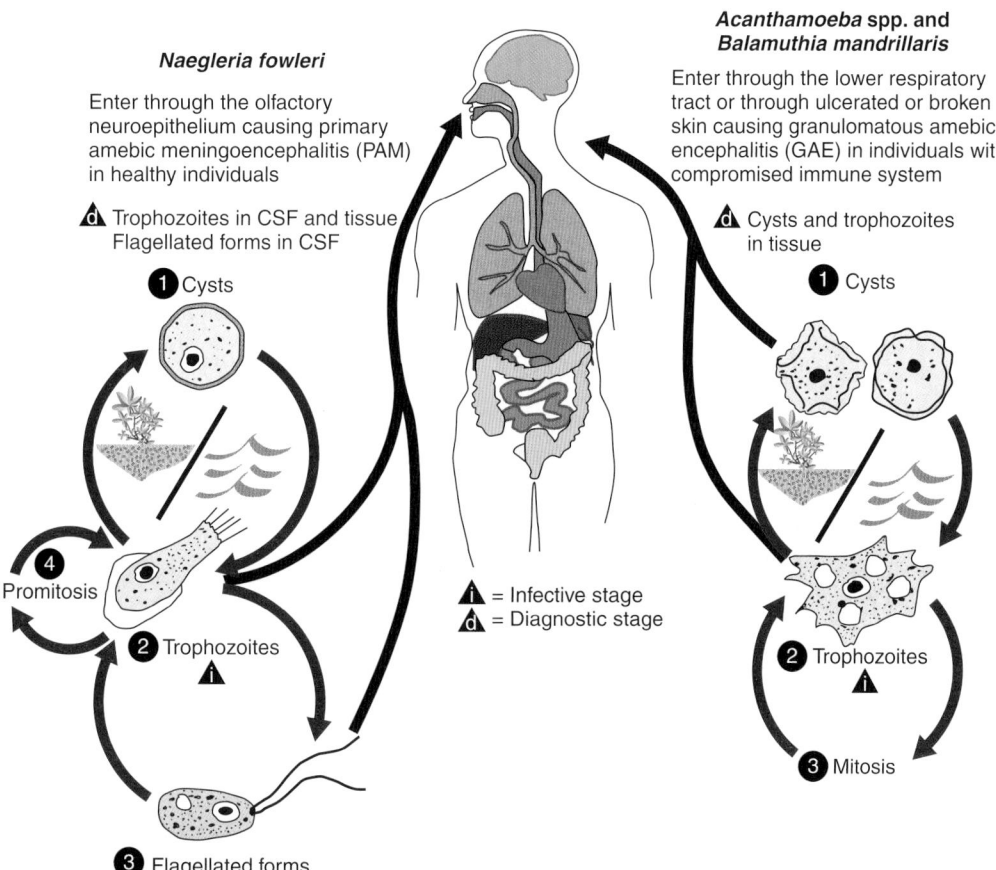

Naegleria fowleri

Enter through the olfactory neuroepithelium causing primary amebic meningoencephalitis (PAM) in healthy individuals

d Trophozoites in CSF and tissue
Flagellated forms in CSF

1 Cysts

4 Promitosis

2 Trophozoites **i**

3 Flagellated forms

Acanthamoeba spp. and Balamuthia mandrillaris

Enter through the lower respiratory tract or through ulcerated or broken skin causing granulomatous amebic encephalitis (GAE) in individuals with compromised immune system

d Cysts and trophozoites in tissue

1 Cysts

2 Trophozoites **i**

3 Mitosis

i = Infective stage
d = Diagnostic stage

• **Fig. 49.1** Life cycles of *Naegleria fowleri, Acanthamoeba* spp., and *Balamuthia,* showing stages and proposed portals of entry. *CSF,* Cerebrospinal fluid. (Courtesy Division of Parasitic Diseases/Centers for Disease Control and Prevention.)

The trophozoites can occur in two forms: amoeboid and flagellate (Table 49.1 and Fig. 49.2). The size ranges from 7 to 35 µm. The diameter of the rounded forms is usually 15 µm. There is a large, central karyosome and no peripheral nuclear chromatin. The cytoplasm is somewhat granular and contains vacuoles. The amoeboid organisms change to the transient pear-shaped flagellate form when transferred from culture or teased from tissue into water and maintained at a temperature of 27°C to 37°C. These flagellate forms do not divide, but when the flagella are lost, the amoeboid forms resume reproduction. Cysts are generally round, measuring 7 to 15 µm with a thick double wall.

Pathogenesis and Spectrum of Disease

PAM caused by *N. fowleri* is an acute, suppurative infection of the brain and meninges (Table 49.1). With extremely rare exceptions, the disease is rapidly fatal in humans. The period between organism contact and onset of symptoms—such as fever, headache, and rhinitis—varies from a few days to 2 weeks. Early symptoms include vague upper respiratory tract distress, headache, lethargy, and occasionally olfactory problems. The acute phase includes sore throat; a stuffy, blocked, or discharging nasal cavity; and severe headache.

Progressive symptoms include pyrexia, vomiting, and stiffness of the neck. Mental confusion and coma usually occur approximately 3 to 5 days before death, which is usually caused by cardiorespiratory arrest and pulmonary edema.

PAM resembles acute bacterial meningitis, and these conditions may be difficult to differentiate. Unfortunately, if the CSF Gram stain is interpreted incorrectly as a false positive, the resulting antibacterial therapy does not affect the amoebae and the patient will usually die within a few days.

Laboratory Diagnosis
Routine Methods

Clinical and laboratory data usually cannot be used to differentiate pyogenic meningitis from PAM. A high index of suspicion is often critical for early diagnosis. Most cases are associated with exposure to contaminated water through swimming or bathing. There is normally an incubation period of 1 day to 2 weeks and then a course of 3 to 6 days, most often ending in death.

Analysis of the CSF may demonstrate a normal or decreased glucose level and increased protein concentration. The leukocyte count will range from several hundred to greater than 20,000/mm³. Although Gram stains and

TABLE
49.1 Free-Living Amoebae Causing Disease in Humans

Morphology[a]

Acanthamoeba

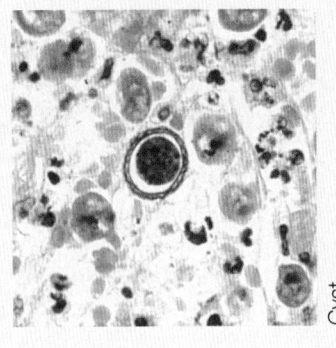

Trophozoite

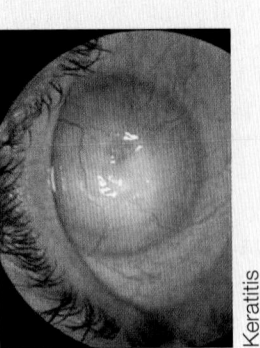

Cyst

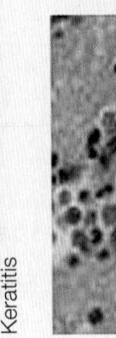

Keratitis

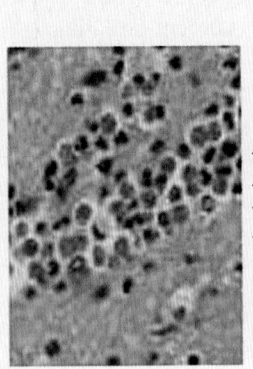

Acanthamoeba in brain

Balamuthia

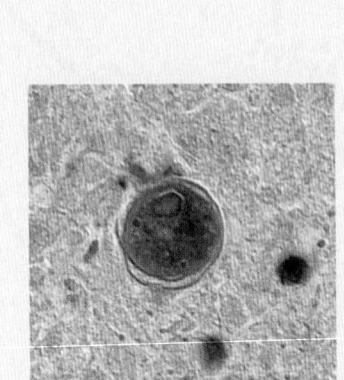

Trophozoite

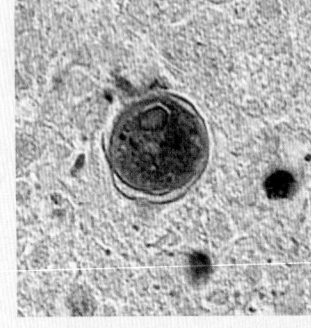

Cyst

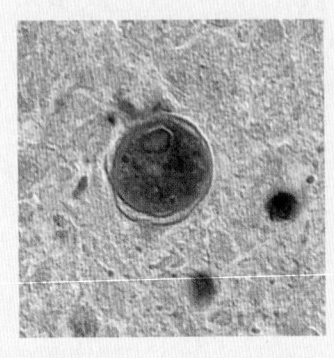

Balamuthia in brain

Naegleria

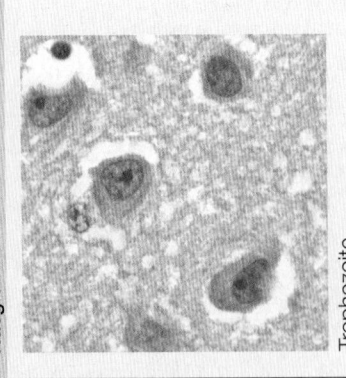

Trophozoite

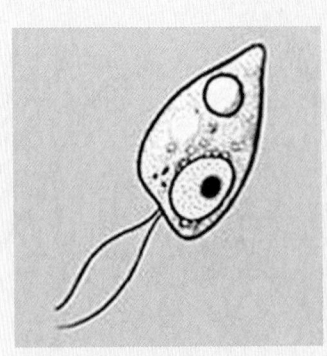

Flagellated form

TABLE 49.1   Free-Living Amoebae Causing Disease in Humans—cont'd

Disease parameter	Acanthamoeba	Acanthamoeba keratitis	Balamuthia	Naegleria
Disease parameter	Granulomatous amebic encephalitis (GAE)	Cutaneous lesions Sinusitis	GAE	Primary amoebic meningoencephalitis (PAM)
General disease description	Chronic, protracted, slowly progressive CNS infection (may involve lungs); generally associated with individuals with underlying diseases	Most common in patients with AIDS, with or without CNS involvement; those receiving immunosuppressive therapy for organ transplantation	Chronic, protracted, slowly progressive CNS infection (may involve lungs); generally associated with individuals with underlying diseases	Rare, but nearly always fatal infection; migration of amoebae to brain through olfactory nerve; symptoms can mimic bacterial meningitis; death usually occurs 3–7 days after onset of symptoms; clinical suspicion based on history critical
Entry into body	Olfactory epithelium, respiratory tract, skin, sinuses	Corneal abrasion	Olfactory epithelium, skin, respiratory tract	Olfactory epithelium
Incubation period	Weeks to months	Days	Weeks to months	Days
Clinical symptoms	Confusion, headache, stiff neck, irritability	Blurred vision, photophobia, inflammation, corneal ring, pain	Slurred speech, muscle weakness, headache, nausea, seizures	Headache, nausea, vomiting, confusion, fever, stiff neck, seizures, coma
Disease pathology	Focal necrosis, granulomas	Corneal ulceration	Multiple necrotic foci, inflammation, cerebral edema	Hemorrhagic necrosis
Diagnostic methods	Brain biopsy, CSF smear/wet prep, culture, indirect immunofluorescence on tissue,[b] PCR[b]	Corneal scrapings or biopsy, stain with calcofluor white, culture, confocal microscopy	Skin lesion biopsy, culture, indirect immunofluorescence of tissue[b]	Brain biopsy, culture on mammalian cells, indirect immunofluorescence of tissue[b]	Brain biopsy, CSF wet prep, culture, indirect immunofluorescence of tissue,[b] PCR[b]

AIDS, Acquired immune deficiency syndrome; *CNS*, central nervous system; *CSF*, cerebrospinal fluid; *PCR*, polymerase chain reaction.

[a]*Acanthamoeba* in brain and *Balamuthia* in brain. Courtesy Dr. Govinda Visvesvara, Centers for Disease Control and Prevention.

[b]Indirect immunofluorescence on tissue and PCR methods available from Centers for Disease Control and Prevention.

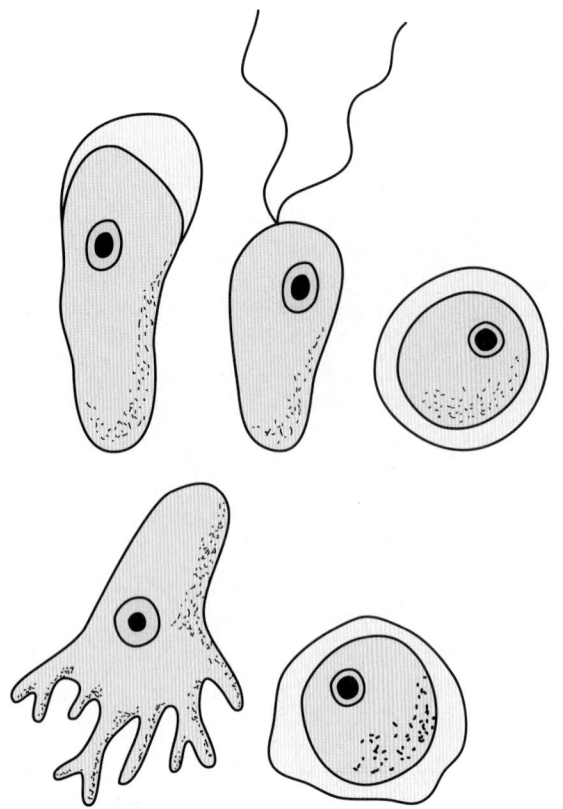

• **Fig. 49.2** *Naegleria fowleri, Acanthamoeba* spp. trophozoites and cysts *(upper row)*. Flagellate and cyst forms of *Naegleria fowleri; (lower row)* trophozoite and cyst of *Acanthamoeba* spp.

bacterial cultures of CSF will be negative, serious complications can occur as the result of incorrect therapy if false-positive Gram stains are reported. CSF may include multiple polymorphonuclear (PMN) cells in the absence of bacteria.

A confirmed diagnosis is made by the identification of amoebae in the CSF or in biopsy specimens. CSF should be placed on a slide under a cover slip and observed for motile trophozoites; smears can be stained with any of the blood smear stains. It is important not to mistake leukocytes for actual organisms or vice versa. This type of misidentification often occurs when a counting chamber is used because the amoebae sink to the bottom and round up; hence, the recommendation is to use a regular microscope slide and cover slip. Depending on the temperature and lag time between specimen collection and examination, motility may vary. Microscope slides may be warmed slightly to improve motility. The most important differential characteristic is the spherical nucleus with a large karyosome.

Specimens should never be refrigerated before examination, and CSF should be centrifuged at a slow speed (250 *g*). If *N. fowleri* is the causative agent, only trophozoites are normally seen, whereas cysts and trophozoites may be present with *Acanthamoeba* spp.

Other Methods

Most cases are diagnosed at autopsy; confirmation of tissue findings must include culture and/or special staining

with monoclonal reagents in indirect fluorescent antibody procedures. Organisms can be cultured on nonnutrient agar plated with nonmucoid strains of *Klebsiella pneumoniae, Klebsiella aerogenes, Enterobacter cloacae*, and *Escherichia coli*. In tissue, the amoebae can be identified using indirect immunofluorescence and immunoperoxidase techniques. Direct fluorescent antibody staining of CSF smears may assist in the identification of *N. fowleri* in the central nervous system (CNS).

Serologic testing currently has no role in the diagnosis of acute PAM, since the time from exposure to the development of symptoms and death is so rapid the immune response is negligible. Nucleic acid methods are available for tracking contaminated environmental sources but are not available in clinical laboratories. Flow cytometry has been used for the identification and differentiation of *N. fowleri* and *Acanthamoeba* species.

Therapy

Although many antimicrobial and antiparasitic drugs have been screened for activity against *N. fowleri,* only a few patients have recovered after receiving intrathecal (injection into the spinal canal) and intravenous injections of amphotericin B or the latter in combination with miconazole. Unfortunately, delay in diagnosis and the fulminant nature of PAM result in few survivors.

Acanthamoeba spp.

General Characteristics

Unlike *N. fowleri, Acanthamoeba* spp. do not have a flagellate stage in the life cycle, only the trophozoite and cyst. Several species of *Acanthamoeba*, including *A. culbertsoni, A. polyphaga, A. castellanii, A. astronyxis, A. hatchetti, A. rhysodes, A. divionensis, A. lugdunensis, A. quina*, and *A. lenticulata,* are implicated in human disease and are not differentiated clinically. These parasites cause GAE primarily in immunosuppressed, chronically ill, or otherwise debilitated individuals. These patients usually have no relevant history involving freshwater exposure. *Acanthamoeba* spp. also cause amoebic keratitis. It is estimated that the incidence in the United States may be one to two cases per million contact lens users.

Motile organisms have spinelike pseudopods; there is a wide organism size range (25 to 40 μm), with the average diameter of the trophozoites being 30 μm. The nucleus has the typical large karyosome, similar to that found in *N. fowleri*. This morphologic characteristic can be seen on a wet preparation.

The cysts are usually round with a single nucleus; they also have a large karyosome, as in the trophozoite nucleus. The double wall is usually visible, with the slightly wrinkled outer cyst wall and a polyhedral inner cyst wall. This cyst morphology is identifiable in organisms cultured on agar plates.

Pathogenesis and Spectrum of Disease
Granulomatous Amoebic Encephalitis

Meningoencephalitis caused by *Acanthamoeba* spp. may present as an acute suppurative inflammation of the brain and meninges similar to *N. fowleri* infection. The incubation period of GAE is unknown; several weeks or months are probably necessary to establish disease. The clinical course tends to be subacute or chronic and is usually associated with trauma or underlying disease and not with swimming. GAE may present with symptoms of confusion, dizziness, drowsiness, nausea, vomiting, headache, lethargy, stiff neck, seizures, and sometimes **hemiparesis.** Unlike PAM caused by *N. fowleri,* both trophozoites and cysts are found throughout the tissue. In addition, dissemination to other tissues—such as the liver, kidneys, trachea, and adrenals—can occur in immunocompromised individuals; additional unusual sites of dissemination include the ear and necrotic bone from a bone graft of the mandible. Some patients, especially those with AIDS, can develop erythematous nodules, chronic ulcerative skin lesions, or abscesses. Biopsies of these lesions should be examined for the presence of *Acanthamoeba* if GAE is suspected.

Keratitis

Acanthamoeba spp. also cause keratitis, uveitis, and corneal ulceration. Clinicians need to consider acanthamebic infection in the differential diagnosis of eye infections that are not responding to bacterial, fungal, or viral therapy. These infections are often caused by direct exposure of the eyes to contaminated materials or solutions. Use of contact lenses is the leading risk factor for keratitis. The use of homemade saline solutions, poor contact lens hygiene, and corneal abrasions are linked to disease transmission. A contact lens can act as a mechanical vector for transport of amoebae present in the storage case onto the cornea. Subsequent multiplication and invasion of the tissue may occur. The pathogenesis of the *Acanthamoeba* infection is due to the migration and adherence between the mannose-binding protein on the organism and the mannose-containing glycoproteins on the mucosal surfaces of the eye or other tissues. The organism releases oxygen radicals and proteases, which destroy connective tissue. Decreased corneal sensation has contributed to the misdiagnosis of *Acanthamoeba* keratitis as herpes simplex keratitis. *Acanthamoeba* keratitis may be present as a secondary or opportunistic infection in patients with herpes simplex keratitis. Unfortunately, as a result, treatment can be delayed for 2 weeks to 3 months.

Cutaneous Infections

Acanthamoeba spp. skin infections appear as hard erythematous nodules or skin lesions. The condition affects immunocompromised patients more often than immunocompetent individuals. The lesions initially appear as purulent papulonodules that develop into indurated nonhealing ulcers. It is unclear if the ulcers are the primary disease or systemic disease following hematogenous spread of the amoebae.

Histologic analysis of the lesions demonstrates extensive tissue necrosis and the presence of both trophozoites and cysts. Cutaneous infections can reach a mortality rate of approximately 75% in the absence of systemic CNS disease.

Laboratory Diagnosis
Routine Methods

The most effective culture approach uses nonnutrient agar plates with Page saline (sodium phosphate, potassium phosphate, sodium chloride, magnesium phosphate, and calcium chloride) and an overlay growth of *Escherichia coli,* on which the amoebae feed. The nonnutrient agar plates and Page saline are available from Hardy Diagnostics, Santa Maria, CA. Amoeba may be detected in as little as 3 days, but negative cultures should be retained for up to 10 days. Amoeba have also been recovered from clinical specimens inoculated to buffered charcoal yeast extract agar (BCYE), tryptic soy agar (TSA) supplemented with 5% horse, rabbit, or sheep blood. Nonnutrient agar overlaid with *Pseudomonas aeruginosa, Klebsiella aerogenes,* or *Stenotrophomonas maltophilia* demonstrates good recovery of both cysts and trophozoites.

Histologic tissue stains are effective. Cysts isolated from cultures can be stained with Gomori silver methenamine, periodic acid–Schiff (PAS), and calcofluor white. Identification of acanthamoebae in ocular samples and other tissues can be difficult, even for trained laboratory professionals; in histologic preparations, the organisms appear similar to keratoplasts as well as neutrophils and monocytes. It has been estimated that up to 70% of clinical *Acanthamoeba* keratitis cases are misdiagnosed as viral keratitis. The average time to diagnosis of keratitis attributable to *Acanthamoeba* infection can average 2.5 weeks longer for noncontact lens wearers than for contact lens users.

Other Methods

CSF or bronchoalveolar lavage (BAL) fluid cytospin preparations can be used to look for amoebae in patients with GAE or respiratory symptoms. The characteristic morphology of the *Acanthamoeba* trophozoites, such as the prominent nucleolus, contractile vacuole, and cytoplasmic vacuoles, can be seen more easily using trichrome or hematoxylin and eosin stains on fixed preparations after cytocentrifugation. The organism may also be cultured on agar plates similarly to *Naegleria* spp. The agar plate should be microscopically examined daily for the presence of amoebae. If an organism is present, the agar should be scraped and inoculated into 1 mL of distilled water and incubated at 37°C and examined periodically for 1 hour. The physician should be informed immediately if an amoeba is present.

In the differential diagnosis of GAE, other space-occupying lesions of the CNS (e.g., toxoplasmosis, tuberculosis, fungal infections, and GAE secondary to *Balamuthia*) must also be considered. Predisposing conditions include Hodgkin disease, diabetes, alcoholism, pregnancy, and corticosteroid therapy. Organisms have also been found in the adrenal gland, brain, eyes, kidneys, liver, pancreas, skin, spleen, thyroid gland, and uterus.

In infections caused by *Acanthamoeba* spp., PAS stains the cyst wall red and methenamine silver stains the cyst black. Normally, *Naegleria* and *Acanthamoeba* isolates are identified to the species level by a reference laboratory, such as the Centers for Disease Control and Prevention (CDC), using indirect fluorescent antibody procedures with a monoclonal or polyclonal antibody.

Therapy
Disseminated Infections

Trophozoites and cysts of *Acanthamoeba* isolates vary in their sensitivity to antimicrobial agents. Successful treatments for keratitis typically consist of a combination of medications. Steroids should not be used to treat cases of GAE, as the medications tend to exacerbate the infection. However, most patients diagnosed with GAE succumb to the infection despite treatment with several drug combinations. *In vitro* testing confirms strain and species differences in sensitivity; however, there is no guarantee that the medications are clinically effective.

Acanthamoeba Keratitis

Prompt treatment of keratitis is essential. Patients should be seen by an ophthalmologist immediately. If the infection is rapidly and properly diagnosed debridement may be sufficient for recovery. If treatment is delayed and the organisms have invaded the cornea or other tissues, therapy may be required for a year or longer. Various prescription eye medications are available.

Balamuthia mandrillaris
General Characteristics

B. mandrillaris is uncommon and was believed to be a harmless soil organism, with no relevance for infecting mammals. Hundreds of cases of human amoebic encephalitis worldwide have been identified, with about half of the cases diagnosed within the United States. Death can occur from a week to several months after the onset of symptoms. Patients eventually die of a massive CNS infection. Genotyping studies indicate that lethal infections caused by *B. mandrillaris* are caused by a single species with a global distribution.

The life cycle is similar to that of *Acanthamoeba* spp.; like *Acanthamoeba* spp., *Balamuthia* does not have a flagellated stage in the life cycle. Both trophozoites and cysts are found in CNS tissue, and their sizes are similar to those of *Acanthamoeba* trophozoites and cysts. It is difficult to differentiate *Balamuthia* from *Acanthamoeba* spp. in tissue sections under a light microscope. The *Balamuthia* trophozoite and cyst is approximately 30 to 120 μm in diameter. Using electron microscopy, the cysts are characterized by three layers in the cyst wall: an outer wrinkled **ectocyst,** a middle structureless **mesocyst,** and an inner thin **endocyst.** Under light microscopy, they appear to have two walls: an outer irregular wall and an inner round wall. In some cases, *Balamuthia* trophozoites in tissue sections appear to have more than one nucleolus in the nucleus. In such cases, it may be possible to distinguish *Balamuthia* amoebae from *Acanthamoeba* organisms based on nuclear morphology, because *Acanthamoeba* trophozoites have only one nucleolus.

Pathogenesis and Spectrum of Disease

The disease is very similar to GAE caused by *Acanthamoeba* spp. The clinical presentation is subacute or chronic and is usually not associated with swimming in freshwater. No characteristic clinical symptoms, laboratory findings, or radiologic indicators have been found to be diagnostic for GAE. The organism produces virulence factors that enhance adhesion to and penetration of the blood-brain barrier. The amoeba causes tissue damage by phagocytosis of cells and the production of toxins and proteases that destroy the extracellular matrices. Whether single or multiple, the lesions in the brain involve mainly the cerebral cortex and subcortical white matter. Generalized symptoms include headache, nausea, vomiting, fever, visual disturbances, dysphagia, seizures, and hemiparesis. The clinical course ranges from a few days to several months. *B. mandrillaris* is larger than human leukocytes, thus making phagocytosis impossible. Instead, in immunocompetent hosts, the immune system attempts to contain them at the portal of entry by mounting a type IV hypersensitivity reaction; however, with rare exceptions, these patients also tend to die with severe CNS disease.

Laboratory Diagnosis

B. mandrillaris does not grow well on *E. coli*–seeded nonnutrient agar plates because, unlike *Naegleria* or *Acanthamoeba*, *B. mandrillaris* does not feed on bacteria. However, these organisms can be cultured in mammalian cell cultures using monkey kidney cells and MRC (human fetal lung fibroblast cells), HEp-2 (human carcinoma cells), and diploid macrophage cell lines. Using human brain microvascular endothelial cells, *B. mandrillaris* has been cultured postmortem from brain and CSF from a case of granulomatous amoebic meningoencephalitis. The organism may be diagnosed by examining blood, CSF, and tissue samples. A cell-free growth medium is also commercially available.

There are two serologic tests that can help confirm the diagnosis of GAE. The indirect immunofluorescence assay (IFA) is a test used to detect antibodies attached to *Balamuthia* amoebae in body tissues. In contrast, immunohistochemistry (IHC) uses specific antibodies against *Balamuthia* to detect the amoebae. Although serum antibodies have been identified in infections, laboratory testing is not routinely available.

Therapy

In vitro studies indicate that *B. mandrillaris* is susceptible to pentamidine isothiocyanate and that patients may benefit from this treatment. Other studies indicate that azithromycin, sulfadiazine, flucytosine, clarithromycin, and miltefosine have amebicidal activity.

Sappinia spp.

Two species of a new free-living amoeba have been identified that may be capable of causing amoebic encephalitis: *S. diploidea* and *S. pedata*. *S. pedata* is the only species that has been clearly associated with human infection. Trophozoites measure approximately 40 to 70 µm and have two nuclei. Cysts have not been identified in human infection but have been visualized in culture. Symptoms of infection may include visual disturbances, headache, and seizures. Computed tomography of the brain may reveal a mass that resembles a tumor. The mass is the site of inflammation and harbors the free-living amoebic trophozoites. Surgical excision followed by antiamebic medications can be used for treatment.

Nucleic Acid Detection (Free-Living Amoebae)

Several isolates for each of the free-living amoebae—*Naegleria, Acanthamoeba,* and *Balamuthia*—have been sequenced. Sequencing of isolates provides information for the development of more specific assays for the identification and treatment of patients with PAM and GAE.

The CDC has developed a real-time polymerase chain reaction (PCR) assay for the simultaneous detection of the three primary free-living amoebae from CSF. This assay has been used successfully to identify amoeba in patient specimens but is not currently available in routine clinical laboratories.

Results Reporting (Free-Living Amoebae)

The presence of any amoebae should be immediately reported to the clinician. Most routine clinical laboratories do not have the technical staff or equipment to identify these organisms and routinely send the specimens to a reference laboratory.

Trichomonas vaginalis

General Characteristics

Infection with *T. vaginalis* is acquired primarily through sexual intercourse, hence the need to diagnose and treat asymptomatic males. The organism is capable of survival for extended periods in a moist environment such as damp towels and underclothes. However, this mode of transmission is thought to be very rare. Infection with *T. vaginalis* occurs worldwide. **Trichomoniasis** is the primary nonviral sexually transmitted disease worldwide, with an estimated annual occurrence of 250 million cases. Infection with *T. vaginalis* has major health consequences for women, including complications in pregnancy, association with cervical cancer, and predisposition to human immunodeficiency virus (HIV) infection.

The life cycle of *T. vaginalis* includes a single trophozoite, which is very similar in morphology to other trichomonads

TABLE 49.2	Characteristics of *Trichomonas vaginalis*
Shape and size	Pear shaped, 7–23 µm long (average, 13 µm); width, 5–15 µm
Motility	Jerky, rapid
Number of nuclei and visibility	1; not visible in unstained mounts
Number of flagella (usually difficult to see)	3–5 anterior, 1 posterior
Other features	Seen in urine, urethral discharge, and vaginal smears; undulating membrane extends half the length of the body; no free posterior flagellum; axostyle easily seen
Infective stage	Trophozoite
Usual location	Vagina (male, urethra)
Striking clinical findings	Leukorrhea, pruritus vulvae (thin white urethral discharge in male)
Other sites of infection	Urethra (prostate in male)
Stage usually recovered during clinical phase	Trophozoite only—no cyst

Trichomonas, wet mount

Trichomonas, Papanicolaou stain

(Table 49.2). The trophozoite is 7 to 23 µm long and 5 to 15 µm wide. The **axostyle** is usually obvious and protrudes through the bottom of the organism, whereas the undulating membrane ends halfway down the side of the trophozoite. There are a large number of granules evident along the axostyle.

Pathogenesis and Spectrum of Disease

Growth of the organism results in inflammation and large numbers of trophozoites in the tissues and the secretions. As the acute infection becomes more chronic, the purulent discharge diminishes, with a decrease in the number of organisms. Symptoms such as vaginal or vulvar pruritus and discharge are often sudden and occur during or after menstruation because of the increased vaginal acidity. Symptoms include vaginal discharge (42%), odor (50%), and edema or erythema (22% to 37%). Complaints also include dysuria and lower abdominal pain.

Between 25% and 50% of infected females may be asymptomatic; they have a normal vaginal pH of 3.8 to 4.2 and normal vaginal microbiota. Even when the infection is in the carrier form, about 50% of infected females will become symptomatic during the following 6 months.

Although vaginitis is the most common finding in females with trichomoniasis, other complications include distention of a fallopian tube with pus, endometritis, infertility, low birth weight, and cervical erosion. There is also an increased association with HIV transmission and cervical dysplasia.

Dysuria, often the earliest symptom, occurs in about 20% of females with vaginal trichomoniasis. Infected males may be asymptomatic, or the infection may be self-limited, be persistent, or result in recurring urethritis. In nonspecific urethritis, *T. vaginalis* has been detected in 10% to 20% of subjects and in 20% to 30% of those, whose sexual partners had vaginitis. Once established, the infection persists for an extended period in females but for only about 10 days or less in males. *T. vaginalis* is the cause of 11% of all cases of nongonococcal urethritis in males.

Respiratory distress has been reported in a full-term normal male infant with *T. vaginalis* with severe respiratory problems after delivery. A wet preparation of thick white sputum demonstrated a few leukocytes and motile flagellates, which were identified as *T. vaginalis*. This study supports previous data confirming that the organism may cause neonatal pneumonia.

Laboratory Diagnosis

Humans are the only natural host for *T. vaginalis,* and organisms reside in the vagina and prostate; they usually do not survive outside the urogenital tract. The parasites feed on the mucosal surface of the vagina, where bacteria and leukocytes are abundant. The preferred pH for good parasitic growth in females is slightly alkaline or acidic (6.0 to 6.3 optimal), not the normal pH (3.8 to 4.2) of the healthy vagina. The organisms can be recovered in urine, in urethral discharge, or after prostatic massage. Often the organisms are recovered in centrifuged urine sediment from both male and female patients.

Wet Mounts

The identification of *T. vaginalis* is often based on the examination of wet preparations of vaginal and urethral discharges, urine, and prostatic secretions. This examination must be performed within 10 to 20 minutes after sample collection; if delayed, the organisms lose their motility and may be missed. Several specimens may need to be examined for detection of the organisms. The sensitivity associated with wet mount examinations varies between 40% and more than 80%. Often, the percent detection from this procedure is quite low, with limited sensitivity and specificity.

Stained Smears

Giemsa or Papanicolaou stain can be used. However, atypical cellular changes can be misinterpreted, particularly on the Papanicolaou smear. The organisms are routinely missed on Gram stains. The number of false-positive and false-negative results reported based on stained smears strongly suggests that confirmation should be accomplished by observation of motile organisms either from the direct wet mount or from appropriate culture media.

Antigen Detection

Several rapid diagnostic tests have been developed, including the OSOM *Trichomonas* rapid immunochromatographic capillary-flow dipstick assay (Genzyme Diagnostics, Cambridge, MA), which is more sensitive than the wet mount. Additionally, an immunofluorescent assay is available—T.VAG DFA (*T. vaginalis* DFA; Chemicon International, Temecula, CA)—that is capable of direct testing of the patient sample.

Nucleic Acid Detection

The use of PCR methods has led to improvements in *T. vaginalis* detection; nonviable organisms and cells and target sequences can be detected. In addition to various culture and transport options, several other products are available, including the Affirm VPIII probe from Becton Dickinson (Cockeysville, MD). The Affirm VPIII detects the three most common organisms associated with vaginal infections: *T. vaginalis, Gardnerella vaginalis,* and *Candida albicans*. An assay approved by the US Food and Drug Administration (FDA) that uses transcription-mediated amplification (Chapter 8) is available for the identification of *T. vaginalis* (Hologic, San Diego, CA). The assay can be automated for testing using either the Panther or Tigris instrumentation. Nucleic acid amplification tests (NAAT) from Cepheid Xpert TV or the GeneXpert system (Sunnyvale, CA) have also been cleared by the FDA for the detection of *T. vaginalis* in specimens from both women and men. A variety of highly sensitive and specific PCR assays are available for the detection of the organism in urine samples. Depending on the patient population, client base, number of requests, and cost, one or more of these options may be appropriate for a particular diagnostic laboratory.

Culture

A convenient plastic envelope method is available that allows immediate examination and culture in one self-contained system. This system is commercially available as the InPouchTV (BIOMED Diagnostics, San Jose, CA) and serves as the specimen transport container, the growth chamber during incubation, and the "slide" during microscopy. Once it is inoculated, it requires no opening for examination, and growth occurs within 5 days. The sensitivity of this system is reported to be superior to that of other available culture methods.

Therapy

Metronidazole remains the recommended option for the treatment of urogenital trichomoniasis and is currently the only drug approved for treatment in the United States. Resistance to both metronidazole and other 5-nitromidazoles has been reported. All sexual partners should be treated simultaneously to prevent reinfection. Tinidazole has also been used for therapy.

Trichomonas tenax

Trichomonas tenax, or oral trichomonas, is commonly found in the oral cavity of humans, dogs, and cats. This parasite colonizes patients with poor oral hygiene and advanced periodontal disease. Transmission is through saliva, droplet spray, and kissing or use of contaminated dishes or drinking water. Trophozoites survive in the body as mouth scavengers that feed on local microorganisms located between the teeth, in tonsillar crypts and pyorrheal pockets, and at the gingival margin around the gums. However, the trophozoites are unable to survive the digestive process.

General Characteristics

Of the three parasites in the genus *Trichomonas*, *T. tenax* is the smallest, measuring only 5 to 14 µm long and 6 to 9 µm wide. The organism can be identified by the long axostyle and tail, four anterior flagella, and an undulating membrane that spans two-thirds the length of the body. The undulating membrane may also resemble small legs. The flagellate has no cyst stage. *T. tenax* may be confused with *T. vaginalis* due to similar morphology. In such cases, the presence of an oral or vaginal parasite should be confirmed.

Pathogenesis and Spectrum of Disease

T. tenax is generally not found in the oral cavity of healthy individuals. It is known to play a pathogenic role in necrotizing ulcerative gingivitis and periodontitis. The organism is also implicated in chronic lung disease. Removal or clearance of the organism results in complete recovery. *T. tenax* is not known to cause specific pathology or disease symptoms. It may be involved in the degradation of periodontal tissue through the secretion of substances such as alkaline phosphatases and the fibronectin cathepsin. The organism appears to primarily worsen preexisting periodontal disease. In rare cases has been reported to cause bronchopulmonary infections in patients with cancer or other lung diseases.

Laboratory Diagnosis

The specimen of choice for the identification of *T. tenax* trophozoites is mouth scrapings. Microscopic examination with bright field or phase contrast microscopy of tartar, the gingival margin of the gums, tonsillar crypts, and pyorrheal pockets of patients suffering from *T. tenax* infections often yields trophozoites. *T. tenax* may be cultured on artificial media, as outlined previously for *T. vaginalis*.

Therapy

Proper oral hygiene in combination with regular dental visits to remove dental plaque prevents colonization.

Toxoplasma gondii

Toxoplasma gondii is a protozoan parasite that infects most species of warm-blooded animals, including humans. Members of the cat family, *Felidae,* are the only known definitive hosts for the sexual stages of *T. gondii* and serve as the main reservoirs of infection. Cats become infected with *T. gondii* through carnivorism or by ingestion of **oocysts.** Outdoor cats are much more likely to become infected than domestic cats that are confined indoors. After the cat has ingested tissue cysts or oocysts, organisms are released and invade epithelial cells of the cat's small intestine. In the small intestine, they undergo an asexual cycle followed by a sexual cycle with the formation of oocysts, which are excreted in the feces. The noninfective oocyst takes 1 to 5 days after excretion to become infective. Cats shed oocysts for 1 to 2 weeks, and large numbers may be shed, often more than 100,000 per gram of feces. Oocysts survive in the environment for several months to more than 1 year and are resistant to disinfectants, freezing, and drying. However, they are killed by heating to 70°C for 10 minutes. The life cycle in the cat takes approximately 19 to 48 days after infection with the oocysts but only 3 to 10 days after the ingestion of meat infected with cysts (e.g., a mouse) (Fig. 49.3).

General Characteristics

There are three infectious stages of *T. gondii*: the **tachyzoites** (in groups or clones), the **bradyzoites** (in tissue cysts), and the sporozoites (in oocysts from cat feces). Tachyzoites rapidly multiply in any cell of the intermediate host and in epithelial cells of the definitive host (cats). Bradyzoites are found within the tissue cysts and usually multiply very slowly. The cyst may contain few to hundreds of organisms, and intramuscular cysts may reach 100 µm in size. The tissue cysts can be found in visceral organs such as the lungs, liver, and kidneys. However, they are more prevalent in the brain, eyes, and skeletal and cardiac muscle. Intact tissue cysts can persist for the life of the host and do not cause an inflammatory response.

Tachyzoites are crescent-shaped and are 2 to 3 µm wide by 4 to 8 µm long (Table 49.3). One end tends to be more rounded than the other is. Giemsa is the stain of choice; the cytoplasm stains pale blue, and the nucleus stains red and is situated toward the broad end of the organism.

Cysts are formed in chronic infections, and the bradyzoites within the cyst wall are strongly PAS positive. During the acute phase, there may be groups of tachyzoites that appear to be cysts; however, they are not strongly PAS positive and have been termed **pseudocysts.**

Pathogenesis and Spectrum of Disease

As the tachyzoites actively grow, increase in number, and eventually rupture from the cell, they invade adjacent cells. This process creates additional lesions. Once the cysts have

Toxoplasmosis
(Toxoplasma gondii)

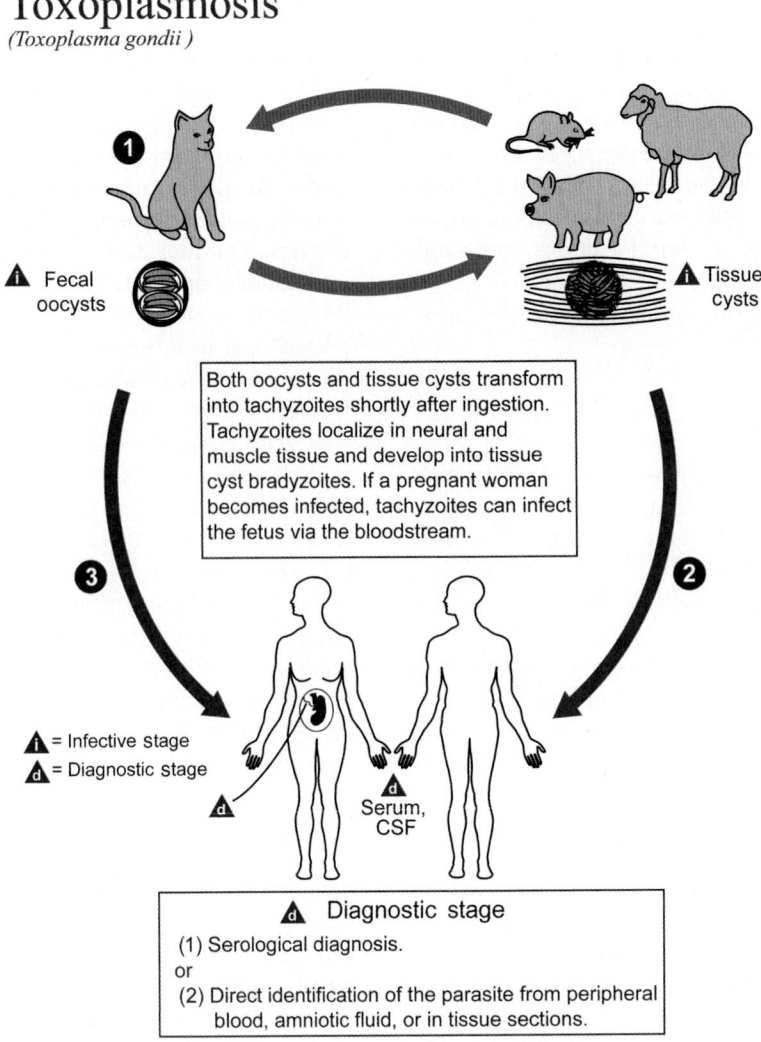

Both oocysts and tissue cysts transform into tachyzoites shortly after ingestion. Tachyzoites localize in neural and muscle tissue and develop into tissue cyst bradyzoites. If a pregnant woman becomes infected, tachyzoites can infect the fetus via the bloodstream.

Fecal oocysts

Tissue cysts

= Infective stage
= Diagnostic stage

Serum, CSF

Diagnostic stage

(1) Serological diagnosis.
or
(2) Direct identification of the parasite from peripheral blood, amniotic fluid, or in tissue sections.

• **Fig. 49.3** An illustration depicting the life cycle of the protozoan *Toxoplasma gondii,* the causal agent for toxoplasmosis. (Photo Courtesy of the Division of Parasitic Diseases/Centers for Disease Control and Prevention.)

been formed, the process becomes quiescent, with little or no multiplication and spread. In immunocompromised or immunodeficient patients, a cyst rupture or primary exposure to the organisms often leads to lesions. The organisms can be disseminated via the lymphatic system and the bloodstream to other tissues.

Toxoplasmosis can be categorized into four groups: (1) acquired in the immunocompetent patient, (2) acquired or reactivated in the immunodeficient patient, (3) congenital, and (4) ocular.

Diagnoses and their interpretations may differ for each clinical category.

Immunocompetent Individuals

In almost all cases, no clinical symptoms are seen during the acute infection. However, 10% to 20% of patients with acute infection may develop painless cervical lymphadenopathy and a flulike illness. This presentation is self-limited, with symptoms resolving within weeks to months. Acute visceral manifestations are present in rare cases. Most

infected patients remain asymptomatic or consider that they have experienced nothing more than a common cold.

Immunocompromised Individuals

Infections in immunocompromised patients can lead to severe complications. Underlying conditions that may affect the disease outcome include Hodgkin disease, non-Hodgkin lymphomas, leukemia, solid tumors, collagen vascular disease, organ transplantation, and AIDS. In the immunocompromised patient, the CNS is primarily involved, but these patients may also have myocarditis or pneumonitis. More than 50% of these patients will show an altered mental state, motor impairment, seizures, abnormal reflexes, and other neurologic sequelae. Toxoplasmosis in patients being treated with immunosuppressive drugs may result from either newly acquired or reactivated latent infection.

In transplant recipients, the disease presentation depends on prior exposure to *T. gondii* by the donor and recipient, the type of organ involved, and the patient's level of immunosuppression. Reactivation of a latent infection or an acute

TABLE 49.3	Morphology of *Toxoplasma gondii* Stages Found in Humans
Stage	**Description**
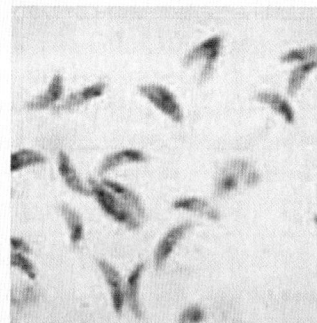 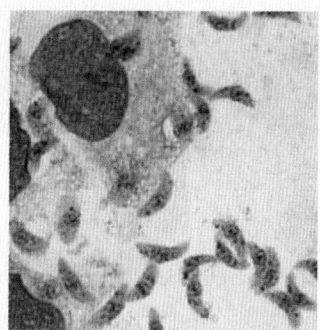 Tachyzoites	Tachyzoites are crescent shaped and are 2–3 µm wide by 4–8 µm long. One end tends to be more rounded than the other is. Giemsa is the stain of choice; cytoplasm stains pale blue; nucleus stains red and is situated toward the broad end of the organism. Tachyzoites are usually seen in early, more acute phases of infection. Tachyzoites rapidly multiply in any cell of the intermediate host (many animals and humans) and in nonintestinal epithelial cells of the definitive host (cats).
Bradyzoites 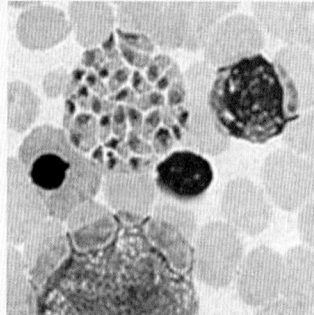 Bone marrow, leukemia patient 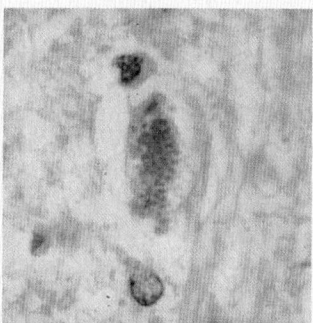 Bradyzoites in tissue	Bradyzoites are found within tissue cysts and multiply very slowly; cyst may contain few to hundreds of organisms, and intramuscular cysts may reach 100 µm in size. Although tissue cysts are seen in visceral organs such as lungs, liver, and kidneys, they are more common in brain, eyes, and skeletal and cardiac muscle.

primary infection acquired directly from the transplanted organ can lead to severe disease. Stem cell transplant (SCT) recipients are particularly susceptible to severe toxoplasmosis, primarily attributable to reactivation of a previously acquired latent infection.

Before the use of highly active antiretroviral therapies (HAARTs), *Toxoplasma* encephalitis (TE) was a life-threatening opportunistic infection among patients with AIDS and was usually fatal if not treated. In AIDS patients with reactivated latent infections, psychiatric manifestations of *T. gondii* may be present, including altered mental status (60%) with delusions, auditory hallucinations, and thought disorders. *T. gondii* enhances HIV-1 replication within reservoir host cells and, at the same time, HIV-1 undermines acquired immunity to the parasite, promoting reactivation of chronic toxoplasmosis.

Congenital Infections

Congenital infection results when the mother acquires a primary infection during pregnancy. Most patients remain asymptomatic during the acute infection. However, congenital infections may be severe if the mother becomes infected during the first or second trimester. At birth or soon thereafter, symptoms in these infants may include retinochoroiditis, cerebral calcification, and occasionally hydrocephalus or microcephaly. Because treatment of the mother may reduce the severity of disease in the infant, prompt and accurate diagnosis is mandatory. Many infants who are asymptomatic at birth will subsequently develop symptoms of congenital toxoplasmosis; however, treatment may help to prevent subsequent sequelae. CNS involvement may not appear until several years later.

Ocular Infections

Ocular toxoplasmosis, an important cause of chorioretinitis, may be the result of congenital or acquired infection; acquired infection is more common than congenital infection. Patients with congenital infection may be asymptomatic until the second or third decade; at that point, cysts may rupture with lesions and develop in the eye. Chorioretinitis is characteristically bilateral in patients with congenital infection but is often unilateral in individuals with acute acquired *T. gondii* infection.

Laboratory Diagnosis

The most common method of diagnosis for toxoplasmosis is serologic testing for *T. gondii*–specific antibodies. Other procedures include PCR; examination of biopsy specimens, buffy coat preparations, or CSF; or isolation of the organism in tissue culture or in laboratory animals. It is important to remember that many individuals have been exposed to *T. gondii* and may have cysts within their tissues. Recovery of organisms from tissue culture or animal inoculation may be misleading because the organisms may be isolated but may not be the etiologic agent of disease. However, two situations in which organism detection may be very significant are (1) tachyzoites in smears and/or tissue cultures inoculated from CSF and (2) tachyzoites in patients with acute pulmonary disease and the demonstration of intracellular and extracellular tachyzoites in Giemsa-stained smears of BAL fluid.

When laboratory personnel decide to initiate *Toxoplasma*-specific antibody testing or switch to a different antibody detection kit, the user must carefully review the manufacturer's package insert and published literature for information on the sensitivity and specificity of the assay.

An in-laboratory comparison of kits should be performed using positive and negative samples confirmed by a toxoplasmosis reference laboratory.

The serologic diagnosis of toxoplasmosis is very complex. A variety of manual and automated assays are available that include enzyme immunoassays, enzyme-linked immunosorbent assays (ELISAs), direct agglutination, an immunosorbent agglutination assay, an indirect IFA, immunocapture, and immunoblot tests.

Nucleic Acid Detection

Nucleic acid–based testing has been successfully used to diagnose congenital toxoplasmosis in amniotic fluid and encephalitis in immunocompromised patients. Although the assay is not commercially available for routine use in clinical laboratories, the test is offered at the Toxoplasma Serology Laboratory in Palo Alto, California.

Therapy

Treatment is recommended for clinically active disease, congenital toxoplasmosis in newborns, pregnant women infected during gestation, chorioretinitis, and symptomatic disease in compromised patients. Therapy is recommended for preventive or suppressive treatment in HIV-infected persons. The currently recommended drugs work primarily against the actively dividing tachyzoite form of *T. gondii* and do not eradicate encysted organisms (bradyzoites).

The most common drug combination used to treat congenital toxoplasmosis consists of pyrimethamine and a sulfonamide (sulfadiazine is recommended in the United States) plus folinic acid in the form of leucovorin calcium to protect the bone marrow from the toxic effects of pyrimethamine. Spiramycin is recommended for pregnant women with acute toxoplasmosis when fetal infection has not been confirmed in an attempt to prevent transmission of *T. gondii* from the mother to the fetus.

In immunosuppressed persons with toxoplasmosis, the combination of pyrimethamine and sulfadiazine plus leucovorin is the preferred treatment. Clindamycin is a second alternative for use in combination with pyrimethamine and leucovorin in those who cannot tolerate sulfonamides. Because relapse often occurs after toxoplasmosis in HIV-infected patients, maintenance therapy with pyrimethamine plus sulfadiazine or pyrimethamine plus clindamycin is recommended. For prophylaxis to prevent an initial episode of toxoplasmosis in *Toxoplasma*-seropositive persons with CD4+ T-lymphocyte counts of less than 100/mL, trimethoprim-sulfamethoxazole is recommended as the first choice, with alternatives consisting of dapsone plus pyrimethamine or atovaquone with or without pyrimethamine. Leucovorin is administered with all regimens, including pyrimethamine. HIV-infected persons who are serologically negative for *Toxoplasma* IgG should be advised to protect themselves from primary infection by eating well-cooked meats and washing their hands after possible soil contact. Cats kept as pets should be fed commercial or well-cooked food, should be kept indoors, and should have their litter boxes changed daily.

Pyrimethamine and sulfadiazine are often used to treat patients with ocular disease. Clindamycin, in combination with other antiparasitic medications, may also be used to treat ocular disease. In addition to antiparasitic drugs, physicians may add corticosteroids to reduce ocular inflammation.

ⓔ Visit the Evolve site for a complete list of procedures, review questions, and case studies.

Bibliography

Andrea SB, Chapin KC: Comparison of Aptima *Trichomonas vaginalis* transcription-mediated amplification assay and BD affirm VPIII for detection of *T. vaginalis* in symptomatic women: performance parameters and epidemiological implications, *J Clin Microbiol* 49(3):866–869, 2011.

Barratt JL, Harkness J, Marriott D, et al.: Importance of nonenteric protozoan infections in immunocompromised people, *Clin Microbiol Rev* 23:795–836, 2010.

Bennett J, Dolin R, Blaser M: *Principles and practice of infectious diseases*, ed 9, Philadelphia, 2020, Elsevier-Saunders.

Booton C, Carmichael JR, Visvesvara GS, et al.: Genotyping of *Balamuthia mandrillaris* based on nuclear 18S and mitochondrial 16S rRNA genes, *Am J Trop Med Hyg* 68:65–69, 2003.

Boyer KM, Holfels E, Roizen N, et al.: Risk factors for *Toxoplasma gondii* infection in mothers of infants with congenital toxoplasmosis: implications for prenatal management and screening, *Am J Obstet Gynecol* 192:564–571, 2005.

Caroll KC, Pfaller MA: *Manual of clinical microbiology*, ed 12, Washington, DC, 2019, ASM Press.

Centers for Disease Control and Prevention: Guidelines for prevention and treatment of opportunistic infections among HIV-exposed and infected children, *MMWR Recommend Rep* 58:1–176, 2009.

Cudmore SL, Delgaty KL, Harward-McClelland SF, et al.: Treatment of infections caused by metronidazole-resistant *Trichomonas vaginalis*, *Clin Microbiol Rev* 17:783–793, 2004.

Dehghan M, Tantbirojn D, Kymer-Davis E, et al.: Neutralizing salivary pH by mouthwashes after an acidic challenge, *J Investig Clin Dent* 8(2):e12198, 2017.

Dubey JP, Lindsay DS, Speer CAL: Structures of *Toxoplasma gondii* tachyzoites, bradyzoites, and sporozoites and biology and development of tissue cysts, *Clin Microbiol Rev* 11:267–299, 1988.

Fallah E, Jafarpour Z, Mahami-Oskouei M, et al.: Molecular characterization of *Acanthamoeba* isolates from surface resting waters in northwest Iran, *Iran J Parasitol* 12(3):355–363, 2017.

Garcia LS: *Diagnostic medical parasitology*, ed 6, Washington, DC, 2016, ASM Press.

Garcia LS: *Practical guide to diagnostic parasitology*, ed 2, Washington, DC, 2009, ASM Press.

Jayasekera S, Sissons J, Tucker J, et al.: Post-mortem culture of *Balamuthia mandrillaris* from the brain and cerebrospinal fluid of a case of granulomatous amoebic meningoencephalitis using human brain microvascular endothelial cells, *J Med Microbiol* 53:1007–1012, 2004.

Kilvington S, Gray T, Dart J, et al.: *Acanthamoeba* keratitis: the role of domestic tap water contamination in the United Kingdom, *Invest Ophthalmol Vis Sci* 45:165–169, 2004.

Marciano-Cabral F, Cabral G: *Acanthamoeba* spp. as agents of disease in humans, *Clin Microbiol Rev* 16:273–307, 2003.

Madarova L, Trnkova K, Feikova S, et al.: A real-time PCR diagnostic method for detection of *Naegleria fowleri*, *Exp Parasitol* 126(1):37–41, 2010.

Maybodi R, Ardakani AH, Bafghi AF, et al.: The effect of nonsurgical periodontal therapy on *Trichomonas tenax* and *Entamoeba gingivalis* in patients with chronic periodontitis, *J Dent* 17(3):171–176, 2016.

Parija SC, Dinoop K, Venugopal H: Management of granulomatous amebic encephalitis: laboratory diagnosis and treatment, *Trop Parasitol* 5(1):23–28, 2015.

Qvarnstrom Y, Visvesvara GS, Sriram R, et al.: Multiplex real-time PCR assay for simultaneous detection of *Acanthamoeba* spp., *Balamuthia mandrillaris,* and *Naegleria fowleri*, *J Clin Microbiol* 44:3589–3595, 2006.

Schuster FL: Cultivation of pathogenic and opportunistic free-living amebas, *Clin Microbiol Rev* 15(3):342–354, 2002.

Schuster FL, Dunnebacke TH, Booton GC, et al.: Environmental isolation of *Balamuthia mandrillaris* associated with a case of amebic encephalitis, *J Clin Microbiol* 41:3175–3180, 2003.

Schuster FL, Visvesvara GS: Free-living amoebae as opportunistic and non-opportunistic pathogens of humans and animals, *Int J Parasitol* 34:1001–1027, 2004.

Schuster FL, Visvesvara GS: Opportunistic amoebae: challenges in prophylaxis and treatment, *Drug Resist Update* 7:41–51, 2004.

Schwebke JR, Burgess D: Trichomoniasis, *Clin Microbiol Rev.* 17:794–803, 2004.

Schwebke JR, Gaydos CA, Davis T: Clinical evaluation of the cepheid xpert TV assay for detection of *Trichomonas vaginalis* with prospectively collected specimens from men and women, *J Clin Microbiol* 56(2):e01091-17, 2018.

Siddiqui R, Khan NA: *Balamuthia* amoebic encephalitis: an emerging disease with fatal consequences. *Microb Pathog* 44(2):89–97, 2008.

Siddiqui R, Khan NA: *Balamuthia mandrillaris*: morphology, biology and virulence, *Trop Parasitol* 5(1):15–22, 2015.

Sohn HJ, Kang H, Seo GE, et al.: Efficient liquid media for encystation of pathogenic free-living amoebae, *Korean J Parasitol* 55(3):233–238, 2017.

Torrey EF, Yolken RH: *Toxoplasma gondii* and schizophrenia, *Emerg Inf Dis* 9:1375–1380, 2003.

Turcekova L, Spisak F, Dubinsky P, Ostro A: Molecular diagnosis of *Toxoplasma gondii* in pregnant women, *Bratisl Lek Listy* 113:307–310, 2012.

Visvesvara GS: Amebic meningoencephalitides and keratitis: challenges in diagnosis and treatment, *Curr Opin Infect Dis* 23:590–594, 2010.

50

Intestinal Nematodes

OBJECTIVES

1. Describe the distinguishing morphologic characteristics and basic life cycle (vectors, hosts, and stages of infectivity) for each of the parasites listed.
2. Define and identify the following parasitic structures when appropriate: mammillated ovum, gravid, rhabditiform larvae, buccal capsule, esophagus, genital primordia, polar hyaline plugs, copulatory bursa, embryonated egg, cutting plates, and filariform larvae.
3. Describe the diseases and mechanism of pathogenicity, including route of transmission, for each of the species listed.
4. Differentiate *Ascaris lumbricoides* adult male and female worms.
5. Define and differentiate direct versus indirect life cycle as related to nematodes and the routes of transmission, including autoinfection and hyperinfections.
6. Identify and differentiate the characteristic morphologies and eggs for *A. lumbricoides, Enterobius vermicularis,* and *Trichuris trichiura.*
7. Compare clinical signs and symptoms, morphologic characteristics, and identification of the hookworm's rhabditiform larvae for *Ancylostoma duodenale* and *Necator americanus.*
8. Compare and contrast the morphologic characteristics and identification of the larval forms of *Strongyloides stercoralis.*
9. List the various methods used to diagnose intestinal nematode infections.
10. Identify the appropriate intestinal nematodes for which the following techniques are useful and explain the principle for each: the Baermann concentration method, agar culture, and Harada-Mori filter paper method for the recovery of intestinal nematodes.

PARASITES TO BE CONSIDERED

Helminths

Nematodes

Intestinal (roundworms)
  Ascaris lumbricoides
  Enterobius vermicularis (pinworm)
  Strongyloides fuelleborni
  Strongyloides stercoralis (threadworm)
  Trichostrongylus spp.
  Trichuris trichiura (whipworm)
Capillaria philippinensis (hookworm)
  Ancylostoma ceylanicum
  Ancylostoma duodenale (Old World)
  Necator americanus (New World)

There are more than 60 species of nematodes known to infect humans. *Ascaris lumbricoides,* hookworms (*Ancylostoma duodenale, Ancylostoma ceylanicum,* and *Necator americanus*), and *Trichuris trichiura* are estimated to infect more than 1 billion people. Nematodes are nonsegmented, elongate, cylindrical worms with a well-developed digestive tract and reproductive system. The adult worms have separate sexes, with the male generally smaller than the female. Most nematodes are diagnosed by finding the characteristic eggs in the stool. The infective stage of the nematodes varies with species; for example, transmission may occur through the ingestion of eggs, whereas others burrow through the skin and migrate to the intestine. The nematodes have very diverse life cycles that result in different routes of transmission and disease symptoms.

Ascaris lumbricoides

General Characteristics

A. lumbricoides is the most common and largest roundworm. The parasite has a worldwide distribution with higher prevalence in the tropical regions. Its eggs are ingested and hatch in the duodenum, penetrate the host's intestinal wall, and migrate to the hepatic portal circulation. The adult worms live and reproduce in the lumen of the small intestine. The ovum is a thick, oval, **mammillated** (outer protrusions) and embryonated egg. The eggs are passed in the feces and become infective 2 to 6 weeks after deposition, depending on the environment. The general life cycle is outlined in Fig. 50.1. The life cycle of *A. lumbricoides* is classified as an **indirect life cycle;** transmission is not via a direct route from one host to the next.

Epidemiology

Geographic distribution is associated with climate and poor sanitation. The eggs of *A. lumbricoides* require a warm, humid environment for the embryonated ovum to mature and become infective. Infection rates are elevated in poverty-stricken areas that have poor sanitation. Transmission is via the fecal-oral route, usually through the ingestion of eggs on contaminated material. *Ascaris* eggs are capable of survival within harsh environmental conditions, including dry or freezing temperatures.

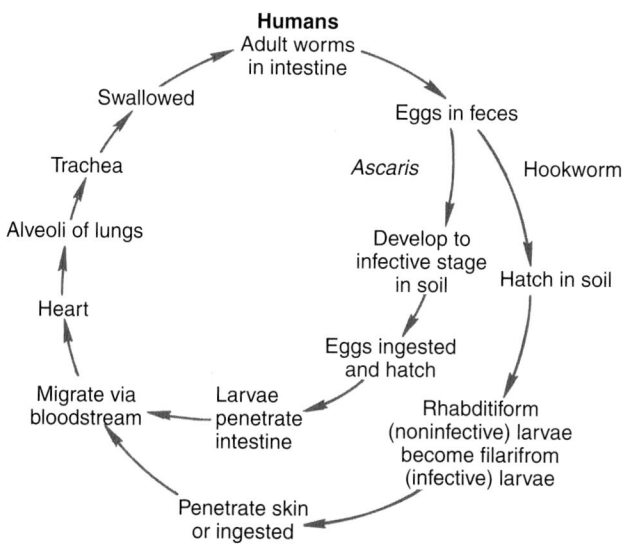

Humans

Adult worms in intestine

Swallowed

Eggs in feces

Trachea

Ascaris   Hookworm

Alveoli of lungs

Develop to infective stage in soil

Hatch in soil

Heart

Eggs ingested and hatch

Migrate via bloodstream

Larvae penetrate intestine

Rhabditiform (noninfective) larvae become filarifrom (infective) larvae

Penetrate skin or ingested

• **Fig. 50.1** Life cycle of *Ascaris lumbricoides* and hookworm (indirect life cycle).

Pathogenesis and Spectrum of Disease

Many *A. lumbricoides* infections are asymptomatic. The presentation of symptoms correlates with the length of infection, the number of worms present, and the overall health of the host. Stool examination findings are typically normal in the absence of previous infection (during the first 40 days). Intestinal symptoms range from mild to severe intestinal obstruction. Some patients will develop pulmonary symptoms due to the migration of larvae through the lungs; such persons present with immune-mediated hypersensitivity pneumonia. The worms may cause an immune condition known as **Löffler syndrome,** characterized by peripheral eosinophilia. Ectopic ascariasis may occur when worms escape the gastrointestinal (GI) tract and enter the appendix or the hepatobiliary or pancreatic ducts and cause an obstruction. Table 50.1 provides a summary of associated diseases.

		TABLE 50.1 Pathogenesis and Spectrum of Associated Diseases

Organism	Pathogenesis	Mode of Transmission and Spectrum of Disease
Ascaris lumbricoides	Attributed to four main factors: 1. Host immune response 2. Effects from larval migration 3. Mechanical disruption and blockage by worms 4. Nutritional deficiency associated with worm burden	Fecal-oral transmission. Reinfection possible. Children and young adolescents have higher infection rates. Pregnant females: unknown effect on unborn fetus. Potential tissue damage from migration to lungs, liver, and immune cell infiltration (pneumonitis). Peripheral eosinophilia (Löffler syndrome). Nutritional impairment in young children. Hepatic ascariasis, including hepatic abscesses and obstructive cholangitis. Intestinal blockage, pancreatic or bile duct. Migration to other tissues may include kidneys, appendix, and pleural cavity.
Enterobius vermicularis	Worm burden may be a single organism to thousands. Rarely migration occurs to nearby tissues.	Fecal-oral or inhalation. Sexual transmission has been reported. Reinfection and autoinfection occur. More common in children and females. Mild nocturnal pruritus. Migration to vagina, uterus, and fallopian tubes where organisms become encapsulated granulomas. Hemorrhagic colitis and inflammation of ileum and colon in homosexual males. Uncommon sites include peritoneal cavity, lungs, liver, urinary tract, and natal cleft.
Strongyloides stercoralis and *Strongyloides fuelleborni*	Varies in severity depending on worm burden and area of body infected. Immune response affects symptoms.	Direct penetration. Chronic and hyperinfection may occur. May remain asymptomatic with peripheral eosinophilia. Cutaneous: • Pruritus and erythema • "Larva currens" tracks under skin from worm migration Pulmonary: • Asymptomatic to pneumonia • Löffler syndrome; shortness of breath and pulmonary infiltrates Intestinal: • Diarrhea, constipation, anorexia, and abdominal pain may occur • Damage to mucosa may occur in heavy infections

TABLE 50.1	Pathogenesis and Spectrum of Associated Diseases—cont'd	
Organism	**Pathogenesis**	**Mode of Transmission and Spectrum of Disease**
Trichostrongylus spp.	Dependent on worm burden.	Diarrhea, anorexia, and general malaise. Damage to intestinal mucosa may occur, resulting in hemorrhage and tissue desquamation. Heavy worm burden may result in anemia and cholecystitis.
Trichuris trichiura	Dependent on worm burden. Mechanical damage to intestinal mucosa and allergic reaction. Migration of parasites.	Fecal-oral transmission. Ingestion of embryonated eggs. Asymptomatic to mild symptoms associated with low worm burden. Heavy infections may result in hemorrhage, weight loss, abdominal pain, blood-tinged stools, and diarrhea. Rectal prolapse and hypochromic anemia in repeated heavy infections in children. Inflammation of mucosa.
Capillaria philippinensis	Dependent on worm burden.	Fecal-oral transmission. Ingestion of larvae-infected seafood such as fish, crab, shrimp, and snails. Malabsorption, fluid loss, and associated loss of electrolytes. Extended infections can result in organ failure and death.
Hookworms: *Ancylostoma duodenale* *Necator americanus* *A. ceylonicum* *A. braziliense* and *A. caninum*	Vary according to life cycle phase and worm burden. Production of proteins that suppress host immune response. Hyaluronidase: facilitates digestion of connective tissue and penetration of epidermis and dermis. Migration of larvae to lungs. Mechanical: attachment, feeding, and anticoagulation production.	Direct penetration. Mild to severe pruritus and potential secondary infections. Ground itch: development of vesicles resulting from erythematous papular rash. Pneumonitis: decreased sensitization compared with *A. lumbricoides* and *S. stercoralis*. Gastrointestinal: • Tissue damage at site of attachment. • Blood loss, anemia. • Acute gastrointestinal phase demonstrates increased eosinophilia. • Increased worm burden may result in death, particularly in young children.
A. duodenale	Period of arrested development.	May be associated with vertical transmission and congenital infections. Eosinophilia peaks in approximately 1 month in gastrointestinal phase.
N. americanus	Proteolytic enzymes that degrade collagen, fibronectin, laminin, and elastin.	Skin-associated symptoms as described for hookworms. Eosinophilia peaks in approximately 2 months in gastrointestinal phase.
A. ceylonicum	Similar to *N. americanus*.	Chronic blood loss that leads to iron-deficiency anemia and protein malnutrition.
A. braziliense	No hydrolytic enzymes. Self-limiting.	Cutaneous larva migrans; organisms remain trapped in the superficial epidermis (up to 10 days), where they migrate to create the pathognomonic serpiginous tunnels.
A. caninum	Secrete various potential allergens; localized allergic reaction.	Eosinophilic enteritis Larvae remain dormant in skeletal muscles and create no symptoms. In some individuals, larvae migrate to the gut and mature into adult worms. Severe recurrent abdominal pain.

Laboratory Diagnosis

Female worms have an extremely high daily output of eggs, making diagnosis relatively easy through the identification of eggs in feces. The large, broadly oval mammillated ova are typically stained brown from bile (Fig. 50.2A). Some eggs are **decorticated,** or lacking the mammillated outer cover (Fig. 50.2B). Infertile eggs may be oval or irregularly shaped, with a thin shell and containing internal granules. Adult worms may also be identified in feces. The adult male worm is smaller (15–31 cm) than the female, with a curved posterior end (Fig. 50.3), and it contains three well-characterized

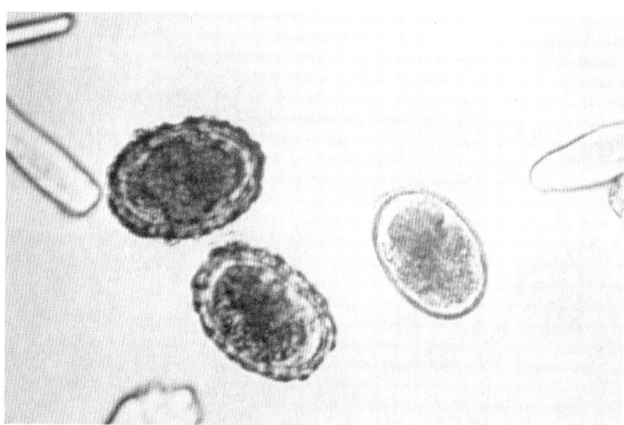

• **Fig. 50.2** *Ascaris lumbricoides* eggs. The ovum on the right is a decorticated example, exhibiting an absent outer layer. Once fertile eggs have embryonated, they become infective after 18 days to several weeks. If ingested, larvae can hatch, causing the intestinal infection known as ascariasis, which infects children more often than adults. (Photo courtesy the Division of Parasitic Diseases/Centers for Disease Control and Prevention.)

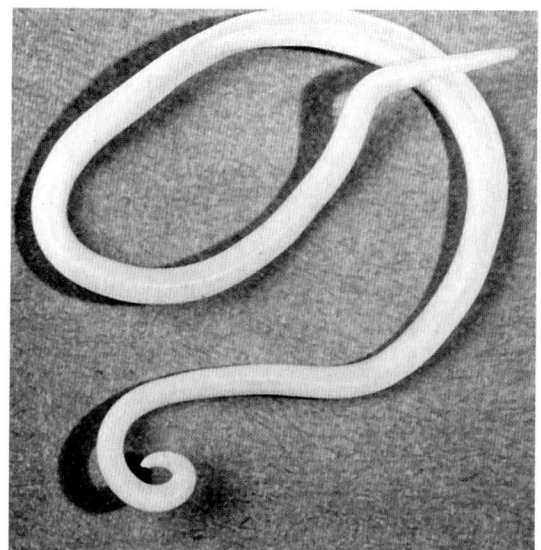

• **Fig. 50.3** *Ascaris lumbricoides* adult male worm. Note the curved posterior end. (Courtesy Dr. Henry Travers, Sioux Falls, SD.)

lips. Larvae may be found in sputum or gastric aspirates because of larval migration during development within the human host. *Ascaris*-specific antibodies may be found (not useful in acute infection and not protective) with serologic studies. Increases in IgE and later IgG may be found. Other diagnostic tests (e.g., polymerase chain reaction [PCR]) have been described for identifying infection with soil-transmitted helminths. However, these are typically used for population-based treatment programs in endemic areas.

Therapy

Anthelmintic treatment is recommended for all infections. Preferred therapy includes oral albendazole or mebendazole.

Prevention

Prevention is managed through proper sanitation and good hygiene.

Enterobius vermicularis

General Characteristics

Enterobius vermicularis (pinworm) has a worldwide distribution and is commonly identified in group settings of children 5 to 10 years of age. The life cycle is considered direct; transmission occurs from an infected host to another individual (Fig. 50.4). During the night, the mature female worm migrates out of the anus of the infected host and lays eggs in the perianal region. The embryonated eggs mature and a third-stage larva develops, resulting in infectivity within hours. Transmission occurs by ingestion or inhalation of eggs. **Retroinfection** may also occur when the eggs hatch and larvae return to the intestine, where they mature.

Epidemiology

Pinworm is more prevalent in school-age children up to about 14 years of age. Infections are associated with institutional crowding and are familial. In adults, pinworm infection is most common in parents aged 30 to 39 years, typically because of transmission from their children aged 5 to 9 years. Overall, males are affected twice as often as females except in people aged 5 to 14 years, when infection is predominantly in females. Transmission is also associated with an increased rate of reinfection within a group or **autoinfection** from hatched larvae.

Pathogenesis and Spectrum of Disease

Infections with *E. vermicularis* are typically asymptomatic. The most common complaint is perianal pruritus (itching) and resultant restless sleep. The movement of the female and the ova cause intense local itching. Ova may survive for up to 3 weeks before hatching. The hatched larvae can then migrate back into the anus and lower intestine, causing retroinfection. Embryonated eggs may be released into the air or onto fomites (e.g., bedding, clothing, toys, paper money) or onto hands and then placed directly into the mouth and swallowed (autoinfection), after which they settle in the small intestines. Occasionally, the parasite may migrate to other nearby tissues, causing pelvic, cervical, or peritoneal granulomas. Table 50.1 summarizes the detail of associated diseases.

Laboratory Diagnosis

Diagnosis is typically by microscopic identification of the characteristic flat-sided ovum (Fig. 50.5). The eggs are best obtained by dabbing the stretched, unwashed perianal folds in the early morning with clear cellophane tape or a

Trichuriasis
(Trichuris trichiura)

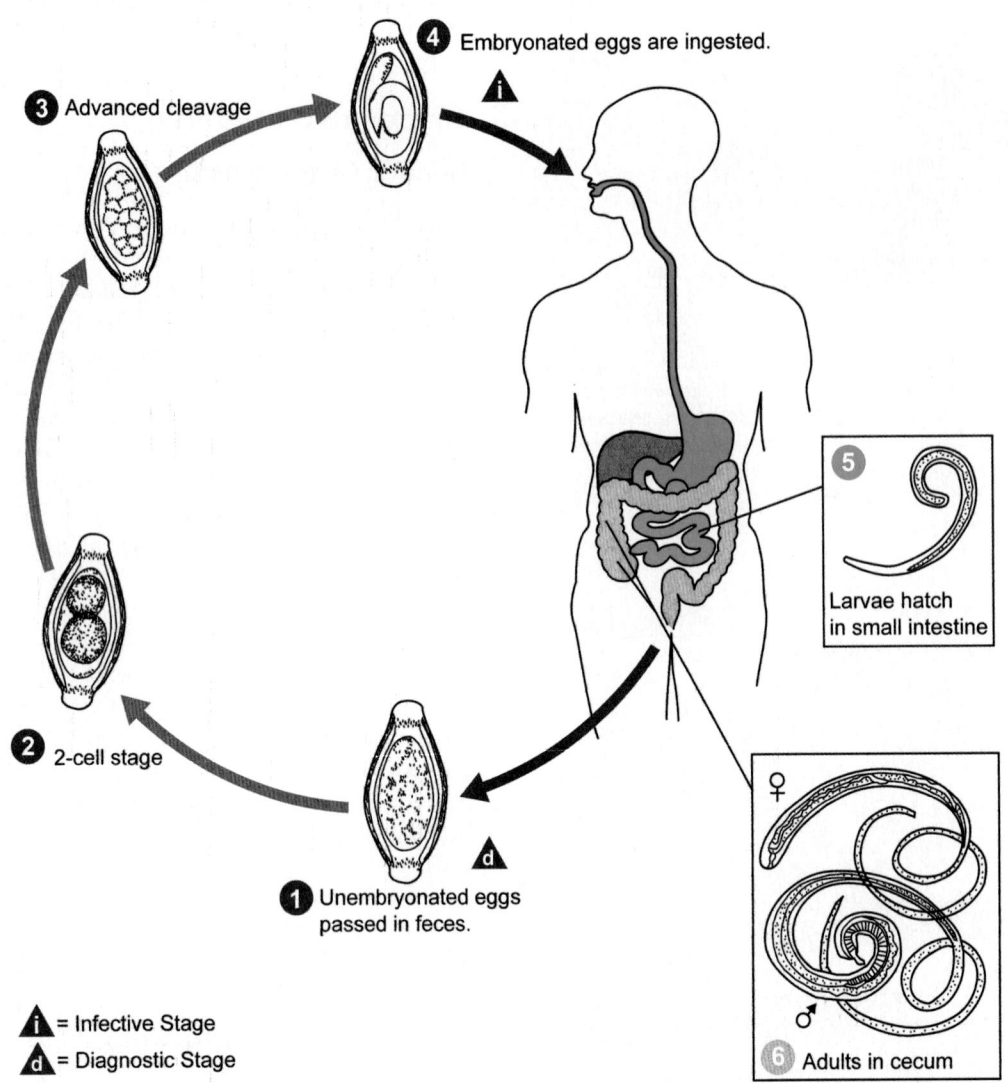

3 Advanced cleavage

4 Embryonated eggs are ingested.

5 Larvae hatch in small intestine

2 2-cell stage

1 Unembryonated eggs passed in feces.

6 Adults in cecum

i = Infective Stage
d = Diagnostic Stage

• **Fig. 50.4** This illustration depicts the direct life cycle of the human whipworm, *Trichuris trichiura,* the causal agent of the disease trichuriasis. (Courtesy the Division of Parasitic Diseases/Centers for Disease Control and Prevention.)

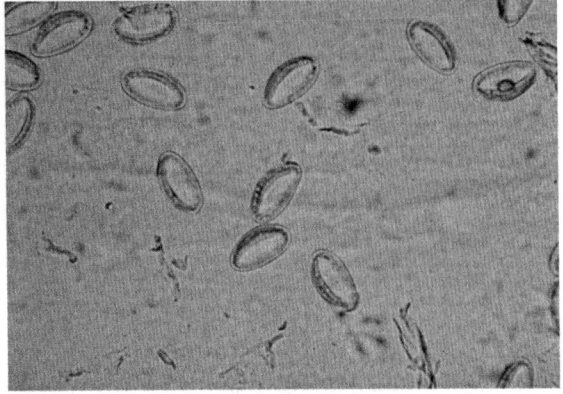

• **Fig. 50.5** *Enterobius vermicularis* eggs (cellophane tape preparation).

commercially available sticky paddle. Eggs are not typically identified in feces, although they may occasionally be found in a stool specimen. Although adult pinworms may be visible, they can easily be confused with small pieces of thread. The female worm is 8 to 13 mm long with a pointed "pin"-shaped tail. In gravid females, almost the entire body is filled with eggs (Fig. 50.6). The males measure only 2 to 5 mm in length, die after fertilization, and may be passed in feces.

Therapy

Anthelmintic therapy with albendazole or mebendazole is generally effective. Pyrantel and piperazine are effective and may be used during pregnancy. Reinfection with

E. vermicularis immediately after the completion of drug therapy is common. Additionally, young pinworms may be resistant to drugs. Successful eradication of pinworm infection requires two doses of medication; an initial dose followed by a subsequent dose 2 weeks later.

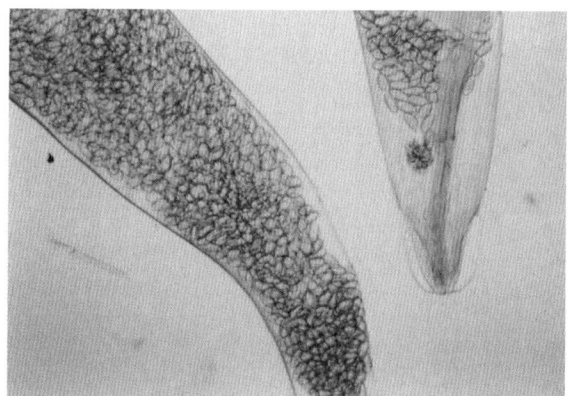

• **Fig. 50.6** *Enterobius vermicularis* gravid female. (Courtesy Dr. Henry Travers, Sioux Falls, SD.)

Prevention

Regular good personal hygiene is the major factor for prevention of continued reinfection and autoinfection.

Strongyloides stercoralis

General Characteristics

Infection with *Strongyloides stercoralis* is less common than that with other intestinal nematodes. The organism is endemic in the tropics and subtropical regions of Asia, Latin America, and Africa. It is estimated that 30 to 100 million people are infected with *Strongyloides* worldwide. A limited geographic distribution exists in the United States and Europe.

S. stercoralis, commonly referred to as the threadworm, may inhabit the intestine or exist as a free-living organism in the soil. The life cycle can be classified as direct, indirect (free-living phase), or autoinfective (Fig. 50.7). The **filariform** (infective) **larvae** penetrate the skin and migrate via the circulatory system to the heart and lungs. The organism

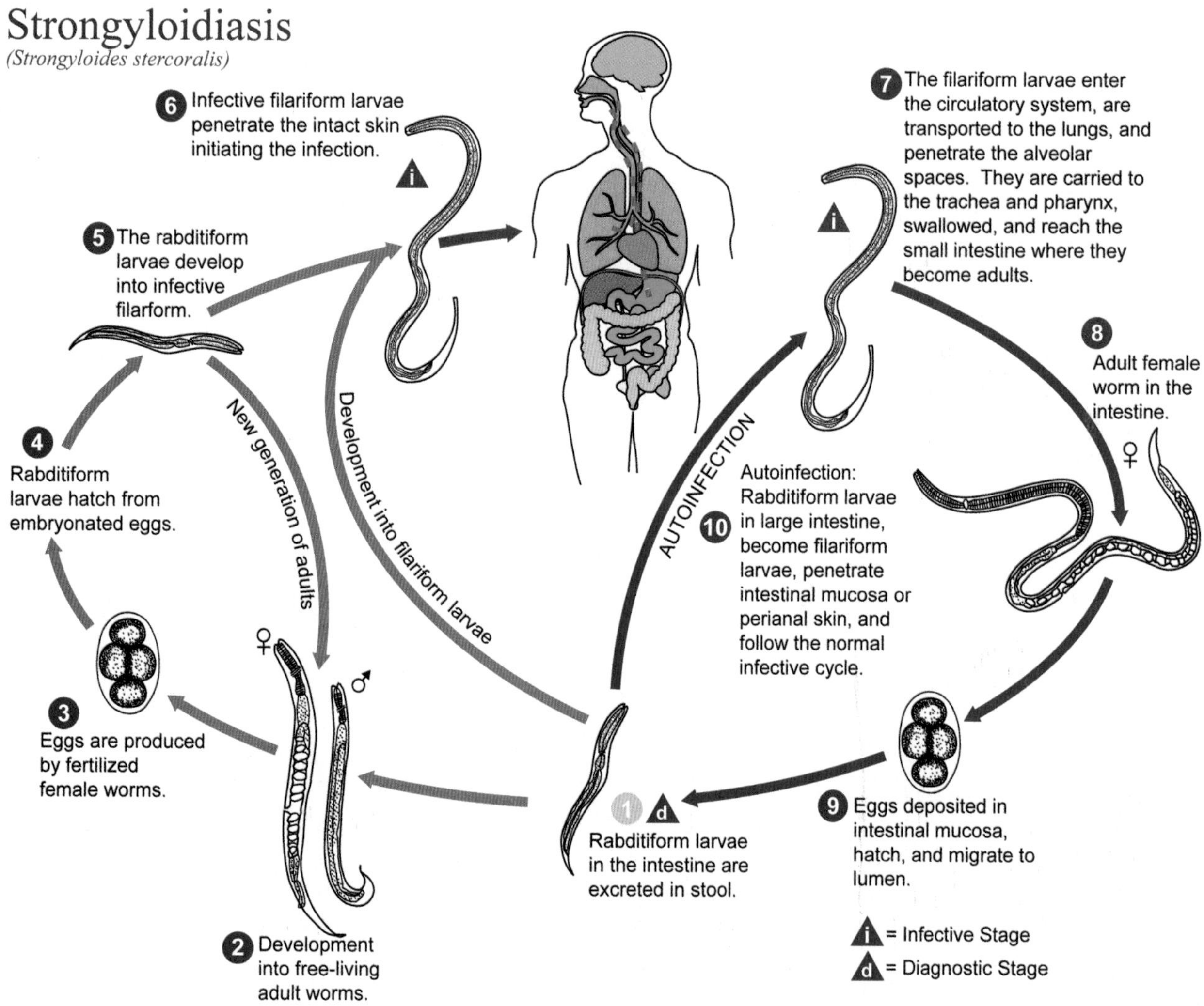

Strongyloidiasis
(Strongyloides stercoralis)

6 Infective filariform larvae penetrate the intact skin initiating the infection.

5 The rabditiform larvae develop into infective filarform.

4 Rabditiform larvae hatch from embryonated eggs.

3 Eggs are produced by fertilized female worms.

2 Development into free-living adult worms.

New generation of adults

Development into filariform larvae

7 The filariform larvae enter the circulatory system, are transported to the lungs, and penetrate the alveolar spaces. They are carried to the trachea and pharynx, swallowed, and reach the small intestine where they become adults.

8 Adult female worm in the intestine.

AUTOINFECTION

10 Autoinfection: Rabditiform larvae in large intestine, become filariform larvae, penetrate intestinal mucosa or perianal skin, and follow the normal infective cycle.

1 **d** Rabditiform larvae in the intestine are excreted in stool.

9 Eggs deposited in intestinal mucosa, hatch, and migrate to lumen.

i = Infective Stage

d = Diagnostic Stage

• **Fig. 50.7** This illustration depicts the life cycle of the parasitic roundworm, *Strongyloides stercoralis*, the causal agent of the parasitic disease strongyloidiasis. (Courtesy the Division of Parasitic Diseases/Centers for Disease Control and Prevention.)

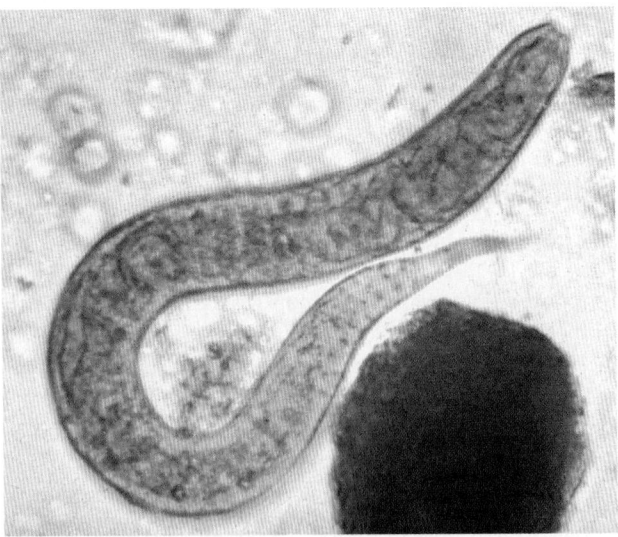

• **Fig. 50.8** *Strongyloides stercoralis* rhabditiform larva, iodine stain.

enters the bronchial tree and then is swallowed; it then lives in the digestive tract and matures into an adult worm. In the intestine, the filariform larvae may also penetrate the mucosa, resulting in autoinfection. The female worm produces eggs by **parthenogenesis** (a form of asexual reproduction in which growth and development occur without fertilization), because parasitic adult male worms are nonexistent. Within the indirect life cycle, the **rhabditiform** (noninfective) **larvae** develop into mature males and egg-producing females (Fig. 50.8). The free-living life cycle may revert to the production of infective larvae at any time.

Epidemiology

S. stercoralis and *S. fuelleborni* are transmitted via direct penetration in endemic areas. Person-to-person transmission of *S. stercoralis* occurs within institutionalized groups, in day care centers, and among homosexual males. *S. fuelleborni* larvae have been identified in breast milk, indicating that a transmammary infection may occur.

Pathogenesis and Spectrum of Disease

Infections may be asymptomatic or consist of a variety of disseminated **strongyloidiasis** syndromes. Reinfection is more commonly associated with immunocompromised patients. Acute infections may develop into a localized, pruritic, erythematous papular rash. Some patients develop a **macropapular** or **urticarial** (red and raised) or **serpiginous** rash on the buttocks, perineum, and thighs. The migration of larvae may cause epigastric pain, nausea, diarrhea, and blood loss. **Hyperinfection,** an increased worm burden within the lungs and intestines, may occur from penetration of the intestine by filariform larvae. Damage to the bowel may also increase the risk of bacterial infection with enteric microorganisms, leading to septicemia or meningitis. Disseminated infections may also result in larvae within the central nervous system, kidneys, and liver.

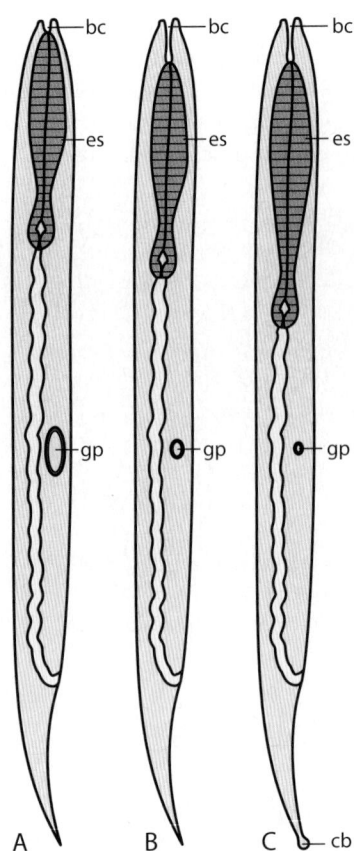

• **Fig. 50.9** Rhabditiform larvae. (A) *Strongyloides*. (B) Hookworm. (C) *Trichostrongylus. bc,* Buccal capsule; *cb,* beadlike swelling of caudal tip; *es,* esophagus; *gp,* genital primordia.

S. fuelleborni, a primate parasite, has been isolated from humans in Africa and Papua New Guinea; infection causes a severe, often fatal systemic illness involving protein-losing enteropathy, which sometimes presents with peritoneal ascites ("swollen belly syndrome"). *S. fuelleborni* follows the same life cycle as *S. stercoralis,* with the important distinction that the eggs (rather than larvae) are passed in the stool. The eggs hatch shortly after passage into the environment, releasing the rhabditiform larvae. Since eggs do not hatch within the host, as with *S. stercoralis,* autoinfection is believed to be impossible. Transmission of *S. fuelleborni* to infants as a result of breastfeeding has been reported. Table 50.1 summarizes the detail of associated diseases.

Laboratory Diagnosis

The rhabditiform larva is the primary diagnostic stage for strongyloidiasis in humans through microscopic examination of stool. The larvae are 250 to 300 μm long; they have a short **buccal capsule,** a large **bulb** on the esophagus, and a prominent **genital primordium** (Fig. 50.9). The filariform larvae are larger (up to 500 μm) and have a notched tail with an esophageal-to-intestinal ratio of 1:1. The eggs, which are rarely identified, are segmented, with a thin shell.

S. stercoralis larvae are most commonly found in human stool specimens. Depending on the fecal transit time through the intestine and the patient's condition, both rhabditiform and rare filariform larvae may be present. If stool examination is delayed, embryonated ova may be found.

Culture of feces for larvae is useful to (1) reveal the presence of parasites when they are too scant to be detected by concentration methods; (2) distinguish whether the infection is due to *S. stercoralis* or hookworm, based on rhabditiform larval morphology, by allowing hookworm egg hatching to occur, thus releasing first-stage larvae; and (3) allow development of larvae into the filariform stage for further differentiation. In the agar culture method, a stool sample is placed on a nutrient agar dish and incubated for 48 hours. The larvae crawl over the top of the agar, leaving tracks in the bacterial growth.

Serologic Testing

Serologic testing is indicated when infection is suspected and the organism cannot be isolated by repeated stool examinations, string test, or duodenal aspirates. A variety of serologic tests are available commercially, including an enzyme immunoassay (EIA), *Strongyloides* IgG EIA (DRG International Inc., Springfield, NJ). The Centers for Disease Control and Prevention also offers a highly sensitive (>95%) cross-reacting enzyme-linked immunosorbent assay (ELISA) with other parasites, including microfilaria, hookworm, *Paragonimus,* and *Echinococcus.* Immunocompromised persons with disseminated strongyloidiasis usually have detectable IgG antibodies despite their immunosuppression, although false-negative results can occur. Cross-reactions in patients with filariasis, schistosomiasis, and ascariasis may also occur, depending on the antigen used. Cross reactivity to sera from *S. fuelleborni*–infected patients probably occurs, but performance has not been evaluated. A positive serologic test result warrants continuing efforts to establish a parasitological diagnosis followed by anthelminthic treatment, as positive serology does not differentiate between past and current infection. Serologic reversion to antibody-negative status is unusual in most strongyloidiasis patients, although antibody levels decrease markedly within 6 months after successful chemotherapy. Thus, serologic monitoring may be useful in the follow-up of treated patients.

Nucleic Acid Detection

Although not available in routine laboratories, real-time PCR methods have been developed that amplify the small subunit of the 18S rRNA, the 18S rRNA, or the cytochrome c oxidase subunit 1 gene. These assays are used to detect DNA in fecal samples and have a demonstrated sensitivity and specificity of 100%. A high-throughput multiplex assay is also available that includes primer and probe pairs for *S. stercoralis* as well as other intestinal nematodes and protozoa.

Additional specimens such as sputum, body fluids, and tissues may be used for the diagnosis of hyperinfection.

Therapy

Ivermectin is the recommended treatment for uncomplicated infections. Albendazole and mebendazole are alternatives but have not proven to be as effective. Thiabendazole has been used to treat children with *S. fuelleborni* swollen belly syndrome. Hyperinfection and disseminated conditions require anthelmintic therapy in combination with broad-spectrum antibiotics to prevent secondary bacterial enteric infections. In addition, patients taking immunosuppressive medications should discontinue their use during infection and treatment. Follow-up examinations are indicated, and treatment should be reinstituted if larvae are identified within 2 weeks after cessation of therapy.

Prevention

Immunocompromised individuals and patients taking immunosuppressive medications should avoid beaches and other areas known to be contaminated.

Trichostrongylus spp.

General Characteristics

Although commonly found in mammals and birds worldwide, approximately 10 different species of *Trichostrongylus* have been found in human infections, including *T. orientalis, T. colubriformis,* and *T. axei.* The worms are small and live in the mucosa of the small intestine. The adult worm has no visible buccal capsule.

Epidemiology

Human infections have been identified in areas within Asia and Africa. Additionally, approximately 70% of the human population in southwestern Iran and a village in Egypt is infected. Infection in humans is acquired by ingestion of plant material contaminated with larvae.

Pathogenesis and Spectrum of Disease

After they are ingested, the larvae mature and migrate through the lungs. Most infections are asymptomatic. Symptoms, when present, are related to the worm burden and the amount of damage within the intestine. Heavy infections can cause GI problems (abdominal pain, diarrhea, anorexia), headache, fatigue, anemia, and eosinophilia. Table 50.1 summarizes the detail of associated diseases.

Laboratory Diagnosis

Laboratory diagnosis includes identification of eggs or hatched larvae in the stool. Eggs are oval, thin-shelled, and

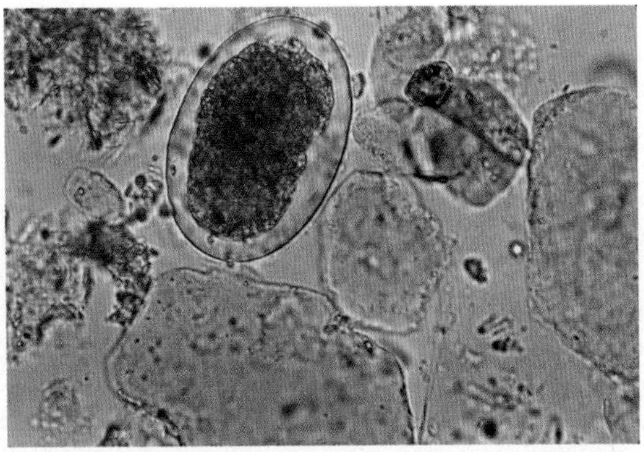

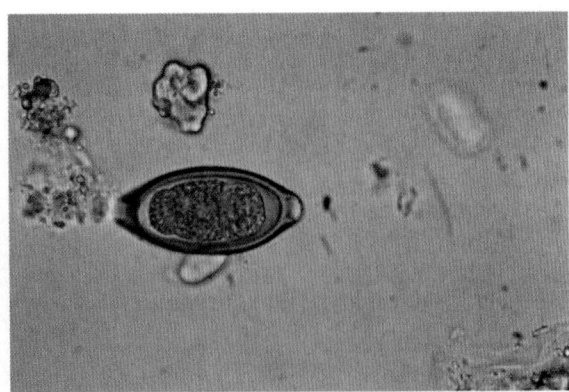

• **Fig. 50.10** *Trichostrongylus* sp. egg. (Courtesy Dr. Henry Travers, Sioux Falls, SD.)

• **Fig. 50.11** *Trichuris trichiura* egg. Note the evident polar hyaline plugs. (Courtesy Dr. Henry Travers, Sioux Falls, SD.)

colorless; they measure 75 to 95 μm in length by 40 to 50 μm in width. Eggs taper at one end and the inner membrane may be wrinkled. The eggs resemble hookworm eggs except that they are slightly longer and more pointed (Fig. 50.10). Patients may have coinfections with hookworm and *S. stercoralis* larvae, so care must be taken to differentiate the two (Fig. 50.9).

Therapy

Anthelmintic agents are recommended, including mebendazole and pyrantel pamoate. Albendazole is the treatment of choice.

Prevention

Thorough washing of plant material, including cultivated vegetables, before handling or ingestion is recommended.

Trichuris trichiura

General Characteristics

T. trichiura, or whipworm, has a worldwide distribution and is usually asymptomatic; however, heavily infected individuals may have symptoms. Unlike other intestinal nematodes discussed in this chapter, there is no tissue migration phase within the life cycle of *T. trichiura*.

Epidemiology

T. trichiura is typically found in moist, warm climates around the world. Infections are relatively common in Asia, Africa, and South America, with some cases identified in the southeastern United States. Often the nematode is identified in coinfections along with *A. lumbricoides* or hookworm in children.

Poor hygiene is associated with increased transmission, especially in children. Humans are infected by ingestion of the embryonated eggs. Larvae are released in the intestine, where they mature into adult worms. Eggs containing the unsegmented **ovum** (diagnostic stage) are then passed in the feces and deposited in the soil. The eggs require a warm, moist environment for embryonation and to become infective to another host.

Pathogenesis and Spectrum of Disease

The pathogenesis and severity of the disease are closely related to the worm burden. The lack of symptoms is related to the life cycle, which does not include a tissue or pulmonary migration stage, resulting in no pulmonary or extra-GI symptoms, as are seen in other nematode infections. Infections range from mild, with a very low worm burden, to severe infections with bleeding and weight loss in heavy worm infestations. Heavy infections, especially in small children, can cause GI problems (abdominal pain, diarrhea, rectal prolapse) and possibly growth suppression. The characteristic whiplike worm buries its threadlike anterior into the intestinal mucosa and feeds on tissue secretions, causing an inflammatory reaction and peripheral eosinophilia. Table 50.1 summarizes the detail of associated diseases.

Laboratory Diagnosis

Diagnosis is typically from the identification of eggs and rarely the adult worm within the feces. An adult female may produce up to 20,000 eggs per day. However, during the lengthy development of mature worms within the intestine, there may be no shedding of eggs for up to 3 months. Eggs appear as brown barrel-shaped structures. They are unembryonated and contain a thick wall with **hyaline polar plugs** at each end (Fig. 50.11). The adult female worm ranges in size from 35 to 50 mm and demonstrates a gradually increasing width from anterior to posterior, with a straight end (Fig. 50.12). The adult male ranges in size from 30 to 45 mm and demonstrates the same broadening morphology with a coiled posterior end. PCR using new sequencing techniques is now available in specialized laboratories.

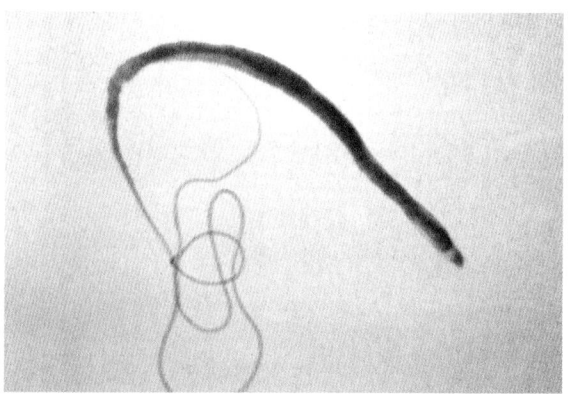

• **Fig. 50.12** Adult female *Trichuris trichiura*. (Courtesy Dr. Henry Travers, Sioux Falls, SD.)

Therapy

Therapy may or may not be indicated, depending on the nutritional status of the host, the length of infection, and the level of worm burden. Anthelmintics such as albendazole are recommended when necessary.

Prevention

Prevention includes practicing proper hygiene and sanitation as well as careful disposal of dirt or soil contaminated with feces.

Capillaria philippinensis

General Characteristics

Capillariasis is a parasitic disease in humans caused by two different species of capillarids: *Capillaria philippinensis* and *Capillaria hepatica* (Chapter 51), a tissue nematode.

C. philippinensis is transferred through the ingestion of infected small freshwater fish and causes intestinal capillariasis. *C. philippinensis* was first recognized as a human parasite in the late 1960s and now has a well-known wide distribution. This parasite is prevalent in the northern Philippines, hence the name *C. philippinensis,* and has also been found in Thailand, Japan, Taiwan, Iran, and Egypt. The parasite reproduces in the gut, resulting in autoinfection and hyperinfection very similar to that observed in *S. stercoralis.*

Epidemiology

C. philippinensis is currently considered a parasite of fish-eating birds, which seem to be the natural definitive host. Human infection is believed to occur from the ingestion of uncooked fish harboring infective larvae. Typically, unembryonated eggs are passed in the stool by birds or humans and become embryonated in the external environment. After the ingestion of raw or undercooked freshwater fish, larvae hatch, penetrate the intestine, and migrate to the tissues. The adult worms reside in the small intestine, where

they burrow into the mucosa. The females deposit unembryonated eggs. Some of these become embryonated in the intestine and release larvae that can cause autoinfection and may cause hyperinfection. In the Philippines, where the organism is prevalent, the people ingest a large spectrum of raw seafood, including fish, shrimp, crabs, and snails. In addition, defecation in the fields or water sources where snails, shrimp, and crabs are collected is common.

Pathogenesis and Spectrum of Disease

C. philippinensis cannot be transmitted human to human and requires an intermediate freshwater fish host. However, adult *C. philippinensis* worms in humans can release eggs that hatch into larvae in the intestine and cause hyperinfection. Initial signs and symptoms of infection include general abdominal pain and diarrhea. Symptoms will vary with the level of worm burden. The larvae are ingested and reside in the small intestine, where they burrow into the mucosa. Because of the parasite's mechanical insertion into the intestinal wall, patients lose weight rapidly, experiencing nausea, vomiting, malabsorption, and fluid loss. Long-term infections lasting weeks to months may result in death attributable to a severe loss of electrolytes, particularly potassium (hypokalemia), and associated organ failure. Table 50.1 summarizes the detail of associated diseases.

Laboratory Diagnosis

Tissue biopsy of the small intestine can be used for the diagnosis of infection with *C. philippinensis*. However, the diagnosis is typically made from the identification of eggs, adult worms, or larvae in stool specimens. The eggs resemble those produced by *T. trichiura*. They are somewhat smaller, with a thick, striated shell and less prominent polar plugs. Female worms produce the characteristic thick-shelled eggs as well as thin-shelled and free larvae.

Therapy

Anthelmintic agents including albendazole and mebendazole are recommended.

Prevention

Adequate preparation and cooking of seafood—including fish, snails, crabs, and shrimp—in endemic areas is encouraged.

Hookworms

Hookworms are known to have a worldwide distribution. The two most common species known to infect humans include *A. duodenale* (Fig. 50.13) and *N. americanus* (Fig. 50.14). Additional hookworm organisms that play a lesser role in human infections include *A. ceylonicum, A.*

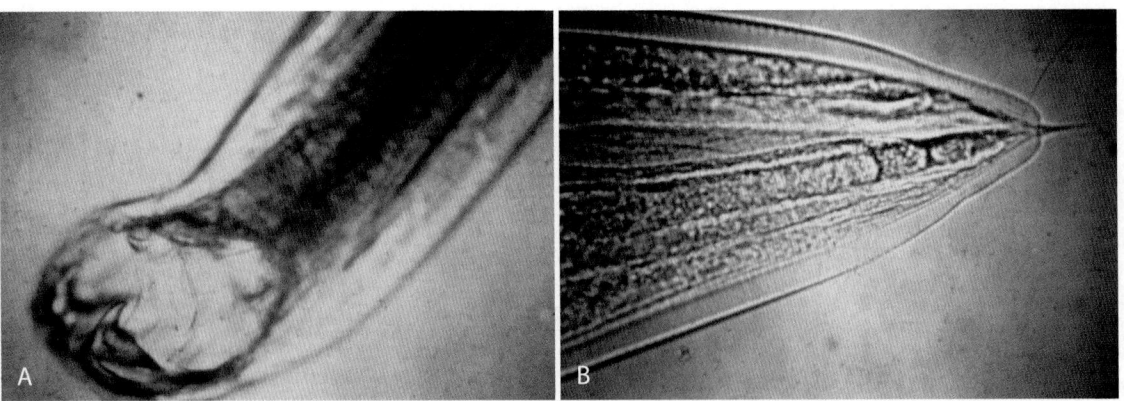

• **Fig. 50.13** (A) *Ancylostoma duodenale* head. (B) Tail; note that it is pointed. (Courtesy Dr. Henry Travers, Sioux Falls, SD.)

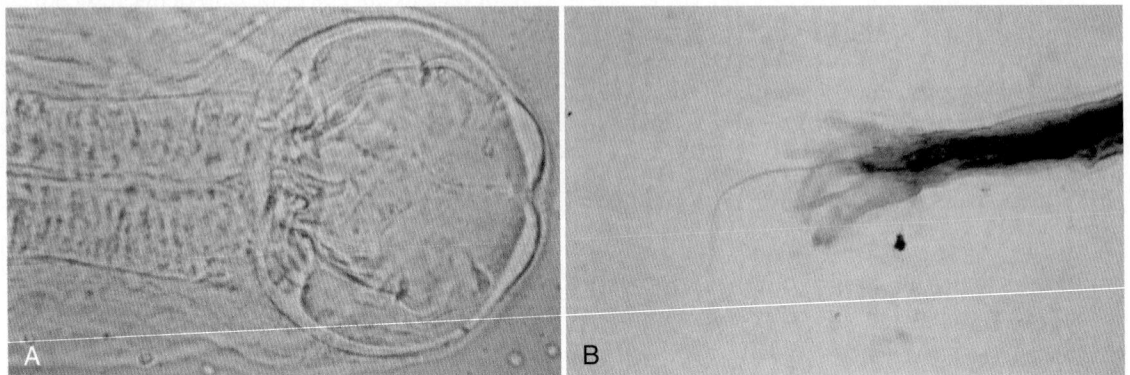

• **Fig. 50.14** (A) *Necator americanus* head; note the evident rounded cutting plates protruding from the head. (B) Copulatory bursa. (Courtesy Dr. Henry Travers, Sioux Falls, SD.)

braziliense, and *A. caninum.* Hookworms are the second most common helminthic infection reported in humans. The eggs and rhabditiform larvae of the species are indistinguishable. Differentiation of the species is based on the morphology of the buccal capsule and the adult male **copulatory bursa** (Fig. 50.14B).

The parasites, infective filariform larvae, penetrate the skin and enter the circulation, where they are capable of breaking through the capillaries and entering the lungs of the host. The larvae migrate up the bronchial tree and over the epiglottis and are swallowed. Upon entering the digestive system, the hookworms attach to the mucosa of the small intestine. Here they secrete anticoagulants and ingest blood as their source of nourishment. The worms mature and eggs are passed in the feces and deposited in soil, where they mature into rhabditiform larvae. The noninfective rhabditiform larvae will then mature into filariform larvae.

Epidemiology

Hookworms are found in areas with moist, warm soil capable of supporting their life cycle. Transmission is generally through direct skin penetration by filariform larvae.

Ancylostoma duodenale

General Characteristics

A. duodenale, or Old World hookworm, is prevalent in southern Europe, northern Africa, Southeast Asia, and South America. The adult male tends to be larger than the adult female of *N. americanus.* They attach to the intestinal mucosa by well-developed mouthparts (Fig. 50.13).

Pathogenesis and Spectrum of Disease

A. duodenale is capable of maturation within the intestine without migrating through the lungs of the host. Table 50.1 summarizes the detail of associated diseases.

Necator americanus

General Characteristics

N. americanus, or New World hookworm, is prevalent in Africa, Southeast Asia, and South and Central America as well as the southeastern United States. It attaches to the intestinal mucosa by well-developed **cutting plates** (Fig. 50.14A).

Pathogenesis and Spectrum of Disease

The major clinical presentation associated with hookworm infections is iron deficiency anemia. Table 50.1 summarizes the detail of associated diseases.

Ancylostoma ceylonicum, Ancylostoma braziliense, and *Ancylostoma caninum*

General Characteristics

A. ceylonicum primarily infects canines and felines but can cause mild hookworm disease in humans. *A. braziliense* is a canine and feline hookworm that, in humans, causes cutaneous larva migrans, or creeping eruption. The condition is generally self-limiting and characterized by the formation of serpiginous burrows as the larvae migrate through the epidermis. *A. caninum* is a canine hookworm that causes eosinophilic enteritis in humans and can causes cutaneous larva migrans.

Pathogenesis and Spectrum of Disease

Hookworm infection gives rise to the following three clinical presentations in humans: (1) classic hookworm disease, a GI infection characterized by chronic blood loss that leads to iron-deficiency anemia and protein malnutrition primarily associated with *N. americanus* and *A. duodenale* and less commonly by the zoonotic species *A. ceylonicum*; (2) cutaneous larva migrans, an infection limited to serpiginous tracks in the skin and most commonly caused by *A. braziliense*; and (3) eosinophilic enteritis, a GI infection characterized by abdominal pain but no blood loss caused by the dog hookworm *A. caninum.*

In cutaneous larva migrans, the infective larvae do not elaborate sufficient concentrations of hydrolytic enzymes to penetrate the junction of the dermis and epidermis. The larvae remain trapped in the epidermis, where they migrate laterally at a rate of 1 to 2 cm/day and create the pathognomonic serpiginous tunnels associated with this condition. Larvae can survive in the epidermis for about 10 days before dying.

In eosinophilic enteritis, *A. caninum* larvae typically enter a human host by penetrating the skin, though infection by oral ingestion is also possible. These larvae probably remain dormant in skeletal muscles and create no symptoms. In some individuals, larvae may reach the gut and mature into adult worms. Why some individuals sustain *A. caninum* development and then respond with a severe localized allergic reaction is unknown. Adult worms secrete various biomolecules that may act as allergens in the intestinal mucosa. Some patients have been reported to experience increasingly severe recurrent abdominal pain.

Laboratory Diagnosis

Hookworms are typically diagnosed by the presence of eggs or rhabditiform larvae in stool specimens. The eggs and

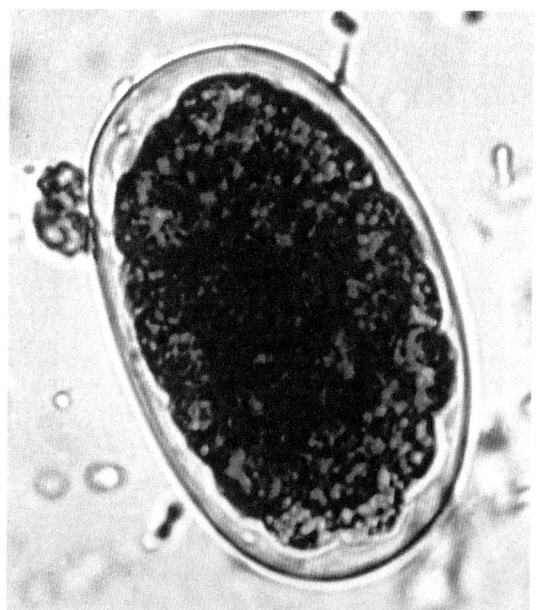

• **Fig. 50.15** Hookworm egg, iodine stain.

larvae of *N. americanus, A. duodenale,* and *A. ceylonicum* are indistinguishable. They are oval and thin-shelled, containing clearly visible four- to eight-cell-stage embryos. There is a characteristic clear space between the shell and the developing embryo (Fig. 50.15). Recovery and identification of eggs on direct smear or from concentration methods is recommended. Eggs may appear distorted on permanently stained smears. The rhabditiform larvae are typically 250 to 300 μm in length with a long buccal capsule and an inconspicuous genital primordium (Fig. 50.16). The larger filariform larvae are approximately 500 μm, with a pointed tail and an esophageal-to-intestinal ratio of 1:4. Both the rhabditiform and filariform larvae must be differentiated from *S. stercoralis.*

Fresh stool stored at room temperature may result in the continued maturation and hatching of larvae. Larvae may be cultured according to the Harada-Mori method previously described in this chapter.

In cases of cutaneous larva migrans, stool examination is not indicated because the larvae remain confined to the skin in almost all cases. In cases of eosinophilic enteritis, no eggs are found, as the adult *A. caninum* worms do not produce eggs in human hosts.

Progress is being made in the development of PCR-based methods for the specific diagnosis of hookworm infection but not available clinically.

Therapy

Anthelmintic agents including albendazole and mebendazole are indicated. However, because of variation in species and geographic distribution, some agents may not be effective in a specific population of parasites, and regional recommendations should be followed because of potential drug tolerance or resistance. Iron supplementation may also be required in severely anemic patients.

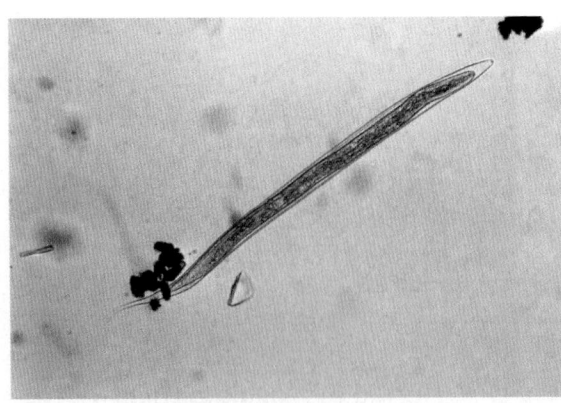

• **Fig. 50.16** Hookworm rhabditiform larvae. (Courtesy Dr. Henry Travers, Sioux Falls, SD.)

Prevention

Contaminated soil and beaches should be avoided. Appropriate footwear such as enclosed shoes should be worn in potentially contaminated areas.

Because of the immunosuppressive activity associated with the production of hookworm proteins, vaccination may be only partially effective. Currently no preventive vaccine exists. However, a protein, ASP-2, secreted by infective larvae of *N. americanus* is being investigated as a potential recombinant vaccine (www.clinicaltrials.gov).

Results and Reporting

Any identification of larvae or eggs in a patient's feces should be reported to the clinician. Treatment is typically recommended in asymptomatic and symptomatic infections. Quantitation of organisms is not required. Because parasite shedding may be intermittent or dependent on specimen quality, a single negative result does not ensure that the patient is not infected, and repeat testing may be necessary.

ⓔ Visit the Evolve site for a complete list of procedures, review questions, and case studies.

Bibliography

Bøås H, Tapia G, Sødahl JA, Rasmussen T, Rønningen KS: *Enterobius vermicularis* and risk factors in healthy Norwegian children, *Pediatr Infect Dis J* 31(9):927–930, 2012.

Carroll KC, Pfaller MA, Landry ML, et al.: *Manual of clinical microbiology*, ed 12, Washington, DC, 2019, ASM.

Garcia LS: *Diagnostic medical parasitology*, ed 6, Washington, DC, 2016, ASM Press.

Genta RM: Predictive value of an enzyme-linked immunosorbent assay (ELISA) for the serodiagnosis of strongyloides, *Am J Clin Pathol* 89:391–394, 1988.

Goncalves MLC, Araujo A, Ferreira LF: Human intestinal parasites in the past: new findings and a review, *Mem Inst Oswaldo Cruz* 98:21041–21210, 2003.

Lamberton PH, Jourdan PM: Human ascariasis: diagnostics update, *Curr Trop Med Rep* 2(4):189–200, 2015.

Page W, Judd J, Bradbury RS: The unique life cycle of *Strongyloides stercoralis* and implications for public health action, *Trop Med Infect Dis* 3(2):53, 2018.

Patsantara GG, Piperaki ET, Tzoumaka-Bakoula C, Kanariou MG: Immune responses in children infected with the pinworm *Enterobius vermicularis* in central Greece, *J Helminthol* 90:337–341, 2016.

Pilotte N, Papaiakovou M, Grant JR, et al.: Improved PCR-based detection of soil transmitted helminth infections using a next-generation sequencing approach to assay design, *PLoS Negl Trop Dis* 10(3):e0004578, 2016.

Strickland GT: *Hunter's tropical medicine and emerging infectious diseases*, ed 8, Philadelphia, 2000, Saunders.

Taniuchi M, Verweij JJ, Noor Z, et al.: High throughput multiplex PCR and probe-based detection with Luminex beads for seven intestinal parasites, *Am J Trop Med Hyg* 84:332–337, 2011.

Watts MR, Robertson G, Bradbury RS: The laboratory diagnosis of *Strongyloides stercoralis*, *Microbiol Aust* 37(1):4–9, 2016.

51

Tissue Nematodes

OBJECTIVES

1. Describe the distinguishing morphologic characteristics and basic life cycle (vectors, hosts, and stages of infectivity) for each of the parasites listed.
2. Describe the diseases and mechanism of pathogenicity, including route of transmission, for each of the species listed.
3. Describe the life cycle of *Trichinella spiralis* in humans and swine, including the infectious form and location of adult worms.
4. Describe trichinosis and disease progression in humans, including body sites affected, peripheral blood presentation, severity of disease, and prognosis.
5. List the various methods used to diagnose tissue nematode infections.
6. Explain the diagnosis and recommended treatment for dracunculosis.
7. Define and differentiate visceral larva migrans, ocular toxocariasis larva migrans, and cutaneous larva migrans.
8. Correlate patient signs, symptoms, and route of transmission with the correct organisms described in this chapter.

PARASITES TO BE CONSIDERED

Helminths
Nematodes (Roundworms)
Tissue
Trichinella britovi
Trichinella murrelli
Trichinella native
Trichinella nelsoni
Trichinella papuae
Trichinella patagoniensis
Trichinella pseudospiralis
Trichinella spiralis
Trichinella zimbabwensis
Neural larva migrans (*Baylisascaris procyonis*)
Visceral larva migrans (*Toxocara canis* or *Toxocara cati*)
Ocular larva migrans toxocariasis (*T. canis* or *T. cati*)
Cutaneous larva migrans (*Ancylostoma braziliense* or *Ancylostoma caninum*)
Capillaria hepatica
Dirofilaria immitis
Dirofilaria hongkongensis
Dracunculus medinensis
Parastrongylus (Angiostrongylus) cantonensis
Parastrongylus (Angiostrongylus) costaricensis
Gnathostoma spinigerum

Tissue nematodes have life cycles similar to those of intestinal nematodes, consisting of five distinct stages including adult male and female worms and four larval stages. These organisms have a worldwide distribution and are predominantly found in the tropics and subtropics. The organisms are transmitted by three routes: biting and subsequent blood-feeding arthropods (filarial worms), as discussed in Chapter 52; ingestion of small freshwater crustaceans; and ingestion of contaminated meat. In most cases, adult worms do not multiply and develop within the human host. Clinical symptoms are dependent on the number of infecting parasites, the tissue invaded, and the host's general health and immune response. Diagnosis is typically by microscopic visualization of the organisms in tissue when appropriate.

Trichinella spp.

General Characteristics

The family *Trichinellidae* contains nine recognized species and three genotypes including *Trichinella spiralis, Trichinella nativa* (T2 and T6), *Trichinella nelsoni, Trichinella murrelli* (T5 and T9), *Trichinella papuae, Trichinella zimbabwensis, Trichinella patagoniensis, Trichinella pseudospiralis,* and *Trichinella britovi* (T3 and T8), all capable of causing trichinosis. The three species with a second genotype are indicated in parentheses. However, *T. spiralis* is the most common human pathogen. The organism is unique compared with other helminths in that all stages of development, including the adult and larval stages, occur within a single host.

Epidemiology

Trichinella occurs worldwide with the cycle maintained in several different mammalian, avian, and reptile species. The primary host serves as the definitive host for the adult worm and the intermediate host for the encysted larvae. Humans acquire the infection by eating undercooked meat that contains the infective encysted larvae. Although this is typically transmitted in pork, human cases have been associated with the ingestion of bear, walrus, and horsemeat as well as the meat of other mammals. The encysted larvae are ingested. When the undercooked meat is digested in the stomach, the larvae are resistant to the gastric pH and pass to the intestine, where they invade the mucosa. In about 1.5 days, the larvae mature and mate, and the female worm begins to release motile larvae. These larvae then migrate to the peripheral bloodstream, lymphatic system, or mesenteric venules and become distributed throughout the body. The larvae then deposit in the striated muscle tissue, where they can continue development and begin to coil, forming nurse cells that nourish the parasite and protect it from the human host's immune response. The nurse cell completes the formation of the cyst within about 2 to 3 weeks, becoming infective. The larvae encyst in the active striated muscle, including the diaphragm, larynx, tongue, jaws, neck, ribs, biceps, and gastrocnemius muscle. The generalized life cycle is depicted in Fig. 51.1. The larvae may remain viable within the cyst for several years. They eventually die, and the encysted capsules become calcified.

Pathogenesis and Spectrum of Disease

Trichinosis is a disease of the muscle caused by infection with the encysted larval form of *Trichinella* spp. (Fig. 51.2). The adult stages reside in the human intestine. The disease ranges from mild to severe depending on the number of parasites present. The intestinal stage lasts approximately 1 week and typically includes mild symptoms of nausea, abdominal discomfort, diarrhea, or constipation. Diarrhea may last as long as 14 weeks with no apparent muscle involvement. The migration of the larvae results in an intense inflammatory response causing periorbital edema, fever, muscle pain or tenderness, headache, and myalgia. A marked peripheral eosinophilia is often present. If the parasitic infection is low, eosinophilia may be the only diagnostic sign evident. Occasionally, splinter hemorrhages may be present below the nails. In addition to the typical infection of the active striated muscle as previously indicated, occasionally larvae migrate into the brain, meninges, and myocardium. However, the larvae do not encyst in these tissues. Brain and meningeal infections result in neurologic symptoms, and infection of the myocardium may result in myocarditis and dysrhythmias, leading to sudden death.

Laboratory Diagnosis

Diagnosis may be difficult because the symptoms may resemble a variety of flulike illnesses. Clinical symptoms that are indicators of trichinosis include fever, muscle pain, gastrointestinal symptoms, facial edema, and eosinophilia as well as subconjunctival, subungual, and retinal hemorrhages. A thorough patient history that includes consumption of laboratory-confirmed parasitized meat or link to a laboratory-confirmed case by exposure to the same common source may help the physician to diagnose the condition in a timely fashion. Identification of encysted larvae through muscle biopsy provides a definitive diagnosis. However, based on location, some tissues may be difficult to access; therefore, the condition may not be diagnosed until a postmortem examination. Histologic examination of formalin-fixed or paraffin-imbedded tissue may be used to visualize

encysted larvae. Occasionally, depending on the length of infection, calcified larvae may be seen in x-rays.

Serologic Testing

Trichinella infections are most often diagnosed in the laboratory based on the detection of antibodies to excretory/secretory *Trichinella* antigen by enzyme-linked immunosorbent assay (ELISA) or indirect immunofluorescence assay (IFA). Serologic diagnosis is sufficient in most cases. Testing is rarely positive in early disease. Patients will present with a specific immunoglobulin G (IgG) antibody response in 3 to 5 weeks after acute illness. A negative serologic test followed by a positive seroconversion is considered a definitive diagnosis.

Nucleic Acid Detection

Molecular species–specific nucleic acid–based amplification assays have been developed. This technique, however, is generally used as confirmatory rather than a screening test due to the high expenditure of labor and time and intensive costs. The direct detection of muscle-stage larvae based upon appropriate examination of muscle biopsies etiologically proves the diagnosis. Furthermore, isolated larvae enable the molecular identification of the *Trichinella* species or genotype—a procedure that is not possible by serology. The disadvantages of this method is that it requires a significant surgical intervention in the affected person, and the sensitivity of the diagnosis depends on the amount of muscle sample tested. Currently these methods are predominantly used in animal epidemiologic studies and have not been implemented within the diagnostic laboratory.

Therapy

Thiabendazole is used during the intestinal phase to reduce the number of potentially infective larvae, and although the encysted larvae cannot be removed, albendazole is used to limit the continued pathologic development of the organism. Supportive measures including analgesics, antihistamines, and steroids, which may be administered to decrease the effects of the generalized inflammatory response.

Prevention

The most effective prevention relies on eating thoroughly cooked meat as well as maintaining good animal husbandry for domestic swine. This is not typically a concern in the United States because of the US Department of Agriculture (USDA) meat inspection requirements and regulations.

Toxocara canis (Visceral Larva Migrans) and *Toxocara cati* (Ocular Larva Migrans)

General Characteristics

Toxocara canis (intestinal ascarid of dogs) and *Toxocara cati* (intestinal ascarid of cats) are the cause of a human syndrome resulting from larval migration within the host.

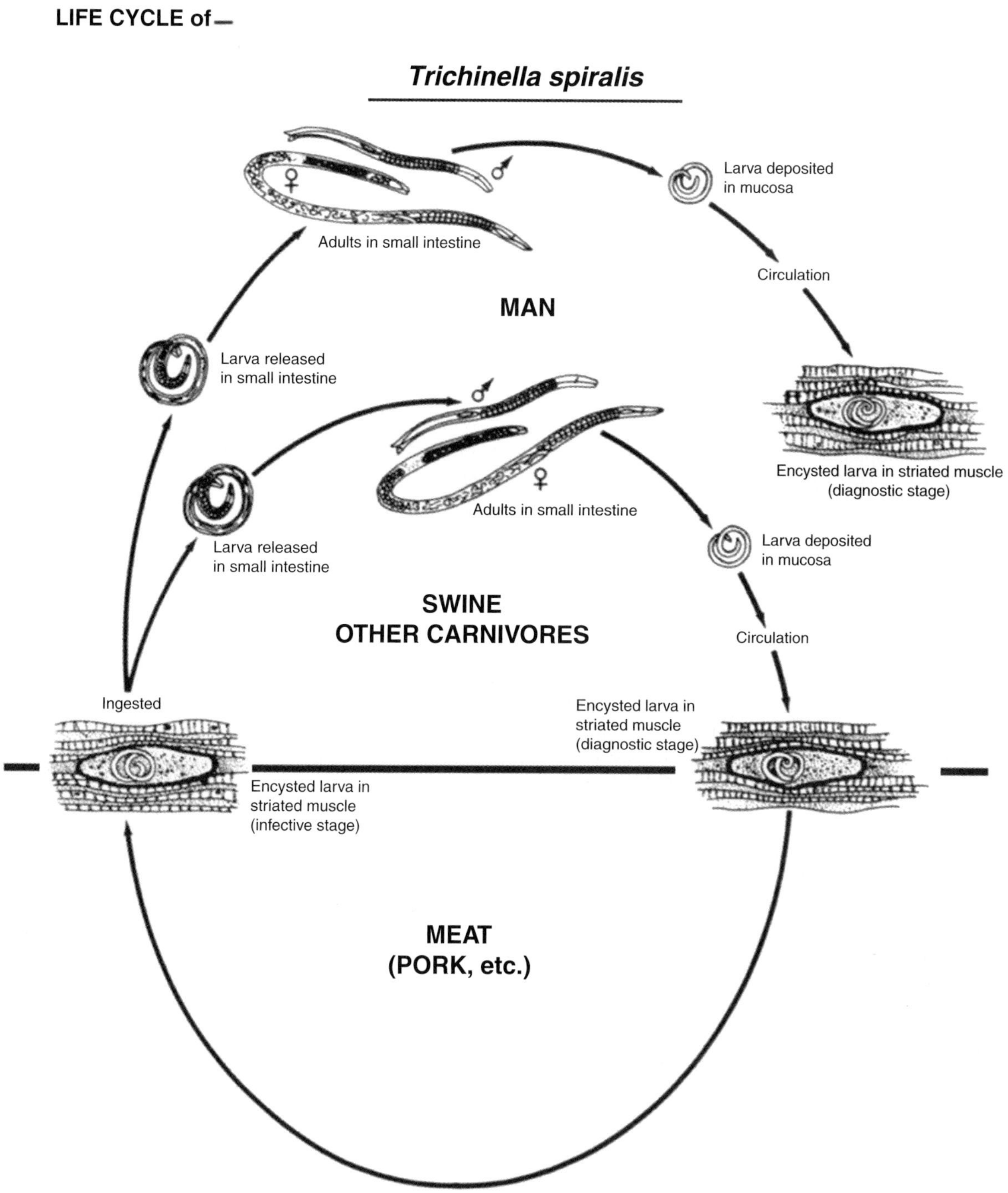

LIFE CYCLE of —

Trichinella spiralis

• **Fig. 51.1** The various life-cycle stages through which the intestinal nematode *Trichinella spiralis* passes as it matures from an egg to its adult form. Trichinellosis is acquired by ingesting meat containing cysts, or encysted larvae, of *Trichinella* spp. organisms. After exposure to gastric acid and pepsin, the larvae are released from the cysts, invading the small bowel mucosa, where they develop into adult worms. (Image Courtesy the Division of Parasitic Diseases/Centers for Disease Control and Prevention.)

Epidemiology

Toxocariasis is a zoonotic disease with worldwide distribution. Humans become infected after the accidental ingestion of the parasite's eggs (Fig. 51.3). The definitive hosts, dogs *(T. canis)* and cats *(T. cati),* pass the larvae transplacentally or lactogenically to their offspring and pass unembryonated eggs in the feces. The eggs mature in 10 to 20 days and then become infective. Once the eggs have been ingested, the larvae are released in the small intestine, penetrate the mucosa, and migrate to the liver, lungs, or other body sites. The adult worms are unable to mature in a human host and

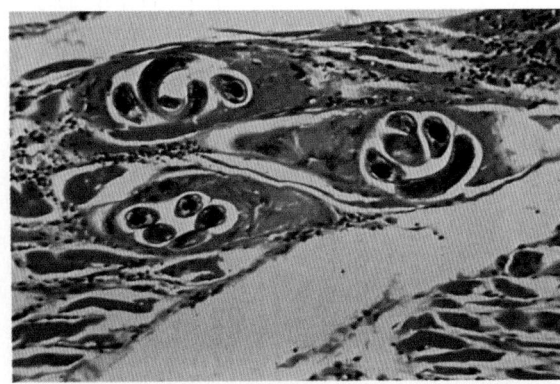

• **Fig. 51.2** Trichinosis; developing *Trichinella* spp. encysted larvae contained within a section of human muscle tissue. (Image Courtesy the Division of Parasitic Diseases/Centers for Disease Control and Prevention.)

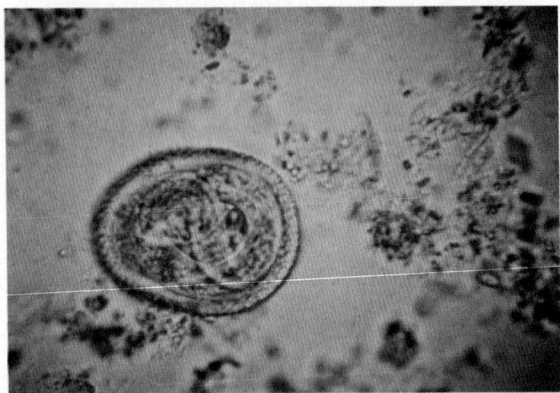

• **Fig. 51.3** *Toxocara canis* egg. Note the rough appearance on the outer surface of the egg. The egg also contains an infectious L2 larva. (Courtesy Dr. Henry Travers, Sioux Falls, SD.)

therefore wander throughout the body, causing the migratory syndromes.

Pathogenesis and Spectrum of Disease

Typically, these infections are mild, but they can sometimes be severe. Severe life-threatening infections occur when there is involvement in the heart, brain, or other vital organs. Disease is more common in young children and may persist for long periods with minimal pathologic manifestations. Larvae that remain in the liver or lungs may become encapsulated in fibrous tissue. **Visceral** (tissue) **larva migrans (VLM)** may result in a high degree of eosinophilia; however, this may be absent in **ocular larva migrans (OLM)**. Symptoms may include fever, hepatomegaly, hyperglobulinemia, pulmonary infiltration, cough, neurologic symptoms, and endophthalmitis. OLM may result in the development of a granulomatous reaction in the retina of the eye. In the **covert or common toxocariasis (CT)** form of toxocariasis, patients exhibit nonspecific symptoms that can be accompanied by eosinophilia and positive *Toxocara* serology. **Neurotoxocariasis (NT)** is caused by invasion of *Toxocara* larvae to the brain and spinal cord, leading to cerebral lesions and

neurologic damage, predominantly in the cerebral and cerebellar white matter with occlusion of cerebral blood vessels. Table 51.1 summarizes the four types of toxocariasis.

Laboratory Diagnosis

Toxocariasis must be differentiated from other migratory helmintic diseases including *Ascaris lumbricoides, Strongyloides stercoralis,* and *Trichinella* spp. A history of exposure to dogs and cats is of importance when an infection with *Toxocara* spp. is being considered. Because humans are an insufficient host for completion of the organism's life cycle, eggs are not passed in the stool. Diagnosis typically requires biopsy of tissue to detect the migrating larvae.

Direct Microscopy

Demonstrating the presence of *Toxocara* larvae in tissue biopsy, cerebrospinal fluid (CSF), or ocular fluids using direct microscopy remains the "gold standard" for the diagnosis of toxocariasis. However, this method is invasive, insensitive, and time consuming. In addition, it can be difficult to distinguish between the larvae of *Toxocara* and those of other ascarids, especially when the larvae are degenerated or when only parts of the larvae are recovered from tissues.

Serologic Testing

Serologic diagnosis has proven effective, particularly in OLM. Aqueous humor–elevated antibody titer specific for *Toxocara* spp., compared with serum levels, is considered diagnostic. Although serologic testing has been useful, it is important to note that antibody titers may vary depending on the location of the infection. A serum titer of 1:8 is considered significant for OLM; 1:32 is significant for VLM.

Nucleic Acid Detection

Molecular techniques have high analytical specificity and shorter turnaround times than other diagnostics. Polymerase chain reaction (PCR)–based assays using a variety of genetic markers have been developed and have enabled the identification and phylogenetic analysis of *T. canis, T. cati,* and other ascarids. PCR-based testing has been utilized to identify *T. canis* larvae collected from human biopsies in OLM and from CSF in neuronal toxocariasis (NT). PCR-based assays, including quantitative real-time PCR (qPCR) and PCR-RFLP have been used for accurate identification and diagnosis of *Toxocara* eggs isolated from feces or soil. The development of loop-mediated isothermal amplification (LAMP) of nucleic acid has provided a rapid and cheap approach for assessing the contamination of soil with *Toxocara* eggs. Molecular methods with improved performance characteristics have the potential to advance the diagnosis of toxocariasis.

Therapy

Effective therapy depends on the location of infection, but several anthelmintic medications have been used, including thiabendazole, ivermectin, albendazole, and

TABLE
51.1 **Characteristics of the Different Clinical Forms of Toxocariasis**

Clinical Syndrome	Primary Population Affected	Primary Affected Sites	Associated Symptoms
VLM	Children age 2–7 years	Liver, heart, lungs, kidneys, and muscle	Fever, respiratory symptoms (such as cough, wheezing, dyspnea, bronchospasm, asthma), hepatomegaly, abdominal pain, vomiting, diarrhea, anorexia, weight loss, fatigue, neurologic manifestations, and pallor
OLM	Children age 5–10 years	Eye	*Toxocara* larval invasion of the peripheral retina and vitreous can cause three major clinical types of OT/OLM syndrome over days to weeks: diffuse nematode endophthalmitis, peripheral inflammatory mass type. In addition, posterior pole granuloma type. In addition, diffuse unilateral subacute neuroretinitis (DUSN), bilateral distal symmetric sensory neuropathy (DSN), and choroidal neovascular membrane formation have been attributed to prolonged *Toxocara* infection. There may be predominant unilateral or uncommon bilateral ocular involvement, characterized by visual impairment, strabismus, leukocoria, solid retinal mass predominantly at the posterior pole, vitreous mass or haze, retinal detachment, cataract, endophthalmitis, papillitis, uveitis, as well as visual loss, vitritis, papillitis, and evanescent outer retinal lesions leading to optic atrophy, retinal-artery narrowing, and diffuse-pigment epithelial degeneration.
CT	Children and adults	No specific site	In adults: breathing difficulties, rash, pruritus, weakness, and abdominal pain, elevated titers of anti-*Toxocara* antibodies, eosinophilia, and elevated total IgE levels
NT (NLM)	Children and adults	Central nervous system	Headache, fever, photophobia, weakness, dorsalgia, confusion, tiredness, visual impairment, epileptic seizures, neuropsychological disturbances, dementia, and depression. Motor impairment can also be observed in clinical NT/NLM cases, such as ataxia, rigor, para- or tetraparesis dysesthesia, urinary retention, and fecal incontinence. Rarely, recognizable neurologic signs of eosinophilic meningitis, encephalitis, myelitis, cerebral vasculitis, epilepsy, neuropsychologic deficits or combined pathological presentations, which may be associated with repeated low-dose infections, or cerebral vasculitis under anthelmintic therapy, optic neuritis, other cranial nerve involvement, and meningoradiculitis. Unlike NT, NLM generally results in rapid progression followed by severe damage, coma, and death.

CT, Covert or common toxocariasis; *DSN*, distal symmetric sensory neuropathy; *OLM*, ocular larva migrans; *NT*, neurotoxocariasis; *NLM*, neuronal larva migrans; *VLM*, visceral larva migrans.

diethylcarbamazine. Antiinflammatory medications including corticosteroids may be used to reduce the pathology associated with inflammation. Photocoagulation has been used to treat OLM. The prognosis is good, even in cases of OLM, with prompt diagnosis and proper treatment.

Prevention

Small children should be kept out of sandboxes and playgrounds frequented by dogs and cats. Sandboxes should be covered when not in use. Encouraging regular hand washing and teaching children to keep dirt out of their mouths will decrease the potential for infection. In addition, regular

deworming of dogs and cats will reduce the spread of infective eggs.

Baylisascaris procyonis (Neural Larva Migrans)

General Characteristics

B. procyonis is found predominantly in raccoons but has now been recognized as causing neural larva migrans (roundworm encephalitis) in more than 100 different species of mammals and birds. Human infections generally result in severe neurologic disease or death.

Epidemiology

The organism can be found in raccoons in North America. The raccoons become infected after ingesting infective eggs or intermediate hosts, rabbits, rodents, or birds infected with encysted larvae. The larvae penetrate the mucosa of the small intestine and mature in the lumen. Humans are accidental intermediate hosts by ingesting eggs that have been released in the raccoon feces into the environment. Reports indicate that the organism has also been identified in domestic dogs and puppies, thus increasing the likelihood of human exposure.

Pathogenesis and Spectrum of Disease

Pathogenesis results from larval migration causing tissue damage and severe inflammatory reactions. Symptoms may include a macular rash on the face and truck, pneumonitis, and hepatomegaly. The larvae invade the eyes (OLM), spinal cord, and brain (NLM). Patients may present with eosinophilic meningoencephalitis or unilateral neuroretinitis. Granulomas have also been identified in the heart, pleura, lungs, large bowel, mesenteric lymph nodes, and other soft tissues. Patients suffering from NLM may experience mild neuropsychological problems progressing to loss of coordination, seizures, coma, and death.

Laboratory Diagnosis

Diagnosis is often made by eliminating other causes related to the presentation of symptoms. Hematologic and CSF examinations are nonspecific. Identification of the migrating larvae, lesions, or larval tracks in the eyes support the diagnosis.

Serologic Testing

Acute and convalescent serum or CSF can be used to detect *B. procyonis* antibodies. Antibodies have been found in asymptomatic family members and other individuals with routine contact with raccoons. Serologic testing is available from the Centers for Disease Control.

Therapy

Systemic corticosteroids and antihelminthic agents have been used to treat infections. Upon diagnosis and at the beginning of treatment the patient has generally already suffered severe neurologic damage.

Ancylostoma braziliense and *Ancylostoma caninum* (Cutaneous Larva Migrans)

General Characteristics

Ancylostoma braziliense and *Ancylostoma caninum* are common hookworms of dogs and cats. The parasites penetrate the skin and cause **cutaneous larva migrans (CLM),** also referred to as creeping eruption.

Epidemiology

Ancylostoma braziliense and *Ancylostoma caninum* are found in warm climates in the southeastern United States. Dogs and cats are the natural definitive host. The infective larvae penetrate the skin of the host and migrate in the circulation. The adult worms reside in the intestine. The eggs are shed in the feces of dogs and cats and undergo maturation in moist, sandy soil of areas protected from desiccation, such as under shady trees and beneath houses. Children are often infected while playing in sandboxes that have been contaminated with dog and cat feces.

Pathogenesis and Spectrum of Disease

The infective larvae penetrate the skin of the human host and migrate through the subcutaneous tissue. The host develops pruritic papules at the site of penetration, followed by serpiginous, vesicular, elevated linear tracks. The larvae will migrate several millimeters each day, forming these continued tracks. The area surrounding the tracks becomes inflamed with marked edema. The patient may present with a peripheral eosinophilia. Infection is typically self-limiting. As the larvae migrate, the host may scratch and scar the tissue, subjecting the host to potential secondary bacterial infections. The signs and symptoms resemble those of infection with similar insect larvae, *S. stercoralis,* and other animal hookworms. Systemic involvement is rare; however, cases of pneumonitis resulting from larval migration into the lungs have been identified. In addition, gastrointestinal discomfort including abdominal pain, diarrhea, and weight loss has been associated with these infections. This condition is referred to as **eosinophilic enteritis.** Table 51.2 summarizes the associated diseases.

Laboratory Diagnosis

Laboratory diagnosis is limited. Evidence of visible tracks and a patient history of possible exposure are usually sufficient. A biopsy (if performed) must be taken 1 to 2 cm ahead of the leading edge of a tract or else the larva may be missed. The patient may present with a peripheral eosinophilia. In systemic cases, larvae may be recovered from sputum, and Charcot-Leyden crystals may be evident.

Therapy and Prevention

Even though CLM is self-limiting, the intense pruritus and risk for infection mandate treatment. Prevention is key and involves avoidance of direct skin contact with fecally contaminated soil. Anthelmintic therapy may include ivermectin or thiabendazole.

Dracunculus medinensis

General Characteristics

Dracunculus medinensis, commonly referred to as the guinea worm, is the cause of a subcutaneous infection known as

TABLE 51.2	Pathogenesis and Spectrum of Associated Diseases	
Organism	Pathogenesis	Mode of Transmission and Spectrum of Disease
Tissue nematodes	Attributed to three main factors: 1. Host immune response 2. Parasitic burden 3. General overall health of host	
Trichinella spp.	Worm burden may be small to several hundred. Migration and deposition of larvae in tissue depends on tissue involved in infection.	Ingestion of poorly cooked meat, particularly domestic swine, but may be found in several mammalian species.
Toxocara canis and Toxocara cati	Migration in host tissue and immune response.	Accidental ingestion of eggs. Mild to severe disease dependent on tissue.
Ancylostoma braziliense or Ancylostoma caninum	Migration, inflammation, and edema. Secondary bacterial infections.	Penetrate skin and migrate in circulation. Pneumonitis may occur. Systemic involvement is rare.
Capillaria hepatica	Dependent on worm burden. Migration of larvae to liver via portal vein and other organs such as lungs and kidneys.	Fecal-oral transmission. Ingestion of embryonated eggs in fecal-contaminated food, water, or soil. Hepatitis, anemia, fever, hypereosinophilia. Extended infection can result in organ failure and death.
Dirofilaria immitis	Pulmonary obstruction, subcutaneous nodules and inflammation. Granulomatous reaction.	Infection upon ingestion by a mosquito during a blood meal. Localized, limited inflammatory reaction.
Dirofilaria hongkongensis	Ocular obstruction and inflammation. Granulomatous reaction.	Infection upon ingestion by a mosquito during a blood meal. Localized; limited inflammatory reaction.
Dracunculus medinensis	Larvae migration, inflammation, and secondary bacterial infections.	Ingestion of infected copepods. Blisters develop where female exits the skin.
Parastrongylus cantonensis	Migration to central nervous system.	Ingestion of infected shrimp, fish, crabs, and frogs. Often self-limiting but may cause meningoencephalitis or meningitis.
Parastrongylus costaricensis	Migration resulting in inflammation and lesions in bowel.	Ingestion of salad contaminated with infected slugs or snails.
Gnathostoma spinigerum	Migration resulting in inflammation.	Ingestion of contaminated fish. Tissue damage based on worm burden and migration pattern.

dracunculiasis. The worm has a characteristic thick cuticle and a large uterus that fills the body cavity and contains **rhabditoid** larvae.

Epidemiology

The parasite was once known to have a worldwide distribution affecting millions of people. In 2008, the World Health Organization in collaboration with governmental groups and other organizations attempted to eradicate the organism. Efforts have reduced the incidence of infection, confining the remaining endemic area to Africa. Humans are infected by the ingestion of freshwater from stagnant ponds containing larvae-infected copepods. The copepods

are digested in the stomach, releasing the larvae. The larvae then penetrate the small intestine and migrate through the thoracic musculature. Both male and female worms mature in approximately 2 to 3 months. The gravid female develops in approximately 10 to 14 months, migrating to the lower extremities. The gravid female produces a blister on the skin; when the host submerges the affected area in water, the blister erupts and releases larvae into the water (Fig. 51.4).

Pathogenesis and Spectrum of Disease

The blisters formed by the gravid female worm cause burning and itching. Systemic symptoms may include

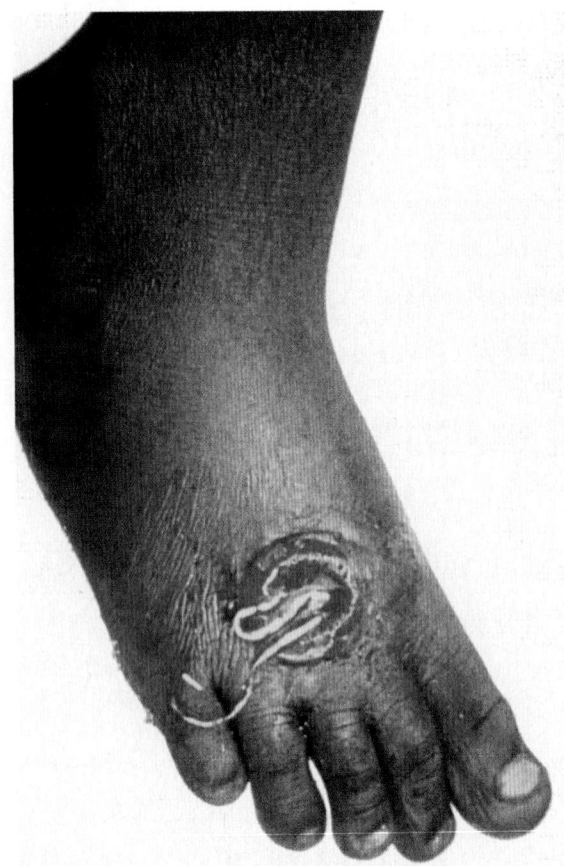

• **Fig. 51.4** *Dracunculus medinensis* emerging from a blister on an infected individual's foot.

fever, nausea, vomiting, diarrhea, headache, urticaria, and eosinophilia. Secondary bacterial infections may occur. In addition, dead worms within the host may be absorbed or may calcify, causing secondary inflammatory symptoms.

Laboratory Diagnosis

Diagnosis is by the identification of larvae or adult worms in clinical specimens. Serology may be used to identify infected patients before there is evidence of blistering and emersion of the worm. No nucleic acid–based tests have yet been developed for the diagnosis of *D. medinensis* infection.

Therapy

Treatment requires removal of the adult worms. The female worms are attached to a stick and slowly retracted from the host by gradual turning of the stick and removal of the worms. Although anthelmintic medications, such as metronidazole or thiabendazole, are not lethal, they are administered to assist with the retraction of the worms. Analgesics and antimicrobials are administered for discomfort and to prevent secondary infections.

Parastrongylus cantonensis (Cerebral Angiostrongyliasis)

General Characteristics

Parastrongylus cantonensis, previously known as *Angiostrongylus* sp., is a filarial worm commonly referred to as the rat lungworm.

Epidemiology

Parastrongylus spp. has a worldwide distribution; however, it remains an endemic health threat mainly in Southeast Asia and the Asian Pacific Islands. Varieties of rodents serve as the definitive host. The adult worms reside in the pulmonary artery and right side of the heart. The eggs shed by the female lodge in the pulmonary capillaries, where the larvae hatch and migrate up the trachea. The larvae are swallowed and passed in the rodent feces. Once released, the larvae infect the intermediate hosts, which are mollusks. The mollusks are consumed by a variety of **paratenic** (not required for the development or life cycle of the parasite) hosts such as shrimp, fish, crabs, and frogs. The rodents then consume the paratenic hosts and the larvae penetrate the intestine, enter the circulation, and migrate to the central nervous system (CNS). After two successive molts, the larvae then reenter the circulation and migrate to the pulmonary artery. Humans are infected by ingestion of either the intermediate or the paratenic host.

Pathogenesis and Spectrum of Disease

The pathogenesis correlates with the worm burden and the site of infection. The larvae may migrate to the CNS, causing meningitis or meningoencephalitis. Symptoms include headache, fever, eosinophilia, eosinophilic meningitis (with cells numbering >10/μL of CSF), increased CSF protein, and neurologic manifestations. Occasionally the larvae may migrate to the eye, causing blindness. Most often, the disease caused by *Parastrongylus* spp. is self-limiting.

Laboratory Diagnosis

Definitive diagnosis relies on histologic identification of the adult female worm, which has a distinctive morphologic appearance with a spiral, winding uterus resembling a barber pole. Highly specific serologic assays are available for patients with elevated eosinophils. Some cross reactivity has been reported between *A. cantonensis* and trichinosis, making diagnosis less specific.

Therapy

Anthelmintic therapy, such as mebendazole, may be helpful. It is important to monitor therapy closely because the therapy may actually exacerbate the inflammatory response of the host and cause more systemic damage. If larvae are located within the eye, surgical removal is recommended.

Parastrongylus costaricensis (Abdominal Angiostrongyliasis)

General Characteristics

Parastrongylus costaricensis is found primarily in the cotton rat and black rat.

Epidemiology

The parasite is endemic in areas of Central and South America, including Mexico and Costa Rica.

Pathogenesis and Spectrum of Disease

The life cycle is very similar to that of *P. cantonensis*. Human infection is typically by ingestion of salad contaminated with excretions from infected slugs or snails. The larvae create inflammatory lesions in the wall of the bowel, resulting in tissue inflammation, necrosis, vomiting, and diarrhea. The patient may experience lower-right-quadrant abdominal pain similar to that manifested in appendicitis. The eggs of *P. costaricensis* may also remain embedded in the tissue of the human host and are not passed in the patient's feces.

Laboratory Diagnosis

Histologic identification of the adult worm, larvae, or eggs in tissue sections results in definitive diagnosis. Patients often present with leukocytosis and eosinophilia. Radiologic imaging may be useful. Currently no molecular tests specific for this infection are available. However, for research purposes, *A. costaricensis* can be identified in tissue by conventional PCR followed by DNA sequencing analysis.

Therapy

Traditional anthelmintic therapy is recommended.

Gnathostoma spinigerum

General Characteristics

Gnathostoma spp., a gastric Spirurida, is found in a variety of mammals worldwide. Dogs and cats serve as the definitive host for *Gnathostoma spinigerum*. Although *G. spinigerum* is the most common species identified in humans, *G. hispidum*, *G. nipponicum*, *G. binucleatum*, *G. procyonis*, *G. binucleatum* and *G. doloresi* have also been associated with infection.

Epidemiology

The adult worms reside in the stomach of the definitive host, where they mate and produce eggs that are passed in the feces. When the feces are deposited in water, the larvae hatch and infect copepods. The larvae mature in the copepods and are then ingested by a variety of intermediate hosts including fish, snakes, and frogs. Inside the intermediate host, the larvae then migrate to the musculature and encyst until the tissue is ingested by the definitive host. The intermediate hosts may serve as a food staple for a paratenic host, such as a bird. Once ingested by the bird, the larvae can remain viable and be passed to the definitive host or to humans. Once in the definitive host, the larvae excyst and penetrate the gastric wall, migrating and maturing in the stomach. Humans act as accidental hosts when they ingest larvae in contaminated fish.

Pathogenesis and Spectrum of Disease

The worms are incapable of maturation within the human host and migrate aimlessly, causing tissue damage and inflammation, thus causing a disease that resembles visceral larva migrans. The infection is not typically fatal; however, it depends on the migration pattern and organs infected. Any organ system can be involved, but the most common manifestation of infection is localized, intermittent, migratory swelling in the skin and subcutaneous tissues. Such swellings may be painful, pruritic, and/or erythematous. In addition, *Gnathostoma* spp. commonly cause a parasitic eosinophilic meningitis due to larval migration into the CNS. Systemic infection is typically associated with peripheral eosinophilia, in which the percentage of eosinophils may exceed 50% of the circulating white blood cells (WBCs).

Laboratory Diagnosis

Identification of the larvae in tissue is definitive for diagnosis. The larval head contains four rows of **cephalic hooklets**, and the body is covered with transverse rows of spines that diminish anteriorly to posteriorly.

Serologic Testing

Both ELISA to detect IgG antibodies and immunoblot testing for neurologic disease has been described; however, these tests are not widely available in the United States and many other countries.

Therapy

Supportive corticosteroid treatment is recommended. Although anthelmintics are not lethal to this organism, they are often recommended. Surgical excision of the larvae is optimal.

Capillaria hepatica

General Characteristics

Capillariasis is a parasitic disease in humans caused by two different species of capillarids: *Capillaria hepatica* and *Capillaria philippinensis* (Chapter 50).

C. hepatica is transferred through the fecal matter of infected animals and can lead to hepatic capillariasis. Infection is rare but has been reported worldwide. Infective eggs hatch in the intestine of the human host, releasing larvae. The larvae migrate via the portal vein to the liver, where humans are considered a terminal host for the parasite.

Epidemiology

C. hepatica is often found in the liver of such animals as small rodents, monkeys, and prairie dogs and can cause cirrhosis in the animal hosts. When these animals are eaten by larger carnivores, capillarid eggs are ingested and passed in the feces. When this fecal matter is deposited in the soil, the eggs become infective in about 30 days. Accidental ingestion of the eggs from contaminated soil occurs in both animals and humans. The eggs hatch and the larvae migrate to the liver and mature into adult worms. The adult worms lay eggs in the liver. Humans are usually infected after ingesting embryonated eggs in fecal-contaminated food, water, or soil.

Pathogenesis and Spectrum of Disease

C. hepatica can be transmitted human to human when eggs are deposited through human fecal matter into the soil. The eggs then become infective in the soil, and humans ingest infective soil directly by eating soil (pica) or consuming it accidentally or indirectly through contaminated food or water. When a human is infected with only one *C. hepatica* worm, there are often no signs or symptoms. The adult worms lay eggs in the liver, resulting in clinical manifestations including hepatitis, anemia, fever, hypereosinophilia, and even death. Larvae may also migrate to the lungs, kidneys, or other organs. Table 51.2 summarizes the associated diseases.

Laboratory Diagnosis

No eggs are excreted in the feces in true human infections. *C. hepatica* can be diagnosed by performing a liver biopsy, needle biopsy, or after death at autopsy to identify the adult worm or eggs.

Therapy

Anthelmintic agents including albendazole and mebendazole are recommended. Steroids have been used with *C. hepatica* infections to help control the inflammation of the liver.

Prevention

Adequate preparation and cooking of seafood—including fish, snails, crabs, and shrimp—in endemic areas is encouraged.

Dirofilaria immitis and Other Species

General Characteristics

The filarial dog heartworm *Dirofilaria immitis* causes human **pulmonary dirofilariasis** worldwide. Although *D. immitis* is the most common species isolated from humans in the United States, additional species infect other mammals. *D. repens* infects wolves, coyotes, and foxes. Other species include *D. ursi* in bears; *D. striata*, wildcats; *D. tenuis*, raccoons; *D. striata*, bobcats and pumas; and *D. subdermata*, porcupines. These organisms are occasionally associated with human infections. *D. repens* is found in cats and dogs in Europe, Africa, and Asia. *Dirofilaria hongkongensis* is a newly identified species from Hong Kong and Asia. The parasite is transmitted by dogs and cats, causes **ocular dirofilariasis**, and is closely related to *D. repens*.

Epidemiology

The adult worms reside in the right ventricle of the heart of the infected mammal. The adult worm releases microfilariae into the bloodstream, which are then ingested by a mosquito. The microfilariae mature into infective larvae in the insect and are then transferred to another host when the mosquito feeds. The larvae migrate through the host, eventually reaching the heart, where they mature into adult worms. Humans are accidental hosts, and the worms are unable to reach maturity. The organisms die and are swept into the pulmonary circulation, where they become lodged in arteries or arterioles. This obstruction of the pulmonary circulation results in thrombosis, infarction, and inflammation. Eventually a wall of fibrous tissue is deposited around the worm, creating a granulomatous reaction. Species of *Dirofilaria* that manifest subcutaneously produce nodules that are often tender and may be fixed or migratory. *D. repens*–associated lesions can occur in a variety of locations, the most typical being exposed sites (e.g., scalp, arms, legs, eyelids, chest), but occasionally lesions have been found in deeper tissue such as the breast, epididymis, spermatic cord, and subconjunctiva. Many reports of *D. tenuis* involve the facial region (e.g., ocular and periocular sites, oral mucosa, cheek) and breast. There are very rare reports of subcutaneous infections with *D. striata*, *D. ursi*, and possibly *D. subdermata* in humans. *D. hongkongensis* larvae migrate to the ocular region and cause recurrent eyelid swelling in both eyes and conjunctival inflammation with watery discharge.

Pathogenesis and Spectrum of Disease

Approximately 50% of patients with dirofilariasis are asymptomatic and present with subcutaneous nodules or lung disease. Symptomatic patients present with generalized symptoms such as cough, chest pain, fever, malaise, chills, and **hemoptysis.** Some patients may present with a peripheral eosinophilia. The respiratory granulomas may be identified radiographically and are typically removed to rule out malignancies. Excision of the nodule or granuloma is typically sufficient treatment, resulting in no long-term pathology.

Laboratory Diagnosis

Definitive diagnosis of the parasite from a nodule may be extremely difficult because of the worm's degeneration in the granuloma. However, the presence of a worm within a pulmonary artery is usually supportive of the diagnosis. Serologic tests are available; however, cross-reactivity may occur with other nematodes; therefore, a negative reaction does not exclude infection. Currently no molecular methods are available in the United States for diagnosis of human dirofilariasis.

Therapy

As previously noted, excision of the granuloma or adult worm is typically sufficient, and additional treatment is not needed.

ⓔ Visit the Evolve site for a complete list of procedures, review questions, and case studies.

Bibliography

Baheti NN, Sreedharan M, Krishnamoorthy T, et al.: Eosinophilic meningitis and an ocular worm in a patient from Kerala, south India, *J Neurol Neurosurg Psychiatry* 79(3):271, 2008.

Bennett J, Dolin R, Blaser M: *Principles and practice of infectious diseases*, ed 9, Philadelphia, 2020, Elsevier-Saunders.

Bussaratid V, Dekumyoy P, Desakorn V, et al.: Predictive factors for *Gnathostoma* seropositivity in patients visiting the Gnathostomiasis Clinic at the Hospital for Tropical Diseases, Thailand during 2000-2005, *Southeast Asian J Trop Med Public Health* 41(6):1316–1321, 2010.

Carroll KC, Pfaller MA, Landry ML, et al.: *Manual of clinical microbiology*, ed 12, Washington, DC, 2019, ASM.

Chen J, Liu Q, Liu GH, et al.: Toxocariasis: a silent threat with a progressive public health impact, *Infect Dis Poverty* 7(1):59, 2018.

Fuller AJ, Munckhof W, Kiers L, et al.: Eosinophilic meningitis due to *Angiostrongylus cantonensis*, *West J Med* 159(1):78–80, 1993.

Gamble HR, Pozio E, Bruschi F, et al.: International Commission on Trichinellosis: recommendations on the use of serological tests for the detection of *Trichinella* infection in animals and man, *Parasite* 11(1):3–13, 2004.

Garcia LS: *Diagnostic medical parasitology*, ed 6, Washington, DC, 2016, ASM Press.

Gottstein B, Pozio E, Nöckler K: Epidemiology, diagnosis, treatment, and control of trichinellosis, *Clin Microbiol Rev* 22(1):127–145, 2009.

Hombu A, Yoshida A, Kikuchi T, et al.: Treatment of larva migrans syndrome with long-term administration of albendazole, *J Microbiol Immunol Infect* 52(1):100–105, 2019.

Intapan PM, Khotsri P, Kanpittaya J, et al.: Immunoblot diagnostic test for neurognathostomiasis, *Am J Trop Med Hyg* 83(4):927–929, 2010.

Leung AK, Barankin B, Hon KLE: Cutaneous larva migrans, *Recent Pat Inflamm Allergy Drug Discov* 11(1):2–11, 2017.

Li CD, Yang HL, Wang Y: *Capillaria hepatica* in China, *World J Gastroenterol* 16(6):698–702, 2010.

Miller CL, Kinsella JM, Garner MM, et al.: Endemic infections of *Parastrongylus (Angiostrongylus) costaricensis* in two species of non-human primates, raccoons, and an opossum from Miami, Florida, *J Parasitol* 92(2):406–408, 2006.

Ogdee JL, Henke SE, Wester DB, et al.: Assessing potential environmental contamination by *Baylisascaris procyonis* eggs from infected raccoons in Southern Texas, *Vector Borne Zoonotic Dis* 17(3):185–189, 2017.

Pradeep RK, Nimisha M, Pakideery V, et al.: Whether *Dirofilaria repens* parasites from South India belong to zoonotic Candidatus *Dirofilaria hongkongensis (Dirofilaria sp. hongkongensis)*? *Infect Genet Evol* 67:121–125, 2019.

Schuster A, Lesshafft H, Talhari S, et al.: Life quality impairment caused by hookworm-related cutaneous larva migrans in resource-poor communities in Manaus, Brazil, *PLoS Negl Trop Dis* 5(11):e1355, 2011.

Simón F, Siles-Lucas M, Morchón R, et al.: Human and animal dirofilariasis: the emergence of a zoonotic mosaic, *Clin Microbiol Rev* 25(3):507–544, 2012.

Veraldi S, Angileri L, Parducci BA, et al.: Treatment of hookworm-related cutaneous larva migrans with topical ivermectin, *J Dermatolog Treat* 3:263, 2017.

Winkler S, Pollreisz A, Georgopoulos M, et al.: Candidatus *Dirofilaria hongkongensis* as causative agent of human ocular filariosis after travel to India, *Emerg Infect Dis* 23(8):1428–1431, 2017.

Wu Z, Nagano I, Pozio E, et al.: The detection of *Trichinella* with polymerase chain reaction (PCR) primers constructed using sequences of random amplified polymorphic DNA (RAPD) or sequences of complementary DNA coding excretory-secretory (E-S) glycoproteins, *Parasitology* 117(Pt 2):173–183, 1998.

Wu Z, Nagano I, Pozio E, et al.: Polymerase chain reaction-restriction fragment length polymorphism (PCR-RFLLP) for the identification of *Trichinella* isolates, *Parasitology* 118(Pt 2):211–218, 1999.

52

Blood and Tissue Filarial Nematodes

OBJECTIVES

1. Describe the distinguishing morphologic characteristics and basic life cycle (vectors, hosts, and stages of infectivity) for each of the parasites listed.
2. Define *microfilariae, hydrocele, chyluria,* and *sheath.*
3. Describe the diseases and mechanism of pathogenicity, including route of transmission, for each of the species listed.
4. Explain periodicity, including nocturnal and diurnal, as it relates to infection with microfilariae and correlate it with the life cycle of the associated arthropod vector.
5. Differentiate the microfilariae based on the presence or absence of a sheath and the arrangement and number of tail nuclei.
6. Describe the two methods of concentrating blood specimens for the identification of organisms within the peripheral blood.
7. Determine the cause of infection based on patient history, signs and symptoms, and laboratory results.

PARASITES TO BE CONSIDERED NEMATODES

Blood and Tissues (Filarial Worms)

Brugia beaveri
Brugia leporis
Brugia malayi
Brugia pahangi
Brugia timori
Dirofilaria spp.
Loa loa
Mansonella ozzardi
Mansonella perstans
Mansonella streptocerca
Onchocerca volvulus
Wuchereria bancrofti

Blood and tissue filarial nematodes are roundworms that infect humans. These organisms are transmitted via a blood-sucking arthropod vector such as a mosquito, midge, or fly. The filarial nematodes infect the subcutaneous tissues, deep connective tissues, body cavities, and lymphatic system. The life cycles of the filarial nematodes are complex (Fig. 52.1). The infective larval stage resides in the insect vector, and the adult worm stage, which is the pathogenic form, resides in humans. When the arthropod vector feeds on a human blood meal, the infective larvae are injected into the bloodstream. The larvae are motile and migrate to the lymphatic vessels. The infective larvae grow and develop into the adult gravid worm in the human host over a period of months. The male and female adult worms mate in the definitive human host. The female worm produces large numbers of larvae called **microfilariae.** Depending on the species, the microfilariae may maintain the egg membrane as a **sheath** or may rupture the egg membrane, resulting in an unsheathed form. These parasites can reside in the host for many years and cause chronic, debilitating conditions and severe inflammatory responses. Identification of the various species is based on the morphology of the microfilaria, the defined circadian rhythm, and the location within the human host. The morphologic characteristics of the microfilariae are important in the identification process and include the presence or absence of the sheath and the presence and arrangement of the nuclei in the worm's tail (Fig. 52.2). A comparison of the morphologic characteristics of the pathogenic filarial worms is depicted in Fig. 52.3. Diagnosis of infection is based on the identification of the microfilariae in the host's blood or tissues.

Wuchereria bancrofti

General Characteristics

Wuchereria bancrofti is transmitted via a mosquito, the *Culex fatigans, Anopheles,* or *Aedes* spp. The adult worm, or microfilaria, has a sheath that stains faintly or not at all. It may grow to approximately 298 μm long and 7.5 to 10 μm wide. The tail is pointed and no nuclei are present (Fig. 52.4).

Epidemiology

W. bancrofti is the most commonly identified species of filarial worms that infect humans. It is widely distributed in the tropics and subtropics, including Africa, South America, Asia, the Pacific Islands, and the Caribbean. The mosquito vectors have complex life cycles that include laying eggs and developing larvae on the surface of a water source. When

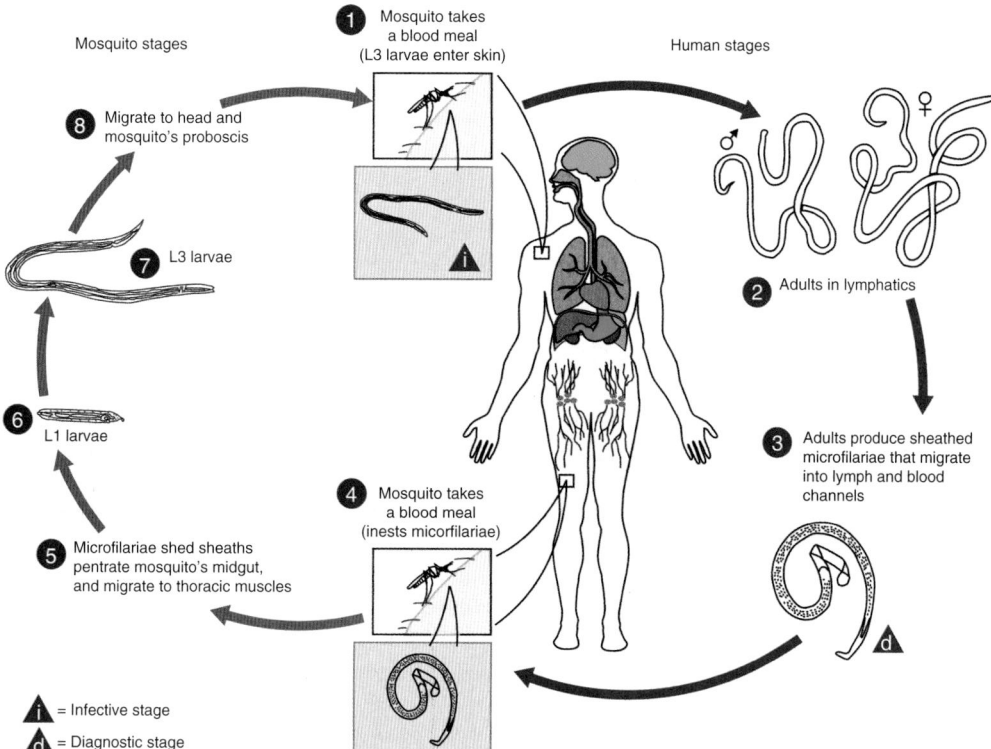

• **Fig. 52.1** Life cycle of *Wucheria bancrofti*. (Courtesy Division of Parasitic Diseases/Centers for Disease Control and Prevention.)

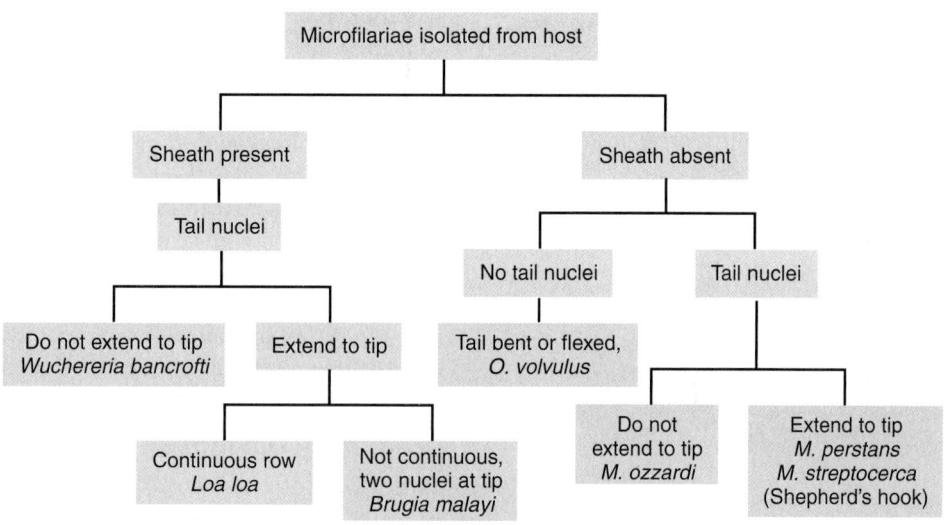

• **Fig. 52.2** Identification of microfilariae.

the larvae mature into adult mosquitos, the males and females will swarm in the evening and mate. The female requires a blood meal to reproduce. The mosquito becomes the intermediate host for the microfilarial parasite. Humans are the definitive host and the reservoir for *W. bancrofti*. The parasite has two forms that demonstrate different periodicities. The nocturnal periodic form is found in the peripheral blood during the night between 10 p.m. and 4 a.m. The second form is found only in the Pacific Islands and is present in the blood at all times, but more frequently during the day in the afternoon hours.

Pathogenesis and Spectrum of Disease

Microfilarial clinical disease varies geographically based on the species of nematode causing the infection. The disease

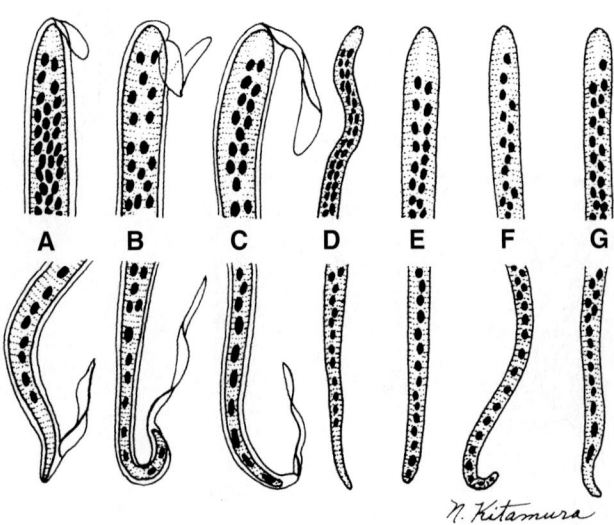

• **Fig. 52.3** Anterior and posterior ends of microfilariae found in humans. (A) *Wuchereria bancrofti.* (B) *Brugia malayi.* (C) *Loa loa.* (D) *Onchocerca volvulus.* (E) *Mansonella perstans.* (F) *Mansonella strepto-cerca.* (G) *Mansonella ozzardi.*

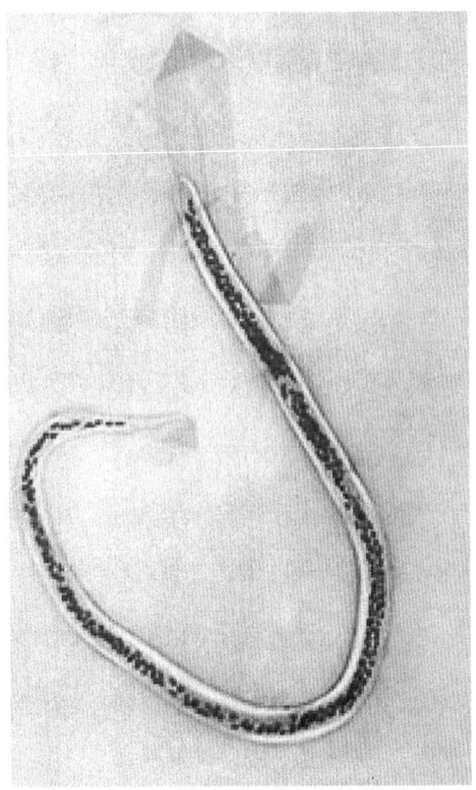

• **Fig. 52.4** Microfilaria of *Wuchereria bancrofti* in thick blood film.

may present as acute or asymptomatic for many years. *W. bancrofti* causes **bancroftian filariasis** and **elephantiasis.** The adult worm resides in the lymphatic vessels distal to the lymph nodes. The presence of organisms within the host results in an immunologic response including inflammation, lymphedema, and hyperplasia. Lymphedema most often occurs in the lower extremities. Elephantiasis is a crippling condition that results from extended periods of filarial

infection. Obstruction of the lymphatic vessels causes fibrosis and a proliferation of dermal and connective tissue, resulting in the wrinkled, dry appearance of an "elephant" extremity. Lymphedema may also occur in the arms, female breasts, and scrotum of infected individuals.

Acute lymphatic filariasis results from worms residing within the lymph nodes. The lymph nodes swell, and lymphangitis may appear peripherally from the infected node. A **hydrocele**—a fluid-filled sac within the scrotum—may form when adult worms block the retroperitoneal or subdiaphragmatic lymphatic vessels. Obstruction of the lymphatic vessels may result in a condition referred to as **chyluria,** which is a result of lymphatic rupture and fluid entering the urine. The urine will appear milky white. Resulting infection and changes in the skin may lead to increased bacterial infections.

Patients residing in tropical regions where filarial parasites are endemic may present with a syndrome referred to as **tropical pulmonary eosinophilia (TPE).** The microfilariae migrate through the pulmonary blood vessels to the lungs, causing an allergic hypersensitivity in the host. The patients develop a strong immune response to the presence of the parasites with an elevated serum immunoglobulin E (IgE) level. Symptoms of TPE include weight loss, low-grade fever, cough and wheezing at night, and lymphadenopathy. Without treatment, patients may develop chronic and progressive respiratory complications leading to death.

Endosymbiont

W. bancrofti, *Brugia* spp., and *Onchocerca volvulus* harbor *Wolbachia* sp., an endosymbiotic alpha-proteobacterium. *Wolbachia* is an obligate intracellular organism.

The parasites require the endosymbiont for larval development, viability, and fertility. The bacteria have been implicated in the pathogenesis of the infection with filarial parasites. The bacterial antigens enhance the host's inflammatory response, leading to increased scarring and damage within the host's lymphatic system. The bacterium is sensitive to tetracycline, doxycycline, azithromycin, and rifampin. Combination antibiotic treatment in conjunction with treatment for the parasite infection improves clearance of the filarial parasite.

Laboratory Diagnosis
Direct Detection

Definitive laboratory diagnosis is based on identification of the parasites in blood, fluids, or tissue. Blood samples should be drawn in accordance with the periodicity of the infection to optimize the likelihood of isolating the infecting organism. Direct examination of blood, urine, hydrocele fluid, or chyle may serve to identify the parasite. The fluid is placed on a slide and air-dried to prevent distortion of the parasite. The specimen should be stained with Giemsa, Wright, or hematoxylin stain and examined microscopically. Ultrasound may be used to visualize the organisms within the tissues.

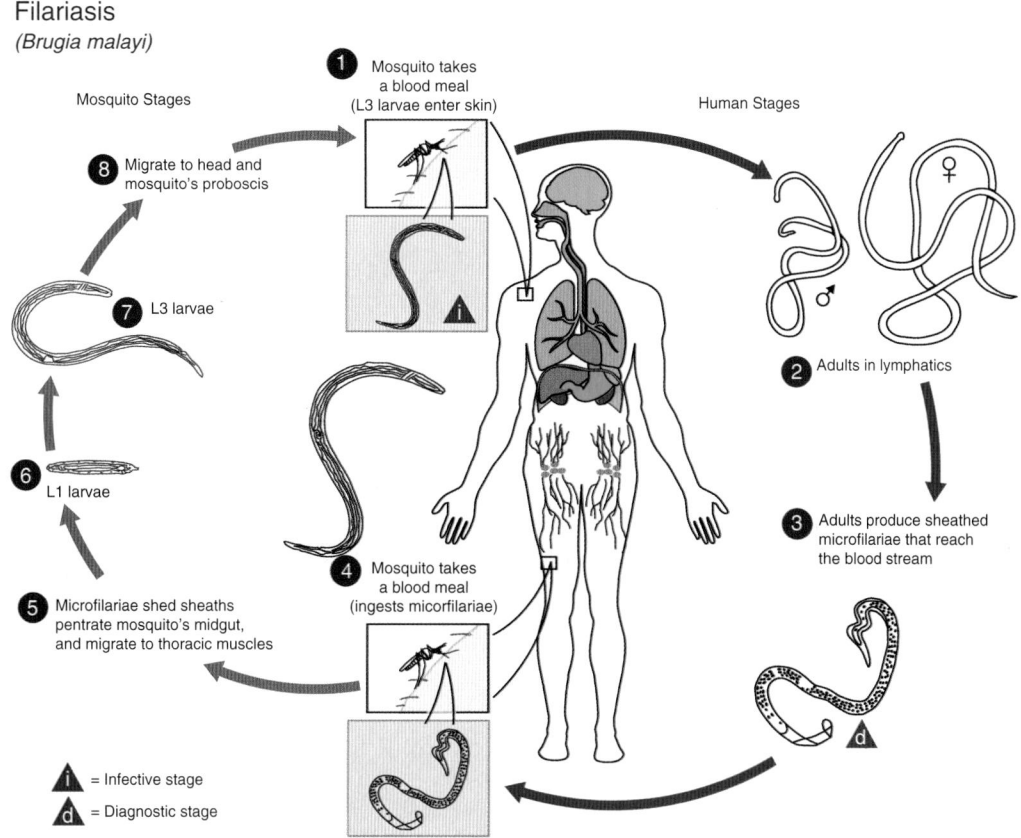

Filariasis
(Brugia malayi)

Mosquito Stages

Human Stages

1 Mosquito takes a blood meal (L3 larvae enter skin)

8 Migrate to head and mosquito's proboscis

7 L3 larvae

6 L1 larvae

5 Microfilariae shed sheaths pentrate mosquito's midgut, and migrate to thoracic muscles

4 Mosquito takes a blood meal (ingests micorfilariae)

2 Adults in lymphatics

3 Adults produce sheathed microfilariae that reach the blood stream

⚠ = Infective stage

d = Diagnostic stage

• **Fig. 52.5** Life cycle of *Brugia* spp. (Courtesy Division of Parasitic Diseases/Centers for Disease Control and Prevention.)

Nucleopore filtration or the **Knott concentration** may be used to increase the likelihood of isolating a filarial parasite from blood. The blood is passed through a polycarbonate filter that contains a 2-μm pore. Distilled water is passed through the filter, lysing the red blood cells and improving visualization of the parasites. The filter is air-dried, stained with Wright or Giemsa, and examined for the presence of microfilaria. The Knott concentration uses centrifugation to concentrate the organisms onto a slide. One milliliter of anticoagulated blood is placed in 9 mL of 2% formalin and centrifuged at 1500 rpm for 1 minute; the sediment is applied to a microscope slide. The slide is stained and examined microscopically. With high-frequency ultrasound, adult worms can sometimes be visualized moving within the lymphatics.

Serologic Testing

Serologic assays that measure antibody response have limited utility in the diagnosis of infections with microfilariae. The antibodies tend to demonstrate a high cross reactivity with other antibodies made in response to a wide variety of parasitic worm infections. The absence of an antibody reaction indicates the lack of infection by a microfilarial species. Laboratory detection of *W. bancrofti*–circulating antigens has demonstrated high specificity (>97%) and sensitivity (from 70% to 80%) in detecting parasitic

infections. The commercial testing formats available are not approved by the US Food and Drug Administration (FDA).

Antigen Detection

A variety of rapid antigen tests are capable of detecting circulating antigens of *W. bancrofti* from whole blood, serum, or plasma. These tests can be used on blood drawn at any time, thus avoiding the need for specimen collection that depends on the periodicity of the microfilariae. Two rapid-format immunochromatographic tests have been shown to be useful and sensitive for the detection of *W. bancrofti* and are being used widely by lymphatic filariasis elimination programs.

Nucleic Acid Detection

Nucleic acid–based methods have been shown to be the most sensitive diagnostic tests for definitive diagnosis of infection with microfilariae. A variety of formats have been developed, including DNA hybridization, polymerase chain reaction (PCR), multiplex PCR, restriction length polymorphism (RFLP), quantitative PCR, and a PCR enzyme-linked immunosorbent assay. These methods can discriminate past and current infection and can be used to monitor therapy. PCR amplification is available in reference laboratories for the rapid diagnosis of an infection with blood microfilariae including *W. bancrofti* and *Brugia* spp. Multiplex PCR-RFLP can differentiate *W. bancrofti, Dirofilaria imminitis, Dirofilaria repens, Brugia pahangi,* and *Brugia malayi* in blood. *B. pahangi* is a common parasite of dogs and cats in Malaysia and has been implicated in human infections. A loop-mediated isothermal application assay has also been developed that may be useful in the field or as a point-of-care diagnostic test. These tests are not currently commercially available.

Brugia malayi and *Brugia timori*

General Characteristics

The *Brugia* spp. are lymphatic filarial parasites resembling *W. bancrofti.* The adult parasites, microfilariae, vary in size (*Brugia timori*, 310 µm long and 5 to 6 µm wide; *Brugia malayi*, 177 to 230 µm long and 5 to 6 µm wide), have a different geographic distribution, and do not typically cause lymphadenitis in the genital regions.

Epidemiology

The *Brugia* spp. are distributed throughout the Far East including China, Indonesia, Korea, Malaysia, Japan, India, and the Philippines. The distribution of *B. timori* is limited to the two islands of Timor, an island of Indonesia. The organism is transmitted via mosquitos included in the genus *Anopheles* and *Mansonia.*

Pathogenesis and Spectrum of Disease

As in infections with *W. bancrofti,* two periodic forms exist. The nocturnal form is the most common and is located near areas of coastal rice fields, whereas the nonperiodic form is associated with infections in areas near swampy forests. The pathogenesis and spectrum of disease is essentially the same as for *W. bancrofti,* with the exception that involvement of the genital lymphatic vessels is predominantly associated with *W. bancrofti.* Urogenital involvement with chyluria does not occur in infections with *Brugia* spp. Clinical disease progresses faster after infection with *B. malayi* than with *W. bancrofti.* Microfilariae may appear in the blood in as little as 3 to 4 months.

Brugia spp. have been implicated in zoonotic infections of dogs, cats, rabbits, and raccoons worldwide. Mosquitos transmit the infection by feeding on an infected animal and then a human host in approximately 2 weeks. Cases of human infection have occurred in the United States in the northeastern region with *B. beaveri. B. beaveri* infect raccoons, bobcats, or mink and *B. leporis* infects rabbit. Clinical disease is typically asymptomatic but may present with a tender region in the cervical, axillary, or inguinal region. The lymphatic mass may contain either a live or a dead worm. If the worm is no longer viable, the mass may be surrounded by a granulomatous reaction.

Laboratory Diagnosis

Definitive diagnosis is generally by identification of microfilariae in the blood of infected individuals. The microfilariae can be distinguished from *W. bancrofti* morphologically. The *B. malayi* microfilariae are sheathed and contain four to five subterminal and two terminal nuclei in the tail. *B. timori* also contains five to eight subterminal and terminal nuclei in the tail, but they are much larger than *B. malayi.* The *B. malayi* sheath will stain bright pink with Giemsa, whereas the *B. timori* sheath does not stain. The microfilariae of *B. timori* tend to be somewhat longer. High-frequency ultrasound has been useful in identifying adult worms in various locations within the patient, such as lymphatic vessels of the legs, inguinal area (groin or lower abdomen), lymph nodes, and female breasts. Nucleic acid–based methods have been developed as previously indicated in the diagnosis of *W. bancrofti* and can differentiate microfilariae.

Therapy

Diethylcarbamazine (DEC) is the treatment of choice for lymphatic filarial parasites including *W. bancrofti* and *Brugia* spp. Additionally, ivermectin and albendazole may be used. Death of the microfilarial worms may result in an increased hypersensitivity reaction requiring the need for treatment with antihistamines to limit the inflammatory symptoms.

Prevention

The use of insect repellent is recommended for travelers in areas where the parasites are endemic. DEC has also been used for prophylactic treatment before travel. Vector control studies in combination with mass drug administration of DEC and ivermectin have successfully decreased the population of the arthropod (insect) vectors and decreased filarial infection in the human hosts.

Loa loa

General Characteristics

Loa loa, commonly referred to as the eye worm, is a microfilaria that circulates in the bloodstream with a diurnal periodicity that peaks in the afternoon between 12:00 p.m. and 2:00 p.m. and resides in the subcutaneous tissue in the human host. The microfilariae may grow up to 300 µm.

Epidemiology

The parasite is found within the rain forests of West and Central Africa. The organism is transmitted through a bite of the tabanid fly or deer fly of the genus *Chrysops.* The female lays her eggs on the leaves of small plants near the water. The larvae feed on small insects and develop in wet soil. The male fly feeds on pollen, and the female feeds on blood.

Pathogenesis and Spectrum of Disease

The organism is often associated with asymptomatic infection. The larvae develop into adult worms in approximately 6 to 12 months but can persist in the human host for up to 17 years. The infection is typically identified when the adult worm is seen migrating within the subconjunctiva of the host. Symptoms associated with infection include episodic **calabar swellings,** which are localized areas of transient angioedema in response to the production of parasitic metabolic products. Predominant swelling on the extremities with inflammation of nearby joints and peripheral nerves may occur. Immune-mediated encephalopathy, nephropathy, and cardiomyopathy may occur.

Laboratory Diagnosis

Infections with *Loa loa* may be asymptomatic for many years before the appearance of microfilariae in the peripheral blood. Therefore patient diagnosis is often made based on the patient's clinical symptoms, including calabar swelling, eosinophilia, and travel or residency in an endemic area.

Direct Detection

Definitive diagnosis is made by identification of adult worms in the eye or in tissue or by identification of microfilariae in the peripheral blood. Microfilariae have a sheath that does not stain with Giemsa. The adult females are larger than the adult males, and the nuclei extend to the tail in an irregularly arranged fashion.

Serologic Testing

As with other filarial infections, serologic assays have limited use for diagnosis. A *Loa*-specific recombinant protein (LLSXP-1) has been used in the development of an enzyme-linked immunosorbent assay (ELISA) and has demonstrated improved specificity but limited sensitivity. A rapid detection test for LLSXP-1 IgG has been developed that demonstrates a sensitivity greater than 90% and a specificity of approximately 95%. Detection of IgG may be useful in confirming the diagnosis in travelers to areas of endemicity in the presence of unexplained eosinophilia and appropriate clinical symptoms.

Nucleic Acid Detection

PCR-based techniques have been developed for the detection of *Loa loa*, with specificities and sensitivities as high as 100% and 95%, respectively. However, these techniques yield negative results during prepatency, the period between initial infection and detectability in the host. These tests also demonstrate false-positive results in individuals with previous *L. loa* infections, as they also detect DNA from dead microfilariae in blood. Real-time qPCR assays have also been developed with high species specificity and sensitivity (96%) for

L. loa. These have been adapted to loop-mediated isothermal amplification (LAMP), allowing the potential for point-of-care and in-field use. A single PCR assay test for loiasis has been approved for diagnostic use in the United States.

Therapy

DEC is the treatment of choice. In heavy infections, inflammation and allergic reactions may occur, requiring the administration of antiinflammatory medications. Allergic responses can result in central nervous system damage, encephalitis, coma, and death.

Prevention

Prophylactic treatment with DEC has been used to prevent infection.

Onchocerca volvulus

General Characteristics

Onchocerca volvulus predominantly resides in tissue nodules within the host. Microfilariae measure approximately 300 μm long by 5 to 9 μm wide.

Epidemiology

O. volvulus is found throughout Africa, Central America, and South America. The parasite is transmitted by the black fly, *Simulium* spp. The black fly lays its eggs in running water where the larvae attach to rocks. The larvae feed on algae and bacteria. The adults emerge as a flying insect. The females require a blood meal, whereas the males are nectar feeders. The flies feed predominantly during the day.

Pathogenesis and Spectrum of Disease

Onchocerciasis, commonly referred to as river blindness, is a result of subcutaneous infection with the parasite. The infections are typically localized to the skin, lymph nodes, and eyes. Skin infections result in pruritus, edema, and erythema. Hypopigmentation or hyperpigmentation can occur after a lengthy infection. Nodules containing the adult worms vary in size and are firm and tender. Lymphadenopathy may be found in the inguinal or femoral regions. Enlargement of the lymph node may result in a condition referred to as "hanging groin," which may develop into a hernia. Onchocercal eye disease may be seen in moderate to heavy infections. Infections of the eye may lead to serious damage and blindness. Mortality increases among adults who experience blindness and systemic infection.

Laboratory Diagnosis
Direct Detection

Definitive diagnosis is made from the identification of the microfilariae from tissue such as in a nodule or skin snip.

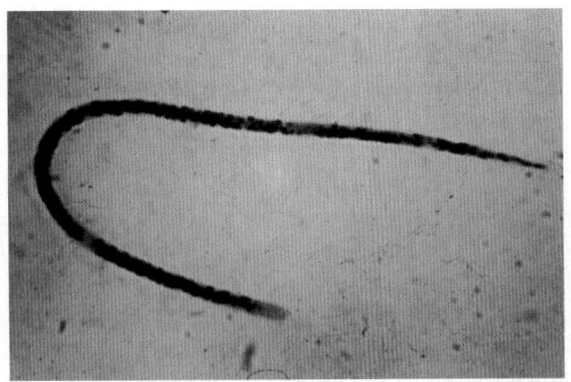

• **Fig. 52.6** Microfilaria of *Onchocerca volvulus*. (Courtesy Dr. Henry Travers, Sioux Falls, SD.)

Skin samples are placed in physiologic buffered saline for up to 24 hours. After incubation, the microfilariae will emerge from the tissue and can be visualized microscopically. Occasionally the microfilariae may be found in blood or urine after treatment. Microfilariae may also be visible in the cornea and the anterior chamber of the eye.

The microfilariae lack a sheath. The tail is tapered, appears bent or flexed, and does not include extension of nuclei to the tip (Fig. 52.6).

Serologic Testing

Although serologic tests generally lack specificity, recombinant ELISAs using multiple antigens have demonstrated increased sensitivity and specificity for the diagnosis of onchocerciasis. A rapid test, the SD Bioline Onchocerciasis, for the detection of an *O. volvulus* antigen known as OV-16, is commercially available. The test is used predominantly for surveillance and elimination of infection but may also be used for the diagnostic confirmation of infection.

Nucleic Acid Detection

PCR amplification assays using material from skin snips or skin scratches provides high sensitivity and specificity; these have been developed, but the limited availability of technical expertise as well as the high cost of the test restrict its use in resource-limited settings and to research laboratories.

Therapy

Ivermectin is the recommended treatment and is effective against both adult worms and microfilariae. However, in Africa, where *O. volvulus* and *L. loa* are coendemic, ivermectin treatment is often associated with encephalopathy in patients with heavy microfilaria infections. Surgical excision of nodules containing adult worms is recommended when they are located on the head. There is evidence that a 6-week course of doxycycline is useful in targeting the endosymbiotic proteobacteria *Wolbachia* spp. This causes sterility in the female adult worms for extended periods, reducing the infection in the host.

Prevention

Black fly larval control using insecticides in endemic areas has been used to assist in the control of transmission of *O. volvulus*. Community-based administration of ivermectin every 6 to 12 months is also being used to interrupt the transmission of the parasite in endemic areas and has been successful for the elimination of the parasite in Latin America.

Mansonella spp. (*M. ozzardi, M. streptocerca, M. perstans*)

General Characteristics

Mansonella spp. are generally not associated with serious infections. The microfilariae of all species are very similar in size, ranging from approximately 200 to 225 μm long and 4 to 6 μm wide.

Epidemiology

Mansonella spp. are distributed throughout varied geographic regions in Africa and South America. *Mansonella ozzardi* is limited to Central and South America and the Caribbean islands. The parasites are transmitted by biting midges of the genus *Culicoides*. The female requires a blood meal for the maturation of eggs and typically bites in the early evening or morning hours. Transmission of *M. ozzardi* has also been associated with bites from the blackfly (*Simulium amazonicum*).

Pathogenesis and Spectrum of Disease

Mansonella streptocerca is found in the skin; however, most infected individuals appear to be asymptomatic. Patients may present with a pruritic or papular rash and pigmentation changes. In addition, lymphadenitis may occur. *Mansonella perstans* resides in the pericardial, pleural, and peritoneal cavities. The location of the *M. ozzardi* adult worms is unknown. Symptomatic patients present with swelling of the arms, face, or other body parts similar to the calabar swelling identified in infections with *L. loa, M. ozzardi*, or *M. perstans* found in the blood.

M. perstans and *M. ozzardi* do not demonstrate periodicity when circulating within the bloodstream. *M. ozzardi* infections are often asymptomatic and therefore are not well characterized. Some infections with *M. ozzardi* demonstrate headache, joint pain, fever, pulmonary symptoms, adenopathy, hepatomegaly, and pruritus.

Laboratory Diagnosis

Laboratory diagnosis for *M. perstans* and *M. ozzardi* is generally made by identifying the microfilariae in blood or other body fluids. *M. perstans* and *M. streptocerca* can be diagnosed by identifying the microfilariae in skin snips.

Mansonella spp. microfilariae do not possess sheaths. *M. streptocerca* and *M. perstans* tails contain nuclei that extend to the end of the tip. The tail of *M. streptocerca* is often referred to as a shepherd's crook. *M. ozzardi* organisms have tails with nuclei that do not extend to the tip.

Nucleic Acid Detection

A few studies have evaluated the use of PCR for the detection of *Mansonella* spp. from venous and capillary blood samples. The tests appear to be more sensitive and specific than microscopy. Currently there are no commercially available nucleic acid tests for *Mansonella* spp.

Therapy

Ivermectin is effective in the treatment of *M. ozzardi* infections. DEC is effective in treating both the adult and microfilarial forms of *M. streptocerca*. Treatment of *M. perstans* infections has not been effective in most cases. However, because of infection with the endosymbiotic bacteria, *Wolbachia* spp., treatment with doxycycline has demonstrated some limited success.

Prevention

Prevention relies on the use of insect repellents and adequate clothing.

Dirofilaria spp. (*D. immitis, D. repens, D. tenuis*)

General Characteristics

Filarial nematodes of the genus *Dirofilaria* cause dirofilariasis. There are many species of *Dirofilaria*, but human infection is most commonly associated with three species, *D. immitis, D. repens,* and *D. tenuis*. Female adult worms grow up to 10 to 12 in in length, whereas males are 4 to 6 in long and have spirally coiled tails. Microfilariae are white, long, and threadlike.

Epidemiology

The definitive natural hosts for these three species are dogs and wild canids, such as foxes and wolves (*D. immitis* and *D. repens*) and raccoons (*D. tenuis*). *D. immitis* is also known as heartworm and is the cause of human dirofilariasis in the eastern and southeastern United States. *D. repens* is the leading cause of human dirofilariasis in Europe and is found in Africa and Asia. *D. tenuis* is found in raccoons in the United States. The adult worms produce microfilariae within the definitive animal host; these circulate in the blood and are ingested by mosquitoes during a blood meal. In mosquitoes, the microfilariae develop into larvae that migrate to the proboscis (the long tubular part of the mosquito's mouth). During a blood meal, the larvae are released into the skin of the human host. The worms are unable to reach maturity in the human host, therefore no microfilariae are detectable. Occasionally larvae will migrate to the pulmonary vessels. Several types of mosquitoes are capable of transmitting *Dirofilaria* infection, including *Aedes, Anopheles,* and *Mansonia*.

Pathogenesis and Spectrum of Disease

Humans and a wide range of other mammals are accidental hosts that play no role in the transmission of *Dirofilaria*. In these hosts, *Dirofilaria* larvae can develop into adult worms but the worms remain sexually immature and no microfilariae are produced.

The number of human dirofilariasis cases reported has increased dramatically in recent years. The worms produce an inconspicuous granulomatous reaction in the subcutaneous tissue, resulting in the formation of a nodule, or they may migrate to the lung, causing human dirofilariasis. Pulmonary infections are usually asymptomatic but may cause chest pain, cough, fever, and pleural effusion. If the worm lodges in the pulmonary artery, an infarct may occur. Eye infections with *Dirofilaria* have been identified in North America, Europe, Australia, Africa, Asia, and the Middle East. These infections present with moderate to severe inflammation, blurred vision, and swelling of the eyes. All *Dirofilaria* examined have contained the *Wolbachia* endosymbiont.

Rarely, *D. immitis* worms have been identified in the brains and testicles of humans.

Laboratory Diagnosis

Dirofilariasis is diagnosed most frequently by the examination of inflammatory lung tissue or skin nodules. The worm's cuticle contains chitin, which can be visualized in tissue sections by staining with calcofluor white.

Therapy

The only method of treatment of human dirofilariasis is surgical removal of the lesion or extraction of the worm. Extraction is not essential, however, as the worms die and are often cleared or sequestered in granulomata without treatment.

Prevention

Routine methods for avoiding mosquito vectors will help to prevent infection.

ⓔ Visit the Evolve site for a complete list of procedures, review questions, and case studies.

Bibliography

Abbas KF, El-Monem SG, Malik Z, et al.: Surgery still opens an unexpected bag of worms! An intraperitoneal live female *Dirofilaria* worm: case report and review of the literature, *Surg Infect*(3)323–325, 2006.

Bennett J, Dolin R, Blaser M: *Principles and practice of infectious diseases*, ed 9, Philadelphia, 2020, Elsevier-Saunders.

Boatin BA, Toé L, Alley ES, et al.: Diagnostics in onchocerciasis: future challenges, *Ann Trop Med Parasitol* 92(suppl 1):S41–S45, 1998.

Boussinesq M: Loiasis, *Ann Trop Med Parasitol* 100(8):715–731, 2006.

Carroll KC, Pfaller MA, Landry ML, et al.: *Manual of clinical microbiology*, ed 12, Washington, DC, 2019, ASM.

Drame PM, Fink DL, Kamgno J, Herrick JA, Nutman TB: Loop-mediated isothermal amplification for rapid and semiquantitative detection of *Loa Loa* infection, *J Clin Microbiol* 52(6):2071–2077, 2014.

Ettinger S, Feldman E: *Textbook of veterinary internal medicine*, ed 7, St Louis, 2010, Saunders.

Fischer P, Wibowo H, Pischke S, et al.: PCR-based detection and identification of the filarial parasite *Brugia timori* from Alor Island, Indonesia, *Ann Trop Med Parasitol* 96:809–821, 2002.

Garcia LS: *Diagnostic medical parasitology*, ed 6, Washington, DC, 2016, ASM Press.

Hamlin KL, Moss DM, Priest JW, et al.: Longitudinal monitoring of the development of antifilarial antibodies and acquisition of *Wuchereria bancrofti* in a highly endemic area of Haiti, *PLoS Negl Trop Dis* 6(12):e1941, 2012, https://doi.org/10.1371/journal.pntd.0001941.

Johnstone C: Heartworm. In *Parasites and parasitic diseases of domestic animals*, Philadelphia, 1998, University of Pennsylvania.

Medeiros JF, Pires Almeida TA, Tavares Silva LB, et al.: A field trial of a PCR-based *Mansonella ozzardi* diagnosis assay detects high-levels of submicroscopic *M. ozzardi* infections in both venous blood samples and FTA card dried blood spots, *Parasit Vectors* 8:280, 2015.

Mishra K, Raj DK, Hazra RK, et al.: The development and evaluation of a single step multiplex PCR method for simultaneous detection of *Brugia malayi* and *Wuchereria bancrofti*, *Mol Cell Probes* 21:355–362, 2007.

Nolan TJ: *Dirofilaria immitis*, Philadelphia, 2004, University of Pennsylvania.

Pani SP, Hoti SL, Elango A, et al.: Evaluation of the ICT whole blood antigen card test to detect infection due to nocturnally periodic *Wuchereria bancrofti* in South India, *Trop Med Int Health* 5:359–363, 2000.

Simón F, López-Belmonte J, Marcos-Atxutegi C, Morchón R, Martín-Pacho JR: What is happening outside North America regarding human dirofilariasis? *Vet Parasitol* 133(2–3):181–189, 2005.

Sunish IP, Rajendran R, Mani TR, et al.: Vector control complements mass drug administration against bancroftian filariasis in Tirukoilur, India, *Bull WHO* 85:138–145, 2007.

Theis JH: Public health aspects of dirofilariasis in the United States, *Vet Parasitol* 133(2–3):157–180, 2004.

Udall DN: Recent updates on onchocerciasis: diagnosis and treatment, *Clin Infect Dis* 44(1):53–60, 2007.

53

Intestinal Cestodes

OBJECTIVES

1. Describe the distinguishing morphologic characteristics, clinical disease, basic life cycle (vectors, hosts, and stages of infectivity), and laboratory diagnosis for the intestinal cestodes included in this chapter.
2. Define and identify (where appropriate) the following parasitic structures: scolex, proglottids, rostellum, hermaphroditic, oncosphere, hexacanth embryo, strobila, bothria, and coracidium.
3. Compare and contrast autoinfection and hyperinfection.
4. List several methods of control and prevention of tapeworm infection.
5. Correlate the life cycles with the specific diagnostic stage(s) for each organism.

PARASITES TO BE CONSIDERED

Intestinal Cestodes (Tapeworms)

Diphyllobothrium latum
Diphyllobothrium nihonkaiense
Diphyllobothrium spp.
Dipylidium caninum
Hymenolepis nana
Hymenolepis diminuta
Taenia asiatica
Taenia crassiceps
Taenia saginata
Taenia solium
Taenia spp.

The intestinal cestodes are commonly referred to as **tapeworms.** Tapeworms have a long, segmented, ribbonlike body with a specialized structure for attachment, or **scolex,** at the anterior end. The adult tapeworm consists of a chain of segments: **proglottids,** which develop posteriorly from the neck region of the scolex forming the body or **strobila.** Proglottids may be classified as immature, mature, or gravid containing the uterus and eggs. The crown of the scolex, the **rostellum,** may be smooth or armed with hooks. The body of the worm (proglottids) varies in the geometric characteristics or number of segments according to the genus and species of the cestode. The mature cestode is **hermaphroditic.** In other words, the organism contains both male and female reproductive organs. Food is absorbed from the host through the worm's **integument,** the outer covering or skin of the organism. Adult worms typically inhabit the small intestine; however, humans may be host to either the adult or the larval forms, depending on the infecting species. Humans infected with a cestode pass the eggs in the feces. The embryo may be visible within the tapeworm egg as an **oncosphere** (larva tapeworm within an embryonic envelope, infective stage) or **hexacanth embryo.** The intermediate host ingests feces containing the adult tapeworm eggs, which further develop into the larva of the cestode. Cestodes generally require one or more intermediate hosts for the completion of their life cycle. Intestinal tapeworm infections are generally asymptomatic. However, if the larval stage develops in human organs outside the intestine, they may cause additional life-threatening complications.

Fresh or preserved stools are the specimens of choice for ova and parasites (O&P) examination and cestode identification. Preserved stool containing adult worms or a string of segments (**strobila**) or the scolex may also be used for diagnosis. Development of serologic testing and molecular assays are more sensitive than stool examination. Although this type of testing may be useful for primary screening, it is most commonly used for confirmation testing for parasitic disease. Chapter 46 describes the methods and specimen requirements in more detail as they relate to parasitology.

Diphyllobothrium latum

General Characteristics

Diphyllobothrium latum, the freshwater broad fish tapeworm, is the largest human tapeworm and the most common species identified within this genus. Adult worms have been known to reach up to 15 m in length, with more than 3000 to 4000 proglottids, and reside within a host for 30 years or more. The proglottids are characteristically wider than long, with a central rosette-shaped uterine structure (Fig. 53.1). The scolex is spatulate and contains two shallow sucking grooves referred to as **bothria** (Fig. 53.2A and B). *Diphyllobothrium* spp. have unembryonated eggs. The eggs are **operculated** (appears as a lid) with a terminal knob, similar to trematode eggs (Fig. 53.2C). The intermediate hosts include crustaceans and freshwater fish.

Epidemiology

Diphyllobothrium is not found in the tropics; it is commonly found worldwide where cool lakes are contaminated

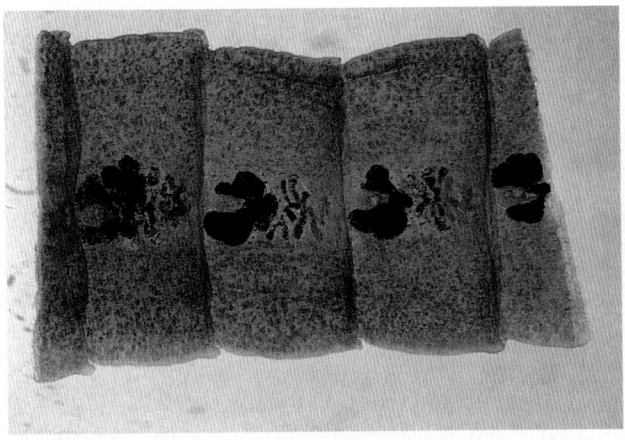

• **Fig. 53.1** Proglottid demonstrating rosette-shaped uterus in *Diphyllobothrium latum.* (Courtesy Division of Parasitic Diseases/ Centers for Disease Control and Prevention.)

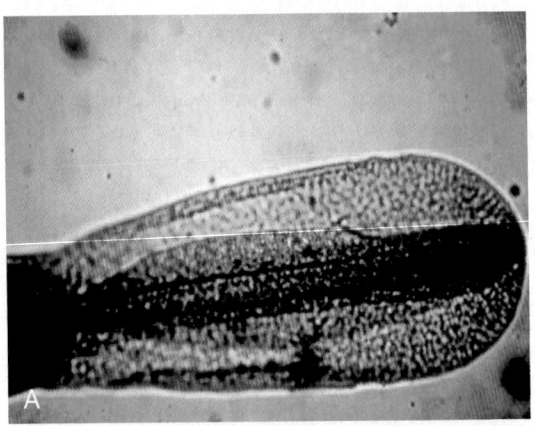

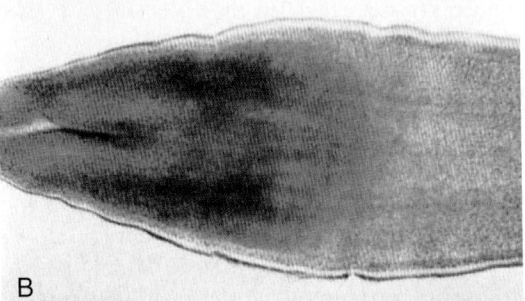

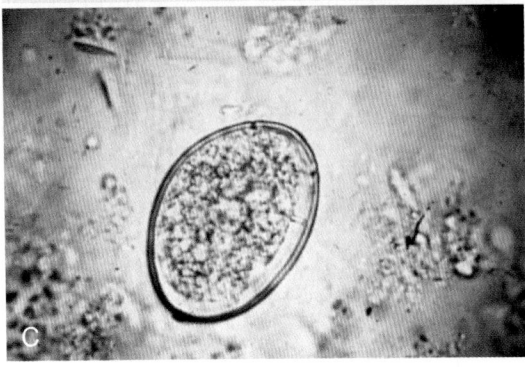

• **Fig. 53.2** (A) *Diphyllobothrium latum* scolex. (B) *D. latum* scolex, bothria visible. (C) *D. latum* ovum. (Courtesy Dr. Henry Travers, Sioux Falls, SD.)

by sewage. *Diphyllobothrium species* can be found wherever freshwater or marine fish are eaten raw, pickled, or marinated. This includes such freshwater fish as burbot, pike, perch, ruff, and salmon. The parasite is found in North America, including the upper Midwest around the Great Lakes, Alaska, and Canada. *D. nihonkaiense*, originally endemic in Japan, is an emerging parasite in other areas of Europe. There are 14 species of *Diphyllobothrium*, all capable of infecting humans. Other species of *Diphyllobothrium* that have been identified in human infection include *D. pacificum* (Southern Pacific coast of South America), *D. cordatum, D. ursi, D. dendriticum* (New Guinea and Australia), *D. lanceolatum, D. dallieae,* and *D. yonagoensis.*

Pathogenesis and Spectrum of Disease

Diphyllobothrium spp. is the only cestode to have an aquatic life cycle (Fig. 53.3). Fish serve as the reservoir host, with humans serving as the definitive host for *D. latum, D. nihonkaiense, D. dendriticum,* and *D. pacificum. D. latum* eggs are found in the feces of infected humans and other fish-eating mammals. Once passed into a water source, such as a lake, the life cycle requires two intermediate hosts. After incubation in freshwater for approximately 2 weeks, the mature eggs release the first larval stage (**coracidium**). The coracidium larva is ciliated and bears six terminal hooks. The coracidium larvae are ingested by copepods. The coracidium larva sheds its epithelium and further develops into a **procercoid** larva (infective form). The fish feed upon the small crustaceans ingesting the procercoid larvae. Within the freshwater fish, the larvae develop into the **plerocercoid** ribbonlike organism with an undivided scolex. The procercoid may pass through multiple paratenic hosts until consumed by a mammal or human. *Diphyllobothrium* infection occurs through the ingestion of infected fish containing the plerocercoid larval form. *Diphyllobothrium latum* and other species mature to an adult tapeworm within the human small intestine. Infection is usually asymptomatic, but mild gastrointestinal symptoms may occur, such as diarrhea, abdominal pain, fatigue, vomiting, or dizziness. Symptoms vary depending on the worm burden and the host's immune response to the organism. The tapeworm nutritional requirements may decrease the host's vitamin B_{12} level, resulting in **pernicious anemia**.

Laboratory Diagnosis

Both eggs and proglottids may be found in the patient's feces. Visualization of the eggs is enhanced using a wet preparation of the patient's stool sample. Diagnosis is made by identification of the ovoid, operculated, yellow-brown eggs (58 to 75 μm × 40 to 50 μm) passed in abundance in the stool. They are sometimes confused with the eggs of *Paragonimus.* The mature gravid proglottids are wider than long (3 mm × 11 mm), often in chains, and contain a rosette-shaped central uterus (Fig. 53.1). *Diphyllobothrium* identification is through assessment of the morphologic characteristics of

Diphyllobothriasis

(Diphyllobothrium spp.)

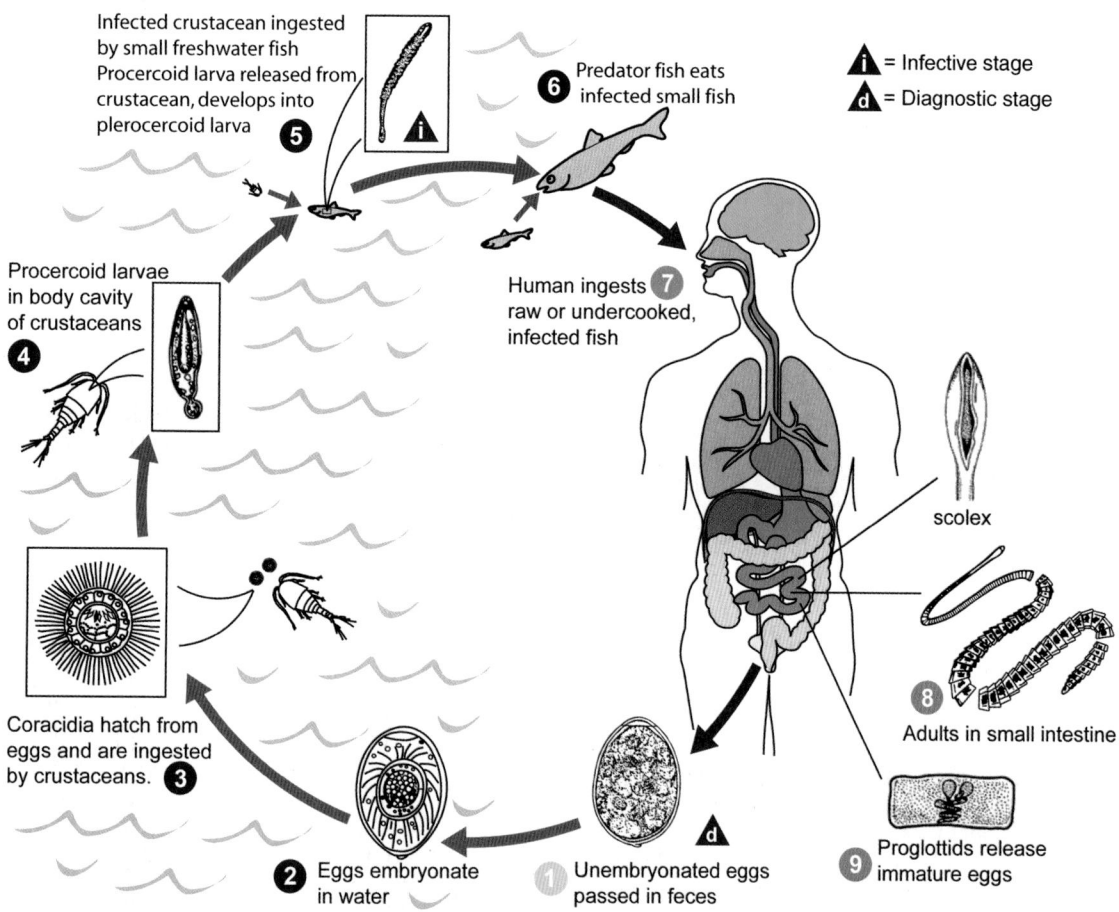

= Infective stage

= Diagnostic stage

Infected crustacean ingested by small freshwater fish Procercoid larva released from crustacean, develops into plerocercoid larva **5**

6 Predator fish eats infected small fish

Procercoid larvae in body cavity of crustaceans **4**

Human ingests **7** raw or undercooked, infected fish

Coracidia hatch from eggs and are ingested by crustaceans. **3**

scolex

8 Adults in small intestine

2 Eggs embryonate in water

1 Unembryonated eggs passed in feces

9 Proglottids release immature eggs

• **Fig. 53.3** Life cycle of *Diphyllobothrium latum*. (Courtesy Division of Parasitic Diseases/Centers for Disease Control and Prevention.)

the proglottids as previously described. Speciation within the genus *Diphyllobothrium* is difficult to impossible using morphological characteristics. Nucleic acid amplification and sequencing is the only reliable tool for speciation. Because all of the species cause similar infections and the therapy is similar, speciation is not necessary for treatment but remains important for epidemiological reasons. Molecular approaches to differential identification of *D. latum* and *D. nihonkaiense* have been successful using restriction fragment length polymorphisms (RFLP) utilizing the ribosomal DNA sequence of the mitochondrial cytochrome c oxidase I (cox1) gene. No serologic tests are available.

Therapy

Humans infected with *Diphyllobothrium* develop little to no protective immunity. Reinfection is common. Treatment with praziquantel or niclosamide is effective and nontoxic. Subsequent stool specimens should be reexamined 6 weeks after treatment. The patient may require a vitamin B_{12} supplement if anemia develops.

Prevention

Prevention simply includes avoiding the consumption of raw fish. The larval stage is destroyed when food is thoroughly cooked at 55°C for 5 minutes or frozen at –20°C for 7 days or flash freezing to –35°C for 15 hours, if the flesh is less than 15 cm thick. Treatment of patients infected with adult tapeworms is indicated to prevent accidental autoinfection. Good hygiene and proper sanitation measures will also prevent reinfection. Treatment of sewage before it enters lakes may help reduce the prevalence of infection.

Dipylidium caninum

General Characteristics

D. caninum, the cat or dog tapeworm (Fig. 53.4), is a double-pored (genital pores) tapeworm consisting of many small proglottids. As the tapeworm matures, the proglottids separate and pass in the stool. They may be recognized based on their characteristic "cucumber seed" appearance when they are wet, as well as their resemblance to a dried grain of rice. Adult tapeworms measure 10 to 70 cm in length. The scolex contains four suckers and an **armed rostellum. Egg packets** may also be found in the feces of the host.

Epidemiology

Infection is common worldwide. In the case of *D. caninum,* human infection is acquired through the accidental

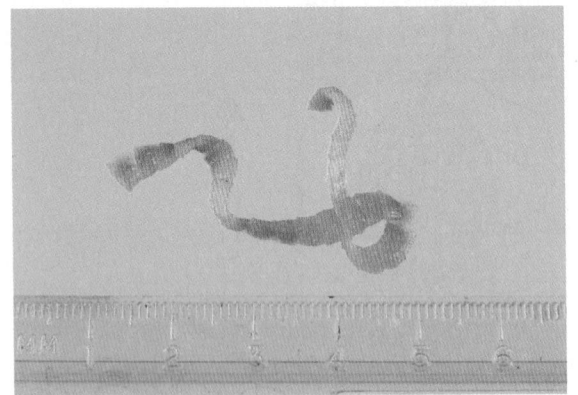

• **Fig. 53.4** *Dipylidium caninum* tapeworm. (Courtesy Dr. Henry Travers, Sioux Falls, SD.)

ingestion of fleas. Infection is most often seen in young children because of close contact with infected pets. The tapeworms are found in both wild and domestic dogs and cats.

Pathogenesis and Spectrum of Disease

Ingestion of an infected flea may result in *D. caninum* infection (Fig. 53.5). The flea is the intermediate host in which infective **cysticercoids** (larval form) develop; humans, dogs and cats are the reservoir hosts. The cysticercoid larval stage is ingested by a dog or cat and develops into cysticercoid **metacestode larvae.** The adult worm develops and matures within the reservoir host. An infected human host will usually pass proglottids in a bowel movement, or they may stick to the skin around the anal area. This may result in misdiagnosis of the infection as *Enterobius vermicularis.* Humans usually have very mild symptoms, such as indigestion, appetite loss, weight loss, perianal itching, persistent diarrhea, and vague abdominal pain. The severity of the disease is dependent on the worm burden. Human infection is usually self-limited.

Laboratory Diagnosis

Symptoms of *Dipylidium* infection are similar to those of pinworm infection; however, the treatments are very

Dipylidium caninum Infection
(*Dipylidium caninum*)

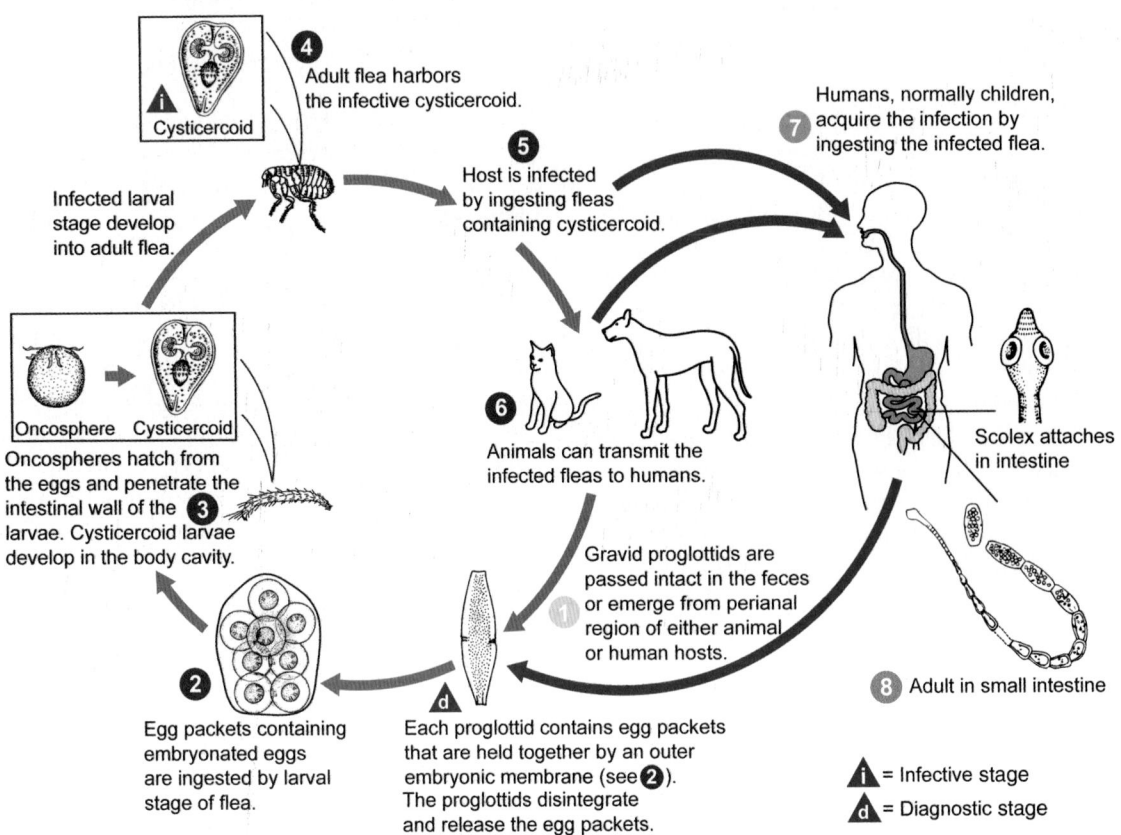

• **Fig. 53.5** Life cycle of *Dipylidium caninum*. (Courtesy Division of Parasitic Diseases/Centers for Disease Control and Prevention.)

different. The laboratory should confirm suspected infections. Proglottids (8 to 23 μm) may be seen in the stool. *D. caninum* is also referred to as the "cucumber seed" tapeworm, as previously described (Fig. 53.6). The first sign of infection may be the appearance of seedlike particles in the stool or undergarments of the patient. These particles are the egg-bearing segments of the tapeworm. Groups of egg packets may be found in the stool (Figs. 53.7E). The adult worms have a scolex with four suckers and a conical/retractile rostellum armed with four to seven rows of small hooklets (Fig. 53.8). Patients may also develop a moderately elevated eosinophilia. Serologic tests are typically performed because of the asymptomatic and self-limiting nature of the infection. Nucleic acid–based testing, testing using RFLP analysis, and hydrolysis probe-based genotyping assays have been developed and validated for genotyping *D. caninum*; currently, however, they are not utilized for clinical diagnostics.

Therapy

Praziquantel and niclosamide are typically effective for treating *D. caninum* infection. The medication causes the tapeworm to dissolve within the intestine. The drugs are generally well tolerated by the patient. Household pets should be treated simultaneously to prevent reinfection.

Prevention

To reduce the risk of infection, flea control of pets in the household will reduce exposure to humans via the intermediate host. Keeping cats indoors will help prevent infection by limiting their exposure to fleas by household cats.

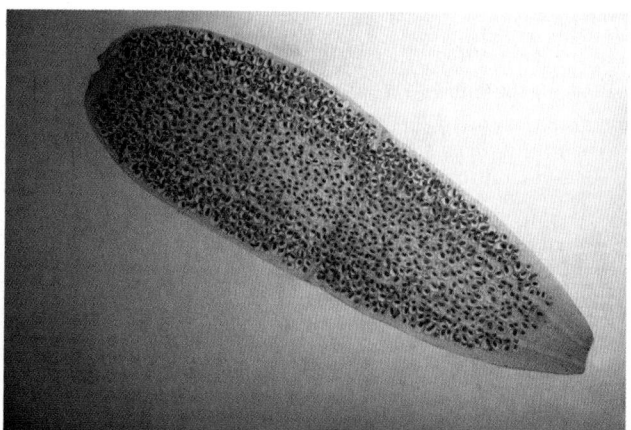

• **Fig. 53.6** This photomicrograph reveals ultrastructural details exhibited by a single *Dipylidium caninum* reproductive proglottid. These *D. caninum* proglottids, which when mature average 12 mm × 3 mm, are pumpkin seed-shaped, are passed with the animal's feces, and often resemble rice grains when dried. Each proglottid contains egg packets that contain 8 to 15 ova, which are held together by an outer embryonic membrane. (Courtesy Division of Parasitic Diseases/Centers for Disease Control and Prevention.)

Hymenolepis nana

General Characteristics

Hymenolepis nana, also known as the dwarf tapeworm, is very small compared with other tapeworms. The organism has a worldwide distribution and may reach up to 4 cm in length. The proglottid contains a scolex with a short-armed rostellum. It is the most common tapeworm. An intermediate host is not required, thus making person-to-person spread possible. An adult dwarf tapeworm can live within the host for approximately 4 to 6 weeks.

Epidemiology

H. nana is generally found in children. Although it is most prevalent in the southern United States, it has a wide distribution—particularly in crowded areas. It is more common in populations living in conditions of poverty or poor hygiene, in daycare centers, and in persons living in institutional settings or prisons.

Pathogenesis and Spectrum of Disease

H. nana has an unusual life cycle; ingestion of the egg can lead to the development of the adult worm in humans, thus bypassing the need for an intermediate host. Humans can serve as both intermediate and definitive hosts. Infection occurs by accidentally ingesting dwarf tapeworm eggs. This happens most commonly through direct fecal-oral transmission or accidental ingestion of an infected arthropod. The worm resides within the upper ileum of the intestinal tract. Once infection occurs, the dwarf tapeworm may reproduce inside the body, thus causing autoinfection. Autoinfection is essentially a reinfection or constant reproduction of the parasite within the host. Massive infection with several thousand worms may follow autoinfection, resulting in hyperinfection. Hyperinfection refers to a large parasitic burden within the host. Autoinfection appears to initiate a cellular and humoral immune response. The immune response will provide the host with some protective immunity. Most patients are asymptomatic. Symptomatic patients may experience weight loss, nausea, and weakness, loss of appetite, diarrhea, and abdominal discomfort. Young children, especially those with a heavy infection, may develop headaches, an itchy perianal area, or have difficulty sleeping.

Laboratory Diagnosis

Adult worms and proglottids are rarely seen in stool specimens. Diagnosis is typically through the identification of eggs in stool specimens. Eggs are characterized by the presence of a thin shell enclosing an embryo (oncosphere) with six hooklets contained within two layers of membrane that is separated from the outer shell. The eggs are spheroidal, pale, and thin-shelled (30 to 47 μm in diameter). The eggs of *H. nana* and *Hymenolepis diminuta* are very similar. However,

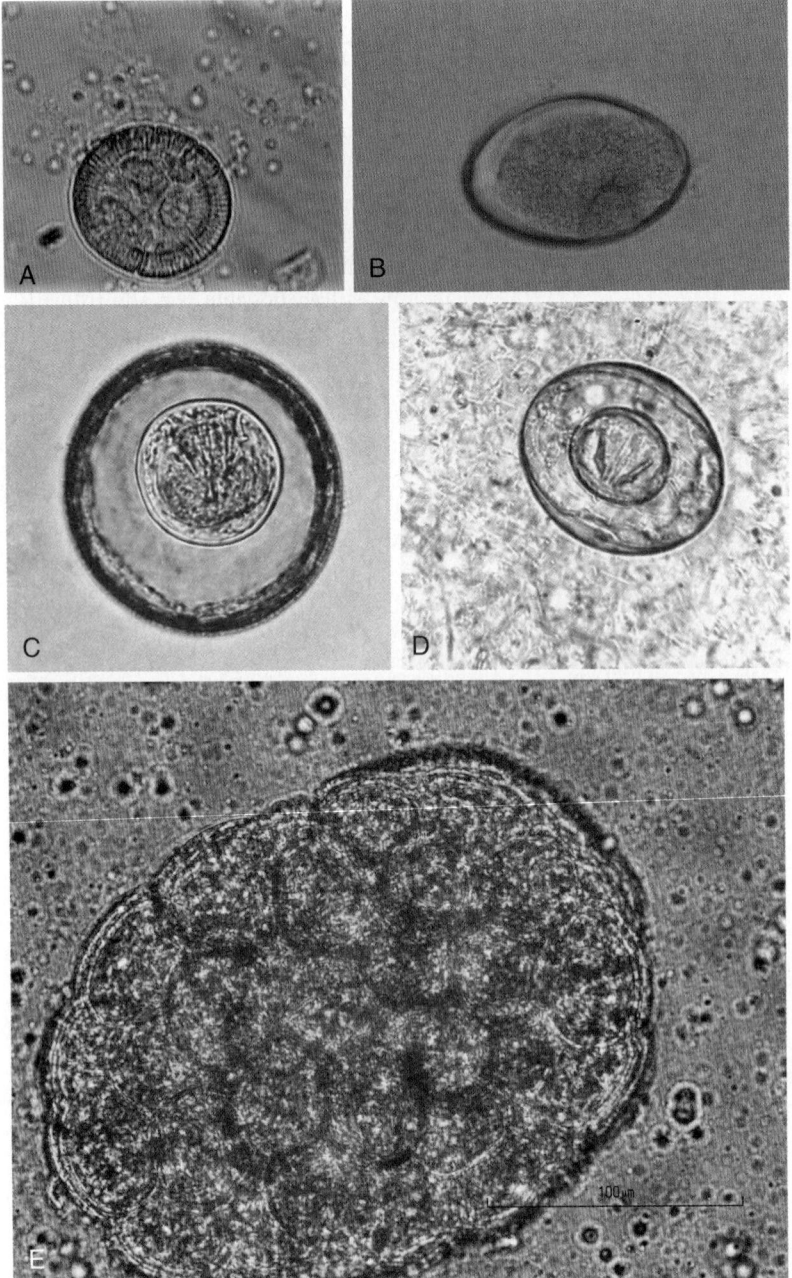

• **Fig. 53.7** (A) *Taenia* spp. egg iodine preparation (400× total magnification). (B) *Diphyllobothrium latum* egg iodine preparation (400× total magnification). (C) *Hymenolepis diminuta* egg. (D) *Hymenolepis nana* egg. (E) *Dipylidium caninum* egg packet iodine preparation (500× total magnification).

H. nana eggs are smaller and have 4 to 8 **polar filaments** present in the space between the oncosphere and the egg-shell (Fig. 53.7). The egg morphology is easily distinguishable in fresh or formalin-fixed fecal samples. It is important to note that eggs are infectious, and therefore unpreserved specimens should be handled carefully. Concentration techniques and repeated examinations will increase the likelihood of detecting light infections. Some patients may demonstrate a low-grade eosinophilia. Nucleic acid–based methods and serological techniques are being developed; however, further evaluation is needed to determine the efficacy and use of these assays in clinical applications.

Therapy

Praziquantel remains the therapy of choice. Niclosamide is also effective and can be repeated with reinfection. Human adults living in endemic areas are provided some immunity as a result of their cellular and humoral immunologic responses.

Prevention

Good hygiene is the best method for control and prevention. Preventing fecal contamination of food and water is the first line of defense. General sanitation measures, along

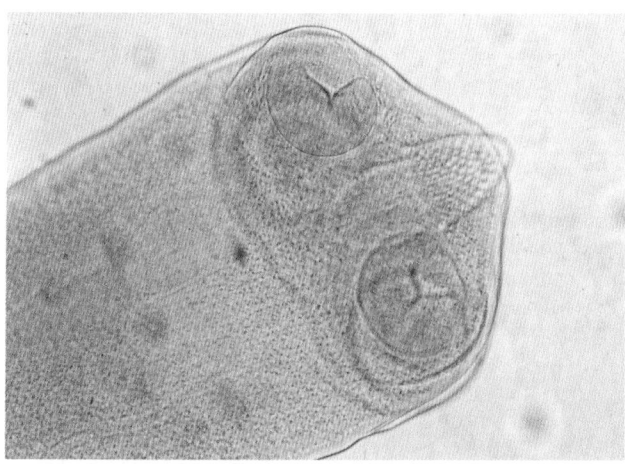

• **Fig. 53.8** *Dipylidium caninum* scolex demonstrating the armed rostellum. (Courtesy Dr. Henry Travers, Sioux Falls, SD.)

with rodent control, are helpful in controlling the flea population.

Hymenolepis diminuta

General Characteristics

H. diminuta, the rat tapeworm, is larger than *H. nana* and can measure 20 to 60 cm in length. Outbreaks of human infection are rare.

Epidemiology

H. diminuta is an uncommon tapeworm in humans and is typically found in rodents, including rats and mice. Rats are typically the natural reservoir. *H. diminuta* can infect humans after contamination of grains and flours with rodent feces.

Pathogenesis and Spectrum of Disease

The life cycle of *H. diminuta* involves insects, similar to the life cycle of *H. nana*. *H. diminuta* rarely infects humans but may do so if a human accidentally ingests an arthropod infected with cysticercoids. Multiple adult worms may mature in the human intestine. Infections are usually well tolerated by the host because of the small size of the organism. Symptoms may include diarrhea, anorexia, nausea, headache, and dizziness. The infection is more common in children, causing mild diarrhea, remittent fever, and abdominal pain.

Laboratory Diagnosis

Proglottids are rarely seen in the stool; diagnosis is made by the identification of eggs. The eggs (70 to 85 μm × 60 to 80 μm) are large, ovoid, yellowish, and moderately thick-shelled. The eggs contain a six-hooked oncosphere with the absence of polar filaments in the space between the oncosphere and the eggshell (Fig. 53.7). The eggs are clearly differentiated from *H. nana* because of the absence of polar filaments. Nucleic acid–based methods and serological techniques are being developed; however, further evaluation is needed to determine the efficacy and use of these assays in clinical applications.

Therapy

H. diminuta is readily treated with praziquantel, although the disease is self-limiting and treatment is often not necessary.

Prevention

Prevention is dependent on controlling the populations of infected mice and rats, along with good hygiene and sanitation.

Taenia solium

General Characteristics

T. solium, the pork tapeworm, is the intestinal cestode capable of causing serious pathologic damage to the human host. Humans serve as the definitive host, whereas pigs serve as the intermediate host. Humans can also serve as the intermediate host. *T. solium* may result in an intestinal infection in which the larvae mature and reside in the small intestine for up to 25 years. The organisms can grow to be 2 to 7 m long and produce more than 1000 proglottids, each containing about 50,000 eggs. **Cysticercosis** (larval forms throughout the body) is the extraintestinal form of the disease and can be much more severe. The disease is life threatening if the organism invades the central nervous system causing neurocysticercosis.

Epidemiology

T. solium has a worldwide distribution. Higher rates of illness have been seen in Latin America, Asia, sub-Saharan Africa, and parts of Oceania. The parasite is found in the United States, typically among immigrants from zones of endemicity. The tapeworm is more prevalent in underdeveloped communities with poor sanitation, and when pork is ingested as undercooked or raw.

Pathogenesis and Spectrum of Disease

T. solium infection can result in the presence of both adult and larval stages in the human host (Fig. 53.9). Infection begins when the intermediate host ingests embryonated eggs in feces. Once the egg is ingested, the hexacanth embryo, armed with three pairs of hooks, is released into the intestine where the embryo penetrates the mucosa. The embryo then matures into a **cysticercus larvae** (containing a fluid-filled bladder) in the tissue. Humans may become infected

Taeniasis

Taenia asiatica, Taenia saginata, Taenia solium

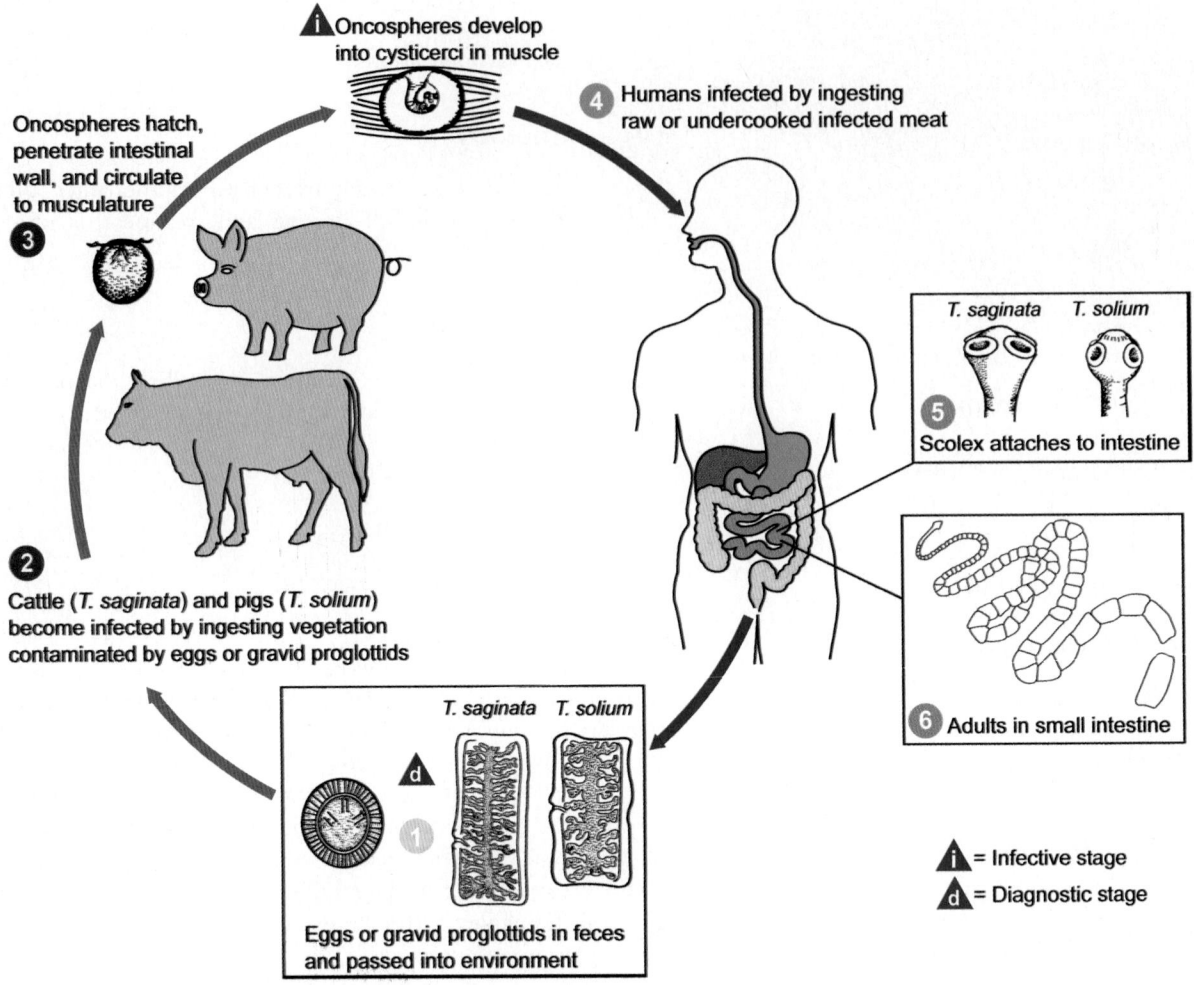

• **Fig. 53.9** Life cycle of *Taenia* spp. (Courtesy Division of Parasitic Diseases/Centers for Disease Control and Prevention.)

when they eat raw or undercooked pork containing embedded larvae with cysts. Pork tapeworm infection is usually caused by ingestion of multiple worms. During ingestion and subsequent digestion of the infected meat, the cysticercus is released and attaches to the mucosa within the small intestine of the human host. The cysticercus matures into an adult worm within approximately 5 to 12 weeks. The eggs are then released in the host's feces. Accidental ingestion of the eggs by the human host may also result in migration of the embryo through the intestine to other areas of the body, including the eyes, brain, muscle, or bone. In addition, the proglottids are motile and may migrate out of the anus. Infection of the adult tapeworm causes few clinical symptoms, although abdominal pain, diarrhea, indigestion, and loss of appetite may be present because of irritation to the mucosa of the intestinal wall. The major complication with *T. solium* is cysticercosis, in which the human host becomes the intermediate host and harbors the larvae in tissues as

previously described. This infection is further discussed in Chapter 74.

Laboratory Diagnosis

Diagnosis of *Taenia* tapeworm infection is through the examination of stool samples. Individuals suspected of infection with *T. solium* should be asked if they have passed any notable tapeworm segments in their stool. Stool specimens should be collected on 3 different days and microscopically examined for the presence of *Taenia* eggs (Fig. 53.7A). Tapeworm eggs can be detected in the stool 2 to 3 months after the tapeworm infection is established. Eggs are round or slightly oval (31 to 43 μm in diameter) and yellow-brown with a thick, striated shell containing a six-hooked oncosphere. Diagnosis is based on the recovery of eggs or proglottids in stool or from the perianal area. *T. solium*, *T. saginata*, and *T. asiatica* cannot be differentiated based on

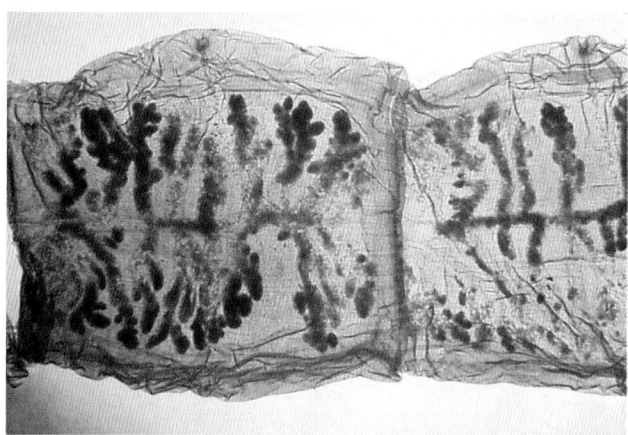

• **Fig. 53.10** This photomicrograph reveals some of the ultrastructural morphology exhibited by a gravid proglottid from a *Taenia solium* tapeworm. The number of primary lateral uterine branches, represented by the dark, India ink-stained irregularities, allows differentiation between the two species. *T. solium* shows 7 to 13 branches on each side. (Courtesy Division of Parasitic Diseases/Centers for Disease Control and Prevention.)

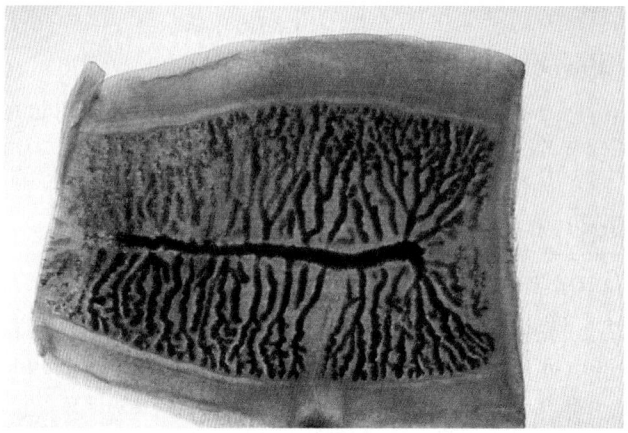

• **Fig. 53.11** This photomicrograph reveals some of the ultrastructural morphology exhibited by a gravid proglottid from a *Taenia saginata* tapeworm. The number of primary lateral uterine branches, represented by the dark, India ink-stained irregularities, allows differentiation between the two species. *T. saginata* shows 15 to 20 branches on each side. (Courtesy Division of Parasitic Diseases/Centers for Disease Control and Prevention.)

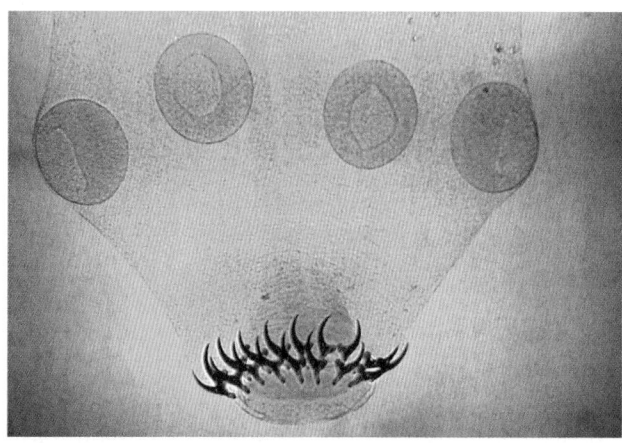

• **Fig. 53.12** This photomicrograph reveals some of the ultrastructural morphology exhibited by the cephalic end of a *Taenia solium*, highlighting the worm's scolex, and its four suckers and two rows of hooks. (Courtesy Division of Parasitic Diseases/Centers for Disease Control and Prevention.)

egg morphology. Speciation requires the examination of gravid proglottids or the scolices. *T. solium* gravid proglottids are longer than wide (19 mm × 17 mm) and may be distinguished from *T. saginata and T. asiatica* according to the number of uterine branches. *T. solium* contains 7 to 13 lateral uterine branches along the proglottid (Fig. 53.10), whereas *T. saginata* and *T. asiatica* contain more than 13 branches. Uterine branches may be visualized by staining the proglottids with India ink (Fig. 53.11). The scolex contains a neck region that is typically short and half the width of the scolex, and differs from that of *T. saginata* by the presence of four suckers with hooks in a double row (Fig. 53.12). The adult worm is usually 3 to 5 m long. Extreme care should be taken when handling infectious stool, because *T. solium* proglottids and eggs are extremely infectious. Additional laboratory findings may include a low-grade eosinophilia, increased serum IgE level, and the presence of atypical lymphocytes in the cerebrospinal fluid.

Serologic assays specific to the adult *T. solium* tapeworm have been developed for the diagnosis of neurocysticercosis. Complement fixation, hemagglutination, enzyme-linked immunosorbent assay (ELISA), and immunoblot can be used for the detection of anticysticercal antibodies in serum, cerebrospinal fluid, and saliva. The enzyme-linked immunoelectrotransfer blot assay is the most effective method for the detection of antibodies, with sensitivity and specificity as high as 100% and 98%, respectively. However, the sensitivity decreases to about 70% in patients with a single cyst or in those with only calcified lesions. ELISA is more reliable when performed in cerebrospinal fluid than in serum, but the accuracy depends on the viability and location of the cysticerci. These advanced serologic tests are not yet commercially available and are generally only available in specialized laboratories. Stool antigen testing detects at least 2 to 3 times more cases of *Taenia* infection than stool microscopy.

Therapy

Adult worms can be eradicated with praziquantel or niclosamide followed by use of a laxative. Expulsion of the scolex must be verified to assume satisfactory treatment.

Prevention

Good hygiene and immediate treatment are essential for the prevention of autoinfection. Pork should be cooked or frozen thoroughly. Cysticerci do not survive temperatures below −10°C or above 50°C. Educational programs concerning the hazards associated with living near human sewage and contaminated drinking water are important in populations at risk. When traveling in countries where food is likely to be contaminated, all raw vegetables and fruits should be washed, peeled, or cooked with clean water before eaten.

Taenia saginata

General Characteristics

T. saginata, or beef tapeworm, has a worldwide distribution and is more common than *T. solium.* The worm can grow 4 to 12 m and contain 1000 to 2000 segments. *T. saginata* may produce 100,000 eggs and live up to 25 years in the human intestine.

Epidemiology

T. saginata has a similar life cycle to that of *T. solium.* Cattle are the intermediate hosts, and humans are infected through the ingestion of cysticerci (larval form with an unarmed scolex) in raw or undercooked beef (Fig. 53.9).

Pathogenesis and Spectrum of Disease

The life cycle of *T. saginata* begins with human ingestion of undercooked or raw meat infected with larvae. The larvae are ingested in the meat and, after digestion, released into the small intestine, where the worm attaches to the mucosa and matures. In about 3 months, the worm may grow up to 4 to 5 m in length, and gravid segments will begin to break off and pass in stool. After deposition of gravid segments in the soil, an intermediate bovine host may ingest the segments. The segments are digested and the eggs hatch, releasing an oncosphere that penetrates the muscle tissue. After penetration of the mucosa, the organisms are carried via the lymphatic vessels and bloodstream throughout the intermediate host. Humans then ingest the infected meat of the intermediate host, as previously indicated. Humans typically are asymptomatic or experience very mild indigestion, loss of appetite, vomiting, and abdominal discomfort. A rare case of severe infection may result in intestinal obstruction and appendicitis. Patients are often unaware of their infection until gravid motile segments are passed in the feces and cause psychological distress.

Laboratory Diagnosis

The stool should be examined for proglottids and eggs; eggs may also be present on anal swabs. The eggs of *T. saginata* are indistinguishable from other *Taenia* spp. The adult worms can reach up to 25 m in length. The uterus of *T. saginata* is longer than wide and typically contains 15 to 18 lateral branches on each side (Fig. 53.11). The scolex has four suckers and is unarmed or does not contain any hooklets (Fig. 53.13). Stool specimens should be handled with care, because the eggs cannot be distinguished from *other Taenia* spp. Slight eosinophilia may develop.

Therapy

Recommended treatment includes praziquantel or niclosamide. Treatment of *T. saginata* can be considered

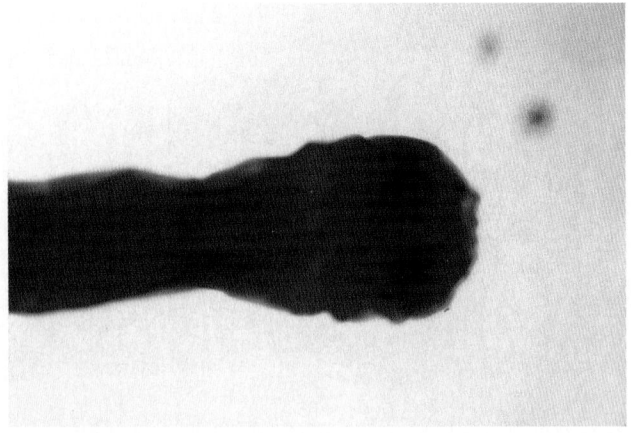

• **Fig. 53.13** Under a low magnification, this photomicrograph highlights the scolex, or head region of the cestode, *Taenia saginata.* (Courtesy Division of Parasitic Diseases/Centers for Disease Control and Prevention.)

successful when no proglottids are passed for 4 consecutive months.

Prevention

Beef should be inspected for cysticerci and thoroughly cooked before it is ingested.

Taenia asiatica

General Characteristics

T. asiatica, or Asian tapeworm, is found primarily in remote areas of the East and Southeast Asian countries to include Taiwan, Indonesia, Korea, Vietnam, the Philippines, Thailand, China, and Japan. The morphology of *T. asiatica*'s gravid proglottids and adult worm is difficult to distinguish from that of *T. saginata.*

Epidemiology

T. asiatica has a similar life cycle to that of *T. solium.* It has been suggested that *T. asiatica* is possibly misdiagnosed as *T. solium* since both species share some of the same hosts, and co-infections are thought to occur more frequently than reported. Pigs, cattle, and goats are the intermediate hosts, and humans are infected through the ingestion of cysticerci (larval form with an unarmed scolex) in raw or undercooked liver from cattle or pork.

Pathogenesis and Spectrum of Disease

The pathogenesis of *T. asiatica* is identical to that of *T. saginata*; which begins with human ingestion of undercooked or raw liver infected with larvae (Fig. 53.9). After penetration of the mucosa, the organisms are carried via the lymphatic vessels and bloodstream throughout the intermediate host. Humans then ingest the infected liver of the intermediate host, as previously indicated. Humans typically are asymptomatic or may experience abdominal pain, nausea, weakness, weight loss, headache, and changes in appetite. Patients are often unaware of their infection until gravid motile segments are passed in the feces. Eosinophilia is seen in some patients.

Laboratory Diagnosis

The stool should be examined for proglottids and eggs; eggs may also be present on anal swabs. The eggs of *T. asiatica* are indistinguishable from those of *T. solium* or *T. saginata*. The uterus of *T. asiatica* is longer than wide and typically contains 12 to 26 lateral branches on each side. The scolex has two rows of rudimentary hooklets that are lost in the mature worm. The adult worm is smaller than *T. saginata*, measuring 4 to 8 m long, and contains fewer proglottids. Stool specimens should be handled with care, because the eggs cannot be distinguished from those of *T. solium* or *T. saginata*.

Therapy

Recommended treatment includes praziquantel or niclosamide, followed by a laxative. Treatment of *T. asiatica* is not usually required; however, if prescribed, it can be considered successful when no proglottids are passed for 4 consecutive months.

Prevention

Pork and beef liver should be inspected for cysticerci and thoroughly cooked before ingested.

Taenia crassiceps

General Characteristics

Taenia crassiceps is a parasitic organism whose adult form infects the intestines of carnivores and has been isolated in human cases of cysticercosis.

Epidemiology

It is commonly found in the Northern Hemisphere, especially throughout Canada and the northern United States. The larval stages of *T. crassiceps* develop subcutaneously or in their body cavities as cysticerci. *T. crassiceps* inhabits the intestines of carnivores. Inside the carnivore, the tapeworm reproduces. The eggs are passed in the feces, with the natural intermediate hosts of this organism usually being small rodents and moles. When the intermediate host is eaten by another carnivore, the parasite's life cycle repeats. Humans serve as intermediate hosts when food or water contaminated with feces from infected hosts is consumed. Close contact with infected domestic dogs has been associated with several human infections.

Pathogenesis and Spectrum of Disease

T. crassiceps rarely infects humans, as a healthy adult human's immune system typically removes the parasite before permanent damage occurs. However, individuals who were infected tended to be immunosuppressed patients. Patients are generally asymptomatic but may present with symptoms, such as headache, nausea, and vomiting. Parasites may accumulate in skeletal muscle and subcutaneous tissue, and some patients present with intraocular infections referred to as ocular larva migrans that can cause serious damage to the eyes, even blindness.

Laboratory Diagnosis

Diagnosis is made by the observation of cysticerci in biopsy or autopsy specimens. Positive ELISA for anticysticercal antibodies helps confirm the diagnosis; however, negative test results do not exclude cysticercosis. The patient may present with eosinophilia.

Therapy

Surgical removal is mandatory for individuals with intraocular cysts. Ocular cysticercosis can be effectively treated with anthelmintics, such as albendazole or praziquantel, and oral corticosteroids for inflammation.

Prevention

Avoid food and water sources that could be contaminated with feces. Animal products consumed should be inspected for cysticerci and thoroughly cooked before ingested.

Nucleic Acid Detection (All Species)

All three species of *Taenia*, and two genotypes of *T. solium*, can be differentiated using nucleic acid base excision sequence scanning thymine-base reader analysis for mitochondrial genes. Polymerase chain (PCR) amplification of the cytochrome oxidase subunit 1 (*cox1*) has been successfully used to identify several *Taenia solium* infections from fixed tissue associated with cases of human cysticercosis. Additional nucleotide sequences used to differentiate the organisms from clinical material include the mitochondrial 12S rRNA, ND1 (NADH dehydrogenase 1), and ITS2 (ribosomal internal transcribed spacer 2). Two additional species were also identified using PCR: *T. serialis* and *T. crassiceps*. *T. serialis* (Chapter 54) was identified in a cystic parasitic larva sample from a subcutaneous sample of a patient's jaw. *T. crassiceps* was identified in sternocleidomastoid muscle of the patient's neck. There have been 12 reported cases of human infection with this species. Four cases of *T. martis* cysticercosis have been identified in human infections.

Ⓔ Visit the Evolve site for a complete list of procedures, review questions, and case studies.

Bibliography

Beugnet F, Labuschagne M, de Vos C, Crafford D, Fourie J: Analysis of *Dipylidium caninum* tapeworms from dogs and cats, or their respective fleas - part 2. Distinct canine and feline host association with two different *Dipylidium caninum* genotypes, *Parasite* 25:31, 2018.

Carroll KC, Pfaller MA, Landry ML, et al.: *Manual of clinical microbiology*, ed 12, Washington, DC, 2019, ASM.

Conlan JV, Vongxay K, Fenwick S, Blacksell SD, Andrew Thompson RC: Does interspecific competition have a moderating effect on *Taenia solium* transmission dynamics in Southeast Asia? *Trends Parasitol* 25:398–403, 2009.

Deplazes P, Eichenberger RM, Grimm F: Wildlife-transmitted *Taenia* and *Versteria cysticercosis* and coenurosis in humans and other primates, *Int J Parasitol Parasites Wildl* 9:342–358, 2019.

Flisser A: State of the art of *Taenia solium* as compared to *Taenia asiatica*, *Korean J Parasitol* 51:43–49, 2013, https://doi.org/10.3347/kjp.2013.51.1.43.

François A, Favennec L, Cambon-Michot C, et al.: *Taenia crassiceps* invasive cysticercosis: a new human pathogen in acquired immunodeficiency syndrome? *Am J Surg Pathol* 22(4):488–492, 1998.

Galán-Puchades MT, Fuentes MV: *Taenia asiatica*: the most neglected human taenia and the possibility of cysticercosis, *Korean J Parasitol* 51(1):51–54, 2013.

Galindo M, Gonzalez MJ, Galanti N: *Echinococcus granulosus protoscolex* formation in natural infections, *Biol Res* 35(3–4):365–371, 2002.

Garcia HH, Del Brutto OH, Nash TE, et al.: New concepts in the diagnosis and management of neurocysticercosis *(Taenia solium)*, *Am J Trop Med Hyg* 72(1):3–9, 2005.

Garcia LS: *Diagnostic medical parasitology*, ed 6, Washington, DC, 2016, ASM Press.

Heldwein K, Biedermann HG, Hamperl WD, et al.: Subcutaneous *Taenia crassiceps* infection in a patient with non-Hodgkin's lymphoma, *Am J Trop Med Hyg* 75(1):108–111, 2006.

Hoberg EP: *Taenia* tapeworms: their biology, evolution and socioeconomic significance, *Microbes Infect* 4(8):859–866, 2002.

Hyneman D: Cestodes. In Baron S, eds: *Medical microbiology*, ed 4, Galveston, TX, 1996, Addison-Wesley.

Jeon HK, Eom KS: Molecular approaches to *Taenia asiatica*, *Korean J Parasitol* 51(1):1–8, 2013.

Jeon HK, Kim KH, Huh S, et al.: Morphologic and genetic identification of *Diphyllobothrium nihonkaiense* in Korea, *Korean J Parasitol* 47(4):369–375, 2009.

Mayta H, Talley A, Gilman RH: Differentiating *Taenia solium* and *Taenia saginata* infections by simple hematoxylin-eosin staining and PCR-restriction enzyme analysis, *J Clin Microbiol* 38:133–137, 2000.

Metwally DM, Al-Enezy HA, Al-Turaiki IM, El-Khadragy MF, Yehia HM, Al-Otaibi TT: Gene-based molecular characterization of cox1 and pnad5 in *Hymenolepis nana* isolated from naturally infected mice and rats in Saudi Arabia, *Biosci Rep* 39(2), 2019, BSR20181224.

Patamia I, Cappello E, Castellano-Chiodo D, Greco F, Nigro L, Cacopardo B: A human case of *Hymenolepis diminuta* in a child from eastern Sicily, *Korean J Parasitol* 48:167–169, 2010.

Roberts L, Schmidt G: *Foundations of parasitology*, ed 8, New York, 2009, McGraw-Hill, pp. 351–352.

Samkari A, Kiska DL, Riddell SW, Wilson K, Weiner LB, Domachowske JB: Dipylidium caninum mimicking recurrent *Enterobius vermicularis* (pinworm) infection, *Clin Pediatr (Phila)*. 47:397–399, 2008.

Schenone H: Praziquantel in the treatment of *Hymenolepis nana* infections in children, *Am J Trop Med Hyg* 29:320, 1980.

Schmid S, Grmm F, Huber M, et al.: JPLL investigator catalog, *Cytopathology* 25(5):340–341, 2013.

Scholz T, Garcia H, Kuchta R, Wicht B: Update on the human broad tapeworm (genus *Diphyllobothrium)*, including clinical relevance, *Clin Microbiol Rev* 22:146–160, 2009.

Sorvillo F, Wilkins P, Shafir S, Eberhard M: Public health implications of cysticercosis acquired in the United States, *Emerg Infect Dis* 17:1–6, 2011.

Sundaram PM, Jayakumar N, Noronha V: Extraocular muscle cysticercosis - a clinical challenge to the ophthalmologists, *Orbit* 23(4):255–262, 2004.

Tappe D, Berkholz J, Mahlke U, et al.: Molecular identification of zoonotic tissue-invasive tapeworm larvae other than *Taenia solium* in suspected human cysticercosis cases, *J Clin Microbiol* 54:172–174, 2016.

Tena D, Simón MP, Gimeno C, et al.: Human infection with *Hymenolepis diminuta*: case report from Spain, *J Clin Microbiol* 36(8):2375–2376, 1998.

Turner JA: Human dipylidiasis (dog tapeworm infection) in the United States, *J Pediatr* 61:763–768, 1962.

Wicht B, Yanagida T, Ito A, et al.: Multiplex PCR for differentiated identification of broadworm tapeworms (cestode: *Diphyllobothrium*) infecting humans, *J Clin Microbiol* 48:311, 2010.

Wiwanitkit V: Overview of *Hymenolepis diminuta* infection among Thai patients, *MedGenMed* 22(6):7, 2004.

54

Tissue Cestodes

OBJECTIVES

1. Describe and compare the life cycles of the tissue cestodes, including reservoir and intermediate hosts.
2. Describe the clinical manifestations and complications of cysticerci in the human host.
3. List the various methods used to diagnose cysticercosis infection.
4. Define and describe the morphologic characteristics of the following: oncosphere, brood capsule, hydatid cyst, and hydatid sand.
5. Describe hydatid disease, including laboratory diagnosis and the best course of treatment.
6. Compare and contrast the pathogenesis and spectrum of disease associated with direct tissue damage versus the immune response to *Echinococcus* spp.
7. Describe the tapeworm that causes coenurosis, including hosts and symptoms of disease.
8. Describe the preventive measures recommended to prevent infection with tissue cestodes.

PARASITES TO BE CONSIDERED

Cestodes (Tapeworms)

Tissue (Larval Forms)
Taenia solium
Echinococcus granulosus complex
    E. granulosus sensu stricto
    E. equinus
    E. ortleppi
    E. canadensis
Echinococcus multilocularis
Echinococcus oligarthrus
Echinococcus vogeli
Taenia multiceps
Taenia serialis
Spirometra mansonoides

Tissue cestodes do not reach the adult stage in the human host. The organisms infect the human in their intermediate or cyst stage. These infections are much more serious than those caused by adult tapeworms. The parasites can cause serious disease or even death. Larval cestodes cause infection after accidental ingestion of eggs excreted from the intermediate host (Table 54.1) and release embryos that migrate and lodge in various organs and tissues in the human body. Diagnosis of larval infections can be problematic.

Taenia solium

General Characteristics

Taenia solium, also known as the pork tapeworm, causes an intestinal infection contracted when a person eats contaminated pork, as discussed in Chapter 53. The adult worm usually causes no clinical disease. Humans may accidentally become the intermediate host by ingesting eggs from human feces. This typically occurs when an individual is already infected with adult *T. solium*. Autoinfection occurs when the individual swallows eggs after improper hand washing. Humans may develop the larval infection, which could result in cysticercosis. Cysticercosis is usually asymptomatic unless larvae invade the central nervous system (CNS), the globe of the eye, or other muscle and tissues.

Epidemiology

T. solium is found worldwide, with a higher incidence in Latin America. The larval form of the infection rarely occurs in the United States but may be found among immigrants from Mexico. After ingestion of *T. solium* eggs, the oncospheres hatch in the intestine and invade the intestinal wall. Once the larvae invade the tissue, the organism is capable of spreading systemically by migration to the brain, liver, and other tissues, causing human cysticercosis. Cysticercosis is defined as larval forms distributed throughout the body. Human cysticercosis may also occur when reverse peristalsis returns gravid segments into the intestine, where the eggs hatch and release oncospheres. Cysticerci develop and may live many years. Cysticerci will eventually die and may calcify, which will aid in diagnosis.

Pathogenesis and Spectrum of Disease

Clinical signs and symptoms depend on the location, viability, and number of the **cysticerci** present. Cysticerci can develop in any organ or tissue of the body. The severity of the symptoms depends on the body site involved; symptoms may not appear for years after the initial infection. The most severe cases are found in the CNS and the eye. Once cysticerci localize in the brain, the organism causes a condition referred to as **neurocysticercosis.** Infection can cause epileptic-type seizures, headaches, mental disturbances, meningitis, or sudden death. Cysticerci can also be

TABLE 54.1 Common Human Parasites, Diagnostic Specimens, Tests, and Positive Findings

Organism	Acquired Infection	Location in Host	Diagnostic Specimen	Diagnostic Test	Positive Specimen	Comments
Tissue cestodes	Source					
Echinococcus granulosus complex	Eggs from dog tapeworm	Liver, lung, etc.	Serum, hydatid cyst aspirate; biopsy	Serology, centrifugation of fluid; histology	Positive serology; hydatid sand, tapeworm tissue	*E. granulosus* (enclosed cyst)
E. oligarthrus	Eggs from a wild dog tapeworm	Definitive: Intestine Intermediate: cysts within various tissues and organs	Serum, scans, biopsy,	Serology, microscopic and confirmation with ELISA and PCR	Tapeworm tissue, positive serology	The cysts resemble those of *E. vogeli*. Exogenous proliferation has not been reported. Unicystic single or multiple metacestodes
E. vogeli	Eggs from a bush dog tapeworm	Definitive: Intestine Intermediate: cysts found primarily in the liver and lungs	Serum, scans, biopsy	Serology, microscopic and confirmation with ELISA and PCR	Tapeworm tissue, positive serology	These cysts are often interconnected and can have multiple chambers, resulting in multichambered cysts as well as endogenous daughter cysts. These proliferating cysts are similar to those of *E. multilocularis*
Echinococcus multilocularis	Eggs from fox tapeworm	CNS, subcutaneous tissues	Serum, scans, biopsy	Serology, films, histology	Positive serology, positive scans, tapeworm tissue	*E. multilocularis* (cyst develops throughout tissue)
Taenia solium (pork)	Eggs from human tapeworm					Small, enclosed cysticerci (cysticercosis)
Taenia multiceps	Eggs from a dog tapeworm	Definitive: Intestine Intermediate: CNS, subcutaneous tissues	Scans, Coenurosis	Biopsy of coenurosis in subcutaneous tissue Serology, confirmation with ELISA and PCR	Positive scans, presence of oncosphere induced coenurosis	Coenurosis most commonly affects the brain, eyes, and subcutaneous tissues
Taenia serialis	Eggs from a dog tapeworm	Definitive: Intestine Intermediate: Various subcutaneous tissues	Scans, coenurosis	Biopsy of coenurosis in subcutaneous tissue	Positive scans, presence of multiple protoscoleces within the coenurosis	Usually identified postmortem
Spirometra mansonoides	Eggs from dog and cat tapeworm	Any organ/tissue in the body	Scans, serum, tissue biopsy	Serology, films, histology, ELISA	Positive serology, positive scans, tapeworm tissue	Adult worm has no scolex, which can help differentiate *Spirometra* from *T. solium*

CNS, Central nervous system; *ELISA,* enzyme-linked immunosorbent assay; *PCR,* polymerase chain reaction.

found in the eye and must be removed to prevent permanent eye damage, including blindness. Much of the damage from cysticercosis is caused by the severe inflammatory host response that occurs after the cysticerci have died. Antibodies are produced and offer the patient secondary immunity.

Laboratory Diagnosis

Cysticercosis can be difficult to diagnose. *T. solium* eggs are found in stools in fewer than half of the patients with cysticercosis. Demonstration of eggs or proglottids in the feces is an indication of *Taenia* infection but does not provide a diagnosis for cysticercosis. Definitive diagnosis usually requires the identification of cysticercus in the tissue. The organism is surgically removed and microscopically examined for the presence of suckers and hooks on the scolex. The cysticercus is round to oval, translucent, and about 5 mm or more in diameter. The organism has a scolex with four suckers and a rostellum with a circle of hooks. Fine-needle aspiration cytology may be helpful in the diagnosis and eliminates the need for surgical biopsy. Diagnosis may also be made using computed tomography (CT) scans and magnetic resonance imaging (MRI). Radiographs may also be useful in detecting calcifying cysticerci within tissue. Ocular cysticercosis may be diagnosed by visual identification of the larval worm. A highly specific and sensitive enzyme-linked immunoelectro-transfer blot assay is available from the Centers for Disease Control and Prevention (CDC). The assay has demonstrated 100% specificity and 98% sensitivity for the identification of antibodies using serum or CSF, primarily for diagnosis of neurocysticercosis. The assay uses purified antigen from *T. solium* containing seven different major glycoproteins. In all patients, regardless of their clinical presentation, the immunoblot assay is slightly more sensitive in serum than in CSF specimens; consequently, there is no need to obtain CSF solely for use in the immunoblot assay. Currently available antibody detection tests for cysticercosis do not distinguish between active and inactive infections and thus have not been useful in evaluating the outcomes and prognoses of treated patients. Nucleic acid–based methods and species-specific polymerase chain reaction (PCR) have been described to differentiate *Taenia* species in CSF, but these are not widely used for clinical laboratory diagnosis of neurocysticercosis.

Therapy

Cysticercosis should be treated with corticosteroids, anticonvulsants, and surgery if deemed appropriate. Treating nonviable cysticerci in the brain of asymptomatic patients has not been proven necessary. Not all patients respond to treatment and not all patients must be treated, because the inflammatory response as a result of the treatment may be more serious than the disease. Symptomatic neurocysticercosis should be managed using treatment that decreases the patient's symptoms. When treatment is suggested, albendazole is the drug of choice. If praziquantel is used, it should be combined with corticosteroids to reduce the inflammatory response and should not be used for ocular or spinal

cord infections. Surgery may be required for ocular, spinal, or brain involvement.

Prevention

Education, meat inspection, and improvement of sanitation measures are the key preventive measures. Other prevention methods are discussed in Chapter 53.

Echinococcus granulosus Complex

General Characteristics

Echinococcus is the smallest of all tapeworms (3 to 9 mm long) with three to five proglottids. It contains a scolex with four suckers and a rostellum with hooks to attach to the intestinal wall. *Echinococcus granulosus sensu lato* can be used as a general term for all of these species and strains. The tapeworm is found in the small intestine of the definitive host, the canine. Eggs are ingested by the intermediate hosts, which include a variety of mammals including sheep (*E. granulosus sensu stricto*), cattle (*E. ortleppi*), moose (*E. canadensis*), horse (*E. equinus*), and humans. Of the several strains of *E. granulosus* that have been identified, the dog-sheep strain is the most common. Regardless of the strain, humans are typically accidental hosts and are considered a dead end, because the life cycle of the organism is unable to continue in a human host. Oncospheres hatch in the intestine of the intermediate host and invade the circulatory system, where they develop into **hydatid cysts.** Disease symptoms vary with the site and size of the cyst. Echinococcosis (**hydatid disease**) results from the presence of one or more cysts, which can develop in any tissue.

Epidemiology

E. granulosus complex is most common in cool, damp areas where the mammalian hosts are prevalent, such as southern South America, Russia, East Africa, and the western United States. The eggs in the definitive host are passed through the feces and contaminate soil, water, or food. The eggs are able to survive freezing conditions and can remain viable within the environment for several years. Adult worms are found only in the definitive canine hosts (Fig. 54.1).

Pathogenesis and Spectrum of Disease

Hydatid disease in humans is potentially dangerous, depending on the size and location of the cyst. Some cysts may remain undetected for many years until they grow large enough to affect other organs. Many people never know they are infected. The cyst is very slow growing in humans. It is usually fluid-filled and has a germinal layer from which many thousands of scolices are budded. These are known as daughter cysts (**brood capsules**), which attach to the germinal layer or free-float in the cyst. The scolices in the hydatid fluid resemble grains of sand and are called **hydatid sand** (Figs. 54.2A and 54.3). The result is a unilocular cyst containing

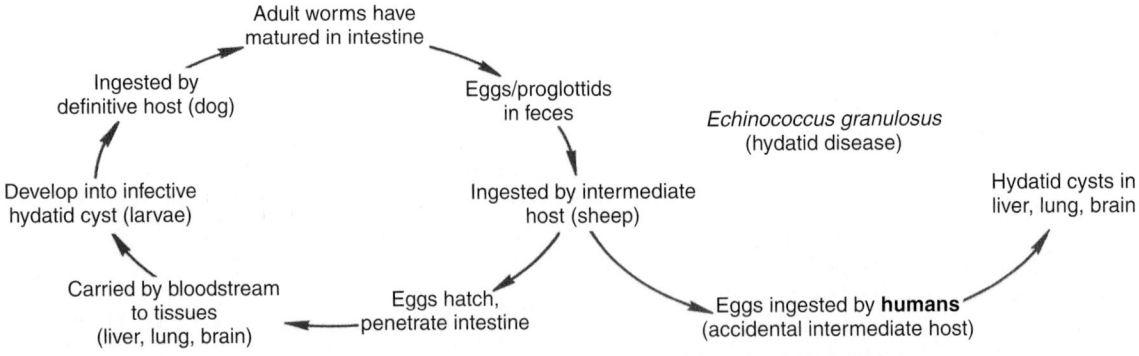

• **Fig. 54.1** Life cycle of *Echinococcus granulosus* (hydatid disease).

future adult worms. The cyst may resemble a slow-growing tumor. Infection in the liver or lungs may be asymptomatic for many years, but the pressure eventually causes noticeable symptoms. Most hydatid cysts occur within the liver. Cysts within the liver cause chronic abdominal pain and allergic reactions and may result in **cholangitis** (infection of the common bile duct) and **cholestasis** (interference with the flow of bile from the liver). Cysts that develop in the lungs may cause infections and abscesses and result in chronic cough, shortness of breath, and chest pain. During the life cycle of the cyst, there may be occasional seepage of fluid into the host tissue and circulation, causing sensitization or activation of the immune response from the presence of the parasite. The rupture and release of the fluid of a hydatid cyst may cause anaphylactic shock as a result of the primary sensitization in a previously asymptomatic individual. If a cyst bursts within the human body, many new cysts may be released that are typically eliminated via the host's cellular immune response. Leaking fluid from a cyst may cause notable eosinophilia.

Laboratory Diagnosis

Clinical symptoms of a slow-growing abdominal tumor with or without eosinophilia are suggestive of infection. Human infection ranges from asymptomatic to severe, including death. Diagnosis of echinococcosis is made through the identification of cysts in the infected organ, accompanied by positive serologic tests. Immunodiagnostic tests can be very helpful in the diagnosis of echinococcal disease and should be used before invasive methods. A variety of serologic tests, including enzyme-linked immunosorbent assay (ELISA) and Western blot serology, are available at the CDC in the United States. However, false-positive reactions may occur in persons with other helminthic infections, cancer, and chronic immune disorders. Negative test results do not rule out echinococcosis because some carriers do not have detectable antibodies. The presence of detectable antibodies in a patient depends on the physical location, integrity, and vitality of the larval cyst. Cysts in the liver are more likely to elicit an antibody response than cysts in the lungs, and, regardless of localization, antibody detection tests are least sensitive in patients with intact hyaline cysts. Cysts in the lungs, brain, and spleen are associated with lowered serodiagnostic reactivity, whereas those in bone appear to regularly stimulate

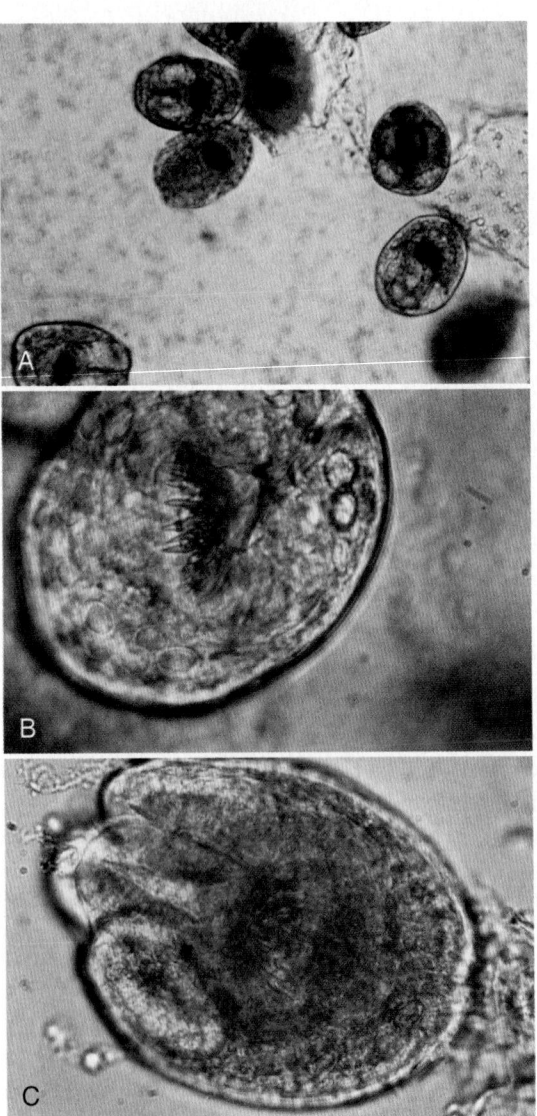

• **Fig. 54.2** (A) *Echinococcus* granules. (B) Ovum. (C) Scolex. (Courtesy Dr. Henry Travers, Sioux Falls, SD.)

a detectable antibody response. Fissuration or rupture of a cyst is followed by an abrupt antibody response. A patient with senescent, calcified, or dead cysts is generally found to be seronegative. Indirect hemagglutination (IHA), indirect fluorescent antibody (IFA) tests, and enzyme immunoassays (EIAs) are sensitive tests for detecting antibodies in serum of patients with cystic disease; sensitivity rates vary from 60% to

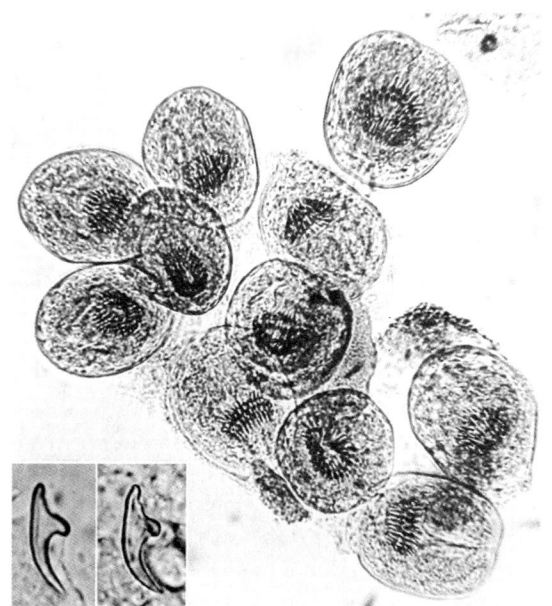

• **Fig. 54.3** *Echinococcus granulosus,* hydatid sand (300×). *(Inset)* Two individual hooklets (1000×).

90%, depending on the characteristics of the cases. At present, the best available serologic diagnosis is obtained by using a combination of tests. EIA or IHA is used to screen all specimens; a positive reaction is confirmed by immunoblot assay or any gel diffusion assay. Although these confirmatory assays give false-positive reactions with sera of 5% to 25% of persons with neurocysticercosis, the clinical and epidemiological presentation of neurocysticercosis is rarely confused with that of cystic echinococcosis.

Antibody responses are also useful in monitoring treatment in some cases. Following successful radical surgery, antibody titers decline and sometimes disappear; titers rise again if secondary cysts develop. Tests for Arc 5 or IgE antibodies appear to reflect antibody decline during the first 24 months postsurgery, whereas the IHA and other tests remain positive for at least 4 years. Consistent declines in antibody titers do not follow chemotherapy. Consequently, the usefulness of serology to monitor the course of disease is limited; imaging techniques provide a more accurate assessment of the patient's condition.

Ultrasound, MRI, and CT have improved the diagnosis and may provide visualization of the fluid-filled cysts. Calcified cysts can be visualized using conventional x-ray. Cysts from different species can also be distinguished by the morphology of the protoscolices, if they are present. Microscopic examination of the cyst fluid for the identification of the scolices can be useful in diagnosis. A 1% eosin stain may be added to the fluid to assist in the visualization and determination of whether the cyst is viable. Nonviable scolices will stain with the eosin; viable scolices will not.

Therapy

PAIR (puncture, aspiration, infection, and reinjection) is used for the inactivation of hydatid sand by injecting the cyst with a cysticidal agent (hypertonic 30% saline, 0.5%

cetrimide, or 70% to 95% ethanol) if surgical removal is not feasible. In other cases, the cysts may be surgically removed after thirty minutes of instillation with one of the previously noted chemical treatments. Albendazole or albendazole plus praziquantel have been used effectively to kill the scolices within the cyst, reduce the size of the cyst, and prevent recurrence. Cystic lesions have been known to resolve in some patients without the need for therapy.

Prevention

Preventive measures include avoiding contact with infected dogs, and deworming animals regularly. Effective control includes educating the population concerning the danger and means of transmission of hydatid disease as well as maintaining good hygiene and practicing safe disposal of dog feces. Slaughtered animals must be disposed of properly to prevent dogs from being exposed to contaminated materials, thus interrupting the *Echinococcus* life cycle.

Echinococcus multilocularis

General Characteristics

Although rarely found in the brains of humans, *Echinococcus multilocularis* causes alveolar hydatid disease, which is a fatal form of **echinococcosis.** It is the most lethal of all helminthic diseases. The cyst is extremely dangerous because it lacks a laminated membrane and develops a series of connected chambers. The chambers contain little or no fluid and rarely contain a scolex. The morphology of the cyst is very similar to that of *E. granulosus,* but the adult organisms are much smaller (1.2 to 3.7 mm). The cysts are very resistant to cold temperatures.

Epidemiology

E. multilocularis is found in Asia, Europe, and northern North America, including areas such as Alaska, Montana, and Minnesota. Foxes, coyotes, and dogs are the definitive host for *E. multilocularis,* whereas rodents are the intermediate host. The parasite is occasionally transmitted to humans through the ingestion of contaminated food or water and by handling infected animals. Fur trappers and veterinarians are at an increased risk of infection because of exposure to infected animals. The life cycle of *E. multilocularis* is essentially identical to that of *E. granulosus.*

Pathogenesis and Spectrum of Disease

Alveolar hydatid disease is a highly lethal, destructive disease. The cyst of *E. multilocularis* grows slowly and may take years to produce clinical symptoms. Many cysts are asymptomatic during the life of the infected individual and are sometimes found during autopsy, surgery, or imaging scans related to other clinical conditions. The severity of symptoms depends on the location of the cyst and the size, as seen with *E. granulosus.* Cysts form primarily in the liver and metastasize to the lung or brain. Cysts in the liver are not restricted with a laminated cyst wall and are capable of expansion into a multicystic structure. This **multilocular** (many chambers) **hydatid cyst** is often mistaken for a hepatic sarcoma, making diagnosis difficult. This disease is often fatal.

Laboratory Diagnosis

Ultrasound, CT, and MRI are used to visualize the cyst and can be supported with serologic testing. Serologic tests, such as ELISA, are sensitive and highly specific. Most patients with alveolar disease have detectable antibodies in serologic tests using heterologous *E. granulosus* or homologous *E. multilocularis* antigens. With crude *Echinococcus* antigens, nonspecific reactions create the same difficulties as described previously with *E. granulosus* complex. However, immunoaffinity-purified *E. multilocularis* antigens (Em2) used in EIA demonstrate positive antibody reactions in more than 95% of alveolar cases. Using a comparison of serologic reactivity to Em2 antigen with that of antigens containing components from both *E. multilocularis* and *E. granulosus* differentiates alveolar from cystic disease. Combining two purified *E. multilocularis* antigens (Em2 and recombinant antigen II/3-10) in a single immunoassay optimizes the sensitivity and specificity. These antigens are commercially available as an EIA kit in Europe, but not in the United States. As in cystic echinococcosis, Em2 tests are more useful for postoperative follow-up than for monitoring the effectiveness of chemotherapy.

Therapy

The most common treatment is to remove the parasite surgically; however, the disease is usually diagnosed late, when it is inoperable and results in a high rate of fatality. Presurgical treatment with albendazole is recommended to reduce the size of the cyst before surgical removal. For inoperable cases, life-long treatment with mebendazole and albendazole has been used successfully and may be the preferred treatment in many cases.

Prevention

Controlling rodents is an important means of prevention, along with educating the public at risk to avoid exposure to infective feces. Practicing good hygiene and periodically deworming household pets are also helpful.

Echinococcus oligarthrus and *Echinococcus vogeli*

General Characteristics

Infections with *E. vogeli* and *E. oligarthrus* are usually known as polycystic echinococcosis (or neotropical polycystic echinococcosis), from the form of the disease that is identified in the intermediate hosts. Because *E. oligarthrus* manifests as a single or discrete cyst in humans, this disease has also been called unicystic echinococcosis.

Epidemiology

Many strains of *Echinococcus* are distributed worldwide; however, *E. vogeli* and E. *oligarthrus* have been found only in Central and South America.

Pathogenesis and Spectrum of Disease

The definitive hosts for *E. vogeli* are bush dogs (*Speothos venaticus*) and the intermediate hosts are South American rodents, especially pacas (*Cuniculus paca*). Dogs, which may be given the entrails from pacas after a hunt, can also act as definitive hosts. The metacestode is found primarily in the liver of the intermediate host, but it can also occur in the lungs and other organs. In pacas, *E. vogeli* cysts are fluid-filled, usually 0.5 cm to 6 cm in diameter, and can occur singly or as aggregates. These cysts are often interconnected and can have multiple chambers. *E. vogeli* undergoes exogenous proliferation in accidental hosts such as primates, resulting in multichambered cysts as well as endogenous daughter cysts. These proliferating cysts, like those of *E. multilocularis*, are invasive. Exogenous proliferation does not seem to occur in the natural host.

The definitive hosts for *E. oligarthrus* are wild felids, and the intermediate hosts are rodents. This species can mature in experimentally infected housecats. In the intermediate host, cysts develop in the muscles, subcutaneous tissues, and internal organs such as the heart and lungs. The cysts resemble those of *E. vogeli* and can reach up to 5 cm in diameter. Exogenous proliferation has not been reported. In human infections, unicystic single or multiple metacestodes were found behind the eye or in the heart.

E. oligarthrus has not been documented in domesticated intermediate mammalian hosts. Two outbreaks caused by *E. vogeli*, one affecting nutrias and the other in nonhuman primates, have been reported in zoos. Orangutans and gorillas developed severe clinical signs including very pendulous abdomens. A number of animals died or had to be euthanized. In pacas, *E. vogeli* does not seem to be symptomatic unless the cysts become very large.

Laboratory Diagnosis

Echinococcus eggs are morphologically indistinguishable from *Taenia* spp., and the tiny proglottids are rarely noticed in feces. ELISAs that detect *Echinococcus* antigens in fecal samples (coproantigen ELISA) can be used to screen definitive hosts. This assay can detect both prepatent and patent infections. A PCR assay designed for fecal samples (copro-DNA assay) is mainly used to confirm the infection or to identify eggs from the feces. *Echinococcus* adults or their proglottids can also be found in the definitive host after purgation with arecoline compounds. *E. oligarthrus* and *E. vogeli* adults usually have three segments. Direct examination of the intestines at necropsy may be used in some circumstances; however, subtle differences are present in the mature proglottids. *E. oligarthrus* is approximately 2 to 3 mm long and *E. vogeli* is 3.9 to 5.6 mm long. In addition to these characteristics, *Echinococcus* species can also be distinguished by PCR followed by sequencing or restriction fragment length polymorphism analysis.

Therapy

In the definitive host, *Echinococcus* spp. can be treated with antihelminthic drugs. Praziquantel, which is effective against both juvenile and adult parasites, is often used. In intermediate hosts, surgery is often the treatment of choice. Long-term antihelminthic treatment may also suppress some cysts. Long-term daily albendazole treatment, after surgical resection of the cyst masses, has suppressed parasite growth in some patients.

Prevention

Preventive measures include avoiding contact with infected dogs and deworming animals regularly. Effective control includes educating the population concerning the danger and routes of transmission associated with the disease as well as maintaining good hygiene and safe disposal of dog feces. Slaughtered animals must be disposed of properly to prevent dogs from being exposed to contaminated materials.

Taenia multiceps and Other Species

General Characteristics

Taenia multiceps is the most common canid tapeworm that causes **coenurosis** in humans. Additional dog tapeworm species, *Taenia crassiceps* and *Taenia serialis,* have also been associated with human coenurosis (Chapter 53). The **coenurus** (larval form) may cause destructive damage or death but is an extremely rare disease in humans. The coenurus cyst is a unilocular cyst that contains a transparent fluid, similar to cysticercus, although the worm has multiple scolices. Daughter cysts may also be seen. The adult tapeworm of *T. multiceps* is 5 to 6 cm long and consists of 200 to 250 segments. The scolex has four suckers and a **proboscis** (tubular appendage) or rostellum with 22 to 32 hooks arranged in two rows.

Epidemiology

T. multiceps is most often found in Africa, although it may be seen in South America, the United States, and Canada. The adult worm is typically found in dogs and other canids. Many animals serve as the intermediate host, such as sheep, cattle, and deer. The animals become infected through the ingestion of eggs while grazing. Humans can also serve as an intermediate host. Human infection occurs from accidental ingestion of dog feces containing the eggs.

Pathogenesis and Spectrum of Disease

The oncosphere hatches and penetrates the intestinal wall of the intermediate host. The embryo is carried via the bloodstream to various parts of the body including the brain, eyes, and CNS, where the organism lodges and the coenurus develops. The coenurus develops into multiple daughter cysts. Symptoms include headache, vomiting, paralysis, and blindness. The coenurus causes a serious disease in sheep and in dogs that have eaten the brains of infected sheep. Infected sheep lose their balance and rotate in circles until they fall (screw disease). The human clinical condition is known as gid, sturdy, or staggers.

Laboratory Diagnosis

Diagnosis is similar to that for *Echinococcus* infection. CT and MRI may be useful for detecting the cysts. Microscopic identification can be used if the cyst has been removed surgically. A serologic test available from the CDC provides additional clinically significant information in combination with imaging studies to establish a diagnosis.

Nucleic acid–based methods have also been used for the diagnosis of *T. multiceps* infections.

Although different serological methods, including ELISA and indirect hemagglutination assay, have been developed to diagnose coenurosis, the antigens used in these assays are natural worm extracts and cannot be produced commercially. Indirect ELISA assays using stable recombinant antigens Tm7 and heat shock protein 70 have been successfully developed for the diagnosis of coenurosis. Although PCR may be useful to detect nucleic acid in CSF, the current complexity of the concentration, extraction, and amplification process prevent routine use in clinical laboratories.

Therapy

Treatment is similar to that for *Echinococcus.* The most common treatment is surgery if possible, although the drugs used for cysticercosis may also be effective against coenurus infection.

Prevention

Dogs associated with sheep and other livestock should not be fed the brain or spinal cord from infected animals and should be dewormed regularly. Good hygiene should be practiced and care taken not to eat or drink anything contaminated with dog feces.

Taenia serialis

General Characteristics

T. serialis has been found in a number of locations, including North America, South America, Europe, and Africa.

Epidemiology

T. serialis, also known as a canid tapeworm, are parasites of carnivores, particularly dogs, with herbivorous animals such as rabbits serving as intermediate hosts. Humans become accidental hosts when eggs are ingested from food or water contaminated with infected dog feces.

Pathogenesis and Spectrum of Disease

Hatching of the *T. serialis* usually occurs only if the eggs have been exposed to gastric secretions. The oncospheres hatch in the intestine, invade the intestinal wall, and are carried in the blood throughout the tissues. Within the tissues, the larvae (called metacestodes) develop into cysticerci or coenuri, which are larvae that group within cysts.

The infection with the metacestode larval form (coenurus) of *T. serialis* is called coenurosis. When humans ingest these eggs from the infected tissue of a definitive host, the eggs develop into coenuri. These coenuri can occur in humans within muscle, brain, eye, or subcutaneous connective tissue. The symptoms are variable, and depend on the location and number of larvae. Coenuri in the skin or subcutaneous tissue usually present as painless nodules. The lesions are often fluctuant and tender. Most subcutaneous nodules manifest on the trunk, sclera, subconjunctiva, neck, shoulders, head, and limbs. Coenuri in the neck may affect movement and swallowing. Clinically, coenuri can mimic lymphomas, lipomas, pseudotumors, or neurofibromas. Coenuri in the CNS cause headache, fever, and vomiting. Localizing neurologic symptoms may also develop, including nerve palsies, Jacksonian epilepsy, pachymeningitis, obstructive or communicating hydrocephalus, and intracranial arteritis with transient hemiparesis. Coenuri in the eye can cause both intraocular and orbital infections, and patients may present with varying degrees of visual impairment. If not removed, coenuri in the eye can result in painful inflammation, glaucoma, and eventual blindness.

Laboratory Diagnosis

Diagnosis is made by the observation of coenuri in tissue biopsy or autopsy specimens. Coenuri are usually readily distinguished from cysticerci by the presence of multiple protoscoleces (infective form of the immature developing scolex).

Therapy and Prevention

Surgical removal or antiparasitic agents can be used to treat coenurus. Oral epsiprantel, praziquantel, or fenbendazole can be used to treat coenuri infection. Discretion should be used when treating this evolving cestode as the dead parasite may cause a significant inflammatory response in the host. The inflammation can be managed with the use of corticosteroids. In many cases surgical removal of the coenurus is a safer option, as leakage of fluid from the cyst during surgery is unlikely to cause a new cyst. Surgical excision is often curative.

Prevention is similar to that for *T. multiceps*. Good hygiene is essential to prevent contamination of food and the environment with feces from infected animals. Proper food preparation is also essential to avoid consumption of infected raw or undercooked meat.

Spirometra mansonoides

General Characteristics

Sparganosis is an infection caused by the plerocercoid larvae of *Spirometra*. The larvae (**spargana**) are white, wrinkled, and ribbon-shaped. They may be 3 mm wide and up to 30 cm long. The sparganum has bothria (longitudinal grooves) instead of suckers. No scolex is present, which can help differentiate *Spirometra* from *T. solium*.

Epidemiology

Spirometra is found worldwide; most human cases of sparganosis are found in Asia. Sparganosis is endemic in animals throughout North America but rare in humans. Adult *Spirometra* live in the intestine of dogs and cats. Eggs are shed in feces, hatch in water, and release free-swimming ciliated coracidia. The coracidia are then ingested by copepods, which become infected. Reptiles, fish, and amphibians ingest infected copepods containing the procercoid (elongated and globular) larvae. The procercoid larvae develop into plerocercoid (pseudosegmented with a scolex) larvae in the second intermediate host. Humans are accidental hosts; they acquire sparganosis after ingestion of contaminated water or by consuming undercooked fish. The life cycle is identical to that of the broad fish tapeworm, *Diphyllobothrium* spp. Humans are unable to serve as the definitive host for *Spirometra*. However, spargana can live up to 20 years in the human host.

Pathogenesis and Spectrum of Disease

Spargana migrate and lodge anywhere in the human body. Clinical symptoms depend on which organs or tissues are involved. Spargana can live for several years before symptoms develop. Sparganosis is usually asymptomatic until the larvae grow and cause an inflammatory reaction. Painful nodules can develop in the tissues. A variety of symptoms may occur, including seizure, weakness, headache, and eye pain that can lead to blindness if left untreated.

Laboratory Diagnosis

Definitive diagnosis is usually made by removal and identification of the sparganum from infected tissue. Serodiagnosis utilizing ELISA methodology can be used to target anti-sparganum IgG antibodies within the blood. ELISA may be positive around 10 to 12 days postinfection and is almost 100% effective at detecting the anti-sparganum antibodies at 14 to 22 days post infection. Clinical history, ELISA, MRI, and CT can all be used together to presumptively diagnose sparganosis. Eosinophilia may also be present.

Therapy

Praziquantel has been used with limited success. Injection of ethanol into the nodule along with surgical removal of the complete sparganum is the treatment of choice.

Prevention

Prevention strategies should include safe drinking water practices and awareness of the dangers of consuming raw fish and amphibians. Water in contaminated areas should be boiled before it is consumed.

ⓔ Visit the Evolve site for a complete list of procedures, review questions, and case studies.

Bibliography

An XX, Yang GY, Wang YW, et al.: Prokaryotic expression of Tm7 gene of *Taenia multiceps* and establishment of indirect ELISA using the expressed protein, *Chin J Vet Sci* 9:99–105, 2011.

Bennett J, Dolin R, Blaser M: *Principles and practice of infectious diseases*, ed 9, Philadelphia, 2020, Elsevier-Saunders.

Blutke A, Hamel D, Hüttner M, et al.: Cystic echinococcosis due to *Echinococcus equinus* in a horse from southern Germany, *J Vet Diagn Invest* 22(3):458–462, 2010.

Budke CM, White Jr AC, Garcia HH: Zoonotic larval cestode infections: neglected, neglected, tropical diseases, *Negl Trop Dis* 3:e319, 2009.

Carroll CL, Connor DH: Sparganosis. In Connor DH, et al.: *Pathology of infectious disease*, Stamford, CT, 1997, Appleton Lange.

Carroll KC, Pfaller MA, Landry ML, et al.: *Manual of clinical microbiology*, ed 12, Washington, DC, 2019, ASM.

Dahniya MH, Hanna RM, Askelou S, et al.: The imaging appearances of hydatid disease at some unusual sites, *Br J Radiol* 74:283–289, 2001.

Eckert J, Deplazes P: Biological, epidemiological, and clinical aspects of echinococcosis, a zoonosis of increasing concern, *Clin Microbiol Rev* 17:107–135, 2004.

El-On J, Shelef I, Cagnano E, et al.: *Taenia multiceps:* a rare human cestode infection in Israel, *Vet Ital* 44:621–631, 2008.

Garcia HH, Evans CA, Nast TE, et al.: Current consensus guidelines for treatment of neurocysticercosis, *Clin Microbiol Rev* 15:747–756, 2002.

Garcia LS: *Diagnostic medical parasitology*, ed 6, Washington, DC, 2016, ASM Press.

Gonzalez LM, Montero E, Harrison LJ, et al.: Differential diagnosis of *Taenia saginata* and *Taenia solium* infection by PCR, *J Clin Microbiol* 38:737–744, 2000.

Horton J: Albendazole for the treatment of echinococcosis, *Fundam Clin Pharmacol* 17:205–212, 2003.

Hu DD, Cui J, Wang L, et al.: Immunoproteomic analysis of the excretory-secretory proteins from *Spirometra mansoni sparganum, Iran J Parasitol* 8(3):408–416, 2013.

Huang X, Xu J, Wang Y, et al.: GP50 as a promising early diagnostic antigen for *Taenia multiceps* infection in goats by indirect ELISA, *Parasit Vectors* 9(1):618, 2016.

Li M-W, Lin H-Y, Xie W-T, et al.: Enzootic sparganosis in Guangdong People's Republic of China, *Emerg Infect Dis* 15(8):1317–1318, 2009.

Liance M, Janir V, Bresson-Hadni S, et al.: Immunodiagnosis of *Echinococcus* infections: confirmatory testing and species differentiation by a new commercial western blot, *J Clin Microbiol* 38:3718–3721, 2000.

Lightowlers MW, Gottstein B: Echinococcosis/hydatidosis: antigens, immunological and molecular diagnosis. In Thompson RCA, Lymbery AJ, editors: *Echinococcus and hydatid disease*, Wallingford, UK, 1995, CAB International, pp 355–410.

McManus DP, Zhang W, Li J, et al.: Echinococcosis, *Lancet* 362:1295–1304, 2003.

Oryan A, Amrabadi O, Sharifiyazdi H, et al.: Application of polymerase chain reaction on cerebrospinal fluid for diagnosis of cerebral coenurosis in small ruminants, *Parasitol Res* 114(10):3741–3746, 2015.

Polat P, Kantarci M, Alper F, et al.: Hydatid disease from head to toe, *Radiographics* 23:475–494, 2003.

Pedrosa I, Saiz A, Arrazola J, et al.: Hydatid disease: radiologic and pathologic features and complications, *Radiographics* 20:795–817, 2000.

Rodriguez S, Wilkins P, Dorny P: Immunological and molecular diagnosis of cysticercosis, *Pathog Glob Health* 106:286–298, 2012.

Spickler, Anna R. *Echinococcosis.* 2011. Available at: http://www.cfsph.iastate.edu/DiseaseInfo/factsheets.php.

Suckow MA, Stevens KA, Wilson RP: *The laboratory rabbit, guinea pig, hamster, and other rodents*, Academic Press, 2012, p 441.

Wang Y, Nie H, Gu X, et al.: An ELISA using recombinant TmHSP70 for the diagnosis of *Taenia multiceps* infections in goats, *Vet Parasitol* 212(3–4):469–472, 2015.

Zhang W, Li J, McManus D: Concepts in immunology and diagnosis of hydatid disease, *Clin Microbiol Rev* 16:18–36, 2003.

55

Intestinal Trematodes

PARASITES TO BE CONSIDERED

Helminths
Trematodes (flukes)
Intestinal
    Echinostoma ilocanum
    Fasciolopsis buski
    Gastrodiscoides hominis
    Heterophyes heterophyes
    Metagonimus yokogawai
    Centrocestus spp.
    Haplorchis spp.
    Stellantchamus spp.
    Pygidiopsis spp.

The intestinal trematodes (flukes) are members of the phylum Platyhelminthes (flatworms), are dorsoventrally flattened, and require at least one intermediate host (a freshwater snail). Human infection occurs by ingestion of **metacercariae** (tailless encrusted larvae) encysted on freshwater vegetation or fish. Most trematodes are hermaphroditic (both ovaries and testes are contained within each adult worm). The parasites are typically identified from eggs shed in the feces.

The adult worms are located in the small intestine, where they lay eggs that may be embryonated or remain unembryonated until shed from the body via feces. The egg continues developing after reaching the water, and a ciliated, free-swimming **miracidium** larva is released. The miracidium enters a snail host and develops into a **redia** (cylindrical larvae), followed by development into tailed **cercariae.** The cercariae emerge from the snail and encyst as a metacercariae on water plants or fish. A human host ingests raw or undercooked plants *(Fasciolopsis buski)*, fish *(Heterophyes, Metagonimus yokogawai),* or freshwater mollusks or fish

(Echinostoma spp.) containing the metacercariae, which excyst in the intestinal tract, attach, and mature into adults. A representative life cycle for *M. yokogawai* is shown in Fig. 55.1.

Echinostoma spp.

General Characteristics

Varieties of species of echinostomes have been reported that infect humans including *E. hortense, E. ilocanum, E. macrorchis, E. perforatum,* and *E. revolutum.* The majority of human infections are caused by *E. ilocanum. E. ilocanum* adult flukes are elongated, leaflike, and approximately 1 cm in length and 0.2 cm in width. Both ends are attenuated, and the posterior end may be slightly pointed. Approximately 50% of adult worms demonstrate 49 to 53 collar spines arranged in alternating rows around the oral sucker. The eggs are passed in the feces of infected patients and are large and oval, with a relatively narrow operculum and small abopercular wrinkles at the posterior end. The eggs measure 89 to 112 μm long and 58 to 69 μm wide.

Epidemiology

Echinostomes infect freshwater mollusks, primarily snails. Infections are common in Russia, Southeast Asia, and the Far East. Rats and dogs serve as reservoir hosts in endemic areas.

Pathogenesis and Spectrum of Disease

Echinostome infections can cause severe clinical manifestations, particularly in cases with heavy worm burdens. Infections can induce mucosal ulceration and bleeding in the duodenum and jejunum through mechanical irritation of the worms (using collar spines, and oral and ventral suckers) leading to severe gastrointestinal discomforts, including epigastric or abdominal pain accompanied by diarrhea, easy fatigue, and malnutrition, for several months' duration.

Patients may appear asymptomatic in light infections and experience mild abdominal pain and diarrhea.

Therapy and Prevention

Praziquantel is the drug of choice for echinostomiasis although it is not included in the US product labeling for

Metagonimiasis
(Metagonimus yokogawai)

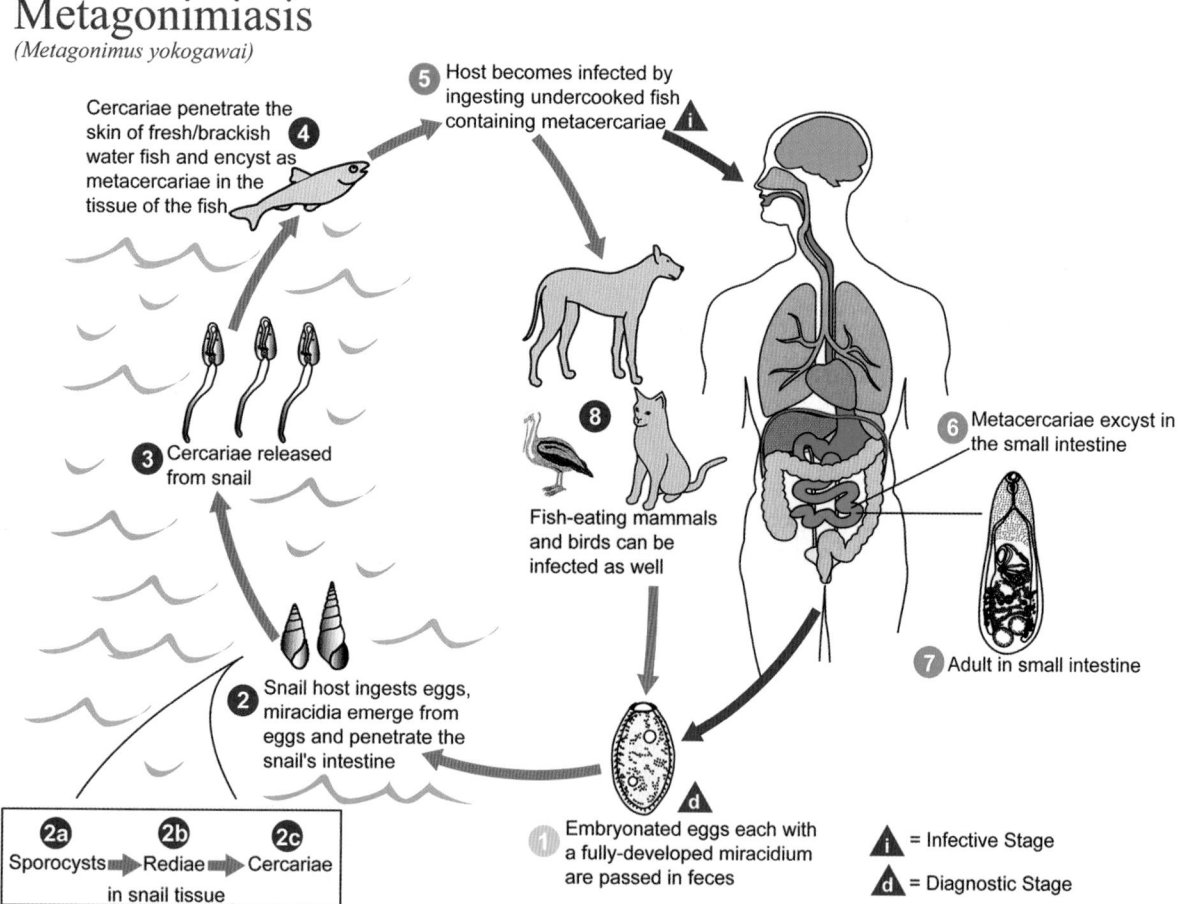

⑤ Host becomes infected by ingesting undercooked fish containing metacercariae **ⓘ**

④ Cercariae penetrate the skin of fresh/brackish water fish and encyst as metacercariae in the tissue of the fish.

③ Cercariae released from snail

⑥ Metacercariae excyst in the small intestine

⑧ Fish-eating mammals and birds can be infected as well

② Snail host ingests eggs, miracidia emerge from eggs and penetrate the snail's intestine

⑦ Adult in small intestine

②a Sporocysts ➡ **②b** Rediae ➡ **②c** Cercariae in snail tissue

① Embryonated eggs each with a fully-developed miracidium are passed in feces **ⓓ**

ⓘ = Infective Stage

ⓓ = Diagnostic Stage

• **Fig. 55.1** This is an illustration of the life cycle of the parasitic trematode, *Metagonimus yokogawai*, the causal agent of metagonimiasis. (Photo Courtesy the Division of Parasitic Diseases/Centers for Disease Control and Prevention.)

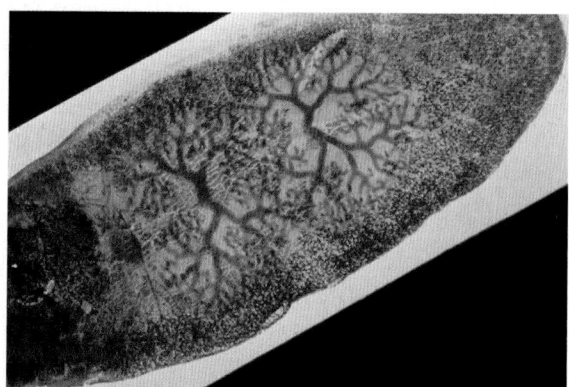

• **Fig. 55.2** Whole mount of *Fasciolopsis buski*. (Courtesy Dr. Henry Travers, Sioux Falls, SD.)

these infections. Although a single dose of 25 mg/kg of praziquantel is the recommended dose for treatment of intestinal fluke infection, echinostome infections can be treated with a slightly lower single oral dose of 10 to 20 mg/kg praziquantel. Proper food preparation and avoiding the consumption of raw, undercooked, or freshly pickled fish prevents infection. Praziquantel is the drug of choice for treatment. In addition, albendazole may also be used.

Fasciolopsis buski General Characteristics

The adults of *F. buski* have an elongated shape and range from 20 to 75 mm long and approximately 8 to 20 mm wide (Fig. 55.2). They have an oral sucker at the anterior end and a ventral sucker located about midway to the posterior end. The eggs, which are indistinguishable from those of *Fasciola hepatica* (Fig. 55.3), are oval and elongated, transparent, and yellow-brown with an operculum (lid) at one end, and they range in size from 130 to 140 mm long and 80 to 85 mm wide and may be unembryonated.

Epidemiology

F. buski is found in Bangladesh, Cambodia, China, India, Indonesia, Laos, Malaysia, Pakistan, Taiwan, Thailand, and Vietnam and is prevalent in school-aged children. Contaminated feces drain into the water from farmland, where feces is used for fertilization, or defecation occurs in or near water sources. Reservoir hosts include pigs, dogs, and rabbits.

F. buski is the largest of the intestinal trematodes, and infection is acquired by ingestion of raw water chestnuts or caltrop (plants with spiny heads or fruit). The definitive host is the pig, and fish-eating wild and domestic animals may

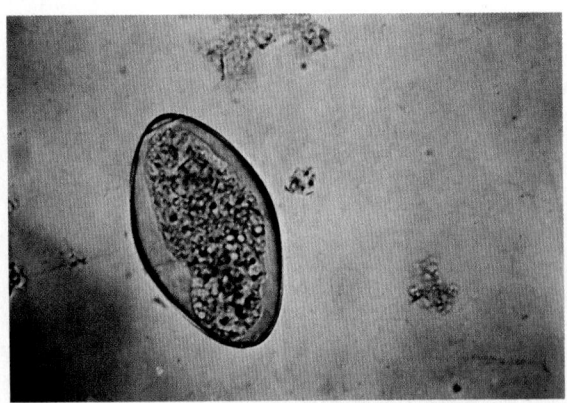

• **Fig. 55.3** *Fasciola* egg. The eggs of *Fasciolopsis buski* and *Fasciola hepatica* are indistinguishable morphologically. (Courtesy Dr. Henry Travers, Sioux Falls, SD.)

serve as reservoir hosts. The water vegetation may become contaminated when feces is used for fertilization or where disposal of farm animal feces is inadequate.

Pathogenesis and Spectrum of Disease

The intestinal attachment site of the adult worms often becomes locally inflamed and ulcerated and may hemorrhage. Moderate to heavy infections may cause abdominal pain, diarrhea, intestinal obstruction, and edema of the abdomen and lower extremities and may result in inadequate absorption of vitamin B_{12}. Eosinophilia is common.

Therapy and Prevention

The current treatment of choice for *F. buski* infection is praziquantel; single dose up to three times a day of niclosamide has been reported to have some *in vitro* efficacy. Infection can be prevented by immersing water plants in boiling water for a few seconds before peeling, and properly cooking water plants and fish before they are eaten. In addition, changes are needed in agricultural practices and health education in the endemic areas.

Gastrodiscoides hominis

General Characteristics

The natural habitat for *G. hominis*, also known as the colonic fluke, is the colon of pigs. The adult worm is vase-shaped and bright pink, averaging 5 to 8 mm long and 3 to 5 mm wide. The anterior region has a prominent oral sucker. The posterior portion is discoidal, and the ventral sucker is close to the posterior end. The tegument is smooth and contains a series of concentric folds bearing numerous tightly packed tubercles. Ciliated and non-ciliated papillae are arranged around the oral sucker on the ventral surface of the worm. Eggs measure approximately 146 by 66 μm, are rhomboidal (parallelogram shape), transparent, and green in color. Each egg contains about 24 vitelline (yolk sac–like) cells and a central unembryonated ovum.

Epidemiology

Human gastrodiscoidiasis is endemic in Southeast Asia, as well as the Philippines, Guyana, India, and Assam. High incidence can be attributed to low standards of sanitation in regions such as rural farms and villages, where night soils are used for fertilizer. Infection in both humans and animals results from the ingestion of contaminated vegetation. Transmission to humans occurs when undercooked or raw infected fish are ingested. Reservoir hosts include rats and deer mice. Humans are an accidental host with pigs serving as the definitive host.

Pathogenesis and Spectrum of Disease

Gastrodiscoidiasis as an infection in the definitive host is usually mild to asymptomatic. Following ingestion by a human host the metacercaria travel through the digestive tract into the duodenum to the cecum, where the larvae self-fertilize and lay eggs. Disease presentation is dependent on the worm burden. Patients may be asymptomatic, but heavy infections cause diarrhea, fever, abdominal pain, colic, malnutrition, and anemia. In severe cases, where there are large numbers of eggs present, papular lesions and desquamation lead to necrosis. Inflammatory reactions can occur in the heart or mesenteric lymphatic system.

Therapy and Prevention

Praziquantel is the treatment of choice for infections. Changes in agricultural practices, health education, and proper hygiene can prevent transmission in the endemic areas. The preferred drug, praziquantel, eliminates the parasite with three doses at 25 mg/kg in 1 day. Prevention of this disease is not difficult when simple sanitary measures are taken. Night soil should never be used as a fertilizer because it could contain any number of parasites. Vegetables should be washed thoroughly, and meat properly cooked.

Heterophyes: Metagonimus yokogawai, Centrocestus spp., Haplorchis spp., Stellantchamus spp., and Pygidiopsis spp.

General Characteristics

There are 22 genera in the family *Heterophyidae*, with six medically relevant genera. *Heterophyes* and *M. yokogawai* are the most prominent. Additional genera included in the family include *Centrocestus* spp., *Haplorchis* spp., *Stellantchamus* spp., and *Pygidiopsis* spp.

Heterophyes heterophyes

Adult *H. heterophyes* worms range in size from 1.0 to 1.7 mm in length and 0.3 to 0.4 mm in width and have a broadly rounded posterior. The adult *H. heterophyes* also has an additional sucker, the genital sucker, which surrounds the genital pore. The eggs are small, yellow-brown, embryonated, and operculated and may have minimal opercular shoulders. Eggs range in size from 26 to 30 mm long and 15 to 17 mm wide and may be indistinguishable from *M. yokogawai*.

Epidemiology

H. heterophyes is distributed throughout China, Egypt, India, Iran, Israel, Japan, Korea, Sudan, the Philippines, Tunisia, and Turkey. Reservoir hosts include cats, dogs, and birds. Snails serve as the intermediate host and a variety of freshwater fish serve as the second intermediate host. This very small trematode is acquired through ingestion of pickled, raw, or inadequately cooked fish.

Metagonimus yokogawai
Adult

M. yokogawai adult worms range in size from 1.0 to 2.5 mm long and approximately 0.4 to 0.8 mm wide. The eggs are small, yellow-brown, embryonated, and operculated, and may have minimal opercular shoulders. Eggs range in size from 26 to 30 mm long and 15 to 17 mm wide and may be indistinguishable from *H. heterophyes*.

Epidemiology

M. yokogawai is found in the Balkans (a cultural region of southeastern Europe), China, Indonesia, Israel, Japan, Korea, Russia, Spain, and Taiwan and is considered the most common intestinal fluke infection in the Far East. Reservoir hosts include cats, dogs, and birds. Freshwater snails serve as the intermediate host, and a variety of freshwater fish serve as the second intermediate host. This very small trematode is acquired through ingestion of pickled, raw, or inadequately cooked fish.

Centrocestus spp.

Adult worms range in size from 280 to 330 μm long and approximately 150 to 180 μm wide. The body is covered in scalelike tegumental spines. The worm has a terminal oral sucker with 32 circumoral spines arranged in two rows and a small ventral sucker. The eggs are oval, yellowish brown, with a distinct operculum. The shell surface appears to have a lattice design. The eggs are approximately 33 μm long and 17 μm wide.

Epidemiology

Centrocestus spp. is an intestinal foodborne trematode that parasitizes birds and mammals, including humans. The species is native to Asia, with worldwide distribution. The primary molluscan intermediate host, *Melanoides* spp., is reported to be present in more than 10 countries throughout Asia and the Americas. Many species of fish are the second intermediate hosts. Metacercariae encyst in the gills of the fish causing pathological developmental delay and death, giving rise to economic losses in the fish farming industry.

Haplorchis spp.

The adult worms of *Haplorchis* are characterized by the presence of a small, armed ventral sucker and a single testis, which differentiates it from *Metagonimus* and *Heterophyes*. A distinct morphological feature of *Haplorchis* is the ventral sucker that has a semi-lunar (half-moon shaped) group of 12 to 16 long, crescentic, and hollow spines and a sinistral (left side) patch of very minute solid spines. The eggs are oval with a convex operculum. The eggs are very similar in shape, size, and morphology to *Opisthorchis viverrini* and cannot be morphologically differentiated.

Epidemiology

Human infections with *Haplorchis* spp. are prevalent in Southeast Asia, including countries located in the Indochina Peninsula, Taiwan, the Philippines, and Egypt. The intermediate host is freshwater snails, *Melania* spp. Fish are the second intermediate hosts, and dozens of species of birds and fish-eating mammals, including dogs, cats, and humans, serve as definitive hosts.

Stellantchamus spp.

The adult flukes are pyriform with a small submedian ventral sucker and an expulsor-type elongated saclike seminal vesicle. Eggs are elongated, ovoid, and slender, from 25.3 to 29.2 μm long and 11.1 to13.4 μm wide.

Epidemiology

Human infections with *Stellantchamus* spp. are prevalent in Southeast Asia, including Korea, Japan, and Kuwait. The intermediate host is the brackish water snail, *Melanoides* spp. The second intermediate hosts are brackish water fish, primarily mullets. Additional freshwater fish, including the half-beaked fish and climbing perch, can also serve as the second intermediate host. Natural definitive hosts include cats, dogs, pigs, rats, humans, and birds.

Pygidiopsis spp.

The adult flukes have a small concave body with a medial ventral sucker. The worm has a unique ventrogenital apparatus (having two groups of spines around the genital pore; 5 to 6 right side and 7 to 9 left side). The two testes are side by side. The worm produces small (19.8 to 22.9 μm long and 11.1 to 13.4 μm wide), ovoid, pyriform eggs with no distinct pattern on the shell.

Epidemiology

Human infections with *Pygidiopsis* spp. are prevalent in Southeast Asia and other regions, including Korea, Japan, Vietnam, and Egypt. The primary intermediate host is the brackish water snail, *Melanoides* spp. The second intermediate host is brackish water fish. The definitive hosts include wolves, cats, dogs, foxes, shrews, rats, pelicans, kites, ducks, and cormorants.

Pathogenicity and Spectrum of Disease

Infections with a small number of worms from any of the heterophyid genera may be asymptomatic. Symptoms in heavy infections may include abdominal pain, diarrhea with a large amount of mucus, and ulceration of the intestinal wall. Eggs may gain entry into the intestinal capillaries and the lymphatic system, where they can be carried to the heart, brain, spinal cord, or other tissues, causing emboli or granuloma formation.

Prevention

Infection can be prevented by avoiding ingestion of raw, inadequately cooked, and pickled or salted fish. The risk of infection could be reduced with improved sanitary conditions and health education programs.

Laboratory Diagnosis

Identification of the intestinal trematodes is made by recovery of eggs, or in rare cases adults, from stool specimens using a sedimentation method such as formalin-ethyl acetate. The sediment may be examined in a wet mount with or without iodine. The eggs of *F. buski* are identical to those of *F. hepatica, E. ilocanum,* and *G. hominis;* and those of *H. heterophyes* and *M. yokogawai* are very similar. Diagnosis of heterophyid infections may also require assessment of symptoms, obtaining a travel history, and/or recovery of adult worms.

Nucleic Acid Detection

Various polymerase chain reaction (PCR) methods have shown potential in detecting intestinal flukes. These methods take advantage of the different types of DNA nucleotide sequence variations demonstrated by the different species within a particular genus. Multiplex qPCR has been developed to detect the presence of the major intestinal parasites known to cause gastroenteritis, including the trematodes *C. sinensis* and *M yokogawai.* The assays reportedly exhibit 100% sensitivity and 100% specificity.

Polymerase chain reaction–restriction fragment length polymorphism (PCR-RFLP) and simple sequence repeat anchored PCR have been reported to be useful in distinguishing species of the *Metagonimus* genus (including *M. yokogawai*). Information derived from RFLP involving specific sites in ribosomal RNA and mitochondrial cytochrome oxidase I (mtCOI) genes may help to differentiate *M. yokogawai* from other Metagonimus species. Six members of the *Heterophyidae* family can be distinguished with PCR assays based on variations in rDNA polymorphisms among the species.

Treatment

The drug of choice for treatment of intestinal trematode infection is praziquantel, an isoquinoline derivative administered orally in three doses for 1 day. There may be some mild side effects, but these usually disappear within 48 hours and may be more severe in those with heavy infections. An alternative drug is niclosamide and is administered for 1 to 2 days.

ⓔ Visit the Evolve site for a complete list of procedures, review questions, and case studies.

Bibliography

Bennett J, Dolin R, Blaser M: *Principles and practice of infectious diseases,* ed 9, Philadelphia, 2020, Elsevier-Saunders.

Bogitsch BJ, Carter CE, Oeltmann TN, editors: *Human parasitology,* ed 3, San Diego, 2005, Academic Press.

Caroll KC, Pfaller MA: *Manual of clinical microbiology,* ed 12, Washington, DC, 2019, ASM Press.

Chai JY, Jung BK: Fishborne zoonotic heterophyid infections: an update, *Food Waterborne Parasitol* 8–9:33–63, 2017.

Chai JY: Echinostomes in humans. In Bernard F, Rafael T, editors: *The biology of echinostomes: from the molecule to the community,* New York, 2009, Springer, pp 147–183.

Chai JY, Shin EH, Lee SH, Rim HJ: Foodborne intestinal flukes in Southeast Asia, *Korean J Parasitol* 47(Suppl):S69–S102, 2009. https://doi.org/10.3347/kjp.2009.47.S.S69.

Chai JY, Sohn WM, Cho J, et al.: *Echinostoma ilocanum* infection in two residents of Savannakhet Province, Lao PDR, *Korean J Parasitol* 56(1):75–79, 2018. https://doi.org/10.3347/kjp.2018.56.1.75.

Dzikowski R, Levy MG, Poore MF, Flowers JR, Paperna I: Use of rDNA polymorphism for identification of heterophyidae infecting freshwater fishes, *Dis Aquat Organ* 59(1):35–41, 2004.

Dada-Adegbola HO, Falade CO, Oluwatoba OA, et al.: *Gastrodiscoides hominis* infection in a Nigerian-case report, *West Afr J Med* 23(2):185–186, 2004.

Fried B, Graczyk TK, Tamang L: Food-borne intestinal trematodiases in humans, *Parasitol Res* 93:159–170, 2004.

Garcia LS: *Diagnostic medical parasitology,* ed 6, Washington, DC, 2016, ASM Press.

Han ET, Shin EH, Phommakorn S, et al.: *Centrocestus formosanus (Digenea: heterophyidae)* encysted in the freshwater fish, *Puntius brevis,* from Lao PDR, *Korean J Parasitol* 46(1):49–53, 2008.

Jeon HK, Lee D, Park H, et al.: Human infections with liver and minute intestinal flukes in Guangxi, China: analysis by DNA sequencing, ultrasonography, and immunoaffinity chromatography, *Korean J Parasitol* 50(4):391–394, 2012.

John DT, Petri WA: *Markell's and Voge's medical parasitology,* ed 9, St Louis, 2006, Elsevier.

Kajugu PE, Hanna RE, Edgar HW, et al.: *Fasciola hepatica:* specificity of a coproantigen ELISA test for diagnosis of fasciolosis in faecal samples from cattle and sheep concurrently infected with gastrointestinal nematodes, coccidians and/or rumen flukes (paramphistomes), under field conditions, *Vet Parasitol* 212(3–4):181–187, 2015.

Keiser J, Utzinger J: Food-borne trematodiases, *Clin Microbiol Rev* 22:466–483, 2009.

Kumchoo K, Wongsawad C, Vanittanakom P, Chai JY, Rojanapaibul A: Effect of niclosamide on the tegumental surface of *Haplorchis taichui* using scanning electron microscopy, *J Helminthol* 81(4):329–337, 2007.

Lee SH, Hwang SW, Chai JY, et al.: Comparative morphology of eggs of heterophyids and *Clonorchis sinensis* causing human infections in Korea, *Korean J Parasitol* 22(2):171–180, 1984.

Lovis L, Mak TK, Phongluxa K, et al.: PCR diagnosis of opisthorchis viverrini and haplorchis taichui infections in a Lao community in an area of endemicity and comparison of diagnostic methods for parasitological field surveys, *J Clin Microbiol* 47(5):1517–1523, 2009.

Quang TD, Duong TH, Richard-Lenoble D, et al.: [Emergence in humans of fascioliasis (from *Fasciola gigantica*) and intestinal distomatosis (from *Fasciolopsis buski*) in Laos], *Sante* 18(3):119–124, 2008.

Won EJ, Kim SH, Kee SJ, et al.: Multiplex real-time PCR assay targeting eight parasites customized to the Korean population: potential use for detection in diarrheal stool samples from gastroenteritis patients, *PloS One* 11(11):e0166957, 2016.

Yang HJ, Guk SM, Han ET, et al.: Molecular differentiation of three species of *Metagonimus* by simple sequence repeat anchored polymerase chain reaction (SSR-PCR) amplification, *J Parasitol* 86(5):1170–1172, 2000.

Yu JR, Chai JY: *Metagonimus*. In Liu D, editor: *Molecular detection of foodborne pathogens*, Boca Raton, FL, 2010, CRC Press, pp 805–812.

56

Liver and Lung Trematodes

OBJECTIVES

1. List the clinically significant trematodes capable of infecting the liver and lungs.
2. Describe the general life cycle of the liver and lung flukes and identify the infective stage for humans.
3. Describe the diagnostic methods used to identify the liver and lung flukes, including the microscopic differentiation of eggs and serologic methods.
4. Describe the pathogenesis of the liver and lung flukes, including location and associated disease manifestations.
5. List the drug of choice for infections with liver and lung flukes.
6. Describe the transmission of the liver and lung flukes and discuss how infection may be prevented.

PARASITES TO BE CONSIDERED

Trematodes (Flukes)

Liver/Lung
Clonorchis sinensis
Opisthorchis felineus
Opisthorchis viverrini
Fasciola gigantica
Fasciola hepatica
Paragonimus africanus
Paragonimus caliensis
Paragonimus heterotremus
Paragonimus kellicotti
Paragonimus mexicanus
Paragonimus miyazakii
Paragonimus skrjabini
Paragonimus uterobilateralis
Paragonimus westermani

The parasites within this chapter are typically food-borne and may have serious economic implications. *Clonorchis* spp., *Opisthorchis* spp., and *Fasciola* spp. live in the biliary ducts of humans. *Paragonimus* spp. are found in the lungs and in other body sites.

The Liver Flukes

General Characteristics

The adults of these trematodes live in the biliary ducts and may be found in the gallbladder in heavy infections. Three of these, *Clonorchis sinensis* (the Chinese liver fluke),

Opisthorchis felineus, and *Opisthorchis viverrini* (the Southeast Asian liver fluke), are elongated and narrow and much smaller than *Fasciola* (the sheep liver fluke). These flukes also all require a freshwater snail as an intermediate host.

Epidemiology and Life Cycle

C. sinensis is distributed throughout China, Japan, Korea, Taiwan, and Vietnam. *O. viverrini* is found in Cambodia, Laos, Thailand, and Vietnam, and *O. felineus* is found in Northern Europe and Asia. Reservoir hosts include dogs and cats. *Fasciola* spp. cause very similar disease, differing primarily in geographic distribution, with *F. hepatica* occurring in Europe and North and South America, and *F. gigantica* in Asia and Africa. *Fasciola* spp. affect the economics of the sheep and cattle industries. Reservoir hosts include dogs, hogs, cats, martens, badgers, minks, weasels, pigs, equines, and rats. Infected feces enter the water system because of improper drainage and unsanitary practices.

The life cycle of the liver flukes is very similar to that of the intestinal flukes. The adult worms produce eggs in the biliary ducts that are then excreted from the body in the feces. The free-swimming miracidium is released from the egg in fresh water and enters the snail host, where it develops into a redia and then cercariae, which leaves the snail and enters the water (Fig. 56.1). The cercariae of *Clonorchis* and *Opisthorchis* are ingested by a second intermediate host, a freshwater fish. The cercariae then encyst and develop into the metacercariae within the intermediate host. The metacercaria is the infective stage for humans. When infected freshwater fish are eaten raw or undercooked, the metacercariae will excyst in the duodenum and then travel to the bile duct, where they mature. The cercariae of *Fasciola* encyst on freshwater vegetation, such as watercress and water chestnuts, and develop into metacercariae. When the infected vegetation is eaten raw, the metacercariae will excyst in the duodenum and then travel to the bile duct and mature. Fig. 56.2 depicts the general life cycles of the liver and lung flukes.

Pathogenesis and Spectrum of Disease

Light infections with *C. sinensis* or *Opisthorchis* spp. are most common and may be asymptomatic. Heavier infections with these flukes may present with fever, abdominal pain, and jaundice. Eosinophilia and increased serum levels of immunoglobulin E (IgE) may occur. Severe infections may cause obstruction of the biliary ducts, resulting in enlargement and tenderness of the liver, cirrhosis, cholecystitis (inflammation of the gallbladder), and cholangiocarcinoma (cancerous growth in bile duct epithelium).

Even light infections with *Fasciola* may cause fever, abdominal pain, nausea, diarrhea, enlargement and tenderness of the liver, jaundice, nonproductive cough, eosinophilia, and elevated serum IgE levels. Leukocytosis, eosinophilia and mild to moderate anemia may also be present. More severe infections may result in obstruction of the biliary ducts, cirrhosis, cholecystitis, and cholangiocarcinoma. During migration in the human body, the larvae may penetrate the peritoneal cavity, and adult flukes may be found in the intestinal walls, lungs, heart, or brain. Many symptoms of infection disappear when the parasite has lodged in the biliary passages resulting in chronic infection. The chronic phase presents with liver abnormalities and eosinophilia. In chronic infections, worms have been identified in the intestinal wall, brain, heart, lungs, and skin.

Laboratory Diagnosis

Identification of the liver flukes is primarily made by recovery of the eggs in feces using a sedimentation method and a wet mount with or without iodine staining.

The adult worms of *Clonorchis* are elongated and narrow and a transparent reddish-yellow color. Adult *Clonorchis* may vary in size from 10 to 25 mm × 3 to 5 mm. The eggs

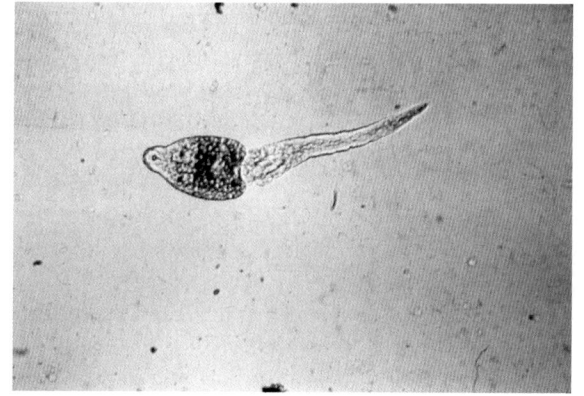

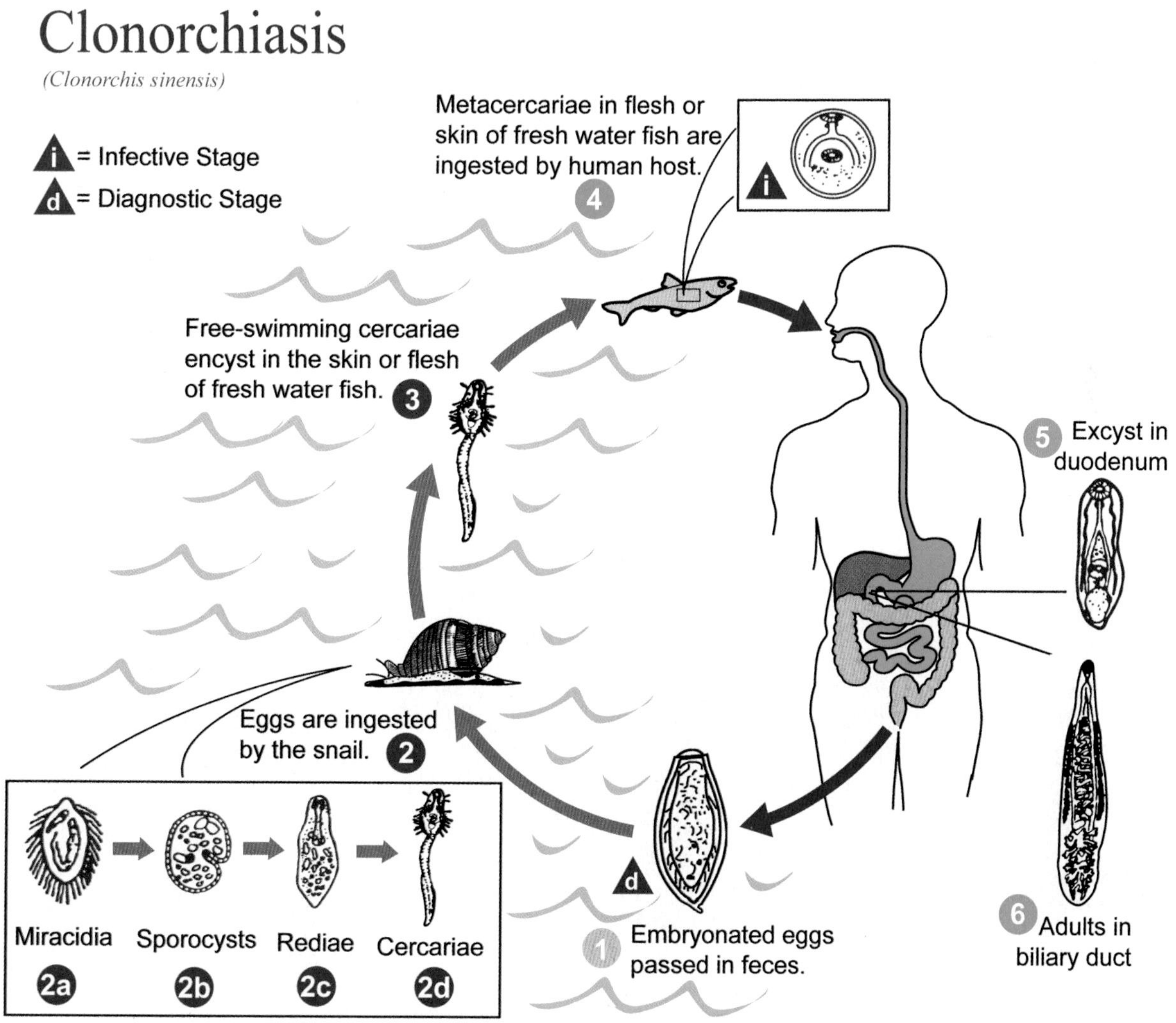

• **Fig. 56.1** Cercaria of a liver fluke. (Photo courtesy Dr. Henry Travers, Sioux Falls, SD.)

Clonorchiasis
(Clonorchis sinensis)

i = Infective Stage

d = Diagnostic Stage

Metacercariae in flesh or skin of fresh water fish are ingested by human host. **4**

Free-swimming cercariae encyst in the skin or flesh of fresh water fish. **3**

5 Excyst in duodenum

Eggs are ingested by the snail. **2**

Miracidia **2a** Sporocysts **2b** Rediae **2c** Cercariae **2d**

d Embryonated eggs passed in feces. **1**

6 Adults in biliary duct

• **Fig. 56.2** Life cycle of the trematode, *Clonorchis sinensis,* the causal agent of clonorchiasis. (Courtesy Division of Parasitic Diseases/Centers for Disease Control and Prevention.)

of *Clonorchis* are 28 to 30 μm × 14 to 18 μm. The eggs have shouldered opercula and a small knob at the end opposite the operculum, are yellow-brown in color, and are embryonated when they leave the body (Fig. 56.3A). Diagnosis is based on microscopic identification of eggs in stool specimens. However, the eggs of *Clonorchis* are practically indistinguishable from those of *Opisthorchis*. The adult fluke can also be surgically recovered.

Like *Clonorchis,* the adult worms of *Opisthorchis* are elongated and narrow and a transparent reddish-yellow color. Adult worms of *Opisthorchis,* however, are much smaller: 5 to 10 mm × 0.8 to 1.9 mm. The adult worm of *O. felineus* is lancet-shaped and is larger than *O. viverrini*. The size of *Opisthorchis* eggs is slightly smaller than *Clonorchis; Opisthorchis* eggs are 19 to 29 μm × 12 to 17 μm. Also like *Clonorchis,* the eggs have shouldered opercula and a small knob at the end opposite the operculum, are yellow-brown in color, and are embryonated when they leave the body (Fig. 56.3). Diagnosis is made by detecting eggs in a duodenal aspirate (bile fluid), the recovery of adult worms, or by clinical history. Eggs are not excreted in patients with biliary obstruction, requiring needle aspiration, surgery, or an autopsy specimen for confirmation.

The adult worm of *Fasciola* is much larger (2 to 5 cm × 0.8 to 1.3 cm) (Fig. 56.3C), with a cephalic cone at the anterior end, that contains the oral sucker. The adult fluke of *F. gigantica* is similar to *F. hepatica*; however, it is somewhat more lancet-shaped and has a less distinct cephalic cone. The eggs are 130 to 150 μm × 70 to 90 μm, operculated, brownish-yellow, and unembryonated when they leave the body. The eggs of *F. gigantica* tend to be somewhat larger (160 to 190 μm by 70 to 90 μm). Because the eggs of *Fasciola* spp. and *Fasciolopsis* are virtually indistinguishable, it may also be necessary to recover eggs from bile specimens or to recover adult worms. The diagnosis of *F. gigantica* is the same as *F. hepatica*; however, eggs may even be less likely to be identified in the stool of infected patients. Definitive identification of *Fasciola* is important, because the treatment is different from that for *Fasciolopsis*. Fig. 55.3 shows the eggs of *Fasciola hepatica,* and Fig. 55.2 is a *Fasciolopsis buski* adult fluke.

Serologic Testing

C. sinensis and *O. viverrini* infections elicit a strong immune response. IgE levels are elevated in infections, and IgM is detectable in acute infections, followed by an increase in IgA and IgG. In chronic infections, the IgA level returns to normal, but IgG and IgM remain elevated. Serological diagnosis has been successful for *C. sinensis*; using ELISA is sensitive and demonstrates low cross-reactivity to related organisms. However, this means of diagnosis is not available for *O. viverrini* due to a lack of standardization and false-positive results; this is caused by cross-reactivity with other parasitic diseases. ELISA has been successful using excretory and secretory antigens from adult worms of *O. felineus* cultivated *in vivo*.

Serologic testing is available for the diagnosis of *Fasciola* spp. Serologic testing can be useful in the acute phase of infection because specific antibodies to *Fasciola* may become detectable 2 to 4 weeks following infection, whereas egg production typically is not apparent until 3 to 4 months after exposure. Serologic testing can also be of value for cases of chronic *Fasciola* infection in persons with low-level or sporadic egg production, as well as in persons with ectopic infection. It may also help rule out pseudofascioliasis associated with ingestion of parasite eggs in sheep or beef liver.

The immune diagnosis of human *F. hepatica* infection includes an enzyme immunoassay (EIA) with excretory-secretory (ES) or recombinant antigens and confirmatory testing of EIA-positive specimens with an immunoblot assay. Enzyme-linked immunosorbent assay (ELISA) serum IgG antibody testing may demonstrate cross-reactivity with other trematodes, such as the schistosomes.

Nucleic Acid Detection

A variety of PCR-based methods including loop-mediated isothermal amplification (LAMP) have been developed for the detection of the liver flukes, including *F. hepatica*. These

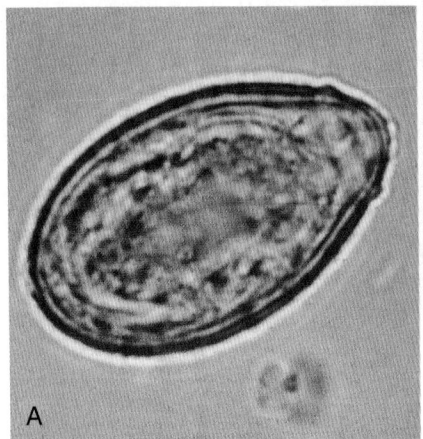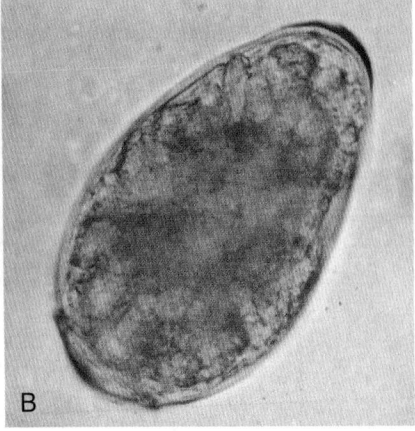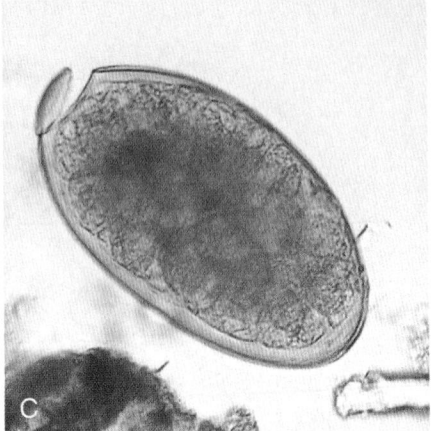

• **Fig. 56.3** Trematode eggs. (A) *Clonorchis sinensis*. (B) *Paragonimus westermani*. (C) *Fasciola hepatica* (note the partially open operculum). (From Centers for Disease Control and Prevention. DPDx-Laboratory Identification of Parasitic Diseases of Public Health Concern.)

methods demonstrate a high sensitivity and specificity for the diagnosis of *F. hepatica* infection in comparison to routine fecal and indirect serological tests. The LAMP detects DNA of *C. sinensis* and *O. viverrini* in freshwater snails, the second intermediate fish hosts, and patient feces. In human fecal samples, LAMP-based technology detects *C. sinensis* in human infection with as low as 1 egg per 100 mg of feces. Further evaluation of the LAMP-based diagnosis test showed a sensitivity of 97.1% and specificity of 100%.

Similar LAMP assays are also available for *O. viverrini*, with the variation of sensitivity and specificity relating to the repetition of different target genes when detecting DNA. A multiplex PCR assay has been used to detect *C. sinensis* and *Opisthorchis* in fish and infected patients in endemic areas. A single-step duplex real-time fluorescence resonance energy transfer (FRET) real-time PCR has been developed to diagnose and differentiate *C. sinensis* and *Opisthorchis* infections in human fecal samples. The assay differentiates the two species with 100% specificity and sensitivity. Despite the clinical utility of nucleic acid methods for the detection of the liver flukes, they are not generally available in routine laboratories, even in endemic regions.

Therapy and Prevention

The drug of choice for treatment of infections with *Clonorchis* and *Opisthorchis* is praziquantel (25 mg/kg) given orally three times per day for 2 days. The drug of choice for the treatment of *Fasciola* spp. is triclabendazole (praziquantel is not as effective). Infections with *Opisthorchis* often require additional treatment with antibiotics due to secondary bacterial infections.

Human infection can be prevented by ensuring that fish and aquatic vegetation are properly cooked before consumption, as well as by the improvement of sanitary conditions, along with good personal hygiene.

The Lung Flukes

General Characteristics

The genus *Paragonimus* contains approximately 15 species known to infect humans. *Paragonimus westermani* is the most common and widely distributed lung fluke. *P. mexicanus* is located in Central and South America, and *P. kellicotti* is found in North and South America. Both are important human pathogens. The adult worms live in the lungs and produce eggs that may be present in sputum, or if expectorated and swallowed may be present in feces. Like other trematodes, a freshwater snail is required as an intermediate host.

Epidemiology and Life Cycle

Paragonimiasis is found primarily in the Far East, in India, the Philippines, China, Japan, Korea, Manchuria, Papua New Guinea, and Southeast Asia, following ingestion of uncooked crabs, crayfish, freshwater shrimp, mussels, and

paratenic hosts. Reservoir hosts for *P. westermani* include dogs and cats, and those for *P. mexicanus* include domestic and wild pigs, dogs, and rodents. Species of *Paragonimus* may also be found in other freshwater crab- or crayfish-eating mammals. *P. kellicotti* is becoming an increasing concern in the United States. It is widely distributed throughout North America and is found in cats, dogs, bobcats, raccoons, foxes, skunks, minks, and coyotes. Transmission in the United States is associated with behavioral activities that include alcohol consumption, dares, and the demonstration of outside survival skills.

The adult worms, encapsulated in the lungs, produce eggs that leave the lung via the bronchioles, stimulating a cough response. The eggs are swallowed and eventually excreted in the feces. Egg size varies with species from approximately 80 to 120 μm long and 45 to 70 μm wide (Fig. 56.3B). The free-swimming miracidium is released from the egg in fresh water and enters the snail host, where it develops into a redia and then cercariae, which leaves the snail and enters the water. The cercariae then enter a second intermediate host, a crab or crayfish, where they encyst and develop into metacercariae. The metacercaria is the infective stage for humans. When infected freshwater crabs and crayfish are eaten raw or undercooked, the metacercariae will excyst in the duodenum and then migrate through the intestinal wall, and eventually through the diaphragm and into the lungs where they encapsulate (usually in pairs) and mature (Fig. 56.2).

Pathogenesis and Spectrum of Disease

Light infections may be asymptomatic. The migration of the metacercariae through muscle and tissue may cause local pain and an immune response to the tissue damage. In the lungs, the immune response causes infiltration of eosinophils and neutrophils. Serum IgE levels are usually elevated. Eventually the adult worms are encapsulated in a granuloma. Presence of the worms in the lungs usually results in a chronic cough, with possible production of blood-tinged sputum. The cough provides a mechanism to transport eggs up into the throat, where they are swallowed and then may be excreted in the feces. The larvae of *P. mexicanus*, *P. skrjabini*, *P. heterotremus*, and *P. hueitungensis* may migrate to other areas of the body, commonly causing subcutaneous or lower abdominal nodules to form. The larvae of *Paragonimus* may enter other sites such as the liver, intestinal wall, muscles, peritoneum, and the brain, where they can cause severe damage. These ectopic infections are generally associated with *P. heterotremus*, *P. mexicanus*, and *P. westermani*. Computed tomography (CT) and magnetic resonance imaging (MRI) may be used to reveal cysts with edema, migration tracks, and nodules in various areas of the body including the brain, liver, and lungs.

Laboratory Diagnosis

The adult worms of *Paragonimus* vary in size, 10 to 25 mm × 3 to 5 mm, and are a reddish-brown color. The eggs of *P. westermani* measure 80 to 120 μm × 45 to 60 μm, and those of *P. mexicanus* are approximately 80 μm × 40 μm. The eggs are unembryonated when they leave the body, operculated with opercular shoulders, thick-shelled, and brownish-yellow. The eggs of *Paragonimus* are similar to those of *Diphyllobothrium* (freshwater fish tapeworm) and can be differentiated by the operculum, opercular shoulders, and thickened shell at the end opposite the operculum.

Paragonimus eggs may be recovered from sputum, pleural effusions, and occasionally in feces using a sedimentation concentration method. The eggs may be observed in a wet mount (with or without iodine stain) (Fig. 56.4). **Charcot-Leyden crystals** may also be observed in sputum or lung tissue specimens. Charcot-Leyden crystals are slender and pointed at both ends. The crystals normally appear colorless and stain purplish to red with trichrome. Elevated levels of eosinophils may be present in whole blood, and elevated IgE levels may be present in serum. Lesions in the lungs may be observed by x-ray.

Serologic Testing

Serologic testing is available in the United States for the diagnosis of *P. westermani* and *P. kellicotti*. EIA tests and immunoblot (IB) assays and hemagglutination tests can be used to diagnose active infections. Antibody levels detected by EIA and IB do decline after chemotherapy and death of the worms. Pleural effusion samples are more suitable for the detection of antibodies than serum. The Division of Parasitic Disease at the Centers for Disease Control and Prevention (CDC) performs serum IgG EIA and immunoblot testing. Cross-reactivity with other species and trematodes may occur.

Nucleic Acid Detection

The conventional immunological diagnosis is sensitive in human paragonimiasis but unsustainable in epidemiological surveys. A LAMP assay has successfully amplified the gene sequence of *P. westermani* eggs in sputum and pleural fluid from patients, as well as metacercariae in freshwater crabs and crayfish. LAMP demonstrates a detection limit of 1 ×

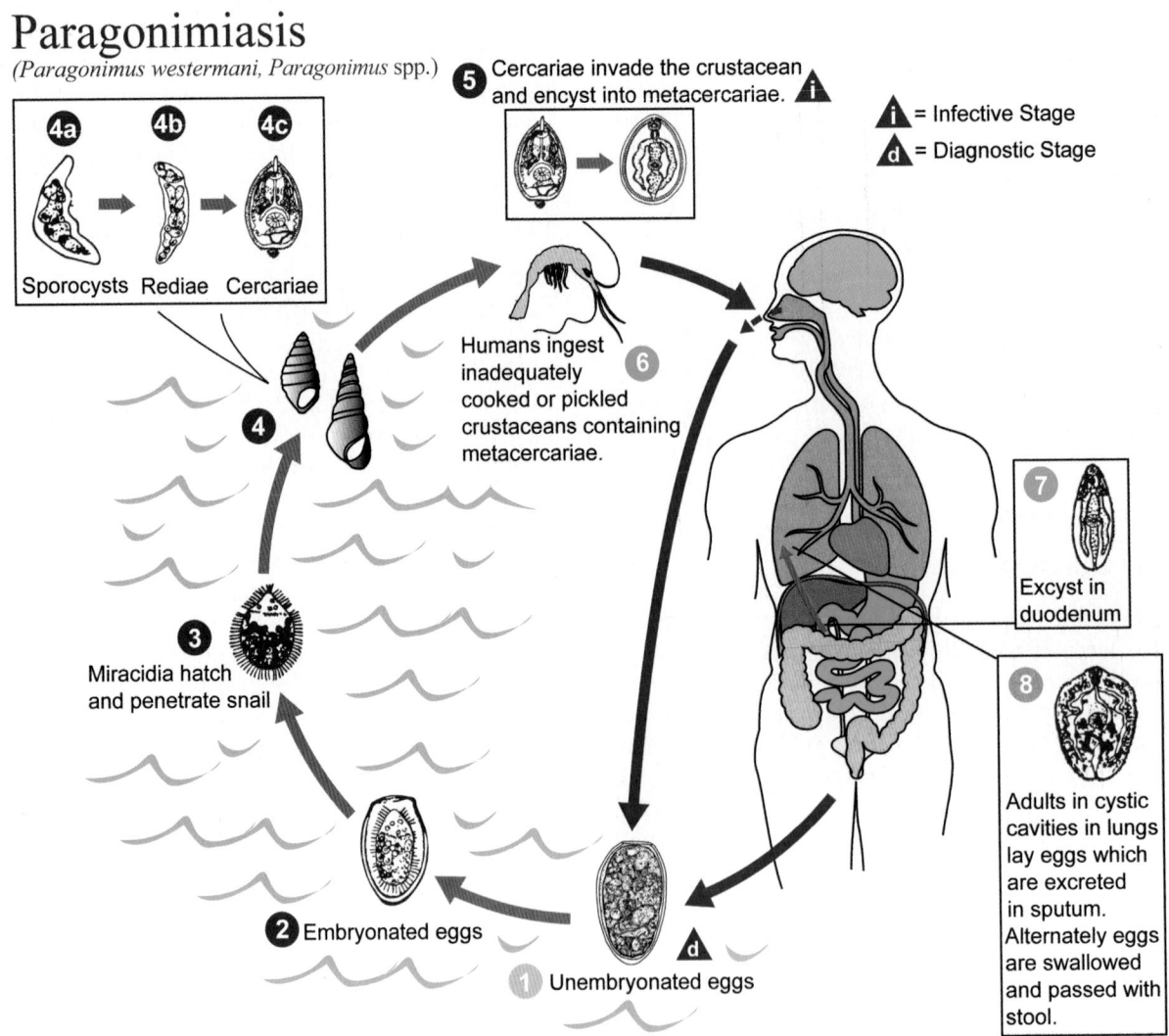

Paragonimiasis
(*Paragonimus westermani, Paragonimus* spp.)

5 Cercariae invade the crustacean and encyst into metacercariae. **i**

i = Infective Stage
d = Diagnostic Stage

4a **4b** **4c**
Sporocysts Rediae Cercariae

Humans ingest inadequately cooked or pickled crustaceans containing metacercariae.

6

7 Excyst in duodenum

4

3 Miracidia hatch and penetrate snail

8 Adults in cystic cavities in lungs lay eggs which are excreted in sputum. Alternately eggs are swallowed and passed with stool.

2 Embryonated eggs

1 Unembryonated eggs **d**

• **Fig. 56.4** Life cycle of the trematode, *Paragonimus westermani*, the causal agent of paragonimiasis. (Courtesy Division of Parasitic Diseases/Centers for Disease Control and Prevention.)

10^{-8} ng/μL, approximately 100 times more sensitive than PCR. The LAMP method also yields positive and negative results coinciding with those from parasitology tests, making it an excellent candidate for field surveys and clinical diagnoses of paragonimiasis.

Treatment and Prevention

The drug of choice for treatment of *Paragonimus* infections is praziquantel given three times a day for 2 to 3 consecutive days. Triclabendazole in a single- or two-dose regimen is also effective but is not available in the United States.

Human infection can be prevented by not eating pickled, raw, or undercooked crabs or crayfish. Crustaceans should be cooked to an internal temperature of 145°F. Care should also be taken to properly clean utensils used in the preparation of these foods. Improvement of sanitary conditions and practices may also help to reduce the prevalence of these infections.

Ⓔ Visit the Evolve site for a complete list of procedures, review questions, and case studies.

Bibliography

Bogitsch BJ, Carter CE, Oeltmann TN, editors: *Human parasitology*, ed 3, San Diego, 2005, Academic Press.

Carroll KC, Pfaller MA, Landry ML, et al.: *Manual of clinical microbiology*, ed 12, Washington, DC, 2019, ASM.

Deng MH, Zhong LY, Kamolnetr O, et al.: Detection of helminths by loop-mediated isothermal amplification assay: a review of updated technology and future outlook, *Infect Dis Poverty* 8(1):20, 2019.

Fried B, Abruzzi A: Food-borne trematode infections of humans in the United States, *Parasitol Res* 106:1263–1280, 2010.

Garcia LS: *Diagnostic medical parasitology*, ed 6, Washington, DC, 2016, ASM Press.

John DT, Petri WA: *Markell's and Voge's medical parasitology*, ed 9, St Louis, MO, 2006, Saunders.

Keiser J, Utzinger J: Food-borne trematodiases, *Clin Microbiol Rev* 22:466–483, 2009.

Shin SH, Hsu A, Chastain HM, et al.: Development of two FhSAP2 recombinant–based assays for immunodiagnosis of human chronic fascioliasis, *Am J Trop Med Hyg* 95(4):852–855, 2016.

Slemenda SB, Maddison SE, Jong EC, et al.: Diagnosis of paragonimiasis by immunoblot, *Am J Trop Med Hyg* 39:469–471, 1988.

Zarrin-Khameh N, Citron DR, Stager CE, et al.: Pulmonary paragonimiasis diagnosed by fine-needle aspiration biopsy, *J Clin Microbiol* 46:2137–2140, 2008.

57

Blood Trematodes

OBJECTIVES

1. List the clinically significant blood trematodes.
2. Describe the general life cycle of the blood trematodes and how human infection occurs.
3. Explain the diagnostic methods used to identify blood trematodes.
4. Differentiate the eggs of the five species of schistosomes.
5. Describe the pathogenesis of the blood trematodes.
6. List the drugs of choice for treatment of blood trematode infections.
7. Describe the natural habitat for blood trematodes and how infection may be prevented.

PARASITES TO BE CONSIDERED

Trematodes

Blood

Schistosoma guineensis
Schistosoma haematobium
Schistosoma intercalatum
Schistosoma japonicum
Schistosoma malayensis
Schistosoma mansoni
Schistosoma mattheei
Schistosoma mekongi
Schistosoma spp.

There are five main species of blood flukes that are primarily associated with disease in humans (known as **schistosomiasis, bilharziasis,** or snail fever), all belonging to the genus *Schistosoma*. These species are *Schistosoma haematobium, Schistosoma mekongi, Schistosoma intercalatum, Schistosoma japonicum* (Oriental blood fluke), and *Schistosoma mansoni*. Seven additional species are rarely associated with human infection and have limited geographic distribution. The blood flukes differ in morphology and life cycle characteristics from the other trematodes. They are similar, however, by requiring a freshwater snail as the intermediate host.

General Characteristics

Unlike the other trematodes, adult schistosomes are not flattened, but are rather long, thin, and rounded in shape. There is an oral sucker surrounding the mouth and a ventral sucker located just slightly below the oral sucker. The adult

male averages 1.5 cm in length and is wider than the female, having a ventral fold that wraps around the female when they mate (Fig. 57.1). The adult female averages 2 cm in length and is very thin.

The eggs of each species are distinct and can be distinguished by size, spine morphology, and sometimes specimen type (Fig. 57.2). The size range for eggs of *S. haematobium* is 110 to 170 μm long by 40 to 70 μm wide, and they have a sharply pointed terminal spine. They are fully embryonated without an operculum. The size range for the eggs of *S. japonicum* is 70 to 100 μm long by 50 to 65 μm wide, and they have a small lateral spine that is sometimes difficult to detect (Fig. 57.3). *S. mekongi* eggs are smaller than those of *S. japonicum*, ranging in size from 50 to 65 μm long by 30 to 55 μm wide. They are fully embryonated without an operculum and have a small lateral spine. The size range for eggs of *S. mansoni* is 115 to 180 μm long by 40 to 75 μm wide, and they have a large lateral spine. *S. mansoni* eggs are inoperculate, immature when released, and take up to 8 to 10 days to develop a miracidium. *S. intercalatum* eggs are fully embryonated without an operculum, have a terminal spine, and range in size from 140 to 240 μm long by 50 to 85 μm wide. *S. intercalatum* eggs resemble those of *S. haematobium* and can be differentiated by Ziehl-Neelsen acid-fast positivity. In addition, *S. intercalatum* eggs are only found in feces, not in urine specimens. Table 57.1 provides a comparison of the schistosome eggs.

One of the main differences between the schistosomes and other trematodes is that instead of being hermaphroditic, there are separate male and female adult worms. In human infection, the adult worms live in either the veins that supply the intestine (*S. japonicum, S. intercalatum, S. mekongi,* and *S. mansoni*) or the veins that supply the urinary bladder *(S. haematobium)*. The eggs are passed from the body in either feces or urine. To reach the inside of the intestine or bladder, the eggs must penetrate the tissue from the veins. This is accomplished via a spine that is distinctive among the major species. The embryonated egg releases the miracidium. once it reaches fresh water, where it enters the snail host and develops into the infectious cercaria. The free-swimming cercariae are capable of penetrating through human skin and do not encyst on aquatic vegetation or within other aquatic wildlife. The cercariae penetrate host tissue until they reach a vein; then they travel to capillaries near the lungs and then to the portal vein of the liver, where they mature. When they are mature, the adult males pair with females and then travel to veins of either the intestine or the bladder, where eggs are produced.

Epidemiology

Schistosomes have a worldwide distribution from Egypt and China to Africa and the Americas. *S. haematobium* is found in Africa and the Arabian Peninsula and has no reservoir hosts. *S. mansoni* and *S. guineensis* are found in Africa, the Arabian Peninsula, and Brazil. Reservoir hosts include wild rodents and marsupials. *S. japonicum* is found in China,

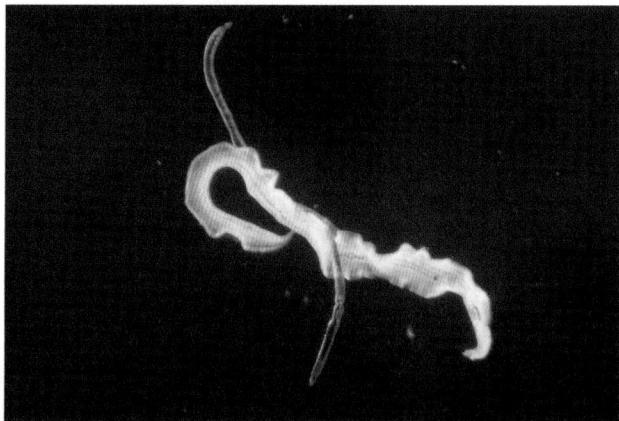

• **Fig. 57.1** This low-power photomicrograph reveals some of the ultrastructural morphology exhibited by coupled male and female *Schistosoma mansoni* parasites. Unlike the flukes, adult schistosomes are either male or female, with the female residing in a gynecophoral canal within the male. Male worms are robust, tuberculate, and measure 6 to 12 mm in length. Females are longer (7 to 17 mm in length) and slender. Adult *S. mansoni* reside in the venous plexuses of the colon and lower ileum and in the portal system of the liver of their host. (Courtesy Division of Parasitic Diseases/Centers for Disease Control and Prevention.)

Indonesia, and the Philippines. Many domestic animals (cats, dogs, cattle, horses, pigs) serve as reservoir hosts, as do some wild animals. *S. mekongi* primarily exists in the lower Mekong River basin in southern Laos, Cambodia, and Thailand. Reservoir hosts include dogs and domestic pigs. *S. intercalatum* and *S. guineensis* are primarily found in central and western Africa. Reservoirs include rodents, marsupials, and nonhuman primates. Human schistosome infection is caused by fecal (and urine) contamination of small bodies of water that favor the growth of the snail hosts. Infection with *S. japonicum* is especially prevalent in areas where humans work in rice paddies.

Reports have indicated that *S. haematobium* is capable of cross-breeding with other species. This phenomenon has been identified between *S. haematobium* and *S. bovis,* as well as between *S. guineensis* and *S. intercalatum.* This is important when considering epidemiology and identification of these parasites

Pathology and Spectrum of Disease

Infection with only a small number of worms may be asymptomatic. A variety of species cause acute toxemic schistosomiasis resembling serum sickness. *S. japonicum* causes significant hepatointestinal disease resulting in portal hypertension and splenic and hepatic enlargement. *S. intercalatum* is primarily associated with rectal schistosomiasis in regions of Africa. *S. haematobium* is the only species that causes urinary schistosomiasis. Quite often, penetration of the skin by cercariae causes localized swelling and itching (cercarial dermatitis). The migration of the larvae through the body may cause transient symptoms of fever, malaise, cough (when they migrate in the lungs), or hepatitis (when in the liver). The adults are able to acquire some host antigens on their outer surface, and so may not elicit an immune response, although the eosinophil count

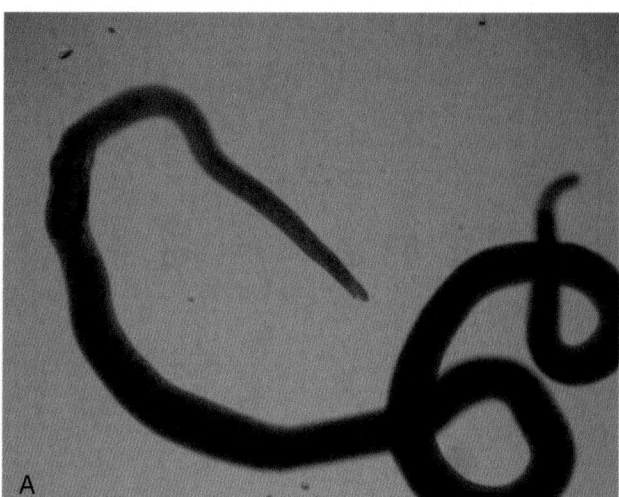
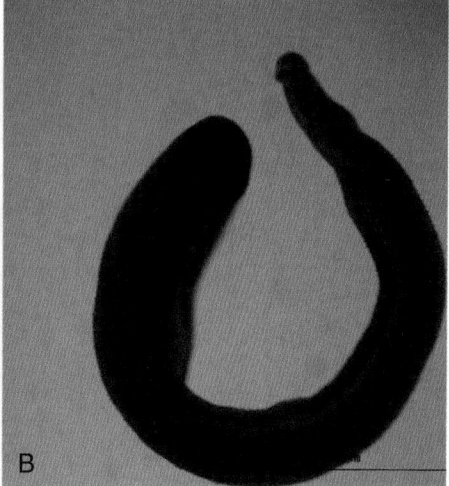

• **Fig. 57.2** (A) *Schistosoma mansoni* adult female; note the long pointed end (400× total magnification). (B) *Schistosoma mansoni* adult male. Males are shorter and wider to accommodate the insertion of the female during copulation. (400× total magnification.)

may be high. Severe tissue damage, with associated pain, fever, and chills, may occur when the eggs travel through tissue to reach the intestines or bladder. There may also be bloody diarrhea or blood in the urine (hematuria). Necrosis, lesions, and granulomas may develop, as well as obstruction of the bowel or ureters. Urinary schistosomiasis may give rise to calcifications in the bladder and renal failure. *S. intercalatum* and *S. guineensis* tend to produce milder symptoms. Eggs are primarily deposited in the colon, resulting in blood and mucus in the stool.

Schistosomiasis

Schistosoma haematobium, S. intercalatum, S. japonicum, S. mansoni, S. mekongi

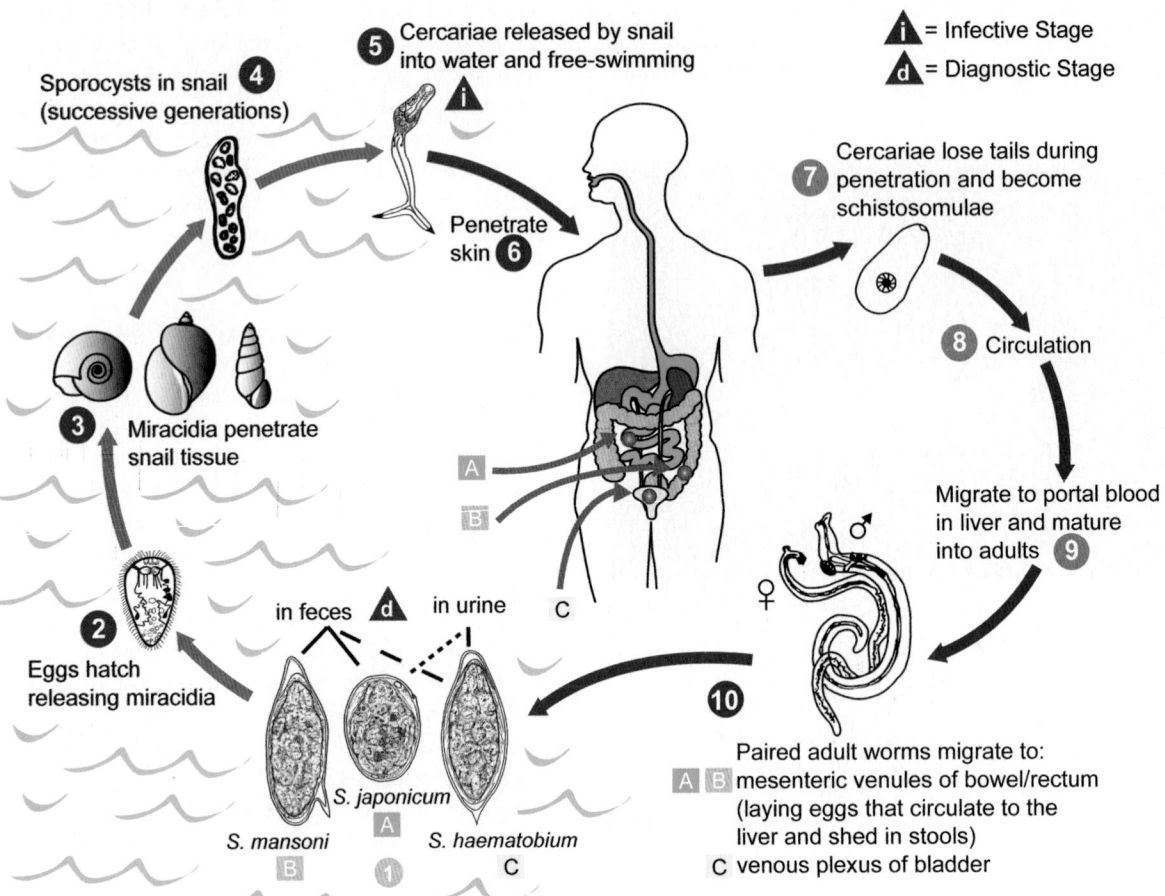

• **Fig. 57.3** This is an illustration depicting the life cycle of flatworms of the genus *Schistosoma*, the causal agents of the parasitic disease schistosomiasis. (Courtesy Division of Parasitic Diseases/Centers for Disease Control and Prevention.)

TABLE 57.1	Diagnostic Characteristics of the Blood Trematodes			
Blood Trematode	**Adult Location**	**Size of Egg**	**Description of Egg**	
Schistosoma haematobium	Veins surrounding bladder	110–170 μm × 40–70 μm	Pointed terminal spine, no operculum, embryonated	
Schistosoma intercalatum/guineensis	Venules of colon	140–240 μm × 50–85 μm	Resembles egg of *S. haematobium,* but acid-fast positive	
Schistosoma japonicum	Venules of small intestine	70–100 μm × 50–65 μm	Small lateral spine, no operculum, embryonated	
Schistosoma mansoni	Venules of large intestine	115–180 μm × 40–75 μm	Large lateral spine, no operculum, embryonated	
Schistosoma mekongi	Venules of small intestine	50–65 μm × 30–55 μm	Resembles egg of *S. mansoni,* but much smaller	

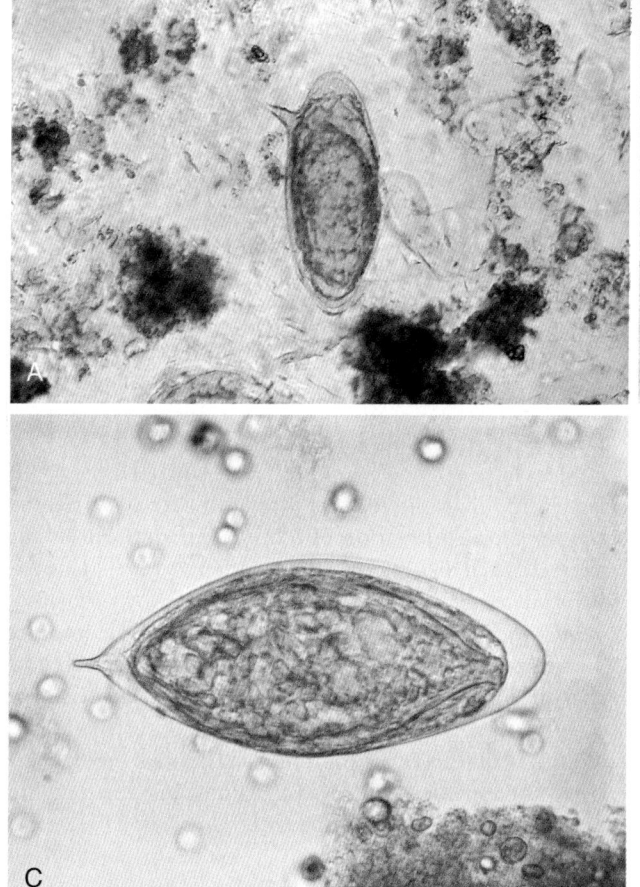

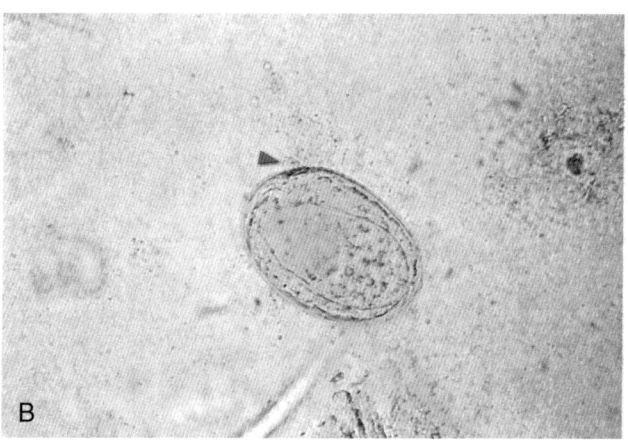

• **Fig. 57.4** (A) *Schistosoma mansoni* egg. (B) *Schistosoma japonicum* egg. The *arrowhead* indicates the presence of the small lateral spine. (C) *Schistosoma haematobium* egg. (Courtesy Division of Parasitic Diseases/Centers for Disease Control and Prevention.)

Penetration of human skin by the cercariae of blood flukes that commonly infect other mammals or aquatic birds may cause a schistosomal dermatitis known as "swimmer's itch." Erythema, edema, and intense itching may develop that usually disappear within 1 week. The cercariae of these species are not able to complete their life cycle by entering the human bloodstream and are destroyed by the host immune system.

Laboratory Diagnosis

The standard method of diagnosis is by the detection of characteristic eggs in feces or rectal biopsy for *S. japonicum, S. mekongi, S. mansoni, S. intercalatum,* and *S. guineensis* (and perhaps *S. haematobium* if these worms have migrated to a bladder vein that is close to the intestine) and in urine (usually concentrated before examination) or bladder tissue biopsy for *S. haematobium.* A wet mount with or without iodine from a sedimentation or concentration method can be examined for eggs. Fig. 57.4A–C provides images of three different schistosome eggs. To optimize recovery of *S. haematobium* in urine, the specimen should be collected between noon and 2 p.m.

Antigen Detection

Two circulating schistosome antigens, the anodic and cathodic antigens, can be detected in the urine of patients with schistosomiasis. A lateral flow rapid detection kit is available for the circulating cathodic antigen and is commercially available. This rapid diagnostic test (RDT) has been used widely in Africa and Brazil but is not FDA approved. Another flow assay is under development for the detection of *S. japonicum* and *S. haematobium.*

Serologic Testing

There are serologic assays that are available for diagnosis of schistosomal IgG antibody (enzyme immunoassay [EIA], enzyme-linked immunosorbent assay [ELISA], and immunoblot), but these methods cannot distinguish between current and previous infections. This type of assay may, however, be useful for travelers who have returned from endemic areas. These assays lack sensitivity and specificity during the early stages of disease, or for detecting persistence of antibodies after treatment for schistosomiasis. These assays are performed at the Division of Parasitic Disease at the Centers for Disease Control and Prevention (CDC) and may be available at some private reference laboratories.

Several nucleic acid–based methods have been developed that demonstrate high sensitivity and specificity using genomic or mitochondrial sequences. In addition, schistosome DNA has been identified in plasma using real-time polymerase chain reaction (PCR). Generally, an etiological method or a simple PCR method cannot distinguish between the species of *Schistosoma*. Repetitive sequences utilizing nested PCR to identify genes located within the parasitic chromosomes aid in detecting schistosomiasis. Various highly repetitive sequences have been successfully used to identify schistosomiasis: *SjR2* for *S. japonicum*, *SM1-7* for *S. mansoni*, and the *Dra I* for *S. haematobium*. In addition, the ribosomal RNA sequences are highly repetitive and conserved in the DNA of schistosomes. Both the 18S and 28S rDNA sequences have been used to detect parasite-derived DNA in fecal, serum, and urine samples in either monoplex or multiplex real-time PCR assays.

Eukaryotic organisms, such as schistosomes, contain mitochondria in their cells. Mitochondria contain their own circular DNA molecule and replicate independently of the cell nucleus in a eukaryotic cell. A novel real-time PCR technique was developed that can identify the nicotinamide adenine dinucleotide hydrogen (NADH) 1 and 2, *nad1* and *nad2*, specific for *S. japonicum*. This method successfully identified *S. japonicum* DNA in human stool samples with low-intensity infections. Another PCR assay has been used to detect the *nad3* in urine samples of patients infected with schistosomes. This approach can accurately differentiate *S. haematobium* from other schistosomes. Additional genes commonly used for identification of *S. japonicum* and *S. mansoni* include *cox2* and *nad6*. A multiplex PCR assay for the cytochrome C oxidase subunit I, *cox1*, of several human schistosomes was developed that can differentiate *S. mansoni*, *S. haematobium*, *S. japonicum*, and *S. mekongi* infections.

Nucleic acid–based tests are highly sensitive and specific; however, costs associated with instrumentation and reagents in endemic areas limit use. Improved methods and tools are needed for broad implementation. Recent reports have shown that loop-mediated isothermal amplification (LAMP), a highly sensitive amplification technique that does not require thermal cycling (and its associated costs and equipment), can detect parasite DNA in a variety of platyhelminth- and nematode-infected hosts, including those with schistosome infections.

Therapy

The drug of choice for treatment of schistosome infections is praziquantel, given in two or three doses daily.

Prevention

Because human infection is through direct penetration by the cercariae, prevention of schistosome infection is more difficult to achieve. Educational programs are required to help people in endemic areas understand how to help prevent infection. Sanitary conditions need to be improved, with proper disposal not only of human waste but also that of domestic animals (in areas with *S. japonicum* and *S. mekongi*). A safe water supply for bathing and washing clothes is also necessary. Various snail control methods have been implemented in endemic regions, but these methods are very costly and would need to be repeated on a regular basis to have the desired effect.

ⓔ Visit the Evolve site for a complete list of procedures, review questions, and case studies.

Bibliography

Bennett J, Dolin R, Blaser M: *Principles and practice of infectious diseases*, ed 9, Philadelphia, 2020, Elsevier-Saunders.

Bogitsch BJ, Carter CE, Oeltmann TN, editors: *Human parasitology*, ed 3, San Diego, 2005, Academic Press.

Carroll KC, Pfaller MA, Landry ML, et al.: *Manual of clinical microbiology*, ed 12, Washington, DC, 2019, ASM.

Garcia LS: *Diagnostic medical parasitology*, ed 6, Washington, DC, 2016, ASM Press.

Gobert GN, Chai M, Duke M, et al.: Copro-PCR-based detection of *Schistoma* eggs using mitochondrial DNA markers, *Mol Cell Probes* 19:250–254, 2005.

Gryseels B, Polman K, Clerinx J, et al.: Human schistosomiasis, *Lancet* 368:1106–1118, 2006.

He P, Song LG, Xie H, et al.: Nucleic acid detection in the diagnosis and prevention of schistosomiasis, *Infect Dis Poverty* 5:25, 2016. https://doi.org/10.1186/s40249-016-0116-y.

John DT, Petri WA: *Markell's and Voge's medical parasitology*, ed 9, St Louis, MO, 2006, Saunders.

Pontes LA, Oliveira MC, Dias-Neto E, et al.: Comparison of a polymerase chain reaction and the Kato-Katz technique for diagnosing infection with *Schistosoma mansoni*, *Am J Trop Med Hyg* 68:652–656, 2003.

Song J, Liu C, Bais S, Mauk MG, Bau HH, Greenberg RM: Molecular detection of schistosome infections with a disposable microfluidic cassette, *PLoS Negl Trop Dis* 9(12):e0004318, 2015. https://doi.org/10.1371/journal.pntd.0004318.

Urbani C, Sinoun M, Socheat D, et al.: Epidemiology and control of *mekongi* schistosomiasis, *Acta Trop* 82:157–168, 2002.

Van Dijk K, Starink MV, Bait A, et al.: The potential of molecular diagnosis of cutaneous ectopic schistosomiases, *Am J Trop Med Hyg* 83:958–959, 2010.

Wichmann D, Panning M, Quack T, et al.: Diagnosing schistosomiasis by detection of cell-free parasite DNA in human plasma, *PLoS Negl Trop Dis* 3:e422, 2009.

Wilson M, Schantz PM, Nutman T, editors: *Molecular and immunological approaches for diagnosis of parasitic infection*, ed 7, Washington, DC, 2006, ASM Press.

58

Overview of Fungal Identification Methods and Strategies

OBJECTIVES

1. Define the terms mycology; saprophytic; dermatophyte; and polymorphic, dimorphic, and thermally dimorphic fungi.
2. Define and differentiate superficial, cutaneous, subcutaneous, and systemic mycoses, including the tissues involved.
3. Differentiate the colonial morphology of yeasts and filamentous fungi (molds).
4. Define and differentiate anamorph, teleomorph, and synanamorph.
5. Describe three ways in which fungi reproduce.
6. List the media used for optimal recovery of fungi, including their incubation requirements.
7. List the common antibacterial agents used in fungal media.
8. Explain and differentiate the characteristic colonial morphology of fungi, including topography (rugose, umbonate, verrucose), texture (cottony, velvety, glabrous, granular, wooly) and surface described (front, reverse).
9. Describe and differentiate the sexual and asexual reproduction of the *Ascomycota*.
10. Define and differentiate rapid, intermediate, and slow growth rates with regard to fungal reproduction and cultivation.
11. Describe the proper method of specimen collection for fungal cultures, including collection site, acceptability, processing, transport, and storage.
12. Give the advantages and disadvantages of using screw-capped culture tubes, compared with agar plates, in the laboratory.
13. Describe the chemical principle and methodologies used to identify fungi, including calcofluor white–potassium hydroxide preparations, hair perforation, cellophane (Scotch) tape preparations, saline/wet mounts, lactophenol cotton or aniline blue, potassium hydroxide, Gram stain, India ink, modified acid-fast stain, periodic acid–Schiff stain (PAS), Wright's stain, Papanicolaou stain, Grocott-Gomori methenamine silver (GMS), hematoxylin and eosin (H&E) stain, Masson-Fontana stain, tease mount, and microslide culture.

Mycology is a specialized discipline in the field of biology concerned with the study of fungi, including their taxonomy, environmental impact, and genetic and biochemical properties. These microorganisms are recognized as important causes of disease, from superficial infections to those that are life threatening and rapidly fatal. Because of the change in patient profiles, particularly the increase in immunocompromised individuals and the increased use of antifungals, a number of fungal species normally found in the environment have been recognized as important causes of human disease. In addition, the implementation of genome-sequencing technology and the ability to identify polymerase chain reaction (PCR)-generated amplicons from nonculturable clinical isolates continually identifies new organisms and increases the understanding of the diversity of fungal infections associated with human disease. It is estimated that more than one billion people worldwide suffer from fungal infections. The modern clinical laboratory, therefore, must provide methods for isolating and identifying the causes of fungal disease. Susceptibility testing of these isolates may also be necessary.

This chapter is designed to assist clinical laboratory professionals and microbiologists with the basics of diagnostic clinical mycology and is not considered inclusive. The field of clinical mycology is rapidly evolving with the implementation of new molecular methods for classification and identification. Therefore, it is often necessary to consult other references for more detailed information within this vast field of study.

Epidemiology

Fungal infections are an increasing threat to individuals. The number of nosocomial, health care–associated, and community-associated infections has increased dramatically. The major factors responsible for the increase in the number of fungal infections are alterations in the host, particularly the growing number of immunocompromised individuals and the increasing use of antifungal medications. Whether associated with the use of antifungal medications, immunosuppressive agents, or serious underlying diseases, these factors may lead to infection by organisms normally nonpathogenic or part of the patient's normal microbiota. These infections may occur in patients with debilitating diseases, such as progressive infection with the human immunodeficiency virus (HIV) or diabetes mellitus or in patients with impaired immunologic function resulting from corticosteroid or antimetabolite chemotherapy. Other common predisposing factors include complex surgical procedures and antibacterial therapy. More than 135,000 valid species of fungi exist, but it is estimated that the number of undiscovered species ranges from 1 to 10 million with about 1000 to 1500 new species identified annually. With the implementation of molecular technology, the number of clinically relevant fungi and pathogenic species will continue to grow. Many of these organisms normally live a **saprophytic** existence (living on dead or decayed organic matter) in nature and persist in the environment.

Fungal infections generally are not communicable in the usual sense, through person-to-person transmission. Humans become accidental hosts for fungi by inhaling spores or through the introduction of fungal elements into tissue by trauma. Except for disease caused by the dimorphic fungi, healthy individuals are relatively resistant to most infections caused by fungi. Classic infections are now appearing in new forms in patients, and the old "harmless" saprophytic molds are implicated in serious diseases. This ability of normally saprophytic fungi to cause disease in patients means that laboratories must be able to identify and report a wide array of fungi.

The primary fungal pathogens appear to have well-defined geographic locations. An example of this is the dimorphic fungi *Coccidioides* spp. *Coccidioides* is usually found only in the Southwest United States in the desert, northern Mexico, and Central America. Opportunistic pathogens such as *Candida* and *Aspergillus* spp. are found all over the world.

General Features of the Fungi

Fungi seen in the clinical laboratory generally can be categorized into two groups based on the appearance of the colonies formed. The **yeasts** are unicellular organisms (Chapter 62) and produce moist, creamy, opaque, or pasty colonies on media, whereas the **filamentous fungi** or **molds** produce multicellular structures (Chapters 59 and 60) and demonstrate fluffy, cottony, woolly, or powdery colonies. Several systemic fungal pathogens that exhibit either a yeast or yeastlike phase and filamentous forms are referred to as **dimorphic.** When dimorphism is temperature-dependent, the fungi are designated as **thermally dimorphic.** In general, these fungi produce a mold form in the environment or when cultured on routine artificial mycology agar at 25°C

to 30°C and are yeastlike in tissue or when cultured on enriched artificial medium at 35°C to 37°C.

The medically important dimorphic fungi are *Histoplasma* sp., *Blastomyces* spp., *Coccidioides* spp., *Cokeromyces recurvatus, Emergomyces* spp., and *Paracoccidioides* spp. Additionally, some of the medically important yeasts, particularly the *Candida* species, may produce yeast forms, pseudohyphae, and/or true hyphae (Chapter 62). Fungi that have more than one independent form or spore stage in their life cycle are called **polymorphic** fungi. The polymorphic features of this group of organisms are not temperature dependent.

Taxonomy of the Fungi

Fungi are composed of a vast array of organisms that are unique compared with plants and animals. They are heterotrophic (saprophytic) and require preformed organic carbon for nutrition. Included among these are the mushrooms, rusts and smuts, molds and mildews, and yeasts. Despite their great variation in morphologic features, most fungi share the following characteristics:

- Chitin in the cell wall
- Ergosterol in the cell membrane
- Reproduction by means of spores, produced asexually or sexually
- Lack of chlorophyll
- Lack of susceptibility to antibacterial antibiotics

Significant changes have resulted in the organization of the groups, taxonomy, and nomenclature within the fungi due to the introduction of molecular methods. Traditionally, the fungi have been categorized based on phenotypic traits, which vary based on temperature, atmospheric conditions, nutrient availability, and humidity, to name a few. Because of this variation, phenotypic classification is unclear, complex, and variable. Molecular analysis of these organisms, which includes extensive DNA sequencing, is now considered the gold standard to determine taxonomic designation and classification. In addition, fungal taxonomy has been complicated by fungi names that describe the sexual (**teleomorph**) or asexual (**anamorph**) stage. This system has become obsolete. The International Botanical Congress adopted a one-fungus, one-name policy, published in the International Code of Nomenclature, Article 59.

The implementation of DNA sequencing for the classification and taxonomy of fungi is not without challenges. As with other microorganisms, fungi have the ability to exchange genetic material and demonstrate evidence of recombination among populations, making speciation difficult. Currently, no standard exists that provides for a definition of the amount of genetic diversity that is allowable, or that limits the species level in taxonomy of fungi. Some clinically relevant fungi have been identified that include **molecular siblings.** A molecular sibling is an organism that cannot be distinguished based on phenotypic, metabolic, and clinical presentation but is recognized as a different

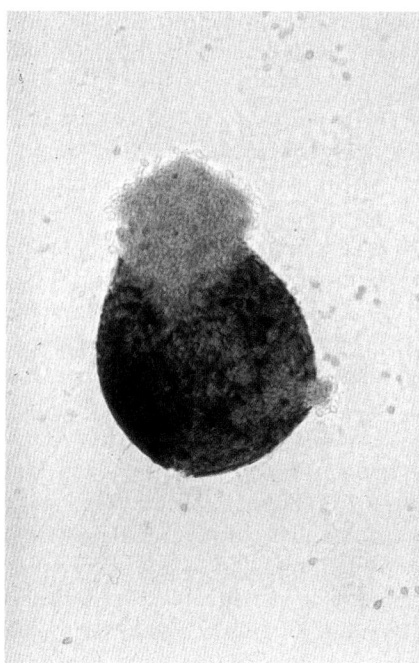

• **Fig. 58.1** A cleistothecium of *Pseudallescheria boydii* that has opened and is releasing numerous ascospores (×750).

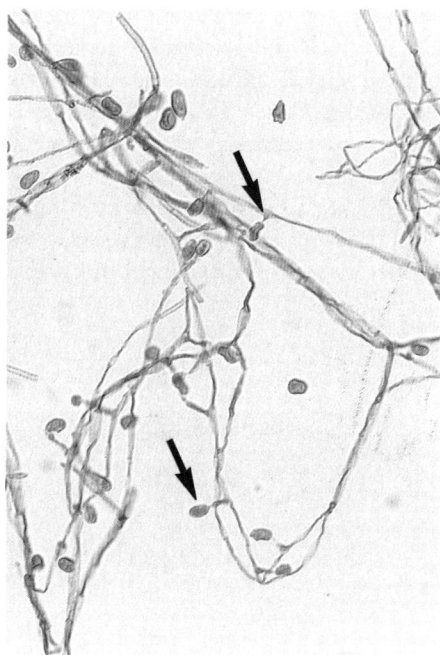

• **Fig. 58.2** *Scedosporium apiospermum* showing asexually produced conidia borne singly on conidiophores (anellophores [arrows]) (×430).

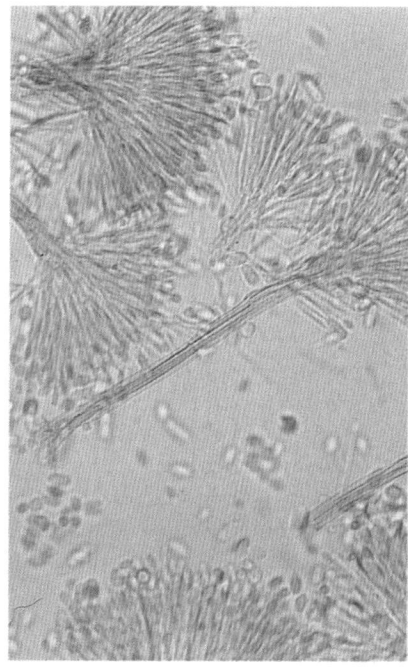

• **Fig. 58.3** Anamorph form of *Pseudallescheria boydii* (×500).

identifications until further studies can be performed on the isolate, including antifungal susceptibility profiles when appropriate.

Historically, the fungi were categorized into three well-established phyla: Zygomycota, Ascomycota, and Basidiomycota. The previous phylum, Zygomycota, contained a very diverse group of organisms. Zygomycota has now been replaced with the subphyla Mucoromycotina and Entomophthoromycotina. The subphyla Mucoromycotina includes the order Mucorales and the genera *Lichtheimia, Mucor, Rhizomucor,* and *Rhizopus*; the Entomophthoromycotina, order Entomophthorales, includes the genera *Basidiobolus* and *Conidiobolus.* These two subphyla include organisms that produce **aseptate** or sparsely **septate hyphae** and exhibit asexual reproduction by **sporangiospores.** Some species may reproduce sexually and form **zygospores** in culture.

The Ascomycota include many fungi that reproduce asexually by the formation of **conidia** (asexual spores) and sexually by the production of **ascospores.** The filamentous ascomycetes are ubiquitous in nature and produce true septate hyphae. They may exhibit a sexual form (teleomorph) but also exist in an asexual form (anamorph) (Figs. 58.1 to 58.3). Fungi that have different asexual forms of the same fungus are called **synanamorphs.** An example of a clinically important fungus that belongs to the phylum Ascomycota is *Histoplasma capsulatum.* Numerous opportunistic fungi such as *Aspergillus,* the atypical fungi, *Pneumocystis,* and yeast such as the *Saccharomyces, Saprochaete,* and *Candida,* also belong to the Ascomycota.

The phylum Basidiomycota includes fungi that reproduce sexually through the formation of **basidiospores** on a specialized structure called the **basidia.** Medically relevant

species based on molecular analysis. Molecular siblings that do not differ in traditional characteristics, including disease presentation, are often considered a **species complex.** The use of the term "complex" does not hold any taxonomic relevance; it provides a system to limit organism identification within the clinical laboratory. Clinical laboratories may choose to report species complexes as preliminary basidiomycetous yeasts include the genera *Cryptococcus, Malassezia, Pseudozyma, Rhodotorula, Sporobolomyces,* and *Trichosporon.* The filamentous Basidiomycetes are uncommon causes of human respiratory and systemic disease in immunocompetent and immunosuppressed patients and are poorly characterized. In addition, several organisms that are pathogenic to humans and have been classified as fungal or parafungal organisms that phenotypically resemble protozoans or yeast and remain unculturable are included in Chapter 61.

Clinical Classification of the Fungi

The complexity associated with the taxonomic classifications of fungi makes the identification of clinically relevant organisms to the species level inherently difficult. For clinicians, dividing the fungi into four categories of mycoses according to the type of infection in combination with macroscopic and microscopic characteristics is used to provide a systematic approach to identification. The clinical categories of fungi are separated as follows:

- **Superficial (cutaneous) mycoses**
- **Subcutaneous mycoses**
- **Systemic mycoses**
- **Opportunistic mycoses**

The superficial, or cutaneous, mycoses are fungal infections that involve hair, skin, or nails without direct invasion of deeper tissue. The fungi in this category include the dermatophytes (agents of ringworm, athlete's foot) and agents of infections such as tinea, tinea nigra, and piedra. All of these infect keratinized tissues.

Some fungi cause infections that are confined to the subcutaneous tissue without dissemination to distant sites.

Examples of subcutaneous infections include chromoblastomycosis, mycetoma, and phaeohyphomycotic cysts (Chapter 60).

Some of the agents of systemic fungal infections include the genera *Blastomyces, Coccidioides, Histoplasma, Cokeromyces, Talaromyces, Sporothrix, Emergomyces,* and *Paracoccidioides.* Infections caused by most of these organisms involve the lungs but also may become widely disseminated and involve any organ system.

Any of the fungi could be considered an opportunistic pathogen in the appropriate clinical setting. The list of uncommon fungi found to cause disease in humans expands every year. Fungi previously thought to be nonpathogenic may be the cause of infections. The infections these organisms cause occur primarily in patients with some type of compromise of the immune system. This may occur secondary to an underlying disease process, such as diabetes mellitus, or prolonged use of an immunosuppressive agent. Although any fungus potentially can cause disease in these patients, the most commonly encountered genera in this group are *Aspergillus, Candida,* and *Cryptococcus,* among others. All of these organisms may cause disseminated (systemic) disease. Some of the dematiaceous fungi may cause deeply invasive phaeohyphomycoses (i.e., produce brown-pigmented structures) in this patient population.

Classification by type of infection allows the clinician to attempt to categorize organisms in a logical fashion into groups by clinical relevance. Table 58.1 presents an example of a classification of infections and their etiologic agents that is useful to clinicians.

The identification of organisms in clinical samples requires examination of the macroscopic and microscopic characteristics of the fungal culture. Although

TABLE 58.1	General Clinical Classification of Pathogenic Fungi		
Cutaneous	**Subcutaneous**	**Opportunistic**	**Systemic**
Superficial mycoses	Chromoblastomycosis	Aspergillosis	Aspergillosis
Tinea	Sporotrichosis	Candidosis	Blastomycosis
Piedra	Mycetoma (eumycotic)	Cryptococcosis	Candidosis
Candidosis	Phaeohyphomycosis	Geotrichosis	Coccidioidomycosis
Dermatophytosis		Mucormycosis	Adiaspiromycosis
		Fusariosis	Emmonsiosis
		Trichosporonosis	Histoplasmosis
		Entomophthoromycosis	Cryptococcosis
		Others[a]	Geotrichosis
			Paracoccidioidomycosis
			Penicilliosis
			Pneumocystosis
			Sporotrichosis
			Pseudoallescheriosis/scedosporiosis
			Mucormycosis
			Entomophthoromycosis
			Fusariosis
			Trichosporonosis

[a]Virtually any fungus may cause disease including systemic infection in a profoundly immunocompromised host.

the macroscopic characteristics may be suggestive of particular genera of fungi, the microscopic characteristics tend to provide a more reliable method for identification. This requires a microscopic examination of the isolate for the appearance of hyphal elements, including the presence, absence, and number of septa. If the hyphae appear to be broad and predominantly **nonseptate** (i.e., cells are not separated by a septum or wall), Mucoromycetes, Basidiobolomycoses, or Entomophthoromycoses should be considered. If the hyphae are septate, they must be examined further for the presence or absence of pigmentation. If a dark pigment is present in the hyphae, the organism is considered to be **melanized** (dematiaceous), and the conidia are then examined for their morphologic features and their arrangement on the hyphae. If the hyphae are nonpigmented, they are considered to be **hyaline.** The fungi are then examined for the type and the arrangement of the conidia produced. The molds are identified by recognition of their characteristic microscopic features.

It is important that the clinical laboratory evaluate the isolation of a fungus from a clinical sample, because it may be regarded as a contaminant acquired during collection, transportation, processing, or incubation. It is important to consider that all contaminating fungi may be considered pathogenic in the appropriate clinical setting. Each isolate should be carefully evaluated on a case-by-case basis.

Pathogenesis and Spectrum of Disease

Fungal infection is caused by either primary pathogens or opportunistic pathogens. Infections caused by primary pathogens can occur in immunocompetent hosts, are not always as virulent, and may lead to subclinical disease. Opportunistic pathogens primarily infect immunocompromised hosts. Opportunistic pathogens include almost any fungus present in the environment. An increase in the identification of opportunistic fungal infections in humans is in large part a result of the immunocompromised nature of the host but also the increasing use of antifungals and improved diagnostic methods. In addition, organism-specific factors, called **virulence factors,** make invading tissues and causing disease easier. Some virulence factors include:

- The organism's size (with inhalation, the organism must be small enough to reach the alveoli)
- The organism's ability to grow at 37°C at a neutral pH
- Conversion of the dimorphic fungi from the mycelial (mold) form into the corresponding yeast or spherule form in the host
- Toxin production

Most of the fungi exist in environmental niches as saprophytic organisms (Table 58.2). Perhaps the fungi that cause disease in humans have developed various mechanisms that allow them to establish disease in the human host. Table 58.3 describes some of the known or speculative virulence factors of the fungi known to be pathogenic for humans.

Laboratory Diagnosis

Collection, Transport, and Culturing of Clinical Specimens

The diagnosis of fungal infections depends entirely on the selection and collection of an appropriate clinical specimen for microscopic analysis and culture. Many fungal infections are similar clinically to mycobacterial infections, and often the same specimen is cultured for both fungi and mycobacteria. If a fungal clinical infection is suspected, the sample should always be cultured on fungal media. If the specimen quantity is insufficient for microscopy and culture, the culture should be performed. Many infections have a primary focus in the lungs; respiratory tract secretions are usually included among the specimens selected for culture. It should be emphasized that dissemination to distant body sites may occur, and fungi may be recovered from nonrespiratory sites.

Proper collection of specimens and rapid transport to the clinical laboratory are crucial to the recovery of fungi. Specimens often contain not only the etiologic agent but also contaminating bacteria or fungi that rapidly overgrow some of the slower-growing pathogenic fungi. The viability of fungi decreases over time. Specimens should be processed within 2 hours of receipt. Most fungal specimens can be maintained at room temperature. If processing of intravascular catheter tips, other medical devices (stents, surgical implants, replacement joints, etc.), lower respiratory tract or urine specimens will be delayed, the samples can be refrigerated for a short time. Dermatologic specimens (skin, hair, nails) are very sensitive to cold temperatures. Yeasts (e.g., *Candida* spp.) commonly are recovered on routine bacteriology media and fungal culture media. A few specific comments concerning specimen collection and culturing are discussed later in this chapter. Additional information on specimen collection is included in Table 5.1.

Lower Respiratory Tract Secretions

Respiratory tract secretions (sputum, induced sputum, bronchial washings, bronchoalveolar lavage, and tracheal aspirations) are perhaps the most common specimens collected for fungal culture. Viscous lower respiratory tract specimens should be pretreated with a mucolytic agent and concentrated by centrifugation. The sediment should then be plated to media without antibiotic and a media containing antibacterial antibiotics to prevent overgrowth by contaminants and ensure optimal recover of fungi. The antifungal agent cycloheximide prevents overgrowth by rapidly growing molds and should be included in at least one of the culture media. As much specimen as possible (0.5 mL) should be used to inoculate each medium. Two fungal organisms commonly isolated from cystic fibrosis (CF) patients include *Candida* spp. and *Scedosporium* spp. Therefore, it is recommended that selective and differential chromogenic medium for the isolation of *Candida* spp. and *Scedosporium*-selective medium containing antifungal

<table>
<tr><td colspan="2">TABLE
58.2</td><td colspan="5">**Summary of Common Pathogens**</td></tr>
</table>

Organism	Natural Habitat	Infectious Form	Mode of Transmission	Common Sites of Infection	Clinical Form
Aspergillus spp.	Ubiquitous, plants	Conidia	Inhalation	Lungs, eyes, skin, nails	Hyphae
Blastomyces spp.	Unknown, possibly soil/wood in moist areas	Probably conidia	Usually inhalation	Lungs, skin, long bones	Yeast
Candida spp.	Human microbiota	Yeast, pseudohyphae, and true hyphae	Direct invasion/dissemination	GI and GU tracts, nails, viscera, blood	Yeast, pseudohyphae, and true hyphae
Coccidioides spp.	Soil of many arid regions	Arthroconidia	Inhalation	Lungs, skin, meninges	Spherules, endospores
Cryptococcus spp.	Bird feces, soil	Yeast[a]	Inhalation	Lungs, skin, meninges	Yeast
Histoplasma capsulatum	Bat and bird feces	Conidia	Inhalation	Lungs, bone marrow, blood	Yeast
Paracoccidioides spp.	Possibly soil, plants	Conidia	Inhalation/trauma	Lungs, skin, mucous membranes	Yeast
Sporothrix spp.	Soil, plants	Conidia/hyphae	Trauma/rarely inhalation	Skin and lymphatics, lungs, meninges	Yeast
Dermatophytes	Human disease, animals, soil	Conidia/hyphae	Contact	Skin, hair, or nails	Hyphae

[a]Possibly the conidia of the teleomorphic stage.
GI, Gastrointestinal; *GU,* genitourinary.

agents dicloran and benomyl should be added to respiratory cultures of CF patients to improve the isolation of these organisms. Specimens may be stored at room temperature if processing is completed within 2 hours; if processing is delayed, specimens should be refrigerated at 4°C.

Sterile Body Fluids Including Cerebrospinal Fluid

Most sterile body fluids are generally collected in heparin blood tubes to prevent clotting. Lysis centrifugation tubes may also be used for the collection of sterile body fluids. Cerebrospinal fluid lumbar puncture tubes collected for culture should be concentrated by centrifugation and the concentrated sediment used to inoculate the culture medium. Cultures should be examined daily. It is recommended that ≥2 mL of specimen should be centrifuged and up to 0.5 mL of sample be inoculated onto each type of fungal culture medium. If less than 1 mL of specimen is submitted for culture, following centrifugation, 1-drop aliquots of the sediment should be placed on several areas on the agar surface. Many laboratories utilize screw-cap tubes containing slants or culture vials to avoid contamination of fungal cultures. Media used for the recovery of fungi from

sterile fluids should contain no antibacterial or antifungal agents. *Cryptococcus* spp., a pathogenic encapsulated yeast associated with meningitis, is inhibited by the antifungal agent cycloheximide.

Once submitted to the laboratory, sterile body fluid specimens should be processed promptly. If prompt processing is not possible, samples should be kept at room temperature. Sterile body fluid specimens should never be refrigerated.

Blood and Bone Marrow

Disseminated fungal infections are a major cause of morbidity and mortality in hospitalized patients, and blood cultures provide an accurate method for determining the cause in many instances. Currently several automated blood culture systems that utilize fungal medium modifications for the isolation of fungi, including the BACTEC (Becton Dickinson, Sparks, MD), BacT/ALERT 3D (bioMérieux, Durham, NC), and VersaTREK (Thermo Scientific, Oakwood Village, OH), are adequate systems for the recovery of yeasts, except *Malassezia* spp.

Laboratories that frequently recover dimorphic fungi and molds from blood or bone marrow are encouraged to use the lysis-centrifugation system, the Isolator. A heparinized syringe or pediatric Isolator tube

TABLE 58.3	Virulence Factors of Medically Important Fungi	
Fungal Pathogen	**Putative Virulence Factor**	
Aspergillus spp.	Elastase-serine protease Proteases Toxins (gliotoxin, fumagillin, helvolic acid) Elastase-metalloprotease Aspartic acid proteinase Aflatoxin Catalase Lysine biosynthesis *p*-aminobenzoic acid synthesis	
Blastomyces spp.	Cell wall alpha-1,3-glucan BAD-1 an adhesion and immune modulator	
Coccidioides spp.	Extracellular proteinases	
Cryptococcus spp.	Capsule Phenoloxidase melanin synthesis Varietal differences	
Dematiaceous fungi	Phenoloxidase melanin synthesis	
Histoplasma capsulatum	Cell wall alpha-1,3-glucan Intracellular growth Thermotolerance CBP, binds calcium	
Paracoccidioides spp.	Estrogen-binding proteins Cell wall components Beta-glucan Alpha-1,3-glucan	
Sporothrix spp.	Thermotolerance Extracellular enzymes	

is recommended for the collection of bone marrow samples. The Isolator has been proven optimal for the recovery of *H. capsulatum* and other filamentous fungi. Special automated fungal media such as the BACTEC MYCO/F lytic medium or BacT/ALERT media may also be used for the isolation of filamentous molds from blood samples. With this system, red blood cells and white blood cells, which may contain the microorganisms, are lysed, and centrifugation concentrates the organisms before culturing. The concentrate is inoculated onto the surface of appropriate culture media, and most fungi are detected within the first 4 days of incubation. However, occasional isolates of *H. capsulatum* may require approximately 10 to 14 days for recovery. In addition to the lysis-centrifugation system, special automated fungal media such as the BACTEC MYCO/F lytic medium or BacT/ALERT media may also be used for the isolation of filamentous molds to improve the recovery from blood. Bone marrow samples should not be placed in automated blood culture media. The optimal temperature for fungal blood cultures is 30°C, and the suggested incubation time is 21 days.

Eye (Corneal Scrapings or Vitreous Humor)

Corneal scrapings collected by a physician should be placed directly onto microscopic slides and inoculated onto noninhibitory media such as Sabouraud dextrose agar, in either an X- or C-shaped pattern. Vitreous humor aspiration should be concentrated by centrifugation, similar to processing a cerebrospinal fluid (CSF) sample, and the sediment should be used for smears and culture. Specimens should be inoculated onto a noninhibitory media, inhibitory mold agar, and brain-heart infusion (BHI) agar with 10% sheep blood. Samples should be processed as soon as possible and stored at room temperature. Media containing cycloheximide should be avoided to prevent inhibition of potential isolates.

Hair, Skin, and Nail Scrapings

Specimens of hair, skin scrapings or biopsies, and nail clippings are usually submitted for dermatophyte culture and are contaminated with bacteria or rapidly growing fungi or both. Samples collected from lesions may be obtained by scraping the skin or nails with a scalpel blade or microscope slide; infected hairs are removed by plucking them with forceps. Only the leading edge of skin lesions should be sampled, because the centers often contain nonviable organisms. These specimens should be placed in a sterile container; they should not be refrigerated. Hair samples may be cut into 1 mm pieces and applied to the medium using a sterile forceps. Skin and nail samples should be cut into smaller pieces, placed on the medium using a sterile forceps and pressed slightly into the agar. **Mycosel agar,** which contains chloramphenicol and cycloheximide, is satisfactory for the recovery of dermatophytes. If infection with *Malassezia furfur* is suspected, olive oil or an olive oil–saturated paper disk should be placed in the first quadrant of the agar plate. Cultures should be incubated for a minimum of 21 days at 30°C before being reported as negative.

Vaginal

Candida spp. are considered normal vaginal flora, and therefore, identification without symptoms is not significant. Vaginal lesions may also be present with histoplasmosis or paracoccidioidomycosis. Vaginal samples should be transported to the laboratory within 24 hours of collection using culture transport swabs. Swabs should be kept moist in sterile tubes. This method of collection provides a specimen suitable for a wet preparation. Both selective and inhibitory agars should be plated. Vaginal cultures should be screened for yeasts using chromogenic agars for *Candida* spp.

Urine

First morning, clean-catch, suprapubic or direct catheterized urine samples are recommended for fungal culture. Urine samples should be processed as soon after collection as possible. The 24-hour urine and Foley catheter samples are unacceptable for culture. Quantitative cultures are not useful. All urine samples should be centrifuged and the sediment cultured using a loop to provide adequate isolation of colonies. Because urine often is contaminated with gram-negative bacteria, media containing antibacterial agents must be used to ensure the recovery of fungi. If processing is completed within 2 hours, samples may remain at room temperature. However, if processing is delayed, specimens should be refrigerated at 4°C. If a urine transport system is used, samples may be stored at room temperature for up to 72 hours.

Tissue

All tissues should be processed before culturing by mincing; it is critical not to grind them. Grinding will disrupt, and may damage, a fungal isolate resulting in no growth; except when *H. capsulatum* is suspected. This pathogen is intracellular, requiring homogenization to release the fungal cells to ensure growth. Tissue pieces should be pressed into the appropriate culture media or partially embedded to provide an oxygen tension gradient, and the cultures should be incubated at 30°C for 21 days (incubation may be extended if clinical suspicion of a mycotic disease is high).

Culture Media and Incubation Requirements

A number of fungal culture media are satisfactory for use in the clinical microbiology laboratory (Table 58.4). Most are adequate for the recovery of fungi. For optimal recovery, a battery of media should be used; the following are recommended:

- Media with and without cycloheximide to prevent the overgrowth of slow-growing fungi by more rapidly growing species. It is important to note that cycloheximide may also be inhibitory to some fungi.
- Media with and without an antibacterial agent (media with an antibacterial agent are used for specimens likely to contain contaminating bacteria; they are not necessary for specimens from sterile sites).
- Inhibitory agar controls bacterial contamination more effectively than Sabouraud dextrose agar.
- Chloramphenicol is an inhibitory agent for the growth of contaminating bacteria; however, it is important to note that it is also inhibitory to *Nocardia* and other aerobic actinomycetes.
- Growth of dimorphic fungi is enhanced on enriched media such as BHI containing antibiotics and 5% to 10% sheep blood. This enhances growth but inhibits sporulation. Once isolated, the fungi should be immediately subcultured to blood-free enriched media for identification.
- Birdseed agar may be used for the cultivation of *Cryptococcus* spp. from CSF, pleural fluid, bone marrow, tissue, and lower respiratory specimens.
- Specific chromogenic agar may be used to identify some species of yeast.
- Additional specialized media may be required for additional fungal isolates that have unique nutritional or incubation requirements.

Agar plates (petri dishes), rectangle agar vials, or screw-capped agar tubes are satisfactory for the recovery of fungi; however, plates or vials are preferred, because they provide better aeration of cultures and a large surface area for better isolation of colonies. Agar plates provide greater ease of handling by laboratory professionals when making microscopic preparations for examination. Agar tends to dehydrate during the extended incubation period required for fungal recovery, but this problem can be minimized by using agar plates or vials containing at least 40 mL of agar and placing them in a humidified incubator. Agar plates should be opened and examined in a certified biologic safety cabinet (BSC). Many laboratories discourage the use of agar plates because of safety considerations; however, the advantages outweigh the disadvantages.

Compared with agar plates, screw-capped culture tubes are more easily stored, require less space for incubation, and are easily handled. In addition, they have a lower dehydration rate, and most laboratory workers believe cultures are less hazardous to handle when in tubes. However, disadvantages, such as relatively poor isolation of colonies, a reduced surface area for culturing, and a tendency to promote anaerobiosis, discourage routine use in most clinical microbiology laboratories. If culture tubes are used, the tube should be as large as possible to provide an adequate surface area for isolation. After inoculation, tubes should be placed in a horizontal position for at least 1 to 2 hours to allow the specimen to absorb to the agar surface and prevent settling at the bottom of the tube.

Cultures should be incubated at room temperature, or preferably at 30°C, for 21 to 30 days before they are reported as negative. A relative humidity in the range of 40% to 50% can be achieved by placing an open pan of water in the incubator. Cultures should be examined at least three times weekly during incubation.

As previously mentioned some clinical specimens are contaminated with bacteria or rapidly growing fungi or both, requiring the use of antifungal and antibacterial agents. The addition of 0.5 μg/mL of cycloheximide and 16 μg/mL of chloramphenicol to media traditionally has been advocated to inhibit the growth of contaminating molds and bacteria, respectively. However, better results have been achieved using a combination of 5 μg/mL of gentamicin and 16 μg/mL of chloramphenicol as antibacterial agents. Ciprofloxacin at a concentration of 5 μg/mL may be used.

Cycloheximide may be added to any of the media that contain or lack antibacterial antibiotics. However, if cycloheximide is included in the battery of culture media, a medium lacking this ingredient should also be included. Pathogenic fungi, such as *Cryptococcus* spp., *Candida krusei* and other *Candida* spp., *Trichosporon* spp., *P. boydii*, and *Aspergillus* spp., are partially or completely inhibited by cycloheximide.

Direct Microscopic Examination

Direct microscopic examination of clinical specimens has been used for many years; however, its usefulness should be reemphasized. Because the mission of a clinical microbiology laboratory is to provide a rapid and accurate diagnosis, the mycology laboratory can provide this service in many cases by direct examination (particularly with the

TABLE 58.4 Fungal Culture Media: Indications for Use

Media	Indications for Use	Media Composition	Mode of Action
Primary Recovery Media			
Brain-heart infusion agar	Primary recovery of saprobic and pathogenic fungi	Brain-heart infusion, enzymatic digest of animal tissue, enzymatic digest of casein, dextrose, sodium chloride	The agar provides a rich medium for bacteria, yeast, and pathogenic fungi.
Brain-heart infusion agar (fungal formulation) with antibiotics	Primary recovery of pathogenic fungi exclusive of dermatophytes	Brain-heart infusion, enzymatic digest of animal tissue, enzymatic digest of casein, dextrose, sodium chloride, 10% sheep blood, antibiotics (chloramphenicol, cycloheximide, and gentamicin)	The agar provides a rich medium for yeast and pathogenic fungi, including systemic dimorphic fungi.
Chromogenic agar	Isolation and presumptive identification of yeast and filamentous fungi	Chromopeptone, Glucose, Chromogen mix, Chloramphenicol	Chromogen mix contains substrates that react with enzymes produced by different organisms that result in the production of characteristic color changes.
Dermatophyte test medium	Primary recovery of dermatophytes; recommended as screening medium	Soy, peptone, dextrose, cycloheximide, gentamicin, chloramphenicol, phenol red	Dermatophytes produce alkaline metabolites, which raise the pH and change the medium from red to yellow.
Inhibitory mold agar	Primary recovery of pathogenic, cycloheximide sensitive fungi exclusive of dermatophytes	Chloramphenicol, casein, dextrose, starch, sodium phosphate, magnesium sulfate, sodium chloride, manganese sulfate	Examine plates for growth. Chloramphenicol inhibits bacterial growth.
Potato flake agar	Primary recovery of saprobic and pathogenic fungi and the stimulation of conidia formation.	Potato flakes, glucose, cycloheximide, chloramphenicol, bromthymol blue	Growth is enhanced by a pH alkaline reaction of fungus. Chloramphenicol and antibiotics inhibit the growth of bacteria and nonpathogenic fungi.
Mycobiotic or mycosel agar	Primary recovery of dermatophytes but may also be used for the recovery of other pathogenic fungi.	Pancreatic digest of soybean meal and dextrose with cycloheximide, chloramphenicol.	Inhibits bacteria and saprophytic fungi
Sabouraud dextrose with brain-heart infusion (SABHI) agar	Primary recovery of saprobic and pathogenic fungi	Sabouraud dextrose, brain-heart infusion agar. With chloramphenicol, cycloheximide, penicillin, and/or streptomycin. 10% sheep blood may be added.	Isolates and enhances growth of all fungi including the yeast phase of dimorphic fungi.
Yeast-extract phosphate agar with ammonia	Primary recovery of pathogenic fungi exclusive of dermatophytes	Yeast extract, dipotassium phosphate, chloramphenicol. 1 drop of ammonium hydroxide is applied to the agar surface prior to inoculation and allowed to diffuse into the medium.	Enhances the recovery and sporulation of *Blastomyces* and *Histoplasma capsulatum* from contaminated specimens
Differential Test Media			
Acetate Ascospore agar	Detection of ascospores in ascosporogenous yeasts (e.g., *Saccharomyces* spp.)	Potassium acetate, yeast extract, dextrose	Potassium acetate is necessary, and yeast extract increases the sporulation of yeasts.

Continued

TABLE 58.4 Fungal Culture Media: Indications for Use—cont'd

Media	Indications for Use	Media Composition	Mode of Action
Christensen's urea agar	Identification of *Cryptococcus, Trichosporon,* and *Rhodotorula* spp. Separation of *Trichophyton mentagrophytes* from *Trichophyton rubrum*	2% urea, phenol red	Produces urease and a change in the pH.
Cornmeal agar with Tween 80 and trypan blue	Differentiation of *Candida* spp. by chlamydospore production	Cornmeal, Tween 80, cornmeal infusion, and trypan blue	Addition of Tween 80 enhances the production of chlamydospores, pseudohyphal and arthrospore formation. The addition of trypan blue provides a contrasting background for observing the morphologic features of yeasts.
Czapek's agar	Differential identification of *Aspergillus* spp.	Sodium nitrate, sucrose, yeast extract	Produces characteristic features of yeast and fungus of any organism that can use sodium nitrate.
Niger seed agar (birdseed agar)	Identification of *Cryptococcus* spp., particularly *Cryptococcus neoformans* and *Cryptococcus gattii*	*Guizotia abyssinica* seeds or niger seeds, dextrose, creatinine, chloramphenicol	*C. neoformans* and *C. gattii* produce the enzyme phenol oxidase, resulting in a brown pigment through metabolism of caffeic acid. Creatinine enhances the melanization of some strains of *C. neoformans.*
Potato dextrose agar	Demonstration of conidia formation and the pigment production by *Trichophyton rubrum;* preparation of microslide cultures and sporulation of dermatophytes	Potato infusion, dextrose, tartaric acid **Note:** Some laboratories use potato flake agar, because it may be more stable.	Carbohydrate and potato infusion promotes the growth of yeasts and molds, and the low pH (tartaric acid) partially inhibits bacterial growth.
Trichophyton agars 1–7	Identification of *Trichophyton* spp.	Dextrose, monopotassium phosphate, magnesium sulfate, amino acids 1. Casamino acids; vitamin free 2. Casamino acids plus inositol 3. Casamino acids plus inositol and thiamine 4. Casamino acids plus thiamine 5. Casamino acids plus niacin 6. Ammonium nitrate 7. Ammonium nitrate plus histidine	*Trichophyton* spp. may be differentiated by growth in the presence of different amino acids.
Yeast fermentation broth	Identification of yeasts by determining fermentation	Yeast extract, peptone, bromcresol purple, and a specific carbohydrate (e.g., dextrose, maltose, sucrose)	Most yeasts produce acid, which is indicated by a change in the solution from purple to yellow as a positive fermenter.
Yeast nitrogen-base agar	Identification of yeasts by determining carbohydrate assimilation	Ammonium sulfate, carbon source (e.g., glucose, sucrose, raffinose)	Assimilation of carbon by yeast cells produces a positive result.

Gram stain) of the clinical specimen submitted for culture. Microbiologists are encouraged to become familiar with the diagnostic features of fungi commonly encountered in clinical specimens and to recognize them when stained by various dyes. This important procedure often can provide the first microbiologic proof of the cause of disease in patients with fungal infection and guide the selection of appropriate media to support growth.

Tables 58.5 and 58.6 present the methods available for direct microscopic detection of fungi in clinical specimens and a summary of the characteristic microscopic features of each. Fig. 58.4 presents photomicrographs of some of the fungi commonly seen in clinical specimens.

Traditionally the potassium hydroxide preparation has been the recommended method for direct microscopic examination of specimens in dermatological samples. Calcofluor white (CW) (Evolve Procedure 58.1) and lactophenol blue (LPCB) bind specifically to polysaccharides, chitin, and cellulose present in fungal cell walls. In addition, LPCB contains lactic acid that aids in the preservation of fungal structures and phenol that acts as a killing agent. Slides prepared using these methods may be observed using fluorescent (CW) or bright-field microscopy (LPCB).

Serologic Testing

Molecular diagnostics may eventually replace the use of serologic testing for the diagnosis of fungal infections. These methods currently lack standardization for performance when taken directly from patient specimens. No commercially available procedures exist for serologic testing of most fungi. However, serology testing is a useful tool for the diagnosis of invasive fungal infections with select organisms, such as *Cryptococcus, Coccidioides, Blastomyces, Histoplasma,* and *Aspergillus* spp.

Antibody testing has proven useful but not for immunocompromised patients, who are incapable of producing a measurable humoral response. Acute and convalescent titers need to be monitored during treatment of the fungal infection.

Immunodiffusion testing is a simple, cost-effective procedure. Although it is 100% specific, it is relatively insensitive and is not used as a screening tool. This test also requires 2 to 3 weeks to exhibit a positive result.

Enzyme immunoassays for both antibody and antigen have been used. These tests are also commonly negative in immunocompromised patients, especially early in the infection.

Point-of-care (POC) testing using lateral flow assay-based devices have the potential to improve the diagnosis of fungal infections, especially in developing countries with limited laboratory resources. POC devices generally are inexpensive and portable while providing rapid and reproducible results that are highly sensitive and specific. Undoubtedly, the development of these devices will be useful in monitoring and detecting fungal antibodies.

(1,3)-β-D-Glucan Detection

(1,3)-β-D-Glucan, a polysaccharide present in the cell wall of some fungi, is found in the blood of patients that have invasive fungal infections. Although detection of the polysaccharide has demonstrated success in the diagnosis and monitoring of fungal meningitis, variation in assay sensitivity and specificity, along with the need for what are considered significant levels in the blood of a patient with fungal infections, indicates further studies are necessary.

Molecular Methods

Phenotypic and biochemical identification methods are extremely time-consuming for the identification of fungal pathogens. One of the most critical risk factors associated with mortality from systemic mycoses is the time to diagnosis, making molecular detection methods ideal in the clinical laboratory. In addition to diagnosis, drug resistance among invasive *Candida* and *Cryptococcus* spp. has increased, requiring the development of new assays to detect drug resistance. Ideally, a molecular direct hybridization assay or amplification assay panel of primers specific for the detection of fungi in clinical specimens would include the most common organisms known to cause disease in immunocompromised patients (including the dimorphic fungi and *Pneumocystis* spp.). The current literature contains references to all of the major human fungal pathogens, describing species and strain-specific primers and probes, yet no commercial methods are available to the clinical laboratory. Sequence-based molecular identification of fungal isolates is a useful diagnostic tool and has resulted in the development of commercial diagnostic assays such as the MicroSEQ D2 rDNA Fungal Sequencing Kit (Thermo Fisher, Grand Island, NY). Currently, DNA sequencing technology, including whole genome sequencing, remains confined to research and reference laboratories due to the large capital investment and expertise required for implementation.

Currently, a few FDA-cleared molecular diagnostic assays are available, which include amplification and hybridization techniques. These assays primarily focus on the identification of *Candida, Cryptococcus, Aspergillus* spp., and the systemic dimorphic fungi.

Matrix-Assisted Laser Desorption Ionization Mass Spectrometry

Matrix-assisted laser desorption ionization time-of-flight mass spectrometry (MALDI-TOF MS) is a biophysical method that significantly reduces the time required to specifically identify fungal organisms. The major disadvantage of this technique is the need to have pure cultures of the clinical isolates for sample preparation, adding days and weeks to the process. The protein profiles for fungi also vary significantly based on environmental and culture conditions, making standardization of the analytical process extremely difficult in fungal identification. The level of fungal organisms, such as yeast in the bloodstream and other clinical fluid samples is generally too low for direct detection by

TABLE
58.5

TABLE 58.5   Summary of Methods Available for Direct Microscopic Detection of Fungi in Clinical Specimens

Method	Use	Time Required	Advantages	Disadvantages
Acid-fast stain and partial acid-fast stain	Detection of mycobacteria and *Nocardia* spp., respectively	12 min	Detects *Nocardia* spp.[a] and some isolates of *Blastomyces* spp.	Tissue homogenates are difficult to observe because of background staining.
Alcian blue or mucicarmine stain.	Mucopolysaccharide stains used to visualize the capsule of *Cryptococcus* spp. in histological tissue sections.	30 min	Detects encapsulated yeast in tissue sections	*Blastomyces dermatitidis* and *Rhinosporidium seeberi* may also react positively with this stain.
Auramine-rhodamine stain	Detection of mycobacteria and *Nocardia* spp., respectively	10 min	Excellent screening tool; sensitive and affordable.	Not as specific for acid-fast organisms as Ziehl-Neelsen stain.
Calcofluor white stain	Detection of fungi	1 min	Can be mixed with KOH; detects fungi rapidly because of bright fluorescence.	Requires use of a fluorescence microscope; background fluorescence prominent, but fungi exhibit more intense fluorescence; vaginal secretions are difficult to interpret. Nonspecific reactions may be observed, such as cotton fibers from swabs and brain tumor biopsies, both falsely resembling branching hyphae.
Gram stain	Detection of bacteria	3 min	Commonly performed on most clinical specimens submitted for bacteriology; detects most fungi.	Some fungi stain well, but others (e.g., *Cryptococcus* spp.) show only stippling and stain weakly in some instances; some isolates of *Nocardia* spp. fail to stain or stain weakly.
India ink (nigrosin) stain	Detection of *Cryptococcus* spp. in CSF	1 min	Diagnostic of meningitis when positive in CSF.	Positive in fewer than 50% of cases of meningitis; not sensitive in non–HIV-infected patients. Artifacts such as erythrocytes, leukocytes, and talc particles from gloves or bubbles may mimic yeast, resulting in false positives.
Lactophenol cotton (aniline) blue wet mount	Most widely used method of staining and observing fungi	1 min	Lactic acid and glycerol preserves structures; slides can be made permanent.	Mechanical treatment dislodges fungal structures.
Potassium hydroxide	Clearing of specimen using 10%–20% KOH to make fungi more readily visible	5 min; if clearing is not complete, an additional 5–10 min is necessary	Rapid detection of fungal elements. 0.1% thimerosal (Sigma Chemical Co.) may be added to preserve the specimen.	Requires experience, because background artifacts are often confusing; clearing of some specimens may require an extended time.
Masson-Fontana stain	Examination of melanin pigment in fungal cell walls	1 h, 10 min	Aids differentiation of melanin and hemosiderin pigments.	Difficult to interpret when only rare granular staining is present.

TABLE 58.5 Summary of Methods Available for Direct Microscopic Detection of Fungi in Clinical Specimens—cont'd

Method	Use	Time Required	Advantages	Disadvantages
Methenamine silver stain	Detection of fungi in histologic section	1 h	Best stain for detecting fungal elements (black) against a pale green or yellow background.	Requires a specialized staining method that is not usually readily available to microbiology laboratories.
Periodic acid–Schiff (PAS) stain	Detection of fungi	20 min; 5 min additional if counterstain is used	Stains fungal elements well; hyphae of molds and yeasts can be readily distinguished.	*Nocardia* spp. do not stain well. Time-consuming and has been replaced in many laboratories by calcofluor white staining procedures.
Toluidine blue O	Rapid detection of *P. jiroveci* from lung biopsy and BAL specimens.	1 min	Quickly performed, easy, rapid results, and cost-effective.	Trophozoites are not discernable.
Wright's stain	Examination of bone marrow or peripheral blood smears	7 min	Detects *Histoplasma capsulatum* and *Cryptococcus* spp.	Most often used to detect *H. capsulatum* and *Cryptococcus* spp. in disseminated disease.

ªPartially acid-fast bacterium.

BAL, Bronchoalveolar lavage; *CSF,* cerebrospinal fluid; *HIV,* human immunodeficiency virus; *KOH,* potassium hydroxide.

MALDI-TOF MS. In addition, proteins and hemoglobin tend to interfere with the spectra analytics making identification problematic. Further clinical studies are needed prior to implementation of direct identification using MALDI-TOF MS for systemic fungal infections. An overview of the technique is discussed in more detail in Chapter 7.

General Considerations for the Identification of Yeasts

Most often yeasts are identified through the use of a combination of differential test media (Fig. 58.5). Identification factors and techniques include the following:
- Colonial morphologic features
- Microscopic morphologic features
- Physiologic studies
- Chromogenic agars (presumptive species identification)
- Rapid commercial yeast identification tests or panels
- Nucleic acid–based methods (direct hybridization or amplification methods)
- Matrix-assisted laser desorption/ionization time-of-flight mass spectroscopy (MALDI-TOF MS)

Several key characteristics can be seen macroscopically. Colonies have a wide variety of colors, shapes, and textures. Chromogenic agar or a combination of rapid tests can be used to differentiate some pathogenic yeast presumptively. Presumptive identification is indicated when the test or combination of tests do not identify characteristics that are unique to that species. The results of these tests must be correlated with the macroscopic and microscopic morphological characteristics and the site of infection (i.e., clinical specimen). Wet preps and lactophenol cotton blue stain can aid microscopic identification by improving the visualization of the fungal reproductive structures. Sexual and asexual characteristics are very important. Often a genus can be determined by the microscopic and macroscopic characteristics. India ink stain is useful when *Cryptococcus* spp. are suspected. Because carbon and nitrogen source differences are the key to differentiating yeasts, many automated and semiautomated commercial systems have been designed with assimilation and fermentation tests. Supplemental testing takes advantage of a limited set of characteristics to further aid identification.

The clinical microbiology laboratory has historically operated under the idea that if the identification of the isolate to the species level is incorrect, the patient will not be adversely affected once the susceptibility is completed. This is problematic, when the specific species identifications are used to determine minimum inhibitory concentrations and breakpoints for treatment for bacterial and fungal infections. Treatment failures, along with the increasing occurrence of resistance to echinocandins, fluconazole, and voriconazole, make accurate identification and susceptibility testing required. Molecular diagnostic techniques, proteomic and genomic, clearly demonstrate more accurate and reliable identification for yeasts than conventional biochemical methods. The use of these methods in the routine clinical laboratory is currently limited by the need for standardization and the expansion of the current databases.

TABLE 58.6	Summary of Characteristic Features of Select Fungi Seen in Direct Examination of Clinical Specimens		
Morphologic Form Found in Specimens	**Organism**	**Size Range (diameter, mm)**	**Characteristic Features**
Yeastlike	*Histoplasma capsulatum*	2–5	Small; oval to round budding cells; often found clustered in histiocytes; difficult to detect when present in small numbers.
	Sporothrix spp.	2–6	Small; oval to round to cigar-shaped; single or multiple buds present; uncommonly seen in clinical specimens.
	Cryptococcus spp.	2–15	Cells exhibit great variation in size; usually spherical but may be football-shaped; buds single or multiple and "pinched off"; capsule may or may not be evident; occasionally, pseudohyphal forms with or without a capsule may be seen in exudates of cerebrospinal fluid.
	Malassezia furfur (in fungemia)	1.5–4.5	Small; bottle-shaped cells, buds separated from parent cell by a septum; emerge from a small collar.
	Blastomyces spp.	8–15	Cells are usually large, double refractile when present; buds usually single; however, several may remain attached to parent cells; buds connected by a broad base.
	Paracoccidioides spp.	5–60	Cells are usually large and are surrounded by smaller buds around the periphery ("mariner's wheel appearance"); smaller cells may be present (2–5 μm) and resemble *H. capsulatum*; buds have "pinched-off" appearance.
Spherules	*Coccidioides* spp.	10–200	Spherules vary in size; some may contain endospores, others may be empty; adjacent spherules may resemble *Blastomyces* spp.; endospores may resemble *H. capsulatum* but show no evidence of budding; spherules may produce multiple germ tubes if a direct preparation is kept in a moist chamber ≥24 h.
	Rhinosporidium seeberi (protozoan [parafungal] pathogen that is studied in mycology)	6–300	Large, thick-walled sporangia containing sporangiospores are present; mature sporangia are larger than spherules of *Coccidioides*; hyphae may be found in cavitary lesions.

TABLE 58.6   Summary of Characteristic Features of Select Fungi Seen in Direct Examination of Clinical Specimens—cont'd

Morphologic Form Found in Specimens	Organism	Size Range (diameter, mm)	Characteristic Features
Yeast and pseudohyphae or hyphae	*Candida* and *Candida dubliniensis*	5–10 (pseudohyphae)	Cells usually exhibit single budding; pseudohyphae, when present, are constricted at the ends and remain attached like links of sausage; hyphae, when present, are septate.
	M. furfur (in tinea versicolor)	3–8 (yeast) 2.5–4 (hyphae)	Short, curved hyphal elements are usually present, along with round yeast cells that retain their spherical shape in compacted clusters; "spaghetti and meatballs."
Pauciseptate hyphae	Mucorales: *Mucor, Rhizopus,* and other genera	10–30	Hyphae are large, ribbonlike, often fractured or twisted; occasional septa may be present; smaller hyphae are confused with those of *Aspergillus* spp., particularly *Aspergillus flavus.*
Hyaline septate hyphae	Dermatophytes, skin and nails	3–15	Hyaline, septate hyphae are commonly seen; chains of arthroconidia may be present.
	Dermatophytes, hair	3–15	Arthroconidia on periphery of hair shaft producing a sheath indicate ectothrix infection; arthroconidia formed by fragmentation of hyphae in the hair shaft indicate endothrix infection. Long hyphal filaments or channels in the hair shaft indicate favus hair infection.
	Aspergillus spp.	3–12	Hyphae are septate and exhibit dichotomous, 45-degree branching; larger hyphae, often disturbed, may resemble those of *Mucorales.*
	Geotrichum spp.	4–12	Hyphae and rectangular arthroconidia are present and sometimes rounded; irregular forms may be present.
	Trichosporon spp.	2–4 by 8	Hyphae and rectangular arthroconidia are present and sometimes rounded; occasionally, blastoconidia may be present.
Dematiaceous septate hyphae	*Bipolaris* spp., *Cladophialophora* spp., *Cladosporium* spp., *Curvularia* spp., *Exophiala* spp., *Exserohilum* spp., *Hortaea werneckii* spp., *Phialophora* spp., and other genera.	2–6	Dematiaceous polymorphous hyphae are seen; budding cells with single septa and chains of swollen rounded cells are often present; occasionally, aggregates may be present in infection caused by *Phialophora* and *Exophiala* spp.
Sclerotic bodies	*Cladophialophora* (formerly *Cladosporium*) *carrionii* *Fonsecaea* spp., *Phialophora verrucosa,* and *Rhinocladiella aquaspersa*	5–20	Brown, round to pleomorphic, thick-walled cells with transverse septations; commonly, cells contain two fission planes that form a tetrad of cells (sclerotic bodies).

Continued

TABLE 58.6	Summary of Characteristic Features of Select Fungi Seen in Direct Examination of Clinical Specimens—cont'd		
Morphologic Form Found in Specimens	Organism	Size Range (diameter, mm)	Characteristic Features
Granules	*Acremonium* spp.	200–300	White, soft granules without a cementlike matrix.
	Aspergillus *Aspergillus nidulans*	500–1000	Black, hard grains with a cementlike matrix at the periphery.
	Curvularia *Curvularia geniculata* *Curvularia lunata*	65–160	White, soft granule without a cementlike matrix.
	Exophiala *Exophiala jeanselmei*	200–300	Black, soft granules, vacuolated, without a cementlike matrix, made of dark hyphae and swollen cells.
	Fusarium *Fusarium verticillioides* (formerly *F. moniliformis*)	200–500	White, soft granules without a cementlike matrix.
	Fusarium solani	300–600	
	Trematosphaeria grisea (formerly *Madurella grisea*)	350–500	Black, soft granules without a cementlike matrix; the periphery is composed of polygonal swollen cells, and the center has a hyphal network.
	Madurella mycetomatis	200–900	Black to brown, hard granules; two types: (1) rust-brown, compact, filled with cementlike matrix; (2) deep brown, filled with numerous vesicles, 6–14 µm in diameter, cementlike matrix in periphery, central area of light-colored hyphae.
	Neotestudina *Neotestudina rosatii*	300–600	White, soft granules with cementlike matrix at the periphery.
	Pseudallescheria *Pseudallescheria boydii*	200–300	White, soft granules composed of hyphae and swollen cells at the periphery in a cementlike matrix.

General Considerations for the Identification of Molds

Filamentous fungi are also identified by a combination of tests (Fig. 58.6). Molds are identified using a combination of the following:

- Growth rate
- Colonial morphologic features
- Microscopic morphologic features

In most cases, the microscopic morphologic features provide the most definitive means of identification. Determination of the growth rate can be most helpful when a mold culture is examined. However, this may have limited value, because the growth rate of certain fungi varies, depending on the amount of inoculum present in a clinical specimen. **Slow growers** form mature colonies in 11 to 21 days, and **intermediate growers** form mature colonies

in 6 to 10 days. **Rapid growers** form mature colonies in 5 days or less.

The growth of *Coccidioides* is often rapid and is hazardous to microbiologists. In general, the growth rate for the dimorphic fungi, *Blastomyces dermatitidis*, *H. capsulatum*, and *P. brasiliensis,* is slow; 1 to 4 weeks usually are required before colonies become visible. In some instances, cultures of *B. dermatitidis*, *Talaromyces marneffei*, and *H. capsulatum* may be detected within 3 to 5 days. This is a somewhat uncommon circumstance, encountered only when large numbers of the organism are present in the specimen. Colonies of *Mucorales* may appear within 24 hours, whereas the other hyaline and melanized (dematiaceous) fungi often exhibit growth in 1 to 5 days. The growth rate of an organism therefore is important, but it must be used in combination with other features before a definitive identification can be made.

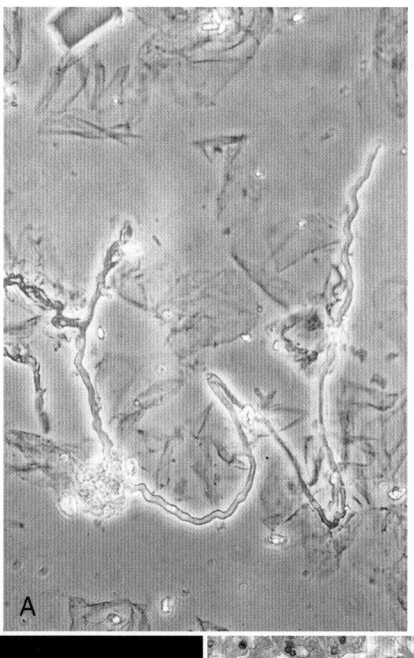

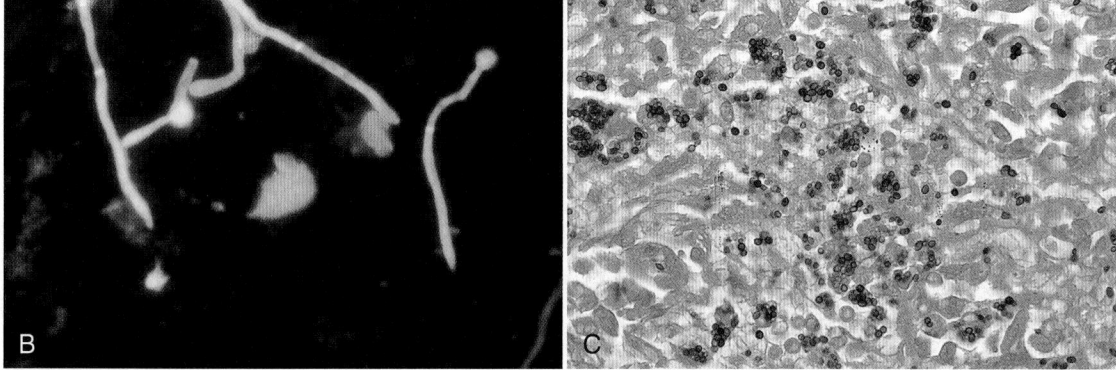

• **Fig. 58.4** Fungi commonly seen in clinical specimens. (A) This potassium hydroxide preparation of a skin scraping from a patient with a dermatophyte infection shows septate hyphae intertwined among epithelial cells. (Phase-contrast microscopy; ×500.) (B) This calcofluor white stain of urine demonstrates *Candida albicans*. (C) The deeply staining, small, uniform yeast cells in this histologic section of lung tissue are typical of *Histoplasma capsulatum*. (Methenamine silver stain; ×430.)

The colonial morphologic features may have limited value for identifying molds because of natural variation among isolates and colonies grown on different culture media. Although common organisms recovered repeatedly in the laboratory may be more easily recognized, colonial morphology is an unreliable criterion that should be used to supplement the microscopic morphologic features of the organism.

The color of the colony and uniformity of the color can be important, along with the presence of diffusible pigments in the media. The examiner must be sure to note the color of both the front and reverse sides of the culture. The colony topography describes the various elevations of the colony on the agar plate. Topography can be described as **verrucose** (furrowed or convoluted), **umbonate** (slightly raised in the center), or **rugose** (furrows radiate out from the center).

The colony's texture should also be noted. Various textures can be seen, such as **cottony** (loose, high aerial mycelium), **velvety** (low aerial mycelium resembling a velvet cloth), **glabrous** (smooth surface with no aerial mycelium), **granular**

(dense, powdery, resembling sugar granules), and **wooly** (high aerial mycelium that appears slightly matted down).

Incubation conditions and culture media must also be considered. For example, *H. capsulatum* appears as a white-to-tan fluffy mold on BHI agar and may have a yeastlike appearance when grown on the same medium containing blood enrichment.

In general, the microscopic morphologic features of the molds are stable and show minimal variation. Definitive identification is based on the characteristic shape, method of reproduction, and arrangement of spores; however, the size of the hyphae also provides helpful information. The large, ribbonlike, **pauciseptate hyphae** of the *Mucorales* are easily recognized; small hyphae, approximately 2 μm in diameter, may suggest the presence of one of the dimorphic fungi or a dermatophyte.

The fungi may be prepared for microscopic observation using several techniques. The procedure traditionally used by most laboratories is the cellophane tape preparation (Evolve Procedure 58.2; Fig. 58.7). It can be prepared

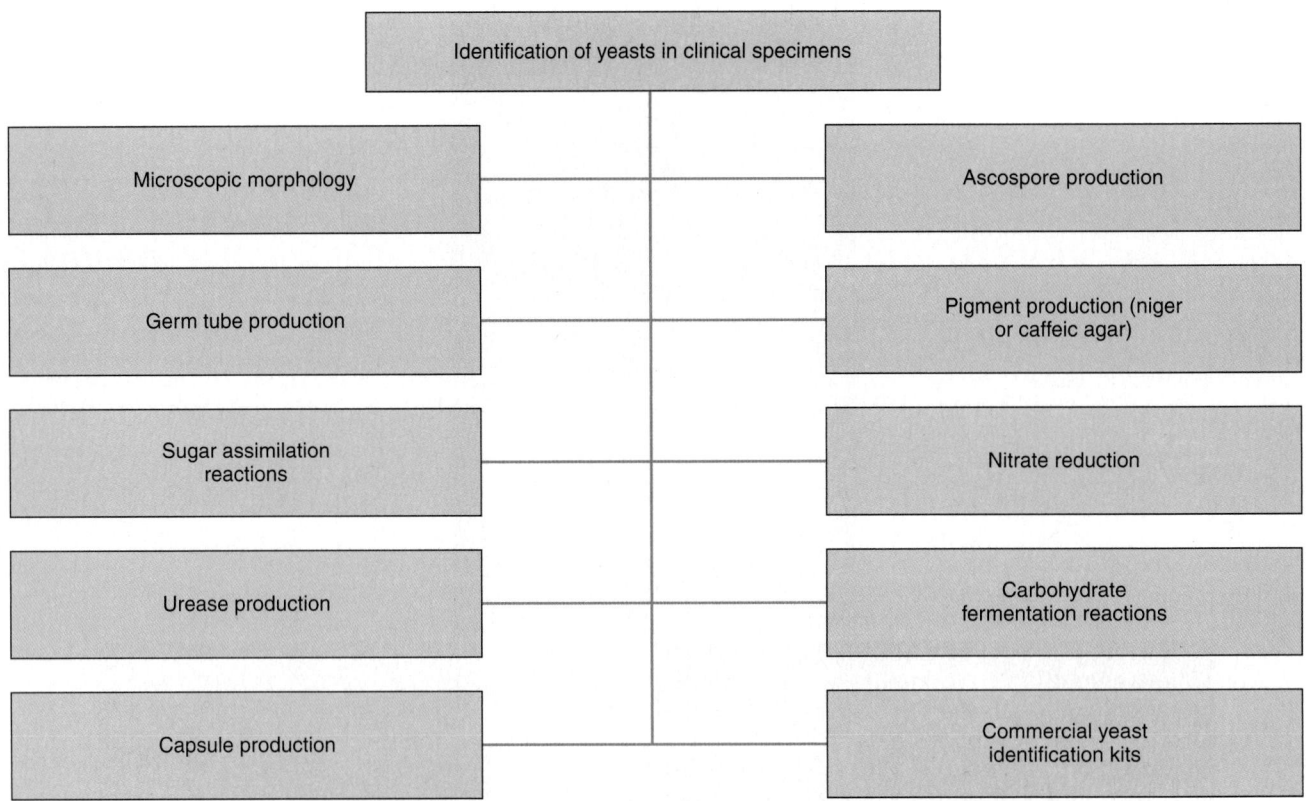

• **Fig. 58.5** Traditional identification of yeasts in clinical specimens. Manual methods, kits, and panels have been predominantly replaced with proteomic and genomic methods.

easily and quickly and often is sufficient to make the identification for most fungi. However, some laboratories prefer the wet mount (Evolve Procedure 58.3; Fig. 58.8) or tease mount (Evolve Procedure 58.4). A microslide culture method (Evolve Procedure 58.5; Fig. 58.9) may be used when greater detail of the morphologic features is required.

General Morphologic Features of the Molds

Specialized types of vegetative hyphae may be helpful for categorizing an organism into a certain group. For example, dermatophytes often produce several types of hyphae, including **antler hyphae,** so named because they are curved, freely branching, and have the appearance of antlers (Fig. 58.10). **Racquet hyphae** are enlarged, club-shaped structures (Fig. 58.11). In addition, certain dermatophytes produce **spiral hyphae** that are coiled or exhibit corkscrewlike turns in the hyphal strand (Fig. 58.12). These structures are not characteristic for any certain group; however, they are found most commonly in dermatophytes.

Some species of fungi (Ascomycota) produce sexual spores in a large, saclike structure called an **ascocarp** (Fig. 58.13). The ascocarp contains smaller sacs, called **asci,** each of which contains four to eight ascospores. This type of sexual reproduction is not commonly seen in the fungi recovered in the clinical microbiology laboratory; most exhibit asexual reproduction. It is possible that all fungi have a sexual form, but

for some species, it has not yet been observed on artificial culture media. **Conidia,** which are produced by most fungi, represent the asexual reproductive cycle. The type of conidia and their morphology and arrangement are important criteria for definitively identifying an organism (Fig. 58.14).

The simplest type of sporulation is the development of a spore directly from the vegetative hyphae. **Arthroconidia** are formed directly from the hyphae by fragmentation through the points of septation (Fig. 58.15). When mature, they appear as square, rectangular, or barrel-shaped thick-walled cells. These result from the simple fragmentation of the hyphae into spores, which are easily dislodged and disseminated into the environment. **Chlamydoconidia** (chlamydospores) are round, thick-walled spores formed directly from the differentiation of hyphae in which there is a concentration of protoplasm and nutrient material (Fig. 58.16). These appear to be resistant resting spores produced by the rounding up and enlargement of the cells of the hyphae. Chlamydoconidia may be **intercalary** (within the hyphae) or **terminal** (on the end of the hyphae).

A variety of other types of spores occur with many species of fungi. Conidia are asexual spores produced singly or in groups by specialized hyphal strands, **conidiophores.** Sometimes the conidia are freed from their point of attachment by pinching off, or **abstriction.** Some conidiophores terminate in a swollen vesicle. From the surface of the vesicle are formed secondary small, **flask-shaped phialides,** which in turn give rise to long chains of conidia. This type of fruiting structure is characteristic of the aspergilli. A single,

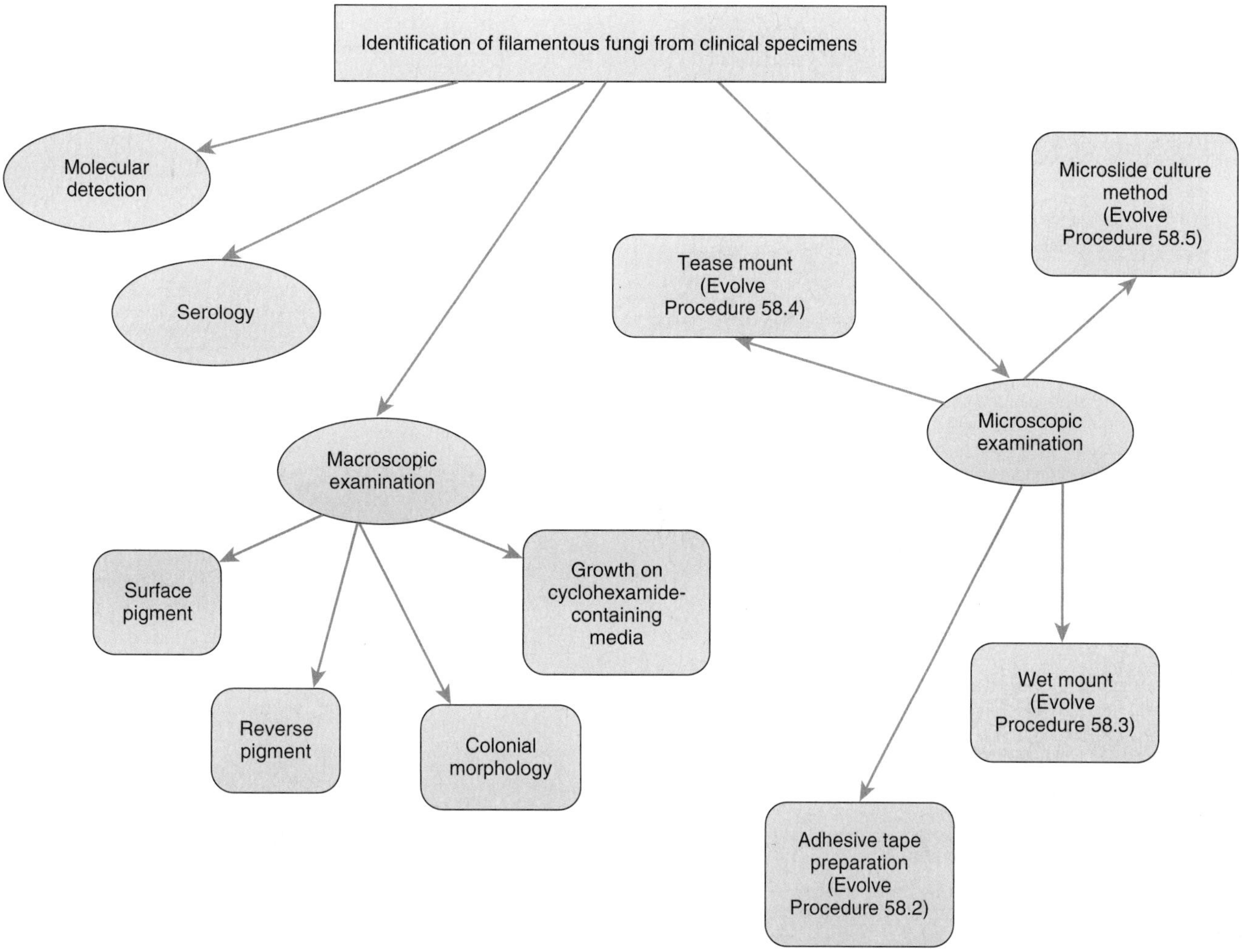

```
                    ┌─────────────────────────────────────────────┐
                    │ Identification of filamentous fungi from      │
                    │ clinical specimens                            │
                    └─────────────────────────────────────────────┘
```

Molecular detection

Serology

Tease mount (Evolve Procedure 58.4)

Microslide culture method (Evolve Procedure 58.5)

Microscopic examination

Macroscopic examination

Surface pigment

Growth on cyclohexamide-containing media

Reverse pigment

Colonial morphology

Wet mount (Evolve Procedure 58.3)

Adhesive tape preparation (Evolve Procedure 58.2)

• **Fig. 58.6** Traditional identification of filamentous fungi from clinical specimens. Some molds may be identified using proteomic and genomic methods.

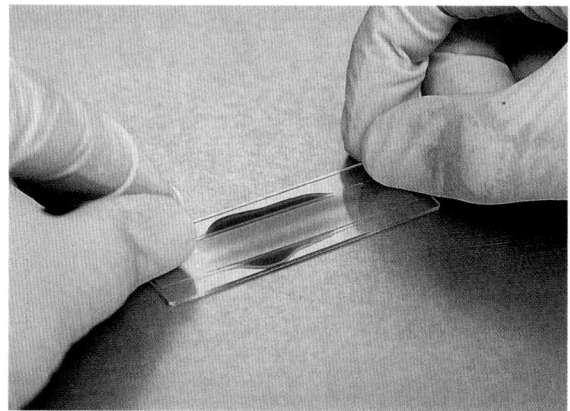

• **Fig. 58.7** Cellophane tape preparation showing placement of tape on slide containing lactophenol cotton or aniline blue.

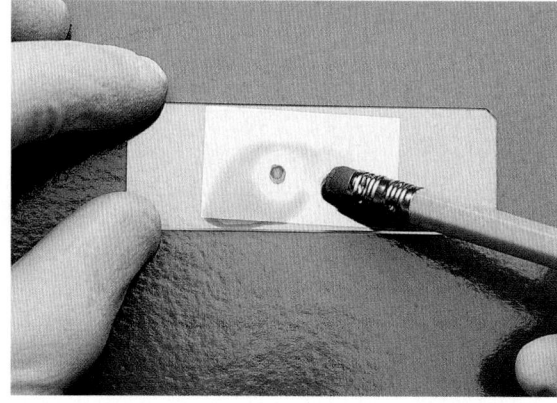

• **Fig. 58.8** Performance of a wet mount showing agar positioned under cover slip before pressure is applied to disperse growth.

simple, slender, tubular conidiophore (**phialide**) that produces a cluster of conidia, held together as a gelatinous mass, is characteristic of certain fungi, including the genus *Acremonium* (Fig. 58.17). In other cases, conidiophores form a branching structure called a **penicillus,** in which each branch terminates in secondary branches (**metulae**)

and phialides, from which chains of conidia are borne (Fig. 58.18). Species of *Penicillium* and *Paecilomyces* are representative of this type of sporulation. Some fungi may produce conidia of two sizes: **microconidia,** which are small, unicellular, round, elliptical, or **pyriform** (pear-shaped), or **macroconidia,** which are large, usually multiseptate, and

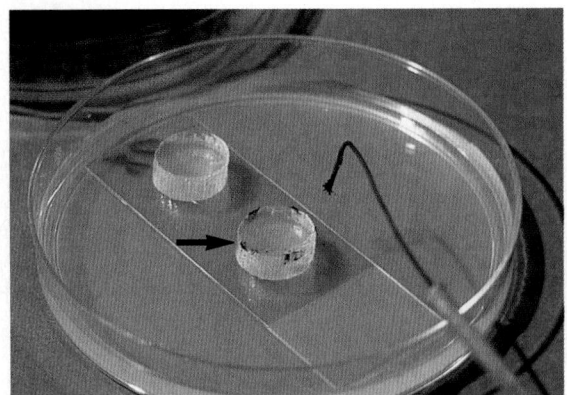

• **Fig. 58.9** Microslide culture showing inoculation of an agar plug *(arrow)*.

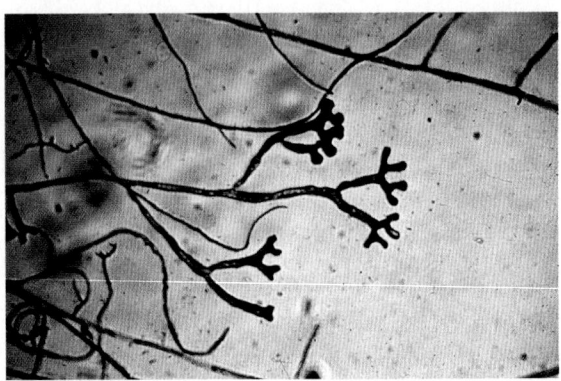

• **Fig. 58.10** Antler hyphae showing swollen hyphal tips, resembling antlers, with lateral and terminal branching (favic chandeliers) (×500).

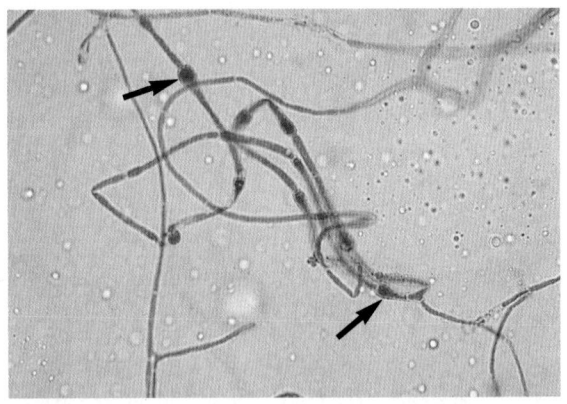

• **Fig. 58.11** Racquet hyphae showing swollen areas *(arrows)* resembling a tennis racquet.

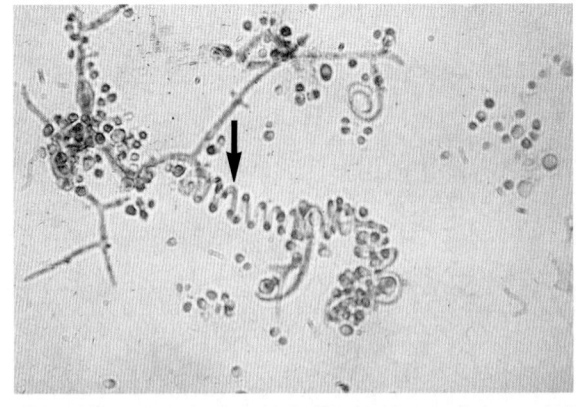

• **Fig. 58.12** Spiral hyphae *(arrow)* showing corkscrewlike turns (×430).

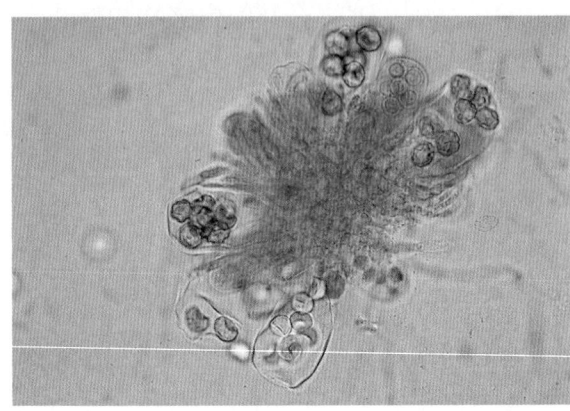

• **Fig. 58.13** Ascocarp showing dark-appearing ascospores (×430).

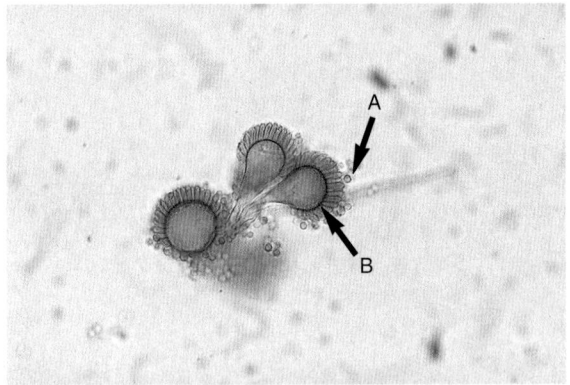

• **Fig. 58.14** Conidia (asexual spores *[A]*) produced on specialized structures (conidiophores *[B]*) of *Aspergillus* (×430).

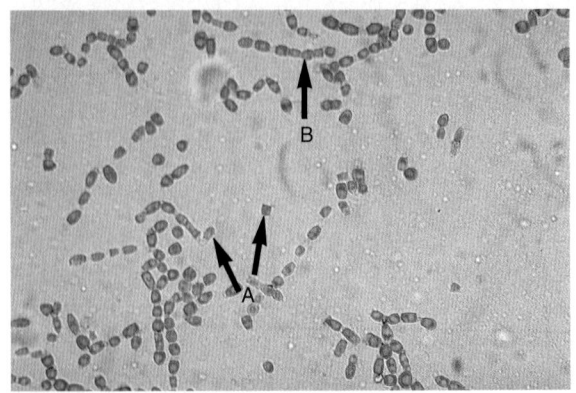

• **Fig. 58.15** Arthroconidia formation *(A)* produced by the breaking down of a hyphal strand *(B)* into individual rectangular units (×430).

club- or spindle-shaped (Fig. 58.19). Microconidia may be borne directly on the side of a hyphal strand or at the end of a conidiophore. Macroconidia are usually borne on a short to long conidiophore and may be smooth or rough-walled. Microconidia and macroconidia are seen in some fungal species and are not specific, except as they are used to differentiate a limited number of genera.

The hyphae of the Mucorales are sparsely septate. Sporulation takes place by progressive cleavage during maturation

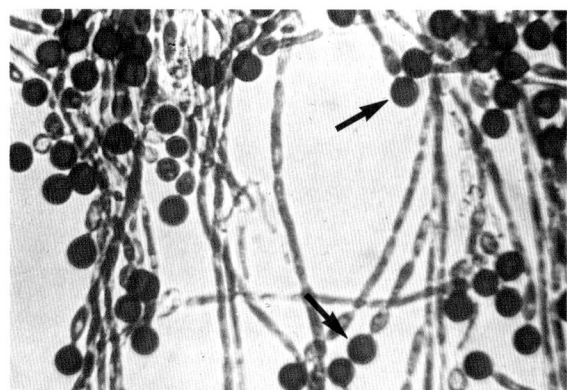

• **Fig. 58.16** Chlamydoconidia composed of thick-walled spherical cells *(arrows)* (×430).

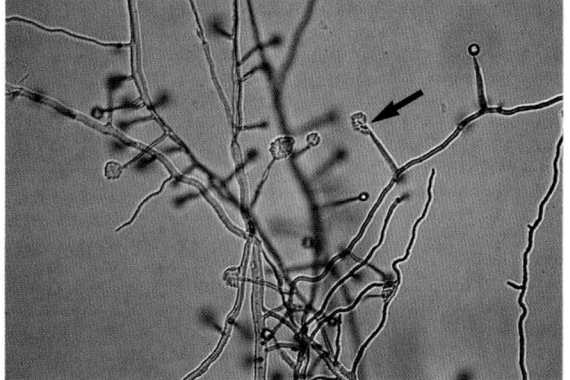

• **Fig. 58.17** Simple tubular phialide with a cluster of conidia at its tip *(arrow)* characteristic of *Acremonium* (×430).

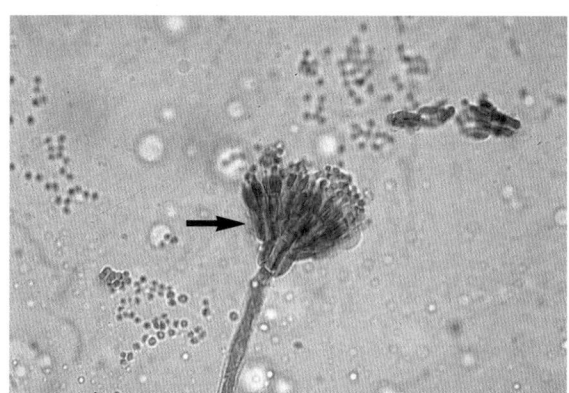

• **Fig. 58.18** Complex method of sporulation in which conidia are borne on phialides produced on secondary branches (metulae *[arrow]*) characteristic of *Penicillium* (×430).

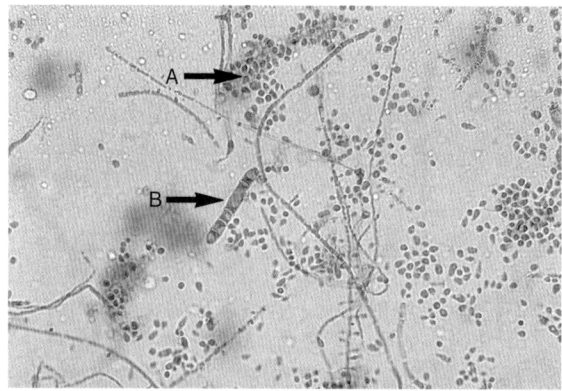

• **Fig. 58.19** In this preparation of a *Trichophyton* species, the numerous, small, spherical microconidia *(A)* are contrasted with a large, elongated macroconidium *(B)* (×430).

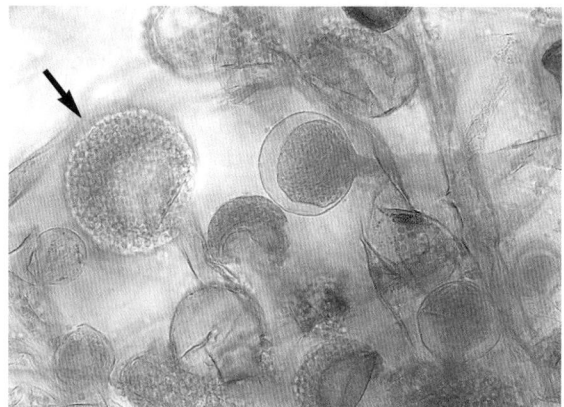

• **Fig. 58.20** Large, saclike sporangia that contain sporangiospores *(arrow)* characteristic of the Mucorales (×250).

in the **sporangium,** a saclike structure produced at the tip of a long stalk (**sporangiophore**). Sporangiospores (spores produced in the sporangium) are produced and released by the rupture of the sporangial wall (Fig. 58.20). In rare cases, some isolates may produce zygospores, rough-walled spores produced by the union of two mating types of a Mucorales; this is an example of sexual reproduction.

Clinical Relevance for Fungal Identification

The question of when and how far to go with the identification of fungi recovered from clinical specimens presents an interesting challenge. The current emphasis on cost containment and the ever-increasing number of opportunistic fungi causing infection in compromised patients prompts consideration of whether all fungi recovered from clinical specimens should be thoroughly identified and reported. The extent of identification of yeasts from various specimen sources is discussed in Chapter 62.

When and how far to proceed in the identification of a mold is a difficult question to answer. Except for obvious plate contaminants, all commonly encountered molds should be identified and reported, if recovered from patients at risk for invasive fungal disease. Immunocompromised patients may have serious or even fatal disease caused by fungi that were once thought to be clinically insignificant. Organisms that fail to sporulate after a reasonable time should be reported as present, but identification is not required if the dimorphic fungi have been ruled out or if the clinician believes the organism is not clinically significant. Ideally, all laboratories should identify all fungi recovered from clinical specimens; however, the limits of practicality and economic considerations play a definite role in the decision-making process. The laboratory director, in consultation with the clinicians, must make this decision after considering the patient population, laboratory practice, and economic implications.

An increasing number of fungi may be isolated in the clinical microbiology laboratory. They are considered environmental microbiota but in reality must be regarded as potential pathogens, because infections with a number of these organisms have been reported. The laboratory must identify and report all organisms recovered from clinical specimens so that their clinical significance can be determined. In many instances, the presence of environmental fungi is unimportant; however, that is not always the case.

Laboratory Safety

Although the handling of fungi recovered from clinical specimens poses risks, a common sense approach to the handling of these specimens protects the laboratory from contamination and workers from becoming infected.

Without exception, mold cultures and clinical specimens must be handled in a class II BSC. Some laboratory professionals believe that mold cultures must be handled in an enclosed BSC equipped with gloves; however, this is not necessary if a laminar flow BSC is used. Yeast cultures may be handled on the bench top. An electric incinerator is suitable for decontaminating a loop used to transfer yeast cultures. Cultures of organisms suspected of being pathogens should be sealed with tape to prevent laboratory contamination and should be autoclaved as soon as the definitive identification is made. If common safety precautions are followed, few problems should occur with laboratory contamination or infection acquired by laboratory personnel.

Prevention

Preventing and controlling fungal infections continue to be a challenge to individuals, researchers, laboratorians, and hospitals. Very few formal recommendations are available to prevent exposure to community-associated fungal infections. Good personal hygiene may be the best course for prevention. However, many strategies can be followed to prevent health care–associated infections. Hospital staff members should be aware of the pathogenesis of fungal infections. Fungi are easily spread in ventilation systems, water, and skin-to-skin contact. Hospitals should follow an infection control plan that includes periodic monitoring of air-handling systems and regular testing for environmental spores. Staff members, patients, and visitors should practice good personal hygiene to minimize exposure to potential fungal infections.

The laboratory also plays an important role in fungal prevention and control. Lack of rapid and specific testing continues to be a factor in a timely diagnosis. Early definitive diagnosis ensures that the appropriate therapy is given promptly and prevents mortality.

ⓔ Visit the Evolve site for a complete list of procedures, review questions, and case studies.

Bibliography

Barenfanger J, Arakere P, Dela Cruz R, et al.: Improved outcomes associated with limiting identification of *Candida* spp. in respiratory secretions, *J Clin Microbiol* 41:5645–5649, 2003.

Beck MR, Dekoster GT, Cistola DP, et al.: NMR structure of a fungal virulence factor reveals structural homology with mammalian saposin B, *Mol Microbiol* 72:344–353, 2009.

Bennett J, Dolin R, Blaser M: *Principles and practice of infectious diseases*, ed 9, Philadelphia, 2020, Elsevier-Saunders.

Bernstein EF, Schuster MG, Stieritz, et al.: Disseminated cutaneous *Pseudallescheria boydii*, *Br J Dermatol* 132:456–460, 1995.

Bille J, Stockman L, Roberts GD, et al.: Evaluation of a lysis-centrifugation system for recovery of yeasts and filamentous fungi from blood, *J Clin Microbiol* 18:469–471, 1983.

Bille J, Edson RS, Roberts GD: Clinical evaluation of the lysis-centrifugation blood culture system for the detection of fungemia and comparison with a conventional biphasic broth blood culture system, *J Clin Microbiol* 19:126–128, 1984.

Brandhorst TT, Gauthier GM, Stein RA, et al.: Calcium binding by essential virulence factor BAD-1 of *Blastomyces dermatitidis*, *J Biol Chem* 280:42156–42163, 2005.

Carroll KC, Pfaller MA, Landry ML, et al.: *Manual of clinical microbiology*, ed 12, Washington, DC, 2019, ASM Press.

Cherniak R, Sundstrom JB: Polysaccharide antigens of the capsule of *Cryptococcus neoformans*, *Infect Immun* 62:1507–1512, 1994.

DeHoog GS, Chaturvedi V, Denning DW, et al.: Name changes in medically important fungi and their implications for clinical practice, *J Clin Microbiol* 53:1056–1062, 2015.

DeHoog GS, Haase G, Chaturvedi V, et al.: Taxonomy of medically important fungi in the molecular era, *Lancet Infect Dis* 13:385–386, 2013.

Hibbett DS, Binder M, Bischoff JF, et al.: A higher-level phylogenetic classification of the fungi, *Mycol Res* 111:509–547, 2007.

Irmenia C, Pagano L, Martino B, et al.: Invasive infections caused by *Trichosporon* species and *Geotrichum capitatum* in patients with hematological malignancies: a retrospective multicenter study from Italy and review of the literature, *J Clin Microbiol* 43:1818–1828, 2005.

Jacobson ES: Pathogenic roles for fungal melanins, *Clin Microbiol Rev* 13:708–717, 2000.

Koneman EW, Church DL, Procop GW, et al.: *Koneman's color atlas and textbook of diagnostic microbiology*, ed 7, Philadelphia, PA, 2017, Wolters Kluwer.

Kwon-Chung KJ, Faser JA, Doering TL, et al.: *Cryptococcus neoformans* and *Cryptococcus gattii*, the etiologic agents of cryptococcosis, *Cold Spring Harb Perspect Med* 4(7):a019760, 2014.

Leber AL: *Mycology and antifungal susceptibility testing, clinical microbiology procedures handbook*, ed 4, Washington, DC, 2016, ASM Press.

Lucas S, da luz Martins M, Flores O, et al.: Differentiation of *Cryptococcus neoformans* varieties and *Cryptococcus gattii* using CAP59-based loop-mediated isothermal DNA amplification, *Clin Microbiol Infect* 16:711–714, 2010.

Madariaga MG, Tenorio A, Proia L: *Trichosporon inkin* peritonitis treated with caspofungin, *J Clin Microbiol* 41:5827–5829, 2003.

Norvell LL: Melbourne approves a new CODE, *Mycotaxon* 116:481–490, 2011.

Procop GW, Roberts GD: Emerging fungal diseases: the importance of the host, *Clin Lab Med* 24:691–719, 2004.

Richardson M, Page I: Role of serological tests in the diagnosis of mold infections, *Curr Fungal Infect Rep* 12:127–136, 2018.

Singh S, Beena PM: Comparative study of different microscopic techniques and culture media for the isolation of dermatophytes, *Indian J Med Microbiol* 21:21–24, 2003.

Steinbach WJ, Schell WA, Miller JL, et al.: *Scedosporium prolificans* osteomyelitis in an immunocompetent child treated with voriconazole and caspofungin, as well as locally applied polyhexamethylene biguanide, *J Clin Microbiol* 41:3981–3985, 2003.

Tomee J, Kauffman HF: Putative virulence factors of *Aspergillus fumigatus*, *Clin Exp Allergy* 30:476–484, 2000.

Vilela R, Mendoza L: Human pathogenic entomophthorales, *Clin Microbiol Rev* 31:e00014–e00018, 2018.

Walsh TJ, Groll A, Hiemenz J, et al.: Infections due to emerging and uncommon medically important fungal pathogens, *Clin Microbiol Infect* 10(Suppl 1):48–66, 2004.

Walsh TJ, Hayden RT, Larone DH: *Larone's medically important fungi: a guide to identification*, ed 6, Washington, DC, 2018, ASM Press.

Wickes BL, Wiederhold NP: Molecular diagnostics in medical mycology, *Nat Commun* 9:5135, 2018.

Wiederhold NP, Gibas CFC: From the clinical mycology laboratory: new species and changes in fungal taxonomy and nomenclature, *J Fungi* 4:138, 2018.

59

Hyaline Molds, Mucorales, Basidiobolales, Entomophthorales, Dermatophytes, and Opportunistic and Systemic Mycoses

OBJECTIVES

1. Describe where Mucorales, Basidiobolales, and Entomophthorales are found, how they are transmitted to humans, and the diseases they cause.
2. Describe the characteristic colony morphology of the Mucorales, Basidiobolales, and Entomophthorales.
3. Outline the tests needed to diagnose a *Trichophyton* species.
4. List the key features that distinguish *Trichophyton rubrum* and *Trichophyton mentagrophytes*.
5. Compare and contrast the ways *Microsporum audouinii* and *Microsporum canis* are spread and the populations at risk.
6. Define ectothrix and endothrix.
7. Explain why diagnosing an opportunistic fungal infection in an immunocompromised patient is difficult.
8. Differentiate mucormycosis and entomophthoromycosis, including the disease presentation, causative agents, predominant patient populations, and treatment.
9. Compare and contrast *Aspergillus* and *Penicillium* spp., both macroscopically and microscopically.
10. Discuss the dimorphic molds in relation to their endemic areas, disease states, and associated diagnostic methods for identification.

HYALINE MOLDS TO BE CONSIDERED

Current Name

Mucorales
Rhizopus spp.
Mucor spp.
Actinomucor sp.
Apophysomyces spp.
Cokeromyces sp.
Lichtheimia spp.
Rhizomucor sp.
Saksenaea spp.
Syncephalastrum sp.
Cunninghamella spp.

Entomophthorales
Conidiobolus spp.

Basidiobolales
Basidiobolus sp.

Dermatophytes
Trichophyton spp.
Microsporum spp.
Epidermophyton sp.

Opportunistic Mycoses
Aspergillus spp.
Fusarium spp.
Geotrichum spp.
Acremonium spp.
Acrophialophora spp.
Arthrographis sp.
Beauveria sp.
Chrysosporium sp.
Coniochaeta spp.
Nannizziopsis sp.
Onychocola sp.
Parengyodontium sp.
Penicillium spp.
Phialemonium spp.
Paecilomyces spp.
Purpureocillium sp.
Rasamsonia spp.
Sarocladium spp. (previously *Acremonium*)
Schizophyllum sp.
Talaromyces spp.
Thermothelomyces sp.

Systemic Mycoses
Blastomyces spp.
Coccidioides spp.
Emergomyces spp.
Emmonsia sp.
Histoplasma capsulatum
Paracoccidioides spp.

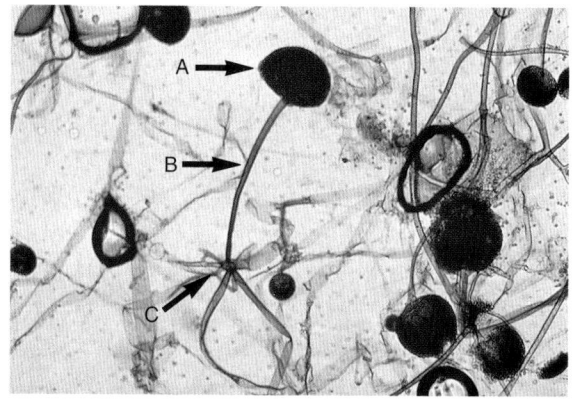

• **Fig. 59.1** *Rhizopus* spp. showing sporangium *(A)* on a long sporangiophore *(B)* arising from pauciseptate hyphae. Note the characteristic rhizoids *(C)* at the base of the sporangiophore (×250).

The Mucorales

General Characteristics

The order Mucorales (Zygomycetes) characteristically produce large, ribbonlike hyphae that are irregular in diameter and contain occasional septa. Because the septa may not be apparent in some preparations, this group sometimes has been characterized as aseptate. The specific identification of these organisms is confirmed by observing the characteristic saclike fruiting structures (sporangia), which produce internally spherical, yellow or brown spores (sporangiospores) (Fig. 59.1). Each sporangium is formed at the tip of a supporting structure (sporangiophore). During maturation, the sporangium becomes fractured, and sporangiospores are released into the environment. Sporangiophores are usually connected to one another by occasionally septate hyphae called **stolons,** which attach at contact points where rootlike structures (**rhizoids**) may appear and anchor the organism to the agar surface. Identification of the Mucorales is partly based on the presence or absence of rhizoids and the position of the rhizoids in relation to the sporangiophores.

Epidemiology and Pathogenesis

Although the Mucorales (*Rhizopus, Mucor, Actinomucor, Cokeromyces, Rhizomucor, Saksenaea, Apophysomyces, Lichtheimia [Absidia], Syncephalastrum,* and *Cunninghamella* spp.) are a less common cause of infection than the aspergilli, they are an important cause of morbidity and mortality in immunocompromised patients, particularly patients with diabetes mellitus. The organisms have a worldwide distribution and are commonly found on decaying vegetable matter or old bread (bread mold) or in soil. The organism is generally acquired by inhalation or ingestion of spores or through percutaneous routes, followed by subsequent development of infection. Once established, the infection is rapidly progressive, particularly in patients with diabetes mellitus who have infections that involve the sinuses. Other immunocompromised patients who are susceptible to infection with

Mucorales include patients with hematologic malignancies such as acute leukemia and stem cell, kidney, and liver transplant patients. Immunocompetent individuals may acquire skin infections with these fungi after traumatic injection with contaminated material. These organisms are also commonly identified as contaminants in the clinical laboratory but are also a source of nosocomial or health care–associated infections.

Spectrum of Disease

Immunocompromised patients are at greatest risk, particularly those who have uncontrolled diabetes mellitus and transplant patients who are undergoing prolonged corticosteroid, antibiotic, or cytotoxic therapy. The organisms that cause **mucormycosis** (an infection caused by Mucorales) have a marked propensity for vascular invasion and rapidly produce thrombosis and necrosis of tissue. One of the most common presentations is the **rhinocerebral form,** in which the nasal mucosa, palate, sinuses, orbit, face, and brain are involved; each shows massive necrosis with vascular invasion and infarction. Perineural invasion also occurs in mucormycoses and is a potential means of retroorbital spread (i.e., invasion into the brain). Other types of infection involve the lungs and gastrointestinal tract; some patients develop disseminated infection. The Mucorales have also caused localized skin infections in immunocompetent patients with severe burns and infections of subcutaneous tissue in patients who have undergone surgery; infection can also be a result of injury and contamination with spores or soil (Fig. 59.2).

Laboratory Diagnosis
Specimen Collection, Transport, and Processing

Blood cultures are not appropriate for diagnosis of mucormycosis. Specimens from deep lesions or tissues and sterile sites should be collected rapidly and aseptically. Sufficient quantity is essential to improve the identification and recovery of the fungal isolate.

Samples collected for the diagnosis of rhinocerebral forms of infection should include nasal discharge or scrapings, sinus aspirate, or a tissue specimen from a vascularized tissue. Respiratory samples may include sputum and bronchoalveolar lavage fluids. However, if these respiratory specimens result in negative results, a transbronchial or percutaneous computed tomography–guided biopsy of pulmonary lesions may be considered. These procedures pose significant risk to the patient and should be considered carefully.

Separate specimens should be collected for the microbiology laboratory and the histology laboratory. Preservatives used for histologic processes, such as formalin, are inhibitory to fungal growth.

Specimens should be transported in sterile containers. Tissue (biopsy specimens) should be moistened by adding a few drops of sterile saline to the container. Specimens should be transported to the laboratory within 2 hours of collection and processed immediately. Mucorales are extremely sensitive to environmental changes. See General

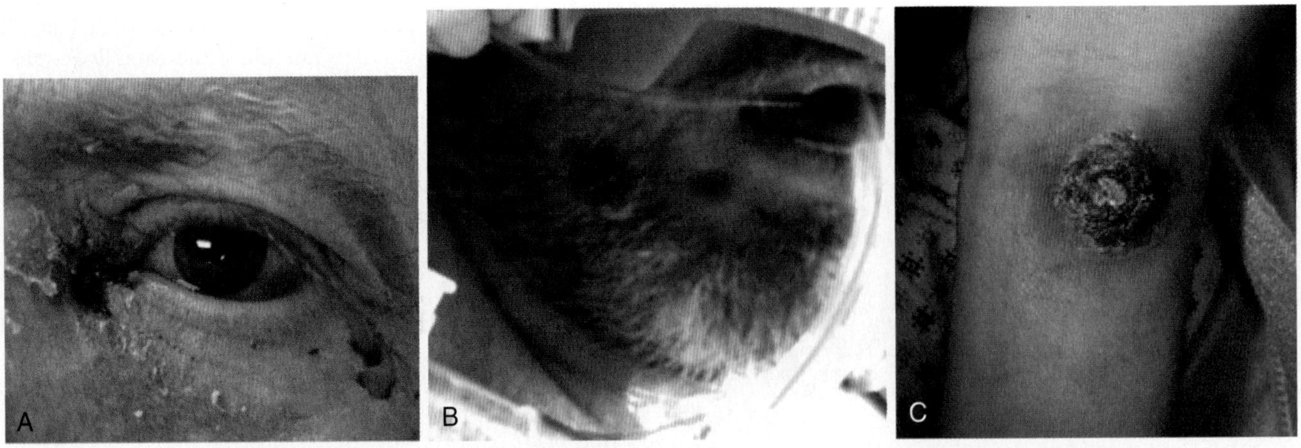

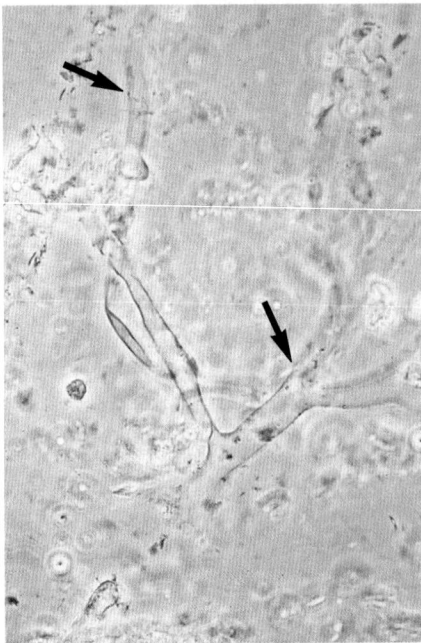

• **Fig. 59.2** Mucormycosis. (A) Orbital involvement in a cancer patient. (B) Necrotic eschar on the hard palate of a cancer patient with rhinocerebral mucormycosis. (C) Chronic nonhealing ulcer after traumatic inoculation. (Courtesy Drs. Gerald Bodey, George Viola, Saud Ahmed, and Mona Shiekh Sroujieh, The University of Texas MD Anderson Cancer Center, Houston, TX.)

Considerations for the Laboratory Diagnosis of Fungal Infections in Chapter 58.

Direct Detection Methods

The diagnosis of mucormycosis is primarily based on direct examination; nucleic acid–based testing; or recovery of the fungus from tissue, body fluids, and exudates.

Stains

A mucormycosis may be diagnosed rapidly by examining tissue specimens or exudate from infected lesions in a calcofluor white and potassium hydroxide preparation. If the sample is too thick, a false negative result may occur because of insufficient dissociation of tissues. It is recommended that the negative slide be maintained overnight and reviewed again the next day. Branching, broad-diameter, predominantly nonseptate hyphae are observed (Fig. 59.3). It is important that the laboratory notify the clinician of these findings, because Mucorales grow rapidly, and vascular invasion occurs at a rapid rate.

Antigen-Protein

Antigen-protein–based assays are not used for the diagnosis of mucormycosis. In addition, beta-D-glucan testing is not useful for diagnosis.

Nucleic Acid–Based Testing

Nucleic acid testing may be performed on formalin-fixed, paraffin-embedded, fresh or frozen tissue samples. Polymerase chain reaction (PCR) amplification of the internal transcribed spacer, as well as seminested PCR of the 18S ribosomal ribonucleic acid (RNA)/deoxyribonucleic acid (DNA) sequence, has been used to confirm identification in samples that have been identified as histopathology positive. A real-time PCR assay has also been developed that amplifies the cytochrome b gene. Nucleic acid purification from formalin-fixed and paraffin-embedded tissues often results in poor quality of extracted DNA. Therefore, fluorescent *in*

• **Fig. 59.3** Phase-contrast microscopy of a potassium hydroxide preparation of sputum. Note the fragmented portions *(arrows)* of broad, predominantly nonseptate hyphae of *Rhizopus* spp.

situ hybridization that does not require DNA extraction or amplification has the potential to improve the identification of the fungi. The technique uses synthetic oligonucleotides specific to the 5.8S and 18S ribosomal ribonucleic acid (rRNA) of the fungi.

PCR amplification of fungal genes from the serum of high-risk patient populations has demonstrated the potential for early diagnosis of mucormycosis before the demonstration of tissue pathology.

Cultivation

Growth media containing high concentrations of carbohydrates inhibits the production of asexual fruiting bodies that are required for the proper identification of the Mucorales species. It is therefore recommended that media such as potato dextrose, 2% malt, and cherry decoction (acidic) agars be used for cultivation. Growth and development of the mycelium in the Mucorales occurs within 24 to 48 hours. Subcultures should be incubated at 27°C to 30°C.

The colonial morphologic features of the Mucorales allow immediate suspicion that an organism belongs to this group. Colonies characteristically produce a fluffy, white to gray or brown hyphal growth that resembles cotton candy and that diffusely covers the surface of the agar within 24 to 96 hours (Fig. 59.4). The hyphae can grow very fast and may lift the lid of the agar plate (also known as a "lid lifter"). The hyphae appear to be coarse. The entire culture dish or tube rapidly fills with loose, grayish hyphae dotted with brown or black sporangia. The different genera and species of Mucorales cannot be differentiated using colonial morphologic features.

Approach to Identification

Mucorales are characterized by the production of branched, nonseptate, wide mycelia (10 to 20 μm). Sexual reproduction occurs by the formation of a thick walled zygospore; however, morphology of the zygospores is not generally useful for routine identification unless the species is homozygous. Asexual reproduction occurs by the formation of sporangiospores in saclike structures termed sporangiophores. The central axis of the sporangia (multispored structure) is termed the **columella (singular)** and a swelling of the sporangiophore below the columellae (plural) is termed the **apophysis.** Some species also produce rhizoids that hold the sporangiophore within the soil or growth substrate. The rhizoids are then connected to a branching root, or stolon.

Rhizopus spp. have mostly unbranched sporangiophores with rhizoids that appear opposite the point where the stolon arises, at the base of the sporangiophore (Fig. 59.1). In contrast, *Mucor* spp. are characterized by sporangiophores that are singularly produced or branched and have a round sporangium at the tip filled with sporangiospores. They do not generally have rhizoids or stolons, which distinguishes this genus from the other genera of the Mucorales (Fig. 59.5). *Lichtheimia* spp. are characterized by the presence of rhizoids that originate between branched or whorled sporangiophores (Fig. 59.6) along the stolons between the rhizoids. The sporangia of *Lichtheimia* spp. are pyriform and have a funnel-shaped area (apophysis) at the junction of the sporangium and the sporangiophore. Usually a septum is formed in the sporangiophore just below the sporangium. *Lichtheimia* produce white, fast-growing wooly colonies that become grayish brown. Other genera that are encountered much less commonly in the clinical laboratory are *Rhizomucor, Actinomucor, Cokeromyces, Syncephalastrum, Saksenaea, Cunninghamella,* and *Apophysomyces* spp. and described in Table 59.1.

Serologic Testing

Serology is not useful for diagnosing mucormycosis. Patients with invasive mucormycosis develop Mucorales-specific

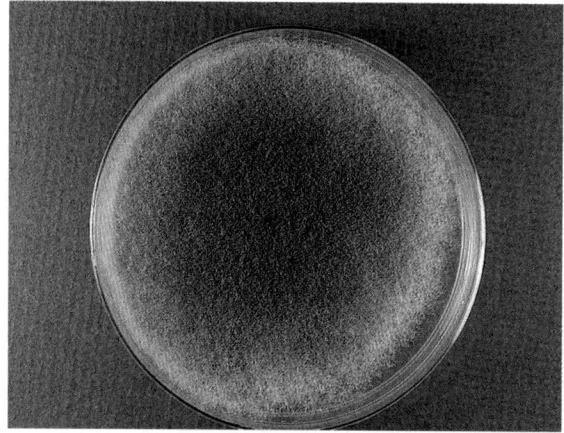

• **Fig. 59.4** *Rhizopus* colony.

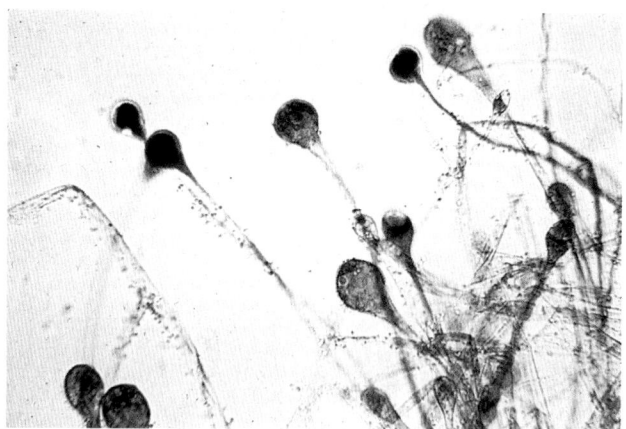

• **Fig. 59.5** *Mucor* spp. showing numerous sporangia without rhizoids (×430).

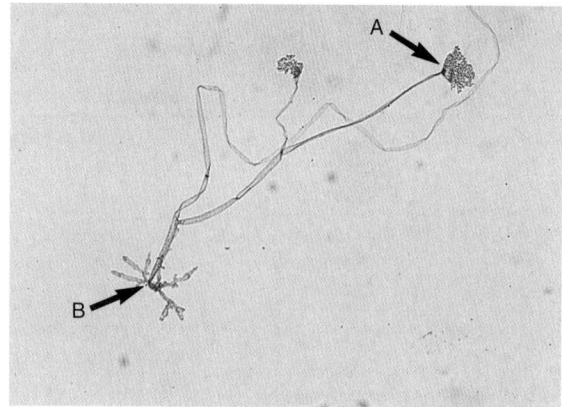

• **Fig. 59.6** *Lichtheimia* spp. *(A)* showing sporangia on long sporangiophores arising from pauciseptate hyphae *(B).* Note that rhizoids are produced between sporangiophores and not at their bases (×250).

T cells that may be used to monitor the course of the disease but not for early diagnosis.

Matrix-Assisted Laser Desorption Ionization Time-of-Flight Mass Spectrometry

Matrix-assisted laser desorption ionization time-of-flight mass spectrometry (MALDI-TOF MS) has been evaluated for the identification of Mucorales. This technique has

TABLE 59.1 Morphological Differentiation of the Mucorales, Entomophthorales, and Basidiobolales

Order/ Genus	Species	Macroscopic Morphology	Microscopic Morphology
Mucorales			
Rhizopus spp.	*R. arrhizus* *R. microsporus* *R. schipperae*	Rapidly produce white cottony colonies that turn brownish to black with the production of sporangiophores. Sporangiophores are unbranched arising singly or in groups, with well-developed rhizoids at the base.	Single or clustered brown sporangiophores. Columellae are ellipsoidal, brown to grey. Sporangiospores are angular and round to ellipsoidal.
Mucor spp.	*M. circinelloides* *M. indicus* *M. irregularis* *M. ramosissimus* *M. velutinosus*	Fast growing white to yellow becoming gray with time. Tall sporangiophores that are simple or branched.	Sporangiospores are hyaline and subspherical to ellipsoidal. *M. circinelloides* rarely produces chlamydospores, and they are absent in *M. ramosissimus*. Columellae are present and some species will demonstrate rhizoids, although it is not typical of the genera.
Actinomucor sp.	*A. elegans*	Growth is slow, colonies appear floccose and white to cream after 7 days becoming brown to beige wooly as they age.	Sporangiophores are hyaline, verticillately branched. Whorls or branches may give rise to secondary branches. Sporangiospores are spherical to ovoidal in a smooth or spiny sporangia, with a subglobose columnella present. Rhizoids and chlamydospores are produced.
Apophysomyces spp.	*A. ossiformis* *A. trapeziformis* *A. variabilis*	Rapid growing white to gray with sporangiophores.	Sporangiophores are smooth-walled, single, unbranched with multispored pyriform sporangia. Columellae are hemispherical, cylindrical, trapezoidal, or ellipsoidal. Apophyses are vase-, bell-, or funnel-shaped.
Cokeromyces sp.	*C. recurvatus*	Slow growing gray to brown.	Long, recurved, twisted stalks arise from terminal vesicles on unbranched sporangiophores. Sporangia are smooth-walled producing spherical sporangiospores. Yeastlike forms are thin- to thick-walled, spherical cells that may produce a ship's wheel appearance similar to *Paracoccidioides brasiliensis* when grown on brain-heart infusion or yeast extract peptone agar.
Lichtheimia spp.	*L. corymbifera* *L. ramosa* *L. ornata*	Fast growing white woolly colonies that become grayish brown with age.	Sporangiophores are highly branched in singles or corymbs from stolons. Rhizoids are present. Sporangia are spherical to pyriform. Columellae are hemispherical to ellipsoidal with a conical apophyses. Sporangiospores are smooth, hyaline, ellipsoidal, cylindrical, or subglobose. Irregular giant cells may be present.
Rhizomucor sp.	*R. miehei* *R. pusillus*	Rapidly growing woolly, gray to brown.	Single or branched sporangiophores on aerial mycelium or stolons. Sporangia are multispored with no apophyses. Sporangiospores are round, hyaline, and smooth-walled.
Saksenaea spp.	*S. erythrospora* *S. oblongispora* *S. vasiformis*	White to gray colonies.	Unbranched sporangiophores with dark (melanized) rhizoids. Flask-shaped sporangia.
Syncephalastrum sp.	*S. racemosum*	Rapid growing white to gray, turns darker with age.	Mostly branched sporangiophores bearing globose vesicles. Smooth-walled sporangia with spherical to ovoid merospores arranged in rows. Rhizoids present.
Cunninghamella spp.	*C. bertholletiae* *C. blakesleeana* *C. echinulate* *C. elegans*	White to dark gray.	Laterally branching sporangiophores with a globose vesicle that bears a 1-spored sporangiola. Sporangiola will become a finely echinulate spherical sporangiospore.
Entomophthorales			
Conidiobolus spp.	*C. coronatus* *C. incongruous* *C. lamprauges*	Fast growing hyaline radially folded. Initially appear waxy and become powdery with age.	Primary conidia are spherical with prominent papilla. Villose conidia appear as the colony ages.
Basidiobolales			
Basidiobolus sp.	*B. ranarum*	Colonies appear as yellow, waxy with radial folds.	Primary conidiophores have swollen apices and discharge spherical conidia. Secondary conidia are pyriform with a knob-like tip. Large aseptate mycelia are produced that break into uninucleate hyphal elements.

demonstrated a high correlation with sequencing methods for the identification of fungal isolates (97%), indicating a potential for use as a routine identification method in the clinical laboratory.

The Entomophthorales and Basidiobolales

General Characteristics

The subdivision Entomophthoromycotina contains more than 250 species distributed worldwide. However, only four species have been identified as significant in clinical samples: Order Entomophthorales; *Conidiobolus coronatus, Conidiobolus lamprauges, Conidiobolus incongruus,* and Order Basidiobolales: *Basidiobolus ranarum.*

Epidemiology and Pathogenesis

The organisms are pathogens of arthropods and animals and are primarily present in the soil, decaying vegetable material, and animal feces. Although there is a worldwide distribution, infections are more commonly identified in warm climates. Infections associated with *Conidiobolus* spp. have been identified in Africa, Madagascar, Mayotte, India, China, Japan, and South America. *B. ranarum* has been associated with infections in India, Myanmar, and Africa. Recent gastrointestinal infections with *B. ranarum* have been identified in the United States. Unlike mucormycosis, **entomophthoromycosis** occurs predominantly in immunocompetent individuals.

Spectrum of Disease

Infections from *B. ranarum,* **basidiobolomycosis** are primarily localized to subcutaneous tissue of the arms, legs, buttocks, trunk, perineum, face, or neck. Disseminated infection is rare. The infection presents as a woody, hard, painless nodule. Gastrointestinal infections have been noted. *Conidiobolus* spp. primarily infect the tissue around the nose and on the face. Infection is believed to be through inhalation of the spores in the nasal cavity or inoculation after trauma. After infection, swelling occurs that extends to the nose, cheeks, eyebrows, upper lip, palate, and pharynx. Rare cases of disseminated infection have occurred in immunocompromised patients.

Laboratory Diagnosis
Specimen Collection, Transport, and Processing

See General Considerations for the Laboratory Diagnosis of Fungal Infections in Chapter 58.

Direct Detection Methods

Direct examination methods should be used as previously described for the Mucorales. The **Splendore-Hoeppli phenomenon** (formation of asteroid bodies), the formation of eosinophilic crystals that appear radiate, starlike, asteroid, or club-shaped around a fungal infection, are associated with hyphae in tissue sections stained with hematoxylin-eosin. This is highly indicative of entomophthoromycosis but can also be observed in other bacterial, fungal, and parasitic infections.

Antigen-Protein
No antigen tests are currently available.

Nucleic Acid–Based Testing
A single polymerase chain amplification assay has been developed for the diagnosis of *Basidiobolus* entomophthoromycosis.

Cultivation
Tissue samples should be sliced or minced and cultivated on potato dextrose agar or Sabouraud agar without cycloheximide. Because of the variation in growth temperatures required for the isolation of the different organisms, cultures should be incubated at 37°C (*Conidiobolus* spp.) with a second culture incubated at 25°C to 30°C (*Basidiobolus* sp.).

Approach to Identification

B. ranarum colonies appear slightly yellow pigmented with radial folds. No aerial hyphae are present. After 7 to 10 days of growth, the culture will produce aseptate mycelia with free uninucleated hyphal elements. Sexual reproduction results in thick-walled zygospores with lateral protuberances or beaks. Primary conidiophores have swollen apices with globose spores that are forcibly discharged from the conidiophores, whereas secondary conidia appear pyriform with a knoblike adhesive tip and are passively discharged.

Conidiobolus spp. is a fast-growing fungus that produces hyaline, radially folded colonies that initially appear waxy and become powdery when mycelia begin to develop. The primary conidia are spherical and have prominent **papilla** (small bumps). **Villose** (hairlike spines) conidia appear as the colony ages. *C. coronatus* can be differentiated from the other species based on the absence of zygospores when grown on potato dextrose agar.

Serologic Testing

No serologic tests are available for the diagnosis of entomophthoromycosis.

The Dermatophytes

General Characteristics

The dermatophytes produce infections involving the superficial areas of the body, including the hair, skin, and nails (**dermatomycoses**). The genera *Trichophyton, Microsporum,* and *Epidermophyton* are the principal etiologic agents of the dermatomycoses. There is significant information based on molecular classification of these organisms that is not fully accepted or approved and therefore has not been majorly restructured in this edition. Table 59.2 includes an overview of the current dermatophytic genus, species,

TABLE 59.2	Dermatophytes		
	Species [Proposed New Name]	**Macroscopic Morphology**	**Microscopic Morphology**
Trichophyton spp.	*T. ajelloi [Arthroderma uncinatum]* *T. concentricum* *T. equinum* *T. erinacei* *T. megninii* *T. mentagrophytes* complex *T. rubrum* *T. schoenleinii* *T. simii* *T. soudanense* *T. terrestre* complex *T. tonsurans* *T. vanbreuseghemii [Arthroderma gertleri]* *T. verrucosum* *T. violaceum*	Species vary from powdery to granular and cottony. Coloration is from white to yellow, or pink. Various reverse colors from white to yellow and red to brown.	Species dependent; macroconidia may or may not be present. Macroconidia are generally pencil or club shaped. Microconidia may be tear dropped or round when present.
Microsporum spp.	*M. audouinii* *M. canis* *M. cookei* complex *[Genus Paraphyton]* *M. ferrugineum* *M. gallinae [Lophophyton gallinae]* *M. gypseum* complex *[Genus Nannizzia]* *M. nanum [Nannizzia nana]* *M. persicolor [Nannizzia persicolor]* *M. praecox [Nannizzia praecox]* *M. racemosum* *M. vanbreuseghemii [Lophophyton gallinae]*	Generally powdery pink to buff with reverse yellow to rose or red-brown.	Macroconidia are generally smooth to rough with tapered ends (rowboat appearance). Microconidia are not present. *M. nanum* macroconidia appear egg-shaped or ellipsoidal.
Epidermophyton sp.	*E. floccosum*	Granular, tan to olive brown with reverse tan to yellow.	Macroconidia are club-shaped (beaver tail) with fewer than 6 cells. Chlamydospores may be present. Microconidia are absent.

proposed nomenclature, and general characteristics. Table 59.3 also includes those routinely isolated in the clinical laboratory.

Epidemiology and Pathogenesis

The dermatophytes break down and utilize keratin as a source of nitrogen. They usually are incapable of penetrating the subcutaneous tissue, unless the host is immunocompromised, and even then, penetration into the subcutis is rare. Species of the genus *Trichophyton* are capable of invading the hair, skin, and nails; *Microsporum* spp. involve only the hair and skin; and *Epidermophyton* sp. involves the skin and nails. Common species of dermatophytes recovered from clinical specimens, in order of frequency, are *Trichophyton rubrum, Trichophyton mentagrophytes, Epidermophyton floccosum, Trichophyton tonsurans, Microsporum canis,* and *Trichophyton verrucosum.* The frequency of recovery of these species may differ by geographic locale. Other geographically limited species are described elsewhere.

Spectrum of Disease

Cutaneous mycoses are perhaps the most common fungal infections of humans. They are usually referred to as **tinea** (Latin for "worm" or "ringworm"). The gross appearance of the lesion is an outer ring of the active, progressing infection, with central healing within the ring. These infections may be characterized by another Latin noun to designate the area of the body involved; for example, **tinea corporis** (ringworm of the body); **tinea cruris** (ringworm of the groin, or "jock itch"); **tinea capitis** (ringworm of the scalp and hair); **tinea barbae** (ringworm of the beard); **tinea unguium** (ringworm of the nail); and **tinea pedis** (ringworm of the feet, or "athlete's foot").

Trichophyton spp.

Members of the genus *Trichophyton* are widely distributed and are the most important and common causes of infections of the feet and nails; they may be responsible for tinea corporis, tinea capitis, tinea unguium, and tinea barbae. They are commonly seen in adult infections, which vary

TABLE 59.3 Characteristics of Dermatophytes Commonly Recovered in the Clinical Laboratory

Dermatophyte	Colonial Morphology	Growth Rate	Microscopic Identification
Microsporum audouinii[a]	Downy white to salmon-pink colony; reverse tan to salmon-pink.	2 weeks	Sterile hyphae; terminal chlamydoconidia, favic chandeliers, and pectinate bodies; macroconidia rarely seen (bizarre shaped if seen); microconidia rare or absent.
Microsporum canis	Colony usually membranous with feathery periphery; center of colony white to buff over orange-yellow; lemon-yellow or yellow-orange apron and reverse.	1 week	Thick-walled, spindle-shaped, multiseptate, rough-walled macroconidia, some with a curved tip; microconidia rarely seen.
Microsporum cookei complex	Velvety to granular with a wine-red reverse	1 week	Thick-walled, rough-walled macroconidia with cellular compartments, no true cross walls; microconidia are teardrop-shaped.
Microsporum gallinae	Flat to velvety with a white surface with pink tinge; red reverse with diffusible pigment	1 week	Smooth to rough-walled macroconidia; thickest cell often at apex; drop-shaped microconidia
Microsporum gypseum	Cinnamon-colored, powdery colony; reverse light tan.	1 week	Thick-walled, rough, elliptical, multiseptate macroconidia; microconidia few or absent.
Epidermophyton floccosum	Center of colony tends to be folded and is khaki green; periphery is yellow; reverse yellowish-brown with observable folds.	1 week	Macroconidia: large, smooth-walled, multiseptate, clavate, and borne singly or in clusters of two or three; microconidia not formed by this species.
Trichophyton mentagrophytes complex	Different colonial types; white, granular, and fluffy varieties; occasional light-yellow periphery in younger cultures; reverse buff to reddish-brown.	7–10 days	Many round to globose microconidia, most commonly borne in grapelike clusters or laterally along the hyphae; spiral hyphae in 30% of isolates; macroconidia are thin-walled, smooth, club-shaped, and multiseptate; numerous or rare, depending on strain.
Trichophyton rubrum	Colonial types vary from white downy to pink granular; rugal folds are common; reverse yellow when colony is young, but wine/red color commonly develops with age.	2 weeks	Microconidia usually teardrop-shaped, most commonly borne along sides of the hyphae; macroconidia usually absent but when present are smooth, thin-walled, and pencil-shaped.
Trichophyton schoenleinii[a]	Irregularly heaped, smooth, white to cream colony with radiating grooves; reverse white.	2–3 weeks	Hyphae usually sterile; many antler-type hyphae seen (favic chandeliers).
Trichophyton tonsurans	White, tan to yellow or rust, suedelike to powdery; wrinkled with heaped or sunken center; reverse yellow to tan to rust red.	7–14 days	Microconidia are teardrop- or club-shaped with flat bottoms; vary in size but usually larger than other dermatophytes; macroconidia rare (balloon forms found when present).
Trichophyton verrucosum	Glabrous to velvety white colonies; rare strains produce yellow-brown color; rugal folds with tendency to skin into agar surface.	2–3 weeks	Microconidia rare, large, and teardrop-shaped when seen; macroconidia extremely rare but form characteristic rat-tail types when seen; many chlamydoconidia seen in chains, particularly when colony is incubated at 37°C.
Trichophyton violaceum[a]	Port wine to deep violet colony, may be heaped or flat with waxy glabrous surface; pigment may be lost on subculture.	2–3 weeks	Branched, tortuous, sterile hyphae; chlamydoconidia commonly aligned in chains.

[a]These organisms are not commonly seen in the United States.

in their clinical manifestations. Most cosmopolitan species are **anthropophilic**, or "human loving"; few are **zoophilic**, primarily infecting animals, and one is geophilic or soil associated. The *T. mentagrophytes* complex includes several zoophilic and anthropophilic species.

Generally, hairs infected with *Trichophyton* organisms do not fluoresce under the ultraviolet (UV) light of a Woods lamp. Fungal elements must be demonstrated inside, surrounding and penetrating the hair shaft or within a skin scraping to diagnose a dermatophyte infection by direct examination. Confirmation requires recovery and identification of the causative organism.

Laboratory Diagnosis

Specimen Collection, Transport, and Processing

See General Considerations for the Laboratory Diagnosis of Fungal Infections in Chapter 58.

Direct Detection Methods

Stains

Calcofluor white or potassium hydroxide preparations reveal the presence of hyaline septate hyphae or arthroconidia (Figs. 58.4 and 59.7). Direct microscopic examination of infected hairs may reveal the hair shaft to be filled with masses of large arthroconidia (4 to 7 μm) in chains, characteristic of an **endothrix** type of invasion. In other instances, the hair shows external masses of spores that ensheathe the hair shaft; this is characteristic of the **ectothrix** type of hair invasion. Hairs infected with *Trichophyton schoenleinii* reveal hyphae and air spaces within the shaft. Evolve Procedure 59.1 describes the hair perforation test used for the differentiation of *Trichophyton* spp.

Antigen-Protein

Antigen-protein–based assays are not useful for the detection or identification of dermatophytes.

Nucleic Acid–Based Testing

Nucleic acid amplification assays for dermatophytes are not routine. Current traditional procedures are more cost effective for superficial infections.

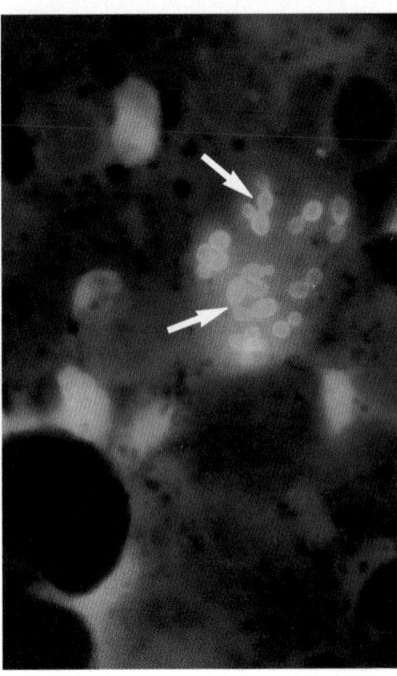

• **Fig. 59.7** Calcofluor white stain of sputum showing intracellular yeast cells of *Histoplasma capsulatum (arrows)*. The cells are 2 to 5 μm in diameter.

Cultivation

Because the dermatophytes generally present a similar microscopic appearance in infected hair, skin, or nails, final identification typically is made by culture. A summary of the colonial and microscopic morphologic features of these fungi is presented in Table 59.2. Fig. 59.8 presents an identification schema useful to the clinical laboratory for identification of commonly encountered dermatophytes. The schema begins with the microscopic features of the dermatophytes that may be visible in the initial examination of the culture. In many instances, the primary recovery medium fails to function as well as a **sporulation medium**. Often the initial growth must be subcultured onto cornmeal agar or potato dextrose agar to induce sporulation.

Approach to Identification

Trichophyton spp.

Microscopically, *Trichophyton* organisms are characterized by smooth, club-shaped, thin-walled macroconidia with three to eight septa ranging from 4 × 8 μm to 8 × 15 μm. The macroconidia are borne singly at the terminal ends of hyphae or on short conidiophores; the microconidia (which may be described as "birds on a fence") predominate and are usually spherical, pyriform (teardrop-shaped), or **clavate** (club-shaped) and 2 to 4 μm (Fig. 59.9). Only the common *Trichophyton* species are described here.

T. rubrum and *T. mentagrophytes* complex are the most common species recovered in the clinical laboratory. *T. rubrum* is a slow-growing organism that produces a flat or heaped-up colony, generally white to reddish, with a cottony or velvety surface. The characteristic cherry-red color is best observed on the reverse side of the colony; however, this is produced only after 3 to 4 weeks of incubation. Occasional strains may lack the deep red pigmentation on primary isolation. Two types of colonies may be produced: fluffy and granular. Microconidia are uncommon in most of the fluffy strains and more common in the granular strains; they occur as small, teardrop-shaped conidia often borne laterally along the sides of the hyphae (Fig. 59.9). Macroconidia are less common, although they are sometimes found in the granular strains, where they appear as thin-walled, smooth-walled, multicelled, cigar-shaped conidia with three to eight septa. *T. rubrum* has no specific nutritional requirements. It does not perforate hair *in vitro* or produce urease.

T. mentagrophytes complex produce two distinct colonial forms: the downy variety recovered from patients with tinea pedis and the granular variety recovered from lesions acquired by contact with animals. The rapidly growing colonies may appear as white to cream-colored or yellow, cottony or downy, and coarsely granular to powdery. They may produce a few spherical microconidia. The granular colonies may show evidence of red pigmentation. The reverse side of the colony is usually rose-brown, occasionally orange to deep red, and may be confused with *T. rubrum*. Granular colonies sporulate freely, with numerous small, spherical

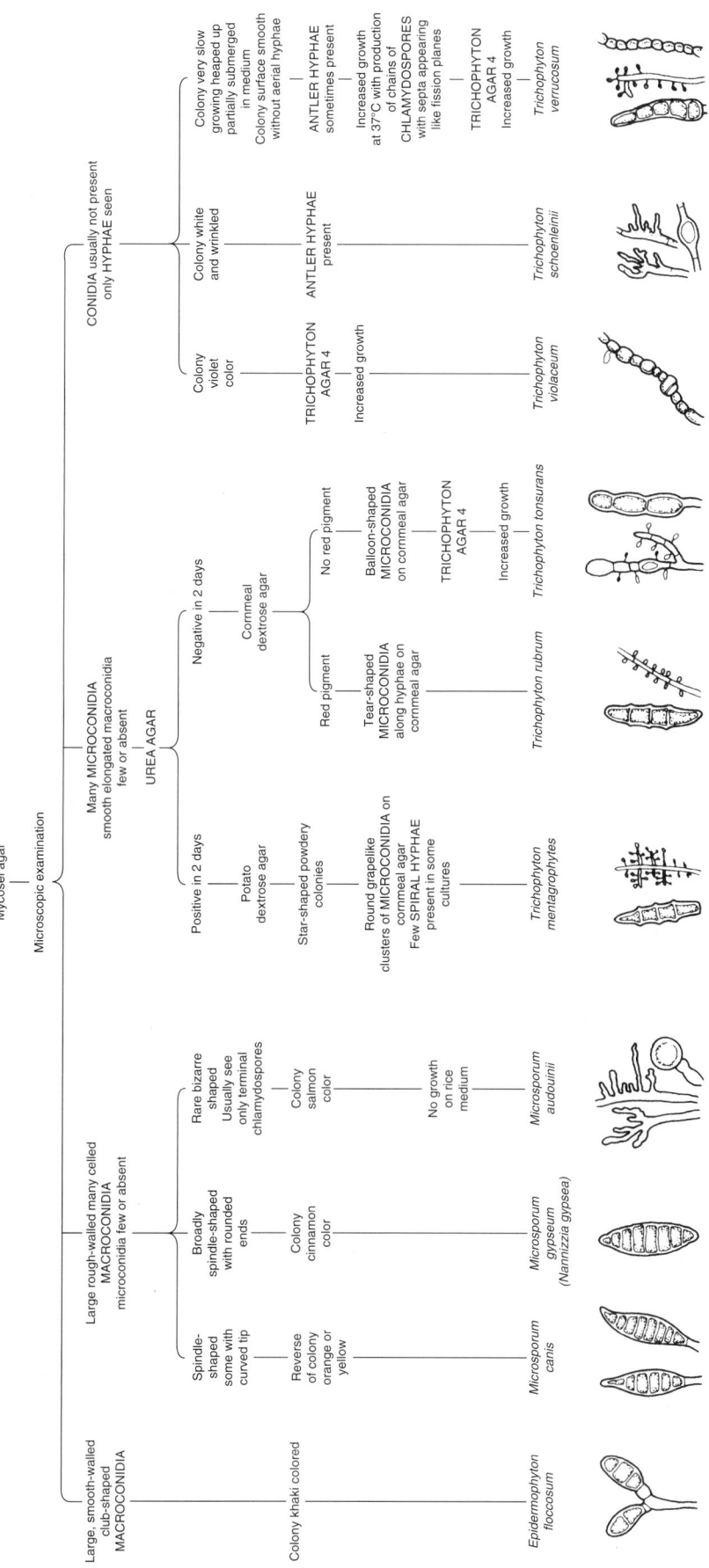

• **Fig. 59.8** Dermatophyte identification schema. (Modified from Koneman EW, Roberts GD. *Practical Laboratory Mycology. 3rd ed.* Baltimore: Williams & Wilkins; 1985.)

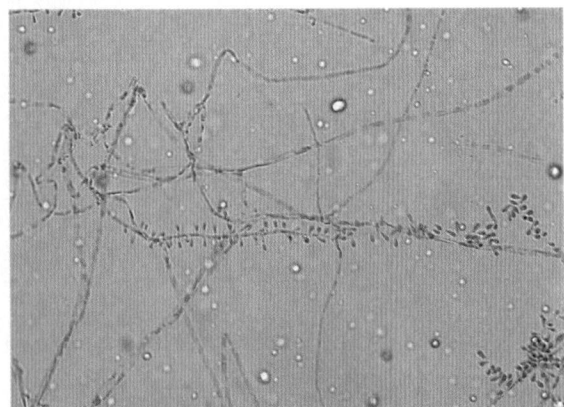

• **Fig. 59.9** *Trichophyton rubrum* showing numerous pyriform microconidia borne singly on hyphae (×750).

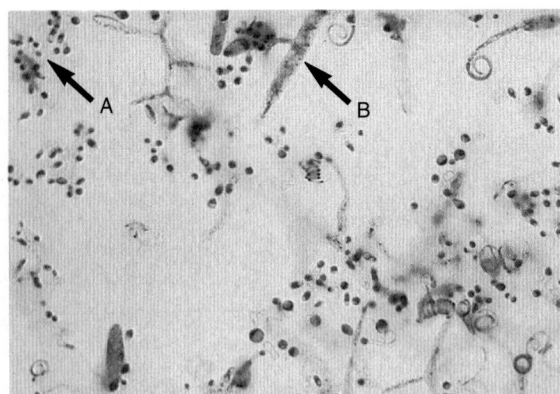

• **Fig. 59.10** *A, Trichophyton mentagrophytes* showing numerous microconidia in grapelike clusters. *B,* Several thin-walled macroconidia also are present (×500).

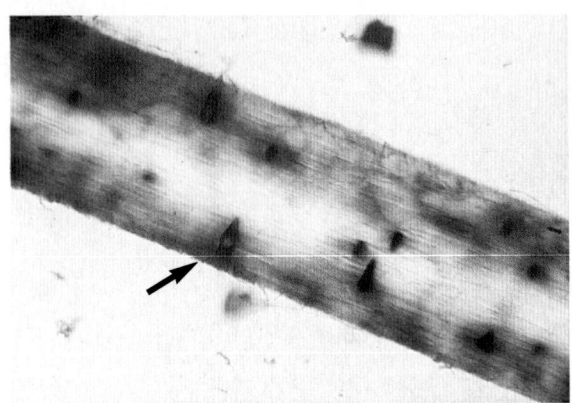

• **Fig. 59.11** Hair perforation by *Trichophyton mentagrophytes.* Wedge-shaped areas *(arrow)* illustrate hair perforation (×100).

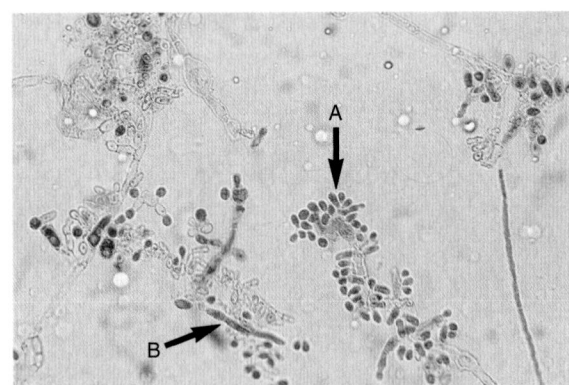

• **Fig. 59.12** *Trichophyton tonsurans* showing numerous microconidia *(A)* that are borne singly or in clusters. A single macroconidium *(B)* (rare) is also present (×600).

microconidia in grapelike clusters and thin-walled, smooth-walled, cigar-shaped macroconidia measuring 6 × 20 μm to 8 × 50 μm, with two to five septa (Fig. 59.10). Macroconidia characteristically exhibit a definite narrow attachment to their base. Spiral hyphae may be found in one third of the isolates recovered.

T. mentagrophytes complex species produce urease within 2 to 3 days after inoculation onto Christensen's urea agar. Unlike *T. rubrum, T. mentagrophytes* complex perforate hair (Fig. 59.11), a feature that may be used to distinguish between the two fungi when differentiation is difficult.

T. tonsurans is responsible for an epidemic form of tinea capitis that commonly occurs in children and occasionally in adults. It has displaced *Microsporum audouinii* as a primary cause of tinea capitis in most of the United States. The fungus causes a low-grade superficial lesion of varying severity and produces circular, scaly patches of **alopecia** (loss of hair). The stubs of hair remain in the epidermis of the scalp after the brittle hairs have broken off, which may give the typical "black dot" ringworm appearance. Because the infected hairs do not fluoresce under a Woods lamp, the physician should carefully search for the embedded stubs, using a bright light.

Cultures of *T. tonsurans* develop slowly and are typically buff to brown, wrinkled, and suedelike in appearance. The colony surface shows radial folds and often develops a crater-like depression in the center with deep fissures. The reverse side of the colony is yellowish- to reddish-brown. Microscopically, numerous microconidia with flat bases are produced on the sides of hyphae. With age, the microconidia tend to become pleomorphic, are swollen to elongated, and are referred to as balloon forms (Fig. 59.12). Chlamydoconidia are abundant in old cultures; swollen and fragmented hyphal cells resembling arthroconidia may be seen. *T. tonsurans* grows poorly on media lacking enrichments (casein agar); however, growth is greatly enhanced by the presence of thiamine or inositol in casein agar.

T. verrucosum causes a variety of lesions in cattle and in humans; it is most often seen in farmers, who acquire the infection from cattle. The lesions are found chiefly on the beard, neck, wrist, and back of the hands; they are deep, pustular, and inflammatory. With pressure, short stubs of hair may be recovered from the purulent lesion. Direct examination of the hair shaft reveals sheaths of isolated chains of large spores (5 to 10 μm in diameter) surrounding the hair shaft (ectothrix) and hyphae within the hair (endothrix). Masses of these conidia may also be seen in exudate from the lesions.

T. verrucosum grows slowly (14 to 30 days); growth is enhanced at 35°C to 37°C and on media enriched with thiamine and inositol. *T. verrucosum* may be suspected when slowly growing colonies appear to embed themselves into the agar surface.

Kane and Smitka[1] described a medium for the early detection and identification of *T. verrucosum*. The ingredients for this medium are 4% casein and 0.5% yeast extract. The organism is recognized by its early hydrolysis of casein and very slow growth rate. Chains of chlamydoconidia are formed regularly at 37°C. Early detection of hydrolysis, the formation of characteristic chains of chlamydoconidia, and the restrictive slow growth rate of *T. verrucosum* differentiate it from *T. schoenleinii,* another slowly growing organism. Colonies are small, heaped, and folded; occasionally they are flat and disk-shaped. At first, they are glabrous and waxy, with a short aerial mycelium. Colonies range from gray and waxlike to bright yellow. The reverse of the colony most often is nonpigmented but may be yellow.

Microscopically, chlamydoconidia in chains and antler hyphae may be the only structures observed microscopically in cultures of *T. verrucosum* (Fig. 58.10). Chlamydoconidia may be abundant at 35°C to 37°C (Fig. 58.16). Microconidia may be produced by some cultures if the medium is enriched with yeast extract or a vitamin (Fig. 59.13). Conidia, when present, are borne laterally from the hyphae and are large and clavate. Macroconidia are rarely formed, vary considerably in size and shape, and are referred to as "rat tail" or "string bean" in appearance.

T. schoenleinii causes a severe type of infection called **favus.** It is characterized by the formation of yellowish cup-shaped crusts, or **scutulae,** on the scalp; considerable scarring of the scalp; and sometimes permanent alopecia. Infections are common among members of the same family. A distinctive invasion of the infected hair, the favic type, is demonstrated by the presence of large, inverted cones of hyphae and arthroconidia at the base of the hair follicle and branching hyphae throughout the length of the hair shaft. Longitudinal tunnels or empty spaces appear in the hair shaft where the hyphae have disintegrated. In calcofluor white or potassium hydroxide preparations, these tunnels are readily filled with fluid; air bubbles may also be seen in these tunnels.

T. schoenleinii is a slowly growing organism (30 days or longer) that produces a white to light-gray colony with a waxy surface. Colonies have an irregular border consisting mostly of submerged hyphae, which tend to crack the agar. The surface of the colony is usually nonpigmented or tan, furrowed, and irregularly folded. The reverse side of the colony is usually tan or nonpigmented. Microscopically, conidia commonly are not formed. The hyphae tend to become knobby and club-shaped at the terminal ends, with the production of many short lateral and terminal branches (Fig. 59.14). Chlamydoconidia are generally numerous. All strains of *T. schoenleinii* may be grown in a vitamin-free medium and grow equally well at room temperature or at 35°C to 37°C.

Trichophyton violaceum causes an infection of the scalp and body and is seen primarily in people living in the Mediterranean region, the Middle and Far East, and Africa. Hair invasion is of the endothrix type; the typical "black dot" type of tinea capitis is observed clinically. Direct microscopic examination of a calcofluor white or potassium hydroxide preparation of the nonfluorescing hairs shows dark, thick hairs filled with masses of arthroconidia arranged in chains, similar to those seen in *T. tonsurans* infections.

Colonies of *T. violaceum* are very slow growing, beginning as cone-shaped, cream-colored, glabrous colonies. Later these become heaped up, verrucous (warty), violet to purple, and waxy in consistency. Colonies may often be described as "port wine" in color. The reverse side of the colony is purple or nonpigmented. Older cultures may develop a velvety area of mycelium and sometimes lose their pigmentation. Microscopically, microconidia and macroconidia generally are not present; only sterile, distorted hyphae and chlamydoconidia are found. In some instances, however, swollen hyphae containing cytoplasmic granules may be seen. Growth of *T. violaceum* is enhanced on media containing thiamine.

Microsporum spp.

Species of the genus *Microsporum* are immediately recognized by the presence of large (8 to 15 μm × 35 to 150 μm),

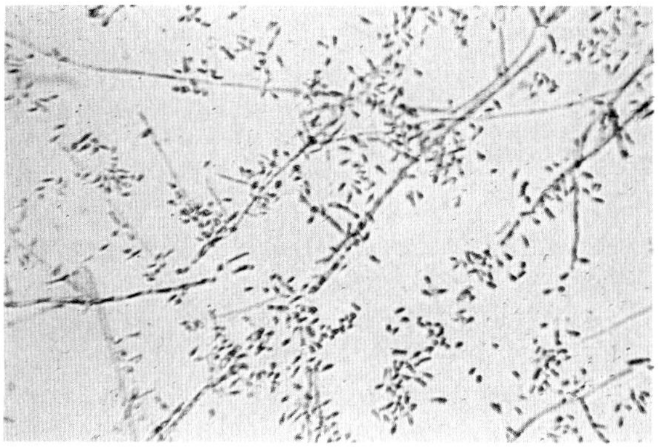

• **Fig. 59.13** *Trichophyton verrucosum* showing microconidia, which are rarely seen (×500).

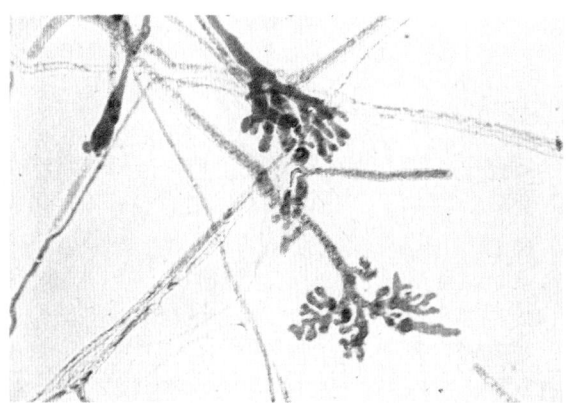

• **Fig. 59.14** *Trichophyton schoenleinii* showing swollen hyphal tips with lateral and terminal branching (favic chandeliers). Microconidia and macroconidia are absent (×500).

spindle-shaped, **echinulate** (covered with small spines), rough-walled macroconidia with thick walls (up to 4 μm) containing four or more septa (Fig. 59.15). The exception is *Microsporum nanum,* which characteristically produces macroconidia with two cells. Microconidia, when present, are small (3 to 7 μm) and club-shaped and are borne on the hyphae, either laterally or on short conidiophores. Cultures of *Microsporum* spp. develop either rapidly or slowly (5 to 14 days) and produce aerial hyphae that may be velvety, powdery, glabrous, or cottony, varying in color from whitish, to buff, to a cinnamon-brown, with varying shades on the reverse side of the colony.

M. audouinii was once the most important cause of epidemic tinea capitis among school children in the United States. This organism is anthropophilic and is spread directly by means of infected hairs on hats, caps, upholstery, combs, or barber clippers. Most infections are chronic; some heal spontaneously, whereas others may persist for several years. Infected hair shafts fluoresce yellow-green under a Woods lamp. Colonies of *M. audouinii* generally grow more slowly than other members of the genus *Microsporum* (10 to 21 days), and they produce a velvety aerial mycelium that is colorless to light gray to tan. The reverse side often appears salmon-pink to reddish-brown. Colonies of *M. audouinii* do not usually sporulate in culture. The addition of yeast extract may stimulate growth and the production of macroconidia in some instances. Most commonly, atypical vegetative forms, such as terminal chlamydoconidia and antler and racquet hyphae, are the only clues to the identification of this organism. *M. audouinii* often is identified as a cause of infection by exclusion of all the other dermatophytes.

M. canis is primarily a pathogen of animals (zoophilic); it is the most common cause of ringworm infection in dogs and cats in the United States. Children and adults acquire the disease through contact with infected animals, particularly puppies and kittens, although human-to-human transfer has been reported. Hairs infected with *M. canis* fluoresce a bright yellow-green under a Woods lamp, which is a useful tool for screening pets as possible sources of human infection. Direct examination of a calcofluor white or potassium

hydroxide preparation of infected hairs reveals small spores (2 to 3 μm) outside the hair. Culture must be performed to provide the specific identification.

Colonies of *M. canis* grow rapidly, are granular or fluffy with a feathery border, white to buff, and characteristically have a lemon-yellow or yellow-orange fringe at the periphery. On aging, the colony becomes dense and cottony and a deeper brownish-yellow or -orange and frequently shows an area of heavy growth in the center. The reverse side of the colony is bright yellow, becoming orange- or reddish-brown with age. In rare cases, strains are recovered that show no reverse-side pigment. Microscopically, *M. canis* shows an abundance of large (15 to 20 μm × 60 to 125 μm), spindle-shaped, multisegmented (four to eight) macroconidia with curved ends (Fig. 59.15). These are thick-walled with spiny (echinulate) projections on their surfaces. Microconidia are usually few in number, but large numbers occasionally may be seen.

Microsporum gypseum complex are free-living fungi of the soil (**geophilic**) that only rarely causes human or animal infection and occasionally may be seen in the clinical laboratory. Infected hairs generally do not fluoresce under a Woods lamp. However, microscopic examination of the infected hairs shows them to be irregularly covered with clusters of spores (5 to 8 μm), some in chains. These arthroconidia of the ectothrix type are considerably larger than those of other *Microsporum* species.

M. gypseum complex species grow rapidly as flat, irregularly fringed colonies with a coarse, powdery surface that appear to be buff or cinnamon colored. The underside of the colony is orange to brownish. Microscopically, macroconidia are seen in large numbers and are characteristically large, are ellipsoidal, have rounded ends, and are multisegmented (three to nine) with echinulated surfaces (Fig. 59.16). Although they are spindle-shaped, these macroconidia are not as pointed at the distal ends as those of *M. canis.* The appearance of the colonial and microscopic morphologic features is sufficient to make the distinction between *M. gypseum* complex and *M. canis.*

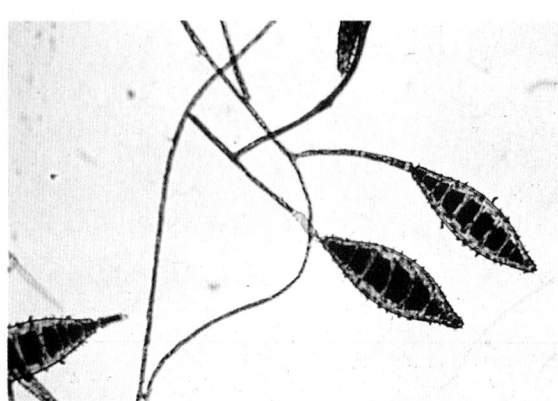

• **Fig. 59.15** Large, rough-walled macroconidia of *Microsporum canis* (×430).

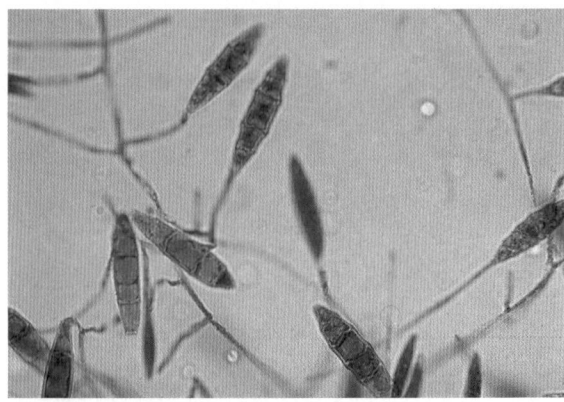

• **Fig. 59.16** *Microsporum gypseum* showing ellipsoidal, multicelled macroconidia (×750).

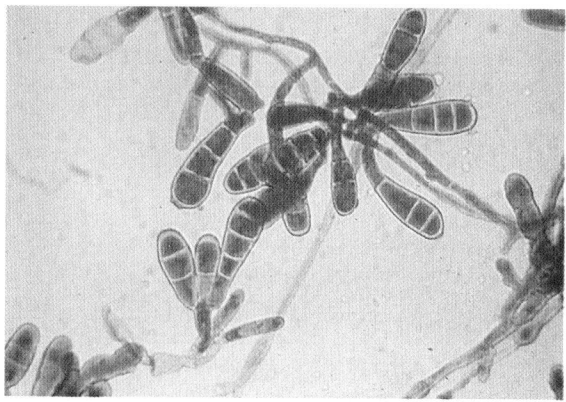

• **Fig. 59.17** *Epidermophyton floccosum* showing numerous smooth, multiseptate, thin-walled macroconidia that appear club-shaped (×1000).

Epidermophyton sp.

E. floccosum, the only member of the genus *Epidermophyton,* is a common cause of tinea cruris and tinea pedis. Because this organism is susceptible to cold, specimens submitted for dermatophyte culture should not be refrigerated before culture, and cultures should not be stored at 4°C. In direct examination of skin scrapings using the calcofluor white or potassium hydroxide preparation, the fungus is seen as fine branching hyphae. *E. floccosum* grows slowly; the growth appears olive-green to khaki, with the periphery surrounded by a dull orange-brown. After several weeks, colonies develop a cottony white aerial mycelium that completely overgrows the colony; the mycelium is sterile and remains so even after subculture. Microscopically, numerous smooth, thin-walled, club-shaped, multiseptate (2 to 4 μm) macroconidia are seen (Fig. 59.17). They are rounded at the tip and are borne singly on a conidiophore or in groups of two or three. Microconidia are absent, spiral hyphae are rare, and chlamydoconidia are usually numerous. The absence of microconidia is useful for differentiating this organism from *Trichophyton* spp.; the morphology of the macroconidia (smooth, thin-walled) is useful for differentiating it from *Microsporum* spp.

Serologic Testing

Serology is not useful for the diagnosis of disease caused by dermatophytes.

The Opportunistic Mycoses

General Characteristics

The tissue-invasive opportunistic mycoses are a group of fungal infections that occur almost exclusively in immunocompromised patients. Opportunistic fungal infections are typically identified in a host compromised by some underlying disease process, such as lymphoma, leukemia, diabetes mellitus, or another defect of the immune system. Many patients, particularly those who undergo some type of transplantation, are placed on treatment with corticosteroids,

cytotoxic drugs, or other immunosuppressive agents to control rejection of the transplanted organ. Many fungi previously believed to be nonpathogenic are now recognized as etiologic agents of opportunistic fungal infections. Because most of the organisms known to cause infection in this group of patients are commonly encountered in the clinical laboratory as **saprobes** (saprophytic fungi), it may be impossible for the laboratorian to determine the clinical significance of these isolates recovered from clinical specimens. Laboratories must identify and report completely the presence of all fungi recovered, because each is a potential pathogen. Many of the organisms associated with opportunistic infections are acquired during construction, demolition, or remodeling of buildings or are hospital-acquired. Other information about the specific clinical aspects of the opportunistic fungal infections is discussed with the individual organism.

Epidemiology and Pathogenesis
Aspergillus spp.

Several *Aspergillus* spp. are among the most commonly encountered fungi in the clinical laboratory (Table 59.4); any are potentially pathogenic in an immunocompromised host, but some species are more commonly associated with disease. There are over 350 species of *Aspergillus* widespread in the environment, where they colonize grain, leaves, soil, and living plants. Conidia of the aspergilli are easily dispersed into the environment, and humans become infected by inhaling them. Assessing the significance of *Aspergillus* organisms in a clinical specimen may be difficult. They are commonly found in cultures of respiratory secretions, skin scrapings, and other specimens.

Pathogenesis and Spectrum of Disease
Aspergillus spp.

Aspergillus spp. can cause disease by ingestion of mycotoxins, traumatic inoculation, or inhalation. *Aspergillus* spp. are capable of causing disseminated infection, as is seen in immunocompromised patients, but also of causing a wide variety of other types of infections, including a pulmonary or sinus fungus ball, allergic bronchopulmonary aspergillosis, external **otomycosis** (a fungus ball of the external auditory canal), mycotic keratitis, **onychomycosis** (infection of the nail and nail bed), sinusitis, endocarditis, and central nervous system (CNS) infection. Most often, immunocompromised patients acquire a primary pulmonary infection that becomes rapidly progressive and may disseminate to virtually any organ.

Fusarium spp. and Other Hyaline Septate Opportunistic Molds

Molecular phylogenetic studies have indicated that organisms that were previously considered individual more accurately represent species complexes containing more than 60 different species. The most commonly isolated organisms within this group are within the *Fusarium solani* species complex, including *F. petroliphilum, F. keratoplasticum, F. falciforme,*

TABLE
59.4 **Clinically Relevant *Aspergillus* spp.**

Species	Macroscopic Morphology	Microscopic Morphology	Seriation
A. fumigatus	Dark blue-green to gray with age; reverse variable	Smooth nonpigmented to green conidiophores short to long with a foot cell at the base; dome shaped vesicle with spherical, rough-walled conidia. Septate hyphae.	Uniseriate; columnar.
A. flavus	Yellow to dark yellow-green	Rough nonpigmented conidiophore; subglobose to globose vesicle; conidia globose (spherical) or ellipsoidal.	Uniseriate and biseriate; loosely radiate or splits into columns with age.
A. nidulans[a]	Dark green, buff to purple-brown; reverse red to purple	Smooth brown conidiophore; hemispherical vesicle; rough, globose conidia; cleistothecia globose and reddish-brown.	Biseriate columnar.
A. niger	Black with white margin, may have yellow surface mycelium; reverse non-pigmented to pale yellow	Smooth nonpigmented to brown conidiophore; globose vesicle; thick-walled brownish-black, rough conidia.	Biseriate radiate that splits into columns with age.
A. terreus	Tan to cinnamon-brown	Smooth, nonpigmented conidiophore; dome-shaped vesicle; smooth subglobose, globose, or elliptical conidia. Single-celled conidia (aleurioconidia) may be present on submerged hyphae.	Biseriate columnar.
A. ustus	Brown-gray or olive-gray; reverse yellow to red or purple	Smooth nonpigmented to brown conidiophore; subglobose to globose vesicle; rough, globose conidia.	Biseriate; radiate to loosely columnar.
A. versicolor	Green to gray or tan with patches of pink or yellow; reverse deep red to variable	Ovate to elliptical vesicle; globose echinulate conidia.	Biseriate; radiate to loosely columnar.

[a]Toxigenic species.

F. solani, F. lichenicola, and *F. neocosmoporiellum.* The second most common group responsible for human disease is the *Fusarium oxysporum* species complex. Additional groups of *Fusarium* spp. that are clinically relevant include the *Fusarium fujikuroi* species complex, *Fusarium incarnatum-Fusarium equiseti* species complex, *Fusarium chlamydosporum* species complex, and the *Fusarium dimerum* species complex.

Infection caused by *Fusarium* spp. and other hyaline septate monomorphic molds is becoming more common, particularly in immunocompromised patients. These organisms are common environmental microbiota and have long been known to cause mycotic keratitis after traumatic implantation into the cornea. Oftentimes infections are associated with the consumption of grains contaminated with trichothecene mycotoxins produced by *F. sporotrichioides* or *F. poae.* Disseminated fusariosis is commonly accompanied by fungemia, which is detected by routine blood culture systems. In contrast, the aspergilli are rarely recovered from blood culture, even in cases of endovascular infection. Necrotic skin lesions are common with disseminated fusariosis. Other types of infection caused by *Fusarium* spp. include sinusitis, wound (burn) infection, allergic fungal sinusitis, and endophthalmitis.

Fusarium spp. are commonly recovered from respiratory tract secretions, skin, and other specimens from patients who show no evidence of infection. Interpretation of culture results rests with the clinician and is often assisted by correlation with histopathology results. *Geotrichum candidum* is an uncommon cause of infection but has been shown to cause wound infections and oral thrush; it is an opportunistic pathogen in immunocompromised hosts. *Acremonium* spp. are also recognized as important pathogens in immunocompromised hosts; these have been associated with disseminated infection, fungemia, subcutaneous lesions, and esophagitis. *Penicillium* spp. includes more than 250 recognized species and are among the most common organisms recovered by the clinical laboratory. In North America, they are rarely associated with invasive fungal disease. However, they may be a cause of allergic bronchopulmonary penicilliosis or chronic allergic sinusitis. *Talaromyces marneffei* is an important and emerging pathogen in Southeast Asia and is discussed further in the section on dimorphic pathogens. Of the *Purpureocillium* species, *Purpureocillium lilacinum* appears to be the most pathogenic species and has been associated with endophthalmitis, cutaneous infections, and arthritis. *Paecilomyces variotii* complex includes five species with *P. variotii* and *P. formosus* being the most important pathogens, causing endocarditis, fungemia, and invasive disease.

A variety of other saprobic fungi are not discussed here in detail and may be encountered in the clinical laboratory but are seen less commonly. Several are included in Table 59.5. Other references are recommended for further information about identification of these organisms.

Laboratory Diagnosis
Specimen Collection, Transport, and Processing
See General Considerations for the Laboratory Diagnosis of Fungal Infections in Chapter 58.

Direct Detection Methods
Stains
Specimens submitted for direct microscopic examination containing organisms in this group demonstrate septate hyphae that usually show evidence of dichotomous branching, often of 45 degrees (Fig. 59.18). In addition, some hyphae may have rounded thick-walled cells. Although often considered to represent an *Aspergillus* species, these

TABLE 59.5 Other Opportunistic Fungal Organisms

Genus	Species	Clinical Significance	Macroscopic Morphology	Microscopic Morphology
Acrophialophora spp.	A. fusispora A. levis A. seudatica	Associated with colonization in cystic fibrosis patients; keratitis, pulmonary infections, and brain abscesses.	Pale white and darken centrally to a gray or brown as the colony ages.	Unbranched, brown echinulate conidiophores, anchored by a foot-cell. Conidia are in chains and may have a distinct band.
Arthrographis sp.	A. kalrae	Rare opportunist that has been recovered from skin, lung, corneal ulcers, and sinusitis.	White, appear creamy, yeastlike on artificial media. Become hyphal and buff with yellow reverse.	Treelike conidiophores with lateral branches; arthroconidia.
Beauveria sp.	B. bassiana	Limited virulence in humans; has been isolated in human cases of keratitis.	Colonies are yellow to white.	Produces solitary conidia sympoidally arranged.
Chrysosporium sp.	C. zonatum	Associated with cases of pneumonia and osteomyelitis.	Colonies are yellow to white.	Produces solitary, usually single-celled aleurioconidia that may be smooth to rough.
Coniochaeta spp.	C. mutabilis C. hoffmannii	Has been isolated in endocarditis and sinusitis in immunocompromised patients.	Colonies are white to salmon, may be moist with darkening black patches.	Phialides are short, stumpy without a basal septum. C. mutabilis forms brown chlamydospores.
Nannizziopsis sp.	N. hominis		White to yellow.	Produces solitary, usually single-celled aleurioconidia. Arthroconidia may be present.
Onychocola sp.	O. canadensis	Associated with onychomycosis.	Raised white to yellow to grayish white.	Two-celled conidia are cylindrical or swollen arthroconidia forming chains.
Parengyodontium sp.	P. album	Identified in cases of endocarditis.		Produces solitary conidia sympoidally arranged.
Phialemonium spp.	P. obovatum	Associated with endocarditis.		
Rasamsonia spp.	R. aegroticola R. eburnea R. piperina	Emerging pathogen in cystic fibrosis patients.		Cuneiform or ellipsoidal conidia.
Sarocladium spp. (previously Acremonium)		Several cases of invasive disease have been reported.		
Schizophyllum sp.	S. radiatum	Allergy related sinusitis and pulmonary disease.		
Thermothelomyces sp.	T. thermophila	Known to cause fatal aortic vasculitis and associated with cerebral abscess and osteomyelitis following traumatic injection.		Produces solitary, usually single-celled aleurioconidia.

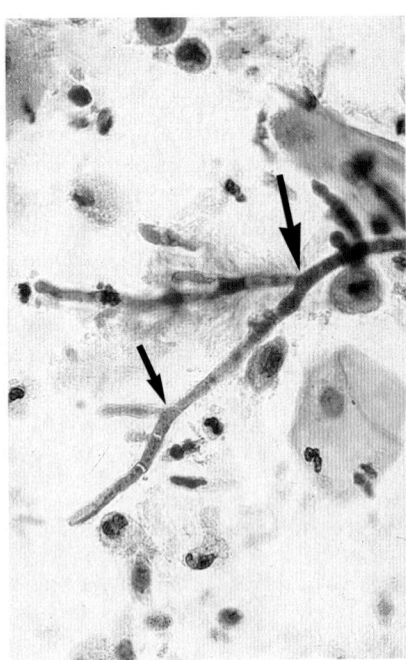

• **Fig. 59.18** Papanicolaou staining of sputum shows the dichotomously branching septate hyphae *(arrows)* of *Aspergillus fumigatus*.

cannot be reliably distinguished from hyphae of *Fusarium* spp., *Pseudallescheria boydii*, or other hyaline molds.

Antigen-Protein

Antigen-protein–based assays are used to monitor patients at high risk for developing invasive fungal infections. One of these assays, the galactomannan (GM) assay, targets GM, a carbohydrate molecule with a mannose backbone that is released from the cell wall of *Aspergillus* spp. *Aspergillus* spp. are the most common source of invasive fungal infections caused by the hyaline septate molds (i.e., **hyalohyphomycosis**). However, the assay may yield false-positive results because of cross-reactivity with other non-*Aspergillus* molds, including *Penicillium, Rhodotorula, Fusarium, Cryptococcus, Blastomyces, Histoplasma capsulatum, Paecilomyces,* and *Alternaria* spp.

The beta-D-glucan assay is designed to detect antigens common to all clinically important fungi. Beta-D-glucan can be detected in the serum of patients infected with systemic aspergillosis. Because the molecule is present in a variety of fungal isolates, the predictive value is not specific to infections with *Aspergillus* spp. It is recommended that the GM and beta-D-glucan assay be used in combination with other diagnostic tests such as nucleic acid amplification for optimal sensitivity and specificity.

Nucleic Acid–Based Tests

Nucleic acid amplification assays are not commonly performed to detect or identify the opportunistic fungi. However, a variety of both broad-range assays (those that detect all fungi) and species-specific assays have been developed and in specialized centers may be used for patient care. These panfungal PCR assays may be used for initial patient

diagnosis followed by DNA sequencing for identification. Multiplex amplification and real-time PCR assays have been developed for the detection of systemic aspergillosis in respiratory specimens, blood, tissue, and CSF. These assays vary significantly in their performance from 60% to 100% specificity and 40% to 100% sensitivity.

Matrix-Assisted Laser Desorption Ionization Time-of-Flight Mass Spectrometry

The use of MALDI-TOF MS for the identification of fungal isolates has the potential to provide quick and accurate species identification. Numerous studies have demonstrated the utility of this technique for the identification of *Aspergillus* spp. and other fungal organisms. The performance of MALDI-TOF MS for the identification of *Aspergillus* spp. has been reported for both young and old colonies with a 98.6% correct identification.

Cultivation

Because aspergilli are commonly recovered, it is imperative that the organism be demonstrated in the direct microscopic examination of fresh clinical specimens or that it be recovered repeatedly from patients with a compatible clinical picture to ensure that the organism is clinically significant. Correlation with biopsy results is the best means of establishing the significance of an isolate. Most *Aspergillus* spp. are susceptible to cycloheximide. Specimens submitted for recovery or subculture of these species should be inoculated onto media that lack this ingredient.

Aspergillus fumigatus is the most commonly recovered species from immunocompromised patients; moreover, it is the species most often seen in the clinical laboratory. *Aspergillus flavus* sometimes is recovered from immunocompromised patients and represents a common isolate in the clinical microbiology laboratory. Recovery of *A. fumigatus* or *A. flavus* from surveillance (nasal) cultures has been correlated with subsequent invasive aspergillosis; however, the absence of a positive nasal culture does not preclude infection. *Aspergillus niger* is commonly seen in the clinical laboratory, but its association with clinical disease is somewhat limited; this organism is a cause of fungus ball and otitis externa. *Aspergillus terreus* is a significant cause of infection in immunocompromised patients, but its frequency of recovery is much lower than that of the previously mentioned species. However, correct identification of *A. terreus* is important because it is innately resistant to amphotericin B.

Approach to Identification

Aspergillus spp.

A. fumigatus is a rapidly growing mold (2 to 6 days) that produces a fluffy to granular, white to blue-green colony. Mature sporulating colonies most often have a blue-green, powdery appearance. Microscopically, *A. fumigatus* is characterized by the presence of septate hyphae and short or long conidiophores with a characteristic "foot cell" at their base. The foot cell is T- or L-shaped at the base of the conidiophore, but it is not a separate cell. The tip of the conidiophore expands into a large, dome-shaped vesicle with bottle-shaped phialides covering the upper half or two thirds of its surface. Long chains of small (2 to 3 μm in diameter), spherical, rough-walled, green conidia form a columnar mass on the vesicle (Fig. 59.19). Cultures of *A. fumigatus* are thermotolerant and able to withstand temperatures up to 45°C.

A. flavus is a somewhat more rapidly growing species (1 to 5 days) that produces a yellow-green colony. Microscopically, vesicles are globose, and phialides are produced directly from the vesicle surface (**uniseriate**) or from a primary row of cells called metulae (**biseriate**). The phialides give rise to short chains of yellow-orange elliptical or spherical conidia that become roughened on the surface with age (Fig. 59.20). The conidiophore of *A. flavus* is also coarsely roughened near the vesicle.

A. niger produces darkly pigmented, roughened spores macroscopically, but microscopically its hyphae are hyaline and septate, as are those of other aspergilli (i.e., it is not melanized). *A. niger* produces mature colonies within 2 to 6 days. Growth begins initially as a yellow colony that soon develops a black, dotted surface as conidia are produced. With age, the colony becomes jet black and powdery, but the reverse remains buff or cream colored; this occurs on any culture medium. Microscopically, *A. niger* shows septate hyphae, long conidiophores supporting spherical vesicles

giving rise to large metulae, and smaller phialides (biseriate), from which long chains of brown to black, rough-walled conidia are produced (Fig. 59.21). The entire surface of the vesicle is involved in sporulation.

A. terreus is less commonly seen in the clinical laboratory; it produces tan colonies that resemble cinnamon. Vesicles are hemispherical, as seen microscopically, and phialides cover the entire surface and are produced from a primary row of metulae (biseriate). Phialides produce globose to elliptical conidia arranged in chains. This species produces larger cells, **aleurioconidia**, which are found on submerged hyphae (Fig. 59.22).

Serologic Testing

The use of serology for *Aspergillus* spp. has been limited to assistance in the diagnosis of chronic or allergic forms of bronchopulmonary aspergillosis and fungus ball.

Serology currently has no value for the diagnosis of disseminated aspergillosis.

Fusarium spp.

Colonies of *Fusarium* spp. grow rapidly, within 2 to 5 days, and are fluffy to cottony and may be pink, purple, yellow, green, or other colors, depending on the species. Microscopically, the hyphae are small and septate

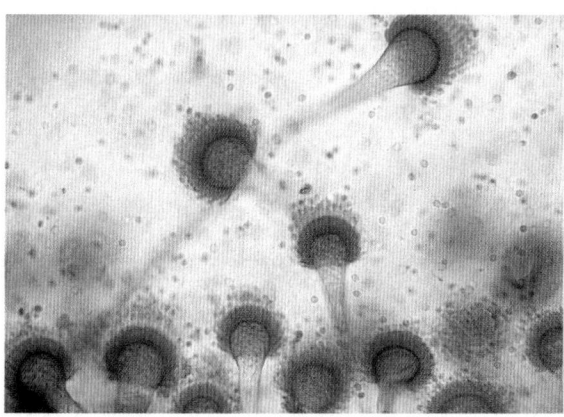

• **Fig. 59.19** *Aspergillus fumigatus* conidiophore and conidia (×400).

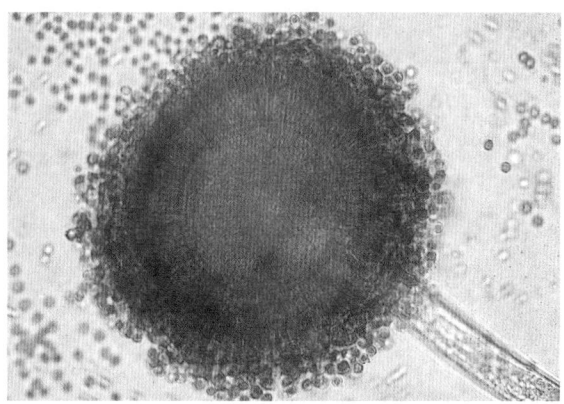

• **Fig. 59.21** *Aspergillus niger* showing a larger spherical vesicle that gives rise to metulae, phialides, and conidia (×750).

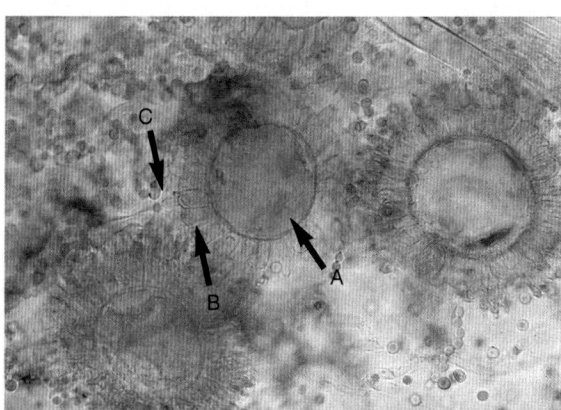

• **Fig. 59.20** *Aspergillus flavus* showing spherical vesicles *(A)* that give rise to metulae *(B)* and phialides *(C)* that produce chains of conidia (×750).

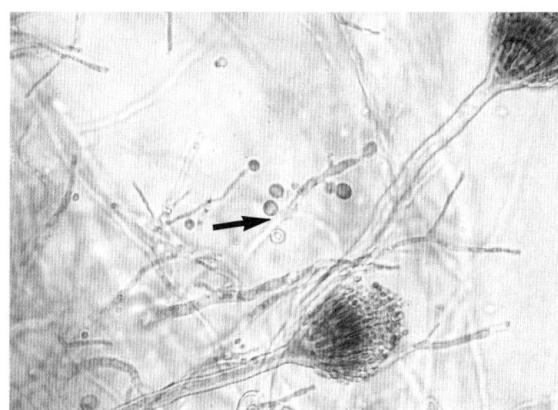

• **Fig. 59.22** *Aspergillus terreus* showing typical head of *Aspergillus* and aleurioconidia *(arrow)* found on submerged hyphae of this species (×500).

and give rise to phialides producing either single-celled microconidia, usually borne in gelatinous heads similar to those seen in *Acremonium* spp. (Fig. 58.17) or large, multicelled macroconidia that are sickle- or boat-shaped and contain numerous septations (Fig. 59.23). Some cultures of *Fusarium* spp. commonly produce numerous chlamydoconidia. The most common medium used to induce sporulation is cornmeal agar. The keys to identification of *Fusarium* spp. are based on growth on potato dextrose agar.

Geotrichum candidum

G. candidum often initially appears as a white to cream-colored, yeastlike colony; some isolates may appear as white, powdery molds. Hyphae are septate and produce numerous rectangular to cylindrical to barrel-shaped arthroconidia (Fig. 59.24). Arthroconidia do not alternate but are contiguous, in contrast to *Coccidioides* spp. (Fig. 59.25). Blastoconidia are not produced.

Acremonium spp.

The *Acremonium* spp. are a polyphyletic group that includes approximately 100 species. Molecular analysis is currently underway and will undoubtedly result in some additional restructuring of this group. Colonies of *Acremonium* spp. are

rapid growing and may appear yeastlike when initial growth is observed. Mature colonies become white to gray to rose or reddish-orange. Microscopically, small septate hyphae that produce single, unbranched, tubelike phialides are observed. Phialides give rise to clusters of elliptical, single-celled conidia contained in a gelatinous cluster at the tip of the phialide (Fig. 58.17). The most frequently encountered species in the United States are *A. kiliense* and *A. schlerotigenum-A. egyptiacum* group.

Penicillium spp. and Talaromyces marneffei

The genus *Penicillium* includes three subgenera: *Aspergilloides*, *Furcatum*, and *Penicillium*. *Talaromyces* is the only species (formerly *Penicillium* sp.) that is considered a true fungal pathogen and not an opportunist. Colonies of *Penicillium* spp. are most commonly shades of green or blue-green, but pink, white, or other colors may be seen. The surface of the colonies may be velvety to powdery because of the presence of conidia. Microscopically, hyphae are hyaline and septate and produce brushlike conidiophores (i.e., penicilli). Conidiophores produce metulae from which flask-shaped phialides producing chains of conidia arise (Fig. 59.26). *T. marneffei* is discussed in the section on hyaline, septate, dimorphic molds.

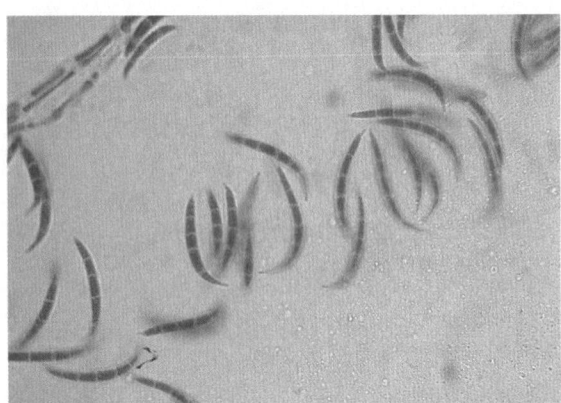

• **Fig. 59.23** *Fusarium* spp. showing characteristic multicelled, sickle-shaped macroconidia (×500).

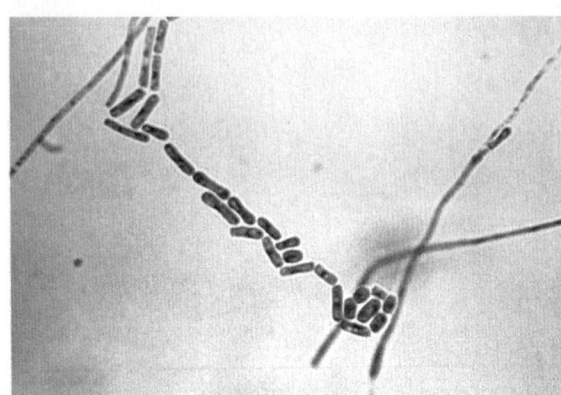

• **Fig. 59.24** *Geotrichum candidum* showing numerous arthroconidia. (Note that arthroconidia do not alternate with a clear (dysjunctor) cell, as in the case of *Coccidioides* (×430).)

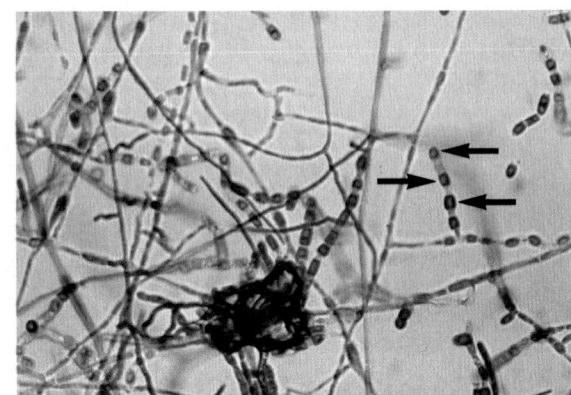

• **Fig. 59.25** Mycelial form of *Coccidioides* spp. showing numerous thick-walled, rectangular, or barrel-shaped *(arrows)* alternate arthroconidia (×500).

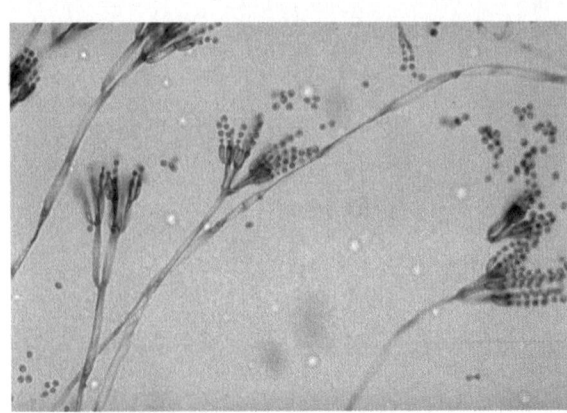

• **Fig. 59.26** *Penicillium* spp. showing typical brushlike conidiophores (penicilli) (×430).

Paecilomyces spp.

Colonies of *Paecilomyces* spp. are often velvety, tan to olive-brown, and somewhat powdery. Microscopically, *Paecilomyces* spp. resemble *Penicillium* spp. in that a penicillus is formed. However, the phialides of *Paecilomyces* spp. are long, delicate, and tapering (Fig. 59.27), in contrast to the more blunted phialides of *Penicillium* spp. The penicillus produces numerous chains of small, oval conidia that are easily dislodged. Single phialides producing chains of conidia may also be present.

Purpureocillium spp.

P. lilacinum exhibits colonies that are considered lilac in color exhibiting shades of lavender to pink. Chlamydospores are absent. The genus demonstrates a slower growth rate than *Paecilomyces* spp. Optimal growth temperature is 25°C to 33°C.

Scopulariopsis spp.

Scopulariopsis brevicaulis, S. asperula, and *S. candida* have been associated with onychomycosis, pulmonary infection, fungus ball, and invasive fungal disease in immunocompromised hosts. Colonies of *Scopulariopsis* spp. initially appear white but later become light brown and powdery. Colonies often resemble those of *M. gypseum.* Microscopically, a *Scopulariopsis* resembles a large *Penicillium* at first glance, because a rudimentary penicillus is produced. **Annellophores** produce the flask-shaped **annelides,** which support the lemon-shaped conidia in chains. Conidia are large, have a flat base, and are rough-walled (Fig. 59.28). The *Scopulariopsis* spp. include both hyaline and dematiaceous species. *Scopulariopsis brumptii* has been reported to have caused a brain abscess in a liver transplant patient and invasive infection in bone marrow recipients. *S. candida* and *S. acremonium* have been identified in association with invasive sinusitis.

Serologic Testing

Serology currently has no value for the diagnosis of the opportunistic disseminated fungal infections discussed.

Systemic Mycoses

As with many other groups of clinically relevant fungi, significant changes have occurred in the classification and taxonomy of these organisms. *H. capsulatum* is now divided into eight clades (biological taxa claiming a common ancestor), or varieties. Seven of these varieties comprise genetically and geographically distinct populations representing a species; however, the *Histoplasma* var. *duboisii,* the African containing clade, demonstrates the same mitochondrial pattern as the *H. capsulatum* var. *capsulatum* of North and South America. *H. capsulatum* is used throughout this section as the primary isolate of interest.

The genera *Blastomyces* and *Coccidioides* have traditionally been representative of single species, *Blastomyces dermatitidis* and *Coccidioides immitis.* More recent characterization has revealed the existence of a subspecies or separate species in the genus *Blastomyces, Blastomyces gilchristii.*

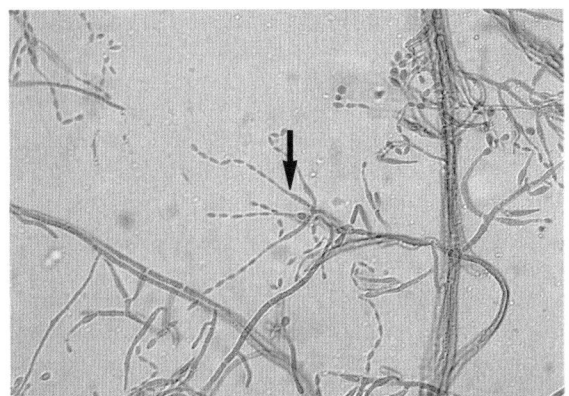

• **Fig. 59.27** *Paecilomyces* spp. showing long, tapering, delicate phialides *(arrow).*

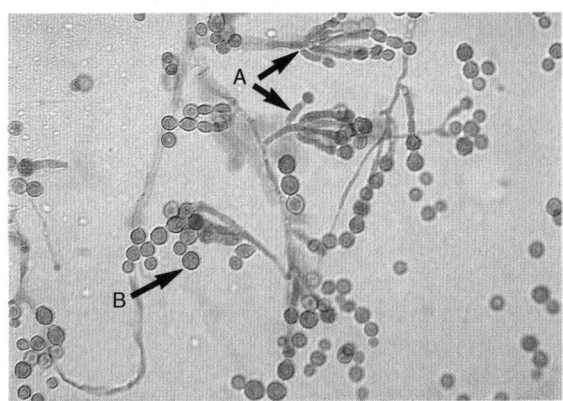

• **Fig. 59.28** *Scopulariopsis* spp. showing a large penicillus *(A)* with echinulate conidia *(B)* (×430).

Polyphasic taxonomic analysis has also revealed a correlation between genotypic characteristics of these organisms and clinical phenotypic presentations. Additional species have now been proposed: *B. percursus, B. parvus* (formerly *Emmonsia parva*), *B. helicus* (formerly *Emmonsia helica*), and *B. silverae.* In addition, *Coccidioides* now comprises two species: *C. immitis* that includes all isolates from California and Washington State and *Coccidioides posadasii,* which comprises all other isolates.

Phylogenetic analysis has indicated that *Paracoccidioides brasiliensis* can be subdivided into at least three distinct species. Several new species are proposed based on geographic regions of endemicity and include *P. lutzii, P. americana, P. restrepiensis,* and *P. venezuelensis.*

The new genus *Emergomyces* contains many of the organisms previously included in the genus *Emmonsia. Emergomyces* includes *Es. pasteurianus* as the type species (previously *Emmonsia pasteuriana*), and four new species: *Es. africanus, Es. orientalis, Es. canadensis,* and *Es. europaeus.* Each species differs in yeast size and geographic distribution.

Emmonsia crescens can be found in the soil and infects humans in North, Central, and South America as well as in Europe, Asia, and Africa. The distribution of disease associated with this fungi is unclear and further analysis is needed.

General Characteristics

Most of the dimorphic fungi produce systemic fungal infections that may involve any of the internal organs of the body, including lymph nodes, bone, subcutaneous tissue, meninges, and skin. The dimorphic fungal pathogens most commonly encountered in North America are *H. capsulatum*, *Blastomyces* spp., and *Coccidioides* spp. *Emmonsia* spp., *Paracoccidioides* spp., and *Emergomyces* spp. are geographically distributed throughout Central and South America. Asymptomatic or subclinical infection is common with *H. capsulatum* and *Coccidioides* and may go unrecognized clinically. These infections may be detectable only by serology or after histopathologic review of tissues removed because of lesions found during a **roentgenographic examination.**

Symptomatic infections may present signs of a mild or more severe but self-limited disease, with positive supportive evidence from cultural or immunologic findings. Patients with disseminated or progressive infection have severe symptoms, with spread of the initial disease, often from a pulmonary locus, to several distant organs. However, some cases of disseminated infection may show little in the way of signs or symptoms of disease for long periods, only to undergo exacerbation later. Immunocompromised patients most often present with disseminated infection, particularly those with advanced human immunodeficiency virus (HIV) infection (i.e., acquired immunodeficiency syndrome [AIDS]) or those receiving long-term corticosteroid therapy.

The classic term systemic mycoses, used to refer to the dimorphic fungi, is somewhat misleading, because other fungi, including *Cryptococcus neoformans* complex, *Candida albicans* complex, and *Aspergillus* spp., may also cause disseminated systemic infections.

Epidemiology

Blastomyces spp.

B. dermatitidis is uncommon as an opportunistic pathogen but may cause aggressive disease in immunocompromised individuals, producing a chronic infection that contains a mixture of suppurative and granulomatous inflammation. The disease (**blastomycosis**) is most commonly found in North America and extends southward from Canada to the Mississippi, Ohio, and Missouri river valleys; Mexico; and Central America. Some isolated cases have also been reported from Africa. The largest numbers of cases occur in the Mississippi, Ohio, and Missouri river valley regions. *B. gilchristii* isolates are primarily localized to northwestern Ontario, Wisconsin, and Minnesota. The exact ecologic niche for this organism in nature has not been determined; however, patients with blastomycosis often have a history of exposure to soil or wood, particularly near waterways. Several outbreaks have been reported and have been related to a common exposure. Blastomycosis is more common in males than in females and seems to be associated with outdoor occupations or activities. The disease also occurs in dogs.

Coccidioides spp.

Coccidioides spp. are found primarily in the desert portion of the southwestern United States and in the semiarid regions of Mexico and Central and South America. Although the geographic distribution of the organism is well defined, infection may be seen in any part of the world because of the ease of travel. The infection (**coccidioidomycosis**) is usually acquired by inhalation of the infective arthroconidia. The infection is not contagious; however, person-to-person spread has been reported from contaminated fomites or through an infected organ donor to a recipient.

Emmonsia spp.

Ea. crescens. are rare causes of human infection. The organism produces a self-limited, localized pulmonary infection that may appear asymptomatic. Diagnosis is generally incidental to other underlying conditions. The organism produces adiaspores, which enlarge but do not reproduce in the patient. The clinical presentation depends on the number of adiaspores inhaled. It is unclear at this time whether the organism demonstrates a species-specific geographic distribution.

Emergomyces spp.

The *Emergomyces* spp. appear as beige, slow growing filamentous colonies at room temperature. The conidiophores are short and unbranched, and they form at right angles to hyaline hyphae. At body temperature, they appear as small oval yeast cells. The organism is endemic in South Africa and transmitted by inhalation. *Emergomyces* spp. is rapidly becoming the most commonly diagnosed dimorphic fungal pathogen.

Histoplasma capsulatum

Outbreaks of **histoplasmosis** have been associated with activities that disperse aerosolized conidia or small hyphal fragments. Infection is acquired through inhalation of these infective structures from the environment. The severity of the disease is generally related directly to the inoculum size and the immunologic status of the host. Numerous cases of histoplasmosis have been reported in people who clean out an old chicken coop or barn that has been undisturbed for long periods and in individuals who work in or clean areas that have served as roosting places for starlings and similar birds. Spelunkers (i.e., cave explorers) are commonly exposed to the organism when it is aerosolized from bat guano in caves. An estimated 500,000 people are infected with *H. capsulatum* annually. The history of exposure often is impossible to document, even though histoplasmosis is perhaps one of the most common systemic fungal infections seen in the Midwest and South in the United States, including areas along the Mississippi River, the Ohio River valley, and the Appalachian Mountains.

Paracoccidioides brasiliensis and *P. lutzi*

Infection caused by *Paracoccidioides* spp. is most commonly found in South America, with the highest prevalences in Brazil, Venezuela, and Colombia. It also has been seen in many other areas, including Mexico, Central America, the Caribbean, and Africa. Occasional imported cases are seen in the United States and Europe. The exact mechanism by which **paracoccidioidomycosis** is acquired is unclear; however, some speculate that it has a pulmonary origin and that it is acquired by inhalation of the organism from the environment. Because mucosal lesions are an integral part of the disease process, it also is speculated that the infection may be acquired through trauma to the oropharynx caused by vegetation commonly chewed by some residents of the endemic areas. The specific ecologic niche of the organism in nature is not known.

Talaromyces marneffei

T. marneffei is a dimorphic pathogenic fungus endemic to Southeast Asia, particularly the Guangxi Zhuang Autonomous Region of the People's Republic of China. *T. marneffei* has been associated with the bamboo rat (*Rhizomys pruinosus*) and the Vietnamese bamboo rat (*Rhizomys sinensis*).

Sporothrix spp.

Sporothrix schenckii has been shown to be a complex of numerous species. Those involved in human infection include *S. schenckii, Sporothrix brasiliensis, Sporothrix globosa,* and *Sporothrix luriei.* *Sporothrix* spp. have a worldwide distribution, and their natural habitat is living or dead vegetation. Humans acquire the infection (**sporotrichosis**) through trauma (thorns, splinters, bites, or scratches), usually to the hand, arm, or leg. The infection is an occupational hazard for farmers, nursery workers, gardeners, florists, and miners; it is commonly known as rose gardener's disease. Infections with *S. brasiliensis* have been transmitted from the bites or scratches of stray cats. Pulmonary sporotrichosis rarely occurs as a result of inhalation of spores.

Pathogenesis and Spectrum of Disease

Traditionally, the systemic mycoses have included only blastomycosis, coccidioidomycosis, histoplasmosis, and paracoccidioidomycosis. Although these fungi are morphologically dissimilar, they have one characteristic in common: dimorphism. Most of these organisms, except for *Coccidioides,* are thermally dimorphic. The dimorphic fungi exist in nature as the mold form, which is distinct from the parasitic or invasive form, sometimes called the tissue form. Distinct morphologic differences may be observed with the dimorphic fungi both *in vivo* and *in vitro,* as discussed later in the chapter.

Blastomyces spp.

Blastomyces spp. commonly produce an acute or chronic suppurative and granulomatous infection. Blastomycosis begins as a respiratory infection and is probably acquired by inhalation of the conidia or hyphal fragments of the organism. The infection may spread and involve secondary sites of infection in the lungs, long bones, soft tissue, and skin.

Coccidioides spp.

Approximately 60% of patients with coccidioidomycosis are asymptomatic and have self-limited respiratory tract infections. However, the infection may become disseminated, with extension to visceral organs, meninges, bone, skin, lymph nodes, and subcutaneous tissue. Fewer than 1% of those who develop coccidioidomycosis ever become seriously ill; dissemination does occur, however, most commonly in individuals of dark-skinned races. Pregnancy also appears to predispose females to disseminated infection. This infection has been known to occur in epidemic proportions. In 1992, an epidemic occurred in northern California, with more than 4000 cases seen in Kern County near Bakersfield. People who visit endemic areas and return to a distant location may present to their local physician; therefore, the endemic mycoses should be considered in the differential diagnosis if the patient has the appropriate travel history. All laboratories should be prepared to deal with the laboratory diagnosis of coccidioidomycosis.

Emergomyces spp.

Es. pasteurianus (previously *Emmonsia*) does not produce **adiaspores** (spores that increase in size inside an animal host) *in vitro* on brain-heart infusion (BHI) agar incubated at 37°C like *Emmonsia* spp. The organism produces cells that resemble budding yeast. Emergomycosis is generally systemic and includes the appearance of widespread cutaneous lesions.

Emmonsia spp.

Nonreplicating *Emmonsia* spp., most notably *Ea. crescens,* produces 25 to 400 µm **adiaspores** *in vitro* on BHI agar incubated at 37°C. In the natural environment the conidia are approximately 2 to 4 µm in diameter but may grow to 500 µm when inhaled into the human lung. The condition associated with inhaled conidia from *Emmonsia* spp. is referred to as **adiaspiromycosis.** The severity of the disease depends on the immunologic status of the patient as well as the inoculum size but may range from asymptomatic to fatal. Symptoms include fever, cough, dyspnea, hemoptysis, weight loss, fatigue, and possible respiratory failure.

Histoplasma capsulatum

H. capsulatum most commonly produces a chronic, granulomatous infection (histoplasmosis) that is primary and begins in the lung and eventually invades the reticuloendothelial system. Approximately 95% of cases are asymptomatic and self-limited, although chronic pulmonary infections occur. The disease can be disseminated throughout the reticuloendothelial system; the primary sites of dissemination are the lymph nodes, liver, spleen, and bone marrow. Infections of the kidneys and meninges are also possible. Resolution of disseminated infection is the rule in immunocompetent hosts, but progressive disease is more common in immunocompromised patients (e.g., patients with AIDS). Ulcerative lesions of the upper respiratory tract may occur in both immunocompetent and immunocompromised hosts.

Paracoccidioides spp.

Paracoccidioides produces a chronic granulomatous infection (paracoccidioidomycosis) that begins as a primary pulmonary infection. It often is asymptomatic and then disseminates to produce ulcerative lesions of the mucous membranes. Ulcerative lesions are commonly present in the nasal and oral mucosa, gingivae, and less commonly the conjunctivae. Lesions occur commonly on the face in association with oral mucous membrane infection. The lesions are characteristically ulcerative, with a serpiginous (snakelike) active border and a crusted surface. Lymph node involvement in the cervical area is common. Pulmonary infection is common, and progressive chronic pulmonary infection is found in approximately 50% of cases. In some patients, dissemination occurs to other anatomic sites, including the lymphatic system, spleen, intestines, liver, brain, meninges, and adrenal glands.

Talaromyces marneffei

T. marneffei commonly infects immunosuppressed individuals. The organism causes either a focal cutaneous or mucocutaneous infection, or it may produce a progressive disseminated and commonly fatal infection. Granulomatous, suppurative, and necrotizing inflammatory responses have been demonstrated. The mode of transmission and the primary source in the environment are unknown, but the bamboo rat has been implicated.

Sporothrix spp.

Sporothrix spp., also dimorphic fungi, are often associated with chronic subcutaneous infections. The primary lesion begins as a small, nonhealing ulcer, often of the index finger or the back of the hand. With time, the infection is characterized by the development of nodular lesions of the skin or subcutaneous tissues at the point of contact and later involves the lymphatic channels and lymph nodes that drain the region. The subcutaneous nodules ulcerate to form an infection that becomes chronic. Only rarely is the disease disseminated. Pulmonary infection may be seen in patients who inhale the spores of *Sporothrix* spp.

Laboratory Diagnosis

Specimen Collection, Transport, and Processing

See General Considerations for the Laboratory Diagnosis of Fungal Infections in Chapter 58.

Direct Detection Methods

Stains

The microscopic morphologic features of the tissue forms, or what has been termed the parasitic forms, of the dimorphic fungi vary with the genus and are described for each.

Blastomyces spp. The diagnosis of blastomycosis may easily be made when a clinical specimen is observed by direct microscopy. *Blastomyces* spp. appear as large, spherical,

thick-walled yeast cells 8 to 15 μm in diameter, usually with a single bud that is connected to the parent cell by a broad base (Figs. 59.29 to 59.31). A smaller form (2 to 8 μm) is seen in rare cases.

Coccidioides spp. In direct microscopic examinations of sputum or other body fluids, *Coccidioides* spp. appear as a nonbudding, thick-walled spherule, 20 to 200 μm in diameter, that contains either granular material or numerous small (2 to 5 μm in diameter), nonbudding endospores (Figs. 59.32 to 59.35). The endospores are freed by rupture of the spherule wall; therefore, empty and collapsed "ghost" spherules may also be present. Small, immature spherules measuring 5 to 20 μm may be confused with *H. capsulatum* or *Blastomyces* spp. Two endospores or immature spherules lying adjacent to one another may give the appearance that

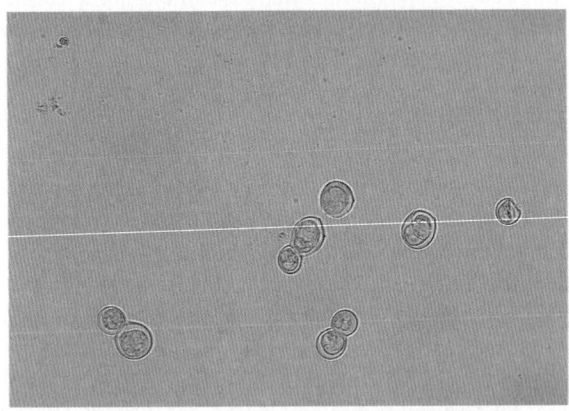

• **Fig. 59.29** *Blastomyces dermatitidis* yeast form showing thick-walled, oval to round, single-budding, yeastlike cells (×500).

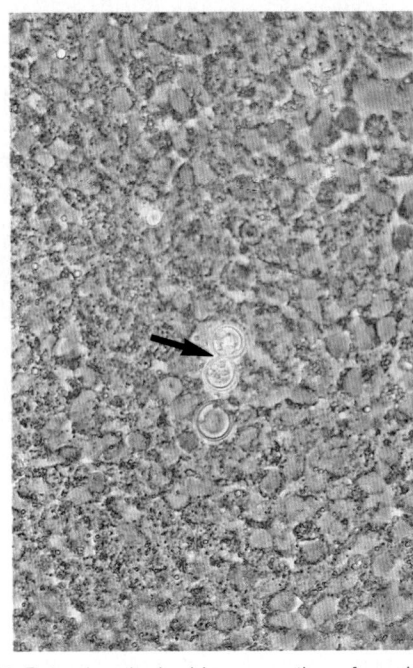

• **Fig. 59.30** Potassium hydroxide preparation of exudate shows a large budding yeast cell with a distinct broad base *(arrow)* between the cells, which is characteristic of *Blastomyces dermatitidis*. (Phase-contrast microscopy.)

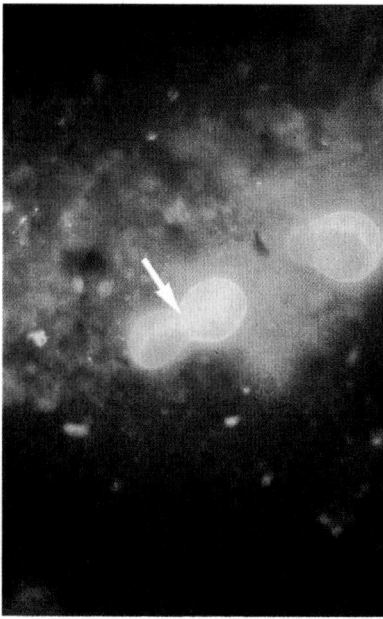

• **Fig. 59.31** Auramine-rhodamine preparation of specimen material from a bone lesion that demonstrates the characteristic broad-based budding yeast *(arrow)* of *Blastomyces dermatitidis.*

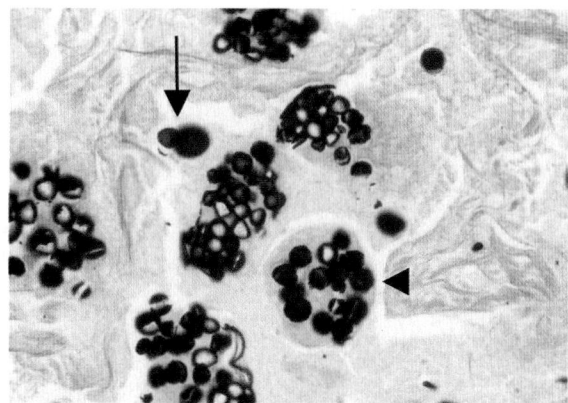

• **Fig. 59.32** Tissue form of *Coccidioides* spp. (i.e., the spherule). The external wall of the spherule does not stain with the silver stain, whereas the internal endospores do stain *(arrowhead)*. Also note how the juxtaposed endospores, which have been released from a spherule that has burst, resemble budding yeast *(arrow)*. (GMS stain; ×400.)

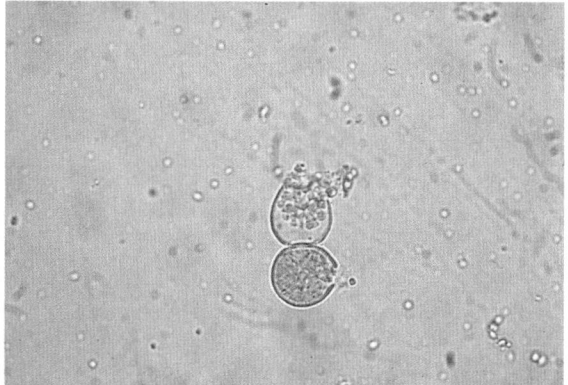

• **Fig. 59.33** Potassium hydroxide preparation of sputum demonstrates two spherules of *Coccidioides* spp. filled with endospores. When these lie adjacent to each other, they may be mistaken for *Blastomyces dermatitidis.* (Bright-field microscopy.)

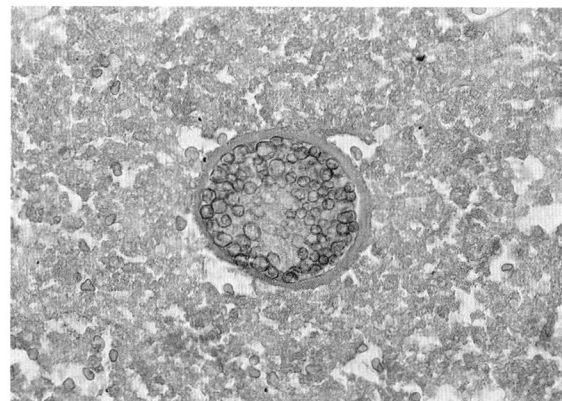

• **Fig. 59.34** Histologic section showing a well-developed spherule of *Coccidioides* spp. that is filled with endospores.

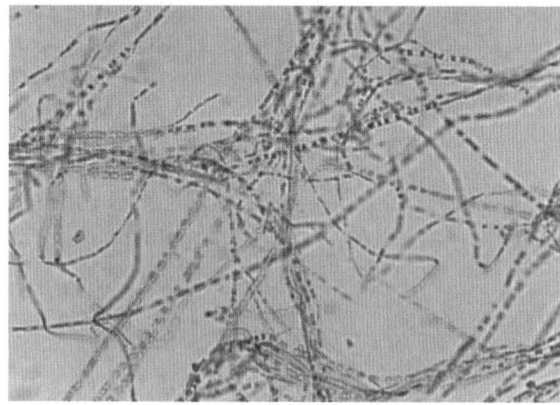

• **Fig. 59.35** *Coccidioides* spp. lactophenol cotton blue preparation from Sabouraud agar demonstrating arthroconidia and barrel shaped cells. (Photo courtesy Anna Hartyunyan, MLS (ASCP), Children's Hospital, Los Angeles, CA.)

budding yeast is present. When identification of *Coccidioides* is questionable, a wet preparation of the clinical specimen may be made using sterile saline, and the edges of the cover glass may be sealed with petrolatum and incubated overnight. When spherules are present, the endospores produce multiple hyphal strands.

***Emergomyces* spp.** *Emergomyces* spp. can be differentiated from *Emmonsia* by the presence of budding yeasts and the absence of adiaspores.

***Emmonsia* spp.** *Emmonsia* spp. have not been successfully cultured from human specimens. Therefore, diagnosis is dependent on the histologic appearance of a thick-walled adiaspore granuloma within the lungs. Unlike *Coccidioides* spp., *Emmonsia* spp. adiaspores do not contain endospores and are typically much larger than spherules. A recent report has indicated that PCR and DNA sequencing may be useful in diagnosing adiaspiromycosis.

Histoplasma capsulatum. Direct microscopic examination of respiratory tract specimens and other similar specimens often fails to reveal the presence of *H. capsulatum*. However, an astute laboratorian may detect the organism when examining Wright- or Giemsa-stained specimens of bone marrow and, in rare cases, peripheral blood.

H. capsulatum is found intracellularly in mononuclear cells as small, round to oval yeast cells 2 to 5 μm in diameter (Fig. 59.36 and Fig. 59.7).

Paracoccidioides brasiliensis. Specimens submitted for direct microscopic examination are important for the diagnosis of paracoccidioidomycosis. Large, round or oval, multiple budding yeast cells (8 to 40 μm in diameter) are usually recognized in sputum, mucosal biopsy specimens, and other exudates. Characteristic multiple budding yeast forms resemble a "mariner's wheel" (Fig. 59.37). The yeast cells surrounding the periphery of the parent cell range from 8 to 15 μm in diameter. Some cells may be as small as 2 to 5 μm but still exhibit multiple buds.

Talaromyces marneffei. Direct examination of infected tissues and exudates reveals that *T. marneffei* produces small, yeastlike cells (2 to 6 μm) that have internal cross-walls; no budding cells are produced (Fig. 59.38). Like *H. capsulatum*, *T. marneffei* may be detected in peripheral blood smears with disseminated disease.

Sporothrix spp. Exudate aspirated from unopened subcutaneous nodules or from open draining lesions often is submitted for culture and direct microscopic examination. Direct examination of this material usually has little diagnostic value, because demonstrating the rare

characteristic yeast forms is difficult. *Sporothrix* usually appear as small (2 to 5 μm in diameter), round to oval to cigar-shaped yeast cells (Fig. 59.39). If stained using the periodic acid-Schiff (PAS) method in histologic section, an amorphous pink material may be seen surrounding the yeast cells (Fig. 59.40).

Antigen-Protein

Immunodiffusion methods (the exoantigen test) may be used to identify isolates of these organisms based on precipitation bands of identity between specific antibodies and fungal antigen extracts. However, these assays have been largely replaced by the more rapid nucleic acid hybridization reactions and automated enzyme immunoassays. Antigen testing is available for *H. capsulatum* and *Blastomyces* in a microtiter plate double antibody sandwich EIA that can detect the antigens in urine, serum, or CSF in disseminated infections. A urinary antigen test is also available for the

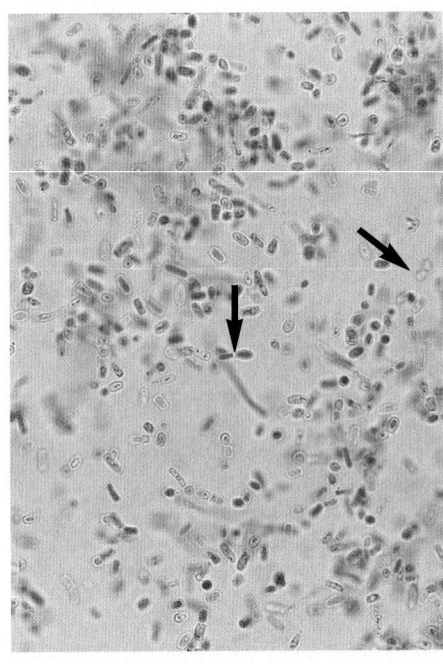
• **Fig. 59.38** *Talaromyces marneffei* and binary fission *(arrows)* (×500).

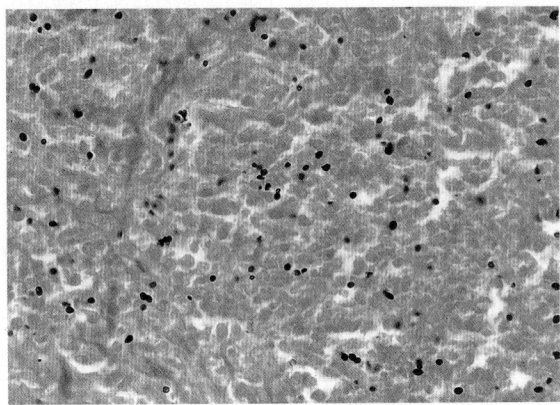
• **Fig. 59.36** These small, oval yeast cells that are relatively uniform in size are characteristic of *Histoplasma capsulatum* (×2000).

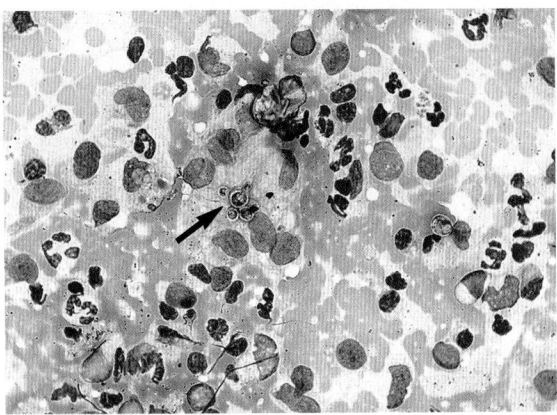
• **Fig. 59.37** *Paracoccidioides brasiliensis* in a bone marrow aspirate shows a yeast cell with multiple buds *(arrow)*.

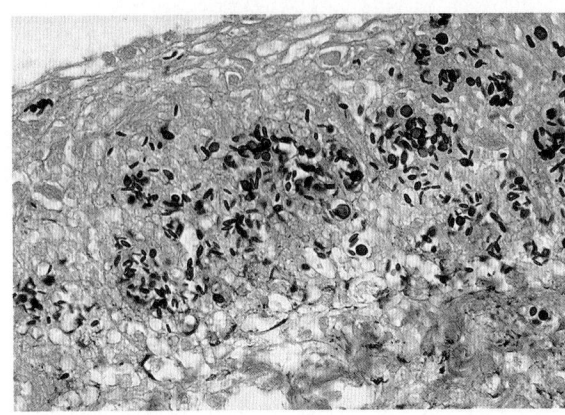
• **Fig. 59.39** The deeply staining bodies in this mouse testis are the yeast forms of *Sporothrix* spp.

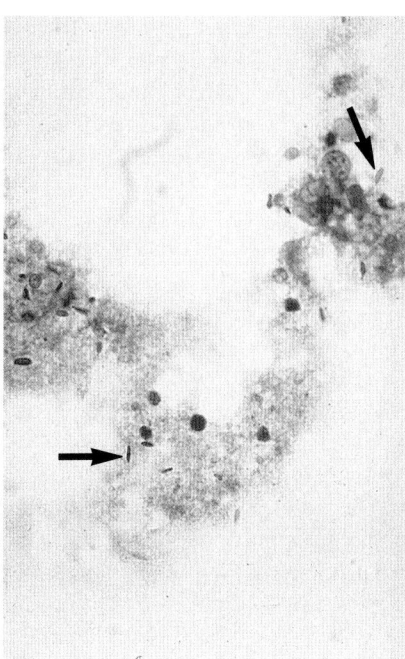

• **Fig. 59.40** Periodic acid-Schiff (PAS) staining of exudate shows the cigar- to oval-shaped yeast cells *(arrows)* of *Sporothrix* spp.

detection of *Coccidioides* spp. Antigen testing is not currently available for the remaining dimorphic fungal pathogens.

Nucleic Acid Testing

Nucleic acid amplification assays are not routinely performed but are available in some reference laboratories and in research settings. A single FDA-approved assay for the detection of *Coccidioides* is available. Real-time or homogeneous, rapid-cycle PCR assays have been described for *H. capsulatum, Blastomyces, Emmonsia, Paracoccidioides,* and *Coccidioides* species. These assays have proven suitable for isolate identification. Reproducibility and specificity of these assays must be thoroughly evaluated for standardization before implementation in clinical laboratories. No molecular tests are available for *Emergomyces* spp.

Cultivation

The dimorphic fungi are regarded as slow-growing organisms, requiring 7 to 21 days for visible growth to appear at 25°C to 30°C. However, exceptions to this rule occur with some frequency. Occasionally cultures of *Blastomyces* and *H. capsulatum* are recovered in as short a time as 2 to 5 days when many organisms are present in the clinical specimen. In contrast, when a small number of colonies of *Blastomyces* and *H. capsulatum* are present, sometimes 21 to 30 days of incubation are required before they are detected. *Coccidioides* is consistently recovered within 3 to 5 days of incubation, but when many organisms are present, colonies may be detected within 48 hours. Cultures of *P. brasiliensis* are commonly recovered within 5 to 25 days, with a usual incubation period of 10 to 15 days. The growth rate, if slow, might lead the laboratorian to suspect the presence of a dimorphic fungus; however, considerable variation in the

time for recovery exists. The exceptions to this slow growth are *Coccidioides* and *T. marneffei,* which may be recovered within 3 to 5 days.

Textbooks present descriptions of the dimorphic fungi that the reader assumes are typical for each particular organism. As is true in other areas of microbiology, variation in the colonial morphologic features also occurs, depending on the strain and the type of medium used. The laboratorian must be aware of this variation and must not rely heavily on colonial morphologic features to identify members of this group of fungi.

The pigmentation of colonies is sometimes helpful but also varies widely; colonies of *Blastomyces* and *H. capsulatum* are described as being fluffy white, with a change in color to tan or buff with age. Some isolates initially appear darkly pigmented, with colors ranging from gray or dark brown to red. On media containing blood enrichment, these organisms may appear heaped, wrinkled, glabrous, neutral in color, and yeastlike; often tufts of aerial hyphae project from the top of the colony. Some colonies may appear pink to red, possibly because of the adsorption of hemoglobin from the blood in the medium. *Coccidioides* is described as fluffy white with scattered areas of hyphae adherent to the agar surface, giving an overall "cobweb" appearance to the colony. However, numerous morphologic forms have been reported, including textures ranging from wooly to powdery and pigmentation ranging from pink-lavender or yellow to brown or buff. The definitive traditional identification method for dimorphic fungus includes observing both the mold and tissue or parasitic forms of the organism. In general, 25°C to 30°C is the optimal temperature for recovery and identification of the dimorphic fungi from clinical specimens. Temperature (35°C to 37°C), certain nutritional factors, and stimulation of growth in tissue independent of temperature are among the factors necessary to initiate the transformation of the mold form to the tissue form. Previously, *Blastomyces* and *H. capsulatum* were identified definitively by the *in vitro* conversion of a mold form to the corresponding yeast form through *in vitro* conversion on a blood-enriched medium incubated at 35°C to 37°C; definitive identification of *Coccidioides* involved conversion to the spherule form by animal inoculation. Except for *Coccidioides,* the conversion of dimorphic molds to the yeast form can be accomplished with some difficulty (Evolve Procedure 59.2). Some reference laboratories may still use the exoantigen test (Evolve Procedure 59.3) to identify the dimorphic pathogens. However, this test requires extended incubation before cultures may be identified.

Blastomyces dermatitidis. *B. dermatitidis* commonly requires incubation for 5 days to 4 weeks or longer at 25°C before growth can be detected. However, it may be detected in as short a time as 2 to 3 days. On enriched culture media, the mold form develops initially as a glabrous or waxy-appearing colony and is off-white to white. With age, the aerial hyphae often turn gray to brown. The waxy, yeastlike appearance is typified on media enriched with blood. Tufts of hyphae often project upward from the colonies, and this has been referred to as the "prickly state" of the organism. However, some isolates appear fluffy on primary recovery and remain so throughout the incubation period. On blood agar at 37°C, colonies are waxy, wrinkled, and yeastlike. Mold-to-yeast conversion usually requires 4 to 5 days.

***Coccidioides* spp.** Cultures of *Coccidioides* are a biohazard to laboratory workers, and strict safety precautions must be followed when cultures are examined. Mature colonies may appear within 2 to 5 days of incubation and may be present on most media, including those used in bacteriology. Laboratory workers are cautioned not to open cultures of fluffy white molds unless they are placed inside a biologic safety cabinet (BSC). Colonies of *Coccidioides* often appear as a delicate, cobweblike growth after 3 to 21 days of incubation. Some portions of the colony exhibit aerial hyphae, whereas in others the hyphae adhere to the agar surface. Most isolates appear fluffy white; however, colonies of varying colors have been reported, ranging from pink to yellow to purple and black. Some colonies exhibit a greenish discoloration on blood agar, and others appear yeastlike, smooth, wrinkled, and tan.

***Emmonsia* and *Emergomyces* spp.** *Emmonsia* spp. produce glabrous, colorless colonies at 25°C that produce yellow to white aerial mycelia over time. Some strains produce orange to gray mycelia. Reverse pigmentation appears gray to grayish-brown. *Emergomyces* spp. appears very similar at 25°C to 30°C and must be differentiated based on the microscopic production of yeastlike cells at 37°C and not adiaspores. Sporulation is enhanced on potato dextrose agar or **Pablum cereal agar.**

The fungi produce conidia from the sides or directly on short stalks that branch from the hyphae. The hyphae may appear swollen and bear peglike structures resulting in the production of secondary conidia in a flowerlike arrangement.

Histoplasma capsulatum. *H. capsulatum* is easily cultured from clinical specimens; however, it may be overgrown by bacteria or rapidly growing molds. A procedure that is useful for recovering *H. capsulatum, B. dermatitidis,* and *Coccidioides* spp. from contaminated specimens (e.g., sputa) uses a yeast extract/phosphate medium and a drop of concentrated ammonium hydroxide (NH_4OH) placed on one side of the inoculated plate of medium. In the past, it was recommended that specimens not be kept at room temperature before culture, because *H. capsulatum* would not survive. The organism survives transit in the mail for as long as 16 days. However, the current recommendation is that specimens be cultured as soon as possible to ensure optimal recovery of *H. capsulatum* and other dimorphic fungi.

H. capsulatum is usually considered a slow-growing mold at 25°C to 30°C and commonly requires 2 to 4 weeks or more for colonies to appear. However, the organism may be recovered in 5 days or less if many yeast cells are present in the clinical specimen. Isolates of *H. capsulatum* have been reported from blood cultures with the Isolator (Alere, Waltham, MA) within a mean time of 8 days. *H. capsulatum* is a white, fluffy mold that turns brown to buff with age. Some isolates ranging

from gray to red have also been reported. The organism also may produce wrinkled, moist, heaped, yeastlike colonies that are soft and cream colored, tan, or pink. Tufts of hyphae often project upward from the colonies, as described for *B. dermatitidis* and *H. capsulatum,* and cannot be differentiated using colonial morphologic features.

Paracoccidioides brasiliensis. Colonies of *P. brasiliensis* grow very slowly (21 to 28 days) and are heaped, wrinkled, moist, and yeastlike. With age, colonies may become covered with a short aerial mycelium and turn tan to brown. The surface of colonies often is heaped with crater formations.

Talaromyces marneffei. At 25°C, *T. marneffei* grows rapidly and produces blue-green to yellowish colonies on Sabouraud agar. A soluble, red to maroon pigment that diffuses into the agar and is often best observed by viewing the reverse of the colony is suggestive of *T. marneffei.* Although the growth rate and colonial morphologic features may help the laboratorian recognize the possibility of a dimorphic fungus, they should be considered in combination with the microscopic morphologic features to make the identification. *T. marneffei* cannot be definitively identified by morphologic features alone; thermal conversion studies or nucleic acid–based testing is needed to confirm the identification of this pathogen.

***Sporothrix* spp.** Colonies of *Sporothrix* spp. grow rapidly (3 to 5 days) and initially are usually small, moist, and white to cream-colored. On further incubation, these become membranous, wrinkled, and coarsely matted, with the color becoming irregularly dark brown or black and the colony becoming leathery in consistency. It is not uncommon for the clinical microbiology laboratory to mistake a young culture of *Sporothrix* spp. for a yeast until the microscopic features are observed.

Approach to Identification
Blastomyces dermatitidis–B. gilchristii
Microscopically, hyphae of the mold form of *Blastomyces* spp. are septate and delicate and measure approximately 2 μm in diameter. Commonly, ropelike strands of hyphae are seen; however, these are found with most of the dimorphic fungi. The characteristic microscopic morphologic features are single, circular to pyriform conidia produced on short conidiophores that resemble lollipops (Fig. 59.41); less commonly, the conidiophores may be elongated. The production of conidia in some isolates is minimal or absent, particularly on a medium containing blood enrichment.

When incubated at 37°C, colonies of the yeast form develop within 7 days and appear waxy, wrinkled, and cream to tan. Microscopically, large, thick-walled yeast cells (8 to 15 μm in diameter) with buds attached by a broad base are seen (Fig. 59.29). Some strains may produce yeast cells as small as 2 to 5 μm, called **microforms.** Although these microforms may be present, a thorough search should reveal more typical yeast forms. During conversion, swollen hyphal forms and immature cells with rudimentary buds are also likely to be present. Because the conversion of *Blastomyces* spp. is easily accomplished, this is feasible in the clinical laboratory; however, this is the most appropriate instance in which mold-to-yeast conversion should be attempted. *Blastomyces* may also be identified by the presence of a specific band (i.e., A band) in the exoantigen test or by nucleic acid probe testing. *H. capsulatum*, *P. boydii*, or *T. rubrum* may occasionally be confused microscopically with *Blastomyces* spp. The site of infection and the relatively slow growth rate of *Blastomyces* spp. and careful examination of the microscopic morphologic features usually differentiate it from these fungi. Identification can also be confirmed using the AccuProbe test (Hologic Inc., San Diego CA) for *Blastomyces*.

Coccidioides spp.

Microscopically, some *Coccidioides* cultures show small, septate hyphae that often exhibit right-angle branches and racquet forms. With age, the hyphae form arthroconidia that are characteristically rectangular to barrel-shaped. The arthroconidia are larger than the hyphae from which they were produced and stain darkly with lactophenol cotton or aniline blue. The arthroconidia are separated by clear or lighter staining, nonviable cells (**dysjunctor cells**). These types of conidia are referred to as **alternate arthroconidia** (Fig. 59.25 and Fig. 59.35). Arthroconidia have been reported to range from 1.5 to 7.5 μm in width and 1.5 to 30 μm in length, whereas most are 3 to 4.5 μm in width and 3 μm in length. Variation has been reported in the shape of arthroconidia, ranging from rounded to square or rectangular to curved; however, most are barrel-shaped. Even if alternate arthroconidia are observed microscopically, definitive identification should be made using nucleic acid probe testing. If a culture is suspected of being *Coccidioides*, it should be sealed with tape to prevent laboratory-acquired infection. Because *Coccidioides* spp. are considered the most infectious of all the fungi, extreme caution should be used in handling cultures of these organisms. Safety precautions include the following:

1. If culture dishes are used, they should be handled only in a Level 3 BSC. Cultures should be sealed with tape if the specimen is suspected to contain *Coccidioides* spp.

2. The use of cotton plug test tubes is discouraged, and screw-capped tubes should be used if culture tubes are preferred. All handling of cultures of *Coccidioides* spp. in screw-capped tubes should be performed inside a BSC.

3. All microscopic preparations for examination should be performed in a Level 3 BSC.

4. Cultures should be autoclaved as soon as final identification is made.

Both species of *Coccidioides* were previously classified as select agents in the United States before removal from the list in 2012.

Other, usually nonvirulent fungi that resemble *Coccidioides* microscopically may be found in the environment. Some molds, such as *Malbranchea* spp., also produce alternate arthroconidia, although these tend to be more rectangular; however, such species must be considered when making the identification. *G. candidum* and *Trichosporon* spp. produce hyphae that disassociate into contiguous arthroconidia; these should not be confused with *Coccidioides* (Fig. 59.42 and Fig. 59.24). The colonial morphologic features of older cultures of these fungi may resemble *Coccidioides* spp., but as noted the arthroconidia are not alternate. It is also important to remember that if confusion in identification does arise, or when occasional strains of *Coccidioides* that fail to sporulate are encountered, identification by exoantigen or nucleic acid testing may be performed. Identification can also be confirmed using the AccuProbe test (Hologic Inc., San Diego CA) for *Coccidioides* spp.

Emmonsia spp. and *Emergomyces* spp.

The typical mold phase for *Emmonsia* and *Emergomyces* spp. was previously described in this chapter; however, culture for conversion to the yeast phase should be grown on **phytone yeast extract agar,** BHI, or BHI with blood at 37°C to 40°C. *Es. pasteuriana* produces yeastlike cells on BHI after approximately 10 days of incubation at 37°C. Other species may require up to 14 days of incubation for the yeast phase to be identified. Some of these organisms may be morphologically indistinguishable. Multilocus gene sequencing may be necessary to fully identify clinical isolates included in these genera.

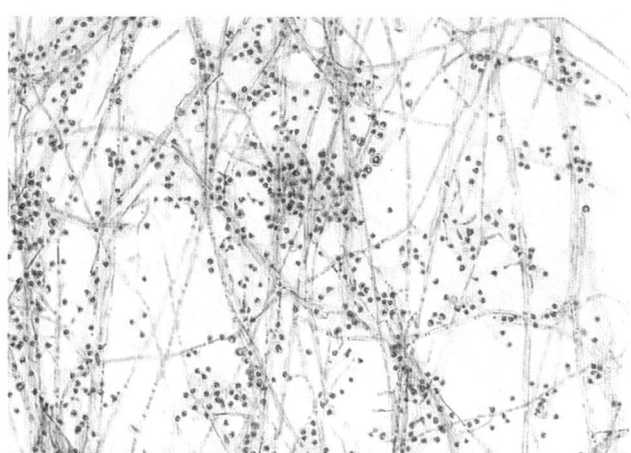

• **Fig. 59.41** The mycelial form of *Blastomyces dermatitidis* shows oval conidia borne laterally on branching hyphae (×1000).

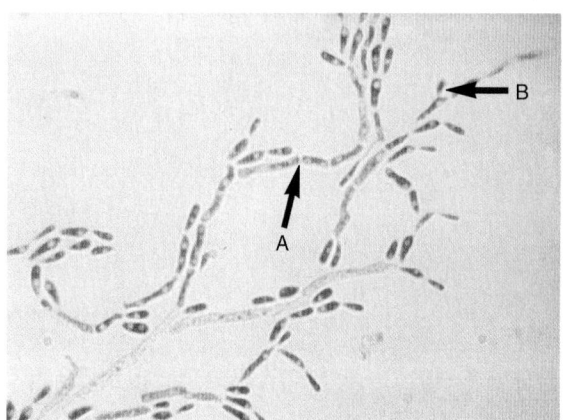

• **Fig. 59.42** *Trichosporon* spp. produce arthroconidia *(A)* and an occasional blastoconidium *(B)*.

Histoplasma capsulatum

Microscopically, the hyphae of *H. capsulatum* are small (approximately 2 μm in diameter) and are often intertwined to form ropelike strands. Commonly, large (8 to 14 μm in diameter) spherical or pyriform, smooth-walled macroconidia are seen in young cultures. With age, the macroconidia become roughened or tuberculate and provide enough evidence to make a tentative identification (Fig. 59.43). The macroconidia are produced either on short or long conidiospores. Some isolates produce round to pyriform, smooth microconidia (2 to 4 μm in diameter), in addition to the characteristic tuberculate macroconidia. Some isolates of *H. capsulatum* fail to sporulate despite numerous attempts to induce sporulation.

Conversion of the mold to the yeast form is usually difficult and is not recommended. Microscopically a mixture of swollen hyphae and small budding yeast cells 2 to 5 μm in diameter should be observed. These are similar to the intracellular yeast cells seen in mononuclear cells in infected tissue. The yeast form of *H. capsulatum* cannot be recognized unless the corresponding mold form is present on another culture or unless the yeast is converted directly to the mold form by incubation at 25°C to 30°C after yeast cells have been observed. Nucleic acid testing is recommended as a definitive means of rapidly identifying this organism.

Paracoccidioides spp.

Microscopically, the mold form is similar to that seen with *B. dermatitidis*. Small hyphae (approximately 2 μm in diameter) are seen, along with numerous chlamydoconidia. Small (3 to 4 μm), delicate, globose or pyriform conidia may be seen arising from the sides of the hyphae or on very short conidiophores (Fig. 59.44). Most often cultures reveal only fine septate hyphae and numerous chlamydoconidia.

After temperature-based conversion on a blood-enriched medium, the colonial morphology of the yeast form is characterized by smooth, soft-wrinkled, yeastlike colonies that are cream to tan. Microscopically, the colonies are composed of yeast cells 10 to 40 μm in diameter surrounded by narrow-necked yeast cells around the periphery, as previously described (Fig. 59.37). If *in vitro* conversion to the yeast form

is unsuccessful, the exoantigen test (Evolve Procedure 59.3) should be used to make the definitive identification of *P. brasiliensis*. There is no commercial DNA probe test available for the identification of *P. brasiliensis*.

Talaromyces marneffei

At 25°C, *T. marneffei* grows rapidly and produces blue-green to yellowish colonies. A soluble red to maroon pigment, which diffuses into the agar, is highly suggestive of *T. marneffei*. At 37°C, conversion of mycelium to the infective, yeastlike form occurs in approximately 2 weeks. Oval, yeastlike cells (2 to 6 μm in diameter) with septa are seen; abortive, extensively branched, and highly septate hyphae may also be present (Fig. 59.38). A variety of laboratory developed nucleic acid tests have been used to identify this organism from clinical samples.

Sporothrix spp.

Microscopically, hyphae are delicate (approximately 2 μm in diameter), septate, and branching. Single-celled conidia 2 to 5 μm in diameter are borne in clusters from the tips of single conidiophores (flowerette arrangement). Each conidium is attached to the conidiophore by an individual, delicate, threadlike structure (**denticle**) that may require examination under oil immersion to be visible. As the culture ages, single-celled, thick-walled, black-pigmented conidia may also be produced along the sides of the hyphae, simulating the arrangement of microconidia produced by *T. rubrum* (sleeve arrangement) (Fig. 59.45).

Because of similar morphologic features, saprophytic species of the genus *Sporotrichum* may be confused with *Sporothrix* spp., and they must be differentiated. During incubation of a culture at 37°C, colonies of *Sporothrix* spp. transform to a soft, cream-colored to white, yeastlike appearance. Microscopically, singly or multiply budding, spherical, oval, or elongate, cigar-shaped yeast cells are observed without difficulty (Fig. 59.46). Conversion from the mold form to the yeast form is easily accomplished and usually occurs within 1 to 5 days after transfer of the culture to a medium containing blood enrichment; most isolates of *Sporothrix* spp. are converted to the yeast form within 12 to 48 hours at 37°C.

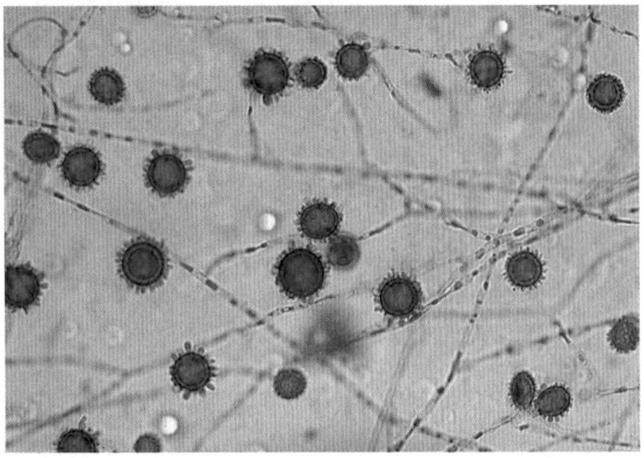

• **Fig. 59.43** The mycelial form of *Histoplasma capsulatum* produces characteristic tuberculate macroconidia (×1000).

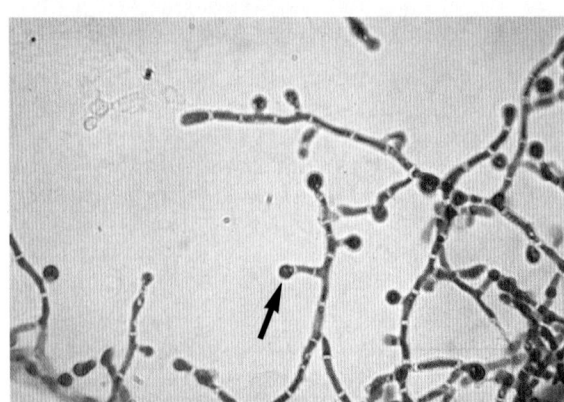

• **Fig. 59.44** Mycelial form of *Paracoccidioides brasiliensis* shows septate hyphae and pyriform conidia singly borne *(arrow)* (×430).

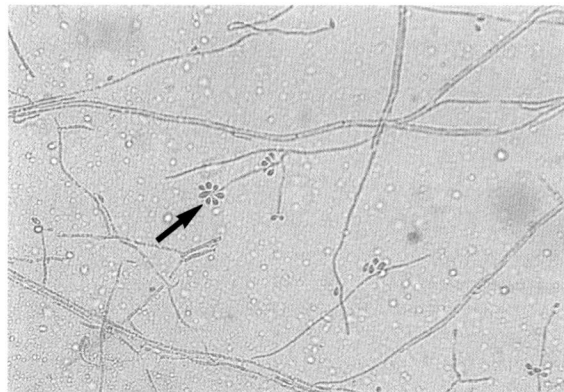

• **Fig. 59.45** The mycelial form of *Sporothrix* spp. demonstrating pyriform to ovoid microconidia in a flowerette morphology at the tip of the conidiophore *(arrow)* (×750).

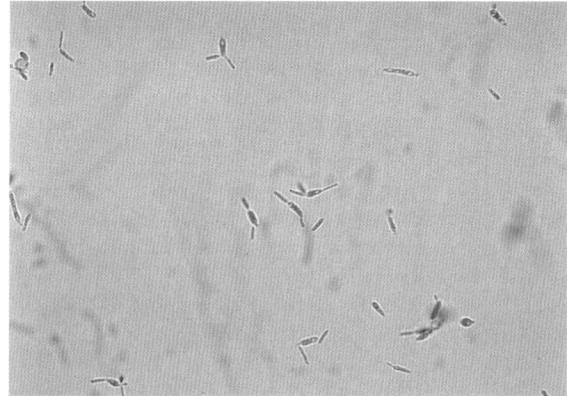

• **Fig. 59.46** The yeast form of *Sporothrix* spp. consists of cigar-shaped and oval budding cells (×500).

Sporotrichum spp. do not produce a yeast form. Molecular sequencing of the 18S rRNA or 28S rRNA along with the calmodulin gene may be required for species identification.

Serologic Testing

Fungal serology includes rapid and useful tests that may aid the diagnosis of systemic fungal infections caused by *H. capsulatum, Paracoccidioides,* and *Coccidioides* species. These tests have also been useful to study the epidemiology of these fungal infections, because even individuals with historically distant, asymptomatic, or subclinical infections often have developed an antibody response to the infecting pathogen. Unfortunately, these tests require detailed preparation and technical expertise. False-negative reactions may occur if serology specimens are drawn in immunocompromised individuals who are unable to produce an antibody response. False-positive reactions may occur because of cross reactivity with other fungi. For example, because the antigens of *H. capsulatum* are similar to those of *B. dermatitidis,* occasionally a specimen from a patient with histoplasmosis demonstrates a positive reaction for *B. dermatitidis* in serologic tests. Serology does not appear to be useful for the diagnosis of blastomycosis, and no tests have been developed for the diagnosis of adiaspiromycosis or emergomycosis.

Two assays, complement fixation and immunodiffusion, have been used together to detect antibodies directed toward *H. capsulatum* and *Coccidioides* spp. In the complement fixation assay, titers of 1:32 or greater indicate active infection with *H. capsulatum.* Titers as low as 1:2 to 1:4 have been identified in patients with coccidioidomycosis. Titers greater than 1:16 usually indicate active disease. Bands of identity form in the immunodiffusion test between known antisera, known fungal antigen, and the antibodies present in the patient's serum. Specific bands of identity are used for serologic detection of particular fungi, whereas nonspecific bands suggest the possibility of an infection by another fungal pathogen. One or two bands of identity, the H protein and M protein bands may occur in patients with histoplasmosis. The presence of both bands indicates active infection. The presence of an M protein band may indicate early or chronic infection. Newer enzyme immunosorbent assays have been developed and demonstrate improved sensitivity and specificity for the identification of histoplasmosis and coccidioidomycosis. A latex agglutination assay has been developed for the presumptive identification of *Coccidioides* infections. However, the test demonstrates a high false positive rate and is not recommended for use with CSF specimens.

ⓔ Visit the Evolve site for a complete list of procedures, review questions, and case studies.

Bibliography

Bailek R, Kern J, Herrmann T, et al.: PCR assays for identification of *Coccidioides posadasii* based on the nucleotide sequence of the antigen 2/proline-rich antigen, *J Clin Microbiol* 42:778–783, 2004.

Bennett J, Dolin R, Blaser M: *Principles and practice of infectious diseases,* ed 9, Philadelphia PA, 2020, Elsevier.

Brown EM, McTaggert LR, Zhang SX, et al.: Phylogenetic analysis reveals a cryptic species *Blastomyces gilchristii,* sp. nov. within the human pathogenic fungus *Blastomyces dermatitidis, PloS One* 8:e59237, 2013.

Carey J, D'Amico R, Sutton DA, et al.: *Paecilomyces lilacinus* vaginitis in an immunocompetent patient, *Emerg Infect Dis* 9: 1155–1158, 2003.

Carroll KC, Pfaller MA, Landry ML, et al.: *Manual of clinical microbiology,* ed 12, Washington, DC, 2019, ASM.

Croxatto A, Prod'hom G, Greub G: Applications of MALDI-TOF mass spectrometry in clinical diagnostic microbiology, *FEMS Microbiol Rev* 36:380–407, 2012.

de Hoog G: In *Atlas of clinical fungi, t.N.a.R. centraal bureau voor schimell cultures,* Spain, 2001, Universita Rovira i Virgili, Utrecht and Reus.

De Carolis E, Posteraro B, Lass-Flori C, et al.: Species identification of *Aspergillus, Fusarium* and *Mucorales* with direct surface analysis by matrix-assisted laser desorption ionization time-of-flight mass spectrometry, *Clin Microbiol Infect* 18:474–484, 2012.

Fleming RV, Walsh TJ, Anaissie EJ: Emerging and less common fungal pathogens, *Infect Dis Clin North Am* 16:915–933, 2002.

Germain G S, Summerbell R: *Identifying filamentous fungi: a clinical handbook,* Belmont, Calif, 1996, Star Publishing.

Gomez-Munoz MT, Fernandez-Barredo S, Martinez-Diaz RA, et al.: Development of a specific polymerase chain reaction assay for the detection of *Basidiobolus, Mycologia* 104:585–591, 2012.

Gutierrez-Rodero F, Moragon M, Ortiz de la Tabla V, et al.: Cutaneous hyalohyphomycosis caused by *Paecilomyces lilacinus* in an immunocompetent host successfully treated with itraconazole: case report and review, *Eur J Clin Microbiol Infect Dis* 18:814–818, 1999.

Heinic GS, Greenspan D, MacPhail LA, et al.: Oral *Geotrichum candidum* infection associated with HIV infection: a case report, *Oral Surg Oral Med Oral Pathol* 73:726–728, 1992.

Heys I, Taljaard J, Orth H: An *Emmonsia* species causing disseminated infection in South Africa, *N Engl J Med* 370:283–284, 2014.

Hussein MR: Mucocutaneous Splendore-Hoeppli phenomenon, *J Cutan Pathol* 35:979–988, 2008.

Kane J, Smitka C: Early detection and identification of *Trichophyton verrucosumm*, *J Clin Microbiol* 8:740–747, 1978.

Kenyon C, Bonorchis K, Corcoran C, et al.: A dimorphic fungus causing disseminated infection in South Africa, *N Engl J Med* 369:1416–1424, 2013.

Khan ZU, Khourshee M, Makar R, et al.: *Basidobolus ranarum* as an etiologic agent of gastrointestinal Zygomycosis, *J Clin Microbiol* 39:2360–2363, 2001.

Kontoyiannis DP, Wessel VC, Bodey GP, et al.: Zygomycosis in the 1990s in a tertiary-care cancer center, *Clin Infect Dis* 30: 851–856, 2000.

Kwon-Chung K, Bennet J. *Medical mycology*, Philadelphia, PA, 1992, Lea & Febiger.

Martagon-Villamil J, Shrestha N, Sholtis M, et al.: Identification of *Histoplasma capsulatum* from culture extracts by real-time PCR, *J Clin Microbiol* 41:1295–1298, 2003.

Meis JF, Kullberg BJ, Pruszczynski M, et al.: Severe osteomyelitis due to the zygomycete *Apophysomyces elegans*, *J Clin Microbiol* 32:3078–3081, 1994.

Modley A, Mosam A, Govender NP, et al.: *Emergomyces africanus*: the mimicking fungus, *Dermatopathology (Basel)* 6(2): 157–162, 2019.

Nucci M: Emerging moulds: *Fusarium, Scedosporium,* and *Zygomycetes* in transplant recipients, *Curr Opin Infect Dis* 16:607–612, 2003.

Odabasi Z, Mattiuzzi G, Estey E, et al.: Beta-D-glucan as a diagnostic adjunct for invasive fungal infections: validation, cutoff development, and performance in patients with acute myelogenous leukemia and myelodysplastic syndrome, *Clin Infect Dis* 39: 199–205, 2004.

Ostrosky-Zeichner L, Alexander BD, Kett DH, et al.: Multicenter clinical evaluation of the (1-3) beta-D-glucan assay as an aid to diagnosis of fungal infections in humans, *Clin Infect Dis* 41:654–659, 2005.

Patel R, Gustaferro CA, Krom RA, et al.: Phaeohyphomycosis due to *Scopulariopsis brumptii* in a liver transplant recipient, *Clin Infect Dis* 19:198–200, 1994.

Persaud SP, Lawton T, Burnham CD, et al.: Comparison of urine antigen assays for the diagnosis of *Histoplasma capsulatum* infection, *J Appl Lab Med* 4(3):370–382, 2019.

Pfeiffer CD, Fine JP, Safdar N: Diagnosis of invasive aspergillosis using a galactomannan assay: a meta-analysis, *Clin Infect Dis* 42:1417–1427, 2006.

Procop GW, Cockerill III FR, Vetter EA, et al.: Performance of five agar media for recovery of fungi from isolator blood cultures, *J Clin Microbiol* 38:3827–3829, 2000.

Schrodl W, Heydel T, Schwartze VU, et al.: Direct analysis and identification of pathogenic *Lichtheimia* species by matrix-assisted laser desorption ionization-time of flight analyzer mediated mass spectrometry, *J Clin Microbiol* 50:419–427, 2012.

Schwartz IS, Govender NP, Sigler L, et al.: *Emergomyces*: the global rise of new dimorphic fungal pathogens, *PLoS Pathog* 15(9):e1007977, 2019.

Skoulidis F, Morgan MS, MacLeod KM: *Penicillium marneffei*: a pathogen on our doorstep? *J R Soc Med* 97:394–396, 2004.

Sun SH, Huppert M, Vukovich KR: Rapid *in vitro* conversion and identification of *Coccidioides immitis*, *J Clin Microbiol* 3:186–190, 1976.

Torres HA, Raad II , Kontoyiannis DP: Infections caused by *Fusarium* species, *J Chemother* 15(Suppl 2):28–35, 2003.

Van Burik JA, Myerson D, Schreckhise RW, Bowden RA: Panfungal PCR assay for detection of fungal infection in human blood specimens, *J Clin Microbiol* 36:1169–1175, 1998.

Walsh TJ, Groll A, Heimenz J, et al.: Infections due to emerging and uncommon medically important fungal pathogens, *Clin Microbiol Infect* 10(Suppl 1):48–66, 2004.

Wang SM, Shieh CC, Liu CC: Successful treatment of *Paecilomyces variotii* splenic abscesses: a rare complication in a previously unrecognized chronic granulomatous disease child, *Diagn Microbiol Infect Dis* 53:149–152, 2005.

Willinger B: Laboratory diagnosis and therapy of invasive fungal infections, *Curr Drug Targets* 7:513–522, 2006.

Woo PC, Leung SY, Ngan A, et al.: A significant number of reported *Absidia corymbifera* (*Lichtheimia corymbifera*) infections are caused by *Lichtheimia ramosa* (syn. *Lichtheimia hongkongensis*): an emerging cause of mucormycosis, *Emerg Microb Infect* 1:e15, 2012.

Zhiyong Z, Mei K, Yanbin L: Disseminated *Penicillium marneffei* infection with fungemia and endobronchial disease in an AIDS patient in China, *Med Princ Pract* 15:235–237, 2006.

60

Dematiaceous (Melanized) Molds

OBJECTIVES

1. Describe the melanized fungi, including natural habitat, transmission, and diseases with signs and symptoms.
2. Identify the site where mycetomas are commonly located and the population or populations at risk of infection.
3. Compare and contrast *Exophiala jeanselmei* and *Exophiala dermatitidis,* including test methods to distinguish between the two.
4. Describe the microscopic and morphologic features of *Pseudallescheria boydii,* including its sexual and asexual forms.
5. Differentiate the diagnostic microscopic features of the molds included in this chapter.

SEPTATE DEMATIACEOUS MOLDS TO BE CONSIDERED

Superficial Infections

Alternaria alternata
Aureobasidium melanogenum
Cladophialophora boppii
Cyphellophora europaea
Cyphellophora laciniata
Cyphellophora pluriseptata
Curvularia spp.
Hortaea werneckii
Neoscytalidium dimidiatum
Piedraia hortae
Scopulariopsis brevicaulis
Triadelphia pulvinata

Cutaneous and Corneal

Alternaria alternata
Alternaria infectoria
Bipolaris oryzae
Cladophialophora boppii
Cladophialophora emmonsii
Cladophialophora saturnica
Cladorrhinum bulbillosum
Cladosporium cladosporioides
Cladosporium oxysporum
Curvularia lunata
Curvularia senegalensis
Curvularia spicifera
Diaporthe longicolla
Diaporthe phaseolorum
Diaporthe phoenicicola

Exophiala bergeri
Exophiala dermatitidis
Exophiala jeanselmei
Exophiala oligosperma
Exophiala xenobiotica
Exserohilum rostratum
Knufia epidermidis
Lasiodiplodia theobromae
Macrophomina phaseolina
Neoscytalidium dimidiatum
Sporothrix pallida

Subcutaneous (Includes Mycetomas)

Alternaria spp.
Cyphellophora suttonii
Cladophialophora bantiana
Curvularia spp.
Diaporthe bougainvilleicola
Diaporthe phaseolorum
Exserohilum spp.
Exophiala spp.
Hongkongmyces pedis
Knoxdaviesia dimorphospora
Lasiodiplodia theobromae
Lomentospora prolificans
Madurella spp.
Neoscytalidium dimidiatum
Ochroconis mirabilis
Phaeoacremonium spp.
Pleurostoma richardsiae
Scedosporium spp.
Scopulariopsis spp.
Trematosphaeria grisea
Veronaea botryose

Systemic Phaeohyphomycosis

Arthrocladium fulminans
Aureobasium pullulans
Cladophialophora bantiana
Cladophialophora modesta
Curvularia spp.
Exserohilum rostratum
Exophiala dermatitidis
Exophiala phaeomuriformis
Exophiala spinifera
Fonsecaea monophora
Fonsecaea pedrosoi
Hormonema dematioides
Lasiodiplodia theobromae
Lomentospora prolificans
Neoscytalidium dimidiatum

SEPTATE DEMATIACEOUS MOLDS TO BE CONSIDERED

Ophiostoma piceae
Phaeoacremonium parasiticum
Phialophora verrucosa
Rhinocladiella mackenziei
Scedosporium spp.
Triadelphia disseminata
Verruconis gallopava

Chromoblastomycosis

Cladophialophora carrionii
Cladophialophora boppii
Cladophialophora samoënsis
Cyphellophora ludoviensis
Phialophora verrucosa
Fonsecaea monophora
Fonsecaea pedrosoi
Fonsecaea pugnacius
Rhinocladiella tropicalis
Rhinocladiella aquaspersa

General Characteristics

The dematiaceous fungi were once only characterized by the dark coloration because of their ability to produce melanin. More recently, organisms, including medically important fungi, have been classified using molecular techniques (Table 60.1). Many of the agents in this chapter cause phaeohyphomycosis or chromoblastomycosis and are known agents of superficial and subcutaneous mycoses that involve the skin and subcutaneous tissues and, less commonly, deeply invasive or disseminated disease. These organisms are ubiquitous in nature and exist as saprophytes and plant pathogens. Humans and animals serve as accidental hosts after traumatic inoculation of the organism into cutaneous and subcutaneous tissues.

In the mycology laboratory, these fungal species often are initially separated by growth rate into the **slow-growing dematiaceous molds,** which may require 7 to 10 days to grow, and the **rapid-growing dematiaceous molds,** which usually grow in less than 7 days. It has been recommended that in medical mycology the term dematiaceous only be applied to rapidly growing members of the Ploesoporales (*Alternaria, Bipolaris, Curvularia, Exoserohilum,* and *Hongkongmyces*). This has not been widely implemented and will take time for all of the changes to be apparent in clinical mycology. When nonsterile body sites are cultured, determining the significance of these organisms is very difficult. If colonies of common saprophytic molds occur near the edge of the plate and are clearly away from the inoculum, they should be considered contaminants unless additional evidence of infection is present.

Epidemiology and Pathogenesis
Superficial Infections

Tinea nigra is a superficial skin infection caused by *Hortaea werneckii,* a halophilic species. It is manifested by blackish brown, macular patches on the palm of the hand or the sole of the foot. Lesions have been compared with silver nitrate staining of the skin. **Black piedra** is a fungal infection of the hair, scalp, and occasionally the axillary and pubic hair caused by the dematiaceous fungus *Piedraia hortae. Neoscytalidium dimidiatum,* a common plant pathogen, causes infections of the skin and nails that may lead to **hyperkeratosis** (thickening of the epidermis). These diseases occur primarily in tropical areas of the world, with cases reported from Africa, Asia, and Latin America. *Phialophora* spp. and *Cyphellophora* spp. have also been known to be the causative agents of mild skin infections and onychomycoses (M & M, Chowdhary 2015).

Several species in the order Chaetothyriales are capable of causing superficial infections in humans including *Cyphellophora* spp., *Phialophora europaea,* and *Knufia epidermidis.* The fungi are typically associated with mild cutaneous skin infections or nail infections.

Mycetoma

A **mycetoma** is a chronic granulomatous infection that usually involves the lower extremities but may occur in any part of the body. The infection is characterized by swelling, purplish discoloration, tumorlike deformities of the subcutaneous tissue, and multiple sinus tracts that drain purulent material containing yellow, white, red, or black granules called grains. The color of the granules is partly dependent on the type of infecting organism. The infection gradually progresses to involve the bone, muscle, or other contiguous tissue and ultimately requires amputation in most progressive cases. Dissemination of the organism may occur but is uncommon. Mycetomas usually are seen among people living in tropical and subtropical regions of the world whose outdoor occupations and failure to wear protective clothing predispose them to trauma.

Two types of mycetomas have been described. Actinomycotic (bacterial) mycetomas are caused by the aerobic actinomycetes, including *Nocardia, Actinomadura,* and *Streptomyces* spp. (The aerobic *Actinomycetes* are described in detail in Chapter 18.) Eumycotic (fungal) mycetomas are caused by a heterogeneous group of fungi that have septate hyphae. Eumycotic mycetomas are subcategorized as white grain mycetomas or black grain mycetomas, a distinction determined by the pigmentation of the infecting agent's hyphae.

Some hyaline septate molds can cause mycetomas; however, the disease is covered in this section because many of the etiologic agents are dematiaceous fungi. Etiologic agents of eumycotic mycetoma to be discussed include *Scedosporium* spp. and *Acremonium* spp., causative agents of white grain mycetomas, and *Exophiala jeanselmei, Curvularia* spp., *Cladophialophora bantiana, Trematosphaeria grisea,* and *Madurella* spp., causative agents of black grain mycetomas.

TABLE 60.1 Classification and Taxonomy of the Clinically Relevant Melanized Fungi

Order	Genera	Species	Characteristics
Botryosphaeria	Lasiodiplodia	L. theobroma	Initially spherical, thick-walled hyaline conidia that brown with age and develop a median septum.
	Macrophomina	M. phaseolina	Dark sclerotic bodies and melanized mycelium.
	Neoscytalidium	N. dimidiatum	Produces arthroconidia in culture.
Calosphaeriales	Pleurostoma	P. ochracea P. repens P. richardsiae	Dark hyphae with pale, tapering phialides that may be single or aggregated in dense brushes; hyaline conidia.
Capnodiales	Cladosporium	C. cladosporioides C. oxysporum C. sphaerospermum	Branching chains of single-celled or septate conidia.
	Hortea	H. werneckii	Yeastlike, aseptate or septate elements.
Chaetothyriales	Anthopsis	Anthopsis sp.	Ampulliform phialides that appear inverted with collarettes.
	Arthrocladium	A. fulminans	Moniliform hyphae and chlamydospore-like structures.
	Cladophialophora	C. bantiana C. carrionii	Long, branched conidial chains and grows at 40°C. Small conidia in branched chains.
	Cyphellophora	C. europaea C. laciniata C. ludoviensis C. pluriseptica C. reptans C. suttonii	Slender, curved, transversely septate conidia.
	Exophiala	E. bergeri E. dermatitidis E. jeanselmei E. oligosperma E. phaeomuriformis E. spinifera E. xenobiotica	Conidia in chains or compacted phialides. *E. dermatitis* is recognized by phialides without collarettes with short annellated zones.
	Fonsecaea	F. compacta F. monophora F. nubica F. pedrosoi F. pugnacius	*Phialophora*-like phialides with collarettes and *Rhinocladiella*-like sympodial conidiophores.
	Knufia	K. epidermidis	Produce phialides, arthroconidia, holoblastic conidia, endoconidia, and yeastlike budding cells in culture.
	Phialophora	P. verrucosa	Darkened funnel-shaped collarettes.
	Rhinocladiella	R. aquaspersa R. atrovirens R. basitona R. mackenziei R. similis R. tropicalis	Sympodial conidiophores with one-celled conidia on denticles.
	Veronaea	V. botryose	Sympodial rachis with denticles, single-septate conidia.
Diaporthales	Diaporthe	D. bougainvilleicola D. longicolla D. phaseolorum D. phoenicicola	Oval to fusoid conidia or thin, curved, or bent elongated conidia.

Continued

TABLE 60.1 **Classification and Taxonomy of the Clinically Relevant Melanized Fungi—cont'd**

Order	Genera	Species	Characteristics
Dothideales	Aureobasidium	A. melanogenum A. pullulans	Budding yeastlike, hyaline and melanized thick-walled hyphae that produce dark brown chlamydospores with age.
	Hormonema	H. dematioides	Produce conidia in a basipetal succession.
Microascales	Knoxdaviesia	K. dimorphospora	Lateral undifferentiated hyphae, epllipsoid, pale brown conidia.
	Lomentospora	L. prolificans	Elongated, annellidic conidiogenous cells and obovoid conidia.
	Microascus	M. brunneosporus M. cinereus M. gracilis	Dark brown to black, globose to ampulliform ascomata, with papilla. Ascospores are ellipsoid or quadrangular. Single or penicillate conidiophores with conidia in basipetal chains.
	Scopulariopsis	S. asperula S. brevicaulis S. candida	Globose or pyriform, black ascomata. Annellides arranged penicillately on conidiophore being single or small groups of stalks, smooth or rough walled conidia in basipetal chains.
	Scedosporium	S. apiospermum S. aurantiacum S. boydii S. dehoogii	Conidiophores with annelides. Conidia are obovoid and become brown with age. Produces laterally on hyphae or short pedicels.
	Triadelphia	T. disseminate T. pulvinata	
Ophiostomatales	Ophiostoma	O. piceae	Subglobose, dark perithecia asci with long necks; yeastlike cells and septate hyphae.
	Sporothrix	S. brasiliensis S. chilensis S. globose S. luriei S. pallida S. schenckii	Conidiophore bear clusters of thin denticles with hyaline, tear-shaped conidia. Subglobose or elongated conidia may also be present.
Pleosporales	Alternaria	A. alternate A. infectoria	Conidia in chains with alternating septa. A. infectoria produces conidia with long apical beaks.
	Bipolaris	B. australiensis B. hawaiiensis B. oryzae B. spicifera	Large ellipsoid to subcylindrical, straight conidia with a distosepta and a dark, flat basal scar.
	Curvularia	C. aeria C. americana C. geniculate C. hominis C. muehlenbeckiae C. lunata C. senegalensis	Elongated conidia that are distoseptate with an asymmetrical swollen middle cell resulting in a curved appearance.
	Exserohilum	E. longirostratum E. mcginnisii E. rostratum	Long, distoseptate conidia with a protruding basal hilum.
	Hongkongmyces	H. pedis	
Sordariales	Madurella	M. mycetomatis	
	Cladorrhinum	C. bulbillosum	Aseptate conidia with intercalary conidiogenous cells with lateral phialide openings.

TABLE 60.1   Classification and Taxonomy of the Clinically Relevant Melanized Fungi—cont'd

Order	Genera	Species	Characteristics
Togniniales	*Phaeoacremonium*	*P. parasiticum* *Phaeoacremonium* spp. (10 additional species)	Warted mycelium and slender, tubular, tapering brown phialides.
Venturiales	*Ochroconis*	*O. mirabilis*	Rust to brown olivaceous colonies that produce 1–3 septate conidia from small, open denticles on sympodial cells.
	Verruconis	*V. gallopava*	Same as *Ochroconis* sp.

Madurella mycetomatis is the most common fungal agent associated with mycetoma. However, nucleic acid–based sequencing of several genes has indicated that multiple additional species exist and are associated with mycetoma. These species have likely been misidentified as *M. mycetomatis* in previous cases and include *Madurella pseudomycetomatis*, *Madurella tropicana,* and *Madurella fahalii.*

Most patients with mycetomas live in tropical regions, but infections can occur in temperate zones. The most common etiologic agent of white grain mycetoma in the United States is caused by *Scedosporium* spp. The organisms associated with mycetoma are saprophytic and commonly found in soil, standing water, and sewage; humans acquire infections through traumatic implantation of the organism into the skin and subcutaneous tissues.

Chromoblastomycosis

Chromoblastomycosis is a chronic fungal infection acquired through traumatic inoculation of an organism, primarily into the skin and subcutaneous tissue. The infection is characterized by the development of a papule at the site of the traumatic insult that slowly enlarges to form warty or tumorlike lesions characterized as resembling cauliflower capable of spreading through the lymphatic system. Secondary infection and ulceration may occur. The lesions usually are confined to the feet and legs but may involve the head, face, neck, and other body surfaces.

Histologic examination of the lesion reveals characteristic **sclerotic bodies,** which are copper-colored, septate cells that appear to be dividing by binary fission and resemble copper pennies. These infections cause hyperplasia of the epidermal layer of the skin, which may be mistaken for squamous cell carcinoma. Fungal brain abscess, known as cerebral chromoblastomycosis, may be caused by the dematiaceous fungi; however, it is more appropriately considered a type of phaeohyphomycosis and is discussed with that disease. Chromoblastomycosis is widely distributed, but most cases occur in tropical and subtropical areas of the world. Occasional cases are reported from temperate zones, including the United States. The infection is seen most often in areas in which agricultural workers do not wear protective clothing and suffer thorn or splinter puncture wounds.

The fungi most often associated with chromoblastomycosis include *Cladophialophora carrionii, Fonsecaea monophora* and *pedrosoi,* and *Phialophora verrucosa.* Additional species of *Cladophialophora* have also been reported as the cause of chromoblastomycosis.

Phaeohyphomycosis

Phaeohyphomycosis is a general term used to describe any infection caused by a dematiaceous organism; it includes molds; brownish, yeastlike cells; pseudohyphae; and hyphae, except those described previously. These infections may be subcutaneous, localized, or systemic, and they may be caused by a number of dematiaceous fungi. They include phaeohyphomycotic cysts, progressive soft tissue infection, brain abscess, sinusitis, endocarditis, mycotic keratitis, pulmonary infection, and systemic infection. Symptoms often include headache, neurologic manifestations, and seizures. The most common fungal isolates associated with neurologic manifestations include *C. bantiana, Rhinocladiella mackenziei, Verruconis gallopava,* and *Exophiala dermatitidis. Alternaria, Exserohilum, Bipolaris, E. jeanselmei, Exophiala spinifera,* and *Curvularia* spp. are also commonly associated with phaeophyomycosis.

Pathogenesis and Spectrum of Disease

The spectrum of disease caused by the dematiaceous fungi ranges from superficial infections (e.g., skin and hair) to emergent, rapidly progressive, and often fatal disease (e.g., brain abscess). The following list, which is not comprehensive, provides the common etiologic agents of diseases that may be caused by dematiaceous fungi (Table 60.2).

- Mycetoma
  - Bacterial: *Nocardia, Actinomadura,* and *Streptomyces* spp.
  - White grain mycetoma: *S. apiospermum* complex and *Acremonium* and *Fusarium* spp.
  - Black grain mycetoma: *Madurella* spp., *E. jeanselmei,* and *Curvularia* spp.
- Chromoblastomycosis: *Cladophialophora, Phialophora,* and *Fonsecaea* spp.
- Phaeohyphomycosis: *E. jeanselmei; E. dermatitidis;* and *Curvularia, Bipolaris, Alternaria,* and *Exserohilum* spp.

- Sinusitis: *Alternaria, Bipolaris, Exserohilum,* and *Curvularia* spp.
- Mycotic keratitis and endophthalmitis: *E. dermatitidis, Bipolaris,* and *Curvularia* spp.
- Brain abscess: *C. bantiana, E. dermatitidis,* and *Bipolaris* spp.

Laboratory Diagnosis

Specimen Collection, Transport, and Processing

See General Considerations for the Laboratory Diagnosis of Fungal Infections in Chapter 58.

TABLE 60.2 Common Isolated Dematiaceous Fungi

Organism	Disease	Site	Tissue Form
Slow-Growing Species			
Cladophialophora spp.	Chromoblastomycosis	Subcutaneous	Sclerotic bodies
	Phaeohyphomycosis	Brain, subcutaneous	Septate hyphae
Verruconis gallopava	Phaeohyphomycosis	Brain, subcutaneous, lungs	Septate hyphae
Exophiala dermatitidis	Phaeohyphomycosis	Brain, eye, subcutaneous, and dissemination	Hyphal fragments and budding yeast
	Pneumonial	Lungs	
Hortaea jeanselmei	Mycetoma phaeomycotic cyst	Subcutaneous	Hyphal fragments and budding yeasts
Hortaea werneckii	Tinea nigra	Skin	Hyphal fragments and budding yeast
Fonsecaea spp.	Chromoblastomycosis	Subcutaneous	Sclerotic bodies
	Phaeohyphomycosis	Brain	Septate hyphae
	Cavitary lung disease	Lungs	Septate hyphae
Phialophora spp.	Chromoblastomycosis	Subcutaneous	Sclerotic bodies
	Phaeohyphomycosis	Subcutaneous	Septate hyphae
	Septic arthritis	Joints	Septate hyphae
Piedraia hortae	Black piedra	Hair	Asci-containing nodules cemented to hair shafts
Madurella spp.	Mycetoma	Subcutaneous	Hyphal fragments
Rapid-Growing Species			
Alternaria spp.	Phaeohyphomycosis	Subcutaneous	Septate hyphae
	Sinusitis	Sinuses	Septate hyphae, possibly fungus ball
	Nasal septal erosion	Nasal septum	Septate hyphae
	Ulcers and onychomycosis	Skin, nails	Septate hyphae
Bipolaris spp.	Phaeohyphomycosis	Subcutaneous, brain, eye, bones	Septate hyphae
	Sinusitis, fungus ball	Sinuses	Septate hyphae; possibly fungus ball
Curvularia spp.	Sinusitis	Sinuses	Septate hyphae; possibly fungus ball
	Phaeohyphomycosis	Subcutaneous, heart valves, eye, and lungs	Septate hyphae
Exserohilum spp.	Phaeohyphomycosis	Subcutaneous	Septate hyphae
Scedosporium spp. (Scedosporium apiospermum complex)	Mycetoma	Subcutaneous	Granules of hyaline hyphae
	Phaeohyphomycosis	Subcutaneous, skin, joints, bones, brain, lungs	Septate, hyaline hyphae

Direct Detection Method

Stains

In general, dematiaceous fungal hyphae are seen in clinical specimens by direct microscopic examination or by histopathologic examination of tissue obtained during surgery or autopsy. The dematiaceous character of the hyphae may not be appreciated if the examination is performed using calcofluor white or fluorescent microscopy alone, without observing the hyphae using traditional transmitted light microscopy. The **Fontana-Masson stain,** 10% silver nitrate and ammonium hydroxide, stains fungal elements brown to black in a red background. This technique improves the detection of melanin granules. The Fontana-Masson stain is useful to detect melanization that may appear as hyaline molds using light microscopy.

Superficial Infections

Direct microscopic examination of a clinical specimen from a patient with tinea nigra may show dematiaceous hyphae and small budding yeast cells and/or hyphal fragments. Portions of hairs from a patient with black piedra are examined in wet mounts using potassium hydroxide (KOH) that is gently heated for nodules composed of cemented mycelium. Crushing the mature nodules reveals oval asci, containing two to eight aseptate ascospores, 19 to 55 μm long by 4 to 8 μm in diameter. The asci are spindle shaped and have a filament at each pole.

Sinusitis associated with fungal infections typically reveal dense masses of pigmented, branched and septate hyphae. The hyphal elements appear as amorphous fungal balls that block the sinus cavities but are not invading the mucosal lining.

Chromoblastomycosis

The laboratory diagnosis of chromoblastomycosis is made easily. Scrapings from crusted lesions added to 10% KOH show **muriform cells** (aggregation of dark brown cells that resemble stones in a stonewall) or sclerotic bodies, which are rounded, brown, 4 to 10 μm in diameter, and have fission planes. They resemble copper pennies (Fig. 60.1).

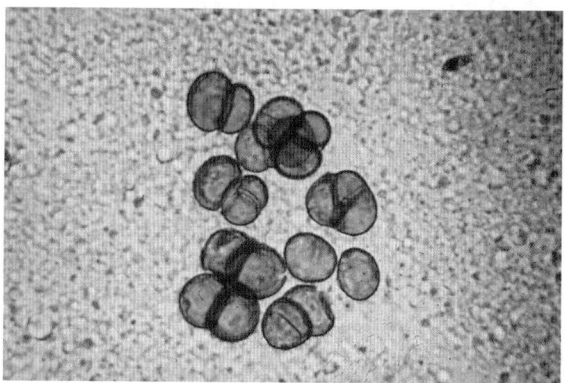

• **Fig. 60.1** Sclerotic bodies from the tissue of a patient with chromoblastomycosis (×400). (From Velasques LF, Restrepo A. Chromomycosis in the toad (*Bufo marinus*) and a comparison of the etiologic agent with fungi causing human chromomycosis. *Sabouraudia* 1975;13:1.)

Mycetoma and Phaeohyphomycosis

Direct examination of clinical specimens from patients with a eumycotic mycetoma or phaeohyphomycosis demonstrates yellowish brown, septate to **moniliform hyphae** (string of beads), with or without budding yeast cells present. The presence of dematiaceous yeasts depends on the fungus. Dematiaceous yeasts are commonly seen in the direct examination of clinical specimens from patients with infections caused by *Exophiala* spp. Macroscopic examination of granules from mycetoma lesions caused by *S. apiospermum* complex reveal them to be white to yellow and 0.2 to 2 mm in diameter. Microscopically, the granules of *S. apiospermum* complex consist of loosely arranged, intertwined septate hyaline hyphae cemented together.

Observation of pigmented hyphae in hematoxylin-eosin or unstained histopathologic sections is presumptive for a diagnosis of dematiaceous fungal disease. The methenamine silver stain used to detect fungal elements in tissues stains fungi black, which makes determining whether they are hyaline septate or dematiaceous septate molds impossible. Fontana-Masson stain, which stains the melanin and melanin-like pigments in the cell walls of these organisms, may be used to confirm the presence of pigmented hyphae in histologic sections. Culture of the specific etiologic agent is necessary for final confirmation.

Serologic Testing

Some serologic and skin tests may be useful for the diagnosis of allergy to dematiaceous fungi. However, serology is not useful for the diagnosis of invasive dematiaceous fungal disease.

Nucleic Acid–Based Tests

Nucleic acid amplification assays can be used for detection or identification of these fungi. Polymerase chain reaction (PCR) tests have been developed for *S. apiospermum* complex, and direct DNA testing is available for *Madurella* spp. from the actual grains. Amplification tests have been developed to detect fungal DNA in normally sterile body fluids such as cerebrospinal fluid and brain tissue in patients with suspected fungal meningitis.

Nucleic acid–based sequencing of ribosomal genes may be used for the identification of fungal isolates. However, sequences should be evaluated carefully by comparison with type strains. In addition, a variety of high-resolution multigene typing systems have been used in recent years primarily for epidemiologic purposes.

Matrix-Assisted Laser Desorption Ionization Time-of-Flight Mass Spectrometry

Matrix-assisted laser desorption ionization time-of-flight mass spectrometry (MALDI-TOF MS) has been successfully used to identify clinically relevant fungal isolates including yeasts and molds. As more application of this technique becomes available in the clinical laboratory, rapid diagnosis of fungal infections will undoubtedly become more accurate, resulting in improved patient prognosis and treatment.

Cultivation

Although dematiaceous molds recovered in the clinical mycology laboratory may represent true pathogens, more often they represent transient microbiota, inhaled spores, or contaminants. Cultures from sterile body sites, if aseptically obtained, should not contain these molds. Cultures should be interpreted in conjunction with the results of the direct examination for fungal elements, corresponding histopathology, and discussion with the clinician to most effectively establish the diagnosis of mycotic infection caused by these organisms.

Superficial Infections

H. werneckii, the causative agent of tinea nigra, may be recovered on common fungal media but grows very slowly. Initial colonies of *H. werneckii* may be olive to black, shiny, and yeastlike (Fig. 60.2) and usually grow within 2 to 3 weeks. As the cultures age, colonies become filamentous, with velvety gray aerial hyphae. *P. hortae,* the causative agent of black piedra, is easily cultured on any fungal culture medium lacking cycloheximide. Colonies of this organism are also very slow growing, appear dark brown to black, and produce aerial mycelium. Some isolates may produce a red to brown diffusible pigment.

Cyphellophora produce slender, curved, one- to three-septate conidia. The conidia are produced on **collarettes.** Cultures are typically melanized without budding cells. *Exophilia,* which is considered a black yeast, demonstrates a high degree of morphologic variability. Colonies initially appear moist and then become wooly or velvety. The conidia are produced from narrow scars or extensions referred to as annelidic. The *Exophilia* are also capable of growth at 40°C and fail to assimilate nitrate. *Phialophora* produce phialides (flask shaped) and have no budding cells.

N. dimidiatum produces a rapidly growing black arthroconidia in culture.

Mycetoma

White Grain Mycetoma. *Scedosporium* spp. grow rapidly (5 to 10 days) on common laboratory media. Initial growth begins as a white, fluffy colony that changes in several weeks to a brownish gray (the so-called mousy gray) colony; the reverse of the colony progresses from tan to dark brown. *Acremonium* spp. that cause mycetomas, such as *Acremonium falciforme,* grow slowly and produce gray colonies.

Black Grain Mycetoma. Colonies of *Madurella* spp. and *E. jeanselmei* (Fig. 60.3) are slow growing, unlike colonies of *Curvularia* spp. Colonies of *Madurella* spp. vary from white (during the early phases of growth) to olive-brown; a brown diffusible pigment is characteristic of this fungus. Colonies of *E. jeanselmei* appear yeastlike and darkly pigmented (olive to black) but in time develop a velvety appearance with the production of aerial hyphae. *Curvularia* spp. produce a fluffy or downy, olive-gray to black colony, and growth is rapid. *T. grisea* forms slow-growing, velvety colonies that appear

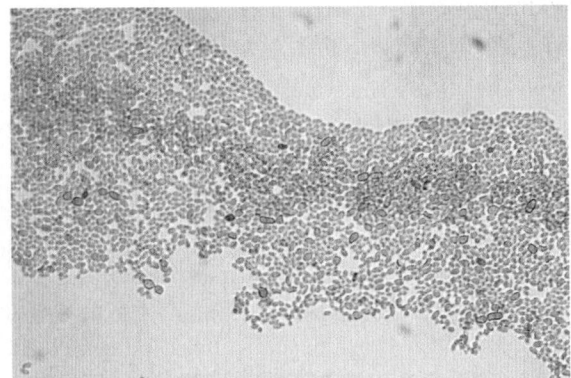

• **Fig. 60.2** Yeast forms of *Hortaea werneckii*.

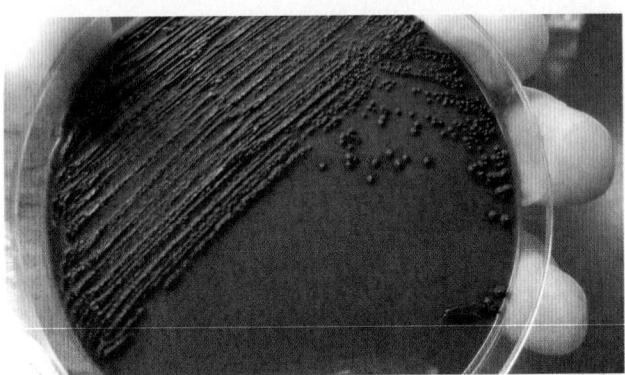

• **Fig. 60.3** *Exophiala jeanselmei* on chocolate agar. (Photo courtesy Brooks Kyle Murillo-Kennedy, Houston, TX.)

smooth or radially furrowed and dark gray or olive-brown to black. The reverse side of the colonies appears black. The hyphae are septate and nonsporulating.

Chromoblastomycosis

The fungi known to cause chromoblastomycosis, *Cladophialophora, Phialophora* spp., and *Fonsecaea* spp., are all dematiaceous. These fungi are slow growing and produce heaped-up, slightly folded, darkly pigmented colonies with a gray to olive to black and velvety or suedelike appearance. The reverse side of the colonies is jet black. Microscopic examination is necessary to identify the pathogenic agent definitively.

Phaeohyphomycosis

The colonies of many of the rapidly growing dematiaceous molds are similar; identification relies on microscopic examination. The colonies of *Alternaria* spp. are rapidly growing, fluffy, and gray to gray-brown or gray-green. *Curvularia* spp. produce rapidly growing colonies that resemble those of *Alternaria* spp. *Bipolaris* spp. produce colonies that are gray-green to dark brown and slightly powdery, as do *Exserohilum* spp.

The colonies of many of the slow-growing dematiaceous molds are also similar to one another and require identification based on microscopic morphology. *E. jeanselmei* and *E. dermatitidis* grow slowly (7 to 21 days) and initially produce shiny, black, yeastlike colonies. *E. derma-titidis* often is mucoid and may be brown, compared with *E. jeanselmei,* but the two organisms are very similar in appearance. Colonies become filamentous and velvety with age because of the production of mycelium. *E. spinifera* produces large, stiff conidiophores. *C. bantiana* produces long, poorly branched conidial chains. The fungus is also capable of growth at 40°C. *R. mackenziei* produces pale brown conidiophores with elongated conidia on denticles (projection or peg) and may produce exophiala-like budding cells in culture. *V. gallopava* produces a rusty-brown to olive colony with one- to three-septate condia on small denticles. The colonial morphology of other slowly growing dematiaceous fungi (e.g., *Fonsecaea* spp.) was described in the previous section.

Approach to Identification
Superficial Infections

H. werneckii is a dematiaceous fungus that produces yeast-like cells that may be one or two celled. Conidia produced by this organism are produced by annellophores (conidia-forming cells that produce conidia-containing transverse rings), which bear successive rings (annelides) that are difficult to see microscopically. The biophysical profile is used to differentiate this fungus from other *Exophiala* spp. In contrast, *P. hortae* usually does not sporulate on routine mycologic media but demonstrates highly septate, dematiaceous hyphae and swollen intercalary cells.

Mycetoma

The specific etiologic agent of a eumycotic mycetoma cannot be determined without culturing the organism. Culture media containing antibiotics should not be used as the sole medium for culturing clinical specimens from a mycetoma, because species of the aerobic actinomycetes are susceptible to antibacterial antibiotics and may be inhibited by these agents.

White Grain Mycetoma: *Scedosporium apiospermum* complex and *Acremonium* spp.

As previously mentioned, white grain mycetoma are hyaline molds that produce septate hyphae. The features described here are useful for identification regardless of the disease process (i.e., mycetoma or hyalohyphomycosis). *S. apio-spermum* complex is also involved in causing a variety of infections elsewhere in the body. These include infections of the nasal sinuses and septum, meningitis, arthritis, endocarditis, mycotic keratitis, external otomycosis, brain abscess, and disseminated invasive infection. Most of these more serious infections occur primarily in immunocompromised patients.

S. apiospermum is the former asexual phase of *Pseudo-allescheria boydii.* A nomenclature transition is currently in progress that would result in a single genus and species name for fungi that demonstrate multiple morphologic forms. The asexually produced conidia of *S. apiospermum* complex are golden brown, elliptical to pyriform and single-celled

and are borne singly from the tips of long or short conidiophores (annellophores) (Fig. 58.2). This anamorph (a fungus that disseminates reproductive structures without meiosis) predominates in cultures from clinical specimens. Another anamorphic form, the *Graphium* stage of *S. apio-spermum* complex, is less common. It consists of clusters of conidiophores with conidia produced at the ends; it has also been referred to as **coremia** (Fig. 58.3). The teleomorphic form of the organism produces brown to black cleistothecia, which are pseudoparenchymatous, saclike structures containing asci and ascospores. When the latter are fully developed, the large (50 to 200 μm), thick-walled cleistothecia rupture, releasing the asci and ascospores (Fig. 58.1).

Another *Scedosporium* species, *Scedosporium prolificans,* has been associated with infections other than mycetomas, such as arthritis or invasive disease in immunocompromised patients. *S. prolificans* differs from *S. apiospermum* in that it produces inflated, flask-shaped annellophores. The obsolete or previous name for *S. prolificans* was *Scedosporium infla-tum,* which more accurately reflects the morphology of the conidiophore. Recognition of this organism also is important, because it is resistant to most if not all the commonly used antifungal agents.

Acremonium spp. develops hyaline hyphae and produces simple, unbranched, erect conidiophores. Single-celled conidia are produced loosely or in gelatinous masses at the tip of the conidiophore (Fig. 58.17). Intercalary and terminal chlamydoconidia may also be produced.

Black Grain Mycetoma: *Exophiala jeanselmei, Curvularia* spp., and *Madurella* spp.

Sterile hyphae are produced when *Madurella* spp. is grown on rich fungal media. Nutritionally poor media may be used to induce sporulation. Long, tapering phialides with collarettes and **sclerotia** may be seen. Temperature tolerance, biochemical hydrolysis, and assimilation studies may be used to differentiate *M. mycetomatis* from *T. grisea.* (See *Phaeohyphomycosis,* later in the chapter, for the description of *E. jeanselmei* and *Curvularia* spp.)

Chromoblastomycosis: *Cladosporium, Phialophora,* and *Fonsecaea* spp.

The taxonomy of the organisms that cause chromoblasto-mycosis is complex. Their identification is based on somewhat distinct microscopic morphologic features. These are polymorphic fungi that may produce more than one type of conidiation. The genus *Cladosporium* includes species that produce long chains of budding, often fusiform, conidia (blastoconidia) that have a dark septal scar.

The genus *Phialophora* includes species that produce short, flask-shaped to tubular phialides, each with a well-developed collarette. Clusters of conidia are produced by the phialides through an apical pore and often remain aggregated near the opening in a gelatinous mass. *Phialophora* spp. produce colonies that are wooly and olive-brown to brownish gray; some strains may appear to have concentric zones of color. Microscopically, hyphae are dematiaceous, and sporulation is

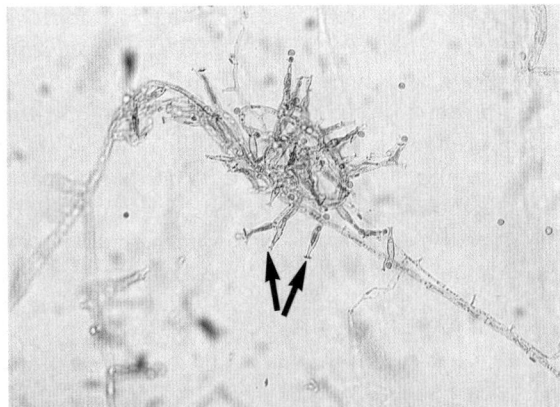

• **Fig. 60.4** *Pleurostomophora richardsiae* (previously *Phialophora richardsiae*) showing phialides with prominent, saucerlike collarette (*arrows*) (×500).

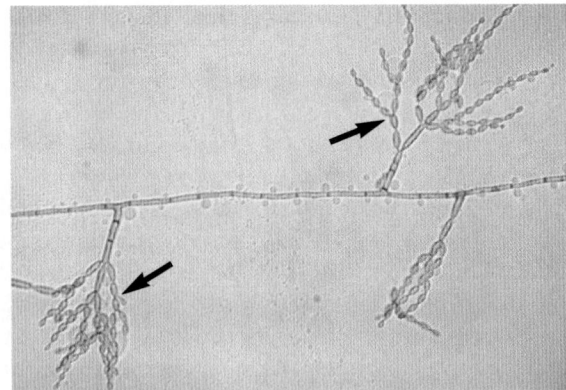

• **Fig. 60.5** *Cladophialophora* spp. showing *Cladophialophora* type of sporulation (*arrows*) with chains of elliptical conidia (×430).

common. *Pleurostomophora richardsiae* (previously *Phialophora richardsiae*) produces phialides with distinct flattened or saucerlike collarettes (Fig. 60.4). In contrast, *P. verrucosa* produces deeper, more cup- or flask-shaped phialides. Pleomorphic phialides may also be seen with these species; however, all produce either or both hyaline elliptical conidia or brown elliptical conidia within the phialides.

The genus *Fonsecaea* includes organisms that exhibit a mixed type of sporulation. The genus produces a distinct *Fonsecaea*-type conidiophore, which somewhat resembles truncated *Cladophialophora*-type sporulation. It may also produce a *Rhinocladiella*-type sporulation, in which single-celled conidia are produced on denticles that arise from all sides of conidiophores (**sympodially**). A mixture of the *Fonsecaea*, *Rhinocladiella*, and *Cladophialophora* types may occur, and phialides with collarettes or *Phialophora*-type sporulation also may be present.

The diagnostic features of the *Cladophialophora*, *Phialophora*, and *Fonsecaea* genera can be summarized as follows:

- *Cladophialophora (C. carrionii)*: *Cladophialophora* type of sporulation with long chains of elliptical conidia (2 to 3 μm × 4 to 5 μm) borne from erect, tall, branching conidiophores (Fig. 60.5).
- *Phialophora* spp.: *P. verrucosa* produces phialides, each with a distinct cup- or flask-shaped collarette (Fig. 60.6); *P. richardsiae* produces phialides with a flattened collarette (Fig. 60.4). Conidia are produced endogenously and occur in clusters at the tip of the phialide.
- *Fonsecaea* spp.: Conidial heads with sympodial arrangement of conidia are seen, with primary conidia giving rise to secondary conidia (Fig. 60.7). *Cladophialophora*-type, *Phialophora*-type, and/or *Rhinocladiella*-type sporulation may also occur.

Phaeohyphomycosis: *Alternaria, Bipolaris, Cladophialophora, Curvularia, Exophiala, Exserohilum,* and *Phialophora* spp.

A useful approach to identification of the dematiaceous molds is first to determine whether single-celled or multicelled conidia are produced. If conidia are produced singly,

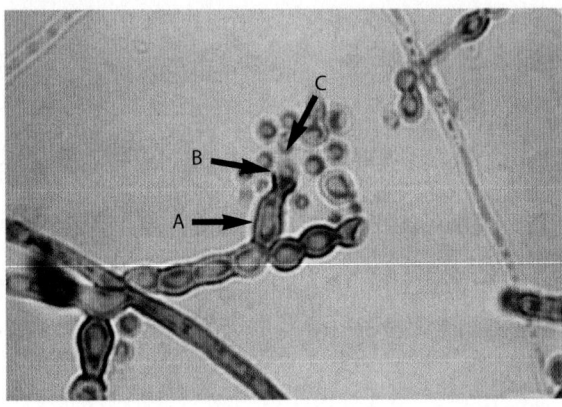

• **Fig. 60.6** *Phialophora verrucosa* showing flask-shaped phialide (*A*) with distinct collarette (*B*) and conidia (*C*) near its tip (×750).

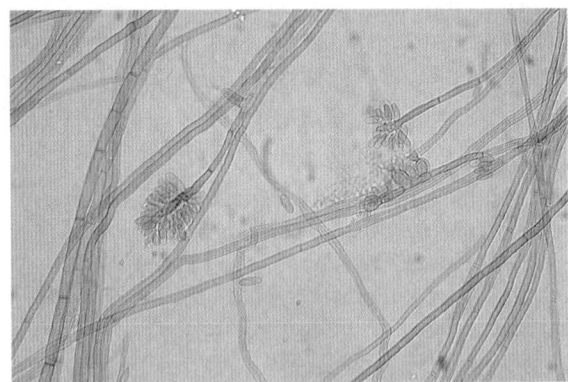

• **Fig. 60.7** Both the *Rhinocladiella* and *Phialophora* types of sporulation may be produced by *Fonsecaea pedrosoi* and are demonstrated here (×430).

the laboratorian should determine whether they are produced individually or in chains (e.g., *Cladophialophora* spp.). In cellophane tape preparations, the chains of conidia produced by *Cladophialophora* spp. are easily disrupted. If multicellular conidia are produced, examining the septation within the conidium is useful. Multicellular conidia with septation in the horizontal axis of the conidium (i.e., the axis perpendicular to the longitudinal axis of the conidium)

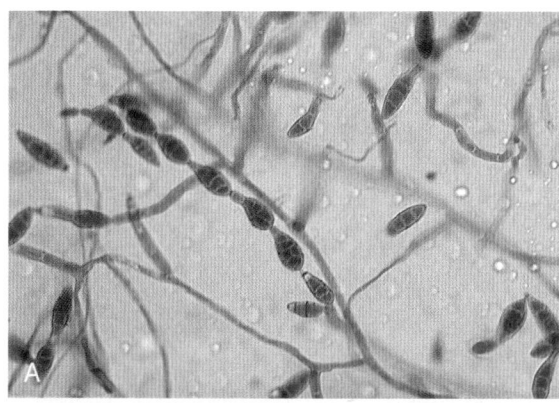

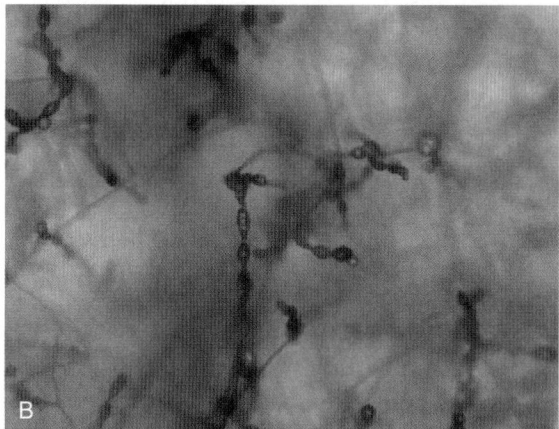

• **Fig. 60.8** (A) *Alternaria* spp. showing chaining multiform dematiaceous conidia with horizontal and longitudinal septa. (B) Microscopic morphology (200× magnification) of *Alternaria* spp. demonstrating growth within Biomed Diagnostics commercially prepared InTray fungal media. The design of the InTray media permits growth and imaging without preparation of microscopic slides, (Photo courtesy Biomed Diagnostics, Inc., White City, OR.)

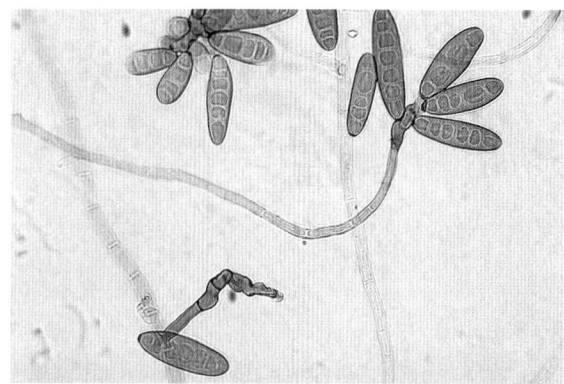

• **Fig. 60.9** *Bipolaris* spp. showing dematiaceous, multicelled conidia produced sympodically from geniculate conidiophores (×430).

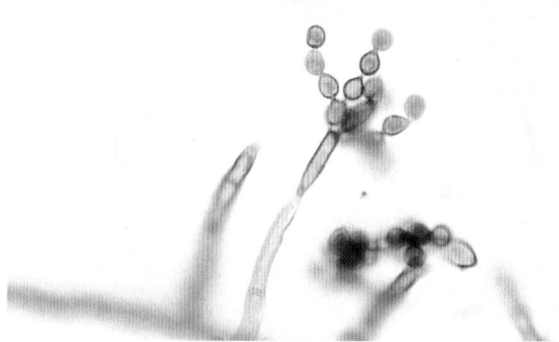

• **Fig. 60.10** *Cladophialophora* spp. showing branching chains of dematiaceous blastoconidia that are easily dislodged during preparation of a microscopic mount (×430).

are characteristic of certain organisms, such as in *Bipolaris* and *Curvularia* spp.; conidia with septation in both the longitudinal and horizontal axes of the conidium are characteristic of other fungi, such as *Alternaria* spp.

***Alternaria* spp.** Microscopically, hyphae are septate and golden-brown pigmented; conidiophores are simple but sometimes branched. Conidiophores bear a chain of large, brown conidia resembling a drumstick and contain both horizontal and longitudinal septa (Fig. 60.8). Observing chains of conidia sometimes is difficult, because they may be dislodged, as the culture mount is prepared.

***Bipolaris* spp.** Hyphae are dematiaceous and septate. However, conidiophores are characteristically bent (**geniculate**) at the locations where conidia are attached; conidia are arranged sympodically and are oblong to **fusoid**. The hilum protrudes slightly (Fig. 60.9). **Germ tubes** are formed at one or both ends, parallel to the long axis of the conidium, when the fungus is incubated in water at 25°C for up to 24 hours (i.e., from both poles, thus the name *Bipolaris*).

***Cladophialophora* spp.** Microscopically, hyphae are septate and brown. Conidiophores are long, branched, and give rise to branching chains of darkly pigmented, budding conidia. Conidia usually are single-celled and exhibit

prominent attachment scars (dysjunctors). The cells that produce the branch points are often referred to as **shield cells** (Fig. 60.10). This organism commonly fails to reveal chains of conidia on wet mounts, because conidia are so easily dislodged.

***Curvularia* spp.** Microscopically, hyphae are dematiaceous and septate. Conidiophores are geniculate (i.e., bent where conidia are attached). Conidia are arranged sympodically and are golden-brown, multicelled, and curved, with a central swollen cell (Fig. 60.11). The end cells are lighter in color than the swollen cell.

***Exophiala* spp.** Only the *Exophiala* species *E. jeanselmei* and *E. dermatitidis* are considered here; although other species exist, they are recovered far less commonly in the clinical laboratory. The microscopic features of young colonies of *Exophilia* spp. exhibit dematiaceous, yeastlike cells (Fig. 60.12). Although these may appear to be budding, close inspection may disclose that the daughter cells are produced by annelides rather than true buds. The microscopic features of young colonies of *Exophilia* spp. exhibit dematiaceous, yeastlike cells. Feltlike, filamentous colonies produce dematiaceous hyphae and conidiophores that are cylindrical and have a tapered tip. Annellations may be visible at the tip, and clusters of oval to round conidia are apparent (Fig. 60.13). Potassium nitrate is

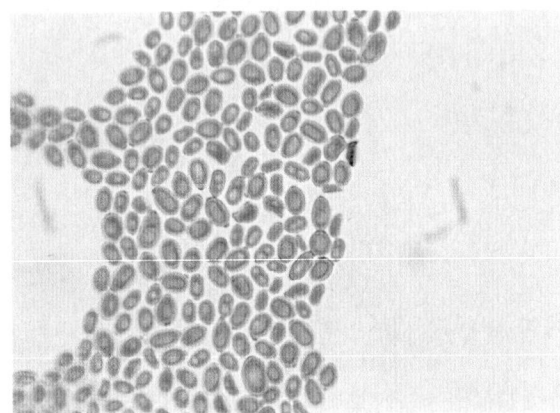

• **Fig. 60.11** *Curvularia* spp. showing twisted conidiophore and curved conidia with a swollen central cell (*arrows*) (×500).

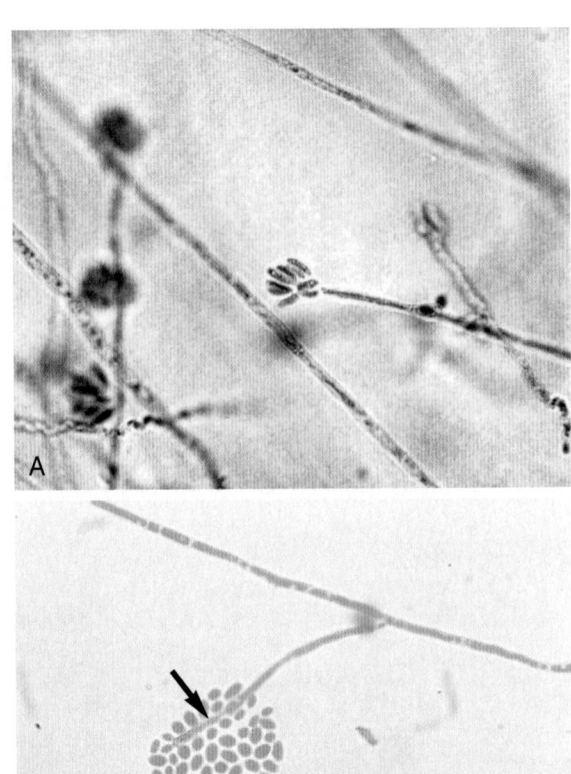

A

B

• **Fig. 60.13** (A) *Exophiala jeanselmei* showing elongated conidiophore (annellophore) with a narrow, tapered tip (×500). (B) *Exophiala dermatitidis* showing elongated tubular annellophores (*arrow*); morphologically very similar to *Exophiala jeanselmei* (×500).

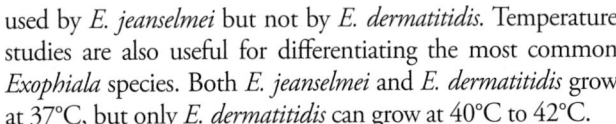

• **Fig. 60.12** *Exophiala dermatitidis* showing dematiaceous, yeast-like cells from a young culture. These forms asexually reproduce via annelides rather than through true budding (blastoconidiation) (×500).

used by *E. jeanselmei* but not by *E. dermatitidis*. Temperature studies are also useful for differentiating the most common *Exophiala* species. Both *E. jeanselmei* and *E. dermatitidis* grow at 37°C, but only *E. dermatitidis* can grow at 40°C to 42°C.

Exserohilum spp. Hyphae are septate and dematiaceous. Conidiophores are geniculate, and conidia are produced sympodically. Conidia are elongate, are ellipsoid to fusoid, and exhibit a prominent **hilum** that is truncated and protruding (Fig. 60.14). The conidia are multicellular, have perpendicular septa, and usually contain five to nine septa.

Antifungal Susceptibilities

Antifungal susceptibilities for melanized fungi for most clinically relevant species are known. However, interpretive breakpoints have not been standardized. Amphotericin B and the azoles have demonstrated clinical effectiveness against infections with melanized fungi. Triazoles, posaconazole, and voriconazole have a broad spectrum of activity against most of these fungi. Occasional treatment

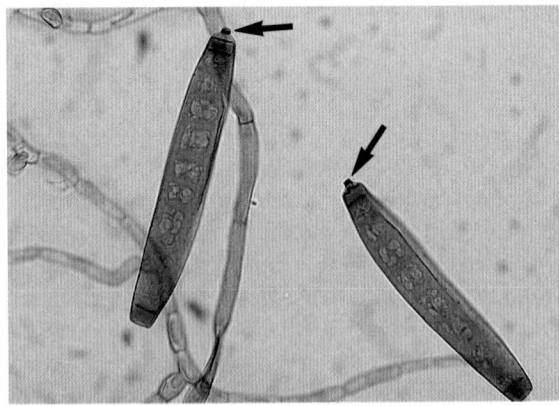

• **Fig. 60.14** *Exserohilum* spp. showing elongated multicelled conidia with prominent hila (*arrows*).

failure of mycetoma has been associated with the use of voriconazole.

ⓔ Visit the Evolve site for a complete list of procedures, review questions, and case studies.

Bibliography

Abd El-Bagi ME, Abdul Wahab O, Al-Thaqafi MA, et al.: Mycetoma of the hand, *Saudi Med J* 25:352, 2004.

Ahmed AO, Van Leeuwen W, Fahal A, et al.: Mycetoma caused by *Madurella mycetomatis:* a neglected infectious burden, *Lancet Infect Dis* 4:566–574, 2004.

Carroll KC, Pfaller MA, Landry ML, et al.: *Manual of clinical microbiology*, ed 12, Washington, DC, 2019, ASM.

Chowdhary A, Perfect J, de Hoog S: Black molds and melanized yeasts pathogenic to humans, *Cold Spring Harb Perspect Med* 5: a019570, 2015.

Gautier M, Ranque S, Normand AC, et al.: Matrix-assisted laser desorption ionization time-of-flight mass spectrometry: revolutionizing clinical laboratory diagnosis of mould infections, *Clin Microbiol Infect* 20:1366–1371, 2014.

Meyer W, Guarro J: Current status of diagnosis of *Scedosporium* infections: what is the impact of new molecular methods? *Curr Fungal Infect Rep* 8:220–226, 2014.

Pang KR, Wu JJ, Huang DB, et al.: Subcutaneous fungal infections, *Dermatol Ther* 17:523–531, 2004.

Sakayama K, Kidani TT, Sugawara YY, et al.: Mycetoma of the foot: a rare case report and review of the literature, *Foot Ankle Int* 25:763–767, 2004.

Tintelnot K, von Hunnius P, de Hoog GS, et al.: Systemic mycosis caused by a new *Cladophialophora* species, *J Med Vet Mycol* 33:349–354, 1995.

61

Atypical and Parafungal Agents

OBJECTIVES

1. Describe the symptoms of *Pneumocystis jirovecii* infection and the cells affected by this organism.
2. List the appropriate specimen types collected for diagnosis of pneumocystis pneumonia.
3. Discuss the laboratory tests used in the diagnosis of *P. jirovecii* infection, including the methodology and biochemical principles.
4. List the diseases and morphologic characteristics used in diagnosing infections of the parafungi *Lacazia loboi*, *Lagenidium* spp., *Pythium insidiosum*, and *Rhinosporidium seeberi*.

GENUS AND SPECIES TO BE CONSIDERED

Current Name	Previous Name
Pneumocystis jirovecii	*Pneumocystis carinii*
Lacazia loboi	
Lagenidium spp.	
Pythium insidiosum	
Rhinosporidium seeberi	

PNEUMOCYSTIS

General Characteristics

In 1999, the name of the organism that causes a pneumonia in immunocompromised humans, commonly called **pneumocystis pneumonia (PCP)**, was changed from *Pneumocystis carinii* to *Pneumocystis jirovecii*. One of the causative organisms for the rodent form of pneumocystis is still called *P. carinii;* the other is *Pneumocystis wakefieldiae*. Although there are currently five recognized species of *Pneumocystis, P. jirovecii* is the only species that is known to infect humans. The organism is an opportunistic, atypical fungus that infects immunocompromised hosts and mostly manifests as PCP. However, transmission from infected patients to immunocompetent health care workers has been reported.

P. jirovecii originally was believed to be a trypanosome. Several factors supported the notion that *P. jirovecii* was a protozoan parasite; its morphology is similar to that of protozoa, and clinically it responds to antiprotozoal drugs but not to antifungal drugs in patients with **pneumocystosis.** Inability to maintain and propagate the organism in routine culture has further limited its characterization, although cultivation is possible under special conditions. *P. jirovecii* exists as three forms in its life cycle: the **trophic form (trophozoite), sporozoite (precyst),** and **ascus (cyst),** which is the diagnostic form.

Although *P. jirovecii* has been shown to be a fungus, it differs from other fungi in various aspects. Its cell membrane contains cholesterol rather than ergosterol. The flexible-walled trophic form is susceptible to osmotic disturbances. In addition, *P. jirovecii* contains only one or two copies of the small ribosomal subunit gene, whereas most other fungi contain numerous copies of this gene. Deoxyribonucleic acid (DNA) sequence analysis of the small ribosomal subunit gene in *P. jirovecii* has disclosed a greater sequence homology with the fungi than with the protozoa. Two independent analyses that compared the DNA sequences of *P. jirovecii* with those of other fungi confirmed the placement of *P. jirovecii* in the fungal kingdom, in the phylum Ascomycota.

Epidemiology

P. jirovecii has a worldwide distribution and most commonly presents as pneumonia in an immunocompromised host. Recently, PCP has been shifting toward non–human immunodeficiency virus (HIV)-infected immunosuppressed patients, such as hematologic malignancy and autoimmunity. The use of powerful immunosuppressive therapies has led to this shift. *Pneumocystis* is transmitted person-to-person via airborne particles. Immunocompetent individuals appear to be the reservoir for *P. jirovecii,* which is transmitted to immunodeficient individuals as a pathogen. Most children by age 2 to 4 years have antibodies to *Pneumocystis,* suggesting acquisition early in life. Vargas et al. showed that *Pneumocystis* DNA was present in 24 of 72 infants, as determined from nasopharyngeal specimens, and that seroconversion occurred in 85% of infants by 20 months of age.

Since the onset of the HIV and acquired immunodeficiency syndrome (AIDS) epidemic in the 1980s, *Pneumocystis* has been defined as the most common opportunistic infection among those with HIV or AIDS in the United States. The introduction of highly active antiretroviral therapy (HAART) for patients with HIV has reduced the incidence of disease. However, PCP remains a significant medical problem because numerous patients with HIV do not respond to therapy, do not comply with therapy, or do not know they are infected.

The results of DNA testing demonstrate the detection of *P. jirovecii* in immunocompetent populations as well as additional groups of patients with chronic underlying disease.

Pathogenesis and Spectrum of Disease

After *P. jirovecii* is inhaled, the trophic form of the pathogen is believed to adhere to type I pneumocytes (thin squamous epithelial cells of the lungs). The organisms replicate extracellularly while bathed in alveolar lining fluid. With successful replication of the organism, the alveolar spaces fill with an eosinophilic foamy material, which can be detected with hematoxylin and eosin staining. This technique does not provide direct staining of the organisms. Methenamine silver or another fungal stain may be used to identify the cyst form of the organism in lung tissue. Infection with the organism and the pathophysiologic changes described result in impaired oxygen-diffusing capacity and hypoxemia. A predominantly interstitial mononuclear inflammatory response is associated with this type of pneumonia. When first described, this pneumonia was known as **interstitial plasma cell pneumonia.**

Symptoms of PCP include a nonproductive cough, low-grade fever, dyspnea, chest tightness, and night sweats. In patients without HIV infection, the underlying conditions most commonly seen as risk factors for this opportunistic infection are asthma, chronic obstructive pulmonary disease (COPD), cystic fibrosis, systemic lupus erythematosus (SLE), pregnancy, rheumatoid arthritis, infection with Epstein-Barr virus, ulcerative colitis, and high-dose corticosteroid therapy. During treatment with an antiretroviral medication, patients show an improvement and an increase in CD4+ cells. However, following a brief period of improvement, the patients begin to deteriorate because of an exaggerated immune response referred to as **immune reconstitution inflammatory syndrome.**

Extrapulmonary infection has been reported in 0.6% to 3% of postmortem samples collected from patients who were diagnosed with *P. jirovecii* pneumonia. Extrapulmonary cysts have been identified in lymph nodes, the spleen, bone marrow, and the liver, predominantly. Additional extrapulmonary sites include the adrenal glands, gastrointestinal tract, genitourinary tract, thyroid, ear, pancreas, eyes, and skin. Multiple sites of infection typically indicate a more rapid disease progression and fatal outcome.

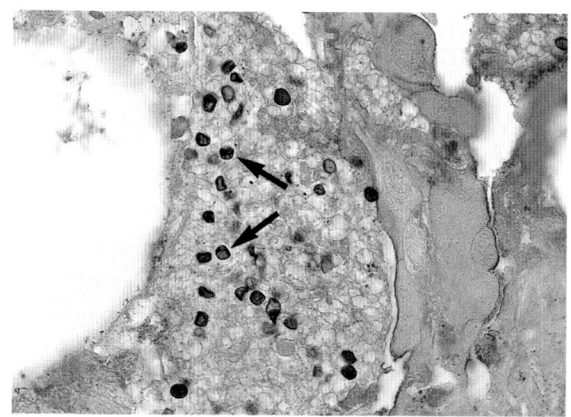

• **Fig. 61.1** Cystic forms of *Pneumocystis jirovecii (arrows)* stain well with methenamine silver and hematoxylin and eosin stain (×500).

Laboratory Diagnosis

Specimen Collection and Transport

Respiratory specimens from the deep portions of the lung, such as bronchoalveolar lavage (BAL), are best for detection of *P. jirovecii*. A sputum specimen submitted for direct examination should be induced sputum obtained by a trained respiratory therapist; otherwise, the rate of false-negative results may be unacceptably high. Additional acceptable respiratory specimens include tracheal aspirates, pleural fluid, transbronchial biopsy, or cellular material from bronchial brushings. Nasopharyngeal and oropharyngeal samples have demonstrated high sensitivity and specificity for the diagnosis of PCP when used in nucleic acid–based testing methods for *P. jirovecii*. Collection for the diagnosis of extrapulmonary pneumocystis requires biopsy of the infected organ and histologic staining.

Specimen Processing

See the following section for specific details for specimen processing required for the various test methods.

Direct Detection Methods
Stains

The diagnosis of *P. jirovecii* pneumonia currently is based on the clinical presentation, radiographic studies, and direct or pathologic examination of respiratory samples or biopsy material. The flexible-walled trophic forms are the predominant morphology of the organism, but these are difficult to visualize. They are somewhat discernible in Giemsa-stained material, but their pleomorphic appearance makes this form of the organism difficult to identify. Giemsa stains the nuclei of all the various life cycle stages as reddish purple with a light blue cytoplasm. A firm-walled cyst also exists, although the cysts are outnumbered by the trophozoites 10 to 1. Cysts are more easily recognized than the trophic form and may be definitively identified using a variety of stains, such as calcofluor white, methenamine silver, and immunofluorescent staining (Fig. 61.1). The cysts are spherical to concave, are uniform in size (4 to 7 μm in diameter), do not bud, and contain distinctive intracystic bodies.

A comparison of the four most common staining methods used for *P. jirovecii* (i.e., Giemsa, immunofluorescent, calcofluor white, and methenamine silver) has demonstrated that immunofluorescent staining (Merifluor *Pneumocystis;* Meridian Bioscience, Cincinnati, OH), Monofluo *P. jirovecii* IFA (Bio-Rad, Hercules, CA), calcofluor white staining (Fungifluor; Polysciences, Warrington, PA), and methenamine silver staining (GMS) and Wright-Giemsa (Diff-Quik; Baxter Scientific, McGaw Park, IL) likely represent the best balance between sensitivity and specificity and have the best overall positive and negative predictive values. The immunofluorescent method showed greater sensitivity than the other three but a smaller negative predictive value. Therefore, if this method is used as a screening tool for the presence of *Pneumocystis*, a confirmatory method should be performed because of the high number of false-positive results.

Direct Detection of (1-3)-Beta-D-Glucan

The ascus (cyst) cell wall component, (1-3)-beta-D-glucan, has been used to successfully diagnose infections with *P. jirovecii*. Other fungi also secrete the molecule but in lower amounts. There are several commercial assays available; however, they are not all Food and Drug Administration (FDA) approved for use within the United States. The Fungitell Assay (Associates of Cape Cod, Falmouth, MA) uses patient serum for the detection of (1-3)-beta-D-glucan. Normal human serum contains low levels of (1-3)-beta-D-glucan (10 to 40 pg/mL) from the commensal yeasts that are present in the alimentary canal and gastrointestinal tract. Therefore values less than 60 pg/mL are considered negative, 60 to 79 pg/mL are indeterminate, and greater than 80 pg/mL are positive. It is important to use additional diagnostic information and confirmatory testing in conjunction with this test, because other yeast or fungi also secrete (1-3)-beta-D-glucan during infection.

Nucleic Acid Detection

A variety of nucleic acid amplification assays for *P. jirovecii* have been developed, including, most recently, real-time polymerase chain reaction (PCR) methods and multiplex assays. However, because of the potential for colonization of immunocompetent populations, positive nucleic acid–based testing results must be directly correlated with the patient's history and clinical presentation. As of this writing, no tests have been FDA approved for use in the United States.

Serologic Testing

Serology is useful for epidemiological purposes but not for the diagnosis.

Cultivation

P. jirovecii is very difficult to cultivate outside the lung; therefore routine culture methods are not performed.

Approach to Identification

See Direct Detection Methods.

Treatment

Trimethoprim-sulfamethoxazole (TMP-SMX) and pentamidine isethionate are the predominant agents used to treat PCP. Both drugs have significant side effects including nephrotoxicity. The use of TMP-SMX is also associated with the development of resistant strains.

Rare Atypical and Parafungal Agents

Lacazia loboi

L. loboi is the causative agent of lobomycosis, a rare granulomatous zoonotic fungal infection mostly of the skin and subcutaneous tissue. The lesions and nodules are described as leprosy-like and generally appear in cooler regions of the body, indicating the pathogen does not grow well at body temperature (37°C). The organism has been found in the soil, on vegetation, and in aquatic animals in tropical and subtropical areas, especially the bottlenose dolphins. The transmission to humans is not known but theorized that infection results from traumatic entry or entry into broken skin from contaminated water. Direct dolphin to human transmission has been reported by an aquarium attendant. Human to human transmission has also been reported.

Laboratory Diagnosis and Treatment

L. loboi can be seen in stained tissue biopsies; the organism itself is uncultivable *in vitro*. Morphologically, the organism resembles *Paracoccidioides brasiliensis* (Chapter 62). Biopsied material will show yeastlike cells and an influx of inflammatory cells. The cells are uniform in size, with a thick outer membrane and appear to be chaining, connected by small tubules. The uniformity in size can help to differentiate from *P. brasiliensis*. Treatment of infection with *L. loboi* is difficult because this organism is resistant to most antifungals; therefore surgical removal is required.

Pythium insidiosum

P. insidiosum is a funguslike, aquatic oomycete organism. The organism is found in the tropical, subtropical, and temperate areas. Isolation of *P. insidiosum* can be performed using mycologic media such as Sabouraud dextrose agar. The organism has two phases, a more funguslike, mycelium-producing phase and a biflagellate zoospore, which is the infectious stage. Zoosporogenesis can be initiated only in water cultures *in vitro*. Infections are thought to be acquired by traumatic injection into the skin or the intestinal tract by traumatic lesions from contaminated aquatic environments. Infective keratitis has also been reported. Person to person transmission has not been observed. Infection with *P. insidiosum* includes cutaneous and subcutaneous lesions with the formation of plaques and ulcers. Orbital infections have also been reported. Vascular pythiosis can be seen more commonly in Thailand, especially in patients with thalassemia.

Laboratory Diagnosis and Treatment

Serologic testing is not specific and therefore not recommended. Tissue samples are used for diagnosis and can be examined by direct microscopy. Samples may be stained with a variety of immunohistochemical stains. Stained skin and tissue samples typically demonstrate hyphal structures that are short or long, sparsely septate, tubular structures and inflammatory cells, especially eosinophils and mast cells. A 10% potassium hydroxide (KOH) preparation may also be used to visualize the hyaline hyphal elements in tissue scrapings.

Culture can be used for the diagnosis of infection with *P. insidiosum*. Small pieces of tissue should be embedded into the mycological media and incubated at 25°C and 37°C for 24 to 48 hours. Specimens received more than 24 hours after collection should be placed in a broth tube and incubated at 37°C. Two percent Sabouraud dextrose agar or broth with or without antibiotics is the most common media used to isolate *P. insidiosum*. However, identification of *P. insidiosum* requires the development of the characteristic oogonia (sexual stage) in culture. This is extremely rare. Nucleic acid–based testing has been used to identify the organism and is recommended over culture. Identification is therefore limited by the lack of availability of the molecular test in clinical laboratories.

Treatment

P. insidiosum do not contain chitin and ergosterol similar to yeasts and fungi; therefore, the organism is resistant to antifungals. Combination antibiotics including minocycline, linezolid, and chloramphenicol have been successfully used to treat keratitis associated with *P. insidiosum*.

Lagenidium spp.

Lagenidium spp. is an emerging oomycete similar to *P. insidiosum* and the causative agent of lagenidiosis. As with *P. insidiosum*, *Lagenidium* spp. has two forms, the mycelial form and the biflagellate zoospore. *Lagenidium* cases have been found in wet areas. The organism is found in crabs, mosquito larvae, nematodes, and other organisms. Person-to-person transmission has not been identified. The organism causes invasive skin, subcutaneous, and arterial infections. Additional infection sites have been also noted: cornea, gastrointestinal tract, and extremities. Systemic infections have also been identified in humans and animals.

Laboratory Diagnosis

The organism can be examined using microscopy and isolated on fungal media similar to *P. insidiosum*. On solid media, *Lagenidium* spp. produces white-yellow submerged colonies. The hyphae have spherical structures, which can be seen at the end of the hyphae in liquid cultures.

Histopathologic staining of the infective sites cannot differentiate between *Lagenidium* or *P. insidiosum*. Morphology is similar, and both initiate localized eosinophilia. The development of the zoospores and the presence of broad, aseptate hyphae in wet mounts, as well as identification by molecular methods, should be used to confirm the presence of *Lagenidium* spp.

Treatment

Lagenidium spp. lack sterols in their cellular membranes and are therefore resistant to antifungal medications.

Rhinosporidium seeberi

R. seeberi is described as a Mesomycetozoea protistal eukaryote. This organism is similar morphologically to the parasitic form of *Coccidioides*. Infections are usually identified in tropical or subtropical areas. The mechanism of transmission is unknown; however, the pathogen can be found in aquatic environments, and resistant spores are present in terrestrial environments. Infection is likely acquired by exposure to resistant spores through breaks in the skin or mucous membranes. Infection results in the formation of painless polyps in the mucosal areas of the nose, eye, larynx, genitalia, and rectum.

Laboratory Diagnosis

Tissue biopsies are the preferred method used for diagnosis. Wet mounts from the polyps demonstrating sporangia and endospores are usually present in cases of rhinosporidiosis. Confirmation of rhinosporidiosis disease is based on the identification of greater than 300 μm spherical sporangia with endospores and a negative fungal culture.

Treatment

R. seeberi is resistant to antifungals. Surgical removal of the infected tissue and polyps can be used, but recurrence is common.

ⓔ Visit the Evolve site for a complete list of procedures, review questions, and case studies.

Bibliography

Caroll KC, Pfaller MA: *Manual of clinical microbiology*, ed 12, Washington, DC, 2019, ASM Press.

Dick MW: *Straminipilous fungi: systematics of the peronosporomycetes, including accounts of the marine straminipilous protists, the plasmodiophorids, and similar organisms*, ed 1, Dordrecht, Netherlands, 2001, Kluwer Academic Publishers.

Gaastra W, Lipman LJA, De Cock AWAM, et al.: *Pythium insidiosum*: an overview, *Vet Microbiol* 146:1–16, 2010.

Giuintuli D, Stringer S, Stringer J: Extraordinary low number of ribosomal RNA genes in *P. carinii*, *J Eukaryot Microbiol* 41:88S, 1994.

Kaplan JE, Hanson D, Dworkin MS, et al.: Epidemiology of human immunodeficiency virus–associated opportunistic infections in the United States in the era of highly active antiretroviral therapy, *Clin Infect Dis* 30(suppl 1):S5–S14, 2000.

Karm MB, Mosadegh L: Extra-pulmonary *Pneumocystis jirovecii* infection: a case report, *Braz J Infect Dis* 18:681–685, 2014.

Maeno S, Yoshinori O, Sunada A, et al.: Successful medical management of *Pythium insidiosum* keratitis using a combination of minocycline, linezolid, and chloramphenicol, *Am J Ophthalmol Case Rep* 15:100498, 2019.

Mendoza L, Newton JC: Immunology and immunotherapy of the infections caused by *Pythium insidiosum*, *Med Mycol* 43:477–486, 2005.

Otieno-Odhiambo P, Wasserman S, Hoving JC: The contribution of host cells to *Pneumocystis immunity*: an update, *Pathogens* 8:52, 2019.

Procop GW, Haddad S, Quinn J, et al.: Detection of *Pneumocystis jirovecii* in respiratory specimens by four staining methods, *J Clin Microbiol* 42:3333–3335, 2004.

Putthia H, Manjuanatha BS, Astekar M, et al.: Palatal rhinosporidiosis: an unusual case report and review of the literature, *J Korean Assoc Oral Maxillofac Surg* 44(6):293–297, 2018.

Seyedmousavi S, Guillot J, Tolooe A, et al.: Neglected fungal zoonoses: hidden threats to man and animals, *Clin Microbiol Infect* 21:416–425, 2015.

Singh CA, Sakthivel P: Rhinosporidiosis, *N Engl J Med* 380(14):1359, 2019.

Spies CFJ, Grooters AM, Lévesque CA, et al.: Molecular phylogeny and taxonomy of *Lagenidium*-like oomycetes pathogenic to mammals, *Fungal Biol* 120:931–947, 2016.

Stringer JR: *Pneumocystis carinii*: what is it, exactly? *Clin Microbiol Rev* 9:489–498, 1996.

Thianprasit M: Human pythiosis, *Trop Dermatol* 4:1, 1990.

Vargas SL, Hughes WT, Santolaya ME, et al.: Search for primary infection by *Pneumocystis carinii* in a cohort of normal, healthy infants, *Clin Infect Dis* 32:855–861, 2001.

White PL, Price JS, Backx M: Therapy and management of *Pneumocystis jirovecii* infection, *J Fungi (Basel)* 4:127, 2018.

62

The Yeasts and Yeastlike Organisms

OBJECTIVES

1. Explain the etiology and epidemiology of *Candida*, *Cryptococcus*, *Trichosporon*, and *Malassezia* spp.
2. Describe the macroscopic phenotypes and microscopic structures used to identify yeasts and yeastlike isolates.
3. Differentiate yeast and yeastlike species based on microscopic, macroscopic, and biochemical test results.
4. Compare and contrast the methods used to identify yeasts, including staining, antigen testing, and biochemical and growth characteristics (i.e., morphology).
5. Diagram an algorithm for identifying the yeasts discussed in this chapter.
6. Describe the limitations associated with the phenotypic and genotypic techniques used for the identification of organisms discussed in this chapter.

GENERA AND SPECIES TO BE CONSIDERED

Apiotrichum sp. (previously *Trichosporon* sp.)
Candida spp.
Cryptococcus spp.
Cutaneotrichosporon spp. (previously *Trichosporon* spp.)
Filobasidium sp. (previously *Cryptococcus* sp.)
Geotrichum sp.
Hannaella sp. (previously *Cryptococcus* sp.)
Malassezia spp.
Naganishia spp. (previously *Cryptococcus* spp.)
Papiliotrema spp. (previously *Cryptococcus* spp.)
Prototheca sp.
Rhodotorula spp.
Saccharomyces sp.
Solicoccozyma sp. (previously *Cryptococcus* sp.)
Saprochaete spp. (previously *Blastoschizomyces* spp.)
Sporobolomyces spp.
Trichosporon spp.
Ustilago spp. (previously *Pseudozyma* spp.)

General Characteristics

Yeasts are eukaryotic, unicellular organisms that are round to oval and range in size from 2 to 60 μm. They are not a formal taxonomic unit, but rather a group of unrelated fungi that demonstrate the unicellular growth form as yeast. The microscopic morphologic features have limited usefulness in helping to differentiate or identify these organisms. The microscopic morphology on cornmeal or RIOT (rice infusion, oxgall, and polysorbate) agar is useful when considered in conjunction with the biophysical profile (i.e., a combination of the biochemical and physical characteristics used in the identification of a microorganism) obtained using a commercial identification system. It is often impossible to differentiate yeasts in direct microscopic and histopathologic examination of clinical specimens, but occasionally particular characteristics are seen that suggest the identification or are **pathognomonic** (i.e., unique) for a specific organism. Important morphologic characteristics that are useful in differentiating yeasts include the size of the cells, the presence or absence of a capsule, the production of chlamydospores, and broad-based or narrow-necked budding. For example, variability in size with evidence of a capsule and narrow-necked budding are features that can be helpful for distinguishing *Cryptococcus* spp. from *Candida* spp. The medically important yeasts discussed in this chapter have been taxonomically classified as *Ascomycota* or *Basidiomycota*.

In general, yeasts reproduce asexually by **blastoconidia** formation (budding) (Fig. 62.1) and sexually by the production of ascospores or basidiospores. The process of budding begins with a weakening and subsequent outpouching of the yeast cell wall. This process continues until the **bud**, or daughter cell, is completely formed. The cytoplasm of the bud is contiguous with the cytoplasm for the original cell. Finally, a cell wall **septum** is created between mother and daughter yeast cells. The daughter cell often eventually detaches from the mother cell, and a residual defect occurs at the budding site (i.e., a **bud scar**).

With certain environmental stimuli, yeast can produce different morphologies. An outpouching of the cell wall that becomes tubular and does not have a constriction at its base is called a **germ tube**; it represents the initial stage of true hyphae formation (Fig. 62.2). Alternatively, if buds elongate, fail to dissociate, and form subsequent buds, **pseudohyphae** are formed; to some, these resemble links of sausage (Fig. 62.3). Pseudohyphae have cell wall constrictions rather than true intracellular septation delineating the fungal cell borders.

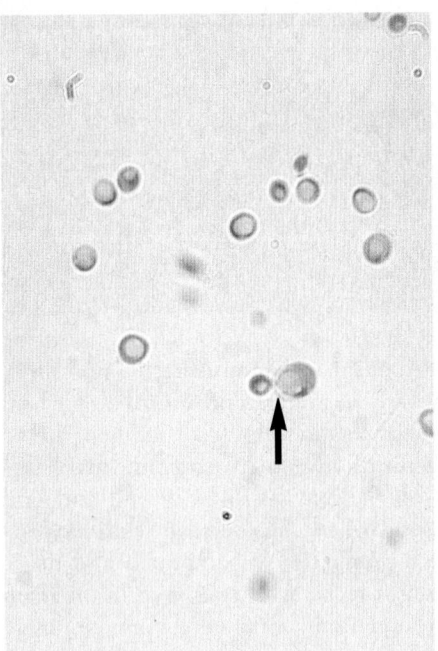

• **Fig. 62.1** Blastoconidia (budding cells *[arrow]*) characteristic of the yeasts.

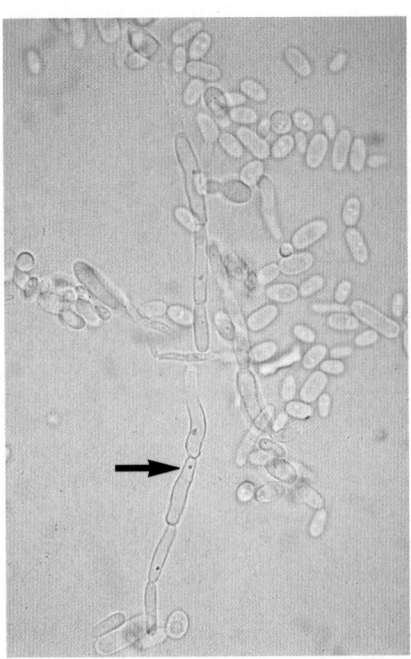

• **Fig. 62.3** Pseudohyphae consisting of elongated cells *(arrow)* with constrictions at attachment.

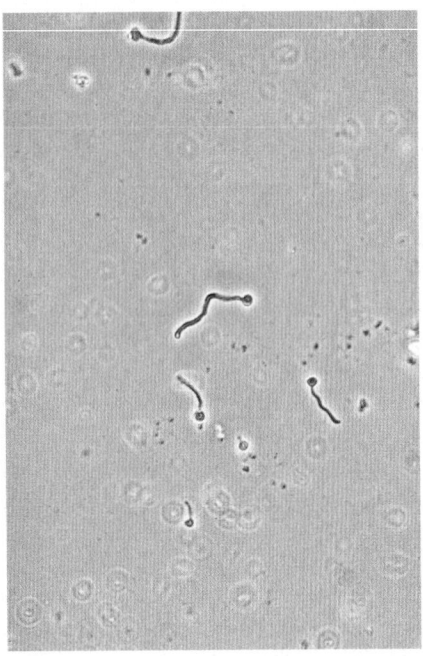

• **Fig. 62.2** Germ tube test for *Candida albicans* showing yeast cells with germ tubes.

Macroscopically, many yeasts may appear as moist, creamy colonies. The yeast may produce a capsule resulting in a shiny or mucoid colonial appearance. Yeast may produce bright pigments, e.g., *Rhodotorula* spp., or appear hyaline or melanized (dematiaceous). Microscopic and macroscopic morphology along with biochemical analysis has been historically used for yeast identification. Commercial databases containing different

phenotypic reactions are often somewhat limited to routinely identify yeasts and can lead to inaccurate results. Most commercial systems can reliably identify commonly encountered organisms, e.g., *C. albicans* complex (*C. albicans, C. africana, C. dubliniensis*) or *C. glabrata.* The worldwide emergence of *Candida auris* presented a global threat as it was often multidrug resistant and no traditional biochemical system could accurately identify the organism. The adoption of matrix-assisted laser desorption ionization time-of-flight mass spectrometry (MALDI-TOF MS) and the decrease in cost of DNA sequencing technology has greatly improved the ability to readily identify infrequently seen organisms in most clinical mycology laboratories. However, not all routine clinical laboratories are equipped with MALDI-TOF MS or other molecular technology. As a result, the commercially available yeast phenotypic identification systems remain available for laboratories of all sizes. Some commercial systems have extensive computer databases that include biochemical profiles of many yeasts. Variations in the reactions of carbohydrates and other substrates utilized are considered in the identification of yeasts provided by these systems.

Commercially available systems can be used in conjunction with some of the less expensive and rapid screening tests that provide presumptive identification of *Cryptococcus* spp. and definitive identification of *Candida albicans.* Chromogenic agar and *C. albicans* peptide nucleic acid fluorescent in situ hybridization (PNA FISH) (AdvanDX, Woburn, MA) are two examples of diagnostic tools that provide rapid characterization for the identification of *C. albicans* (Fig. 62.4). Because some laboratories continue

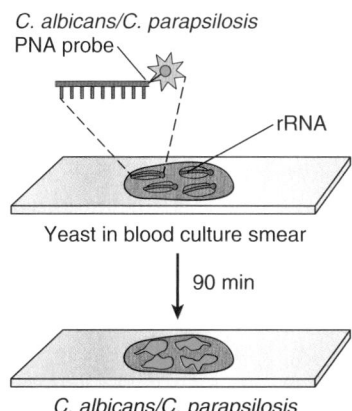

C. albicans/C. parapsilosis
PNA probe

rRNA

Yeast in blood culture smear

90 min

C. albicans/C. parapsilosis

• **Fig. 62.4** The AdvanDx (Woburn, MA) Yeast Traffic Light PNA FISH qualitative nucleic acid hybridization assay for identification of *Candida* on positive blood smears.

to use conventional systems, the information presented in this section discusses rapid screening methods for presumptive identification of yeasts, commercial identification systems, and a conventional schema for identifying commonly encountered yeast.

The number of fungal infections caused by yeasts and yeastlike fungi has increased significantly. This can be attributed to patients living longer with chronic health conditions (i.e., diabetes). Most of these infections have been caused by various *Candida* spp. However, other yeasts also cause significant disease, particularly in immunocompromised hosts (i.e., recipients of hematopoietic stem cell and solid organ transplants). In addition to causing disease in immunocompromised patients, infections are common in postsurgical patients, trauma patients, and patients with long-term indwelling catheters. Some of these yeasts are resistant to commonly used antifungal agents, which emphasizes the need for prompt, appropriate identification and, in some cases, antifungal susceptibility testing. Unfortunately, antifungal susceptibility testing (Chapter 63) is not as widely performed in most clinical laboratories compared to susceptibility testing for bacteria.

Epidemiology

Yeast are ubiquitous in the environment and often are part of the microbiota of both humans and animals. Immunocompromised patients are particularly susceptible to infection from yeasts that are members of the endogenous human microbiota, particularly the skin, upper respiratory, gastrointestinal (GI), and genitourinary tracts. Health care–associated infections can contribute to the increased development of pathogenic yeast infections because of person-to-person transmission.

Candida spp.

The genus *Candida* contains more than 200 species. *Candida* spp. are the yeast identified most commonly in the

mycology laboratory and responsible for most opportunistic fungal infections. Currently *Candida* spp. are the fourth most common cause of hospital-acquired bloodstream infections (BSIs), and nonalbicans *Candida* species cause two-thirds of invasive infections in the United States. According to data from the CDC Emerging Infections Program, in some geographic locations, *C. glabrata* complex species are frequently isolated. Yeast infection mortality rates can exceed 50% or more in patients with severe candidemia. Ninety-five percent of all invasive *Candida* infections are attributed to *C. albicans* complex, *C. glabrata* complex (*C. glabrata*, *C. bracarensis*, *C. nivariensis*), *C. tropicalis*, *C. parapsilosis* complex (*C. parapsilosis*, *C. orthopsilosis*, *C. metapsilosis*), and *C. krusei*.

Differentiating among the *Candida* spp. in the clinical mycology laboratory is vital as susceptibility to antifungal agents can no longer be reliably predicted due to mutations in drug targets and the acquisition of resistance determinants.

Cryptococcus spp.

Cryptococcus spp. are a basidiomycetous yeast. *Cryptococcus neoformans* and *C. gattii* complex was historically divided into five serotypes. Serotype A has been referred to as *C. neoformans* var. *grubii*, and serotype D as *C. neoformans* var. *neoformans*. Serotypes B and C were the distinct species *C. gattii*. Based on molecular diagnostics the group has been reorganized. The name *C. neoformans* has been retained to describe the species formerly designated *C. neoformans* var. *grubii*, and the new species *C. deneoformans* refers to those serotype D isolates (formerly *C. neoformans* var. *neoformans*). The *C. gattii* complex is composed of five cryptic species: *C. gattii*, *C. deuterogattii*, *C. tetragattii*, *C. decagattii*, and *C. bacillisporus*. An increasing number of non-*C. neoformans* species have also been increasingly isolated from human infections, and many have been reclassified into other genera as discussed in this chapter.

Standard biochemical laboratory tests do not differentiate *C. neoformans* from *C. deneoformans* or the five species in the *C. gattii* complex. *C. neoformans* is widely distributed in nature, and aerosolization is a prerequisite to most infections. *C. neoformans* can infect many organisms including amoebas, flies, other insects, nematodes, and a variety of animals such as dolphins, koalas, and cats. *C. neoformans* is the most commonly isolated species in immunocompromised hosts worldwide, and *C. deneoformans* is more commonly isolated in Europe. These two species are found in pigeon or other bird excreta. *C. gattii* complex occasionally is isolated from immunocompromised patients; however, more infections are identified in immunocompetent individuals in areas where the organisms are endemic. The natural habitat for *C. gattii* complex are gum trees and other plants in temperate and subtropical regions.

Filobasidium sp., Hannaella sp., Naganishia spp., Papiliotrema spp., and Solicoccozyma sp.

The organisms in this group are all non-*C. neoformans* species that have been reclassified and are occasionally isolated from a variety of serious human infections. *Filobasidium uniguttulatum* (previously *Cryptococcus uniguttulatus*) has been associated with ventriculitis and meningitis. *Hannaella luteolus* (previously *Cryptococcus luteolus*) has been known to cause tenosynovitis, requiring more than a year of antifungal treatment. The genus *Naganishia* includes four organisms previously included in the *Cryptococcus* genus: *N. adeliensis* (*C. adeliensis*), *N. albidus* (*C. albidus*), *N. diffluens* (*C. diffluens*), and *N. liquefaciens* (*C. liquefaciens*). The genus *Papiliotrema* includes the previous *Cryptococcus* species, *C. laurentii* and *C. flavescens*. And lastly, *Cryptococcus terreus* is now included in the genus *Solicoccozyma*. These organisms are opportunistic pathogens, and like *Cryptococcus* spp. the reservoir and transmission for the organisms is contaminated excreta from pigeons and other birds. *F. uniguttulatum* has also demonstrated resistance to common antifungal agents including azoles and flucytosine. The nomenclature changes and reorganization have the potential to result in misdiagnosis in the clinical laboratory and treatment failures in the highly susceptible immunocompromised patient populations.

Geotrichum sp.

Geotrichum candidum can be isolated as normal human microbiota and is considered an opportunistic pathogen. The organism is commonly isolated from respiratory infections in immunocompromised individuals.

Malassezia spp.

Malassezia are included in the *Basidiomycota* and are found on the skin of humans and animals. There are more than 15 species of *Malassezia* spp. The organism causes several superficial skin diseases as well as pulmonary and bloodstream infections. Many of the species are lipophilic. *M. furfur, M. globosa, M. obtuse, M. pachydermatis, M. slooffiae*, and *M. sympodialis* are the more commonly isolated species in the clinical laboratory.

Prototheca spp.

The *Prototheca* spp. are considered achlorophyllous algae but are included here as a yeastlike organism because the clinical presentation is fungal-like and they are often confused with yeast. The genus includes six species that are ubiquitous in nature. *Prototheca wickerhamii* and *P. zopfii* are the two species more commonly isolated in the clinical laboratory. An increasing number of *Prototheca* spp. systemic infections are becoming more prevalent in immunocompromised patients.

Rhodotorula spp.

The genus *Rhodotorula* contains numerous species that are ubiquitous in the environment. The organisms are normal inhabitants of the skin and can be found in many different environments from food and beverages to salt and freshwater including bathtubs, showers, and swimming pools. There have been several changes to the taxonomic distribution of species, and it will undoubtedly continue to evolve. Currently there are several species that are clinically relevant including *R. dairenensis, R. glutinis*, and *R. mucilaginosa*.

Saccharomyces sp.

Saccharomyces cerevisiae has long been considered nonpathogenic and rarely associated with human disease. However, recent use of probiotic prophylaxis for treatment of antibiotic-associated diarrhea and contact with health foods containing the organism has resulted in the reports of increasing infections associated with the organism. The organism has also been transmitted in health care settings and is able to persist in the environment. Person-to-person transmission is possible resulting in colonization and infection in immunocompromised individuals.

Saprochaete spp.

Saprochaete (previously *Blastoschizomyces*) belongs to the Ascomycetous yeasts. *Saprochaete* spp. are typically found in the environment in regions where the summers are hot and dry with warm, wet winters. The organisms may also be isolated as normal human microbiota from the skin, respiratory, and GI tract. Although the genus contains approximately 12 valid species, *S. capitata* is the most common clinically isolated species. Infections have been primarily identified in immunocompromised patients.

Sporobolomyces spp.

The organisms within the genus *Sporobolomyces* are also environmental organisms that can be found in aquatic habitats such as freshwater lakes, in association with plants, mammals, or birds. Many of the species have been reassigned to other genera using molecular techniques. However, the three species that are clinically significant have been retained in the *Sporobolomyces* spp. (i.e., *S. holosaticus, roseus*, and *S. salmonicolor*).

Trichosporon spp., Apiotrichum spp., and Cutaneotrichosporon spp.

The genus *Trichosporon* has been reorganized with several species being moved to the related genera, *Apiotrichum* and *Cutaneotrichosporon*. Many of these organisms are associated with cutaneous and systemic infections that can result in high mortality rates. The organisms are also often isolated in health care–associated infections.

Ustilago spp.

Ustilago spp. (previously *Pseudozyma*) are emerging pathogens and typically found in the environment as plant pathogens. They have been referred to as smuts that cause significant damage to agricultural crops. There are six recognized species that have been isolated from blood specimens and associated with disseminated infection. The organisms are primarily transmitted to humans by the inhalation of spores from the environment. As with other fungal infections, infected patients are typically immunocompromised, thrombocytopenic, and neutropenic.

Pathogenesis and Spectrum of Disease

Candida albicans Complex

The *C. albicans* complex is composed of three species: *C. albicans, C. dubliniensis,* and *C. africana. C. albicans sensu stricto* is the major pathogen of the *Candida* genus and is commonly identified in the clinical laboratory. **Candidiasis** is a clinical syndrome caused by a *Candida* spp. It may include oroesophageal candidiasis, **intertriginous candidiasis** (in which skin folds are involved), **paronychia** (an infection of the tissues surrounding the nails), onychomycosis (an infection of the nail and the nail bed), respiratory infections, vulvovaginitis, pulmonary infection, eye infection, candidemia, endocarditis, meningitis, or disseminated infection. **Thrush,** an infection of the mucous membranes in the mouth, is considered a localized infection. Thrush can be seen in newborns, patients with HIV infection, individuals with diabetes, and patients undergoing chemotherapy. Creamy patches or colonies appear on the tongue and mucous membranes. *Candida* spp. may be recovered from the oropharynx, GI tract, genitourinary tract, and skin.

The clinical significance of the organisms recovered from respiratory tract secretions is difficult to determine, because *Candida* spp. are considered part of the normal oropharyngeal microbiota in humans. Invasive candidiasis has increased in incidence because of the increase in patients with compromised immunity, expansion of critical care units and outpatient clinics, and delayed therapy. Invasive candidiasis and hematogenous spread has resulted in an increase in BSIs, osteomyelitis, endocarditis, endophthalmitis, meningitis, peritonitis, myositis, and pancreatitis. Meningitis has increased in pediatric cases in association with several risk factors, including gestational age, administration of antimicrobials, central vascular catheterization, parenteral nutrition, and the use of antacids. In addition, an increased *C. albicans* carriage rate

has been identified in health care workers. Simultaneous recovery of the same species of yeast from several body sites, including urine, is a good indicator of disseminated infection and fungemia.

The pathogenesis of *Candida* infections is extremely complex and probably varies with each species. Adhesion of organisms to the epithelium of the GI or urinary tract is a crucial factor for colonization with *Candida* spp. Three distinct aspartyl proteases have been described in *C. albicans,* and strains with high levels of proteases have been shown to have an increased ability to cause disease in experimental animal models. Hydrophobic molecules on the surface of *Candida* spp. also appear to be important in pathogenesis, and a strong correlation exists between adhesion and surface hydrophobicity. The yeast also possesses several adhesions that are linked to the β-1,6-glucans of the fungal cell wall. These adhesions are referred to as agglutinin-like sequences (ALS) and are designated ALSp1-7 or ALSp9. Expression of the adhesions varies with the fungal morphology and the site of infection. These adhesions can also interact with each other forming aggregations and facilitate the formation of biofilm. Clinical isolates appear to be adapted to form intricate polymicrobial biofilms with pathogenic bacteria such as *Staphylococcus aureus.* This is associated with the yeasts' ability to undergo phenotypic switching (i.e., the ability to produce pseudohyphae and hyphae). *C. albicans* can switch to a filamentous form (Fig. 62.5), permitting other pathogenic organisms to imbed in the filaments and form a polymicrobial matrix or biofilm. The ability of *C. albicans* to phenotypically switch to a filamentous form is common in patients who are neutropenic, suggesting that chemicals or cytokines produced play a role in the suppression of this phenotype. In addition, commensal strains of *C. albicans* are no longer capable of forming hyphae. *C. albicans* has also been shown to produce a toxin, candidalysin, a cytolytic peptide secreted by the yeast hyphae. This toxin initiates an inflammatory response and initiates epithelial invasion by the yeast. *C. albicans* produces over 225 proteins that facilitate tissue invasion, immune evasion, nutrient acquisition, and other pathogenic mechanisms. Significant research regarding the human microbiome has also uncovered a coevolutionary relationship with the maintenance of the normal human microbiota on mucosal surfaces and the immune system. This dynamic interaction will undoubtedly provide further insight into the fine balance between *C. albicans* and other *Candida* spp. as a commensal versus a pathogen.

Nonalbicans *Candida*

The other *Candida* spp. (also called nonalbicans *Candida*), once believed to not cause disease, are now recognized as agents of infection in certain patient populations. *C. tropicalis* and *C. auris* appear to possess some of the same

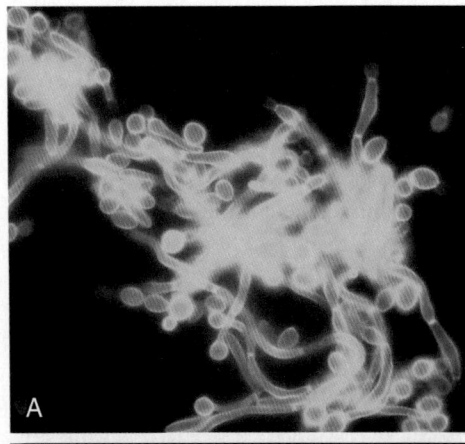

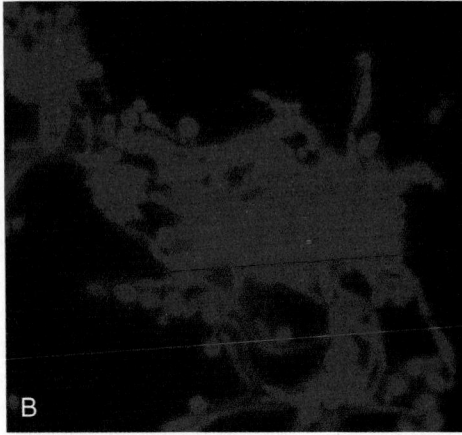

• **Fig. 62.5** (A) Calcofluor white fluorescent stain of *Candida albicans* (×100) after growth in human serum at 37°C in conjunction with methicillin-resistant *Staphylococcus aureus*, demonstrating phenotypic switching to the filamentous form. Apparent shadowing are areas of imbedded growth of *S. aureus*. (B) Same specimen stained with Texas red. Note the areas from *A* that appear filled in with staining with Texas red because of the presence of a polymicrobial growth with *C. albicans* and *S. aureus*. (Photo courtesy Amanda Graves, BS, MLS [ASCP], Palm Coast, FL.)

virulence factors as *C. albicans*. *C. auris* is also resistant to fluconazole. Numerous species of nonalbicans *Candida* are routinely isolated in association with human infection. The other most common are *C. glabrata* complex, *C. krusei, C. tropicalis,* and *C. parapsilosis* complex. The incidence of infection with *C. glabrata* is higher in older adults than in young adults and children. *C. glabrata* has also demonstrated resistance to common antifungal drugs such as fluconazole and the echinocandins. *C. glabrata* has been isolated from serious infections including endocarditis, meningitis, and disseminated disease. *C. tropicalis* has been shown to be prevalent in patients with hematologic malignancies, especially those who are neutropenic. Because *C. krusei* is intrinsically resistant to the azole class of antifungals, fluconazole, identification of this species is essential to proper clinical management of the patient. *C. parapsilosis* complex is the primary cause of fungemia in the neonatal intensive care unit (NICU). *C. parapsilosis* complex organisms are also the second most commonly isolated *Candida* spp. in positive blood cultures.

A variety of other *Candida* spp. have been identified in infections and should be considered when evaluating an isolated culture of yeast. These include *C. blankii, C. catenulata, C. ciferrii, C. eremophila, C. dubliniensis, C. inconspicua, C. fabianii, C. famata, C. glaebosa, C. guilliermondii, C. haemulonii, C. kefyr, C. lambica, C. lipolytica, C. lusitaniae, C. norvegensis, C. pelliculosa, C. pulcherrima, Candida rugosa* complex, *C. utilis,* and *C. zeylanoides*.

Cryptococcus neoformans

Cryptococcosis is an acute, subacute, or chronic fungal infection that has several manifestations. *C. neoformans, C. deneoformans,* and members of the *C. gattii* complex are considered the major human pathogens. Differences in the infections by *Cryptococcus* spp. appear to be dependent on the host immune status and not the species of yeast. Immune clearance of *C. neoformans* is very efficient in immunocompetent individuals. However, in immunocompromised hosts, especially those deficient in CD4 T cells, the organism travels to the central nervous system, where the yeast can cause cryptococcal meningitis. Patients with a moderately compromised immune system or who are early in the disease process of cryptococcal fungemia may present without concomitant meningitis. Disseminated cryptococcosis and cryptococcal meningitis is well recognized in patients with AIDS and remains an important cause of morbidity and mortality in these patients in resource-poor countries that do not have access to highly active antiretroviral therapy.

Patients with disseminated infection may have painless papular skin lesions that may ulcerate. Other, less common manifestations of cryptococcosis include endocarditis, hepatitis, renal infection, and pleural effusion. The clinical significance of *Cryptococcus neoformans* is somewhat difficult to assess. However, given the severity of disease it can cause, its presence in clinical specimens should be considered significant. In many instances, the clinical symptoms are suppressed by corticosteroid therapy, which is a risk factor for disease. Cryptococcal infection is strongly associated with such debilitating disease as leukemia, lymphoma, and the immunosuppressive therapy that may be required for these and other underlying diseases. In some cases, the presence of the organism in clinical specimens precedes the symptoms of underlying disease. In addition, the introduction of antiretroviral therapy has lowered the incidence of infection rates and death from cryptococcal meningitis in AIDS patients. This treatment has resulted in a paradox, in that as the patient's immune response improves, it can trigger an exaggerated inflammatory response known as immune reconstitution inflammatory syndrome (IRIS). IRIS remains a clinical challenge. Early treatment with ART in cases of cryptococcal meningitis seem to exacerbate the infection and may result in rapid death. The key seems to be the ability to diagnose cryptococcal meningitis early and administer antifungals to reduce the fungal burden in conjunction with immune modulators to block the influx of macrophages to the CNS, preventing IRIS.

Cryptococcus spp. can exhibit a very characteristic polysaccharide capsule. The capsule collapses and protects the yeast from desiccation under dry conditions. The capsule is believed to help the organism survive passage through the pigeon gut before it is excreted. The reduction in the yeast's cell size caused by capsular collapse places the organism in the ideal size range for alveolar deposition in the human host. In addition, the polysaccharide capsule contains compounds that phagocytes do not recognize which prevents clearing of the organism. Acapsular strains of *Cryptococcus*, which possess a very reduced capsule, are more easily phagocytized by inflammatory cells and removed from infected host.

Phenoloxidase, an enzyme found in *C. neoformans*, is responsible for melanin production. Melanin has been demonstrated to act as a virulence factor by making the organism resistant to leukocyte attack. Evidence also has been presented that increased melanin production can decrease immune system functions, such as lymphocyte proliferation and tumor necrosis factor production. *C. neoformans* also produces a wide variety of enzymes including lipases, proteases, and urease. Urease catalyzes the degradation of urea into CO_2 and ammonia promoting adhesion and potentially exerting a toxic effect on the tight junctions of the blood brain barrier to facilitate invasion. The production of urease also promotes the accumulation of immature dendritic cells, making phagocytosis of the pathogen ineffective. *C. gattii* can modulate the host's immune system by reducing the inflammatory response and evading the immune system completely by altering expression of capsular antigens very similarly to *C. neoformans*. *Cryptococcus* spp. undergo bisexual reproduction. During *Cryptococcus* sexual reproduction, yeast cells undergo a morphological transition to a hyphal form. However, unlike the other cryptococcal species, *C. deneoformans* is capable of very robust unisexual reproduction in the absence of the opposite mating type. Studies have demonstrated that this is regulated by the highly complex calcineurin pathway. This pathway differs slightly in the different *Cryptococcus* spp. and regulates virulence, stress response, and temperature sensitivity. Further studies of this complex system in the various species will lead to a better understanding of the organism's physiology, response to the host immune system, and disease progression. This may lead to novel antifungals that can be used to prevent and treat cryptococcal infections. It is important to note that although there appears to be a different pathobiology associated with *C. deneoformans* than either *C. neoformans* or *C. gattii*, they are all treated the same by primary health care providers.

Filobasidium sp., *Hannaella* sp., *Naganishia* spp., *Papiliotrema* spp., and *Solicoccozyma* sp.

Increasing incidence of infections with the non-*C. neoformans* organisms has been reported in patients with a history of impaired immunity. The clinical manifestations are similar to *C. neoformans* and *C. gattii*, including central nervous system invasion and fungaemia. Additional presentations include reports of pulmonary, GI, ocular, and cutaneous infections.

Malassezia spp.

Malassezia furfur causes tinea versicolor, a skin infection characterized by superficial, brownish, scaly areas on light-skinned individuals and lighter areas on dark-skinned people. The lesions occur on the smooth surfaces of the body, namely the trunk, arms, shoulders, and face. The disorder has a worldwide distribution. *M. furfur* is also a cause of disseminated infection in infants and young children and in adults receiving lipid replacement therapy. *Malassezia sloofiae, Malassezia globosa, Malassezia sympodialis,* and occasionally *Malassezia restricta* have also been recovered from skin lesions associated with pityriasis versicolor. *M. furfur* and *M. pachydermatis* have been associated with fungemia in immunocompromised patients.

Geotrichum and *Prototheca* spp.

Infection with *Geotrichum candidum* is often isolated from patients with impaired immunity. The organism has been isolated from blood, respiratory, GI, oropharyngeal, skin, and vaginal specimens. However, it is important to note it is considered normal microbiota and therefore isolation should be interpreted with care. Disseminated infection with *G. candidum* has been reported.

Prototheca spp. infections are often a result of traumatic inoculation to the eye or subcutaneous tissue. The organism has been associated with cutaneous and subcutaneous tissue infections, keratitis, and systemic prototheca. Organisms have also been isolated from patients in the absence of disease.

Rhodotorula spp. and *Sporobolomyces* spp.

A resident microbiota of the human skin, *Rhodotorula* spp. resemble *Cryptococcus* spp., appearing as round, oval-shaped, budding yeasts that produce capsules. *Rhodotorula* are associated with cases of human infection, including septicemia, meningitis, peritonitis, and peritoneal dialysis.

Sporobolomyces is included here as it produces a salmon-colored to coral pigment that can be easily confused with *Rhodotorula* on artificial media. As a ubiquitous, environmental organism, *Sporobolomyces* has been associated with rare cases of fungemia and meningitis in immunocompromised patients. Additional reported clinical manifestations include dermatitis and allergic alveolitis. Three species, *Sporobolomyces holsaticus, Sporobolomyces roseus,* and *Sporobolomyces salmonicolor,* have been associated with human infections.

Saccharomyces cerevisiae

Saccharomyces cerevisiae is the common yeast that is used in baking and the preparation of a variety of food products and is a component in probiotics. The yeast has been linked to human-to-human transmission in association with health foods and baking. Probiotics contain live organisms and are used to prevent and treat antibiotic-associated diarrhea including infection with *Clostridioides difficile,* inflammatory bowel disease, and malabsorption syndrome. Infections have been reported that are the result of intestinal translocation by *S. cerevisiae* and venous catheter contamination in the health care setting. *Saccharomyces* sp. has been isolated from cases of thrush, vulvovaginitis, empyema, and BSIs.

Saprochaete spp.

Saprochaete spp. is an emerging pathogen that is often isolated from patients with debilitating disease such as leukemia, renal transplants, ambulatory dialysis, and osteomyelitis. Isolation is typically from the blood of immunocompromised patients who are neutropenic. The organism has also been isolated in the normal microbiota of the human skin and GI tract.

Trichosporon spp., *Cutaneotrichosporon* spp., and *Apiotrichum* sp.

Trichosporonosis is caused by a variety of *Trichosporon* spp. that have undergone changes in nomenclature based on DNA sequence comparisons. There are approximately 37 valid species with 5 organisms (*Trichosporon inkin, Trichosporon ovoides, Cutaneotrichosporon asahii, C. mucoides,* and *Apiotrichum loubieri*) primarily associated with human disease almost exclusively in immunocompromised patients, particularly those with leukemia. Skin lesions accompanied by fungemia are common. Endocarditis, endophthalmitis, and brain abscess have been reported. *C. asahii* is the most common organism isolated from systemic infections and invasive trichosporonosis. These organisms occasionally are recovered from respiratory tract secretions, skin, the oropharynx, and the stool of patients with no evidence of infection and may represent transient colonization of those individuals.

    White piedra, an uncommon fungal infection of immunocompetent patients, is found in both tropical and temperate regions of the world. It is characterized by the development of soft, yellow or pale brown aggregations around hair shafts in the axillary, facial, genital, and scalp regions of the body. The organisms that cause this disease typically invade the cortex of the hair, causing damage.

Ustilago spp.

Ustilago spp. are primarily associated with infections in patients with one or more risk factors including neutropenia, chemotherapy, thrombocytopenia, or the presence of an indwelling catheter. Several species have been isolated from systemic infections as well as from respiratory and pleural fluids and a brain abscess.

Laboratory Diagnosis

Specimen Collection, Transport, and Processing

See General Considerations for the Laboratory Diagnosis of Fungal Infections in Chapter 58.

Stains
Candida spp.
Direct microscopic examination of clinical specimens containing *Candida* organisms reveals budding yeast cells (blastoconidia) 2 to 4 μm in diameter and/or pseudohyphae (Fig. 62.6) showing regular points of constriction, resembling links of sausage. True septate hyphae (filamentation) may also be produced by *C. albicans, C. africana,* and *C. dubliniensis.* The blastoconidia, hyphae, and pseudohyphae are strongly gram positive. The approximate number of such forms should be reported, because the presence of large numbers in a fresh clinical specimen may have diagnostic significance. Microscopically, *C. glabrata* blastoconidia are notably smaller (at 1 to 4 μm) than those of other medically significant *Candida* spp.

Cryptococcus spp.
Traditionally, the India ink preparation has been a widely used method for the rapid detection of *Cryptococcus* spp. in clinical specimens including CSF, urine, and other body fluids. This method is still used as a rapid and inexpensive assessment tool and has considerable diagnostic value in resource-poor settings. This method delineates the large capsule of *Cryptococcus* spp., because the ink particles cannot penetrate the capsular polysaccharide material. Although useful, many laboratories have replaced the India ink with the more sensitive latex agglutination test that detects cryptococcal antigen (CAD).

    Microscopic examination of other clinical specimens, including respiratory secretions, can be difficult to use if they contain a lot of cellular material and debris. *Cryptococcus* spp. appear as a spherical, single- or multiple-budding, thick-walled yeast 2 to 15 μm in diameter. The organism is usually surrounded by a wide, refractile polysaccharide

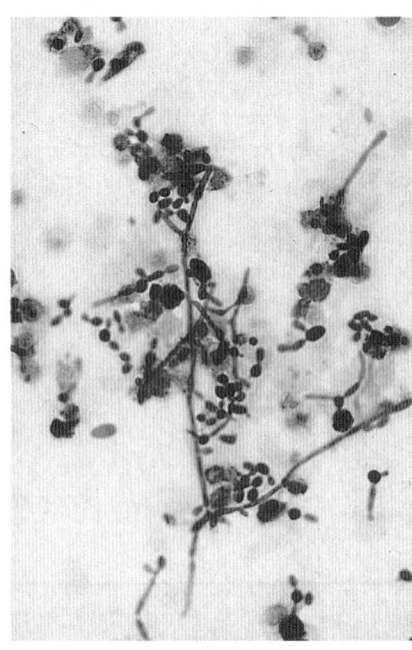

• **Fig. 62.6** Periodic acid–Schiff (PAS) staining of urine demonstrates blastoconidia and pseudohyphae of *Candida albicans.*

capsule (Fig. 62.7). Perhaps the most important characteristic of *Cryptococcus* spp. is the extreme variation in the size of the yeast cells; this is unrelated to the amount of polysaccharide capsule present. It is important to remember that not all isolates of *Cryptococcus* exhibit a discernible capsule.

Malassezia spp.

Malassezia spp. are often detected through direct microscopic examination of skin scrapings. The organism is easily recognized as oval- or bottle-shaped cells that exhibit monopolar budding in the presence of a cell wall with a septum at the site of the bud scar. Small hyphal fragments also are observed (Fig. 62.8); the morphology is commonly described as "spaghetti and meatballs." In cases of fungemia, the morphologic form seen in direct examination of blood cultures is small yeasts without the presence of pseudohyphae.

Trichosporon spp., *Cutaneotrichosporon* spp., and *Apiotrichum* sp.

Microscopic examination of clinical specimens that contain *Trichosporon* spp., *Cutaneotrichosporon*, and *Apiotrichum* spp. reveals hyaline hyphae, numerous round to rectangular arthroconidia, and occasionally a few blastoconidia. Usually hyphae and arthroconidia predominate. In white piedra, white nodules are removed and observed using the potassium hydroxide (KOH) preparation after light pressure is applied to the coverslip to crush the nodule. Hyaline hyphae 2 to 4 μm wide and arthroconidia are found in the preparation of the cementlike material that binds the hyphae together. The organism may be identified in culture by the presence of true hyphae, blastoconidia, and arthroconidia

in conjunction with a positive urease (Fig. 59.40). Although *Cutaneotrichosporon asahii* may be distinguished from other organisms by its biophysical profile (carbohydrate and substrate utilization), these organisms are likely best distinguished at the species level with molecular tools, such as DNA sequencing.

Other Organisms Resembling Yeasts (*Geotrichum*, *Prototheca*, and *Ustilago* spp.)
Antigen Detection

Most systemic fungal infections may be detectable using a common fungal cell wall antigen, beta-1,3-glucan. Several commercial kits as well as automated instrumentation is available for the detection of the fungal antigen in blood samples. *Cryptococcus* spp. do not contain beta-1,3-glucan, and the test has performed poorly in the detection of *Saprochaete* spp.

The CAD test for *C. neoformans* may be performed on cerebrospinal fluid or serum. In many laboratories this assay has replaced the use of India ink to screen for *C. neoformans*. It should be noted that *Trichosporon* spp. produce an antigen similar to that of *C. neoformans*. Sera from patients who have trichosporonosis often yield false-positive CAD tests when latex agglutination methods are used.

In addition, a variety of commercial kits are available for the detection of carbohydrate and protein antigens associated with disseminated *Candida* spp. infections. Sensitivity and specificity vary across systems for these assays. Some correlation with successful antifungal therapy has been reported for the COBAS FARA II analyzer (Roche Diagnostic Systems, Indianapolis, IN) and the test for the fungal antigen D-arabinitol. Specificity of the assays can be

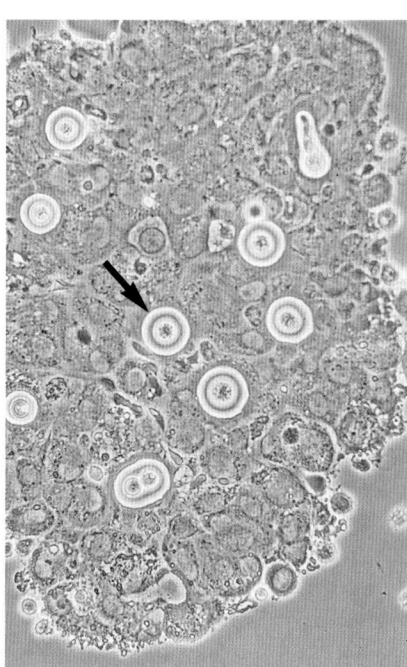

• **Fig. 62.7** Potassium hydroxide preparation of pleural fluid shows the encapsulated, variably sized, spherical yeast cells *(arrow)* of *Cryptococcus neoformans* (phase-contrast microscopy).

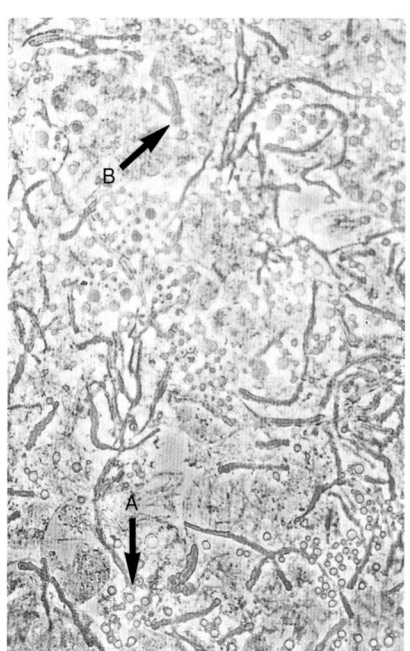

• **Fig. 62.8** Potassium hydroxide preparation of a skin scraping from a patient with tinea versicolor demonstrates spherical yeast cells *(A)* and short hyphal fragments *(B)* of *Malassezia furfur.* (Phase-contrast microscopy; ×500.)

improved by the addition of a secondary antigen or in parallel with serological tests for *Candida*-specific antibodies.

Nucleic Acid Detection

Nucleic acid amplification tests (NAATs) have been developed for a variety of yeast species. The US Food and Drug Administration (FDA) has approved several commercially available PNA FISH kits for the detection of *Candida* spp. from positive blood cultures (Fig. 62.4). The assay can detect *C. albicans* complex, *C. tropicalis, C. glabrata*, and *C. parapsilosis* complex. The assay uses fluorescein-labeled PNA probes that target the species-specific 16S rRNA on blood smears made from positive blood cultures. The slides are then reviewed with a fluorescent microscope. The PNA FISH assay has a demonstrated sensitivity and specificity of 100%. All positive tests should be subcultured to ensure that no other yeasts are present.

Additional multiplex PCR assays are also available to detect yeast in positive blood cultures that integrate nucleic acid extraction, amplification detection, and analysis. The BioFire FilmArray (bioMérieux, Durham, NC) includes detection for *C. albicans, C. glabrata, C. krusei, C. parapsilosis*, and *C. tropicalis* in approximately one hour. The Luminex xTAG PCR assay (Luminex Molecular Diagnostics, Ontario, Canada) can detect 23 different fungi including *Candida* spp. in a single sample using microsphere technology.

The FDA-approved Affirm VPIII (Becton Dickinson, Franklin Lakes, NJ) DNA probe assay is available for the direct detection of *Candida* spp. The assay detects *Candida* spp., *Gardnerella vaginalis*, and *Trichomonas vaginalis* nucleic acids in vaginal samples. The T2 *Candida* panel (T2 Biosystems, Lexington, MA) uses a magnetic resonance-based system for the detection of *C. albicans, C. tropicalis, C. glabrata, C. krusei*, and *C. parapsilosis* in whole blood samples. The assay is intended for use in seriously ill patients for rapid and early detection of fungemia.

Cultivation

Candida spp.

The colonial and microscopic morphologic features of *Candida* spp. have little value for making a definitive identification. Most *Candida* spp. produce smooth, creamy white colonies, but some produce dry, wrinkled, dull colonies. In 50% of autopsy-proven cases of invasive candidiasis, organisms could not be isolated from blood culture bottles. Blood culture systems, such as the automated BACTEC (Becton Dickinson, Franklin Lakes, NJ) and BacT/ALERT (BioMérieux, Durham, NC), have increased the recovery of *Candida* spp.

Cryptococcus spp.

C. neoformans is easily cultured on routine fungal culture media without cycloheximide. The organism is inhibited by the presence of cycloheximide at 25°C to 30°C. For optimal recovery of *C. neoformans* from cerebrospinal fluid,

a 0.45-mm membrane filter should be used with a sterile syringe. The filter is placed on the surface of the culture medium and is removed at daily intervals so that growth under the filter can be visualized. An alternative to the membrane filter technique is culture after centrifugation.

Colonies of *C. neoformans* usually appear on culture media within 1 to 5 days. The growth begins as a smooth, white to tan colony that may be mucoid to creamy (Fig. 62.9). It is important to recognize the colonial morphology on different culture media, because variation does occur; for example, on inhibitory mold agar, *C. neoformans* appears as a golden yellow, nonmucoid colony. Textbooks typically characterize the colonial morphology as being *Klebsiella*-like because of the large amount of polysaccharide capsule present. Most isolates of *C. neoformans* do not have large capsules and may not have the typical mucoid appearance.

Trichosporon spp., Cutaneotrichosporon spp., and Apiotrichum sp.

Colonies of the organisms included in these three genera vary in their morphology; however, most are cream-colored, heaped, dry to moist, and wrinkled. Some may appear white, dry, and powdery.

Malassezia spp.

Malassezia spp. are infrequently cultured in the clinical laboratory. Of the 14 valid species, 13 are recognized as being lipid dependent. Recovery of the organism is not required to establish a diagnosis in skin infections, and it is seldom attempted for this purpose. Cultivation requires an agar medium enriched with natural long chain fatty acids (olive oil). The colonies are small compared with the colonies of *C. albicans* and are creamy and white to off-white. Some specialized culture media, for example modified Dixon agar, are available and will support the cultivation of *Malassezia* spp. without the addition of olive oil.

Approach to Identification

The historical approach to yeast identification has consisted of evaluating the carbohydrate and substrate utilization

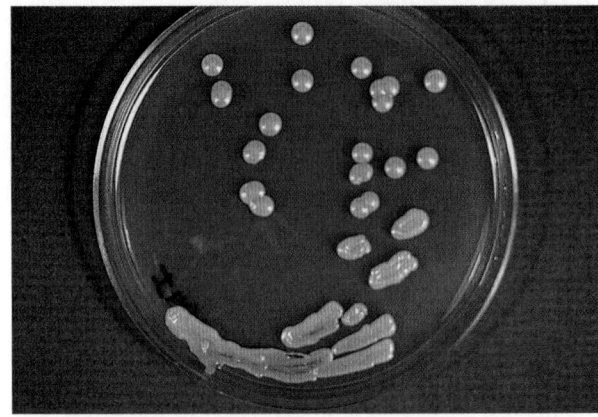

• **Fig. 62.9** Colonies of *Cryptococcus neoformans* appear shiny and mucoid because of the presence of a polysaccharide capsule.

profile with a commercial identification system and observing the microscopic morphology in a cornmeal or RIOT agar preparation. This latter aspect is particularly important for discovering any errors in identification that may have been made by the commercial system. For example, if a commercial system designates an isolate as *C. glabrata* but pseudohyphae are seen in the cornmeal preparation, additional testing is needed to identify the isolate correctly, as *C. glabrata* does not produce pseudohyphae. It is extremely important that all additional tests be performed on pure cultures. If a culture is prepared from a nonsterile site, it may also be contaminated with bacteria. Cultures can be purified by subculturing to a Sabouraud dextrose agar plate with antibiotics or treated with hydrochloric acid (HCl). The HCl procedure is completed by inoculating a colony to three 5-mL tubes of Sabouraud glucose broth. Then 1 N HCl is added to each tube: four drops to the first tube, two drops to the second tube, and one drop to the third tube. Following incubation at 25°C for 24 to 48 hours, 0.1 mL of the broth cultures are subcultured to Sabouraud dextrose agar. In addition, if more than one yeast is present, subculturing to chromogenic media may be useful. An overall general scheme for yeast identification is provided in Fig. 62.10.

Candida spp.

C. albicans complex may be identified by the production of germ tubes or chlamydoconidia (Fig. 62.11; also see Fig. 62.2). Other *Candida* spp. are most commonly identified by the utilization of specific substrates and the fermentation or assimilation of carbohydrates. For instance, *C. glabrata* ferments and assimilates glucose and trehalose, whereas *C. tropicalis* ferments and assimilates sucrose and maltose. Another method of identifying *C. albicans* and differentiating it from other *Candida* spp. is based on the presence of chlamydoconidia (Fig. 62.11) on cornmeal agar containing 1% Tween 80 and trypan blue incubated at room temperature for 24 to 48 hours. The morphologic features of yeasts on cornmeal agar containing Tween 80 often allow tentative identification of select species (Table 62.1).

Colonies that appear starlike or possess feetlike projections on agar, as previously described on blood agar, may be identified as *C. albicans*. However, this method is not as sensitive, and requires a longer incubation of 24 to 48 hours. In addition, species such as *Trichosporon* spp. may also appear as colonies with the pseudohyphal fringe within 18 to 24 hours of incubation on blood agar. A Gram stain of the isolate would provide a means of differentiation of the isolate as *Trichosporon* spp. by the characteristic presence of arthroconidia.

Germ Tube Test

The germ tube test (Evolve Procedure 62.1) is a simple and economical method used in the clinical laboratory to identify *C. albicans*. Approximately 80% of the yeasts recovered from clinical specimens are *C. albicans*, and results of the germ tube test are available within 3 hours.

Germ tubes appear as early hyphal-like extensions that are produced without a constriction at the point of origin

from the yeast cell (Fig. 62.3). *C. dubliniensis* and *C. africana* also produce germ tubes. Although *C. dubliniensis* and *C. africana* are infrequently encountered in clinical specimens, supplemental biochemical or morphologic testing may be needed to differentiate them from *C. albicans*. *C. tropicalis* produces what have been called "pseudo–germ tubes," which are constricted at the base or point of germ tube origin on the yeast cell. Unless this is recognized, and the laboratorian has developed the skills to distinguish between germ tubes and pseudo–germ tubes, *C. tropicalis* isolates may be misidentified as *C. albicans*.

C. albicans produces beta-galactose aminidase and L-proline aminopeptidase. Other *Candida* spp. may produce one of the enzymes but not both. Assays such as BactiCard *Candida* (Remel Laboratories, Lenexa, KS) can be used to detect these enzymes. All rapid enzymatic screening methods are sensitive and specific for rapid identification of *C. albicans*, including the BactiCard, Murex *C. albicans*-50, Albicanssure, and the API 20C AUX yeast identification systems. Compared with the germ tube test, these tests require less time (5 to 30 minutes). Overall, these methods provide a rapid and objective alternative to the germ tube test.

Cryptococcus neoformans

Diagnosis has been historically made by the identification of encapsulated yeast in the spinal fluid using India ink. Cryptococcal meningitis is a serious condition that requires rapid diagnostic testing. One rapid CrAg test (IMMY, Norman, OK, United States) is a lateral flow immunoassay that can be used to qualitatively identify antigen and perform a quantitative titer. This test can be performed directly on serum or cerebrospinal fluid. Results are readily available after a short 10-minute incubation step. If grown in culture, *C. neoformans* may be presumptively identified based on rapid urease production and failure to utilize inorganic nitrate. Final identification of *C. neoformans* usually is based on substrate utilization patterns and pigment production on niger seed (thistle or birdseed) agar (Fig. 62.12).

Rapid Urease Test

The rapid urease test (Evolve Procedure 62.2) is a useful tool for screening for urease-producing yeasts recovered from respiratory secretions and other clinical specimens. Alternatives to this method include use of a heavy inoculum placed on the tip of the slant on Christensen's urea agar and subsequent incubation at 35°C to 37°C. In many instances, a positive reaction occurs within several hours; however, 1 to 2 days of incubation may be required. Interestingly, strains of *Rhodotorula* spp., some *Candida* spp., and *Trichosporon* spp. hydrolyze urea over time, so a distinction should be made between a traditional urease test, which takes an overnight incubation, and the rapid urease test.

Rapid Trehalose Test

The rapid trehalose test can be used for presumptive identification of *C. glabrata*. This test should be used in conjunction with microscopic morphology (small cell size)

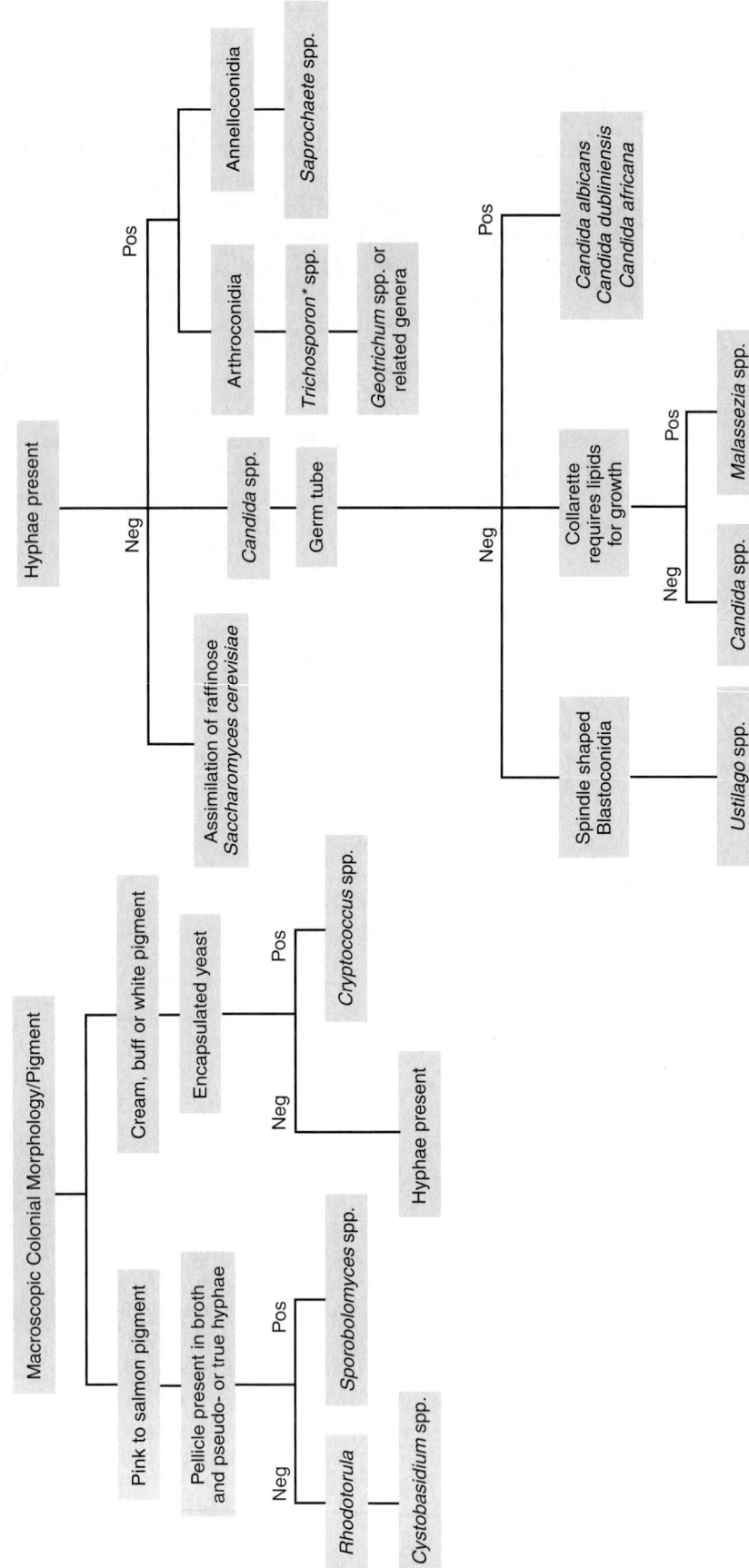

• **Fig. 62.10** General schema for the identification of yeast. *Also includes *Apiotrichum* and *Cutaneotrichosporon*.

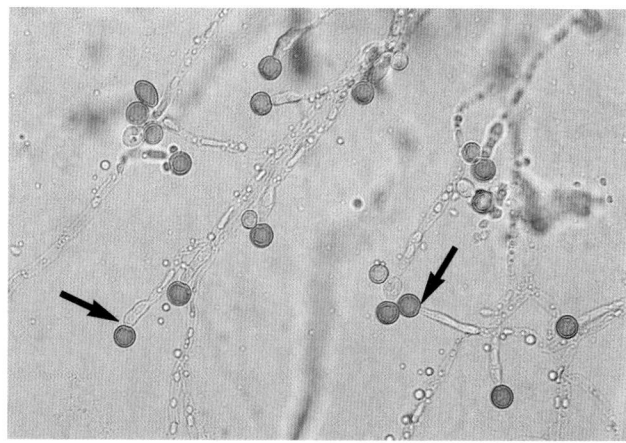

• **Fig. 62.11** Chlamydoconidia of *Candida albicans* (arrows).

and the failure to produce a germ tube. In addition, correlation of appearance on CHROMagar enhances and improves identification. The rapid trehalose test has also been combined with maltose hydrolysis in a 30-second dipstick assay.

Trichosporon spp., Cutaneotrichosporon spp., and Apiotrichum sp.

Organisms within these genera are indicated in the presence of predominate contiguous arthroconidia that are rectangular, often with rounded ends, along with septate hyaline hyphae. Blastoconidia are sometimes present but are not seen in all cultures. Positive urease production differentiates these genera from *Saprochaete* and *Geotrichum* spp. Final identification is based on the characteristic substrate utilization.

Malassezia spp.

M. furfur may be recovered from the blood of patients who have fungemia. Growth in the presence of a long-chain fatty acid, in conjunction with the "bowling pin" or "pop bottle" morphology, is sufficient for identification. *Malassezia* spp. that do not require long-chain fatty acid supplementation can be identified using substrate utilization analysis and cornmeal agar morphology.

Commercial Yeast Identification Systems

Commercial yeast identification systems have provided laboratories with standardized test methods. The methods are rapid, providing results within 24 to 72 hours. The systems provide an identification based on a database of thousands of yeast biotypes that considers the variation in substrate utilization patterns. The manufacturers also provide computer consultation services to the laboratory for the identification of isolates that produce an atypical result. Although these systems are powerful tools, they should not be used as the sole method of identification; traditionally, they are most effectively used in conjunction with yeast morphology on routine media.

Multiple Species Identification Systems
API-20C AUX

The API-20C AUX yeast identification system (bioMérieux, Marcy l'Etoile, France) has an extensive data set of all commercial systems available. The system consists of a strip that contains 20 microcapsules, 19 of which contain dehydrated carbohydrates for determining assimilation test profiles of yeasts. Reactions are compared with growth (turbidity) in the first cupule, which lacks a carbohydrate substrate. Reactions are read, and results are converted to a seven-digit biotype profile number. Most of the yeasts are identified within 48 hours; however, some *Cryptococcus* and *Trichosporon* spp. may require up to 72 hours. The API-20C AUX yeast identification system, as well as all other commercially available products, requires that the microscopic morphologic features of yeast grown on cornmeal agar containing 1% Tween 80 and trypan blue be correlated with the substrate utilization patterns.

MicroScan Rapid Yeast Identification Panel

The MicroScan Yeast Identification Panel (Beckman Coulter Inc., Brea, CA) is a 96-well, microtiter plate containing 27 dehydrated substrates. It was introduced as an alternative to the API-20C AUX yeast identification system. It uses chromogenic substrates to assess specific enzyme activity, which can be detected within 4 hours. Specific enzyme profiles have been generated for many of the yeasts commonly encountered in the clinical microbiology laboratory.

Vitek Biochemical Cards

The Yeast Biochemical Card (bioMérieux, Durham, NC) is a 30-well, disposable plastic card that contains conventional biochemical tests and negative controls. It is used with the Vitek 2 system. Evaluation of this system showed an overall accuracy of identification near 100% compared with API-20C AUX. Fewer than one fourth of the yeasts required additional biochemical or morphologic tests to confirm the identification. Of all correctly identified yeasts, more than half were reported within 24 hours of incubation.

Chromogenic Agars

Chromogenic agar is a differential medium useful for the recovery of *Candida* organisms in clinical specimens, differentiation of *Candida* spp., and isolation of colonies. Distinct enzymes of different *Candida* spp. react with chromogenic substrates to yield a characteristic colony color. When used with colonial morphologic features, the colored growth on the agar based on enzymatic substrates can provide a presumptive identification. Many of these agars can be used for the identification of *C. albicans, C. tropicalis, C. krusei*, and *C. glabrata*. All manufacturer directions should be followed closely, as differences in temperatures and incubation times can alter the appearance of the colonies.

Matrix-Assisted Laser Desorption Ionization Time-of-Flight

Both commercially available MALDI identification systems the Biotyper CA System (Bruker Daltonics) and the Vitek

TABLE 62.1 Characteristic Microscopic Features of the Commonly Encountered Yeast and Yeastlike Organisms on Cornmeal Tween 80 Agar

Organism	Arthroconidia/Blastoconidia	Pseudohyphae or Hyphae
Candida albicans complex	Spherical clusters at regular intervals on pseudohyphae	Chlamydoconidia present on hyphae
Candida auris	Round to oval, elongated	Pseudohyphal-like forms
Candida dubliniensis	Ovoid budding yeast cells	Chlamydoconidia present on hyphae
Candida glabrata complex	Small, spherical, and tightly compacted	None produced
Candida kefyr	Elongated, lie parallel to pseudohyphae	Pseudohyphae present but not characteristic
Candida krusei	Elongated; clusters occur at septa of pseudohyphae	Branched pseudohyphae
Candida lusitaniae	Blastoconidia, may appear in short chains	Short, curved pseudohyphae with blastoconidia formed at or between septa
Candida parapsilosis complex	Present but not characteristic	Sagebrush or "shaggy star" appearance; large (giant) hyphae present
Candida rugose complex	Elongated blastoconidia, may be in chains	Pseudohyphae present
Candida tropicalis	Produced randomly along hyphae or pseudohyphae	Pseudohyphae present but not characteristic
Cryptococcus spp.	Round to oval, vary in size, separated by a capsule	Rare; usually not seen
Geotrichum candidum	Rectangular arthroconidia	Coarse true hyphae
Malassezia spp.	Yeastlike cells that are phialides with small collarettes; budlike structures on a broad base	Hyphal elements are generally absent, but rudimentary forms may be present
Prototheca spp.	Sporangia of various sizes containing endospores; budding does not occur	No hyphae
Rhodotorula spp.	Round to oval-shaped, multilateral budding cells with capsules	Rudimentary pseudohyphae may be present
Saccharomyces spp.	Large round to oval with multilateral budding	Rudimentary short pseudohyphae sometimes present
Saprochaete capitatus	Round to oval budding yeastlike cells, few arthroconidia and annelloconidia	Hyphae and pseudohyphae with annellides clustered on the tips
Sporobolomyces spp.	Oval to ellipsoidal cells, blastoconidia; ballistoconidia can produce satellite colonies	Pseudohyphae with blastoconidia on sterigmata (protrusion), true hyphae may be present
Trichosporon, spp.[a]	Numerous arthroconidia, resembling *Geotrichum* spp.; blastoconidia may appear singly or in short chains	May be present but difficult to find, septate hyphae and pseudohyphae
Ustilago spp.	Elongate, irregular, spindle or bean-pod shaped yeastlike cells	Short hyphae with clamp connections may be observed

[a]*Trichosporon, Apiotrichum,* and *Cutaneotrichosporon* spp.

MS (bioMérieux) can identify yeast and fungal isolates with excellent accuracy. See Chapter 7 for more information. MALDI-TOF requires that isolates be cultured overnight and then processed using a standardized extraction procedure. Several studies report the correct identification of yeast to the species level up to approximately 98% compared with traditional culture methods. In addition, some laboratories require the direct isolation of organisms from blood culture systems without subculturing to another medium to facilitate identification, though these methods are not FDA approved and require rigorous independent validation and verification by the individual laboratory. Both Bruker and bioMérieux continuously improve their FDA-cleared databases by adding spectra of additional strains (increasing species diversity) as well as incorporating new species.

Cornmeal Agar Morphology

Cornmeal agar morphology can be used to determine whether the yeast produces blastoconidia, arthroconidia,

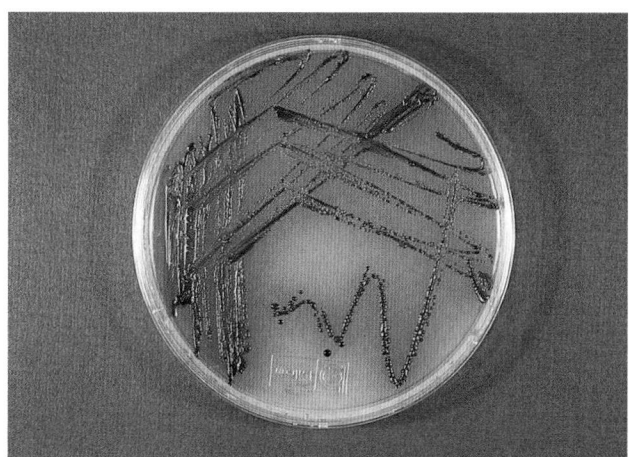

• **Fig. 62.12** *Cryptococcus neoformans* colonies are brown when grown on niger seed agar.

pseudohyphae, true hyphae, and/or chlamydoconidia (Evolve Procedure 62.3). Cornmeal agar morphology can be used to detect characteristic chlamydoconidia produced by *C. albicans*. Microscopic morphology on cornmeal agar can be used to differentiate *Cryptococcus, Saccharomyces, Candida, Geotrichum,* and *Trichosporon*. The morphologic features of the common *Candida* spp. are distinct enough to provide a presumptive identification. This can be accomplished for *C. albicans, C. glabrata, C. krusei, C. parapsilosis, C. tropicalis,* and *C. kefyr,* keeping in mind that numerous other species, uncommonly recovered in the clinical laboratory, might resemble microscopically any of the species.

Cornmeal agar morphology is less useful for identification of the uncommonly encountered yeasts. It should be used as an additional test in conjunction with a commercial yeast identification system.

Carbohydrate Utilization

Carbohydrate utilization patterns are the historical conventional methods for the definitive identification of yeasts recovered in a clinical laboratory. Various methods have been advocated for use in determining carbohydrate utilization patterns by clinically important yeasts. Evolve Procedure 62.4 provides a method for determining carbohydrate utilization.

Once the carbohydrate utilization profile has been obtained, reactions may be compared with those listed in tables in most mycology laboratory manuals. In most instances, carbohydrate utilization tests provide definitive identification of the yeast, and additional tests are unnecessary. Some laboratories prefer carbohydrate fermentation tests, which are simply performed using purple broth containing different carbohydrate substrates. In general, carbohydrate fermentation tests are unnecessary and are not recommended for routine use.

Phenoloxidase Detection Using Niger Seed Agar

Use of a simplified *Guizotia abyssinica* (niger seed) medium is a definitive method for detecting phenoloxidase production by yeasts (Evolve Procedure 62.5). Most isolates of *C. neoformans* readily produce phenoloxidase; however, some do not. In addition, in some instances, cultures of *C. neoformans* have been shown to contain both phenoloxidase-producing and phenoloxidase-deficient colonies in the same culture.

If conventional methods are used, all criteria, including urease production, carbohydrate utilization, and the phenoloxidase test, must be met before a final identification of *C. neoformans* is made.

Nucleic Acid Sequencing Methods

Nucleic acid sequencing provides more accuracy than conventional biochemical methods within 12 hours following colony isolation. Multiple genes are needed to develop reproducible, specific, and sensitive sequence data for standardization of identification. Methods including conventional Sanger DNA sequencing, pyrosequencing, and whole genome sequencing will undoubtedly improve the accuracy of classification and identification of yeast and yeastlike organisms as techniques improve for use in the clinical laboratory.

ⓔ Visit the Evolve site for a complete list of procedures, review questions, and case studies.

Bibliography

Abdelhamed AM, Zhang SX, Watkins T, et al.: Multicenter evaluation of *Candida* QuickFISH BC for identification of *Candida* species directly from blood culture bottles, *J Clin Microbiol* 53:1672–1676, 2015.

Alexander BD, Ashley ED, Reller LB, et al.: Cost savings with implementation of PNA FISH testing for identification of *Candida albicans* in blood cultures, *Diagn Microbiol Infect Dis* 54:277–282, 2006.

Aubertine CL, Rivera M, Rohan SM, et al.: Comparative study of the new colorimetric VITEK 2 yeast identification card versus the older fluorometric card and of CHROMagar *Candida* as a source medium with the new card, *J Clin Microbiol* 44:227–228, 2006.

Bader O, Weig M, Taverne-Ghadwal L, et al.: Improved clinical laboratory identification of human pathogenic yeasts by matrix-assisted laser desorption ionization-time-of-flight spectrometry, *Clin Microbiol Infect* 17:1359–1365, 2011.

Barenfanger J, Arakere P, Dela Cruz R, et al.: Improved outcomes associated with limiting identification of *Candida* spp. in respiratory secretions, *J Clin Microbiol* 41:5645–5649, 2003.

Bennett J, Dolin R, Blaser M: *Principles and practice of infectious diseases*, ed 9, Philadelphia, 2020, Elsevier-Saunders.

Berenguer J, Buck M, Witebsky F, et al.: Lysis-centrifugation blood cultures in the detection of tissue-proven invasive candidiasis: disseminated versus single-organ infection, *Diagn Microbiol Infect Dis* 17:103–109, 1993.

Bille E, Dauphin B, Leto J, et al.: MALDI-TOF MS Andromas strategy for routine identification of bacteria, mycobacteria, yeasts, *Aspergillus* spp. and positive blood cultures, *Clin Microbial Infect* 18:1117–1125, 2012.

Calderone RA: Introduction and historical perspectives. In Calderone R, editor: *Candida and candidiasis*, Washington, DC, 2002, ASM Press.

Campuzano A, Wormley FL: Innate immunity against *Cryptococcus*, from recognition to elimination, *J Fungi (Basel)* 4(1):33, 2018.

Carroll KC, Pfaller MA, Landry ML, et al.: *Manual of clinical microbiology*, ed 2, Washington, DC, 2019, ASM Press.

Chalupovaa J, Rausa M, Sedlarovab M, et al.: Identification of fungal microorganisms by MALDI-TOF mass spectrometry, *Biotechnol Adv* 32:230–241, 2012.

Chan KS, Deepak RN, Tan MG, et al.: Abbreviated identification of *Candida albicans* by the presence of a pseudohyphal fringe ("spiking" appearance)—some caveats, *J Med Microbiol* 60:687–688, 2011.

Cherniak R, Sundstrom JB: Polysaccharide antigens of the capsule of *Cryptococcus neoformans*, *Infect Immun* 62:1507–1512, 1994.

Clancy CJ, Pappas PG, Vasquez J, et al.: Detecting infections rapidly and easily for candidemia trial, Part 2 (DIRECT2): a prospective, multicenter study of the T2 *Candida* panel, *Clin Infect Dis* 66:1678–1686, 2018.

Cleveland AA, Harrison LH, Farley MM, et al.: Declining incidence of candidemia and the shifting epidemiology of *Candida* resistance in two US metropolitan areas, 2008-2013: results from population-based surveillance, *PloS One* 10:e0120452, 2015.

Cortegiani A, Misseri G, Fasciana T, et al.: Epidemiology, clinical characteristics, resistance, and treatment of infections by *Candida auris*, *J Intensive Care* 6:69, 2018.

Damji R, Mukherji A, Mussani F: *Sporobolomyces salmonicolor*: a case report of a rare cutaneous fungal infection, *SAGE Open Med Case Rep* 7:2050313X19844154, 2019.

De Almeida JN, Favero Gimenes VM, Francisco EC, et al.: Evaluating and improving Vitek MS for identification of clinically relevant species of *Trichosporon* and closely related genera *Cutaneotrichosporon* and *Apiotrichum*, *J Clin Microbiol* 55(8):2439–2444, 2017.

Ellepola ANB, Hurst SF, Ellie CM, et al.: Rapid and unequivocal differentiation of *Candida dubliniensis* from other *Candida* species using species-specific DNA probes: comparison with phenotypic identification methods, *Oral Microbiol Immunol* 18:379–388, 2003.

Ellepola ANB, Morrison CJ: Laboratory diagnosis of invasive candidiasis, *J Microbiol* 43:65–84, 2005.

Freydière AM, Parant F, Noel-Baron F, et al.: Identification of *Candida glabrata* by a 30-second trehalase test, *J Clin Microbiol* 40:3602–3605, 2002.

Frerydiere AM, Robert T, Ploton C, et al.: Rapid Identification of *Candida glabrata* with a new commercial test, GLABRATA RTT, *J Clin Microbiol* 41:3861–3863, 2003.

Fu C, Donadio N, Cardenans ME, et al.: Dissecting the roles of the calcineurin pathway in unisexual reproduction, stress responses, and virulence in *Cryptococcus deneoformans*, *Genetics* 208(2):639–653, 2018.

Guiver M, Levi K, Oppenheim BA, et al.: Rapid identification of *Candida* species by TaqMan PCR, *J Clin Pathol* 54:362–366, 2001.

Hagen F, Khayhan K, Theelen B, et al.: Recognition of seven species in the *Cryptococcus gattii/Cryptococcus neoformans* species complex, *Fungal Genet Biol* 78:16–48, 2015.

Heelan J, Siliezar D, Coon K: Comparison of rapid testing methods for enzyme production with the germ tube method for presumptive identification of *Candida albicans*, *J Clin Microbiol* 34:2847–2849, 1996.

Hunter-Ellul L, Schepp ED, Lea A, et al.: A rare case of *Cryptococcus luteolus*-related tenosynovitis, *Infection* 42(4):771–774, 2014.

Hsu MC, Chen KW, Lo HJ, et al.: Species identification of medically important fungi by use of real-time LightCycler PCR, *J Med Microbiol* 52:1071–1076, 2003.

Jarvis JN, Percival A, Bauman S, et al.: Evaluation of a novel point-of-care cryptococcal antigen test on serum, plasma, and urine from patients with HIV-associated cryptococcal meningitis, *Clin Infect Dis* 53:1019–1023, 2011.

Jin WY, Jang SJ, Lee MJ, et al.: Evaluation of VITEK 2, Microscan, and Phoenix for identification of clinical isolates and reference strains, *Diagn Microb Infect Dis* 70:442–447, 2011.

Kathavade RJ, Kura MM, Valand AG, et al.: *Candida tropicalis*: its prevalence, pathogenicity and increasing resistance to fluconazole, *J Med Microbiol* 59:873–880, 2010.

Kathuria S, Singh PK, Sharma C, et al.: Multidrug-resistant *Candida auris* misidentified as *Candida haemulonii*: characterization by matrix-assisted laser desorption ionization–time of flight mass spectrometry and DNA sequencing and its antifungal susceptibility profile variability by Vitek 2, CLSI broth microdilution, and etest method, *J Clin Microbiol* 53:1823–1830, 2015.

Kreger-Van Rij N: *The yeasts: a taxonomic study*, New York, NY, 1984, Elsevier.

Kronstad JW, Attarian R, Cadieux B, et al.: Expanding fungal pathogenesis: *Cryptococcus* breaks out of the opportunistic box, *Nat Rev Microbiol* 9:193–203, 2011.

Masuda M, Hirose N, Ishikawa T, et al.: *Prototheca miyajii* sp. nov., isolated from a patient with systemic protothecosis, *Int J Syst Evol Microbiol* 66(3):1510–1520, 2016.

Liguori G, Di Onofrio V, Lucariello A, et al.: Oral candidiasis: a comparison between conventional methods and multiplex polymerase chain reaction for species identification, *Oral Microbiol Immunol* 24:76–78, 2009.

Liguori G, Galle F, Lucariello A, et al.: Comparison between multiplex PCR and phenotypic systems for *Candida* spp. identification, *New Microbiol* 33:63–67, 2010.

Lockhart SR: Current epidemiology of Candida infection, *Clin Microbiol Newsl* 36:131, 2014.

Lockhart SR, Iqbal N, Cleveland AA, et al.: Species identification and antifungal susceptibility testing of *Candida* bloodstream isolates from population-based surveillance studies in two U.S. cities from 2008 to 2011, *J Clin Microbiol* 50:3435–3442, 2012.

Loiex C, Wallet F, Sendid B, et al.: Evaluation of VITEK 2 colorimetric cards versus fluorometric cards for identification of yeasts, *Diagn Microbiol Infect Dis* 56:455–457, 2006.

Meya DB, Manabe YC, Boulware DR, et al.: The immunopathogenesis of cryptococcal immune reconstitution inflammatory syndrome-understanding a conundrum, *Curr Opin Infect Dis* 29(1):10–22, 2016.

Murray CK, Beckius ML, Green JA, et al.: Use of chromogenic medium in the isolation of yeasts from clinical specimens, *J Med Microbiol* 54:981–985, 2005.

Murray MP, Zinchuk R, Larone DH: CHROMagar *Candida* as the sole primary medium for isolation of yeasts and as a source medium for the rapid-assimilation-of-trehalose test, *J Clin Microbiol* 43:1210–1212, 2005.

Neely LA, Audeh M, Phung NA, et al.: T2 magnetic resonance enables nanoparticle-mediated rapid detection of candidemia in whole blood, *Sci Transl Med* 5:182ra54, 2013.

Oliveira K, Haase G, Kurtzman C, et al.: Differentiation of *Candida albicans* and *Candida dubliniensis* by fluorescent *in situ* hybridization with peptide nucleic acid probes, *J Clin Microbiol* 39:4138–4141, 2001.

Paliwal DK, Randhawa HS: Evaluation of a simplified *Guizotia abyssinica* seed medium for differentiation of *Cryptococcus neoformans*, *J Clin Microbiol* 7:346–348, 1978.

Pan W, Liao W, Hagen F, et al.: Meningitis caused by *Filobasidium uniguttulatum*: case report and overview of the literature, *Mycoses* 55(2):105–109, 2012.

Pande A, Non LR, Romee R, Santos CAQ: *Pseudozyma* and other non-*Candida* opportunistic yeast bloodstream infections in a large stem cell transplant center, *Transpl Infect Dis* 19(2), 2017, https://doi.org/10.1111/tid.12664.

Pfaller MA, Diekema DJ, Gibbs DL, et al.: Geographic variation in the frequency of isolation and fluconazole and voriconazole susceptibilities of *Candida glabrata:* an assessment from the ARTEMIS DISK global antifungal surveillance program, global antifungal surveillance group, *Diagn Microbiol Infect Dis* 67:162–171, 2010.

Pfaller MA, Diekema DJ, Gibbs DL, et al.: Results from the ARTEMIS DISK Global Antifungal Surveillance Study, 1997 to 2007: a 10.5-year analysis of susceptibilities of *Candida* species to fluconazole and voriconazole as determined by CLSI standardized disk diffusion, Global Antifungal Surveillance Group, *J Clin Microbiol* 48:1366–1377, 2010.

Pfaller MA, Houston A, Coffmann S: Application of CHROMagar *Candida* for rapid screening of clinical specimens for *Candida albicans, Candida tropicalis, Candida krusei,* and *Candida (Torulopsis) glabrata, J Clin Microbiol* 34:58–61, 1996.

Pfaller MA, Moet GJ, Messer SA, et al.: *Candida* bloodstream infections: comparison of species distribution and resistance to echinocandin and azole antifungal agents in intensive care unit (ICU) and non-ICU settings in the SENTRY Antimicrobial Surveillance Program (2008-2009), *Int J Antimicrob Agents* 38:65–69, 2011.

Romanio MR, Coraine LA, Maielo VP, et al.: *Saccharomyces cerevisiae* fungemia in a pediatric patient after treatment with probiotics, *Rev Paul Pediatr* 35(3):361–364, 2017.

Rigby S, Procop GW, Haase G, et al.: Fluorescence *in situ* hybridization with peptide nucleic acid probes for rapid identification of *Candida albicans* directly from blood culture bottles, *J Clin Microbiol* 40:2182–2186, 2002.

Silva S, Negri M, Henriques M, et al.: *Candida glabrata, Candida parapsilosis* and *Candida tropicalis:* biology, epidemiology, pathogenicity and antifungal resistance, *FEMS Microbiol Rev* 36:288–305, 2012.

Spyridoula-Angeliki N, Kichik N, Brown R, et al.: *Candida albicans* interactions with mucosal surfaces during health and disease, *Pathogens* 8(2):53, 2019.

St Germain G, Beauchesne D: Evaluation of the MicroScan rapid yeast identification panel, *J Clin Microbiol* 29:2296–2299, 1991.

Tan GL, Peterson EM: CHROMagar *Candida* medium for direct susceptibility testing of yeast from blood cultures, *J Clin Microbiol* 43:1727–1731, 2005.

Tham R, Erbas B, Dharmage SC, et al.: Outdoor fungal spores and acute respiratory effects in vulnerable individuals, *Environ Res* 178:108675, 2019, https://doi.org/10.1016/j.envres.2019.108675.

Trofa D, Gacser A, Nosanchuk JD, et al.: *Candida parapsilosis,* an emerging fungal pathogen, *Clin Microbiol Rev* 21:606–625, 2008.

Van Herendael BH, Bruynseels P, Bensaid M, et al.: Validation of a modified algorithm for the identification of yeast isolates using matrix-associated laser desorption ionization time-of-flight mass spectrometry (MALDI-TOF MS), *Eur J Clin Microbiol* 31:841–848, 2012.

Walsh TJ, Hayden RT, Larone DH: *Larone's medically important fungi: a guide to identification,* ed 6, Washington, DC, 2018, ASM Press.

Wang Y, Aisen P, Casadevall A: *Cryptococcus neoformans* melanin and virulence: mechanism of action, *Infect Immun* 63:3131–3136, 1995.

Wiesner DL, Boulware DR: *Cryptococcus*-related immune reconstitution inflammatory syndrome (IRIS): pathogenesis and its clinical implications, *Curr Fungal Infect Rep* 5(4):252–261, 2012.

Wilson DA, Joyce MJ, Hall LS, et al.: Multicenter evaluation of a *C. albicans* peptide nucleic acid fluorescent *in situ* hybridization probe for characterization of yeast isolates from blood cultures, *J Clin Microbiol* 43:2909–2912, 2005.

Wu Y, Du PC, Li WG, et al.: Identification and molecular analysis of pathogenic yeasts in droppings of domestic pigeons in Beijing, China, *Mycopathologia* 174(3):203–214, 2012.

Zaragoza O: Basic principles of the virulence of *Cryptococcus, Virulence* 10(1):490–501, 2019.

Zilberberg MD, Shorr AF, Kollef MH, et al.: Secular trends in candidemia-related hospitalization in the United States, 2000-2005, *Infect Control Hosp Epidemiol* 29:978–980, 2008.

Zilberberg MD, Kollef MH, Arnold H, et al.: Inappropriate empiric antifungal therapy for candidemia in the ICU and hospital resource utilization: a retrospective cohort study, *BMC Infect Dis* 10:150, 2010.

63

Antifungal Susceptibility Testing, Therapy, and Prevention

OBJECTIVES

1. Name the documents that contain the current guidelines for antifungal susceptibility testing.
2. Identify three circumstances in which antifungal susceptibility testing may be valuable.
3. List three areas of concern that complicate interpretive guidelines.
4. Explain how amphotericin B is produced, how it is administered, and its most significant adverse reaction.
5. Describe the mechanism of action of flucytosine and the drug's therapeutic use.
6. Identify three echinocandins and describe their mechanism of action.

Antifungal Susceptibility Testing

Antifungal susceptibility testing (AFST) is designed to provide information that helps the physician select the appropriate antifungal agent to treat a specific infection. Although AFST perhaps has not advanced as far as methods for determining the susceptibility of bacteria to antimicrobial agents, significant progress has been made. As with performing antimicrobial susceptibility testing, it is imperative to utilize standardized methods to ensure reproducibility between clinical microbiology laboratories. Only by doing so will the laboratory be able to communicate and report accurate test results to guide clinicians in therapeutic decision making.

The Clinical Laboratory Standards Institute (CLSI) sets the standards for AFST. The current guidelines for these tests are provided in the following four documents, which are available on the CLSI website (www.clsi.org):

- M27-A3, *Reference Method for Broth Dilution Antifungal Susceptibility Testing of Yeasts,* Approved Standard. This document covers requirements for use of the broth microdilution method. The standards for susceptibility testing are very specific about the inoculum size, test medium, incubation time and temperature, and end point of yeasts that cause invasive fungal infections.

- M27-S4, *Reference Method for Broth Dilution Antifungal Susceptibility Testing of Yeasts,* Fourth Informational Supplement. This document provides species-specific breakpoints against different antifungal agents.
- M38-A2, *Reference Method for Broth Dilution Antifungal Susceptibility Testing of Filamentous Fungi,* Approved Standard. This standard is a microdilution method for molds that cause invasive and cutaneous infections.
- M44-A2, *Method for Antifungal Disk Diffusion Susceptibility Testing of Yeasts and Molds* (M51-A), Approved Guideline. This standard provides methodology for disk diffusion testing for *Candida* spp., including quality control and interpretation guidelines.

It must be emphasized that the methodology and interpretation of antifungal susceptibility tests continue to evolve, and the laboratory should check for updated standards on a regular basis. Antifungal susceptibility tests are costly and time-consuming, but they may have value in the following circumstances:

- Determining antifungi grams for specific fungi in an institution
- Aid in the management of patients with candidemia, especially those caused by non-albicans *Candida* spp.
- Aid in the management of patients with invasive candidiasis

CLSI considers the previously published breakpoints for itraconazole and 5-flucytosine to all *Candida* spp. obsolete. Breakpoints are published as species-specific for fluconazole, voriconazole, and the echinocandins.

Isolates of the same species may exhibit differences in minimal inhibitory concentrations (MICs) because of previous exposure to antifungal agents or acquisition of a genetic mechanism of resistance. CLSI's most recent interpretative guidelines should be followed whenever possible, as they contain species-specific breakpoints.

The preferred medium for the performance of broth dilution AFST is RPMI 1640 (Roswell Park Memorial Institute 1640). The specific formulation contains the reducing agent glutathione without bicarbonate, high concentrations of vitamins, and phenol red as the pH indicator. The desired

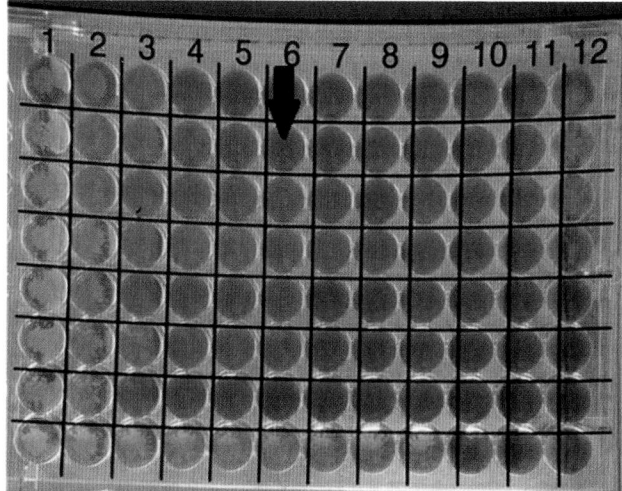

• **Fig. 63.1** A Sensititre YeastOne YO9 (Thermo Fisher Scientific) panel inoculated with *Candida krusei* ATCC 6258. The panel contains alamar blue as a growth indicator. The minimal inhibitory concentrations (MICs) are interpreted as the first blue well. In the example, the MIC for micafungin is 0.25 µg/mL.

pH range for the medium for accurate testing is between 6.9 and 7.1. The recommended buffer to use for adjusting pH is MOPS [3-(N-morpholino) propanesulfonic acid] (final concentration 0.165 mol/L for pH 7.0). Overnight cultures of pure *Candida* isolates grown on Sabouraud dextrose or potato dextrose agar are selected and used to prepare a suspension in 0.85% saline or sterile water equivalent to a 0.5 McFarland turbidity standard. The organism is then diluted 1:100 to make a working stock suspension followed by a subsequent a 1:20 dilution from the working stock in RPMI 1640 broth medium. AFST plates are incubated for 24 hours in ambient air in a 35°C incubator. If there is inadequate growth in the growth control well for the isolate being tested, the plate is incubated for an additional 24 hours. Susceptibility testing for *Cryptococcus neoformans* should be incubated for 70 to 74 hours before interpreting results.

In addition to manual broth dilution susceptibility testing, commercial panels are also available. The Sensititre Yeast-One YO9 (Thermo Fisher Scientific) is a 96-well microtiter plate containing nine antifungal agents and can be used for testing *Candida* spp., *Cryptococcus* spp., and *Aspergillus* spp. (Fig. 63.1). The panel contains an alamar blue indicator that can be used to visually interpret MIC results.

Any laboratory that is not equipped to perform CLSI methods, or validated equivalent methods, for susceptibility of clinically important fungal isolates should send the isolates to a reference laboratory for testing. At a minimum an azole agent and an echinocandin should be tested, as azole resistance varies among *Candida* spp.

Antifungal Therapy and Prevention

Numerous antifungal agents have been developed; however, few newer agents are on the horizon. The increasing number of immunosuppressed patients and the expansion of drug resistance of microorganisms make the development and appropriate use of antifungal agents two of the most important areas in microbiology and infectious diseases. This section is meant to provide an overview to commonly used antifungal agents; it is by no means comprehensive.

Azole Antifungal Drugs

The azole group of antifungal agents consists of the imidazoles and the triazoles. These compounds contain six carbon ring structures with conjugated double bonds, chloride residues, and five carbon ring structures that contain at least two nitrogen molecules. Traditionally used agents in this group include fluconazole, itraconazole, and ketoconazole. The newer triazoles are voriconazole, posaconazole, and, most recently, isavuconazole. Azole antifungal agents disrupt the integrity of the fungal cell membrane by interfering with the synthesis of ergosterol.

Fluconazole

Fluconazole, a triazole, is exceptionally soluble in water, which allows either oral or intravenous administration. Fluconazole typically has excellent activity against most *Candida* spp. and *Cryptococcus* spp.; therapeutic levels are easily reached in the central nervous system. There have been reports of resistance in *C. albicans* after short-term treatment in mucosal or deep-seated forms of invasive candidiasis and in *C. neoformans* in patients with AIDS after long-term therapy. Side effects of fluconazole therapy are usually minimal. The susceptibility of *C. glabrata* to fluconazole is not predictable. Isolates of *C. glabrata* may be susceptible at higher doses of drug administration, that is, susceptible dose-dependent (SDD) or resistant to fluconazole. The emerging pathogen, *C. auris*, has also demonstrated resistance to fluconazole. Other notable yeasts or yeastlike fungi resistant to fluconazole are *C. krusei* and *Rhodotorula* spp. In addition, the antifungal has no activity against *Aspergillus* spp., *Fusarium* spp., or Mucorales molds.

Itraconazole

Itraconazole has a spectrum of activity that is similar to ketoconazole but is better tolerated. In addition, itraconazole has been shown to be effective in cases of aspergillosis, onychomycosis, oropharyngeal/esophageal candidiasis, and infections caused by the systemic fungal pathogens, e.g., *Blastomyces, Histoplasma, Paracoccidioides, Talaromyces,* and *Sporothrix* spp. histoplasmosis. Itraconazole may have limited activity against *C. neoformans*. Adverse reactions principally include gastrointestinal disturbances; however, vestibular disturbances, edema, and skin irritations have been reported.

Ketoconazole

Ketoconazole is an imidazole that is available orally for systemic infections, but the main use is as a topical agent. It is useful in mild cases of paracoccidioidomycosis and is an alternative to amphotericin B for infections caused by *Blastomyces, Coccidioides, Sporothrix,* or *Histoplasma* spp. Ketoconazole may be used if prolonged oral therapy for chronic mucocutaneous candidiasis is needed. *In vivo*, ketoconazole is fungistatic because fungicidal levels are not achievable with therapeutic concentrations. Adverse reactions include transient elevations in liver enzymes; nausea; and dose-related gynecomastia, decreased libido, and oligospermia in males. There are several other anti-fungals that are less toxic and therefore other alternatives are generally used except in resource-limited environments.

Voriconazole

Voriconazole has an expanded spectrum of activity compared with itraconazole. In addition to the uses described previously for itraconazole, voriconazole demonstrates useful activity against some *Fusarium* strains as well as activity against *Scedosporium* spp., *Candida* spp. *C. neoformans*, and *Trichosporon* spp. The Mucorales are resistant to voriconazole. This agent is often used as salvage therapy for severe cases of *Coccidioides* meningitis and with other dimorphic fungi, including *Blastomyces, Histoplasma*, and *Talaromyces* spp. Elevated liver enzymes may occur, as may transient visual disturbances, which can significantly alarm the patient if the individual is not forewarned.

Posaconazole

Posaconazole was originally available as an oral triazole structurally similar to voriconazole with activity against *Candida* spp., *Aspergillus* spp., *C. neoformans, Trichosporon,* and the Mucorales. The antifungal is also now available as an intravenous formulation that can be used in treatment of seriously ill patients. The antifungal appears less effective against *Fusarium* spp. and *Scedosporium* spp. It is commonly prescribed as prophylaxis to prevent invasive *Aspergillus* and *Candida* infections in high-risk patients including hematopoietic stem cell transplant recipients with graft-versus-host disease or those with neutropenia following chemotherapy for hematologic malignancies. Posaconazole is also very effective in systemic infections with the thermally dimorphic fungi.

Isavuconazole

Isavuconazole is a triazole available as an oral or parenteral agent and is primarily used for the treatment of invasive aspergillosis (IA) or invasive mucormycosis (IM). There is documentation, however, that panazole-resistant isolates of *Aspergillus fumigatus* are also resistant to isavuconazole. Common side effects include nausea, diarrhea, headache, increased liver enzymes, and peripheral edema. Considering the favorable outcomes for IA and IM infections, use of isavuconazole was investigated for candidemia and invasive candidiasis; however, the results of that study were unable to demonstrate noninferiority of isavuconazole relative to caspofungin for the primary treatment of candidemia and invasive candidiasis.

Echinocandins

The echinocandins (anidulafungin, caspofungin, micafungin) are semisynthetic lipopeptide antifungal agents that inhibit the 1,3-beta-D-glucan synthase that is involved in fungal cell wall synthesis. The drug is effective against *Candida* spp., including strains that are resistant to fluconazole. They are typically used for the prophylaxis and treatment of *Candida* spp. infections in adult and pediatric patients. The echinocandins are only available as intravenous medications. In addition to the treatment of candidiasis, they are also effective against *Aspergillus* spp. They are ineffective against fungi that lack 1,3-beta-D-glucan, including *C. neoformans, Trichosporon* spp., *Fusarium* spp., and the Mucorales. Side effects are minimal.

Polyene Macrolide Antifungals

Polyene macrolide antifungal agents consist of a group of complex organic molecules, most of which contain multiple, conjugated, double-bond, and one- to three-ring structures. This group includes many of the most commonly used antifungal agents, such as amphotericin B, the colloidal and liposomal preparations of amphotericin B, nystatin, and griseofulvin.

Amphotericin B

Amphotericin B is produced by the actinomycete *Streptomyces nodosus*. It is commonly infused intravenously to treat deep-seated fungal infections, e.g., IA, and those caused by *Candida* spp., *Cryptococcus* spp., and members of the Mucorales. Amphotericin B binds the ergosterol component of the fungal cell membrane and alters the selective permeability of this membrane. The most significant adverse reaction associated with amphotericin B therapy is renal insufficiency. The liposomal amphotericin B formulation diminishes this adverse reaction. Although amphotericin B is active against a wide variety of fungi, resistant organisms exist that the laboratory must be able to identify. Clinical failures in cases treated with amphotericin B include infections caused by *Pseudallescheria boydii, Scedosporium prolificans, Aspergillus terreus, Trichosporon* spp., and most cases involving *Fusarium* spp. CLSI has not published clinical breakpoints for any *Candida* spp. against amphotericin B. Instead, they publish an epidemiologic cutoff value (ECV) based on the MIC distribution for the organism against the drug in question. For *Candida* spp., the amphotericin B ECV has been set at ≥4 µg/mL. *Candida* isolates with MICs at or above this cutoff are presumed to contain some acquired mechanism of resistance.

Nystatin

Nystatin, an antifungal agent produced by *Streptomyces noursei,* is not absorbed in the gastrointestinal tract. It is principally used locally to treat oral or vulvovaginal candidiasis. The toxicity of this drug is prohibitive to parenteral use.

Griseofulvin

Griseofulvin is an antifungal antibiotic produced predominantly by *Penicillium griseofulvum*. Its mechanism of action consists of binding microtubular proteins, which are required for mitosis. Griseofulvin is an oral agent used to treat dermatophytoses, which are not responsive to azole antifungal therapy. Headache, gastrointestinal disturbances, and photosensitivity are a few of the adverse reactions that limit the usefulness of this drug.

5-Fluorocytosine (Flucytosine)

Flucytosine is a pyrimidine base, which is fluorinated in the fifth position. Flucytosine is metabolized to 5-fluorouracil, which is incorporated into fungal ribonucleic acid (RNA). This subsequently inhibits protein synthesis. Flucytosine is also metabolized into fluorodeoxyuridine monophosphate, a potent inhibitor of DNA synthesis. Flucytosine and amphotericin B act synergistically and have been used in combination therapy for treating infections caused by *Candida* spp. and *Cryptococcus* spp. Side effects and the emergence of resistance among *Candida* spp. and *C. neoformans* occurs in approximately 2% to 3% of all isolates.

Allylamines
Terbinafine and Naftifine

Terbinafine and naftifine are synthetic allylamines that are highly lipophilic, allowing them to accumulate in the skin, nails, and fatty tissue. The drugs interfere with fungal cell wall synthesis and are effective topical treatments for infections. Terbinafine is available as an oral or topical medication, whereas naftifine is only available in topical form. These antifungals are typically used in dermatophyte infections, and the development of resistance is rare even after prolonged exposure.

Selenium Sulfide

Selenium sulfide shampoos, available commercially, provide antifungal activity against *Malassezia furfur*, the causative agent of tinea versicolor. Additionally, selenium sulfide is sporicidal for *Trichophyton tonsurans*.

ⓔ Visit the Evolve site for a complete list of procedures, review questions, and case studies.

Bibliography

Carroll KC, Pfaller MA, Landry ML, et al.: *Manual of clinical microbiology*, ed 12, Washington, DC, 2019, ASM.

Deorukhkar SC, Saini S: Echinocandin susceptibility profile of resistant *Candida* species isolated from blood stream infections, *Infect Disord Drug Targets.* 2016;16(1):63-68. Available at: http://www.ncbi.nlm.nih.gov/pubmed/26648186. Accessed December 12, 2015.

Korting HC, Kiencke P, Nelles S: Comparable efficacy and safety of various topical formulations of terbinafine in tinea pedis irrespective of the treatment regimen: results of a meta-analysis, *Am J Clin Dermatol* 8:357–364, 2007.

Kullberg BJ, Viscoli C, Pappas PG, et al.: Isavuconazole versus caspofungin in the treatment of candidemia and other invasive candida infections: the ACTIVE trial, *Clin Infect Dis* 68:1981–1989, 2019.

Lass-Florl C, Griff K, Mayr A, et al.: Epidemiology and outcome of infections due to *Aspergillus terreus:* 10-year single centre experience, *Br J Haematol* 131:201–207, 2005.

Mayr A, Aigner M, Lass-Florl C: Anidulafungin for the treatment of invasive candidiasis, *Clin Microbiol Infect* 17(suppl 1):1–12, 2011.

O'Sullivan AK, Weinstein MC, Pandya A, et al.: Cost-effectiveness of posaconazole versus fluconazole for prevention of invasive fungal infections in U.S. patients with graft-versus-host disease, *Am J Health Syst Pharm* 69:149–156, 2012.

Perea S, Patterson TF: Antifungal resistance in pathogenic fungi, *Clin Infect Dis* 35:1073–1080, 2002.

Pfaller MA, Messer SA, Woosley LN, et al.: Echinocandin and triazole antifungal susceptibility profiles for clinical opportunistic yeast and mold isolates collected from 2010 to 2011: application of new CLSI clinical breakpoints and epidemiological cutoff values for characterization of geographic and temporal trends of antifungal resistance, *J Clin Microbiol* 8:2571–2581, 2013.

Pfaller MA, Diekema DJ: Rare and emerging opportunistic fungal pathogens: concern for resistance beyond *Candida albicans* and *Aspergillus fumigatus*, *J Clin Microbiol* 4:4419–4431, 2004.

Scott LJ: Micafungin: a review of its use in the prophylaxis and treatment of invasive *Candida* infections, *Drugs* 72:2141–2165, 2012.

Solovieva E, Olsufyeva EN, Preobrazhenskaya MN: Chemical modifications of antifungal polyene macrolide antibiotics, *Russ Chem Rev* 80:103–126, 2011.

Wolf DG, Falk R, Hacham M, et al.: Multidrug-resistant *Trichosporon asahii* infection of nongranulocytopenic patients in three intensive care units, *J Clin Microbiol* 39:4420–4425, 2001.

64

Overview of the Methods and Strategies in Virology

OBJECTIVES

1. Describe the physical components that make up a virion, and list a function for each component.
2. Define the viral infectious cycle, including naming the six steps in this process.
3. Explain viral tropism and provide a specific example related to a human pathogen.
4. Define the properties used to classify viruses and how these properties can be used to predict infection before a confirmed laboratory result.
5. Explain the general steps in viral pathogenesis (e.g., of a respiratory virus).
6. List some of the reasons for the increase in demand for clinical viral services in the field of infectious disease diagnostics.
7. Name some of the equipment necessary to set up a clinical virology laboratory and give the function of each piece.
8. List some of the viruses associated with the following clinical specimens: throat or nasopharyngeal swab or aspirate, urine, stool, lesion, blood, bone marrow, and stool or rectal swab.
9. List some of the most commonly used laboratory tests for detecting the following viruses: enterovirus, herpes simplex virus, influenza virus, norovirus, and respiratory syncytial virus (RSV).
10. Describe the Tzanck test procedure and list the viruses for which the test is used.
11. Define monolayer, primary cells, semicontinuous (low passage) cells, and continuous cells. Explain the incubation conditions for routine cell cultures.
12. Explain the types of cell lines used in viral cell culture; describe their similarities and differences, and how cytopathic effects (CPEs) are rated when reading cell cultures.
13. Describe a shell vial cell culture and explain its advantages over conventional cell culture.
14. Define the hemadsorption procedure and name the viruses for which the test is used.
15. Name the virus family capable of establishing viral latency in the human dorsal nerve root ganglion and explain the possible consequence of the latency.
16. Name the preferred tissue type of cell culture for growth of the following viruses: influenza A virus, varicella-zoster virus, herpes virus, and cytomegalovirus (CMV).
17. Associate an appropriate viral pathogen with the following viral syndromes: infant croup, infant bronchiolitis, adult gastroenteritis, parotitis, infectious mononucleosis, and meningitis.
18. Outline the benefits of mass spectrometry for viral pathogen identification versus other viral detection methods.

The survival of viral infectious agents depends on their ability to infect and reside in a living organism. These tiny organisms are believed to have evolved alongside humans and in conjunction with the domestication of animals. Throughout history, evidence shows that viruses are able to survive when stable host populations are available to provide a means for continued propagation. Viruses that established a long-term relationship with their host (i.e., did not kill the host immediately upon infection) were the first to become adapted and coevolve with the host species. Some of these earliest viruses in humans were believed to be retroviruses, such as the herpes viruses and papillomaviruses, which will be discussed in more detail in this chapter and Chapter 65.

A **virus** is an obligate intracellular parasite, that is among the smallest of all infectious agents and capable of infecting an animal, insect, plant, or bacterial cell. Viruses are found in every ecosystem. As strict obligate intracellular parasites, they are incapable of replication without a living host cell. Virus types are very specific, and each has a limited number of hosts it can infect; this is referred to as **viral tropism.**

Much is still unknown about the origins of viral agents, although most speculation indicates that viruses affecting humans established themselves in the human population via direct transmission of an animal virus to a human. Transmission of viruses from animals to humans still occurs, as demonstrated in the more recent viral outbreaks associated with the severe acute respiratory syndrome (SARS), West Nile, and influenza A H5 viruses, as well as the 2009 H1N1 virus, formerly known as the "swine flu." The influenza virus has been known to infect humans since the 1700s in Italy and has proven to be one of the deadliest viruses to affect humans. The virus was named to indicate disease resulting from the "influence" of miasma (bad air).

The emergence of a new viral disease across a very large geographic region (worldwide) with prolonged human-to-human transmission is called a **pandemic.** Most of the pandemics recorded had been caused by an influenza virus. Influenza virus pandemics result when the virus undergoes a **genetic shift**, and the reassortment of genes combines with those of another organism, usually an animal. The resulting virus emerges as a completely new or "novel" virus. The genetic changes in viral genomes may result from **antigenic shift** (major changes that result in novel viral antigens) and/or **antigenic drift** (minor changes that occur continuously over time as the virus replicates). One of the most deadly influenza outbreaks was the Spanish flu pandemic of 1918 to 1919. This pandemic was associated with infection with a novel influenza virus of avian origin. After a period of adaptation in humans, the virus emerged in pandemic form and was responsible for more than 50 million deaths worldwide, including 500,000 in the United States. What was so different about this pandemic was that it affected young and healthy individuals, not just the very young or very old. The more recent influenza pandemic of the 20th century was associated with a human influenza virus in which genes reassorted in combination with an avian influenza virus. The most recent pandemic began in December 2019 and is caused by SARS-CoV-2, also known as COVID-19. This is a novel coronavirus originating in Wuhan, China and causes an acute respiratory distress syndrome, an extreme proinflammatory response, and multiorgan dysfunction.

Protection from viral infection has been successful for some viral pathogens. Vaccination (immunization) has proven to be a valuable tool in the control of viral diseases such as yellow fever and rabies and has been instrumental in the eradication of one of the most lethal viruses, smallpox. However, many viral diseases such as influenza, acquired immunodeficiency syndrome (AIDS), and hepatitis continue to pose challenges in treatment, prevention, and control.

The science of clinical virology has seen a rapid expansion in the past few years as new and emerging pathogenic viruses continue to evolve. The science of virology will continue to evolve, and clinicians will continue to rely on the laboratory scientist for the development and implementation of testing to diagnose, treat, and prevent viral disease.

General Characteristics

Viral Structure

Virus particles, referred to as **virions**, consist of two or three parts:

- An inner nucleic acid core, consisting of either ribonucleic acid (RNA) or deoxyribonucleic acid (DNA)
- A protein coat that surrounds and protects the nucleic acid (the **capsid**)
- In some of the larger viruses, a lipid-containing envelope that surrounds the virus

Because enveloped viruses are very susceptible to drying and destruction in the environment, they typically are transmitted by direct contact, such as respiratory, sexual, or parenteral contact. This prevents exposure to the environment and successful propagation of the viral agent to another susceptible host. Viruses that do not have an envelope are often referred to as **"naked" viruses.** Naked viruses are very resistant to environmental factors. Because of their stability, they typically are transmitted by the fecal-oral route. Many viruses have **glycoprotein spikes** extending from their surface. The term **nucleocapsid** is often used to describe the nucleic acid genome surrounded by a symmetric protein coat (Fig. 64.1).

The function of the nucleic acid genome is to encode the proteins required for viral penetration, transmission, and replication. The viral genome structure determines the mechanism for viral replication. A variety of viral genome structures exist, including (+) sense–strand RNA, (–) sense–strand RNA, and DNA genomes. In addition, viral genomes may be single- or double-stranded molecules. The structural implications of variation in genome organization are discussed in more detail in the section on viral replication.

The viral capsid protects the viral genome and is responsible for the tropism to specific cell types in naked viruses. Viral capsids typically are composed of repeating structural subunits referred to as **capsomeres.** The capsomeres associate to form the capsid and a characteristic symmetric structure. The most common capsid structures geometrically form a helical or icosahedral structure (Fig. 64.1). Icosahedral capsids are cubical and have 20 flat sides; irregularly shaped capsids usually assume a helical form and are spiral-shaped.

As mentioned, in some viruses the nucleocapsid is enclosed in a lipid envelope. The envelope is responsible for viral entry into the host cell (Fig. 64.1). During the infectious process, enveloped virions bud from a host cell's cytoplasmic, nuclear, or endoplasmic reticular membrane, and a portion of the membrane remains attached to the virion as the viral envelope. Inserted into this viral envelope are viral proteins, such as hemagglutinin (HA), neuraminidase, or glycoprotein spikes. The glycoprotein spikes assist in stabilization of attachment for the lipid envelope and for attachment to the host cell to facilitate viral entry. Some enveloped viruses also contain a **matrix protein** that lies between the envelope and the nucleocapsid. The matrix protein may have enzymatic activities or biologic functions related to infection, such as inhibition of host-cell transcription.

Viruses that cause disease in humans range from approximately 20 to 300 nm. Even the largest viruses, such as the poxviruses, cannot be detected with a light microscope, because they are less than one fourth the size of a staphylococcal cell (Fig. 64.2). Virus particles can be visualized using an electron microscope. This assists in the classification of viruses based on structural components.

Virus Taxonomy

Viral taxonomy is determined by the International Committee on Taxonomy of Viruses (ICTV) of the Virology Division of the International Union of Microbiological Societies. The ICTV report indicates that viral taxonomy consists of 14 Orders (name ending in -virales), 150 Families (-viridae), 79 Subfamilies (-virinae), 1019 Genera (-virus), and 5560 Species. Classification of viral species can be problematic and therefore is often polythetic; that is, the members of a group share common characteristics but may not

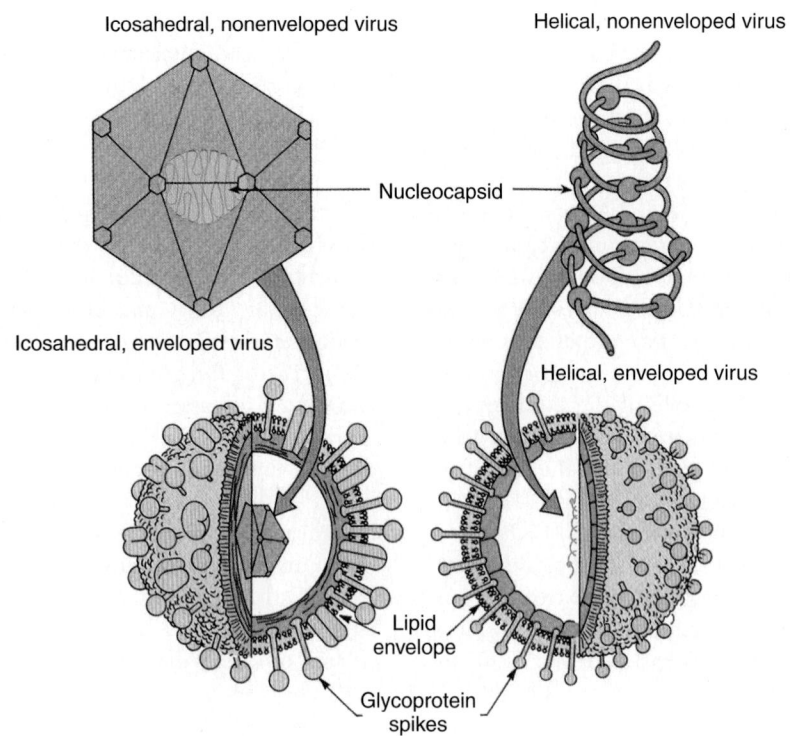

• **Fig. 64.1** A viral particle. Enveloped and nonenveloped virions have an icosahedral or irregular (usually helical) shape. (Modified from Murray PR, Drew WL, Kobayashi GS, et al, eds. *Medical Microbiology,* St Louis: Mosby; 1990.)

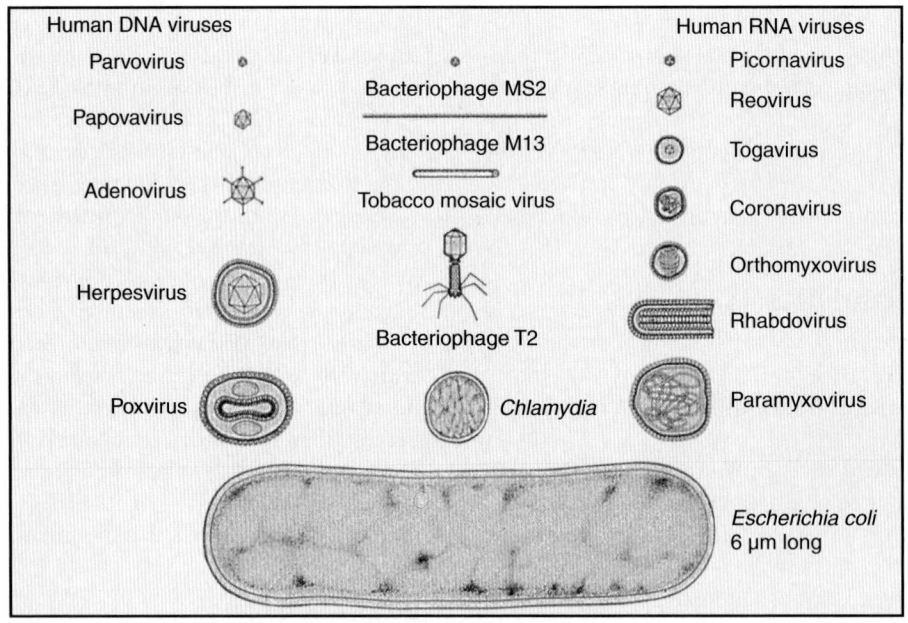

• **Fig. 64.2** Relative sizes of representative viruses, bacteriophages (bacterial viruses), and bacteria, including chlamydia. *DNA,* Deoxyribonucleic acid; *RNA,* ribonucleic acid. (From Murray PR, Drew WL, Kobayashi GS, et al, eds. *Medical Microbiology,* St Louis: Mosby; 1990.)

have a single defining characteristic. In addition, some viral families currently are not assigned to an order, and some species are not assigned to a family.

Complex viral taxonomy incorporates a variety of categories, including information related to host range, transmission, disease pathology, antigenicity, and viral particle properties, such as size, envelope, capsid structure, physical properties, genome type, and configuration. For simplicity purposes, many texts limit viral classification to three basic properties: (1) viral morphology; (2) method of

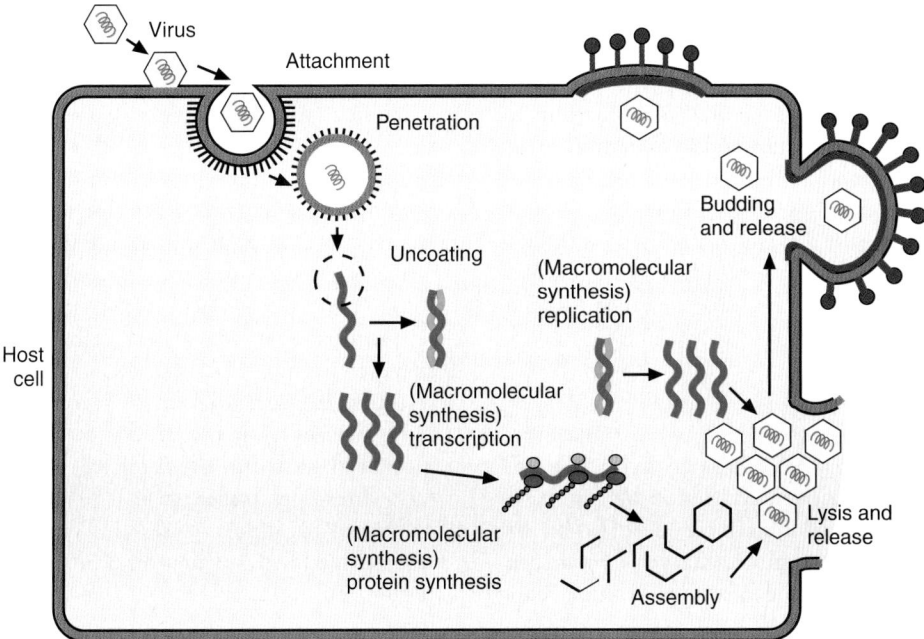

• **Fig. 64.3** The viral infectious cycle. (Modified from Murray PR, Drew WL, Kobayashi GS, et al., eds. *Medical Microbiology,* St Louis: Mosby; 1990.)

replication, including genome organization (whether the genome is RNA or DNA and single- or double-stranded); and (3) presence or absence of a lipid envelope. The phrase "means of replication" refers to the strategy the virus uses to duplicate the viral genome. For example, **enteroviruses** have single-stranded RNA genomes that synthesize additional strands of RNA, whereas **retroviruses** make RNA molecules in a two-step process by first synthesizing DNA, which subsequently is converted to RNA.

Characterization of viral genomes has increasingly improved because of advances in molecular techniques. Sequencing of viral nucleic acids, including entire DNA or RNA genomes, has become a routine procedure in the clinical research setting and has specific applications in the clinical diagnostic laboratory as well. Next-generation sequencing for the monitoring of viral therapy, resistance testing, outbreak management, characterization, and surveillance will continue to evolve. This is not without challenges to the clinical laboratory including the need for technical expertise, the cost of instrumentation, data analysis, and interpretations.

Viral Replication

Viruses are strict intracellular parasites that rely upon components of the host cell to replicate, and therefore are capable of replication only within a host cell. The six steps of virus replication, called the **infectious cycle,** proceed as follows (Fig. 64.3):

1. **Attachment,** also referred to as adsorption, is the first step of the infectious cycle. It involves recognition of a suitable host cell and specific binding between viral capsid proteins (often the glycoprotein spikes) and the carbohydrate receptor of the host cell. Each type of virus specifically recognizes and attaches to a specific type of host cell, allowing infection of some tissues but not others (viral tropism, as described previously).

2. **Penetration** (also referred to as virus entry) is the process by which viruses enter the host cell. One mechanism of penetration involves fusion of the viral envelope with the host cell membrane. This method not only provides a mechanism for internalizing the virus, but also leads to fusion between the infected host cell and additional nearby host cells, forming multinucleated cells called **syncytia.** Detection of syncytia can be used to determine the presence of virus in cell cultures or stained smears of clinical specimens. Other mechanisms of viral penetration include phagocytosis by host cells (endocytosis) or injection of viral nucleic acids into the host cell.

3. **Uncoating** occurs once the virus has been internalized. It is the process by which the capsid is removed; this may be by degradation of viral enzymes or host enzymes or by simple dissociation. Uncoating is necessary to release the viral genome for delivery of the viral DNA or RNA to its intracellular site of replication in the nucleus or cytoplasm.

4. **Macromolecular synthesis** involves the production of nucleic acids and protein polymers. Viral transcription leads to the synthesis of messenger RNA (mRNA), which encodes early and late viral proteins. Early proteins are nonstructural elements, such as enzymes, and late proteins are structural components. In addition, replication of viral nucleic acid is necessary to synthesize genomes that are incorporated into progeny virus particles. The mechanics of macromolecular synthesis varies depending on the organization of the viral genome (i.e., positive or negative sense RNA, single- or double-stranded nucleic acid genome).

5. **Viral assembly** is the process by which structural proteins, genomes, and in some cases viral enzymes are assembled into virus particles. Envelopes are acquired during viral "budding" from a host cell membrane. Nuclear endoplasmic reticulum and cytoplasmic membranes are common areas for budding. Acquisition of an envelope is the final step in viral assembly.

6. **Release** of intact virus particles occurs after cell lysis (**lytic virus**) or by virus particle **budding** from cytoplasmic membranes. Release by budding may not result in rapid host cell death, as does release by cell lysis.

Epidemiology

Viruses are transmitted from person to person by the respiratory, fecal-oral, and sexual contact routes; by trauma or injection with contaminated objects or needles; by tissue transplants (including blood transfusions); by arthropod or animal bites; and during gestation (transplacental transmission).

Pathogenesis and Spectrum of Disease

Once introduced into a host, the virus infects susceptible cells and the infectious cycle begins. Viral infections may produce one of three characteristic clinical presentations: (1) **acute viral infection,** displaying evident signs and symptoms; (2) **latent infection,** which has no visible signs and symptoms, but the virus is still present in the host cell in a **lysogenic state** (inserted into the host genome in a resting state) or maintained as a nuclear or cytoplasmic **episome;** and (3) **chronic or persistent infection,** in which low levels of virus are detectable and the degree of visible signs or symptoms varies.

After viral infection at a local, often mucosal site, **viremia** may occur (viruses disseminated in peripheral blood), which may serve to inoculate secondary target tissues distant from the primary site of infection. Secondary viremia may occur in a variety of tissues, such as the skin, salivary glands, kidneys, brain, and other central nervous system (CNS) tissues including the meninges. After peripheral dissemination, symptomatic disease may ensue. Disease resolves when specific antibody and cell-mediated immune mechanisms prevent continued replication, spread of the virus, and associated host immune responses (i.e., inflammation). Tissue is damaged during lysis of virus-infected cells or by immunopathologic mechanisms directed against the virus that are also destructive to neighboring tissue. Most DNA-containing viruses, such as those in the herpesvirus group, remain latent in host tissues with no observable signs or symptoms of disease. Retroviruses and most DNA viruses establish a latent state after primary infection. During the latent state, the viral genome is often integrated into the host cell's chromosome and no viral replication occurs. Latent viruses can reactivate silently, resulting in viral replication and shedding but no clinical symptoms, or they can reactivate and cause symptomatic, even fatal, disease. Reactivation may accompany immune suppression, resulting in the recurrence of clinically apparent disease.

Occasionally, pathogenic viruses stimulate an immune reaction that cross-reacts with antigenically similar components of the host tissues, resulting in impairment to host function; this is called **autoimmune pathogenesis.** When present, it occurs well after the acute viral infection has resolved and after antibodies are generated in response to viral antigens; this process takes several weeks to occur. In some cases, viral infection can promote **transformation** or **immortalization** of host cells through expression of specific viral proteins that affect the cell cycle, ultimately resulting in dysregulation or uncontrolled cell proliferation. Viruses with the ability to stimulate uncontrolled growth of host cells are referred to as **oncogenic viruses** (also known as **oncoviruses**). Several high-risk subtypes of human papillomaviruses (HPV) are oncogenic and are responsible for dysregulation of normal epithelial differentiation leading to cervical cancer and certain types of oral cancer.

The diverse variety of pathogenic mechanisms associated with viral infections is illustrated in the spectrum of disease caused by the measles virus. After replication in the upper respiratory tract and subsequent viremia, the virus infects many susceptible cell types throughout the body, including endothelial cells in capillaries of the skin. This is accompanied by local inflammation and results in the characteristic rash of measles. The immune system of immunocompetent individuals eradicates the virus, resolving the infection, resulting in lifelong immunity to reinfection. In some, antibody produced in response to the measles infection cross reacts with tissue in the CNS, causing a post-infectious encephalitis. In others, slow but continuing replication of damaged virus in the brain gives rise to **subacute sclerosing panencephalitis (SSPE).** In severely immunocompromised individuals, ongoing primary infection is not aborted by the usual immune mechanisms, and the outcome is death (Fig. 64.4).

Prevention and Therapy

Vaccines are a safe and reliable method for prevention of many disease-causing viruses. Immunizations are available for some human disease-causing viruses. In some cases, the vaccine produces a life-long immunological response that protects the individual from disease. Widespread vaccinations also provide population-level benefits, referred to as **herd immunity**, that protects individuals who are unable to be vaccinated due to age, allergies, or other health condition. Loss of herd immunity due to declines in vaccination rates can have severe consequences as demonstrated by recent outbreaks of measles across the United States. From January to April 2019, the Centers for Disease Control (CDC) reported 465 cases of measles in 19 states, from a virus that was completely eradicated endemically in the year 2000, as indicated by a zero incidence of cases over a 12-month period or longer.

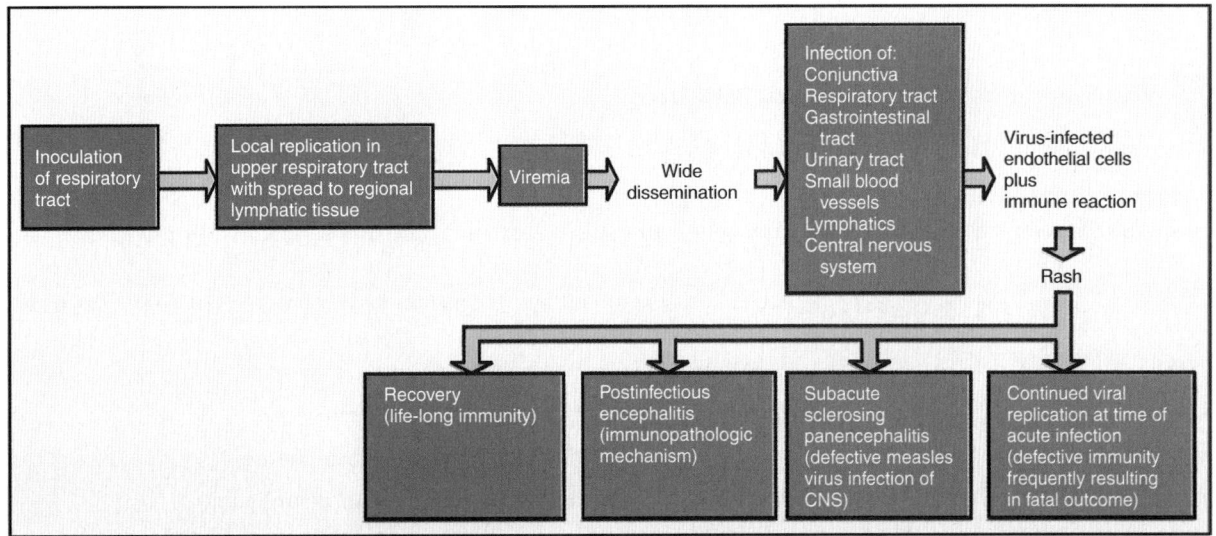

• **Fig. 64.4** Viral pathogenesis is illustrated by the mechanisms through which the measles virus spreads in the body. *CNS,* Central nervous system. (From Murray PR, Drew WL, Kobayashi GS, et al., eds. *Medical Microbiology,* St Louis: Mosby; 1990.)

However, for viruses for which there are no available vaccines, effective prevention involves regular, thorough hand washing and avoiding contact with others during episodes of evident signs of disease, such as fever, cough, diarrhea, and respiratory distress. For sexually transmitted viruses, prevention may also involve the use of condoms (male and female versions) during vaginal, anal, or oral sex.

Antiviral Agents

An increased understanding of viral structure and replication has improved the availability of therapeutic agents for the treatment of viral infections. More than 70 antiviral drugs are formally licensed for clinical use in the United States, and more than half of these are used in the combination treatment, termed **antiretroviral therapy (ART),** of human immunodeficiency virus (HIV) infections. Antivirals also are used in the treatment of hepatitis C virus (HCV), herpes viruses (herpes simplex virus [HSV], varicella-zoster virus [VZV], and cytomegalovirus [CMV]), hepatitis B virus (HBV), respiratory syncytial virus (RSV), and the influenza viruses. (Antiviral agents are reviewed in more detail in Chapter 65.)

Viruses That Cause Human Diseases

Hundreds of viruses that cause disease in humans are included in five orders: Bunyavirales, Herpesvirales, Mononegavirales, Nidovirales, and Picornavirales. The infections range in severity from completely asymptomatic to rapidly killing the human host. Individual viruses may cause several different diseases, and conversely, many viruses may cause the same disease, all of which complicates the understanding of viral disease in humans. For example, viruses that can cause encephalitis include HSV, many

arboviruses, rabies virus, HIV, measles virus, and others. However, HSV also can cause pharyngitis, genital infection, conjunctivitis, and encephalitis. Viruses that are important human pathogens and the viral syndromes they cause are summarized in Table 64.1. Specific viral agents and their role in human disease are discussed in Chapter 65.

Laboratory Diagnosis

Designing a Clinical Virology Laboratory

The demand for clinical virology laboratory services has skyrocketed due to the introduction of virus-specific antiviral drugs; the commercial availability of reagents; the development of rapid diagnostic techniques using conventional methods such as enzyme immunoassays (EIAs); the ready availability of cell lines for virus detection in cell cultures; and the widespread use of nucleic acid amplification tests for detecting viral infections. Ironically, improved medical care, in the form of organ transplantation and immune suppression with cancer therapy, has resulted in an increased number of patients with viral disease. When these factors are considered along with the appearance of emerging and re-emerging viral pathogens that are threatening local and world populations (e.g., SARS, avian influenza, Crimean-Congo fever, Ebola, Lassa, Nipah, Rift Valley fever, Zika, African Swine fever), laboratory diagnosis of viral infection becomes far more important than in previous years.

When determining which virology tests to offer, each clinical laboratory should decide whether the test is required for the appropriate care of the patient population and whether techniques are available that provide an accurate, cost-effective test result. Viral diseases that require laboratory diagnosis include sexually transmitted diseases, diarrhea, respiratory disease in adults and children, aseptic

TABLE 64.1 Viral Syndromes and Common Viral Pathogens

Viral Syndrome	Viral Pathogens
Infants and Children	
Upper respiratory tract infection	Rhinovirus, coronavirus, parainfluenza, adenovirus, respiratory syncytial virus, influenza
Pharyngitis	Adenovirus, coxsackie A, herpes simplex virus, Epstein-Barr virus, rhinovirus, parainfluenza, influenza
Croup	Parainfluenza, respiratory syncytial virus, metapneumovirus
Bronchitis	Parainfluenza, respiratory syncytial virus, metapneumovirus
Bronchiolitis	Respiratory syncytial virus, parainfluenza, metapneumovirus
Pneumonia	Respiratory syncytial virus, adenovirus, influenza, parainfluenza
Gastroenteritis	Rotavirus, adenovirus 40-41, calicivirus, astrovirus
Congenital and neonatal disease	HSV-2, echovirus, and other enteroviruses, CMV, parvovirus B19, VZV, HIV, hepatitis viruses, Zika
Adults	
Upper respiratory tract infection	Rhinovirus, coronavirus, adenovirus, influenza, parainfluenza, Epstein-Barr virus
Pneumonia	Influenza, adenovirus, sin nombre virus (hantavirus), severe acute respiratory syndrome (SARS), coronavirus
Pleurodynia	Coxsackie B
Gastroenteritis	Noroviruses
Cervical cancer and certain types of oral cancer	Human papillomavirus
All Patients	
Parotitis	Mumps, parainfluenza
Myocarditis/pericarditis	Coxsackie B and echoviruses
Keratitis/conjunctivitis	Herpes simplex virus, VZV, adenovirus, enterovirus 70
Pleurodynia	Coxsackie B
Herpangina	Coxsackie A
Febrile illness with rash	Echoviruses and coxsackie viruses
Infectious mononucleosis	Epstein-Barr virus and CMV
Meningitis	Echoviruses and coxsackie viruses, mumps, lymphocytic choriomeningitis, HSV-2
Encephalitis	HSV-1, togaviruses, bunyaviruses, flaviviruses, rabies, enteroviruses, measles, HIV, JCV
Hepatitis	Hepatitis A, B, C, D (delta agent), E, and non-A, B, C, D, E
Hemorrhagic cystitis	Adenovirus, BK virus
Cutaneous infection with or without rash	HSV-1 and HSV-2, VZV, enteroviruses, measles, rubella, parvovirus B-19, human herpes virus 6 and 7, HPV, poxviruses, including smallpox, monkeypox, molluscum contagiosum, and orf
Hemorrhagic fever	Ebola, Marburg, Lassa, yellow fever, dengue, and other viruses
Generalized, no specific target organ	HIV-1, HIV-2, HTLV-1

CMV, Cytomegalovirus; *HIV,* human immunodeficiency virus; *HPV,* human papillomavirus; *HSV-1,* herpes simplex virus type 1; *HSV-2,* herpes simplex virus type 2; *HTLV-1,* human T-lymphotropic virus type 1; *JCV,* JC virus; *VZV,* varicella-zoster virus.

meningitis, arbovirus encephalitis, congenital diseases, hepatitis, and infections in immunocompromised individuals.

Laboratory scientists in a clinical virology laboratory must be familiar with cell culture, EIA, immunofluorescence methods, molecular methods (e.g., polymerase chain reaction [PCR] and next generation sequencing), and mass spectrometry (MS) in addition to other common laboratory techniques (Table 64.2). Large equipment needed for a full-service virology laboratory includes a laminar flow biologic safety cabinet (BSC), fluorescence microscope, inverted bright field microscope, refrigerated centrifuge, incubator, refrigerator and freezer, roller drum for holding cell culture tubes during incubation, and enzymes for molecular testing instrumentation (Figs. 64.5 to 64.7). In addition, many clinical laboratories are becoming more automated with high-throughput instruments and robotic fluid handlers. This trend in automation is likely to continue with the goal of streamlining workflow, decreasing turn-around times, and improving service offerings.

Standard precautions and Biosafety Level 2 (BSL-2) conditions are needed for community and most nonretroviral laboratories. Regulatory requirements include standard microbiologic practices, training in biosafety, protective clothing and gloves, limited access, and decontamination of all infectious waste.

Many viruses are too dangerous and should never be propagated in a BSL-2 laboratory because of the risk of accidental exposure and lack of effective therapies, including influenza H5N1, SARS coronavirus, hemorrhagic fever viruses, and smallpox. Specialized high-containment laboratories (BSL-3 and BSL-4) exist at government facilities and some academic institutions that are dedicated and equipped to work with such agents, but they are generally not routinely used for clinical diagnostic purposes.

Specimen Selection and Collection
General Principles

Specimen selection depends on the specific disease syndrome, viral agents suspected, and time of year. Selecting a specimen based on symptoms is confusing, because most viruses enter through the upper respiratory tract and infect tissues that may produce symptoms distant from the primary inoculation site. For example, aseptic meningitis, caused by infection with various types of enterovirus (EV), may be identified by detecting virus in the throat, on a rectal swab, or in cerebrospinal fluid (CSF) specimens. Pharyngitis and gastrointestinal symptoms may not be among the patient's complaints upon clinical presentation.

Specimen selection based on the suspected viral agent is also complicated by the fact that similar clinical syndromes can be caused by many different viruses. When specimens required for identification of a specific virus are collected without thorough consideration of other possible viral and nonviral agents, additional important etiologic agents may be missed.

Selection of the appropriate type of specimen is one of the keys to a correct test result. Selection should include the proper specimen source and the correct sample volume and timing of collection. This information should be reviewed institutionally on an annual basis and made available to clinicians.

Appropriate specimen selection dictates that the specimen type and suspected viruses should be included on the requisition. The laboratory should always be notified if rare agents representing a danger to laboratory workers are suspected (e.g., SARS coronavirus, H5N1 avian influenza virus, hemorrhagic fever viruses). Serum for serologic testing may be necessary, and some viral diseases are more common during specific months. Table 64.3 presents specimens for the diagnosis of viral diseases, noting trends in seasonality.

Specimens for the detection of virus should be collected as early as possible after the onset of symptomatic disease. Virus may no longer be present as early as 2 days after the appearance of symptoms. However, other factors, such as the patient's immune status or age, the type of virus, and the amount of systemic involvement, may play a role in the length of time viral shedding is evident, allowing effective laboratory detection. Certain viruses, such as West Nile virus, produce a brief, low viremia and undetectable levels at the onset of symptoms. Recommendations for collection of various specimens are summarized in this section.

In addition to the type of specimen and collection method, validated devices or containers can enhance the recovery and detection of the viral agent. Swab specimens should not contain chemicals or other compounds that may be toxic to cultured cells and therefore are unsuitable for viral specimen collection. Calcium alginate swabs interfere with nucleic acid-based tests, the recovery of some enveloped viruses, and fluorescent-antibody tests and therefore should not be used.

Throat, Nasopharyngeal Swab, or Aspirate

In general, nasopharyngeal aspirates are superior to throat or nasopharyngeal swabs for recovering viruses; however, swabs are considerably more convenient. This is because most respiratory viruses replicate in the ciliated epithelial cells of the posterior nasopharynx. Throat swabs are acceptable for the recovery of EVs, adenoviruses, and HSV and for use in highly sensitive nucleic acid amplification tests (NAATs) whereas nasopharyngeal swabs or aspirate specimens are preferred for the detection of RSV and influenza and parainfluenza viruses. Rhinovirus detection requires a nasal specimen. Throat specimens are collected with a dry, sterile swab by passing the swab over the inflamed, vesiculated, or purulent areas on the posterior pharynx. The swab should not be touched to the tongue, buccal mucosa, teeth, or gums. Swabs should be polyester, Dacron, or rayon with plastic or aluminum shafts. Calcium alginate impairs the recovery of enveloped viruses, interferes with fluorescent-antibody tests, and are inhibitory to some NAATs. Flocked swabs made from nylon fiber are designed to optimize specimen absorption and release of respiratory epithelial cells for direct fluorescent testing of respiratory viruses. Nasopharyngeal secretion specimens are collected by inserting a swab

TABLE 64.2 **Diagnostic Methods for the Detection and Identification of Viruses**

Virus	NAAT	Culture	Antigen	Antibody	Pathology	Comments
Adenoviruses	P	A	P	A	A	NAAT is the most sensitive and can be used to monitor viral load. Antigen assays may be used for ocular, enteric, or respiratory adenoviruses.
Arboviruses	P, SP	SP	A	P, SP	NA	NAAT and antibody testing are useful in acute infection. Culture requires BSL-3 or BSL-4. NAAT not available except for West Nile virus.
Coronaviruses (SARS-CoV, SARS-CoV-2, Middle Eastern respiratory syndrome [MERS])	P, SP	SP	SP	SP	NA	NAAT and antibody testing, SARS-CoV and MERS testing is only available in public health or research laboratories. SARS-CoV-2 testing is available as an Emergency Use Authorization method in most large laboratories.
Cytomegalovirus (CMV)	P	A	A	P	A	NAAT most sensitive and can be used to determine viral load. IgM screen for recent infection and IgG to determine immune status.
Enteroviruses and parechoviruses	P	A	NA	NA	NA	NAAT more sensitive, preferred for CNS infections.
Epstein Barr virus (EBV)	P	NA	A	P	A	Serology is the preferred test for primary infection. NAAT is useful for monitoring viral load.
Filoviruses (Ebola or Marburg), and arenaviruses (lymphocytic choriomeningitis virus [LCMV], Lassa virus [LASV], others)	SP	SP	SP	P, SP	SP	NAAT is recommended. BSL-4 required for culture, except for LCMV.
Hantaviruses	SP	SP	SP	P	NA	NAAT and serology equally useful. BSL-4 required for culture.
Hepatitis A virus	NA	NA	NA	P	NA	Serology is standard testing.
Hepatitis B virus	P	NA	P	P	NA	Serology is used for diagnosis and monitoring course of infection. NAAT is used to monitor therapy and for genotype determination.
Hepatitis C virus	P	NA	A	P	NA	Serology used for diagnosis. NAAT confirms active infection and monitoring therapy. Genotype determination can be used to identify drug regimen and duration of therapy.
Hepatitis D virus	P	NA	P	P	NA	Testing confined to reference laboratories.
Hepatitis E virus	P, SP	NA	NA	P	NA	Serology is the standard diagnostic test. NAAT is required for transplant patients.
Herpes simplex virus	P	NA	NA	A	NA	NAAT is preferred method, especially in CSF. Serology is used to determine immune status.
Human immunodeficiency virus (HIV)	P	SP	P	P	NA	Serology is primary diagnostic method. NAAT are used to guide therapy and monitor response.

Continued

TABLE 64.2 Diagnostic Methods for the Detection and Identification of Viruses—cont'd

Virus	NAAT	Culture	Antigen	Antibody	Pathology	Comments
Human T-cell lympho-tropic virus (HTLV)	A	ND	NA	P	A	Serology is the primary diagnostic method. NAAT is useful when serology is indeterminate.
Influenza viruses	P	A	P	ND	ND	NAAT is the most sensitive. Serology is useful for epidemiological studies.
Noroviruses	P	NA	SP	NA	NA	NAAT is primarily recommended.
Parainfluenza viruses	P	A	P	NA	NA	NAAT is more sensitive and recommended.
Parvovirus B19	P	NA	SP	P	A	Serology is used in immunocompetent patients. NAAT is the test recommended in immunocompromised patients.
Rabies virus	SP	SP	SP	P	P, SP	Testing is completed in public health laboratories. NAAT and culture can be completed on saliva, CSF, and tissue. Serology is used to monitor antibody titers following vaccination.
Respiratory syncytial virus (RSV)	P	A	P	NA	NA	NAAT is the most sensitive. Rapid antigen testing may be useful in pediatric patients.
Rotaviruses	P	NA	P	NA	NA	Antigen testing has been routine; however, NAAT gastroenteritis panels are now more widely available.
Varicella zoster virus (VZV)	P	A	P	A	A	NAAT is the most sensitive. Serology is useful in determining immunity and can be used in CNS vasculopathy.

A, Alternative testing where the clinical utility may be limited to specific infections, clinical sample types, or other clinical indications; *BSL,* biosafety level; *CNS,* central nervous system; *NA,* test is not available, not generally used, or for research use only; *P,* preferred test for routine clinical diagnostics; *SARS,* severe acute respiratory syndrome; *SP,* testing is limited to public health laboratories or other specialized laboratory due to specialized testing or biosafety concerns.
Modified from Carroll KC, Pfaller MA, Landry ML, et al. *Manual of Clinical Microbiology.* 12th ed. Washington, DC: ASM; 2019.

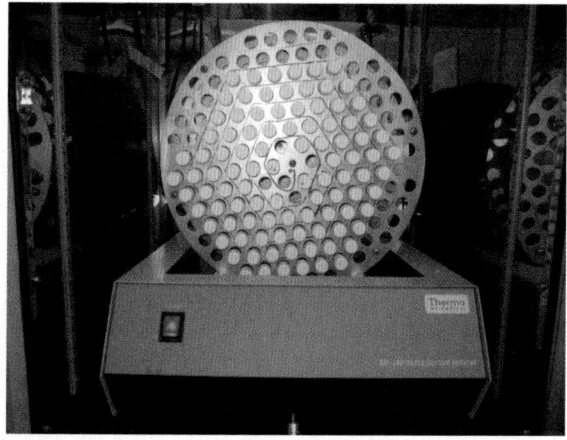

• **Fig. 64.5** Roller drum used to hold cell culture tubes during incubation. Slow rotation continually bathes the cells in the medium.

with a flexible shaft through the nostril into the nasopharynx or by washing and collecting the secretions by rinsing with a bulb syringe and 3 to 7 mL of buffered saline. The saline is squirted into the nose by squeezing the bulb and aspirated with small tubing that is inserted into the other nostril when the bulb or suction is released. Self-collected foam nasal swabs have demonstrated improved sensitivity over nasal washes for the detection of several viruses from respiratory viruses by NAAT.

Bronchial and Bronchoalveolar Washes

Washings and lavage fluid collected during bronchoscopy are excellent specimens for detecting viruses that infect the lower respiratory tract, especially influenza viruses and adenoviruses. Sputum may be acceptable for identification of viral pathogens using NAATs. Respiratory fluids or swabs in viral transport media should be centrifuged to remove contaminating materials. The supernatant can be used for culture. Further clarification may be completed using filtration. This process may result in the removal of virus infected cells and reduce the recovery of viral agents from the sample. It is not necessary to remove contamination in samples for antigen and nucleic acid testing.

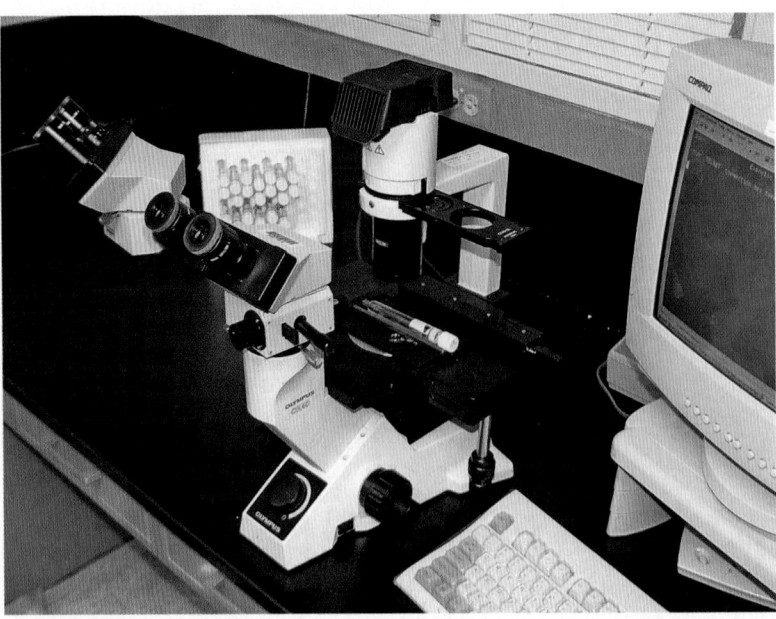

• **Fig. 64.6** Inverted microscope used to examine cell monolayers growing attached to the inside surface beneath the liquid medium. Note that the objective is under the glass test tube, facilitating observation of the cell monolayer.

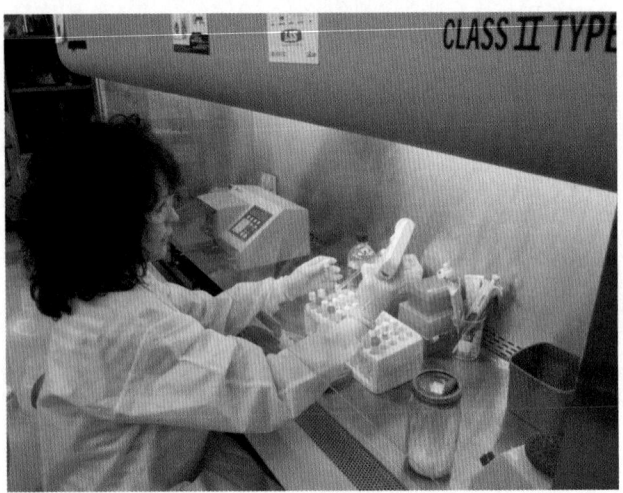

• **Fig. 64.7** Class II biologic safety cabinet used in a clinical virology laboratory.

Rectal Swabs and Stool Specimens

Stool and rectal swabs of fecal specimens are used to detect rotavirus, enteric adenoviruses (serotypes 40 and 41), and EVs. Many agents of viral gastroenteritis do not grow in cell culture and require antigen or NAAT for detection. In general, stool specimens are preferable to rectal swabs and should be required for rotavirus and enteric adenovirus testing. Rectal swabs are acceptable for detecting EVs in patients suspected of having an enteroviral disease, such as aseptic meningitis. The rectal swab is inserted 3 to 5 cm into the rectum and rotated against the mucosa to obtain feces. The swab should then be placed in appropriate transport media. A stool sample is preferred over a rectal swab because of the potential for decreased viral recovery from a small sample size. Five to 10 mL of freshly passed diarrheal stool or stool collected in a diaper from young infants is sufficient and preferred for rotavirus and enteric adenovirus detection.

Due to bacterial contamination of stool, centrifugation, filtration, or both are necessary for cell cultures for the recovery of viral agents.

Urine

CMV, mumps, rubella, and measles viruses, polyomaviruses, and adenoviruses can all be detected in urine, though these viruses are often shed intermittently or in low numbers. Viral recovery may be increased by processing multiple (two to three) specimens in parallel. Improved recovery results with a minimum specimen volume of 10 mL. The urine pH and contaminating bacteria may interfere with viral replication. Virus recovery in cell culture is improved by centrifugation or filtering to remove contaminants and neutralizing the pH with a 7.5% solution of sodium bicarbonate or diluting the sample with viral transport media. Ambient storage of urine should be minimized for NAAT. Nucleic acids are rapidly degraded in urine due to the low pH and high urea content. Extraction of nucleic acids is required prior to testing to prevent inhibition by additional substances commonly found in urine samples.

Skin and Mucous Membrane Lesions

EVs, HSV, VZV, and in rare cases CMV or pox viruses can be detected in vesicular lesions of the skin and mucous membranes. Once the vesicle has ulcerated or crusted, detection of the virus is difficult using culture, antigen, or NAAT.

Collection of fluid specimens from vesicles can be completed using a capillary pipette, syringe, or swab placed in viral transport media. A tuberculin syringe can be used to

TABLE 64.3   Specimens for Diagnosis of Viral Diseases

Disease Categories and Probable Viral Agent	Season of Most Common Occurrence	Throat/ Nasopharynx	Stool	CSF	Urine	Other
Respiratory						
Adenoviruses	Y	++++				
Influenza virus	W	++++				
Parainfluenza virus	Y	++++				
Respiratory syncytial virus (RSV)	W	++++				
Metapneumovirus	W	++++				
Rhinoviruses	Y					Nasal (+++)
SARS coronavirus	W	++++				
Sin nombre virus	SP, S					Serum
Dermatologic and Mucous Membrane						
Vesicular						
Enterovirus	S, F	++	+++			Vesicle fluid or scraping
Herpes simplex virus[a]	Y					Vesicle fluid or scraping
Varicella-zoster virus[a]	Y	++				Vesicle fluid or scraping
Monkeypox	Y					Vesicle fluid or scraping
Exanthematous						
Enterovirus	S, F	+++	++			
Measles	Y	++			++	Serum
Rubella	Y				++	Serum
Parvovirus	Y					Serum, amniotic fluid
Pustular/Nodular						
Molluscum contagiosum, orf	Y					Tissue
Warts Papillomavirus	Y					Tissue/cells, thin-prep cervical
Meningoencephalitis/Encephalitis						
Arboviruses	S, F					CSF and serum
Enteroviruses	S, F	+++		++	++++	
Herpes simplex virus	Y			++++		Brain biopsy
Lymphocytic choriomeningitis	Y					Serum
Mumps virus	Y					Serum
HIV	Y					Brain biopsy
Polyomavirus (JC virus)	Y					Brain biopsy
Rabies virus	Y					Corneal cells, brain
Gastrointestinal Disease						
Adenoviruses (serotypes 40–41)	Y		++++			Stool
Noroviruses	S		++++			Stool
Rotavirus	W, SP		++++			Stool

TABLE 64.3	Specimens for Diagnosis of Viral Diseases—cont'd					
Disease Categories and Probable Viral Agent	Season of Most Common Occurrence	Throat/ Nasopharynx	Stool	CSF	Urine	Other
Dermatologic and Mucous Membrane						
Congenital and Perinatal						
Cytomegalovirus	Y				+++	Serum
Enteroviruses	S, F	+++		+++	+++	
Herpes simplex virus	Y					Vesicle fluid
Parvovirus	Y					Amniotic fluid, liver tissue
Rubella	Y				++	Serum
Zika	Y				++++	Serum (+++)
Eye (Ocular Disease)						
Adenoviruses	Y	++				Conjunctival swab or scraping
Herpes simplex virus	Y					Conjunctival swab or scraping
Varicella-zoster virus	Y					Conjunctival swab or scraping
Posttransplantation Syndrome						
Cytomegalovirus	Y				++	Blood (++++) tissue (++++)
Epstein-Barr virus	Y					Blood, tissue
Human herpesvirus-6 (HH6)	Y					Blood
Herpes simplex	Y					Tissue (+++)
BK virus	Y				++++	
Myocarditis, Pericarditis, and Pleurodynia						
Coxsackie B	S, F	+++		++		Pericardial fluid (++++)
Hemorrhagic Fevers						
Ebola/Marburg viruses	Y					Tissue, respiratory secretions, and serum
Lassa fever virus	Y	+++			+	Serum and throat washes
Hepatitis						
Hepatitis	Y					Blood

aDirect fluorescent antibody studies are available for herpes simplex virus and varicella-zoster virus.
Specimens indicated beside specific viruses should be obtained if that specific virus is suspected (++++, most appropriate; +, least appropriate).
CSF, Cerebrospinal fluid; F, fall; HIV, human immunodeficiency virus; S, summer; SARS, severe acute respiratory syndrome; SP, spring; W, winter; Y, year-round.

aspirate fluid from the vesicle. The needle is flushed with a viral transport medium prior to aspiration. Cleaning the area with an antiseptic such as an iodophor or alcohol may inactivate the virus. Antisepsis should therefore be performed after the aspiration of the sample, If the sample is collected using a swab, the vesicle should be unroofed (remove the crust) with a sterile needle or scalpel. The swab should be rolled over the base and margin of the lesion to collect virally infected epithelial cells and placed in viral transport media. Caution should be taken to not cause bleeding, as antibodies present in the blood may neutralize the virus interfering with cultivation. Samples may be used for culture, antigen, or NAAT.

Sterile Body Fluids Other Than Blood

Sterile body fluids, especially CSF and pericardial and pleural fluids, may contain EVs, HSV, VZV, influenza viruses, or

CMV. These specimens are collected aseptically by the physician and sent to the laboratory for processing. CSF samples collected by lumbar puncture for NAAT should not be centrifuged prior to nucleic acid extraction. Extraction should be completed prior to testing to eliminate antibodies, proteins, and other potential inhibitors of molecular amplification enzymes. CSF and other sterile body fluids are not diluted with viral transport media as it may cause false negative results. In addition, fluid specimens contaminated with blood may inhibit viral cultivation due to the presence of antibodies.

Viral infections may occur during pregnancy that may cause serious disease in the fetus or newborn. Amniotic fluid is collected by amniocentesis. NAAT is the most common method used for accurate diagnosis of congenital CMV infections, VZV, or parvovirus B19. If testing is delayed, the nucleic acids should be extracted and refrigerated up to 48 hours or frozen at –70°C. The samples may also be used for culture, but sensitivity is significantly lower than NAAT.

Blood serum, plasma, purified peripheral blood leukocytes, and whole blood may be used for viral detection. Viral culture of blood is used primarily to detect CMV; however, HSV, VZV, EVs, and adenovirus occasionally may be encountered. CMV viremia is associated with peripheral blood leukocytes. Five to ten milliliters of anticoagulated blood collected in a whole blood tube is needed. Heparinized or ethylenediaminetetraacetic acid (EDTA) anticoagulated blood is acceptable for CMV detection. Leukocyte fractionation should occur within 8 hours of collection. Density gradient methods that include centrifugation are commercially available for the removal of erythrocytes that would be inhibitory to viral replication in culture.

EDTA and citrated blood should be used for samples collected for nucleic acid testing, because other anticoagulants may interfere with the enzyme functions required for NAATs. Serum may be used for serologic tests and nucleic acid assays. If whole blood is used for NAAT, heme and the metabolic precursors for heme must be removed prior to testing. Many commercial extraction protocols include the reagents and processes to remove these components.

Dried Blood Spots

Dried blood samples can be used for the detection of viral antibodies as well as NAAT. Samples can be collected from a capillary finger stick and air dried for 2 hours. Once dried, the sample is placed in a hermetically sealed bag or container containing a desiccant to avoid exposure to moisture and prevent the growth of any contaminating bacteria. Samples may be transported at room temperature, refrigerated, or frozen at –20°C or lower.

Bone Marrow

Bone marrow for virus detection should be added to a sterile tube with anticoagulant. Heparin or EDTA anticoagulants are acceptable for culture. EDTA or ACD (anticoagulant citrate dextrose solution) should be used if the specimen is intended for nucleic acid testing. Specimens are collected by aspiration and should be processed for the fractionation of leukocytes as soon as possible. Bone marrow specimens for NAAT may be refrigerated if processing is delayed. Freezing and thawing will result in cell lysis releasing heme and other cellular components that are inhibitory to NAATs. Nucleic acids must be extracted prior to NAAT methods.

Tissue

Tissue specimens are especially useful for detecting viruses that commonly infect the lungs (CMV, influenza virus, adenovirus, sin nombre virus), brain (HSV), and gastrointestinal tract (CMV). Other viruses may be identified from the liver, lymph nodes, kidney, spleen, or cardiac tissue. Specimens are collected during surgical procedures. Fresh tissue is required for culture and is preferred for nucleic acid assays, but formalin-fixed and paraffin-embedded tissues may be used after removal of the paraffin (deparaffinization) and extraction. The stability of nucleic acids in tissue varies with viral and tissue type. Samples should be transported to the laboratory on wet ice or frozen. Tissue should be minced and digested with proteolytic enzymes prior to nucleic acid extraction. Fresh tissue for viral cultivation should be homogenized in viral transport media and centrifuged to remove unwanted cellular debris. The supernatant is then used to inoculate the viral culture.

Genital Specimens

Genital specimens often are required for detection of HSV and HPV. Genital lesions or ulcerations should be collected and processed as previously described for skin lesions and placed in appropriate viral transport media. Cervical specimens may be collected using a swab or brush and placed in viral transport media. Most manufactured endocervical or liquid-based cytology devices are appropriate for nucleic acid testing. Following the manufacturer's recommended protocols is essential when processing such specimens. Anal specimens should be collected using a Dacron swab moistened with saline and transported in liquid cytology media for the detection of HPV.

Oral

Some viral infections are transmitted in oral secretions and can be detected from oral mucosal cells, saliva, glandular duct salvia, or oral mucosal transudates. These samples can be used for culture or NAATs. Salivary gland fluid may also be used for the detection of viral antibodies including secretory IgA, IgM, and IgG. Samples are collected using a sputum collection device, swab, or spatula and placed in transport media.

Serum for Antibody Testing

Acute and convalescent serum specimens may be needed to detect antibody to specific viruses. Acute specimens should be collected as soon as possible after the appearance of symptoms. The convalescent specimen is collected a minimum of 2 to 3 weeks after the acute specimen. In both cases, an appropriate specimen is 3 to 5 mL of serum collected by venipuncture. Serum can be stored for hours or days at 4°C or for weeks or months at −20°C or lower before testing. Testing for virus-specific IgM should be completed before freezing whenever possible, because IgM may form insoluble aggregates upon thawing, producing a false-negative result.

Specimen Transport and Storage

Ideally all specimens collected for detection of virus should be processed immediately. Specimens for viral isolation should not be allowed to sit at room or higher temperature. Specimens should be kept cool (4°C) and immediately transported to the laboratory. If a delay in transport is unavoidable, the specimen should be refrigerated, not frozen, until processed. Every attempt should be made to process the specimen within 12 to 24 hours of collection. Under unusual circumstances, specimens may need to be held for several days before processing and should be stored based on specimen type as previously indicated in this chapter.

If a commercial kit is used for viral identification (e.g., nucleic acid testing), the specimens should be transported and stored according to the manufacturer's instructions.

Commercially prepared transport media are useful for maintaining viral stability. They are used to transport small volumes of fluid specimens, small tissues and scrapings, and swab specimens, especially when contamination with microbial flora is expected. Transport media contain protein (e.g., serum, albumin, or gelatin) to stabilize the viral agents and antimicrobials to prevent overgrowth of bacteria and fungi. Penicillin (500 units/mL) and streptomycin (500 to 1000 µg/mL) have been used traditionally; however, a more potent mixture is composed of vancomycin (20 µg/mL), gentamicin (50 µg/mL), and amphotericin (10 µg/mL). If serum is added as the protein source, fetal calf serum is recommended, because it is less likely to contain inhibitors, such as antibodies. Examples of successful transport media include Stuart's medium; Amie's medium; Leibovitz-Emory medium; Hanks' balanced salt solution (HBSS); Eagle's tissue culture medium; and the commercially available M4, M5, and universal transport media. Respiratory and rectal and stool specimens can be maintained in modified Stuart's medium, modified HBSS, or Leibovitz-Emory medium containing antimicrobials.

Specimen Processing
General Principles

Specimens for viral culture should be processed immediately upon receipt in the laboratory. This may be accomplished by combining bacteriology and virology processing responsibilities. Although the threat of cell culture contamination in the past dictated separation of virology procedures, the addition of broad-spectrum antimicrobials to cell cultures has significantly reduced the possibility of cross-contamination with bacteria and fungi. In most laboratories, processing with other microbiology specimens allows viral cultures to be processed 7 days a week. If delays must occur, specimens should be stored in a viral transport medium at 4°C as

described previously. Delay in the processing of fluid specimens requires dilution in a transport medium (1:2 to 1:5) before storage.

In addition to patient identification and demographics, each specimen for virus isolation or identification should be accompanied by a requisition that provides (1) the source of the specimen; (2) the clinical history or viruses suspected; and (3) the date and time of specimen collection. If this information is not available, a call for additional details should be made to the requesting physician or to the person caring for the patient.

Viral specimens should be processed in a BSL-2 or BSL-3 dependent on suspected viral agent. (Fig. 64.7). This protects specimens from contamination by the processing technologist and protects those in the laboratory from infectious aerosols created when specimens are manipulated. When patient cell cultures are manipulated, such as during inoculation or feeding (exchange of cell culture medium), only one patient sample or series of cell culture tubes should be open at one time. Aerosols and microsplashes contribute to cross-contamination of cultures, especially during viral respiratory season when a high percentage of specimens are positive for influenza virus, RSV, and other viruses.

Processing virology specimens for culture is not complicated (Table 64.4). In general, any primary specimen or swab specimen that may be contaminated with bacteria or fungi should be added to a viral transport medium. Normally sterile body fluids can be inoculated directly to cell culture. Sterile body fluid specimens, whether in viral transport medium or not, should be vortexed immediately before inoculation to break up virus-containing cells and resuspend the inoculum. Adding sterile glass beads to the transport medium helps break up cell clumps and release virus from cell aggregates. This may not be necessary, because some commercially available mediums already contain beads. Grossly contaminated or potentially toxic specimens, such as minced or ground tissue, can be centrifuged ($1000 \times g$ for 15 minutes) and the virus-containing supernatant may be used as the inoculum. Each viral cell culture tube should be inoculated with 200 to 400 µL of specimen. If insufficient specimen is available, the specimen obtained should be diluted with a viral transport medium to increase the volume. Excess specimen can be stored at −70°C in the event the initial culture is contaminated. A set of uninoculated cultures should be maintained simultaneously for continual monitoring of sterility and contamination throughout the process.

Contaminated specimens can be reprocessed with an antibiotic-containing viral transport medium if they were not originally handled in this manner, or they can be filtered using a disposable 0.22 to 0.45 µm filter, and the filtrate can be recultured. In practice, virus is rarely detected in culture from most specimens requiring reprocessing. When these specimens are processed, the specimen should be allowed to adsorb in an incubator at 35°C to 37°C for 30 to 60 minutes; 1 to 1.5 mL of maintenance medium should be added, and the tubes returned to the incubator, preferably

TABLE
64.4 **Laboratory Processing of Viral Specimens for Cell Culture**

Source	Specimen	Processing[a]	Cells for Detection of Common Viruses
Blood	Anticoagulated blood	Separate leukocytes (Evolve Procedure 64.1).	PMK, HDF, HEp-2
Cerebrospinal fluid (CSF)	1 mL CSF	Inoculate directly.	PMK, HDF, HEp-2
Stool or rectal swab	Pea-sized aliquot of feces	Place in 2 mL of viral transport medium vortex. Centrifuge at 1000× g for 15 min and use supernatant fluid for inoculum.	PMK, HDF, HEp-2
Genital, skin	Vesicle fluid or scraping	Emulsify in viral transport medium.	HDF
Miscellaneous	Swab, fluids	Emulsify in viral transport medium. Fluid, inoculate directly.	PMK, HDF, HEp-2
Respiratory tract	Nasopharyngeal secretions, throat swab, respiratory tract washings, sputum	Dilute with viral transport medium.	PMK, HDF, HEp-2
Tissue	Tissue in sterile container	Mince with sterile scalpel and scissors and gently grind. Prepare 20% suspension in viral transport medium. Centrifuge at 1000× g for 15 min and use supernatant fluid for inoculum.	PMK, HDF, HEp-2
Urine	Midstream specimen	Clear: Inoculate directly. Turbid: Centrifuge at 1000× g for 15 min and use supernatant fluid for inocula.	HDF, HEp-2 (if adenovirus suspected)

[a]All inocula into tissue culture tubes are 0.25 mL volumes.
HDF, Human diploid fibroblast; *HEp-2*, human epidermoid; *PMK*, primary monkey kidney.

in a roller rack in a rotating drum. Blood for viral culture requires special processing to isolate leukocytes, followed by inoculation into cell culture tubes (Evolve Procedure 64.1). Rapid shell vial cell cultures are used to detect many viruses. (Handling and examination of cell cultures after inoculation with specimen are discussed later in this chapter.)

Specimens used for NAAT may need to be processed and the extraction of nucleic acids may be necessary prior to storage to prevent degradation of nucleic acids as previously described in this chapter.

Processing Based on Requests for Specific Viruses

Arboviruses

Arboviruses are a group of viruses that are transmitted by mosquitoes, ticks, or other arthropods resulting in a spectrum of disease, from mild viral syndrome to encephalitis. There are several viral antigen tests available for use in the field in endemic areas. Positive field tests should be confirmed using either serologic or NAATs. Diagnosis of arbovirus encephalitis, such as Eastern, Western, Venezuelan,

St. Louis, and California encephalitis; and La Crosse, West Nile, and Zika virus infection requires detection of virus-specific IgM antibody in serum or a rise in IgG antibody titer in paired sera. Detection of virus-specific IgM in CSF is available for most agents. Culture of arboviruses for diagnostic purposes is not practical.

Several types of NAAT for some agents are available through state public health laboratories, specialized reference and academic laboratory. NAATs may be less sensitive than serodiagnosis because the virus and the viral nucleic acid are only detectable for brief periods during infection. In addition, the efficiency of the extraction and purification of the target RNA can significantly impact the sensitivity of the assay.

Cytomegalovirus

CMV can be detected in clinical specimens using conventional cell culture, shell vial assay, antigenemia immunoassay, or NAAT methods. CMV produces **cytopathic effects (CPEs)** in diploid fibroblast cells in 3 to 28 days, averaging

7 days. Sensitivity of the CMV shell vial assay is equivalent to conventional cell culture, and results are available within 16 hours. The antigenemia immunoassay uses monoclonal antibody in an indirect immunoperoxidase enzymatic reaction or indirect immunofluorescent stain to detect CMV protein (pp65) in peripheral blood leukocytes. The antigenemia assay requires 2 to 4 hours and includes the sedimentation and separation of leukocytes, counting of leukocytes, and a standardized density smear preparation, followed by staining and counting of infected (fluorescing) cells (Evolve Procedure 64.2). Results are reported as the number of positive leukocytes per total number of leukocytes in the smear. Several quantitative CMV PCR testing platforms are also available for detection and quantitation of CMV viremia. Molecular assays have replaced the antigenemia assay in some laboratories. The quantitation of CMV-DNA is the best predictor of CMV disease. It is essential in the diagnosis of disease in immunocompromised patients. CMV DNA can be detected in whole blood, peripheral blood leukocytes, plasma, and serum by PCR. Qualitative assays may also be useful in unique cases including the use of saliva, urine, tissue, amniotic fluid, or fetal blood for the diagnosis of congenital infection and aqueous or vitreous humor for the detection of CMV retinitis. A negative qualitative result is highly predictive of the absence of systemic CMV disease or tissue-invasive infection. Although there seems to be some agreement between antigenemia assays and quantitative CMV DNA assays, there are differences because the assays measure different features of the virus. Because of the variation between samples, patient populations, and thresholds for predicting disease in different laboratories, it is important for the laboratory to monitor the relative changes in a specific patient using the same assay and specimen type over time. Molecular methods are essential in establishing criteria for patients developing disease, monitoring therapy, and predicting viral resistance.

Enteroviruses and Parechoviruses

Molecular sequencing of viruses has effectively redefined the organization and classification of viruses traditionally included in this group. Some of the viruses initially included in the EVs have now been reclassified as parechovirus (PeV). Both the EVs and PeVs are capable of causing many localized and systemic infections. These viruses can be detected using conventional cell culture and NAATs. A combination of human and primate cell lines are used to isolate EV and PeV viruses, although no single cell line supports the growth of all viruses. To reduce waste and provide availability when needed, frozen "ready cells" (Diagnostic Hybrids, Athens, OH) may be used. Ready cells may be stored for up to 5 months and demonstrate comparable results as fresh cells. Presumptive diagnosis is based on CPEs. Confirmation or definitive diagnosis is accomplished using commercially available FA stains.

NAAT is the preferred method for the detection and diagnosis of infections with EV and PeV. Some viruses fail to grow in cell culture or propagation methods are unknown.

In addition, NAAT detection for EVs has improved patient care, demonstrating a clear correlation of improved outcomes when comparing time to result and length of hospital stays. This is significant in cases of EV septic meningitis. There are FDA approved real-time assays available for the detection of EV in CSF for the detection of meningitis, including the Cepheid Xpert and the BioFire Meningitis/Encephalitis (ME) Panel.

Epstein-Barr Virus

Serologic tests are useful in the diagnosis of Epstein-Barr virus (EBV)–associated diseases, including infectious mononucleosis, and remains the method of choice. There are a variety of assays available that differ in the methodology, antigens, and antibody isotype included in the test. Isolation of EBV (in cultured B lymphocytes) is not routinely performed in clinical laboratories. Cellular tropism of EBV in the peripheral blood in patients with high, persistent viral loads are being examined using cell phenotyping and flow cytometry. These assays are currently not available in routine diagnostic laboratories.

NAAT is used for quantitative direct detection of EBV DNA. The World Health Organization has approved an international standard for EBV which is a whole virus preparation produced by the National Institute for Biological Standards and Controls (United Kingdom). This standard should be extracted in the same matrix as the clinical sample simultaneously to properly quantitate the viral DNA in the patient sample. Although the creation of an international standard has reduced the variability associated with the use of molecular methods in the diagnosis of EBV infections, other limitations remain including the variability in commercial reagents and gene targets used in the assays. Patient results with low viremia tend to show the greatest variation in results. It is therefore recommended that viral DNA values should be at least threefold to be considered significant to changes in viral replication. If the assay values are very close or near the limit of detection of the specific assay, viral load changes may only be significant if greater than 5-fold differences are noted. Extraction, contamination, and inhibition controls should also be included in the assay along with the EBV standard.

Hepatitis Viruses

Disease or asymptomatic carriage caused by hepatitis A, B, C, D, and E viruses is detected using serology, antigen detection, or NAAT. Even though hepatitis viruses are not routinely cultured, a variety of diagnostic tests are available for the detection of antibody and antigen. Hepatitis A, usually transmitted through contaminated food and water, is diagnosed by screening for the IgM antibody using serologic methods. HAV RNA can be detected in blood and stool and is useful in the diagnosis of early infections especially in cases with questionable serologic results. Hepatitis B produces acute and chronic infection and is associated with hepatocellular carcinoma; it is transmitted parenterally and by tattooing, acupuncture, sexual contact, and perinatal infection.

Several HBV-specific antigens can be detected in a patient during infection. The diagnosis of hepatitis B infection uses a combination of antigen and antibody detection and NAAT. Serologic diagnosis of hepatitis B infection is made through the quantitation of antibody that includes the antibody to the surface, core, and e antigens. The first marker to appear in acute infection is the hepatitis B surface antigen (HBsAg); as the infection resolves, HBsAg disappears and hepatitis B surface antibody (HBsAb) appears. NAAT are used to quantify HBV DNA to evaluate infections and monitor patients with chronic infections during treatment. In addition, there are patients who are infected with immune escape mutants that do not test positive by serological methods requiring HBV DNA testing to exclude low-level carrier states. Molecular methods are used to determine HBV DNA levels and to assist in establishing the stage of disease as well as monitoring patients on anti-viral therapy.

Hepatitis C is an RNA virus transmitted by blood transfusion, intravenous drug abuse, hemodialysis, and contaminated instruments, such as body piercing and tattooing devices. HCV infection becomes chronic in more than 80% of patients. The diagnosis is typically made by antibody detection followed by HCV RNA NAAT to determine the status of viral replication. The detection of HCV viral RNA is the primary determining factor to diagnose chronic infection. HCV RNA can also be measured quantitatively by PCR to assess the patient's response to antiviral therapies. HDV infection can be detected using serologic screening assays. A positive result may indicate acute or chronic infection and should be followed by an HDV RNA test. HEV RNA detection and quantification by PCR is the gold standard for the diagnosis of acute infection.

Herpes Simplex and Herpes B Virus

HSV type 1 and 2 cause a variety of infections including gingivostomatitis, fever, oral lesions, genital lesions, and lymphadenopathy. Herpes B virus is very similar to HSV in terms of structure, morphology, and viral replication and can cause serious illness including myelitis and encephalitis with a mortality rate of greater than 70% if left untreated. HSV grows rapidly in most cell lines. MRC-5 or mink lung fibroblast cell lines are recommended, along with a continuous cell line such as A-549. Ready cells, as previously described, are also available for the cultivation of herpes viruses. Fifty percent of genital HSV isolates are detected within 24 hours and 100% within 3 to 5 days. Cultures should be examined daily and finalized if negative after 5 days of incubation. The enzyme-linked viral-induced system (ELVIS; Diagnostic Hybrids, Athens, OH) is a special shell vial system available for detection of HSV in 24 hours. When the cells become infected with HSV, they accumulate beta-galactosidase. After incubation, the shell vial is fixed and stained with substrate for beta-galactosidase, resulting in a visible blue color change that can be viewed using an inverted microscope. This technique is described in more detail later in this chapter. In addition, type-specific serology tests, such as HerpeSelect (Focus Diagnostics, Cypress, CA) are also available.

NAAT are the most sensitive methods for the detection of HSV. There are a variety of qualitative and quantitative FDA approved molecular HSV assays available. Molecular detection is extremely useful in the detection of virus in CSF. Viral quantification can be used to monitor response to antiviral therapy in severe infections such as HSV encephalitis and neonatal infections. Molecular methods for the detection of HSV are preferentially used in many laboratories; however, conventional culture remains useful in the diagnosis of herpes in mucocutaneous, genital, and ocular lesions.

Human Immunodeficiency Virus and Other Retroviruses

HIV type 1 (HIV-1) is detected using serologic methods (i.e., antibody or antigen) and molecular methods (reverse transcriptase PCR [RT-PCR]). HIV-1 enzyme-linked immunosorbent assay (ELISA) antibody tests also detect antibody to HIV type 2 (HIV-2). The ELISA screening test is no longer confirmed with an HIV-1–specific Western blot test or with an ELISA for HIV-2 followed by an HIV-2–specific Western blot test. Recently infected patients may test as a false negative or indeterminate result using these methods. In addition, HIV-2 may be misidentified as HIV-1 in serologic methods. The current recommendation is to test for HIV-1 and HIV-2 using a combination anti-HIV-1 and HIV-2 and HIV-1 p24 antigen immunoassay. All reactive specimens should then be tested using an immunoassay that specifically differentiates HIV-1 and HIV-2. Samples that are reactive on the initial screening assay but are negative or indeterminate on the follow-up immunoassay are then subjected to nucleic acid-based testing for resolution. Recently infected patients who have not seroconverted or newborn babies with maternal antibody can be identified as HIV-infected using sensitive RT-PCR assays. HIV infection can also be monitored in those receiving antiviral therapy using quantitative molecular testing with plasma specimens, CD4+ T-lymphocyte determinations, and an antiretroviral resistance assay. Successful antiviral therapy should reduce the HIV plasma viral load to undetectable levels. These assays can also be used as prognostic indicators and to determine infectiousness.

Rapid point of care HIV immunoassays are not available for use following occupational blood or body fluid exposure or for pregnant women during labor when HIV status is unknown. These assays are either immunoconcentration methods or lateral flow assays. Home testing systems include the OraQuick in-home HIV test (OraSure Technologies, Bethlehem, PA). The test provides results within 20 minutes using an oral fluid sample. A positive result does not indicate definitive infection with HIV. CDC recommends early detection and testing by qualified personnel for the management of infection and appropriate follow-up testing. Home testing does not replace professional diagnosis and patient care.

Human lymphotropic viruses type 1 (HTLV-1) and type 2 (HTLV-2) are associated with very different disease presentations. HTLV-1 is associated with the development of adult T-cell leukemia/lymphoma (ATLL) and myelopathy/ tropical spastic paraparesis (HAM/TSP), whereas HTLV-2 has not been definitively associated with malignancies (however, it has been associated with a neurological disease that resembles HAM/TSP with a slower progression and milder disease). HTLV-3 and HTLV-4 have been identified in a few individuals residing in Cameroon and has not spread locally or globally. NAAT are the preferred method for the determination of infection status, confirmation of serologic results, identifying tissue distribution, and distinguishing the different HTLV viral groups. All blood donors and patients with relevant clinical signs and symptoms should be screened for antibodies to HTLV-1 and HTLV-2. Western Blot is still utilized as a confirmatory test following a positive test for HTLV ½ by serological screening immunoassays. If the Western Blot is indeterminant or untypeable based on viral glycoproteins, then peripheral blood mononuclear cells should be completed using type-specific PCR.

Influenza A and B Viruses

Influenza A and B viruses can be detected using conventional cell culture, shell vial culture, membrane EIA, immunochromatographic assays, fluoroimmunoassays, indirect and direct staining of respiratory tract secretions using FA methods (Fig. 64.8), and RT-PCR. PMK cells demonstrate improved detection compared with other cell lines. The median time to detection, using hemadsorption at day 2 or 3, is approximately 3 days. FA staining is used to confirm and type isolates as A or B. Nearly all positive influenza samples demonstrate detectable virus after 1 week of incubation. NAAT is commonly used for the detection and characterization of influenza viruses. RT-PCR is the current recommended method of detection in most laboratories due to the rapid detection of the virus in clinical specimens with a sensitivity that is equal to or exceeds that of culture-based methods. Several multiplex respiratory panels are also available that include the influenza viruses. Multiplex assays may be less sensitive than a monospecific molecular assay. In addition, several CLIA-waived point-of-care molecular methods are available that can be used in outpatient settings. The molecular point of care assays has demonstrated improved sensitivity over serologic-based rapid antigen tests.

Pediatric Respiratory Viruses

Influenza and parainfluenza viruses, RSV, and adenoviruses should be considered in specimens from hospitalized infants and children younger than 10 years of age with suspected viral lower respiratory tract disease. All viruses can be detected by fluorescent staining of respiratory secretions or rapid cell culture (shell vial). If direct fluorescent staining is used, cell culture confirmation of all negatives should be examined for children suspected of having viruses other than RSV. Many laboratories use R-Mix cells in a rapid shell vial format to detect respiratory viruses (Box 64.1). This approach mixes two cell lines (human lung carcinoma A549 and mink lung fibroblast Mv1Lu cells; Diagnostic Hybrids, Athens, OH) in a single shell vial. Two R-Mix

shell vial tubes are inoculated for each specimen. After an 18- to 24-hour incubation, the cell mixture from one tube is stained with a pooled antibody reagent designed to detect all common respiratory viruses. Positive (fluorescent) specimens have the second tube scraped, spotted onto eight-well slides, and stained with individual antibody reagents to identify the specific virus.

If conventional cell culture is used, influenza and parainfluenza viruses are detected in PMK cells by CPEs or hemadsorption. Fluorescent staining is used for confirmation and typing. Adenovirus and RSV are detected in HEp-2 cell culture and confirmed, if necessary, by fluorescent staining. FA staining, conducted by experienced personnel, is equivalent to culture in sensitivity and should be used for single specimens or small batches. Conventional ELISA also is accurate and recommended for large batches of specimens.

Specimens from infants or young children sent for RSV detection should be tested by a rapid, nonculture RSV test. These rapid diagnostic tests (RDTs) come in different formats and may be called dipstick immunoassays, lateral flow immunoassays, or membrane ELISAs. Although these RDTs and related testing methods can be less sensitive than culture, results are available quickly (typically less than 20 minutes) and easily making these methods convenient for testing in an emergency room, urgent care clinic, doctor's office, or pharmacy.

NAAT methods have demonstrated an increased sensitivity and successful diagnosis for RSV over other methodologies. In addition, numerous multiplex molecular systems are also commercially available that include respiratory viral pathogens. These rapid assays have the potential to improve care by decreasing the length of stay and shorten the duration of antimicrobial antibiotic administration.

Gastroenteritis Viruses

Immunoassays including microplate EIAs, latex agglutination and rapid membrane-based immunochromatographic assays are commercially available for rotaviruses and enteric adenovirus types 40 and 41. Other viruses, such as astroviruses and caliciviruses that include noroviruses, do not cause life-threatening diarrheal disease; screening is not routinely used for astrovirus. A single norovirus assay, Ridascreen Norovirus 3rd Generation EIA (R-Biopharm AG. Darmstadt, Germany), is FDA licensed for the preliminary identification of norovirus in outbreak situations.

NAAT methods are the method of choice for the rapid detection of gastroenteritis causing viruses. Several monoplex and multiplex assays are commercially available for the detection of gastroenteritis causing viruses including rotavirus, noroviruses, sapovirus, astrovirus, and the enteric adenoviruses.

TORCH

TORCH is an acronym for *Toxoplasma,* rubella, CMV, and HSV. Testing for these agents and for other viral causes of infection in newborns is appropriate during pregnancy. Transplacental infection can result in congenital defects and postnatal complications. CMV is frequently associated with congenital infections.

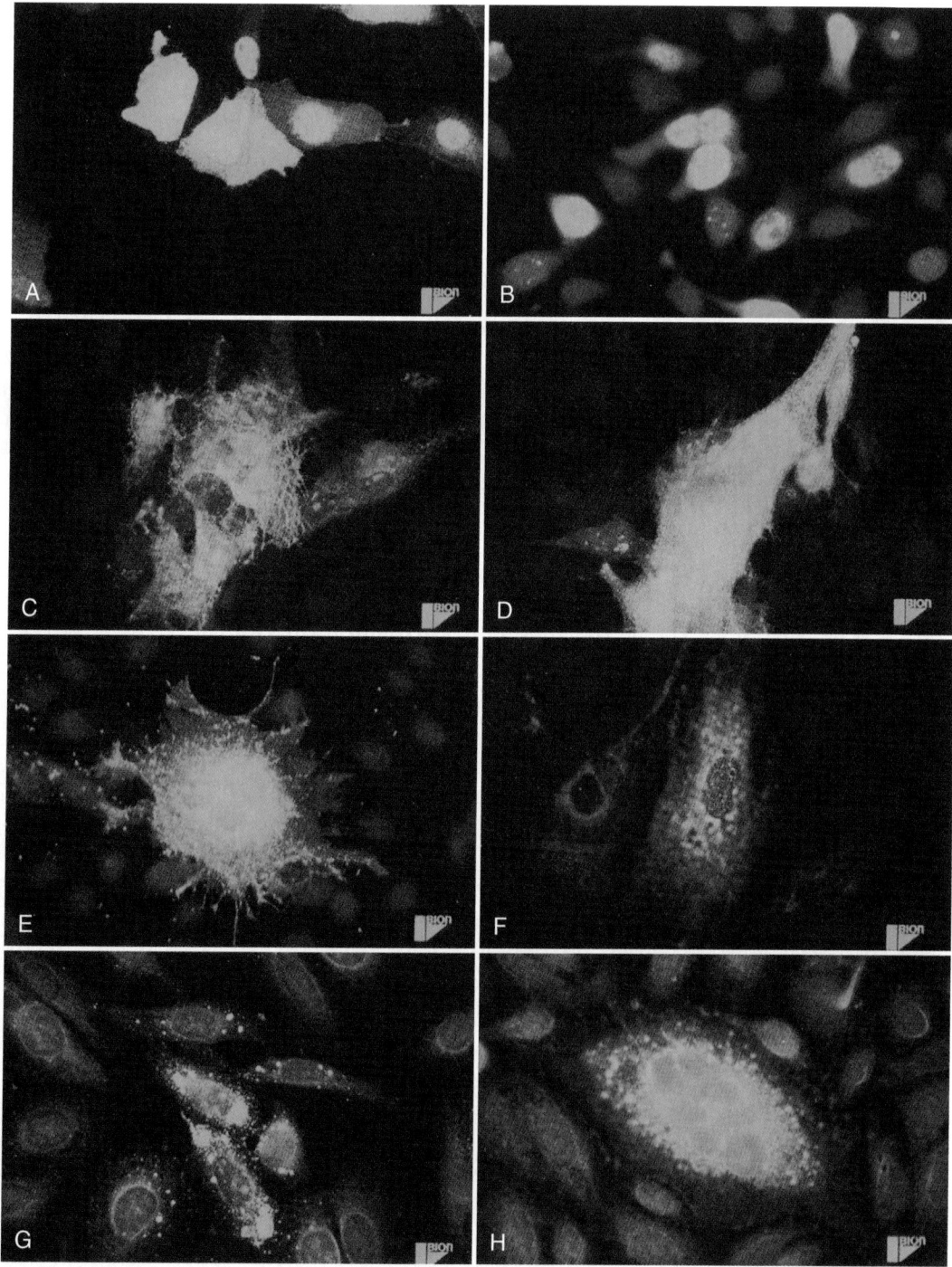

• **Fig. 64.8** Fluorescent antibody staining of virus-infected cells. (A) Influenza virus. (B) Adenovirus. (C) Varicella-zoster virus. (D) Herpes simplex virus. (E) Respiratory syncytial virus. (F) Parainfluenza virus. (G) Mumps virus. (H) Measles virus. (Courtesy Bion Enterprises, Park Ridge, IL.)

A blanket request for TORCH assays should be avoided when possible, especially in specimens from newborns. Clinical presentation in the newborn may be characteristic for one or two of the viral agents, and tests for these agents should be pursued.

Varicella-Zoster Virus

VZV causes chickenpox (varicella) and shingles (zoster). **Varicella** (a vesicular eruption) is the clinical presentation associated with a primary VZV infection. VZV, a DNA virus, establishes latency in the dorsal nerve root ganglions. Months to years later, during periods of relative immune suppression, VZV reactivates to cause zoster. **Zoster** is a modified or limited form of varicella, localized to a specific **dermatome,** the cutaneous area served by the infected nerve ganglion. Virus is present in the vesicular fluid and in the cells at the base of the vesicle. Material for viral detection should be collected from newly formed vesicles. Once the

Purpose

To rapidly detect respiratory viruses (influenza A and B viruses; respiratory syncytial viruses; parainfluenza virus types 1, 2, and 3; and adenovirus) using shell vial cell culture and fluorescent antibody staining.

Principle

A shell vial incubated for 24–48 h is stained with a pool of fluorescently conjugated antibodies capable of reacting with common respiratory viruses. If the result is positive, a second shell vial is scraped and applied as multiple spots to a microscope slide for staining with individual antibody conjugates, each specific for a different virus.

Specimen

Lower respiratory tract secretions (sputum, endotracheal or bronchial washes, bronchoalveolar lavages), lung tissue, or nasopharyngeal secretions. Throat swabs and specimens are not recommended.

Materials

- R-Mix shell vials containing a mixture of human lung carcinoma and mink lung cells (Diagnostic Hybrids, Athens, OH)
- Centrifuge
- Incubator
- Fluorescent microscope
- Monoclonal antibody screening reagent pool
- Specific virus monoclonal antibody staining reagents (all conjugated to fluorescein isothiocyanate [FITC])

Methods

1. Thaw, wash, and add refeed medium to cells in shell vials.
2. Inoculate specimen to two duplicate vials.
3. Centrifuge shell vials at 700× g for 1 h.
4. Incubate at 35°C–37°C for 24–48 h.
5. Stain one vial with monoclonal antibody pool screening reagent; if the result is positive, scrape the other shell vial and spot onto an eight-well slide.
6. Stain with specific monoclonal staining reagent to detect the specific virus present.

Interpretation

Report the specific virus detected with specific monoclonal staining reagent. If no fluorescence is detected with the monoclonal pool screening reagent, report as "No Respiratory Viruses Detected."

Procedure Notes

R-Mix shell vials should be screened and stained at 24 h for influenza A and B viruses. Respiratory syncytial viruses; parainfluenza virus types 1, 2, and 3; and adenovirus require 48 h of incubation for maximum sensitivity.

vesicle has opened and crusted over, detection is unlikely. Virus can be detected by staining cells from the base of the vesicles, by culturing cells and vesicular fluid, or by NAAT testing of fluid and cells.

A stained smear of cells from the base of a skin vesicle used to detect VZV or HSV inclusions is referred to as a

Tzanck test (described previously). Giemsa, Papanicolaou (Pap), or another suitable cytologic staining method may be used for the Tzanck test, which detects typical multinucleated giant cells and inclusions (Fig. 64.9A). FA staining also can be used to detect VZV in Tzanck smears. Traditionally, a diploid fibroblast cell culture (e.g., MRC-5) has been used to detect VZV, which requires up to 28 days before visible CPEs is produced. The shell vial assay reduces the detection time to 48 hours and significantly increases sensitivity, identifying virus that fails to produce CPEs in conventional cell culture. Comparison of FA staining of Tzanck smears, conventional cell culture, rapid shell vial culture, and PCR testing shows PCR to be the most sensitive method of detection for VZV. NAAT have improved the diagnosis of VZV disease in the CNS, disseminated infections in immunocompromised patients, and herpes zoster in patients who do not develop the characteristic rash. Qualitative as well as quantitative assays are now available that are highly sensitive and can be performed in many routine diagnostic laboratories. In addition, VZV is included in a variety of multiplex PCR assays, including the BioFire Film Array ME panel.

Virus Detection Methods

Cytology and Histology

A readily available technique for detecting virus is cytologic or histologic examination for characteristic viral inclusions. This involves the morphologic study of cells or tissue, respectively. **Viral inclusions** are intracellular structures formed by aggregates of virus or viral components in an infected cell or abnormal accumulations of cellular materials resulting from virus-induced metabolic disruption. Inclusions occur in single or syncytial cells. **Syncytial cells** are aggregates of cells fused to form one large cell with multiple nuclei. Pap- or Giemsa-stained cytologic smears may be examined for inclusions or syncytia. Inclusions resulting from infection with CMV, adenovirus, parvovirus, papillomavirus, and molluscum contagiosum virus can be detected by histologic examination of tissue stained with hematoxylin and eosin or Pap (Fig. 64.9B through F). Less commonly, inclusions characteristic of measles and rabies viruses are detected by examining stained tissues (Fig. 64.9G and H). Rabies virus inclusions in brain tissue are called **Negri bodies**. Cytology and histology are less sensitive than culture but were historically used for viruses that are difficult or dangerous to isolate in the laboratory, such as parvovirus and rabies virus, respectively. However, due to the advancement and improvements in the development of NAATs, molecular assays are now available and recommended for the rapid detection of the rabies virus and the B19V parvovirus.

Immunodiagnostics (Antigen Detection)

High-quality, commercially available viral antibody reagents have led to the development of fluorescent antibody, EIA, latex agglutination, and immunoperoxidase tests that detect viral antigen in patient specimens.

Direct and indirect immunofluorescent methods are used. Direct immunofluorescent testing involves the use of

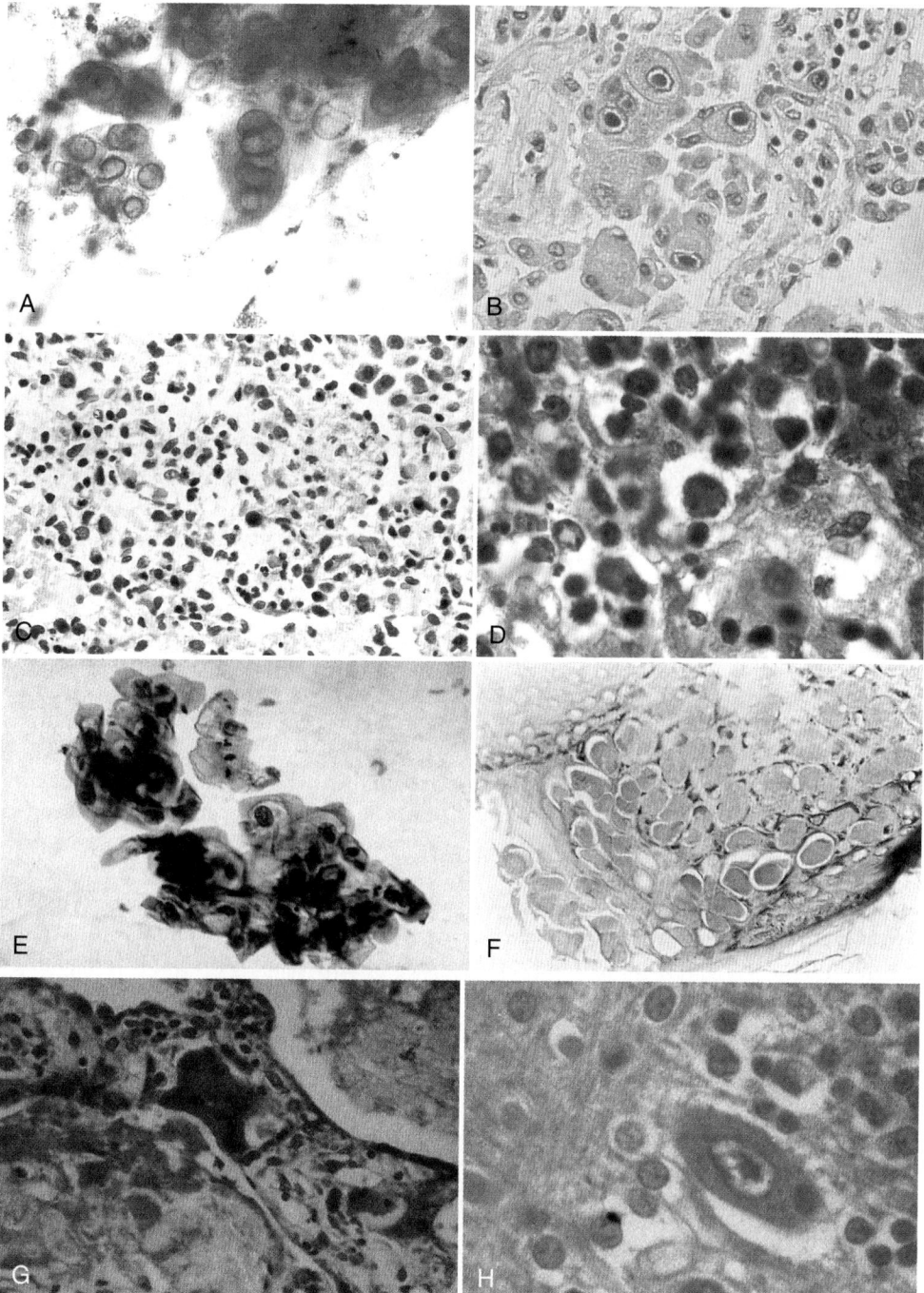

• **Fig. 64.9** Viral inclusions. (A) Papanicolaou-stained smear showing multinucleated giant cells typical of herpes simplex or varicella-zoster viruses. (B) Hematoxylin and eosin (HE)–stained lung tissue containing intranuclear inclusion within enlarged cytomegalovirus–infected cells. (C) HE-stained lung tissue containing epithelial cells with intranuclear inclusions characteristic of adenovirus. (D) HE-stained liver from stillborn fetus showing intranuclear inclusions in erythroblasts (extramedullary hematopoiesis) resulting from parvovirus infection. (E) Papanicolaou stain of exfoliated cervicovaginal epithelial cells showing perinuclear vacuolization and nuclear enlargement characteristic of human papillomavirus infection. (F) HE-stained epidermis filled with molluscum bodies, which are large, eosinophilic, cytoplasmic inclusions resulting from infection with molluscum contagiosum virus. (G) HE-stained cells infected with measles virus. (H) HE-stained brain tissue showing oval, eosinophilic rabies cytoplasmic inclusion (Negri body). (E and F, From Murray PR, Kobayashi GS, Pfaller MA, et al, eds. *Medical Microbiology.* 2nd ed. St Louis: Mosby; 1994.)

a labeled antiviral antibody; the label is usually fluorescein isothiocyanate (FITC), which is layered over a specimen suspected of containing a homologous virus. The indirect immunofluorescent procedure is a two-step test in which unlabeled antiviral antibody is added to the slide, followed by a labeled (FITC) antiglobulin (also called a secondary antibody) that binds to the first-step antibody bound to virus in the specimen. Direct immunofluorescence is generally more rapid and specific than indirect immunofluorescence but less sensitive. The increased sensitivity of indirect immunofluorescence results from signal amplification that occurs with the addition of the second antibody. Signal amplification decreases specificity by increasing nonspecific background fluorescence.

Direct immunofluorescence is best suited to situations in which large quantities of virus are suspected or when high-quality, concentrated monoclonal antibodies are used, such as for the detection of RSV in a specimen or the identification of viruses growing in cell culture.

Indirect immunofluorescence should be used when lower quantities of virus are suspected, such as detection of respiratory viruses in specimens from adult patients. High-quality monoclonal antibodies improve the sensitivity and specificity of immunofluorescence testing.

Strict criteria for the interpretation of fluorescent patterns must be used. This includes standard interpretation of fluorescent intensity (Table 64.6) and recognition of viral inclusion morphology. Nuclear and cytoplasmic staining patterns are typical for influenza virus, adenovirus, and the herpes viruses; cytoplasmic staining is typical for RSV, parainfluenza, and mumps viruses; and staining within multinucleated giant cells is typical of measles virus or the herpes viruses (Figs. 64.9 and 64.10). False-positive staining can occur with specimens containing yeasts, certain bacteria, mucus, or leukocytes. Leukocytes, which contain Fc receptors for antibody, also can cause nonspecific binding of antibody conjugates. To verify the medical laboratorian's ability to interpret FA tests, every laboratory should perform viral culture or some alternative detection method along with immunofluorescence until in-house performance has been established.

The most useful immunofluorescent stains in the clinical virology laboratory are those for RSV, influenza and parainfluenza viruses, adenovirus, HSV, VZV, and CMV. A pool of antibodies can be used to screen a specimen for multiple viruses. A positive screen is tested with each individual reagent to identify the exact virus. Screening pools have been used successfully to detect respiratory viruses in specimens from children. Such pools are less sensitive when used with specimens from adults because of the lower numbers of viral particles typically found in the specimens.

EIA methods used in clinical virology include solid-phase ELISA and the membrane-bound ELISA. Solid-phase ELISA is performed in a small test tube or microtiter tray. Breakaway strips of microtiter wells are available for low-volume test runs. The remaining unused wells can be saved for future testing. Membrane ELISA tests, also known as

lateral flow immunoassays or RDTs have been developed for low-volume testing and for cases in which rapid results are needed. They can be performed by individuals with minimal training and usually require less than 20 to 30 minutes to complete. The membrane method uses a handheld reaction chamber with a cellulose-like membrane. The specimen and reagents are applied to the membrane. After a short incubation period, a chromogenic (color) reaction occurs on the surface of the membrane and is read visually. Built-in controls on the same membrane provide convenient monitoring of the test procedure. The most used EIAs for antigen detection are those for RSV (solid-phase and membrane), rotavirus (solid-phase and membrane), and influenza viruses (membrane).

Advantages of EIAs includes the use of relatively stable reagents and results that can be interpreted qualitatively (positive or negative) or quantitatively (titer or degree of positive reaction). It is important to note that EIAs commonly have an indeterminate or borderline interpretative category. This result implies that low levels of viral antigen or background interference prevented a clear-cut positive or negative result. Such results usually require repeat testing of a second specimen to prevent false negative results due to interference with the test method or to detect a rise in antigen level. ELISAs are sensitive and simple to perform and can be easily automated. However, specimen quality cannot be evaluated; that is, the number of cells cannot be assessed, as can be determined microscopically with fluorescent immunoassays.

Immunoperoxidase staining and latex agglutination are additional techniques used to detect viral antigens. Immunoperoxidase staining is commonly used to stain histologic sections for virus but is less popular than immunofluorescence staining in clinical virology laboratories. Latex agglutination is an easy and inexpensive method but lacks sensitivity compared with ELISA and fluorescent immunoassays.

Enzyme-Linked Virus-Inducible System

The ELVIS, previously mentioned for HSV detection, uses a baby hamster kidney (BHK) cell culture system with a cloned (added) beta-galactosidase gene that is expressed only when cells are infected with a virus. In the ELVIS-HSV test system (Diagnostic Hybrids, Athens, OH), the genetically engineered BHK cells are attached to the wells of a multiwell microtiter plate. After inoculation of the specimens and overnight incubation, growth of HSV results in the production of the beta-galactosidase enzyme by the BHK cells. Beta-galactosidase serves as the "reporter" molecule. When cells are fixed and stained for beta-galactosidase activity, positive staining indicates the presence of HSV type 1 (HSV-1) or HSV type 2 (HSV-2). Wells that do not contain HSV do not stain.

Nucleic Acid Based Methods

During the past two decades, the introduction of nucleic acid detection techniques into the clinical virology laboratory has resulted in a major shift in testing strategy. With the use of both nucleic acid detection and amplification-based systems, in conjunction with automated nucleic acid isolation techniques for sample preparation, nearly all virology laboratories use commercial or in-house molecular assays, and some laboratories advocate for the complete reliance on molecular detection over viral culture. These technologic improvements make it possible to generate results within 2 to 6 hours because they do not rely upon viral culture techniques. Nucleic acid detection can be accomplished using nucleic acid probes, which are short segments of DNA that hybridize with complementary viral DNA or RNA segments. The probe is labeled with a fluorescent or chromogenic tag that allows detection using nucleic acid hybridization. The probe reaction can occur *in situ*, such as in a paraffin-embedded tissue thin section; in liquid; or in

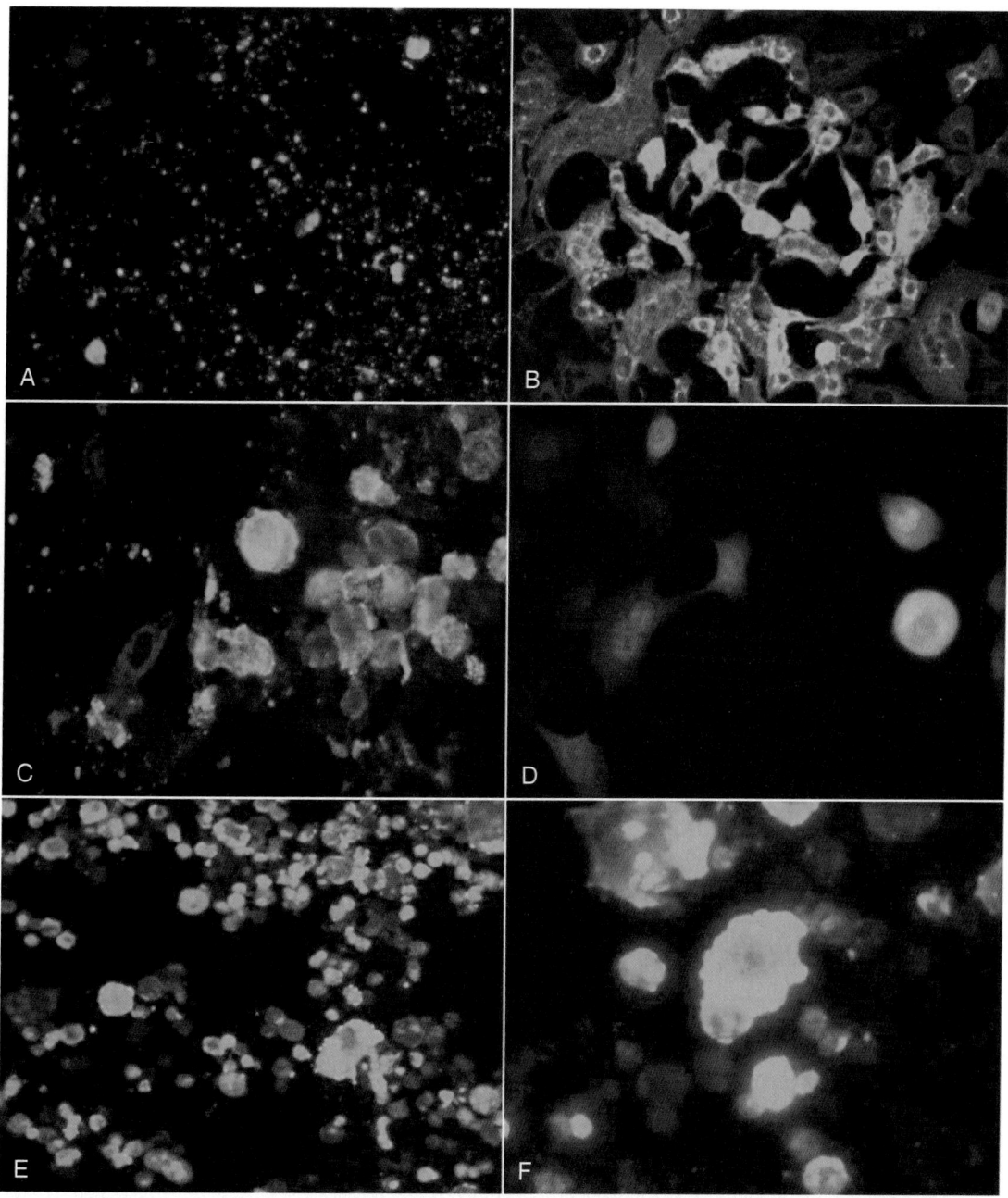

• **Fig. 64.10** (A) Rhesus monkey kidney (RMK) cells infected with respiratory syncytial virus (RSV) at 400×, stained with Light Diagnostics RSV MoAb. Fluorescence is seen in the cytoplasm and associated with syncytia. Cytoplasmic staining is often punctate with small inclusions. (B) Herpes simplex virus (HSV) I–infected Vero cell control slide at 200× stained with Pathfinder HSV 1 MoAb DFA assay. Fluorescent staining is cytoplasmic. (C) Influenza B–infected RMK cells at 400×. Stained with Light Diagnostics Influenza B MoAb. Fluorescence is nuclear, cytoplasmic, or both. Nuclear staining is uniformly bright, and the cytoplasmic staining is often punctate with large inclusions. (D) HSV II–infected A549 cells at 200× stained with Pathfinder HSV II MoAb DFA assay. Fluorescence may stain the cytoplasm, the nucleus, or both depending on the stage of the infection cycle. When infected cells are rounded, staining may appear nuclear because of the cytoplasm covering the nucleus. (E) HSV II–infected A549 cells at 200×. (F) HSV II–infected A549 cells at 400×. Picture shows the multinucleated "giant" cells characteristic of HSV II cytopathogenic effect (CPE).

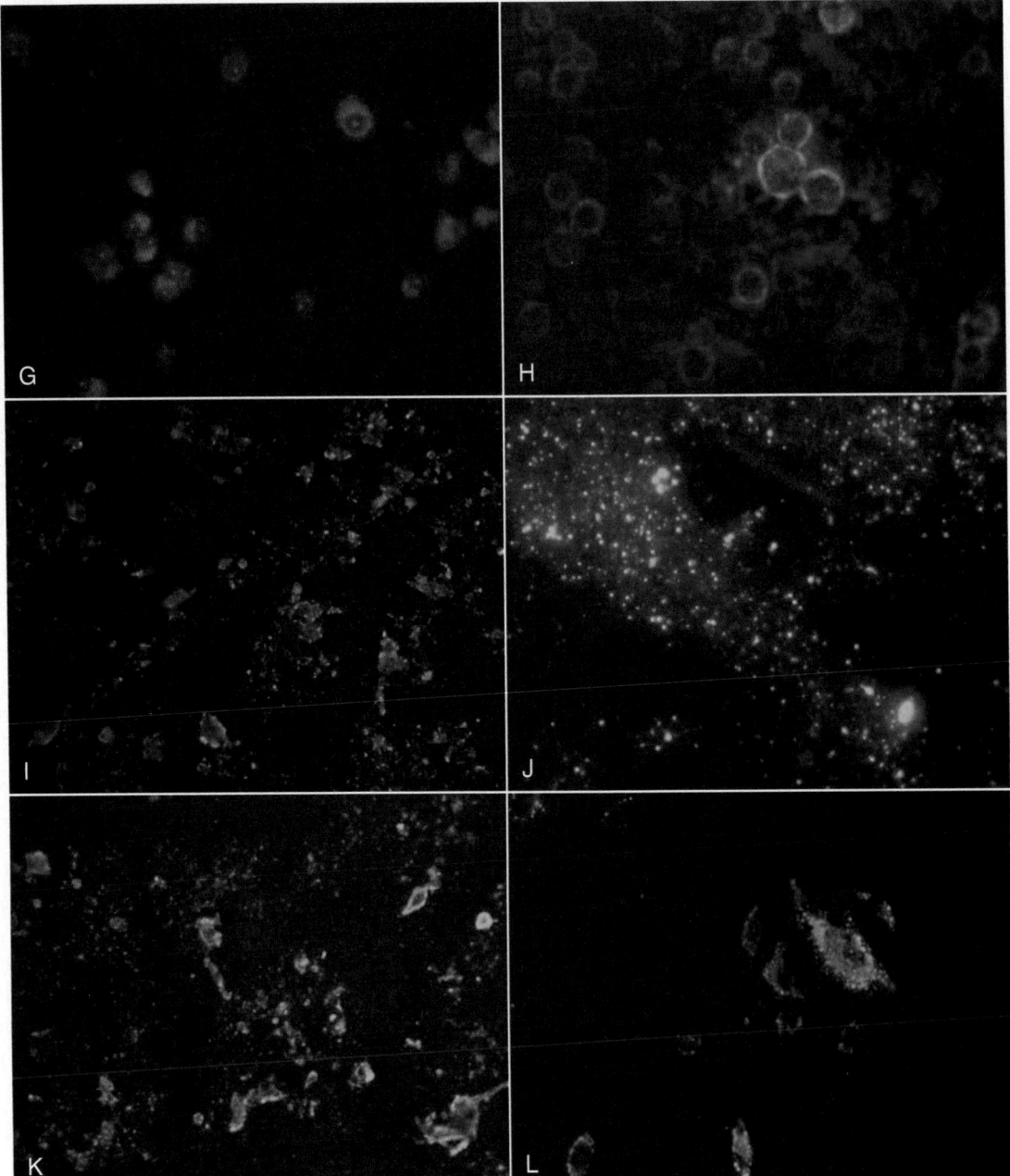

• **Fig. 64.10 cont'd** (G) Uninfected cells, no fluorescence seen. (H) Adenovirus–infected RMK cells at 400×. Stained with LD Adenovirus MoAb. Fluorescence is nuclear, cytoplasmic, or both. Shows the characteristic rounding of infected cells. (I) Parainfluenza 2–infected RMK cells at 200×. Stained with LD Parainfluenza 2 MoAb. Fluorescence is confined to the cytoplasm, and staining is punctate with irregular inclusions. (J) Rabies-positive brain tissue using Fujirebio conjugated MoAb at 400×. Bright apple-green fluorescence of particles ranging in size and morphology from "dust particles" to prominent cytoplasmic inclusion "Negri bodies." (K) Parainfluenza 3–infected RMK cells at 200×. Stained with LD Parainfluenza 3 MoAb. In a typical staining pattern, fluorescence is confined to the cytoplasm and staining is punctate with irregular inclusions. (L) Mumps IgM Bion IFA Control Slide at 200×. Stained with Bion Mumps IgM MoAb. Antigen/antibody complexes are visualized by conjugation with fluorescent stain.

a reaction vessel or on a membrane surface. A DNA probe test used to detect papillomavirus DNA in a smear of cervical cells is illustrated in Fig. 64.11. Nucleic acid probes are most useful when the amount of virus is relatively abundant; viral culture is slow or not possible; and the available immunoassays lack sensitivity or specificity.

When there are too few DNA target fragments in the original specimen to be detected by a nucleic acid probe, then the targets can be amplified using molecular techniques such as PCR to increase the nucleic acid copies within a detectable range. These and other molecular techniques are described in more detail in Chapter 8. The PCR reaction with ensuing

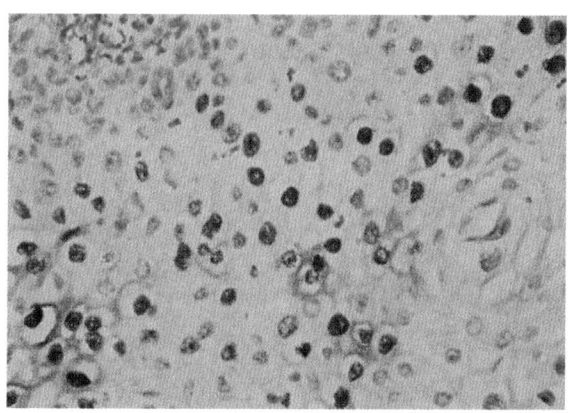

• **Fig. 64.11** Smear of cervical cells stained with probe for papillomavirus deoxyribonucleic acid (DNA). Dark-staining cells contain viral DNA. (Courtesy Children's Hospital Medical Center of Akron, Akron, OH.)

amplicon identification has been automated and made very rapid. Quantitative PCR testing, or real-time PCR, is illustrated in Fig. 64.12. In real-time PCR, target amplification and detection occur simultaneously in the same tube; with conventional PCR, amplification and product detection take place separately. The PCR product can be detected as it is produced; novel fluorogenic probes or fluorescent dyes are used to monitor the reaction and detect the PCR product as it accumulates. This requires special thermal cyclers with precision optics that can monitor the fluorescent emission from the sample wells.

The PCR can be used similarly to amplify and detect RNA viruses by using the reverse transcriptase (RT) enzyme. The first step in reverse transcription (RT-PCR) includes making a complementary DNA strand of the RNA segment in question. The usual PCR steps used to multiply the DNA target are then performed, leading to DNA amplicons that, when identified, signify the presence of the original RNA sequence. The rapid appearance and broad application of molecular diagnostics require the introduction and use of standardized materials and external quality control programs. In addition, the use of universal internal controls throughout the procedure ensures accuracy. Several new multiplex assays and microassays capable of detecting multiple viruses in a single reaction have been developed. These assays are particularly useful for the diagnosis of respiratory pathogens and are described in more detail in Chapter 65. Advances in the direct detection of viral particles by NAAT has provided rapid detection of viruses in less than 1 hour. This has resulted in a decreased need for viral culture for the diagnosis and management of viral diseases. In addition, FDA approved quantitative nucleic acid viral load testing in blood is improving. CLIA-waived NAATs have been introduced that include closed system devices with results available in 20 to 30 minutes for infectious agents such as influenza A and B and RSV and 60 minutes for multiple viruses and bacterial pathogens in a single sample in multiplex syndrome panels.

Cell Culture

Conventional Cell Culture

Viruses are strict intracellular parasites, requiring a living cell for multiplication and reproduction. To detect virus

using living cells, suitable host cells, cell culture media, and techniques in cell culture maintenance are necessary. Host cells, referred to as **cell cultures** (referred to by some as **tissue cultures**), originate as a few cells and grow into a **cell monolayer** (single confluent layer) on the sides of glass or plastic test tubes. The cells are kept moist and are supplied with nutrients by keeping them continuously immersed in a cell culture medium. Cell cultures are routinely incubated in a roller drum that holds cell culture test tubes tilted 5 to 7 degrees while they slowly revolve (0.5 to 1 rpm) at 35°C to 37°C (Fig. 64.5). Cell culture tubes can be incubated in a stationary rack rather than a roller drum. Rapidly growing viruses, such as HSV, appear to be equally detected using either of the two methods. Comparative studies are not available for most viruses.

Metabolism of growing cells in a closed tube results in the production of carbon dioxide and acidification of the growth medium. To counteract the pH decrease, a bicarbonate buffering system is used in the culture medium to keep the cells at physiologic pH (7.2). Phenol red, a pH indicator that remains red at physiologic pH, yellow at acidic pH, and purple at alkaline pH, is added to monitor the pH of the medium. Once inoculated, cell cultures are incubated for 1 to 4 weeks, depending on the suspected viral agents. Periodically the cells are inspected microscopically with an inverted light microscope for the presence of virus, indicated by areas of rounded, dead, or dying cells (the CPE). The degree of CPEs is graded from 1+ to 4+; 1+ involves 25% of the cell monolayer; 2+ involves 50%; 3+ involves 75%; and 4+ involves 100% of the cell monolayer.

Virus-induced CPE also presents two other important considerations: the rate at which CPE progresses and whether the type of cell culture in which the virus grows may be used for presumptive identification. An example of rate can be seen with HSV, in which CPE progresses rapidly to involve the entire cell monolayer. In contrast, two other herpes viruses, VZV and CMV, grow slowly, mainly in human diploid fibroblasts (HDFs), and CPE progresses over several days or weeks. The fact that the cell culture type may serve as an indicator of the presumptive identification can be seen with poliovirus and echovirus. Poliovirus and echovirus produce similar CPE in primary rhesus monkey kidney (RMK) cells, but echovirus does not induce CPE in continuous cell lines, whereas poliovirus does. A trained virologist can determine whether CPE is a result of viral growth or is nonspecific because of cell toxicity from the addition of the specimen, contamination with bacteria or fungi, or simply old culture cells. Inoculation into fresh cells should amplify viral effects and dilute toxic effects.

Two kinds of media, **growth medium** and **maintenance medium,** are used for cell culture. Both are prepared with Eagle's minimum essential medium (EMEM) in Hanks' or Earle's balanced salt solution (HBSS or EBSS, respectively) and include antimicrobials to prevent bacterial contamination. HBSS has a better buffering capacity with carbon dioxide (CO_2), whereas EBSS has a better buffering capacity in ambient air. Added antimicrobials typically include vancomycin

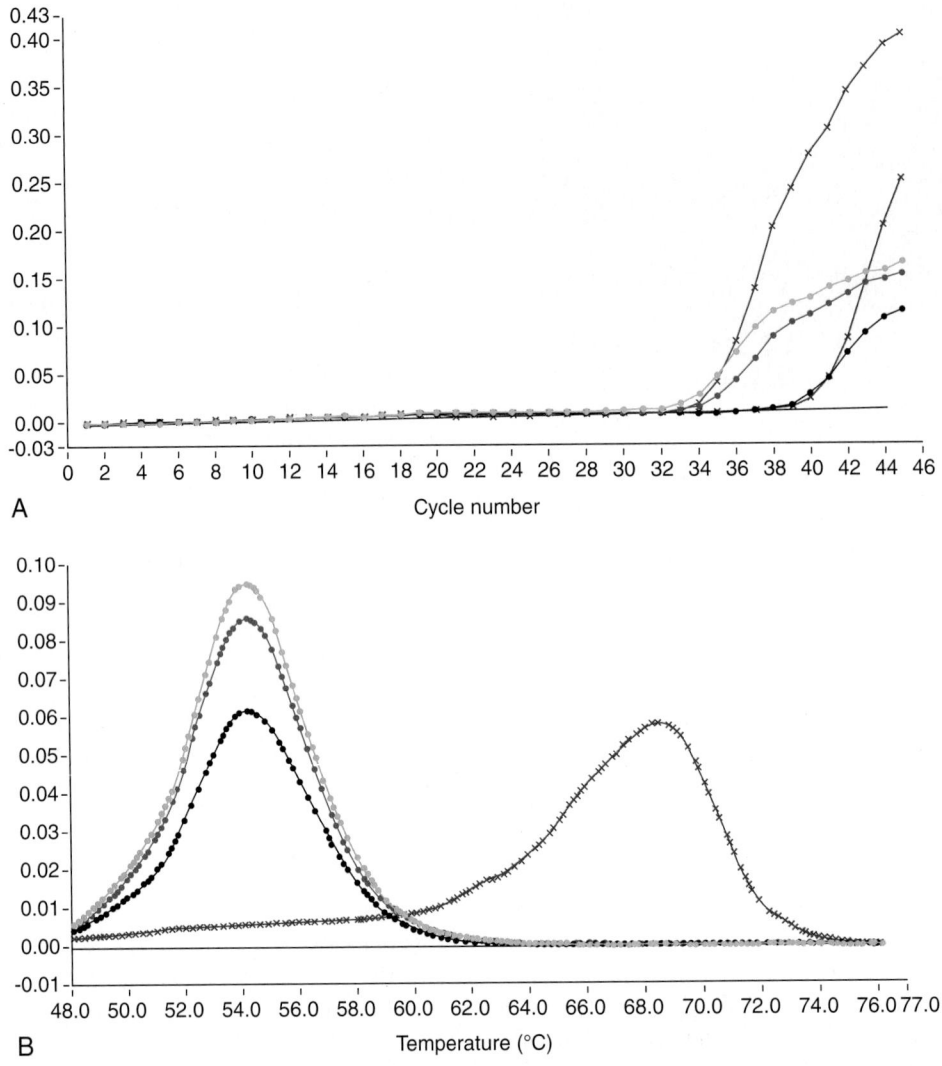

• **Fig. 64.12** Real-time polymerase chain reaction (PCR) detection of herpes simplex virus (HSV). *Black, red,* and *light green lines* represent three different HSV type 1 (HSV-1) viruses. *Pink* and *dark green lines* represent two different HSV type 2 (HSV-2) viruses. (A) Cycle crossover detection of HSV-1 and HSV-2 amplicons, with all viruses detected between cycles 34 and 40. (B) Melt curve confirmation of the presence of HSV-1 and HSV-2 viruses. HSV-1 amplicons melt at approximately 54°C (three HSV-1 viruses confirmed), and HSV-2 amplicons melt at approximately 68°C (one HSV-2 virus confirmed).

(10 µg/mL), gentamicin (20 µg/mL), and amphotericin (2.5 µg/mL). Growth medium is a serum-rich nutrient medium (10% fetal, newborn, or agammaglobulinemic calf serum) designed to support rapid cell growth. This medium is used to initiate the growth of cells when cell cultures are prepared in-house or to feed purchased cell cultures that have incomplete cell monolayers. **"Feeding"** refers to the removal of old medium, followed by the addition of fresh culture medium.

Maintenance medium is similar to growth medium but contains less serum (0% to 2%) and is used to keep cells in a steady state of metabolism. Fetal, newborn, or agammaglobulinemic calf serum is used to avoid inhibitors of virus replication, such as specific antibodies, and because it is free of mycoplasmas present in the serum of older animals.

Several kinds of cell cultures are routinely used for isolation of viruses. A cell culture becomes a **cell line** once it has been passed, or subcultured, *in vitro.* Cell lines are classified as primary, diploid (semicontinuous), or continuous. **Primary cell lines** have been passed only once or twice since harvesting (e.g., PMK cells). Further passage of primary cells, such as after experimental immortalization (e.g., through HPV E6/E7 oncoprotein expression), results in a cell line that will replicate indefinitely but typically has decreased receptivity to viral infection. **Diploid cell lines** remain virus-sensitive through 20 to 50 passages. Human dermal fibroblasts (HDFs), such as lung fibroblasts, are a commonly used diploid cell line. **Continuous cell lines,** such as human epidermoid carcinoma (HEp-2) cells, can be passed and remain sensitive to virus infections indefinitely. Unfortunately, most viruses do not grow well in continuous cell lines. Most clinically significant viruses can be recovered using one cell culture type from each group. A combination commonly used by clinical laboratories is RMK cells, MRC-5 lung fibroblast cells, and HEp-2 cells or A-549 cells (Table 64.5).

TABLE 64.5 Cell Culture Isolation and Identification of Common Clinically Encountered Viruses

Virus	PMK	HEp-2	HDF	CPE Description	Rate of Growth (days)	Identification and Comments
Adenovirus	++[a]	+++	++	Rounding and aggregation of infected cells in grapelike clusters	2–10	Confirm by FA test; serotype by cell culture neutralization
Cytomegalovirus (CMV)	–	–	++++	Discrete, small foci of rounded cells	5–28	Distinct CPEs sufficient to identify; confirm by FA test
Enterovirus	++++	+	++	Characteristic refractile angular or tear-shaped CPEs; progresses to involve entire monolayer	2–8	Confirm by FA test; stable at pH 3
Herpes simplex (HSV)	+	++++	++++	Rounded, swollen refractile cells; occasional syncytia, especially with HSV-2; rapidly involves entire monolayer	1–3 (may take up to 7)	Distinct CPEs sufficient to identify; confirm by FA test
Influenza	++++	–	±	Destructive degeneration with swollen, vacuolated cells	2–10	Detect by hemadsorption or hemagglutination with guinea pig RBCs; identify by FA test
Mumps	+++	±	±	CPEs usually absent; syncytia occasionally seen	5–10	Detect by hemadsorption with guinea pig RBCs; confirm by FA test
Parainfluenza	+++	–	–	CPEs usually minimal or absent	4–10	Detect by hemadsorption with guinea pig RBCs; identify by FA test
Respiratory syncytial virus (RSV)	+	+++	+	Syncytia in HEp-2 cells	3–10	Distinct CPEs in HEp-2 cells sufficient for presumptive identification; confirm by FA test
Rhinovirus	++	–	+++	Characteristic refractile rounding of cells; in PMK, CPE is identical to that produced by enteroviruses	4–10	Labile at pH 3; growth optimal at 32°C–33°C
Varicella-zoster virus	–	–	++	Discrete foci of rounded, swollen, refractile cells; slowly involves entire monolayer	5–28	Confirm by FA test

[a]Relative sensitivity of cell cultures for recovering the virus: –, None recovered; ±, rare strains recovered; +, few strains recovered; ++++, ≥80% of strains recovered.
CPEs, Cytopathic effects; *FA,* fluorescent antibody; *HDF,* human diploid fibroblast; *HEp-2,* human epidermoid; *PMK,* primary monkey kidney; *RBCs,* red blood cells.

Inoculated cell cultures should be incubated immediately at 35°C. After allowing virus to adsorb to the cell monolayer for 12 to 24 hours, the remaining inoculum and culture medium commonly are removed and replaced with fresh maintenance medium. This prevents most inoculum-induced cell culture toxicity and improves virus recovery. Incubation should be continued for 5 to 28 days, depending on the suspected agent (Table 64.5). Maintenance medium should be changed periodically (usually once or twice weekly) to provide fresh nutrients to the cells.

Blind passage refers to passing cells and fluid to a second cell culture tube. Blind passage is used to detect viruses that may not produce CPE in the initial culture tube but produce CPE when the "beefed-up" inoculum is passed to a second tube. Cell cultures that show nonspecific or ambiguous CPE are also passed to additional cell culture tubes. Toxicity, which causes ambiguous CPE, is diluted during passage and should not appear in the second cell culture tube. In both cases, passage is performed by scraping the monolayer off the sides of the tube with a pipette or disrupting the monolayer by vortexing with sterile glass beads added to the culture tube, followed by inoculation of 0.25 mL of the resulting suspension into a new cell culture. Blind passage is less commonly used, because the added time and expense do not justify detection of a few additional isolates after extended incubation in two cell culture tubes.

Shell Vial Cell Culture

The **shell vial** cell culture is a rapid modification of conventional cell culture. Virus is detected more quickly using the shell vial technique, because the infected cell monolayer is stained for viral antigens produced soon after infection and before the development of CPEs. Viruses that normally take days to weeks to produce CPEs can be identified within 1 to 2 days by detecting early produced viral antigens. A shell vial culture tube, a 15 mm × 45 mm 1-dram vial, is prepared by adding a round coverslip to the bottom of the tube, covering with growth medium, and adding appropriate cells (Fig. 64.13). During incubation, a cell monolayer forms on top of the coverslip. Shell vials should be used 5 to 9 days after the cells have been added. Shell vials can be purchased with the monolayer already formed. Specimens are inoculated onto the shell vial cell monolayer by low-speed centrifugation. This enhances viral infectivity for reasons that are not well understood. Coverslips are stained using virus-specific immunofluorescent conjugates. The presence and visualization of characteristic fluorescing inclusions are used to confirm the presence of an infecting virus (Fig. 64.14). The shell vial procedure for detecting CMV is presented in detail in Evolve Procedure 64.3.

The shell vial culture technique can be used to detect most viruses that grow in conventional cell culture. It is best used for viruses requiring relatively long incubation before producing CPEs, such as CMV and VZV. The advantage of the shell vial procedure over traditional cell culture is speed; most viruses are detected within 24 hours. The disadvantage is that only a single type of virus can be detected per shell vial. For example, a specimen that might contain influenza A or B or adenovirus would need to be inoculated to three separate shell vials so that each vial could be stained with a separate virus-specific conjugate. Other strategies pool antibody for detection of many viruses with a single vial. Additional vials from positive specimens are then stained with individual conjugates to identify the specific virus present. The shell vial procedure with mixed cell types used to detect seven different respiratory viruses is outlined in Box 64.1.

Identification of Viruses Detected in Cell Culture

Viruses are most often detected in cell culture by the recognition of CPEs. Virus-infected cells change their usual morphology and eventually lyse or detach from the glass surface while dying. Viruses have distinct CPEs, just as colonies of bacteria on agar plates have unique morphologies (Fig. 64.15). CPEs may be quantitated as indicated in Table 64.6. Preliminary identification of a virus frequently can be made based on the cell line that supports viral replication, how quickly the virus produced CPE, and a description of the CPEs (Table 64.5). Experienced virologists can presumptively identify

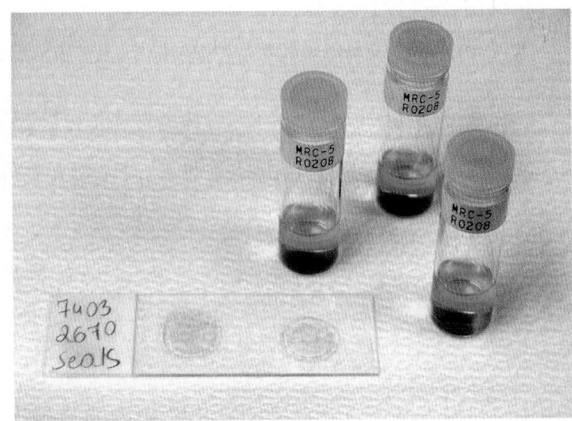

• **Fig. 64.13** Shell vial cell culture tubes and stained coverslips. At the bottom of each shell vial tube under the culture medium is a round coverslip with a cell monolayer on the top surface. After incubation, the coverslip is removed, stained, and placed on a microscope slide for fluorescence viewing. Note that two stained coverslips are on the glass slide.

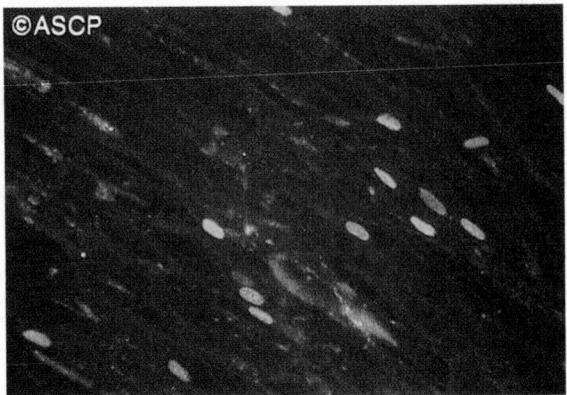

• **Fig. 64.14** Typical fluorescing nuclei of human diploid fibroblast cells infected with cytomegalovirus as seen in the shell vial assay. (Courtesy Bostick CC. Laboratory detection of CMV. Microbiology Tech Sample No MB-3; 1992.)

TABLE 64.6	Quantitation of Cell Culture Cytopathic Effects
Quantitation	**Interpretation**
Negative	Uninfected monolayer
Equivocal (±)	Atypical alteration of monolayer involving few cells
1+	1%–25% of monolayer exhibits cytopathic effects (CPEs)
2+	25%–50% of monolayer exhibits CPEs
3+	50%–75% of monolayer exhibits CPEs
4+	76%–100% of monolayer exhibits CPEs

most viruses isolated in clinical laboratories based on these criteria. When confirmation or definitive identification is required, additional testing can be performed. Some viruses that produce little or no CPE (e.g., influenza, parainfluenza, and mumps viruses) can be detected by hemadsorption, because infected cells contain viral hemadsorbing glycoproteins in their outer membranes. The addition of guinea pig red blood cells (RBCs) to the cell culture tube, followed by a wash to remove nonadsorbed RBCs, results in a ring of RBCs around infected cells (Fig. 64.15G). Cell cultures demonstrating hemadsorption can be stained with fluorescent-labeled antisera to identify the specific hemadsorbing virus present. Detailed procedures for culture confirmation by FA staining and hemadsorption for the detection of influenza and parainfluenza viruses are presented in Evolve Procedures 64.4 and 64.5.

Matrix-Assisted Desorption Ionization Time-of-Flight Mass Spectrometry

While already a mainstay in clinical laboratories for identification of microbial and fungal pathogens, **mass spectrometry** has also emerged as an important tool for viral detection when combined with PCR amplification or viral culture. MS is an analytical technique that precisely measures the mass of proteins or DNA fragments in a sample. Benefits of MS include rapid, accurate, and specific analysis of proteins, oligonucleotides, and carbohydrates. When used following PCR, MS analysis provides precise measurement of the amplicon mass generated during the PCR reaction. This exact mass measurement allows determination of the base composition of the amplified DNA and deconvolution of that information into potential sequences based on comparison against well-constructed databases of logical possibilities. Furthermore,

the use of multiple broad-range and specific PCR primers supports detection of unknown viral species, evaluation of strain relatedness, and identification of resistance genes from a single specimen making this a very powerful diagnostic technique. When used following culture (limited to cultivable viruses), MS analysis of the viral proteome (nucleocapsid, glycoproteins, etc.) can be used in pathogen identification as well as improving scientific understanding of viral infection and pathogenesis. Limitations of MS for viral diagnostics include the heavy reliance upon known reference databases for comparison of spectral signatures to establish a positive identification of one or more pathogens present in a sample. In addition, the presence of unwanted proteins or biological materials can impede MS analysis.

There are a variety of commercially available matrix-assisted laser desorption ionization time-of-flight mass spectrometry (MALDI-TOF MS) systems on the market today that exist as standalone fully- or semi-automated instruments. Manufacturers include Agilent, bioMérieux, Bruker, Sciex, Shimadzu, Thermo Fisher Scientific, and Waters, just to name a few. Again, an important barrier in adopting MS in clinical settings has been demonstrating to the FDA that tests have been validated in real-world clinical settings. However, the enormous potential of MALDI-TOF MS to provide rapid, nontargeted bacterial and viral detection continues to drive development and adoption of this technology in clinical laboratories.

Serologic Testing
General Principles

Viral serologic methods are used primarily to determine a patient's immune status and to confirm the patient's

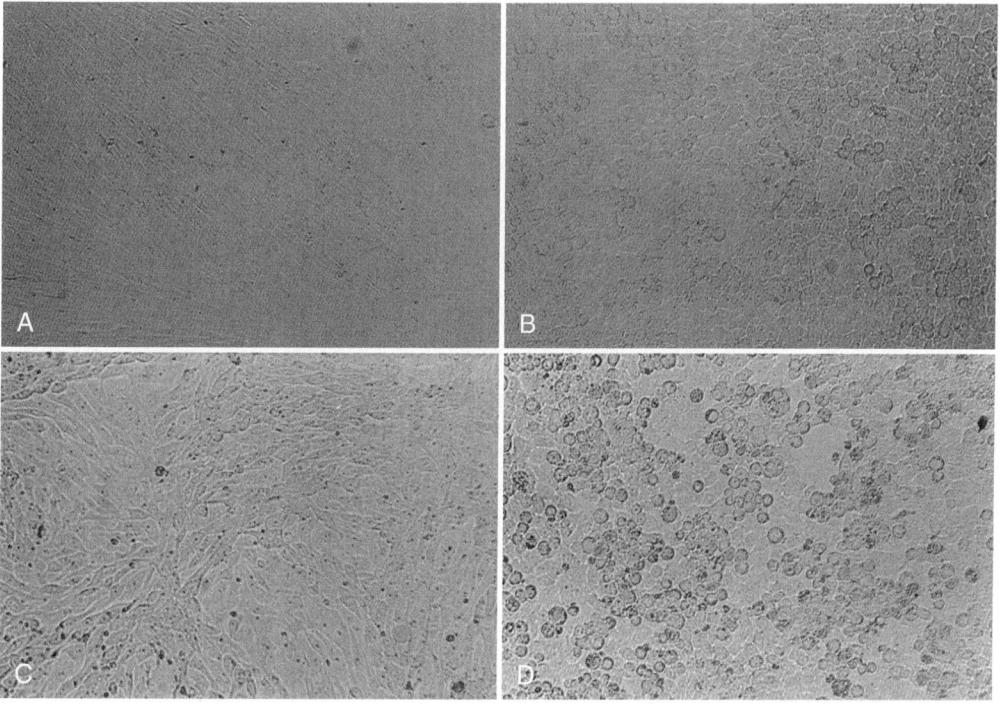

• **Fig. 64.15** Cell culture morphology and viral cytopathic effects. (A) Normal human diploid lung fibroblast cells (HDF). (B) Normal HEp-2 cells. (C) Normal primary monkey kidney cells (PMK). (D) HEp-2 cells infected with adenovirus.

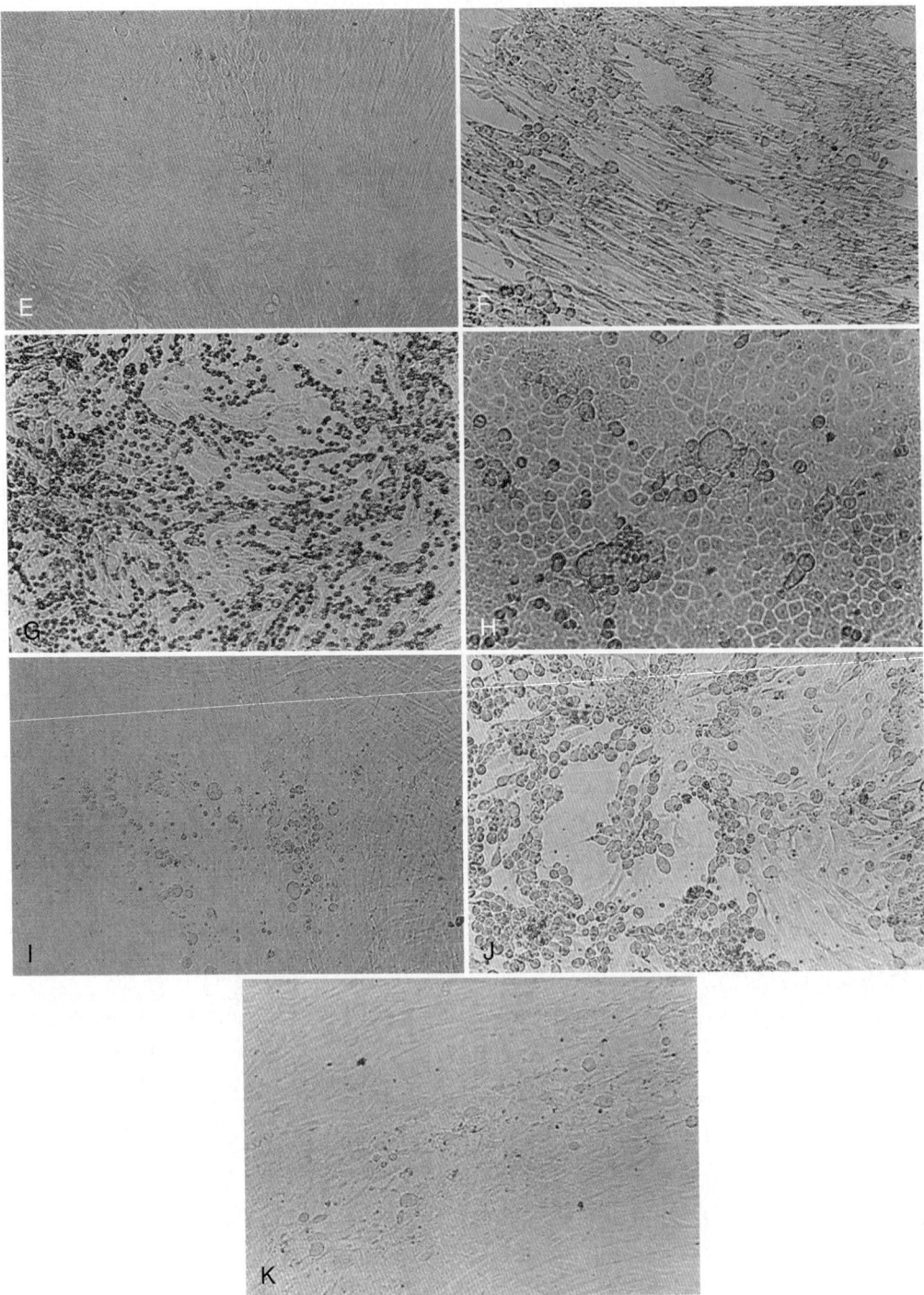

• **Fig. 64.15 cont'd** (E) HDF cells infected with cytomegalovirus. (F) HDF cells infected with herpes simplex virus. (G) PMK cells infected with hemadsorbing virus, such as influenza, parainfluenza, or mumps, plus guinea pig erythrocytes. (H) HEp-2 cells infected with respiratory syncytial virus. (I) HDF cells infected with rhinovirus. (J) PMK cells infected with echovirus. (K) HDF cells infected with varicella-zoster virus. (From US Department of Health, Education, and Welfare, Public Health Service, Centers for Disease Control, Atlanta, GA.)

diagnosis when the virus cannot be cultivated in cell culture or detected readily by immunoassay or molecular methods.

In most viral infections, IgM is undetectable 1 to 4 months after the acute infection resolves, but detectable levels of IgG remain for the life of the patient. If a patient is infected with an antigenically similar virus or the original strain has remained latent and reactivates later, virus-specific IgG and IgM antibody levels may increase. The secondary IgM response may be difficult to detect; however, a significant IgG rise in titer (fourfold) is typically apparent in immunocompetent patients.

An immune status check measures whether a virus has previously infected a patient. A positive result with a sensitive, virus-specific IgG test indicates past infection. Some immune status tests include methods that can detect both IgG and IgM; these are used to identify recent or active infections.

To diagnose active disease, two approaches are helpful. Detection of virus-specific IgM in an acute-phase specimen collected at least 7 to 14 days after the onset of symptoms indicates current or very recent disease. Detection of a fourfold (or equivalent increase if twofold dilutions are not tested) antibody titer rise between acute and convalescent sera also indicates current or recent disease. Acute-phase serum should be collected as soon as possible after the onset of symptoms. The convalescent specimen should be collected 2 to 3 weeks after the acute-phase specimen. If a single post-acute serum, collected between acute and convalescent times, or a convalescent specimen is all that is available for testing, an extremely high, virus-specific IgG titer may suggest infection. The exact titer specific for active disease, if known at all, varies with each testing method and virus. In general, titers high enough to be diagnostic are unusual, and single specimens should not be tested. A reasonable policy would involve using IgM tests, where available, and performing IgG tests only on paired acute and convalescent specimens. IgG tests are not needed on the first, acute specimen until receipt of the convalescent specimen. This eliminates useless testing of single specimens when a second sample is never submitted for analysis.

Many serologic methods are or have been routinely used to detect antiviral antibody. Prominent among these are ELISA, indirect immunofluorescence, anticomplement immunofluorescence (ACIF), and Western immunoblotting. An advantage of ELISA is that it can be used to detect IgM-specific antibodies free of common interfering factors, particularly through use of an antibody-capture technique. Indirect immunofluorescence is best used for individual specimens or small-batch testing.

Immunofluorescence also can be used to detect virus-specific IgM; however, it requires prior separation and elimination of the IgG fraction, which if present can result in both false-positive and false-negative results. IgM and IgG can be separated by ion exchange chromatography; by immune precipitation; or with an IgG inactivation reagent, such as Gullsorb (Meridian Bioscience), a reagent containing an antihuman IgG reagent (caprine) capable of neutralizing up to 15 mg/mL of IgG antibody in human serum.

IgG indirect FA testing is subject to false-positive results because of antibody-Fc receptors that occur in cells infected with virus. Indirect immunofluorescence antibody (IFA) testing is performed using virus-infected substrate cells fixed to a microscope slide. When the substrate cells are overlaid with patient serum, the Fc portion of the antibody molecule binds to these receptors. Fluorescent-labeled antiglobulin attaches to both homologous antibody (bound to viral antigen) and to Fc-bound antibody. Subsequent fluorescence of Fc-bound antibody results in a false-positive or falsely

elevated reading. To prevent this complication, the ACIF test can be used. Because fluorescent-labeled complement binds only to antigen-antibody complexes, the nonspecific antibody attached by Fc receptors, which is complement free, does not fluoresce. Western immunoblotting is also used for viral antibody detection. Because complex antigens are separated into individual components during the Western blot procedure, and positive or negative reactions are observed with each of these components, the Western blot provides a more specific result than other serologic tests, such as EIA.

False-positive and false-negative results can occur when testing for virus-specific IgM antibodies. False-positive results occur when rheumatoid factor, an anti-IgG/IgM-type globulin, combines with homologous or virus-specific IgG present in the patient specimen. Labeled anti-IgM combines with either bound virus-specific IgM or rheumatoid factor, causing falsely positive fluorescence. False-negative IgM test results occur when high levels of strongly binding homologous IgG antibodies prevent binding of IgM molecules, decreasing or eliminating IgM-specific fluorescence. Both problems can be eliminated by testing the IgG-free serum fraction.

Immune Status Testing

Immune status tests are used to determine if patients have been infected with (or vaccinated for) a virus in the past, conferring lifelong immunity to reinfection. Rubella antibody immune status testing is used for women of childbearing age. A positive result (presence of IgG antibody) indicates past infection or immunization and implies that congenital infection will not occur during subsequent pregnancies. Absence of IgG antibody implies susceptibility to infection and should prompt rubella vaccination if the woman is not pregnant. Varicella and measles assays are used most commonly for assessing the immune status in health care workers. Those with no IgG antibody must avoid infected patients and receive a booster or secondary vaccination. CMV immune status is useful for organ transplant donors and recipients and premature babies hospitalized in newborn intensive care nurseries who are likely to receive blood transfusions. Transplant recipients are also susceptible to life-threatening CMV infection. Knowing the CMV status of the donor and recipient enables the physician to monitor the transplant patient and when necessary to treat the patient. Newborns whose mothers were never infected with CMV are susceptible to serious, primary CMV infection that can be transmitted in white blood cells (WBCs) during blood transfusion. CMV-negative babies should receive only CMV-negative blood.

Serology Panels

In some cases, testing for antibody to an individual virus is less helpful than using a battery of antigens to test for antibody to many viruses. The use of a combination of serologic tests to diagnose a clinical syndrome may be useful when the viruses under consideration cannot be cultured;

specimens of infected tissue are not available (e.g., brain tissue); antiviral agents have been administered; or the patient is convalescing and isolation of virus is unlikely. In most cases, some but not all viruses in a panel may require testing. Consultation with the patient's physician can narrow the list of potential viral agents that may be the cause of the infection.

Preservation and Storage of Viruses

Clinical virology laboratories must have a method for storing and retrieving viruses, along with an accurate inventory

system from which to identify and locate stored viruses. Isolates should be kept as control strains and, in rare instances, for epidemiologic investigations or clinical research applications. Public health laboratories may use current EV or influenza virus strains for typing. Viruses can be stored by freezing at –70°C or in liquid nitrogen. Freezing at –70°C is more practical for clinical laboratories. A method for preserving and storing viruses by freezing is described in Evolve Procedure 64.6.

ⓔ Visit the Evolve site for a complete list of procedures, review questions, and case studies.

Bibliography

Balfour Jr HH: Drug therapy, *N Engl J Med* 340:1255–1268, 1999.

Baron EJ, Miller JM, Weinstein MP, et al.: A guide to utilization of the microbiology laboratory for diagnosis of infectious diseases: 2013 recommendations by the Infectious Diseases Society of America (IDSA) and the American Society for Microbiology (ASM), *Clin Infect Dis* 57:1–100, 2013.

Calderaro A, Arcangeletti MC, Rodighiero I, et al.: Identification of different respiratory viruses, after a cell culture step, by matrix assisted laser desorption/ionization time of flight mass spectrometry (MALDI-TOF MS), *Sci Rep* 6:36082, 2016.

Carr J, Gyorfi T: Human papillomavirus, *Clin Lab Med* 20:235–255, 2000.

Carroll KC, Pfaller MA, Landry ML, et al.: *Manual of clinical microbiology*, ed 12, Washington, DC, 2019, ASM.

Centers for Disease Control and Prevention: *Manual for the Surveillance of Vaccine-Preventable Diseases*. Available at: https://www.cdc.gov/vaccines/pubs/surv-manual/index.html.

Cockerill FR: Application of rapid-cycle real-time polymerase chain reaction for diagnostic testing in the clinical microbiology laboratory, *Arch Pathol Lab Med* 127:1112–1120, 2003.

Constantine N, Zhao R: Molecular-based laboratory testing and monitoring for human immunodeficiency virus infections, *Clin Lab Sci* 18:263–270, 2005.

Debiasi RL, Tyler KL: Molecular methods for diagnosis of viral encephalitis, *Clin Microbiol Rev* 17:903–925, 2004.

De Carolis E, Vella A, Vaccaro L, et al.: Application of MALDI-TOF mass spectrometry in clinical diagnostic microbiology, *J Infect Dev Ctries* 8:1081–1088, 2014.

De Clercq E: Antiviral drugs in current clinical use, *J Clin Virol* 30:115–133, 2004.

Espy MJ, Uhl JR, Sloan M, et al.: Real-time PCR in clinical microbiology: applications for routine laboratory testing, *Clin Microbiol Rev* 19:165–256, 2006.

Flint SJ, Enquist LW, Krug RM, et al.: *Principles of virology: molecular biology, pathogenesis and control*, ed 2, Washington, DC, 2004, ASM Press.

Forbes BA: Introducing a molecular test into the clinical microbiology laboratory: development, evaluation, and validation, *Arch Pathol Lab Med* 127:1106–1111, 2003.

Gavin PJ, Thomson RB: Review of rapid diagnostic tests for influenza, *Clin Appl Immunol Rev* 4:151–172, 2003.

Griffith JT Rohde RE. Ebola: implications for the clinical laboratory. Accessed July 2, 2015. Available at: http://www.ascls.org/images/publications/journals/Ebola_virus_manuscript.pdf.

Harris KR, Dighe AS: Laboratory testing for viral hepatitis, *Am J Clin Pathol* 118(suppl 1):S18–S25, 2002.

Johnson FB: Transport of viral specimens, *Clin Microbiol Rev* 3:120–131, 1990.

Kowalski RP, Karenchak LM, Shah C, et al.: ELVIS: a new 24-hour culture test for detecting herpes simplex virus from ocular samples, *Arch Ophthalmol* 120:960–962, 2002.

Lauer GM, Walker BD: Hepatitis C virus infection, *N Engl J Med* 345:41–52, 2001.

Lee WM: Hepatitis B virus infection, *N Engl J Med* 337:1733–1745, 1997.

Lefkowitz EJ, Davison AJ, Sabanadozovic S, et al. *Online (10th) Report of the International Committee on Taxonomy of Viruses*. Available at: https://talk.ictvonline.org/ictv-reports/.

Lesprit P, Scieux C, Lemann M, et al.: Use of the cytomegalovirus (CMV) antigenemia assay for the rapid diagnosis of primary CMV infection in hospitalized adults, *Clin Infect Dis* 26:646–650, 1998.

Liang TJ, Rehermann B, Seeff LB, et al.: Pathogenesis, natural history, treatment, and prevention of hepatitis C, *Ann Intern Med* 132:296–305, 2000.

McGowin CL, Rohde RE, Redwine G: More than just a test result: molecular screening of human papilloma virus for contemporary management of cervical cancer risk, *Clin Lab Sci* 27:43–46, 2014.

McGowin CL, Rohde RE, Whitlock GC: Other pathogens of significant public health concern. In Hu P, Hedge M, Lennon PA, editors: *Modern clinical molecular techniques*, New York, NY, 2012, Springer Press, pp 225–241.

McIntosh K, McAdam AJ: Human metapneumovirus: an important new respiratory virus, *N Engl J Med* 350:431–433, 2004.

Milholland MT, Castro-Arellano I, Suzán G, et al.: Global diversity and distribution of hantaviruses and their hosts, *EcoHealth* 15:163–208, 2018, https://doi.org/10.1007/s10393-017-1305-2.

Miller NS, Yen-Lieberman B, Poulter MD, et al.: Comparative clinical evaluation of the IsoAmp HSV Assay with ELVIS HSV culture/ID/typing test system for the detection of herpes simplex virus in genital and oral lesions, *J Clin Virol* 54:355–358, 2012.

Niesters HG: Molecular and diagnostic clinical virology in real-time, *Clin Microbiol Infect* 10:5–11, 2004.

Ozenci V, Patel R, Ullberg M, et al.: Demise of polymerase chain reaction/electrospray ionization-mass spectrometry as an infectious disease diagnostic tool, *Clin Infect Dis* 66:452–455, 2018.

Paltiel DA, Walensky RP: Home HIV testing: good news but not a game changer, *Ann Intern Med* 157:744–746, 2012.

Petersen LR, Marfin AA: West Nile virus: a primer for the clinician, *Ann Intern Med* 137:173–179, 2002.

Pigott DC: Hemorrhagic fever viruses, *Crit Care Clin* 21:765–783, 2005.

Poon LL, Guan Y, Nicholls JM, et al.: The aetiology, origins, and diagnosis of severe acute respiratory syndrome, *Lancet Infect Dis* 4:663–671, 2004.

Rohde RE, Mayes BC: Molecular diagnosis and epidemiology of rabies. In Hu P, Hedge M, Lennon PA, editors: *Modern clinical molecular techniques*, New Edition, New York, NY, 2012, Springer Press.

Rivers MN, Alexander JL, Rohde RE, Rush PJ: Hantavirus pulmonary syndrome (HPS) in Texas, 1993–2006, *South Med J* 102:36–41, 2009.

Schiffman M, Castle PE: Human papillomavirus epidemiology and public health, *Arch Pathol Lab Med* 127:930–934, 2003.

Schmaljohn C, Hjelle B: Hantaviruses: a global disease problem, *Emerg Infect Dis* 3:95–104, 1997.

Schubert S, Kostrzewa M: MALDI-TOF MS in the microbiology laboratory: current trends, *Curr Issues Mol Biol* 23:17–20, 2017.

Sejvar JJ, Chowdary Y, Schomogyi M, et al.: Human monkeypox infections: a family cluster in the Midwestern United States, *J Infect Dis* 190:1833–1840, 2004.

Singhal N, Kumar M, Kanauja PK, et al.: MALDI-TOF mass spectrometry: an emerging technology for microbial identification and diagnosis, *Front Microbiol* 6:791, 2015.

Storch GA: Diagnostic virology, *Clin Infect Dis* 31:739–751, 2000.

Thomson RB, Bertram H: Laboratory diagnosis of central nervous system infections, *Infect Dis Clin North Am* 15:1047–1071, 2001.

Van Helvoort T: When did virology start? *ASM News* 62:142–145, 1996.

Wilson PJ, Rohde RE, Oertli E, et al.: *Rabies: clinical considerations and exposure evaluations*, St. Louis, MO, 2019, Elsevier.

Warrell MJ, Warrell DA: Rabies and other lyssavirus diseases, *Lancet* 363:959–969, 2004.

Wilder-Smith A, Schwartz E: Dengue in travelers, *N Engl J Med* 353:924–932, 2005.

Writing Committee of the World Health Organization Consultation on Human Influenza A/H5: Avian influenza A (H5N1) infection in humans, *N Engl J Med* 353:1374–1385, 2005.

65

Viruses in Human Disease

Viruses in Human Disease

Viruses of medical importance to humans comprise 10 families of deoxyribonucleic acid (DNA) viruses and 21 families of ribonucleic acid (RNA) viruses. This chapter examines the specific families of viruses, including the diseases and the symptoms associated with the viral infection. Tables 65.1 and 65.2 divide the virus families according to the makeup of the viral genome, either RNA or DNA, and are a quick reference for the viruses.

Adenoviridae

Adenoviruses are large (70 to 90 nm), icosahedral, nonenveloped, single double-stranded, linear DNA viruses. This virus was first isolated from cultures of human adenoids and tonsils in the early 1950s, hence the name **adenovirus.**

TABLE 65.1 Major Families of Medically Important Deoxyribonucleic Acid Viruses

Virus Families (in Order of Increasing Size)	Size (nm)	Envelope	Capsid Symmetry	Genome Structure	Viruses
Parvoviridae	~22	No	Icosahedral	SS	Parvovirus B19 virus Human bocaviruses Human bufavirus Parv4
Papillomaviridae	~55	No	Icosahedral	DS Circular	Human papillomaviruses
Polyomaviridae	40–45	No	Icosahedral	DS Circular	John Cunningham (JC) and BK (renal transplant patient initials) polyoma-viruses Merkel cell polyomavirus Trichodysplasia spinulosa polyomavirus
Hepadnaviridae	42	Yes	Pleomorphic	DS Incomplete circular	Hepatitis B virus
Adenoviridae	70–90	No	Icosahedral	DS	Human adenoviruses (85 serotypes)
Herpesviridae	120–300	Yes	Icosahedral	DS	Herpes simplex viruses type 1, 2 Varicella-zoster Cytomegalovirus Epstein-Barr Human herpesvirus (HHV-6, HHV-7, and HHV-8 (KSHV)
Poxviridae	200–450	Yes	Oval or brick-shaped	DS	Variola Vaccinia Orf Molluscum contagiosum Monkey-pox viruses

DS, Double-stranded; *KSHV,* Kaposi sarcoma-associated virus; *SS*, single-stranded.

The adenoviruses belong to the family *Adenoviridae* and are widely distributed in nature. However, only members of the genus *Mastadenovirus,* referred to as adenoviruses, cause human infection. Currently, 85 serotypes of human adenoviruses have been described. Based on molecular methods, types 52 to 85 are defined as genotypes. Genotypes can be more closely associated with types of virulence and clinical symptoms. Differentiation of serotype and genotype is not necessary unless there is a specific property that is clinically significant such as an observable difference in the immunological response based on virulence of the virus. In addition, within genotypes, molecular variants have been identified as subtypes or genome types and are designated with lowercase letters after the numbered type. These types are then divided into seven species, A through G, with species B subdivided into two subspecies (B1 and B2); virus types are then numbered within the species classification. The viruses can cause a broad range of disease in humans. Respiratory and gastrointestinal diseases are the most common clinical manifestation associated with adenovirus infection.

Adenoviruses cause less than 5% of all acute respiratory disease in the general population; however, they account for up to 15% of all acute diarrheal infections in children.

By the age of 10 years, most children have been exposed to and infected with at least one of the adenovirus species. In addition, adenovirus F-type 40 and 41 cause gastroenteritis in infants and young children, and other types are associated with conjunctivitis and keratitis. Small outbreaks of gastroenteritis associated with adenovirus A, types 12, 18, 31, and 16, have also been reported. Although respiratory and gastrointestinal diseases are most common, disseminated disease in multiple organ systems may develop in compromised hosts. Infections are frequent and severe in pediatric hematopoietic stem cell transplant patients. Infections in these patients may present as a sepsislike condition with infection of multiple organisms resulting in mortality greater than 80%. Recently, several adenovirus types have also been linked to obesity and adipogenesis.

Transmission of the virus may occur primarily by the respiratory route, as an aerosolized droplet or as an airborne particle, or by a fecal-oral route. Respiratory disease caused by adenovirus is usually acquired through contact with contaminated respiratory secretions, stool, or fomites. The virus is very stable and can remain viable for weeks at variable temperatures on surfaces and in liquid solutions. The incubation period for respiratory disease is 2 to 14 days and

TABLE 65.2					
Major Families of Medically Important Ribonucleic Acid Viruses					
Virus Families (in Order of Increasing Size)	**Size (nm)**	**Envelope**	**Capsid Symmetry**	**Genome Structure**	**Important Members**
Arenaviridae	7–10	Yes	Spherical	SS (–) Circular segmented	Lymphocytic choriomeningitis virus Lassa fever virus Lujo virus Machupo virus Guanarito virus Sabia virus Chapare virus
Astroviridae	28–30	No	Starlike	SS (+)	Gastroenteritis-causing astroviruses
Picornaviridae	~30	No	Icosahedral	SS (+)	Cardioviruses Polioviruses (coxsackie viruses) Parechoviruses, enteroviruses Hepatitis A virus Rhinoviruses
Hepeviridae	32–34	No	Icosahedral	SS (+)	Hepatitis E virus
Calciviridae	30–38	No	Icosahedral	SS (+)	Norovirus Sapovirus
Flaviviridae	40–50	Yes	Icosahedral	SS (+)	Arboviruses Yellow fever Dengue West Nile Zika Japanese encephalitis, and St. Louis encephalitis nonarboviruses: hepatitis C virus
Togaviridae	60–70	Yes	Icosahedral	SS (+)	Rubella virus Alpha viruses
Reoviridae	~70	No "Rota" or wheel-shaped virus	Icosahedral "Rota" or wheel-shaped virus	DS 11 segments	Rotavirus Colorado tick fever
Orthomyxoviridae	80–120	Yes	Spherical, pleomorphic	SS (–) 8 segments	Human influenza virus types A, B, C Swine and avian influenza viruses
Hantaviridae	80–120	Yes	Spherical, pleomorphic	SS (–) 3 segments	Hantaan (*sin nombre*) viruses
Retroviridae	100–150	Yes	Icosahedral	SS (+) diploid	Human HIV 1 & 2 Human T-cell lymphotropic virus (HTLV 1 & 2)
Coronaviridae	120–160	Yes	Helical, crown-shaped virus	SS (+)	Coronavirus (CoV) types 1–3 CoV type 4 (SARS) virus MERS-CoV, SARS-CoV-2 (COVID-19)
Pneumoviridae	100–1000	Yes	Spherical, pleomorphic	SS (–)	Respiratory syncytial virus Human metapneumovirus
Rhabdoviridae	~180 X 75	Yes	Helical, bullet-shaped virus	SS (–)	Rabies virus
Filoviridae	Varies	Yes	Complex, pleomorphic, rodlike	SS (–)	Marburg virus Ebola virus
Paramyxoviridae	150–350	Yes	Spherical, pleomorphic	SS (–)	Mumps Measles (rubeola) Parainfluenza viruses Respiratory syncytial viruses

DS, Double-stranded; (+), positive-sense strand; (–), negative-sense strand; *SS*, single-stranded.

3 to 10 days for gastroenteritis. Common upper respiratory tract infections caused by adenovirus include colds, tonsillitis, pharyngitis, pharyngoconjunctival fever, and sometimes croup (viral infection of the larynx). Infections of the eye and conjunctivitis often accompany respiratory infection, and in children, otitis media (ear infection) is often a complication of the respiratory disease. Lower respiratory tract infections can be quite severe in children, and adenovirus pneumonia is often fatal in infants and young children.

A unique feature of the adenoviruses is the ability to cause severe, acute respiratory disease epidemics in military recruits, often resulting in considerable morbidity and mortality. A highly effective vaccine to control outbreaks is approved for military personnel between the ages of 17 and 50 for types 4 and 7.

Adenoviruses can be detected from a variety of specimens depending on the clinical presentation and test requirements. See Chapter 64 for an overview of specimen types used for the identification of viral infections.

Direct detection of adenoviruses targets viral antigens using monoclonal antibodies (mAbs). Assay formats include immunofluorescence (IF), enzyme immunoassay (EIA), latex agglutination, and lateral-flow immunochromatographic (IC) assays. Nucleic acid amplification tests (NAATs) for adenovirus have become the most popular diagnostic method because of the reduced detection time and increased sensitivity over traditional cell culture. NAATs have been used to detect adenovirus in all specimen types. Quantitative real-time polymerase chain reaction (PCR) on plasma, peripheral blood mononuclear cells, or whole blood is used for the detection and determination of adenovirus viremia in compromised patients to predict current and disseminated disease. These assays have also been applied to other samples (such as stool) in efforts to improve care in hematologic stem cell transplant patients. Transplant centers routinely screen and monitor adenovirus viremia in patients months after transplantation.

Adenoviruses can be cultured using various epithelial cell lines, such as A-549, HEp-2, KB, and He-La cells. Growth is usually apparent in traditional cell culture 2 to 5 days after inoculation. Adenovirus produces a characteristic grapelike cluster cytopathic effect (CPE). Rapid cell culture (i.e., shell vials) using centrifugation reduces detection time but is less sensitive than conventional tube culture. A confirmatory follow-up test is performed using an indirect fluorescent antibody (IFA) technique or EIA. Culture may still be used to detect types that may be missed by direct methods or for identification and typing of novel viruses in epidemiologic studies.

Arenaviridae

Arenaviruses, of the family *Arenaviridae,* include 43 spherical, enveloped RNA viruses that have T-shaped glycoprotein spikes 7 to 10 nm long surrounding the surface membrane of the virion. The viruses can readily infect a variety of mammalian species, especially rodents and bats, often resulting in a deleterious effect on the reservoir rodent host. Human transmission usually occurs through inhalation of aerosols of infected rodent excrement (urine, saliva, feces, nasal secretions) or by direct contact with infected rodents. Ectoparasites have also been implicated in transmission to humans. Health care–related transmission has been reported for Lassa and Machupo viruses. Disease in humans has been associated with nine arenaviruses, which clinically display a broad range of symptoms, from asymptomatic (no symptoms) to fever, prostration, headache, and vomiting, to the more severe cases of meningitis and hemorrhagic fever.

Arenaviruses are classified into Old World (OW) and New World (NW) groups based upon serotyping and phylogenetic analysis. The OW arenaviruses capable of causing disease in humans include the prototypic lymphocytic choriomeningitis virus (LCMV) and the highly pathogenic Lassa fever virus (first detected in Lassa, Nigeria). LCMV has been identified in cases of aseptic meningitis in Europe and the Americas. LCMV can occur in rural and urban areas with high rodent populations and has been acquired from pet hamsters. It has also been linked to at least 10 human deaths following organ transplantation from LCMV-infected individuals. Lassa has been associated with hemorrhagic fever, shock, and death in 5% to 15% of symptomatic patients (80% of cases are asymptomatic), killing approximately 5000 people each year. Lassa fever virus is a significant cause of morbidity and mortality in West Africa, where economic resources are limited. Capillary leak and widespread organ involvement, accompanied by shock, respiratory distress, and/or hemorrhage, are responsible for most deaths from Lassa fever. Other, less commonly reported arenaviruses may also cause hemorrhagic fever, including LuJo virus, which caused a Lassa fever–like outbreak in South Africa, and Junin virus, associated with Argentine hemorrhagic fever. Isolated arenavirus outbreaks have also been caused by Machupo virus (MACV) in Bolivia, Guanarito virus (GTOV) in Venezuela, Sabia virus in Brazil, and Chapare virus in Bolivia.

Arenavirus infection is diagnosed using enzyme-linked immunosorbent assay (ELISA)-based serologic tests or reverse transcriptase polymerase chain reaction (RT-PCR) to detect viral nucleic acid. An antigen capture ELISA for the quantitative detection of arenavirus in serum and tissue culture supernatants has been used for early detection and identification. Viral isolation using cell culture is not routinely recommended. Cell culture for viral isolation has proven to be unreliable because of inconsistent sensitivity. In addition, handling cultures and specimens puts laboratory personnel at high risk. Samples and cultures containing LCMV require Biosafety Level (BSL) 3 facilities, and Lassa fever virus requires a BSL 4 laboratory. Serologic diagnosis is also difficult, because the immunologic antibody response is delayed for several days and often weeks after symptomatic illness. Multiplex RT-PCR assays have been developed to detect several arenaviruses and are becoming more widely available in the acute care or routine clinical laboratory setting.

Astroviridae

Astroviruses, so called because of their characteristic starlike surface structure, are small (28 to 30 nm), round, nonenveloped, single-stranded, positive-sense RNA viruses associated with gastroenteritis. Transmission occurs via the fecal-oral route through close contact with infected individuals or contaminated fomites. Astroviruses are more commonly associated with pediatric infections, military troops, and nursing home and immunocompromised patients. Gastroenteritis caused by astroviruses are usually mild and self-limiting. A number of antigen detection tests have been developed for the detection of astroviruses in stool but are not available for use in the United States. A multiplex NAAT, the FilmArray gastrointestinal panel (bioMerieux BioFire Diagnostics, Salt Lake City, UT) can be used to detect astroviruses from stool samples.

Caliciviridae

Caliciviruses are small (30 to 38 nm), rounded, nonenveloped, single-stranded, positive RNA viruses that cause acute gastroenteritis in humans. Caliciviruses have been previously recognized as major animal pathogens and have a broad host range and disease manifestation. The viruses cause respiratory disease in cats, a vesicular disease in swine, and a hemorrhagic disease in rabbits. Not until the 1990s did the taxonomic status of noroviruses (formerly known as Norwalk-like viruses, named after Norwalk, OH) result in classification in the family *Caliciviridae.*

Members of the *Norovirus* and *Sapovirus* genera are the primary cause of viral gastroenteritis in humans and are referred to as the **human caliciviruses** (HuCVs). Previously called "Norwalk-like viruses" and "Sapporo-like viruses," the viruses were named after their prototype strains, the Norwalk virus and the Sapporo virus, respectively. These viruses are referred to as the norovirus and sapovirus. The HuCVs are further classified into genogroups, and within the genogroups, into genetic clusters. Human isolates in the norovirus genogroup include genogroups I, II, and IV and in the sapovirus genogroup, I, II, IV, and V.

Roughly 685 million cases of gastroenteritis are caused by norovirus each year, making it the most common cause of acute gastroenteritis worldwide. Among these cases, approximately 200 million occur in children under the age of 5, resulting in an estimated 50,000 to 70,000 or more childhood deaths every year, mostly in developing countries. Yet the impact of norovirus infection can be felt in both low- and high-income countries, where it is a major public health concern due to its ability to cause large outbreaks in semi-closed environments, such as cruise ships, nursing homes, schools, summer camps, hospitals, and restaurants. Several factors contribute to the rapid spread of infection: fecal-oral transmission, the low infectious dose (fewer than 100 virus particles), and the virus's high environmental stability. Noroviruses are easily transmitted in food, water, person to person, or in airborne droplets of vomitus. The virus persists

in water despite treatment processes. Worldwide norovirus infection is estimated to cost nearly $65 billion in direct health care costs and lost productivity every year.

Norovirus infections cause moderate to severe gastroenteritis; the clinical symptoms include nausea, abdominal cramps, vomiting, and watery diarrhea. Symptoms usually occur after a 1- to 2-day incubation period and continue for approximately 1 to 3 days. Vomiting occurs more often in children than in adults. Infection with sapovirus causes mild to moderate gastroenteritis with symptoms similar to norovirus; however, sapoviruses more frequently cause disease in infants and toddlers than in school-age children, whereas norovirus infections are common to all age groups. Maximum viral shedding in the feces occurs early, at the onset of clinical symptoms, but viral shedding can occur for up to 2 to 3 weeks after cessation of the clinical symptoms. As a result, control of viral transmission is problematic, and infection does not confer long-lasting immunity.

Norovirus cannot be cultivated using cell culture. The most widely used identification method is RT-PCR. Commercially available ELISA kits that use mAbs or hyperimmune sera are also available to detect norovirus but demonstrate lower sensitivity and specificity than RT-PCR. Multiplex NAATs, the Verigene Enteric Pathogens Nucleic Acid Test (Luminex Corporation, Austin, TX) and the FilmArray gastrointestinal panel (bioMerieux BioFire Diagnostics, Marcy I Etoile, France) can be used to detect noroviruses from stool samples. The FilmArray also detects sapoviruses.

Coronaviridae

The family *Coronaviridae* includes the genera *Alphaletovirus, Alphacoronavirus, Betacoronavirus, Deltacoronavirus,* and *Gammacoronavirus,* collectively referred to as coronaviruses (CoVs). This family contains many species of both human and animal origin. Once considered a harmless virus causing the "common cold," the CoVs cause a wide variety of disease in animals and birds. In general, CoVs are pleomorphic, roughly spherical, very large (120 to 160 nm across), enveloped linear positive-stranded RNA viruses. The prefix "corona" results from the viral structure and the crownlike surface projections on the external surface of the virus that can be seen with electron microscopy. Most of the human respiratory CoVs cause colds and occasionally pneumonia in adults. Together the rhinoviruses (RVs) and CoVs cause more than 55% of the common colds in the human population. CoVs are found in a wide range of domestic and wild mammals and birds. A variety of species and subspecies occur worldwide; they are characterized by frequent recombination and the formation of distinct genotypes.

Three specific genotypes known to infect humans belong to the genus *Betacoronavirus* and emerged as a result of recombination events and zoonotic transmission, including the severe acute respiratory syndrome–related coronavirus (SARS-CoV), the Middle East respiratory syndrome–related coronavirus (MERS-CoV) and the COVID-19, also known as SARS-CoV-2. Viral transmission is person-to-person via contaminated respiratory secretions or aerosols. The virus is present in the highest concentration in the nasal passages, where it infects the nasal epithelial cells. CoVs are believed to cause diarrhea in infants, based on the presence (as seen with electron microscopy) of coronavirus-like particles in the stool of symptomatic patients.

CoVs are generally associated with upper respiratory tract infection and occasional lower respiratory tract infection in patients of all ages. Some animal CoVs are known to cause acute gastroenteritis in humans.

Severe respiratory disease associated with CoVs is characterized by a rapid onset of high fever, followed by a dry cough and dyspnea. The severe respiratory syndrome follows an incubation period of approximately 2 to 7 days after the appearance of the initial symptoms (fever, headache, myalgia, and malaise). The illness progresses to severe respiratory distress, requiring the patient to be hospitalized for supportive care and mechanical ventilation. The period of maximum infectivity and highest viral loads in the upper airways of patients begins in the second week of illness, during the time the patients often were severely ill. This poses a high risk of transmission to health care workers during this period.

COVID-19 emerged as a new human CoV in December of 2019, when local outbreaks of a CoV-like severe respiratory disease was reported in individuals who had frequented a Hunan seafood and animal market in Wuhan, China. COVID-19 rapidly became a worldwide pandemic, with nearly 70,000 cases reported within the first month, resulting in a fatality rate of 2% to 3%. Within approximately 5 months, 185 countries worldwide reported widespread human infections with the virus, and an alarming fatality rate. SARS-CoV-2 has nucleic acid similarity to two bat-derived SARS–like CoVs of bat origin, SL-CoVZC45 and SL-CoVZXC21. COVID-19 resulted in asymptomatic to mild to severe acute respiratory disease, cardiac abnormalities, coagulopathies, and immune syndromes that posed significant treatment difficulties. Symptoms could include anything from a headache, high fevers, body aches, shortness of breath, low oxygen saturation, diarrhea, dry cough, anosmia (loss of smell), and dysgeusia (distortion of taste), As a novel virus, the race for effective treatment and a vaccine was initiated in numerous labs across the globe.

All CoVs pose a significant diagnostic challenge, with very low levels of CoV in the respiratory tract during the early phase of disease. Although antigen detection is available for some CoVs, the technique lacks sensitivity compared with nucleic acid–based testing. Molecular testing by RT-PCR remains the recommended method for laboratory diagnosis. Several commercially available multiplex assays are available for the rapid detection of the human endemic species of CoV. During the COVID-19 outbreak, the Centers for Disease Control (CDC) released an emergency use authorization (EUA) RT-PCR diagnostic panel. CDC as well as other commercial manufacturers also produced multiple RT-PCR diagnostic panels capable of detecting SARS-CoV-2,

influenzae A, and influenzae B. CDC released an EUA for the detection of antibodies to COVID-19 to determine the general overall infection rate in the United States and to evaluate commercial serological tests available for laboratory diagnostics. Although nucleic acid testing by RT-PCR is the most useful diagnostic test available, the CoVs are capable of growth in cell culture using either the Vero-CCL81 or the Vero-E6 cell line. The characteristic viral CPE appears as a rapid cell rounding, refractivity, and detachment. BSL 3 or higher is required for propagation and manipulation of cell cultures containing this virus.

Throughout the pandemic treatment options for SARS-CoV-2 improved as information relative to the biology and pathology of the virus became available. No drug has been proven to be an effective therapy for COVID-19; however, several clinically available drugs were repurposed for use in treating COVID-19, and new experimental treatments were authorized by the FDA under the emergency use authorization during the pandemic. The standard of care for patients primarily focused on supportive measures, managing fever and potential preventative care using the repurposed or experimental treatments. Chloroquine and hydroxychloroquine were initially being tested as an antiviral medication in several studies. However, the therapeutic index appeared to be very narrow and several adverse effects associated with the drug including life-threatening toxicity, cardiomyopathy, arrhythmias, and hemolytic anemias were identified, and the use of the drug was terminated. Remdesivir, a nucleoside analog that inhibits viral RNA synthesis, which was developed by Gilead Sciences (Foster City, CA) for treatment of Ebola, is only available as an intravenous medication. The use of remdesivir improves the patient's respiratory symptoms when administered during either a 5- or 10-day treatment. Patients receiving remdesivir should be monitored daily for potential liver toxicity. If the patient's liver enzymes are elevated (alanine aminotransferase and aspartate aminotransferase) and continue to rise, remdesivir should be discontinued. In addition to a variety of other antiviral medications, treatments often include drugs that inhibit or reduce the effects of proinflammatory cytokines that have been associated with the development of severe pneumonia, a high risk of multiorgan failure and death. Interleukin-6 (IL-6) was identified as being 10-fold higher in patients with severe COVID-19 infection and those that were critically ill. Because most laboratories are unable to measure IL-6 levels, C-reactive protein (CRP), is used as a marker for IL-6, as IL-6 inhibitors rapidly reduce the levels of CRP. Tocilizumab, a human monoclonal antibody to IL-6, has been used to treat COVID-19, resulting in the reduced use of supplemental oxygen and improvement in clinical symptoms. The FDA also approved the emergency use of convalescent plasma in patients with COVID-19. Convalescent plasma is obtained from patients who are eligible to donate blood, have had no symptoms of COVID-19 for at least 14 days and no longer test positive for SARS-CoV-2 RNA by RT-PCR. The use of convalescent plasma demonstrated a reduction in hospital stays and reduction in mortality. In addition to these treatments, several commercial biotechnology companies actively pursued the development and manufacturing of human SARS-CoV-2 antibodies for use in clinical trials for the treatment of disease. Vaccine development and clinical trials were underway by a variety of manufacturers across the globe at the time of this writing.

The COVID-19 pandemic has posed a significant challenge to health care systems not only in the United States but throughout the global community. Health systems lacked the supply chain necessary to provide adequate personal protective equipment to health care workers, testing supplies for COVID-19 as well as general medical and diagnostic laboratory supplies and highlighted the shortage of medical laboratory science professionals. Undoubtedly, the evolution of the recent pandemic has and will continue to identify new methods and approaches to the diagnosis, treatment, and management of infectious disease now and in the future.

Filoviridae

The *Filoviridae* family of viruses currently includes five genera: the *Cuevavirus, Ebolavirus, Marburgvirus, Striavirus,* and *Thamnovirus.* Ebola virus and Marburg virus are considered the most pathogenic and virulent of all the hemorrhagic fever viruses. As a family, **filoviruses** are pleomorphic, long rodlike, enveloped, nonsegmented, single-stranded, negative-sense RNA viruses. The filamentous morphology appears in many forms or configurations, such as the number 6, U, or circular. Marburg hemorrhagic fever virus displays the characteristic "shepherd's hook" morphology. The term **viral hemorrhagic fever** is used to describe a severe multisystem syndrome in which multiple organ systems are affected throughout the body. The patient's vascular system becomes damaged, and the body's ability to regulate itself is impaired. Infection with the Marburg or Ebola virus, endemic in Africa, results in severe hemorrhage, vomiting, abdominal pain, myalgia, pharyngitis, conjunctivitis, and proteinuria, and it is often fatal. Human case fatality rates for Ebola virus disease (EVD) can exceed 80%; the toll for Marburg virus infection is much lower, with a case fatality rate of 23% to 25%. These diseases have no cure or well-established drug treatment.

Ebola virus is named after a river in Zaire (now the Democratic Republic of the Congo), where it was first identified. The genus *Ebolavirus* has five subspecies, based on the location where the viral strain was first identified: *Zaire ebolavirus, Sudan ebolavirus, Tai Forest ebolavirus* (formerly referred to as *Cote d'Ivoire ebolavirus* or Ebola–Ivory Coast), *Bundibugyo ebolavirus,* and *Reston ebolavirus.* All of the Ebola subspecies cause disease in humans and nonhuman primates (i.e., chimpanzees, gorillas, and monkeys) except for *Reston ebolavirus,* which causes disease only in nonhuman primates. Infections are acute, with no carrier state, and humans become ill after contact with an infected animal, usually a primate. Transmission of the virus is rapid.

Individuals caring for the sick who come in contact with the patient's secretions quickly develop symptoms.

Ebola outbreaks have elicited worldwide response, with the World Health Organization (WHO) declaring a Public Health Emergency of International Concern. The largest outbreak occurred in West Africa (Guinea, Liberia, and Sierra Leone) in 2014 to 2015 with 28,616 confirmed, probable, and suspected cases and 11,310 reported deaths. Subsequent outbreaks have occurred in the Democratic Republic of Congo in 2017 and again in 2019, which continues to claim lives (1396 deaths among 2071 total patients, as of June 10, 2019). This outbreak appears to be spreading into Uganda.

Treatment options for EVD are limited but have increased significantly following the recent outbreaks. Supportive care, such as fluid replacement therapy, that is carefully managed and monitored by trained health workers improves chances of survival. Other treatments being used to help people survive EVD include kidney dialysis, blood transfusions, repurposed pharmaceuticals (favipiravir), mAb biologics, blood/plasma replacement therapy, and vaccines. Of the biologics, two mAb cocktails are currently in various stages of clinical trials, including ZMapp (Leafbio, San Diego, CA) and MIL 77 (MabWorks, Allston, MA) MIL 77 has already been prescribed to treat EVD patients under compassionate use guidelines. Blood/plasma replacement therapies utilize whole blood or plasma from recovered (convalescent) EVD patients and the antibodies contained therein to confer some degree of immune protection to the recipient. Phase II/III convalescent plasma and whole blood trials are ongoing in Sierra Leone and Guinea. In addition, there are at least 15 Ebola vaccines being developed and in various stages of human clinical trials, according to the WHO. The first to emerge from Phase III clinical trials is rVSV-ZEBOV (NewLink Genetics and Merck Vaccines USA in collaboration with the Public Health Agency of Canada), which works by replacing a gene from a harmless virus known as vesicular stomatitis virus (VSV) with a gene encoding an Ebola virus surface protein. Clinical trial results indicate that rVSV-ZEBOV offers substantial protection against EVD, with no cases occurring in vaccinated individuals 10 days or more after vaccination. Vaccination strategies involving rVSV-ZEBOV, although not yet licensed, are currently being used through emergency authorization to control the Ebola outbreak in the Democratic Republic of Congo. Recognizing the urgent need for a vaccine, large consortiums such as the Partnership for Research on Ebola Vaccinations (PREVAC) have been assembled to include research and academic institutions, health authorities and scientists from Ebola-affected countries, pharmaceutical companies, nongovernment organizations, and national public health officials with the goal of enhancing Ebola research activities to prevent or respond effectively to the next potential Ebola outbreak. PREVAC conducted randomized, double-blind studies of rVSV-ZEBOV with and without a boost, and another two-dose vaccination process, referred to as a **heterologous prime-boost** with Ad26,

ZEBOV, and MVA-BN-Filo. The rVSV-ZEBOV is now a US Food and Drug Administration (FDA)-approved vaccine for Ebola (Johnson and Johnson, in collaboration with Bavarian Nordic).

The natural animal reservoir for the Ebola and Marburg viruses has never been determined, although the animal source is believed to be native to Africa. Disease outbreaks in monkeys have occurred in the United States in research facilities. Several monkeys housed in separate cages became ill simultaneously. Laboratory workers working in these facilities were also infected and developed antibodies but never developed symptoms of the disease. Reston ebolavirus is known to have caused infections through aerosolization of secretions.

RT-PCR is used to identify the Ebola and Marburg viruses. Electron microscopy is also available in some research facilities. Cell culture is available in laboratories with BSL 4 facilities. Antibody production occurs after an Ebola virus infection, and an antigen-capture ELISA is available to detect IgM and IgG antibodies to Ebola virus. Seven diagnostics have been approved for Emergency Use Assessment and Listing procedure (EUAL) by WHO including the OraQuick Ebola Rapid Antigen Test Kit (OraSure Technologies, Inc., Bethlehem, PA), SD Q Line Ebola Zaire Ag (SD Biosensor Inc. Gyeonggi-do, Republic of Korea), Xpert Ebola Test (Cepheid, Sunnyvale, CA), LiferiverTM Ebola Virus (EBOV) Real Time RT-PCR Kit (Shanghai ZJ BioTech Co., Ltd., Goettingen, Germany), and RealStar Filovirus Screen RT-PCR Kit (Altona Diagnostics GmbH, Hamburg, Germany).

Flaviviridae

The **flaviviruses** (family *Flaviviridae*) are small (40 to 50 nm), single-stranded, nonsegmented, positive-sense RNA, enveloped, icosahedral viruses. The name is derived from the Latin word *flavus,* which means "yellow." The first disease identified in this group was yellow fever, which causes yellow jaundice in humans. The family includes four genera: *Flavivirus, Hepacivirus, Pegivirus,* and *Pestivirus.* Most members of the genus *Flavivirus* are also known as **arboviruses**, which are arthropod-borne and primarily transmitted via mosquitoes, causing diseases such as Zika fever, yellow fever, dengue, West Nile viral encephalitis, and Japanese and St. Louis encephalitis. Hepatitis C virus (HCV) is a flavivirus but not an arbovirus.

Yellow Fever

In the jungle habitat, monkeys serve as the reservoir for the yellow fever virus, and the vector is a mosquito. In urban outbreaks, humans can serve as the reservoir, as long as the mosquito vector is present.

The yellow fever virus primarily infects liver cells, resulting in fever, jaundice, and hemorrhage. Transmission through the mosquito bite is followed by a 3- to 6-day incubation period. The onset of symptoms is sudden and includes fever,

rigors, headache, and backache. The patient's clinical condition progresses rapidly, and the patient becomes intensely ill with nausea, vomiting, facial edema, dusky pallor, swollen bleeding gums, and hemorrhagic tendencies that cause black vomit, melena (black tarry feces), and ecchymoses (bruising). Mortality rates range from 5% to 50%; when death occurs, it is usually within 6 to 7 days after the onset of symptoms but rarely after 10 days. The characteristic yellow jaundice typically is seen in convalescing patients. Prevention in urban areas depends on elimination of the yellow fever vector, the mosquito, *Aedes aegypti.* The current vaccine is very effective at preventing infection.

Diagnosis of yellow fever infection is often a result of correlation of the patient's clinical symptoms with the patient's location and travel history. Laboratory testing on serum or cerebrospinal fluid (CSF) is available for detection of virus-specific antibodies or neutralizing antibodies. Serologic testing is also available using IgM-capture ELISA, microsphere-based immunoassays (MIAs), and IgG ELISA. In fatal cases of yellow fever, patient tissues may be sent to reference laboratories for nucleic acid amplification, histopathology, and cell culture. A single NAAT, the FTD Tropical Fever Africa Yellow Fever multiplex assay, is available from Mikrogen Diagnostik, Germany.

Dengue

Dengue virus is the most prevalent arbovirus in the world, with incidence rates growing dramatically in recent decades, putting nearly half of the world's population at risk. By some estimates, there are more than 390 million people infected each year, most of which are asymptomatic. Some degree of clinical disease (mild to severe) is evident in roughly 100 million of these cases. Prior to 1970, the virus was endemic only to Latin America, Puerto Rico, and Mexico, but since has expanded its range to more than 100 countries in Africa, the Americas, the Eastern Mediterranean, South-East Asia and the Western Pacific and is the leading cause of illness and death in the tropics and subtropics. Most cases reported in the United States (more than 90%) are travel related. Humans are the main reservoir for this virus, and person-to-person transmission occurs through a mosquito vector. Control methods for dengue are focused on control of the mosquito vector and early detection, which, with access to proper medical care, lowers fatality rates below 1%.

Dengue virus has four serotypes that cause a variety of clinical manifestations, including nonlethal fever, arthritis, and rash. Infection with one serotype confers immunity only to the infecting serotype. Subsequent infection with one of the three remaining serotypes may result in immune-enhanced disease in the form of severe hemorrhagic fever or dengue shock syndrome. Of the more than 390 million cases of dengue fever, 500,000 cases result in dengue hemorrhagic fever, causing approximately 25,000 deaths annually. Dengue normally affects adults and older children. The infection begins with a sudden onset of fever, severe headache, chills, and general myalgia. Often a macropapular rash may be visible on the trunk of the body that then spreads to the face and extremities. No vaccine is available for dengue, although a live-attenuated vaccine has shown efficacy in clinical trials for seropositive individuals. Laboratory diagnosis is based on the presence of virus-specific IgM antibody, a fourfold rise in specific IgG antibody, or a positive RT-PCR amplification for dengue genomic sequences. Multiple monoplex and multiplex NAATs are available for the diagnosis and detection of the dengue virus.

West Nile Virus

West Nile virus (first isolated in the West Nile district of Uganda), a flavivirus closely related to the Japanese and St. Louis encephalitis viruses, is endemic in Africa, Israel, Europe, the United States, Canada, Mexico, Central America, South America, and some Caribbean islands. The virus accounts for the largest number of cases of viral encephalitis in the United States.

West Nile virus is maintained in a bird-mosquito cycle. Birds are the natural reservoir for the virus. Many species of mosquitos and birds have been identified as being able to be infected with the West Nile virus. Amplification of virus during warm months results in the death of bird hosts, most commonly crows, ravens, and jays. Bridge mosquitos (those that bite both humans and birds) are responsible for transmission to humans; as the viral population increases in birds, more humans become infected. Interestingly, West Nile virus also has been transmitted person-to-person through blood transfusions, tissue transplantation, and via human breast milk. Infection is accompanied by fever, headache, body aches, joint pains, vomiting, diarrhea, rash, leukopenia, and/or malaise in roughly 1 out of every 5 cases, while progression to encephalitis or meningitis can occur in roughly 1 out of every 150 cases.

Laboratory diagnosis typically involves detection of IgM antibody to West Nile virus in the patient's serum or CSF. Several commercial kits are available for detection of West Nile IgM- and IgG-specific antibodies using ELISA or IFA methods. A variety of monoplex (and a single multiplex) NAATs are available for the detection of West Nile virus. Nucleic acid amplification testing has also been successful in detecting the arbovirus from the tissues of fatal cases and has also been used to detect the virus from the tissues of birds. Additionally, similar molecular testing has been used to detect West Nile virus in mosquito pools. West Nile mosquito surveillance has become increasingly important in the attempt to control this disease.

Zika Virus

Zika virus was first identified in Uganda in 1947 in monkeys and 5 years later in humans in Uganda and nearby countries. Since then, outbreaks of Zika virus disease have occurred in Africa, the Americas, Asia, and the Pacific. In May 2015, the Pan American Health Organization (PAHO) issued an alert regarding a Zika virus outbreak in Brazil with reports

of neuropathy, myelitis, and Guillain-Barre syndrome, a rare autoimmune disorder impacting the peripheral nervous system that leads to weakness, numbness, tingling, and can eventually cause paralysis in adults and children. Shortly thereafter, reports of pregnant women giving birth to babies with defects such as microencephaly and other congenital malformations (now known as congenital Zika syndrome) were linked to Zika virus; other poor pregnancy-associated outcomes were also reported. There is no specific treatment for Zika. Patients are recommended to push fluids to prevent dehydration, get plenty of rest, and take acetaminophen (Tylenol) to reduce fever and pain.

Transmission of Zika virus occurs from infected mosquitos (*Aedes* spp.), mother to fetus during pregnancy, sexual contact, transfusion of blood and blood products, and organ transplantation. Zika virus has been detected in whole blood, serum, plasma, urine CSF, semen, saliva, and amniotic fluid. Laboratory diagnosis is typically performed using whole blood, serum, and/or urine. If a patient is presenting with onset of symptoms less than 7 days, then nucleic acid testing (NAAT) is recommended. If a patient is presenting with onset of symptoms ≥7 days, then IgM serological testing and/or NAAT is recommended. When using NAAT beyond the 7-day window, negative results may be misleading, because viremia drops rapidly approximately 7 days after onset of symptoms and may not be detected by the test at the lower end of sensitivity, producing a false-negative test result. Several serologic and NAAT tests are commercially available for the diagnosis and detection of the Zika virus.

Hepatitis C Virus

The HCV causes hepatitis (inflammation of the liver). Worldwide, an estimated 177.5 to 185 million people are infected and carriers of HCV; about 2.4 million of those live in the United States. The virus can cause both acute and chronic disease, ranging in severity from a mild illness lasting a few weeks to a serious, lifelong illness. Acute infection with HCV progresses to a chronic infection in 50% to 90% of infected individuals (Fig. 65.1). The acute infection with HCV often goes undiagnosed, because it is often asymptomatic. When clinical illness is present, it is generally mild. Chronic infection with HCV is an important cause of liver disease and is associated with the development of cirrhosis (scarring of the liver), severe liver damage, and liver cancers such as hepatocellular carcinoma. There are currently no vaccines for hepatitis C. Treatment of acute disease generally involves monitoring by a physician and surveillance for chronic disease progression. Chronic hepatitis C treatments have gotten much better in recent years with more than 13 single or combination therapies currently FDA-approved. Most of these treatments involve an 8- to 12-week course of oral therapy (pills) and can cure over 90% of people with few side effects.

The virus is transmitted predominantly by exposure to infected blood, such as during intravenous drug use,

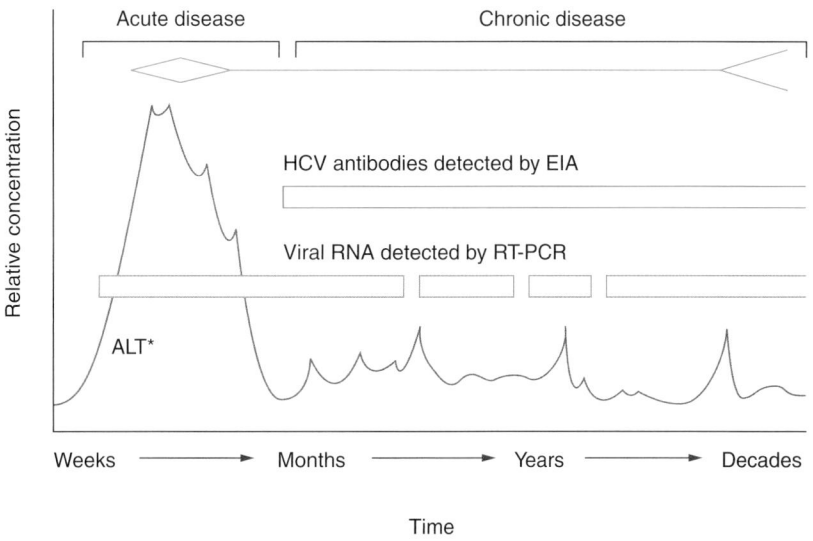

Acute disease   Chronic disease

HCV antibodies detected by EIA

Viral RNA detected by RT-PCR

ALT*

Weeks → Months → Years → Decades

Time

*Alanine aminotransferase marker for liver necrosis.

• **Fig. 65.1** Time course of immune response and disease caused by hepatitis C virus *(HCV)*. *EIA*, Enzyme immunoassay; *RNA*, ribonucleic acid; *RT-PCR*, reverse transcriptase polymerase chain reaction.

needle-stick injuries in health care settings, and contaminated blood products. The screening of blood products for HCV has virtually eliminated the risk of transmission through administration of contaminated blood products. Less efficient modes of transmission include sexual contact with infected partners, acupuncture, tattooing, body piercing, and sharing of personal hygiene products that have come into contact with blood (i.e., razors and toothbrushes).

HCV disease is identified with screening antibody tests, anti-HCV EIA, and NAAT. HCV NAATs are useful for diagnosis of acute infections in seronegative patients. Chronic disease is often diagnosed using serologic screening tests followed by HCV RNA NAAT to demonstrate viral replication. In addition, quantitative NAAT is used to determine the amount of virus in the blood to monitor antiviral therapy. Finally, viral genotyping using molecular techniques is available for identifying genotypes that do not respond appropriately to therapy. The full benefits of modern laboratory testing, including the application of molecular methods, has significantly improved the recognition, monitoring, and treatment of HCV disease. A variety of serologic and NAAT platforms are commercially available for the detection and monitoring of HCV infection.

Hantaviridae

The hantaviruses, in the family *Hantaviridae*, are fairly large (80 to 120 nm) spherical or pleomorphic, enveloped, single-stranded, segmented RNA viruses. Hantaviruses were previously included in the family of *Bunyaviridae*. However, unlike the bunyaviruses, which are transmitted by arthropods (arboviruses), the hantaviruses are rodent-borne and transmitted through exposure (inhalation) to aerosolized rodent excreta. Rodents develop a chronic infection that

results in shedding of the virus in saliva, feces, and urine. Disruption of animal excreta by vacuuming, sweeping, or shaking rugs aerosolizes infected particles, which are then inhaled. Evidence indicates that the chance of inhaling these particles is greater in indoor, poorly ventilated spaces than through outdoor exposure.

Hantavirus pulmonary syndrome (HPS) was originally discovered in 1993 in the Four Corners area of the southwestern United States (Arizona, New Mexico, Colorado, and Utah) during an outbreak of an unexplained pulmonary illness among several young, healthy people who died from acute respiratory failure. HPS begins with generalized symptoms that include headache, fever, and body aches, typically after an incubation period of 11 to 32 days. Subsequently, the symptoms become much more severe, leading to hemorrhagic fever, kidney disease, and acute respiratory failure. The deer mouse *(Peromyscus maniculatus)* is the primary host for the hantavirus, referred to as the *sin nombre* virus (SNV). Transmission of the virus from rodent to human is the only documented mode of human infection.

Since the discovery of SNV, several hantaviruses that cause HPS have been discovered throughout the United States. The Bayou virus, carried by the rice rat *(Oryzomys palustris),* was first identified in a patient from the state of Louisiana. The cotton rat *(Sigmodon hispidus)* is the carrier of the Black Creek Canal virus, identified in a patient from Florida. The white-footed mouse *(Peromyscus leucopus)* has been implicated in a case of a hantavirus infection called the New York-1 virus. Additional cases of HPS stemming from related hantaviruses have been documented in Argentina, Brazil, Canada, Chile, Paraguay, and Uruguay, making HPS a panhemispheric disease. Currently there is no vaccine for hantavirus, and therapeutics are only in experimental stages.

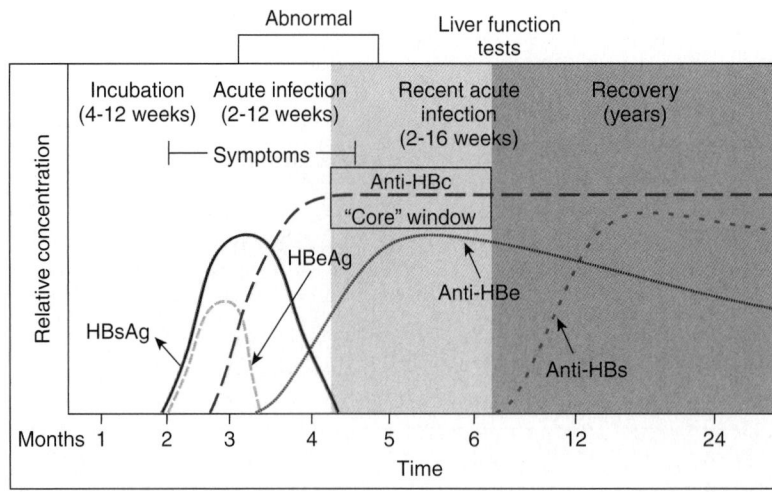

• **Fig. 65.2** Time course of antigenemia and immune response in a patient demonstrating recovery from acute hepatitis B *(HB)* infection.

Laboratory diagnosis relies on the identification of hantavirus using a NAAT from serum, whole blood, bronchoalveolar lavage fluid, or tissue. Hantavirus RNA is generally detectable within 3 to 10 days following the development of symptoms. The circulation of variation RNA genome types in any geographic location can complicate the use of NAAT. In order to address this, the CDC has developed a pan-hantavirus assay that is capable of detecting the highly conserved genomic L segment. This is only useful in genetically similar species and only during the acute phase of the illness during viremia. Viral RNA may be undetectable by the time the patient is hospitalized.

In addition to NAAT, diagnosis also relies on the use of serologic assays for hantavirus-specific IgM or IgG antibody. By the time symptoms have appeared, all patients have formed hantavirus-specific IgM antibody, and most have also developed hantavirus-specific IgG antibody. ELISA is usually the method of choice for diagnosis. The assay is available at the CDC, many state public health laboratories, and some commercial reference laboratories.

Hepadnaviridae

Hepatitis B virus (HBV) is the prototype virus of the *Hepadnaviridae* family (*hepa-* from hepatitis and *dna* from the genome type). The virus has long been recognized as a significant cause of liver damage associated with morbidity and mortality. Other mammalian and avian hepadnaviruses are known to exist. **Hepadnaviruses** are pleomorphic, enveloped viruses containing circular, partially double-stranded DNA that replicates through an RNA intermediate. Replication occurs by means of reverse transcription and then DNA replication.

Although a successful vaccine against HBV exists, the number of humans infected with HBV worldwide is nearly 400 million, and approximately 50 million new cases occur annually. Humans are the only source of the virus. Percutaneous exposure to blood or blood products

is the primary route of transmission. However, the virus may also be contracted through perinatal or sexual contact. HBV is a relatively heat-stable virus and can retain its infectivity in drying blood and other bodily fluids for several days. HBV infection previously was associated with blood transfusion, but this is now rare because of the routine screening of blood products and widespread vaccination program.

The incubation period for an acute HBV infection usually is 1 to 3 months but may be considerably longer. The initial symptoms of acute infection often are nonspecific, much like mild, flulike symptoms (Fig. 65.2). Many cases are asymptomatic, especially in children. The infection presents as an acute or chronic hepatitis with a pathologic effect on the liver, resulting in self-limited or fatal outcomes. Fatal disease is most likely to occur in people coinfected with the hepatitis D virus (delta agent), a deficient RNA virus capable of replication in cells infected with HBV. Chronic HBV infection remains a significant worldwide cause of liver cirrhosis and hepatocellular carcinoma despite the availability of an effective vaccine.

Because of the generality of HBV symptoms and the similarities it shares with other causative agents of hepatitis, clinicians rely extensively on the laboratory for confirmation of the clinical diagnosis of acute or chronic infection and identification of the virus. Laboratory diagnosis typically uses a combination of NAAT and immunoassays. Several commercial types of serologic and NAAT tests are available. Immunoassays are available for specific identification of viral antigens or antibodies (viral markers) in a patient's blood. The most common type of immunoassay uses the EIA format. Most of the commercially available serologic assays demonstrate excellent specificity and sensitivity. HBV is not cultivatable *in vitro*.

Hepatitis B surface antigen (HBsAg) is the most reliable marker for identifying HBV infection. The antigen becomes evident in the patient's serum weeks before any biochemical evidence associated with liver damage (biochemical liver assays may show only minimal elevation). HBsAg remains in the serum during the acute and chronic stages of hepatitis B. The presence of HBsAg 6 months after acute infection indicates that the patient is a chronic carrier. IgM (anti-HBcAg) to hepatitis B core antigen (HBcAg) appears early in the course of disease, during the acute infection. Anti-HBsAg (antibody to surface antigen) indicates the patient is in convalescence or previously vaccinated and has developed immunity. The presence of HBeAg (hepatitis B e antigen) indicates high infectivity and a chronic carrier state.

The best indication of active viral replication and a high state of infectivity is the presence of HBV DNA in the serum. Viral DNA may be detected by a number of NAATs, including PCR. A number of user-friendly molecular assays that provide a quick turnaround time are widely available and are characterized by high analytical sensitivity and specificity. Also, detection of HBV DNA in serum is used to resolve questionable serologic results. Quantitation of viral DNA is helpful in the initial evaluation of the patient's condition and for predicting the patient's response to treatment. Molecular methods for the detection and quantitation of HBV DNA differ significantly in the limit of detection, dynamic range, and detection method used. The WHO established an International HBV DNA standard to improve the standardization of the diagnostic assays and results.

Hepeviridae

Hepatitis E virus (HEV) is the type species of the genus *Hepevirus* in the family *Hepeviridae*. Previously classified in the family of caliciviruses, HEV is a small (32 to 34 nm), nonenveloped virus with a single-stranded RNA genome. There are four other members of this virus family known to cause enlarged liver and spleen disease in chickens, pigs, wild boar, monkeys, and rodents. Several genetic and antigenic variants or strains of HEV exist and are referred to as genotypes. The different viral strains are common to different geographic locations. Genotype 3 is the strain found in the United States. HEV has also been isolated from swine worldwide and from wild deer in Japan. HEV is not endemic in the United States and other developed areas of the world.

The primary mode of transmission is the consumption of water contaminated with animal feces. There is a potential for transmission from animals to humans, also known as zoonotic infection. HEV infection results in an acute and generally self-limiting viral hepatitis. Infection typically begins with nonspecific symptoms common to many viral illnesses, such as fever, headache, nausea, and stomach pain. The first signs of a potential hepatitis infection are dark urine, pale feces, and yellow discoloration of the skin and sclera (i.e., jaundice). However, not all patients develop jaundice. The liver of infected individuals typically is enlarged and tender. Most infected patients do not progress to a long-term carrier status.

This virus is well established in developing countries as a cause of hepatitis clinically similar to infection with the hepatitis A virus (HAV). It differs from HAV in that the virus can cause an exceptionally high fatality rate among pregnant women. Fulminant hepatitis develops rapidly and is fatal in approximately 30% of women when infected during the third trimester of pregnancy. The reason for this high rate of mortality among pregnant women is not known. Women should take all possible precautions to avoid exposure to HEV while pregnant, including refraining from traveling to areas of the world where HEV is endemic, such as India and Pakistan.

Two vaccines for HEV have been developed; however, only one, HEV 239, is licensed for use in humans; it is currently only available in China. The three-dose vaccine has been shown to demonstrate protective antibodies across all HEV genotypes and is 97% effective in preventing symptomatic acute hepatitis.

Clinical diagnosis of HEV infection is important not only to control outbreaks but also for clinical management of the disease. During patient diagnosis, it is imperative to rule out the other types of hepatitis that can cause a more serious form of disease. With HEV infection, liver function tests (LFTs) typically demonstrate increased levels of serum bilirubin, aspartate aminotransferase (AST), and alanine aminotransferase (ALT) at the time of disease onset. Detection and quantification of HEV RNA in blood, stool, and other body fluids is considered the "gold standard" for the diagnosis of acute infection. There are a variety of NAATs commercially available for the detection and quantification of HEV RNA. The diagnosis can be confirmed using serologic testing. High levels of both IgM and IgG antibodies are produced at disease onset. Although the high levels of IgG confer lifetime immunity to those infected with hepatitis A, whether the antibodies produced in HEV infection do the same is not known. A variety of commercial immunoassays are available that vary in sensitivity and specificity, primarily because of the antigenic variability of the virus. Cell culture systems for HEV are rare and limited to genotype 3 and 4 strains. Cell culture systems are used for research studies and are not used in clinical diagnostics.

Herpesviridae

The *Herpesviridae* family includes nine different viruses capable of infecting humans. The word *herpes* is derived from the Greek word meaning "to creep" and was historically used to describe the spreading, ulcerative skin lesions typically seen in a herpes simplex virus (HSV) infection. **Herpes viruses** are large (120 to 300 nm), double-stranded DNA, enveloped, icosahedral viruses. The virion consists of four components: the nucleic acid core, the capsid, the tegument, and the envelope. The **tegument,** an asymmetric structure made of a fibrous material, surrounds the capsid and contains 20 different proteins. These proteins enter the host cell upon fusion of the envelope and cell membrane and initiate the viral replication cycle.

Nine human herpes group viruses have been described. Herpes viruses are widely disseminated among animal species. However, the zoonotic forms of most herpes do not infect humans, except for herpes B virus from nonhuman primates. Herpes B virus causes a severe, usually fatal encephalitis in humans. Human herpes viruses (HHVs) include HSV types 1 and 2 (HSV-1 and HSV-2), varicella-zoster virus (VZV), Epstein-Barr virus (EBV), and cytomegalovirus (CMV). More recently detected herpes viruses include HHV types 6 (HHV-6), 7 (HHV-7), and 8 (HHV-8). HHV-6 and HHV-7 are lymphotropic viruses acquired early in life. HHV-8, Kaposi sarcoma–associated herpes virus (KSHV), causes a tumor of the connective tissue. HHV-6 and HHV-7 are associated with the childhood disease roseola (**exanthem subitum**). The disease is characterized by a short period of fever and a skin rash.

A unique feature of the herpes virus family is their hallmark characteristic of latency, or the virus's ability to reside in the infected host while staying in a repressed state. Reactivation of the virus can be caused by various stimuli, including fever, emotional stress, exposure to ultraviolet (UV) light, or axonal injury. Recurrence of viral replication at subsequent times results in disease that may be present differentially as a result of the host's immune response. Viruses in this family are capable of viral recurrence or reactivation. HSV-1 may reactivate, causing mucous membrane disease or life-threatening encephalitis. Encephalitis caused by HSV is the most common viral encephalitis, with 2.3 million cases reported annually. HSV-2 reactivates, causing mucous membrane vesicles or aseptic meningitis. VZV reactivates as localized lesions (shingles). EBV reactivates, causing asymptomatic shedding of virus in the oropharynx or as disseminated disease in immunocompromised patients. As does EBV, CMV recurs symptomatically in compromised hosts as a pathogen in many tissues (e.g., heart, gastrointestinal tract, lung, brain). HHV-6 and HHV-7 also cause reactivation disease in compromised hosts.

Herpesviruses

HSV-1 and HSV-2 share several viral characteristics, including a variable host range, a short replication cycle, rapid spread in cell culture, efficient destruction of infected cells, and the ability to establish latency in the sensory ganglia of the central nervous system (CNS). These viruses affect individuals of all ages and are the cause of a wide variety of disease, including mucous membrane and skin lesions and ocular, visceral, and CNS disease. HSV-1 and HSV-2 are transmitted during close personal contact; HSV-1 infection occurs at the oropharyngeal mucosa and genital sites, and HSV-2 infection occurs at genital sites. The clinical presentation of primary genital HSV-1 cannot be distinguished from HSV-2. Primary HSV-1 infection usually occurs by the time a child reaches the age of 5 years, and more than 50 million people in the United States are believed to have oral herpes. A subset of primary infections, approximately 10% to 15%, actually result in clinical disease.

The defining characteristic associated with herpes infection is the recurrence of ulcerative anogenital skin lesions after the primary infection. More than 50% of infected individuals have a recurrent episode of a lesion outbreak within 1 year after initial infection. HSV-1 is associated with mucosal lesions that resemble small vesicles that last 4 to 7 days. The lesions from HSV-1 and HSV-2 are referred to as **herpes labialis, facialis,** or **febrilis; orolabial lesions** are commonly referred to as cold sores or fever blisters. In women, HSV-2 produces vesicles on the mucosal membranes, labia, and vagina. In men, vesicles form on the shaft of the penis, the prepuce (foreskin), and the glans penis. Systemic symptoms often accompany the primary infection in women, including fever, headache, malaise, and generalized myalgias.

HSV-1 is the most commonly reported viral CNS infection and usually occurs as a result of viral neurotropic spread through the olfactory bulb. This type of infection often occurs in infants and immunocompromised patients. Without treatment, mortality rates associated with HSV infection may be as high as 80%. After appropriate treatment, the mortality rate typically is reduced to 15% in newborns and 20% in other patients. Even when treated, individuals who survive often suffer neurologic, lasting effects, experiencing difficulties in memory, cognition, and personality disorders.

Laboratory diagnosis of herpes infection is available using a variety of diagnostic methodologies. The virus can be detected using direct antigen testing or nucleic acid amplification assays (PCR) and paired serologic assays of acute and convalescent serum specimens. Direct antigen detection is a rapid, sensitive, and an inexpensive method for diagnosis. The antigen present in the lesion is mixed with HSV-specific antibody. If the viral antigen is present, it forms a complex with the antibody that can be identified using IF or immunoperoxidase (IP) staining. Immunostaining methods are less expensive than culture and DNA amplification and require less expertise than culture. This same type of reaction can be applied in an immunoassay, usually ELISA. Immunoassay offers the additional benefit of adaptability to automation.

Nucleic acid testing for the herpes virus is more widely used and is more sensitive than cell culture and antigen detection. Molecular amplification can be especially beneficial for rapid diagnosis and treatment of herpes viral encephalitis. Both qualitative and quantitative molecular assays are commercially available from a variety of manufacturers for the identification and diagnosis of herpes viral infection.

Cell culture success is highly dependent on the sample collection procedure and the quality of the specimen. The herpes lesion or vesicle should be punctured, and the vesicular fluid absorbed with a swab, making sure to swab the base of the vesicle. Samples should be inoculated into cell culture within 1 hour after collection. If this is not possible, the swab should be placed in viral transport media and either refrigerated (4°C) or frozen at −70°C to preserve the specimen until it can be properly processed and inoculated into cell culture. Herpes is readily grown in cell culture using A-549, MRC-5, or Vero cell lines. The virus is fast-growing and typically produces a characteristic rounding, refractile CPE within 5 days using traditional cell culture and 1 to 2 days using shell vial culture after inoculation. The use of either cell culture method has been replaced in most laboratories by NAAT methods.

The herpes B virus is very similar to HSV and is generally detectable as soon as 6 hours post-infection. The virus is transmitted to humans via animal bites, mucosal or eye exposures, breaks in the skin, needle sticks, and potentially through contaminated aerosols. Symptoms of infection occur within 3 to 5 days including a vesicular lesion, erythema, edema, lymphangitis, and lymphadenopathy. This is followed by fever, myalgia, vomiting, cramping, and neurologic symptoms that progress to paralysis, respiratory distress, seizures, and death in 10 days to 6 weeks. NAAT is the preferred method of diagnosis. Antibodies to herpes B virus cross-react with HSV-1 and HSV-2, requiring careful interpretation if used for diagnosis. Herpes B virus can be cultivated in monkey kidney and chick embryo cells and demonstrates CPE similar to HSV.

Varicella-Zoster Virus

VZV causes a classic childhood disease, chicken pox, and is characterized by the appearance of a maculopapular rash. Before the introduction of the vaccine for VZV, more than 90% of the adults in the United States demonstrated immunity to VZV as a result of childhood infection. Virus transmission is increased during the inclement months, because individuals are typically in close proximity, spending more time indoors. The virus is transmitted person to person via respiratory secretions.

VZV infects the conjunctiva or mucosa of the upper respiratory tract and then travels to the lymph nodes. Four to 6 days after the initial infection, infected T cells enter the bloodstream and cause a primary viremia. The infected T cells invade the liver, spleen, and other organs, causing a second round of infection. A secondary viremia ensues, 14 days after the initial infection. This secondary wave infects cells in the skin, causing the characteristic vesicular rash of chicken pox. Symptoms at the onset of infection are usually general and include fever and malaise that appear before the onset of the maculopapular rash on the patient's trunk and scalp. The lesions usually crust over in 1 to 2 days but do not resolve for approximately 3 weeks. After the acute viral replication in the skin, VZV affects the sensory ganglia in the CNS, where it establishes latency; that is, the virus "hides" in the CNS, which is not subject to vigorous immune surveillance. After a period of latency, the virus may initiate another acute infectious cycle. This reactivation produces the characteristic recurrent disease known as **shingles,** which occurs predominately in immunocompetent people older than 45 years. Shingles follows an anatomic route around the torso along the dorsal ganglia as the virus spreads cell to cell along the neurons to epithelial cells in the skin. This condition results in vesicular lesions similar to those produced during the primary infection. Shingles may be accompanied by a painful condition known as **postherpetic neuralgia.** This condition causes a chronic, debilitating pain that can persist long after other symptoms of shingles have resolved. This pain is believed to be caused by VZV destruction of neurons.

Laboratory diagnosis is not recommended for uncomplicated cases of VZV infection in healthy children or adults. However, in certain situations, such as infection in an immunosuppressed patient or neonate, laboratory diagnosis of VZV may be beneficial.

The virus produces inclusions and giant cells. The traditional method for identifying VZV was to scrape the base of a fresh vesicular lesion and stain the scrapings with Tzanck, Giemsa, or hematoxylin-eosin stain to identify the inclusions or giant cells. This method is complicated by the fact that HSV also produces inclusion bodies. An additional rapid method for identification of VZV is direct identification of viral antigens. Samples of vesicle epithelial cells are collected, and smears are prepared and stained with fluorescent, dye-conjugated, mAbs to VZV and then observed with a fluorescent microscope. This is a fairly rapid method, because it can be performed within hours of receiving the specimen. However, interpretation and sensitivity can be questionable if not enough epithelial cells are collected.

VZV can grow in cell culture. The virus produces a characteristic CPE of small clusters of ovoid cells in fibroid cells such as MRC-5, HF, and A549. However, the virus grows slowly, and positivity of the culture may take 7 to 10 days. Shell vial cultures are a simplified method of detecting VZV compared with regular cell culture. Shell vials use cover slips with MRC-5 cells attached in a monolayer across the surface. After inoculation, the cover slip is fixed with acetone after 3 and 6 days of viral growth. The cover slip is stained with fluorescein isothiocyanate–conjugated (FITC) monoclonal IgG antibody specific for VZV. Positive specimens exhibit a cytoplasmic, apple-green fluorescence when viewed under a fluorescent microscope. Serologic assays for VZV IgG and IgM antibodies are also available to determine the patient's immune status. Several commercial ELISAs are available for detection and quantitation of VZV antibodies.

Molecular diagnostic testing for VZV has become the standard platform for the detection and diagnosis of VZV disease, replacing conventional methods of identifying the virus. It is especially useful in the rapid diagnosis of neurological disease associated with VZV, including cerebellitis, aseptic meningitis, and encephalitis. Molecular methods can detect multiple HHVs in a single clinical specimen using multiplex PCR. Multiple NAAT VZV assays are commercially available including multiplex automated DNA microarray methods for high-throughput detection of multiple herpes viruses, including VZV, in clinical samples. Molecular diagnostics also can quantitate viral VZV DNA in the blood. Molecular testing is useful for monitoring patients considered high risk for severe VZV infection.

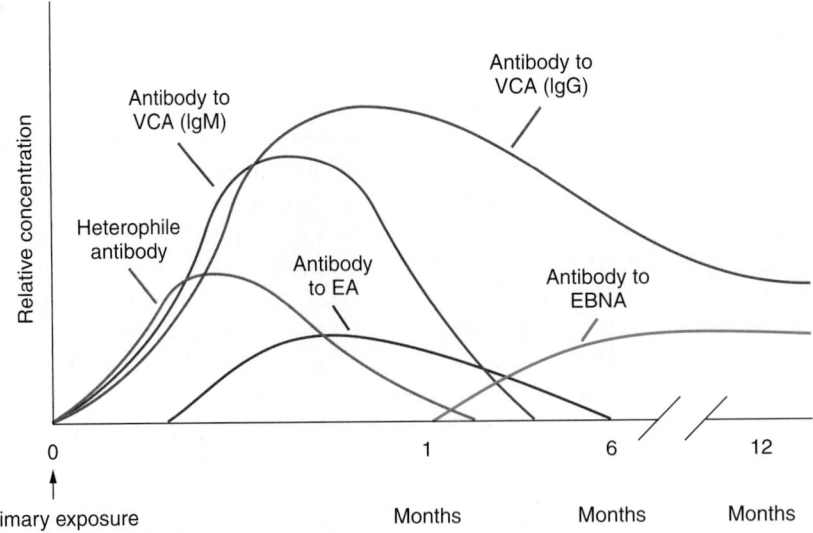

• **Fig. 65.3** Time course of immune response to Epstein-Barr (EBV) infection. *EA,* Early antigen; *EBNA,* Epstein-Barr nuclear antigen; *VCA,* viral capsid antigen.

Epstein-Barr Virus

EBV was discovered four decades ago during a search for the cause of Burkitt lymphoma, a disease that predominately affects children in Africa. EBV is responsible for the disease **infectious mononucleosis (IM).** The virus, which is transmitted in the saliva of infected patients, typically affects adolescents and young adults. The major symptoms include fever, sore throat, headache, malaise, and fatigue. Lymphadenopathy (swollen lymph nodes) and splenomegaly may occur during the disease. Mononucleosis typically is diagnosed through serologic methods that detect antibodies to EBV (Fig. 65.3). Nonspecific heterophile antibodies (also referred to as **Paul-Bunnell antibodies**) appear early on during the disease, making the diagnosis difficult. Antibody production to the virus typically follows the classic immune response, resulting in specific IgM production followed by IgG production. Antibody (IgM) to the **viral capsid antigen (VCA)** appears within 4 weeks after infection. This is followed by IgG and IgA antibody to the **early antigen (EA),** indicating acute or recent infection. Both the EA-IgG and IgA may be undetectable after approximately 6 months. Some Anti-EA IgG antibodies may persist in the patient's serum for life. These persistent antibodies typically are elevated in patients with Burkitt lymphoma. The final diagnostic serologic marker is the antibody to the **nuclear antigen (EBNA)** that appears within 1 month of infection and peaks approximately 6 to 12 months after infection. In addition to Burkitt lymphoma, other cancers have been associated with EBV infection (e.g., nasopharyngeal carcinoma). EBV is recognized as an important agent in the development of lymphoma or other lymphoproliferative disorders in transplant recipients.

Molecular assays have become instrumental in the diagnosis of herpes viruses. A variety of EBV DNA assays are available commercially. The method and sample matrix used is dependent on the suspected clinical syndrome. Quantitative assays for the detection and diagnosis of EBV infection are preferred over qualitative in order to determine the risk for the patient in progressing to EBV-associated disorders. Detection of EBV DNA and microRNAs (small noncoding RNAs involved in gene regulation) in nasopharyngeal brushings has been used for the diagnosis of EBV associated nasopharyngeal carcinoma. The prediction for the development of EBV-associated posttransplant lymphoproliferative disorder (PTLD) can be determined by monitoring EBV DNA loads shortly after transplantation. Monitoring viral loads and reducing immunosuppressive medications has reduced the incidence of EBV associated PTLD. In order to assist in the standardization of molecular methods for the detection and monitoring of EBV DNA, the WHO approved the use of a whole EBV preparation that was created by the National Institute of Biological Standards and Controls, United Kingdom.

Cytomegalovirus

CMV infection is a common cause of congenital birth defects. The virus is included in the TORCH panel for disease screening in infants. (TORCH is an acronym for toxoplasma, rubella, CMV, and HSV-1). Besides being the cause of congenital infection in infants, CMV has been found to cause an IM–like illness in immunocompromised patients. The disease can be extremely serious in immunosuppressed organ transplant recipients. CMV can be identified using viral cell culture, serologic tests for IgM and IgG antibodies, direct antigen detection, and nucleic acid testing. Although the virus grows in cell culture using human fibroblasts, it is a slow-growing virus that requires 1 to 2 weeks of incubation before CPE is evident, providing a diagnosis within 24 to 48 hours. CMV antigenemia (Chapter 64 and

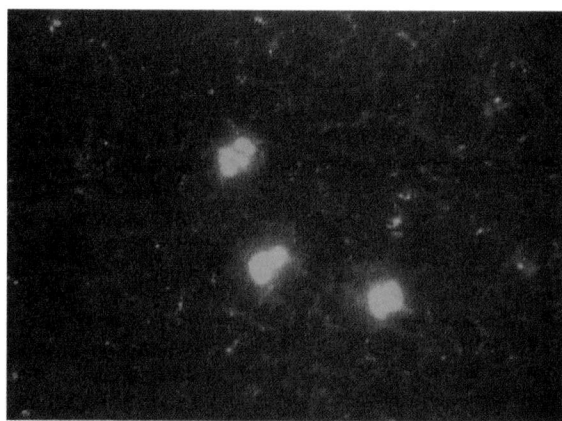

• **Fig. 65.4** Typical fluorescing white blood cells containing cytomegalovirus (CMV) antigen, as seen in the CMV antigenemia stain.

Evolve Procedure 64.2) is routinely used to monitor therapy for CMV infection. A positive CMV antigenemia result is shown in Fig. 65.4.

Molecular qualitative and quantitative PCR amplification have replaced the antigenemia assay in most clinical laboratories. A variety of assays are available for the detection of CMV DNA and mRNA in both monoplex and multiplex panels. NAATs are used for the identification and detection of CMV DNA in immunocompromised patients, including patients with acquired immune deficiency syndrome (AIDS), transplant recipients, and patients with congenital infections, as well as for monitoring the efficiency of antiviral therapy. Viral load measured using CMV DNA is considered the best predictor for the development of CMV-associated disease. Comparative analyses of CMV antigenemia and CMV DNA quantitation demonstrate general agreement when used to monitor disease syndromes.

Orthomyxoviridae

The influenza virus is a member of the family *Orthomyxoviridae*. The **orthomyxoviruses** are large (80 to 120 nm), pleomorphic, spherical, enveloped, single-stranded, segmented, negative-sense RNA viruses. Of all the respiratory viruses known to infect humans, influenza is the cause of the greatest number of serious acute illnesses; more than 200,000 hospitalizations and more than 30,000 deaths occur in the United States every year. Although three types of influenza viruses are known to infect humans (A, B, and C), type C usually causes subclinical infections or mild respiratory disease. Influenza virus A, influenza virus B, and influenza virus C can be distinguished based on the antigenic differences in the **matrix protein (M)** and the **nucleoprotein (NP)**. Influenza virus A is further subdivided based on the major surface glycoproteins, **hemagglutinin (HA)** and **neuraminidase (NA).** Influenza A naturally infects many bird species, swine, seals, felines, and horses. Influenza B and C are only known to infect humans.

Projecting from the envelope of the virion are the two major surface glycoproteins, HA and NA. The HA proteins are rod-shaped spikes that enable viral attachment to sialic acid–containing cellular receptors. Once attached to the receptors, the virus can initiate infection. The NA proteins are mushroom-shaped spikes. They facilitate the release of mature virions from infected cells and assist in viral movement through mucus to adjacent cells. Eighteen different HA molecules and 11 different NA molecules have been identified. All of the different viral protein antigenic types can be found in the avian species. Various subtypes of both influenza A and B can cause global epidemics and pandemics following the emergence of a novel HA strain that can be transmitted readily from person to person. One example, influenza A H3N2, is a highly pathogenic virus. Infection with H3N2 results in greater mortality than infection with influenza A H1N1 or influenza B.

A unique property of influenza A and influenza B is the organization of the viral genome. It is composed of an eight-part, segmented RNA genome, each segment essentially serving as a single gene. This property, combined with the influenza viruses' unique ability to alter their HA and NA antigens, results in the production of an antigenically different virus from year to year. This is termed antigenic drift. Antigenic drift is a continuous, gradual form of change in the viral genome during replication. Antigenic drift occurs in all viral influenza types.

Influenza A undergoes a seasonal antigenic drift every year, making the formulation of an effective vaccine challenging. Antigenic shift is a much more dramatic change in the viral genome and only occurs with influenza A viruses. Antigenic shift occurs when a circulating influenza A strain acquires a completely new, or novel, subtype. This phenomenon occurs when two different strains of influenza virus simultaneously infect a single host. During viral replication the segmented genome of the influenza virus may reassort, mixing segments from the different strains during the infection, resulting in a unique antigenic combination. Avian influenza and human influenza reassortment of genes have been the cause of several pandemics throughout history. Often swine act as the intermediate, or "mixing vessel," for these reassortment events. Viruses from avian and human origin can infect and replicate in the swine respiratory epithelium. When these reassortments occur, a virus emerges against which the population does not have immune protection because of the new antigenic structure. When this happens, a pandemic (global outbreak) can occur if the virus is able to sustain human-to-human transmission. Often pandemics result in high rates of human mortality with significant social, infrastructure, and economic consequences. Enhanced surveillance for the pandemic strain of influenza H1N1 was preceded by the appearance of the avian influenza, commonly referred to as the "bird flu," circulating in Asia. This influenza strain stems from the avian population. The influenza virus (H5N1) is a highly pathogenic avian influenza that has reassorted multiple times with other avian influenza strains capable of causing disease in poultry and other birds. Despite the high prevalence of H5N1 among avian populations, human infection remains low, and the low transmissibility suggests a natural barrier to cross-species infection. Most human infections are acquired as a result of contact with infected poultry raised inside or outside the home. The case fatality rate for this disease is close to 60%. This virus has significantly affected the worldwide economy. It has caused the death and destruction of more than 500 million wild and domestic birds worldwide and resulted in losses to the poultry industry of more than $10 billion. Other avian influenza A virus subtypes are also of concern, including H7N7 in commercial poultry farms in the Netherlands, which has been associated with respiratory illness. H7N9 has emerged in poultry markets in China and has been associated with human infections.

Influenza normally is transmitted person to person through inhalation of aerosolized droplets of infected secretions. The incubation period is 1 to 4 days, with rapid onset of symptoms, including fever, nonproductive cough, sore throat, rhinitis, headache, malaise, and myalgia. The illness usually resolves within a week, although some symptoms may persist longer. Gastrointestinal symptoms, including watery diarrhea, vomiting, and abdominal pain, may occur in the absence of respiratory symptoms.

Bacterial coinfections are common with influenza, possibly because of viral NA-induced changes in the respiratory epithelium that allow increased bacterial adherence or decreased mucociliary clearance. Clusters of fatal methicillin-resistant *Staphylococcus aureus* (MRSA) infections secondary to seasonal influenza A have been reported in otherwise healthy children and adults.

Testing for influenza can be completed by viral culture, detection of viral nucleic acid or antigen, and serology. Optimal testing requires proper collection and timing of specimens, and both high-throughput and point of care testing is available. Virus is shed 3 to 5 days after the onset of symptoms. Optimal specimens are collected from the posterior nasopharynx. The epithelium of the nasopharynx usually contains high titers of virus and large amounts of infected cells. A variety of other respiratory samples, including nasal aspirates, nasal wash, throat swabs, and throat washes, may be used for viral identification. The samples should be placed in viral transport media and may be stored at 4°C for up to 5 days. If the sample must be stored longer, it should be stored in a freezer at −70°C until processed.

RT-PCR is the new gold standard for the identification of respiratory viruses. The technique is effective when specimens are compromised, such as when they are collected late in the course of the disease or when appropriate collection and transportation requirements have not been met. Sensitivity has proven to be equal to or better than that of cell culture. A variety of NAATs are commercially available for the identification and characterization of influenza A, B, and C. In addition, multiplex respiratory panels are also available that include influenza A, B, and various subtypes. However, multiplex assays may demonstrate reduced sensitivity in comparison to monoplex assays. DNA microarray assays have been developed to identify and differentiate viral subtypes; however, they are expensive, and are only available in specialized laboratories.

Cell culture is available for influenza virus using a variety of cell lines. Primary monkey kidney (PMK) cell lines and Madin-Darby canine kidney (MDCK) cell lines have demonstrated a consistent season-to-season isolation frequency of influenza virus. Sometimes the influenza viruses fail to produce a CPE in traditional cell culture, requiring additional testing by hemadsorption with guinea pig red blood cells (RBCs) for viral detection. Cell cultures are reviewed every 1 to 3 days and screened by hemadsorption. Cells that demonstrate 4+ CPE can be used for further characterization. Follow-up confirmatory methods include immunofluorescent assays (IFAs). Rapid shell vials can be used to detect virus in 24 to 72 hours, using type-specific mAbs. Shell vials cannot be used to produce virus for subsequent viral studies.

Papillomaviruses

Papillomaviruses are small (~55 nm), nonenveloped, circular, double-stranded DNA viruses. These viruses are abundant in nature and cause infections in humans, dogs, cattle, monkeys, and many other species. The *Papillomaviridae* family includes the HPVs. HPVs cause human warts. They exhibit a tissue tropism for either cutaneous or mucosal tissue. The viruses have not been cultivated in cell culture, which prevents the production of type-specific antigens and corresponding typing antisera. HPVs are divided into more than 200 genotypes based on the viral DNA sequences. Much attention has been focused on the more than 40 sexually transmitted genotypes and their role in the pathogenesis of cancer. The International Agency for Research on Cancer has designated 12 HPV types as oncogenic or high risk for the development of cancer. The various HPV genotypes have differing cellular tropisms, resulting in defined variation in the clinical presentation of the warts. For example, HPV-1 is associated with plantar warts; HPV-2 and HPV-4 are associated with common warts of the hands; and HPV-6, HPV-11, and others are associated with genital warts. Anogenital warts are associated with HPV types 6 and 11 and rarely associated with cancer. HPV types 6 and 11 are also associated with oral and upper respiratory tract warts. Oral and respiratory warts can be associated with cancer. Morbidity does occur in nonmalignant cases due to the need for surgical removal, damage to vocal cords, and potential respiratory obstruction. HPV high-risk genotypes cause cervical, vulvar, vaginal, squamous cell oropharynx, anal, and penile cancer. Approximately 95% of all cervical cancers are HPV positive. HPV-16 and 18 cause more than 70% of the cases.

HPV infection is the most prevalent sexually transmitted viral disease in the United States. Infection is detected using histopathologic or cytologic examination of cutaneous biopsy or cells, respectively, and DNA probe assays for identification of specific genotypes in infected epithelial cells. A single, liquid-based cytology sample can be used for cytology and genotyping. NAATs are used for screening and the management of cervical disease. Several commercial nucleic acid–based HPV assays currently are commercially available in the United States. The assays vary in the method of amplification, signal or target; the detected nucleic acid, RNA or DNA; the level of genotyping included in the assay; and the level of technical complexity. There are currently no commercial assays available to monitor viral load for HPV. The quantification is difficult to reproduce due to the variation in viral copy number (amount of nucleic acid) unevenly distributed throughout the tissue. Next-generation sequencing of HPV is available in research laboratory settings. However, to utilize this technology in clinical applications advances in the HPV consensus sequence and database management (bioinformatics) is required and has the potential to improve HPV diagnosis and management in the future. Three vaccines for HPV are currently licensed by the FDA: Cervarix (Glaxo Smith Kline, Brentford, Middlesex, United Kingdom), Gardasil, and Gardasil-9 (Merck & Co., Inc, Whitehouse Station, NJ), all of which protect against the two most common carcinogenic types, HPV 16 and 18. Gardasil also protects against HPV types 6 and 11, which are responsible for more than 90% of anogenital warts. Gardasil-9 further protects against several lower-risk HPV types (31, 33, 45, 52, and 58) known to be associated with cervical and most HPV-induced oral cancers.

Paramyxoviridae

The *Paramyxoviridae* family includes many pathogenic viruses. Many of these viruses are identified more often in young children, including measles, mumps, Nipah virus, and parainfluenza viruses. **Paramyxoviruses** do not have a segmented genome, as do the orthomyxoviruses, and therefore do not undergo antigenic shift. Paramyxoviruses are large (150 to 350 nm) pleomorphic, spherical or filamentous, enveloped negative-sense, single-stranded, RNA viruses, and all members of this group can cause respiratory disease.

Human parainfluenza viruses are important pathogens in children. Viral infection may present as either croup or other upper respiratory diseases in children and adults. The paramyxoviruses are second only to respiratory syncytial virus (RSV) in causing bronchiolitis and pneumonia in infants and young children. The parainfluenza virus has four subtypes; parainfluenza 1 is the most common cause of croup, and parainfluenza 3 is second in prevalence to RSV as a disease of infants and very young children. Most children have had an infection with parainfluenza 3 by 2 years of age. Parainfluenza 3 is most often associated with severe disease and fatalities. Parainfluenza 4 causes all of the same respiratory infections associated with the other types, except croup. Parainfluenza 1 and 3 are also associated with severe pulmonary infections in adults, often requiring hospitalization. Parainfluenza viruses are also associated with significant morbidity and mortality in immunocompromised patients.

Parainfluenza viral infection is acquired through inoculation of mucous membranes of the respiratory tract with infectious secretions transmitted on fomites or as large, droplet aerosols. Parainfluenza virus can live up to 10 hours

on varying surfaces. Laboratory identification is accomplished through the use of direct detection of the parainfluenza using NAATs. There are a variety of monoplex and multiplex panels that are capable of detecting all four types of parainfluenza. Molecular methods have improved sensitivity over serologic or cell culture methods and are particularly useful in rapid diagnosing of infections in immunocompromised patients. Cell culture, using primary or continuous cell lines, followed by confirmatory testing using IFA, DFA, or other methods of antigen detection can also be used but has been replaced by molecular methods in most clinical laboratories.

Mumps is an acute, self-limiting disease characterized by **parotitis** (inflamed salivary gland) accompanied by a high temperature (fever) and fatigue. The mumps virus is transmitted through droplets and contact with contaminated fomites. Humans are the only known reservoir for the virus. Despite the implementation of a trivalent vaccine for measles, mumps, and rubeola in the late 1960s, infections with the mumps virus continue to be on the rise. Research studies have identified new circulating mumps virus strains based on a comparative genomic analysis. This indicates that the current vaccine may not provide adequate protection and may need reformulation. The average incubation period for infection is approximately 16 to 18 days followed by the development of nonspecific respiratory symptoms, slightly elevated temperature and the characteristic enlargement of one or both of the parotid glands. Patients have been reported to develop meningoencephalitis, orchitis, oophoritis, polyarthritis, and pancreatitis as complications following initial infection.

Laboratory diagnosis is generally made by the detection of viral RNA in oral fluid, CSF, saliva, throat, or urine specimens using molecular methods. NAATs are generally more sensitive than viral isolation in culture. There are currently no FDA-cleared molecular assays commercially available for the identification of mumps in clinical samples; however, the CDC has developed and standardized two assays to be used for the identification of the virus. Traditional cell culture can be used, but CPE characterized by rounded and multinucleated giant cells requires 6 to 8 days of incubation and may not appear at all. Rapid shell vial culture can detect pre-CPE within 24 to 48 hours following inoculation. Previous vaccination for the mumps virus may also lower the probability of isolating the virus in cell culture. Therefore, it is important to note that failure to isolate the virus does not rule out infection.

Measles Virus

The measles (rubeola) virus is a pleomorphic, enveloped, nonsegmented single-stranded, negative-sense RNA virus that causes an acute, generalized infection often accompanied by a characteristic rash. The hallmark rash of measles infection is referred to as **Koplik spots,** which are bluish white spots with a red halo located on the buccal or labial mucosa. These spots are found on the inner lip or opposite the lower molars in the mouth. The virus is transmitted from person to person through aerosols and infects the mucosal cells of the respiratory tract.

Measles is one of six classic childhood diseases capable of causing a rash or skin eruption (exanthem). The other diseases that cause an exanthem are scarlet fever (which is caused by a bacterium, group A streptococcus); **rubella** (German measles), referred to as **atypical scarlet fever; erythema infectiosum** (or **fifth disease,** caused by parvovirus B-19); and **roseola** (caused by HHV-6). The illness begins with a cough, coryza, conjunctivitis, and fever. As the symptoms increase over the next several days the Koplik spots develop, before the erythematous rash appears. The rash presents as macules that appear on the forehead or behind the ears, spreading to the trunk, then to the arms and legs. Measles can be fatal as a result of immunosuppression and disseminated CNS complications including encephalomyelitis and subacute sclerosing panencephalitis (SSPE). Infection during pregnancy can result in congenital malformations in the unborn fetus.

Since the introduction of the live attenuated childhood trivalent vaccine against measles, mumps, and rubella (MMR), measles infections are rare in the United States and Europe. However, new outbreaks are becoming more common in the United States because of an increase in the number of unvaccinated individuals. In just the first 4 months of 2019, the CDC reported 465 cases in 19 states, from a virus that was completely eradicated endemically in the year 2000, marked by zero cases over a 12-month period or longer. These viruses continue to circulate and remain a common illness in developing countries. Mortality rates from measles infections can be as high as 20%, as a result of contributing factors such as poor hygiene and malnutrition. These viruses are often brought into the United States by travelers or people from other countries. The potential for an outbreak arises when infected individuals come in contact with unvaccinated individuals, and prompt laboratory investigation of suspect cases is required.

Diagnostic testing for these viruses involves serologic analysis of patient serum for IgM and IgG antibodies and nucleic acid detection. NAAT for viral RNA and nucleic acid sequencing is the only way to distinguish a vaccine reaction from a wild-type viral infection, although IgG avidity assays are also available, which can assist in ruling in a case of measles. For measles cell culture, the specimens of choice are respiratory, oropharynx, conjunctiva, or blood specimens. These viruses are also shed in the urine; therefore, urine specimens can be examined for their presence.

Parvoviridae

Parvoviruses (the Latin term *parvus* means "small") have a wide distribution among warm-blooded animals. Viruses that only cause disease in animals are referred to as **epizootic**. Parvoviruses are small (~22 nm) nonenveloped, icosahedral, linear, single-stranded DNA viruses. At least five different parvoviruses are known to infect humans, with parvovirus B19 being the best characterized. The additional viruses that infect humans include the human bocaviruses, Parv4, human bufavirus, and nonpathogenic adeno-associated virus. Parvovirus B19 is transmitted by close contact through respiratory droplets. The replication of parvovirus B19 in human cells is largely restricted to erythroid progenitor cells, adult bone marrow, and fetal liver cells (the site of erythropoiesis during fetal development). Important diseases associated with parvovirus B-19 infection are fifth disease (the fifth of the childhood exanthems), aplastic crisis in patients with underlying hemoglobinopathies, and fetal infection (hydrops fetalis) resulting from transplacental inoculation. Parvovirus causes a biphasic illness in humans. The first phase, marked by fever, malaise, myalgia, and chills, corresponds to peak levels of virus and destruction of erythroblasts. This phase, when mild, may be overlooked or considered a nonspecific viral disease. The second phase involves rash and arthralgia, which occur after the virus has disappeared but at a time when parvovirus-specific antibody can be detected. This is consistent with the appearance of the rash caused by immune complex deposition in the capillaries of the skin. IgM antibodies appear within 7 days after infection, followed by IgG at approximately 14 days.

Laboratory diagnosis is accomplished using NAAT for the detection of B19 DNA in clinical samples. Molecular methods are extremely sensitive. B19 DNA is easily identified and can be detected months even years following the patient's complete recovery. This necessitates the use of quantitative PCR to distinguish recent or current infection from past infections with the virus. Parvovirus B19 cannot be propagated in traditional cell culture, because the virus can only be grown in erythroid progenitor cells. Therefore, cell culture has not been used for viral propagation outside of the research laboratory. Parvovirus-specific IgM or virus-specific IgG antibody testing with paired acute and convalescent sera can be helpful in the diagnosis of infection. Immunoassays are generally sensitive and specific, and a variety of commercial assays are available.

Picornaviridae

Picornaviruses are small (~30 nm; from the Italian word *piccolo,* meaning "small"), nonenveloped, single-stranded positive-sense RNA viruses. They are among the simplest of the RNA viruses, with a highly structured capsid that has limited surface elaboration. This family of viruses includes the enteroviruses, RVs, parechovirus and cardioviruses, and HAV.

Enteroviruses, Parechoviruses, and Polioviruses

Enterovirus infections are among the most common human viral infections, and although these infections often are mild, the viruses also can cause serious disease. Enteroviruses are responsible for a variety of diseases and conditions, including aseptic meningitis, paralytic poliomyelitis, and encephalitis, in addition to respiratory illness, myocarditis, and pericarditis. Enteroviruses are the most common cause of **aseptic meningitis,** an inflammation of the brain parenchyma, and have been isolated from more than 40% of patients with this disease.

Before the development of the polio vaccine, the polio enterovirus was responsible for paralytic poliomyelitis around the world.

The enteroviruses originally were divided into poliovirus, coxsackie virus, and echovirus groups based on similarity of characteristics in cell culture and disease in humans. Classification based on these criteria resulted in the definition of 67 serogroups of enterovirus. Genetic diversity among these viruses, recognized through the application of modern molecular techniques, dictates that newly characterized strains be given enterovirus-type designations rather than serotype status in one of the three original groups. The molecular and serotype designations provide an improved classification system because of the previously poor disease- and phenotype-based classification system. Human enteroviruses have now been reclassified into seven species, human enteroviruses A to D and RVs A to C. The echoviruses are genetically different from the other enteroviruses and have been renamed HPeV1 and HPeV2. The parechovirus is now classified into two species, PeV A and PeV B. Additional recombinant viruses are continuing to be identified using next generation sequencing.

The enteroviruses and parechoviruses are found worldwide and are transmitted by the respiratory and fecal-oral routes. Therefore, the primary site for viral infection is the respiratory epithelium or the gastrointestinal tract. The five most common viruses associated with endemic infection include enteroviruses type E9, E13, E30, and CVB5 and account for more than 48% of reported cases. Only 3.3% of enterovirus infections have been associated with death. Most infections with both enteroviruses and parechoviruses are asymptomatic. Both viruses also cause a mild viral syndrome that manifests as an acute nonspecific febrile illness with or without a rash. The most serious condition associated with infection is aseptic meningitis. The enteroviruses cause more than 80% of the cases of aseptic meningitis in the United States. HPeV3 has also been identified in association with aseptic meningitis and neonatal sepsis. Systemic disease can cause an infection in any organ system. Poliomyelitis, inflammatory damage to the anterior horn cells of the spinal cord, was traditionally associated with polio virus (PV). However, acute flaccid myelitis (AFM), associated with PV infection, is now more commonly identified in infections with nonpolio enteroviruses (NPEVs), PeVs and circulating vaccine-derived polio viruses (cVDPVs). These cVDPVs are derived from the previous live vaccine (Oral Sabin) used to prevent polio, which have regained their ability to cause poliomyelitis. Several NPEVs are also known to cause AFM. Neonatal systemic disease is associated with EV and PeV acquired *in utero*, perinatally or postnatally within 2 weeks. Finally, respiratory syndromes including pneumonia, bronchiolitis, and lower respiratory disease may be associated with enteroviral infections in young children and infants.

Specimens for the diagnosis of enteroviral infections depend on the clinical signs and symptoms present. Specimens of choice for detecting enterovirus are stool specimens or rectal swabs, throat swabs or nasopharyngeal washings, and CSF. For cases of acute hyperemia conjunctivitis, conjunctival swabs or tears can be used. Serum or plasma may also be used in cases of aseptic meningitis or neonatal sepsis.

NAAT are the preferred method for the diagnosis and identification of EV and PeV. Although both can be readily grown in cell culture and produce a characteristic CPE of visible cell rounding and shrinking, as well as refractility and cell degeneration, the technique has little clinical value due the lengthy incubation times of 10 to 21 days for viral isolation. Molecular methods for the identification of these viruses are sensitive, specific, rapid, and clinically useful for decreasing length of stay during hospitalization. Prior to being tested by nucleic acid–based methods, viral RNA must be extracted to eliminate RNases in the sample and degradation of the viral RNA. Both monoplex and multiplex molecular platforms are commercially available and FDA-cleared for the identification of both EV and PeV.

Serologic testing for the presence of IgM, IgA, or IgM antibodies with ELISA can be used for suspect cases of enterovirus infection, including myocarditis and congenital infections in pregnant women, as well as an epidemiologic tool in enterovirus outbreaks.

Rhinovirus

RV is the cause of the common cold. Similar to other members of the *Picornaviridae*, RVs are small (20 to 27 nm), nonenveloped, icosahedral single-stranded, positive-sense RNA viruses. RVs have been classified as three separate species, A to C. There are approximately 166 recognized serotypes of RVs. It is also important to note that a previous infection with one serotype of RV does not confer immunity to a subsequent infection with a different serotype.

The virus's name reflects the fact that the primary infection and replication site is the epithelial cells in the nose. RVs are responsible for more than 50% of viral colds and cause more upper respiratory viral infections than any other virus. Although typically mild, RV infections can cause complications such as otitis media and sinusitis and can exacerbate previously existing conditions such as asthma, chronic obstructive pulmonary disease (COPD), and cystic fibrosis, in which the risk of severe lower respiratory disease is significantly increased, and morbidity can result. Considerably more cases of lower respiratory tract disease in adults are caused by RV than was previously known. Infection occurs by person-to-person transmission of infected respiratory secretions. Infection usually occurs through self-inoculation through the eyes or nose and also occurs through contact with infectious aerosols. Symptoms usually begin 2 to 3 days after exposure. The clinical presentation includes a profuse, watery nasal discharge frequently accompanied by symptoms of headache, malaise, sneezing, nasal congestion, sore throat, and cough. Illness generally lasts 10 days to 2 weeks.

Confirmation of RV infection is rarely required for clinical reasons, because the infection is typically self-limiting. However, the specimen of choice for diagnosis is nasal secretions. NAAT is generally used for detection of RV because of the fast turnaround times and increased sensitivity. As with numerous other viral respiratory pathogens, several commercial monoplex and multiplex assays are available for the detection of RV infections.

Culture can be performed for RV using human cell lines such as MRC-5, human embryonic lung fibroblast strains WI-38, and human embryonic kidney (HEK) cells. CPE usually occurs 1 to 4 days after inoculation. CPE appears as large and small round refractile cells in the fibroblast cell line. The RVs grow best or exclusively at lower temperatures (30°C); therefore, detection in clinical virology laboratories often is unlikely because typical incubation temperatures for viral cell culture are 35°C to 37°C. If required, cell culture conditions should resemble the physiologic environment in the nasal passages, including a pH of 7 and a temperature of 33°C to 35°C. An acid treatment of the clinical sample before culture inoculation can be used to distinguish RV growth from acid-stable enteroviruses. However, this test is not readily available in clinical laboratories because of its complexity and long turnaround time. IFA cannot be used to confirm RV in cell culture, because no mAbs or antigen detection assays are available.

Hepatitis A Virus

HAV, another member of the picornaviruses, causes an infectious nonchronic hepatitis. HAV is usually transmitted through contaminated food or water or household contact with an infected person. Other transmission routes include sharing of contaminated needles (illicit drug use), travel to endemic countries, and homosexual male intercourse. The virus is significantly different from the other picornaviruses based on the liver tissue tropism, high thermal stability, and viral assembly. HAV is a small, icosahedral, single-strand, positive-sense RNA virus that produces two forms of fully infectious viral particles. One form is a small (27 nm), non-enveloped virion that is shed in the feces, and the second is a much larger (50 to 110 nm) virion that is enveloped and circulates in the peripheral bloodstream. Transmission is fecal-oral through the ingestion of contaminated food or water, close contact between infected individuals and less frequently, by anal sexual contact, IV drug use, and contaminated blood products.

NAAT can be used to detect the HAV RNA in blood and stool before clinical symptoms are apparent. Nucleic acid–based testing is useful in establishing early infection. A variety of quantitative and qualitative molecular methods are commercially available for the detection of HAV RNA in clinical samples. HAV is the only hepatitis group of viruses capable of growth in cell culture. A serologic assay to identify the IgM or IgG are available for diagnosis of HAV infection (Fig. 65.5). False-positive HAV IgM results do occur following resolution of the infection and in the

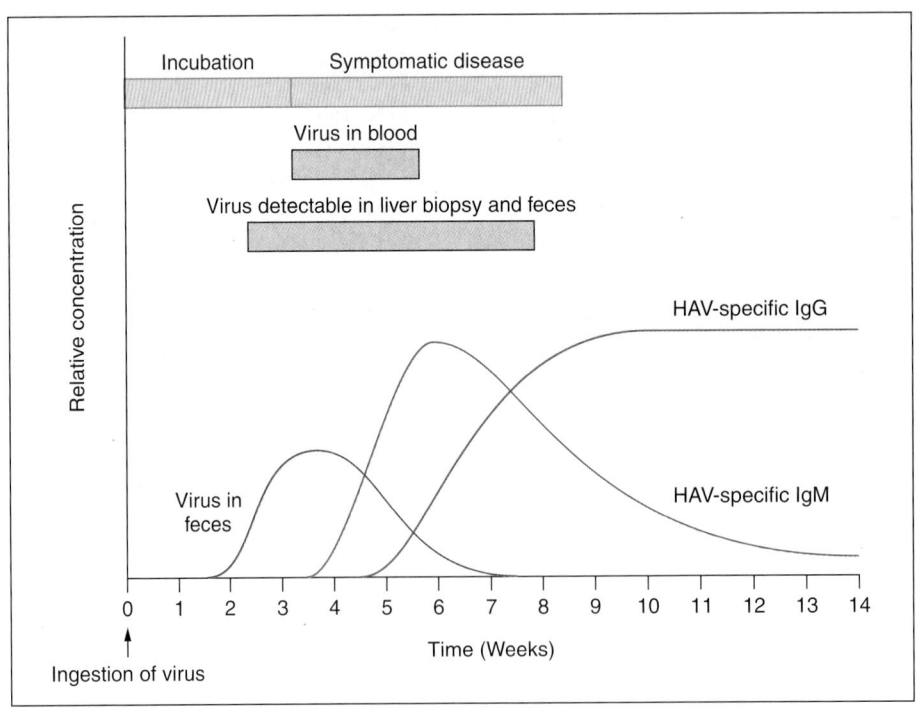

• **Fig. 65.5** Time course of disease and immune response to hepatitis A virus *(HAV)*. (Modified from Murray PR, Kobayashi GS, Pfaller MA, et al., eds. *Medical Microbiology*. 2nd ed. St Louis: Mosby; 1994.)

absence of HAV IgG. A vaccine against this virus for adults and for children older than 2 years of age became available during the 1990s.

Pneumoviridae

The *Pneumoviridae* includes RSV and the human metapneumovirus (HMPVs). RSV is an enveloped, single-stranded, nonsegmented, negative-sense RNA virus. Transmission occurs via respiratory secretions. RSV causes bronchiolitis in young children and is the most significant cause of acute lower respiratory tract infection in children younger than 5 years of age worldwide. The virus is also capable of causing a high rate of morbidity and mortality in adults older than 65 years. According to the CDC, each year in the United States, RSV is responsible for more than 14,000 deaths and approximately 180,000 hospitalizations. The virus contains a surface protein called **F (fusion) protein**. F protein mediates host cell fusion into syncytial cells, which are a hallmark of RSV infection and so named because of the CPE syncytia formation in monolayer cell culture. RSV immune serum prevents severe RSV bronchiolitis during the early months of life in susceptible newborns at risk for RSV disease and those with underlying medical conditions, especially in premature children with underdeveloped lungs.

Diagnostic testing for RSV also is performed using rapid direct antigen testing, nucleic acid detection, and cell culture. Rapid antigen direct tests (RADTs) are simple, waived tests and can be completed within 30 minutes. A variety of RADTs are commercially available; however, the sensitivity is relatively low and can result in false negative results. Multiple monoplex and multiplex platforms for the detection of RSV in respiratory samples are available from commercial manufacturers. The assays also demonstrate an increased sensitivity over RADTs and the rapid diagnosis of infections has improved patient care by reducing the length of stay and duration of antibiotic administration in health care facilities. Cell culture remains the gold standard for the isolation of the virus. Cell culture is not affected by viral mutations that can result in false negatives when using NAAT. However, cell culture requires propagation of cell lines and much higher technical expertise. Several respiratory viruses including parainfluenza virus 3 and the measles virus produce similar CPE. Cell culture requires confirmation with RSV type-specific IF for identification.

HMPV is closely related to RSV. It is a large (150 to 600 nm), enveloped, single stranded, nonsegmented, negative-sense RNA virus. The virus is ubiquitous and infects all age groups. In infections in children, this virus appears to be less common than RSV but more common than parainfluenza virus, making it an important, medically relevant infectious agent. The virus causes bronchiolitis and pneumonia in infants and most likely lower respiratory tract disease in older adults. In infants 6 to 12 months of age, infection with metapneumovirus is likely to show an increase in lower airway involvement. The virus is considered the second or third most common cause of hospitalization for lower airway

disease in pediatric patients. Like RSV, metapneumovirus is associated with winter epidemics that vary in severity from year to year. Isolation of metapneumovirus from cell culture is difficult because the virus is very slow to grow and often takes longer than 2 weeks to develop detectable CPE. RADTs are available that are highly specific but have low sensitivity in comparison to NAAT. However, they are frequently used in combination with molecular methods due to their cost, low complexity, and rapid turnaround time. Nucleic acid testing for viral RNA is considered the gold standard for HMPV. There are a variety of FDA-cleared platforms and assays available for the detection of HMPV simultaneously with other respiratory viruses. This is clinically significant in the diagnosis of HMPV because the symptoms are very nonspecific, and it allows the detection of coinfections. Approximately 42% of pediatric HMPV cases were identified to be coinfections with other respiratory viruses. Isolation of the virus using conventional or shell vial culture techniques are of little utility in the clinical laboratory. The virus grows poorly or not at all in most cell lines used for the isolation of respiratory viruses. The CPE is also nondistinctive, requiring specific identification of the virus using mAb (IFA) or nucleic acid (RNA) amplification.

Polyomaviridae

The **polyomaviruses** are small (40 to 45 nm), icosahedral, nonenveloped, circular, double-stranded DNA viruses that have been isolated from many species, including humans. There are 14 different human polyomaviruses (HPyVs) that have been characterized. The first human viruses included the JC (John Cunningham) JCPyV and the BK (renal transplant patient with the initials B.K.) BKPyV viruses, named with the initials of the patients from whom the viruses were first isolated. There are four subtypes of BKPyV, I to IV, and seven subtypes of JCPyV. The subtypes, or genotypes, of the viruses are distributed throughout the world and associated with different human populations and geographic distribution. Infection with these viruses usually occurs during childhood and appears to have little clinical significance. It is believed that the viruses are transmitted through respiratory or oral secretions. Other polyomaviruses, WUPyV, MCPyV, and KIPyV, have been detected in respiratory infections. These viral infections include latent states in the kidney and B lymphocytes and can result in symptomatic reactivation during periods of immune suppression.

Immunocompromised individuals almost always present with the pathologic effects of infections caused by the polyomaviruses. JCPyV virus reactivates, resulting in disease in the CNS; BKPyV virus causes a hemorrhagic cystitis. The MCPyV, which causes Merkel cell carcinoma, is associated with a high percentage of tumors and has also been detected in respiratory specimens. Trichodysplasia spinulosa, a rare skin disease, has been diagnosed in immunocompromised individuals associated with TSPyV infection.

Laboratory diagnosis is generally performed in routine laboratories using NAATs for the detection and quantitation of HPyVs. These assays are very challenging to develop due to the genetic variability of genotypes among these viruses. There are currently no FDA cleared or approved assays available for the identification of polyomaviruses, although some laboratories have developed testing methodologies. The WHO has approved a BKPyV standard produced by the National Institute for Biological Standards and both BKPyV and JCPyV control materials are commercially available from the American Type Culture Collection, Manassas, VA. *In situ* hybridization using BKPyV or JCPyV in conjunction with immunohistochemical staining can be used to identify virus HPyVs in tissue for the diagnosis of clinical disease; however, these methodologies are not available in routine laboratories. Both BKPyV and JCPyV can be isolated in cell culture; however, this method is not used in clinical diagnostic laboratories and is confined to research settings.

Poxviridae

The **poxviruses** are the largest and most complex of all viruses. The virions consist of a double-stranded DNA genome. The virions appear as oval or brick-shaped structures 200 to 450 nm in length. Because of their large size, poxvirus virions may be visualized through a light microscope.

One of the most feared viruses of history, smallpox, is a member of this family. Smallpox played a crucial role in demonstrating the importance of vaccination to protect against disease. Smallpox is known to infect only humans and exists as two distinct subtypes. Variola major, which caused the most severe disease (case fatality rate of 30%), occurred mainly in Asia; variola minor was associated with less severe disease and case fatality rates of 0.1% to 2%. As a result of an intensive vaccination campaign, WHO declared naturally occurring variola virus eradicated in 1980. The variola virus no longer circulates in nature. The virus is feared as a possible biologic weapon, and testing capability for this organism is maintained by hundreds of Laboratory Response Network (LRN) laboratories throughout the nation. All known stocks of the virus are held at two WHO collaborating laboratories: the CDC in Atlanta, Georgia, and the State Center of Virology and Biotechnology (VECTOR) in Koltsovo, Russia. Since the eradication of smallpox in 1980, most vaccination campaigns against this virus have stopped, and most of the world's population lacks any protective immunity against this disease or any related poxviruses.

Besides the smallpox virus, 10 other poxviruses are capable of infecting humans. Except for the smallpox virus and the molluscum contagiosum (MCV) virus, most of these are zoonoses, or infections that result from contact with animals. Fortunately, other than monkeypox (MPXV) and the eradicated smallpox virus (VARV), none of these viruses can sustain human-to-human transmission. The viruses normally are acquired through abrasions of the skin and contact with an infected animal, or in the case of human monkeypox, through the oropharynx, nasopharynx, or

abrasions on the skin. Poxvirus replicates in the epidermal cells and causes change in the cellular structure, characterized by the "pocks" on the skin. Poxvirus infection can take one of two courses: it can cause a localized infection at the site of inoculation, with little spread from the original site of inoculation, or it can cause a fulminant, systemic infection that spreads the virus throughout the body, resulting in an increased mortality rate. The second type of infection is associated with variola virus (smallpox) and monkeypox. MPXV is indistinguishable from smallpox infection except that it lacks the same level of mortality and transmissibility. The monkeypox virus is found in the tropical rain forests of Africa. The host reservoir consists of one or more rodent species.

After the individual is exposed to the virus, symptoms of fever and headache occur first, followed by the development of a rash and lymphadenopathy. The rash typically first appears on the face, beginning as **macules** (small, round changes in skin color), progressing to **papules** (slightly elevated with no fluid), to **vesicles** (containing a bubble of fluid), and then **pustules** (containing purulent material consisting of necrotic inflammatory cells). Depending on the severity of the disease, the illness can last 2 to 4 weeks.

Another member of the poxvirus family is the MCV, which causes single or small clusters of lesions. Its only host is humans, and infection occurs either nonsexual, through direct contact or fomites, or sexually, through intimate contact. Usually a self-limiting disease in healthy individuals, molluscum contagiosum can cause a more severe form of disease in immunocompromised patients, resulting in large lesions, especially on the face, neck, scalp, and upper body.

Orf is another member of the poxvirus family and is transmitted from sheep to humans through human direct contact with infected sheep. This virus causes single or multiple nodules, usually on the hands. These nodules may be painful and may be accompanied by symptoms such as low-grade fever and lymph node swelling. The infection usually resolves in 4 to 6 weeks without further complication, although autoinoculation of the eye can have more serious consequences. An orf diagnosis is made through direct examination of the nodule, along with epidemiologic evidence of a recent history of contact with sheep or lambs.

Direct antigen detection for the poxviruses is not routinely performed in diagnostic laboratories. However, a RADT, the Tetracore Orthopox BioThreat assay, which uses a lateral flow system is available to detect the presence of virus in clinical specimens. The CDC has a pan-poxvirus PCR assay that can be used to screen clinical specimens for poxviruses other than avian species. Many national laboratories and LRN laboratories in the United States use NAAT for rapid response to diagnose polyomavirus infections and rule out smallpox.

Reoviridae

The **reoviruses** were first isolated from respiratory and enteric specimens and therefore are referred to as

respiratory-enteric-orphan viruses (reoviruses). The term "orphan" originally was included in the description of the virus as a result of the absence of an associated disease when the viruses were first described. Reoviruses infect most mammalian species and are readily detected in water contaminated with animal feces. Common human pathogens of this family include the rotaviruses and the agent of Colorado tick fever. Rotaviruses are medium-sized (70 nm) nonenveloped, double-stranded, segmented RNA viruses composed of three concentric protein shells: the outer shell, the inner shell, and the core. This triple-layered icosahedral protein capsid gives the virus a wheel-like or "rota" appearance. Based on the proteins present in these shells, rotavirus is further classified into seven distinct groups, A through G; groups A, B, and C cause human disease. Rotavirus is now recognized as the major causative agent of infantile severe gastroenteritis throughout the world. Gastroenteritis caused by rotavirus can occur in children of all ages but is most common in infants from 6 months to 3 years old. The disease is characterized by sudden onset of vomiting, followed by explosive, watery diarrhea and moderate to high fever, often accompanied by dehydration. The severity of the disease often is worse for children in developing countries because of malnutrition and limited or delayed health care. Rotaviruses are transmitted by the fecal-oral route, although airborne transmission has been suspected as the cause of nosocomial infections and outbreaks in nursing homes, hospitals, and day care centers. Rotavirus occurs more frequently in the winter months in temperate climates.

Many methods of laboratory testing are available for the diagnosis of rotavirus. Rotavirus can be detected directly in the stool using ELISA, latex agglutination, IC, RT-PCR, and cell culture. The latex agglutination test and IC platforms offer rapid results with limited laboratory equipment, an advantage in developing countries where resources are limited. A variety of nucleic acid monoplex and multiplex gastroenteritis panels are available for the diagnosis of rotavirus infection. Rotavirus is difficult to cultivate from human specimens. Viral isolation is not normally attempted.

Retroviridae

The retrovirus family *Retroviridae* constitutes a large group of viruses that primarily infect vertebrates. **Retroviruses** are enveloped RNA viruses, and each virion contains two identical copies of single-stranded RNA. The viral nucleic acid strands are surrounded by the structural proteins that form the nucleocapsid and the matrix shell. On the outer surface of the nucleocapsid and matrix protein is the lipid envelope derived from the host cell membrane. Proteins that mediate adsorption and penetration into the host cell membrane are inserted into the viral envelope. Retroviruses are unique, because the virus particle is packaged with the reverse transcriptase enzyme. Reverse transcriptase allows the viral RNA genome to be replicated into DNA and then RNA rather than directly into RNA.

Amino acid sequencing of the reverse transcriptase protein divides the retrovirus family into groups. The human immunodeficiency viruses types 1 and 2 (HIV-1 and HIV-2) are members of this family, as are the human T cell lymphoma viruses types 1 and 2 (HTLV-1 and HTLV-2). HIV-1 (Fig. 65.6) is the more aggressive virus and is responsible for the AIDS pandemic. AIDS is the end stage of a process in which the immune system and its ability to control infections and malignant proliferation is destroyed. The virus has an affinity for the CD4+ surface marker of T lymphocytes. As the number of CD4+ T lymphocytes decreases, the risk and severity of opportunistic infections increases. Some of the most common opportunistic infections associated with HIV infection include disseminated coccidioidomycosis, cryptococcosis, cryptosporidiosis, histoplasmosis, recurrent pneumonia, and pneumocystis pneumonia. Current CDC recommendations for the detection of HIV begins with an initial FDA-approved antigen-antibody combination immunoassay. Reactive specimens with the initial antigen-antibody combination immunoassay should be then tested with an FDA-approved antibody immunoassay that differentiates HIV-1 antibodies from HIV-2 antibodies. Finally, specimens that are reactive on the initial antigen-antibody combination immunoassay and nonreactive or indeterminate on the HIV-1/HIV-2 antibody differentiation immunoassay should be tested with an FDA-approved HIV-1 NAT. For a quick reference guide to this algorithm, see Fig. 65.7. However, the detection of viral nucleic acids using qualitative molecular methods can be useful in diagnosing acute HIV-1 infection and neonatal infections. Diagnosis of HIV infection in babies born to HIV-positive mothers is problematic because of maternal IgG in the baby's blood; therefore, PCR for identification of viral DNA or RNA is recommended. HIV RNA viral load assays are also used to measure the quantity of HIV-1 present in plasma as a prognostic indicator, to monitor treatment and determine infectious status of patients. Clinical management of infected individuals involves the use of highly active antiretroviral therapy (HAART) and depends on the measurement of CD4+ lymphocytes and the viral load. Genome sequencing is used to establish susceptibility to antiviral agents.

HTLVs are fairly large (80 to 100 nm) and enveloped; they contain two positive-sense strand RNA genomes. HTLV-1 is endemic in the Caribbean, Africa, South and Central America, Melanesia, and Japan. However, only a small percentage of people infected (fewer than 4%) develop symptoms and disease. HTLV-1 is associated with two major diseases, adult T-cell leukemia/lymphoma and myelopathy/tropical spastic paresis. The average time from infection to the development of adult T-cell leukemia is approximately 40 years.

Cell-to-cell contact and TAX-induced (HTLV-1 oncoprotein referred to as TAX) clonal expansion of infected cells are the major avenues for viral replication, making detection of the virus difficult. As a result, serologic detection has remained the gold standard for diagnosis. Qualitative

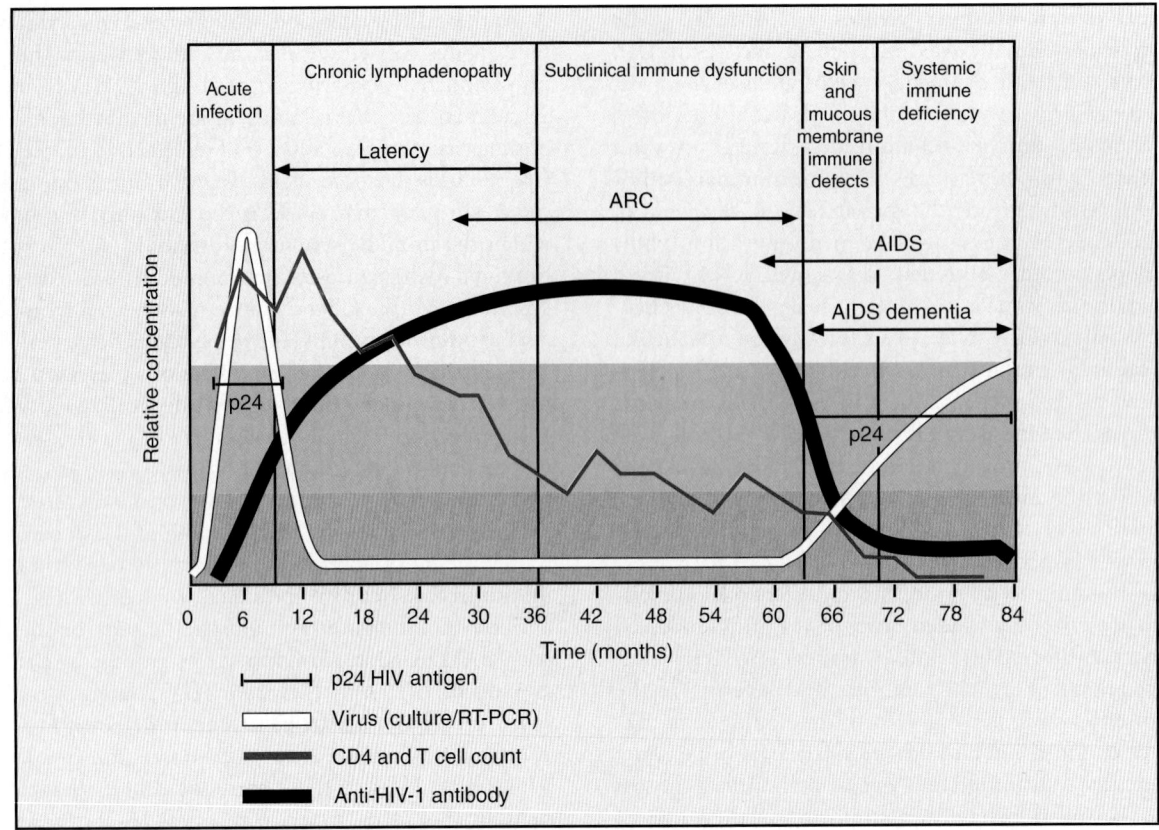

• **Fig. 65.6** Usual time course of immune response, viremia, and disease resulting from untreated human immunodeficiency virus type 1 (HIV-1) infection. *AIDS,* Acquired immune deficiency syndrome; *ARC,* AIDS-related complex; *RT-PCR,* reverse transcriptase polymerase chain reaction. (Redrawn from Murray PR, Kobayashi GS, Pfaller MA, et al. *Medical Microbiology.* 2nd ed. St Louis: Mosby; 1992.)

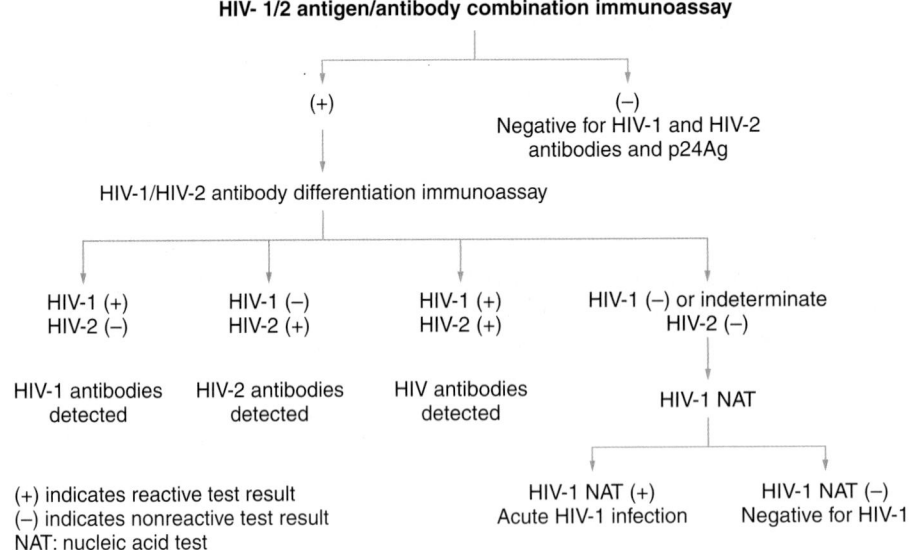

• **Fig. 65.7** Diagram of the Centers for Disease Control and Prevention recommended diagnostic algorithm that replaces the use of the Western blot test in the confirmation of HIV infection.

PCR has been used to distinguish HTLV-1 and HTLV-2 infection. Molecular methods are also useful in determining infection status, comparison with serologic results, and determining tissue distribution of the viruses.

Rhabdoviridae

The family *Rhabdoviridae* includes many viruses that result in acute, fatal viral encephalitis. **Rhabdoviruses** infect plants, arthropods, fish, and mammals. The bullet-shaped virion consists of single-stranded RNA with a helical nucleocapsid surrounded by a lipid bilayer envelope. Spikelike projections approximately 10 nm long extend from the surface of the lipid bilayer. The rabies lyssavirus (RABV) is a neurotropic virus that infects all mammals; with very few exceptions, infection terminates in the death of the infected mammal. The RABV is transmitted through the saliva of infected animals, usually by a bite. After inoculation, the virus may initially multiply in the musculoskeletal tissue or invade the peripheral nerves or nerve endings directly. After infection of the nerve cells, the viral genome progresses centripetally transneuronally, through retrograde axoplasmic flow to the CNS. In the CNS it proceeds from first-order neurons to second-order neurons. The neurons are the site of viral replication, mainly in the brain and spinal cord; from there the virus spreads to peripheral nerves and to some nonnervous tissue, including the salivary glands. After a variable incubation period, human disease usually begins with generalized symptoms of malaise, fever, fatigue, anorexia, and headache. Commonly (and characteristically for this disease) symptoms include pain and sometimes tingling at the site of exposure, which can be the first "rabies-specific" symptom. After this prodromal phase, behavioral changes may start to manifest, followed by rapidly progressing neurologic symptoms that lead to coma and death.

Only six cases of survival of a rabies infection have been documented worldwide. These cases include patients who survived without any complications; other patients have experienced significant neurologic impairment. There is no definitive treatment for rabies once clinical signs and symptoms are present. Updated protocol and statistics related to patient treatment and survival are maintained by the Medical College of Wisconsin and can be accessed at https://www.mcw.edu/departments/pediatrics/divisions/infectious-diseases/rabies-registry-website. In the United States today, human fatalities associated with rabies typically occur in people who fail to seek medical assistance, usually because they were unaware of their exposure. This is particularly common with bat bites, which can be as small as a hypodermic needle.

Animal rabies presents similar to human rabies. After the prodromal phase of the disease, a period of increased excitation occurs, with or without aggression. Clinical presentations of rabies often are described as "furious" or "dumb"; the furious type is associated with heightened aggression and agitation, and the dumb type with lethargy and paralysis.

Rabies is diagnosed by postmortem examination of brain tissue using a direct IFA. Specific sections of the brain are examined for the rabies antigen using fluorescent-tagged mAbs and a fluorescent microscope. Prompt, accurate diagnosis of rabies infections in animals is important to ensure the success of post-exposure prophylaxis for human victims of animal bites and injuries. Despite molecular technological advances, NAAT testing is not used in the routine diagnostic laboratory for the detection of RABV. The CDC has developed a RT-PCR assay for the detection of RABV in human antemortem and confirmatory postmortem animal testing procedures.

Togaviridae

The **togaviruses** (*Togaviridae* family) includes rubella virus and the alpha viruses, a large group of mosquito-borne arboviruses. Rubella is found only in the human population and is transmitted through direct contact with nasopharyngeal secretions or by congenital transmission. Rubella, sometimes called the "German measles," is usually a benign disease characterized by fever and rash. Before the trivalent vaccine, MMR, was developed, rubella was an epidemic disease. A risk associated with this disease is exposure and infection of pregnant women. The virus can infect the developing fetus, causing multiple congenital anomalies. Intrauterine infection during the first trimester may result in low birth weight, mental retardation, deafness, congenital heart disease, and neurologic defects. Infection that occurs later in pregnancy may result in splenomegaly or osteomyelitis, among other birth defects. Fetal infection can be prevented through vaccination of all women before pregnancy.

The alphaviruses are medium-sized (60 to 70 nm), enveloped, nonsegmented, positive-sense strand RNA arboviruses. In arbovirus infections, mosquitoes infect a vertebrate host (e.g., birds and rodents); the virus multiplies (amplifies) in this host and is picked up and passed along in subsequent mosquito bites. Humans are infected incidentally and are not amplifiers of the virus; rather, they are dead-end hosts, unable to pass on the virus to other humans or animals. Human disease varies from asymptomatic infection to fatal encephalitis and includes Eastern, Western, and Venezuelan equine encephalitides. Togavirus disease is diagnosed through detection of specific serum IgG and IgM antibodies. A variety of NAATs are available for the detection of some arboviruses; however, many are only available in specialized reference laboratories. Virus isolation is not practical in clinical laboratories.

Prions in Human Disease

Exposure to prions (infectious proteins) can lead to transmissible **spongiform encephalopathies,** a group of uncurable and fatal neurodegenerative disorders of humans and other animals. The most common of the prion diseases in humans, but still relatively rare in incidence (approximately 1 case per million persons per year worldwide), is

Creutzfeldt-Jakob disease (CJD). Even more rare but often publicized in media outlets is **bovine spongiform encephalopathy (BSE),** otherwise known as mad cow disease. Clinically, CJD, BSE, and other spongiform encephalopathies are very diverse in presentation and include behavioral and personality changes, depression, and a range of psychotic symptoms. The molecular bases of BSE and CJD are similar in that, physiologically, all prion diseases are the result of protein misfolding and subsequent propagation of the misfolded protein state within tissues. Aggregates of misfolded proteins form amyloid fibers, ultimately resulting in the formation of tissue plaques. Therefore, similar to viruses but in contrast to bacterial and eukaryotic pathogens, prions are not characterized as living organisms. Most prion disease in humans arises sporadically; some are due to mutations, and others are caused by zoonotic or iatrogenic transmission. However, during disease development, misfolded proteins can induce the misfolding of properly folded proteins within a tissue, which then in turn continue the process of accumulation and dissemination of the aberrant protein. The prion protein aggregates are very stable within the cell, and mass accumulation of the misfolded proteins ultimately leads to cell death and tissue damage.

Prion disease can be diagnosed using a variety of techniques and information, including clinical presentation, family history, brain tissue studies, analysis of CSF, genetic testing, magnetic resonance imaging (MRI), and electroencephalograms. However, autopsy remains the gold standard for definitive diagnosis, disease classification, and determining disease origin.

(e) Visit the Evolve site for a complete list of procedures, review questions, and case studies.

Bibliography

Agnandji ST, Huttner A, Zinser ME, et al.: Phase 1 trials of rVSV Ebola vaccine in Africa and Europe—preliminary report, *N Engl J Med* 374:1647–1660, 2016.

Alexander LN, Seward JF, Santibanez TA, et al.: Vaccine policy changes and epidemiology of poliomyelitis in the United Sates, *J Am Med Assoc* 292:1696–1701, 2004.

Baron EJ, Miller JM, Weinstein MP, et al.: A guide to utilization of the microbiology laboratory for diagnosis of infectious diseases: 2013 recommendations by the Infectious Diseases Society of America (IDSA) and the American Society for Microbiology (ASM), *Clin Infect Dis* 57:1–100, 2013.

Bartsch SM, Lopman BA, Ozawa S, et al.: Global economic burden of norovirus gastroenteritis, *PloS One* 11:e0151219.

Binda S, Mammoliti A, Primache V, et al.: Pp65 antigenemia plasma real-time PCR and DBS test in symptomatic and asymptomatic cytomegalovirus congenitally infected newborns, *BMC Infect Dis* 10:24–28, 2010.

Cabral F, Arruda LB, de Araujo ML, et al.: Detection of T-cell lymphotropic virus type 1 in plasma samples, *Virus Res* 163:87–90, 2012.

Carroll KC, Pfaller MA, Landry ML, et al.: *Manual of clinical microbiology,* ed 12, Washington, DC, 2019, ASM.

Centers for Disease Control and Prevention: Outbreak of severe acute respiratory syndrome: worldwide, 2003, *Morb Mortal Wkly Rep* 52:226–228, 2003.

Centers for Disease Control and Prevention: Resurgence of wild poliovirus type 1 transmission and consequences of importation: 21 countries, 2002-2005, *Morb Mortal Wkly Rep* 55:145–150, 2006.

Centers for Disease Control and Prevention: Revised US surveillance case definition for severe acute respiratory syndrome (SARS) and update on SARS cases: United States and worldwide, December, 2003, *Morb Mortal Wkly Rep* 52:1202–1206, 2003.

Centers for Disease Control and Prevention. *Quick Reference Guide – Laboratory Testing for the Diagnosis of HIV Infection: Updated Recommendations.* June 27, 2014. Available at: https://doi.org/10.15620/cdc.23447. Accessed January 25, 2016.

Centers for Disease Control and Prevention. *Rabies in the U.S. – Public Health Importance of Rabies.* Available at: https://www.cdc.gov/rabies/location/usa/index.html. Accessed July 17, 2019.

Centers for Disease Control and Prevention. *CDC 2019-Novel Coronavirus (2019-nCoV) Real-Time RT-PCR Diagnostic Panel, CDC-006-00019, Revision: 02 CDC/DDID/NCIRD/ Division of Viral Diseases Effective.* July 13, 2020. Accessed March 15, 2020.

Centers for Disease Control and Prevention. *Serology Testing for Covid-19 at CDC.* Available at: https://www.cdc.gov/coronavirus/2019-ncov/lab/serology-testing.html. Accessed May 8, 2020.

Cockerill FR: Application of rapid-cycle real-time polymerase chain reaction for diagnostic testing in the clinical microbiology laboratory, *Arch Pathol Lab Med* 127:1112–1120, 2003.

Constantine N, Zhao R: Molecular-based laboratory testing and monitoring for human immunodeficiency virus infections, *Clin Lab Sci* 18:263–270, 2005.

Debiasi RL, Tyler KL: Molecular methods for diagnosis of viral encephalitis, *Clin Microbiol Rev* 17:903–925, 2004.

De Clercq E: Antiviral drugs in current clinical use, *J Clin Virol* 30:115–133, 2004.

Dufresne AT, Gromeier M: Understanding polio: new insights from a cold virus, *Microbe* 1:13, 2006.

Espy MJ, Uhl JR, Sloan M, et al.: Real-time PCR in clinical microbiology: applications for routine laboratory testing, *Clin Microbiol Rev* 19:165–256, 2006.

First Ebola vaccine approved. *Nat Biotechnol.* 2020;38(1):6. https://doi.org/10.1038/s41587-019-0385-7.

Flint SJ, Enquist LW, Krug RM, et al.: *Principles of virology: molecular biology, pathogenesis and control,* ed 12, Washington, DC, 2004, ASM Press.

Griffith JT, Rohde RE: Ebola: implications for the clinical laboratory, *Clin Lab Sci,* 2014, Available at: http://www.ascls.org/images/publications/journals/Ebola_virus_manuscript.pdf. Accessed 2 July 2015.

Havelaar AH, Kirk MD, Torgerson PR, et al.: World Health Organization global estimates and regional comparisons of the burden of foodborne disease in 2010, *PLoS Med* 12:e1001923, 2015.

Henao-Restrepo AM, Camacho A, Longini IM, et al.: Efficacy and effectiveness of an rVSV-vectored vaccine in preventing Ebola virus disease: final results from the Guinea ring vaccination, open-label, cluster-randomized trial (Ebola Ça Suffit!), *Lancet* 389:505–518, 2017.

Henrickson KJ: Parainfluenza viruses, *Clin Microbiol Rev* 16:242–264, 2003.

Kahn JS: Epidemiology of human metapneumovirus, *Clin Microbiol Rev* 19:546–557, 2006.

Lai CC, Shih TP, Ko WC, et al.: Severe acute respiratory syndrome coronavirus 2 (SARS-CoV-2) and coronavirus disease-2019 (COVID-19): the epidemic and the challenges, *Int J Antimicrob Agents* 55:105924, 2020.

Lauer GM, Walker BD: Hepatitis C virus infection, *N Engl J Med* 345:41–52, 2001.

Lévy Y, Lane C, Piot P, et al.: Prevention of Ebola virus disease through vaccination: where we are in 2018, *Lancet* 392:787–790, 2018.

Lopman BA, Steele D, Kirkwood CD, et al.: The vast and varied global burden of norovirus: prospects for prevention and control, *PLoS Med* 13:e1001999, 2016.

McGowin CL, Rohde RE, Redwine G: More than just a test result: molecular screening of human papilloma virus for contemporary management of cervical cancer risk, *Clin Lab Sci* 27:43–46, 2014.

McGowin CL, Rohde RE, Whitlock GC: Other pathogens of significant public health concern. In Hu P, Hedge M, Lennon PA, editors: *Modern clinical molecular techniques*, (new edition), New York, NY, 2012, Springer Press.

McIntosh K, McAdam AJ: Human metapneumovirus: an important new respiratory virus, *N Engl J Med* 350:431–433, 2004.

Milholland MT, Castro-Arellano I, Suzán G, et al.: Global diversity and distribution of Hantaviruses and their hosts, *EcoHealth* 15:163–208, 2018, https://doi.org/10.1007/s10393-017-1305-2.

Nainan OV, Xia F, Vaughan G, et al.: Diagnosis of hepatitis A virus infection: a molecular approach, *Clin Microbiol Rev* 19:63–79, 2006.

Niesters HGM: Molecular and diagnostic clinical virology in real-time, *Clin Microbiol Infect* 10:5–11, 2004.

Pigott DC: Hemorrhagic fever viruses, *Crit Care Clin* 21:765–783, 2005.

Poon LL, Guan Y, Nicholls JM, et al.: The aetiology, origins, and diagnosis of severe acute respiratory syndrome, *Lancet Infect Dis* 4:663–671, 2004.

Rohde RE, Mayes BC: Molecular diagnosis and epidemiology of rabies. In Hu P, Hedge M, Lennon PA, editors: *Modern clinical molecular techniques* (new edition), New York, NY, 2012, Springer Press.

Rohde RE, Wilson PJ, Mayes BC, et al.: Rabies: methods and guidelines for assessing a clinical rarity, *Am Soc Clin Path. 2004 Microbiology No. MB-4 Tech Sample* 21–29, 2004.

Rivers MN, Alexander JL, Rohde RE, Rush PJ: Hantavirus pulmonary syndrome (HPS) in Texas, 1993-2006, *South Med J* 102:36–41, 2009.

Rubin J, David D, Willoughby Jr RE, et al.: Applying the Milwaukee Protocol to treat canine rabies in Equatorial Guinea, *Scand J Infect Dis* 41:372–380, 2009.

Sahu KK, Mishra AJ, Lal A: Comprehensive update on current outbreak of novel coronavirus infection (2019-nCoV), *Ann Transl Med* 8(6):393, 2020.

Schiffman M, Castle PE: Human papillomavirus epidemiology and public health, *Arch Pathol Lab Med* 127:930–934, 2003.

Storch GA: Diagnostic virology, *Clin Infect Dis* 31:739–751, 2000.

Thomson RB, Bertram H: Laboratory diagnosis of central nervous system infections, *Infect Dis Clin North Am* 15:1047–1071, 2001.

Vijayvargia P, Garrigos ZE, Almeida NEC, et al.: Treatment considerations for COVID-19, a critical review of the evidence (or lack thereof), *Mayo Clin Proc* 95(7):1454–1466, 2020.

Voss JD, Atkinson RL, Dhurandhar NV: Role of adenoviruses in obesity, *Rev Med Virol* 25:379–387, 2015.

Wilder-Smith A, Schwartz E: Dengue in travelers, *N Engl J Med* 353:924–932, 2005.

World Health Organization: *Fact Sheet Dengue and Severe Dengue.* April 15, 2019. Available at: https://www.who.int/news-room/fact-sheets/detail/dengue-and-severe-dengue. Accessed 16 June 2019.

World Health Organization: *Situation Report on the Ebola Outbreak in North Kivu, 45.* 2019. Available at: https://www.who.int/ebola/en/. Accessed 12 June 2019.

Wilson PJ, Rohde RE, Oertli E, et al.: *Rabies: clinical considerations and exposure evaluations*, St. Louis, MO, 2019, Elsevier.

Writing Committee of the World Health Organization Consultation on Human Influenza A/H5: Avian influenza A (H5N1) infection in humans, *N Engl J Med* 353:1374–1385, 2005.

66

Antiviral Therapy, Susceptibility Testing, and Prevention

OBJECTIVES

1. Define antiviral resistance and explain what may lead a health care provider to believe that resistance to antiviral therapy is occurring.
2. Define antiviral susceptibility testing and list some of the factors that may vary the end results of testing.
3. Explain the lack of standardization of protocols for antiviral susceptibility testing.
4. Define the criteria that determine whether antiviral susceptibility testing should be performed.
5. Explain the difference between phenotypic and genotypic antiviral susceptibility testing.
6. Name some of the types of phenotypic susceptibility testing and list some of the advantages and disadvantages of this method of susceptibility testing.
7. Describe the methodology of genotypic susceptibility testing and list some of the illnesses for which it is used.
8. List the reasons for drug susceptibility testing for individuals infected with the human immunodeficiency virus (HIV).
9. List the vaccinations used to prevent influenza infection. Also, explain why this vaccine must be reformulated every year and why ongoing surveillance of influenza isolates is crucial to the global vaccination program.
10. Define antigenic shift and antigenic drift as relevant to influenza virus.
11. Name the two classes of antiviral medications used to treat and prevent influenza. Also, list the four antiviral medications that have been approved by the US Food and Drug Administration (FDA) and briefly explain their mode of action and resistance.
12. Define immune prophylaxis. Distinguish disease immunity developed by active immunization and by immune prophylaxis.
13. Describe the process of global eradication of viral diseases. Identify a viral disease that has been globally eradicated, and identify other viral diseases currently considered for eradication.

Antiviral Therapy

Antiviral therapy has expanded over the past several years as a treatment for a number of viral infections. Antiviral agents approved by the US Food and Drug Administration (FDA) are active against one or more viruses (Table 66.1). The viruses that are targeted for treatment include human immunodeficiency virus type 1 and 2 (HIV-1 and HIV-2), human herpes viruses, hepatitis viruses B and C (HBV and HCV), and influenza A and B. Although most of the population is susceptible to such treatments, overuse of these agents has led to the emergence of drug-resistant strains, especially in immunocompromised patients. Drug resistance typically results from mutations that alter the molecular targets of the drug. Ribonucleic acid (RNA) viruses mutate more frequently than deoxyribonucleic acid (DNA) viruses because of the infidelity or error rate associated with RNA polymerases. Resistance has been known to develop against all agents and may be detected *in vitro* by using antiviral susceptibility testing. Testing for viral susceptibility is now considered the standard of practice for the management of viral infections and proper patient care. Virology laboratories are increasingly being asked to perform *in vitro* testing of antiviral agents when a patient's infection fails to respond to antiviral therapy; however, testing for antiviral resistance is not currently available in many clinical settings. This chapter provides an overview of the viral diseases in which antiviral resistance has emerged, the need for *in vitro* susceptibility testing, and the phenotypic and genotypic susceptibility testing methods currently available.

Antiviral Resistance

Antiviral resistance means that a virus has changed in such a way that the antiviral drug is less effective in preventing illness. Antiviral resistance is indicated if a patient is taking an antiviral drug that has been proven *in vitro* to be effective against a virus, but the patient shows no improvement and continues to deteriorate clinically. **Drug resistance** must be distinguished from clinical resistance. With **clinical resistance,** the viral infection fails to respond to the antiviral therapy because of factors other than a change in the virus; such factors may include the patient's immunologic status, the pharmacokinetics of the antiviral drug in the individual patient,

TABLE 66.1 Antiviral Agents

Virus	Mode of Action	Target	Examples of Common Drugs
CMV	Nucleoside analog	Viral DNA	Ganciclovir or valganciclovir
CoV (COVID-19)	Nucleoside analog Nonnucleoside RNA polymerase inhibitor	Viral RNA RNA Polymerase	Remdesivir Favipiravir
HIV[a]	Nucleoside analog Nucleotide reverse transcriptase inhibitor Nonnucleoside analog Protease inhibitor Fusion (entry) inhibitor	Viral DNA Viral DNA Reverse transcriptase Viral protease Virus, host cell membrane	Efavirenz (nonnucleoside analog) Tenofovir disoproxil fumarate (nucleotide reverse transcriptase inhibitor) Emtricitabine (nucleoside analog) Atazanavir (protease inhibitor)
HSV/VZV	Nucleoside analog Pyrophosphate analog	Viral DNA DNA polymerase	Acyclovir (Zovirax) Foscarnet (Foscavir)
Hepatitis B	Nucleoside analog Nucleotide analog	Reverse transcriptase DNA polymerase	Lamivudine Adefovir dipivoxil
Influenza A	Inhibit penetration and uncoating of virus	Host cell membrane	Amantadine, imantadine
Influenza A and B	Prevent release of virus	Neuraminidase inhibitors	Zanamivir, oseltamivir, and peramivir
RSV	Inhibit expression of viral mRNA and protein synthesis	Viral mRNA	Ribavirin
HCV	Inhibit expression of viral mRNA; increase resistance to virus Nucleotide analog	Viral mRNA or neighboring host cells Inhibitor of HCV polymerase	Ribavirin Sofosbuvir
Picornaviruses (enteroviruses and rhinoviruses)	Inhibit attachment and uncoating of virus	Binds to virus	Pleconaril

[a]Many antiretroviral drugs in different mechanistic classes are available to design treatment regimens. See the most recent information for treatment: https://www.hiv.gov/hiv-basics/staying-in-hiv-care/hiv-treatment/hiv-treatment-overview.
CMV, Cytomegalovirus; *DNA,* deoxyribonucleic acid; *HCV,* hepatitis C virus; *HIV,* human immunodeficiency virus; *HSV,* herpes simplex virus; *mRNA,* messenger ribonucleic acid; *RSV,* respiratory syncytial virus; *VZV,* varicella-zoster virus.

and, if a combination of drugs is administered, potential antagonism and interference with the absorption of one or more drugs. Other patient factors that also affect the success of drug therapy include nonadherence to or intolerance to a specific drug and prescriptive errors, such as inappropriate doses or route of administration. In addition, infections in immunocompromised patients may fail to respond to therapy that has proven effective in immunocompetent individuals.

The final result of antiviral susceptibility testing is determined by many variables, and these variables also hinder the standardization of antiviral susceptibility testing. Some of these variables include the following:
• Cell line used to grow the virus
• Inoculum viral titer
• Culture incubation time
• Concentration range of the antiviral drug tested
• Reference strains

• Assay method
• End-point criteria
• Calculation of the end-point
• Interpretation of the end-point

Each of these categories in turn has variables that affect the final results. For example, if the inoculum quantity is too large, a susceptible isolate may appear resistant; if the inoculum quantity is too small, the isolate may appear susceptible. The complexity of all these variables makes it imperative that established control strains also be tested when antiviral susceptibility testing is performed. Controls should include both drug-resistant and drug-susceptible isolates that have been well characterized. Several research laboratories across the nation can provide reference and drug-resistant strains of a virus for susceptibility testing; they include the National Institute of Allergy and Infectious Diseases AIDS Research and Reference Reagent Program (niaid.nih.gov) and the American Type Culture Collection (atcc.org). Pharmaceutical companies may also maintain control strains.

Methods of Antiviral Susceptibility Testing

The purpose of antiviral susceptibility testing is to evaluate new antiviral chemoprophylaxis, to test for cross resistance or cross reactivity to alternate agents, and to determine how frequently drug-resistant viral mutations occur.

The two general types of antiviral susceptibility testing are phenotypic testing and genotypic testing. **Phenotypic susceptibility assays** measure viral replication in the presence of antiviral agents; they measure the inhibitory effect of an antiviral agent on the entire virus population in a clinical isolate. **Genotypic susceptibility assays** use polymerase chain reaction (PCR) to detect genes known to be responsible for resistance, coupled with molecular sequencing to determine whether genome alterations associated with resistance have occurred. These assays use the virus's nucleic acid to determine whether the virus has mutations capable of causing viral drug resistance. Alternately, a combination of the two general types of antiviral susceptibility, known as a **virtual phenotype resistance assay,** may be performed. This assay is a characterization of the patient's virus genotype compared with a database that includes paired genotypic and phenotypic information. This information is then used to estimate the most likely phenotype of the patient's virus. The success of this approach varies with the virus type and antiviral drugs examined.

Each of these types of susceptibility testing has unique properties that can be used to complement each other. Phenotypic assays are better used to assess the combined effect of multiple-resistance mutations on drug susceptibility, but they are labor intensive, are expensive, and have lengthy turnaround times. Genotypic assays have a shorter turnaround time and are less expensive than phenotypic assays, but they can detect only defined viral mutations that may or may not result in a drug-resistant phenotype.

Phenotypic Assays

Phenotypic assays use a variety of end-point measurements to determine whether a virus is inhibited by an antiviral drug or demonstrates drug resistance. Some of these end-point measurements include a reduction in the number of plaques, inhibition of viral DNA synthesis, a reduction in the yield of a viral structural protein, or a reduction of the enzymatic activity of a functional protein. As mentioned, an advantage of phenotypic assays is that they are much better for assessing the combined effect of multiple-resistance mutations on drug susceptibility. This has been useful for assaying viruses such as HBV, HIV-1, and human cytomegalovirus (HCMV), which acquire resistance mutations in multiple genes. The disadvantages of phenotypic assays are that they are labor intensive, expensive, and require weeks to perform.

Plaque Reduction Assay

The **plaque reduction assay (PRA)** is the standard method of antiviral susceptibility testing against which new methods are compared. CLSI has developed standardized PRA protocols for antiviral susceptibility testing for HSV. This test is based on the principle of inhibition of viral plaque formation in the presence of an antiviral agent. The concentration of antiviral drug that inhibits plaque formation by 50% is the **IC50**; that is, the 50% inhibitory concentration and 50% effective concentration.

Dye Uptake Assay

The **dye uptake (DU) assay** has been used for years in the susceptibility testing of HSV. When the virus is in the presence of an antiviral drug, only cells that are alive and viable take up a vital dye called **neutral red.** After infection with HSV, the relative amount of dye bound to viable cells compared with that bound to uninfected cells determines the extent of the viral lytic activity. The drug concentration that inhibits viral lytic activity by 50% is the IC50. This assay is also used for other herpes viruses, including cytomegalovirus (CMV) and varicella-zoster virus (VZV).

Enzyme Immunoassay

The enzyme immunoassay (EIA) uses spectrophotometric analysis to quantitatively measure the amount of viral activity. The concentration of antiviral agent that reduces the amount of absorbance by 50% compared with the absorbance values of a viral control is the IC50. This method of susceptibility testing has been used for influenza A, HSV, and VZV.

Neuraminidase Inhibition Assay

The **neuraminidase (NA) inhibition assay** is used to detect NA inhibition resistance when the drugs oseltamivir and zanamivir are used to treat influenza A and influenza B infections. Oseltamivir and zanamivir act by inhibiting the influenza viral protein NA. Resistance to these drugs is measured by incubating cultured influenza isolates containing NA with varying concentrations of the drugs. A fluorogenic substrate is then added, allowing the fluorescence to be quantitated by a fluorimeter. The IC50 is calculated by comparing the activity of viral NA to a control reaction that does not use any NA inhibitors.

Recombinant Virus Assays

A **recombinant virus assay (RVA)** monitors the phenotypic behavior of specific genes in the virus genome in the presence of the antiviral drug. One of the first RVA assays measured HIV-1 resistance to protease and reverse transcriptase inhibitors. An artificial genetic construct that includes a vector nucleic acid molecule with a reporter, as well as the patient's gene of interest, is recombined into a **chimeric molecule.** This is then **cotransfected** into a susceptible cell line. The chimeric structure, or **pseudovirus,** can then be tested *in vitro* in the presence of antiviral drugs. The chimeric molecule emits light from the reporter during viral replication. If the virus is susceptible to the antiviral, the light emission will decrease, indicating a potential effective treatment against the viral gene that has been introduced into the recombinant structure.

Genotypic Susceptibility Assays

Genotypic susceptibility assays use PCR to detect genes known to be responsible for resistance, coupled with genetic sequencing to determine whether genome alterations associated with resistance have occurred. Genotypic assays use DNA Sanger sequencing, pyrosequencing, and next-generation sequencing by automated sequencers; PCR amplification and single nucleotide polymorphism (SNP) multiplex assays for allelic discrimination; and *in vitro* reverse hybridization line probe assays (LIPAs). These assays are rapid, because isolation of the virus in culture is not necessary for testing.

The response to an antiviral agent is also measured by quantitative monitoring of the viral load (by means of the nucleic acid concentration) in the patient's blood. Such testing is common in patients infected with HBV, HCV, and CMV. Genotypic assays have been used to identify mutations in the VZV thymidine kinase (TK) and DNA polymerase genes resulting in antiviral resistance. The viral load in genotypic susceptibility assays should diminish significantly after addition of an antiviral agent to which the virus is susceptible. Using molecular testing (e.g., quantitative PCR) to measure the amount of virus in serum is a surrogate test for resistance to antiviral agents. The viral load rises quickly when resistance appears.

Pyrosequencing

DNA sequencing is among the most important testing methods for the study of biologic entities. Pyrosequencing is a sequence-based detection method that allows rapid, accurate quantification of sequence variation. It allows rapid acquisition of short reads (100 to 200 bp) of genomic sequence to identify known mutations. It is based on the technology of detection of released pyrophosphate (PPi) during DNA synthesis. (See Chapter 8 for more information of pyrosequencing.) In a sequence of enzymatic reactions, a polymerase enzyme catalyzes the addition of nucleotides into a nucleic acid chain. A PPi molecule is released and converted to adenosine triphosphate (ATP) by the ATP enzyme sulfurylase. Visible light is produced when a luciferin molecule is oxidized during the luciferase reaction. The visible light or signal strength generated is proportional to the number of nucleotides incorporated into the final product.

Two types of pyrosequencing methods are available: the solid-phase pyrosequencing and liquid-phase pyrosequencing. Solid-phase pyrosequencing involves a three-enzyme system that uses immobilized DNA, and a washing step is performed to remove excess substrate after each nucleotide addition. In liquid-phase pyrosequencing, a fourth nucleotide-degrading enzyme (made from potato) is added. The advantage of the liquid-phase system is that it eliminates the need for solid support and the intermediate washing step, allowing the reaction to be performed in a single tube.

Because of its rapid, accurate quantification of sequence variation, pyrosequencing is an adaptable tool that can be used for a wide range of applications. Automation with pyrosequencing is made possible by the liquid-phase methodology. Pyrosequencing signals are quantitative, which allows many people to be screened through examination of the allelic frequency in a population. This technique also is used taxonomically to group different organisms into strains or subtypes, and it can be applied to bacteria, yeasts, and viruses. The technique can be applied to the resequencing of PCR-amplified disease genes for mutation screening. It also is used to screen clinical isolates for the genes that confer resistance to antiviral therapy, such as for analysis of influenza specimens for the adamantine resistance mutation. There are no FDA cleared or approved pyrosequencing methods for use in antiviral susceptibility testing.

Next Generation Sequencing

Next generation sequencing platforms are increasingly becoming used for the diagnosis of emerging viral agents, molecular epidemiology, and drug resistance testing. These methods depend on the development of large databases of information that include the drug-resistant mutations and their association with viral phenotype, treatment, and clinical outcomes. This process will require continued development of resistance databases and automation. See Chapter 8 for more information on whole-genome next generation sequencing (WG-NGS).

Human Immunodeficiency Virus

Patients infected with HIV commonly develop resistance to the antiretroviral drugs, which often results in treatment failure. Genotypic testing is recommended for baseline screening of all newly diagnosed patients. Testing for antiretroviral resistance is crucial to the assessment of a regimen of drugs intended to suppress HIV replication and to test for cross resistance to alternative antiretroviral drugs. The US Department of Health and Human Services and a European panel of experts have developed guidelines and established protocols to monitor patients with acute and chronic HIV infection. Susceptibility testing should proceed as follows:
1. Before the initiation of therapy
2. When antiretroviral regimens are changed in cases of treatment failure
3. When suboptimal viral load reduction is seen after beginning or changing therapy

A single FDA-cleared assay is also available for HIV-1 genotyping, the ViroSeq HIV-1 system (Abbott Diagnostics, Abbott Park, IL). This method uses a PCR amplification followed by Sanger sequencing of the protease and reverse transcription gene. A variety of specialized and large reference laboratories have developed laboratory developed tests (LDTs) for the detection of antiviral mutations for various drugs used to treat HIV.

Genotypic susceptibility testing has become a routine component of the management of patients infected with HIV. Genotypic assays for mutations that confer resistance are useful because of their rapid turnaround time.

Influenza

Currently, two main approaches are used in health care to control the spread of influenza: vaccination and the use of antiviral drugs. The influenza virus has the unique capability of being able to change its antigenic makeup; this mechanism, known as antigenic drift, occurs with all three types of influenza virus (A, B, and C). Influenza A shows the greatest rate of antigenic change. Antigenic drift is caused by sequential point mutations in the hemagglutination (HA) or NA genes that arise during viral ribonucleoprotein (RNP) replication and immune selection, giving rise to new strains; this gives the virus the ability to reinfect "nonimmune" susceptible hosts each season. Another phenomenon, antigenic shift, is manifested only by the influenza A virus. It involves complete reassortment of the segmented viral genome during a coinfection with a nonhuman animal, which results in major antigenic change and periodic worldwide outbreaks (pandemics) of a never-before circulated type of influenza A virus. Influenza B undergoes antigenic change very slowly.

Antigenic drift requires the reformulation of the influenza vaccine each year to ensure maximum efficacy against the currently circulating strains of influenza A and influenza B. This is accomplished by global surveillance of the yearly influenza epidemics to evaluate the strains that are circulating and provide early detection of viruses that may have pandemic potential. The World Health Organization (WHO) coordinates an influenza surveillance program in more than 80 countries. In the United States, the surveillance program established by the Centers for Disease Control and Prevention (CDC) includes monitoring of pneumonia and influenza deaths above a calculated "**epidemic threshold.**" It also includes tallying pediatric deaths, assessment of weekly virology data, and typing of influenza virus isolates submitted by reference laboratories. This extensive surveillance system provides the data for determining and predicting the influenza strains likely to be circulating in the upcoming winter. Vaccine components are chosen annually by WHO based on the analysis and typing of these strains. The summer months are used to manufacture the vaccine so that it is ready for distribution to health care providers in early autumn. In the United States, the vaccine is prepared from viruses grown in embryonated chicken eggs. The vaccine may be a trivalent vaccine containing two influenza A strains with the newest HA and NA surface antigens and a current type B strain or a quadrivalent vaccine containing antigens to two influenza A and two influenza B strains.

Several types of vaccine are used to prevent influenza infection: the inactivated influenza vaccine (IIV3), the live attenuated influenza virus vaccine (LAIV), and the recombinant hemagglutinin vaccine (RIV). The IIV3 is a noninfectious vaccine (Afluria) administered intramuscularly for individuals 5 years and older or using a high-pressure jet injector for individuals 18 years through 64 years of age. The IIV3 vaccines may be trivalent containing influenza A (H1NA), A (H3N2), and B or quadrivalent containing influenza B viruses from two lineages (B/Victoria and B/Yamagata). A high dose flu vaccine referred to as Fluzone-High is a trivalent vaccine that contains four times more antigen than the standard inactivated flu vaccine. Fluzone-High dose is specifically licensed for patients 65 years of age and older. An additional trivalent inactivated virus vaccine, Fluad, is also available for patients 65 years of age and older. Fluad contains the adjuvant MF59, which increases the patient's immune response to the vaccine providing improved protection from influenza infection. There are at least four quadrivalent flu vaccines available that are either egg based or cell based on recombinant vaccines. There are many vaccine options available; however, everyone that is 6 months of age or older should receive an annual influenza vaccine.

The LAIV contains live whole infectious virus. The LAIV causes shedding of the virus that is detectable in rapid antigen assays for about a week. The LAIV is also quadrivalent and contains the same strains as the IIV quadrivalent vaccine. The RIV contains 45 µg of baculovirus-expressed, recombinant hemagglutinin for A (H1NA) and A (H3N2) and an influenza B strain. The strains included in vaccines are reviewed twice annually by the WHO.

Two classes of antiviral drugs, the adamantanes (M2 protein inhibitors) and the NA inhibitors, currently are used to treat influenza infections. The adamantanes, which include the drugs amantadine and rimantadine, were the first class of antiviral, antiinfluenza drugs developed. The drugs function by blocking the virion M2 ion channel, which prevents the virus from uncoating. This class of drugs is effective only at treating cases of influenza A; it has never had any effect on influenza B infections. The NA inhibitors include the drugs zanamivir (Relenza), oseltamivir (Tamiflu), and peramivir. Peramivir was approved for use in 2014; however, it is only available as an intravenous injection and is given in a single dose for uncomplicated influenza. These drugs inhibit the viral protein NA, which prevents release of the virus from infected cells. The NA inhibitors are used to treat both influenza A and influenza B infections, although oseltamivir has been reported to have lower efficacy against influenza B. Both classes of drugs have proven to be most effective when administered within 48 hours of symptoms. The drugs shorten the duration of the infection and reduce complications.

The need for effective influenza antiviral susceptibility surveillance has increased around the world, and its importance is validated by the emergence of universal resistance to the adamantine antiviral therapy for influenza A (H3N2). Samples of viruses collected from around the United States and worldwide are studied to determine whether they are resistant to any of the four influenza antiviral drugs approved by the FDA. The CDC, in collaboration with state public health departments and WHO, conduct ongoing surveillance and perform testing of influenza viruses to monitor the development of antiviral resistance. The number of domestic and global surveillance sites are being increased, and the data from this surveillance are used to make public health policy recommendations on the use of antiviral medications. The CDC is constantly improving the methods for rapid detection and monitoring antiviral resistance. Several LDTs including real-time assays, high-resolution melt RT-PCR, SNP analysis using capillary electrophoresis, and real-time allelic discrimination assays have been developed for influenza susceptibility testing. Sanger and pyrosequencing assays are also used to identify resistance mutations in the NA gene. Laboratory methods for testing are constantly being improved, and the number of laboratories capable of antiviral resistance testing is increasing.

Antiviral resistance to the M2 protein inhibitors develops in about 30% of patients following a few days of therapy. Natural resistance has also emerged in influenza A H3N2 and H1N1. Because of the high prevalence of drug-resistant strains, these antivirals are no longer recommended for treatment in the United States. Resistance mutations to the neuraminidase inhibitors depend on the influenza type (A or B) and subtype (N1 or N2). This requires ongoing genotypic and phenotypic surveillance and susceptibility testing. Genotypic assays are generally used for clinical management and surveillance, whereas enzymatic assays are used for surveillance and characterizing novel NA variants.

Prevention of Other Viral Infections

Vaccination

Control of many viral diseases has been accomplished by vaccination. Since Jenner developed the first vaccine against smallpox 200 years ago, attenuated-live or inactivated-dead viral vaccines have been used successively to prevent yellow fever, poliomyelitis, measles, mumps, rubella, hepatitis B, and influenza (Table 66.2). Smallpox was eliminated in 1977 by an effective vaccination program. Additional vaccines continue to appear. New smallpox vaccines with fewer side effects are being developed to prevent outbreaks in the event of bioterrorism. A live-attenuated varicella (chickenpox) vaccine is now recommended for all children, and an inactivated hepatitis A vaccine is available for travelers and others entering areas of higher endemicity. Rotavirus vaccines are approved by the FDA and are now available. Recombinant vaccines are also available for the prevention of HPV infection.

Immune Prophylaxis and Therapy

Immune prophylaxis is used to prevent serious viral infection in patients who are immunocompromised or

TABLE 66.2	Examples of Vaccines for Preventing Viral Diseases	
Disease	**Type of Vaccine**
Yellow fever	Attenuated-live
Polio virus (PV)	Inactivated
Measles	Attenuated-live
Mumps	Attenuated-live
Rubella	Attenuated-live
Hepatitis B (HBV)	Inactivated and recombinant
Influenza	Attenuated-live, inactivated, and recombinant
Smallpox virus (VARV)	Attenuated-live
Chickenpox (VZV)	Attenuated-live
Hepatitis A virus (HAV)	Inactivated
Human papilloma virus (HPV)	Recombinant
Rabies virus (RABV)	Inactivated
Rotavirus (RV)	Attenuated-live

VARV, Variola virus; *VZV,* varicella-zoster virus.

functionally compromised. Instead of actively immunizing an individual with an antiviral vaccine, limited protection can be conferred by intramuscular inoculation of human immunoglobulin. Pooled human immunoglobulin contains antibody against all common viruses. Specific high-titered immunoglobulin can be collected from patients recovering from a specific infection to ensure maximum antibody levels. Immune prophylaxis should be considered an emergency procedure. Table 66.3 lists immune prophylaxis available for viral infections.

Passive immunoprophylaxis of respiratory syncytial virus (RSV) infection in infants younger than 2 years who have underlying lung disease resulting from premature birth or congenital heart disease is particularly effective at preventing life-threatening bronchiolitis and pneumonia in this patient group. The drug, palivizumab (Synagis), is a manufactured antibody to RSV. It is used in certain infants and young children to prevent RSV infections of the bronchioles and lungs; it cannot be used to treat a child that already is symptomatic because of an RSV infection.

Passive immunization occasionally is effective as therapy for viral infection (Table 66.3). Therapy with immune serum for some hemorrhagic fevers, such as Lassa fever, has also been successful in reducing mortality associated with the disease.

Eradication

Global eradication of a viral disease has occurred only with smallpox. Factors that result in eradication of any viral

<table>
</table>

TABLE 66.3	Immune Prophylaxis or Therapy for Viral Diseases
Disease	**Circumstances of Use**
Prophylaxis	
Hepatitis A virus (HAV)	Traveler to developing country
Hepatitis B virus (HBV)	Newborns of infected mothers or unimmunized laboratory worker after needlestick
Rabies virus (RABV)	After bite from potentially rabid animal
Measles	Unimmunized close contact with infected individual
Varicella-zoster virus (VZV)	Newborns of infected mothers at time of delivery
Respiratory	Infants younger than 2 years of age with underlying lung syncytial disease virus
Therapy	
CoV (COVID-19)	Immunomodulators such as tocilizumab an IL-6 inhibitor are used reduce potential cytokine storms and other immune related damage in severe to critical cases.
Lassa fever	During disease to reduce severity

disease include no animal reservoir, a lack of recurrent infectivity, one or few stable serotypes, and an effective vaccine. Viral diseases currently considered candidates for eradication include measles and poliomyelitis. Poliomyelitis has been known and feared by humans for thousands of years. Infection with the poliovirus causes an acute flaccid paralysis that can affect the ability to breathe. The disease was often seen in children. In the mid-1950s, Jonas Salk developed the first polio vaccine from dead virus, and in 1960, Sabin developed an oral polio vaccine using a live-attenuated virus. These developments allowed the United States to launch a massive vaccination program against polio, and the last case of indigenous polio was reported in the United States in 1979 (other reports of polio cases were a result of vaccination or occurred in individuals who had emigrated from other countries).

In 1988, WHO resolved to eradicate acute paralytic poliomyelitis from the rest of the world and staged a massive vaccination campaign to accomplish this. WHO has continued this effort with many collaborating agencies as the Polio Global Eradication Initiative. Detailed information and updates can be located at http://polioeradication.org/polio-today/. The strategies to eradicate the disease include surveillance of acute flaccid paralysis, routine vaccination with the oral polio vaccine, and supplementary immunization activities.

Ⓔ Visit the Evolve site for a complete list of procedures, review questions, and case studies.

Bibliography

Balfour HH: Drug therapy, *N Engl J Med* 340:1255–1268, 1999.
Carroll KC, Pfaller MA, Landry ML, et al.: *Manual of clinical microbiology*, ed 12, Washington, DC, 2019, ASM.
Centers for Disease Control and Prevention. *Preventing Seasonal Flu with Vaccination*. http://www.cdc.gov/flu/protect/vaccine/index.htm. Accessed July 30, 2019.
Constantine N, Zhao R: Molecular-based laboratory testing and monitoring for human immunodeficiency virus infections, *Clin Lab Sci* 18:263–270, 2005.
De Clercq E: Antiviral drugs in current clinical use, *J Clin Virol* 30:115–133, 2004.
Hayden FG, Shindo N: Influenza virus polymerase inhibitors in clinical development, *Curr Opin Infect Dis* 32(2):176–186, 2019.
Lee N, Hurt AC: Neuraminidase inhibitor resistance in influenza: a clinical perspective, *Curr Opin Infect Dis* 31(6):520–526, 2018.
Lee W: Hepatitis B virus infection, *N Engl J Med* 337:1733–1745, 1997.
Levine AJ: *Viruses*, New York, NY, 1991, Scientific American Library.
Liang TJ, Rehermann B, Seeff L, et al.: Pathogenesis, natural history, treatment, and prevention of hepatitis C, *Ann Intern Med* 132:296–305, 2000.

McSharry J, Lurain N, Drusanao G, et al.: Rapid ganciclovir susceptibility assay using flow cytometry for HCMV isolates, *Antimicrob Agents Chemother* 42:2326–2331, 1998.
Niesters HG: Molecular and diagnostic clinical virology in real-time, *Clin Microbiol Infect* 10:5–11, 2004.
Polio Global Eradication Initiative. *Polio Today*. Available at: http://polioeradication.org/polio-today/. Accessed July 30, 2019.
Ronaghi M: Pyrosequencing sheds light on DNA sequencing, *Genome Res* 11(1):3–11, 2001.
Sagnelli E, Starace M, Minichini C, et al.: Resistance detection and re-treatment options in hepatitis C virus-related liver diseases after DAA-treatment failure, *Infection* 46(6):761–783, 2018.
Specter S, Hodinka RL, Young SA, et al.: *Clinical virology manual*, ed 4, Washington, DC, 2009, ASM Press.
Storch GA: Diagnostic virology, *Clin Infect Dis* 31:739–751, 2000.
Vijayvargia P, Garrigos ZE, Almeida NEC, et al.: Treatment considerations for COVID-19, a critical review of the evidence (or lack thereof), *Mayo Clin Proc* 95(7):1454–1466, 2020.
Wong SK, Li A, Lanctot KL, et al.: Adherence and outcomes: a systematic review of palivizumab utilization, *Expert Rev Respir Med* 12(2):27–42, 2018.

67

Bloodstream Infections

OBJECTIVES

1. Identify and describe some of the medical consequences that occur when the bloodstream is infected by microorganisms.
2. Name the most common causes of bacterial bloodstream infection and explain the routes of transmission and source of infection.
3. Define the following bloodstream infections: bacteremia, fungemia, and septicemia.
4. List the most common fungi associated with bloodstream infections and the population of patients most often affected by this type of infection.
5. Explain what causes mortality in most cases of parasitic bloodborne infections.
6. Differentiate between intravascular and extravascular bloodstream infections.
7. Define continuous bacteremia and provide an example.
8. Describe the development of infective endocarditis, including the contributing factors and the microorganisms that are the primary cause for the condition.
9. Define mycotic aneurysms and suppurative thrombophlebitis and describe the causes for these conditions.
10. Explain the pathogenic features of *Staphylococcus epidermidis* that make it uniquely suited for causing catheter-related infections.
11. Explain the importance of collection parameters associated with blood cultures for suspected cases of bloodstream infections, including collection time, the number of cultures, and the volume of blood required.
12. List and briefly describe some of the blood culture systems available to the microbiologist, including the self-contained systems, the lysis centrifugation systems, and instrument-based systems.
13. List some of the most common causes of bloodstream infection associated with the blood cultures from HIV-infected patients.
14. Define the acronym HACEK and describe the type of bloodborne infections these organisms are most often associated with.
15. Outline the guidelines used to determine whether agents isolated from blood cultures are true pathogens or probable contaminants.

Invasion of the bloodstream by microorganisms constitutes one of the most serious situations in infectious disease. Microorganisms present in the circulating blood—whether continuously, intermittently, or transiently—are a threat to every organ in the body. The suffix –emia is derived from the Greek word meaning "blood" and refers to the presence of a substance in the blood; **bacteremia** refers to the presence of bacteria in the blood, **viremia** refers to the presence of a virus in the bloodstream, **parasitemia** refers to the presence of a parasite in the blood (Chapters 48, 52, and 57), and **fungemia** refers to the presence of fungi in the bloodstream. **Sepsis** or **septicemia** therefore indicates organisms are present in the blood, producing an infection and reproducing within the bloodstream. Invasion of the bloodstream resulting from any organism can have serious immediate consequences, including shock, multiple organ failure, **disseminated intravascular coagulation (DIC),** and death. According to the Centers for Disease Control and Prevention (CDC), the incidence of sepsis or bloodstream infections has nearly doubled in the past decade. It is one of the leading causes of death in the United States and one of the most expensive conditions to treat in a hospital, accounting for approximately 20% of all intensive care unit (ICU) admissions and the leading cause of ICU noncardiac mortality. Timely detection and identification of bloodborne pathogens are two of the most important functions of the microbiology laboratory. This includes traditional culture-based methods as described previously in Chapter 7 as well as newer rapid detection methods such as nucleic acid–based testing (Chapter 8) or chemotaxonomic methods such as matrix-assisted laser desorption ionization time-of-flight mass spectrometry (MALDI-TOF MS), also included in Chapter 7. To combat the rising incidence of sepsis, algorithms for diagnosis and treatment of sepsis are being instituted to reduce mortality. These algorithms include microbiologic testing, clinical chemistry (lactate, procalcitonin, and other biochemical markers), delivering fluids for hydration, and initiating rapid treatment with broad spectrum antibiotics.

953

General Considerations

The successful recovery of microorganisms from blood by the laboratory depends on many, often complex, factors: the type of sepsis, the specimen collection method, the blood volume, the number and timing of blood cultures and the use of supportive diagnostic information, the interpretation of results, and the type of patient population being served by the laboratory. All these parameters must be considered in the development of the diagnostic protocol within the laboratory to maximize the detection and recovery of microorganisms and ensure quality patient care. Bloodstream infections dramatically increase health care costs and mortality. The definition and delineation of the clinical syndromes associated with bloodstream infections have been standardized by the American College of Chest Physicians and the Society for Critical Care Medicine. Sepsis, a systemic response to infection, previously referred to as the **systemic inflammatory response syndrome (SIRS),** is now further defined to include sepsis associated with **hypoperfusion** or **hypofunction** (decreased function) or new organ dysfunction or abnormal performance (**severe sepsis**) or hypotension (**septic shock**). Despite the advances in laboratory diagnostics and medical treatment, there remain no clear, reliable laboratory-based criteria for the absolute prediction of a patient's response and outcome associated with a bloodstream infection.

Etiology

As previously mentioned, all major groups of microbes can be present in the bloodstream during many diseases.

Bloodstream infections are classified as **health care–associated infections (HAIs),** including **device-associated infections (DAIs)** such as **central line–associated bloodstream infections (CLA-BSIs),** or **community-acquired bloodstream infections (CA-BSIs).** A health care–associated bloodstream infection is defined as a positive blood culture that occurs 2 days or longer after admission to the health care facility. Conversely a CA-BSI is defined as an infection that occurs in the community or before 2 days of admission to the facility or hospitalization. Although the definition seems clear, the changes in patient demographics (the increasing numbers of immunocompromised individuals) and the changes in health care delivery associated with outpatient clinics for the treatment of cancer, acquired immune deficiency syndrome (AIDS), and other debilitating diseases makes the distinction difficult.

CA-BSIs can be subdivided into two groups: patients who are being treated with serious comorbid conditions such as cancer or diabetes or have immunosuppression (AIDS or immunosuppressive therapy associated with organ transplants) that require permanent intravenous (IV) devices, surgical treatments, or hemodialysis and those patients without any previous underlying condition who simply acquire an infection related to a localized or foci of infection, such as an abscess. The difference between the

> ### • BOX 67.1 Organisms Commonly Isolated From Blood Cultures
>
> *Staphylococcus aureus*
> *Escherichia coli*
> *Staphylococcus epidermidis*
> Other coagulase-negative staphylococci
> *Enterococcus* spp.
> *Candida albicans*
> *Pseudomonas aeruginosa*
> *Klebsiella pneumoniae*
> Viridans streptococci
> *Streptococcus pneumoniae*
> *Enterobacter cloacae*
> *Proteus* spp.
> Beta-hemolytic streptococci
> Anaerobic bacteria: *Bacteroides* and *Clostridium* spp.

two groups is that patients in the second group are typically infected with antibiotic-susceptible organisms, whereas patients with comorbid conditions typically are infected with antibiotic-resistant organisms.

As previously mentioned, all major groups of microbes can be present in the bloodstream during many diseases. However, HAIs are most often associated with the presence of an intravascular catheter or other device, surgical site infection, or invasive procedure in an anatomic site that contains microorganisms (microbiota) such as the gastrointestinal tract. Most cases of severe sepsis are associated with either bacterial or fungal organisms that are acquired from the patient's normal microbiota.

Bacteria

The organisms most commonly isolated from blood include *Staphylococcus aureus, Streptococcus pneumoniae,* and *Escherichia coli.* Other organisms associated with bloodstream infections are likely to be inhabitants of the health care environment and/or colonize the skin, oropharynx, and gastrointestinal tract of patients. The most common cases of secondary sepsis associated with a primary site of infection are identified in patients with lung or abdominal infections. Some of the most common, clinically significant organisms isolated from blood cultures are listed in Box 67.1. In general, the number of fungi and coagulase-negative staphylococci has increased, whereas the number of clinically significant anaerobic isolates has decreased.

Localized anatomic infections may lead to bacteremia or **toxemia** (circulating bacterial products) that stimulate a systemic inflammatory response. For example, *Neisseria meningitidis* is capable of growth in the bloodstream inducing DIC, severe sepsis, and eventually septic shock. Of importance, the laboratory isolation of certain bacterial species from blood can indicate the presence of an underlying, occult, or undiagnosed neoplasm. Alterations in local conditions at the site of a neoplasm may allow the bacteria to proliferate and seed the bloodstream. Another possible mechanism is reduced killing of bacterial cells by the host phagocytes. Organisms associated with neoplastic disease include *Clostridium septicum, Clostridium tertium,* and other uncommonly isolated clostridial species; *Streptococcus gallolyticus (S. bovis* group); *Aeromonas hydrophila* subsp. *hydrophilia; Plesiomonas shigelloides;* and *Campylobacter* spp. Finally, if *Streptococcus anginosus* group (*S. anginosus, Streptococcus constellatus,* and *Streptococcus intermedius*) bacteria are isolated from blood, the possibility of an abscess should be considered.

Fungi

Fungemia (the presence of fungi in blood) is usually a serious condition, occurring primarily in immunosuppressed patients and in those with serious or terminal illness. *Candida albicans* is by far the most common species isolated from bloodstream infections; however, a variety of species have been identified. *Candida* spp. infection is often associated with long-term hospitalization, intravascular catheters, diabetes, and other malignancies and correlates with the length of hospitalization. *Candida* spp. can form biofilm (an extracellular polysaccharide material) that permits hematogenous spread of the organism and provides a high level of antibiotic resistance (Chapter 62). *Malassezia furfur* can often be isolated in patients, particularly neonates, receiving lipid-supplemented parenteral nutrition.

Except for *Histoplasma,* which multiply in leukocytes (white blood cells), fungi do not invade blood cells, but their presence in the blood usually indicates a focus of infection elsewhere in the body. Fungi in the bloodstream can disseminate to all organs of the host, where they may grow, invade normal tissue, and produce toxic products. Fungi gain entrance to the circulatory system via loss of integrity of the gastrointestinal or other mucosa; through damaged skin; from primary sites of infection, such as the lung or other organs; or by means of intravascular catheters.

Systemic fungal infections begin as pneumonia and may disseminate from the lungs, which serve as the portal of entry. Arthroconidia of *Coccidioides* spp. and microconidia of *Histoplasma capsulatum* and *Blastomyces dermatitidis* are ingested by alveolar macrophages in the lung. These macrophages carry the fungi to nearby lymph nodes, usually the hilar nodes. The fungi multiply within the node tissue and ultimately are released into the circulating blood, from which they can seed other organs or are destroyed by the body's defenses. Molds are particularly insensitive to host defenses such as antibody and phagocytic cells because of their large size and their sterol-containing cell wall structure.

Parasites

Eukaryotic parasites may be found transiently in the bloodstream as they migrate to other tissues or organs. Their presence, however, cannot be considered consistent with a state of good health. For example, tachyzoites of the parasite *Toxoplasma gondii* may be found in circulating blood. They invade cells within lymph nodes and other organs, including the lungs, liver, heart, brain, and eyes. The resulting cellular destruction accounts for the manifestations of

toxoplasmosis. Also, microfilariae are seen in peripheral blood during infection with *Mansonella, Loa loa, Wuchereria,* or *Brugia.*

Malarial parasites invade host erythrocytes and hepatic parenchymal cells. The significant anemia and subsequent tissue **hypoxia** (reduction in oxygen levels) may result from destruction of red blood cells by the parasite. Vascular trapping of normal erythrocytes by the infected red blood cells, which are less flexible and tend to clog small capillaries, is a major cause of morbidity. The host's immunologic response is to remove the parasites and damaged red blood cells; the immune response may also have deleterious effects.

Parasites in the bloodstream are usually detected by direct visualization, however some specialized laboratories have developed nucleic acid-based tests that include polymerase chain reaction (PCR) and direct probe methods that are particularly useful when there is a low parasitemia or the identification of the organism is questionable by microscopy (Chapter 48). Those parasites for which traditional diagnosis is predominantly dependent on observation of the organism in peripheral blood smears include *Plasmodium, Trypanosoma,* and *Babesia.* Patients with malaria or filariasis may display a periodicity in their episodes of fever that allows the physician to time the collection of blood for microscopic examination intended for optimal detection. Rapid serologic methods and molecular methods are currently used to detect malaria, babesiosis, and trypanosomiasis. These tests are described in Chapter 48.

Viruses

Although many viruses do circulate in the peripheral blood at some stage of disease, the primary pathology relates to infection of the target organ or cells. Those viruses that preferentially infect blood cells are Epstein-Barr virus (invades lymphocytes), cytomegalovirus (invades monocytes, polymorphonuclear cells, and lymphocytes), and human immunodeficiency virus (HIV) (involves CD4+ T lymphocytes and macrophages) and other human retroviruses that attack lymphocytes. The pathogenesis of viral diseases of the blood is the same as that for viral diseases of any organ; by diverting the cellular machinery to create new viral components or by other means, the virus may prevent the host cell from performing its normal function. The cell may be destroyed or damaged by viral replication, and immunologic responses of the host may also contribute to the pathogenesis.

Although many viral diseases have a viremic stage, recovery of virus particles or detection of circulating viruses is used in the diagnosis of only a few diseases. Chapter 64 discusses the recovery of viruses from blood in greater detail.

Types of Bacteremia

Bacteremia may be transient, continuous, or intermittent. Most people have experienced **transient** (asymptomatic and a result of a procedure associated with a nonsterile anatomic site) bacteremia; teething infants and people having dental procedures have had oral microbiota gain entry to the bloodstream through breaks in the gums. Other conditions in which bacteria are transiently present in the bloodstream include manipulation of infected tissues, devices or instrumentation inserted through contaminated mucosal surfaces, and surgery involving nonsterile sites. These circumstances may also lead to significant septicemia, although normally the bacteria are cleared from the blood by scavenging leukocytes, resulting in no infection. Septicemia can occur when the bacteria multiply more rapidly than the immune system is capable of killing and removing the organism.

In septic shock, bacterial endocarditis, and other endovascular infections, organisms are released into the bloodstream at a constant rate (**continuous bacteremia**). Also, during the early stages of specific infections, including typhoid fever, brucellosis, and leptospirosis, bacteria are continuously present in the bloodstream. Septic shock typically presents in two clinical stages: vasoconstriction and low cardiac output followed by vasodilation resulting in increased vascular resistance and cardiac output that causes systemic organ damage.

In most other infections, such as in patients with undrained abscesses, bacteria can be found **intermittently** (periodically present at various time intervals) in the bloodstream. Of note, the causative agents of meningitis, pneumonia, pyogenic arthritis, and osteomyelitis are often recovered from blood during the early course of these diseases. In the case of intermittent seeding of the blood from a sequestered focus of infection, such as an abscess, bacteria are released into the blood approximately 45 minutes before a febrile episode.

The symptoms of sepsis or septicemia are fever, chills, and malaise; these are caused by the presence of the invading microorganism and the toxins produced by these microorganisms. The older the patient is, the greater the risk and the rate of mortality because of septicemia.

Types of Bloodstream Infections

The two major categories of bloodstream infections are **intravascular** (those that originate within the cardiovascular system) and **extravascular** (those that result from bacteria entering the blood circulation through the lymphatic system from another site of infection). Of note, other organisms, such as fungi, may also cause intravascular or extravascular infections. However, because bacteria account for most significant vascular infections, these types of bloodstream infections are discussed in more detail. Factors contributing to the initiation of bloodstream infections are immunosuppressive agents, widespread use of broad-spectrum antibiotics that suppress the normal microbiota and allow the emergence of resistant strains of bacteria, invasive procedures that allow bacteria access to the interior of the host, more extensive surgical procedures, and prolonged survival of debilitated and seriously ill patients.

Intravascular Infections

Intravascular infections include infective endocarditis, mycotic aneurysm, suppurative thrombophlebitis, and IV

catheter–associated bacteremia. Because these infections are within the vascular system, organisms are present in the bloodstream at a constant rate (i.e., a continuous bacteremia). These infections in the cardiovascular system are extremely serious and considered life threatening.

Endocarditis

The development of **infective endocarditis** (infection of the endocardium most commonly caused by bacteria) is believed to involve several independent events. Cardiac abnormalities, such as congenital valvular diseases that lead to turbulence in blood flow or direct trauma from IV catheters, can damage cardiac endothelium. This damage to the endothelial surface results in the deposition of platelets and fibrin. If bacteria transiently gain access to the bloodstream (this can occur after an innocuous procedure such as brushing the teeth) after alteration of the capillary endothelial cells, the organisms may stick to and then colonize the damaged cardiac endothelial cell surface. After colonization, the surface will rapidly be covered with a protective layer of fibrin and platelets. This protective environment is favorable to further bacterial multiplication. This web of platelets, fibrin, inflammatory cells, and entrapped organisms is called a **vegetation** (Fig. 67.1). The resulting vegetation ultimately seeds bacteria into the blood at a slow but constant rate.

The primary causes of infective endocarditis are the viridans streptococci, comprising several species (Box 67.2). These organisms are normal inhabitants of the oral cavity, often gaining entrance to the bloodstream because of gingivitis, periodontitis, or dental manipulation. Heart valves, especially those that have been previously damaged, present convenient surfaces for attachment of these bacteria. *Streptococcus sanguis* and *Streptococcus mutans* are commonly isolated in streptococcal endocarditis. Gram-negative bacilli, known as the HACEK group, *Aggregatibacter aphrophilus, Actinobacillus actinomycetemcomitans, Cardiobacterium* spp., *Eikenella corrodens,* and *Kingella kingae,* can also be associated with endocarditis.

With the ever-increasing use of IV catheters, arterial lines, and vascular prostheses, organisms considered normal or health care–associated inhabitants of the human skin can gain access to the bloodstream and attach to various surfaces, including heart valves and vascular endothelium. It has been estimated that more than 200,000 health care–associated bloodstream infections occur annually in the United States in adults and children. Most of these infections are caused by the use of intravascular catheters. *Staphylococcus epidermidis* and other coagulase-negative staphylococci have been increasingly implicated as the cause of infection associated with intravascular catheters. *S. epidermidis* is the most common etiologic agent identified in prosthetic valve endocarditis, with *S. aureus* being the second most common. *S. aureus* is an important cause of septicemia without endocarditis and is found in association with other foci, such as abscesses, wound infections, and pneumonia, as well as sepsis related to indwelling intravascular catheters.

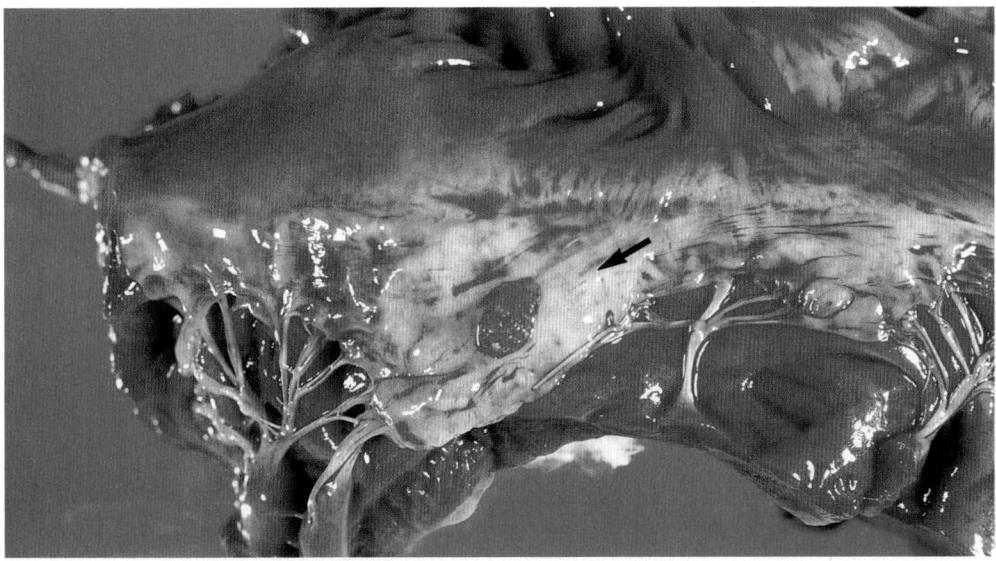

• **Fig. 67.1** Vegetations of bacterial endocarditis. *Arrow* indicates the vegetations. (Courtesy Celeste N. Powers, MD, PhD, Virginia Commonwealth University Medical Center, Medical College of Virginia Campus, Richmond, VA.)

• BOX 67.2 Agents of Infective Endocarditis

Aggregatibacter aphrophilus
Viridans streptococci[a]
　Abiotrophia spp. and *Granulicatella* spp. (previously referred to as nutritionally deficient streptococci)
Enterococcia
Streptococcus bovis
Staphylococcus aureus[a]
Staphylococci (coagulase-negative)
Enterobacterales
Pseudomonas spp. (usually in drug users)
Haemophilus spp.
Unusual gram-negative bacilli (e.g., *Actinobacillus, Cardiobacterium, Eikenella, Coxiella burnetii*)
Yeast
Other (including polymicrobial infectious endocarditis)

[a]Most common organisms associated with native valve endocarditis in non–drug-using adults.

Mycotic Aneurysm and Suppurative Thrombophlebitis

Two other intravascular infections, mycotic aneurysms and suppurative thrombophlebitis, result from damage to the endothelial cells lining blood vessels. With respect to mycotic aneurysm, an infection causes inflammatory damage and weakening of an arterial wall; this weakening causes a bulging of the arterial wall (i.e., aneurysm) that can eventually rupture. The etiologic agents are similar to those that cause endocarditis.

Suppurative thrombophlebitis is an inflammation of a vein wall. The pathogenesis of this intravascular infection involves an alteration in the vein's endothelial lining followed by clot formation. The site is then seeded with organisms, thereby establishing a primary site of infection. Suppurative thrombophlebitis represents a common complication of hospitalized patients caused by the increasing use of IV catheters.

Intravenous Catheter–Associated Bacteremia. IV catheters are an integral part of the care for many hospitalized patients. For example, central venous catheters are used to administer fluids, blood products, medications, antibiotics, and nutrition and for hemodynamic monitoring. Unfortunately, a major consequence of these medical devices is colonization of the catheter by either bacteria or fungi, which can lead to catheter infection and a serious bloodstream infection. This consequence is a major source of health care–associated illness and death.

IV catheter–associated bacteremia (or fungemia) is believed to occur primarily by two routes (Fig. 67.2). The first route involves the movement of organisms from the catheter entry site through the patient's skin and down the external surface of the catheter to the catheter tip within the bloodstream. After arriving at the tip, the organisms multiply and may cause a bacteremia. The second way that IV catheter–associated bacteremia may occur is by migration of organisms along the inside of the catheter (the lumen) to the catheter tip. The catheter's hub, where the tubing connects into the IV catheter, is considered the site at which organisms gain access to the patient's bloodstream through the catheter lumen. The most common etiologic agents for IV catheter–associated bloodstream infections, regardless of the route of infection, are organisms found on the skin (Box 67.3). Certain strains of *Staphylococcus* spp. appear to be uniquely suited for causing catheter-related infections because of their ability to produce a biofilm or slime that consists of complex polysaccharides believed to help the organism adhere to the catheter's surface. The initial attachment of *Staphylococcus* spp. to the catheter's polystyrene surface is related to a cell surface protein. Once attached, the organism proliferates, subsequently forming a biofilm. Uncommon routes of IV catheter–tip infection include contaminated fluids or bloodborne seeding from another infection site.

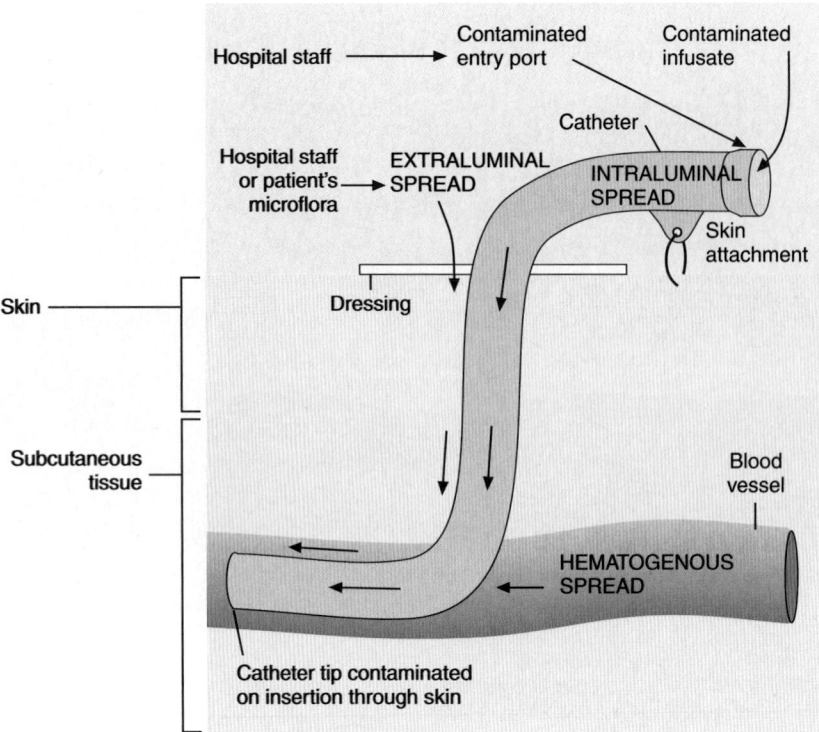

• **Fig. 67.2** Possible routes by which microorganisms gain access to the bloodstream to cause intravenous catheter–associated bacteremia. (Modified from Elliott TS. PHLS communicable disease report: line-associated bacteremias. *CDR Review*. 1993;3:R91.)

• **BOX 67.3   Common Agents of Intravenous Catheter–Associated Bacteremia**

Staphylococcus epidermidis
Other coagulase-negative staphylococci
Staphylococcus aureus
Enterobacterales
Pseudomonas aeruginosa
Candida spp.
Corynebacterium spp.
Other gram-negative rods

Extravascular Infections

Except for intravascular infections, bacteria usually enter the circulation through the lymphatic system. Most cases of clinically significant bacteremia are a result of extravascular infection. When organisms multiply at a local site of infection such as the lung, they are drained by the lymphatics and reach the bloodstream. In most individuals, organisms in the bloodstream are effectively and rapidly removed by the reticuloendothelial system in the liver, spleen, and bone marrow and by circulating phagocytic cells. Depending on the extent of immunologic control of the infection, the organism may be circulated more widely, thereby causing a bacteremia or fungemia.

The most common portals of entry for bacteremia are the genitourinary tract (25%), respiratory tract (20%), abscesses (10%), surgical wound infections (5%), biliary tract (5%), miscellaneous sites (10%), and uncertain sites (25%). For the most part, the probability of bacteremia occurring from an extravascular site depends on the site of infection, its severity, and the organism. For example, any organism producing meningitis is likely to produce bacteremia at the same time. Of importance, certain organisms causing extravascular infections commonly invade the bloodstream; some of these organisms are listed in Table 67.1. In addition to these organisms, many other bacteria and fungi that cause extravascular infections are also capable of invading the bloodstream. Whether these organisms invade the bloodstream depends on the host's ability to control the infection and the organism's pathogenic potential. Some of the organisms associated with potential bloodstream infections from a localized site include members of the Enterobacterales, *S. pneumoniae, S. aureus, Neisseria gonorrhoeae,* anaerobic cocci, *Bacteroides, Clostridium, Klebsiella,* beta-hemolytic streptococci, and *Pseudomonas*. These are only some of the organisms commonly isolated from blood. Almost every known bacterial species and many fungal species have been implicated in extravascular bloodstream infections.

Clinical Manifestations

As previously discussed, bacteremia may indicate the presence of a focus of disease, such as intravascular infection, pneumonia, or liver abscess, or it may represent transient release of bacteria into the bloodstream. Septicemia or sepsis indicates a condition in which bacteria or their products (toxins) are causing harm to the host. Unfortunately,

	TABLE 67.1	Organisms Commonly Associated With Bloodstream Invasion From Extravascular Sites of Infection

Organism	Extravascular Site of Infection
Anaerobic organisms	Wound, soft tissue
Brucella spp.	Reticuloendothelial system
Candida albicans	Genitourinary tract
Chlamydia pneumoniae	Respiratory
Clostridium spp.	Wound, soft tissue
Coagulase negative staphylococci	Wound, soft tissue
Enterobacterales (*E. coli, Klebsiella* spp., *Enterobacter* spp., *Proteus* spp., *Enterococcus* spp.)	Genitourinary tract infections, CNS
Haemophilus influenzae	Meninges (CNS), epiglottitis, periorbital region, respiratory
Legionella spp.	Respiratory
Listeria monocytogenes	Meninges (CNS)
Neisseria meningitidis	Meninges (CNS)
Pseudomonas aeruginosa	Wound, soft tissue, CNS
Salmonella enterica Typhi	Small intestine, regional lymph nodes of the intestine, reticuloendothelial system
Streptococcus pneumoniae	Meninges (CNS), respiratory
Streptococcus pyogenes	Wound, soft tissue
Staphylococcus aureus	Wound, soft tissue, meninges (CNS)

CNS, Central nervous system.

clinicians often use the terms bacteremia and septicemia interchangeably. Signs and symptoms of an SIRS may include fever or hypothermia (low body temperature), chills, hyperventilation (abnormally increased breathing leading to excess loss of carbon dioxide from the body) and subsequent respiratory alkalosis (a condition caused by the loss of acid leading to an increase in pH), skin lesions, change in mental status, and diarrhea. Sepsis is a form of SIRS with an identifiable infection. SIRS is classified as severe sepsis once the infection leads to organ or tissue damage and dysfunction. More serious manifestations include hypotension or shock, DIC, and major organ system failure. The syndrome known as septic shock, as previously mentioned, is characterized by fever, acute respiratory distress, shock, renal failure, intravascular coagulation, and tissue destruction and can be initiated by either exotoxins or endotoxins. Septic

shock is mediated by the production of cytokines from activated mononuclear cells, such as tumor necrosis factor and interleukins.

Shock is the gravest complication of septicemia. In septic shock, the presence of bacterial products and the host's response act to shut down major host physiologic systems. Clinical manifestations include a drop in blood pressure, increase in heart rate, functional impairment in vital organs (brain, kidney, liver, and lungs), acid-base alterations, and bleeding problems. Gram-negative bacteria contain a substance in their cell walls, called endotoxin, which has a strong effect on several physiologic functions. This substance, a lipopolysaccharide (LPS) that composes part of the cell wall structure (Chapter 2), may be released during the normal growth cycles of bacteria or after the destruction of bacteria by host defenses. Endotoxin (or the core of the LPS, lipid A) has been shown to mediate numerous systemic reactions, including a febrile response, and the activation of complement and certain blood-clotting factors. Although gram-positive bacteria do not contain the lipid A endotoxin, many produce **exotoxins** (bacterial products secreted into the environment), and the effects of their presence in the bloodstream may be equally devastating to the patient.

DIC is a disastrous complication of sepsis. DIC is characterized by numerous small blood vessels becoming clogged with blood clots and bleeding because of the depletion of coagulation factors. DIC can occur with septicemia involving any circulating pathogen, including parasites, viruses, and fungi, although it is most commonly a consequence of gram-negative bacterial sepsis.

Immunocompromised Patients

One of the greatest challenges facing microbiologists is the handling of blood cultures from immunocompromised patients. The number of immunocompromised patients has steadily increased in recent years in large part as the result of advances in medicine. People undergoing organ transplantation, elderly persons, individuals with malignant disease (e.g., malignancies and cancer), and those receiving therapy for the malignancy are examples of immunosuppressed patients. AIDS has also contributed to the increase in the number of immunocompromised or immunosuppressed individuals. The marked immunosuppression brought about by infection with the HIV in patients with AIDS is a result of this virus' profound impairment of cellular immunity. Patients with AIDS have the greatest diversity of pathogens recovered from blood, including mycobacterial species, *Bartonella henselae, Corynebacterium jeikeium, Shigella flexneri,* unusual *Salmonella* spp., *H. capsulatum, Cryptococcus* spp., and cytomegalovirus.

As is typically observed in other hospitalized patients, organisms such as gram-positive aerobic bacteria (e.g., *S. aureus, Enterococcus*) and gram-negative aerobic bacteria (e.g., Enterobacterales, *Pseudomonas aeruginosa*) are common causes of bloodstream infections in immunocompromised patients. In addition, bloodstream infections in immunocompromised patients are commonly caused by either unusual pathogens whose recovery from blood requires special techniques or by organisms normally considered contaminants when isolated from blood cultures. Therefore microbiologists must be aware of the potential pathogenicity of organisms in immunosuppressed patients that are typically considered as probable blood culture contaminants. Without this knowledge, aerobic gram-positive rods isolated from blood cultures may be dismissed as contaminating diphtheroids, when, in fact, the organism is *C. jeikeium,* known to cause bacteremia in immunosuppressed patients. Microbiologists must be familiar with the unusual pathogens isolated from blood cultures obtained from immunocompromised patients and organisms that require special techniques for isolation (some of the special considerations are covered later in this chapter).

Detection of Bacteremia

Mortality rates associated with bloodstream infection range from 30% to 50%. Because bacteremia typically represents a life-threatening infection, the prompt detection and recovery of microorganisms from blood is of paramount importance. However, even with the advanced improvement in laboratory diagnostic methods, approximately 30% of all blood culture isolates do not have a directly linked identifiable source of infection. This leads to difficulties in the effective diagnosis and treatment of bloodstream infections.

To detect bloodstream infections, a patient's blood must be obtained by aseptic venipuncture and then incubated in culture media. Bacterial growth can be detected using techniques ranging from manual (in underdeveloped countries) to automated methods. After sufficient growth the organism's phenotypic (biochemical profile), nucleic acid, or protein spectrum is identified as a specific organism, and if it is considered pathogenic or treatment is necessary for the patient, the organism is then tested for susceptibility to various antimicrobial agents.

Specimen Collection
Preparation of the Site

Because blood culture media have been developed as enrichment broths to encourage the multiplication of as few as a single organism, these media will enhance growth of contaminating organisms, including normal microbiota of human skin. Therefore careful skin preparation before collecting the blood sample is of paramount importance to reduce the risk of introducing contaminants into blood culture media.

The vein from which the blood is to be drawn must be chosen before the skin is disinfected. If a patient has an existing IV line, the blood should be drawn below the existing line; blood drawn above the line will be diluted with fluid being infused. It is less desirable to draw blood through a vascular shunt or catheter because these prosthetic devices are difficult to decontaminate completely and may be colonized with a microbial biofilm within the vasculature of the patient.

Antisepsis
Once a vein is selected, the skin site is defatted (fat removal) with 70% isopropyl alcohol, and an antiseptic is applied to kill surface and subsurface bacteria. Regardless of the antiseptic used, it is critical to follow the manufacturer's recommendation for the length of time the antiseptic can remain on the skin. Available data indicate that iodine tincture (iodine in alcohol) and chlorhexidine are equivalent for skin preparation before drawing blood cultures. The steps necessary for drawing blood for culture are given in Evolve Procedure 67.1, which can be found on the Evolve site.

As part of ongoing quality assurance, laboratories should determine the rate of blood culture contamination by clinically evaluating patients' conditions in conjunction with the organism isolated from culture. Laboratories that recover contaminants at rates greater than 3% should suspect improper phlebotomy techniques and should institute measures to educate the phlebotomists in proper skin preparation methods. Higher infection rates may occur in specialty hospitals or long-term centers for critically ill patients.

Precautions
Standard precautions require that phlebotomists wear gloves for blood drawing. Because blood for culture must be obtained aseptically, it is important that contaminated surfaces that might come in contact with the venipuncture site be disinfected. For example, if the site must be touched after preparation, the phlebotomist must disinfect the gloved fingers used for palpation. Also, if the rubber stopper or septum of the container into which blood is to be inoculated (e.g., test tubes or commercial culture bottles) is potentially contaminated, the phlebotomist must disinfect the septum.

Specimen Volume
Adults
For many years, it has been recognized that most bacteremia in adults have a low number of colony-forming units (CFU) per milliliter (mL) of blood. For example, in several studies, fewer than 30 CFU/mL of blood were commonly found in patients with clinically significant bacteremia. Therefore a sufficient sample volume is critical for the successful detection of bacteremia.

There is a direct relationship between the volume of blood and an increased probability that the laboratory will isolate the infecting organism. Therefore collection of two to four sets of cultures using 10 to 20 mL of blood per culture may be required to properly identify and diagnose bloodstream infections in adults.

Children
It is not safe to take large samples of blood from children, particularly infants. The optimal volume of blood required for successful identification of organisms from infants and children has not been clearly delineated. Similar to adults, this patient population has low-level (small numbers of organisms) bacteremia or fungemia. Considering the low levels of circulating organisms in infants and children and based on

the premise that it is safe to obtain as much as 4% to 4.5% of a patient's known total blood volume for culture and the relationship between blood volume and patient weight, for infants and small children, only 1 to 5 mL of blood should be drawn for culture. In addition, blood volumes drawn for culture should be closely monitored and reduced as necessary in anemic patients. Blood culture bottles are available that are designed specifically for pediatric patients. Because blood specimens from septic children may yield fewer than 5 CFU/mL of the organism, quantities less than 1 mL may not be adequate to detect pathogens. Nevertheless, smaller volumes should still be cultured, because high levels of bacteremia (more than 1000 CFU/mL of blood) are detected in some infants. If a bloodstream infection is suspected, all the blood should be placed in an aerobic pediatric bottle, because young patients are at a much lower risk of infection by anaerobic organisms.

Number of Blood Cultures

Because periodicity of microorganisms in the bloodstream may be characteristic for some diseases, continuous for some and random in others, patterns of bacteremia must be considered in establishing standards for the timing and number of blood cultures. If the volume of blood is adequate, usually two or four sets of blood cultures are sufficient to achieve the optimum blood culture sensitivity. A single blood culture is not sufficient for ruling out infection, whereas a second blood culture frequently establishes the diagnosis in at least 80% to 90% of patients. Three separate blood collections of 16 to 20 mL each, and an additional blood culture or two taken on the second day, if necessary, detects most etiologic agents (96% to 98%) in the bloodstream. The rate of recovery reaches nearly 100% for the detection of pathogens following four blood cultures; however, it is important to consider all factors including clinical diagnosis and other patient conditions when considering the large amount of blood sample required for optimal testing. This presumes use of a culture system adequate for growth of the organism involved, which often entails extending the incubation period.

Timing of Collection

The timing of cultures is not as important as other factors in patients with intravascular infections, because organisms are released into the bloodstream at a constant rate. Because the timing of intermittent sepsis is unpredictable, it is generally accepted that three or four blood cultures should be spaced an hour apart. However, in most cases, no significant difference in the yield between multiple blood cultures obtained simultaneously or those obtained at intervals has been demonstrated. The overall volume of blood cultured is more critical to increasing organism yield than timing.

Regardless, blood should be transported immediately to the laboratory and placed into the incubator or instrument as soon as possible. With blood culture instrumentation, a delay beyond 2 hours can delay the detection of positive cultures.

Miscellaneous Matters

Anticoagulation

Blood drawn for culture must not be allowed to clot. If the infecting organism becomes entrapped within a clot, its presence may go undetected. Thus, blood drawn for culture may be either inoculated directly into the blood culture broth media or into a sterile blood collection tube containing an anticoagulant for transport to the laboratory for subsequent inoculation. Heparin, ethylenediaminetetraacetic acid (EDTA), and citrate inhibit numerous organisms and are not recommended for use. Sodium polyanethol sulfonate (SPS) in concentrations of 0.025% to 0.03% is the best anticoagulant available for blood cultures. As a result, the most commonly used preparation in blood culture media today is 0.025% to 0.05% SPS. In addition to its anticoagulant properties, SPS also inactivates lysozyme, is anticomplementary and antiphagocytic and interferes with the activity of some antimicrobial agents, notably aminoglycosides. SPS, however, may inhibit the growth of a few microorganisms, such as some strains of *Neisseria* spp., *Gardnerella vaginalis, Streptobacillus moniliformis,* and all strains of *Peptostreptococcus anaerobius.* Because of the inhibitory effect of SPS on some organisms in conjunction with the necessity for an additional step to transfer the blood to the ultimate culture bottles that increases the risk of exposure to bloodborne pathogens as well as contamination, using collection tubes instead of direct inoculation into culture bottles may compromise organism recovery. For these reasons, the use of intermediate collection tubes is discouraged.

Dilution

In addition to the volume of blood collected and type of medium chosen, the dilution factor for the blood in the medium must be considered. To conserve space and materials, it is desirable to combine the largest feasible amount of blood from the patient (usually 10 mL) with the smallest amount of medium that will still encourage the growth of bacteria and dilute out or inactivate the antibacterial components of the blood. Traditionally, a 1:10 ratio of blood to medium was required for successful bacterial growth; however, several new commercial media containing resins or other additives have demonstrated enhanced recovery with as low as a 1:4 ratio. For this purpose, a 1:4 ratio of blood to unmodified medium has been found to be adequate in conventional blood cultures. All commercial blood culture systems (discussed later in this chapter) specify the appropriate dilution.

Blood Culture Media

The diversity of organisms recovered from blood requires an equally diverse and large number of media to enhance the growth of these organisms. Basic blood culture media contain a nutrient broth and an anticoagulant. Several different broth formulations are commercially available. Most blood culture bottles available commercially contain trypticase soy broth. More specialized broth bases include Columbia, brain heart infusion, *Brucella* broth, or other enriched media.

Types of Blood Culture Bottles

The addition of penicillinase to blood culture media for inactivation of penicillin has been largely superseded by the availability of a resin-containing medium that inactivates most antibiotics nonselectively by adsorbing them to the surface of the resin particles. Resin-containing media may enhance isolation of staphylococci, particularly when patients are receiving bacteriostatic drugs. The BACTEC system (Becton Dickinson Microbiology Systems, Sparks, MD) offers several resin-containing media. In addition to resin-containing media, BacT/ALERT has a blood culture bottle with supplemented brain-heart infusion (BHI) broth containing activated charcoal particles that significantly increase the yield of microorganisms over standard blood culture media. In addition, resins or charcoal may be added to commercial media to absorb and inactivate antimicrobial agents in the patient's blood sample. Care should be exercised when interpreting Gram stains from resin- and charcoal-containing bottles. The additives may be confused with gram-positive organisms. In addition to the traditional BacT/ALERT culture media, bioMérieux now offers next generation Fastidious Antimicrobial Neutralization Plus media (FAN^{R}Plus). The media are supplemented with Adsorbent Polymeric Beads that neutralize antimicrobials but provide clearer Gram stains.

In general, each blood culture set includes a blood culture bottle designated for aerobic recovery and one for anaerobic recovery of bacteria. Because of the decline in the proportion of positive blood cultures yielding anaerobic bacteria coupled with the increasing pressure for laboratories to be cost effective, some investigators have recommended laboratories discard this routine practice of processing all blood samples aerobically and anaerobically. It has been proposed that anaerobic cultures should be selectively performed, and, in place of the anaerobic blood culture, a second aerobic bottle be included. Depending on the patient population served by the laboratory, numbers of blood cultures submitted, and personnel and financial resources, the laboratory may have one or more methods available to ensure detection of the broadest range of organisms in the least possible time.

Culture Techniques

Special blood culture broth systems are available for the isolation of mycobacteria. The systems are useful in detecting disseminated infections caused by *Mycobacterium tuberculosis* and no tuberculosis mycobacteria.

Conventional Blood Cultures
Incubation Conditions
The atmosphere in commercially prepared blood culture bottles is usually at a low oxidation-reduction potential, permitting the growth of most facultative and some anaerobic organisms. Constant agitation of the bottles during the first 24 hours of incubation enhances the growth of most aerobic bacteria.

Self-Contained Manual Culture Systems

A modification of the biphasic blood culture medium is the BD BBL Septi-Chek system (Becton Dickinson Microbiology Systems, Sparks, MD) consisting of a conventional blood culture broth bottle with an attached chamber containing a slide coated with agar or several types of agars. Special media for isolation of fungi and mycobacteria are also available. To subculture, the entire broth contents are allowed to contact the agar surface by inverting the bottle, a simple procedure that does not require opening the bottle or using needles. The bottles should be tipped at least twice weekly to wash the liquid culture over the agar coated slide to culture any organisms that are growing in the broth. The large volume of broth subcultured and the enclosed method provide faster detection for many organisms than is possible with conventional systems. The Septi-Chek system appears to enhance the recovery of *S. pneumoniae,* but such biphasic systems do not efficiently recover anaerobic isolates, therefore requiring a second anaerobic bottle.

The Signal Blood Culture System (Thermo Fisher Scientific, Waltham, MA), is a single one-bottle system that can be used to isolate common aerobic, anaerobic, and microaerophilic organisms from both adults and pediatrics. The bottle contains 80 mL of broth and a detection chamber. The bottles are agitated and incubated at 35 to 37°C. When an organism begins to metabolize, the CO_2 formed by the microorganism increases pressure within the bottle pushing some of the blood specimen broth mixture through a needle that extends from the liquid into the Signal Detection Chamber. The presence of fluid in the detection chamber indicates a positive culture and can then be removed for additional testing such as Gram-stain or plating to solid media.

Both manual blood culture systems should be examined daily for growth. Growth within blood/broth is indicated by turbidity (visible using reflected or transmitted light), hemolysis, CO_2 (gas production), or visual growth on the surface or as flocculation.

Lysis Centrifugation

The Isolator/Isostat System Press and Rack (Alere, Waltham, MA) is a lysis centrifugation system that includes a hand-operated press used to apply a cap to the tube and is commercially available. The Isolator consists of a stoppered tube containing saponin to lyse blood cells and SPS as an anticoagulant (Fig. 67.3). After centrifugation, the supernatant is discarded, the sediment containing the pathogen is vigorously vortexed, and the entire sediment is plated to solid agar. Benefits of this system include rapid and improved recovery of filamentous fungi, the presence of actual colonies for direct identification and susceptibility testing after initial incubation, the ability to quantify the CFU present in the blood, rapid detection of polymicrobial infections, dispensing with the need for a separate antibiotic-removal step, the ability to choose special media for initial culture setup based on clinical impression (e.g., direct plating onto media supportive of *Legionella* spp. or *Mycobacterium* spp.),

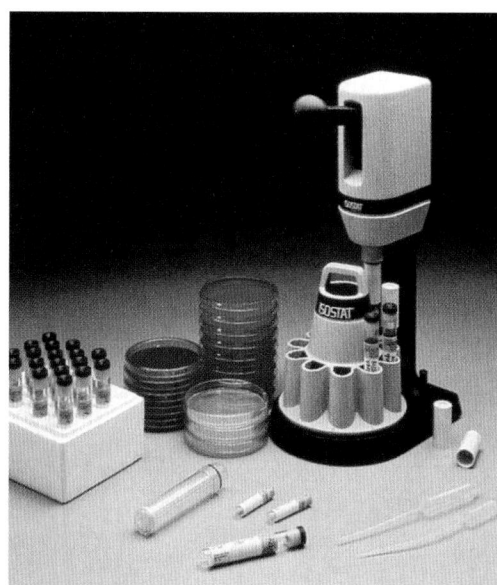

• **Fig. 67.3** Lysis centrifugation blood culture (Isolator/Isostat System, Alere, Waltham, MA) uses vacuum-draw collection tubes with a lysing agent and special apparatus (Isostat Press) to facilitate removal of the supernatant without the use of needles.

and potential enhanced recovery of intracellular microorganisms caused by lysis of host cells. Possible limitations of the system seem to be a relatively high rate of plate contamination and a decreased ability to detect certain bacteria, such as *S. pneumoniae, Listeria monocytogenes, Haemophilus influenzae,* and anaerobic bacteria, compared with conventional systems. If a mixed infection is suspected, an additional blood culture collection tube should be inoculated simultaneously.

Instrument-Based Systems

During these times of cost constraints in health care and a corresponding requirement for clinically relevant care, the development of improved instrumentation for blood cultures has improved the identification of the pathogens improving patient care. Instruments are capable of rapid and accurate detection of organisms in blood specimens. By using newer instrumentation, laboratories processing a large volume of blood cultures also provide results cost effectively.

BACTEC Systems

Many laboratories use the BACTEC system (Becton Dickinson Microbiology Systems, Sparks, MD), which measures the production of carbon dioxide (CO_2) by metabolizing organisms. Blood or sterile body fluid for routine culture is inoculated into bottles containing appropriate substrates.

The BACTEC blood culture systems are fully automated with the incubator, shaker, and detector all in one instrument. These fully automated blood culture systems use fluorescence to measure CO_2 released by organisms; a gas-permeable fluorescent sensor is on the bottom of each vial. As CO_2 diffuses into the sensor and dissolves in water present in the sensor matrix, hydrogen (H^+) ions are generated.

These H^+ ions cause a decrease in pH, which, in turn, increases the fluorescent output of the sensor. There is continuous monitoring of each bottle, and detection is external to the bottle.

BacT/ALERT Microbial Detection System

Other laboratories use the BacT/ALERT System (bioMérieux, Durham, NC), which measures CO_2-derived pH changes with a colorimetric sensor in the bottom of each bottle. The sensor is separated from the broth medium by a membrane permeable to CO_2. As organisms grow, they release CO_2, which diffuses across the membrane and is dissolved in water present in the matrix of the sensor. As CO_2 is dissolved, free hydrogen ions are generated. These free hydrogen ions cause a color change in the sensor (blue to light green to yellow as the pH decreases); a sensor in the instrument reads this color change.

Versa TREK System

The Versa TREK system (Thermo Scientific, TREK Diagnostics, Cleveland, OH) uses a unique agitation system during blood culture inoculation. The aerobic media bottles each contain a small magnetic stir bar that enhances oxygenation during incubation. Like the other systems, this is also a continuously monitoring instrument.

Non–Culture Based Methods for the Identification of Bacteremia or Sepsis

Because blood culture systems are insensitive to rapid detection of bacteremia or sepsis, several biochemical markers have been used as indicators or biomarkers for diagnosis or prognosis in cases of bacteremia and sepsis. These biomarkers include chemicals made by or released into the bloodstream, such as beta-D-glucan, or galactomannan produced by fungal organisms to human interleukins (IL-10 and IL-1Ra), other immune response related molecules (i.e., presepsin, IL-6, monocyte chemoattractant protein), and physiological indicators including C-reactive protein, lactate, or procalcitonin. Procalcitonin assays have been widely used to monitor patients in clinical settings to assist in the identification of pathogens, predict mortality, and monitor the use of antibiotics and reduce the duration of therapy in bloodstream infections. Interleukins and other immune response related molecules rapidly rise when blood stream infections are present and can assist in the differentiation of other inflammatory conditions. The enzymatic detection of beta-D-glucan or enzyme immunoassays for circulating mannans are becoming increasingly used for the detection of invasive systemic fungal infections. In addition, various nucleic acid-based systems are also widely used for the direct detection of viral, fungal, and bacterial pathogens in the bloodstream.

Procalcitonin is secreted by the thyroid gland and neuroendocrine cells of the lungs and intestines. It is normally found in serum concentrations of less than 0.1 ng/mL in healthy individuals. Both the lung and intestinal cells

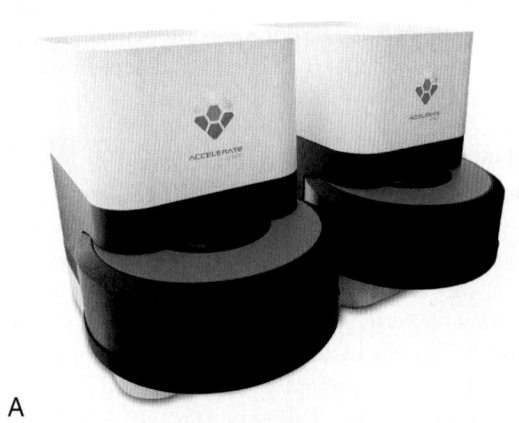
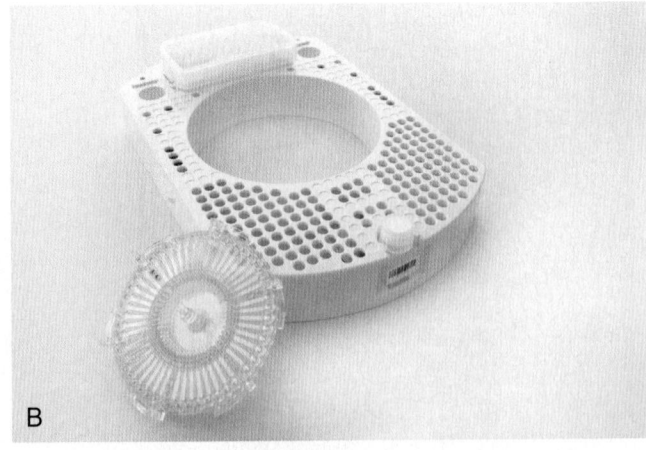

• **Fig. 67.4** (A) FDA-approved combination identification and antibiotic sensitivity system, the Accelerate Pheno system (Accelerate Diagnostics Inc, Tucson AZ). (B) Sample cartridge.

increase the production of procalcitonin in response to inflammation resulting in a rapid increase in the serum of up to 400 times the normal value or greater than 4 ng/mL. The values of procalcitonin in the serum have also been used as a prognostic indicator for bacterial infection in the presence of inflammation and the progression to severe sepsis. A serum level of less than 0.5 ng/mL indicates no risk of infection, 0.5 to 2.0 ng/mL moderate risk of infection, and 2 to 10 ng/mL indicates a high risk of infection and progression to severe sepsis.

The T2Candida system (T2 Biosystems, Inc., Lexington, MA) is a magnetic resonance assay combined with nucleic acid amplification of five major *Candida* species. The system can be utilized to identify invasive *Candida* species in adults as well as small-volume blood specimens from pediatric patients within 5 hours.

Two FDA-cleared nucleic acid systems, the Verigene assay (Luminex, Austin, TX) and the BioFire FilmArray Blood Culture Identification panel (bioMérieux, Inc, Durham, NC), have demonstrated reported concordance with clinical results from 86% to 100% depending on the infectious agent. The BioFire FilmArray Blood Culture Identification Panel, or BCID, contains 27 targets that include yeast and gram-positive and gram-negative bacteria commonly isolated from bloodstream infections. In addition, the assay detects three antibiotic resistance genes associated with bloodstream infections: *mec A*, methicillin resistance; *vanA/B*, vancomycin resistance; and *KPC*, carbapenem resistance. The Verigene assay has separate assays for gram-positive (11 different species or genera) and gram-negative (9 different species or genera) organisms along with the detection of antimicrobial resistance genes including *mec A* and *vanA/B* in gram-positive organisms and extended-spectrum beta-lactamase (ESBL) and carbapenemase in gram-negative organisms.

Although most of the bloodstream infections are monomicrobic, polymicrobic infections do occur. The sensitivity for the detection of multiple pathogens directly from the bloodstream is limited. In addition, the nucleic acid-based methods require a follow-up culture to complete antimicrobial sensitivity testing. An FDA-approved combination system, the Accelerate Pheno system (Accelerate Diagnostics Inc, Tucson AZ), does not require a separate culture following identification of the bloodstream pathogen (Fig. 67.4). The system combines the identification of pathogens directly from the blood specimen within approximately 90 minutes followed by the antimicrobial sensitivity results in about 7 hours from the same sample. The system uses electrochemistry and proprietary gel technology to separate microorganisms from the matrix of molecules in the blood specimen. The cells are concentrated using electrokinetic concentration technology. The cells are captured in a flow cell and positioned for image capture and analysis as the organisms grow. The antibiotic sensitivity reports the minimal inhibitory concentration using morphokinetic cellular images by digital microscopy every 10 minutes in real time. The Accelerate Pheno system identifies 14 bacteria that include gram-positive and gram-negative pathogens and two *Candida* species from blood specimens with a reported approximate specificity and sensitivity of 98%.

Matrix-Assisted Laser Desorption Ionization Time-of-Flight Mass Spectrometry

MALDI-TOF MS has been successfully used to identify many organisms indirectly following pure colony isolation from blood cultures (Chapter 7). However, the antibiotic sensitivity testing requires additional overnight incubation and analysis prior to reporting to the primary care provider. Direct microorganism identification from blood cultures using MALDI-TOF has been successful but reports indicate that it has not improved the methods to complete antimicrobial sensitivity testing nor shortened the duration of antimicrobial therapy for patients with bloodstream infections.

Intravenous Catheter–Associated Infections

The insertion of an IV catheter during hospitalization is common practice. Infection, either locally at the catheter insertion site or sepsis caused by bacteremia, is one of the most common complications of catheter placement. IV catheters are easily contaminated by normal skin microbiota, as well as colonized by microorganisms capable of forming mono- or polymicrobial biofilms on the surface of the catheter tip. Because the skin of all patients is colonized with normal microbiota that are also common pathogens in catheters, techniques used to diagnose catheter-related infections attempt to quantitate bacterial growth. Diagnosis of an IV catheter–related bacteremia (or fungemia) is difficult, because there are often no signs of infection at the catheter insertion site, and the typical signs and symptoms of sepsis can overlap with other clinical manifestations; even the finding of a positive blood culture does not identify the catheter as the source. To date, various methods, such as semiquantitative cultures, Gram stains of the skin entry site, and culture of IV catheter tips following catheter removal are used to monitor potential IV catheter–associated infections. The terminal end of the IV catheter is removed and rolled several times across a blood agar plate. The tip is then removed from the agar plate and placed in enrichment broth. Both the plate and enrichment broth are incubated at 37°C for 18 to 24 hours. After inoculation, the blood agar plates are examined, and any isolates are identified according to the laboratory protocol. The enrichment broth may be subcultured to blood agar and anaerobic media for further analysis and potential detection of intraluminal colonization.

Handling Positive Direct Detection and Indirect Detection From Culture

Most laboratories use a broth-based automated blood culture method. When a positive culture is indicated according to the automated detection system including nucleic acid–based direct detection systems, a Gram-stained smear of an air-dried drop of the direct sample or blood culture medium should be performed. Methanol fixation of the smear preserves bacterial and cellular morphology, which may be especially valuable for detecting gram-negative bacteria among red cell debris. As soon as a morphologic description can be tentatively assigned to an organism detected in blood, the physician should be contacted and given all available information. Determining the clinical significance of an isolate is the physician's responsibility. If no organisms are seen on microscopic examination of a bottle that appears positive, the blood culture should be reincubated. In a patient, with high white blood cell counts, the cellular metabolism can create the production of metabolites including CO_2, causing a false-positive reaction in the automated systems.

Direct Rapid Tests from Blood Culture Bottles

Numerous rapid tests for identification and presumptive antimicrobial susceptibilities can be performed from the broth blood culture if a monomicrobic infection is suspected (based on microscopic evaluation). A suspension of the organism that approximates the turbidity of a 0.5 McFarland standard, obtained directly from the broth or by centrifuging the broth and resuspending the pelleted

bacteria, can be used to perform either disk diffusion (qualitative) or broth dilution (quantitative) antimicrobial susceptibility tests. These suspensions may also be used to perform preliminary tests such as coagulase, thermostable nuclease, esculin hydrolysis, bile solubility, antigen detection by fluorescent-antibody stain or agglutination procedures for gram-positive bacteria, oxidase, and commercially available rapid identification kits for gram-negative bacteria. Presumptive results must be verified with conventional procedures using pure cultures.

In the event of possible future studies (e.g., additional susceptibility testing), isolates from blood cultures may be stored by freezing at –70°C in 10% skim milk. A commercial preservation system, Microbank beads, is available for the preservation and storage of bacterial and fungal isolates (Pro-Laboratory Diagnostics, Austin, TX). The vials contain pretreated beads and a cryopreservative solution that improves storage of microorganisms. Storing an agar slant of the isolate under sterile mineral oil at room temperature is a good alternative to freezing. It may be necessary to compare separate isolates from the same patient or isolates of the same species from different patients months after the bacteria were isolated.

Interpretation of Blood Culture Results

Because of the increasing incidence of blood and vascular infection caused by bacteria normally considered avirulent, indigenous microbiota of a healthy human host, interpretation of the significance of growth of such bacteria in blood cultures has become increasingly difficult. On one hand, contaminants may lead to unnecessary antibiotic therapy, additional testing and consultation, and increased length of hospital stay. Costs related to false-positive blood culture results (i.e., contaminants) are associated with 40% higher charges for IV antibiotics and microbiology testing. On the other hand, failure to recognize and appropriately treat indigenous microbiota can have dire consequences. Guidelines that can assist in distinguishing probable pathogens from contaminants are as follows:

- Probable contaminant
  - Growth of *Bacillus* spp., *Corynebacterium* spp., *Propionibacterium* spp., or *Cutibacterium* spp. in one of several cultures
    - Note: *Bacillus anthracis* must be ruled out before dismissing *Bacillus* species as a probable contaminant.
  - Growth of multiple organisms from one of several cultures (polymicrobial bacteremia is uncommon)
  - The clinical presentation or course is not consistent with sepsis
  - The organism causing the infection at a primary site of infection is not the same as that isolated from the blood culture
- Probable pathogen
  - Growth of the same organism in repeated cultures obtained either at different times or from different anatomic sites

- Growth of certain organisms in cultures obtained from patients suspected of endocarditis, such as enterococci, or gram-negative rods in patients with clinical gram-negative sepsis
- Growth of certain organisms such as members of Enterobacterales, *S. pneumoniae,* gram-negative anaerobes, and *Streptococcus pyogenes*
- Isolation of commensal microbiota from blood cultures obtained from patients suspected to be bacteremic (e.g., immunosuppressed patients or those with prosthetic devices)
- Type(s) of isolates recovered from other body sites and response to therapy.

Special Considerations for Other Relevant Organisms Isolated From Blood

The organisms discussed in this section require somewhat different conditions for their successful recovery from blood culture samples. Most of these organisms are rarely isolated from blood. Therefore it is important for the physician to notify the laboratory of remarkable patient history, such as travel abroad. It is also important the laboratory be aware of organisms isolated from blood cultures that are considered potential agents for bioterrorist attacks. These bacteria include *B. anthracis, Francisella tularensis, Brucella* spp., and *Yersinia pestis.* Finally, in addition to the organisms discussed later that require special conditions for isolation from blood, several organisms are unable to grow on artificial media and are best diagnosed by alternative methods such as serology or nucleic acid amplification assays; these organisms are listed in Box 67.4.

HACEK Bacteria

As mentioned earlier in the chapter, the term HACEK refers to a group of fastidious, gram-negative bacilli including *A. aphrophilus, A. actinomycetemcomitans, C. hominis, E. corrodens,* and *K. kingae.* Recovery of these organisms from blood cultures is usually associated with infective endocarditis. Other fastidious organisms, such as *Capnocytophaga* spp., *Rothia dentocariosa, Flavobacterium* spp., and *Chromobacterium* spp., may also be isolated from blood cultures. Continuous monitoring blood culture systems have indicated that almost all bloodstream infections with these

---

• BOX 67.4 Microorganisms That Cause Bloodstream Infections but Do Not Grow on Artificial Media

Coxiella burnetii
Chlamydia spp. (*C. pneumoniae* and *C. psittaci*)
Rickettsia spp.
Tropheryma whipplei

---

organisms, including endocarditis, were detected within 5 days of incubation.

Campylobacter and *Helicobacter* spp.

Several species of *Campylobacter* and *Helicobacter* are occasionally isolated from blood cultures, usually growing within the 5-day incubation protocol. However, these organisms are small, thin, curved, gram-negative rods that may only be visualized using an AO stain after detection by continuous monitoring instruments. Because of the fastidious nature of these organisms, appropriate media and atmospheric conditions for subculture from blood culture bottles must be used (Chapter 33).

Fungi

Many fungi, particularly yeast, can be recovered in standard blood culture media if the bottle is incubated at the appropriate temperature and has been vented and agitated to allow sufficient oxygenation for fungal growth. However, some fungi may grow slowly and poorly in these media, which best support bacterial growth. Optimal isolation of fungi in blood cultures is achieved with either agitated incubation of a commercial biphasic system, such as the Septi-Chek, or by using the lysis centrifugation system. Manufacturers of media for automated blood culture systems have developed specific media for fungal isolation. These media formulas have dramatically increased the numbers of fungi isolated from patients with fungemia and have shortened the incubation time required for detection of the fungi. An increasing incidence of bloodstream infections with invasive *Candida* spp. and polymicrobial infections of *C. albicans* in combination with *S. aureus* has become a significant concern. Both organisms have demonstrated an increasing resistance to antimicrobials, posing serious treatment difficulties and increased mortality rates. Blood specimens for detecting fungemia are collected in the same manner as for bacterial culture.

Mycobacterium spp.

Patients with HIV infection can have disseminated infection with species of nontuberculous mycobacteria, predominantly *Mycobacterium avium* complex. HIV infections along with multidrug-resistant strains of *Mycobacterium* spp. result in high rates of mortality. Extra-pulmonary disease can become disseminated by entering the bloodstream and being carried to multiple sites throughout the body. Rapidly growing nontuberculosis species of *Mycobacterium* are also more frequently identified in bloodstream infections in immunocompromised patients.

Special media, such as Middlebrook 7H9 broth with 0.05% SPS or BHI broth with 0.5% polysorbate 80, with or without a Middlebrook 7H11 agar slant, enhances the recovery of *Mycobacterium* spp. In addition, the isolator system may also be used for growth of *Mycobacterium* spp.

The broth-based systems for the detection of *Mycobacterium* bloodstream infections provide a mechanism for continued monitoring, prevent cross-contamination, and provide a safer environment for laboratory personal. Despite the advantages, mycobacterial bloodstream infections can go undetected in automated broth culture systems.

Brucella spp.

Brucellosis is a common disease in many developing countries but is uncommon in developed countries. Because brucellosis may be included in the differential diagnosis of many infections, microbiologists should be prepared to process blood cultures suspected of having *Brucella;* blood cultures are positive in 70% to 90% of patients with brucellosis. Septicemia occurs primarily during the first 3 weeks of illness. Special handling may be required for recovering *Brucella* spp. from blood, because these organisms are fastidious, often slow-growing, intracellular parasites. Best recovery is obtained with *Brucella* broth or trypticase soy broth. The use of biphasic media may enhance growth, or the Isolator system may allow release of intracellular bacteria.

The use of continuous monitoring systems has enhanced recovery of *Brucella* spp. For example, the use of the BACTEC instruments makes possible the diagnosis of more than 95% of positive cultures within a 5-day period without routine subcultures of negative vials.

Spirochetes
Borrelia spp.

Visualization in direct preparations is diagnostic for 70% of cases of relapsing fever, a febrile disease caused by *Borrelia recurrentis*. Organisms may be seen in direct wet preparations of a drop of anticoagulated blood diluted in saline as long, thin, unevenly coiled spirochetes that seem to push the red blood cells around as they move. Thick and thin smears of blood, prepared as for malaria testing and stained with Wright's or Giemsa stain, are also sensitive for the detection of *Borrelia*.

Blood cultures using standard bacterial blood cultures incubated for 2 to 3 weeks have been successful for the identification of *B. burgdorferi*. Detection can be enhanced by periodically sampling culture aliquots and using nucleic acid amplification techniques.

Leptospira spp.

Leptospirosis can be diagnosed by isolating the causative spirochete from blood during the first 4 to 7 days of illness. Leptospires will grow 1 to 3 cm below the surface, usually within 2 weeks. The organisms remain viable in blood with SPS for 11 days, allowing for transport of specimens from distant locations. Direct dark-field examination of peripheral blood is not recommended, because many artifacts are present that resemble spirochetes. If blood must be shipped to a reference laboratory for culture, blood may be collected in heparin, oxalate, or citrate tubes and maintained at ambient temperature. One to two drops of blood are inoculated into semisolid oleic acid–albumin medium at the patient's bedside. Various commercial mediums are available, such as Fletcher's medium (BD Diagnostics, Sparks, MD). Multiple cultures are recommended to improve recovery of the organisms. *Leptospira* spp. do not grow well in conventional blood culture systems; molecular assays may improve detection of the organism, as may the use of serologic markers for rapid diagnosis. (Further information about *Borrelia* and *Leptospira* is provided in Chapter 45.)

Granulicatella and *Abiotrophia* spp.

Granulicatella spp. and *Abiotrophia* spp., previously known as nutritionally variant streptococci, are unable to multiply without the addition of 0.001% pyridoxal hydrochloride (also called thiol or vitamin B_6). These streptococci have been associated with bacteremia and endocarditis. Although human blood introduced into the blood culture medium provides enough of the pyridoxal to allow the organisms to multiply in the bottle, standard sheep blood agar plates may not support their growth. Subculturing the broth to a 5% sheep blood agar plate and either overlaying a streak of *S. aureus* or dropping a pyridoxal disk to produce the supplement generally allows colonies of the streptococci to grow as tiny satellites next to the streak. Some commercial media may be supplemented with enough pyridoxal (0.001%) to support growth of nutritionally variant streptococci.

Mycoplasma spp.

Invasive and systemic disease from *Mycoplasma* spp., including *M. hominis* and oral commensals are likely more prevalent than diagnosed. The use of automated blood culture continuously monitoring systems is not recommended for detection of *Mycoplasma* spp. The organisms are inhibited by SPS, the anticoagulant used in most automated blood culture media.

Bartonella spp.

Bartonella spp. have been reported to cause bacteremia and endocarditis in both immunocompetent and immunocompromised patients. *B. henselae* has also been linked to cat-scratch disease, a common infectious disease in the United States. Cat-scratch disease is characterized by a persistent necrotizing inflammation of the lymph nodes. Biphasic or broth culture systems may be used for the isolation of *Bartonella* spp., however the organisms rarely reach a high level of turbidity or activate the CO_2 detector in automated systems. Serology remains the most reliable method for diagnosis of *Bartonella* bacteremia.

ℯ Visit the Evolve site for a complete list of procedures, review questions, and case studies.

Bibliography

Accelerate Phenotest BC. Timing is everything for some patients. Available at: http://acceleratediagnostics.com/products/accelerate-phenotest-bc/. Accessed June 1, 2019.

Adler H, Baumlin N, Frie R: Evaluation of acridine orange staining as a replacement of subcultures for BacT/ALERT-positive, Gram stain-negative blood cultures, *J Clin Microbiol* 41:5238–5239, 2003.

Agan BK, Dolan MJ: Laboratory diagnosis of *Bartonella* infections, *Clin Lab Med* 22:937–962, 2002.

Ani C, Farshidpanah S, Bellinghausen S, et al.: Variations in organism-specific severe sepsis mortality in the United States: 1999-2008, *Crit Care Med* 43:65–77, 2015.

Aziz H, Ross LL, Conway-Klaassen J, Tille P: Role of the microbiology laboratory in the diagnosis of sepsis, *Int J Biomed Lab Sci (IJBLS)* 9(No.1):7–14, 2020.

Aziz H, Ross LL, Tille P, Conway-Klaassen: Rapid identification of pathogens recovered from blood stream infections, *Int J Biomed Lab Sci (IJBLS)* 9(No.1):15–22, 2020.

Barenfanger J, Drake C, Lawhorn J, et al.: Comparison of chlorhexidine and tincture of iodine for skin antisepsis in preparation for blood sample collection, *J Clin Microbiol* 42:2216–2217, 2004.

Baron EJ, Weinstein MP, Dunne WM, et al.: Blood cultures IV. In Baron EJ, editor: *Cumitech 1C*, Washington, DC, 2005, American Society for Microbiology.

Beckman M, Washam MC, DeBurger B, et al.: Reliability of the verigene system for the identification of Gram-positive bacteria and detection of antimicrobial resistance markers from children with bacteremia, *Diagn Microbiol Infect Dis* 93(3):191–195, 2019.

Beebe JL, Koneman EL: Recovery of uncommon bacteria from blood: association with neoplastic disease, *Clin Microbiol Rev* 8:336–356, 1995.

Bhatt M, Sarangi G, Paty BP, et al.: Biofilm as a virulence marker in *Candida* species in nosocomial bloodstream infection and its correlation with antifungal resistance, *Indian J Med Microbiol* 33(Suppl 1):S112–S114, 2015.

Calfee DP, Farr BM: Comparison of four antiseptic preparations for skin in the prevention of contamination of percutaneously drawn blood cultures: a randomized trial, *J Clin Microbiol* 40:1660–1665, 2002.

Carroll KC, Pfaller MA, Landry ML, et al.: *Manual of clinical microbiology*, ed 12, Washington, DC, 2019, ASM.

Centers for Disease Control and Prevention: Guidelines for the prevention of intravascular catheter-related infections, *Morb Mortal Wkly Rep* 51(RR-10):1–32, 2002.

Cockerill FR, Wilson JW, Vetter EA, et al.: Optimal testing parameters for blood cultures, *Clin Infect Dis* 38:1724–1730, 2004.

Conway-Klaassen J, Tille P, Aziz H: The use of biomarkers in the diagnosis and management of sepsis, *Int J Biomed Lab Sci (IJBLS)* 9(No.1):23–31, 2020.

Decker SO, Kruger A, Wilk H, et al.: New approaches for the detection of invasive fungal diseases in patients following liver transplantation-results of an observational clinical pilot study, *Langenbeck's Arch Surg* 404:309–325, 2019.

Fernandez-Guerrero ML, Ramos J, Soriano F: Mycoplasma hominis bacteraemia not associated with genital infections, *J Infect* 39:91–94, 1999.

Galeski DF, Edwards J, Matthew K, Kallen J, et al.: Benchmarking the incidence and mortality of severe sepsis in the United States, *Crit Care Med* 5:1167–1174, 2013.

Giri S, Kindo AJ: A review of *Candida* species causing blood stream infection, *Indian J Med Microbiol* 30:270–278, 2012.

Godinez-Vidal AR, Veronica RH, Montero-Garcia PJ, et al.: Evaluation of the serum procalcitonin level as an indicator of severity and mortality in abdominal sepsis due to secondary peritonitis, *Cir Cir* 87(3):255–259, 2019.

Lamey JR, Eschenbach DA, Mitchell SH, et al.: Isolation of mycoplasmas and bacteria from the blood of postpartum women, *Am J Obstet Gynecol* 143:104–112, 1982.

Levett PN: Usefulness of serologic analysis as a predictor of the infecting serovar in patients with severe leptospirosis, *Clin Infect Dis* 36:447–452, 2003.

Levett PN, Morey RE, Galloway RL, et al.: Detection of pathogenic leptospires by real-time quantitative PCR, *J Med Microbiol* 54:45–49, 2005.

Maggi RG, Duncan AW, Breitschwerdt EB: Novel chemically modified liquid medium that will support the growth of seven *Bartonella* species, *J Clin Microbiol* 43:2651–2655, 2005.

Mathur P, Tak V, Gunjiyal J, et al.: Device-associated infections at a level-1 trauma centre of a developing nation: impact of automated surveillance, training and feedbacks, *Indian J Med Microbiol* 33:51–62, 2015.

Mermel LA, Farr BM, Sheretz RJ, et al.: Guidelines for the management of intravascular catheter-related infections, *Clin Infect Dis* 32:1249–1272, 2001.

Mermel LA, Maki DG: Detection of bacteremia in adults: consequences of culturing an inadequate volume of blood, *Ann Intern Med* 119:270–272, 1993.

Meyer RD, Clough W: Extragenital *Mycoplasma hominis* infections in adults: emphasis on immunosuppression, *Clin Infect Dis* 17(Suppl 1):S243–S249, 1993.

Morris AJ, Wilson ML, Mirrett S, et al.: Rationale for selective use of anaerobic blood cultures, *J Clin Microbiol* 31:2110–2113, 1993.

Needlestick Safety, Prevention Act, Oliveri S, Trovato L, Betta P, et al.: *Malassezia furfur* funganemia in a neonatal patient detected by lysis-centrifugation blood culture method: first case reported in Italy, *Mycoses* 54:638–640, 2011.

Osthoff M, Gurtler N, Bassetti S, et al.: Impact of MALDI-TOF MS-based identification directly from positive blood cultures on patient management: a controlled clinical trial, *Clin Microbiol Infect* 23(2):78–85, 2017.

Pancholi R, Carroll KC, Buchan BW, et al.: Multicenter evaluation of the accelerate PhenoTest BC kit for rapid identification and phenotypic antimicrobial susceptibility testing using morphokinetic cellular analysis, *J Clin Microbiol* 56(4):e01329-17, 2018.

Payne M, Champagne S, Lowe C, et al.: Evaluation of the FilmArray blood culture identification panel compared to direct MALDI-TOF MS identification for rapid identification of pathogens, *J Med Microbiol* 67(9):1253–1256, 2018.

Pfaller MA, Diekema DJ: Twelve years of fluconazole in clinical practice: global trends in species distribution and fluconazole susceptibility of bloodstream isolates of *Candida*, *Clin Microbiol Infect* 10(Suppl 1):11–23, 2004.

Potjo M, Theron AJ, Cockeran R, et al.: Interleukin-10 and interleukin-1 receptor antagonist distinguish between patients with sepsis and systemic inflammatory response syndrome (SIRS), *Cytokine* 12:227–233, 2019.

Pradier M, Boucher A, Robineau O, et al.: *Mycobacterium mucogenicum* bacteremia: major role of clinical microbiologists, *BMC Infect Dis* 18:646, 2018.

Rhee C, Gohil S, Klompas M: Regulatory mandates for sepsis care—reasons for caution, *N Engl J Med* 18:1673–1676, 2014.

Salzman MB, Rubin LG: Intravenous catheter-related infections, *Adv Pediatr Infect Dis* 10:337–368, 1995.

Schuetz P, Bretscher C, Bernasconi L, et al.: Overview of procalcitonin assays and procalcitonin-guided protocols for the management of patients with infections and sepsis, *Expert Rev Mol Diagn* 17:593–601, 2017.

Tille P, Aziz H, Conway-Klaassen: Septicemia: an extreme host response to a global healthcare problem, *Int J Biomed Lab Sci (IJBLS)* 9(No.1):1–6, 2020.

Tille P, Rohde R, Reagan J, Felkner M, Mitchell AH: The perfect storm: emerging trends and pathogens in healthcare, *Clin Lab Sci* 29(1):32–38, 2016.

Walsh TJ, Katragkou A, Chem T, et al.: Invasive candidiasis in infants and children: recent advances in epidemiology, diagnosis and treatment, *J Fungi (Basel)* 5:11, 2019.

Wenzel RP, Edmond MB: The impact of hospital-acquired bloodstream infections, *Emerg Infect Dis* 7:174–177, 2001.

Wisplinghoff H, Bischoff T, Tallent SM, et al.: Nosocomial bloodstream infections in U.S. hospitals: analysis of 24,179 cases from a prospective nationwide surveillance study, *Clin Infect Dis* 39:309–317, 2004.

Wisplinghoff H, Seifert H, Tallent SM, et al.: Nosocomial bloodstream infections in pediatric patients in United States hospitals; epidemiology, clinical features and susceptibilities, *Pediatr Infect Dis J* 22:686–691, 2003.

Yagupsky P: Detection of *Brucellae* in blood cultures, *J Clin Microbiol* 37:3437–3442, 1999.

68

Infections of the Lower Respiratory Tract

General Considerations

Anatomy

The **respiratory tract** can be divided into two major areas: the **upper respiratory tract** consists of all structures above the larynx, whereas the **lower respiratory tract** follows airflow below the larynx through the trachea to the bronchi and bronchioles and then into the alveolar spaces where gas exchange occurs (Fig. 68.1). The respiratory and gastrointestinal tracts are the two major connections between the interior of the body and the outside environment. The respiratory tract is the pathway through which the body acquires fresh oxygen and removes unneeded carbon dioxide. It begins with the nasal and oral passages, which humidify inspired air, and extends past the nasopharynx and oropharynx to the **trachea** and then into the lungs. The trachea divides into **bronchi,** which subdivide into **bronchioles,** the smallest branches that terminate in the **alveoli.** Some 300 million alveoli are estimated to be present in the lungs; these are the primary microscopic gas exchange structures of the respiratory tract.

Familiarization with the anatomic structure of the thoracic cavity ensures proper specimen collection from various sites in the lower respiratory tract for processing by the laboratory. The **thoracic cavity,** which contains the heart and lungs, has three partitions separated from one another by **pleura** (Fig. 68.1). The lungs occupy the right and left pleural cavities, whereas the **mediastinum** (space between the lungs) is occupied mainly by the esophagus, trachea, large blood vessels, and heart.

Pathogenesis of the Respiratory Tract: Basic Concepts

Microorganisms primarily cause disease by a limited number of pathogenic mechanisms (Chapter 3). Because these mechanisms relate to respiratory tract infections, they are discussed briefly. Encounters between the human body and microorganisms occur many times each day. However, establishment of infection after such contact tends to be the exception rather than the rule. Whether an organism is successful in establishing an infection depends not only on the organism's ability to cause disease (pathogenicity) but also on the human host's ability to prevent the infection.

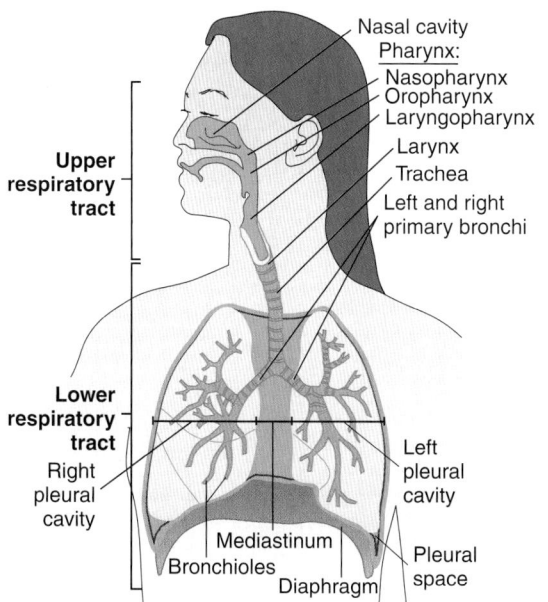

• **Fig. 68.1** Anatomy of the respiratory tract, including upper and lower respiratory tract regions.

Host Factors

The human host has several mechanisms that nonspecifically protect the respiratory tract from infection that includes the conducting airways and the lower respiratory tract. In the conducting airways these mechanisms include the nasal hairs, convoluted passages, and the mucous lining of the nasal turbinates (long curled bones within nasal cavity); secretory IgA, IgM, IgG, and nonspecific antibacterial substances (lysozyme, lactoferrin, secretory leukocyte proteinase inhibitor) in respiratory secretions; the cilia and mucous lining of the trachea; sharp-angled branching of airways; and reflexes such as coughing, sneezing, and swallowing. These mechanisms prevent foreign objects or organisms from entering the bronchi and gaining access to the lungs, which remain sterile in the healthy host. Aspiration of minor amounts of oropharyngeal material, as occurs often during sleep, plays an important role in the pathogenesis of many types of pneumonia. Once particles escape the mucociliary sweeping activity and enter the alveoli, phagocytes, such as dendritic cells and alveolar macrophages ingest them and carry them to the lymphatics. Additional nonspecific mechanisms of the lower respiratory tract include the chemical nature of the alveolar fluid (surfactant, fibronectin, immunoglobulins, complement, free fatty acids, and iron-binding proteins), and bronchus-associated lymphoid tissue (BALT).

In addition to these nonspecific host defenses, normal microbiota of the nasopharynx and oropharynx help prevent colonization by pathogenic organisms of the upper respiratory tract. Normal bacterial microbiota prevents the colonization of pathogens by competing for the same space and nutrients as well as production of **bacteriocins** and metabolic products that are toxic to invading organisms. Some of the bacteria that can be isolated as part of the indigenous human microbiome of healthy hosts, as well as many

---

• BOX 68.1   Organisms Present in the Nasopharynx and Oropharynx of Healthy Humans

Possible Pathogens

Acinetobacter spp.
Viridans streptococci, including *Streptococcus anginosus* group
Beta-hemolytic streptococci
Streptococcus pneumoniae
Staphylococcus aureus
Neisseria meningitides
Mycoplasma spp.
Haemophilus influenzae
Haemophilus parainfluenzae
Moraxella catarrhalis
Candida albicans
Herpes simplex virus
Enterobacterales
Mycobacterium spp.
Pseudomonas spp.
Burkholderia cepacia
Filamentous fungi
Klebsiella ozaenae
Eikenella corrodens
Bacteroides spp.
Peptostreptococcus spp.
Actinomyces spp.
Capnocytophaga spp.
Actinobacillus spp., *Actinobacillus actinomycetemcomitans*
Aggregatibacter aphrophilus
Entamoeba gingivalis
Trichomonas tenax

Rare Pathogens

Nonhemolytic streptococci
Micrococci
Corynebacterium spp.
Coagulase-negative staphylococci
Neisseria spp., other than *Neisseria gonorrhoeae* and *Neisseria meningitides*
Lactobacillus spp.
Veillonella spp.
Spirochetes
Rothia dentocariosa
Leptotrichia buccalis
Selenomonas
Wolinella
Rothia mucilaginosus (formerly *Stomatococcus mucilaginosus*)
Campylobacter spp.

---

species that may cause disease under certain circumstances and are often isolated from the respiratory tracts of healthy persons, are listed in Box 68.1. Under certain circumstances and for unknown reasons, these colonizing organisms can cause disease—perhaps because of previous damage by a viral infection, loss of some host immunity, or physical damage to the respiratory epithelium (e.g., from smoking). Differentiation of normal microbiota of the respiratory tract is important for determining the importance of an isolate in the clinical laboratory. Colonization does not always represent an infection. It is important to differentiate colonization from infection based on the specimen source, number of organisms present, and presence or quantity of white blood cells. Organisms isolated from normally sterile sites in the respiratory tract by sterile methods that prevent contamination with normal microbiota should be definitively identified and reported to the clinician.

Microorganism Virulence Factors

Organisms possess traits or produce products that promote colonization and subsequent infection in the host. The **virulence**, or disease-producing capability of an organism, depends on several factors including adherence, production of toxins, amount of growth or proliferation, tissue damage, avoiding the host immune response, and ability to disseminate.

Adherence

For any organism to cause disease, it must first gain a foothold within the respiratory tract to grow to sufficient numbers to produce symptoms. Therefore, most etiologic agents of respiratory tract disease must first adhere to the mucosa of the respiratory tract. The presence of normal microbiota and the overall state of the host affect the ability of microorganisms to adhere. Surviving or growing on host tissue without causing overt harmful effects is termed colonization. Except for those microorganisms inhaled directly into the lungs, all etiologic agents of disease must first colonize the respiratory tract before they can cause harm.

Streptococcus pyogenes possess specific adherence factors such as fimbriae comprising molecules such as lipoteichoic acids and M proteins. These molecules appear as a thin layer of fuzz surrounding the bacteria. *Staphylococcus aureus* and certain viridans streptococci are other bacteria that possess these lipoteichoic acid adherence complexes. Many gram-negative bacteria (which do not have lipoteichoic acids), including Enterobacterales, *Legionella* spp., *Pseudomonas* spp., *Bordetella pertussis*, and *Haemophilus* spp., also adhere by means of proteinaceous fingerlike surface fimbriae. Viruses possess either a hemagglutinin (influenza and parainfluenza viruses) or other proteins that mediate their epithelial attachment.

Toxins

Certain microorganisms are almost always considered to be etiologic agents of disease if they are present in any numbers in the respiratory tract because they possess virulence factors that are expressed in every host. These organisms are listed in Box 68.2. The production of extracellular toxin (exotoxins) was one of the first pathogenic mechanisms discovered among bacteria. *Corynebacterium diphtheria, Corynebacterium ulcerans,* and *Corynebacterium pseudotuberculosis* are classic examples of a bacteria that produce disease through the action of an extracellular toxin. Once the organism colonizes the upper respiratory epithelium, it produces a toxin that is disseminated systemically, adhering preferentially to central nervous system cells and muscle cells of the heart. Systemic disease is characterized by myocarditis, peripheral neuritis, and local disease that can lead to respiratory distress. Growth of toxigenic *Corynebacterium*

• BOX 68.2 **Respiratory Tract Pathogens**

Definite Respiratory Tract Pathogens

Corynebacterium spp. (toxin-producing)
Mycobacterium tuberculosis
Mycoplasma pneumoniae
Chlamydia trachomatis
Chlamydia pneumoniae
Bordetella pertussis
Legionella spp.
Pneumocystis jiroveci
Nocardia spp.
Histoplasma capsulatum
Coccidioides spp.
Cryptococcus spp. (may also be recovered from patients without disease)
Blastomyces dermatitidis
Viruses (respiratory syncytial virus, coronaviruses, human metapneumovirus, adenoviruses, enteroviruses, hantavirus, herpes simplex virus, influenza and parainfluenza virus, rhinoviruses, severe acute respiratory syndrome)

Rare Respiratory Tract Pathogens

Francisella tularensis
Bacillus anthracis
Yersinia pestis
Burkholderia pseudomallei
Coxiella burnetii
Chlamydia psittaci
Brucella spp.
Salmonella spp.
Pasteurella multocida
Klebsiella rhinoscleromatis
Varicella-zoster virus (VZV)
Parasites

spp. causes necrosis and sloughing of the epithelial mucosa, producing a "diphtheritic (pseudo) membrane," which may extend from the anterior nasal mucosa to the bronchi or may be limited to any area between—most often the tonsillar and peritonsillar areas. The membrane may cause sore throat and interfere with respiration and swallowing. Although nontoxic strains of *Corynebacterium* spp. can cause local disease, it is much milder than disease associated with toxigenic strains.

Some strains of *Pseudomonas aeruginosa* produce a toxin similar to diphtheria toxin. Whether this toxin contributes to the pathogenesis of respiratory tract infection with *P. aeruginosa* has not been established. *B. pertussis,* the agent of whooping cough, also produces toxins. The role of these toxins in production of disease is not clear. They may act to inhibit the activity of phagocytic cells or to damage cells of the respiratory tract. *S. aureus* and beta-hemolytic streptococci produce extracellular enzymes capable of damaging host cells or tissues. Extracellular products of staphylococci aid in the production of tissue necrosis and the destruction of phagocytic cells and contribute to the abscess formation associated with infection caused by this organism. Although *S. aureus* can be recovered from throat specimens, it has not been proven to cause pharyngitis. Enzymes of streptococci, including hyaluronidase, allow rapid dissemination of the bacteria. Many other etiologic agents of respiratory tract infection also produce extracellular enzymes and toxins.

Microorganism Growth

In addition to adherence and toxin production, pathogens cause disease by merely growing in host tissue, interfering with normal tissue function, and attracting host immune effectors, such as neutrophils and macrophages. Once these cells begin to attack the invading pathogens and repair the damaged host tissue, an expanding reaction ensues with more nonspecific and immunologic factors being attracted to the area, increasing the amount of host tissue damage. Respiratory viral infections usually progress in this manner, as do many types of pneumonias (inflammation and accumulation of fluid in the alveoli), such as those caused by *Streptococcus pneumoniae, S. pyogenes, S. aureus, Haemophilus influenzae, Neisseria meningitidis, Moraxella catarrhalis, Mycoplasma pneumoniae, Mycobacterium tuberculosis,* and most gram-negative bacilli.

Avoiding the Host Response

Another virulence mechanism present in various respiratory tract pathogens is the ability to evade host defense mechanisms. *S. pneumoniae, N. meningitidis, H. influenzae, Klebsiella pneumoniae,* mucoid *P. aeruginosa, Cryptococcus* spp., and others possess polysaccharide capsules that serve both to prevent engulfment by phagocytic host cells and to protect somatic antigens from being exposed to host immunoglobulins. The capsular material is produced in such abundance by certain bacteria, such as pneumococci, that soluble polysaccharide antigen particles can bind host antibodies, blocking them from serving as opsonins. Vaccine consisting of capsular antigens provides host protection to infection, indicating that the capsular polysaccharide is a major virulence mechanism of *H. influenzae, S. pneumoniae,* and *N. meningitidis.*

Some respiratory pathogens evade the host immune system by multiplying within host cells. *Chlamydia trachomatis, Chlamydia psittaci, Chlamydia pneumoniae,* and all viruses replicate within host cells. They have evolved methods for being taken in by the "nonprofessional" phagocytic cells of the host to where they thrive within the intracellular environment. Once within these cells, the organism is protected from host humoral immune factors and other phagocytic cells. This protection lasts until the host cell becomes sufficiently damaged that the organism is then recognized as foreign by the host and is attacked. A second group of organisms that cause respiratory tract disease comprises organisms capable of survival within phagocytic host cells (usually macrophages). Once inside the phagocytic cell, these respiratory tract pathogens can multiply. *Legionella, Pneumocystis jiroveci,* and *Histoplasma capsulatum* are some of the more common intracellular pathogens.

M. tuberculosis is the classic representative of an intracellular pathogen. In primary tuberculosis, the organism is carried to an alveolus in a **droplet nucleus,** a tiny aerosol particle containing tubercle bacilli. Once phagocytized by alveolar macrophages, organisms are carried to the nearest lymph node, usually in the hilar or other mediastinal chains (bronchopulmonary lymph nodes). In the lymph node, the organisms slowly multiply within macrophages. Ultimately, *M. tuberculosis* destroys the macrophage and is subsequently taken up by other phagocytic cells. Tubercle bacilli multiply to a critical mass within the protected environment of the macrophages, which are prevented from accomplishing phagosome-lysosome fusion capable of destroying the bacteria. Having reached a critical mass, the organisms spill out of the destroyed macrophages, through the lymphatics, and into the bloodstream, producing mycobacteremia and carrying tubercle bacilli to many parts of the body. In most cases, the host immune system reacts sufficiently at this point to kill the bacilli; however, a small reservoir of live bacteria may be left in areas of normally high oxygen concentration, such as the apical (top) portion of the lung. These bacilli are walled off, and years later, an insult to the host, either immunologic or physical, may cause breakdown of the focus of latent tubercle bacilli, allowing active multiplication and disease (secondary tuberculosis). In certain patients with primary immune defects, the initial bacteremia seeds bacteria throughout a compromised host, leading to **disseminated** or **miliary tuberculosis.** Growth of the bacteria within host macrophages and histiocytes in the lung causes an influx of more effector cells, including lymphocytes, neutrophils, and histiocytes, eventually resulting in **granuloma** formation, then tissue destruction and cavity formation. The lesion consists of a semisolid, amorphous tissue mass resembling semisoft cheese, from which it received the name **caseating necrosis** (death of cells or tissues). The infection can extend into bronchioles and bronchi from which bacteria are disseminated via respiratory secretions and coughing. Aerosolized droplets are produced by coughing and contain organisms that are inhaled by the next susceptible host. Other portions of the patient's lungs may become infected as well through aspiration (inhalation of a fluid or solid).

Diseases of the Lower Respiratory Tract

Bronchitis

Acute

Acute bronchitis is characterized by acute inflammation of the tracheobronchial tree. This condition may be part of, or preceded by, an upper respiratory tract infection such as influenza (the "flu") or the common cold. Most infections occur during the winter when acute respiratory tract infections are common.

The pathogenesis of acute bronchitis has no specific documented cause but appears to be a mixture of viral cytopathic events and a response by the host immune system. Regardless of the cause, the protective functions of the bronchial epithelium are disturbed, and excessive fluid accumulates in the bronchi. Depending on the source of infection, destruction of the bronchial epithelium may be either extensive (e.g., influenza virus) or minimal (e.g., rhinovirus colds).

TABLE 68.1	Major Causes of Acute Bronchitis	
Bacteria	**Viruses**	
Bordetella pertussis, Bordetella parapertussis, Mycoplasma pneumoniae, Chlamydia pneumoniae	Influenza virus, adenovirus, rhinovirus, coronavirus (other less common viruses: respiratory syncytial virus, human metapneumovirus, coxsackie A21 virus)	

• BOX 68.3 **Viral Agents That Cause Bronchiolitis**

Respiratory syncytial virus
Parainfluenza viruses, types 1–3
Rhinoviruses
Adenoviruses
Influenza viruses
Enteroviruses
Human metapneumovirus

Clinically, bronchitis is characterized by cough, variable fever, and sputum production. **Sputum** (pus from the lungs) is often clear at the onset but may become **purulent** as the illness persists. Bronchitis may manifest as **croup** (a clinical condition marked by a barking cough or hoarseness).

The value of microbiologic studies to determine the cause of acute bronchitis in otherwise healthy individuals has not been established. Acute bronchitis is often caused by infection with viral agents, such as influenza and respiratory syncytial virus (RSV). Less than 10% of acute bronchitis is caused by bacterial pathogens including *M. pneumoniae, B. pertussis,* and *C. pneumoniae.* The bacterium *B. pertussis* (Chapter 36) is often associated with bronchitis in infants and preschool children (Table 68.1). The best specimen for diagnosis of pertussis is a deep nasopharyngeal specimen; nasopharyngeal aspirates are more sensitive than swabs in younger patients (infants and young children). Swabs should be dacron or rayon.

Chronic Versus Acute

Chronic bronchitis is a common condition affecting about 10% to 25% of adults. This disease is defined by clinical symptoms in which excessive mucus production leads to coughing up sputum on most days during at least 3 consecutive months for more than 2 successive years. Cigarette smoking, infection, and inhalation of dust or fumes are important contributing factors. Acute bronchitis is not related to long-term injury causing damage to the lungs but is typically a result of an infectious process.

Patients with chronic bronchitis can suffer from acute flare-ups of infection, but determination of the cause of the infection is difficult. Potentially pathogenic bacteria, such as nonencapsulated strains of *H. influenzae, S. pneumoniae,* and *M. catarrhalis,* are frequently cultured from the bronchi of these patients. Because of chronic colonization, it is difficult to incriminate one of these organisms as the specific cause of an acute infection in patients with chronic bronchitis. Although the role of bacteria in acute infections in these patients is questionable, viruses are frequent causes.

Bronchiolitis

Bronchiolitis, the inflammation of the smaller diameter bronchiolar epithelial surfaces, is an acute viral lower respiratory tract infection that primarily occurs during the first 2 years of life. Characteristic clinical manifestations include an acute onset of wheezing and hyperinflation as well as cough, rhinorrhea (runny nose), tachypnea (rapid breathing), and respiratory distress. The disease is primarily associated with viral infections including human metapneumovirus and RSV. RSV accounts for 40% to 80% of cases of bronchiolitis and demonstrates a marked seasonality; the etiologic agents of bronchiolitis are listed in Box 68.3. Like other viral infections, bronchiolitis shows a marked seasonality in temperate climates with a yearly increase in cases during winter to early spring.

Initially, the virus replicates in the epithelium of the upper respiratory tract, but in infants it rapidly spreads to the lower respiratory tract. Early inflammation of the bronchial epithelium progresses to necrosis. Symptoms such as wheezing may be related to the type of inflammatory response to the virus and other host factors. For the most part, patients are managed based on clinical parameters, with the laboratory having a role in cases that require hospitalization; a specific viral cause can be identified in many infants by viral isolation from respiratory secretions, preferably from a nasal wash (Chapter 64).

Pneumonia

Pneumonia (inflammation and accumulation of fluid in the lower respiratory tract involving the lung's airways and supporting structures) is a major cause of illness and death. There are two major categories of pneumonias: those considered community-acquired pneumonia (patients are believed to have acquired their infection outside the hospital setting) and those including hospital- or ventilator-associated (patients are believed to have acquired their infection within hospital setting, usually at least 2 days following admission) or health care–associated (affects only patients hospitalized in an acute care hospital for 2 or more days within 90 days of infection from a long-term care facility; or patients who have received recent intravenous antibiotic therapy, chemotherapy, or wound care within 30 days of the current infection; or who have attended a hospital, hemodialysis clinic, or other outpatient clinic) pneumonia. Nevertheless, once a microorganism has successfully invaded the lung, disease can follow, affecting the alveolar spaces and their supporting structure, the interstitium, and the terminal bronchioles.

Pathogenesis

Organisms can cause infection of the lung by four possible routes: by upper airway colonization or infection that subsequently extends into the lung, by aspiration of organisms (thereby avoiding the upper airway defenses), by inhalation of airborne droplets containing the organism, or by seeding of the lung via the blood from a distant site of infection. Viruses cause primary infections of the respiratory tract and inhibit host defenses that, in turn, can lead to a secondary bacterial infection. For example, viruses may destroy respiratory epithelium and disrupt normal ciliary activity. Presumably, the growth of viruses in host cells disrupts the function of the latter and encourages the influx of nonspecific immune effector cells, exacerbating the damage. Damage to host epithelial tissue by virus infection is known to predispose patients to secondary bacterial infection.

Aspiration of oropharyngeal contents is important in the pathogenesis of many types of pneumonia. Aspiration may occur during a loss of consciousness such as during anesthesia or a seizure, or after alcohol or drug abuse, but other individuals, particularly geriatric patients, may also develop **aspiration pneumonia.** Neurologic disease or esophageal pathology and periodontal disease or gingivitis are other important risk factors. Aided by gravity and often by loss of some host nonspecific protective mechanisms, organisms reach lung tissue, where they multiply and attract host inflammatory cells. Other mechanisms include inhalation of aerosolized material and hematogenous seeding. The buildup of cell debris and fluid contributes to the loss of lung function and thus to the pathology.

Furthermore, regarding the pathogenesis of hospital-associated, health care–associated, and ventilator-associated pneumonias, health care devices, the environment, and the transfer between the patient and staff or other patients can serve as sources of pathogens causing pneumonia. The primary routes for bacterial entry into the lower respiratory tract are by aspiration of oropharyngeal organisms or leakage of secretions containing bacteria around an endotracheal tube. For these reasons, intubation and mechanical ventilation significantly increase the risk of pneumonia (6- to 21-fold). In addition, bacterial and viral biofilm in the endotracheal tube with subsequent spread to distal airways may be important in the pathogenesis of ventilator-associated pneumonia.

Clinical Manifestations

The symptoms suggestive of pneumonia include fever, chills, chest pain, and cough. In the past, pneumonias were classified into two major groups: (1) typical or acute pneumonias (e.g., *S. pneumoniae*) and (2) atypical pneumonias, based on whether the cough was productive or nonproductive of mucoid sputum. However, analysis of symptoms of pneumonia caused by the atypical pneumonia pathogens (*M. pneumoniae, Legionella pneumophila, M. tuberculosis, Francisella tularensis, C. psittaci, Coxiella burnetii,* and *C. pneumoniae*) has revealed no significant differences from those symptoms of patients with typical bacterial pneumonias. Because of this overlap in symptoms, it is important to consider all possible etiologies associated with the patient's clinical presentation.

Some patients with pneumonia exhibit no signs or symptoms related to their respiratory tract (i.e., some only have fever). Therefore, physical examination of the patient, chest radiography, patient history, and clinical laboratory findings are important. In addition to respiratory symptoms, 10% to 30% of patients with pneumonia complain of headache, nausea, vomiting, abdominal pain, diarrhea, and myalgias.

Epidemiology and Etiologic Agents

As previously mentioned, there are two major categories of pneumonias: those considered community-acquired pneumonias and hospital-, ventilator-, or health care–associated pneumonias (HCAPs). Because the epidemiology and causes can differ, these categories are discussed separately. Pneumonia in an immunocompromised patient is addressed separately in this chapter. Emerging viral infections associated with severe acute respiratory syndrome (SARS and COVID-19) and influenza outbreaks (H1N1) are typically associated with upper respiratory infections but may lead to serious lower respiratory infections in young, elderly, or immunocompromised patients. See Chapter 65 for detailed information related to these emerging viral infectious diseases and diagnostic recommendations.

Community-Acquired Pneumonia

Community-acquired pneumonia may be caused by bacteria, fungi, viruses, or protozoans. Because symptoms are often nonspecific, empirical antibiotic therapy is typically administered before the identification of the etiologic agent. The cause of acute pneumonia is strongly dependent on age. More than 80% of the cases of pneumonia in infants and children are caused by viruses, compared with less than 10% to 20% of the cases of pneumonia in adults.

Children. Community-acquired pneumonia in children is a common and potentially serious infection. Determining the cause of pneumonia is challenging because the lungs are rarely sampled directly, and sputum is difficult to obtain from children. Among previously healthy patients 2 months to 5 years old, RSV, human metapneumovirus, parainfluenza, influenza, and adenoviruses are the most common etiologic agents of lower respiratory tract disease. Children are less likely to develop bacterial pneumonia, usually caused by *H. influenzae, S. pneumoniae,* or *S. aureus.* Neonates may acquire lower respiratory tract infections with *C. trachomatis* or *P. jiroveci* (which likely indicates an immature immune system or an underlying immune defect).

M. pneumoniae and *C. pneumoniae* are the most common causes of bacterial pneumonia in school-age children (5 to 14 years of age). The four most common causes of community-acquired viral pneumonia in children include influenza, RSV, parainfluenza, and adenovirus. The agents associated with health care–associated (nosocomial) outbreaks in children include the influenza virus, RSV, and adenovirus. Mixed viral and bacterial infections have been documented in 35% of patients, with most of these (81%) being mixed viral-bacterial infections. In addition, the time of onset of hospital- or ventilator-associated pneumonia is an important epidemiologic variable and risk factor: early-onset pneumonia (defined as occurring within the first 4 days of hospitalization) usually carries a better prognosis, being more likely to be caused by antibiotic-sensitive bacteria, whereas late-onset pneumonia (5 days or more) is more likely to be caused by multidrug-resistant organisms and is associated with increased patient morbidity and mortality.

Young Adults. The most common etiologic agent of lower respiratory tract infection among adults younger than 30 years of age is *M. pneumoniae,* which is transmitted via close contact. Contact with secretions seems to be more important than inhalation of aerosols for transmission and infection. After contact with respiratory mucosa, *Mycoplasma* can adhere to and colonize respiratory mucosal cells. Both a protein adherence factor and gliding motility determine virulence. *Mycoplasma* attach to the cilia of respiratory mucosal cells; once there, they multiply and destroy ciliary function. Attachment and cytotoxins produced by the organisms induce cell damage. *C. pneumoniae* is the third most common agent of lower respiratory tract infection in young adults, following mycoplasmas and influenza viruses; it also affects older individuals. *Chlamydia* spp., intracellular pathogens capable of disrupting cellular function and causing respiratory disease, are similar to viral pathogens.

The epidemiology and treatment of community-acquired and hospital-acquired pneumonia have changed dramatically because of improvements in diagnostics, antimicrobial therapy, and supportive care modalities. The changes in the organization of health care has made the distinction between community-acquired, hospital-acquired, and HCAP less clear. However, pneumonia remains an important cause of morbidity and mortality in elderly patients. The American Thoracic Society and the Infectious Disease Society of America guidelines have suggested that patients who have been hospitalized in the last 90 days, reside in a nursing home or long-term care facility, or have had recent intravenous antibiotic therapy or hemodialysis be classified as a patient with HCAP. Patients with HCAP have a higher incidence of cardiopulmonary and neurodegenerative diseases, cancer, chronic kidney disease, chronic obstructive pulmonary disease, and immunosuppression than elderly patients with community-acquired pneumonia. Both populations become infected with various organisms. The organisms most frequently responsible for community-acquired pneumonia include *S. pneumoniae, H. influenzae, M. pneumoniae, C. pneumoniae, M. catarrhalis,* and *Legionella* spp. The increasing use of the pneumococcal vaccine has decreased the incidence of pneumococcal *(S. pneumoniae)* pneumonia. Factors that contribute to the onset of pneumonia include decreased mucociliary function, cough reflex, level of consciousness, periodontal disease, and general mobility. Patients with health care–associated infections are more frequently colonized with gram-negative bacilli and other multidrug-resistant pathogens, perhaps because

of poor oral hygiene, decreased saliva, or decreased epithelial cell turnover. The microorganisms associated with these infections, in addition to those previously mentioned, may include methicillin-resistant *S. aureus* (MRSA), *P. aeruginosa,* a variety of Enterobacterales, *Acinetobacter* spp., anaerobic bacteria, carbapenamase-resistant *Klebsiella pneumoniae,* and extended-spectrum beta-lactamase–resistant Enterobacterales (ESBLS). According to the Infectious Diseases Society of America (IDSA), the decision to hospitalize a patient or to treat him or her as an outpatient is possibly the single most important clinical decision made by physicians during illness. This decision in turn impacts the subsequent site of treatment (home, hospital, or intensive care unit), intensity of laboratory evaluation, antibiotic therapy, and cost. Thus the IDSA has developed management guidelines for community-acquired pneumonia in adults based on a three-step process: (1) assessment of preexisting conditions that might compromise safety of home care, (2) quantification of short-term mortality (referred to as the pneumonia port severity index [PSI] and based on a prediction rule derived from more than 14,000 patients) with subsequent assignment of patients to five risk classes (classes I through V), and (3) clinical judgment. The PSI, however, is not useful for patients in nursing homes or other health care facilities. It is therefore essential to properly assess the severity of the disease in cases of community-acquired and HCAP in elderly patients in a manner that clearly includes the three major management guidelines as outlined by the IDSA.

Pneumonia secondary to aspiration of gastric or oral secretions is common. The most common agents include oral anaerobes such as black-pigmented *Prevotella* and *Porphyromonas* spp., *Prevotella oris, Prevotella buccae, Prevotella disiens, Bacteroides* spp., fusobacteria, and anaerobic or microaerophilic streptococci. The most common aerobic isolates associated with community-acquired aspiration pneumonia are *Streptococcus* spp. and *H. influenzae.* The anaerobic infectious agents possess many factors, such as extracellular enzymes and capsules enhancing their ability to produce disease. It is their presence, however, in an abnormal site within a host producing lowered oxidation-reduction potential secondary to tissue damage that contributes to their pathogenicity. *S. aureus,* various Enterobacterales (*Serratia marcescens, Escherichia coli, Acinetobacter* spp., and *K. pneumoniae*), and *Pseudomonas* may also be acquired by aspiration; *Legionella* spp., *M. catarrhalis, C. pneumoniae,* meningococci, and other agents may also be implicated. Pneumonia is the leading cause of death among patients with health care–associated (nosocomial) infections with as high as 50% mortality among patients in intensive care units. Some of these pneumonias are secondary to sepsis, and some are related to contaminated inhalation therapy equipment, particularly for intubated patients. Hospitalized patients or long-term care patients may experience asymptomatic colonization of the upper airway that results in aspiration of microorganisms into the lower respiratory tract. In addition to those organisms previously listed, these patients are more prone to infections with the multidrug-resistant strains of bacteria (ESBLS and MRSA), including *Providencia stuartii, Morganella morganii, E. coli, Proteus mirabilis, K. pneumoniae, Enterobacter* spp., and *S. aureus.*

Adults (Viral Pneumonia)

Adults contract an estimated 100 million cases annually of community-acquired viral pneumonia caused by influenza, adenovirus, enteroviruses (coxsackieviruses and rhinoviruses), coronaviruses (SARS-CoV-2), human metapneumovirus, parainfluenza, and RSV, particularly during epidemics. Influenza-associated viral pneumonia poses an increased risk for pregnant women of approximately four to nine times greater than that of the general public, with the greatest risk associated with the third trimester. RSV is considered the third most common cause of community-acquired pneumoniae with a higher percentage of the deaths occurring in patients over the age of 65. Similar to RSV, human metapneumovirus has been associated with outbreaks in long-term care facilities. After viral pneumonia, secondary bacterial disease is commonly caused by beta-hemolytic streptococci, *S. aureus, M. catarrhalis, H. influenzae,* and *C. pneumoniae.* Other agents that may be considered depending on the geographic location and clinical presentation are viruses in the hantavirus group, the most common of which is sin nombre virus, as well as SARS-CoV-2 and MERS (Chapter 65).

Of these agents, influenza virus, RSV, SARS-CoV-2, and adenovirus have been implicated in health care–associated outbreaks. The time of onset of hospital-, health care–, or ventilator-associated pneumonia is an important epidemiologic variable and risk factor.

Adults (Fungal Pneumonia)

Unusual causes of acute lower respiratory tract infection in adults include *Actinomyces* and *Nocardia* spp. Other agents may rarely be recovered from sputum and include the agents of plague, tularemia, melioidosis *(Burkholderia pseudomallei), Brucella, Salmonella, Coxiella burnetii* (Q fever), *Bacillus anthracis, Pasteurella multocida,* and certain parasitic agents such as *Paragonimus westermani, Entamoeba histolytica, Ascaris lumbricoides,* and *Strongyloides* spp. (the latter may cause fatal disease in immunosuppressed patients). A high index of suspicion by the clinician is usually a prerequisite to a diagnosis of parasitic pneumonia in the United States. Psittacosis should be ruled out as a cause of acute lower respiratory tract infection in patients who have had recent contact with birds. Among the fungal causes, *H. capsulatum, Blastomyces dermatitidis, Coccidioides immitis, Cryptococcus* spp., and, occasionally, *Aspergillus* spp. may cause acute pneumonia. Therefore, occupational history and any exposure to animals are important in suggesting specific potential infectious agents.

Chronic Lower Respiratory Tract Infections

M. tuberculosis is the most likely etiologic agent of chronic lower respiratory tract infection, but fungal infection and anaerobic pleuropulmonary infection may also run a subacute or chronic course. Mycobacteria other than *M. tuberculosis* may also cause such disease, particularly *Mycobacterium avium* complex and *Mycobacterium kansasii.* Although possible causes of acute, community-acquired lower respiratory tract infections, fungi and parasites are more commonly isolated from patients with chronic disease. *Actinomyces* and *Nocardia* may also be associated with gradual onset of symptoms. *Actinomyces* is usually associated with an infection of the pleura or chest wall, and *Nocardia* may be isolated along with an infection caused by *M. tuberculosis.* The pathogenesis of many of the infections caused by agents of chronic lower respiratory tract disease is characterized by the requirement for breakdown of cell-mediated immunity in the host or the ability of these agents to avoid being destroyed by host cell-mediated immune mechanisms. This may be caused by an effect on macrophages, the ability to mask foreign antigens, sheer size, or some other factor, allowing microbes to grow within host tissues without eliciting an overwhelming local immune reaction.

Cystic fibrosis (CF) is a genetic disorder that leads to persistent bacterial infection in the lung, causing airway wall damage and chronic obstructive lung disease. Eventually, a combination of airway secretions and damage leads to poor gas exchange in the lungs, cardiac malfunction, and subsequent death. Patients with CF may present as young adults with chronic respiratory tract disease or, more commonly, as children with gastrointestinal problems and stunted growth. *S. aureus* is the most prevalent bacterial pathogen. *H. influenzae* is also often identified from the upper airway of young children with CF. A very mucoid *Pseudomonas,* characterized by production of copious amounts of extracellular capsular polysaccharide, can be isolated from the sputum of almost all patients with CF who are older than 18 years of age, becoming more prevalent with increasing age after 5 years. Even if CF has not been diagnosed, isolation of a mucoid *P. aeruginosa* from sputum should alert the clinician to the possibility of underlying disease. Microbiologists should always report this unusual morphologic feature. In addition to mucoid *Pseudomonas* and *S. aureus,* patients with CF are likely to harbor *H. influenzae; S. pneumoniae; Stenotrophomonas maltophilia; Achromobacter xylosoxidans; Ralstonia* spp.; *Cupriavidus* spp.; *Pandoraea* spp.; *E. coli;* strains of *Burkholderia cepacia* complex; fast-growing mycobacteria *(Mycobacterium abscessus);* RSV; influenza; and fungi including *Aspergillus, Scedosporium* spp., and *Exophiala dermatitidis.* In addition, because of the viscous mucous plugs associated with CF, several anaerobic organisms and normal oral microbiota have been detected in the lungs of CF patients, including *Prevotella, Veillonella, Actinomyces,* and *Fusobacterium. Gemella* and *Rothia mucilaginosa* have been identified and associated with poor outcomes in CF patients. Using advanced diagnostic molecular methods, additional organisms have also been identified in chronic polymicrobial CF infections, including viridans streptococci, *Streptococcus constellatus, Streptococcus milleri, Streptococcus intermedius,* and *Streptococcus anginosus* group.

Lung abscess is usually a complication of acute or chronic pneumonia. In these circumstances, organisms infecting the lung cause localized destruction of the lung parenchyma (functional elements of the lung). Symptoms associated with lung abscess are similar to those of acute and chronic pneumonia, except symptoms fail to resolve with treatment.

Immunocompromised Patients

Patients With Neoplasms. Patients with cancer are at high risk to become infected because of either granulocytopenia or other defects in phagocytic defenses, cellular or humoral immune dysfunction, damage to mucosal surfaces and the skin, and various medical procedures such as blood product transfusion. In these patients, the nature of the malignancy often determines the cause (Table 68.2), and pneumonia is a frequent clinical manifestation.

TABLE 68.2	Examples of Infectious Agents Commonly Associated With Certain Malignancies
Malignancy (Site and Type of Infections)	**Pathogens**
Acute nonlymphocytic leukemia (pneumonia, oral lesions, cutaneous lesions, urinary tract infections, hepatitis, most often sepsis without obvious focus)	Enterobacterales *Pseudomonas* Staphylococci *Corynebacterium jeikeium* *Candida* *Aspergillus* *Mucor* Hepatitis C and other non-A, non-B
Acute lymphocytic leukemia (pneumonia, cutaneous lesions, pharyngitis, disseminated disease)	Streptococci (all types) *Pneumocystis jiroveci* Herpes simplex virus Cytomegalovirus Varicella-zoster virus
Lymphoma (disseminated disease, pneumonia, urinary tract infections, sepsis, cutaneous lesions)	*Brucella* *Candida* (mucocutaneous) *Cryptococcus* spp. Herpes simplex virus (cutaneous) Varicella-zoster virus Cytomegalovirus *Pneumocystis jiroveci* *Toxoplasma gondii* *Listeria monocytogenes* Mycobacteria *Nocardia* *Salmonella* Staphylococci Enterobacterales *Pseudomonas* *Strongyloides stercoralis*
Multiple myeloma (pneumonia, cutaneous lesions, sepsis)	*Haemophilus influenzae* *Streptococcus pneumoniae* *Neisseria meningitides* Enterobacterales *Pseudomonas* Varicella-zoster virus *Candida* *Aspergillus*

Transplant Recipients. For successful organ transplantation, the recipient's immune system must be suppressed. As a result, these patients are predisposed to infection. Regardless of the type of organ transplant (heart, renal, bone marrow, lung, liver, pancreas), most infections occur within 4 months after transplantation. Major infections can occur within the first month but are usually associated with infections carried over from the pretransplant period. Pulmonary infections are of great importance in this patient population. Some of the most common causes of pneumonia include *S. aureus, S. pneumoniae, H. influenzae, P. jiroveci,* and cytomegalovirus. In addition, other organisms such as *Cryptococcus* spp., *Aspergillus* spp., *Candida* spp., *Nocardia* spp., and others can cause life-threatening pulmonary infection.

Patients With Human Immunodeficiency Virus. Patients who are infected with human immunodeficiency virus (HIV) are at high risk for developing pneumonia. As discussed in the previous chapter, opportunistic infections because of severe immunodeficiency are a major cause of illness and death among these patients. In the United States the most common opportunistic infection among patients with acquired immune deficiency syndrome (AIDS) is *P. jiroveci* pneumonia. Although *P. jiroveci* is a major pulmonary pathogen, other organisms must be considered in this patient population, including *M. tuberculosis* and *M. avium* complex, as well as common bacterial pathogens such as *S. pneumoniae* and *H. influenzae*. In addition to these common pathogens, many other organisms can cause lower respiratory tract infections, including *Nocardia* spp., *Rhodococcus equi* (a gram-positive, aerobic, pleomorphic organism), and *Legionella* spp. Additional opportunistic respiratory infections occur from viral agents such as cytomegalovirus and herpes simplex virus (HSV) (Chapter 65).

Pleural Infections

If an organism infecting the lung subsequently gains access to the pleural space via an abnormal passage (**fistula**), the patient may develop an **empyema** (pus in a body cavity such as the pleural cavity). Symptoms in these patients are insidious, because early during disease they are related to the primary infection in the lung. Once enough purulent exudate is formed, typical physical and radiographic findings indicative of an empyema are produced.

Laboratory Diagnosis of Lower Respiratory Tract Infections

Specimen Collection and Transport

Although rapid determination of the etiologic agent is of paramount importance in managing pneumonia, the responsible pathogen is not identified in as many as 50% of patients, despite extensive diagnostic testing. Unfortunately, no single test can identify all potential lower respiratory tract pathogens. Refer to Table 5.1 for an overview of the methods used to collect, transport, and process specimens from the lower respiratory tract.

Sputum

Expectorated

The examination of expectorated sputum has been the primary means of determining the causes of bacterial pneumonia. However, lower respiratory tract secretions will be contaminated with upper respiratory tract secretions, especially saliva, unless they are collected using an invasive technique. For this reason, sputum is among the least clinically relevant specimens received for culture in microbiology laboratories, even though it is one of the most numerous and time-consuming specimens.

Good sputum samples depend on thorough health care worker education and patient understanding throughout all phases of the collection process. Food should not have been ingested for 1 to 2 hours before expectoration, and the mouth should be rinsed with saline or water just before expectoration. Patients should be instructed to provide a deep-coughed specimen. The material should be expelled into a sterile container, with an attempt to minimize contamination by saliva. Specimens should be transported to the laboratory immediately. Even a moderate amount of time at room temperature can result in the loss of viable infectious agents and the recovery of pathogens.

Induced

Patients unable to produce sputum may be assisted by respiratory therapists, who use postural drainage and thoracic percussion to stimulate production of acceptable sputum. Before specimen collection, patients should brush the buccal mucosa, tongue, and gums with a wet toothbrush. As an alternative, an aerosol-induced specimen may be collected for the isolation of mycobacterial or fungal agents. Induced sputum is also recognized for its high diagnostic yield in cases of *P. jiroveci* pneumonia. Aerosol-induced specimens are collected by allowing the patient to breathe aerosolized droplets, using an ultrasonic nebulizer containing 10% 0.85% NaCl or until a strong cough reflex is initiated. Lower respiratory secretions obtained in this way appear watery, resembling saliva, although they often contain material directly from alveolar spaces. These specimens are usually adequate for culture and should be accepted in the laboratory without prescreening. Obtaining such a specimen may obviate the need for a more invasive procedure, such as bronchoscopy or needle aspiration.

The gastric aspirate is used exclusively for isolation of acid-fast bacilli and may be collected from patients who are unable to produce sputum, particularly young children. Before the patient wakes up in the morning, a nasogastric tube is inserted into the stomach and contents are withdrawn (on the assumption that acid-fast bacilli from the respiratory tract were swallowed during the night and will be present in the stomach). The relative resistance of mycobacteria to acidity allows them to remain viable for a short period. Gastric aspirate specimens must be delivered to the

laboratory immediately so that the acidity can be neutralized. Specimens can be neutralized and then transported if immediate delivery is not possible.

Endotracheal or Tracheostomy Suction Specimens

Patients with tracheostomies are unable to produce sputum in the normal fashion, but lower respiratory tract secretions can easily be collected in a Lukens trap (Fig. 68.2). Tracheostomy aspirates or tracheostomy suction specimens should be treated as sputum by the laboratory. Patients with tracheostomies rapidly become colonized with gram-negative bacilli and other nosocomial pathogens. Such colonization per se is not clinically relevant, but these organisms may be aspirated into the lungs and cause pneumonia. Culture results should be correlated with clinical signs and symptoms.

Bronchoscopy

Bronchoscopy specimens include bronchoalveolar lavage (BAL), bronchial washing, bronchial brushing, and transbronchial biopsies. The diagnosis of pneumonia, particularly in HIV-infected and other immunocompromised patients, often necessitates the use of more invasive procedures. Fiberoptic bronchoscopy has dramatically affected the evaluation and management of these infections. With this method, the bronchial mucosa can be directly visualized and collected for biopsy, and the lung tissue can be sent for transbronchial biopsy for the evaluation of lung cancer and other lung diseases. Although transbronchial biopsy is

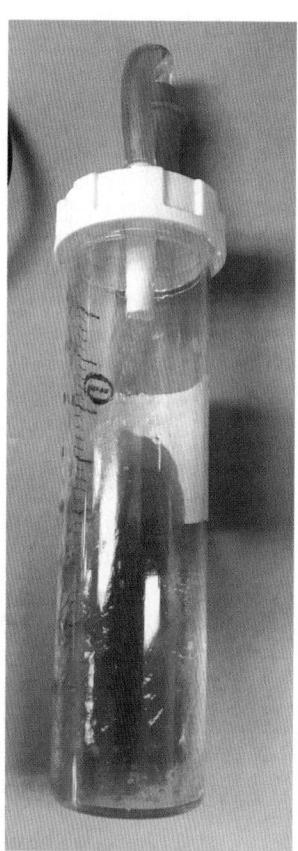

• **Fig. 68.2** Tracheal secretions received in the laboratory in a Lukens trap.

important, the procedure is often associated with significant complications such as bleeding. The sample should be transported in sterile 0.85% saline.

During bronchoscopy, physicians obtain bronchial washings or aspirates, BAL samples, protected bronchial brush samples, or specimens for transbronchial biopsy. Bronchial washings or aspirates are collected by inserting a small amount of sterile physiologic saline into the bronchial tree and withdrawing the fluid. These specimens will be contaminated with upper respiratory tract microbiota such as viridans streptococci and *Neisseria* spp. Recovery of potentially pathogenic organisms from bronchial washings should be attempted.

A deep sampling of desquamated host cells and secretions can be collected through bronchoscopy and BAL. Lavages are especially suitable for detecting *Pneumocystis* cysts and fungal elements. During this procedure, a high volume of saline (100 to 300 mL) is infused into a lung segment through the bronchoscope to obtain cells and protein of the pulmonary interstitium and alveolar spaces. It is estimated that more than 1 million alveoli are sampled during this process. The value of this technique in conjunction with quantitative culture for the diagnosis of most major respiratory tract pathogens, including bacterial pneumonia, has been documented. Scientists have found significant correlation between acute bacterial pneumonia and greater than 10^3 to 10^4 bacterial colonies per milliliter of BAL fluid. BAL has been shown to be a safe and practical method for diagnosing opportunistic pulmonary infections in immunosuppressed patients. At bedside, nonbronchoscopic "mini BAL" using a Metras catheter has been introduced; typically, 20 mL or less of saline is instilled.

Another type of respiratory specimen is obtained via a protected catheter bronchial brush as part of a bronchoscopy examination. Specimens obtained by this moderately invasive collection procedure are suited for microbiologic studies, particularly in aspiration pneumonia. Protected specimen brush bristles collect from 0.001 to 0.01 mL of material. An overview of the collection process is shown in Fig. 68.3. Upon receipt, contents of the bronchial brush may be suspended in 1 mL of broth solution with vigorous vortexing and inoculated onto culture media using a 0.01-mL calibrated inoculating loop. Some researchers have indicated that specimens obtained via double-lumen–protected catheters are suitable for both anaerobic and aerobic cultures. Colony counts of at least 1000 organisms per milliliter in the broth diluent (or 10^6/mL in the original specimen) have been considered to correlate with infection. All facets of the bronchoscopic procedure—such as order of sampling, use of anesthetic, and rapidity of plating—should be rigorously standardized.

Transtracheal Aspirates

Percutaneous transtracheal aspirates (TTAs) are obtained by inserting a small plastic catheter into the trachea via a needle previously inserted through the skin and cricothyroid membrane. This invasive procedure, although somewhat uncomfortable for the patient and not suitable for all patients (it cannot be used in uncooperative patients, in patients with bleeding tendency, or in patients with poor oxygenation), reduces the likelihood that a specimen will be contaminated by upper respiratory tract microbiota and diluted by added fluids, provided care is taken to keep the catheter from being coughed back up into the pharynx. Although this technique is rarely used, anaerobes, such as *Actinomyces* and those associated with aspiration pneumonia, can be isolated from TTA specimens.

Other Invasive Procedures

When **pleural empyema** is present, thoracentesis may be used to obtain infected fluid for direct examination and culture. This constitutes an excellent specimen that accurately reflects the bacteriology of an associated pneumonia. Laboratory examination of such material is discussed in Chapter 76. Blood cultures, of course, should always be obtained from patients with pneumonia.

For patients with pneumonia, a thin needle aspiration of material from the involved area of the lung may be performed percutaneously. If no material is withdrawn into the syringe after the first try, approximately 3 mL of sterile saline can be injected and then withdrawn into the syringe. Patients with emphysema, uremia, thrombocytopenia, or pulmonary hypertension may be at increased risk of complications (primarily pneumothorax [air in the pleural space] or bleeding) from this procedure. The specimens obtained are very small in volume, and protection from aeration is usually impossible. This technique is more frequently used in children than in adults.

The most invasive procedure for obtaining respiratory tract specimens is the open lung biopsy. Performed by surgeons, this method is used to procure a wedge of lung tissue. Biopsy specimens are extremely helpful for diagnosing severe viral infections, such as herpes simplex pneumonia, for rapid diagnosis of *Pneumocystis* pneumonia, and for other hard-to-diagnose or life-threatening pneumonias.

Specimen Processing
Direct Visual Examination

Lower respiratory tract specimens can be examined by direct wet preparation for parasites and special procedures for *Pneumocystis*. Fungal elements can be visualized under phase microscopy with 10% potassium hydroxide, under ultraviolet light with calcofluor white, or using periodic acid-Schiff–stained smears.

For most other evaluations, the specimen must be fixed and stained. Bacteria and yeasts can be recognized on Gram stain. One of the most important uses of the Gram stain, however, is to evaluate the quality of expectorated sputum received for routine bacteriologic culture. A portion of the specimen consisting of purulent material is chosen for the stain. The smear can be evaluated adequately even before it is stained, thus negating the need for Gram stain of specimens later judged unacceptable. An acceptable specimen yields fewer than 10 squamous epithelial cells per low-power field

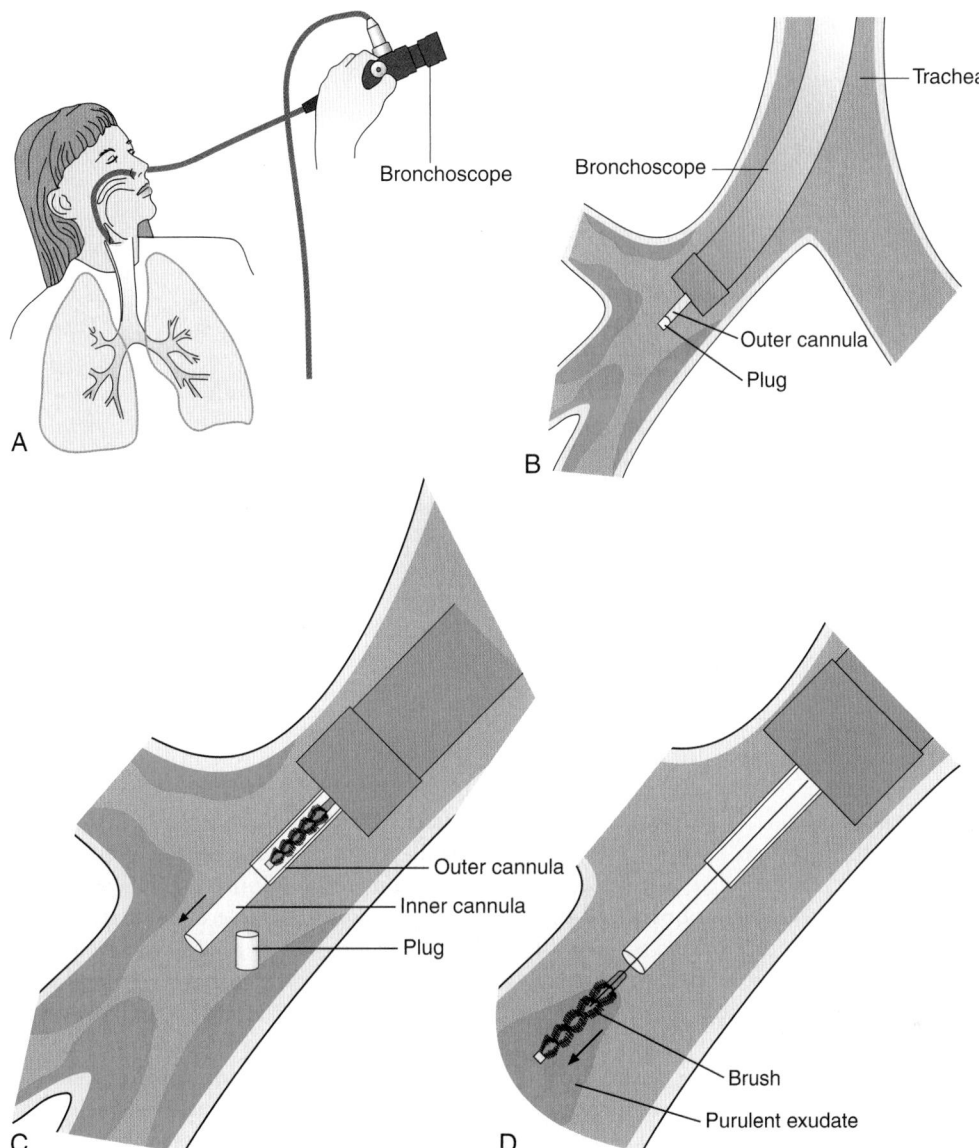

• **Fig. 68.3** Overview for obtaining a protected catheter bronchial brush during a bronchoscopy examination. (A) The bronchoscope is introduced into the nose and advanced through the nasopharyngeal passage into the trachea. The bronchoscope is then inserted into the lung area of interest. (B) A small brush that holds 0.001 to 0.01 mL of secretions is placed within a double cannula. The end of the outermost tube or cannula is closed with a displaceable plug made of absorbable gel. The cannula is inserted to the proper area. (C) Once in the correct area, the inner cannula is pushed out, dislodging the protective plug as it is extruded. (D) The brush is then extended beyond the inner cannula, and the specimen is collected by "brushing" the involved area. The brush is withdrawn into the inner cannula, which is withdrawn into the outer cannula to prevent contamination by upper airway organisms as it is removed.

(100×). The number of white blood cells may not be relevant, because many patients are severely neutropenic, and specimens from these patients will not show white blood cells on Gram stain examination. On the other hand, the presence of 25 or more polymorphonuclear neutrophils (PMNs) per 100× field, together with few squamous epithelial cells, implies an excellent specimen (Fig. 68.4). Samples that contain predominantly upper respiratory tract material should be rejected. Previously, only expectorated sputa were suitable for rejection based on microscopic screening. However, endotracheal aspirates (ETAs) from mechanically ventilated adult patients can be screened by Gram stain. Criteria used to reject ETAs from adult patients include greater than 10 squamous epithelial cells per low-power field or no organisms seen under oil immersion (1000×). In *Legionella* pneumonia, sputum may be scant and watery, with few or no host cells. Such specimens may be positive by direct fluorescent antibody (DFA) stain and culture, and they should not be subjected to screening procedures. Conversely, sputum from patients with CF should be screened. A throat swab is an acceptable specimen from patients with CF in selected clinical settings and should be processed in a similar

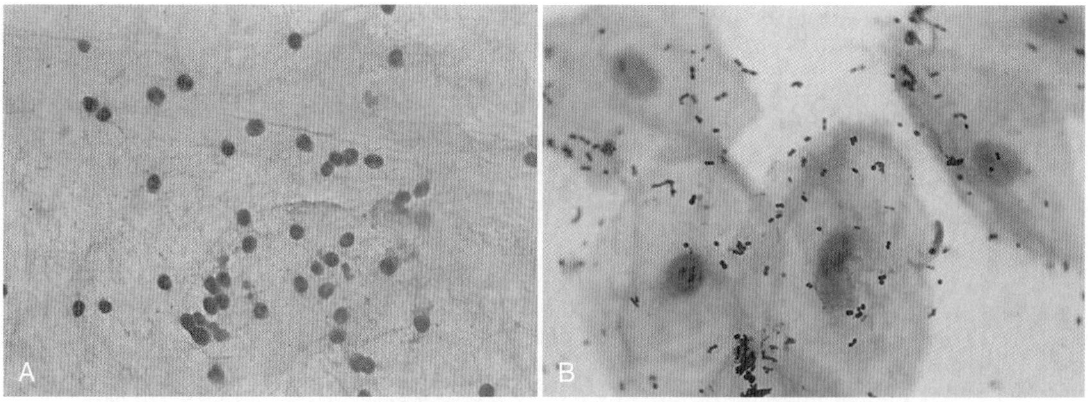

• **Fig. 68.4** Gram stain of sputum specimens. (A) This specimen contains numerous polymorphonuclear leukocytes and no visible squamous epithelial cells, indicating that the specimen is acceptable for routine bacteriologic culture. (B) This specimen contains numerous squamous epithelial cells and rare polymorphonuclear leukocytes, indicating an inadequate specimen for routine sputum culture.

manner as CF sputum. Staining of respiratory samples is useful and should be compared with culture results to reveal errors in procedures, specimen collection, and transport or specimen identification.

Respiratory secretions may need to be concentrated before staining. The cytocentrifuge instrument has been used successfully for this purpose, concentrating the cellular material in an easily examined monolayer on a glass slide. As an alternative, specimens are centrifuged, and the sediment is used for visual examinations and cultures. For screening purposes, the presence of **ciliated columnar bronchial epithelial cells, goblet cells,** or pulmonary macrophages in specimens obtained by bronchoscopy or BAL indicates a specimen from the lower respiratory tract.

In addition to the Gram stain, respiratory specimens may be stained for acid-fast bacilli with either the classic Ziehl-Neelsen or the Kinyoun carbolfuchsin stain. Auramine or auramine-rhodamine is also used to detect acid-fast organisms. Because they are fluorescent, these stains are more sensitive than the acid-fast formulas and are preferable for rapid screening. Slides may be restained with the classic stains directly over the fluorochrome stains if all the immersion oil has been removed carefully with xylene. All the acid-fast stains will reveal *Cryptosporidium* spp. if they are present in the respiratory tract, as may occur in immunosuppressed patients. These patients are often at risk of infection with *P. jiroveci.* Although the modified Gomori methenamine silver stain has been traditionally used to recognize *Nocardia, Actinomyces,* fungi, and parasites, it takes approximately 1 hour of the technologist's time to perform, is technically demanding, and is not suitable as an emergency procedure. A rapid stain, toluidine blue O, has been used in many laboratories with some success. Toluidine blue O can be used to stain *Pneumocystis, Nocardia asteroides,* and some fungi. A monoclonal antibody stain is the optimum stain for *Pneumocystis* (Chapter 58) for less invasive specimens such as BAL and induced sputa.

DFA staining has been used to detect *Legionella* spp. in lower respiratory tract specimens. Sputum, pleural fluid, aspirated material, and tissues are all suitable specimens. Because there are so many different serotypes of legionellae, polyclonal antibody reagents and a monoclonal antibody directed against all serotypes of *L. pneumophila* are used. Because of low sensitivity (50% to 75%), DFA results should not be relied on in lieu of culture. Rather, *Legionella* culture, DFA or urinary antigen, and serology should be performed for optimum sensitivity. See Chapter 34 for details regarding detection of *Legionella* spp.

Commercially available DFA reagents are also used to detect antigens of numerous viruses, including herpes simplex, cytomegalovirus, adenovirus, influenza viruses, and RSV (Chapter 64), but have been replaced in most laboratories by direct nucleic acid amplification testing. Commercial suppliers of reagents provide procedure information for each of these tests. Monoclonal and polyclonal fluorescent stains for *C. trachomatis* are available and may be useful for staining respiratory secretions of infants with pneumonia. Several molecular amplification techniques (Chapter 8) for the direct detection of respiratory pathogens have been described. Amplification assays are also available for the direct detection of *M. tuberculosis* on smear-positive specimens (Chapter 42).

Rapid direct detection from respiratory samples is now available using nucleic acid–based methods. The xTAG Respiratory Viral Panel (RVP) (Luminex Corporation, Austin, TX) can be used for the simultaneous detection of influenza (four types), RSV, human metapneumovirus, and adenovirus from nasopharyngeal swabs. In addition, the FilmArray Respiratory Panel (bioMérieux, Durham, NC) can detect upper respiratory tract infections associated with coronavirus (four types), adenovirus, influenza (five types), rhinovirus, parainfluenza virus (four types), enterovirus, human metapneumovirus, RSV, *B. pertussis, M. pneumoniae,* and *C. pneumoniae* in approximately 1 hour directly from patient samples. Smaller molecular panels are also available, such as the real-time multiplex amplification kit for influenza A and B and RSV (Hologic, San Diego, CA). During the COVID-19 (SARS-CoV-2) outbreak in 2020, the

Centers for Disease Control and Prevention (CDC) released an emergency use authorization (EUA) RT-PCR diagnostic panel. The CDC as well as other commercial manufacturers also produced multiple RT-PCR diagnostic panels capable of detecting SARS-CoV-2, influenzae A, and influenzae B. The *illumigene* (Meridian Bioscience, Inc., Cincinnati, OH) manufacturers produce a variety of nucleic acid–based tests that use isothermal loop-mediated amplification. All but the COVID-19 EUA diagnostic tests, the previously mentioned methods are Food and Drug Administration (FDA)-approved. Diagnostic microbiology is rapidly evolving, and the availability of nucleic acid–based testing continues to expand and evolve quickly. The rapid detection of respiratory pathogens using molecular diagnostics has significantly decreased the turnaround time for the diagnosis of infections. High-throughput nucleic acid sequencing can be used to identify most respiratory pathogens in a specimen for diagnosis. However, there are extensive limitations for the implementation of this technology in the clinical laboratory due to computational and bioinformatics needs. It is important when considering the use of a nucleic acid–based assay that the laboratory consider their patient population, including severity of illness, immune status, and transplant histories. In addition, matrix-assisted laser desorption ionization time-of-flight mass spectrometry (MALDI-TOF MS) may be used for organism identification depending on the type of organism isolated. See organism-specific chapters for information on MALDI-TOF MS.

Routine Culture

Most of the commonly sought etiologic agents of lower respiratory tract infections are isolated on routine media: 5% sheep blood agar, MacConkey agar for the isolation and differentiation of gram-negative bacilli, and chocolate agar for *Haemophilus* and *Neisseria* spp. Because of contaminating normal oral microbiota, sputum specimens, specimens obtained by bronchial washing and lavage, tracheal aspirates, and tracheostomy or endotracheal tube aspirates are not inoculated to enrichment broth or incubated anaerobically. Only specimens obtained by percutaneous aspiration (including transtracheal aspiration) and protected bronchial brush are suitable for anaerobic culture; the latter must be completed quantitatively for proper interpretation (refer to prior discussion). Transtracheal and percutaneous lung aspiration material may be inoculated to enriched thioglycollate as well as to solid media. For suspected cases of Legionnaires disease, buffered charcoal-yeast extract (BCYE) agar and selective BCYE should be inoculated. Plates should be streaked in four quadrants to provide a basis for objective semiquantitation to define the amount of growth. After 24 to 48 hours of incubation, the numbers and types of colonies are recorded. For *Legionella* cultures, colonies form on the selective agar after 3 to 5 days at 35°C.

Sputum specimens from patients known to have CF should be inoculated to selective agar, such as specific chromogenic agar, for recovery of *S. aureus* and selective horse blood–bacitracin, incubated anaerobically and aerobically, for

recovery of *H. influenzae* that may be obscured by the mucoid *Pseudomonas* on routine media. The use of a selective medium for *B. cepacia,* such as PC or OFPBL agars, is also necessary.

For interpretation of culture results on those specimens contaminated by normal oropharyngeal microbiota (e.g., expectorated and induced sputum, bronchial washings), growth of the predominant aerobic and facultative anaerobic bacteria is reported. To ensure optimum culture reporting, conditions must be well defined in terms of an objective grading system for streaked plates. Finally, the clinical significance of culture findings depends not only on standardized and appropriate laboratory methods but also on how specimens are collected and transported, other laboratory data, and the patient's clinical presentation.

Numerous bacterial agents that cause lower respiratory tract infections are not detected by routine bacteriologic culture. Mycobacteria, *Chlamydia, Nocardia, B. pertussis, Legionella,* and *M. pneumoniae* require special procedures for detection; this also applies to viruses and fungi. Optimal recovery for *M. tuberculosis* requires multiple specimens for acid-fast staining, culture, and at least one sample for nucleic acid–based testing as recommended by the Centers for Disease Control and Prevention. Refer to the appropriate chapter section for more information regarding these organisms. Finally, one must keep in mind those potential agents for bioterrorist attack, such as *B. anthracis, F. tularensis,* and *Yersinia pestis,* that might be recovered from respiratory specimens (Chapter 79).

ⓔ Visit the Evolve site for a complete list of procedures, review questions, and case studies.

Bibliography

American Thoracic Society and the Infectious Diseases Society of America: Guidelines for the management of adults with hospital-acquired, ventilator-associated, and healthcare-associated pneumonia, *Am J Respir Crit Care Med* 171:388–416, 2005.

Badell E, Guillot S, Tulliez M, et al.: Improved quadruplex real-time PCR assay for the diagnosis of diphtheria, *J Med Microbiol* 68(10):1455–1465, 2019.

Bartlett JG, Dowell SF, Mandell LA, et al.: Practice guidelines for the management of community-acquired pneumonia in adults, *Clin Infect Dis* 31:347–382, 2000.

Bennett J, Dolin R, Blaser M: *Principles and practice of infectious diseases,* ed 9, Philadelphia, PA, 2020, Elsevier.

Boivin G, Abed Y, Pelletier G, et al.: Virological features and clinical manifestations associated with human metapneumovirus: a new paramyxovirus responsible for acute respiratory tract infections in all age groups, *J Infect Dis* 186:1330–1334, 2002.

Broughton WA, Middleton III RM, Kirkpatrick MB, et al.: Bronchoscopic protected specimen brush and bronchoalveolar lavage in the diagnosis of bacterial pneumonia, *Infect Dis Clin North Am* 5:437–452, 1991.

Caliendo AM: Enhanced diagnosis of *Pneumocystis carinii*: promises and problems, *Clin Microbiol Newsl* 18:113, 1996.

Campbell S, Forbes BA: The clinical microbiology laboratory in the diagnosis of lower respiratory tract infections, *J Clin Microbiol* 49:S30–S33, 2011.

Cantral DE, Tape TG, Reed EC, et al.: Quantitative culture of bronchoalveolar lavage fluid for the diagnosis of bacterial pneumonia, *Am J Med* 95:601–607, 1993.

Carroll KA: Laboratory diagnosis of lower respiratory tract infections: controversy and conundrums, *J Clin Microbiol* 40:3115–3120, 2002.

Carroll KC, Pfaller MA, Landry ML, et al.: *Manual of clinical microbiology*, ed 12, Washington, DC, 2019, ASM.

Cesario TC: Viruses associated with pneumonia in adults, *Clin Pract* 55:107–113, 2012.

Cilloniz C, Dominedo C, Torres A: An overview of guidelines for the management of hospital-acquired and ventilator-associated pneumonia caused by multi-drug resistant Gram-negative bacteria, *Curr Opin Infect Dis* 32:656–662, 2019, https://doi.org/10.1097/QCO.0000000000000596.

Denny F, Clyde WJ: Acute lower respiratory tract infections in non-hospitalized children, *J Pediatr* 108:635–646, 1989.

Doring G, Parameswaran IG, Murphy TF: Differential adaptation of microbial pathogens to airways of patients with cystic fibrosis and chronic obstructive pulmonary disease, *FEMS Microbiol Rev* 35:124–146, 2010.

Falcone M, Blasi F, Menichetti F, et al.: Pneumonia in frail older patients: an up to date, *Intern Emerg Med* 7:415–424, 2012.

Kuo CC, Jackson LA, Campbell LA, et al.: *Chlamydia pneumoniae* (TWAR), *Clin Microbiol Rev* 8:451–461, 1995.

Lee JM, Lee JH, Kim YK: Laboratory impact of rapid molecular tests used for the detection of respiratory pathogens, *Clin Lab* 64(9):1545–1551, 2018.

Lentino JR: The nonvalue of unscreened sputum specimens in the diagnosis of pneumonia, *Clin Microbiol Newsl* 9:70, 1987.

Maabar M, Davison AJ, Vučak M, et al.: DisCVR: rapid viral diagnosis from high-throughput sequencing data, *Virus Evol* 5(2):vez033, 2019.

Marrie TJ: Community-acquired pneumonia, *Clin Infect Dis* 18:501–513, 1994.

Marrie TJ, Durant H, Bates L: Community-acquired pneumonia requiring hospitalization: a 5-year prospective study, *Rev Infect Dis* 11:586–599, 1989.

McIntosh K: Community-acquired pneumonia in children, *N Engl J Med* 346:429–437, 2002.

Morris AJ, Tanner DC, Reller RB: Rejection criteria for endotracheal aspirates from adults, *J Clin Microbiol* 31:1027–1029, 1993.

Navarro D, Garcia-Maset L, Gimenao C, et al.: Performance of the Binax NOW *Streptococcus pneumoniae* urinary antigen assay for diagnosis of pneumonia in children with underlying pulmonary diseases in the absence of acute pneumococcal infection, *J Clin Microbiol* 42:4853–4855, 2004.

Niederman MS, Bass Jr JB, Campbell GD, et al.: Guidelines for the initial management of adults with community-acquired pneumonia: diagnosis, assessment of severity, and initial antimicrobial therapy, *Am Rev Respir Dis* 148:1418–1426, 1993.

Roson B, Fernandez-Sabe N, Carratala J, et al.: Contribution of a urinary antigen assay (Binax NOW) to the early diagnosis of pneumococcal pneumonia, *Clin Infect Dis* 38:222–226, 2004.

Sadeghi E, Matlow A, MacLusky I, et al.: Utility of Gram stain in evaluation of sputa from patients with cystic fibrosis, *J Clin Microbiol* 32:54–58, 1994.

Stuckey-Schrock K, Hayes BL, George CM: Community-acquired pneumonia in children, *Am Fam Physician* 86:661–667, 2012.

Thoulouze MI, Alcover A: Can viruses form biofilms? *Trends Microbiol* 19:257–262, 2011.

Tollemar J: Prophylaxis against fungal infections in transplant recipients: possible approaches, *BioDrugs* 11:309–318, 1999.

Tsolia MN, Psarras S, Bossios A, et al.: Etiology of community-acquired pneumonia in hospitalized school-age children: evidence for high prevalence of viral infections, *Clin Infect Dis* 39:681–686, 2004.

69

Upper Respiratory Tract Infections and Other Infections of the Oral Cavity and Neck

OBJECTIVES

1. Explain the anatomy and structures of the upper respiratory tract, including the three parts of the pharynx.
2. Identify the principal causative organism of pharyngitis; name other organisms capable of causing pharyngitis.
3. Define the following conditions: laryngitis, epiglottis, and parotitis. List the etiologic organisms associated with these conditions.
4. Explain the pathogenic mechanisms (virulence factors) associated with *Streptococcus pyogenes* pharyngitis.
5. Define Vincent angina and peritonsillar abscesses. What organism do they share as the causative agent of disease?
6. Describe the disease process caused by pharyngeal infection with *Corynebacterium diphtheriae*; name the hallmark symptom of this infection and list the complications associated with infection.
7. Differentiate between stomatitis and thrush and explain the testing process for each disease.
8. Outline the steps used in the culture of specimens for the isolation of *S. pyogenes*.
9. Explain the signs and symptoms and pathogenic mechanisms associated with disease caused by *Bordetella pertussis*. What special requirements are needed to detect this organism in culture?
10. List three types of periodontal infections that require culture to identify the causative agent of infection; name the bacteria associated with these infections.
11. Explain the unique characteristics of group C and G streptococci and explain how they contribute to their pathogenesis.

General Considerations

Anatomy

The respiratory tract is generally divided into two regions, the upper and the lower.

The upper respiratory tract includes all the structures down to the larynx: the sinuses, throat, nasal cavity, epiglottis, and larynx; the throat is also called the **pharynx.** These anatomic structures are shown in Fig. 69.1.

The pharynx is a tubelike structure that extends from the base of the skull to the esophagus (Fig. 69.1). Made of muscle, this structure is divided into three parts:

- **Nasopharynx**—portion of the pharynx above the soft palate
- **Oropharynx**—portion of the pharynx between the soft palate and epiglottis
- **Laryngopharynx**—portion of the pharynx below the epiglottis that opens into the larynx

The oropharynx and nasopharynx are lined with stratified squamous epithelial cells that are teeming with normal microbiota. The tonsils are contained within the oropharynx; the larynx is located between the root of the tongue and the upper end of the trachea.

Pathogenesis

An overview of the pathogenesis of respiratory tract infections is presented in Chapter 68. It is important to keep in mind that upper respiratory tract infections may spread and become more serious because the mucosa (mucous membrane) of the upper tract is continuous with the mucosal lining of the sinuses, eustachian tube, middle ear, and lower respiratory tract.

Diseases of the Upper Respiratory Tract, Oral Cavity, and Neck

Upper Respiratory Tract

Diseases of the upper respiratory tract are named according to the anatomic sites involved. Most of these infections are self-limiting, and most infections are of viral origin.

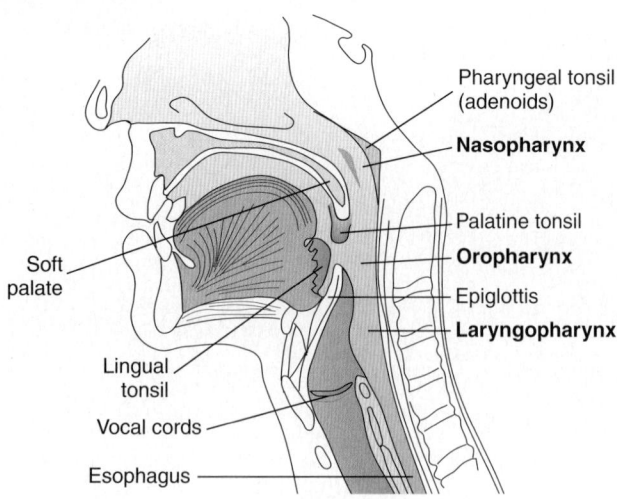

• **Fig. 69.1** The pharynx, including its three divisions and nearby structures.

Laryngitis

Acute laryngitis is usually associated with the common cold or influenza syndromes. Characteristically, patients complain of hoarseness and lowering or deepening of the voice. Acute laryngitis is generally a benign illness.

Acute laryngitis is almost exclusively associated with viral infection. All the major respiratory viruses have been associated with laryngitis; however influenza and parainfluenza viruses, rhinoviruses, adenoviruses, coronavirus, and human metapneumovirus are the most common etiologic agents. If examination of the larynx reveals an exudate or membrane on the pharyngeal or laryngeal mucosa, streptococcal infection, mononucleosis, or diphtheria should be suspected (see the discussion about miscellaneous infections caused by other agents, presented later in this chapter). *Haemophilus influenzae* is the most frequent microorganism recovered from patients with bacterial laryngitis. Chronic laryngitis, although less commonly associated with infectious agents, may be caused by bacteria or fungal isolates. Infections have been identified that are associated with methicillin-resistant *Staphylococcus aureus* (MRSA), *Bordetella pertussis, Mycoplasma pneumoniae,* and *Candida* spp.

Laryngotracheobronchitis

Another clinical syndrome closely related to laryngitis is acute **laryngotracheobronchitis,** or **croup.** Croup is a relatively common illness in young children, primarily those younger than 3 years of age. Of significance, croup can represent a potentially more serious disease if the infection extends downward from the larynx to involve the trachea or even the bronchi. Illness is characterized by variable fever; inspiratory stridor (difficulty in moving enough air through the larynx); hoarseness; and a harsh, barking, nonproductive cough. These symptoms last for 3 to 4 days, although the cough may persist for a longer period. In young infants, severe respiratory distress and fever are common symptoms.

Similar to the etiologic agents of laryngitis, viruses are a primary cause of croup; parainfluenza viruses are the major etiologic agents. In addition to parainfluenza viruses, influenza viruses, respiratory syncytial virus, and adenoviruses can also cause croup.

Other agents capable of causing croup, though not as frequently, include *M. pneumoniae,* rhinoviruses, and enteroviruses.

Epiglottitis

Epiglottitis is an infection of the epiglottis (elastic cartilage flap covering the entrance to the trachea) and other soft tissues above the vocal cords. Infection of the epiglottis can lead to significant edema (swelling) and inflammation resulting in respiratory distress or failure. Infected individuals typically present with fever, difficulty in swallowing because of pain, drooling, and respiratory obstruction with inspiratory stridor. Epiglottitis is a potentially life-threatening disease, because the patient's airway can become completely obstructed (blocked) if not treated.

In contrast to laryngitis, epiglottitis is usually associated with bacterial infections. In the past, 2- to 4-year-old children were typically infected with *H. influenzae* type b as the primary cause of epiglottitis. However, because of the common use of *H. influenzae* type b conjugated vaccine, the typical patient is now an adult that presents with a sore throat. Other organisms implicated are *Streptococcus pneumoniae, Streptococcus pyogenes, Staphylococcus aureus,* and *Neisseria meningitidis.* Diagnosis is established on clinical grounds, including the visualization of the epiglottis, which appears swollen and bright red in color. Bacteriologic culture of the epiglottis is contraindicated because swabbing of the epiglottis may lead to respiratory obstruction. Additional bacterial pathogens identified in cases of epiglottitis include *H. parainfluenzae, Klebsiella pneumoniae,* and *Pseudomonas aeruginosa.* Immunocompromised patients and patients receiving immunosuppressive therapy or antibiotics may experience epiglottitis caused by *Candida* spp. Viral agents including herpes simplex virus type 1 (HSV-1), influenzae B, and parainfluenzae type 3 may cause epiglottitis infection.

Pharyngitis, Tonsillitis, and Peritonsillar Abscesses
Pharyngitis and Tonsillitis

Pharyngitis (sore throat) and **tonsillitis** are common upper respiratory tract infections that affect both children and adults. Acute pharyngitis is an illness that commonly causes people to seek medical care.

Clinical Manifestations. Infection of the pharynx is associated with pharyngeal pain. Visualization of the pharynx reveals erythematous (red) and swollen tissue. Depending on the infectious agent, either inflammatory exudate (fluid with protein, inflammatory cells, and cellular debris), vesicles (small, blisterlike sacs containing liquid) and mucosal ulceration, or nasopharyngeal lymphoid hyperplasia (swollen lymph nodes) may be observed.

Pathogenesis. Pathogenic mechanisms differ and depend on the organism causing the pharyngitis. For example, some organisms directly invade the pharyngeal mucosa (e.g., *Arcanobacterium haemolyticum*), others elaborate toxins and other virulence factors at the site (e.g., *Corynebacterium diphtheriae*), and still others invade the pharyngeal mucosa and elaborate toxins and other virulence factors (e.g., *S. pyogenes*). Pathogenic mechanisms are reviewed in Part III according to various organism groups. Many cases of acute pharyngitis are associated with viral infections, are self-limiting, and require no medical treatment.

Epidemiology and Etiologic Agents. Most cases of pharyngitis occur during the colder months (winter to early spring) and often accompany other infections, primarily those caused by viruses. Patients with respiratory tract infections caused by influenza types A and B, parainfluenza, coxsackie A, rhinoviruses, or coronaviruses typically complain of a sore throat. Pharyngitis, often with ulceration, is also commonly found in patients with infectious mononucleosis caused by either Epstein-Barr virus (EBV) or cytomegalovirus (CMV). Although less common, pharyngitis caused by adenovirus or HSV is clinically severe and results in extensive destruction of the mucosal lining (cytopathology) of the pharynx. Finally, acute retroviral syndrome caused by human immunodeficiency virus 1 (HIV-1) may be associated with acute pharyngitis.

Although different bacteria can cause pharyngitis or tonsillitis, the primary cause of bacterial pharyngitis is *S. pyogenes* (or group A beta-hemolytic streptococci). Viral pharyngitis and pharyngitis or tonsillitis caused by other agents must be differentiated from that caused by *S. pyogenes*. Pharyngitis resulting from *S. pyogenes* is treatable with penicillin and a variety of other antimicrobials, whereas viral infections are not. In addition, treatment is of importance, because infection with *S. pyogenes* can lead to complications such as **acute rheumatic fever** and **glomerulonephritis.** These complications are referred to as **poststreptococcal sequelae** (diseases that follow a streptococcal infection) and are primarily immunologically mediated; these sequelae are discussed in greater detail in Chapter 14. *S. pyogenes* may also cause pyogenic infections (suppurations) of the tonsils, sinuses, and middle ear, or cellulitis as secondary pyogenic sequelae after an episode of pharyngitis. Accordingly, streptococcal pharyngitis is usually treated to prevent both the suppurative (pus forming) and nonsuppurative sequelae, as well as to decrease morbidity.

Although bacteria other than group A streptococci may cause pharyngitis, this occurs less often. Large colony isolates primarily of groups C and G streptococci (classified as *Streptococcus dysgalactiae* subsp. *equisimilis*) are pyogenic streptococci with similar virulence traits as *S. pyogenes*; symptoms of pharyngitis caused by these agents are also similar to *S. pyogenes*. These agents have been associated with poststreptococcal sequelae, namely glomerulonephritis and rheumatic fever. In addition, glomerulonephritis has been reported after infection with *S. equi* subsp. *zooepidemicus*. Studies have demonstrated that these streptococci

TABLE 69.1	Examples of Bacteria That Can Cause Acute Pharyngitis and Tonsillitis
Organism	**Disease**
Streptococcus pyogenes	Pharyngitis/tonsillitis/ rheumatic fever/scarlet fever
Group C and G beta-hemolytic streptococci	Pharyngitis/tonsillitis
Arcanobacterium haemolyticum	Pharyngitis/tonsillitis/rash
Fusobacterium necrophorum	Pharyngitis/tonsillitis
Neisseria gonorrhoeae	Pharyngitis/tonsillitis/ disseminated disease
Corynebacterium ulcerans	Pharyngitis
Mycoplasma pneumoniae	Pneumonia/bronchitis/ pharyngitis
Yersinia enterocolitica	Pharyngitis/enterocolitis
Human immunodeficiency virus-1	Pharyngitis/acute retroviral disease

can exchange genetic information with *S. pyogenes* and thus potentially obtain virulence factors usually associated with *S. pyogenes* such as M proteins, streptolysin O, and superantigen genes. *A. haemolyticum* is also a cause of pharyngitis among adolescents. Examples of agents that can cause pharyngitis or tonsillitis are listed in Table 69.1.

Although *H. influenzae, S. aureus,* and *S. pneumoniae* are commonly isolated from nasopharyngeal and throat cultures, they have not been shown to cause pharyngitis. Carriage of any of these organisms, as well as *N. meningitidis,* may have clinical importance for some patients. Cultures of specimens obtained from the anterior nares often yield *S. aureus.* The carriage rate for this organism is especially high among health care workers, and 10% to 30% of the general population can be colonized with this microbe, depending on the population characteristics. Bacterial pharyngitis may also be attributed to infection with *C. diphtheriae, Fusobacterium necrophorum,* and *Neisseria gonorrhoeae.* Viral pharyngitis may be caused by adenoviruses, coronaviruses, EBV, HIV, and influenza.

Vincent angina, also called **acute necrotizing ulcerative gingivitis,** or **trench mouth,** is a mixed bacterial-spirochetal infection of the gingival edge. The infection is relatively rare today, but it is considered a serious disease because it is often complicated by septic jugular thrombophlebitis, bacteremia, and widespread metastatic infection. Adults are affected more commonly than children; poor oral hygiene is a predisposing factor. Multiple anaerobes, especially *F. necrophorum,* are implicated in this syndrome. Although Gram stain of a throat specimen is usually not predictive, in those patients with symptoms suggestive of Vincent angina, Gram stain reveals numerous fusiform, gram-negative bacilli and spirochetes.

• BOX 69.1	Viral Agents That Can Cause Rhinitis
Rhinoviruses	>156 types
Coronaviruses	5 types
Adenoviruses	57 types
Parainfluenza and influenza viruses	5 and 3 types
Respiratory syncytial virus	2 types
Metapneumovirus	2 types
Other viruses: Bocavirus and Entero- virus	

Peritonsillar Abscesses

Peritonsillar abscesses are generally considered a complication of tonsillitis. This infection is most common in children older than 5 years of age and in young adults. It is important to treat these infections, because they can spread to adjacent tissues, as well as erode into the carotid artery to cause an acute hemorrhage. The predominant organisms isolated in peritonsillar abscesses include non–spore-forming anaerobes, such as *Fusobacterium* (especially *F. necrophorum*), *Bacteroides* (including the *Bacteroides fragilis* group), and anaerobic cocci. *S. pyogenes* and viridans streptococci may also be involved.

Rhinitis

Rhinitis (common cold) is an inflammation of the nasal mucous membrane or lining. Depending on the host response and the etiologic agent, rhinitis is characterized by variable fever, increased mucous secretions, inflammatory edema of the nasal mucosa, sneezing, and watery eyes. With rare exceptions, rhinitis is typically associated with viral infections (20% to 25%); some of these agents are listed in Box 69.1. Rhinitis is common because of the large number of different causative viruses, and reinfections may occur. Bacterial agents associated with rhinitis (10% to 15%) include *Chlamydia pneumoniae, M. pneumoniae,* and group A streptococci.

Miscellaneous Infections Caused by Other Agents

Corynebacterium diphtheriae

Pharyngitis caused by *C. diphtheriae* is less common than streptococcal pharyngitis. After an incubation period of 2 to 4 days, diphtheria usually presents as pharyngitis or tonsillitis. Patients are often febrile and complain of sore throat and malaise (body discomfort). The hallmark for diphtheria is the presence of an exudate or membrane that is usually on the tonsils or pharyngeal wall. The gray-white membrane is a result of the action of diphtheria toxin on the epithelium at the site of infection. Complications are common with diphtheria and are usually seen during the last stage of the disease (paroxysmal stage). The most feared complications are those involving the central nervous system, such as seizures, coma, or blindness. Information as to how this organism causes disease is discussed in Chapter 68. Additional specifics regarding this organism are provided in Chapter 16.

Bordetella pertussis

Although mass immunization programs have greatly reduced the incidence of pertussis, substantial numbers of cases (because of outbreaks and regional epidemics) still occur. An increase in the number of identifiable cases may be a result of improved awareness and diagnostic methods, such as nucleic acid–based testing. In addition, the lack of vaccinations of young children has also caused an increase in infections. It is important for laboratories to be capable of detecting, isolating, and identifying the organism either by culture or nucleic acid–based methods, or the specimen should be referred to a reference laboratory.

Characteristically, pertussis, or whooping cough, is a prolonged disease (lasting as long as 6 to 8 weeks) marked by paroxysmal (sudden or intense) coughing.

After an incubation period of 7 to 13 days, a patient with symptomatic infection develops upper respiratory symptoms, including a dry cough, fever, runny nose, and sneezing. After about 2 weeks, this may progress to spells of paroxysmal coughing. As these episodes worsen, the characteristic whoop, caused by attempted inspiration through an epiglottis undergoing spasm, begins. Vomiting may occur, and usually a lymphocytosis is present. This phase of the illness may last as long as 6 weeks. Bacterial culture for *B. pertussis* is effective using nasopharyngeal specimens during the first 2 weeks when symptoms are evident. Amplification and polymerase chain reaction (PCR) may demonstrate positive results within 4 weeks of the onset of symptoms. However, positive results should be interpreted with caution and in correlation with patient signs and symptoms. More information regarding *B. pertussis* is provided in Chapter 36.

Klebsiella spp.

Rhinoscleroma is a rare form of chronic granulomatous infection of the nasal passages, including the sinuses and occasionally the pharynx and larynx. Associated with *Klebsiella rhinoscleromatis,* the disease is characterized by nasal obstruction appearing over a long period, caused by tumor-like growth with local extension. *Klebsiella ozaenae* causes another uncommon condition called **atrophic rhinitis (ozena),** characterized by a chronic, mucopurulent nasal discharge that is often foul smelling. It is caused by secondary, low-grade anaerobic infection.

These two tissue-destructive diseases are transmitted person-to-person through exposure to infected nasal secretions and occur more frequently in tropical climates.

Oral Cavity

Stomatitis

Stomatitis is an inflammation of the mucous membranes of the oral cavity. HSV is the primary agent of this disease, in which multiple ulcerative lesions are seen on the oral mucosa. These lesions are painful and can be found in the mouth and in the oropharynx. Herpetic infections of the oral cavity are prevalent among immunosuppressed patients. Stomatitis has also been associated with *Kingella kingae,* treponemes, and infection with the measles virus.

Thrush

Candida spp. can also invade the oral mucosa. Immunosuppressed patients, including very young infants, may develop oral candidiasis, called **thrush.** Oral thrush can extend to produce pharyngitis or esophagitis, a common finding in patients with acquired immunodeficiency syndrome and in other immunosuppressed patients. Thrush is suspected if whitish patches of exudate on an area of inflammation are observed on the buccal mucosa, tongue, or oropharynx. Oral mucositis or pharyngitis in a granulocytopenic patient may be caused by Enterobacterales, *S. aureus,* or *Candida* spp. and is manifested by erythema, sore throat, and possibly exudate or ulceration. Although typically considered nonpathogenic, the yeast *Saccharomyces cerevisiae* has been reported to cause thrush.

Periodontal Infections

The three dental problems that may require culture and identification in a clinical laboratory include (1) root canal infections, with or without periapical abscess; (2) orofacial odontogenic infections, with or without osteomyelitis (inflammation of a bone) in the jaw; and (3) perimandibular space infections. Oral bacteria are clearly important in other dental processes, such as caries (destruction of the mineralized tissues of the tooth; a cavity), periodontal (tissues in, around, and supporting the tooth) disease, and localized juvenile periodontitis, but clinical laboratories are not involved in culturing in such cases.

Etiologic Agents

The bacteriology is similar in all these infections and involves primarily anaerobic bacteria and streptococci except for perimandibular space infections, which may also involve staphylococci and *Eikenella corrodens.* The streptococci are microaerobic or facultative and are usually alpha-hemolytic (particularly the *Streptococcus anginosus* group—see Chapter 13); they are found in 20% to 30% of dental infections.

Members of the *B. fragilis* group are found in root canal infections, orofacial odontogenic infections, and bacteremia secondary to dental extraction. Anaerobic cocci (both *Peptostreptococcus* and *Veillonella*), pigmented *Prevotella* and *Porphyromonas,* the *Prevotella oralis* group, and *Fusobacterium* are also associated with each of the three conditions mentioned, as well as in postextraction bacteremia. Infection with *Actinomyces israelii* may complicate oral surgery.

Salivary Gland Infections

Acute suppurative parotitis (inflammation of the salivary glands located under the cheek in front of and below the external ear) is seen in very ill patients, especially those who are dehydrated, malnourished, elderly, or recovering from surgery. It is associated with painful, tender swelling of the parotid gland; purulent drainage may be evident at the opening of the duct of the gland in the mouth. *S. aureus* is the major pathogen, but on occasion Enterobacterales, other gram-negative bacilli, and oral anaerobes may play a role in infection. Chronic bacterial parotitis has been described involving *S. aureus* or mixed oral aerobes and anaerobes. Less often, other salivary glands may be involved with a bacterial infection, usually because of ductal obstruction.

The mumps virus is traditionally the major viral agent involved in parotitis; however, since the advent of childhood vaccination, infection with mumps virus is rarely diagnosed. Influenza virus and enteroviruses may also cause this syndrome. Viral parotitis is typically diagnosed using serology. Infrequently, *Mycobacterium tuberculosis* may involve the parotid gland in conjunction with pulmonary tuberculosis.

Neck

Infections of the deep spaces of the neck are potentially serious, because they may spread to critical structures such as major vessels of the neck or to the mediastinum, leading to mediastinitis, purulent pericarditis, and pleural empyema. Oral microbiota is commonly responsible for these types of infections. Accordingly, the predominant organisms are anaerobes, primarily *Peptostreptococcus,* various *Bacteroides, Prevotella, Porphyromonas, Fusobacterium* spp., and *Actinomyces.* Streptococci, chiefly of the viridans variety, are also important. *S. aureus* and various aerobic, gram-negative bacilli may be recovered, particularly from patients developing these problems in the hospital.

Scrofula is a tuberculous infection in the cervical lymph nodes that may be associated with *Mycobacterium scrofulaceum* or *Mycobacterium avium* complex. *Mycobacterium avium* complex is a heterogenous group comprising *M. avium* and *Mycobacterium intracellulare* (Chapter 42). The characteristic signs and symptoms include painless swelling of the lymph nodes with the rare appearance of fever or ulcerations. Diagnosis may require bacterial culture of the lymph nodes, computed tomography (CT) of the neck, biopsy, and chest x-ray.

Diagnosis of Upper Respiratory Tract Infections

Collection and Transport of Specimens

Sterile, dacron, or rayon swabs with plastic shafts are suitable for collecting most upper respiratory tract microorganisms. Flocked swabs may also be used when available. If the swab remains moist, no further precautions need to be taken for specimens cultured within 4 hours of collection. After that period, transport medium is required to maintain viability and prevent overgrowth of contaminating organisms. Swabs for detection of group A streptococci (*S. pyogenes*) are the only exception. This organism is highly resistant to desiccation and remains viable on a dry swab for as long as 48 to 72 hours. Throat swabs are also adequate for recovery of adenoviruses and herpes viruses, *C. diphtheriae, Mycoplasma, Chlamydia,* and *Candida* spp. Transport media is required for the isolation of *Mycoplasma* and *Chlamydia* to ensure viability. Recovery of *C. diphtheriae* is enhanced by culturing both the throat and nasopharynx.

Nasopharyngeal swabs are better suited for recovery of *B. pertussis; Neisseria* spp.; and several viruses, including respiratory syncytial virus, parainfluenza virus, and the other viruses causing rhinitis. Optimum conditions for the collection and transport of specimens for viral detection or culture are described in Chapter 64. Although swabs made of calcium alginate are commonly used to collect nasopharyngeal specimens (excluding those specimens for chlamydia or viral culture), nasopharyngeal secretions collected by either aspiration or washing will improve recovery for *Bordetella* spp., because a larger amount of material is obtained.

The type of swab used for collection is very important. For example, cotton swabs should never be used for culture, because fibers contain fatty acids on the surface, which are capable of killing *Bordetella.* Calcium alginate or dacron swabs are acceptable for obtaining nasopharyngeal swab specimens; calcium alginate is optimal for culture. However, if nucleic acid–based testing is to be performed, dacron or rayon swabs on plastic shafts are preferred. Specimens for culture of *B. pertussis* ideally should be inoculated directly to fresh media at the patient's bedside. If this is not possible, transport for less than 2 hours in 1% casamino acid medium at room temperature is acceptable. If specimens are plated on the day of collection, Amie's transport medium with charcoal is acceptable. If specimens are plated more than 24 hours after collection, Regan-Lowe or Jones-Kendrick transport medium is optimal; both contain charcoal, starch, and nutrients as well as cephalexin. If lengthy delays in transport are expected, transport of specimens in Regan-Lowe medium at 4°C is recommended.

Direct Visual Examination or Detection

A Gram stain of material obtained from upper respiratory secretions or lesions may not improve diagnosis. Yeastlike cells can be identified, which are helpful in identifying thrush, and the characteristic pattern of fusiform and spirochetes of Vincent angina may be visualized. Gram crystal violet (allowed to remain on the slide for 1 minute before rinsing with tap water) and the Gram stain can be used to identify the spirilla and fusiform bacilli of Vincent angina. However, if crystal violet is used, the smear should be very thin, because everything will be intensely gram positive, making a thick smear difficult to read. Additionally, spirilla and bacilli may be stained using a dilute solution of carbol fuchsin.

For causes of pharyngitis, Gram stains are unreliable. Direct smears of exudate from membranelike lesions used to differentiate diphtheria from other causes are also not reliable or recommended.

Fungal elements, including yeast cells and pseudohyphae, may be visualized with a 10% potassium hydroxide (KOH)

preparation, calcofluor white fluorescent stain, or periodic acid-Schiff (PAS) stain. Numerous studies have demonstrated that nucleic acid–based amplification tests (NAAT) for *B. pertussis* in nasopharyngeal secretions are superior to culture. A wide variety of commercial systems are available for the detection of *B. pertussis* nucleic acid. Various methods, including fluorescent antibody stain reagents, enzyme immunoassays (EIAs), and NAAT, are also commercially available to detect numerous viral agents (Chapter 64).

Improvement in the development of rapid methods for detecting group A streptococcal antigen or nucleic acid has obviated the need for culture of pharyngeal specimens. At least 40 commercial products are available to identify group A streptococcal antigens using membrane EIA or latex agglutination techniques. Although the specific procedures vary with the EIA kit, several generalizations can be made. Throat swabs are incubated in an acid reagent or enzyme to extract the group A–specific carbohydrate antigen. Dacron swabs seem to be most efficient at releasing antigen, although other types of swabs may yield acceptable results. In laboratory comparisons between a rapid antigen detection method and conventional culture methods for detecting the presence of group A streptococci in throat swabs, the commercial kits have shown relatively acceptable (62% to more than 90%) sensitivity and specificity. Specimens with a negative direct antigen test for group A streptococci should be cultured (requires collection of specimen with two swabs) or confirmed using a nucleic acid method. Group A streptococci can be directly detected from pharyngeal specimens by nucleic acid–based testing using different molecular assay formats. The commercially available assay (Group A Strep Direct Test [GAS Direct], Hologic Inc., Bedford, MA) uses a nonisotopic, chemiluminescent, single-stranded deoxyribonucleic acid (DNA) probe complementary to the ribosomal ribonucleic acid (rRNA) target of the group A streptococcus. The assay detects organisms directly from swab specimens by lysing the bacterial cells before amplification. Dacron swabs are acceptable for use with this assay. Sensitivities of the Hologic GAS Direct test range from 91.7% to 99.3% compared with culture. A rapid-cycle real-time PCR method, the Light Cycler Strep-A (Roche Applied Science, Indianapolis, IN), also detects *S. pyogenes* directly from throat swabs. Using this technology, 32 samples (including controls) can be tested per run in about 1.5 hours. Isothermal DNA amplification is also available for the detection of group A streptococcus from throat swabs (Illumigene Group A Streptococcus, Meridian Bioscience, Inc., Cincinnati, OH) and demonstrates sensitivity equal to the GAS. See Chapter 8 for more information on isothermal DNA amplification.

Culture

Streptococcus pyogenes (Beta-Hemolytic Group A Streptococci)

Because the primary cause of bacterial pharyngitis in North America is *S. pyogenes,* most laboratories routinely screen throat cultures for this organism. Throat culture

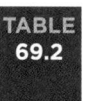

TABLE 69.2 Medium and Atmosphere for Incubation of Cultures to Recover Group A Streptococci From Pharyngeal Specimens

Media	Atmosphere of Incubation
Sheep blood agar	Anaerobic
Sheep blood agar with coverslip over the primary area of inoculation	Aerobic
Sheep blood agar with trimethoprim-sulfamethoxazole	5%–10% CO_2 or anaerobic

has historically been considered the gold standard for the diagnosis of *S. pyogenes*. Group A streptococci are usually beta-hemolytic; less than 1% are nonhemolytic. Three variables must be taken into consideration regarding successful culture of group A streptococci from pharyngeal specimens: medium, atmosphere, and duration of incubation. There are four recommended combinations of media and atmosphere of incubation for throat specimens; these are listed in Table 69.2. Regardless of the medium and atmosphere of incubation used, culture plates should be incubated for at least 48 hours before reporting as negative for group A streptococci.

Drawbacks to culture include an extended incubation time of 24 to 48 hours for visible colony formation with additional manipulations of the beta-hemolytic organisms for definitive identification (Chapter 14). If sufficient numbers of pure colonies are not available for identification, a subculture requiring additional incubation is necessary. By placing a 0.04-unit differential bacitracin filter paper disk, available commercially, directly on the area of initial inoculation, presumptive identification of *S. pyogenes* can be made after overnight incubation (all of group A and a very small percentage of group B streptococci are susceptible). However, use of the bacitracin disk in the primary area of inoculation reduces the sensitivity and specificity of culture and identification of *S. pyogenes*. Sometimes growth of too few beta-hemolytic colonies or overgrowth of other organisms makes interpretation difficult. Therefore using the bacitracin disk as the only method of identification of *S. pyogenes* is not recommended. New selective agars, such as streptococcal selective agar, have been developed that suppress the growth of almost all normal microbiota and beta-hemolytic streptococci except for groups A and B and *A. haemolyticum*. Direct antigen or nucleic acid detection tests or the PYR test (Chapter 12) can also be carried out on isolated beta-hemolytic colonies.

Corynebacterium diphtheriae

If diphtheria is suspected, the physician must communicate this information to the clinical laboratory. Because streptococcal pharyngitis is included in the differential diagnosis of diphtheria and because dual infections do occur, cultures for *C. diphtheriae* should be plated onto sheep blood agar or streptococcal selective agar, as well as onto special media for

recovery of this agent. These special media include a Loeffler agar slant and a cystine-tellurite agar plate. Chapter 16 discusses the identification of the organism. Recovery of this organism is improved when culturing specimens from the throat and nasopharynx of potentially infected patients. In addition to culture, rapid toxigenicity assays, including immunoassays and NAAT, may be used to assist in the diagnosis. Caution should be used when interpreting molecular assays, because positive results have been associated with related species of corynebacteria.

Bordetella pertussis

Freshly prepared Bordet-Gengou agar was the first medium developed for isolation of *B. pertussis* or *B. parapertussis*. However, because it was inconvenient to use, other media were subsequently developed (Chapter 36). Regan-Lowe or charcoal horse blood agar is now recommended for use in diagnostic laboratories. Because the organisms are extremely delicate, specimens should be plated directly onto media, if possible. The yield of positive isolations from clinical cases of pertussis seems to vary from 20% to 98% depending on the stage of disease, previous treatment of the patient, age of the patient, and laboratory techniques. Because of the limitations associated with culture and serologic diagnostic methods, significant effort has been put into developing nucleic acid amplification methods. Nucleic acid–based diagnostic tests for the direct detection of *B. pertussis* and *B. parapertussis* genes by various PCR procedures, including real-time PCR, have replaced direct fluorescent antibody methods (DFA) in the clinical laboratory.

Neisseria spp.

Specimens received in the laboratory for isolation of *N. meningitidis* (for detection of carriers) or *N. gonorrhoeae* should be plated to a selective medium, either modified Thayer-Martin or Martin-Lewis agar. After 24 to 48 hours of incubation in 5% to 10% carbon dioxide, typical colonies of *Neisseria* spp. may be visible. Nucleic acid–based methods have replaced enzyme-linked immunosorbent assay systems for rapid diagnosis of *N. gonorrhoeae* and *N. meningitidis* (Chapter 39).

Epiglottitis

Clinical specimens from cases of epiglottitis (swabs obtained by a physician) should be plated to sheep blood agar, chocolate agar (for recovery of *Haemophilus* spp.), and a streptococcal selective medium. Refer to Table 5.1 for an overview of the methods used to collect, transport, and process different specimens from the upper respiratory tract.

Diagnosis of Infections in the Oral Cavity and Neck

Collection and Transport

It is important to prevent or minimize contamination with oral microbiota when collecting oral and dental material for diagnosis of infection. For collection of material from root canal infection, the tooth is isolated by means of a rubber dam. A sterile field is established, the tooth is swabbed with 70% alcohol, and after the root canal is exposed, a sterile paper point is inserted, removed, and placed into semisolid, nonnutritive, anaerobic transport medium. Alternatively, needle aspiration can be used if sufficient purulent material is present. Completely defining the microbiota of such infections is beyond the scope of routine clinical microbiology laboratories.

Specimens from neck space infections can usually be obtained with a syringe and needle or by biopsy during a surgical procedure. Transport must be under anaerobic conditions.

Direct Visual Examination

All material submitted for culture should be smeared and examined by Gram stain and other appropriate techniques for fungi (i.e., calcofluor white, KOH, or PAS stains), if requested.

Culture

Infections such as peritonsillar abscesses, oral and dental infections, and neck space infections usually involve anaerobic bacteria. The anaerobes involved typically originate in the oral cavity and are often more delicate than anaerobes isolated from other clinical material. Very careful methods are required to provide optimal specimens for anaerobic cultivation, as well as collection and transport for the recovery and identification of the etiologic agents. See Chapter 40 for more information related to anaerobic organisms.

ⓔ Visit the Evolve site for a complete list of procedures, review questions, and case studies.

Bibliography

Bennett J, Dolin R, Blaser M: *Principles and practice of infectious diseases*, ed 9, Philadelphia, PA, 2020, Elsevier.

Bourbeau PP: Role of the microbiology laboratory in diagnosis and management of pharyngitis, *J Clin Microbiol* 41:3467–3472, 2003.

Bourbeau PP, Heiter BJ: Use of swabs without transport media for the gen-probe group a strep direct test, *J Clin Microbiol* 42:3207–3211, 2004.

Cambier M, Janssens M, Wauters G: Isolation of *Arcanobacterium haemolyticum* from patients with pharyngitis in Belgium, *Acta Clin Belg* 47:303–307, 1992.

Carroll KC, Pfaller MA, Landry ML, et al.: *Manual of clinical microbiology*, ed 12, Washington, DC, 2019, ASM.

Cloud JL, Hymas W, Carroll KC: Impact of nasopharyngeal swab types on detection of *Bordetella pertussis* by PCR and culture, *J Clin Microbiol* 40:3838–3840, 2002.

Hallander HO, Reizenstein E, Renemar B, et al.: Comparison of nasopharyngeal aspirates with swabs for culture of *Bordetella pertussis*, *J Clin Microbiol* 31:50–52, 1993.

Kellogg JA: Suitability of throat culture procedures for detection of group a streptococci and as reference standards for evaluation of streptococcal antigen kits, *J Clin Microb* 28:165–169, 1990.

Liakos T, Kaye K, Rubin AD: Methicillin-resistant *Staphylococcus aureus* laryngitis, *Ann Otol Rhinol Laryngol* 119:590–593, 2010.

McGowan KL: Diagnostic tests for pertussis: culture vs. DFA vs. PCR, *Clin Microbiol Newsl* 24:143–149, 2002.

Moulis G, Martin-Blondel G: Scrofula, the king's evil, *Can Med Assoc J* 184:1061, 2012.

Sachse S, Seidel P, Gerlach D, et al.: Superantigen-like gene(s) in human pathogenic *Streptococcus dysgalactiae*, subsp. *equisimilis*: genomic localization of the gene encoding streptococcal pyrogenic exotoxin G (spe Gdys), *FEMS Immunol Med Microbiol* 34:159–167, 2002.

70

Meningitis and Other Infections of the Central Nervous System

OBJECTIVES

1. Describe the anatomy of the central nervous system (CNS), and list the anatomic structures that compose it.
2. Define meninges; name the three separate layers and describe their function.
3. Define the cerebrospinal fluid and list its functions.
4. Describe the routes of infection for the CNS.
5. Explain the host defense mechanisms that protect the central nervous system from infection.
6. Define meningitis, and describe the two major types of meningitis, including the etiologic agents.
7. Discuss the cause of acute meningitis, and explain the host predisposing factors for neonates; identify the most commonly associated bacterial pathogens.
8. Discuss how the advent of the *Haemophilus influenzae* type b (Hib) vaccine in the United States has helped to prevent pediatric cases of meningitis.
9. Compare acute and chronic meningitis; outline the distinguishing symptoms and cerebrospinal fluid (CSF) findings for each, including cell counts and chemistry laboratory results.
10. Explain the disease processes for encephalitis and meningoencephalitis.
11. Discuss two ways that meningoencephalitis infections, brain abscesses, or other CNS infections are caused by parasites; identify the associated infecting organisms and the population of patients at increased risk for developing these conditions.
12. Explain the collection, transport, and specimen storage requirements for CSF; include specimen processing and the appropriate distribution of specimen throughout the laboratory.
13. List the culture media used to identify the causative agent of meningitis in bacterial, mycobacterial, and fungal infections; what incubation conditions are required for each type of organism?
14. Describe the use of advanced technologies including matrix-assisted laser desorption ionization time-of-flight mass spectrometry (MALDI-TOF MS), and nucleic acid–based testing in the direct diagnosis of CNS infections.

General Considerations

Anatomy

Diagnosis of an infection involving the central nervous system (CNS) is of critical importance. Most clinicians consider infection in the CNS to be a medical emergency. An understanding of the basic anatomy and physiology of the CNS is helpful for the microbiologist to ensure appropriate specimen processing and interpretation of laboratory results.

Coverings and Spaces of the Central Nervous System

The central nervous system consists of the brain and the spinal cord. Because of the vital and essential role of the CNS in the body's regulatory processes, the brain and spinal cord have two protective coverings: an outer covering consisting of bone and an inner covering of membranes called the **meninges.** The outer bone covering encases the brain (i.e., cranial bones or skull) and spinal cord (i.e., the vertebrae). The meninges are a collective term for the three distinct membrane layers surrounding the brain and spinal column:
- **Dura mater**—outermost membrane layer
- **Arachnoid mater**—middle layer
- **Pia mater**—innermost membrane layer

The pia mater and the arachnoid membrane are collectively called the **leptomeninges.** The portion of the arachnoid that covers the top of the brain contains arachnoid villi, which are special structures that absorb the spinal fluid and allow it to pass into the blood.

Between and around the meninges are spaces that include the **epidural, subdural,** and **subarachnoid spaces.** The relative location of the meninges and spaces to one another in the brain are depicted in Fig. 70.1. The location and nature of the meninges and spaces are summarized in Table 70.1.

Cerebrospinal Fluid

Cerebrospinal fluid (CSF) surrounds the brain and spinal cord and has several functions. The CSF provides cushioning and buoyancy for the bulk of the brain, reducing the effective weight of the brain by a factor of 30. CSF carries essential metabolites into the neural tissue and cleanses the tissues of wastes as it circulates around the brain, ventricles, and spinal cord. Every 3 to 4 hours, the entire volume of CSF is exchanged. The amount of CSF in humans depends on the developmental age of the individual, reaching a volume of approximately 150 mL by 5 years of age. In addition to these functions, CSF provides a means by which the brain monitors changes in the internal environment.

CSF is found in the subarachnoid space (Table 70.1) and within cavities and canals of the brain and spinal cord. There are four large, fluid-filled spaces within the brain referred to as **ventricles.** Specialized secretory cells, called the **choroid plexus,** produce CSF. The choroid plexus is located centrally within the brain in the third and fourth ventricles. Approximately 23 mL of CSF are contained within these ventricles in an adult. The fluid travels around the outside areas of the brain within the subarachnoid space, driven primarily by the pressure produced initially at the choroid plexus (Fig. 70.2). By virtue of its circulation, chemical and

cellular changes in the CSF may provide valuable information about infections within the subarachnoid space.

Routes of Infection

One of the most important defense mechanisms of the CNS is the **blood-brain barrier.** The blood-brain barrier functions to maintain homeostasis in the brain by restricting the flow of chemical constituents from the blood to the CNS. For the CNS to become infected with a bacterium, parasite, or virus, the blood-brain barrier must be penetrated.

Organisms may gain access to the CNS through several primary routes:

- Hematogenous spread: This is followed by entry into the subarachnoid space through the choroid plexus or through other blood vessels of the brain. This is the most common route of infection for the CNS.
- Direct spread from an infected site: The extension of an infection close to or contiguous with the CNS can occasionally occur; examples of such infections include otitis media (infection of middle ear), sinusitis, and mastoiditis.
- Anatomic defects in CNS structures: Anatomic defects as a result of surgery, trauma, or congenital abnormalities can allow microorganisms easy and ready access to the CNS.
- Travel along nerves leading to the brain (direct intraneural): This is the least common route of CNS infection and occurs with organisms such as rabies virus, which travels along peripheral sensory nerves, and herpes simplex virus.

Diseases of the Central Nervous System
Meningitis

Infection within the subarachnoid space or throughout the leptomeninges is called **meningitis.** Based on the host's response to the invading microorganism, meningitis is divided into two major categories: purulent and aseptic meningitis.

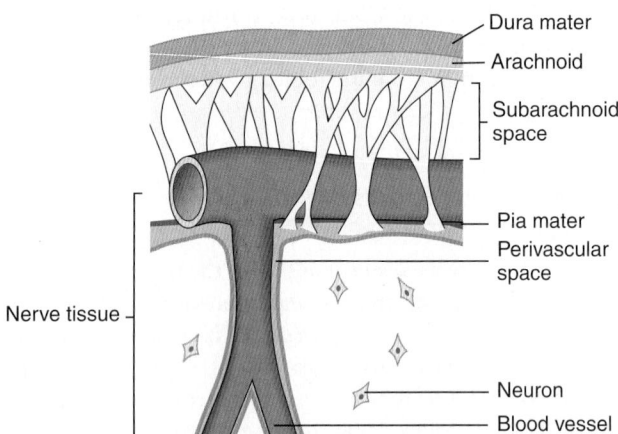

Dura mater
Arachnoid
Subarachnoid space
Pia mater
Perivascular space
Nerve tissue
Neuron
Blood vessel

• **Fig. 70.1** Cross-section of the brain showing the important membrane coverings and spacing and other key structures.

TABLE 70.1	Inner Coverings (Meninges) of the Brain, Spinal Cord, and Surrounding Spaces		
Anatomic Structure	**Relative Location**	**Key Features**	
Epidural space	Outside the dura mater yet inside the skull	Cushion of fat and connective tissues	
Dura mater	Outermost membrane	Membrane that adheres to the skull; white fibrous tissue	
Subdural space	Between the dura mater and the arachnoid membrane	Cushion of lubricating serous fluid	
Arachnoid membrane	Between the dura mater and pia mater	Delicate, cobweblike membrane covering the brain and spinal cord	
Subarachnoid space	Beneath the arachnoid membrane	Contains a significant amount of cerebrospinal fluid in an adult (~125–150 mL)	
Pia mater	Beneath the subarachnoid space	Adheres to the outer surface of the brain and spinal cord; contains blood vessels	

Purulent Meningitis

A patient with **purulent meningitis** typically has a marked, acute inflammatory exudative CSF containing large numbers of polymorphonuclear cells (PMNs). The underlying CNS tissue, in particular the ventricles, is often involved. If the ventricles become involved, this process is referred to as **ventriculitis.** Bacterial organisms are usually the cause of these infections.

Pathogenesis. The outcome of a host-microbe interaction depends on the characteristics of both the host and the microorganism. As previously indicated, an important host defense mechanism within the CNS is the blood-brain barrier; this barrier involves the choroid plexus, arachnoid membrane, and the cerebral microvascular endothelium. The unique structural properties of the vascular endothelium, such as the continuous intercellular tight junctions, provide a barrier minimizing the passage of infectious agents into the CSF. The normal function of the vascular endothelium includes regulating the transport of nutrients into and out of the CSF, including low-molecular-weight plasma proteins, glucose, and electrolytes.

The host's age and other underlying factors contribute to whether an individual is predisposed to the development of infectious meningitis. Neonates have the highest infection rate for meningitis, because of the immature neonatal immune system, the increased permeability of the

blood-brain barrier in newborns, and the presence of colonizing bacteria in the female vaginal tract that can pass to the infant during childbirth. The most common bacterial pathogens responsible for meningitis in newborns are group B streptococci, *Escherichia coli,* and *Listeria monocytogenes.* Before the advent of the *Haemophilus influenzae* type b (Hib) vaccine in the United States in 1985, Hib was a common cause of meningitis in children 4 months to 5 years of age. Because of the incorporation of Hib into childhood immunization programs, childhood Hib disease has dramatically declined not only in the United States, but worldwide.

Among young adults, *Neisseria meningitidis* is typically the agent that is associated with meningitis. *N. meningitidis* has been identified in epidemics among young adults in crowded conditions (e.g., military recruits and college dormitories). There are two types of meningococcal vaccines (vaccines for *N. meningitidis*) available in the United States: meningococcal conjugate vaccines (for young adults 11 to 12 years of age), with a booster recommended at the age of 16, and serogroup B meningococcal vaccines (16 to 35 years of age). *Streptococcus pneumoniae* is a common cause of meningitis in young children and the elderly; often this meningitis develops from bacteremia or from infection of the sinuses or middle ear. There are two pneumococcal vaccines (vaccines for *S. pneumoniae*) that are recommended currently in the United States. The pneumococcal conjugate

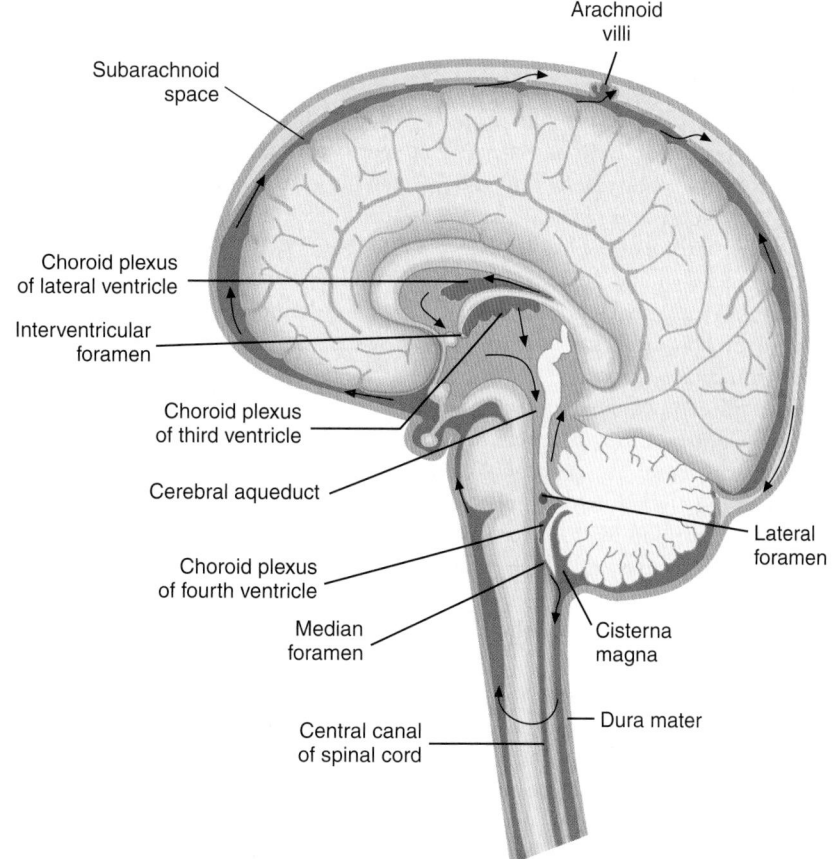

• **Fig. 70.2** Flow of cerebrospinal fluid (CSF) through the brain. CSF originates in the choroid plexus and then flows through the ventricles and subarachnoid space and into the bloodstream.

vaccine (PCV13) protects against infection from 13 different serotypes of *S. pneumoniae* and is used for vaccination of children and adults. The second vaccine, pneumococcal polysaccharide vaccine (PPSV), provides protection from 23 serotypes of *S. pneumoniae,* including those associated with serious life-threatening infections. This vaccine is recommended for adults 65 years of age and older or anyone over the age of 19 years who has long-term health problems or is immunocompromised.

Because the respiratory tract is the primary portal of entry for many etiologic agents of meningitis, factors that predispose adults to meningitis are often the same factors that increase the likelihood for the development of pneumonia or other respiratory tract colonization or infection. Alcoholism, splenectomy, diabetes mellitus, prosthetic devices, and immunosuppression contribute to increased risk. Finally, patients with prosthetic devices, particularly CNS and ventriculoperitoneal shunts, are at increased risk for developing meningitis.

For organisms to reach the CNS (primarily by the blood-borne route), host defense mechanisms must be overcome. Most cases of meningitis are a result of bacteria that share a similar pathogenesis. The successful meningeal pathogen must first sequentially colonize and cross host mucosal epithelium, then enter and thrive within the bloodstream. The most common causes of meningitis possess the ability to evade host defenses at each of these levels. For example, clinical isolates of *S. pneumoniae* and *N. meningitidis* secrete IgA proteases capable of destroying the host's secretory IgA, thereby facilitating bacterial attachment to the epithelium. In addition, all the most common etiologic agents of bacterial meningitis possess an antiphagocytic capsule that allows the organisms to evade destruction by the host immune system.

Organisms appear to enter the CNS by interacting and subsequently breaking down the blood-brain barrier at the level of microvascular endothelium. One of the least understood processes in the pathogenesis of meningitis is how organisms cross this barrier into the subarachnoid space. Nevertheless, there appear to be specific bacterial surface components, such as pili, polysaccharide capsules, and lipoteichoic acids, which facilitate adhesion of the organisms to the microvascular endothelial cells and subsequent penetration into the CSF. Organisms can enter (1) through loss of capillary integrity by disrupting tight junctions of the blood-brain barrier, (2) through transport within circulating phagocytic cells, or (3) by crossing the endothelial cell lining within endothelial cell vacuoles. After gaining access, the organism multiplies within the CSF, a site initially free of antimicrobial antibodies or phagocytic cells.

Clinical Manifestations. Meningitis can be classified as either an acute or a chronic disease in the onset and overall progression within the host. It is important to note that not all patients will present with the classic signs and symptoms associated with CNS infection discussed in this chapter. One example is the presence of seizures. Seizures may assist in the differentiation of meningitis from encephalitis. Seizures are generally a late clinical manifestation in meningitis and

an early indicator in encephalitis. Computed tomography (CT) of the head and neck should be completed prior to a CSF lumbar puncture in immunocompromised patients, patients with a decreased level of consciousness, or focal neurological defects to rule out noninfectious disease.

Acute. Classical symptoms of acute meningitis include fever, stiff neck, headache, nausea and vomiting, neurologic abnormalities, and change in mental status.

In acute bacterial meningitis, the CSF usually contains large numbers of inflammatory cells ($>1000/mm^3$), primarily PMNs. The CSF shows a decreased glucose level relative to the serum glucose level and an increase in protein concentration. In a healthy individual, the normal CSF glucose level is 0.6 of the serum glucose level and ranges from 45 to 100 mg/dL; the CSF protein range in an adult is 15 to 50 mg/dL; newborn CSF protein ranges run as high as 170 mg/dL, with an average of 90 mg/dL.

The sequelae of acute bacterial meningitis in children are common and serious. Seizures occur in 20% to 30% of patients, and other neurologic changes are common. Acute sequelae include cerebral edema, hydrocephalus, cerebral herniation, and focal neurologic changes. Permanent deafness can occur in 10% of children who recover from bacterial meningitis. Other subtle physiologic and psychological sequelae may also follow an episode of acute bacterial meningitis.

Chronic. Chronic meningitis is common in patients who are immunocompromised, although this is not always the case. Patients experience an insidious onset of disease, with some or all the following symptoms: fever, headache, stiff neck, nausea and vomiting, lethargy, confusion, and mental deterioration. Symptoms may persist for a month or longer before treatment is sought. The CSF usually manifests an abnormal number of white blood cells (usually lymphocytic), elevated protein, and decrease in glucose content (Table 70.2). The pathogenesis of chronic meningitis is similar to that of acute disease.

Epidemiology and Etiologic Agents of Acute Meningitis. The cause of acute meningitis depends on the age of the patient. Most cases in the United States occur in children younger than 5 years of age. Before 1985, *H. influenzae* type b was the most common infectious agent in children between 1 month and 6 years of age within the United States. Ninety-five percent of all cases were caused by *H. influenzae* type b, *N. meningitidis,* and *S. pneumoniae.* In 1985, the first Hib vaccine, a polysaccharide vaccine, was licensed for use in children 18 months of age or older but was not efficacious in children younger than 18 months. However, the widespread use of conjugate vaccine, Hib polysaccharide-protein conjugate, in children as young as 2 months of age, has significantly affected the incidence of invasive *H. influenzae* type b disease; the total number of annual cases of *H. influenzae* disease has decreased significantly in the United States and Europe and the number of cases of *H. influenzae* meningitis by 94%. However, the risks for meningococcal and pneumococcal diseases resulting from agents other than *H. influenzae* have remained

TABLE 70.2	Guidelines for Interpretation of Results After Hematologic and Chemical Analysis of Cerebrospinal Fluid From Children and Adults (Excluding Neonates)				
Clinical Setting	Leukocytes (mm³)	Predominant Cell Type	Protein	Glucose[a]
Normal	0–5	None	15–50 mg/dL	45–100 mg/dL
Viral infection	2–2000 (mean of 80)	Mononuclear[b]	Slightly elevated (50–100 mg/dL) or normal	Normal
Purulent infection	5–20,000 (mean of 800)	Polymorphonuclear	Elevated (>100 mg/dL)	Low (<45 mg/dL), but may be normal early during disease
Tuberculosis and fungi	5–2000 (mean of 100)	Mononuclear	Elevated (>50 mg/dL)	Normal or often low (>45 mg/dL)

[a]Must consider cerebrospinal fluid (CSF) glucose level in relation to blood glucose level. Normally, the CSF glucose serum ratio is 0.6, or 50%–70% of the blood glucose normal value.
[b]About 20%–75% of cases may have PMN leukocytosis early during infection.

level. Children older than 6 years are less likely to develop meningitis, but the risk for meningitis infection increases when the child reaches early adulthood. As previously mentioned, neonates have the highest incidence of acute meningitis, with a concomitant increased mortality rate (as high as 20%). Organisms causing disease in the newborn are different from those that affect other age groups; many of them are acquired by the newborn during passage through the mother's vaginal vault. Neonates are likely to be infected with, in order of incidence, group B streptococci, *Escherichia coli,* other gram-negative bacilli, and *Listeria monocytogenes;* occasionally other organisms may be involved. For example, *Elizabethkingia meningoseptica* and *Elizabethkingia anopheles* are both associated with severe cases of neonatal meningitis. These organisms are normal inhabitants of water in the environment and may be transmitted from mother to fetus or acquired as a nosocomial infection.

Important causes of meningitis in adults, in addition to the meningococcus in young adults, include pneumococci, *L. monocytogenes,* and, less commonly, *Staphylococcus aureus* and various gram-negative bacilli (*E. coli, Klebsiella* spp., *Serratia marcescens, Pseudomonas aeruginosa, Acinetobacter* spp., and *Salmonella* spp.). Meningitis caused by the latter organisms results from hematogenous seeding from various sources, including urinary tract infections. Spirochetal meningitis or neurosyphilis can be caused by dissemination of *Treponema pallidum* early in the infectious process. CSF abnormalities may occur in up to 9% of patients who are seronegative for syphilis and may overlap in clinical presentation, including asymptomatic, meningeal, meningovascular, parenchymatous, and gummatous. Although *Naegleria fowleri* is the primary cause of meningoencephalitis, additional genera may also be associated with infection, including *Acanthamoeba* and *Balamuthia. Parastrongylus cantonensis* is the most common cause of eosinophilic meningitis or encephalitis. The nematode larvae invade the CSF directly from the bloodstream and mature into adult worms migrating throughout the brain. Additional organisms

capable of causing eosinophilic meningitis include *Paragonimus westermani, Gnathostoma* spp. (myeloencephalitis), *Baylisascaris procyonis* (neural larva migrans [NLM]), and *Taenia solium.*

Aseptic Meningitis

Aseptic meningitis is usually viral and is characterized by an increase of lymphocytes and other mononuclear cells (pleocytosis) in the CSF; bacterial and fungal cultures are negative. This contrasts with bacterial meningitis, which is characterized by purulence and the PMN cell response in the CSF. However, viral meningitis may mimic bacterial meningitis with an increase in PMNs within the first 24 hours followed by a transition to a lymphocytic pleocytosis. Aseptic meningitis is usually self-limiting, with symptoms that may include fever, headache, stiff neck, nausea, and vomiting.

In addition to the increase of lymphocytes and other mononuclear cells in the CSF, the glucose level remains normal, whereas the protein CSF level may remain normal or may be slightly elevated. Aseptic meningitis can also be a symptom for syphilis and some other spirochete diseases (e.g., leptospirosis and Lyme borreliosis). Stiff neck and CSF pleocytosis may also be associated with other disease processes, such as malignancy.

Enteroviruses are currently the leading cause of aseptic meningitis. Infants and young children are the most common population susceptible to infection. Additional viral agents associated with aseptic meningitis include herpes simplex virus (HSV); varicella-zoster-virus (VZV); cytomegalovirus (CMV); Epstein-Barr virus (EBV); and human herpesviruses 6, 7, and 8. The mumps virus may contribute to aseptic meningitis cases in nonimmunized populations.

Encephalitis/Meningoencephalitis

There are over 100 different pathogens capable of causing encephalitis. Encephalitis is an acute inflammation of the brain parenchyma and is usually caused by direct viral invasion. Concomitant meningitis occurring with encephalitis is known as **meningoencephalitis**, and the cellular infiltrate present in the CSF is typically lymphocytic rather than PMNs.

The host response to these CNS infections can differ somewhat from those associated with purulent or aseptic meningitis. Early during viral encephalitis, or when considerable tissue damage occurs as a part of encephalitis, the nature of the inflammatory cells found in the CSF may be no different from that associated with bacterial meningitis; cell counts, however, are typically much lower.

Viral Encephalitis

Viral encephalitis, which cannot always be distinguished clinically from meningitis, is common in the warmer months. The primary agents are enteroviruses (coxsackie viruses A and B and echoviruses), mumps virus, herpes simplex virus, and arboviruses (West Nile virus, togavirus, bunyavirus, equine encephalitis, St. Louis encephalitis, and other encephalitis viruses). Herpes simplex virus is the most common virus associated with viral encephalitis in developed countries. Other viruses—such as measles, cytomegalovirus, lymphocytic choriomeningitis, Epstein-Barr virus, hepatitis, varicella-zoster virus, rabies virus, myxoviruses, and paramyxoviruses—are less commonly encountered. Any preceding viral illness and exposure history are important considerations in establishing a cause by clinical means.

West Nile virus is the most common flavivirus reported in the United States with cases identified in all 48 contiguous states. Neuroinvasive infection with West Nile presents with symptoms of headache, fever, and a change in consciousness along with altered mental status. Examination of the CSF shows an increase in leukocytes with a marked increase in lymphocytes. Chemistries demonstrate an elevated protein count and normal glucose levels. Definitive diagnosis requires testing for the presence of the IgM antibody to West Nile in the serum or CSF, and because IgM does not cross the blood-brain barrier, presence of IgM antibody to West Nile in the CSF is a strong indicator for CNS infection. Polymerase chain reaction (PCR) can also be used to test for West Nile infection, but because West Nile infections have a transient and low viremia, results must be interpreted with caution. A negative result does not necessarily rule out West Nile infection.

Involvement of the nervous system in patients who are infected with the human immunodeficiency virus (HIV) is common. HIV is a neurotropic (attracted to nerve cells) virus capable of entering the CNS by macrophage transport and is the cause of various neurologic syndromes. As HIV-infected individuals become progressively more immunosuppressed, the CNS becomes a target for opportunistic pathogens, such as cytomegalovirus, BK virus, and JC (John Cunningham) virus, which can produce meningitis or encephalitis. BK virus is named after the initials of the first renal transplant patient where the virus was identified in association with clinical disease.

Parasitic Infections

Parasites can cause meningoencephalitis, brain abscess (see the following discussion), or other CNS infection via two routes. A rare but devastating meningoencephalitis is caused by the free-living amoeba *N. fowleri*, which invades the brain via direct extension from the nasal mucosa. These organisms are acquired during swimming or diving in natural, stagnating freshwater ponds and lakes. Although *N. fowleri* is the primary cause of meningoencephalitis, additional genera may also be associated with infection including *Balamuthia* spp. and *Acanthamoeba* spp. (granulomatous amebic encephalitis); *Sappinia pedata*, is now a confirmed human parasitic pathogen linked to the development of encephalitis.

Other parasites reach the brain via hematogenous spread. Toxoplasmosis, caused by an intracellular parasite that destroys brain parenchyma, is a common CNS affliction in HIV-infected patients with acquired immune deficiency syndrome (AIDS). *Entamoeba histolytica* and *Strongyloides stercoralis* have been identified in brain tissue, and the larval form of *T. solium* (the pork tapeworm), referred to as a cysticercus, can travel to the brain via the bloodstream and encyst within the brain tissue. Amoebic brain infection and cysticercosis cause changes in the CSF that are similar to meningitis.

Parastrongylus cantonensis is the most common cause of eosinophilic meningitis. The nematode larvae invade the CSF directly from the bloodstream and mature into adult worms migrating throughout the brain. Additional organisms capable of causing eosinophilic meningitis include *Gnathostoma* spp., *Baylisascaris procyonis*, *Paragonimus westermani*, and *T. solium*. Symptoms include headache and visual disturbances. Approximately 50% of the patients' experience vomiting and moderate fever. Approximately 10% to 20% of patients infected with *Trichinella spiralis* may exhibit CNS involvement with a mortality rate of 50% if untreated. Symptoms can mimic meningitis or encephalitis.

Brain Abscess

Brain abscesses (localized collections of pus in a cavity formed by the breakdown of tissue) may occasionally cause changes in the CSF and clinical symptoms similar to meningitis. Brain abscesses result from contiguous infection of the sinuses, middle ear, or mastoids (25% to 50%), hematogenously (15% to 30%), or through direct inoculation as a result of trauma or surgery (8% to 19%). Brain abscesses may rupture into the subarachnoid space, producing severe meningitis with a high mortality rate. If anaerobic organisms or viridans streptococci are recovered from CSF cultures, the diagnosis of brain abscess should be considered; however, CSF culture is typically negative in brain abscess. Patients who are immunosuppressed or who have diabetes with ketoacidosis may present with a rapid progressive fungal infection (phycomycosis) of the nasal sinuses or palatal region capable of traveling directly to the brain. The complex polymicrobial infections isolated from brain abscesses are far too extensive to list.

Shunt Infections

Information and studies related to infections involving CSF shunts is limited. The organisms reported to be most commonly associated with infections include coagulase-negative staphylococcus, *S. aureus*, *Propionibacterium acnes*, and viridians group streptococci. A few gram-negative rods have been identified, including *P. aeruginosa*, *Klebsiella* spp., *E. coli*, and *S. marcescens*. Positive cultures are most often associated with shunt tip cultures, shunt valves, and cerebral ventricle fluid.

Laboratory Diagnosis of Central Nervous System Infections

Meningitis

Except in unusual circumstances, a lumbar puncture (spinal tap) is one of the first steps in the diagnosis of a patient with suspected CNS infection, in particular, meningitis. Refer to Table 5.1 to review the procedure for collecting, transporting, and processing specimens obtained from the central nervous system.

Specimen Collection and Transport

CSF is collected by aseptically inserting a needle into the subarachnoid space (lumbar puncture), at the lumbar spine region between L3, L4, or L5. Three or four tubes of CSF should be collected into sterile collection tubes that contain no additives. The tubes are numbered sequentially in the order in which they were collected along with the patient's name. When processing the CSF collection tubes in the laboratory, tube 1 is used for chemistry studies, glucose and protein count, and immunology studies, because these tests are least affected by the presence of blood cells or bacteria introduced as a result of the spinal tap procedure; tube 2 is used for culture, allowing a larger proportion of the total fluid to be concentrated, which can facilitate the detection of infectious agents present in low numbers; tubes 3 and 4 are used for cell count and differential, because these tubes are least likely to contain cells introduced by the collection procedure. If a small capillary blood vessel is inadvertently broken during the spinal tap, blood cells picked up from this source will usually be absent from the last tube collected; comparison of counts between tubes 1 and 3 or 4 is occasionally needed if a traumatic tap is suspected or to differentiate a traumatic bloody tap from a true subarachnoid hemorrhage. In a traumatic tap, the red blood cells will be unevenly distributed among the three tubes, with the heaviest concentration of red blood cells in tube 1 and diminishing amounts in all subsequent tubes. In an intracranial hemorrhage, the red blood cells will be evenly distributed among all the tubes. If only one tube of CSF is collected, it should be submitted to microbiology first. The volume of CSF that can be collected is based on the volume available in the patient (adult versus neonate) and the opening pressure of the CSF when the needle first punctures the subarachnoid space. An elevated pressure requires the CSF fluid to be withdrawn more slowly, which may prevent the collection of a larger volume. The volume of CSF is critical for detecting certain microorganisms, such as mycobacteria and fungi. A minimum of 5 to 10 mL is recommended for detecting these agents by centrifugation and subsequent culture. When the laboratory receives an inadequate volume of CSF, the physician should be consulted regarding the order of priority for laboratory tests. Processing too little specimen lowers the sensitivity of laboratory tests, which may lead to false-negative results. This is potentially more harmful to patient care than performing an additional lumbar puncture to obtain the necessary amount of sample.

CSF should be hand-delivered immediately (≤15 minutes at room temperature) to the laboratory. Certain agents, such as *S. pneumoniae*, may not be detectable after an hour or longer. Specimens for microbiology studies should never be refrigerated; if not rapidly processed, CSF should be incubated (35°C) or left at room temperature. One exception to this rule involves CSF for viral studies. These specimens may be refrigerated for as long as 48 hours after collection or frozen at −70°C if a longer delay is anticipated until they are processed and inoculated into culture media. CSF for viral studies should never be frozen at temperatures above −70°C. CSF samples for viral identification should also not be added to transport media as they do not require antimicrobials to suppress other microorganisms. In addition, dilution using transport media may cause false-negative results. If not processed immediately, CSF specimen for hematology studies can be refrigerated, whereas the CSF for chemistry and serology can be frozen (−20°C).

Information gathered from specimen analysis should be promptly relayed to the clinician, who can directly affect therapeutic outcome. Such specimens should be processed immediately upon receipt in the laboratory (STAT) and results reported to the physician as soon as possible.

Initial Processing

Initial processing of CSF for bacterial, fungal, or parasitic studies includes centrifugation of all specimens with a volume greater than 1 mL for least 15 minutes at 1500×*g*. CSF specimens collected for viral nucleic acid–based tests should not be centrifuged prior to nucleic acid extraction, as most viral nucleic acid will be cell associated. Specimens in which cryptococci or mycobacteria are suspected require special handling. (Discussions of techniques for culturing CSF for mycobacteria and fungi are found in Chapters 42 and 58, respectively.) If less than 1 mL of CSF is available, the specimens should be Gram stained and plated directly to blood, chocolate agar, and primary fungal isolation media, when appropriate. For bacterial culture, the supernatant is removed to a sterile tube, leaving approximately 0.5 mL of fluid. For fungal culture, the supernatant should not be removed unless a portion is required for cryptococcal antigen testing. The remaining fluid is used to suspend the sediment for visual examination or culture. Mixing of the sediment after the supernatant has been removed is critical for bacterial culture. Forcefully aspirating the sediment up and down into a sterile pipette several times will adequately disperse the organisms that remained adherent to the bottom of the tube after centrifugation. Laboratories that use a sterile pipette to remove portions of the sediment from underneath the supernatant will miss a significant number of positive specimens. The supernatant can be used to test for the presence of antigens, for rapid diagnostic tests (vertical flow immunochromatography), to test for *N. meningitidis,* or for chemistry evaluations (e.g., protein, glucose, lactate, C-reactive protein). As a safeguard, the laboratorian should keep the supernatant even if it has no immediate use.

Cerebrospinal Fluid Laboratory Results

As previously mentioned, CSF is also removed for analysis of cells, protein, and glucose. Ideally, the glucose content of the peripheral blood is determined simultaneously for comparison with CSF levels. General guidelines for the interpretation of results are shown in Table 70.2.

Because the results of hematologic and chemical tests directly relate to the probability of infection, communication between the physician and the microbiology laboratory is essential. The diagnosis of acute bacterial meningitis can be excluded in patients with normal fluid parameters in almost all cases, precluding further expensive and labor-intensive microbiologic processing beyond a standard smear and culture (which must be included in all cases). One exception is a patient infected with *Listeria monocytogenes.* Forty percent of patients with listeriosis demonstrate a positive CSF culture for isolation of the organism; however, the CSF may demonstrate normal cell counts and the Gram stain may not show any bacteria. *L. monocytogenes* can present as meningitis, encephalitis, abscess, or ventriculitis. Similar criteria have been used to exclude performance of smear and culture for tuberculosis and syphilis serology on CSF specimens.

Visual Detection of Etiologic Agents

After centrifugation, the resulting CSF sediment may be visually examined for the presence of cells and organisms.

Stained Smear of Sediment

Gram stain must be performed on all CSF sediments. False-positive smears have resulted from inadvertent use of contaminated slides. Therefore use of alcohol-dipped and flamed or autoclaved slides is recommended. After thoroughly mixing the sediment, a heaped drop is placed on the surface of a sterile or alcohol-cleaned slide. The sediment should never be spread out on the slide surface, because this increases the difficulty of finding small numbers of microorganisms. The drop of sediment is allowed to air dry, is heat or methanol fixed, and is stained by either Gram stain (Fig. 70.3) or acridine orange. The acridine orange fluorochrome stain may allow faster examination of the slide under high-power magnification (400×) and thus a more thorough examination. The brightly fluorescing bacteria will be easily visible. All suspicious smears can be stained using the Gram

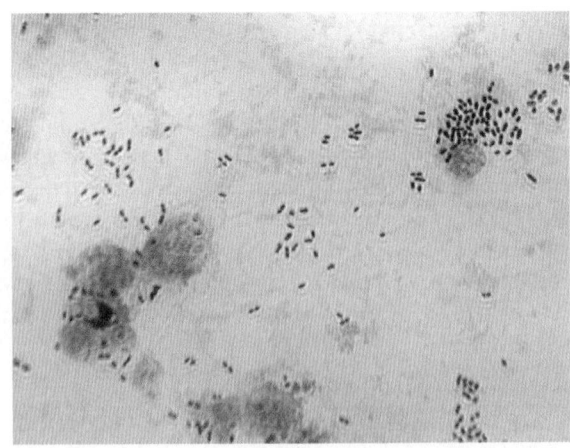

• **Fig. 70.3** Gram stain of cerebrospinal fluid showing white blood cells and many gram-positive diplococci. This specimen subsequently grew *Streptococcus pneumoniae.*

stain (directly over the acridine orange) to confirm the presence and morphology of organisms.

Using a cytospin centrifuge to prepare slides for staining has also been found to be an excellent alternative procedure. This method for preparing smears for staining concentrates cellular material and bacterial cells up to a 1000-fold. By centrifugation, a small amount of CSF (or other body fluid) is concentrated onto a circular area of a microscopic slide (Fig. 70.4), fixed, stained, and then examined.

The presence or absence of bacteria, inflammatory cells, and erythrocytes should be reported after examination. Based on demographic and clinical patient data and Gram stain morphology, the cause of most bacterial meningitis cases can be presumptively determined within the first 30 minutes after receipt of the specimen.

Wet Preparation

Amoebas are best observed by examining thoroughly mixed sediment as a wet preparation under phase-contrast microscopy. If a phase-contrast microscope is not available, observing under light microscopy with the condenser closed slightly can be used as an alternative. Amoebas are identifiable by their typical slow, methodical movement in one direction via pseudopodia. The organisms may require a little time under the warm light of the microscope before they begin to move. Organisms must be distinguished from motile macrophages, which occasionally occurs in CSF. If a wet preparation is suspicious, a trichrome stain can assist in the differentiation of amoebas from somatic cells. The pathogenic amoebas can be cultured on a lawn of *K. pneumoniae* or *E. coli* (Chapter 46).

India Ink Stain

The large polysaccharide capsule of *Cryptococcus* spp. allows these organisms to be visualized by the India ink stain. However, latex agglutination testing for capsular antigen is more sensitive and extremely specific. Lateral flow assays are now available for the primary screening of CSF for suspected cases of cryptococcal meningitis. Antigen testing is

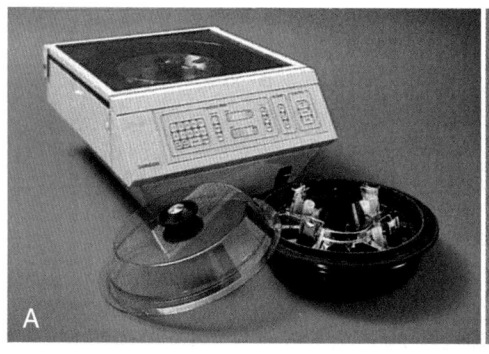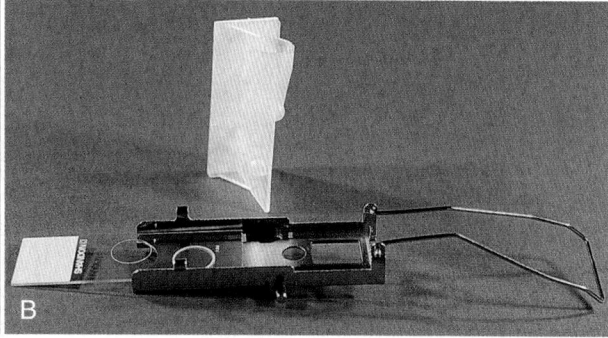

• **Fig. 70.4** (A) Cytocentrifuge. (B) Device used to prepare the concentrated smears of material from body fluid specimens such as cerebrospinal fluid by cytocentrifugation. (A, Courtesy Cytospin 2, Shandon, Inc., Pittsburgh, PA.)

recommended over the use of an India ink stain. Furthermore, strains of *Cryptococcus* spp. that infect patients with AIDS may not possess detectable capsules, making culture essential. To perform the India ink preparation, a drop of CSF sediment is mixed with one-third volume of India ink. The India ink can be protected against contamination by adding 0.05 mL thimerosal (Merthiolate, Sigma Chemical Co., St. Louis, MO) to the stain. After mixing the CSF and ink to make a smooth suspension, a coverslip is applied to the drop, and the preparation is examined under high-power magnification (400×) for characteristic encapsulated yeast cells, which can be confirmed by examination under oil immersion. Inexperienced microbiologists must be careful not to confuse white blood cells with yeast. The presence of encapsulated buds, smaller than the mother cell, is diagnostic.

Direct Detection of Etiologic Agents

Antigen

Commercial reagents and kits are available for the rapid detection of antigen in the CSF; the following sections review the methodologies used; for more detailed specifics, refer to Chapter 9.

Bacteria. Rapid antigen detection from CSF has been largely accomplished by the techniques of latex agglutination (Chapter 9). All commercial agglutination systems use the principle of an antibody-coated particle capable of binding to specific antigen, resulting in macroscopically visible agglutination. The soluble capsular polysaccharide found in the common etiologic agents of meningitis, including the group B streptococcal polysaccharide, are well suited to serve as bridging antigens. The agglutination assays may contain either a polyclonal or monoclonal antibody or an antigen from an infectious agent.

In general, the commercial systems have been developed for use with CSF, urine, or serum, although results with serum have not been as diagnostically useful as those with CSF. Soluble antigens from *Streptococcus agalactiae* and *H. influenzae* may concentrate in the urine. Urine, however, seems to produce a higher incidence of nonspecific reactions than either serum or CSF. The manufacturers' directions must be followed for performance of antigen detection test

systems for different specimen types. Although some of the systems require pretreatment of samples (usually heating for 5 minutes), not all manufacturers recommend pretreatment. The reagents, however, may yield false positives or cross reactions if the specimen is not pretreated. Interference by rheumatoid factor and other substances, more often present in body fluids other than CSF, has also been reported. The rapid extraction of antigen procedure (REAP; Evolve Procedure 70.1) has been shown to effectively reduce a substantial portion of nonspecific and false-positive reactions, at least for tests performed with latex particle reagents. This procedure is recommended for laboratories that use commercial body fluid antigen detection kits. Some commercial systems have an extraction procedure included in the protocol.

Based on the findings of several studies, only a limited number of clinically useful situations warrant bacterial antigen testing (BAT). Examples include CSF specimens from previously treated patients and Gram stain–negative CSF specimens with abnormal parameters (elevated protein, decreased glucose, or an abnormal white blood cell count). The assays are not substitutes for properly performed smears and cultures. Some of the assays demonstrate a decreased sensitivity and specificity. Considering these limitations, practice guidelines for the diagnosis and management of bacterial meningitis do not recommend routine use of BAT.

***Cryptococcus* spp.** Reagents for the detection of the polysaccharide capsular antigen of *Cryptococcus* spp. are available commercially. CSF specimens that yield positive results for cryptococcal antigen should be tested with a second latex agglutination test for rheumatoid factor. The commercial test systems incorporate rheumatoid factor testing in the protocol. A positive rheumatoid factor test renders the cryptococcal latex test uninterpretable, and the results should be reported as such, unless the rheumatoid factor antibodies have been inactivated. Undiluted specimens used in latex agglutination assays or enzyme immunoassays containing large amounts of capsular antigen may yield a false-negative reaction caused by a prozone phenomenon. Patients with AIDS may have an antigen titer more than 100,000, requiring many dilutions to reach an end-point. Serial dilution protocols are useful for monitoring a patient's response to treatment, as well as for initial diagnosis.

Lateral flow assays are now available (the IMMY cryptococcal LFA [Abacus ALS, Meadowbrook, Queensland, Australia]), and demonstrate superior sensitivity to latex agglutination assays. In addition, the turn-around time for results is shorter, and they can be used on urine samples and capillary blood samples.

Nucleic Acid Detection

Traditional methods, including Gram stain and culture, can take several days to identify the etiological agent associated with CSF infections resulting in prolonged antimicrobial therapies and lengthened hospital stays. With the introduction of amplification technologies, such as PCR, many reports in the literature recommend the application of nucleic acid–based technologies for the diagnosis of CNS infections caused by various microorganisms. Published data indicate that nucleic acid–based assays demonstrate increased sensitivity and specificity compared with presently available techniques, particularly of CNS infections caused by herpes simplex virus and enteroviruses. PCR testing for HSV, EBV, CMV, and enterovirus in CNS infections has a sensitivity nearing 100%.

The FilmArray meningitis/encephalitis panel (BioFire Diagnostics, Salt Lake City, UT) is a US Food and Drug Administration (FDA)-cleared, multiplex panel that detects 14 pathogens including 6 bacterial, 1 fungal, and 7 viral infectious agents. It is estimated that up to 50% of cases of encephalitis and 60% of cases of meningitis fail to identify an etiological agent. Delays in treatment may result in increased morbidity and mortality, and unnecessary treatment promotes the development of antibiotic resistance and increased health care costs. However, a retrospective study by Dack and colleagues indicates that the use of the BioFire FilmArray does not significantly reduce the length of stay or antimicrobial treatment associated with meningitis. This may be due to factors that include clinicians concerned with other health care–associated risks and continuing antimicrobial therapy in the presence of negative results. A significant advantage to using traditional culture methods in combination with nucleic acid–based testing is the identification of CSF infections that include more than one infectious pathogen. Although a low percentage, the FilmArray ME panel has been reported to identify several cases of coinfections when routine testing resulted in the identification of a single pathogen. Examples include bacterial and fungal pathogens such as *H. influenzae* and *L. monocytogenes*, *Cryptococcus* spp. and *S. pneumoniae*, *N. meningitidis,* and *S. pneumoniae*. Other coinfections included viral agents such as HSV-1 and HHV-6, CMV, and VZV, or combination bacterial viral infection with *H. influenzae* and HHV-6 or a combination fungal and viral infection with *Cryptococcus* spp. and HSV-1. Other advanced techniques are continually being developed, including an advanced fragment PCR based analysis capable of identifying 22 different pathogens associated with meningitis or encephalitis by F. Long et al. PCR analysis has also been successfully used to diagnose neurosyphilis. Additional multiplex laboratory developed tests not only include bacterial, fungal, and viral agents, but others also include the detection of the free-living amoebic parasites *Balamuthia mandrillaris* and *Acanthamoeba*. The successful detection of parasites in CNS using these assays has not demonstrated sufficient clinical sensitivity and false positive results. The identification of parasitic pathogens in the CNS using nucleic acid testing requires extensive development and evaluation. Although nucleic acid–based testing does not appear to decrease length of stay or the use of antimicrobials associated with bacterial, fungal, and viral pathogens, the diagnostic sensitivity and specificity, along with the identification of pathogens that are not detected by traditional methods and the identification of rare co-infections, are significant and support the use of nucleic acid–based testing in the diagnosis and treatment of CSF infections. A variety of nucleic acid–based testing methods are now currently available.

Next generation sequencing, although not widely available in routine clinical laboratories, has been used to identify pathogens in undiagnosed infectious encephalitis. Reports include the identification of astrovirus and neuroleptospirosis both in immunocompromised patients, HSV-1, HSV-2, and *Brucella* sp. in multiple cases of neurobrucellosis. The diagnosis of neurobrucellosis is significantly challenging as the signs and symptoms are extremely nonspecific and resemble other infectious diseases including tuberculosis, syphilis, Lyme disease, and *Cryptococcus* spp. infection. Traditional methods for the diagnosis of neurobrucellosis demonstrate a very low sensitivity; 28% demonstrate positive blood cultures and 15% show positive CSF cultures. These cases indicate a significant important step in the rapid and accurate diagnosis for patients of unexpected diagnoses in suspected cases of CNS infections using next generation sequencing.

Matrix-Assisted Laser Desorption Ionization Time-of-Flight Mass Spectrometry

Matrix-assisted laser desorption ionization time-of-flight mass spectrometry (MALDI-TOF MS) requires growth of the organism before application and spectral analysis. Studies are currently underway to determine the efficiency for the direct detection of microorganisms in CSF in cases of bacterial meningitis. A study by Bishop et al., using fresh CSF samples, demonstrated a sensitivity of 76.2% for the identification of gram-negative bacilli postneurosurgical meningitis; however, for gram-positive cocci postsurgical and community-acquired meningitis, only a single sample was identified correctly. The interpretation of direct specimen Gram stains, followed by culture or nucleic acid–based testing, remain the gold standard for directing empirical antibiotic treatment of patients in suspected cases of meningitis, encephalitis, and other CNS infections.

Culture

Most cases of bacterial meningitis are caused by a single organism and require a limited number of culture media.

Bacteria and Fungi

Routine bacteriologic media should include a chocolate agar plate, 5% sheep blood agar plate, and an enrichment broth, usually thioglycolate without indicator. The chocolate agar plate is needed to recover fastidious organisms, most notably *H. influenzae,* which are unable to grow on blood agar plates; the use of the blood agar plate aids in the recognition of *S. pneumoniae*. After vortexing the sediment and preparing smears, several drops of the sediment should be inoculated to each medium. Plates should be incubated at 37°C in 5% to 10% carbon dioxide (CO_2) for at least 72 hours. If a CO_2 incubator is not available, a candle jar or an automated environmental vacuum system can be used to create a CO_2-enriched atmosphere. The broth should be incubated in air at 37°C for at least 5 to 10 days. The broth cap must be loose to allow free exchange of air. If organisms morphologically resembling anaerobic bacteria are seen on the Gram stain or if a brain abscess is suspected, an anaerobic blood agar plate may also be inoculated. These media will support the growth of almost all bacterial pathogens and several fungi.

The symptoms of chronic meningitis that prompt a physician to request fungal cultures are the same as those for tuberculous meningitis. Cultures for mycobacteria are addressed in Chapter 42. For CSF fungal cultures, two drops of the well-mixed sediment should be inoculated onto Sabouraud dextrose agar or other non–blood-containing medium and brain-heart infusion with 5% sheep blood. Fungal media should be incubated in room air at 30°C for 4 weeks. If possible, two sets of media should be inoculated, with one set incubated at 30°C and the other at 35°C.

Parasites and Viruses

Conditions for the culture of free-living amoebae and viral agents are discussed in Chapters 46 and 64, respectively. The physician must notify the laboratory to culture these agents.

Brain Abscess/Biopsies

Specimen Collection, Transport, and Processing. Whenever possible, biopsy specimens or aspirates from brain abscesses should be submitted to the laboratory under anaerobic conditions. Several devices are commercially available to transport biopsy specimens under anaerobic conditions. Swabs are not considered an optimum specimen, but if used to collect abscess material they should be sent in a transport device that maintains an anaerobic environment.

Biopsy specimens should be minced in sterile saline before plating and smear preparation. This processing should be kept to a minimum to reduce oxygenation.

Abscess and biopsy specimens submitted for culture should be inoculated onto 5% sheep blood and chocolate agar plates. Plates should be incubated in 5% to 10% CO_2 for 72 hours at 35°C. In addition, an anaerobic agar plate and broth with an anaerobic indicator, vitamin K, and hemin should be inoculated and incubated in an anaerobic environment at 35°C. Anaerobic culture plates are incubated for a minimum of 72 hours but are examined after 48 hours of incubation. Anaerobic broths should be incubated

for a minimum of 5 days. If a fungal cause is suspected, fungal media, such as brain-heart infusion with blood and antibiotics or inhibitory mold agar, should be inoculated.

ⓔ Visit the Evolve site for a complete list of procedures, review questions, and case studies.

Bibliography

Albright RE, Christenson RH, Emlet JL, et al.: Issues in cerebrospinal fluid management: acid-fast bacillus smear and culture, *Am J Clin Pathol* 95:418–423, 1991.

Albright RE, Graham CB, Christenson RH, et al.: Issues in cerebrospinal fluid management: CSF venereal disease research laboratory testing, *Am J Clin Pathol* 95:397–401, 1991.

Al Masalma MA, Lonjon M, Richet H, et al.: Metagenomic analysis of brain abscesses identifies specific bacterial associations, *Clin Infect Dis* 54:202–210, 2011.

Bennett J, Dolin R, Blaser M: *Principles and practice of infectious diseases*, ed 9, Philadelphia, PA, 2020, Elsevier.

Bishop B, Geffen Y, Plaut A, et al.: The use of matrix-assisted laser desorption/ionization time-of-flight mass spectrometry for rapid bacterial identification in patients with smear-positive bacterial meningitis, *Clin Microbiol Infect* 24(2):171–174, 2018.

Carroll KC, Pfaller MA: *Manual of clinical microbiology*, ed 12, Washington, DC, 2019, ASM Press.

Castro R, Aguas MJ, Batista T, et al.: Detection of *Treponema pallidum* sp. *pallidum* DNA in cerebral spinal fluid by two PCR techniques, *J Clin Lab Anal* 30(5):628–632, 2016.

Centers for Disease Control and Prevention: *Epidemic/epizootic West Nile virus in the United States: guidelines for surveillance, prevention and control–3rd revision*, 2003, Available at www.cdc.gov/ncidod/dvbid/westnile/resources/wnvguidelines2003.pdf.

Conen A, Walti LN, Merlo A, et al.: Characteristics and treatment outcome of cerebrospinal fluid shunt-associated infections in adults: a retrospective analysis over an 11-year period, *Clin Infect Dis* 47:73–82, 2008.

Culbreath K, Melanson S, Gale J, et al.: Validation and retrospective clinical evaluation of quantitative 16S rRNA gene metagenomics sequencing assay for bacterial pathogen detection in body fluids, *J Mol Diagn* 21:913–923, 2019, https://doi.org/10.1016/j.jmoldx.2019.05.002.

Dack K, Pankow S, Abla E: Contribution of the BioFire FilmArray meningitis/encephalitis panel. Assessing antimicrobial duration and length of stay, *Kans J Med* 12(1):1–3, 2019.

Fan S, Ren H, Wei Y, et al.: Next-generation sequencing of the cerebral spinal fluid in the diagnosis of neurobrucellosis, *Int J Infect Dis* 67:20–24, 2018.

Garcia LS: *Diagnostic medical parasitology*, ed 6, Washington DC, 2016, ASM Press.

Guan H, Shen A, Lv X, et al.: Detection of virus in CSF from the cases with meningoencephalitis by next-generation sequencing, *J Neurovirol* 22(2):240–245, 2016.

Hariharan S: BK virus nephritis after renal transplantation: a review, *Kidney Int* 69:655–662, 2006.

Hayward RA, Shapiro MF, Oye RK: Laboratory testing on cerebrospinal fluid: a reappraisal, *Lancet* 1:1–4, 1987.

Huang C, Morse D, Slater B, et al.: Multiple-year experience in the diagnosis of viral central nervous system infections with a panel of polymerase chain reaction assays for detection of 11 viruses, *Clin Infect Dis* 39:630–635, 2004.

Korimbocus J, Scaramozzino N, Lacroix B, et al.: DNA probe array for the simultaneous identification of herpesviruses, enteroviruses, and flaviviruses, *J Clin Microbiol* 43:3779–3787, 2005.

Liesman RM, Strasburg AP, Heitman AK, et al.: Evaluation of a commercial multiplex molecular panel for diagnosis of infectious meningitis and encephalitis, *J Clin Microbiol* 56(4):e01927–17, 2018.

Lindsey NP, Lehman JA, Staples E, et al.: West Nile virus and other arboviral diseases-United States, 2013, *Morb Mortal Wkly Rep* 63(24):521–526, 2014.

Long F, Kong M, Wu S, et al.: Development and validation of an advanced fragment-analysis based assay for the detection of 22 pathogens in the cerebrospinal fluid of patients with meningitis and encephalitis, *J Clin Lab Anal* 33(3):e22707, 2019.

Mongkolrattanothai K, Naccache SN, Bender JM, et al.: Neurobrucellosis: unexpected answer from metagenomic next-generation sequencing, *J Pediatric Infect Dis Soc* 6(4):393–398, 2017.

Onyango CO, Loparev V, Lidechi S, et al.: Evaluation of a Taqman array card for detection of central nervous system infections, *J Clin Microbiol* 55(7):2035–2044, 2017.

Parkkinen J, Korhonen TK, Pere A, et al.: Binding sites in the rat brain for *Escherichia coli* S fimbriae associated with neonatal meningitis, *J Clin Invest* 81:860–865, 1988.

Piquet AL, Lyons JL: Infectious meningitis and encephalitis, *Semin Neurol* 36(4):367–372, 2016.

Plaut AG: The IgA1 proteases of pathogenic bacteria, *Annu Rev Microbiol* 37:603–622, 1983.

Poppert S, Essig A, Stoehr B, et al.: Rapid diagnosis of bacterial meningitis by real-time PCR and fluorescence *in situ* hybridization, *J Clin Microbiol* 43:3390–3397, 2005.

Schwartz MN: Bacterial meningitis—a view of the past 90 years, *N Engl J Med* 351:1826–1828, 2004.

Segawa S, Sawai S, Murata S, et al.: Direct application of MALDI-TOF mass spectrometry to cerebralspinal fluid for rapid pathogen identification in a patient with bacterial meningitis, *Clin Chim Acta* 435:59–61, 2014.

Smith LP, Hunter Jr KW, Hemming VG, et al.: Improved detection of bacterial antigens by latex agglutination after rapid extraction from body fluids, *J Clin Microbiol* 20:981–984, 1984.

Strasinger S, DiLorenzo M: *Urinalysis and body fluids*, ed 5, Philadelphia, PA, 2008, FA Davis.

Tarai B, Das P: FilmArray meningitis/encephalitis (ME) panel, a rapid molecular platform for diagnosis of CNS infections in a tertiary care hospital in North India: one-and-half-year review, *Neurol Sci* 40(1):81–88, 2019.

Tunkel AR, Hartman BJ, Kaplan SL, et al.: Practice guidelines for the management of bacterial meningitis, *Clin Infect Dis* 39:1267–1284, 2004.

van de Beek D, de Gan J, Spanjaard L, et al.: Clinical features and prognostic factors in adults with bacterial meningitis, *N Engl J Med* 351:1849–1859, 2004.

Virji M, Alexandrescu C, Ferguson DJ, et al.: Variations in the expression of pili: the effect on adherence of *Neisseria meningitidis* to human epithelial and endothelial cells, *Mol Microbiol* 6:1271–1279, 1992.

Virji M, Kayhty H, Ferguson DJ, et al.: The role of pili in the interactions of pathogenic *Neisseria* with cultured human endothelial cells, *Mol Microbiol* 5:1831–1841, 1991.

Wilhelm C, Ellner JJ: Chronic meningitis, *Neurol Clin* 4:115–141, 1986.

Walsh TJ, Hayden RT, Larone DH: *Larone's medically important fungi: a guide to identification*, ed 6, Washington, DC, 2018, ASM Press.

71

Infections of the Eyes, Ears, and Sinuses

OBJECTIVES

1. Describe the anatomy of the eye, including naming the external and internal structures.
2. Name the three tissues, outer to inner, of the eyeball.
3. Differentiate normal flora of the eye and potential pathogens.
4. Describe the defense mechanisms of the eye for protection from infective agents.
5. Define the following diseases of the eye: blepharitis, hordeolum, conjunctivitis, keratitis, uveitis, and endophthalmitis.
6. List the common types of eye infections, the associated etiologic agents, and the at-risk patient population for each.
7. Define keratitis, and identify the organisms associated with the infection, the virulence factors, and the antimicrobial-resistant properties for each.
8. Define endophthalmitis, explain how it is contracted, and identify the etiologic agents.
9. Explain mycotic endophthalmitis and list the risk factors that may predispose an individual to this type of infection.
10. Define a periocular infection, and list some of the associated infectious agents and the different types of clinical presentations of the infection.
11. Identify the anatomic parts of the ear, and list the structures associated with each region within the ear.
12. Define the external ear infections acute externa otitis and chronic externa otitis; list the potential pathogens.
13. Define otitis media; differentiate acute and chronic otitis media and name the most commonly encountered pathogens and the age group most often affected by this disease.
14. Explain the laboratory method used to culture the eye and the ear, including appropriate media; describe collection and transportation requirements.
15. Differentiate acute and chronic sinusitis.
16. Explain why the organisms that cause otitis media are often the same ones responsible for sinusitis.
17. List the collection methods and culture media used for cases of sinusitis.
18. Correlate signs and symptoms of infection with the results of laboratory diagnostic procedures for the identification of the etiologic agent associated with infections of the eye, ear, and sinuses.

Eyes

Anatomy

Eye (ocular) infections can be divided based on the area of the eye infected. The external structures of the eye—eyelids, conjunctiva, sclera, and cornea—are depicted in Fig. 71.1. The eyeball comprises three layers. From the outside in, these tissues are the sclera, choroid, and retina. The **sclera** is a tough, white, fibrous tissue (i.e., "white" of the eye). The anterior (toward the front) portion of the sclera is the **cornea,** which is transparent and has no blood vessels. A mucous membrane, called the **conjunctiva,** lines each eyelid and extends onto the surface of the eye itself. The **choroid** is the vascular layer of the eye that contains the connective tissue. The **retina,** the innermost layer of the eye, contains light-sensitive cells that transmit signals and images to the optical nerve.

Only a small portion of the eye is exposed to the environment; about five-sixths of the eyeball is enclosed within bony orbits shaped like four-sided pyramids. The large interior space of the eyeball is divided into two sections: the anterior and posterior cavities (Fig. 71.1). The anterior cavity is filled with a clear and watery substance called **aqueous humor;** the posterior cavity is filled with a soft, gelatin-like substance called **vitreous humor.**

Infections can occur in the eye's **lacrimal** (pertaining to tears) system. The major components of the lacrimal apparatus include the lacrimal gland, lacrimal canaliculi (short channel), and lacrimal sac.

Resident Microbiota

Rather sparse indigenous microbiota is present in the conjunctival sac. *Staphylococcus epidermidis* and *Lactobacillus* spp. are the most common organisms; *Cutibacterium acnes* may also be present. *Staphylococcus aureus* is found in less than 30% of individuals, and *Haemophilus influenzae* colonizes 0.4% to 25%. *Moraxella catarrhalis,* various Enterobacterales, and various streptococci (*Streptococcus pyogenes, Streptococcus pneumoniae,* other alpha-hemolytic and

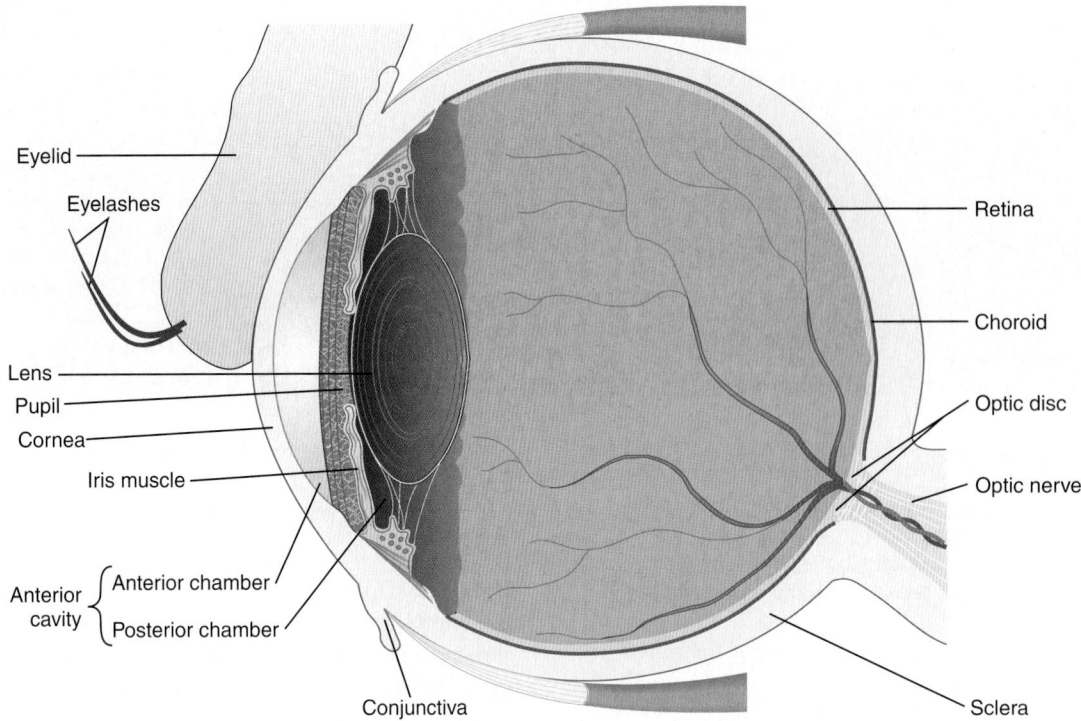

• **Fig. 71.1** Key anatomic structures of the eye. (Modified from Thibodeau GA, Patton KT. *Anatomy and Physiology.* 2nd ed. St Louis: Mosby; 1993.)

gamma-hemolytic forms) are found in a very small percentage of individuals.

Diseases

The eye and its associated structures are uniquely predisposed to infection by various microorganisms. The major infections of the eye are listed in Table 71.1, along with a brief description of the disease.

Pathogenesis

The eye has several defense mechanisms. The eyelashes prevent the entry of foreign material into the eye. The lids blink 15 to 20 times per minute, during which time secretions of the lacrimal glands and goblet cells wash away bacteria and foreign matter. Lysozyme and immunoglobulin A (IgA) are secreted locally and serve as part of the eye's natural defense mechanisms. Also, the eyes themselves are enclosed within the bony orbits. The delicate intraocular structures are enveloped in a tough collagenous coat (sclera and cornea). If these barriers are broken by a penetrating injury or ulceration, infection may occur. Infection can also reach the eye via the bloodstream from another site of infection. Finally, because three of the four walls of the orbit are contiguous with the paranasal (facial) sinuses, sinus infections may extend directly to the periocular orbital structures.

Epidemiology and Etiology of Disease

Blepharitis and Hordeolum

Blepharitis may appear as a bump on the eyelid that is red and swollen, resembling a pimple. Most bumps on the

eyelid are caused by an inflamed oil gland on the edge of the eyelid and are a form of **hordeolum**—more commonly referred to as a **stye.** A stye is more of an acute infection, whereas blepharitis tends to present as a chronic condition that can cause conjunctivitis, functional tear deficiency, or corneal inflammation and infection. Bacteria, viruses, and occasionally lice or *Demodex* mites can cause blepharitis, an infection of the eyelid surrounding the eye. Although occasionally isolated from surfaces surrounding the healthy eye, *S. aureus* and *S. epidermidis* are the most common infectious agents associated with the development of a stye and blepharitis in developed countries. Symptoms include burning, itching, the sensation of the presence of a foreign body, and crusting of the eyelids.

Viruses can also cause a vesicular (blisterlike) eruption of the eyelids. Herpes simplex virus (HSV) produces vesicles on the eyelids that typically crust and heal with scarring within 2 weeks. Unfortunately, once this vesicular stage has resolved, the lesions can be confused with bacterial blepharitis.

Finally, the pubic louse *Phthirus pubis* has a predilection for eyelash hair. The presence of this organism produces irritation, itch, and swelling of the lid margins (edges).

Conjunctivitis

Bacterial **conjunctivitis,** commonly referred to as "pink eye," is the most common type of ocular infection and may be caused by allergies, bacterial, parasitic, fungal, or viral infection. The principal causes of acute conjunctivitis in a normal host are listed in Table 71.1. Age-related factors are key in the identification of the etiologic agent. Neonatal conjunctivitis (ophthalmia neonatorum) occurs within

TABLE 71.1 Infections of the Eye

Infection	Description	Bacteria	Viruses	Fungi	Parasites
Blepharitis	Inflammation of the margins (edges) of the eyelids (eyelids, eyelashes, or associated pilosebaceous glands or meibomian glands); symptoms include irritation, redness, burning sensation, and occasional itching. Condition is typically bilateral.	*Staphylococcus aureus, Pseudomonas aeruginosa, Capnocytophaga ochracea*	Herpes simplex virus (HSV)	*Malassezia furfur, Blastomyces* sp.	*Phthirus pubis, Leishmania donovani, Demodex* mites
Conjunctivitis	Inflammation of the conjunctiva; symptoms vary according to the etiologic agent, but most patients have swelling of the conjunctiva, inflammatory exudates, and burning and itching.	*Streptococcus pneumoniae, Haemophilus influenzae, S. aureus, Haemophilus* spp., *Chlamydia trachomatis, Neisseria gonorrhoeae, Streptococcus pyogenes, Moraxella* spp., *Corynebacterium* spp., *P. aeruginosa*	Adenoviruses, HSV, varicella zoster, Epstein-Barr virus (EBV), influenza virus, paramyxovirus, rubella, human immunodeficiency virus (HIV) enterovirus, coxsackie A, variola (smallpox), SARS-CoV-2	*Candida* spp., *Blastomyces* spp., *Sporothrix schenckii, Rhinosporidium seeberi*	*Leishmania* spp., *Microsporidia* spp., *Loa loa, Demodex* (mites)
Keratitis	Inflammation of the cornea; although there are no specific clinical signs to confirm infection, most patients complain of pain and usually some decrease in vision, with or without discharge from the eye.	*S. aureus, S. epidermidis, S. pneumoniae, S. pyogenes,* viridans streptococci, *Enterococcus faecalis, Peptostreptococcus, P. aeruginosa,* Enterobacterales, *Moraxella lacunata, Bacillus* spp., *Mycobacterium* spp., spirochetes, *C. trachomatis*	HSV, adenoviruses, varicella zoster, vaccinia, Epstein-Barr, rubeola, enteroviruses, and coxsackie virus	*Fusarium, Aspergillus* spp., *Candida* spp., *Acremonium, Alternaria, Penicillium, Bipolaris, Nosema, Vittaforma, Encephalitozoon* spp.	*Acanthamoeba* spp., *Onchocerca volvulus, Leishmania brasiliensis, Trypanosoma* spp.
Keratoconjunctivitis	Infection involving both the conjunctiva and cornea; ophthalmia neonatorum is an acute conjunctivitis or keratoconjunctivitis of the newborn caused by either *N. gonorrhoeae* or *C. trachomatis*.	Refer to agents for keratitis/conjunctivitis	Refer to agents for keratitis/conjunctivitis	Refer to agents for keratitis	*Toxoplasma gondii, Toxocara*
Chorioretinitis and uveitis	Inflammation of the retina and underlying choroid or the uvea; infection can result in loss of vision.	*Mycobacterium tuberculosis, Treponema pallidum, Borrelia burgdorferi*	Cytomegalovirus, HSV	*Candida* spp.	*T. gondii, Toxocara, Treponema pallidum, Brucella* spp.

Continued

TABLE 71.1

TABLE 71.1 **Infections of the Eye—cont'd**

Infection	Description	Bacteria	Viruses	Fungi	Parasites
Endophthal-mitis	Infection of the aqueous or vitre-ous humor. This infection is usually caused by bacteria or fungi, is rare, develops suddenly, and progresses rapidly, often lead-ing to blindness. Pain, especially while moving the eye, and decreased vision are prominent features.	S. aureus, S. epidermi-dis, S. pneumoniae, other streptococcal species, P. aeru-ginosa, Klebsiella pneumoniae, other gram-negative organ-isms, Nocardia spp.	HSV, varicella zoster	Candida spp., Aspergil-lus spp., Fusarium spp.	Toxocara, Oncho-cerca volvulus
Lacrimal infections, canaliculitis	A rare, chronic inflammation of the lacrimal canals in which the eyelid swells and there is a thick, mucopurulent discharge.	Actinomyces, Propioni-bacterium propioni-cum			
Dacryocystis	Inflammation of the lacrimal sac that is accompanied by pain, swelling, and tenderness of the soft tissue in the medial canthal region.	S. pneumoniae, S. aureus, S. pyogenes, H. influenzae		C. albicans, Aspergillus spp.	
Dacryoadenitis	Acute infection of the lacrimal gland; these infections are rare and can be accompanied by pain, redness, and swelling of the upper eyelid and conjunctival discharge.	S. pneumoniae, S. aureus, S. pyogenes			

Note: This table is not intended to be all-inclusive for the infectious agents capable of causing eye infections.

4 weeks following birth, caused by bacterial, viral, chlamydial, or toxic reactions to chemicals. In neonates, neisserial and chlamydial infections are common and are acquired during passage through an infected vaginal canal. With the common practice of instilling antibiotic drops into the eyes of newborns in the United States, the incidence of gonococcal and chlamydial conjunctivitis has dropped dramatically. However, *Chlamydia trachomatis* remains responsible for one of the most important types of conjunctivitis, referred to as **trachoma.** Trachoma is one of the leading causes of blindness in the world, primarily in underdeveloped countries.

In children, the most common causes of bacterial conjunctivitis include *H. influenzae, S. pneumoniae,* and perhaps *S. aureus, S. pneumoniae,* and *Haemophilus aegyptius*

have been isolated from conjunctivitis epidemics. *Corynebacterium* spp. colonize the lids and conjunctiva and are the overall leading cause of conjunctivitis. Inflammation of the conjunctiva is characterized by redness, itching, and discharge, and the condition is highly contagious; it can be transferred from one eye to the other by rubbing the infected eye and can be easily transferred to other individuals.

Numerous other bacteria may also cause conjunctivitis. For example, diphtheritic conjunctivitis may occur in conjunction with diphtheria elsewhere in the body. *Moraxella lacunata* produces a localized conjunctivitis with little discharge from the eye. Distinctive clinical pictures may also occur with conjunctivitis caused by *Mycobacterium tuberculosis, Francisella tularensis, Treponema pallidum,* and *Yersinia enterocolitica.*

Fungi may be responsible for this type of infection as well, often in association with a foreign body that has been introduced into the eye or an underlying host immunologic problem. Fungi including *Candida* spp., *Blastomyces* spp., and *Sporothrix schenckii* have been associated with conjunctivitis. However, these infections are uncommon.

Parasitic conjunctivitis has been associated with *Leishmania* spp., cryptosporidium, fly larvae, and nematodes such as *Loa loa*. Parasites that are known to infect the lid margin or lashes, such as lice and mites, may cause conjunctivitis as a subsequent reaction to blepharitis caused by the organism.

In adults, the cause of conjunctivitis is usually viral, with adenovirus being the most common viral cause; 20% of such infections in children resulted from adenoviruses in one large US study, and 14% of infections in adult patients were caused by adenoviruses in another study. Adenovirus types 3, 4, and 7A are common. Most viral conjunctivitis is self-limited but is highly contagious, with the potential to cause major outbreaks. Worldwide, enterovirus 70 and coxsackievirus A24 are responsible for outbreaks and epidemics of acute hemorrhagic conjunctivitis. A coxsackievirus A24 variant has been reported with several outbreaks of hemorrhagic conjunctivitis in several countries. Patients can develop systemic symptoms including fever, fatigue, and limb pain; however, severe complications and death are rare. A lateral flow immunochromatographic cartridge test, the AdenoPlus (Rapid Pathogen Screening, Inc., Sarasota, FL), is available for the detection of ocular adenovirus infections. The test includes a built-in sampling pad that can be used to collect fluid by touching the eye. The assay demonstrates an 85% sensitivity and a 98% specificity, when compared with polymerase chain reaction (PCR). Negative results using the AdenoPlus should be confirmed by real-time PCR to avoid false negatives that would result in continued infection and damage to the eye.

Keratitis

Keratitis (corneal infection) may be caused by a variety of infectious agents, usually after some type of trauma to the ocular surface. Keratitis should be regarded as an emergency, because corneal perforation and loss of the eye can occur within 24 hours when organisms such as *Pseudomonas aeruginosa*, *S. aureus*, or HSV are involved. Bacteria account for 65% to 90% of corneal infections.

In the United States, *S. aureus*, *S. pneumoniae*, and *P. aeruginosa* account for more than 80% of all bacterial corneal ulcers. Many culture-positive cases are now being recognized as polymicrobial. A toxic factor known as **exopeptidase** has been implicated in the pathogenesis of corneal ulcer produced by *S. pneumoniae*. With *P. aeruginosa* and *Neisseria gonorrhoeae*, proteolytic enzymes are responsible for the corneal destruction. Gonococcus may cause keratitis during inadequately treated conjunctivitis. *Acinetobacter*, which may look identical microscopically to gonococcus and is resistant to penicillin and many other antimicrobial agents, can cause corneal perforation. Many other bacteria, several viruses other than HSV, and many fungi may cause

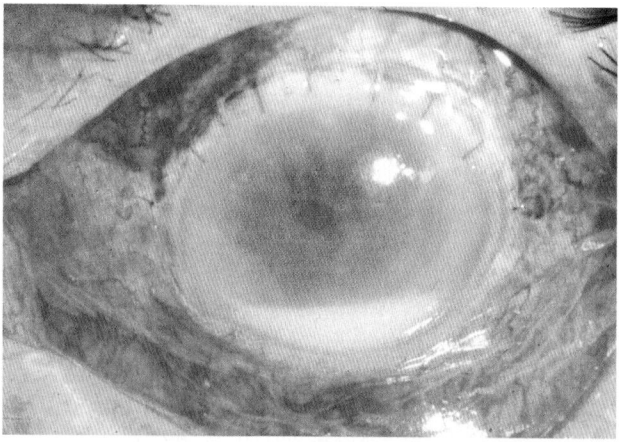

• **Fig. 71.2** Endophthalmitis. (Courtesy Donald J. D'Amico.)

keratitis. Risk factors associated with the development of fungal keratitis caused by *Candida* spp. include epithelial ulceration, topical corticosteroid use, corneal transplants, and the use of soft contact lenses. Fungal keratitis may also result as a complication of trauma.

Although still unusual, a previously rare etiologic agent of corneal infections has become more common in users of soft and extended-wear contact lenses. *Acanthamoeba* spp., free-living amoebae, can survive in improperly sterilized cleaning fluids and be introduced into the eye with the contact lens. The fungus *Fusarium* is an infectious disease associated with contact lens use or contact lens solutions. This genus of fungus is ubiquitous and can be found in soil and tap water and on many plants; fungal keratitis is rare but is usually associated with trauma to the eye from an object contaminated with plant matter. This infection can be serious and can lead to the loss of vision. Other bacterial and fungal causes of infection have also been traced to inadequate cleaning of lenses.

Additional parasites are also associated with keratitis in different geographical regions, including the microfilariae *Onchocerca volvulus*, *Leishmania* spp., microsporidia, and trypanosomes. It is important to consider potential coinfections with other organisms, as that will decrease the effectiveness of the treatment and may result in the loss of vision.

Endophthalmitis

Surgical trauma, nonsurgical trauma (uncommonly), and hematogenous spread from distant sites of infection are the typical routes of transmission for **endophthalmitis** (Fig. 71.2). The infection may be limited to specific tissues within the eye or may involve all the intraocular contents. Bacteria are the most common infectious agents responsible for endophthalmitis.

After surgery or trauma, evidence of the disease is usually identified within 24 to 48 hours. Postoperative infection involves primarily normal microbiota from the ocular surface. Although *S. epidermidis* and *S. aureus* are responsible for most cases of endophthalmitis after cataract removal, any bacterium, including those considered to be saprophytic,

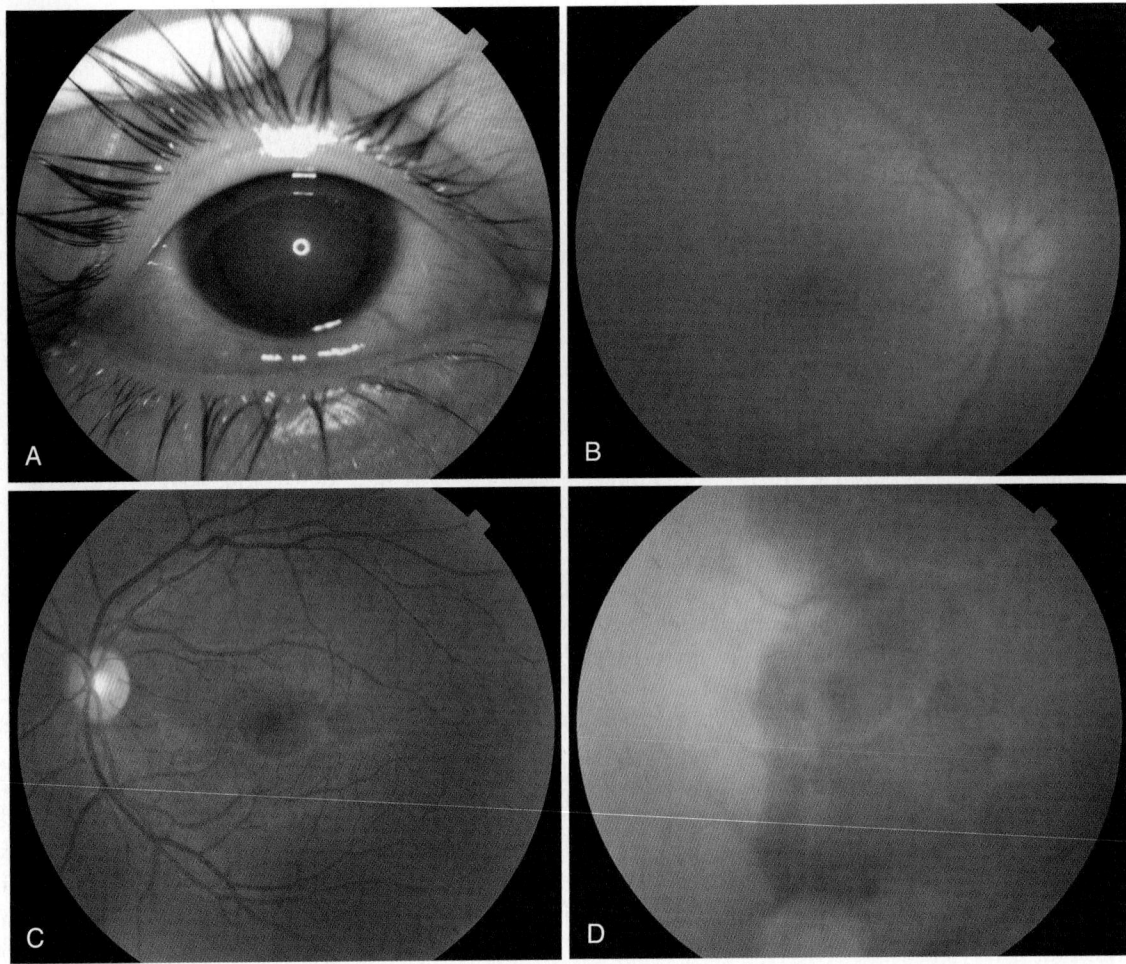

• **Fig. 71.3** Acute retinal necrosis caused by herpes simplex. (A) External view. (B) Limited funduscopic view. (C) Funduscopic view of the normal unaffected eye. (D) View of peripheral retina demonstrating peripheral necrotizing retinitis and vasculitis (whitening and hemorrhage).

may cause endophthalmitis. In hematogenous endophthalmitis, a septic focus elsewhere is usually evident before the onset of the intraocular infection. *Bacillus cereus* has caused endophthalmitis in people addicted to narcotics and after transfusion with contaminated blood. Endophthalmitis associated with meningitis may involve various organisms, including *H. influenzae*, streptococci, and *Neisseria meningitidis*. *Nocardia* endophthalmitis may follow pulmonary infection with this organism.

Mycotic infection of the eye has increased significantly since the 1980s because of the increased use of antibiotics, corticosteroids, antineoplastic chemotherapy, addictive drugs, and hyperalimentation (overeating). Fungi generally considered to be saprophytic are important causes of postoperative endophthalmitis (Table 71.1). Endogenous mycotic endophthalmitis is most often caused by *Candida albicans*. High-risk patients include those with diabetes or some other chronic underlying disease. Exogenous *Candida* spp. endophthalmitis is uncommon but may develop following surgical procedures, trauma, or keratitis. *Aspergillus* or *Fusarium* species may also be associated with trauma-related infections. Other causes of hematogenous ocular

infection include *Aspergillus, Cryptococcus, Coccidioides, Sporothrix,* and *Blastomyces.*

Endophthalmitis may be a result of viral or parasitic infections. Viral causes of endophthalmitis include HSV (Fig. 71.3), varicella (herpes) zoster virus (VZV), cytomegalovirus, and measles viruses. The most common parasitic agent associated with endophthalmitis is *Toxocara. Toxoplasma gondii* is a well-known cause of **chorioretinitis.** Thirteen percent of patients with cysticercosis (*Taenia solium*) have ocular involvement. Onchocerca usually produces keratitis, but intraocular infection also occurs.

Periocular

Canaliculitis, one of three infections of the lacrimal apparatus (Table 71.1), is an inflammation of the lacrimal canal and is usually caused by *Actinomyces* or *Propionibacterium propionicum.* Infection of the lacrimal sac (**dacryocystitis**) may involve numerous bacterial and fungal agents; the major causes are listed in Table 71.1. **Dacryoadenitis** is an uncommon infection of the lacrimal gland characterized by pain of the upper eyelid with erythema and often involves pyogenic bacteria such as *S. aureus* and streptococci.

Chronic infections of the lacrimal gland occur in tuberculosis, syphilis, leprosy, and schistosomiasis. Acute inflammation of the gland may occur during mumps and infectious mononucleosis.

Orbital cellulitis is an acute infection of the orbital contents and is most often caused by bacteria. This is a potentially serious infection because it may spread posteriorly to produce central nervous system complications. Most cases involve spread from contiguous sources such as the paranasal sinuses. In children, bloodborne bacteria, notably *H. influenzae*, may lead to orbital cellulitis. *S. aureus* is the most common etiologic agent; *S. pyogenes* and *S. pneumoniae* are also common. Anaerobes may cause cellulitis secondary to chronic sinusitis, primarily in adults. Mucormycosis of the orbit is a serious, invasive fungal infection seen particularly in patients with diabetes who have poor control of their disease, patients with acidosis from other causes, and patients with malignant disease receiving cytotoxic and immunosuppressive therapy. *Aspergillus* may produce a similar infection in the same settings but also can cause mild, chronic infections of the orbit.

Surgical techniques involving the ocular implantation of prosthetic or donor lenses have resulted in increasing numbers of iatrogenic (resulting from the activities of a physician) infections. Isolation of *C. acnes* may have clinical significance in such situations, in contrast to many other sites in which it is usually considered to be a contaminant. Nontuberculous mycobacterial periocular infections have become increasingly important in patients with systemic disease. These infections are more prevalent in immunocompromised patients.

Uveitis

The **uvea** is the pigmented, middle layer of the eye that is between the cornea-sclera and the retina. Inflammation of the uvea is termed **uveitis. Retinitis,** inflammation of the retina, is also considered in this section, even though it is technically a separate structure from the uvea. There are approximately 70 to 115 cases per 100,000 individuals who are annually affected by uveitis in the United States. More than 50% of cases of uveitis are idiopathic; however, the condition may be caused by an autoimmune reaction, infection, or trauma.

Infectious uveitis typically is a result of hematogenous spread of the agent of infection. The eye has a blood-eye barrier similar to the blood-brain barrier that must be breached for an infection to occur. Inflammation causes this barrier to break down, resulting in infection. The most common causes for uveitis include herpes viruses (HSV, VZV, and cytomegalovirus) and *Toxoplasma* spp.

Other Infections

Opportunistic infections in human immunodeficiency virus (HIV)–infected individuals can involve the eye. Systemic infections that involve the eye include cytomegalovirus, *Pneumocystis jiroveci, Cryptococcus neoformans, Mycobacterium avium* complex, and *Candida* spp. Most often the retina, choroid, and optic nerve are infected with these agents, resulting in significant visual morbidity (unhealthy condition) if left untreated. However, because of the widespread use of highly active antiretroviral therapy capable of assisting in immune system recovery and lowering the viral load in patients with HIV infection, the incidence of acquired immune deficiency syndrome (AIDS) and related ophthalmic infections has declined sharply.

Laboratory Diagnosis
Specimen Collection and Transport

Cell cultures for the isolation of *C. trachomatis* have been replaced by nucleic acid–based testing methods. Cell culture is only performed in specialized laboratories for antimicrobial susceptibility. Purulent material from the surface of the lower conjunctival sac and inner canthus (angle) of the eye is collected on a sterile swab for cultures. Both eyes should be cultured separately. Chlamydial cultures are taken with a dry calcium alginate swab and placed in a 2-SP (2-sucrose phosphate) transport medium.

For patients with keratitis, an ophthalmologist collects scrapings of the cornea with a heat-sterilized platinum spatula. For bacterial isolation, multiple inoculations with the spatula are made to blood agar, chocolate agar, an agar for the isolation of fungi, thioglycollate broth, and an anaerobic blood agar plate. Other special media may be used if indicated. Corneal specimens for culture of HSV and adenovirus are placed in viral transport media. Recently the collection of two corneal scrapes (one used for Gram stain and the other transported in brain-heart infusion medium and used for culture) was determined to provide a simple method for diagnosis of bacterial keratitis.

Cultures of endophthalmitis specimens are inoculated with material obtained by the ophthalmologist from the anterior and posterior chambers of the eye, wound abscesses, and wound dehiscence (splitting open). Lid infection material is collected on a swab in the conventional manner. For microbiologic studies of canaliculitis, material from the lacrimal canal should be transported under anaerobic conditions. Aspiration of fluid from the orbit is contraindicated in patients with orbital cellulitis. A patient history of sinusitis in association with orbital cellulitis is an indication for obtaining an otolaryngologist's assistance in the collection of material from the maxillary sinus by **antral puncture.** Blood cultures should also be obtained. Tissue biopsy is essential for the microbiologic diagnosis of mucormycosis. Because cultures are usually negative, the diagnosis is made by histologic examination.

Direct Visual Examination

All material submitted for culture should be smeared and examined directly by Gram stain or other appropriate microscopic techniques. In bacterial conjunctivitis, polymorphonuclear leukocytes predominate; in viral infection, the host cells are primarily lymphocytes and monocytes. Specimens in which *Chlamydia* is suspected can be stained immediately with monoclonal antibody conjugated to fluorescein for the detection of elementary bodies or inclusions. Using histologic stains, basophilic intracytoplasmic inclusion bodies are seen in epithelial cells. Cytologists and anatomic pathologists usually perform these tests. Direct examination of conjunctivitis specimens using histologic methods (Tzanck smear; a scraping from the lesion for collection of cells) may reveal multinucleated epithelial cells typical of herpes viral infections. However, DFA stains available for both HSV and VZV are recommended for rapid diagnosis of viral infections. In patients with keratitis, scrapings may be examined using Gram, Giemsa, periodic acid-Schiff (PAS), and methenamine silver stains. If *Acanthamoeba* or other amoebae are suspected, corneal scrapings or a corneal biopsy should be kept at room temperature (24°C to 28°C) and a direct wet preparation should be examined for motile trophozoites, and a trichrome stain should be added to the regimen. For this diagnosis, however, culture is by far the most sensitive detection method for the identification of the organism. In patients with endophthalmitis, the specimen is examined using Gram, Giemsa, PAS, and methenamine silver stains. When submitted in large volumes of fluid, ophthalmic specimens must be concentrated by centrifugation before additional studies are performed.

Nucleic Acid Testing Methods

In general, for nucleic acid testing methods, the manufacturer provides specific directions and/or specific collection vials or transport media. All collection, processing, and transport should follow the manufacturer's recommended protocols.

Other Nonculture Methods

Although acute and convalescent serologic tests for viral agents might be used in the event of epidemic conjunctivitis, they typically are not performed, because the infections are self-limited. Enzyme-linked immunosorbent assay (ELISA) tests and DFA staining are available for the detection of *C. trachomatis*. An ELISA test of aqueous humor is available for the diagnosis of *Toxocara* infection. Finally, nucleic acid–based methods have replaced most of these methods and are used for the diagnosis of viral and chlamydial keratoconjunctivitis, along with other ophthalmic infections, including uveitis.

Culture

Because of the constant washing action of the tears, the number of organisms recovered from cultures of eye infections may be relatively low. Unless the clinical specimen is obviously purulent, using a relatively large inoculum and a variety of media is recommended to ensure recovery of the etiologic agent. Conjunctival scrapings placed directly onto media yield the best results. At a minimum, blood and chocolate agar plates should be inoculated and incubated under increased carbon dioxide tension (5% to 10% CO_2). Because potential pathogens may be present in an eye without causing infection, it can be very helpful to culture both eyes. If a potential pathogen grows in cultures of the infected and the uninfected eye, the organism may not be causing the infection; however, if the organism only grows in culture from the infected eye, it is most likely the causative agent. When *M. lacunata* is suspected, Loeffler medium may prove useful; the growth of the organism often leads to proteolysis and pitting of the medium, although nonproteolytic strains may be isolated. If diphtheritic conjunctivitis is suspected, Loeffler or cystine-tellurite medium should be used. For more serious eye infections, such as keratitis, endophthalmitis, and orbital cellulitis, a reduced anaerobic blood agar plate, a medium for the isolation of fungi, and a liquid medium such as thioglycolate broth should always be included. The diagnosis of endophthalmitis typically requires a culture of the vitreous; vitreous washings typically yield positive cultures better than more invasive techniques. Invasive techniques for the collection of vitreous include either a needle aspirate or vitrectomy. A **vitrectomy** is a surgical procedure that simultaneously cuts and collects some vitreous fluid. Blood cultures are also important in serious eye infections.

Specimen cultures for *Chlamydia* and viruses should be inoculated to appropriate media from transport broth.

For *Chlamydia* isolation, cycloheximide-treated McCoy cells should be used; for viral isolation the use of human embryonic kidney, primary monkey kidney, and Hep-2 cell lines is recommended.

Ears

Anatomy

The ear is divided into three anatomic parts: the external, middle, and inner ear. Important anatomic structures are depicted in Fig. 71.4.

The middle ear is part of a continuous system including the nares, nasopharynx, auditory tube, and mastoid air spaces. These structures are lined with respiratory epithelium (e.g., ciliated cells, mucus-secreting goblet cells).

Resident Microbiota

The normal microbiota within the external ear canal is rather sparse, similar to flora of the conjunctival sac. Pneumococci (*S. pneumoniae*), *C. acnes*, *S. aureus*, and Enterobacterales are somewhat more common. *P. aeruginosa* is found on occasion. *Candida* spp. (non–*C. albicans*) are also common.

Diseases, Epidemiology, and Etiology of Disease

Otitis Externa (External Ear Infections)

Otitis externa is similar to skin and soft tissue infection. Two major types of external otitis exist: acute or chronic. **Acute external otitis** may be localized or diffuse. Acute localized disease occurs in the form of a pustule or furuncle and typically is caused by *S. aureus*. Erysipelas caused by group A streptococci may involve the external ear canal and the soft tissue of the ear. Acute diffuse otitis externa

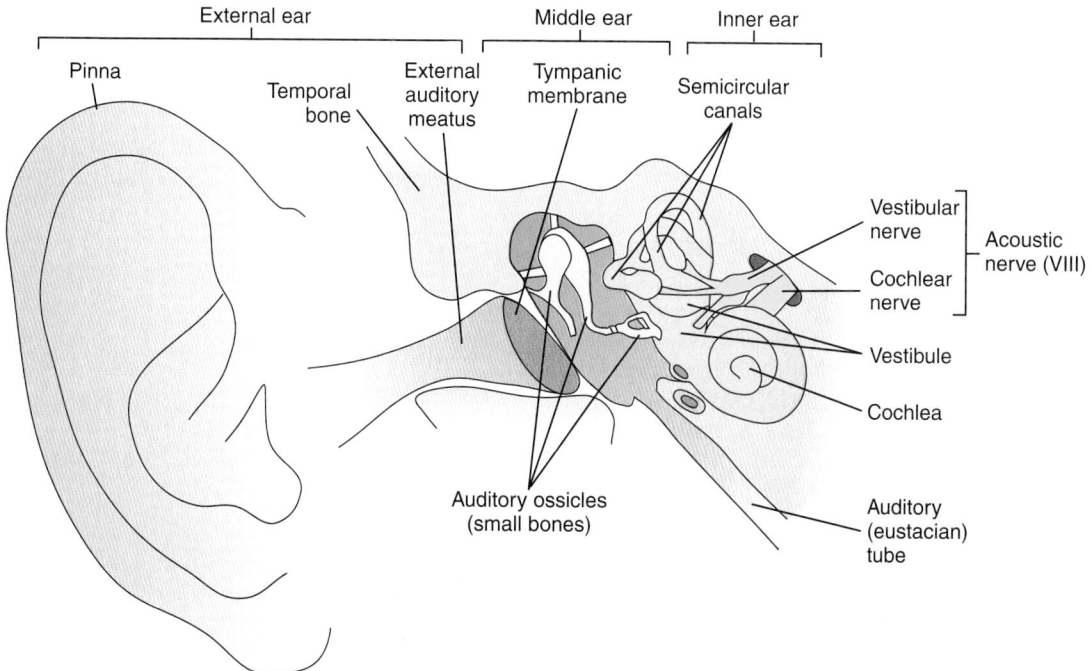

• **Fig. 71.4** The ear. (Modified from Thibodeau GA, Patton KT. *Anatomy and Physiology*. 2nd ed., St Louis: Mosby; 1993.)

(swimmer's ear) is related to maceration (softening of tissue) of the ear from swimming or hot, humid weather. Gram-negative bacilli, particularly *P. aeruginosa*, play an important role. A severe, hemorrhagic external otitis caused by *P. aeruginosa* is difficult to treat and has occasionally been related to hot tub use.

Chronic otitis externa results from the irritation of drainage from the middle ear in patients with chronic, suppurative otitis media and a perforated eardrum. **Malignant otitis externa** is a necrotizing infection that spreads to adjacent areas of soft tissue, cartilage, and bone. If allowed to progress and spread into the central nervous system or vascular channel, a life-threatening condition may develop. *P. aeruginosa*, in particular, and anaerobes are commonly associated with this process. Malignant otitis media is seen in patients with diabetes who have blood vessel disease of the tissues overlying the temporal bone in which poor local perfusion of tissues results in an environment conducive for invasion by bacteria. On occasion, external otitis can extend into the cartilage of the ear, usually requiring surgical intervention. Certain viruses may infect the external auditory canal, the soft tissue of the ear, or the tympanic membrane; influenza A virus is a suspected, but not an established, cause. VZV may cause painful vesicles within the soft tissue of the ear and the ear canal. Viral agents such as influenza and bacterial agents are typically associated with acute otitis media (*S. pneumoniae, H. influenzae,* and *M. catarrhalis*). *Mycoplasma pneumoniae* is rarely associated with this condition.

Otitis Media (Middle Ear Infections)

In children (in whom **otitis media** is most common), pneumococci and *H. influenzae* are the usual etiologic agents in acute disease. Group A streptococci (*S. pyogenes*), *M. catarrhalis, S. aureus,* gram-negative enteric bacilli, and anaerobes are also associated with middle ear infections. Viruses, chiefly respiratory syncytial virus (RSV), coronaviruses, enteroviruses, rhinoviruses, and influenza viruses, have been recovered from the middle ear fluid of children with acute or chronic otitis media. *C. trachomatis* and *M. pneumoniae* have occasionally been isolated from middle ear aspirates. Otitis media with effusion (fluid) is considered a chronic sequela of acute otitis media. A slowly growing organism, *Alloiococcus otitis,* is a pathogen that has been isolated from patients with otitis media with effusion.

Chronic otitis media yields a predominantly anaerobic flora, with *Peptostreptococcus* spp., *Bacteroides fragilis* group, *Prevotella melaninogenica* (pigmented, anaerobic, gram-negative rods), *Porphyromonas,* other *Prevotella* spp., and *Fusobacterium nucleatum* as the principal pathogens; less common are *S. aureus, P. aeruginosa, Proteus* spp., and other gram-negative facultative bacilli. Table 71.2 summarizes the major causes of ear infections.

The **mastoid** is a portion of the temporal bone (lower sides of the skull) containing the mastoid sinuses (cavities). **Mastoiditis** is a complication of chronic otitis media in which organisms find their way into the mastoid sinuses. To prevent the further spread of this infection to the central nervous system, a **mastoidectomy** is performed.

Pathogenesis

Local trauma, the presence of foreign bodies, or excessive moisture can lead to otitis externa (external ear infections).

TABLE 71.2	Major Infectious Causes of Ear Infection
Disease	**Common Causes**
Otitis externa	Acute: *Staphylococcus aureus, Streptococcus pyogenes, Pseudomonas aeruginosa;* other gram-negative bacilli
	Chronic: *P. aeruginosa;* anaerobes
Otitis media	Acute *Streptococcus pneumoniae; Haemophilus influenzae; Moraxella catarrhalis; S. pyogenes;* respiratory syncytial virus; influenza virus; coronaviruses, enteroviruses, rhinoviruses
	Chronic: Anaerobes

Note: This table is not intended to be all-inclusive for the infectious agents capable of causing ear infections.

Occasionally, an infection from the middle ear can extend by purulent drainage to the external ear.

Anatomic or physiologic abnormalities of the auditory tube can predispose individuals to develop otitis media. The auditory tube is responsible for protecting the middle ear from nasopharyngeal secretions, draining secretions produced in the middle ear into the nasopharynx, and ventilating the middle ear and equilibrating air pressure with the external ear canal. If any of these functions become compromised and fluid develops in the middle ear, infection may occur. To illustrate, if a person has a viral upper respiratory infection, the auditory tube becomes inflamed and swollen. This inflammation and swelling may, in turn, compromise the auditory tube's ventilating function, resulting in a negative, rather than a positive, pressure in the middle ear. This change in pressure can then allow for potentially pathogenic bacteria present in the nasopharynx to enter the middle ear.

Laboratory Diagnosis

Specimen Collection and Transport

Although middle ear infection, or otitis media, is usually not diagnosed by culture, culture can be used for the laboratory diagnosis of external otitis; the external ear should be cleansed with a mild germicide such as 1:1000 aqueous solution of benzalkonium chloride to reduce the numbers of contaminating skin microbiota before obtaining the specimen. Material from the ear, especially that obtained after spontaneous perforation of the eardrum or by needle aspiration of middle ear fluid (**tympanocentesis**), should be collected by an otolaryngologist, using sterile equipment. Specimens from the mastoid are generally taken on swabs during surgery, although actual bone is preferred. Specimens should be transported anaerobically.

Direct Visual Examination

Material aspirated from the middle ear or mastoid is also examined directly for bacteria and fungi. The calcofluor white or PAS stains can reveal fungal elements. Methenamine silver stains have the added efficiency of staining most bacterial and fungal organisms and several parasitic species.

Culture and Nonculture Methods

Ear specimens submitted for culture should be inoculated to blood, MacConkey, and chocolate agars. Anaerobic cultures should also be set up on those specimens obtained by tympanocentesis or those obtained from patients with chronic otitis media or mastoiditis. Because cultures of middle ear effusions are culture positive for only 20% to 30% of patients, conventional and nucleic acid–based test methods have been used to detect the common middle ear pathogens.

Sinuses

Anatomy

The sinuses, like the mastoids, are unique, air-filled cavities within the head (Fig. 71.5). The sinuses are normally sterile. These structures, as well as the eustachian tube, the middle ear, and the respiratory portion of the pharynx, are lined by respiratory epithelium. The clearance of secretions and contaminants depends on normal ciliary activity and mucous flow.

Diseases

The pathogens associated with otitis media are the same ones associated with **sinusitis**; bacteria from the nose and throat make their way to the inner ear and sinuses. Acute sinusitis usually develops during a cold or influenza illness and tends to be self-limited, lasting 1 to 3 weeks, and is usually more prevalent in winter and spring. Acute sinusitis is often difficult to distinguish from the primary illness. Symptoms include purulent nasal and postnasal discharge, a feeling of pressure over the sinus areas of the face, cough, and a nasal quality to the voice. Fever is sometimes present.

Occasionally, acute sinusitis persists and reaches a chronic state in which bacterial colonization occurs and the condition no longer responds to antibiotic treatment. Ordinarily, surgery or drainage is required for successful management. Patients with chronic sinusitis may have acute exacerbations (flare-ups). Other complications include local extension into the orbit, skull, meninges, or brain, and development of chronic sinusitis.

Pathogenesis

Most cases of acute sinusitis are believed to be bacterial complications following a viral respiratory infection. The exact mechanisms involved are unknown. About 5% to 10% of acute maxillary sinus infections result from infection originating from a dental source. The maxillary sinuses are close to the roots of the upper teeth, providing a mechanism for dental infections to extend into the sinuses. The primary

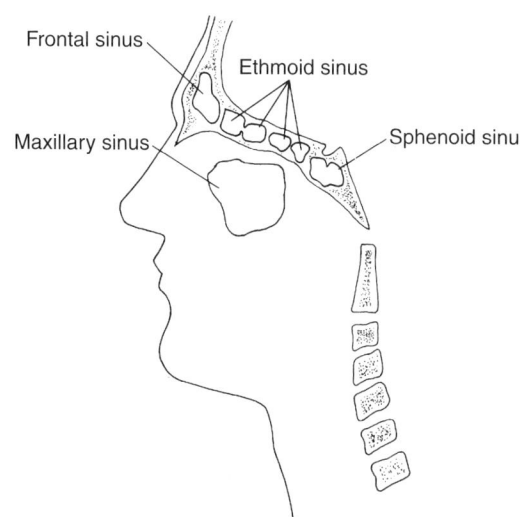

• **Fig. 71.5** Location of the paranasal sinuses. (From Milliken ME, Campbell G. *Essential Competencies for Patient Care*. St Louis: Mosby; 1985.)

TABLE 71.3	Major Infectious Causes of Acute Sinusitis	
Age Group	**Common Causes**
Young adults	*Haemophilus influenzae, Streptococcus pneumoniae, Streptococcus pyogenes, Moraxella catarrhalis*
Children	*S. pneumoniae, H. influenzae, M. catarrhalis*, rhinovirus

Note: This table is not intended to be all-inclusive for the infectious agents capable of causing sinusitis.

problems associated with the development of chronic sinusitis include inadequate drainage, impaired mucociliary clearance, and mucosal damage.

Epidemiology and Etiology of Disease

Although difficult to assess, the actual incidence of acute sinusitis parallels that of acute upper respiratory tract infections (i.e., being most prevalent in the fall through spring).

Most studies of the microbiology of acute sinusitis are associated with maxillary sinusitis, because it is the most common type and specimen collection is available through puncture and aspiration. Acute viral sinusitis is one of the most common causes of respiratory tract infection and, in most cases, resolves without treatment. However, published estimates indicate that 0.5% to 2% of cases of acute viral sinusitis in adults are complicated by bacterial sinusitis. This scenario is even more common in children. Bacterial cultures are positive in about three-fourths of patients. Studies

have indicated that *S. pneumoniae* and *H. influenzae* are the major bacterial pathogens in adults with acute sinusitis; other species such as beta-hemolytic and alpha-hemolytic streptococci, *S. aureus*, and anaerobes have also been cultured but less commonly. The predominant bacterial organisms associated with chronic sinusitis include *S. pneumoniae, H. influenzae*, and *M. catarrhalis*; less commonly, isolated organisms include anaerobic streptococci, *Prevotella* spp., and *Fusobacterium* spp. Fungal pathogens such as *Aspergillus, Fusarium*, and *C. albicans* have also been identified in cases of chronic sinusitis using culture and nucleic acid–based test methods.

The major causes of acute sinusitis are summarized in Table 71.3. *M. catarrhalis* has been isolated in chronic sinusitis in children.

Laboratory Diagnosis

In most cases, a diagnosis can be made based on physical findings, history, radiograph studies, and other imaging techniques such as magnetic resonance imaging. However, if a laboratory diagnosis is needed, an otolaryngologist collects a specimen from the maxillary sinus by puncture and aspiration or during surgery. Sinus drainage is unacceptable for smear or culture, because this material will be contaminated with aerobic and anaerobic normal respiratory microbiota; sinus washings or aspirates surgically collected are the specimens of choice. Gram-stained smears and aerobic and anaerobic cultures should be performed on each specimen. Aerobic culture media should include blood, chocolate, and MacConkey agar.

Matrix-Assisted Laser Desorption Ionization Time-of-Flight Mass Spectrometry

Matrix-assisted laser desorption ionization time-of-flight mass spectrometry (MALDI-TOF MS) may be used to identify pathogens from these infections directly from pure colony isolates. The limitations of identification, however, rely on technical expertise in sample preparation and the limitations of the current database (Chapter 7).

ⓔ Visit the Evolve site for a complete list of procedures, review questions, and case studies.

Bibliography

Bennett J, Dolin R, Blaser M: *Principles and practice of infectious diseases*, ed 9, Philadelphia, PA, 2019, Elsevier.

Bernardes TF, Bonfioli AA: Blepharitis, *Semin Ophthalmol* 25: 79–83, 2010.

Carbonnelle E, Grohs P, Jacquier H, et al.: Robustness of two MALDI-TOF mass spectrometry systems for bacterial identification, *J Microbiol Methods* 89:133–136, 2012.

Carroll KC, Pfaller MA, Landry ML, et al.: *Manual of clinical microbiology*, ed 12, Washington, DC, 2019, ASM.

Cramer L, Emara DM, Gadre AK: Mycoplasma an unlikely cause of bullous myringitis, *Ear Nose Throat J* 91:E30–E31, 2012.

Creemers-Schild D, Gronthoud F, Spanjaard L, et al.: *Fusobacterium necrophorum*, an emerging pathogen of otogenic and paranasal infections? *New Microbes New Infect* 2:52–57, 2014.

Finegold SM, Flynn MJ, Rose FV, et al.: Bacteriologic findings associated with chronic bacterial maxillary sinusitis in adults, *Clin Infect Dis* 35:428–433, 2002.

Hendolin PH, Paulin L, Ylikoski J: Clinically applicable multiplex PCR for four middle ear pathogens, *J Clin Microbiol* 38:125–132, 2000.

Henry CR, Flynn HW, Miller D, et al.: Infectious keratitis progressing to endophthalmitis: a 15-year study of microbiology, associated factors, and clinical outcomes, *Ophthalmology* 119:2443–2449, 2012.

Holtz KK, Townsend KR, Furst JW, et al.: An assessment of the AdenoPlus Point-of-Care test for diagnosing Adenoviral conjunctivitis and its effect on antimicrobial stewardship, *Mayo Clin Proc Innov Qual Outcomes* 1(2):170–175, 2017.

Kaye SB, Rao PG, Smith G, et al.: Simplifying collection of corneal specimens in cases of suspected bacterial keratitis, *J Clin Microbiol* 41:3192–3197, 2003.

Kim ST, Choi JH, Jeon HG, et al.: Comparison between polymerase chain reaction and fungal culture for the detection of fungi in patients with chronic sinusitis and normal controls, *Acta Otolaryngol* 125:72–75, 2005.

Lynn WA, Lightman S: The eye in systemic infection, *Lancet* 364:1439–1450, 2004.

Marciano-Cabral F, Cabral G: *Acanthamoeba* spp. as agents of disease in humans, *Clin Microbiol Rev* 16:273–307, 2003.

Moorthy RS, Valluri S, Rao NA: Nontuberculous mycobacterial ocular and adnexal infections, *Surv Ophthalmol* 57:202–235, 2012.

Palmu AA, Herva E, Savolainen H, et al.: Association of clinical signs and symptoms with bacterial findings in acute otitis media, *Clin Infect Dis* 38:234–242, 2004.

Piccirillo JF: Clinical practice. Acute bacterial sinusitis, *N Engl J Med* 351:902–910, 2004.

Roels P: Ocular infections of AIDS: new considerations for patients using highly active anti-retroviral therapy (HAART), *Optometry* 75:624–628, 2004.

Sande M, Gwaltney JM: Acute community-acquired bacterial sinusitis: continuing challenges and current management, *Clin Infect Dis* 39:S151–S158, 2004.

Skevaki CL, Galani IE, Pararas MV, et al.: Treatment of viral conjunctivitis with antiviral drugs, *Drugs* 71:331–347, 2011.

Solomon AW, Peeling RW, Foster A, et al.: Diagnosis and assessment of trachoma, *Clin Microbiol Rev* 17:982–1011, 2004.

Zhang L, Zhao N, Huang X, et al.: Molecular epidemiology of acute hemorrhagic conjunctivitis caused by coxsackie A type 24 variant in China, 2004-2014, *Sci Rep* 7:45202, 2017. Accessed October 20, 2019.

72

Infections of the Urinary Tract

OBJECTIVES

1. Describe the anatomy and identify the structures of the male and female urinary tracts.
2. Name the organisms that colonize the urethra and are considered normal microbiota.
3. Explain how the female urinary tract anatomy may predispose females to urinary tract infections.
4. Differentiate between community-acquired urinary tract infections and hospital- and health care–associated urinary tract infections.
5. List the routes of transmission that allow bacteria to invade and cause a urinary tract infection.
6. Name the physical and chemical properties of urine that contribute to its role in the body's defense mechanism against the bacteria capable of causing urinary tract infections.
7. Explain host and microbial factors that determine whether bacteria will be able to colonize and cause a urinary tract infection.
8. Name the properties bacteria possess that predispose them to have greater pathogenicity in causing urinary tract infections.
9. Define the five major types of urinary tract infections: pyelonephritis, cystitis, urethritis, acute urethral syndrome, and asymptomatic bacteriuria.
10. Compare complicated and uncomplicated urinary tract infections.
11. Explain the collection methods for urine specimens, including clean catch midstream urine, straight catheterized urine, a suprapubic bladder aspiration, and an indwelling catheter collection.
12. Describe the urine-screening methods available to determine bacteriuria and pyuria.
13. Explain the nitrate reductase test, the leukocyte esterase test, and the catalase test regarding their urine-screening capability.
14. Name the media required for urine cultures.
15. Explain the proper methodology for plating and interpreting a quantitative urine culture.
16. Correlate signs and symptoms with the results of laboratory diagnostic procedures for the identification of the etiologic agent associated with infections of the urinary tract.

General Considerations

Anatomy

The urinary tract consists of the kidneys, ureters, bladder, and urethra (Fig. 72.1). The function of the urinary tract is to make and process urine. Urine is an ultrafiltrate of blood that consists mostly of water but also contains nitrogenous wastes, sodium, potassium, chloride, and other analytes. Urine is normally a sterile fluid. Often, **urinary tract infections (UTIs)** are characterized as being either **upper (U-UTI)** or **lower (L-UTI)** based primarily on the anatomic location of the infection: the lower urinary tract encompasses the bladder and urethra, and the upper urinary tract encompasses the ureters and kidneys. Upper UTIs affect the ureters (**ureteritis**) or the renal parenchyma (**pyelonephritis**). Lower UTIs may affect the urethra (**urethritis**), the bladder (**cystitis**), or the prostate in males (**prostatitis**). Symptomatic L-UTIs and asymptomatic U-UTIs do not rule out the possibility that the infectious agent may also be affecting the upper urinary tract.

The anatomy of the female urethra is of importance to the pathogenesis of UTIs. The female urethra is relatively short compared with the male urethra and lies in close proximity to the warm, moist, perirectal region, which is teeming with microorganisms. Because of the shorter urethra, bacteria can reach the bladder more easily in the female host; thus UTIs are primarily a disorder in females. In males, the incidence of UTIs increases after the age of 60 years, when the enlargement of the prostate interferes with the removal of urine from the bladder.

UTIs can also be classified as **uncomplicated** or **complicated.** An uncomplicated UTI indicates that there are no structural or neurological abnormalities associated with the urinary tract. A complicated UTI indicates a history of persistent, recurring infections that may be a result of physiological factors that predispose the patient to infection. This may include previous kidney failure, obstruction, kidney transplant, immunosuppression, or urinary retention.

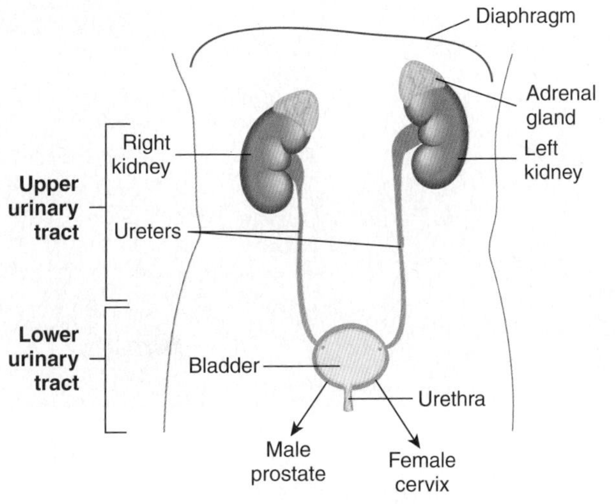

• **Fig. 72.1** Overview of the anatomy of the urinary tract. (From Potter PH, Perry AG. *Fundamentals of Nursing*. St Louis: Mosby; 1985.)

Resident Microbiota of the Urinary Tract

The urethra has resident microbiota that colonize its epithelium in the distal portion; these organisms are lactobacilli, corynebacteria, enterococci, and coagulase-negative staphylococci (Box 72.1). Potential pathogens, including gram-negative aerobic bacilli (primarily Enterobacterales) and occasional yeasts, are also present as transient colonizers. All areas of the urinary tract above the urethra in a healthy human were previously considered sterile. There is increasing evidence that the urinary bladder may be protected by normal microbiota. Urine is typically sterile, but noninvasive methods for collecting urine must rely on a specimen that has passed through a contaminated milieu. Therefore, quantitative cultures for the diagnosis of UTIs have been used to discriminate among contamination, colonization, and infection.

Infections of the Urinary Tract

Epidemiology

UTIs are among the most common bacterial infections that lead patients to seek medical care. It has been estimated that more than 7 million outpatient visits, 1 million visits to the emergency department, and 100,000 hospital stays every year in the United States are a result of UTIs. Approximately 60% of all females and 5% of all males will have a UTI at some time during their lives. Of note, UTIs are also the most common hospital- and health care–associated infection.

The exact prevalence of UTIs is age- and sex-dependent. During the first year of life, UTIs occur in less than 2% in males and females. The incidence of UTIs among males remains relatively low after 1 year of age and until approximately 60 years of age, when enlargement of the prostate interferes with emptying of the bladder. Extensive studies have shown that the incidence of **bacteriuria** (presence of

---

> • **BOX 72.1** Resident Microbiota of the Urethra
>
> Coagulase-negative staphylococci (excluding *Staphylococcus saprophyticus*)
> Viridans and nonhemolytic streptococci
> Lactobacilli (adult females)
> Diphtheroids (*Corynebacterium* spp.)
> Nonpathogenic (saprobic) *Neisseria* spp. (adult women)
> Anaerobic cocci
> *Propionibacterium* spp. (adult patients)
> Commensal *Mycobacterium* spp.
> Commensal *Mycoplasma* spp.
> Yeasts (pregnant, adult females)

bacteria in urine) among females 5 through 17 years of age is 1% to 3%. The prevalence of bacteriuria in females increases gradually with time to as high as 10% to 20% in older females. In females between 20 and 40 years of age who have had UTIs, as many as 50% may become reinfected within 1 year. The association of UTIs with sexual intercourse may also contribute to this increased incidence, because sexual activity increases the chances of bacterial contamination of the female urethra. Finally, because of anatomic and hormonal changes that favor the development of UTIs, the incidence of bacteriuria increases during pregnancy. These infections can lead to serious infections in both the mother and fetus. Estrogen deficiency in postmenopausal females, resulting in a decrease in normal vaginal microbiota (in particular, lactobacilli), is associated with recurrent UTIs.

UTIs are important complications of diabetes, renal disease, renal transplantation, and structural and neurologic abnormalities that interfere with urine flow. In 40% to 60% of renal transplant recipients, the urinary tract is the source for the primary occurrence of bacteremia, and in these patients, the recurrence rate is about 40%. In addition, UTIs are a leading cause of gram-negative sepsis in hospitalized patients and are the origin for about half of all health care–associated infections caused by urinary catheters.

Etiologic Agents

Community-Acquired

Escherichia coli is by far the most common cause of uncomplicated community-acquired UTIs. At the molecular level, *E. coli*, designated uropathogenic *E. coli* (UPEC), which causes UTIs, is sufficiently different from other types of *E. coli*. *E. coli* O25-H4 has emerged as a significant urinary tract pathogen in community-acquired infections. Other bacteria commonly isolated from patients with UTIs are *Klebsiella* spp., other Enterobacterales, *Staphylococcus saprophyticus*, and enterococci. More than 95% of uncomplicated UTIs are caused by a single bacterial species. In more complicated UTIs, particularly in recurrent infections, the relative frequency of infection caused by *Proteus, Pseudomonas, Klebsiella*, and *Enterobacter* spp. increases. In addition, community-acquired UTIs are increasingly associated with multidrug-resistant organisms such as extended beta-lactamase-resistant *E. coli*.

Hospital- and Health Care–Associated

The hospital or health care environment plays an important role in determining the organisms involved in UTIs. Hospitalized patients are most likely to be infected by antibiotic-resistant *E. coli*, *Klebsiella* spp., *Proteus* spp., staphylococci, enterococci, other Enterobacterales, *Pseudomonas aeruginosa*, *Enterobacter* spp., and *Candida* spp. The introduction of a foreign body into the urinary tract, especially one that remains in place for an extended period (e.g., Foley catheter), carries a substantial risk of infection, particularly if obstruction is present. Approximately 35% of all health care–associated infections are UTIs. Eighty percent of those infections are associated with the use of an indwelling catheter. In addition, highly antibiotic-resistant microorganisms such as extended-beta-lactamase–producing organisms (ESBL); Amp C beta-lactamase-, carbapenemase-producing Enterobacterales, and *Acinetobacter* spp. are increasingly identified in health care–associated UTIs. It is also not unusual to identify multiple bacterial species or infectious agents in complicated UTIs, due to repeat medical procedures and previous treatment with antibiotics. Consequently, UTI is the most common health care–associated infection in the United States, and the infected urinary tract is the most common source of bacteremia.

Miscellaneous

Other less commonly isolated agents are other gram-negative bacilli, such as *Acinetobacter* and *Alcaligenes* spp., other *Pseudomonas* spp., *Citrobacter* spp., *Gardnerella vaginalis*, *Aerococcus urinae*, and beta-hemolytic streptococci. Bacteria such as mycobacteria (predominantly in patients who are human immunodeficiency virus [HIV]-positive), *Chlamydia trachomatis*, *Ureaplasma urealyticum*, *Mycoplasma hominis*, *Campylobacter* spp., *Haemophilus influenzae*, *Leptospira*, and certain *Corynebacterium* spp. (e.g., *C. renale*) are rarely recovered from urine. In addition, *Actinobaculum schaalii* (vaginal and skin microbiota) and other *Actinobaculum* spp. may be dismissed as normal microbiota or overlooked in urine cultures because of these organisms' slow growth rate. Because renal transplant recipients are immunosuppressed, these patients not only suffer from common uropathogens but are also susceptible to opportunistic infections with unusual pathogens. A study involving renal transplant recipients showed that for culture-negative urine, amplification of regions in bacterial 16S ribosomal ribonucleic acid (rRNA) and subsequent analysis by high-performance liquid chromatography detected the presence of several known uropathogens as well as unusual agents. For example, urine specimens from renal transplant recipients or infants may contain *Listeria monocytogenes* associated with a systemic infection. *Salmonella* spp. may be recovered during the early stages of typhoid fever; their presence should be immediately reported to the physician. If anaerobes are suspected, the physician should perform a percutaneous bladder tap unless urine can be obtained from the upper urinary tract by another means (e.g., from a nephrostomy tube). Communication by the clinician to the laboratory that such an agent is suspected is important for detecting such agents. In patients with "sterile pyuria," Gram stain may reveal unusual organisms with distinctive morphology (e.g., *H. influenzae*, anaerobes). The presence of any organisms on smear that do not grow in culture is an important clue to the cause of the infection. The laboratory can then take the action necessary to optimize chances for recovery.

As previously noted, *Candida* spp. may be isolated from patients with other debilitating disease (i.e., diabetes or urinary tract obstructions) and are associated with immunosuppressive therapy or immunosuppressive conditions and antibiotic treatment. Additional fungi capable of causing systemic infections that may also be identified in urine samples include *Blastomyces dermatitidis*, *Coccidioides immitis*, *Cryptococcus neoformans*, and *Histoplasma capsulatum*. The identification of a fungal isolate in a urine specimen should be carefully evaluated and reported to the attending clinician.

In general, viruses and parasites are not usually considered urinary tract pathogens. However, adenovirus has been implicated as the causative agent in hemorrhagic cystitis in pediatric patients. *Trichomonas vaginalis* may occasionally be observed in urinary sediment, and *Schistosoma haematobium* can lodge in the urinary tract and release eggs into the urine.

Pathogenesis
Routes of Infection

Bacteria can invade and cause a UTI via three major routes: **ascending, hematogenous,** and **lymphatic pathways.** Although the ascending route is the most common course of infection in females, ascent in association with instrumentation (e.g., urinary catheterization, cystoscopy) is the most common cause of health care–associated UTIs in both sexes. For UTIs to occur by the ascending pathway, enteric gram-negative bacteria and other microorganisms that originate in the gastrointestinal tract must be able to colonize the vaginal cavity or the periurethral area. Once these organisms gain access to the bladder, they may multiply and then pass up the ureters to the kidneys. UTIs occur more often in females, at least partially because of the short female urethra and its proximity to the anus. As previously mentioned, sexual activity can increase the chances of bacterial contamination of the female urethra. In addition, postmenopausal women are more susceptible to uropathogens due to the deficiency in estrogen and the loss of protective lactobacilli in the vaginal tract.

In most hospitalized patients, UTI is preceded by urinary catheterization or other manipulation of the urinary tract. The pathogenesis of catheter-associated UTI is not fully understood. It is certain that soon after hospitalization, patients become colonized with bacteria endemic to the institution—often gram-negative aerobic and facultative bacilli carrying resistance markers. These bacteria colonize the patient's skin, gastrointestinal tract, and mucous membranes, including the anterior urethra. With the insertion of a catheter, the bacteria may be pushed along the urethra into the bladder or, with an indwelling catheter, may migrate along the track between the catheter and the urethral mucosa, gaining access to the bladder. It is estimated that approximately 10% to 30% of catheterized patients will develop **bacteriuria** (presence of bacteria in urine).

UTIs may also occur by the hematogenous, or blood-borne, route. Hematogenous spread usually occurs as a result of bacteremia. Any systemic infection can lead to seeding of the kidney, but certain organisms, such as *Staphylococcus aureus* or *Salmonella* spp., are particularly invasive. Although most infections involving the kidneys are acquired through the ascending route, yeast (usually *Candida albicans*), *Mycobacterium tuberculosis*, *Salmonella* spp., *Leptospira* spp., or *S. aureus* in the urine may indicate pyelonephritis acquired via hematogenous spread or the descending route. Hematogenous spread accounts for less than 5% of UTIs and rarely occurs with gram-negative bacilli.

Finally, increased pressure on the bladder can cause lymphatic flow into the kidneys, resulting in UTI. However, evidence for the significance of this potential route is insufficient, indicating that the ascending route remains the major mechanism for the development of UTI.

The Host-Pathogen Relationship

Many individuals (females) are colonized in the vaginal or periurethral area with organisms originating from the gastrointestinal tract, yet they do not develop urinary infections. Whether an organism is able to colonize and then cause a UTI is determined in large part by a complex interplay of host and microbial factors.

In most cases, the host defense mechanisms can eliminate the organisms. Urine itself is inhibitory to some of the urethral microbiota, such as anaerobes. In addition, if urine has a low pH, high or low osmolality, high urea concentration, or high organic acid content, even organisms capable of growth in the urinary tract may be inhibited. If bacteria do gain access to the bladder, the constant flushing of contaminated urine from the body either eliminates bacteria or maintains their numbers at low levels. Clearly, any interference with the act of normal voiding, such as mechanical obstruction resulting from kidney stones or strictures, will promote the development of UTI. Also, the bladder mucosal surface has antibacterial properties. If the infection is not eradicated, the site of infection remains in the superficial mucosa; deep layers of the bladder are rarely involved.

In addition to the previously described host defenses, a valvelike mechanism at the junction of the ureter and bladder prevents the reflux (backward flow) of urine from the bladder to the upper urinary tract. Therefore, if the function of these valves is inhibited or compromised in any way, such as by obstruction or congenital abnormalities, urine reflux provides a direct route for organisms to reach the kidney. Hormonal changes associated with pregnancy and their effects on the urinary tract increase the chance for urine reflux to the upper urinary tract.

Activation of the host immune response by uropathogens also plays a key role in fending off infection. For example,

bacterial contact with urothelial cells initiates an immune response via a variety of signaling pathways. Bacterial lipopolysaccharide (LPS; Chapter 2) activates host cells to ultimately release cytokines such as tumor necrosis factor and interferon-gamma. In addition, bacteria can activate the complement cascade, leading to the production of biologically active components such as opsonins, as well as augment the host's adaptive immune response. Host factors that lead to host susceptibility or resistance to uropathogens have been identified. For example, a glycoprotein synthesized exclusively by epithelial cells in a specific anatomic location in the kidney, referred to as **Tamm-Horsfall protein (THP)** or **uromodulin,** serves as an antiadherence factor by binding to *E. coli*–expressing type 1 fimbriae (discussed later). **Defensins,** a group of small antimicrobial peptides, are produced by a variety of host cells such as macrophages, neutrophils, and cells in the urinary tract and attach to the bacterial cell, eventually causing the organism's death.

Although many microorganisms can cause UTIs, most cases are a result of infection by a few organisms. To illustrate, only a limited number of serogroups of *E. coli* (01, 02, 04, 06, 07, 08, 075, 0150, 018ab) cause a significant proportion of UTIs. Numerous investigations indicate that UPEC possesses virulence factors that enhance their ability to colonize and invade the urinary tract. Some of these virulence factors include increased adherence to vaginal and uroepithelial cells by bacterial surface structures (adhesins), pili (P [PAP] type 1), and multiple types of fimbriae; the production of alpha-hemolysin (inhibits the production of protective cytokines), cytotoxic necrotizing factor (CNF), an autotransported protease (Sat), aerobactin (iuc), and a siderophore receptor (iroN); and resistance to serum-killing activity. Also, genome sequences of UPEC strains have been determined, indicating that several potential virulence factor genes associated with the acquisition and development of UTIs are encoded on pathogenicity islands (e.g., hemolysins and *E. coli* P fimbriae). By definition, pathogenicity islands (Chapter 3) contain genes that are associated with virulence and are absent from avirulent (not typically found in fecal strains) or less virulent strains of the same species. UPEC strains are a major cause of community-acquired UTIs.

The importance of adherence in the pathogenesis of UTIs has also been demonstrated with other species of bacteria. Once introduced into the urinary tract, *Proteus* strains appear to be uniquely suited to cause significant disease in the urinary tract. Data indicate that these strains can facilitate their adherence to the mucosa of kidneys. Also, *Proteus* is able to hydrolyze urea via urease production. The species *Proteus mirabilis* accounts for approximately 77% of the urinary isolates. Hydrolysis of urea results in an increase in urine pH that is directly toxic to kidney cells and stimulates the formation of kidney stones. Similar findings have been made with *Klebsiella* spp. *S. saprophyticus* also adheres better to uroepithelial cells than *S. aureus* or *S. epidermidis*.

Other bacterial characteristics may be important in the pathogenesis of UTIs. Motility may be important for organisms to ascend to the upper urinary tract against the flow of urine and cause pyelonephritis. Some organisms demonstrate greater production of capsular K antigen (K1, K5, and K12); this antigen protects bacteria from being phagocytized.

Finally, despite numerous host defenses and even antibiotic treatments that can effectively sterilize the urine, a significant proportion of patients have recurrent UTIs. Studies show that uropathogens can invade superficial epithelial cells in the bladder and replicate, forming large foci of intracellular organisms. This invasion of bladder epithelial cells triggers the host immune response, which in turn causes the superficial cells to exfoliate within hours after infection. Although this exfoliation is considered a host defense mechanism by eliminating infected cells, intracellular organisms can reemerge from the bladder epithelial cells and invade the underlying, new superficial layer of epithelial cells, consequently persisting within the urinary tract. It has been reported that intracellular bacteria mature into numerous, large protrusions on the bladder surface they referred to as "pods." This bacterial organization—in which the intracellular bacteria are embedded in a fibrous, polysaccharide-rich matrix resembling that of a biofilm—may help further explain the persistence of bladder infections despite strong host defenses.

Types of Infection and Their Clinical Manifestations

UTI encompasses a broad range of clinical entities that differ in terms of clinical presentation, degree of tissue invasion, epidemiologic setting, and requirements for antibiotic therapy. There are several types of UTIs: urethritis, ureteritis, asymptomatic bacteriuria, cystitis, the urethral syndrome, and pyelonephritis. Uncomplicated infections occur primarily in otherwise healthy females and occasionally in male infants and adolescent and adult males. Most uncomplicated infections respond readily to antibiotic agents to which the etiologic agent is susceptible. Complicated infections occur in both sexes. In general, individuals who develop complicated infections often have certain risk factors. Some of these risk factors are listed in Box 72.2. In general, complicated infections are more difficult to treat and have greater morbidity (e.g., kidney damage, bacteremia) and mortality compared with uncomplicated infections. UTIs identified in pregnant women, men, children,

• BOX 72.2 Risk Factors Associated With Complicated Urinary Tract Infections

Underlying diseases that predispose the kidney to infection (e.g., diabetes, sickle cell anemia)
Kidney stones
Structural or functional abnormalities of the urinary tract (e.g., a tipped bladder)
Indwelling urinary catheters

and hospitalized patients or patients in other health care–associated settings (e.g., cancer outpatient clinics) may be considered complicated infections. The organisms associated with these infections are commonly highly resistant to many antimicrobials.

The clinical presentation of UTIs may vary, ranging from asymptomatic infection to pyelonephritis (infection of the kidney and its pelvis). Some UTI symptoms may be nonspecific, and the symptoms of lower UTIs may be considerably similar to those of upper UTIs.

Urethritis

Symptoms associated with urethritis (infection of the urethra), **dysuria** (painful or difficult urination), and frequency are similar to those associated with other lower UTIs. Urethritis is a common infection. Because *C. trachomatis, Neisseria gonorrhoeae,* and *T. vaginalis* are common causes of urethritis and considered to be sexually transmitted, urethritis is discussed as a sexually transmitted disease in Chapter 73.

Ureteritis

Inflammation or infection within the ureters (ureteritis) is considered in combination with kidney infections. UTI within the ureters indicates that organisms have begun or are in the process of ascending into the kidneys and should be treated similarly to prevent further infection.

Asymptomatic Bacteriuria

Asymptomatic bacteriuria or **asymptomatic UTI** is the isolation of a specified quantitative count of bacteria in an appropriately collected urine specimen obtained from a person without symptoms or signs of urinary infection. Asymptomatic bacteriuria is common, but its prevalence varies widely with age, gender, and the presence of genitourinary abnormalities or underlying diseases. For example, the prevalence of bacteriuria increases with age in healthy females from as low as about 1% among school-age females to at least 20% among females 80 years of age or older living in the community, whereas bacteriuria is rare in healthy young males. Because its clinical significance was controversial (asymptomatic bacteriuria precedes UTI but does not always lead to asymptomatic infection), guidelines have been published for the diagnosis and treatment of asymptomatic bacteriuria in adults older than 18 years of age. The foundation of these guidelines rests on the premise that screening of asymptomatic subjects for bacteriuria is appropriate if bacteriuria has adverse outcomes that can be prevented by antimicrobial therapy. Thus, screening and treatment for asymptomatic bacteriuria are recommended for pregnant females (because of the risk of progression to severe symptomatic UTI and possible harm to the fetus), males undergoing transurethral resection of the prostate, and individuals undergoing urologic procedures for which mucosal bleeding is anticipated. In contrast, screening for or treatment of asymptomatic bacteriuria is not recommended for premenopausal, nonpregnant females; diabetic females;

older persons living in the community; older institutionalized adults; persons with spinal cord injury; or catheterized patients while the catheter is in place.

Cystitis

Typically, patients with cystitis (infection of the bladder) complain of dysuria, frequency, and urgency (compelling need to urinate). These symptoms are a result not only of inflammation of the bladder but also of multiplication of bacteria in the urine and urethra. Often, there is tenderness and pain over the area of the bladder. In some individuals, the urine is grossly bloody. The patient may note urine cloudiness and a bad odor. Because cystitis is a localized infection, fever and other signs of systemic illness are usually not present.

Acute Urethral Syndrome

Another UTI is **acute urethral syndrome.** Patients with this syndrome are primarily young, sexually active females, who experience dysuria, frequency, and urgency but yield fewer organisms than 10^5 colony-forming units of bacteria per milliliter (CFU/mL) urine on culture. The criterion of greater than 10^5 CFU/mL of urine is highly indicative of infection in most patients with UTIs. Almost 50% of all females who seek medical attention for complaints of symptoms of acute cystitis fall into this group. Although *C. trachomatis* and *N. gonorrhoeae* urethritis, anaerobic infection, genital herpes, and vaginitis account for some cases of acute urethral syndrome, most of these females are infected with organisms identical to those that cause cystitis but in numbers less than 10^5 CFU/mL of urine. A cutoff of 10^2 CFU/mL, rather than 10^5 CFU/mL, must be used for this group of patients, but concomitant pyuria (presence of eight or more leukocytes per cubic millimeter on microscopic examination of uncentrifuged urine) must also be present. Approximately 90% of these females have pyuria, an important discriminatory feature of infection.

Pyelonephritis

Pyelonephritis refers to inflammation of the kidney parenchyma, calices (cup-shaped division of the renal pelvis), and pelvis (upper end of the ureter that is located inside the kidney) and is usually caused by bacterial infection. Pyelonephritis may appear as an acute or chronic condition. Acute pyelonephritis presents with enlarged kidneys that contain surface abscesses. Chronic pyelonephritis presents with scarring on one or both kidneys and interstitial fibrosis on the pelvic wall. An inflammatory infiltrate of white blood cells, predominantly lymphocytes, is typically present. In addition, the tubules in the kidneys may either be dilated or constricted and contain **colloid casts** (crystalized mucous secretions). The typical clinical presentation of an upper UTI includes fever and flank (lower back) pain and, frequently, lower tract symptoms (frequency, urgency, and dysuria). Patients can also exhibit systemic signs of infection such as vomiting, diarrhea, chills, increased heart rate, and lower abdominal pain. Of significance, 40% of patients with acute pyelonephritis are bacteremic. Acute papillary necrosis of one or more renal pyramids (cone-shaped tissue) may occur as a complication associated with pyelonephritis.

Urosepsis

Approximately 25% of sepsis cases (severe blood infection) are a result of **urosepsis,** a systemic infection that may develop from community-, hospital-, or health care–associated UTIs. Urosepsis is defined as evidence of a UTI and two or more additional signs including an elevated temperature (>38°C), an elevated heart rate (>90 beats/min), an increased respiratory rate (>20 breaths/min or a PCO_2 of <32 mm Hg), or an abnormal white blood cell count (>12,000/mm^3, <4000/mm^3, or >10% neutrophilic band forms). Early diagnosis and treatment of UTIs are essential in preventing urosepsis.

Laboratory Diagnosis of Urinary Tract Infections

As previously mentioned, because noninvasive methods for collecting urine must rely on a specimen that has passed through a contaminated milieu, quantitative cultures for the diagnosis of UTI are used to discriminate between contamination, colonization, and infection. Refer to Table 5.1 for a quick reference for collecting, transporting, and processing urinary tract specimens.

Specimen Collection

Prevention of contamination by normal vaginal, perineal, and anterior urethral microbiota is the most important consideration for the collection of a clinically relevant urine specimen.

Clean-Catch Midstream Urine

The least invasive and preferred routine collection procedure, the clean-catch midstream urine specimen collection, must be performed carefully for optimal results, especially with female patients. Good patient education is essential. Guidelines for proper specimen collection should be prepared on a printed card (bilingual, if necessary), with the procedure clearly described and preferably illustrated to help ensure patient compliance. The patient should be instructed to wash their hands before cleaning the periurethral area, wiping from front to back three times, each time with a clean sterile gauze pad soaked with a mild detergent to prevent contamination. Of importance, the patient should also be instructed to rinse well with two or more sponges soaked in sterile distilled water to remove the detergent, which may be bacteriostatic. Once cleansing is completed, the patient should retract the labial folds or glans penis, begin to void, and then collect a midstream urine sample. Studies show that uncleansed, first-void specimens from males are as sensitive as (but less specific than) midstream urine specimens. Sterile bags may be used for infants and children.

Straight Catheterized Urine

Although slightly more invasive, urinary catheterization provides a method for the collection of uncontaminated urine from the bladder in uncooperative patients or patients unable to void because of other underlying physiologic conditions. Either a physician or another trained health professional performs this procedure. Risk exists, however, that urethral organisms will be introduced into the bladder with the catheter.

Suprapubic Bladder Aspiration

After preparation of the skin, urine is withdrawn directly into a syringe through a percutaneously inserted needle during **suprapubic bladder aspiration,** thereby ensuring a contamination-free specimen. The bladder must be full before the procedure is performed. This collection technique may be indicated in certain clinical situations, such as pediatric practice, when urine is difficult to obtain. If good aseptic techniques are used, this procedure can be performed with little risk in premature infants, neonates, small children, and pregnant women and other adults with full bladders.

Indwelling Catheter

Patients who are housed in hospitals and long-term care facilities and those treated in other health care–associated settings such as outpatient clinics for cancer and transplant patients are more frequently required to use indwelling urinary catheters. These patients are very likely to develop bacteriuria, which predisposes them to more severe infections. Specimen collection from patients with indwelling catheters requires scrupulous aseptic technique. Health care workers who manipulate a urinary catheter in any way should wear gloves. The catheter tubing should be clamped off above the port to allow the collection of freshly voided urine. The catheter port or wall of the tubing should then be cleaned vigorously with 70% ethanol, and urine should be aspirated via a needle and syringe; the integrity of the closed drainage system must be maintained to prevent the introduction of organisms into the bladder. Specimens obtained from the collection bag are inappropriate, because organisms can multiply there, obscuring the true relative numbers. Cultures should be obtained when patients are ill; routine monitoring does not yield clinically relevant data.

Specimen Transport

Because it is an excellent supportive medium for the growth of most bacteria, urine must be immediately refrigerated or preserved. Bacterial counts in refrigerated (4°C) urine remain constant for as long as 24 hours. Urine transport tubes (BD Urine Culture Kit [Becton Dickinson Vacutainer Kits, Franklin Lakes, NJ]) containing boric acid, sodium borate, and sodium formate have been shown to preserve bacteria without refrigeration for as long as 48 hours when more than 10^5 CFU/mL (100,000 organisms per milliliter) are present in the initial urine specimen. The system may inhibit the growth of certain organisms, and it must be used

with a minimum of 3 mL of urine. Boric acid products preserve bacterial viability in urine in the absence of antibiotics. For patients from whom colony counts of organisms of less than 100,000/mL might be clinically significant, plating within 2 hours of collection is recommended. The kit provides a convenient method for preserving and transporting urine from remote areas where refrigeration is not practical.

Screening Procedures

As many as 60% to 80% of all urine specimens received for culture by the acute care medical center laboratory may contain no etiologic agents of infection or contain only contaminants. Procedures developed to quickly identify those urine specimens that will be negative on culture and circumvent excessive use of media, technical staff, and the overnight incubation period are discussed in this section. A reliable screening test for the presence or absence of bacteriuria provides physicians important same-day information that a conventional urine culture may take a day or longer to provide. Many screening methods have been advocated for use in detecting bacteriuria and/or pyuria.

Red blood cells or erythrocytes identified in the urine, **hematuria,** may also indicate UTI, but this occurs in a variety of other physiologic disorders. White blood cell casts in urine are strong evidence of pyelonephritis but can also be associated with renal disease in the absence of infection. In addition, elevated levels of protein (<2 g in 24 hours) in a urine sample may also indicate a UTI.

Gram or Methylene Blue Stain

A differential Gram stain or basic nondifferential methylene blue stain of urine is an easy, inexpensive means to provide immediate information as to the nature of the infecting organism (bacteria or yeast) to guide empiric therapy. After a drop of well-mixed urine is allowed to air dry, the smear is fixed, stained, and examined under oil immersion (1000×) for the presence of 1 or 5 bacteria per oil immersion field (OIF). The performance characteristics of the urine Gram stain are not well defined, in that different criteria have been used to define a positive result (1 or 5 bacteria per OIF). Using either 1 or 5 bacteria/OIF has a sensitivity of 96% and 95%, respectively, and a specificity of 91% when correlated with significant bacteriuria (>10^5 CFU/mL—extrapolated as one bacterium per microscopic field in an uncentrifuged sample). The absence of bacteria in a stained sediment from a centrifuged sample (5 minutes at 2000 rpm) indicates the probability that the specimen contains less than 10^4 bacteria/mL. The Gram stain should not be relied on for detecting polymorphonuclear leukocytes in urine, because leukocytes deteriorate quickly in urine that is not fresh or not adequately preserved. Many microbiologists have not adopted Gram stain examination of urine specimens because of its unreliability in detecting lower yet clinically significant numbers of organisms and because of its labor intensity. If used, urine Gram stain should be limited to patients with acute pyelonephritis, patients with invasive

UTIs, or other patients for whom immediate information is necessary for appropriate clinical management.

Pyuria

Pyuria (10 leukocytes/mm^3, using a hematocytomer from a clean-catch midstream specimen) is the hallmark of inflammation, and the presence of polymorphonuclear neutrophils (PMNs) can be detected and enumerated in uncentrifuged specimens. This method of screening urine correlates well with the number of PMNs (neutrophils) excreted per hour, the best indicator of the host's state. Patients with more than 300,000 PMNs excreted into the urine per hour are likely to have a current infection. The standard urinalysis (usually completed in the laboratory hematology or chemistry sections) includes an examination of the centrifuged sediment of urine for enumeration of PMNs, results of which do not correlate well with either the PMN excretion rate or the presence of infection. Pyuria also can be associated with other clinical diseases, such as vaginitis, and therefore is not specific for UTIs.

Indirect Indices

Screening tests commonly detect bacteriuria or pyuria by examining for the presence of bacterial enzymes or PMN enzymes rather than the organisms or PMNs themselves.

Nitrate Reductase (Griess) Test

The nitrate reductase (Griess) test looks for the presence of urinary nitrite, an indicator of UTI. Nitrate-reducing enzymes that are produced by the most common urinary tract pathogens reduce nitrate to nitrite. This test has been incorporated onto a urinary dipstick that also tests for leukocyte esterase—an enzyme produced by PMNs (discussed next). Liquid-chromatography tandem mass spectrometry (LC-MS/MS) has been used to screen urine for the presence of nitrate and nitrite for the diagnosis of UTIs. This test is not sensitive to variations in urine chemistry and has a demonstrated specificity (91%) and sensitivity (95%), which is greater than using the nitrate reductase test.

Leukocyte Esterase Test

As previously mentioned, evidence of a host response to infection is the presence of PMNs in the urine. Because inflammatory cells produce leukocyte esterase, a simple, inexpensive, and rapid method that measures this enzyme has been developed. Studies have shown that leukocyte esterase activity correlates with hemocytometer chamber counts. The nitrate reductase and leukocyte esterase tests have been incorporated into the urinary dipstick. Numerous manufacturers sell these strips commercially, and the strips are one of the most widely used enzymatic tests. Although the sensitivity of the combination strip is higher than either test alone, the sensitivity of this combination screening is not great enough to recommend its use as a standalone test in most circumstances. Of note, the leukocyte esterase test is not sensitive enough for determining pyuria in patients with acute urethral syndrome.

Catalase

The Accutest Uriscreen (JANT Pharmacal Corp., Encino, CA) is another rapid urine-screening system based on the detection of catalase present in human somatic cells and in most bacterial species that commonly cause UTIs except for streptococci and enterococci. Approximately 1.5 to 2 mL of urine is added to a tube containing dehydrated substrate. Hydrogen peroxide is added to the urine, and the solution is mixed gently. The formation of bubbles above the liquid surface is interpreted as a positive test. Visible results are available in approximately 2 minutes.

Automated and Semiautomated Systems

Automated screening systems offer a large throughput with minimal labor and a rapid turnaround time compared with conventional cultures.

Various automated or semiautomated urine-screening systems are commercially available, such as the Iris Urinalysis System (Beckman-Coulter, Inc., Brea, CA), and can analyze a urine or body fluid sample in one instrument. The instrument analyzes both the microscopic components and the urine chemistries by combining technology of both types of analyzers into one automated system. The Iris System uses a flow-imaging microscopy method to capture individual images of each particle identified in the specimen and then classifies the particle using Auto-Particle Recognition (APP) software. Siemens Medical Solutions USA, Inc. (Malvern, PA) manufactures a wide range of CLINITEK automated/semiautomated urine analyzers that include point-of-care to high-throughput walkaway instruments. In addition, the Sysmex UN-2000 (Lincolnshire, IL) uses flow cytometry and specific fluorescent dyes for the physical and chemical identification of organisms and other particles in urine samples. Various studies have indicated that automated urinalysis instrumentation has demonstrated limitations and continue to recommend manual microscopic analysis of urine samples for the diagnosis of UTI.

General Comments Regarding Screening Procedures

In general, screening methods are insensitive at levels below 10^5 CFU/mL. Therefore, they are not acceptable for urine specimens collected by suprapubic aspiration, catheterization, or cystoscopy. Screening methods may also fail to detect a significant number of infections in symptomatic patients with low colony counts (10^2 to 10^3 CFU/mL), such as young, sexually active females with acute urethral syndrome. Further complicating the laboratory's decision as to whether to adopt a screening method is whether screening results will be used to rule out infection in asymptomatic patients. Under these circumstances, testing for pyuria is essential.

Therefore, given the importance of the 10^2 CFU/mL count and the PMN count, no screening test should be used indiscriminately. Selecting a screening method largely depends on the laboratory and the patient population being served by the laboratory. For example, there will be a cost advantage in screening urine in laboratories that receive many culture-negative specimens. On the other hand, urine from patients with symptoms of UTI plus a selected group expected to have asymptomatic bacteriuria should be cultured. For example, patients in their first trimester of pregnancy should be cultured, because these patients might appear asymptomatic but have a covert infection and become symptomatic later; UTIs in pregnant females may lead to pyelonephritis and the likelihood of a premature birth. Other situations in which patients with no symptoms of UTI might be cultured include the following:

- Bacteremia of unknown source
- Urinary tract obstruction
- Follow-up after removal of an indwelling catheter
- Follow-up of previous therapy

Other factors that must be considered when selecting a rapid urine screen include accuracy, ease of test performance, reproducibility, turnaround time, and whether bacteriuria or pyuria is detected.

Urine Culture

Inoculation and Incubation of Urine Cultures

Once it has been determined that a urine specimen should be cultured for isolation of the common agents of UTI, a measured amount of urine is inoculated to each of the appropriate media. The urine should be mixed thoroughly before plating. The plates can be inoculated using a calibrated loop designed to deliver a known volume, either 0.01 or 0.001 mL of urine. These loops, made of platinum, plastic, or other material, can be obtained from laboratory supply companies.

The calibrated loop that delivers the larger volume of urine (0.01 mL) is recommended to detect lower numbers of organisms in certain specimens. For example, urine collected from catheterization, nephrostomies, ileal conduits, and suprapubic aspirates should be plated with the larger calibrated loop. The communication of pertinent clinical history to the laboratory is essential so that appropriate processing can be performed.

The choice of media to inoculate depends on the patient population served and the microbiologist's preference. The use of a 5% sheep blood agar plate and a MacConkey agar plate allows the detection of most gram-negative bacilli, staphylococci, streptococci, and enterococci. To save cost and somewhat streamline culture processing, many laboratories use an agar plate split in half (biplate); one side contains 5% sheep blood agar and the other half contains MacConkey or Eosin Methylene Blue agar (Fig. 72.2).

In some circumstances, enterococci and other streptococci may be obscured by heavy growth of Enterobacterales. Because of this possibility, some laboratories add a selective plate for gram-positive organisms, such as Columbia colistin-nalidixic acid agar (CNA) or Enterococcosel Agar (Bile Esculin Azide Agar, Becton-Dickinson, Sparks, MD). Although some discriminatory capability may be added, cost is also added to the procedure. In addition

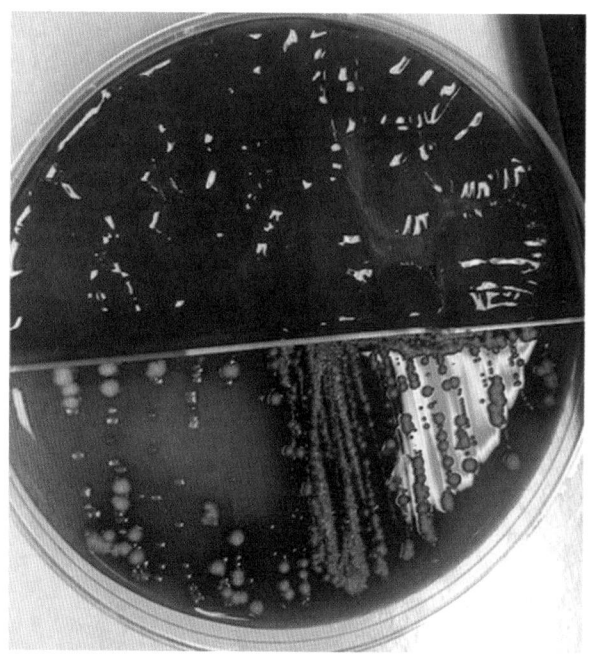

• **Fig. 72.2** *Cronobacter sakazakii* isolated from a urinary sample on a 5% sheep blood agar/eosin methylene blue biplate.

to increased cost, inclusion of plated media selective for gram-positive organisms generally provides no or limited additional information. Many European laboratories use cystine-lactose electrolyte-deficient (CLED) agar. CLED agar does not contain sodium chloride, inhibiting the characteristic swarming of *Proteus* spp., but still supports adequate growth of most common urinary pathogens. In recent years, chromogenic media have been introduced and become commercially available from several manufacturers, allowing more specific direct detection and differentiation of urinary tract pathogens on primary plates, such as BD CHROMagar (Becton Dickson, Heidelberg, Germany). This medium uses enzymatic reactions to identify *E. coli* and *Enterococcus* without additional confirmatory testing from urine specimens and provides presumptive identification of *S. saprophyticus*, *Streptococcus agalactiae*, *Klebsiella-Enterobacter-Serratia*, and the *Proteus-Morganella-Providencia* groups.

Before inoculation, urine is mixed thoroughly, and the top of the container is then removed. The calibrated loop is inserted vertically into the urine in a cup. Otherwise, more than the desired volume of urine will be taken up, potentially affecting the quantitative culture result (Fig. 72.3). A widely used method is described in Evolve Procedure 72.1. Once inoculated, the plates are streaked to obtain isolated colonies (Fig. 72.4).

Once plated, urine cultures are incubated overnight at 35°C. Incubation for a minimum of 24 hours is typically necessary to detect uropathogens. Thus, some specimens inoculated late in the day cannot be read accurately the next morning. These cultures should either be reincubated until the next day or interpreted later in the day when a full 24-hour incubation has been completed.

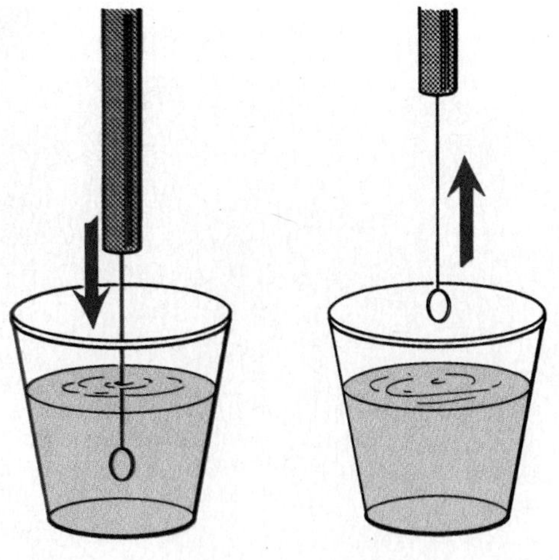

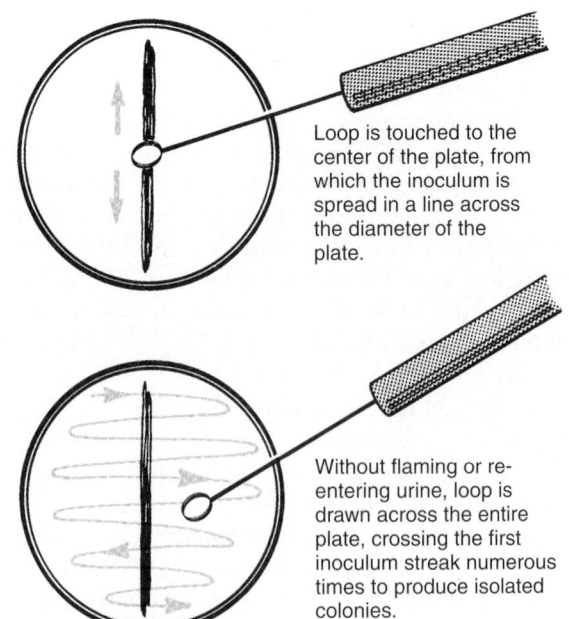

• **Fig. 72.3** Method for inserting a calibrated loop into urine to ensure that the proper amount of specimen adheres to the loop.

Loop is touched to the center of the plate, from which the inoculum is spread in a line across the diameter of the plate.

Without flaming or re-entering urine, loop is drawn across the entire plate, crossing the first inoculum streak numerous times to produce isolated colonies.

• **Fig. 72.4** Method for streaking with calibrated urine loop to produce isolated colonies and countable colony-forming units.

Interpretation of Urine Cultures

As previously mentioned, UTIs may be completely asymptomatic, produce mild symptoms, or cause life-threatening infections. Of importance, the criteria most useful for microbiologic assessment of urine specimens is dependent not only on the type of urine submitted (e.g., voided, straight catheterization) but the clinical history of the patient (e.g., age, sex, symptoms, antibiotic therapy).

One major problem in interpreting urine cultures arises because urine cultures collected by the voided technique may be contaminated with normal microbiota, including Enterobacterales. Determining what colony count represents true infection from contamination is of utmost importance and is related to the patient's clinical presentation. Several studies have proposed the use of different cutoffs in colony counts based on clinical presentation; an example of one such set of guidelines is given in Table 72.1.

Ideally, the clinician caring for the patient should provide the laboratory with enough clinical information to allow specimens from different patient populations to be identified. These specimens could then be selectively processed using the guidelines in Table 72.1. However, because microbiology laboratories frequently receive little or no clinical information about patients, questions have been raised as to whether these cutoffs are practical and realistic for routine laboratory use. Further complicating urine culture interpretation is the increasing difficulty in distinguishing between infection and contamination as the criterion for a positive culture is lowered from 10^5 CFU/mL to 10^2 CFU/mL. Because of these issues, many laboratories establish their own interpretative criteria for urine cultures based on the type of urine submitted (e.g., clean-catch midstream, catheterized, or surgically obtained specimens such as suprapubic aspirates). Variations in interpretative guidelines occur from one laboratory to another, but some generalities can be made; these are listed in Table 72.2. Some examples of urine culture results are shown in Fig. 72.5 to illustrate some of these interpretations. See the Evolve site for a semi-quantitative procedure for the inoculation of urine cultures.

In addition to the previously described guidelines, a pure culture of *S. aureus* is significant regardless of the number of CFUs, and antimicrobial susceptibility tests are performed. The presence of yeast in any number is reported to physicians, and pure cultures of yeast may be identified to the species level. In all urine, regardless of the extent of final workup, all isolates should be enumerated (e.g., three different organisms present at 10^3 CFU/mL), and those present in numbers greater than 10^4 CFU/mL should be described morphologically (e.g., non–lactose fermenting gram-negative rods).

ⓔ Visit the Evolve site for a complete list of procedures, review questions, and case studies.

TABLE 72.1 Criteria for Classification of Urinary Tract Infections by Clinical Syndrome

Category	Clinical	Laboratory Results
Acute, uncomplicated UTI in females	Dysuria, urgency, frequency, suprapubic pain No urinary symptoms in last 4 weeks before the current episode No fever or flank pain	≥10 WBC/mm^3 ≥10^3 CFU/mL uropathogens[a] in CCMS urine
Acute, uncomplicated pyelonephritis	Fever, chills Flank pain on examination Other diagnoses excluded No history or clinical evidence of urologic abnormalities	≥10 WBC/mm^3 ≥10^4 CFU/mL uropathogens in CCMS urine
Complicated UTI and UTI in males	Any combination of symptoms listed above. One or more factors associated with complicated UTI[b]	≥10 WBC/mm^3 ≥10^5 CFU/mL uropathogens in CCMS urine
Asymptomatic bacteriuria: female patients	No urinary symptoms	± >10 WBC/mm^3 ≥10^5 CFU/mL in two CCMS cultures >24 h apart
Asymptomatic bacteriuria: male patients	No urinary symptoms	± >10 WBC/mm^3 ≥10^3 CFU/mL (suggestive) ≥10^5 CFU/mL (definitive) in one CCMS

[a]Uropathogens: Organisms that commonly cause UTIs.
[b]Factors associated with complicated UTI include any UTI in a male patient, indwelling or intermittent urinary catheter, more than 100 mL of postvoid residual urine, obstructive uropathy, urologic abnormalities, azotemia (excess urea in the blood, even without structural abnormalities), and renal transplantation.
CCMS, Clean-catch midstream urine; CFU, colony-forming unit; UTI, urinary tract infection; WBC, white blood cells.
Data from Stamm WE. Criteria for the diagnosis of urinary tract infection and for the assessment of therapeutic effectiveness. Infection 20(suppl 3):S151, 1992; and Bennett J, Dolin R, Blaser M. Principles and Practice of Infectious Diseases. 8th ed. Philadelphia: Elsevier-Saunders; 2015.

TABLE 72.2 Suggested Interpretative Guidelines for Urine Cultures

Result	Specific Specimen Type/Associated Clinical Condition, if Known	Workup
≥10^4 CFU/mL of a single potential pathogen or for each of two potential pathogens	CCMS urine/pyelonephritis, acute cystitis, asymptomatic bacteriuria, or catheterized urines	Complete[a]
≥10^3 CFU/mL of a single potential pathogen	CCMS urine/symptomatic male patients or catheterized urine or acute urethral syndrome	Complete
≥ Three organism types with no predominating organism	CCMS urine or catheterized urine	None; because of possible contamination, ask for another specimen
Either two or three organism types with predominant growth of one organism type and <10^4 CFU/mL of the other organism type(s)	CCMS urine	Complete workup for the predominating[b] organism(s); description of the organism(s)
≥10^2 CFU/mL of any number of organism types (set up with a 0.001- and 0.01-mL calibrated loop)	Suprapubic aspirates, any other surgically obtained urine (including ileal conduits, cystoscopy specimens)	Complete

[a]A complete workup includes identification of the organism and appropriate susceptibility testing.
CCMS, Clean-catch midstream urine; CFU, colony-forming unit.
[b]Predominant growth is 10^4 to 10^5 CFU/mL or more.

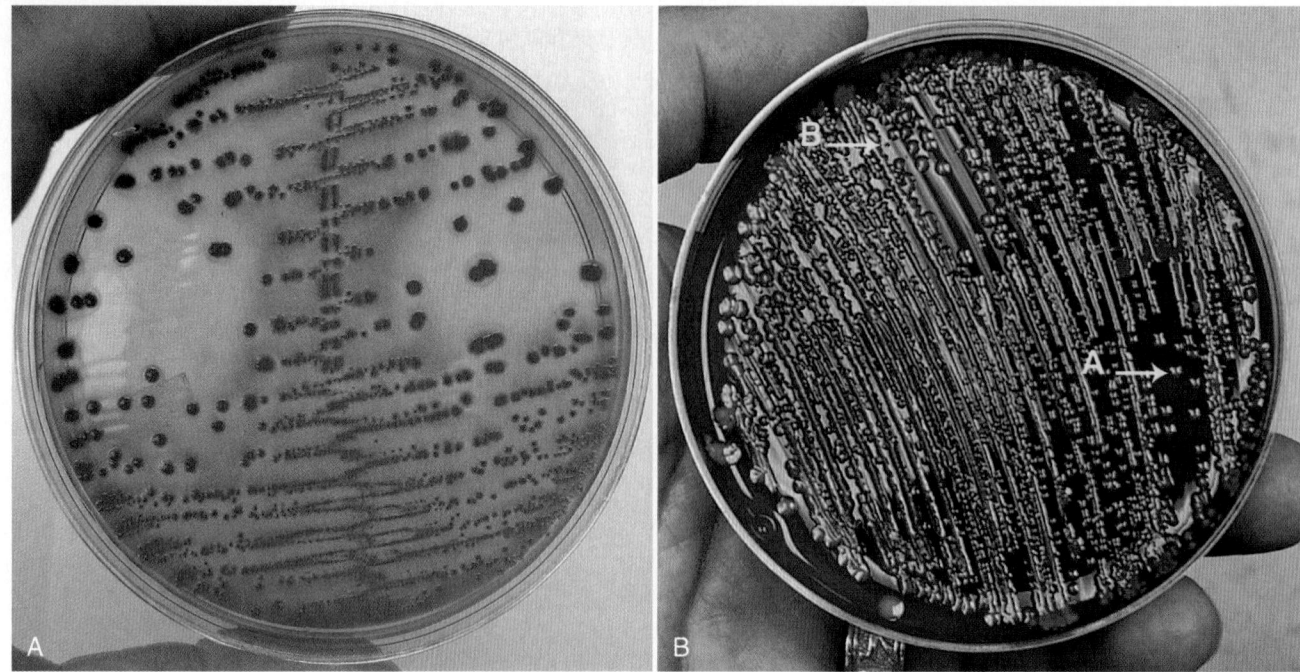

• **Fig. 72.5** Culture results illustrating some of the various interpretative guidelines. (A) Growth of 10^5 CFU/mL or more of a lactose-fermenting gram-negative rod in a clean-catch midstream (CCMS) urine sample from a patient with pyelonephritis; complete workup would be done. (B) Growth of 10^5 CFU/mL or more of a lactose-fermenting gram-negative rod (*arrow A*) and less than 10^4 CFU/mL of another organism type (*arrow B*) from a CCMS urine; only the organism with a colony count of at least 10^4 to 10^5 CFU/mL would be worked up completely. *CFU*, Colony-forming units.

Bibliography

Anderson AC, Martin SM, Hultgren SJ: Host subversion by formation of intracellular bacterial communities in the urinary tract, *Microbes Infect* 6:1094–1101, 2004.

Bartosova K, Kubicek Z, Franekova J, et al.: Analysis of four automated urinalysis systems compared to reference methods, *Clin Lab* 62(11):2115–2123, 2016.

Bennett J, Dolin R, Blaser M: *Principles and practice of infectious diseases*, ed 9, Philadelphia, PA, 2020, Elsevier.

Bernard MS, Hunter KF, Moore KN: A review of strategies to decrease the duration of indwelling urethral catheters and potentially reduce the incidence of catheter-associated urinary tract infections, *Urol Nurs* 32:29–37, 2012.

Carroll KC, Pfaller MA: *Manual of clinical microbiology*, ed 12, Washington, DC, 2019, ASM Press.

Chao MR, Shih YM, Hsu YW, et al.: Urinary nitrite/nitrate ratio measured by isotope-dilution LC-MS/MS as a tool to screen for urinary tract infections, *Free Radic Biol Med* 93:77–83, 2016.

Churchill D, Gregson D: Screening urine samples for significant bacteriuria in the clinical microbiology laboratory, *Clin Microbiol Newsl* 26:179, 2004.

Domann E, Hong G, Imirzalioglu C, et al.: Culture-independent identification of pathogenic bacteria and polymicrobial infections in the genitourinary tract of renal transplant recipients, *J Clin Microbiol* 41:5500–5510, 2003.

Foxman B, Brown P: Epidemiology of urinary tract infections: transmission and risk factors, incidence, and costs, *Infect Dis Clin North Am* 17:227–241, 2003.

Kucheria R, Dasgupta P, Sacks SH, et al.: Urinary tract infections: new insights into a common problem, *Postgrad Med J* 81:83–86, 2005.

Kunin CM, White LV, Hua TH: A reassessment of the importance of "low-count" bacteriuria in young women with acute urinary symptoms, *Ann Intern Med* 119:454–460, 1993.

Nicolle LE, Bradley S, Colgan R, et al.: Infectious Diseases Society of America guidelines for the diagnosis and treatment of asymptomatic bacteriuria in adults, *Clin Infect Dis* 40:643–654, 2005.

Nosseir SB, Lind LR, Winkler HA: Recurrent uncomplicated urinary tract infections in women: a review, *J Womens Health* 21:347–354, 2012.

Parham NJ, Pollard SJ, Chaudhuri RR, et al.: Prevalence of pathogenicity island IICFT073 genes among extraintestinal clinical isolates of *Escherichia coli*, *J Clin Microbiol* 43:2425–2434, 2005.

Pezzlo M: Detection of urinary tract infections by rapid methods, *Clin Microbiol Rev* 1:268–280, 1988.

Pezzlo M, York MK: Urine cultures. Section 3.12. In Isenberg HD, editor: *Clinical microbiology procedures handbook*, vol. 1. Washington, DC, 2004, American Society for Microbiology.

Sharda N, Bakhtar O, Thajudeen B, et al.: Manual urine microscopy versus automated urine analyzer microscopy in patients with acute kidney injury, *Lab Med* 45(4):e152–e155, 2014.

Stamm WE: Criteria for the diagnosis of urinary tract infection and for the assessment of therapeutic effectiveness, *Infection* 20(Suppl 3):S151–S154, 1992.

Stevens M: Evaluation of questor urine screening for bacteriuria and pyuria, *J Clin Pathol* 46:817–821, 1993.

Venuti K, Cabrera C, Burkett LS, et al.: Impact of menopausal status on uropathogen prevalence and antimicrobial resistance profiles, *Female Pelvic Med Reconstr Surg*, 2019. https://doi.org/10.1097/SPV.0000000000000778.

Wagenlehner FM, Pilatz A, Weidner W: Urosepsis—from the view of the urologist, *Int J Antimicrob Agents* (Suppl 38):51–57, 2011.

Wilson ML, Gaido L: Laboratory diagnosis of urinary tract infections in adult patients, *Clin Infect Dis* 38:1150–1158, 2004.

73

Genital Tract Infections

General Considerations

Anatomy

Familiarity with the anatomic structures is important for appropriate processing of specimens from genital tract sites and interpretation of microbiologic laboratory results. The key anatomic structures for the female and male genital tract in relation to other important structures are shown in Fig. 73.1.

The female reproductive system consists of two main parts: the **uterus** and the **ovaries.** The uterus produces vaginal and uterine secretions and is the location where the human fetus grows and matures during reproduction. The ovaries connect to the uterus and the fallopian tubes. The ovaries produce the female eggs that pass through the fallopian tubes and will imbed in the uterus when fertilized by the male sperm. The uterus connects to the vaginal opening through the cervix.

The male reproductive system, unlike the female, consists of several organs that are located external to the abdominal cavity. The main organs consist of the **penis** and the **testes** that produce the semen and sperm for fertilization of the female egg. The sperm is stored in a small gland coiled around the testis, the **epididymis.** The **prostate gland** surrounds the ejaculatory duct and produces semen, prostatic fluid, and seminal fluid.

Resident Microbiota

The lining of the human genital tract consists of a mucosal layer of transitional (cells capable of undergoing shape change or transitions), columnar (ciliated and longer than wide), and squamous epithelial (thin and flat) cells. Various species of commensal bacteria colonize these surfaces, causing no harm to the host except under abnormal circumstances. The colonization of the surface by resident microbiota produces a biologic barrier preventing the adherence of pathogenic organisms. Normal urethral microbiota includes coagulase-negative staphylococci and corynebacteria, as well as various anaerobes. The **vulva** and penis, especially the area underneath the **prepuce** (foreskin) of the uncircumcised male, may harbor *Mycobacterium smegmatis* along with other gram-positive bacteria.

The microbiota of the female genital tract varies with the pH and estrogen concentration of the mucosa, which depend on the host's age. Prepubescent and postmenopausal females primarily harbor staphylococci and corynebacteria (the same microbiota present on surface epithelium); whereas females of reproductive age may harbor large numbers of facultative bacteria, such as Enterobacterales, streptococci, and staphylococci, as well as anaerobes, such as lactobacilli, anaerobic non–spore-forming bacilli and cocci, and clostridia. Lactobacilli are the predominant organisms in secretions in normal, healthy vaginas. The lactobacilli present in vaginal secretions metabolize glucose to lactic acid, resulting in a pH of approximately 4.0. The acidic pH coupled with the organism's ability to produce hydrogen peroxide prevents infection by exogenous sexually transmitted pathogens. Many women carry group B beta-hemolytic

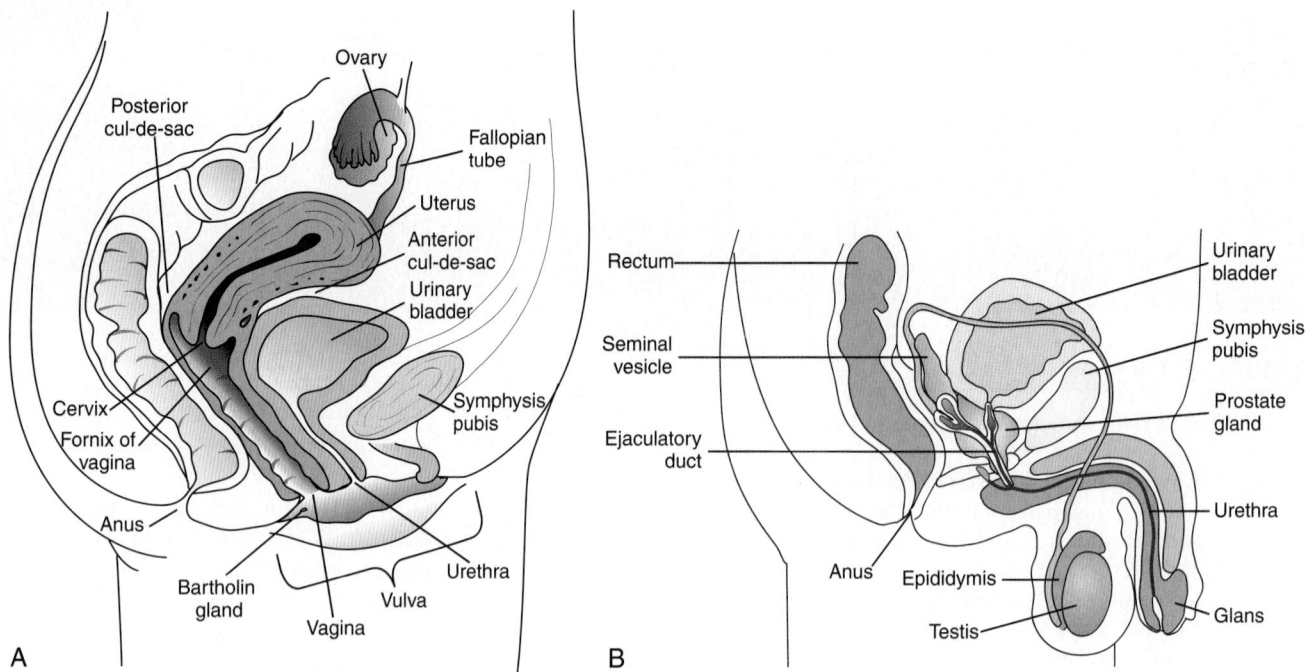

• **Fig. 73.1** Location of key anatomic structures of the female (A) and male (B) genital tracts in relation to other major anatomic structures.

streptococci *(Streptococcus agalactiae),* which may be transmitted to the neonate. Although yeasts (acquired from the gastrointestinal tract) may be transiently recovered from the female vaginal tract, they are not considered normal microbiota.

Sexually Transmitted Diseases and Other Genital Tract Infections

Genital tract infections may be classified as endogenous or exogenous. Exogenous infections may be acquired as people engage in sexual activity, and these infections are referred to as **sexually transmitted diseases (STDs).** In contrast, endogenous infections result from normal genital microbiota.

Female genital tract infections can be divided into **lower genital tract** (vulva, vagina, and cervix) and **upper genital tract** (uterus, fallopian tubes, ovaries, and abdominal cavity) infections. Lower genital tract infections are commonly acquired by sexual or direct contact. Although the organisms that cause lower genital tract infections are not usually part of the normal genital tract microbiota, some organisms normally present in very low numbers can increase sufficiently to cause disease. Upper genital tract infections are frequently an extension of a lower tract infection in which organisms from the vagina or cervix travel into the uterine cavity and on through the endometrium to the fallopian tubes and ovaries. Similarly, an organism can spread along contiguous mucosal surfaces in the male from a lower genital tract site of infection (i.e., urethra) and cause infection in a reproductive organ, such as the epididymis.

Genital Tract Infections

Sexually Transmitted Diseases and Other Lower Genital Tract Infections

Lower genital tract infections may be acquired either through sexual contact with an infected partner or through nonsexual means. These infections are some of the most common infectious diseases.

Epidemiology and Etiologic Agents

STDs or sexually transmitted infections (STIs) are major public health problems in all populations and socioeconomic groups worldwide. The incidence and spread of STDs are greatly influenced by numerous factors, such as the availability of multiple sexual partners, the presence of asymptomatic infection, the frequent movement of people within populations, and increasing affluence.

The number of microorganisms that can cause genital tract infections is large. These organisms are diverse, representing all four major groups of microorganisms: bacteria, viruses, fungi, and parasites. The major causes of genital tract infections are listed in Table 73.1.

Routes of Transmission

Although genital tract infections can be caused by members of the patient's genital microbiota (endogenous infections), the overwhelming majority of lower genital tract infections are sexually transmitted.

Sexually Transmitted

Chlamydia trachomatis (CT), *Neisseria gonorrhoeae* (GC), *Trichomonas vaginalis,* human immunodeficiency virus

TABLE 73.1 Major Causes of Genital Tract Infections and Sexually Transmitted Diseases

Frequency	Disease	Agent	Organism Group
More Common	Genital and anal warts (condyloma); cervical dysplasia; cancer	Human papillomavirus	Viruses
	Vaginitis	*Gardnerella/Mobiluncus, Trichomonas vaginalis, Candida albicans*	Bacteria, parasites, fungi
	Urethritis/cervicitis (also acute salpingitis, acute perihepatitis, urethritis, pharyngitis)	*Neisseria gonorrhoeae, Chlamydia trachomatis, Ureaplasma urealyticum*	Bacteria
	Herpes genitalis (genital/skin ulcers)	Herpes simplex virus type 2 (less commonly type 1)	Viruses
	AIDS	Human immunodeficiency virus (HIV)	Viruses
	Hepatitis (acute and chronic infection)	Hepatitis B virus	Viruses
Less Common	Lymphogranuloma venereum	*C. trachomatis* (L-1, L-2, L-3 serovars)	Bacteria
	Granuloma inguinale	*Klebsiella granulomatis* (Donovania)	Bacteria
	Syphilis	*Treponema pallidum*	Bacteria
	Chancroid	*Haemophilus ducreyi*	Bacteria
	Scabies, mites	*Sarcoptes scabiei*	Ectoparasites
	Pediculosis pubis, "crabs" infestation	*Phthirus pubis*	Ectoparasites
	Enteritis (homosexuals/proctitis)	*Giardia duodenalis, Entamoeba histolytica, Shigella* spp., *Salmonella* spp., *Enterobius vermicularis, Campylobacter* spp., *Helicobacter* spp.	Bacteria, parasites
	Molluscum contagiosum	Poxlike virus	Viruses
	Heterophile-negative mononucleosis, congenital infections	Cytomegalovirus	Viruses

(HIV), *Treponema pallidum, Ureaplasma urealyticum, Mycoplasma hominis,* other mycoplasmas, herpes simplex virus (HSV), and others may be acquired during sexual activity. In addition, other agents that cause genital tract disease and may be sexually transmitted include adenovirus, hepatitis B, human T-cell lymphotropic virus (HTLV), coxsackie virus, molluscum contagiosum virus (a member of the poxvirus group), the human papillomaviruses (HPVs) of genital warts (condylomata acuminata; types 6, 11, and others) and those associated with cervical carcinoma (predominantly types 16 and 18, but numerous others are also implicated), *Klebsiella granulomatis,* and ectoparasites, such as scabies and lice. Some of these agents are not routinely isolated from clinical specimens. Infections with more than one agent may occur; therefore, dual or concurrent infections should always be considered.

An individual's sexual habits and practices dictate potential sites of infection. Homosexual practices and increasingly common heterosexual practices of anal-genital or oral-genital intercourse allow for transmission of a genital tract infection to other body sites, such as the pharynx or anorectic region. In addition, these practices have required that other gastrointestinal and systemic pathogens also be considered etiologic agents of STDs. The intestinal protozoa *Giardia duodenalis, Entamoeba histolytica,* and *Cryptosporidium* spp. are significant causes of STDs, especially among homosexual populations. In the same group of patients, fecal pathogens, such as *Salmonella, Shigella, Campylobacter,* and *Microsporidium* are often transmitted sexually. Oral-genital practices may provide an opportunity for *N. meningitidis* to colonize and infect the genital tract. In fact, *N. meningitidis* is increasingly being recognized as a pathogen associated with urethritis. Outbreaks with *N. meningitidis* have been predominately identified in heterosexual males. Viruses shed in secretions or present in blood (cytomegalovirus [CMV]; hepatitis B, and possibly C and E; other non-A, non-B hepatitis viruses; HTLV type I [HTLV-I]; and HIV) are spread by sexual practices.

Certain infections that are sexually transmitted occur on the surface epithelium of or near the lower genital tract. The major pathogens of these types of infections include HSV, *Haemophilus ducreyi,* and *T. pallidum.*

Other Routes

Organisms may also be introduced into the genital tract by instrumentation, presence of a foreign body, or chemical or immunologic processes that cause irritation and can subsequently cause infection. These infections are often a result of infection with the same organisms capable of causing skin or wound infections. Infection can also be transmitted from mother to infant either *in vivo* or during delivery. For example, transplacental infection may occur with syphilis, HIV, CMV, or HSV. Infection in the newborn can also be acquired during delivery by direct contact with an infectious lesion or discharge in the mother and a susceptible mucous membrane, such as the eye in the infant. STDs such as HSV, *C. trachomatis,* and *N. gonorrhoeae* may be transmitted from mother to newborn in this manner. Other organisms, such as group B streptococci, *Escherichia coli,* and *Listeria monocytogenes* originating from the mother may also be transmitted to the infant before, during, or after birth. (Infections in the fetus and newborn are discussed later in this chapter.)

Clinical Manifestations

Clinical manifestations of lower genital tract infections are as varied and diverse as the etiologies.

Asymptomatic

Although symptoms of genital tract infections generally cause the patient to seek medical attention, a patient with an STD—especially a female—may be free of symptoms (i.e., asymptomatic). For example, gonorrhea *(N. gonorrhoeae)* or chlamydia *(C. trachomatis)* infection is usually obvious in males because of a urethral discharge, yet females with either or both infections may have either minimal symptoms or no symptoms at all. Also, the primary lesion of syphilis (chancre) can be unremarkable and go unnoticed by the patient. Therefore, the lack of symptoms does not guarantee the absence of disease. Unfortunately, these asymptomatic individuals can serve as reservoirs for infection and unknowingly spread the pathogen to other individuals. Asymptomatic infections in females caused by *N. gonorrhoeae* or *C. trachomatis* that go untreated can lead to serious sequelae, such as **pelvic inflammatory disease** (PID) or infertility.

Dysuria

Although a common presenting symptom associated with urinary tract infection, dysuria (painful urination) can also result from an STD caused by organisms such as *N. gonorrhoeae, C. trachomatis,* and HSV.

Urethral Discharge

The presence of an inflammatory exudate at the tip of the urethral meatus is generally observed in males; the symptoms of urethral infection in females are not commonly localized. Most males complain of discomfort at the penile tip as well as dysuria. Urethritis (swelling and irritation of the urethra) may be gonococcal, caused by *N. gonorrhoeae,* or nongonococcal. Nongonococcal urethritis (NGU) can be caused by common urinary tract infection isolates, adenoviruses, *C. trachomatis, T. vaginalis* (less frequently), and genital mycoplasmas, such as *M. hominis, Mycoplasma genitalium,* and *U. urealyticum.*

Lesions of the Skin and Mucous Membranes

Numerous organisms can cause genital lesions that are diverse in both their appearance and their associated symptoms (Fig. 73.2) but are most often associated with STDs. The agents and their features of infection are summarized in Table 73.2. Some of these infections, such as genital herpes (caused by HSV) or genital warts (caused by HPVs and discussed in Chapter 65), are common; whereas others, such as lymphogranuloma venereum and granuloma inguinale, are uncommon in the United States. Genital skin and mucous membrane infections are often polymicrobial, making the diagnosis difficult. In addition, the characteristics of the lesions may vary from one type of infectious process to another for the same organisms. For example, specific HPV genotypes infect mucosal cells in the cervix and anus. The virus can cause a progressive spectrum of abnormalities classified as low-grade and high-grade **squamous intraepithelial neoplasia** (the process of rapid cell growth that is faster than normal and continues to grow—i.e., a tumor) and in some cases, progress to invasive cervical or anal cancer.

The patient's history of behavior and other relevant clinical information are important when attempting to identify the infectious agent associated with the lesion. For example, recurrent genital lesions and periods of **dysesthesias** (pain when touched) with intermittent outbreaks suggests infection with HSV 1 or 2. The virus remains inactive within the nerve ganglia during asymptomatic periods and then reemerges after an illness or other physiologic stress placed on the host. A patient's medication history may also attribute to the eruption of a genital lesion. An individual who has recently completed antibiotic therapy for an unrelated condition who has sexual contact with a partner infected with *Candida albicans* may be more susceptible to infection. In addition, patients who have underlying autoimmune diseases, such as Crohn disease or HIV infection, are more susceptible to other infections and the development of genital lesions.

Vaginitis

Inflammation of the vaginal mucosa, called **vaginitis,** is a common clinical syndrome accounting for approximately 10 million office visits each year. Females who present with vaginal symptoms often complain of an abnormal discharge and additional symptoms, such as an offensive odor or itching. **Vulvitis,** local irritation of external genitalia, may be associated with vaginitis. The three most common causes of vaginitis in premenopausal females are vaginal candidiasis, bacterial vaginosis (BV) (group B streptococci, *E. coli,* and enterococci), and trichomoniasis.

C. albicans causes about 80% to 90% of the cases of vaginal candidiasis; other species of *Candida* account for the remaining cases. Yeast can be carried vaginally in small

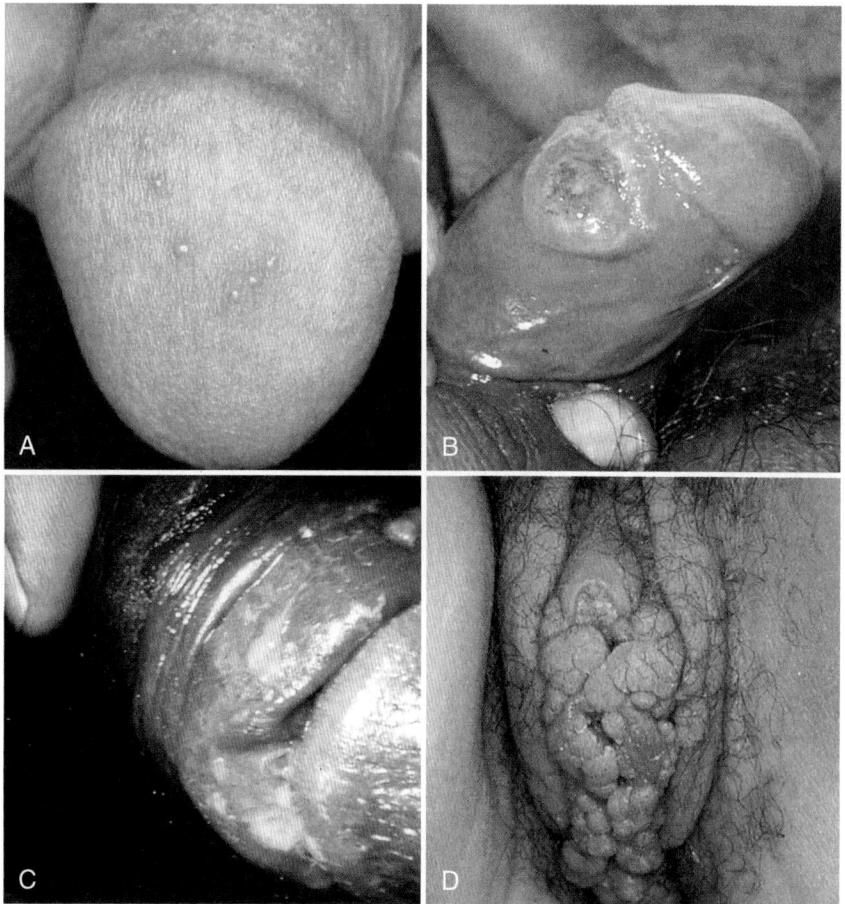

• **Fig. 73.2** Genital lesions of the skin and mucous membranes that are sexually transmitted. (A) Genital herpes showing vesicular lesions. (B) Typical chancre of primary syphilis. (C) Early chancroid lesion of the penis. (D) Condyloma acuminatum. (From Farrar WE, Wood MJ, Innes JA, et al. *Infectious Diseases Text and Color Atlas*. 2nd ed. London: Gower Medical Publishing; 1992.)

numbers and produce no symptoms. Most patients experiencing candidiasis complain of perivaginal itching, often with little or no discharge. Irritating symptoms such as erythema are also associated with candidiasis. Discharge is classically thick and "cheesy" in appearance (Fig. 73.3). Nonalbicans infections are more commonly associated with infections because of the increased use of topical antifungal genital creams and ointments.

Vaginal infection with *T. vaginalis,* a protozoan parasite, produces a profuse, slightly offensive, yellow-green discharge; patients commonly complain of itching. Additional symptoms may include dysuria and **dyspareunia** (persistent genital pain during intercourse). Some patients will present with a strawberry-appearing vaginal mucosa because of capillary dilation. The pH of the vaginal secretions will also typically increase to higher than 4.5, and numerous leukocytes and motile trophozoites may be present. About 25% of females carrying trichomonads are asymptomatic.

In addition to vaginitis caused by these two organisms, there is a third type referred to as **bacterial vaginosis** (BV). Initially, BV was thought to be associated with *Gardnerella vaginalis* infection, but *G. vaginalis* was isolated from 40% of women without vaginitis. Therefore, the presence of *G.*

vaginalis should not be considered diagnostic for BV. BV is polymicrobial in etiology, involving *G. vaginalis* and other facultative and anaerobic organisms. The exact mechanism for the onset of BV is unknown, although it appears to be associated with a reduction in lactobacilli and hydrogen peroxide production, a rise in the vaginal pH, and the overgrowth of BV-associated organisms. Synergistic activity of various anaerobic organisms, including *Prevotella* spp., *Porphyromonas* spp., *Bacteroides* spp., *Peptostreptococcus* spp., *Mobiluncus* spp. (curved, motile rods), and *Mycoplasma* spp., as well as *G. vaginalis,* seems to contribute to the pathology of BV. BV is characterized by perivaginal irritation that is considerably milder than trichomoniasis or candidiasis and is usually associated with a foul-smelling discharge, often described as having a "fishy" odor. This odor is a result of products of bacterial metabolism (polyamines) being volatilized by vaginal fluids. Some patients also complain of abdominal discomfort. Dysuria and dyspareunia are rare. It appears that BV and trichomoniasis frequently coexist. Because BV can recur in the absence of sexual re-exposure and other settings (e.g., non–sexually active females or virgins), BV is not exclusively sexually transmitted. BV also increases a female's risk of acquiring HIV, is associated with

TABLE 73.2	**Summary of Common Causes of Genital Lesions of the Skin and Mucous Membranes**		
Agent	**Disease**	**Lesion**	**Major Associated Symptoms**
Herpes simplex virus	Genital herpes	Papules, vesicles (blisters), pustules, or ulcers	Multiple lesions that are usually painful and tender, can recur (Fig. 73.2A).
Treponema pallidum	Primary syphilis	Genital ulcer (chancre)	Usually a single lesion, painless; lesion has even edges, represents the first of three stages of syphilis (Fig. 73.2B).
Haemophilus ducreyi	Chancroid	Papule that becomes pustular and ulcerates (chancroid); multiple ulcers may develop	Ulcer is deeply invasive, tender, painful, and purulent in appearance; edges of lesion are ragged (Fig. 73.2C).
Chlamydia trachomatis serotype L1, L2, and L3	Lymphogranuloma venereum	Small ulcer or vesicle that heals spontaneously without leaving a scar	After lesion heals, painful, swollen lymph nodes (lymphadenopathy) develop 2–6 weeks later; fever and chills; severe lymphatic obstruction and lymphedema can develop.
Klebsiella	Granuloma inguinale	Single or multiple subcutaneous nodules	Indolent and chronic course; nodules enlarge granulomatis and erode through the skin, producing a deep red, sharply defined ulcer that is painless.
Human papillomavirus	Condylomata acuminate (primary genotypes 6 and 11)	Genital warts	Warts have a cauliflower-like appearance; usually multiple lesions that can be flat or elevated; usually asymptomatic apart from physical presence (Fig. 73.2D).
	Condylomata planum (primary genotypes 16, 18, 31, 33)	Flat, genital warts	Cervical warts that must be visualized by using a magnifying lens after the application of acetic acid (called colposcopy); infections can cause neoplasias that, in some cases, can progress to cervical cancer.

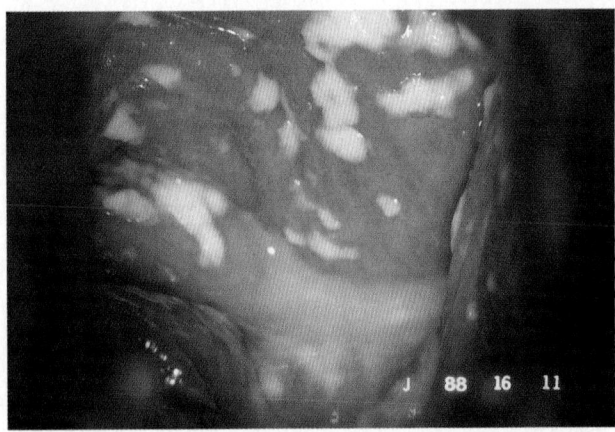

• **Fig. 73.3** Vulvovaginal candidiasis. Visible adherent white patches with surrounding erythema on the cervical mucosa.

increased complications in pregnancy, and may be involved in the pathogenesis of PID.

Although uncommon, there are other infectious causes of vaginitis. Three are briefly mentioned here because Gram stain of vaginal secretions may be helpful. The clinical syndrome referred to as **desquamate inflammatory vaginitis** resembles a bacterial vaginitis. The syndrome manifests in premenopausal patients with a diffuse, exudative vaginitis with massive vaginal cell exfoliation, purulent vaginal discharge, and an occasional vaginal and cervical spotted rash.

Laboratory findings include an elevated pH (>5.0) of vaginal secretions. Also, numerous polymorphonuclear cells, an increased number of parabasal cells, the absence of gram-positive bacilli, and their replacement by occasional gram-positive cocci may be observed on direct Gram stain (Fig. 73.4). Basal cells appear because of the extensive exfoliation of epithelial cells. Symptoms associated with another disorder, lactobacillosis, resemble those of candidiasis and often follow antifungal therapy. Gram stain or wet mount typically reveals many very long lactobacilli. These predominately anaerobic lactobacilli are 40 to 75 μm in length and are significantly longer than the average normal microbiota lactobacillus (5 to 15 μm). Finally, preexisting lesions caused by other diseases may become secondarily infected with a mixed anaerobic microbiota of fusobacteria and spirochetes. This is referred to as **fusiform-spirochete disease;** this infection can progress rapidly. Gram stain examination reveals inflammatory cells in conjunction with gram-negative fusiform bacterial morphotypes and spirochetes.

Cervicitis

Polymorphonuclear neutrophils (PMNs) are normally present in the endocervix; however, an abnormally increased number of PMNs may be associated with **cervicitis** (inflammation of the cervix). Therefore, a purulent discharge from the endocervix can be observed in some cases of cervicitis. The endocervix is the site from which *N. gonorrhoeae* is

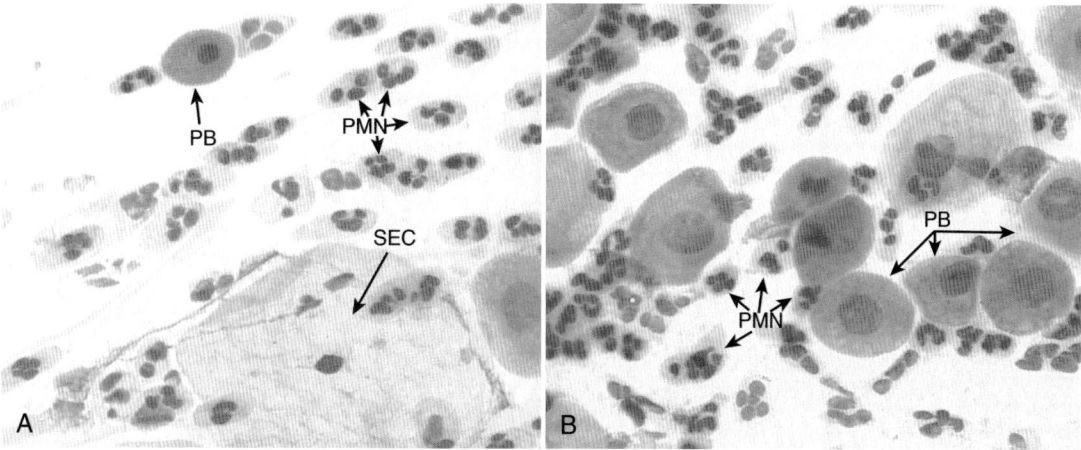

• **Fig. 73.4** Gram stain of vaginal secretions from a patient with desquamate inflammatory vaginitis. (A) Numerous polymorphonuclear cells (*PMNs*), a squamous epithelial cell (*SEC*), a parabasal cell (*PB*), and the absence of lactobacilli are observed. (B) Numerous PMNs, several PBs, and the absence of lactobacilli are observed.

most frequently isolated in females with gonococcal infections. In patients presenting with cervicitis, *C. trachomatis* and *M. genitalium* can also be isolated; chlamydia has not been associated with cervicitis. Patients are often infected with both *N. gonorrhoeae* and *C. trachomatis*. Because most females with cervicitis caused by gonococci or chlamydia are asymptomatic, and cervical abnormalities are either subtle or absent in these patients, an appropriate laboratory diagnosis to detect these organisms must be performed.

HSV and HPV can also infect the cervix. In females with herpes cervicitis, the cervix is friable (bleeds easily) and may have ulcers. Affected patients may also have lower abdominal pain.

Anorectal Lesions

As previously mentioned, because of the homosexual practice and increasingly common heterosexual practice of anal-genital intercourse, sites of infection in addition to those in the genital tract must be considered. The anorectum and pharynx are commonly infected with the classic STDs, including anal warts and cancer caused by HPV, as well as other viruses and parasites. Patients with symptoms of **proctitis** (inflammation of the rectum) caused by *N. gonorrhoeae* or *C. trachomatis* complain of itching, mucopurulent anal discharge, anal pain, bleeding, and **tenesmus** (painful straining during a bowel movement). Anorectal infection caused by HSV is associated with severe anal pain, rectal discharge, tenesmus, and systemic signs and symptoms, such as fever, chills, and headaches.

In HIV-infected individuals and other immunocompromised patients, these infections tend to last longer, are more severe, and are more difficult to treat compared with infection in immunocompetent individuals. Anorectal lesions are common in HIV-infected patients and include anal **condylomata**, anal abscesses, and ulcers. Anal abscesses and ulcers can be caused by various organisms, including CMV, *Mycobacterium avium* complex, HSV, *Campylobacter* spp., and *Shigella*, as well as traditional etiologic agents of STDs.

Bartholinitis

In adult females, the Bartholin gland is a 1-cm mucus-producing gland on each side of the vaginal orifice. Each gland has a 2-cm duct that opens on the inner surface of the labia minora. If infected, this duct can become blocked and result in a Bartholin gland abscess (**Bartholinitis**). Although *N. gonorrhoeae* and *C. trachomatis* can cause infection, anaerobic and polymicrobic infections originating from normal genital microbiota are more common.

Infections of the Reproductive Organs and Other Upper Genital Tract Infections

Besides the lower genital tract, infections can occur in the reproductive organs of both males and females.

Females

Infection of the female reproductive organs (i.e., uterus, fallopian tubes, ovaries, and even the abdominal cavity) can occur. The organisms spread as they ascend from lower tract sites of infection. Organisms may also be introduced to the reproductive organs by surgery, instrumentation, or during childbirth.

Pelvic Inflammatory Disease

PID is an infection that results when cervical microorganisms travel upward to the endometrium (inner membrane of the uterus), fallopian tubes, and other pelvic structures. This infection can produce one or more of the following inflammatory conditions: **endometritis, salpingitis** (inflammation of the fallopian tubes), localized or generalized peritonitis, or abscesses involving the fallopian tubes or ovaries. Patients with PID often have intermittent abdominal pain and tenderness, vaginal discharge, dysuria, and possibly systemic symptoms, such as fever, weight loss, and headache. Serious complications, such as permanent scarring of the fallopian tubes and infertility, can arise if PID is untreated.

TABLE 73.3	Common Etiologic Agents of Prenatal and Neonatal Infections	

Time of Infection[a]	Route of Infection	Common Agents
Prenatal	Transplacental	Bacteria: *Listeria monocytogenes*, *Treponema pallidum*, *Borrelia burgdorferi* Viruses: cytomegalovirus (CMV), rubella, HIV, parvovirus B19, enteroviruses Parasites: *Toxoplasma gondii*, *Plasmodium* spp.
	Ascending	Bacteria: group B streptococci, *Escherichia coli*, *L. monocytogenes*, *Chlamydia trachomatis*, genital mycoplasmas Viruses: CMV, herpes simplex virus (HSV)
Natal	Passing through the birth canal	Bacteria: group B streptococci, *E. coli*, *L. monocytogenes*, *N. gonorrhoeae*, *C. trachomatis* Viruses: CMV, HSV, enteroviruses, hepatitis B virus, human immunodeficiency virus (HIV)
Postnatal	All the aforementioned routes, from the nursery environment, or from maternal contact (e.g., breastfeeding)	All agents listed previously and various organisms from the nursery environment, including gram-negative bacteria and viruses, such as respiratory syncytial virus

[a]Some newborns develop infections during the first 4 weeks of postnatal life. Infections may be delayed manifestations of earlier prenatal (before birth), natal, or postnatal (after birth) acquisition of pathogens.

Infection with *N. gonorrhoeae* or *C. trachomatis* in the lower genital tract can lead to PID if a female is not adequately treated. Other organisms, such as anaerobes, gram-negative rods, streptococci, and mycoplasmas, may ascend through the cervix, particularly after parturition (childbirth), dilation of the cervix, or abortion. The presence of an intrauterine device (IUD) is associated with a slightly higher rate of PID. Such infections caused by *Actinomyces* have been associated with the use of IUDs.

Infections After Gynecologic Surgery

After gynecologic surgery, such as a vaginal hysterectomy, patients frequently develop postoperative infections including pelvic cellulitis or abscesses. The major pathogens include normal human microbiota: aerobic gram-positive cocci, gram-negative bacilli, anaerobes such as *Peptostreptococcus* spp., and genital mycoplasmas.

Infections Associated With Pregnancy

Infections can also occur in females during pregnancy (prenatal) or after the birth (postpartum) of a child. These infections may, in turn, be transmitted to the infant; they are not only capable of compromising the mother's health but also the health of the developing fetus or neonate.

While developing within the uterus, the fetus is protected from most environmental factors, including infectious agents. The human immune system does not become fully competent until several months after birth. Immunoglobulins that cross the placental barrier, primarily immunoglobulin G (IgG), protect the newborn from many infections until the infant begins to produce immunoglobulins of his or her own in response to antigenic stimuli. This unique environmental niche, however, does expose the vulnerable fetus to pathogens present in the mother.

• BOX 73.1 Organisms Commonly Isolated in Chorioamnionitis

Anaerobic bacteria
Genital mycoplasmas
Group B streptococci
Escherichia coli

Prenatal infections (those that occur any time before birth) may be acquired hematogenously or by ascending genital tract routes from mother to infant. If the mother has a bloodstream infection, organisms can reach and cross the placenta, with possible spread of infection to the developing fetus. Organisms that can cross the placenta are listed in Table 73.3. Alternatively, organisms can also infect the fetus by the ascending route from the vagina through torn or ruptured fetal membranes. **Chorioamnionitis** is an infection of the uterus and its contents during pregnancy. This infection is commonly acquired when organisms spread from the vagina or cervix after premature or prolonged rupture of the membranes, or during labor. Organisms that are commonly isolated from amniotic fluid are listed in Box 73.1. Other maternal infections associated with adverse pregnancy outcomes that are not generally sexually transmitted include parvovirus B19, rubella, and *L. monocytogenes*.

Males

Infections in male reproductive organs can also occur and include epididymitis, prostatitis, and orchitis (testicular swelling). **Epididymitis,** an inflammation of the epididymis, is commonly seen in sexually active men. Patients complain of fever and pain and swelling of the testicle. Patients may also present with dysuria and a urethral discharge. There are two general types of epididymitis: nonspecific bacterial epididymitis caused by aerobic gram-negative rods, enterococci, or *Pseudomonas* spp.; and sexually transmitted epididymitis most commonly associated with *N. gonorrhoeae* and *C. trachomatis*. However, bacterial epididymitis is typically associated with an underlying genitourinary abnormality that requires surgery or urethral catheterization. Infections may also be caused by enteric bacteria and coagulase-negative staphylococci in males over 35 years of age and in homosexual males; these infections are often associated with obstruction by the prostate gland.

Prostatitis is a term to clinically describe adult male patients who have perineal, lower back, or lower abdominal pain, urinary discomfort, or ejaculatory complaints. Prostatitis is caused by both infectious and noninfectious means. Bacteria can cause an acute or chronic prostatitis. Patients with acute bacterial prostatitis have dysuria and urinary frequency—symptoms typically associated with lower urinary tract infection. These patients frequently have systemic signs of illness, such as fever. Chronic bacterial prostatitis is an important cause of persistent bacteriuria in males leading to recurrent bacterial urinary tract infections. The common causes of these infections are similar to the bacterial causes of lower urinary tract infections, such as *E. coli*, *Pseudomonas* spp., and other enteric organisms.

Finally, inflammation of the testicles, **orchitis**, is uncommon and generally acquired by the blood-borne dissemination of viruses. Mumps is associated with most cases. Patients exhibit testicular pain and swelling after infection. Infections range from mild to severe. In addition, **epididymo-orchitis** may occur after infection of the epididymis. Organisms typically isolated from bacterial orchitis include staphylococci, streptococci, *E. coli*, *Klebsiella pneumoniae*, and *Pseudomonas aeruginosa*.

Gonorrhea

Gonorrhea is a common STI caused by the bacterium *N. gonorrhoeae*. The infection may be spread by direct contact with secretions within the mouth, vagina, penis, or perianal region. The organism reproduces in warm, moist areas of the body including the urethra of males and females, fallopian tubes, uterus, and cervix.

Symptoms occur 2 to 5 days after infection in females. Males may not display symptoms for up to 1 month after infection. Symptoms in females include a vaginal discharge, pain and frequency on urination, sore throat, abdominal pain, fever, and painful sexual intercourse. Males experience pain and frequency during urination, a penile discharge, red or swollen urethra, and tenderness in the testes. The characteristics of the urethral discharge may vary from cloudy to clear and is therefore an unreliable indicator for gonococcal urethritis in males.

Gonorrhea can be directly diagnosed by Gram staining a sample of urethral discharge, cervical specimens, or joint fluids. *N. gonorrhoeae* is a gram-negative diplococcus with a characteristic kidney bean shape on Gram stain. The detection of intracellular diplococci in male secretions

is diagnostic for *N. gonorrhoeae*. Extracellular diplococci in females is an indication of normal genital microbiota; however, intracellular diplococci indicate the presence of pathogenic organisms. Definitive diagnosis in females must include confirmation by culture. Infection with *N. gonorrhoeae* can lead to increased complications, including PID and gonorrheal ophthalmia neonatorum (eye infections) in newborns. *N. meningitidis* has been increasingly associated with urethritis.

Nongonococcal urethritis (NGU) is most commonly associated with *C. trachomatis* infection. Additional organisms that may be isolated from specimens in cases of NGU include *U. urealyticum* and *M. genitalium*.

Syphilis

Syphilis is an STD that is caused by the bacterium *T. pallidum*. The organism is transmitted from person to person through direct contact with infected lesions on the external genital area, vagina, anus, or rectum. Syphilis may also be transmitted from mother to baby during pregnancy.

Many individuals can be infected and remain asymptomatic for years, making the control of this disease difficult. The disease is characterized by three stages: primary, secondary, and tertiary (also referred to as late or latent syphilis). Direct diagnosis may be accomplished by dark-field microscopy of material from an infectious lesion. However, serology provides a more accurate and reliable method for diagnosis. (See Chapter 45 for a more detailed description of the disease and laboratory diagnosis.)

Laboratory Diagnosis of Genital Tract Infections

Lower Genital Tract Infections

Urethritis, Cervicitis, and Vaginitis

Specimen Collection

This discussion focuses on those specimens submitted for culture or direct examination. Procedures for the collection and transport of specimens for detection of agents by other noncultural methods (e.g., detection of infectious agents using nucleic acid–based tests) should be followed according to the respective manufacturer's instructions. (Refer to Table 5.1 for a review of collection, transport, and processing of genital tract specimens.)

Urethral. Urethral discharge may occur in both males and females infected with pathogens, such as *N. gonorrhoeae*, *N. meningitidis*, and *T. vaginalis*. The presence of infection is more likely to be asymptomatic in females, because the discharge is usually less profuse and may be masked by normal vaginal secretions. *U. urealyticum* can also be isolated from male urethral discharge.

A small urogenital swab designed expressly for collection of such specimens should be used. These swabs are made of cotton or rayon, treated with charcoal to adsorb material toxic to gonococci, and wrapped tightly over one end of a thin wire shaft. Cotton- or rayon-tipped swabs on a thin wire may also be used to collect specimens for isolation of mycoplasmas and chlamydiae. Calcium alginate swabs are generally more toxic for HSV, gonococci, chlamydia, and mycoplasmas than treated cotton swabs. Because dacron swabs are least toxic, they are recommended for viral specimens. Dacron-tipped swabs on plastic shafts are also acceptable for chlamydiae and genital mycoplasmas.

To obtain a urethral specimen, a swab is inserted approximately 2 cm into the urethra and rotated gently before withdrawing. Because chlamydiae are intracellular pathogens, it is important to remove epithelial cells (with the swab) from the urethral mucosa. Separate swabs for cultivation of gonococci, chlamydiae, and ureaplasma are required. When profuse urethral discharge is present, particularly in males, the discharge may be collected externally without inserting a sampling device into the urethra. However, a urethral swab for chlamydiae must be collected on males. A few drops of first-voided urine have also been used successfully to detect gonococci in males.

Because *T. vaginalis* may be present in urethral discharge, material for culture should be collected by swab, as described, and another specimen collected on a swab and placed into a tube containing 0.5 mL of sterile physiologic saline. This specimen should be delivered to the laboratory immediately. Direct wet mounts and cultures for *T. vaginalis* can be performed from this second specimen. Commercial media for culture of *Trichomonas* are available. The first few drops of voided urine make a suitable specimen for recovery of *Trichomonas* from infected males, if it is inoculated into culture media immediately. Alternatively, material may be smeared onto a slide for a fluorescent antibody stain. Plastic envelopes for direct examination and subsequent culture are also available (InPouch TV, BIOMED, White City, OR); sensitivity of this system is superior to other available methods, and organism viability is maintained up to 48 hours. In addition, several other techniques are available, including enzyme immunoassay, latex agglutination tests, and the Affirm VPIII probe (Becton Dickinson, Cockeysville, MD). Nucleic acid–based test methods are the most sensitive for the detection and identification of *T. vaginalis* directly in clinical specimens.

N. gonorrhoeae may be detected from clinical specimens using a variety of nucleic acid–based methods using a DNA probe that hybridizes to organismal ribosomal ribonucleic acid (rRNA). Fully automated systems for complete sample processing are available that reduce technical time. These tests are rapidly evolving and widely used for quick detection of *N. gonorrhoeae* from vaginal, urethral, thin-prep, and urine specimens. *N. meningitidis* should be considered when a urethral Gram stain indicates the presence of gram-negative intracellular diplococci and a nonculture based test, such as nucleic acid amplification test (NAAT), is negative for the presence of *N. gonorrhoeae*.

Cervical and Vaginal. Organisms that cause purulent vaginal discharge (vaginitis) include *T. vaginalis,* gonococci, *Candida* spp. and, rarely, beta-hemolytic streptococci. The same organisms that cause purulent infections in the urethra may also infect the epithelial cells in the cervical opening (os), as can HSV. Mucus is removed by gently rubbing the area with a cotton ball. The urethral swab is inserted into the cervical canal and rotated and moved from side to side for 30 seconds before removal.

Swabs are handled as previously described for urethral swabs for isolation of *Trichomonas* and gonococci. Chlamydiae cause a mucopurulent cervicitis with discharge. Endocervical specimens are obtained after the cervix has been exposed with a speculum, which allows visualization of vaginal and cervical architecture, and after ectocervical mucus has been adequately removed. The speculum is moistened with warm water, because many lubricants contain antibacterial agents. Because normal vaginal secretions contain great quantities of bacteria, care must be taken to prevent or minimize contamination of swabs for culture by contact with these secretions. A small, nylon-bristled cytology brush, or Cytobrush, may be used to ensure that cellular material is collected. Collection may result in patient discomfort and bleeding.

In addition to cervical specimens, which are particularly useful for isolating herpes, gonococci, mycoplasmas, and chlamydiae, vaginal discharge specimens may be collected. Organisms likely to cause vaginal discharge include *Trichomonas,* yeast, and the agents of BV. Swabs for diagnosis of BV are dipped into the fluid that collects in the posterior fornix of the vagina.

Genital tract infections caused by sexually transmitted agents in children (preadolescents) are most often the result of sexual abuse. Because of medico-legal implications, the laboratory should treat specimens from such patients with extreme care, carefully identifying and documenting all isolates. Although nucleic acid–based testing methods are available for the identification of organisms associated with sexual abuse cases, culture remains the preferred method of detection for *C. trachomatis* and *N. gonorrhoeae* in medico-legal cases. In addition, cultivation of the isolate may be required to link the specific isolate to the perpetrator using epidemiologic studies. It is important to follow the current rules and regulations of each state for the collection and processing of isolates in these situations.

Because it is impossible to exclude contamination with vaginal microbiota, obtaining swabs of Bartholin gland exudate is not recommended. Infected Bartholin glands should be aspirated with needle and syringe after careful skin preparation, and cultures should be evaluated for anaerobes and aerobes.

Transport. Swabs collected for isolation of gonococci may be transported to the laboratory in modified Stuart's or Amie's charcoal transport media and held at room temperature until inoculated to culture media. Good recovery of gonococci is possible if swabs are cultured within 12 hours of collection. Material that must be held longer than 12 hours should be inoculated directly to one of the commercial systems designed for recovery of gonococci, described later in this chapter.

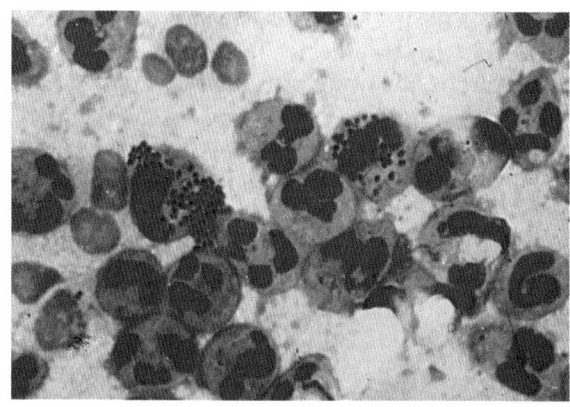

• **Fig. 73.5** Gram-negative intracellular diplococci, which are diagnostic for gonorrhea in urethral discharge and presumptive for gonorrhea in vaginal discharge.

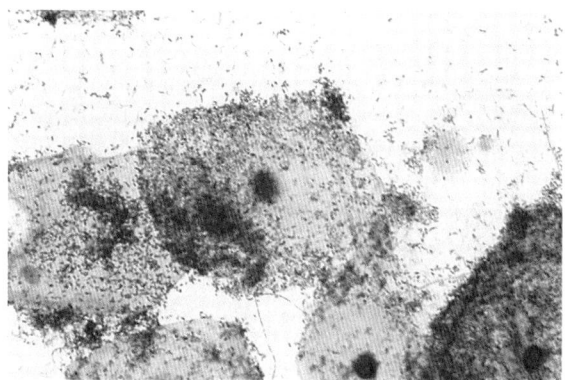

• **Fig. 73.6** Clue cells in vaginal discharge suggestive of bacterial vaginosis.

Swabs for isolation of chlamydiae and mycoplasmas are transported in specific transport media containing antibiotics and other essential components. Specimens for chlamydia culture should be transported on ice. (Specimens transported at room temperature should be inoculated within 15 minutes of collection.) Specimens can be stored at 4°C for up to 24 hours. If culture inoculation will be delayed more than 24 hours, specimens should be quick-frozen in a dry ice and 95% ethanol bath and stored at −70°C until cultured. If collected and transported in specific transport media, specimens for genital mycoplasma culture may be transported on ice or at room temperature. If not in genital mycoplasma transport media, specimens should be transported on ice to suppress the growth of contaminating microbiota.

Direct Microscopic Examination

In addition to culture, urethral discharge may be examined by Gram stain for the presence of gram-negative intracellular diplococci (Fig. 73.5), usually indicative of gonorrhea in males. After inoculation to culture media, the swab is rolled over the surface of a glass slide, covering an area of at least 1 cm². Specimens collected from within the urethra may contain small cuboidal epithelial cells with a large nucleus. Numerous PMNs, more than four per oil immersion field, will also be visible in acute urethritis. If the Gram stain is characteristic of normal skin or genital microbiota, cultures of urethral discharge need not be performed. Urethral smears from females may also be examined. If extracellular organisms resembling *N. gonorrhoeae* are seen, the microbiologist should continue to examine the smear for intracellular diplococci. Presumptive diagnosis can be useful when decisions are to be made regarding immediate therapy, but confirmatory cultures or an alternative nonculture method should always be performed on specimens from females. Some strains of *N. gonorrhoeae* are sensitive to the amount of vancomycin present in selective media. If suspicious organisms seen on smear fail to grow in culture, reculture on chocolate agar without antibiotics may be warranted and *N. meningitidis* should also be considered. In addition, a Gram stain that contains numerous PMNs without intracellular gram-negative diplococci may also be suggestive of NGU.

Fluorescein-conjugated monoclonal antibody reagents are sensitive and specific for visualization of the inclusions of *C. trachomatis* in cell cultures or elementary bodies in urethral and cervical specimens containing cells. Reagents for direct staining of specimens are available commercially in complete collection and test systems, but the increased technologist time required limits the usefulness of this method for laboratories that receive many specimens, except as a confirmatory test for other antigen detection systems with borderline results. In some studies, the sensitivity of visual detection of chlamydia with these reagents has been similar to that of culture. False-positive results should not occur if at least 10 morphologically compatible fluorescing elementary bodies are seen on the smear. No direct visual methods exist for detection of mycoplasmas, but nucleic acid–based assays are the most sensitive for diagnosis of these fastidious organisms.

Direct microscopic examination of a wet preparation of vaginal discharge provides the simplest rapid diagnostic test for *T. vaginalis* and can be examined immediately. Motile trophozoites of *Trichomonas* can be visualized in a routine wet preparation in two thirds of cases or a direct fluorescent antibody (DFA) stain, Merifluor (chlamydia) (Meridian Diagnostics, Cincinnati, OH) may be used. Positive findings on a wet mount are diagnostic for trichomoniasis, but results are often negative in males.

Budding cells and pseudohyphae of yeast can also be easily identified in wet preparations by adding 10% potassium hydroxide (KOH) to a separate preparation, thereby dissolving host cell protein and enhancing the visibility of fungal elements.

BV, characterized by a foul-smelling discharge, can be diagnosed microscopically or clinically. The discharge is primarily sloughed epithelial cells, many of which are completely covered by tiny, gram-variable rods, and coccobacilli. These cells are called **clue cells** (Fig. 73.6). The absence of inflammatory cells in the vaginal discharge is another sign of BV. Although *G. vaginalis* has been historically associated with the syndrome and can be cultured on a human blood bilayer plate, culture is not recommended for diagnosis of BV. A clinical diagnosis of BV is dependent on the presence of three or more of the following criteria: homogeneous, gray discharge; clue cells seen on wet mount or Gram stain; a pH higher than 4.5; and an amine or fishy odor elicited by the addition of a drop of 10% KOH to the discharge on a slide or on the speculum.

BV may be differentiated from other vaginal infection by Gram stain (Fig. 73.7). A grading system for Gram stains of vaginal discharge has been developed (see Evolve Procedure 73.1). This system is based on the presence or absence of certain bacterial morphologies. Typically, in patients with BV, lactobacilli are either absent or few in number, whereas curved, gram-variable rods (*Mobiluncus* spp.) or *G. vaginalis* and *Bacteroides* morphotypes predominate. The Gram stain is more sensitive and specific than either the wet mount for detection of clue cells or culture for *G. vaginalis,* and the smear can be saved and reexamined later.

Culture

Samples for isolation of gonococci may be inoculated directly to culture media, obviating the need for transport medium. Commercially produced systems have been developed for this purpose, and many clinicians inoculate standard plates directly if convenient access to an incubator is available. Modified Thayer-Martin medium is most often used, although New York City (NYC) medium has the added advantage of supporting the growth of mycoplasmas and gonococci. The specimen swab is rolled across the agar with constant turning to expose all surfaces to the medium.

Specimens must be inoculated to additional media for isolation of yeast, streptococci, and mycoplasmas. Yeast grows well on Columbia agar base with 5% sheep blood and colistin and nalidixic acid (CNA), although more selective media are available. Most yeast and streptococci also grow on standard blood agar; thus, adding special fungal media, such as Sabouraud brain-heart infusion agar (SABHI), is unwarranted.

A specimen from the lower vagina followed by the rectum using the same swab at 35 to 37 weeks' gestation, reliably predicts the presence of group B streptococci at delivery. The swab should be transported to the laboratory in a nonnutritive transport medium, such as Amie's or Stuart's, without charcoal and then inoculated into a recommended selective broth medium, such as Todd-Hewitt broth supplemented either with gentamicin and nalidixic acid or with CNA referred to as LIM broth. Selective enrichment broths are subcultured to agar the next day to isolate and identify group B streptococci. In addition, the presence of group B streptococci in urine in any concentration from a pregnant female is a marker for heavy genital tract colonization. Any quantity of group B streptococci in urine from pregnant women should be worked up in the laboratory (Chapter 72).

T. vaginalis may be cultured in Diamond's medium (available commercially) or plastic envelopes inoculated with discharge material. Culture techniques are most sensitive. A commercially available biphasic genital mycoplasma culture system (Mycotrim-GU, Irvine Scientific, Santa Ana, CA) can be used to culture *Mycoplasma* spp. and *U. urealyticum,* although commercially prepared media are not as sensitive as fresh media. *M. genitalium* may not grow on commercial media because of the presence of thallium acetate.

Nonculture Methods

Various nonculture methods may be used to diagnose genital tract diseases, including serology, latex agglutination, nucleic acid hybridization and amplification assays, and enzyme immunoassays. Most assays detect a single or possibly two genital tract pathogens and are commercially available. These methods are described in more detail in chapters relating to individual pathogens.

As previously discussed, BV involves several organisms. Although the Gram stain offers high sensitivity and specificity, it is not immediately available. Currently, commercial laboratory tests are available to aid in the diagnosis of BV, but not all are available in the United States; a test for sialidase (OSOM BVBLUE, Sekisui Diagnostics, Framingham, MA) in conjunction with measuring pH has been reported to be

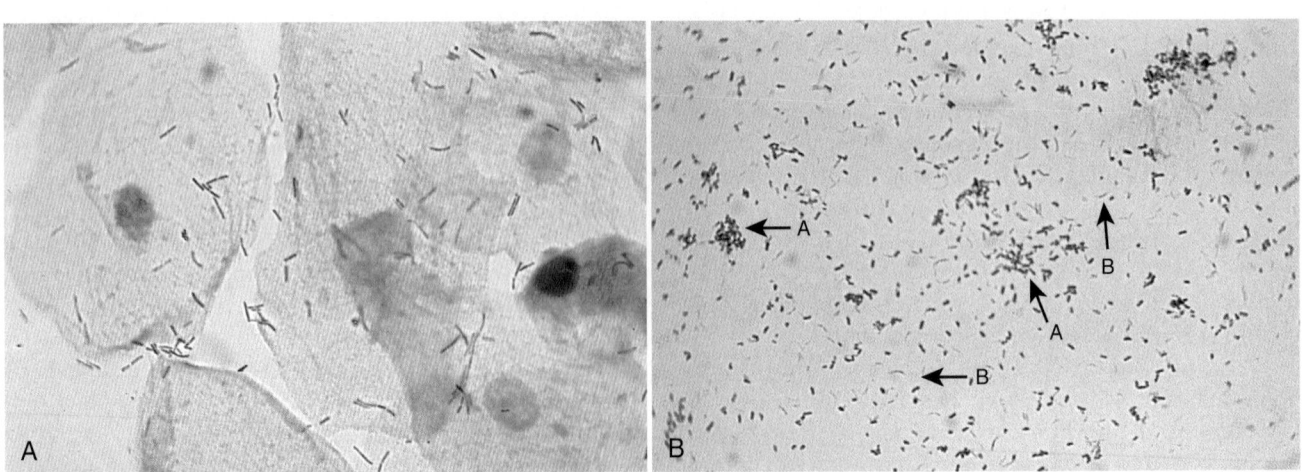

• **Fig. 73.7** (A) Predominance of lactobacilli in Gram stain from healthy vagina. (B) Absence of lactobacilli and presence of *Gardnerella vaginalis (A arrows)* and *Mobiluncus* spp. *(B arrows)* morphologies.

a rapid, highly sensitive, and specific means to diagnose BV. Sialidases are secreted from anaerobic gram-negative rods, such as *Bacteroides* and *Prevotella* as well as *Gardnerella,* and play a role in bacterial nutrition, cellular interactions, and immune response evasion, which in turn improves the ability of bacteria to adhere to, invade, and destroy mucosal tissue. A hybridization assay (Affirm VP III Microbial Identification Test; Becton Dickinson Microbiology Systems, Burlington, NC) is commercially available to diagnose BV, as well as genital tract infections caused by *Candida* spp. and *T. vaginalis.* Once the appropriate reagents and specimen are added to special trays, the entire hybridization assays are then performed using instrumentation (Fig. 73.8). Evaluations indicate this system is sensitive and specific.

In addition to microscopic examination, NAAT should be performed on vaginal, cervical, or urine specimens when cervicitis is suspected. A variety of assays are available for the detection of associated pathogens, such as the automated Aptima Combo 2 Assay (Fig. 73.9). This assay is a transcription-mediated amplification (TMA) test that utilizes target capture for the *in vitro* qualitative detection and differentiation of rRNA from *C. trachomatis* and/or *N. gonorrhoeae* using the Panther System (Hologic) as a testing platform.

Genital Skin and Mucous Membrane Lesions

External genital lesions are usually either vesicular or ulcerative. Causes of lesions can be determined by physical examination, histologic or cytologic examination, and microscopic examination or culture of exudate. Gram staining is typically not useful for the identification of organisms and the evaluation of genital lesions because of the presence of contaminating normal microbiota.

Vesicles in the genital area are almost always attributable to viruses, and herpes simplex is the most common cause. Epithelial cells from the base of a vesicle may be spread onto the surface of a slide (Tzanck smear) and examined for the typical multinucleated giant cells of HSV by staining with Wright-Giemsa stain or immunofluorescent antibody stains for viral antigens. NAATs are recommended for HSV testing that provide excellent sensitivity. Additionally, or alternatively, the material may be transported for culture of the virus as outlined in Evolve Procedure 73.2. Specimens positive for HSV will typically demonstrate cytopathic effect (changes in cell morphology) within 48 hours. Cultures have been largely replaced by NAATs.

Several commercial fluorescein-conjugated monoclonal and polyclonal antibodies directed against herpetic antigens of either type 1 or 2 are available. When fluorescent antibody–stained lesion material containing enough cells is viewed under ultraviolet light, the diagnosis can be made in 70% to 90% of patients. Laboratories that routinely process genital material for herpes should be using immunofluorescent staining reagents when a rapid answer is desired; otherwise, culture, which is generally positive in 2 days. Nonfluorescent markers, such as biotin-avidin-horseradish peroxidase or alkaline phosphatase, have also been conjugated to these specific antibodies, often allowing for earlier detection of herpes-infected cells in tissue culture monolayers.

Serologic assays are currently available to distinguish HSV 1 and HSV 2 and have been modified that allow the use of these tests in a clinic setting.

Lesions caused by HPV are typically characterized using the Papanicolaou smear (Pap) or a biopsy. These methods lack specificity, and, therefore, positive smears should be confirmed with a nucleic acid–based test such as hybrid capture or polymerase chain reaction.

Material from lesions suggestive of syphilis should be examined by dark-field or fluorescent microscopy. Dark-field microscopy is not useful for the differentiation of pathogenic from nonpathogenic treponemes. A two-step serologic test using the rapid plasma reagin (RPR), Venereal Disease Research Laboratory (VDRL), or unheated serum reagin (USR) test—followed by a confirmatory test—is the recommended procedure for the diagnosis of syphilis.

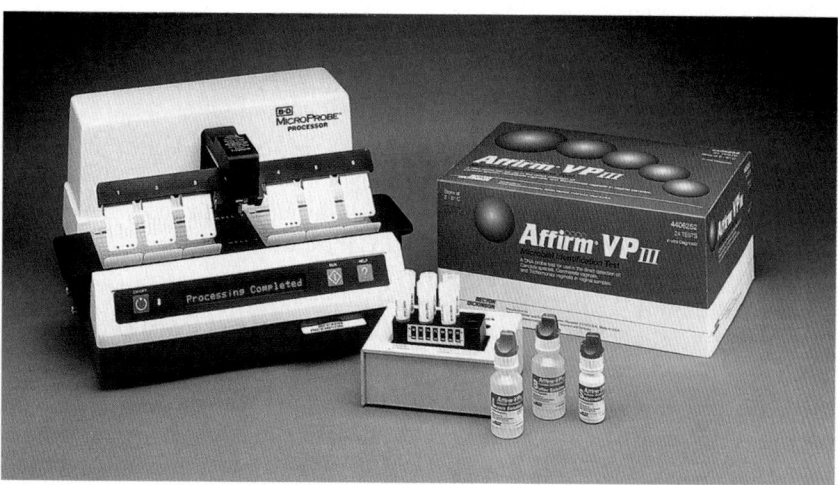

• **Fig. 73.8** Affirm VP III Microbial Identification Test used to differentiate the three major causes of vaginitis/bacterial vaginosis from a single sample within 1 hour. (Courtesy Becton Dickinson Microbiology Systems. Affirm is a trademark of Becton Dickinson and Co.)

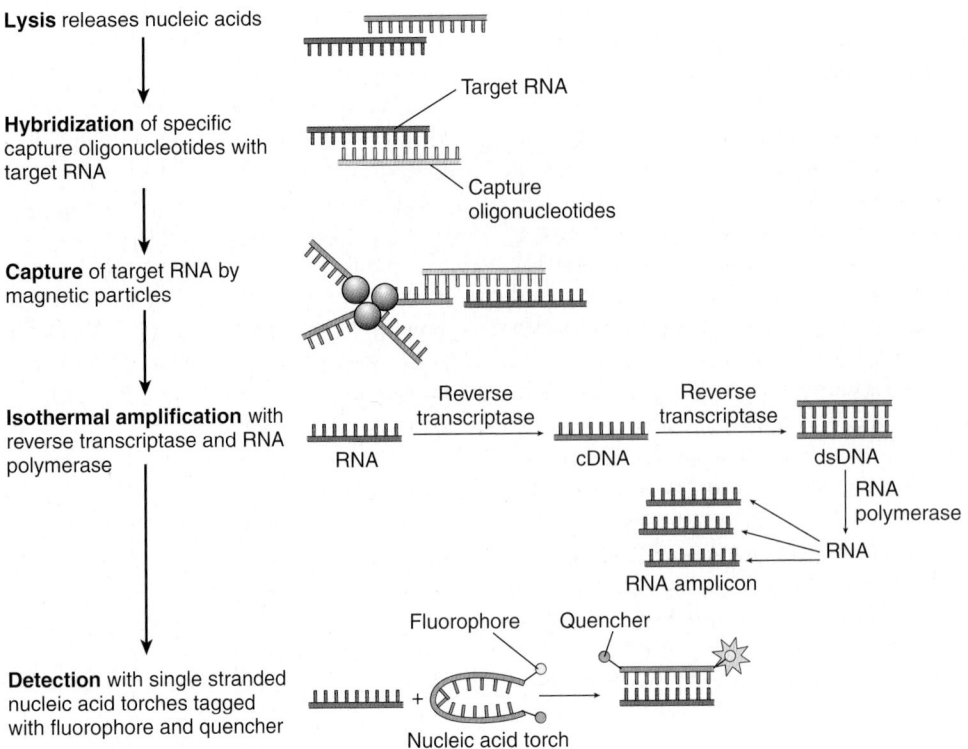

Lysis releases nucleic acids

Hybridization of specific capture oligonucleotides with target RNA

Target RNA

Capture oligonucleotides

Capture of target RNA by magnetic particles

Isothermal amplification with reverse transcriptase and RNA polymerase

Reverse transcriptase

Reverse transcriptase

RNA

cDNA

dsDNA

RNA polymerase

RNA

RNA amplicon

Detection with single stranded nucleic acid torches tagged with fluorophore and quencher

Fluorophore

Quencher

Nucleic acid torch

• **Fig. 73.9** The Aptima Combo 2 Assay is a transcription-mediated amplification (TMA) test that utilizes target capture for the *in vitro* qualitative detection and differentiation of ribosomal RNA (rRNA) from *Chlamydia trachomatis* (CT) and/or *Neisseria gonorrhoeae* (GC) using the Panther System (Hologic) as a testing platform. *NAAT,* Nucleic acid amplification test. (Adapted from teaching materials, courtesy Jim Flanigan, American Society for Clinical Laboratory Science.)

(These procedures are described in Chapter 45.) NAAT have also been developed for the detection of *T. pallidum.*

All lesions suspected of infectious etiology may be Gram stained in addition to the procedures described. The smear of lesion material from a patient with chancroid may show many small, pleomorphic, slender, gram-negative rods and coccobacilli arranged in chains and groups referred to as a "school of fish," characteristics of *H. ducreyi.* However, culture has been shown to be more sensitive for diagnosis of this agent. Material collected on cotton or dacron swabs may be transported in modified Stuart's medium. Specimens should be inoculated to culture media within 1 hour of collection. A special agar, consisting of Mueller-Hinton–based chocolate agar enriched with 1% IsoVitaleX (Becton-Dickinson, Franklin Lakes, NJ) and vancomycin (3 mg/mL), has yielded good isolation if cultures are incubated in 5% to 7% carbon dioxide in a moist atmosphere, such as a candle jar. *H. ducreyi* grows best at 33°C. NAAT have also been developed for the detection of *H ducreyi.*

Granuloma inguinale *(K. granulomatis)* (Fig. 73.8) is diagnosed by staining a crushed preparation of a small piece of biopsy tissue obtained from the edge of the base of the ulcer with Wright's or Giemsa stain and finding characteristic **Donovan bodies** (bipolar staining rods within macrophages). No acceptable media for isolation of *K. granulomatis* are available.

Buboes

Buboes, swollen lymph glands in the inguinal (pelvic) region, are often evidence of a genital tract infection. Buboes are common in patients with primary syphilis, genital herpes, lymphogranuloma venereum, and chancroid. Patients with acquired immune deficiency syndrome (AIDS) may show generalized lymphadenopathy. Other diseases that are not sexually transmitted, such as plague, tularemia, and lymphoma, can also produce buboes. Material from buboes may be aspirated for microscopic examination and culture. Isolation by cell culture or the identification of *C. trachomatis* using nucleic acid–based test methods is considered diagnostic.

Infections of the Reproductive Organs
Pelvic Inflammatory Disease

PID is often caused by the same organisms that cause cervicitis or by organisms that make up the normal microbiota of the vaginal mucosa. Diagnosis is often made based on signs and symptoms. Because of the profuse normal microbiota of the vaginal tract, specimens must be collected in such a way as to prevent vaginal microbiota contamination. Aspirated material collected by needle and syringe represents the best specimen. If this cannot be obtained at the time of surgery or laparoscopy, collection of intrauterine contents using a protected suction curetting device or double-lumen sampling device inserted through the cervix is also acceptable. **Culdocentesis** (aspiration of fluid in the cul-de-sac), after decontamination of the vagina by povidone-iodine, is satisfactory but rarely practiced today.

Aspirated material should be placed into an anaerobic transport container. The presence of mixed anaerobic microbiota, gonococci, or both, can be rapidly detected from a Gram stain. Direct examination with fluorescent monoclonal antibody stain may also detect chlamydiae. All specimens should be inoculated to media that allow the recovery of anaerobic, facultative, and aerobic bacteria, gonococci, fungi, mycoplasmas, and chlamydiae. All material collected from normally sterile body sites in the genital tract should be inoculated to chocolate agar and placed into a suitable broth, such as thioglycollate, in addition to the other types of media noted. If only specimens obtained on routine swabs inserted through the cervix are available, cultures should be performed for detection of gonococci and chlamydiae.

Miscellaneous Infections

Infections of the male prostate, epididymis, and testes are usually bacterial. Uropathogens, such as *E. coli*, *P. aeruginosa*, and *Enterococcus* spp. cause more than 60% of acute bacterial prostatitis. In younger males, chlamydia and *N. gonorrhoeae* predominates as the cause of sexually transmitted epididymitis and possibly of prostatitis. Orchitis, or inflammation of the testes, can be caused by the same uropathogens as the other conditions as well as viral infections. The mumps virus is the cause of most cases of viral orchitis. Urine or discharge collected via the urethra is the specimen of choice unless an abscess is drained surgically or by needle and syringe. The first few milliliters of voided urine may be collected before and after prostatic massage to try to pinpoint the anatomic site of the infection. Cultures are inoculated to support the growth of anaerobic, facultative, and aerobic bacteria, as well as gonococci.

Infections of Neonates and Human Products of Conception

Suspected infections acquired by the fetus because of a maternal infection that crosses the placenta (congenital infection) can be diagnosed culturally or serologically in the newborn. Because maternal IgG crosses the placenta, serologic tests are often difficult to interpret (Chapter 9). Nucleic acid testing for viruses included in the *Herpesviridae* are more widely used and are more sensitive than cell culture and antigen detection. Although HSV, varicella-zoster virus (VZV), enteroviruses, and CMV can be cultured easily—as can most bacterial agents—rubella and parvovirus B19 are more difficult to culture. Nasal and urine specimens offer the greatest yield for viral isolation, although blood,

cerebrospinal fluid, and material from a lesion can also be productive. Systemic neonatal herpes without lesions may be difficult to diagnose unless tissue biopsy material is examined, because the viruses may not be present in cerebrospinal fluid or blood. Bacteria and fungi can be isolated from lesions, blood, and other normally sterile sites.

Determining the presence of fetal immunoglobulin M (IgM) directed against the agent in question establishes the serologic diagnosis of congenital infection. Until recently, ultracentrifugation was required for separation of IgM from IgG, the only definitive means of preventing false-positive results caused by maternal IgG or fetal rheumatoid factor. Ion-exchange chromatography columns, antihuman IgG, and bacterial proteins that bind to IgG, are commercially available for removing cross-reactive IgG and rheumatoid factor to obtain more homogeneous IgM for differentiation of fetal antibody. Indirect fluorescent antibody and enzyme-linked immunosorbent assay (ELISA) test systems are commercially available to detect IgM against *T. gondii*, rubella, CMV, HSV, and VZV. Interference by rheumatoid factor is still a consideration in most commercial IgM test systems (Chapter 9). The ability to detect viral inclusions in tissue, conjunctiva scrapings, and vesicular lesions, traditionally performed with Giemsa stain, has been improved because of the availability of monoclonal and polyclonal fluorescent antibody reagents, which are described in the chapters that discuss individual agents.

Infections that infants can acquire as they pass through an infected birth canal or that are related to difficult labor, premature birth, premature rupture of the membranes, or other events include the following:
- HSV and CMV
- Gonorrhea
- Group B streptococcal sepsis
- Chlamydial conjunctivitis and pneumonia
- *E. coli* or other neonatal meningitis

In the laboratory, these infections are diagnosed by direct detection, including NAATS or culturing for the agents when possible, or by performing serologic tests. The appropriate specimens (e.g., cerebrospinal fluid, serum, pus, tracheal aspirate) should be examined and inoculated immediately. Routine body surface cultures of infants in intensive care have not been shown to be helpful for predicting subsequent disease. The use of viral cell culture methods has been replaced in most laboratories by NAAT methods.

Finally, certain infectious agents are known to cause fetal infection and even abortion. For example, *L. monocytogenes,* the causative agent of mild flulike symptoms in the mother, can cause extensive disease and abortion of the fetus if infection occurs late in the pregnancy. Therefore, isolation of the organism from the placenta and from tissues of the fetus is important.

ⓔ Visit the Evolve site for a complete list of procedures, review questions, and case studies.

Bibliography

Anderson MR, Klink K, Cohrssen A: Evaluation of vaginal complaints, *JAMA* 291:1368–1379, 2004.

Bennett J, Dolin R, Blaser M: *Principles and practice of infectious diseases*, ed 9, Philadelphia, PA, 2020, Elsevier.

Carroll KC, Pfaller MA: *Manual of clinical microbiology*, ed 12, Washington, DC, 2019, ASM Press.

Clarridge JE, Shawar R, Simon B: *Haemophilus ducreyi* and chancroid: practical aspects for the clinical microbiology laboratory, *Clin Microbiol Newsl* 12:137–141, 1990.

Creatsas G, Deligeoroglou E: Microbial ecology of the lower genital tract in women with sexually transmitted diseases, *J Med Microbiol* 61:1347–1351, 2012.

Curry A, Williams T, Penny ML: Pelvic inflammatory disease: diagnosis, management, and prevention, *Am Fam Physician* 100(6):357–364, 2019.

Fredricks DN, Fiedler TL, Marrazzo JM: Molecular identification of bacteria associated with bacterial vaginosis, *N Engl J Med* 353:1899–1911, 2005.

Hammerschlag MR, Guillen CD: Medical and legal implications of testing for sexually transmitted infections in children, *Clin Microbiol Rev* 23:493–506, 2010.

Hillier SL, Krohn MA, Rabe LK, et al.: Normal vaginal flora, H_2O_2-producing lactobacilli and bacterial vaginosis in pregnant women, *Clin Infect Dis* 16(Suppl 4):S273–S281, 1993.

Johnson RE, Newhall WJ, Rapp JR, et al.: Screening tests to detect *Chlamydia trachomatis* and *Neisseria gonorrhoeae* infections—2002, *MMWR* 51(RR-15):1–38, 2002.

Kellogg JA, Seiple JW, Klinedinst JL, et al.: Comparison of cytobrushes with swabs for recovery of endocervical cells and for Chlamydiazyme detection of *Chlamydia trachomatis*, *J Clin Microbiol* 30:2988–2990, 1992.

Nugent RP, Krohn MA, Hillier SL: Reliability of diagnosing bacterial vaginosis is improved by a standardized method of Gram stain interpretation, *J Clin Microbiol* 29:297–301, 1991.

Schmid GP, Faur YC, Valu JA, et al.: Enhanced recovery of *Haemophilus ducreyi* from clinical specimens by incubation at 33°C versus 35°C, *J Clin Microbiol* 33:3257–3259, 1995.

Schrag S, Gorwitz R, Fultz-Butts K, et al.: Prevention of perinatal group B streptococcal disease, revised guidelines from CDC, *MMWR Recomm Rep* 51(RR-11):1–22, 2002.

Sobel JD: What's new in bacterial vaginosis and trichomoniasis? *Infect Dis Clin North Am* 19:387–406, 2005.

Wilson J: Managing recurrent bacterial vaginosis, *Sex Transm Infect* 80:8–11, 2004.

Wood JC, Lu RM, Peterson EM, et al.: Evaluation of mycotrim-GU for isolation of *Mycoplasma* species and *Ureaplasma urealyticum*, *J Clin Microbiol* 22:789–792, 1985.

74

Gastrointestinal Tract Infections

OBJECTIVES

1. Describe the general anatomy of the gastrointestinal tract and the relationship to transmission of infectious disease.
2. Differentiate normal human microbiota from pathogenic organisms and describe the relative numbers of organisms distributed throughout the gastrointestinal tract.
3. Identify nonbacterial agents of infection of the gastrointestinal tract and name their associated diseases.
4. Describe innate immunity as it relates to the gastrointestinal tract, including physical, chemical, and bacterial components.
5. Differentiate infections of the upper and lower gastrointestinal tract based on clinical manifestations including watery diarrhea and bloody diarrhea (dysentery).
6. Identify the major cause for antimicrobial therapy–associated diarrhea and the proper laboratory diagnostic procedure for identification, including the toxin assay.
7. Identify the most common causes for watery diarrhea, dysentery, pseudomembranous colitis, and infant botulism.
8. Describe the bacterial pathogenic mechanisms associated with gastrointestinal disease, including the presence and function of enterotoxins, attachment, and invasion mechanisms.
9. Determine the adequacy of a specimen based on collection, transport, and specimen type for the diagnosis of gastrointestinal infections.
10. Define the following media, including the organisms identified and the chemical properties associated with the selection and differentiation within the media: MAC, SMAC, EMB, HEK, XLD, SS, and Campy.
11. List the organisms and microbial products that can be detected by nonculture methods.
12. Explain how the use of culture independent methods affects the surveillance and trends in diagnostic testing and antimicrobial sensitivity patterns for epidemiological purposes.
13. Correlate patient signs and symptoms with laboratory results for the identification of the gastrointestinal pathogen.

Anatomy

We are all connected to the external environment through our gastrointestinal (GI) tract (Fig. 74.1). What we swallow enters the GI tract and passes through the esophagus into the stomach, through the small and large intestines, and finally to the anus. During passage, fluids and other components are added to this material as secretory products of individual cells and as enzymatic secretions of glands and organs, and they are removed from this material by absorption through the gut epithelium.

The major components of the GI tract are listed in Box 74.1. The nature of the epithelial cells lining the GI tract varies with each portion. The lining of the GI tract is called the **mucosa.** Because of the differing nature of the mucosal surfaces of various segments of the bowel, specific infectious disease processes tend to occur in each segment.

The wall of the small intestine has folds that have millions of tiny, hairlike projections called **villi.** Each villus contains an arteriole, venule, and lymph vessel (Fig. 74.2). The function of villi is to absorb fluids and nutrients from the intestinal contents. Epithelial cells lining the surface of villi have a surface resembling a fine brush, referred to as a **brush border.** The brush border is formed by nearly 2000 microvilli per epithelial cell. Intestinal digestive enzymes are produced in brush border cells toward the top of the villi. Villi and microvilli help make the small intestine the primary site of digestion and absorption by significantly increasing the surface area; more than 90% of physiologic net fluid absorption occurs here. Mucus-secreting **goblet cells** are found in large numbers of villi and intestinal crypts.

Similar to the small intestine, the large intestine is composed of several segments (Box 74.1). The wall of the large intestine consists of **columnar epithelial cells,** many of which are mucus-producing goblet cells. In contrast to the small intestine, there are no villous projections into the lumen. The remaining excess fluid within the GI tract is resorbed through the cells lining the large intestine before waste is finally discharged through the rectum.

In addition to the previously discussed components of the GI tract, numerous other organs and structures are either located in the main digestive organs or open into them. These accessory organs and structures include the salivary glands, tongue, teeth, liver, gallbladder, and pancreas. Except for the teeth and salivary glands, these organs are illustrated in Fig. 74.1.

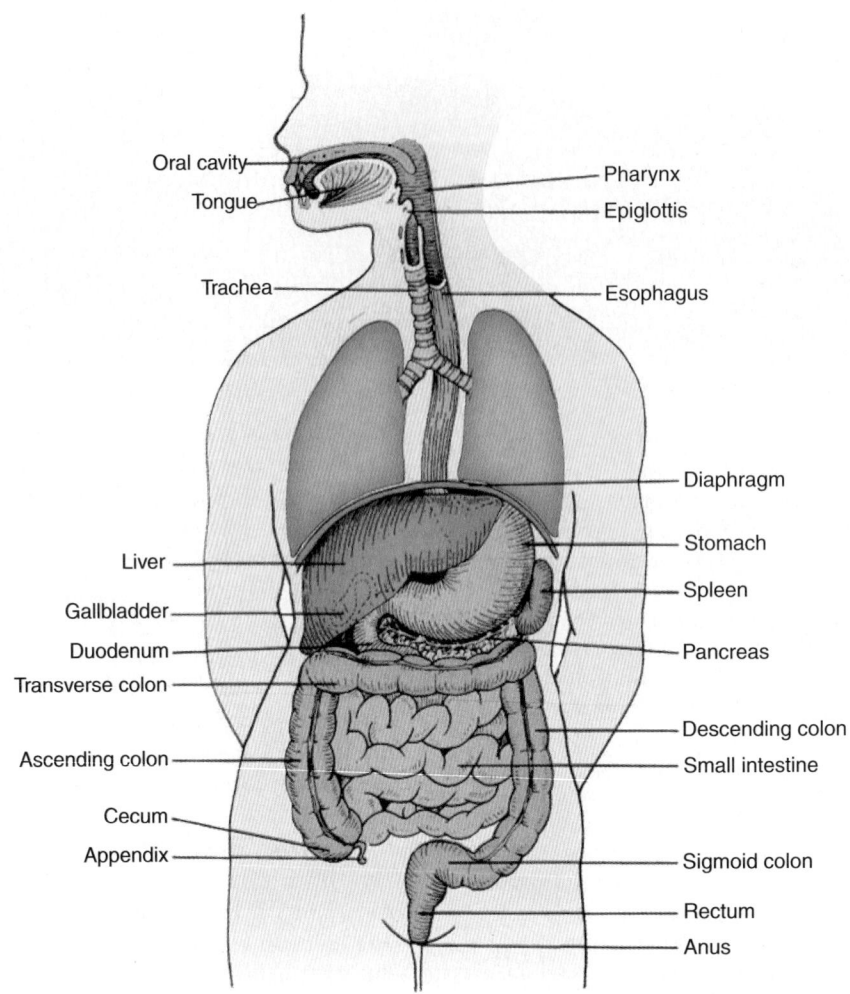

• **Fig. 74.1** General anatomy of the gastrointestinal tract. (From Broadwell DC, Jackson BS. *Principles of Ostomy Care*. St Louis: Mosby; 1982.)

Resident Gastrointestinal Microbiome

The GI tract contains vast, diverse normal microbiota. Although the acidity of the stomach prevents any significant colonization in a normal host under most circumstances, many species can survive passage through the stomach to become resident within the lower intestinal tract. Normally, the upper small intestine contains only sparse microbiota (bacteria, primarily streptococci; lactobacilli; and yeasts; 10^1 to 10^3/mL), but in the distal ileum, counts are about 10^6 to 10^7/mL, with Enterobacterales and *Bacteroides* spp. predominantly present.

The GI microbiome assists in the maintenance of a healthy environment and physiologic status of the host by providing essential vitamins and nutrients, influencing the natural and adaptive immune response as well as protecting the mucosal surface. An individual's GI microbiota varies according to the host genetics; nutritional status; previous or current antimicrobial, antifungal, or other chemotherapeutic agents; age; and the geographic region. Infants

usually are colonized by normal human epithelial microbiota, such as staphylococci, *Corynebacterium* spp., and other gram-positive organisms (bifidobacteria, clostridia, lactobacilli, streptococci), within a few hours of birth. Over time, the content of the intestinal microbiota changes. The normal microbiota of the adult large bowel (colon) is established relatively early in life and consists predominantly of anaerobic species, including *Bacteroides, Clostridium, Peptostreptococcus, Bifidobacterium,* and *Eubacterium*. Aerobes, including *Escherichia* spp., other Enterobacterales, enterococci, and streptococci, are outnumbered by anaerobes 1000:1. The number of bacteria per gram of stool within the bowel lumen increases steadily as material approaches the sigmoid colon (the last segment). Eighty percent of the dry weight of feces from a healthy human consists of bacteria, which can be present in numbers as high as 10^{11} to 10^{12} colony-forming units (CFU)/g of stool.

All regions in the GI tract from the oral cavity to the anus contain three major bacterial phyla: *Bacteroidetes, Firmicutes,* and *Proteobacteria*. However, variations in the predominant

Mouth
Oropharynx
Esophagus
Stomach
- *Fundus:* enlarged portion of the stomach to the left and above the opening of the esophagus into the stomach
- *Body:* central part of the stomach
- *Pylorus:* lower portion of the stomach
Small intestine
- *Duodenum:* uppermost division; attached to pyloric end of the stomach
- *Jejunum:* midsection of the small intestine
- *Ileum:* lower portion of the small intestine
Large intestine
- Cecum
- Colon
  Ascending colon: lies on the right side of the abdomen and extends up to the lower portion of the liver; the ileum joins the large intestine at the junction of the cecum and the ascending colon
  Transverse colon: passes horizontally across the abdomen
  Descending colon: lies on the left side of the abdomen in a vertical position
  Sigmoid colon: extends downward, subsequently joining the rectum
- Rectum
- Anal canal

phyla occur throughout the locations within the GI tract. The upper GI tract consists primarily of the bacterial families *Veillonellaceae, Pseudomonadaceae,* and *Streptococcaceae,* whereas the lower GI tract consists primarily of *Lachnospiraceae, Bacteroidaceae,* and *Ruminococcaceae.* There are differences in the reported populations of the normal microbiota that appear to be geographical in nature; more studies are needed as the details associated with a healthy normal GI tract microbiome is unraveled. This information may be useful for the development of appropriate measures in the prevention and treatment of autoimmune diseases, GI illness, and other disease syndromes through dietary intervention and the use of probiotics.

Gastroenteritis

Worldwide, diarrheal diseases are the ninth leading cause of death; about 48 million enteric infections occur each year. These infections cause significant morbidity and death, particularly in elderly people and children younger than 5 years of age. It has been estimated that nearly 1.7 billion cases of childhood diarrheal diseases, particularly in developing countries, occur globally each year. Even in developed countries, significant morbidity occurs as a result of diarrheal illness. Although acute diarrheal syndromes are usually self-limited, some patients with infectious diarrhea require diagnostic studies and treatment.

Pathogenesis

Similar to the pathogenesis of urinary tract infections, the host and the invading microorganism possess key features that determine whether an enteric pathogen is able to cause microbial diarrhea.

Host Factors

The human host has numerous defenses that normally prevent or control disease produced by enteric pathogens. For example, the acidity of the stomach effectively restricts the number and types of organisms that enter the lower GI tract. Normal peristalsis helps move organisms toward the rectum, interfering with their ability to adhere to the mucosa. The mucous layer coating the epithelium entraps microorganisms and helps propel them through the gut. The normal microbiota prevents colonization by potential pathogens.

Mucous membranes line the GI tract, as well as the respiratory and urogenital tracts. These membranes are exposed to the external environment in the form of food, water, and air. These membranes contain multiple cell types; some are secreting or absorbing cells that perform physiologic functions of the membrane, whereas others serve as protective barriers. For example, sets of specialized cells called **follicles** are part of the mucous membrane lining the GI tract and serve a protective function. Collections of follicles are called **Peyer patches.** Follicles contain M cells, macrophages, and B and T cells. As a result of the collective action of the follicle components after uptake and processing of the bacteria or antigens, secretory immunoglobulin A (sIgA) is released. Phagocytic cells and sIgA within the gut help destroy etiologic agents of disease, as do eosinophils, which are particularly active against parasites. Follicles and Peyer patches are found in the small and large intestines.

Other factors that determine the progression and potential invasion by pathogenic organisms include the host's personal hygiene and age. An initial step in the pathogenesis of enteric infections is ingestion of the pathogen. Most enteric pathogens, including bacteria, viruses, and parasites, are transmitted by the **fecal-oral route.** Enteric infections can be spread by contamination of food products or drinking water and then subsequent ingestion. The age of the host also plays a role in whether disease is established. For example, diarrheal infections caused by rotavirus or enteropathogenic *Escherichia coli* tend to affect young children.

Finally, the normal intestinal microbiome is an important factor in the host protection from the introduction of a potentially harmful microorganism. Whenever a reduction in normal microbiota occurs as a result of antibiotic treatment or some host factor, resistance to GI infection is significantly reduced. The most common example of the protective effect of normal microbiota is the development of the syndrome **pseudomembranous colitis (PMC).** This inflammatory disease of the large bowel is caused by the toxins of the anaerobic organism *Clostridioides difficile* and occasionally

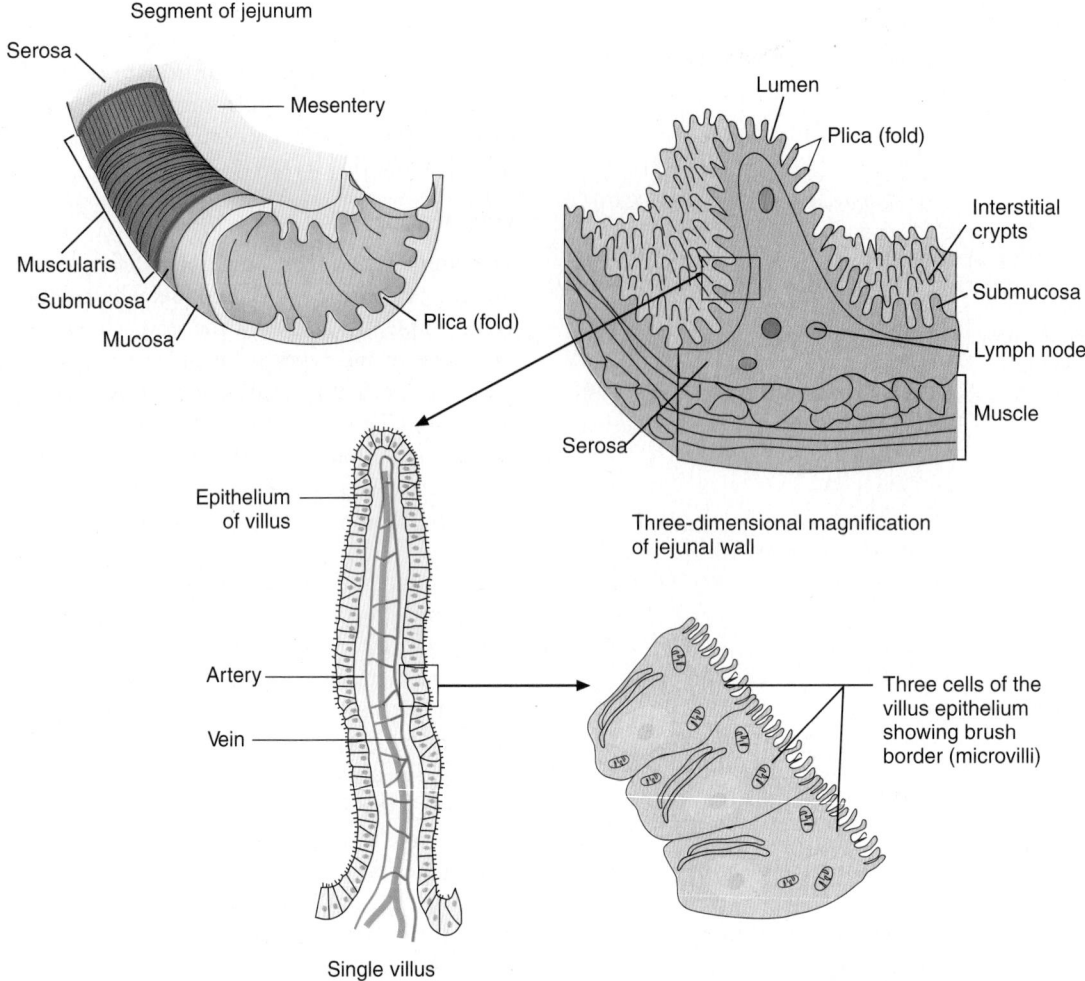

• **Fig. 74.2** Wall of the small intestine. Villi cover the folds of the mucosal layer; in turn, each villus is covered with epithelial cells.

other clostridia and perhaps even *Staphylococcus aureus.* The inflammatory disease seldom occurs except after antimicrobial or antimetabolite treatment that has altered the normal microbiota. Almost every antimicrobial agent and several cancer agents have been associated with the development of PMC. *C. difficile,* usually acquired from the hospital environment, is suppressed by normal microbiota. When the normal microbiota is reduced, *C. difficile* can multiply and produce its toxins. This syndrome is also known as **antibiotic-associated colitis (AAC).** Other microorganisms that may gain a foothold when released from selective pressure of normal microbiota include *Candida* spp., staphylococci, *Pseudomonas* spp., and various Enterobacterales.

Microbial Factors

The ability of an organism to cause GI infection depends not only on the susceptibility of the human host to the invading organism but also on the organism's virulence traits. To cause GI infection, a microorganism must possess one or more factors that allow it to overcome host defenses or it must enter the host at a time when one or more of the innate defense systems are inactive. For example, certain stool pathogens are able to survive gastric acidity only if

the acidity has been reduced by bicarbonate, other buffers, or by medications for ulcers (e.g., cimetidine, ranitidine, H_2 blockers). Pathogens ingested with milk have a better chance of survival because milk neutralizes stomach acidity. Organisms such as *Mycobacterium tuberculosis, Shigella, E. coli* O157:H7, and *C. difficile* (a spore-forming bacterium) can withstand exposure to gastric acids and thus require much smaller infectious doses than do acid-sensitive organisms such as *Salmonella.*

Primary Pathogenic Mechanisms

Because the normal adult GI tract receives up to 8 L of ingested fluid daily, plus the secretions of the various glands that contribute to digestion (salivary glands, pancreas, gallbladder, stomach), of which all but a small amount must be resorbed, any disruption of the normal flow or reabsorption of fluid will profoundly affect the host. Depending on how they interact with the human host, enteric pathogens may cause disease in one or more of the following three ways:
• Changing the delicate balance of water and electrolytes in the small bowel, resulting in massive fluid secretion. In many cases, this process is mediated by enterotoxin production. This is a noninflammatory process.

TABLE 74.1 Examples of Microorganisms That Cause Gastrointestinal Infection for Each Primary Pathogenic Mechanism

Mechanism	Examples of Microorganisms
Toxin Production	
Enterotoxin	*Vibrio cholera*
	Noncholera vibrios
	Shigella dysenteriae type 1
	Enterotoxigenic *Escherichia coli*
	Salmonella spp.
	Clostridioides difficile (toxin A)
	Aeromonas
	Campylobacter jejuni subsp. *jejuni*
Cytotoxin	*Shigella* spp.
	C. difficile (toxin B)
	Entamoeba histolytica
	Enterohemorrhagic *Escherichia coli*
Neurotoxin	*Clostridium botulinum*
	Clostridium perfringens
	Staphylococcus aureus
	Bacillus cereus
Attachment within or close to mucosal cells/adherence	Enteropathogenic *E. coli*
	Enterohemorrhagic *E. coli*
	Cryptosporidium parvum
	Cystoisospora belli
	Rotavirus
	Hepatitis A, B, C
	Noroviruses
Invasion	*Shigella* spp.
	Enteroinvasive *E. coli*
	Entamoeba histolytica
	Neobalantidium coli
	C. jejuni subsp. *jejuni*
	Plesiomonas shigelloides
	Yersinia enterocolitica
	Edwardsiella tarda

- Causing cell destruction or a marked inflammatory response after invasion of host cells and possible cytotoxin production, usually in the colon.
- Penetrating the intestinal mucosa, with subsequent spread and multiplication in lymphatic or reticuloendothelial cells outside of the bowel; these infections are considered systemic infections.

Examples of microorganisms for each of these pathogenic mechanisms are listed in Table 74.1.

Toxins

Enterotoxins. **Enterotoxins** alter the metabolic activity of intestinal epithelial cells, resulting in an outpouring of electrolytes and fluid into the lumen. They act primarily in the jejunum and upper ileum, where most fluid transport takes place. The stool of patients with enterotoxic diarrheal disease involving the small bowel is profuse and watery, and blood or polymorphonuclear neutrophils are not prominent features.

The classic example of an enterotoxin is that of *Vibrio cholerae* (Fig. 74.3). This toxin consists of two subunits, A and B. The A subunit is composed of one molecule of A_1, the toxic moiety, and one molecule of A_2, which binds an A_1 subunit to five B subunits. The B subunits bind the toxin to a receptor (a ganglioside, an acidic glycolipid) on the intestinal cell membrane. Once bound, the toxin acts on adenylate cyclase enzyme, which catalyzes the transformation of adenosine triphosphate (ATP) to cyclic adenosine monophosphate (cAMP). Increased levels of cAMP stimulate the cell to actively secrete ions into the intestinal lumen. To maintain osmotic stabilization, the cells then secrete fluid into the lumen. The fluid is drawn from the intravascular fluid store of the body. Patients therefore can become dehydrated and hypotensive rapidly. *V. cholerae* inhabits sea and stagnant water and is spread in contaminated water. The organisms have been isolated from coastal waters of several states, and sporadic cases of cholera occur in the United States. Additional information about *V. cholerae* is provided in Chapter 25.

Other organisms also produce a cholera-like enterotoxin. A group of vibrios similar to *V. cholerae* but serologically different, known as the noncholera vibrios, produce disease clinically identical to cholera, affected by a very similar toxin. The heat-labile toxin (LT) elaborated by certain strains of *E. coli*, called enterotoxigenic *E. coli* (ETEC), is similar to cholera toxin, sharing cross-reactive antigenic determinants. The enterotoxins of some *Salmonella* spp. (including *Salmonella enterica* subsp. *arizonae*), *Vibrio parahaemolyticus*, the *Campylobacter jejuni* subsp. *jejuni*, *C. jejuni* subsp. *doylei*, *Clostridium perfringens*, *C. difficile*, *Bacillus cereus*, *Aeromonas*, *Shigella dysenteriae*, and many others also cause positive reactions in at least one of the tests for enterotoxin (discussed later). The exact contribution of these enterotoxins to the pathogenicity of most stool pathogens remains to be elucidated.

Certain strains of *E. coli*, in addition to producing an LT similar to cholera toxin, also produce a heat-stable toxin (ST) with other properties. Although ST also promotes fluid secretion into the intestinal lumen, its effect is mediated by activation of guanylate cyclase, resulting in increased levels of cyclic guanylate monophosphate (GMP), which yields the same net effect as increased cAMP. Tests for ST include commercial immunoassays for the detection of Shiga toxin or serotyping for the O157 lipopolysaccharide. There are several Food and Drug Administration (FDA)-approved assays for the detection and diagnosis of STEC, *Salmonella*, and *Shigella*/EIEC (Chapter 19). In addition, there are chromogenic agars for the visual detection of O157:H7 after direct inoculation as a primary culture medium.

Cytotoxins. **Cytotoxins,** which constitute the second category of toxins, disrupt the structure of individual intestinal epithelial cells. When destroyed, these cells slough from the surface of the mucosa, leaving it raw and unprotected. The secretory or absorptive activities of the cells no longer function properly. The damaged tissue evokes a strong inflammatory response from the host, further inflicting

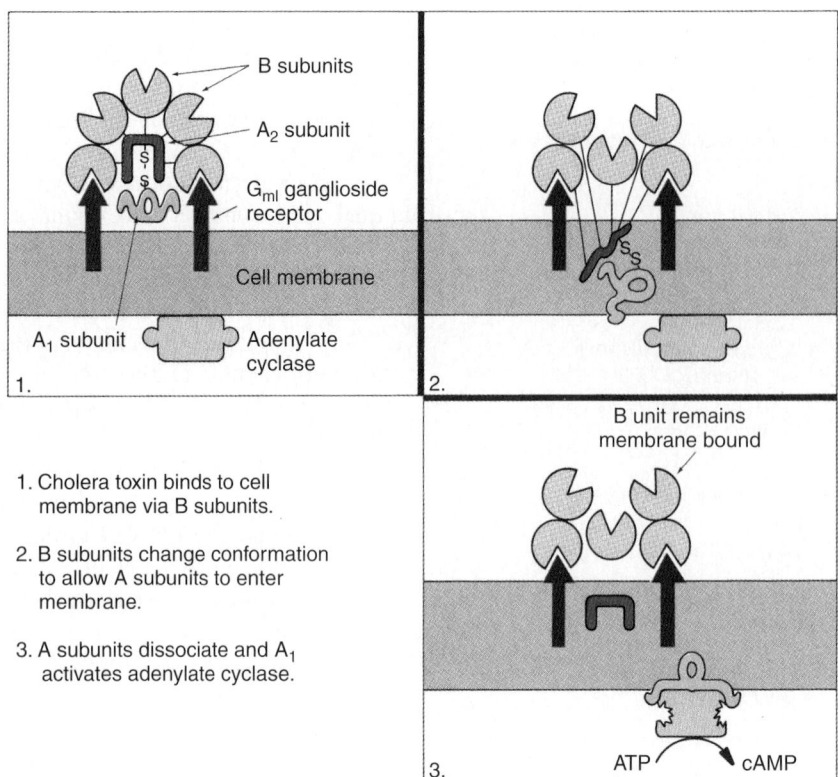

B subunits

A₂ subunit

G_{ml} ganglioside receptor

Cell membrane

A₁ subunit

Adenylate cyclase

1.

2.

B unit remains membrane bound

3.

ATP   cAMP

1. Cholera toxin binds to cell membrane via B subunits.

2. B subunits change conformation to allow A subunits to enter membrane.

3. A subunits dissociate and A₁ activates adenylate cyclase.

• **Fig. 74.3** The structure and action of cholera toxin.

tissue damage. Numerous polymorphonuclear neutrophils and blood are often seen in the stool, and pain, cramps, and tenesmus (painful straining during a bowel movement) are common symptoms. The term **dysentery** refers to this destructive disease of the mucosa, almost exclusively occurring in the colon. Cytotoxin has not yet been shown to be the sole virulence factor for any etiologic agent of GI disease, because most agents produce a cytotoxin in conjunction with other factors.

E. coli strains seem to possess virulence mechanisms of many types. Some strains produce a cytotoxin capable of destroying epithelial cells and blood cells. Certain strains produce a cytotoxin that affects Vero cells (African green monkey kidney cells) and resemble the cytotoxin produced by *S. dysenteriae* (Shiga toxin); such strains of *E. coli* are associated with hemorrhagic colitis and after infection result in sequelae such as hemolytic-uremic syndrome (HUS) and thrombotic thrombocytopenia purpura (TTP). These strains of *E. coli* are referred to as enterohemorrhagic *E. coli,* also referred to as serotoxigenic. See Chapter 19 for more information related to toxigenic *E. coli.* Table 74.2 summarizes the key pathogenic features of the primary groups of diarrheagenic *E. coli.*

C. difficile produces a cytotoxin, the presence of which is a most useful marker for diagnosis of PMC. *S. dysenteriae, S. aureus, C. perfringens,* and *V. parahaemolyticus* produce cytotoxins that contribute to the pathogenesis of diarrhea, although they may not be essential for the initiation of disease. Other vibrios, *Aeromonas hydrophila, Entamoeba histolytica,* and *C. jejuni* subsp. *jejuni,* the most common cause

of GI disease in many areas of the United States, have been shown to produce cytotoxins.

C. difficile toxigenic strains produce two protein exotoxins, referred to as toxin A and toxin B. Both toxins bind to receptors on the brush border of the intestinal epithelium and are then internalized. Once inside the cell, both toxins modify proteins that are involved in the regulation of the actin cytoskeleton. This affects actin polymerization, causing disturbances and separation of the cell-to-cell tight junctions, rupturing the cells and causing mucosal damage.

S. dysenteriae produces a very potent cytotoxin referred to as type 1. This toxin is also produced by various strains of *E. coli* (STEC). The cytotoxin is an A₁-B₅ protein toxin. The toxin targets the GB3 (globotriaosylceramide) membrane receptor; the toxin becomes internalized and is transported into the endoplasmic reticulum (ER) and to the nuclear membrane. The A subunit of the toxin is then able to cleave the 28S ribosomal ribonucleic acid (rRNA) interfering with protein synthesis that results in host cell death. The ultimate effect is vascular damage to the endothelial surface, bloody diarrhea, and potentially HUS.

Bacteria are not the only toxin-producing organisms capable of causing cellular pathology within the GI tract. *E. histolytica* produces a phospholipase A and pore-forming peptides that upon direct contact with phagocytic cells result in direct cell death, reducing effective clearing of the protozoan parasite.

Neurotoxins. Food poisoning, or **intoxication,** may occur as a result of ingesting toxins produced by microorganisms. The microorganisms usually produce their toxins

TABLE 74.2	Overview of the Primary Groups of *Escherichia coli* That Cause Diarrhea in Humans		
Type	**Primary Mode of Pathogenesis**	**Other Comments**
Enterotoxigenic (ETEC)	Produces heat-labile (LT) or heat-stable (ST) entero-toxins; genes of both toxins reside on a plasmid; LTs are closely related in structure and function to cholera toxin; STs result in net intestinal fluid secretion by stimulating guanylate cyclase.	Common cause of traveler's diarrhea; infects all ages.
Enteroaggregative (EAEC)	Binds to small intestine cells via fimbriae encoded by a large molecular weight plasmid, forming small clumps of bacteria on the cell surface; other plasmid-borne virulence factors include structured pilin, a heat-stable enterotoxin, novel antiag-gregative protein, and a heat-labile enterotoxin, all believed to be the cause of the associated diarrhea.	Infects primarily young children.
Enteroinvasive (EIEC)	Pathogenesis has yet to be totally elucidated; stud-ies suggest that mechanisms by which diarrhea results are virtually identical to those of *Shigella* spp.	Very difficult to distinguish from *Shigella* spp. and other *E. coli* strains.
Enteropathogenic (EPEC)	Initially attaches in the colon and small intestine and then becomes intimately adhered to intestinal epithelial cells, subsequently causing the loss of enterocyte microvilli (effacement); genes for attachment/effacement reside in a cluster on the bacterial chromosome (i.e., pathogenicity island).	Diarrhea in infants, particularly in large urban hospitals.
Enterohemorrhagic (STEC)	Attaches to and effaces gut epithelial cells in a simi-lar manner as EPEC; in addition, STEC elaborates Shiga toxins.	Although many outbreaks are caused by *E. coli* O157:H7, other serotypes have been implicated in outbreaks and sporadic cases. Gene recombination among strains makes classifi-cation difficult.
	Produce one or more Shiga toxins referred to as verocytotoxins. Attaches to and effaces gut epithelial cells in a similar manner as EPEC.	O157 STEC serotypes; contains most common serotypes O157:H7 and nonmotile O157: NM. There are more than 150 non-O157 serotypes that have been isolated from patients with diarrhea or hemolytic-uremic syndrome.

in foodstuffs before they are ingested; thus, the patient ingests preformed toxin. Strictly speaking, these syndromes are not GI infections but rather intoxications; because they are acquired by ingestion of microorganisms or their products, they are considered in this chapter. Particularly in staphylococcal food poisoning and botulism, the caus-ative organisms may not be present in the patient's bowel (Box 74.2).

Bacterial agents of food poisoning that produce neu-rotoxins include *S. aureus* and *B. cereus.* Toxins produced by these organisms cause vomiting, independent of other actions on the gut mucosa. Staphylococcal food poisoning is one of the most commonly reported categories of food-borne disease. The organisms grow in warm food, primar-ily meat or dairy products, and produce the toxin. Onset of disease is usually within 2 to 6 hours of ingestion. *B. cereus* produces two toxins, one of which is preformed and is called the **emetic toxin,** because it produces vomiting. The second type, probably involving several enterotoxins, causes diarrhea. Often acquired from eating rice, *B. cereus* has also

been associated with cooked meat, poultry, vegetables, and desserts.

Perhaps the most common cause of food poisoning is type A *C. perfringens,* which produces a neurotoxin in the host after ingestion. As a result, a relatively mild, self-limited (usually 24-hour) gastroenteritis occurs, often in outbreaks in hospitals. Meats and gravies are typical foods associated with this type of food poisoning.

One of the most potent neurotoxins is produced by the anaerobic organism *Clostridium botulinum.* This toxin pre-vents the release of the neurotransmitter acetylcholine at the cholinergic nerve junctions, causing **flaccid** (rag doll) **paralysis.** The toxin acts primarily on the peripheral nerves but also on the autonomic nervous system. Patients exhibit descending symmetric paralysis and ultimately die of respi-ratory paralysis unless they are mechanically ventilated. In most cases, adult patients who develop botulism have ingested the preformed toxin in food (home-canned tomato products and canned, cream-based foods are often impli-cated), and the disease is considered intoxication, although

C. botulinum has been recovered from the stools of many adult patients. A relatively recently recognized syndrome, **infant botulism,** is a true GI infection. In adults, the normal microbiota probably prevents colonization by *C. botulinum,* whereas the organism can multiply and produce toxin in the infant bowel. Infant botulism is not uncommon; babies acquire the organism by ingestion, although the source of the bacterium is not always clear. Because an association has been found with honey and corn syrup, infants younger than 9 months of age should not be fed honey. The effect of the toxin is the same whether ingested in food or produced by growing organisms within the bowel.

Attachment. An organism's ability to cause disease can also depend on its ability to colonize and adhere to the bowel. To illustrate, ETEC must be able to adhere to and colonize the small intestine, as well as produce an enterotoxin. These organisms produce an adherence antigen, called **colonization factor antigen (CFA).** Certain strains of *E. coli* referred to as the enteropathogenic *E. coli* (EPEC) attach and then adhere to the intestinal brush border. This localized adherence is mediated by the production of pili. After attaching, EPEC disrupts normal cell function by effacing the brush epithelium, thereby causing diarrheal disease. This complete process is referred to as **attachment and effacement.** Genes responsible for the initial adherence of ETEC, STEC, and EPEC to intestinal epithelial cells reside on a transmissible plasmid. STEC has the same ability to attach to intestinal epithelial cells and cause effacement. In addition, STEC produces a Shiga toxin that spreads to the bloodstream, causing systemic damage to vascular endothelial cells of various organs, including kidney, colon, small intestine, and lung. STEC is believed to have arisen because of an EPEC strain that became infected with a bacteriophage carrying the Shiga toxin gene (Fig. 74.4).

Giardia duodenalis, a parasite, has increasingly become more common as an etiologic agent of GI disease in the United States. Excreted into fresh water by natural animal hosts such as the beaver, the organism can be acquired by drinking stream water or even city water in some localities, particularly in the Rocky Mountain region. The organism, a flagellated protozoan, adheres to the intestinal mucosa of the small bowel by means of a ventral sucker, destroying the mucosal cells' ability to participate in normal secretion and absorption. No evidence indicates invasion or toxin production.

Cryptosporidium and *Cystoisospora* spp., parasitic etiologic agents of diarrhea in animals and poultry and more recently recognized as causing human disease, probably also act by adhering to intestinal mucosa and disrupting function. Cryptosporidium are often seen in the diarrhea of patients with acquired immunodeficiency syndrome (AIDS), as well as in travelers' diarrhea, daycare epidemics, and diarrhea in people with animal exposure. *Cryptosporidium* and *Cystoisospora* spp. may cause severe, protracted diarrhea in AIDS patients. Other coccidian parasites, such as microsporidia, produce diarrhea by destroying intestinal cell function.

Origins of STEC

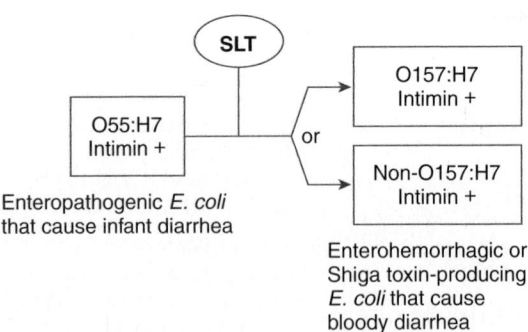

• **Fig. 74.4** It appears that the presence of enterohemorrhagic *Escherichia coli* (STEC) strain O157:H7 was not simply overlooked before 1982. *E. coli* O157:H7 strains are closely related to a Shiga toxin–negative enteropathogenic *E. coli* (EPEC) strain O55:H7. It is proposed that this EPEC strain O55:H7 became infected by a bacteriophage that encoded Shiga toxin (*SLT*); it is now recognized that at least 25 different virulence-associated genes may be associated with STEC and are classified into five "seropathotypes" A through E.

Invasion. After initial and essential adherence to GI mucosal cells, some enteric pathogens can gain access to the intracellular environment. Invasion allows the organism to reach deeper tissues, access nutrients for growth, and possibly avoid the host immune system.

In the case of diarrhea caused by *Shigella,* the primary mechanism of disease production consists of (1) the triggering and directing by *Shigella* entry into colonic epithelial cells by genes located on a plasmid, and once internalized, (2) the rapid multiplication of *Shigella* in the submucosa and lamina propria and the organism's intracellular and extracellular spread to other adjacent colonic epithelial cells. Once in the host cell cytoplasm, *Shigella* spp. cause apoptosis and release of the cytokines interleukin (IL)-1 and IL-8. The inflammatory response to these cytokines damages the colonic mucosa and exacerbates (aggravates) the infection. The genes for invasiveness are located on a large invasion plasmid. These activities lead to extensive superficial tissue destruction. If these two steps do not occur, the clinical presentation of classic dysentery does not develop (Table 74.3). The entry process is illustrated in Fig. 74.5.

Salmonellae interact with the apical (top) microvilli of colonic epithelial cells, disrupting the brush border. Similar to *Shigella, Salmonella* spp. also stimulate the host cell to internalize through rearrangements of host actin filaments and other cytoskeleton proteins. Once the whole bacteria are internalized within endocytic vesicles of the host epithelial cell, organisms begin to multiply within the vacuoles. In contrast to *Shigella* spp. that use the colonic mucosal epithelium as a site of multiplication, certain serotypes of *Salmonella,* such as *S. enterica* serovar Typhi, use the colonic epithelium as a route to gain access to the submucosal layers, mesenteric lymph nodes, and subsequently the bloodstream. The entry of *Salmonella* is a complex process involving several essential genes, as well as environmental conditions of the host cell; this process is still being delineated. Many virulence factors for invasion of salmonellae

TABLE 74.3 Types of Enteric Infections

Pathogenic Mechanism	Major Symptoms	Examples of Etiologic Agents
Upsetting of fluid and electrolyte balance/noninflammatory	Watery diarrhea No fecal leukocytes No fever	*Vibrio cholerae* Rotavirus Noroviruses Enteric adenoviruses Enterotoxigenic *Escherichia coli* *Giardia duodenalis* *Bacillus cereus*
Invasion and possible cytotoxin production/inflammatory (dysentery)	Dysenteric-like diarrhea (mucus, blood, white cells) Fever Fecal leukocytes	*Shigella* spp. Enteroinvasive *E. coli* *Salmonella* spp. *Entamoeba histolytica*
Penetration with subsequent access to the bloodstream (enteric fever)	Signs of systemic infection (headache, malaise, sore throat) Fever	*Salmonella enterica* serotype Typhi *Yersinia enterocolitica*

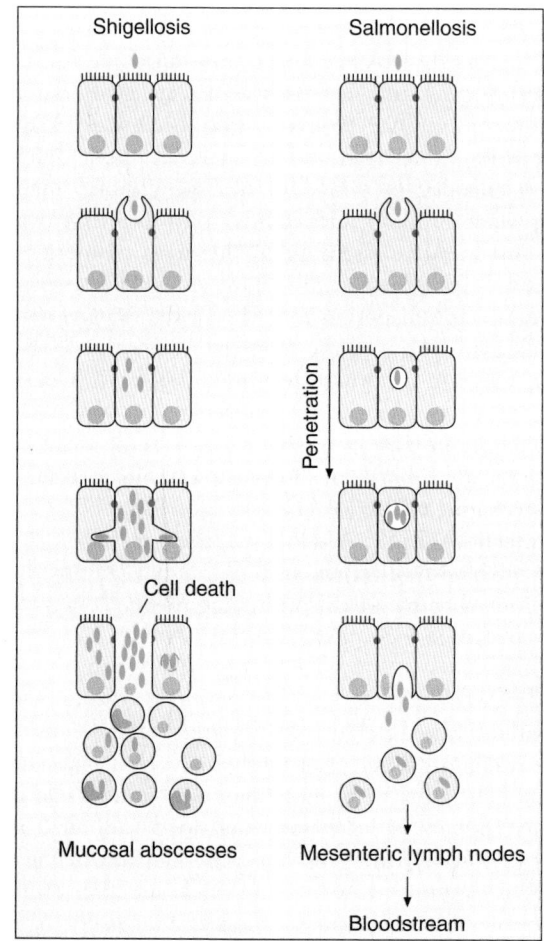

• **Fig. 74.5** The invasion of *Shigella* and *Salmonella* into intestinal epithelial cells. (Republished with permission of Oxford University Press from Sensonetti PJ. *Reviews of Infectious Diseases.* 1991;13[4].)

into nonphagocytic cells as well as their ability to cause systemic infections by surviving in phagocytic cells and replicating within the *Salmonella*-containing vesicle in a variety of eukaryotic cells are determined by chromosomal genes, many of which are located within pathogenicity islands. Invasiveness is also believed to contribute to the pathogenesis of disease associated with species of vibrios, campylobacters, *Yersinia enterocolitica*, *Plesiomonas shigelloides*, and *Edwardsiella tarda*.

Certain parasites, particularly *E. histolytica* and *Neobalantidium coli*, invade the intestinal epithelium of the colon. The ensuing amoebic dysentery is characterized by blood and numerous white blood cells, and the patient experiences cramping and tenesmus. Other parasites acquired by ingestion, such as *Trichinella*, may cause transient bloody diarrhea and pain during migration through the intestinal mucosa to their preferred sites within the host.

Other organisms selectively destroy absorptive cells (e.g., villus tip cells) in the mucosa, disrupting their normal cell function and thereby causing diarrhea. Rotaviruses and Norwalk-like viruses are both visualized by electron microscopy within the absorptive cells at the ends of the intestinal villi, where they multiply and destroy cellular function. As a result, the villi become shortened, and inflammatory cells infiltrate the mucosa, further contributing to the pathologic condition. In addition to these viral agents, hepatitis A, B, and C and occasionally enteric adenoviruses have been associated with diarrheal symptoms in patients.

Miscellaneous Virulence Factors
Other virulence traits appear to be involved in the development of GI infections and include characteristics such as motility, chemotaxis, and mucinase production. Also, the possession of certain antigens, such as the Vi antigen of

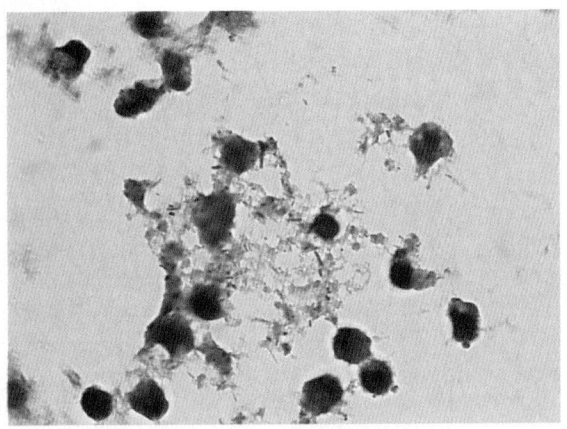

• **Fig. 74.6** Wright's stain of stool from a patient with shigellosis showing moderate numbers of polymorphonuclear cells.

S. enterica serotype Typhi and certain cell wall components, are also associated with virulence.

Clinical Manifestations

The clinical symptoms experienced by a patient are largely dependent on how the enteric pathogen causes disease. To illustrate, patients infected with an enteric pathogen that upsets fluid and electrolyte balance have no fecal leukocytes present in the stool and experience watery diarrhea; fever is usually absent or mild. Although nausea, vomiting, and abdominal pain may also be present, the dominant feature is intestinal fluid loss. In contrast, patients infected with an enteric pathogen that causes significant cell destruction and inflammation have fecal leukocytes present in the stool (Fig. 74.6). Their diarrhea is often characterized by the presence of mucus and blood; in many of these patients, fever is a prominent component of their disease, as are abdominal pain, cramps, and tenesmus. Finally, patients who become infected with a pathogen capable of penetrating the intestinal mucosa of the small intestine without producing enterocolitis and then subsequently spreading and multiplying at other sites will present with signs and symptoms of a systemic illness such as headache, sore throat, malaise, and fever; diarrhea in these patients is not a prominent feature and is absent or mild in many cases. Features of these three types of enteric infections are summarized in Table 74.3.

Epidemiology

GI infections occur in numerous epidemiologic settings. Awareness of these different settings is important because knowledge of an epidemiologic setting can help provide a basis for the diagnosis and clues to possible causes. When this knowledge is combined with clinical findings, the cause of the infection can often be narrowed to three or four organisms.

Institutional Settings

Diarrheal illness can be a major problem in institutional settings such as daycare centers, hospitals, and nursing homes. Because individual hygiene is often difficult to maintain in these settings, coupled with the presence of several organisms with relatively low infecting doses such as *Shigella* and *G. duodenalis,* numerous outbreaks of diarrheal illness caused by various organisms have been reported. Organisms such as *Shigella, C. jejuni* subsp. *jejuni, G. duodenalis, Cryptosporidium,* and rotaviruses have been reported to cause outbreaks in daycare centers. Of significance, these infections can be spread to family members. Similarly, outbreaks caused by these organisms, as well as hemorrhagic *E. coli* O157:H7, have been reported in nursing homes and other extended-care facilities.

Health care–associated (nosocomial) diarrheal illness is also a problem for patients and personnel in outpatient clinics, extended care facilities, and hospitals. Rotaviruses, adenoviruses, and coxsackie viruses have also been identified in health care–associated settings. In addition to these organisms, *C. difficile* is a major enteric pathogen that has been identified in outbreaks in hospitals and other settings, including nursing homes and extended-care facilities. This organism is a hardy pathogen that readily survives on **fomites** (inanimate objects) such as floors, bed rails, call buttons, and doorknobs and on the hands of hospital personnel caring for the patient. Of clinical concern is the emergence of a strain of *C. difficile* with increased virulence and fluoroquinolone resistance. By partial deletions in a toxin regulatory gene, *tad,* these isolates can produce 16- to 23-fold more toxin A and B. In addition, a separate binary toxin has been described that is encoded by *cdtA* and *cdtB* genes; *cdtB* mediates cell surface binding and cellular translocation, whereas *cdtA* disrupts the assembly of the actin filament, causing cell death. These strains have emerged as a cause of geographically dispersed outbreaks of *C. difficile*–associated disease. Many of the reported cases caused by these strains were in otherwise healthy patients with minimal or no exposure to a health care setting. *C. difficile* is the most common pathogen isolated in patients with antibiotic-associated diarrhea. However, **antibiotic-associated hemorrhagic colitis (AAHC)** is not linked to *C. difficile* infection (CDI). AAHC symptoms include a sudden onset of bloody diarrhea and abdominal cramps during antibiotic therapy. Toxin-producing *Klebsiella oxytoca* has been identified as a causative agent of AAHC.

Traveler's Diarrhea

Individuals who travel into developing geographic areas with poor sanitation are at particularly high risk for developing diarrhea. In areas with poor sanitation, enteric pathogens heavily contaminate the water and food. Although many types of enteric pathogens can cause diarrhea in travelers, ETEC is a leading cause in Asia, Africa, and Latin America, accounting for about 50% of cases. *Salmonella, Shigella, Campylobacter* spp., vibrios, rotavirus, and Norwalk virus can also cause diarrhea in travelers, depending on the area or country they visit.

Foodborne and Waterborne Outbreaks

The Centers for Disease Control and Prevention indicate that more than 48 million cases of foodborne illness are reported in the United States each year. Eating raw or undercooked fish, shellfish, or meats and drinking unpasteurized milk increases the risks of certain bacterial, parasitic, and viral infections. Many foodborne outbreaks can be traced to poor hygienic practices of food handlers such as not washing hands after using the toilet; hepatitis A, Norwalk virus, and *Salmonella* are a few examples of infectious agents and organisms that have contaminated food during preparation by a food handler and caused diarrheal disease. The number of cases of salmonellosis has gradually increased, with many of these infections associated with eating raw or undercooked eggs. Also, the potential for widespread dissemination of foodborne pathogens has increased because of factors such as the tendency to eat outside the home, the export and import of food sources worldwide, and travel.

In addition to foodborne outbreaks of GI tract infections, waterborne outbreaks of diarrheal disease caused by *G. duodenalis* and *Cryptosporidium* have been traced to inadequately filtered surface water. Recreational waters, including swimming pools, can also become contaminated with enteric pathogens such as *Shigella* and *G. duodenalis* because of poor toilet facilities or practices. Box 74.2 provides a listing of the more common GI syndromes, incubation period, and organisms associated with foodborne and waterborne illness.

Immunocompromised Hosts

GI tract infections in individuals infected with human immunodeficiency virus (HIV) and other patients who are immunosuppressed, such as organ transplant recipients or individuals receiving chemotherapy, are a diagnostic challenge for the clinician and microbiologist. For example, cytotoxic chemotherapy or antibiotic therapy may predispose patients to develop *C. difficile* colitis.

Diarrhea is a common clinical manifestation of infection with HIV. Numerous pathogens and opportunistic pathogens have been identified and are believed to cause recurrent or chronic diarrhea. Commonly reported etiologic agents include the following:

- Species of *Salmonella, Shigella,* and *Campylobacter*
- Cytomegalovirus
- *Cryptosporidium, Cystoisospora belli*
- Microsporidia
- *E. histolytica*
- *Mycobacterium* spp.
- *G. duodenalis*

Etiologic Agents

Many microorganisms can cause enteric infections. A discussion of each organism is beyond the scope of this chapter. Rather, these organisms are addressed in Parts III through VI of the textbook. Table 74.4 summarizes the general characteristics of the more common agents of enteric infections.

BOX 74.2 Foodborne and Waterborne Gastrointestinal Syndromes

General Symptoms	Incubation/ Occurrence	Etiology
Nausea and vomiting	1–8 hours	*Staphylococcus aureus*
		Bacillus cereus
Abdominal cramps and diarrhea	8–16 hours	*Clostridium perfringens*
		B. cereus
Fever, abdominal cramps, and diarrhea	6–48 hours	*Salmonella*
		Shigella
		Vibrio
		Campylobacter
		Escherichia coli (STEC)
		Yersinia enterocolitica
Abdominal cramps and watery diarrhea	16–72 hours	*Listeria monocytogenes*
		E. coli (ETEC)
		Vibrio
Vomiting and nonblood diarrhea	10–51 hours	Noroviruses
Fever, abdominal cramps, with or without diarrhea	1–11 days	*Y. enterocolitica*
Bloody diarrhea with low fever	3–8 days	STEC
Paralysis	18–36 hours	*Clostridium botulinum*[a]
Persistent diarrhea	1–3 weeks	Parasitic
		Cryptosporidium
		Giardia
		Cyclospora
Systemic illness		*Vibrio vulnificus*
		Vibrio spp.
		Toxoplasma gondii
		Trichinella spp.

[a]Approximately 50% of patients will present with nausea and vomiting, and 20% with diarrhea; others may demonstrate constipation.

Other Infections of the Gastrointestinal Tract

Besides causing disease in the small and large intestine, microorganisms can also infect other sites of the GI tract, as well as the GI tract's accessory organs.

TABLE 74.4 General Characteristics of Agents of Enteric Infections

Organism	Common Sources or Predisposing Condition	Distribution	Clinical Presentation	Predominant Pathogenic Mechanism	Fecal Leukocytes
Arcobacter spp.	Foodborne	Unknown	Watery diarrhea or chronic	Unknown	Unknown
Bacillus cereus	Meats, vegetables, rice	Worldwide	Intoxication: vomiting or watery diarrhea	Ingestion of preformed toxin (food poisoning)	−
Clostridium botulinum	Improperly preserved vegetables, meat, fish	Worldwide	Neuromuscular paralysis	Ingestion of preformed toxin (food poisoning)	−
Staphylococcus aureus	Meats, salads, dairy products	Worldwide	Intoxication: vomiting	Ingestion of preformed toxin (food poisoning)	−
Clostridium perfringens	Meats, poultry	Worldwide	Watery diarrhea	Ingestion of organism followed by toxin production	−
Aeromonas	Water	Worldwide	Watery diarrhea, dysentery, and chronic diarrhea	Heat-labile cytotoxic enterotoxin (*alt* gene) and/or heat-stable cytotoxic enterotoxin (*ast* gene)	−
Campylobacter spp.	Water, poultry, milk	Worldwide	Dysentery	Invasion	+
Clostridioides difficile	Antimicrobial therapy; immunosuppression, underlying gastrointestinal disease, health care–associated exposure	Worldwide	Dysentery	Enterotoxin and cytotoxin	+/−
Diarrheagenic *Escherichia coli*					
Enteropathogenic (EPEC)		Worldwide	Watery diarrhea	Adherence/invasion without multiplication	−
Enterotoxigenic (ETEC)	Food, water	Worldwide—more prevalent in developing countries	Watery diarrhea	Enterotoxin	−
Enteroinvasive (EIEC)	Food	Worldwide	Dysentery	Invasion, enterotoxin	+
Enterohemorrhagic (STEC)	Meats	Worldwide	Watery, often bloody diarrhea	Cytotoxin	−/+
Plesiomonas shigelloides	Fresh water, shellfish	Worldwide	Watery, invasive dysentery-like, and subacute/chronic	Enterotoxins: *in vitro* Demonstration of cholera-like toxin, thermostable and thermolabile toxins, beta-hemolysins and cytotoxins	+/−
Salmonella spp. (nontyphoidal)	Food, water	Worldwide	Dysentery	Invasion	+

TABLE 74.4 General Characteristics of Agents of Enteric Infections—cont'd

Organism	Common Sources or Predisposing Condition	Distribution	Clinical Presentation	Predominant Pathogenic Mechanism	Fecal Leukocytes
Salmonella enterica serovar Typhi	Food, water	Tropical, developing countries	Enteric fever	Penetration	+ (monocytes, not PMNs)
Shigella spp.	Food, water	Worldwide	Dysentery	Invasion	+
Shigella dysenteriae	Water	Tropical, developing countries	Dysentery	Invasion, cytotoxin	+
Vibrio cholerae	Water, shellfish	Asia, Africa, Middle East, South and North America (along coastal areas)	Watery diarrhea	Enterotoxin, cytotoxin	−/+
Yersinia enterocolitica	Milk, pork, water	Worldwide	Watery diarrhea, and/or enteric fever	Invasion, penetration	−
Giardia duodenalis	Food, water	Worldwide	Watery diarrhea	Unknown—impaired absorption	−
Cryptosporidium parvum	Animals, water	Worldwide	Watery diarrhea	Adherence	−
Entamoeba histolytica	Food, water	Worldwide (more common in developing countries)	Dysentery	Invasion, cytotoxin	−/+ (amoebae destroy the white cells)
Rotavirus	Person-to-person; viral shedding often occurs during subclinical presentation and after cessation of diarrhea	Worldwide	Watery diarrhea	Mucosal damage leading to impaired absorption in small intestine; can be life-threatening	−
Enteric adenoviruses	Day care settings and health care–associated settings (hospitals); immunocompromised patients, particularly hematopoietic stem cell transplant recipients	Worldwide	Sporadic cases; chronic watery or subclinical presentation	Unknown	−
Astroviruses	Unknown	Worldwide	Pediatric gastroenteritis or asymptomatic in all ages; watery diarrhea	Unknown	−
Noroviruses (Caliciviruses)	Shellfish, salads Immunohematology ABH secretors and Lewis histo-blood groups serve as viral receptors	Worldwide	Watery diarrhea	Mucosal damage leading to impaired absorption in small intestine	−

ABH, A, B, and H, blood group antigens; *PMN*, Polymorphonuclear cells.

Esophagitis

Infections of the mucosa of the esophagus (**esophagitis**) can cause painful or difficult swallowing or the sensation that something is lodged in the throat while swallowing. Individuals who have esophagitis usually have local or systemic underlying illnesses such as hematologic malignancies or HIV infection, or they are receiving immunosuppressive therapy. The most common etiologic agents are *Candida* spp. (primarily *C. albicans*), herpes simplex virus, and cytomegalovirus.

Diagnosis of esophagitis is primarily based on the appearance of *Candida* spp. on a smear collected by an endoscopic brushing or biopsy of the esophagus. The smears may be examined by Gram stain, calcofluor white, or silver stain. Samples may also be submitted for histologic examination or viral culture.

Gastritis

Gastritis refers to inflammation of the gastric mucosa. This illness is associated with nausea and upper abdominal pain; vomiting, burping, and fever may also be present. A curved organism called *Helicobacter pylori* is seen on the surface of gastric epithelial cells of patients with gastritis. The organism is recovered from gastric biopsy material obtained endoscopically but not from stool. After acute infection, *H. pylori* can persist for years in most individuals, with many remaining asymptomatic. *H. pylori* is also the causative agent of peptic ulcer disease and a significant risk factor for the development of stomach cancer.

Proctitis

Proctitis is the inflammation of the rectum (distal portion of the large intestine). Common symptoms associated with proctitis are itching and a mucous discharge from the rectum; if the infection progresses, ulcers and abscesses may form in the rectum. Most infections are sexually transmitted through anal intercourse. *Chlamydia trachomatis,* herpes simplex, *Treponema pallidum,* and *Neisseria gonorrhoeae* are the most common etiologic agents.

Miscellaneous

Unusual agents and those that have not been cultured, such as mycobacteria that may be associated with Crohn disease and the bacterium associated with Whipple disease, *Tropheryma whipplei,* are also candidates as etiologic agents of GI disease. *T. whipplei* forms intracellular clusters within vacuoles of phagocytic cells or as extracellular bacteria. The organism is widespread in the environment and is associated with a high rate of human colonization. The human immune response generally results in clearance of the organism unless there is an immune deficiency resulting in predisposition for disease. Whipple disease typically occurs years after initial infection with *T. whipplei,* resulting in chronic diarrhea and migratory arthralgia of the joints. Central nervous system damage may occur, resulting in poor prognosis and antibiotic treatment failure.

Occasionally, stool cultures from patients with diarrheal disease yield heavy growth of organisms such as enterococci, *Pseudomonas* spp., or *Klebsiella pneumoniae,* not usually found in such numbers as normal microbiota. Only anecdotal evidence suggests that these organisms contribute to the pathogenesis of the diarrhea. Agents of sexually transmitted disease may cause GI symptoms when they are introduced into the colon via sexual intercourse. *Mycobacterium intracellulare* may be sexually transmitted, resulting in systemic disease in patients with AIDS. The pathogenesis of infections resulting from *Blastocystis hominis* (a possible coccidian etiologic agent of human diarrheal disease) is not well documented, although these organisms are associated with GI symptoms. Epidemiologic studies indicate that the organism is likely the pathogen when present in high numbers in the presence of GI disease and the absence of other etiologic agents.

Laboratory Diagnosis of Gastrointestinal Tract Infections

Specimen Collection and Transport

If enteric pathogens are to be detected by the laboratory, adherence to appropriate guidelines for specimen collection and transport is imperative (see Table 5.1 for a quick guide to specimen collection, transport, and processing). Stool (feces) specimens and rectal swabs are often submitted for the identification of the pathogen associated with diarrhea or food poisoning. If an etiologic agent is not isolated with the first culture or visual examination, two additional specimens should be submitted to the laboratory over the next few days. Because organisms may be shed intermittently, collection of specimens at different times over several days enhances recovery. Certain infectious agents, such as *Giardia,* may be difficult to detect, requiring the processing of multiple specimens over weeks, duodenal aspirates (in the case of *Giardia*), or additional alternative methods.

General Comments

Stool specimens submitted for the identification of enteric pathogens and delivered to the laboratory within 30 minutes may be collected in a clean plastic container. The samples should not be contaminated with urine, barium, or toilet paper. Rectal swabs should be placed in transport medium such as Stuart's. Stool for direct wet-mount examination, *C. difficile* toxin assay, and ELISA or the latex agglutination test for rotavirus must be sent to the laboratory without any added preservatives or liquids. Volume of a liquid stool at least equal to 1 teaspoon (5 mL) or a pea-sized piece of formed stool is necessary for most procedures. Nucleic acid–based GI panels for the identification of enteric pathogens including viral agents should be collected as described by the manufacturer.

Stool Specimens for Bacterial Culture

If a delay longer than 2 hours is anticipated for stools for bacterial culture, the specimen should be placed in transport medium. The Cary-Blair transport medium preserves the viability of intestinal bacterial pathogens, including *Campylobacter* and *Vibrio* spp. However, the media produced by different manufacturers can vary. Most workers recommend reducing the agar content of Cary-Blair medium from 0.5% to 0.16% (modified) for maintenance of *Campylobacter* spp. Buffered glycerol transport medium does not maintain these bacteria. Additional transport media, such as alkaline peptone water, is preferred for the isolation of *V. cholerae.* Several manufacturers produce a small vial of Cary-Blair with a self-contained plastic scoop suitable for collecting samples.

Because *Shigella* spp. are sensitive to environmental factors, a transport medium of equal parts of glycerol and 0.033 M phosphate buffer (pH 7.0) increases the viability of *Shigella* compared with Cary-Blair. For this purpose, maintaining the glycerol transport medium at refrigerator or freezer temperatures also improves recovery.

If a patient did not enter the hospital with GI symptoms but develops diarrhea more than 3 days after admission, careful consideration of the potential etiologic agent being an enteric pathogen or virus other than *C. difficile* is unlikely. However, community-acquired CDI does occur after hospital discharge or another outpatient treatment. Therefore, outpatient samples submitted for culture or nucleic acid testing for *C. difficile* should not be rejected. However, if initial testing is negative, repeat testing is not warranted.

Stool Specimens for Ova and Parasites

For detection of ova and parasites, specimen preservation with a fixative is recommended for visual examination (Chapter 46).

Stool Specimens for Viruses

Stools for virus culture must be refrigerated if they are not inoculated into cell cultures within 2 hours. A rectal swab, transported in modified Stuart's transport medium or another viral transport medium, is adequate for recovery of most viruses from feces. See Chapter 64 for more information regarding the collection and transport of specimens for viral culture. Samples collected for use in nucleic acid–based testing should follow the manufacturer's recommended procedures.

Miscellaneous Specimen Types

Other specimens that may be obtained for diagnosis of GI tract infection include duodenal aspirates. These samples should be examined immediately using direct microscopy for the presence of motile protozoan trophozoites, cultured for bacteria, and placed into polyvinyl alcohol (PVA) fixative for subsequent parasitic examination. The laboratory should be informed in advance so that the specimen can be processed and examined efficiently.

The string test has proved useful for diagnosing duodenal parasites, such as *Giardia,* and for isolating *S. enterica* serotype Typhi from carriers and patients with acute typhoid fever. This test is still used in underdeveloped countries worldwide. The patient swallows a weighted gelatin capsule containing a tightly wound length of string, which is left protruding from the mouth and taped to the cheek. After

a predetermined period, during which the capsule reaches the duodenum and dissolves, the string, now covered with duodenal contents, is retracted and delivered immediately to the laboratory. The microbiologist strips the mucus and secretions attached to the string and deposits some material on slides for direct examination and some material into fixative for preparation of permanent stained mounts. The microbiologist also inoculates some material to appropriate media for isolation of bacteria.

Direct Detection of Agents of Gastroenteritis in Feces

Wet Mounts

A direct wet mount of fecal material, particularly with liquid or unformed stool, is the fastest method for detecting motile trophozoites of *Dientamoeba fragilis, Entamoeba, Giardia,* and other intestinal parasites. Occasionally the larvae or adult worms of other parasites may be visualized. Experienced observers can also see the refractile forms of *Cryptosporidium* and many types of cysts on the direct wet mount, including *Cyclospora cayetanensis,* a parasite that is associated with the consumption of contaminated food such as raspberries. If present in sufficient numbers, the ova of intestinal parasites can be seen.

Examination of a direct wet mount of fecal material containing blood or mucus, with the addition of an equal portion of Loeffler methylene blue, is helpful for detection of leukocytes, which occasionally aids in differentiating among the various types of diarrheal syndromes. Infectious inflammatory diarrhea caused by enteric pathogens will present as leukocyte-positive, whereas secretory diarrhea associated with toxin-producing organisms, viruses, and protozoans will present as leukocyte-negative. In addition, fecal leukocytes degrade rapidly and may make identification and quantification difficult. Another commercially available test detects lactoferrin, which is a glycoprotein released from neutrophil granules into the stool sample. This assay demonstrates improved sensitivity and specificity compared with detection of intact WBCs. A sample that appears lactoferrin-positive is considered positive for the presence of fecal leukocytes. Under phase-contrast and dark-field microscopy, the darting motility and curved forms of *Campylobacter* may be observed in a warm sample. Water or saline, which will immobilize *Campylobacter,* should not be used. However, for practical reasons most laboratories do not use a wet mount.

Stains

Feces may be Gram stained for detection of certain etiologic agents. For example, many thin, comma-shaped, gram-negative bacilli may indicate *Campylobacter* infection (if vibrios have been ruled out). In addition, polymorphonuclear cells may also be detected. An acid-fast stain can be used to detect *Cryptosporidium* spp., mycobacteria, and *Cystoisospora* spp. Examination of fixed fecal material for parasites by trichrome or other stains is covered in Chapter 46. A permanent stained preparation should be made from all stool specimens received for detection of parasites.

Antigen Detection

Enzyme immunoassays (EIAs) can detect numerous microorganisms capable of causing GI tract infections. For example, EIAs are commercially available to detect *E. coli* O157:H7 and *Campylobacter* spp., the presence of the Shiga toxins produced by STEC, or the presence of *C. difficile* toxins A or A and B. In addition, rotavirus is detected using a solid-phase EIA procedure. EIA methods are also available for detection of antigens of *Cryptosporidium* and *G. duodenalis* as well as *E. histolytica*. EIA methods have also been evaluated for detection of certain bacterial pathogens. Laboratory diagnosis of *C. difficile* uses EIA or latex agglutination kits coupled with glutamate dehydrogenase (GDH) and A/B toxin in a combination assay.

Nucleic Acid Testing

The development of amplification techniques has led to numerous publications for the direct detection of many enteric pathogens, including all major organism groups—bacteria, viruses, and parasites. Nucleic acid–based testing is available for a large variety of pathogens such as *C. difficile*, *Campylobacter* spp., staphylococci, and enterococci including antibiotic-resistant determinants and additional viral agents associated with GI disease. It is important to note that some studies indicate that concordance between phenotypic and molecular diagnostic panels vary. The accuracy for the detection of *Salmonella* spp. in nucleic acid testing methods has been shown to not be as effective as traditional methods. In addition, failure to maintain cultures of GI isolates that have been identified using nucleic acid–based methods presents a new challenge. The organism itself is not available for susceptibility testing if required, which is very important for certain bacterial pathogens (e.g., *Shigella*) for which susceptibility patterns vary. This is reducing the amount of epidemiological data available to monitor trends and patterns in antibiotic sensitivity patterns in GI pathogens. The implementation of whole genome sequencing for molecular epidemiology in diagnostic laboratories will improve the gaps that have been created by using culture independent methods for the diagnosis of GI infections.

Culture of Fecal Material for Isolation of Etiologic Agents

Bacteria

Fecal specimens for culture should be inoculated to several media for maximal yield, including solid agar and broth. The choice of media is based on the requirements of the clinician, the geographic region, the patient population, known endemic infectious agents, and the laboratory. Recommendations for a standardized selection of media are included in this section; however, each laboratory should consider the factors previously listed to determine the most efficient isolation and diagnostic methods offered in the facility.

Organisms for Routine Culture

Stool received for routine culture in most clinical laboratories in the United States should be examined for the presence of *Campylobacter*, *Salmonella*, and *Shigella* spp. under all circumstances. Detection of *Aeromonas* and *Plesiomonas* spp. should be incorporated into routine stool culture procedures. The cost of doing a stool examination on every patient for all potential enteric pathogens is prohibitive. The decision as to what other bacteria are routinely cultured should consider the incidence of GI tract infections caused by etiologic agents in the area served by the laboratory. For example, if the incidence of *Y. enterocolitica* gastroenteritis is high enough in the area served by the laboratory, then this agent should also be sought routinely. Similarly, because of the increasing prevalence of disease caused by *Vibrio* spp. in individuals living in high-risk areas of the United States (sea coast), laboratories in these localities may routinely look for these organisms. Conversely, unless a patient has a significant travel history, a laboratory located in the Midwestern United States should not routinely look for these organisms except by special request. Protocols for culture of enterohemorrhagic *E. coli* (e.g., *E. coli* O157:H7) vary greatly; based on incidence of disease, laboratories routinely use non–culture-based methods for this organism when cases of severe diarrhea are implicated. Selective or screening media to detect *E. coli* O157:H7 also vary greatly, including using a 1% sorbitol-containing medium (most O157:H7 *E. coli* are sorbitol-negative), a specific trypticase blood agar (Unipath GmbH, Wesel, Germany), Ramba CHROM (Gibson Laboratories, LLC, Lexington, KY), CHROMagar (BD Diagnostics, Franklin Lakes, NJ), or Rainbow Agar O157 (Bio-log, Inc., Hayward, CA).

Routine Culture Methods

An in-depth discussion regarding culture of all enteric pathogens is beyond the scope of this chapter. Because U.S. laboratories are routinely using non–culture-based methods for the identification of enteric bacterial pathogens, laboratories should consider performing reflux cultures on enteric pathogens for further characterization, changing trends in diagnostic practices, and surveillance studies. As culture independent methods evolve, including whole genome sequencing availability, diagnostic practices will continue to evolve, and the need for culturing these organisms may not be necessary. Laboratories should routinely examine stools for the presence of *Salmonella*, *Shigella*, and *Campylobacter* spp., therefore, culture of these organisms is addressed. Culture conditions for all other pathogens, including viruses, are covered in Parts III, IV, and VI. Specimens received for detection of the most commonly isolated Enterobacterales and *Salmonella* and *Shigella* spp. should be plated to a supportive medium, a slightly selective and differential medium, and a moderately selective medium.

Blood agar (tryptic soy agar with 5% sheep blood) is an excellent general supportive medium. Blood agar medium allows growth of yeast species, staphylococci, and enterococci, in addition to gram-negative bacilli. The absence of normal gram-negative fecal microbiota or the presence of significant quantities of organisms such as *S. aureus*, yeasts, and *Pseudomonas aeruginosa* can be evaluated. The use of blood agar also provides colonies for oxidase testing. Several colonies that do not resemble *Pseudomonas* spp. from the third or fourth quadrant should be routinely screened for production of cytochrome oxidase. If numerous colonies are present, *Aeromonas, Vibrio,* or *Plesiomonas* spp. should be suspected.

The slightly selective agar should support growth of most Enterobacterales, vibrios, and other possible pathogens; MacConkey agar works well. Some laboratories use eosin-methylene blue (EMB), which demonstrates a slight increase in inhibition of contaminating microorganisms. All lactose-negative colonies should be tested further, ensuring adequate detection of vibrios and pathogenic Enterobacterales. Lactose-positive vibrios (*V. vulnificus*), pathogenic *Escherichia* spp. (particularly *E. coli*), some *Aeromonas* spp., and *Plesiomonas* spp. may not be distinctive on MacConkey agar.

***Salmonella* and *Shigella*.** Maximum recovery of *Salmonella* and *Shigella* is obtained when inoculating an enrichment broth in addition to primary direct plating of specimens. The selective enrichment using selenite broth is commonly used for both organisms. Gram-negative broth may also be used in some laboratories as an enrichment media for the isolation of *Shigella* spp. Selenite-F broth can be used for the isolation and enrichment of *Salmonella* spp. Selenite broth base with mannitol is used for *S. enterica* serotype Typhi and *S. enterica* serotype Paratyphi. The specimen should also be inoculated to a moderately selective agar such as Hektoen enteric (HE), xylose-lysine deoxycholate (XLD) media, or CHROMagar *Salmonella*. HE and XLD are used in many laboratories because both *Salmonella* and *Shigella* can be isolated using these agars. Cultures suspected of isolation for *S. enterica* serotype Typhi should include a highly selective medium such as brilliant green agar or bismuth sulfite agar. These media inhibit growth of most Enterobacterales, allowing *Salmonella* and *Shigella* spp. to be detected. Colony morphologies of lactose-negative, lactose-positive, and H$_2$S-producing organisms are illustrated in Fig. 74.7. All these media are incubated at 35°C to 37°C in ambient air and examined at 24 and 48 hours for suspicious colonies.

***Campylobacter*.** Cultures for isolation of *C. jejuni* and *Campylobacter coli* should be inoculated to a combination of at least two selective agars containing antimicrobial agents that suppress the growth of normal microbiota. The introduction of a blood-free, charcoal-containing medium containing selective antibiotic components has improved recovery of most enteropathogenic *Campylobacter* spp. There are two primary formulations commercially available: charcoal cefoperazone deoxycholate agar (CCDA) and charcoal-based selective medium (CSm). Blood-containing medium, Skirrow medium, and Campy-CVA (cefoperazone, vancomycin, amphotericin) are also available. *Brucella* broth base has yielded less satisfactory recovery of *Campylobacter* spp. Blood-free formulations are reported to have better performance for the isolation of *Campylobacter* spp. from stool specimens. Commercially produced agar plates for isolation of campylobacters are available from several manufacturers. These plates are incubated in a microaerophilic atmosphere at 42°C and examined at 24 and 48 hours for suspicious colonies. Culture methods for other campylobacters associated with GI disease, such as *C. hyointestinalis* subsp. *hyointestinalis* and *C. fetus* subsp. *fetus,* are provided in Chapter 33.

Enrichment Broths. As previously indicated, enrichment broths are sometimes used for enhanced recovery of *Salmonella, Shigella, Campylobacter,* and *Y. enterocolitica,* although *Shigella* usually does not survive enrichment. Gram-negative broth (Hajna GN) or selenite F broth yields good recovery for most routine cultures. Enrichment broths for Enterobacterales should be incubated in air at 35°C for 6 to 8 hours, and then several drops should be subcultured to at least two selective media. Stool specimens would be inoculated to broth initially along with plating to primary culture media; those broths that test negative (demonstrate no growth) could be discarded without subculturing. Campy-thioglycollate enrichment broth increases the yields of positive cultures for *Campylobacter* spp., although it is not necessary for routine use. Enrichment broth for *Campylobacter* is refrigerated overnight or for a minimum of 8 hours before a few drops are plated to *Campylobacter* agar and incubated at 42°C in a microaerophilic atmosphere.

Laboratory Diagnosis of *Clostridioides difficile*–Associated Diarrhea

The definitive diagnosis of *C. difficile*–associated diarrhea is based on clinical criteria combined with laboratory testing. Visualization of a characteristic pseudomembrane or plaque on colonoscopy is diagnostic for PMC and, with the appropriate history of prior antibiotic use, meets the criteria for diagnosis of antibiotic-associated PMC. Additional patient risk factors should also be considered for potential diagnosis for CDI, such as advanced age (>65 years), immunosuppression or other severe underlying GI disease, use of proton pump inhibitors, and exposure to a health care setting. No single laboratory test will establish the diagnosis unequivocally. Two major types of tests are available for routine use: culture for direct detection of the organism and detection of cytotoxin (toxin A, B, or both) by cell culture cytotoxicity neutralization or EIA. In addition, most laboratories are using nucleic acid–based testing methods. Some of the commercially available nucleic acid–based assays include BD Gene Ohm (BD Diagnostics, La Jolla, CA), Cepheid Xpert (Cepheid, Sunnyvale, CA), FilmArray (Bio-Fire Diagnostics Inc., Salt Lake City, UT), Roche LightCycler (Roche Applied Science), and ProGastro (Hologic, San Diego, CA). Nucleic acid–based testing demonstrates high sensitivity and specificity for the diagnosis of *C. difficile*–associated diarrhea. Diagnosis of a CDI should include a method to identify the organism and a method to assess the toxin status including immunoassay for either toxin A or B, cell culture cytotoxicity, or a nucleic acid method for the detection of toxin B. This prevents an incorrect diagnosis of clinical disease and administration of unnecessary medications or antibiotics in a patient colonized with a nontoxigenic strain.

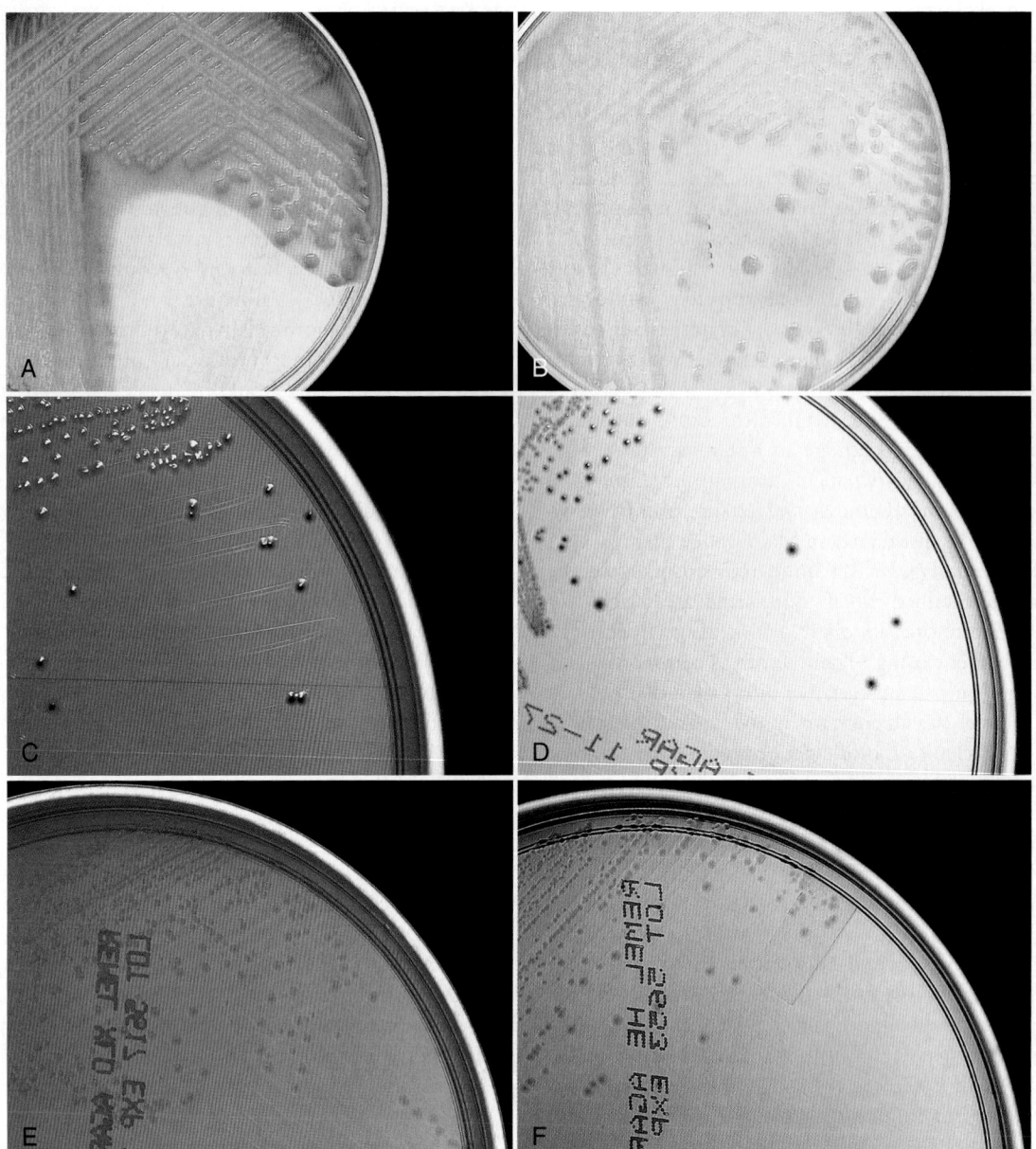

• **Fig. 74.7** Colonies of a lactose-positive organism growing on xylose-lysine deoxycholate (XLD) agar (A) and Hektoen enteric (HE) agar (B). Colonies of *Salmonella enteritidis* (lactose-negative) growing on XLD (C) and HE agar (D). (Note how both agars detect H_2S production.) Colonies of *Shigella* (lactose-negative) growing on XLD (E) and HE agar (F).

(e) Visit the Evolve site for a complete list of procedures, review questions, and case studies.

Bibliography

Bennett J, Dolin R, Blaser M: *Principles and practice of infectious diseases*, ed 9, Philadelphia, PA, 2020, Elsevier-Saunders.

Buvens G, Pierard D: Low prevalence of STEC autotransporter contributing to biofilm formation (Sab) in verocytotoxin-producing *E. coli* isolates of humans and raw meats, *Eur J Clin Microbiol Infect Dis* 31:1463–1465, 2012.

Carroll KC, Pfaller MA, Landry ML, et al.: *Manual of clinical microbiology*, ed 12, Washington, DC, 2019, ASM.

Gavin PJ, Thomson RB: Diagnosis of enterohemorrhagic *Escherichia coli* infection by detection of Shiga toxins, *Clin Microbiol Newsl* 26:49, 2004.

Goldenberg SD, Cliff PR, French GL: Glutamate dehydrogenase for laboratory diagnosis of *Clostridium difficile* infection, *J Clin Microbiol* 48:3050–3051, 2010.

Herwaldt BL, Beach MJ: The return of *Cyclospora* in 1997: another outbreak of cyclosporiasis in North America associated with imported raspberries, *Ann Intern Med* 130:210–220, 1999.

Kaye SA, Obrig TG: Pathogenesis *of E. coli* hemolytic-uremic syndrome, *Clin Microbiol Newsl* 18:49, 1996.

Kehl SC: Role of the laboratory in the diagnosis of entero-hemorrhagic *Escherichia coli* infections, *J Clin Microbiol* 40:2711–2715, 2002.

Kellner T, Parsons B, Chui L, et al.: Comparative evaluation of enteric bacterial culture and a molecular multiplex syndromic panel in children with acute gastroenteritis, *J Clin Microbiol* 57(6):e00205–e00219, 2019. https://doi.org/10.1128/JCM.00205-19.

Loo VG, Poirier L, Miller MA, et al.: A predominantly clonal multi-institutional outbreak of *Clostridium difficile*-associated diarrhea with high morbidity and mortality, *N Engl J Med* 353:2442–2449, 2005.

MacKenzie AM, Orrbine E, Hyde L, et al.: Performance of the ImmunoCard STAT! *E. coli* O157:H7 test for detection of *Escherichia coli* O157:H7 in stools, *J Clin Microbiol* 38:1866–1868, 2000.

Marder EP, Cieslak PR, Cronquist AB, et al.: Incidence and trends of infections with pathogens transmitted commonly through food and the effect of increasing use of culture-independent diagnostic tests on surveillance-foodborne diseases active surveillance network, 10 U.S. Sites, 2013-2016, *MMWR Morb Mortal Wkly Rep* 66(15):397–403, 2017.

McDonald LC, Killgore GE, Thompson A, et al.: An epidemic, toxin gene-variant of *Clostridium difficile*, *N Engl J Med* 353:2433–2441, 2005.

Novicki TJ, Daly JA, Mottice SL, et al.: Comparison of sorbitol MacConkey agar and a two-step method which utilizes enzyme-linked immunosorbent assay toxin testing and a chromogenic agar to detect and isolate enterohemorrhagic *Escherichia coli*, *J Clin Microbiol* 38:547–551, 2000.

O'Horo JC, Jones A, Sternke M, et al.: Molecular techniques for diagnosis of *Clostridium difficile* infection: systematic review and meta-analysis, *Mayo Clin Proc* 87:643–651, 2012.

Redondo N, Carroll A, McNamara E: Molecular characterization of *Campylobacter* causing human clinical infection using whole-genome sequencing: virulence, antimicrobial resistance and phylogeny in Ireland, *PloS One* 14(7):e0219088, 2019. https://doi.org/10.1371/journal.pone.0219088.

Sansonetti PJ: Genetic and molecular basis of epithelial cell invasion by *Shigella* species, *Rev Infect Dis* 13(Suppl 4):S285–S292, 1991.

Schmidt H, Hensel M: Pathogenicity islands in bacterial pathogenesis, *Clin Microbiol Rev* 17:14–56, 2004.

Voth DE, Ballard JD: *Clostridium difficile* toxins: mechanisms of action and role in disease, *Clin Microbiol Rev* 18:247–263, 2005.

Vuik F, Dicksved J, Lam SY, et al.: Composition of the mucosa-associated microbiota along the entire gastrointestinal tract of human individuals, *United European Gastroenterol J* 7(7):897–907, 2019.

Wilkins TD, Bartlett JG: *Clostridium difficile* testing: after 20 years, still challenging, *J Clin Microbiol* 41:531–534, 2003.

Zollner-Schwetz I, Hogenauer C, Joainig M, et al.: Role of *Klebsiella oxytoca* in antibiotic-associated diarrhea, *Clin Infect Dis* 47:e74–e78, 2008.

75

Skin, Soft Tissue, and Wound Infections

General Considerations

The skin serves as a barrier between the internal organs and the external environment. Skin is subjected to frequent trauma and therefore is at risk of infection. In addition, manifestations visible on the surface of the skin can provide clues for the identification of an internal systemic disease.

Anatomy of the Skin

The skin is divided into two distinct layers: the **epidermis** (the outermost layer), and the **dermis.** The subcutaneous tissue beneath the dermis connects the skin to underlying structures (Fig. 75.1). The epidermis is made up of stratified squamous epithelium. **Hair follicles, sebaceous glands** (oil-producing), and **sweat glands** open to the skin surface through the epidermis. The dermis is composed of dense connective tissue rich in blood and nerve endings, and some hair follicles and sebaceous glands originate here. The **subcutaneous tissue** contains loose connective tissue and is rich in fat. Deeper hair follicles and sweat glands originate in this layer. Below the subcutaneous layer are thin **fascial membranes** (sheets or bands of fibrous tissue) covering muscles, ligaments, and other connective tissue.

Function of the Skin

The skin is the body's largest and thinnest organ. It forms a self-repairing and protective boundary between the body's internal environment and the external environment. Skin plays a crucial role in the control of body temperature, excretion of water and salts, synthesis of important chemicals and hormones, and as a sensory organ. The skin has an important protective function because of the composition of the outermost layer of the epidermis, which is composed of cells containing **keratin,** a water-repellent protein. The skin's normal microbiota, pH, and chemical defenses (high salt and acidic environment) also help prevent colonization by many pathogens. Examples of resident microbiota are listed in Box 75.1, although variation can occur among people.

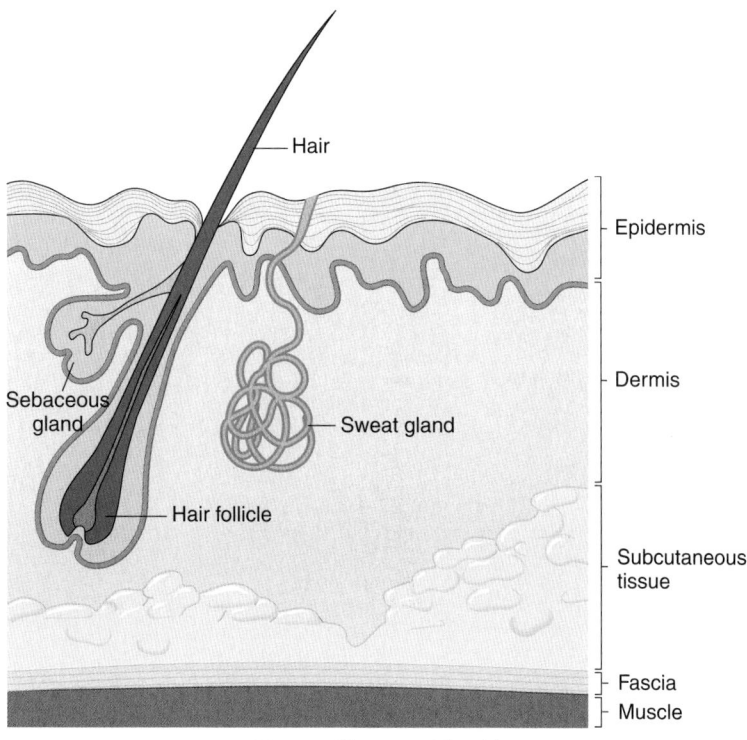

• **Fig. 75.1** Diagram of the skin.

Diphtheroids
Staphylococcus epidermidis
Other coagulase-negative staphylococci
Cutibacterium acnes

Prevalence, Etiology, and Pathogenesis

Approximately 15% of all patients who seek medical attention have either some skin disease or a skin lesion, many of which are infectious. Various bacteria, fungi, parasites, and viruses may be involved. These infections can include one or several causative agents. Because of the diversity of etiologic agents and the potential complexity of these infections, only the most common infections involving the skin and subcutaneous tissues will be addressed.

Skin infections can arise from the invasion of certain organisms from the external environment through breaks in the skin or from organisms that reach the skin through the blood as part of a systemic disease. In some infections, such as staphylococcal scalded-skin syndrome, toxins produced by the bacteria cause skin lesions. In others, lesions are a result of the host's immune response to microbial antigens.

Because of the diversity of etiologic agents, clinicians will often rely on the appearance of skin lesions for diagnostic clues to determine the required laboratory testing. The physical characteristics of the lesions can indicate the need for smear, culture, biopsy, or surgical procedures. Some of the terms most commonly used to describe manifestations of skin infections are provided in Table 75.1. Fig. 75.2 shows examples of some skin lesions.

Skin and Soft Tissue Infections

Infections of the Epidermis and Dermis

Numerous infections of the skin may occur. Several of the most common are discussed here.

Infections in or Around Hair Follicles

Folliculitis, furuncles, and **carbuncles** are localized abscesses either in or around hair follicles. These infections are distinguished from one another based on size and the extent of involvement in subcutaneous tissues. Table 75.2 summarizes each infection's respective clinical features. For the most part, these infections are precipitated by blockage of the hair follicle with skin oils (**sebum**) or because of minor trauma resulting from friction, such as that caused by clothes rubbing against the skin. *Staphylococcus aureus* is the most common etiologic agent for all three infections. Members of the Enterobacterales, *Malassezia furfur*, and *Candida* spp. may also cause folliculitis. Outbreaks of folliculitis caused by *Pseudomonas aeruginosa* have been reported to be associated with the use of whirlpools, swimming pools, and hot tubs.

Infections in the Keratinized Layer of the Epidermis

Because of their ability to utilize the keratin in the epidermal cells, the dermatophyte fungi are significant and well-suited pathogens for infection. Unlike the previously discussed infections, dermatophytes do not invade the deeper layers of

TABLE
75.1   **Manifestations of Skin Infections**

Term	Description	Possible Etiologic Agents (Infections)
Macule	A circumscribed (limited), flat discoloration of the skin	Dermatophytes *Treponema pallidum* (secondary syphilis) Viruses, such as enteroviruses (exanthems rashes)
Papule	An elevated, solid lesion ≤5 mm in diameter	Human papillomavirus types 3 and 10 (flat warts) Pox virus (molluscum contagiosum) *Sarcoptes scabiei* (scabies) *Staphylococcus aureus, Pseudomonas aeruginosa*, etc. (folliculitis)
Nodule	A raised, solid lesion >5 mm in diameter	*Corynebacterium diphtheriae* *Sporothrix schenckii* Miscellaneous fungi (subcutaneous mycoses) *Mycobacterium marinum* *Nocardia* spp. *S. aureus* (furuncle)
Pustule	A circumscribed, raised, pus-filled (leukocytes and fluid) lesion	*Candida* spp. Dermatophytes Herpes simplex virus *Neisseria gonorrhoeae* (gonorrhea) *S. aureus* (folliculitis) *S. aureus* or group A streptococci (impetigo) Varicella-zoster virus (chickenpox)
Vesicle	A circumscribed, raised, fluid-filled (blisterlike) lesion ≤5 mm in diameter	Herpes simplex virus Varicella-zoster virus (chickenpox and shingles)
Bulla	A circumscribed, raised, fluid-filled lesion >5 mm in diameter	Clostridial species (necrotizing gas gangrene) Herpes simplex virus Other gram-negative bacilli *S. aureus* (bullous impetigo and scalded-skin syndrome) *Vibrio vulnificus* and other *Vibrio* spp.
Scales	Dry, horny, platelike lesions	Dermatophytes (tinea)
Ulcer	A lesion with loss of epidermis and dermis	*Bacillus anthracis* (cutaneous anthrax) Bowel microbiota (decubiti) *Haemophilus ducreyi* (chancroid) *T. pallidum* (chancre of primary syphilis)

Adapted from Lazar AJF. *Robbins Basic Pathology.* 8th ed. St Louis: Saunders; 2007.

skin. Because keratin is also present in hair and nails, these fungi may also cause superficial infections at these sites (see Chapter 60 for more information).

Infections in the Deeper Layers of the Epidermis and Dermis

Most infections in the deeper layers of the epidermis and dermis result from the inoculation of microorganisms by traumatic breaks in the skin. These superficial skin infections usually do not require surgical intervention. Table 75.3 summarizes these infections. In most instances, these infections resolve with local care and only occasionally require antimicrobial therapy.

Cutaneous ulcers usually involve a loss of epidermal and part of the dermal tissues. In contrast, **nodules** are inflammatory foci in which the epidermal and dermal layers remain largely intact. Various bacteria and fungi can cause ulcerative or nodular skin lesions after direct traumatic inoculation. Examples of these causative agents include *Bacillus anthracis, Corynebacterium diphtheriae, Mycobacterium marinum, Nocardia* spp., and *Sporothrix schenckii.*

Infections of the Subcutaneous Tissues

Infections of the subcutaneous tissues may manifest as **abscesses, ulcers,** or **boils.** The most common etiologic agent of subcutaneous abscesses in healthy individuals is *S. aureus.* Many subcutaneous abscesses are polymicrobial. To a large degree, the organisms isolated from these abscesses depend on the site of infection. For example, anaerobes are commonly isolated from abscesses of the perineal, inguinal, and buttock area, whereas nonperineal infection is commonly caused by a polymicrobial infection containing facultative organisms.

Progressive synergistic gangrene, or **Meleney ulcer,** is a slowly progressive infection of the subcutaneous tissue that usually begins as an ulcer after trauma or surgery. The infection leads to subcutaneous necrosis and enlargement of a

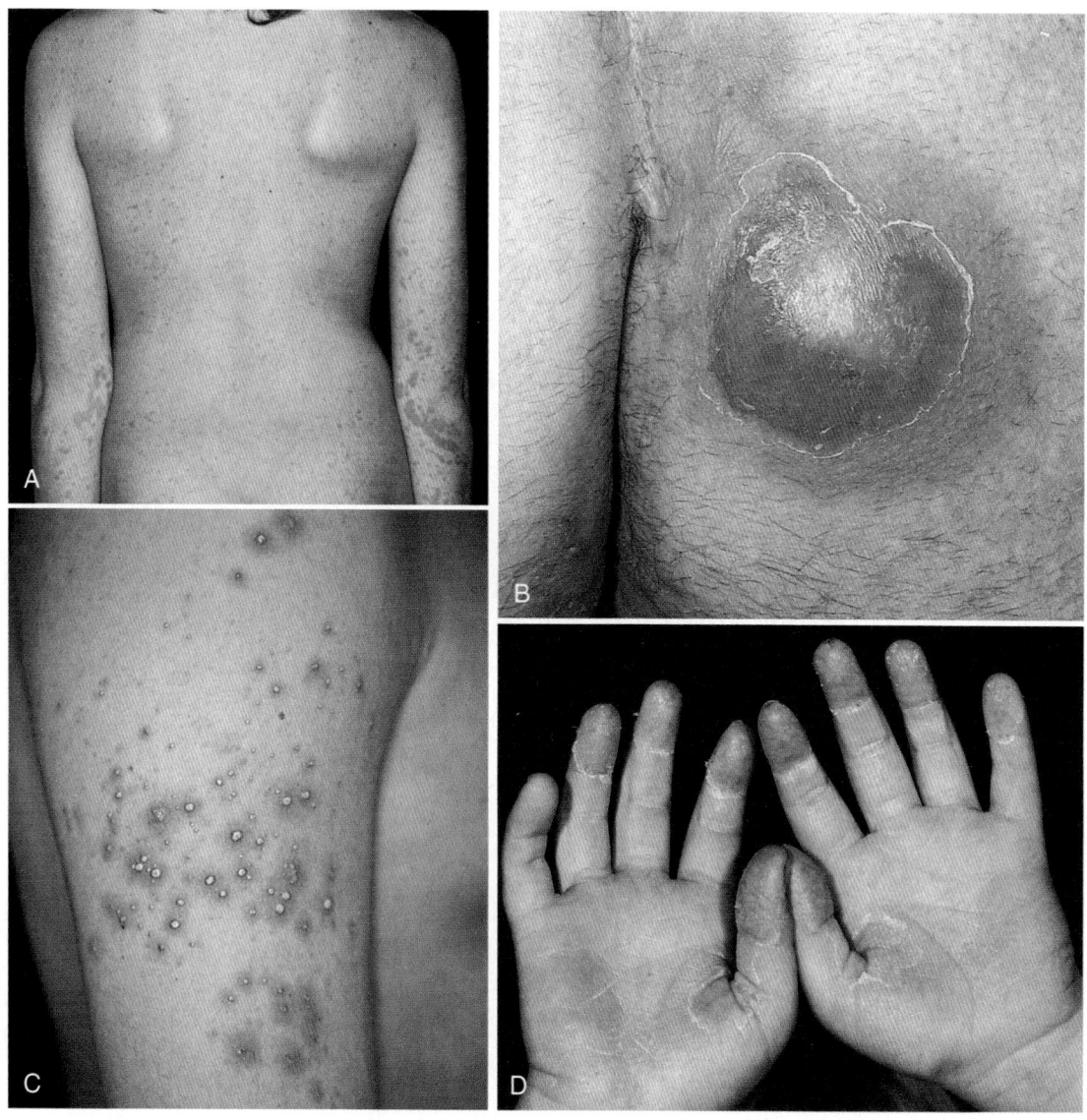

• **Fig. 75.2** (A) Viral maculopapular rash. (B) Furuncle. (C) Folliculitis caused by *Staphylococcus aureus* showing numerous pustules. (D) Desquamation (shedding or scaling) of the skin resulting from scarlet fever caused by group A streptococci. (A and D, From Habif TB. *Clinical Dermatology: A Color Guide to Diagnosis and Therapy.* 3rd ed. St Louis: Mosby; 1996.)

TABLE 75.2	Infections Involving Hair Follicles
Infection	**Skin Manifestations**
Folliculitis (minor infection of hair follicles)	Papules or pustules that are pierced by a hair and surrounded with redness
Furuncle (boil)	Abscess that begins as a red nodule in a hair follicle that ultimately becomes painful and full of pus
Carbuncle	Furuncles that coalesce and spread more deeply to the dermis and subcutaneous tissues; they usually have multiple sites, which drain to the skin surface (sinuses)

visible ulcer. This is a true polymicrobial infection in which microaerophilic streptococci grow synergistically with *S. aureus.* The infection may also include other facultative or anaerobic organisms.

In many instances, infections of the epidermis and dermis extend deeper and become subcutaneous infections and may even reach the fascia or muscle. For example, **erysipelas** (Fig. 75.3) can develop into subcutaneous **cellulitis** and eventually **necrotizing fasciitis.** Similarly, folliculitis can readily develop into a subcutaneous abscess or carbuncle that can extend to the fascia. Cellulitis can also extend to the subcutaneous tissues (Fig. 75.4). Anaerobic cellulitis is associated with the production of large amounts of gas by organisms that may be present in the subcutaneous tissue. This type of infection is most often located in the extremities and is particularly common among patients with

TABLE 75.3 Infections of the Epidermal and Dermal Layers of the Skin

Infection	Key Features of Infection	Etiologies	Other Comments
Erysipelas	Primarily involves the dermis and most superficial parts of the subcutaneous tissue; lesions are painful, red, swollen, and indurated; patients are febrile, and regional lymphadenopathy (swollen glands) is often present; lesion has a marked, well-demarcated, raised border (Fig. 75.3)	Group A streptococci (*Streptococcus pyogenes* [sometimes groups B, C, or G streptococci])	Infants, children, and elderly individuals are most affected; primarily a clinical diagnosis
Erythrasma	Chronic infection of the keratinized layer of the epidermis; lesions are dry, scaly, itchy, and reddish brown	*Corynebacterium minutissimum*—possible cause	Common in diabetics; resembles dermatophyte infection
Erysipeloid	Purplish-red, nonvesiculated skin lesion with an irregular, raised border; the lesions itch and burn; fever and other systemic symptoms are uncommon	*Erysipelothrix rhusiopathiae*	Uncommon; considered an occupational disease
Impetigo	Erythematous (red) lesions that may be bullous (less common) or nonbullous	Nonbullous—group A streptococci (*S. pyogenes*) Bullous—*Staphylococcus aureus*	
Cellulitis	Diffuse, spreading infection involving the deeper layers of the dermis; lesions are ill-defined, flat, painful, red, and swollen; patients have fever, chills, and regional lymphadenopathy (Fig. 75.4)	Commonly: Group A streptococci and other streptococci, *S. aureus* Less common: *Aeromonas* spp., *Vibrio* spp., and *Haemophilus influenzae* (typically affects young children)	Primarily a clinical diagnosis
Dermatophytoses	Superficial fungal infections of the skin and its appendages (i.e., ringworm, athlete's foot, jock itch, and infections of nails and hair)	*Epidermophyton, Microsporum,* and *Trichophyton* spp.	
Hidradenitis	Chronic infection of obstructed apocrine (sweat) glands in the axillar, genital, or perianal areas with intermittent discharge of often foul-smelling pus	*S. aureus, Streptococcus anginosus* group, anaerobic streptococci, and *Bacteroides* spp.	
Infected pilonidal tuft cyst or hairs	Pain and swelling; redness	Anaerobes, including *Bacteroides fragilis* group, *Prevotella, Fusobacterium,* anaerobic gram-positive cocci, and *Clostridium* spp.	

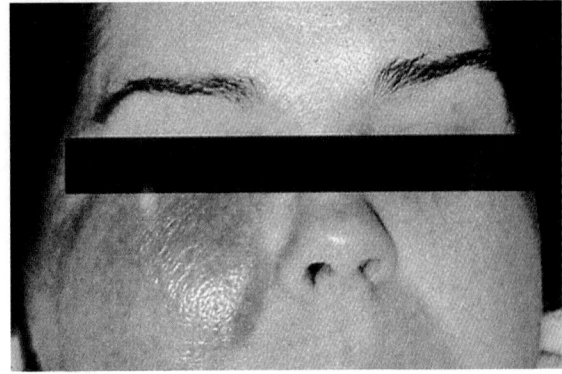

• **Fig. 75.3** Erysipelas caused by group A streptococci.

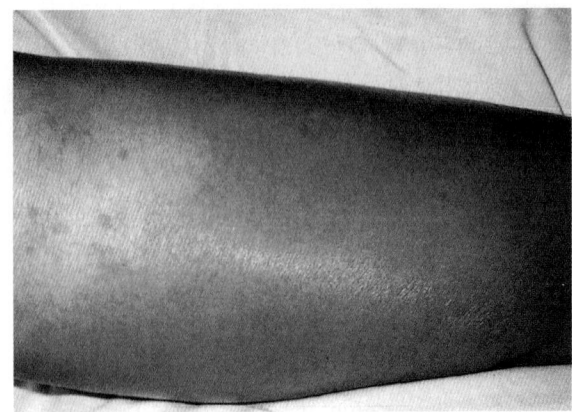

• **Fig. 75.4** Cellulitis. (From Farrar WE, Wood MJ, Innes JA, et al. *Infectious Diseases: Text and Color Atlas.* 2nd ed. London: Mosby-Wolfe; 1992.)

diabetes. The infection may involve the neck, abdominal wall, perineum, connective tissue, or other areas. Anaerobic cellulitis may also occur as a postoperative condition. The onset and spread of the lesion are usually slow, and patients may not immediately show obvious systemic effects. The causative agents in deep tissue infections are almost always a mixture of aerobic, facultative, and anaerobic organisms. Common aerobic, facultative organisms include *Escherichia coli,* alpha-hemolytic and nonhemolytic streptococci, and *S. aureus.* However, group A streptococci and other members of the Enterobacterales may be encountered as well. The anaerobes are typically found in greater numbers and in more varieties and include *Peptostreptococcus* spp., *Bacillus fragilis* group strains, *Prevotella* spp., *Porphyromonas* spp., other anaerobic gram-negative bacilli, and clostridia. Bacteremia is not usually present.

Infections of the Muscle Fascia and Muscles

There are several uncommon, yet serious or potentially serious, forms of deep and often extensive soft tissue and skin infections.

Necrotizing Fasciitis

Necrotizing fasciitis is a serious infection that is relatively uncommon. The basic pathology involves infection of the fascia overlying the muscles, often with involvement of the overlying soft tissue. At the fascial level, no barrier exists to prevent the spread of infection, so fasciitis may extend widely and rapidly to involve large areas of the body in a short amount of time. There are three distinct types of necrotizing fasciitis based on the bacteriological agents involved in the infection. Type I is polymicrobial and typically involves *Bacteroides* or *Peptostreptococcus* in combination with one or more facultative organism, such as group A streptococci or Enterobacterales. Type II is generally a monomicrobic infection with group A streptococci but may be associated with another species, often *S. aureus.* Type III is a result of infection with marine gram-negative pathogens, such as *Aeromonas hydrophilia* or *Vibrio* spp. Necrotizing fasciitis is most often acute and can affect any area of the body.

Progressive Bacterial Synergistic Gangrene

Progressive bacterial synergistic gangrene is usually a chronic necrotic condition of the skin most often encountered as a postoperative complication, particularly after abdominal or thoracic surgery or other medical procedures and devices, such as a colostomy (opening that connects the colon to the abdominal wall). The lesions may be extensive and, with involvement of the abdominal wall, may lead to **evisceration** (extrusion of the internal organs). As the name implies, this is a synergistic polymicrobial infection with microaerophilic streptococci and *S. aureus.* Other organisms may also be present, including anaerobic streptococci, *Proteus* spp., other gram-negative bacilli, or other facultative and anaerobic bacteria. This type of infection is uncommon. Cultures should be taken from the advancing outer edge

of the lesion (not the central portion of the wound). This prevents missing cultivation of microaerophilic streptococci that may be involved in the infection.

Myositis

Myositis (inflammation of muscle) can be caused by a variety of organisms. The nature of the pathologic process is variable, sometimes involving extensive necrosis of muscle or focal collections of suppuration (pus) in muscle (**pyomyositis**). This may occur because of a penetrating wound, vascular insufficiency in an extremity, or another contiguous infection. The most common cause of acute bacterial myositis from hematogenous spread is *S. aureus.* Categories of bacterial myositis include pyomyositis, psoas abscess (pus in the iliopsoas muscle compartment), *S. aureus* myositis, group A streptococcal necrotizing myositis, group B streptococcal myositis, clostridial gas gangrene, and nonclostridial myositis. Serious vascular problems resulting from loss of blood supply may lead to death of muscle tissue, leading to a secondary infection (vascular gangrene). Organisms that cause myositis or other muscle pathology are listed in Box 75.2.

Wound Infections

Besides skin and soft tissue infections, wound infections occur primarily from breaks in the skin because of complications associated with surgery, trauma, and bites, or from diseases that interrupt the mucosal or skin surface.

• BOX 75.2   Organisms Producing Myositis or Other Muscle Pathology

Clostridium perfringens
Clostridium novyi
Clostridium septicum
Clostridium histolyticum
Clostridium sordellii
Clostridium sporogenes
Paraclostridium bifermentans (previously *Clostridium*)
Bacillus spp.
Aeromonas spp.
Peptostreptococcus spp.
Microaerobic streptococci
Bacteroides spp.
Enterobacterales
Staphylococcus aureus
Group A streptococci (*Streptococcus pyogenes*)
Pseudomonas spp.
Vibrio vulnificus
Mycobacterium tuberculosis
Salmonella enterica serotype Typhi
Legionella spp.
Rickettsia spp.
Viruses
Trichinella spp.
Taenia solium
Toxoplasma gondii

Microbial biofilms have also increased the length and chronicity of wound infections.

Postoperative Infections

Surgical site infections are among the most common health care–associated infections. Sources of surgical wound infections can include the patient's normal microbiota or organisms present in the hospital environment. These organisms are introduced to the patient by medical procedures or underlying disease or trauma (e.g., burns). The nature of the infecting organism depends on the patient's underlying condition and the location of the medical treatment or procedure. The most common organism involved in postoperative infections is *S. aureus*. Surgical procedures in the colorectal or other lower gastrointestinal areas have the highest incidence of postoperative infections because of the presence of intestinal bacteria. These infections are most likely to be caused by enteric gram-negative bacteria, anaerobes, and enterococci. Principal pathogens are listed in Box 75.3.

Bites

Bite wounds can be the result of human teeth, as well as a large variety of domestic or wild animals. The infectious agents associated with the bite may come from the environment, the victim's normal skin microbiota, and the oral flora of the biter. This makes the variety of potential infectious agents quite diverse. Human bite (Fig. 75.5) infections can be attributed to occlusion bites or closed-fist injuries. Not surprisingly, the most commonly isolated organisms are normal oral microbiota. Most frequently isolated are viridans streptococci (particularly *Streptococcus anginosus*), *S. aureus*, and *Eikenella corrodens*. Common anaerobes isolated include *Prevotella*, *Fusobacterium*, *Veillonella*, and *Peptostreptococcus* species. These infections are usually polymicrobial and contain both aerobic and anaerobic organisms.

• BOX 75.3 Organisms Encountered in Postoperative Wound Infections

Staphylococcus aureus
Coagulase-negative staphylococci
Streptococcus pyogenes
Streptococcus anginosus group streptococci (*Streptococcus anginosus, Streptococcus constellatus, Streptococcus intermedius*)
Microaerophilic streptococci
Enterococci
Proteus, Morganella, and *Providencia* spp.
Other Enterobacterales
Escherichia coli
Pseudomonas spp.
Candida spp.
Bacteroides spp.
Prevotella and *Porphyromonas* spp.
Fusobacterium spp.
Clostridium spp.
Peptostreptococcus spp.
Non–spore-forming, anaerobic, gram-positive bacilli

Animal bites account for approximately 1% of all emergency room visits in the United States. The most common animal bites are from domestic cats and dogs. Bites from these animals (Fig. 75.6) usually are infected with organisms commonly found in the animal's oral and nasal fluids. The most commonly isolated aerobes are *Pasteurella, Streptococcus, Neisseria,* and *Staphylococcus* species. The most commonly isolated anaerobes are *Fusobacterium, Bacteroides,* and *Porphyromonas* species. Similar to human bites, animal bite wound infections are usually polymicrobial and include aerobes and anaerobes. Other far less common animal bites may also become infected. Rat bite infections are usually caused by *Streptobacillus moniliformis*. Snakebites may become infected with *A. hydrophilia.*

Burns

Burns are a significant cause of mortality due to hospital-associated infections; 42% to 65% of deaths in burn patients are associated with infection. Infected burn wounds may be associated with many organisms, causing significant mortality, and may interfere with the success of skin grafts. Bacteria cause 70% of burn wound infections, 20% to 25% are caused

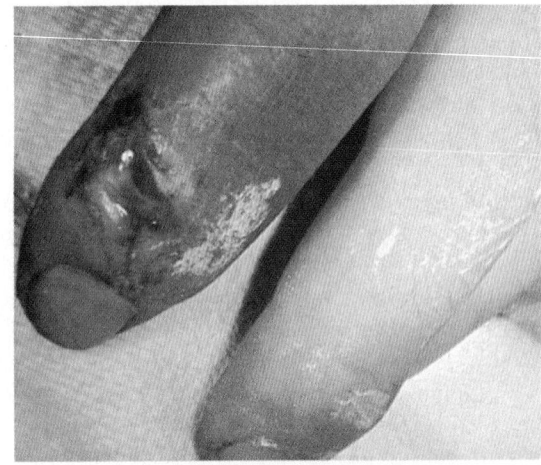

• **Fig. 75.5** Human bite infection.

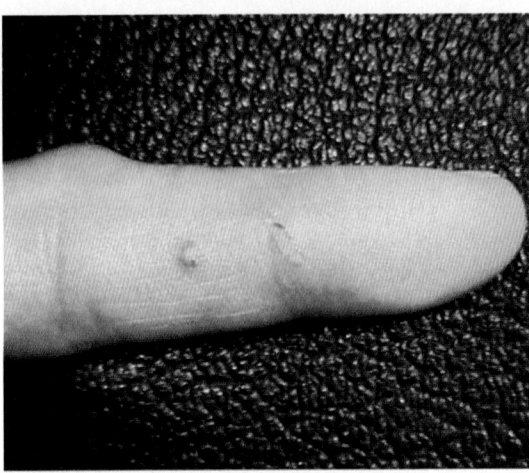

• **Fig. 75.6** Animal bite infection caused by *Pasteurella* spp.

by fungi, and anaerobic organisms and viruses cause 5% to 10%. Burn wound infections can commonly be identified as four types: **impetigo;** surgical infections; cellulitis; bacteremia and invasive, systemic infections. Factors that contribute to the development of infection include loss of the skin barrier, coagulated proteins and other microbial nutrients, loss of vascularity of the wound, dehydration of surrounding tissue, and the inflammatory response of the patient's immune system. Gram-positive organs tend to be isolated from early infections, whereas the incidence of infection with gram-negative organisms increases with the length of hospitalization. The organisms isolated most often from burns include *S. aureus, P. aeruginosa,* enterococci, *Enterobacter* spp., and *E. coli.* Other organisms, such as fungi (e.g., *Candida* spp., *Aspergillus niger, Fusarium* spp., and *Mucor* spp.) and viruses may also be involved in invasive burn infections. The risk of infections with multidrug-resistant organisms also increases with the length of stay for burn patients. These organisms include *P. aeruginosa, Acinetobacter baumannii, Stenotrophomonas maltophilia,* and *S. aureus.*

Special Circumstances Regarding Skin and Soft Tissue Infections

In addition to the infections previously discussed, other circumstances can cause skin and underlying soft tissue to become infected. Some of these infections are associated with an immunocompromised host; others are manifestations of systemic infection.

Infections Related to Vascular and Neurologic Problems

Frequently, a patient with infections associated with vascular or neurologic problems has diabetes mellitus. These patients have a high risk of developing infections, especially in their lower extremities. The excess glucose present in their blood can result in impaired microvascular circulation and peripheral motor neuropathy, leading to an increased risk of infection. Any skin-damaging injury or surgery greatly increases that risk. In addition, because of the complications associated with impaired circulation and neuropathy, the infected tissue of a diabetic patient does not heal as rapidly as that of a healthy individual. An estimated 25% of adults with diabetes will develop a foot infection, and the risk increases with age. Foot infections can lead to amputations and greatly increased mortality. Periodically, an acute cellulitis and lymphangitis may be associated with chronic, low-grade infection, thereby making control of the patient's diabetes difficult. Peripheral vascular disease unrelated to diabetes may also predispose a patient to skin and soft tissue infections, but usually these infections are easier to manage because there is no associated neuropathy.

Foot infections in diabetic patients can accelerate dramatically, producing devastating consequences without proper treatment. Therefore, appropriate techniques used to obtain a microbiologic sample are critical. Culture of aspirated fluid or pus, not surface swabbing, is more likely to

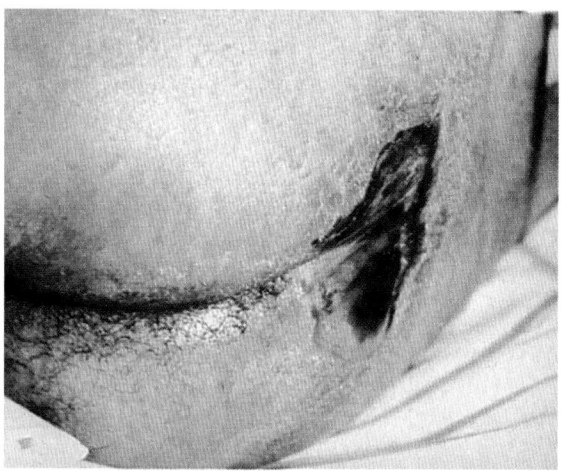

• **Fig. 75.7** Sacral decubitus ulcer.

yield a causative agent—particularly if taken from a deep pocket within the wound. In addition, culture of debrided infected tissue improves the diagnosis of these infections. The most common bacteria isolated from mild to moderate diabetic foot infections include *S. aureus,* group B streptococci, members of the Enterobacterales, and anaerobes. More severe infections are usually polymicrobial. Extension of the infection into the underlying bone produces a difficult-to-manage osteomyelitis. Definitive diagnosis of this infection requires a specimen of bone obtained during open or percutaneous biopsy.

Venous insufficiency may also predispose an individual to infection, again primarily in the lower extremities (often in the calf or lower leg rather than the foot). Infections related to poor blood supply often involve *S. aureus* and group A streptococci. Those with open ulcers may become colonized with Enterobacterales and *P. aeruginosa.* Anaerobes are also frequently involved in these infections, as a result of the blood supply creating anaerobic conditions. Anaerobes that may be involved include *Bacteroides fragilis* group, *Prevotella, Porphyromonas, Peptostreptococcus* and, less commonly, *Clostridium* species.

Another common type of infection in this general category, especially in the elderly or chronically ill, bedridden patient, is infected **decubitus ulcer** (pressure sore; Fig. 75.7). Anaerobic conditions are present in the lesions as a result of tissue necrosis. Most of these lesions are located near the anus or on the lower extremities. Because these patients are relatively helpless and have limited mobility, the ulcers may become contaminated with gastrointestinal bacteria, leading to chronic infection. These conditions contribute to further death of tissue and extension of the decubitus ulcer. Bacteremia is a possible complication; *B. fragilis* group is often involved, as are clostridia and other enteric bacteria. Health care–associated pathogens, such as *S. aureus* and *P. aeruginosa,* may also be recovered.

Sinus Tracts and Fistulas

Sometimes, a deep-seated infection will develop a channel, called a **sinus tract,** to the skin surface. The sinus tract will

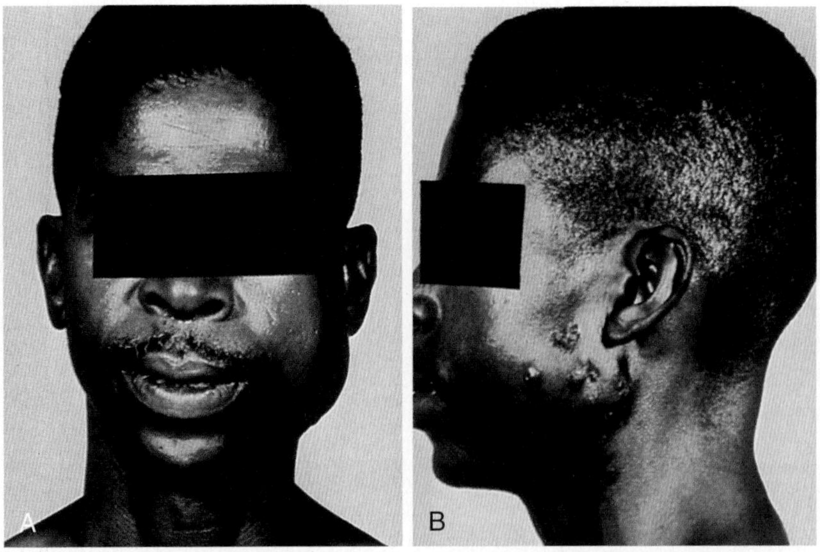

• **Fig. 75.8** Actinomycosis. (A) Note "lumpy jaw." (B) Side view. Note sinuses in skin of face and neck.

drain fluid and pus onto the skin. The infections involved are often chronic and may include osteomyelitis. The organisms commonly involved in sinus tract formation with an underlying osteomyelitis include *S. aureus,* various members of the Enterobacterales, *P. aeruginosa,* anaerobic gram-negative bacilli, and anaerobic gram-positive cocci. In the case of actinomycosis (Fig. 75.8), with or without bone involvement, the organisms involved include *Actinomyces* spp., *Aggregatibacter actinomycetemcomitans, Propionibacterium propionicum, Prevotella* or *Porphyromonas* species, and other non–spore-forming anaerobes. Chronic draining sinuses may also be found in patients with tuberculosis and atypical mycobacterial infection, *Nocardia* infection, and infections associated with implanted foreign bodies. Curetting or biopsy specimens from the debrided, cleansed sinus should be used for culture.

Abnormal channels connecting epithelial surfaces, either between two internal organs or between an organ and the skin epithelium, are known as **fistulas.** Infections associated with fistulas often pose insurmountable problems in terms of collecting a meaningful specimen because the organ involved may contain indigenous microbiota. Examples include perirectal fistulas from the small bowel to the skin associated with Crohn disease or chronic intraabdominal infection. When the bowel is involved, cultures for specific organisms, such as mycobacteria or *Actinomyces,* are useful. An attempt should always be made to rule out specific associated underlying causes, such as tuberculosis, actinomycosis, and malignancy. A biopsy should be performed in these situations.

Systemic Infections and Skin Manifestations

Cutaneous manifestations of systemic infections, such as bacteremia or endocarditis, may be important clues for the clinician. These represent an opportunity for direct detection or culture for the presence of an organism. For example, a scraping of **petechiae** (tiny red hemorrhagic spots in the skin) from patients with meningococcemia may demonstrate the presence of gram-negative diplococci. In other patients, the skin lesion may represent a metastatic infection. In *Vibrio vulnificus* sepsis, dramatic-appearing cutaneous ulcers with **necrotizing vasculitis** or **bullae** may be seen. In some patients, skin lesions may represent a noninfectious complication of a local or systemic infection, such as scarlet fever or toxic shock syndrome. Various organisms involved in systemic infections capable of producing cutaneous lesions are listed in Box 75.4.

Laboratory Diagnostic Procedures

Infections of the Epidermis and Dermis

For many of the infections of the epidermis and dermis, such as impetigo, folliculitis, cellulitis, and erysipelas, diagnosis is generally based on clinical observations. Table 75.3 provides the key features and etiologic agents of these infections.

Erysipeloid

In **erysipeloid,** usually the Gram stain or culture of superficial wound drainage is negative. However, culture of a full-thickness skin biopsy taken at the margin of the lesion can confirm the clinical diagnosis.

Superficial Mycoses and Erythrasma

If a dermatophyte infection is suspected, the lesion is cleaned, and scrapings are obtained from the active border of the lesion. These scrapings should be treated with 10% potassium hydroxide and examined for the presence of hyphae. The specimen may also be cultured if necessary (Chapter 59). A Woods lamp examination of the skin lesions for tinea versicolor may show golden-yellow fluorescence.

Erythrasma, which is caused by infection with *Corynebacterium minutissimum,* can be diagnosed by making smears from the lesion revealing gram-positive pleomorphic

Viridans streptococci
Staphylococcus aureus
Enterococci
Group A and other beta-hemolytic streptococci
Neisseria gonorrhoeae
Neisseria meningitidis
Haemophilus influenzae
Pseudomonas aeruginosa
Pseudomonas spp.
Listeria monocytogenes
Vibrio vulnificus
Salmonella enterica serotype Typhi
Mycobacterium tuberculosis
Mycobacterium leprae
Treponema pallidum
Leptospira spp.
Streptobacillus moniliformis
Bartonella bacilliformis
Bartonella henselae
Rickettsia spp.
Candida spp.
Cryptococcus spp.
Blastomyces dermatitidis
Coccidioides immitis
Histoplasma capsulatum

bacilli. If necessary, skin scrapings may be cultured in media containing serum. A Woods lamp examination of the skin lesions may reveal a coral red fluorescence resulting from the production of porphyrin by *C. minutissimum.*

Erysipelas and Cellulitis

As previously mentioned, diagnosis of erysipelas and cellulitis can generally be made based on clinical observation. Swab specimens from bullae, pustules, or ulcers may be cultured. Culturing of needle aspiration or punch biopsy specimens is not recommended and rarely informative. Blood cultures are also typically negative.

Vesicles and Bullae

These fluid-filled lesions characteristically involve specific organisms (Table 75.1). Material in a blisterlike lesion may vary from **serous** (resembling serum) **fluid** to **serosanguineous** (composed of serum and blood) **fluid** or **hemorrhagic** (bloody) **fluid.** Large bullae may permit withdrawal of fluid by needle and syringe aspiration. Specimens from tiny vesicles may need to be collected with a swab. The clinician can usually anticipate whether the lesion is viral or bacterial and may even suspect an organism. Specimens should be submitted for viral or bacterial culture based on the clinical presentation.

Bullous lesions are often associated with sepsis, requiring the collection of blood for nucleic acid testing or cultures. Gas gangrene caused by *Clostridium perfringens* and other clostridia is characterized by bronzed skin with bullous lesions. Gram stain of the fluid from the lesions typically reveals gram-positive bacilli.

Infections of the Subcutaneous Tissue

Proper collection and transport of specimens are important factors in the laboratory diagnosis of all infections. Specimen collection for the diagnosis of subcutaneous tissue infection is particularly difficult, because many of these lesions are open and readily colonized by nosocomial pathogens that may not be involved in the systemic underlying infection. The most reliable specimens for determining the etiology of ulcers and nodules are those obtained from the base of the ulcer or nodule after removal of overlying debris, or by surgical biopsy of deep tissues, avoiding contact with the superficial layers of the lesion. A Gram stain of the specimen should be performed, and material aerobically cultured on blood and MacConkey agar. If fungi, *Nocardia* spp., or mycobacterial infection is suspected, appropriate fungal media or mycobacterial media should be used. These culture methods are addressed in greater detail in Chapters 42 and 59, respectively.

Similar challenges exist in collecting material for culture from sinus tracts. The material should be obtained from the deepest portion of the sinus tract. If systemic symptoms, such as fever, are present, blood cultures should also be collected. A Gram stain should be routinely performed. Cultures should be inoculated to recover both facultative and anaerobic bacteria in the same manner as for surgical wounds. Nucleic acid–based assays may be used to directly identify organisms, such as *S. aureus,* in wound infections. In addition, when deep tissue or bone infections are suspected and yield negative culture results, molecular assays may aid in the identification of the infectious agent.

Infections of the Muscle Fascia and Muscles

Blood cultures should always be collected from patients with significant **myonecrosis.** Transport of material (tissue is recommended, followed by purulent material, and then a swab) should be under anaerobic conditions. Gram stains should be routinely performed. Cultures should be inoculated to recover both facultative and anaerobic bacteria in the same manner as for surgical wounds.

Wound Infections
Postoperative

Because anaerobic bacteria are involved in many of these infections, specimen collection should be completed carefully to avoid indigenous microbiota. Specimen transport in anaerobic conditions is essential. Unusual organisms associated with postsurgical wound infections, such as *Mycoplasma hominis, Mycobacterium chelonae, Mycobacterium fortuitum,* fungi, and even *Legionella* spp., should not be overlooked. A Gram-stained smear of material submitted for culture should be examined. Exudates from superficial wounds should routinely be inoculated to blood, MacConkey, and Colistin-nalidixic acid (CNA) agars, as well as an enrichment broth. Material from deep wounds should be inoculated onto media for both anaerobic and aerobic cultures. More detailed information regarding the processing of specimens for anaerobic cultures is presented in Chapters 40 and 41.

Bites

Bite wound infections usually involve relatively small lesions and minimal exudate. A swab specimen for aerobic culture and one in anaerobic transport media should be collected. Surrounding skin should be thoroughly disinfected before the specimen is obtained. The best material for culture is purulent exudate aspirated from the depth of the wound or samples obtained during surgery involving incision and drainage or **debridement** (removal of all dead and necrotic tissue). Gram-stained smears should be prepared and examined. For aerobic cultures, a minimum of blood, MacConkey, and chocolate agar should be inoculated.

Burns

For many burn patients, diagnosis of infection is based on clinical symptoms, signs, and examination of the burn wound. When possible, cultures should be performed on any purulent wound exudates, and blood cultures should also be collected. Surface specimens should be collected with a moistened sterile swab using a minimal amount of pressure. Sometimes a quantitative or semiquantitative culture (Evolve Procedure 75.1) of a tissue biopsy specimen is used for infection surveillance, or to identify the most prevalent organism in a polymicrobial infection. This type of culture is reported in colony-forming units (CFUs) per gram of tissue, with a result of 10^5 CFUs/g or more indicative of a potentially serious infection.

ⓔ Visit the Evolve site for a complete list of procedures, review questions, and case studies.

Bibliography

Bailey E, Kroshinsky D: Cellulitis: diagnosis and management, *Dermatol Ther* 24:229–239, 2011.

Bennett J, Dolin R, Blaser M: *Principles and practice of infectious diseases*, ed 9, Philadelphia, PA, 2020, Elsevier-Saunders.

Capoor MR, Sarabahi S, Tiwari VK, et al.: Fungal infections in burns: diagnosis and management, *Indian J Plast Surg* 43:S37–S42, 2010.

Carroll KC, Pfaller MA: *Manual of clinical microbiology*, ed 12, Washington, DC, 2019, ASM Press.

Crum-Cianflone NF: Bacterial, fungal, parasitic, and viral myositis, *Clin Microbiol Rev* 21:473–494, 2008.

Humphreys H: Preventing and controlling the risk of post-operative surgical-site infections, *Eur Infect Dis* 2:110–112, 2008.

Hurlow JJ, Humphreys GJ, Bowling FL, et al.: Diabetic foot infection: a critical complication, *Int Wound J* 15(5):814–821, 2018.

Hurt JB, Maday KR: Management and treatment of animal bites, *JAAPA* 4:27–31, 2018.

Lachiewicz AM, Hauck CG, Weber DJ, et al.: Bacterial infections after burn injuries: impact of multidrug resistance, *Clin Infect Dis* 65(12):2130–2136, 2017.

Lazar AJF: The skin. In: *Robbins basic pathology*, ed 8, St. Louis, MO, 2007, Saunders.

Levy PY, Fenollar F: The role of molecular diagnostics in implant-associated bone and joint infection, *Clin Microbiol Infect* 18:1168–1175, 2012.

Lipsky BA: Medical treatment of diabetic foot infections, *Clin Infect Dis* 39(Suppl 2):S104–S114, 2004.

Mayhall CG: The epidemiology of burn wound infections: then and now, *Clin Infect Dis* 37:543–550, 2003.

Mena KD, Gerba CP: Risk assessment of *Pseudomonas aeruginosa* in water, *Rev Environ Contam Toxicol* 201:71–115, 2006.

Murphy E: Microbiology of animal bites, *Clin Microbiol Newsl* 30:47–50, 2008.

Oehler RL, Velez AP, Mizrachi M, et al.: Bite-related and septic syndromes caused by cats and dogs, *Lancet Infect Dis* 9:439–447, 2009.

Polavarapu N, Ogilvie MP, Panthaki ZJ: Microbiology of burn wound infections, *J Craniofac Surg* 19:899–902, 2008.

Salkind AR, Rao KC: Antibiotic prophylaxis to prevent surgical site infections, *Am Fam Physician* 83:585–590, 2011.

Sankar RU, Biswas R, Raja S, et al.: Brain abscess and cervical lymphadenitis due to *Paraclostridium bifermentans*: a report of two cases, *Anaerobe* 51:8–11, 2018.

Talan AD, Abrahamian FM, Moran GJ, et al.: Clinical presentation and bacteriologic analysis of infected human bites in patients presenting to emergency departments, *Clin Infect Dis* 37:1481–1489, 2003.

Williams DT, Hilton JR, Harding KG: Diagnosing foot infection in diabetes, *Clin Infect Dis* 39(Suppl 2):S83–S86, 2004.

76

Normally Sterile Body Fluids, Bone and Bone Marrow, and Solid Tissues

OBJECTIVES

1. Describe the five main cavities of the human body; also name the membranes associated with these cavities and state the function of these membranes.
2. Define each of the following body cavity fluids and explain the diagnostic culture methods for each: pleural fluid, pericardial fluid, peritoneal fluid, joint fluid, and dialysis fluid.
3. Define parietal and visceral pleura.
4. Define cellulitis; name the etiologic agents of this illness and explain the associated risk factors for the development of disease.
5. Define pleural effusion; explain the difference between exudative pleural effusion and transudative pleural effusion.
6. Explain when a pleural effusion becomes an empyema and what medical condition contributes to the development of an empyema?
7. Define pericarditis and myocarditis; explain the physical conditions that may contribute to the accumulation of pericardial fluid.
8. Define peritonitis; differentiate between primary and secondary peritonitis.
9. Name the etiologic agents most commonly isolated from primary peritonitis cases in children, adults, sexually active females, and immunocompromised patients.
10. Define osteomyelitis; explain how this infection is transmitted, the diagnostic method, and the organisms most commonly responsible for this type of infection.
11. Explain the process for culturing organisms from the following specimens: bone, tissue, and bone marrow.
12. Correlate patient signs and symptoms with laboratory results to identify the etiologic agent associated with the body fluid, bone and bone marrow, and other solid tissue infection.

The human body is divided into five main body cavities: cranial, spinal, thoracic, abdominal, and pelvic. Each cavity is lined with membranes, and within the body wall and these membranes, or **between** the membranes and organs, are small spaces filled with minute amounts of

fluid. The purpose of this fluid is to bathe the organs and membranes, reducing friction between organs.

Bacteria, fungi, viruses, or parasites can invade any body tissue or sterile body fluid site. Although from different areas of the body, all specimens discussed in this chapter are considered normally sterile. Therefore, even one colony of a potentially pathogenic microorganism may be significant. (Refer to Table 5.1 for a quick guide regarding collection, transport, and processing of specimens from sterile body sites.)

Specimens From Sterile Body Sites

Fluids

In response to infection, fluid may accumulate in any body cavity. Infected solid tissue often presents as cellulitis or with abscess formation. Areas of the body from which fluids are typically sent for microbiologic studies (in addition to blood and cerebrospinal fluid [Chapters 67 and 70]) are listed in Table 76.1. In general, peritoneal, pleural, and pericardial fluids may be cultured in aerobic and anaerobic blood culture bottles. This method should not be used if a polymicrobial infection is suspected, as some organisms can overgrow fastidious or other slow-growing organisms resulting in incomplete identification of the pathogens.

Pleural Fluid

Lining the entire thoracic cavity (Chapter 68) of the body is a serous membrane called the **parietal pleura.** Covering the outer surface of the lung is another membrane called the **visceral pleura** (Fig. 76.1). Within the pleural space between the lung and chest wall is a small amount of fluid called **pleural fluid** that lubricates the surfaces of the pleura (the membranes surrounding the lungs and lining of the chest cavity). Normally, equilibrium exists among the pleural membranes, but in certain disease states, such as cardiac, hepatic, or renal disease, excess amounts of this fluid can be produced and accumulates in the pleural space; this is known as a **pleural effusion.** Pleural effusions can either be exudative or transudative. **Exudative pleural effusions** are caused by inflammation, infection, and cancer, whereas **transudative effusions** result from systemic changes, such as congestive heart failure.

Normal pleural fluid contains few or no cells and has a consistency similar to serum, but with a lower protein count. Pleural fluid containing numerous white blood cells is indicative of infection. Pleural fluid specimens are collected by **thoracentesis,** a procedure in which a needle is inserted through the chest wall into the pleural space and the excess fluid aspirated. This fluid is then submitted to the laboratory as thoracentesis fluid, pleural fluid, or empyema fluid. The fluid, or effusion, can then be analyzed for cell count, total protein, glucose, lactate dehydrogenase, amylase, cytology, nucleic acid testing, and culture. The total protein and glucose results determine whether the effusion is transudate or exudate. The patient's serum or plasma glucose level is needed to compare with the results indicated in the body fluid. Several characteristics can be used to determine whether a fluid is a transudate or exudate (Table 76.2).

When effusions are extremely purulent (i.e., full of pus), the effusion is referred to as an **empyema.** Empyema often arises as a complication of pneumonia, but other infections near the lung (e.g., subdiaphragmatic infection) may seed

TABLE 76.1	Microbiology Laboratory Body Fluid Collection Sites	
Body Area	**Fluid Name(s)**
Thorax	Thoracentesis or pleural or empyema fluid
Abdominal cavity	Paracentesis or ascitic or peritoneal fluid
Joint	Synovial fluid
Pericardium	Pericardial fluid

TABLE 76.2	Pleural Fluid Effusion Characteristics	
	Transudate	**Exudate**
Appearance	Clear	Cloudy
Specific gravity	<1.015	>1.015
Total protein	<3.0 mg/dL	>3.0 mg/dL
LD fluid/serum ratio	<0.6	>0.6
Cholesterol	<60 mg/dL	>60 mg/dL
Cholesterol fluid/ serum ratio	<0.3	>0.3
Bilirubin fluid/ serum ratio	<0.6	>0.6
Total protein fluid/ serum ratio	<0.5	>0.6
White blood cells	<1000/μL (all white blood cell types, all <50%)	>1000/μL
Red blood cells	<10,000/μL = because of traumatic tap	>100,000/μL
Clotting	Will not clot	May clot

Modified from Strasinger SK, Di Lorenzo MS. *Urinalysis and Body Fluids.* 5th ed. Philadelphia: F.A. Davis; 2008.

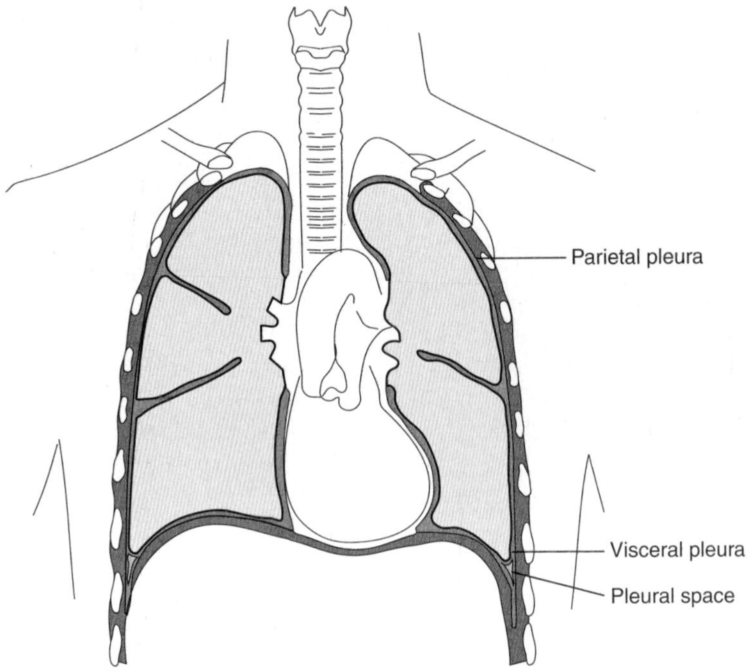

• **Fig. 76.1** The location of the pleural space in relation to the parietal and visceral pleura and the rest of the respiratory tract.

Parietal pleura

Visceral pleura

Pleural space

microorganisms into the pleural cavity. It has been estimated that 50% to 60% of patients develop empyema as a complication of pneumonia.

Peritoneal Fluid

The **peritoneum** is a large, moist, continuous sheet of serous membrane lining the walls of the abdominal-pelvic cavity and the outer coat of the organs contained within the cavity (Fig. 76.2). In the abdomen, these two membrane linings are separated by a space called the **peritoneal cavity,** which contains or abuts the liver, pancreas, spleen, stomach, and intestinal tract, bladder, and fallopian tubes and ovaries. The kidneys occupy a retroperitoneal (behind the peritoneum) position. Within the healthy human peritoneal cavity is a small amount of fluid that maintains the surface moisture of the peritoneum. Normal **peritoneal fluid** contains as many as 300 white blood cells per milliliter, but the protein content and specific gravity of the fluid are low. During an infectious or inflammatory process, increased amounts of fluid accumulate in the peritoneal cavity, a condition called **ascites.** Most cases of ascites are caused by liver disease, and in severe cases, the abdomen is often distended. The fluid can be collected for testing by **paracentesis** (the insertion of a needle into the abdomen and removal of fluid). The peritoneal or ascites fluid can then be analyzed for amylase, protein, albumin, cell count, nucleic acid testing, culture, and cytology. Often ascitic fluid contains an increased number of inflammatory cells and an elevated protein level.

Agents of infection gain access to the peritoneum through a perforation of the bowel, through infection within abdominal viscera, by way of the bloodstream, or by external inoculation (as in surgery or trauma). On occasion, as in pelvic inflammatory disease (PID), organisms travel through the natural channels of the fallopian tubes into the peritoneal cavity.

Primary Peritonitis

Peritonitis results when the peritoneal membrane becomes inflamed and can be either primary or secondary. **Primary peritonitis** (spontaneous bacterial peritonitis) is rare and results when infection spreads from the blood and lymph nodes with no apparent evidence of infection. The organisms likely to be recovered from patient specimens with primary peritonitis vary with the patient's age. The most common etiologic agents in children are *Streptococcus pneumoniae* and group A streptococci, Enterobacterales, other gram-negative bacilli, and staphylococci. In adults, *Escherichia coli* is the most common bacterium, followed by *Klebsiella pneumoniae, S. pneumoniae,* other streptococci species (including enterococci), and other Enterobacterales. Polymicrobic peritonitis is unusual in the absence of bowel perforation or rupture. Among sexually active young women, *Neisseria gonorrhoeae* and *Chlamydia trachomatis* are common etiologic agents of peritoneal infection, often in the form of a **perihepatitis** (inflammation of the surface of the liver, called **Fitz-Hugh–Curtis syndrome**). Tuberculous peritonitis

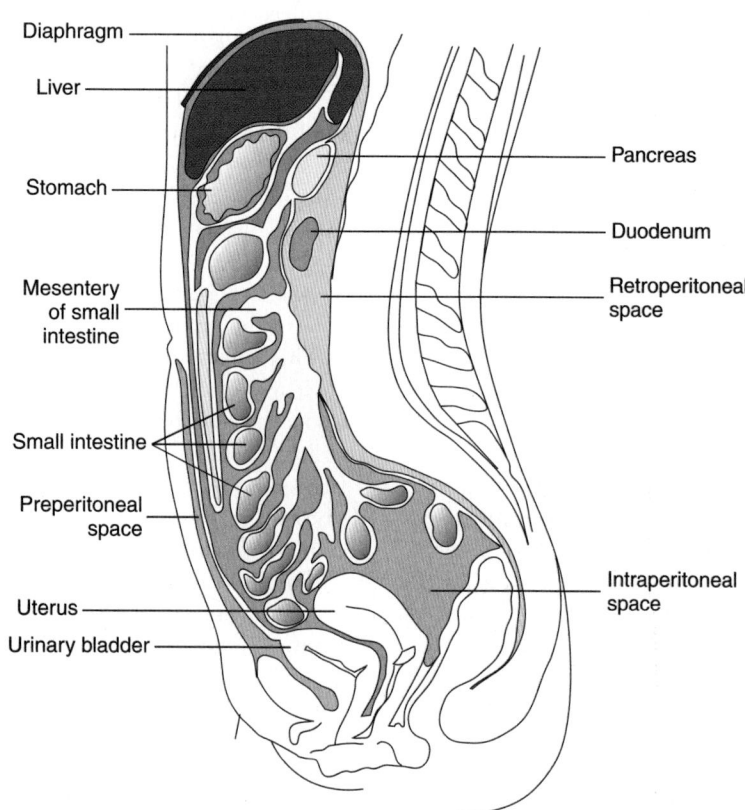

• **Fig. 76.2** The abdominal cavity. The retroperitoneal and preperitoneal spaces are considered as extraperitoneal (outside) spaces. (Modified from Thibodeau GA. *Anatomy and Physiology.* St Louis: Mosby; 1993.)

occurs uncommonly in the United States and is more likely to be found among individuals who have recently traveled to South America, Southeast Asia, or Africa. Tuberculous peritonitis can occur from direct entry into the peritoneal cavity from the lymph nodes, intestine, or genital tract from patients with active disease. However, more often it is a result of hematogenous dissemination from the lungs. Fungal causes of peritonitis are not common, but *Candida* spp. may be recovered from immunosuppressed patients and patients receiving prolonged antibacterial therapy.

Secondary and Tertiary Peritonitis

Secondary peritonitis is a complication of a perforated viscus (organ), surgery, traumatic injury, loss of bowel wall integrity after a destructive disease (e.g., ulcerative colitis, ruptured appendix, carcinoma), obstruction, or a preceding infection (liver abscess, salpingitis, septicemia). The nature, location, and etiology of the underlying process govern the agents recovered from peritoneal fluid. With PID as the background, gonococci, anaerobes, or chlamydiae are isolated. With peritonitis or intraabdominal abscess, anaerobes generally are found in peritoneal fluid, usually together with Enterobacterales and enterococci or other streptococci. In patients whose bowel microbiota has been altered by antimicrobial agents, more resistant gram-negative bacilli and *Staphylococcus aureus* may be encountered. Because anaerobes outnumber aerobes in the bowel by 1000-fold, it is not surprising that anaerobic organisms play a prominent role in intraabdominal infection, perhaps acting synergistically with facultative bacteria. The organisms likely to be recovered include *E. coli,* the *Bacteroides fragilis* group, enterococci and other streptococci, *Bilophila* spp., other anaerobic gram-negative bacilli, anaerobic gram-positive cocci, and clostridia.

Tertiary peritonitis is considered when a patient with peritonitis and systemic symptoms of sepsis persists following treatment for either primary or secondary peritonitis. This condition is more common in immunosuppressed and critically ill patients. Pathogens typically isolated in these cases include organisms, such as coagulase negative staphylococci, enterococci, Enterobacterales, anaerobes, or *Candida* spp.

Peritoneal Dialysis Fluid

More than 900,000 patients with end-stage renal disease are maintained on **continuous ambulatory peritoneal dialysis (CAPD).** One in every 10 American adults, totaling more than 20 million, suffer from some type of chronic kidney disease. In this treatment, fluid is injected into the peritoneal cavity and subsequently removed, which allows exchange of salts and water and removal of various wastes in the absence of kidney function. Because the dialysate fluid is injected into the peritoneal cavity via a catheter, the break in the skin barrier places the dialysis patient at significant risk for infection. The average incidence of peritonitis in these patients is up to two episodes per year, per patient. Peritonitis is diagnosed by the presence of two

of the following: cloudy dialysate, abdominal pain, or a positive culture from dialysate. Although white blood cells are usually plentiful (a value of leukocytes >100/mL is usually indicative of infection), the number of organisms is usually too low for detection on Gram stain of the peritoneal fluid sediment unless a concentrating technique is used; fungi are more readily detected. Many recent studies show that improved sensitivity can be achieved by using automated blood culture systems in which 10 mL of fluid is inoculated into culture bottles. Rapid detection of pathogens has also been successful using polymerase chain reaction (PCR) and 16s rRNA sequencing. The sensitivity associated with 16s rRNA sequencing varies significantly due to the inability to distinguish organisms due to high genetic similarity and should be used in conjunction with culture.

Most infections originate from the patient's normal skin microbiota; *Staphylococcus epidermidis* and *S. aureus* are the most common etiologic agents, followed by streptococci, aerobic or facultative gram-negative bacilli, *Candida* spp., *Corynebacterium* spp., and others. The oxygen content of peritoneal dialysate is usually too high for the development of anaerobic infection. Among the gram-negative bacilli isolated, *Pseudomonas* spp., *Acinetobacter* spp., and the Enterobacterales are commonly observed.

Pericardial Fluid

The heart and contiguous major blood vessels are surrounded by the **pericardium,** a protective tissue. The area between the **epicardium**—which is the membrane surrounding the heart muscle—and the pericardium is called the **pericardial space,** and normally contains 15 to 20 mL of clear fluid. If an infectious agent is present within the fluid, the pericardium may become distended and tight, and eventually **tamponade** (interference with cardiac function and circulation) can ensue. Up to 500 mL of fluid can accumulate during infection, which may seriously complicate cardiac function.

Agents of **pericarditis** (inflammation of the pericardium) are usually viruses, especially coxsackie virus. Bacterial pericarditis usually occurs during a severe systemic infection. Parasites, certain fungi, and noninfectious causes are also associated with this disease.

Myocarditis (inflammation of the heart muscle itself) may accompany or follow pericarditis. The pathogenesis of disease involves the host inflammatory response contributing to fluid buildup, as well as cell and tissue damage. Common causes of myocarditis include viral infections with coxsackie virus, echoviruses, or adenovirus. The most common etiologic agents of pericarditis and myocarditis are listed in Box 76.1. Other bacteria, fungi, and parasitic agents have been recovered from pericardial effusions.

Patients who develop pericarditis resulting from agents other than viruses are often immunocompromised or suffering from a chronic disease. An example is infective endocarditis, in which a myocardial abscess develops and then ruptures into the pericardial space.

• BOX 76.1 Common Etiologic Agents of Pericarditis and Myocarditis

Viruses

Enteroviruses (primary coxsackie A and B and, less commonly, echoviruses)
Adenoviruses
Influenza viruses

Bacteria (Relatively Uncommon)

Mycoplasma pneumoniae
Chlamydia trachomatis
Mycobacterium tuberculosis
Staphylococcus aureus
Streptococcus pneumoniae
Enterobacterales and other gram-negative bacilli

Fungi (Relatively Uncommon)

Coccidioides immitis
Aspergillus spp.
Candida spp.
Cryptococcus spp.
Histoplasma capsulatum

Parasites (Relatively Uncommon)

Entamoeba histolytica
Toxoplasma gondii

• BOX 76.2 Most Commonly Encountered Etiologic Agents of Infectious Arthritis

Bacterial

Staphylococcus aureus
Beta-hemolytic streptococci
Streptococci (other)
Haemophilus influenzae
Haemophilus spp. (other)
Bacteroides spp.
Fusobacterium spp.
Neisseria gonorrhoeae
Pseudomonas spp.
Salmonella spp.
Pasteurella multocida
Moraxella osloensis
Kingella kingae
Moraxella catarrhalis
Capnocytophaga spp.
Corynebacterium spp.
Clostridium spp.
Finegoldia spp.
Eikenella corrodens
Actinomyces spp.
Mycobacterium spp.
Mycoplasma spp.
Ureaplasma urealyticum
Borrelia burgdorferi

Fungal

Candida spp.
Cryptococcus spp.
Coccidioides immitis
Sporothrix schenckii

Viral

Hepatitis viruses
Rubella
Other viruses (rarely)

Joint Fluid

Arthritis is an inflammation in a joint space. Infectious arthritis may involve any joint in the body. Infection of the joint usually occurs secondary to hematogenous spread of bacteria or, less often, fungi as a direct extension of infection of the bone. It may also occur after injection of material, especially corticosteroids, into joints or after insertion of prosthetic material (e.g., total hip replacement). Although infectious arthritis usually occurs at a single site (monoarticular), a preexisting bacteremia or fungemia may seed more than one joint to establish polyarticular infection, particularly when multiple joints are diseased, such as in rheumatoid arthritis. In bacterial arthritis, the knees and hips are the most commonly affected joints in all age groups.

In addition to active infections associated with viable microorganisms within the joint, sterile, self-limited arthritis caused by antigen-antibody interactions may follow an episode of infection, such as meningococcal meningitis. When an etiologic agent cannot be isolated from an inflamed joint fluid specimen, either the absence of viable agents or inadequate transport or culturing procedures may be the cause. For example, even under the best circumstances, *Borrelia burgdorferi* is isolated from the joints of fewer than 20% of patients with Lyme disease. Nonspecific test results, such as increased white blood cell count, decreased glucose, or elevated protein, may indicate that an infectious agent is present but is inconclusive.

Overall, *S. aureus* is the most common etiologic agent of septic arthritis, accounting for approximately 70% of infections. In adults younger than 30 years of age, however, *N. gonorrhoeae* is commonly isolated. *Haemophilus influenzae* has been the most common agent of bacteremia in children younger than 2 years of age; consequently, it has been the most common cause of infectious arthritis in these patients, followed by *S. aureus.* The widespread use of *H. influenzae* type B vaccine has contributed to a change in this pattern. Streptococci, including groups A *(Streptococcus pyogenes)* and B *(Streptococcus agalactiae),* pneumococci, and viridans streptococci, are prominent among bacterial agents associated with infectious arthritis in patients of all ages. Among anaerobic bacteria, *Bacteroides,* including *B. fragilis,* may be recovered as well as *Fusobacterium necrophorum,* which usually involves more than one joint during sepsis. Among people living in certain endemic areas of the United States and Europe, infectious arthritis is a prominent feature associated with Lyme disease. Chronic monoarticular arthritis is commonly caused by mycobacteria, *Nocardia asteroides,* and fungi. Some of the more common etiologic agents of infectious arthritis are listed in Box 76.2.

These agents act to stimulate a host inflammatory response, which is initially responsible for the pathology of the infection. Arthritis is also a symptom associated with infectious diseases caused by certain agents, such as *Neisseria meningitidis,* group A streptococci (rheumatic fever), and *Streptobacillus moniliformis,* in which the agent cannot be recovered from joint fluid. Presumably, antigen-antibody complexes formed during active infection accumulate in a joint, initiating an inflammatory response that is responsible for the ensuing damage.

Infections in prosthetic joints are usually associated with somewhat different etiologic agents than those in natural joints. After insertion of the prosthesis, organisms that gained access during the surgical procedure slowly multiply until they reach a critical mass and produce a host response. This may occur long after the initial surgery; approximately half of all prosthetic joint infections occur more than 1 year after surgery. Normal skin bacteria are the most common etiologic agents, with *S. epidermidis,* other coagulase-negative staphylococci, *Corynebacterium* spp., and *Cutibacterium* spp. being the most prevalent. However, *S. aureus* is also a major pathogen in this infectious disease. Alternatively, organisms may reach joints during hematogenous spread from distant, infected sites.

Arthritis caused by viral agents usually occurs simultaneously with the systemic illness and may be the result of direct entry to the joint or a host immune-mediated response. Viral arthritis is associated with Parvovirus B19, Alphaviruses such as Chikungunya, rubella, hepatitis viruses B and C, HIV-1, and HTLV-1.

Diagnosis of joint infections requires an aspiration of joint fluid for culture and microscopic examination. Inoculating the fluid directly into blood culture bottles may prevent the fluid from clotting. Some of the fluid may be Gram-stained and inoculated onto blood, as well as chocolate and anaerobic media. The use of AFB (acid-fast bacteria) and fungal media must also be considered.

Bone

Bone Marrow Aspiration or Biopsy

Diagnosis of diseases, including brucellosis, histoplasmosis, blastomycosis, tuberculosis and leishmaniasis, can sometimes be made by detection of the organisms in bone marrow. *Brucella* spp. can be isolated on culture media, as can fungi, but parasitic agents must be visualized in smears or sections made from bone marrow material. Bone marrow aspirates are not likely to assist in the identification of most bacterial diseases. Many transplant centers will submit bone marrow aspirates in lysis centrifugation tubes or sterile containers for bacterial culture. If sterile containers are received, the sample should be placed in a blood culture bottle and incubated in the automated instrument. Many of the etiologic agents associated with disseminated infections in patients with human immunodeficiency virus (HIV) may be visualized or isolated from bone marrow. Some of these organisms include cytomegalovirus, *Cryptococcus neoformans,* and *Mycobacterium avium* complex.

Bone Biopsy

A small piece of infected bone is occasionally sent to the microbiology laboratory to identify the etiologic agent of **osteomyelitis** (infection of bone). Patients develop osteomyelitis from hematogenous spread of an infectious agent, invasion of bone tissue from an adjacent site (e.g., joint infection, dental infection), breakdown of tissue caused by trauma or surgery, or lack of adequate circulation followed by colonization of a skin ulceration with microorganisms. Once established, infections in bone may progress toward chronicity, particularly if blood supply is insufficient in the affected area.

S. aureus, seeded during bacteremia, is the most common etiologic agent of osteomyelitis among patients of all age groups. The toxins and enzymes produced by this bacterium, as well as its ability to adhere to smooth surfaces by expressing high-affinity adhesions to components of the bone matrix and producing a protective glycocalyx coating, contribute to the organism's pathogenicity. Osteomyelitis in younger patients is often associated with a single agent. Such infections are usually of hematogenous origin. Other organisms recovered from hematogenously acquired osteomyelitis include coagulase negative staphylococci, *Finegoldia, Salmonella* spp., *Haemophilus* spp., Enterobacterales, *Pseudomonas* spp., *F. necrophorum,* and various fungi. *S. aureus* or *P. aeruginosa* is often recovered from patients with drug addictions. Parasites or viruses are rarely, if ever, etiologic agents of osteomyelitis.

Bone biopsies from infections that have spread to a bone from a contiguous source or that are associated with poor circulation, especially in patients with diabetes, are likely to yield multiple isolates. Gram-negative bacilli are increasingly common among hospitalized patients; a break in the skin (surgery or intravenous line) may precede establishment of gram-negative osteomyelitis. Breaks in skin from other causes, such as a bite wound or trauma, also may be the initial event leading to underlying bone infection. For example, a human bite may lead to infection with *Eikenella corrodens,* whereas an animal bite may result in *Pasteurella multocida* osteomyelitis. Poor oral hygiene may lead to osteomyelitis of the jaw with *Actinomyces* spp., *Capnocytophaga* spp., and other oral microbiota, particularly anaerobes. Pigmented *Prevotella* and *Porphyromonas, Fusobacterium,* and *Finegoldia* spp. are often involved. A pelvic infection in females may result in a mixed aerobic and anaerobic osteomyelitis of the pubic bone.

Patients with neuropathy (pathologic changes in the peripheral nervous system) in the extremities—notably patients with diabetes, who may have poor circulation, may experience an unrecognized or notable trauma. They develop ulcers on the feet that do not heal, become infected, and may eventually progress to involve underlying bone. These infections are usually polymicrobial, involving anaerobic and aerobic bacteria. *Prevotella* or *Porphyromonas,* other gram-negative anaerobes, including the *B. fragilis* group, *Finegoldia* spp., *S. aureus,* and group A and other streptococci are common agents.

Nucleic acid–based testing, such as PCR, is useful in determining the infectious organism associated with the patient's condition and can be used for rapid diagnosis in conjunction with traditional culture.

• BOX 76.3 **Infectious Agents in Tissue Requiring Special Media**

Actinomyces spp.
Brucella spp.
Legionella spp.
Bartonella henselae (cat-scratch disease bacilli)
Systemic fungi
Mycoplasma spp.
Mycobacterium spp.
Viruses

Solid Tissues

Pieces of tissue are removed from patients during surgical or needle biopsy procedures or may be collected at autopsy. Any agent of infection may cause disease in tissue, and laboratory practices should be adequate to recover bacteria, fungi, and viruses and detect the presence of parasites. Fastidious organisms (e.g., *Brucella* spp.) and agents of chronic disease (e.g., systemic fungi and mycobacteria) may require special media and long incubation periods for isolation. Some agents requiring special supportive or selective media are listed in Box 76.3. In addition, some organisms may be visualized using histopathology, such as *Treponema pallidum*, *Klebsiella granulomatous*, or *Spirillum minus*. DNA sequencing and other nucleic acid–based methods are useful in the detection of organisms that cause genital ulcers or organisms that are found in complex biofilms.

Laboratory Diagnostic Procedures

Specimen Collection and Transport

Requirements for the collection and transport of specimens from sterile body sites vary because of the numerous types of specimens that can be collected and submitted to the laboratory for testing. For all specimens, the recommended procedures and transport systems for molecular detect varies and manufacturer directions should be followed accordingly.

Fluids and Aspirates

Most specimens (pleural, peritoneal, pericardial, and synovial fluids) are collected by aspiration with a needle and syringe. Collecting pericardial fluid is not without risk to the patient, because the sample is collected from the cavity immediately adjacent to the heart. Collection is performed by needle aspiration with electrocardiographic monitoring or as a surgical procedure. Laboratory personnel should be alerted in advance of the procedure, ensuring that the appropriate media, tissue culture media, and stain procedures are available immediately.

Body fluids from sterile sites should be transported to the laboratory in a sterile tube or airtight vial. Between 1 and 5 mL of specimen is adequate for isolation of most bacteria,

but the larger the specimen, the better, particularly for isolation of *Mycobacterium tuberculosis* and fungi; at least 5 mL should be submitted for recovery of these organisms. Ten milliliters of fluid are recommended for the diagnosis of peritonitis. Anaerobic transport vials are available from several sources. These vials are prepared in an oxygen-free atmosphere and are sealed with a rubber septum or short stopper through which the fluid is injected. Transportation of fluid in a syringe capped with a sterile rubber stopper is not recommended. Most clinically significant anaerobic bacteria survive adequately in aerobic transport containers (e.g., sterile, screw-capped tubes) for short periods if the specimen is purulent and of adequate volume. However, collection in anaerobic transport media is recommended, and procedures vary in different laboratories. Specimens received in anaerobic transport vials should be inoculated to routine aerobic (an enriched broth, blood, chocolate, and sometimes MacConkey agar plates) and anaerobic media as quickly as possible. Specimens for recovery of fungi or mycobacteria may be transported in sterile, screw-capped tubes. At least 5 to 10 mL of fluid are required for adequate recovery of small numbers of organisms. If gonococci or chlamydia are suspected, additional aliquots should be sent to the laboratory for smears and appropriate cultures.

Percutaneous catheters are placed during many surgical procedures to prevent the accumulation of exudate and blood at the operative site. Often, the laboratory receives drainage fluids from these catheters for culture when signs and symptoms suggest infection. However, culture of such fluid is potentially misleading when the fluid becomes contaminated within the catheter or collection device, or when the fluid does not originate from a site of the infection. Direct aspiration of potentially infected fluid collections, rather than catheter drainage fluid, should be submitted for culture for the assessment of deep tissue infections in patients.

With respect to pericardial, pleural, synovial, and peritoneal fluids, the inoculation of blood culture broth bottles at the bedside or in the laboratory may be beneficial. An additional specimen should be submitted to the laboratory for a Gram stain. The specimen in the blood culture bottle is processed as a blood culture, facilitating the recovery of small numbers of organisms and diluting out the effects of antibiotics. Citrate or sodium polyanetholesulfonate (SPS) may be used as an anticoagulant. Specimens collected by percutaneous needle aspiration (paracentesis) or at the time of surgery should be inoculated into aerobic and anaerobic blood culture bottles as soon as possible.

Fluid from patients receiving CAPD can be submitted to the laboratory in a sterile tube, urine cup, or the original bag. The bag is entered with a sterile needle and syringe to withdraw fluid for culture. Fluid should be directly inoculated into blood culture bottles (20 mL recommended [10 mL in each of two culture bottles]). Numerous studies

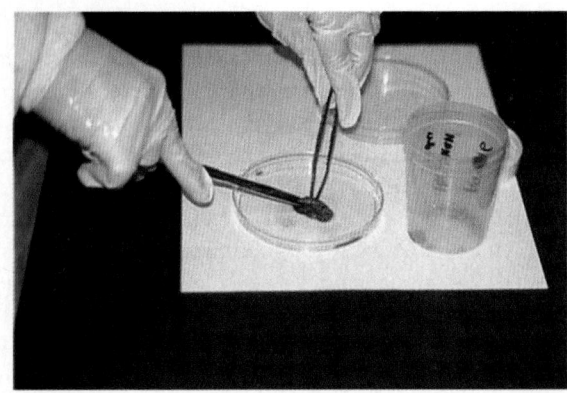

• **Fig. 76.3** Mincing a piece of tissue for culture using sterile forceps and scissors. Note: Perform this procedure in a biosafety cabinet.

indicate that in addition to blood culture bottles, an adult Isolator tube is a sensitive and specific method for culture.

Bone

Bone marrow is typically aspirated from the interstitium of the iliac crest. Usually, this material is not processed for routine bacteria as previously indicated, because blood cultures are equally useful, and false-positive cultures for skin bacteria (*S. epidermidis*) are common. Some laboratories report good recovery from bone marrow material injected into a pediatric Isolator tube (ISOLATOR 1.5 mL, Alere, Waltham, MA) as a collection and transport device. The lytic agents within the Isolator tube are believed to lyse cellular components, presumably freeing intracellular bacteria for enhanced recovery. Bone removed at surgery or by percutaneous biopsy is sent to the laboratory in a sterile container.

Tissue

Tissue specimens are obtained after careful preparation of the skin. It is critical that biopsy specimens be collected aseptically and submitted to the microbiology laboratory in a sterile container; a wide-mouthed, screw-capped bottle or plastic container is recommended. Anaerobic organisms survive within infected tissue long enough to be recovered from culture. A small amount of sterile, nonbacteriostatic saline may be added to keep the specimen moist. Because homogenizing with a tissue grinder can destroy some organisms by the shearing forces generated during grinding, it is often best to use sterile scissors and forceps to mince larger tissue specimens into small pieces suitable for culturing (Fig. 76.3). *Legionella* spp. may be inhibited by saline. A section of lung should be submitted without saline for *Legionella* isolation.

If anaerobic organisms are of concern, a small amount of tissue can be placed into a loosely capped, wide-mouthed plastic tube and sealed into an anaerobic pouch system, which also seals in enough moisture for survival of organisms in tissue until the specimen is plated. The surgeon should take responsibility for seeing that a second specimen is submitted to anatomic pathology for histologic studies.

Formaldehyde-fixed tissue is not useful for recovery of viable microorganisms, although some organisms can be recovered after very short periods of time. Material from draining sinus tracts should include a portion of the tract's wall obtained by deep curettage. Tissue from infective endocarditis should contain a portion of the valve and vegetation if the patient is undergoing valve replacement.

In some cases, contaminated material may be submitted for microbiologic examination. Specimens, such as tonsils or autopsy tissue, may be surface cauterized with a heated spatula or blanched by immersing in boiling water for 5 to 10 seconds to reduce surface contamination. The specimen may then be dissected with sterile instruments to permit culturing of the specimen's center, which will not be affected by the heating. Alternatively, larger tissues may be cut in half with sterile scissors or a blade, and the interior portion cultured for microbes.

Because surgical specimens are obtained at great risk and expense to the patient, and because supplementary specimens cannot be obtained easily, it is important that the laboratory save a portion of the original tissue (if enough material is available) in a small amount of sterile broth in the refrigerator and at –70°C (or, if necessary, at –20°C) for at least 4 weeks in case additional studies are indicated. If the entire tissue must be ground up for culture, a small amount of the suspension should be placed into a sterile tube and refrigerated.

Specimen Processing, Direct Examination, and Culture

Fluids and Aspirates

Techniques for laboratory processing of sterile body fluids are similar except for those previously discussed that are directly inoculated into blood culture bottles. Clear fluids may be concentrated by centrifugation or filtration, whereas purulent material can be inoculated directly to media. A body fluid received in the laboratory that is already clotted must be homogenized to release trapped bacteria and minced or cut to release fungal cells. Either processing of such specimens in a motorized tissue homogenizer or grinding them manually in a mortar and pestle or glass tissue grinder allows better recovery of bacteria. Hand grinding is often preferred, because motorized grinding can generate considerable heat and thereby kill microorganisms in the specimen. Grinding may lyse fungal elements; therefore, it is not recommended with specimens processed for fungi. Small amounts of whole material from a clot should be aseptically cut with a scalpel and placed directly onto media for isolation of fungi.

All fluids should be processed for direct microscopic examination. In general, if one organism is seen per oil immersion field, at least 10^5 organisms per milliliter of specimen are present. Often only a few organisms are present in normally sterile body fluids. Organisms must be concentrated in body fluids. For microscopic examination, cytocentrifugation (Fig. 70.4) should be used to prepare

Gram-stained smears, because organisms can be further concentrated up to 1000-fold. Body fluids should be concentrated by either filtration or high-speed centrifugation. Once the sample is concentrated, the supernatant is aseptically decanted or aspirated with a sterile pipette, leaving approximately 1 mL of liquid in which to thoroughly mix the sediment. Vigorous vortexing or drawing the sediment up and down into a pipette several times is required to adequately suspend the sediment. This procedure should be carried out in a biologic safety cabinet. The suspension is used to inoculate media. Direct potassium hydroxide (KOH) or calcofluor white preparations for fungi, and acid-fast stain for mycobacteria, can also be performed. (See Chapter 6 for detailed descriptions related to the preparation of smears for staining procedures.)

Specimens for fungi should be examined by direct wet preparation or by preparing a separate smear for periodic acid-Schiff (PAS) staining in addition to Gram stain. Either 10% KOH or calcofluor white is recommended for visualization of fungal elements from a wet preparation. In addition to hyphal forms, material from the thoracic cavity may contain spherules of *Coccidioides* or budding yeast cells.

Lysis of leukocytes before concentration of CAPD effluents can significantly enhance recovery of organisms. Filtration of CAPD fluid through a 0.45-mm pore membrane filter allows a greater volume of fluid to be processed and usually yields better results. Because the numbers of infecting organisms may be low (less than one organism per 10 mL of fluid), a large quantity of fluid must be processed. Sediment obtained from at least 50 mL of fluid has been recommended. If the specimen is filtered, the filter should be cut aseptically into three pieces: one of which is placed on chocolate agar for incubation in 5% carbon dioxide, one on MacConkey agar, and the other on a blood agar plate for anaerobic incubation.

If fluids have been concentrated by centrifugation, the resulting sediment should be inoculated to an enrichment broth, blood, and chocolate agars. Because these specimens are from normally sterile sites, selective media are inadvisable, because they may inhibit the growth of some organisms. Appropriate procedures for the isolation of anaerobes, mycobacteria, fungi, *Chlamydia* spp., and viruses should be used when such cultures are clinically indicated.

Bone

Clotted bone marrow aspirates or biopsies must be homogenized or ground to release trapped microorganisms. Specimens are inoculated to the same media as for other sterile body fluids. A special medium for enhancement of growth of *Brucella* spp. and incubation in 10% carbon dioxide may be needed. A portion of the specimen may be inoculated directly to fungal media. Sections are also made from biopsy material (bone) for fixation, staining, and examination (usually by anatomic pathologists) for the presence of mycobacterial, fungal, or parasitic agents. With respect to obtaining specimens from patients suspected of having osteomyelitis, cultures taken from open wound sites above infected bone,

or material taken from a draining sinus leading to an area of osteomyelitis, may not reflect the actual etiologic agent of the underlying osteomyelitis. Cultures of bone samples obtained during wound debridement surgery appear to be more useful for directing antibiotic therapy for better clinical outcome.

Diagnosis of prosthetic (artificial) joint infections is often difficult. Unfortunately, there is no universally accepted definition for the diagnosis of infection in the absence of microbiologic evidence, because clinical symptoms such as pain do not differentiate infection from mechanical joint failure. There is no standardized approach to the laboratory diagnosis of these infections, and published data are conflicting. Further complicating the diagnosis is that the most common bacteria causing prosthesis infections are common skin contaminants such as coagulase-negative staphylococci. Some studies have reported that culture is relatively insensitive, possibly because of the organisms residing in biofilms, whereas PCR assays were able to detect most pathogens associated with prosthetic joint infections. Five or six operative bone specimens should be submitted for culture and three or more should yield the isolation and identification of the same organism for a definite diagnosis of infection. However, a study using PCR and culture using multiple media types and prolonged incubation found that appropriate culture was adequate to exclude bacterial infection in hip prostheses, and PCR did not enhance diagnostic sensitivity for infection.

Normal bone is difficult to break up; however, most infected bone is soft and necrotic. Grinding the specimen in a mortar and pestle may break off some pieces. Small shavings from the most necrotic-looking areas of the bone specimen may sometimes be scraped off aseptically and inoculated onto media. Pieces should be placed directly into media for recovery of fungi. Small bits of bone can be ground with sterile broth to form a suspension for bacteriologic and mycobacterial cultures. If anaerobes are to be recovered, all manipulations are best performed in an anaerobic chamber. If such an environment is unavailable, microbiologists should work quickly within a biosafety cabinet to inoculate prereduced anaerobic plates and broth with material from the bone.

Solid Tissue

Tissue should be manipulated in a laminar flow biologic safety cabinet. Processing tissue within an anaerobic chamber is even better. The microbiologist should cut through the infected area (which is often discolored) with a sterile scalpel blade. Half of the specimen can be used for fungal cultures and the other half for bacterial cultures. Both types of microbial agents should be considered in all tissue specimens. Some samples should also be sent to surgical pathology for histologic examination. Specimens should be processed for viruses or acid-fast bacilli when requested. Material that is to be cultured for parasites should be finely minced or teased before inoculation into broth. Direct examination of stained tissue for parasites is often performed in the anatomic pathology laboratory. Imprint cultures of tissues may yield bacteriologic results identical to homogenates and may help differentiate microbial infection within the tissue's center from surface colonization (growth only at the edge). Additional media can be inoculated for incubation at lower temperatures, which may facilitate recovery of certain systemic fungi and mycobacteria.

Tissue may also be inoculated to tissue culture cells for isolation of viruses. Brain, lung, spinal fluid, and blood are generally good specimens for viral isolation. Tissue may be examined by immunofluorescence for the presence of herpes simplex virus, varicella-zoster virus, cytomegalovirus, or rabies viral particles. Lung tissue should be examined by direct fluorescent antibody test for *Legionella* spp.

The tissues of all fetuses, premature infants, and babies who have died of an infectious process should be cultured for *Listeria*. Specimens of the brain, spinal fluid, blood, liver, and spleen are most likely to contain the organism.

(e) Visit the Evolve site for a complete list of procedures, review questions, and case studies.

Bibliography

Ahmadi SH, Neela V, Hamat RA, et al.: Rapid detection and identification of pathogens in patients with continuous ambulatory peritoneal dialysis (CAPD) associated peritonitis by 16s rRNA gene sequencing, *Trop Biomed* 30(4):602–607, 2013.

Atkins BL, Athanasou N, Deeks JJ, et al.: Prospective evaluation of criteria for microbiological diagnosis of prosthetic-joint infection at revision arthroplasty, *J Clin Microbiol* 36:2932–2939, 1998.

Bennett J, Dolin R, Blaser M: *Principles and practice of infectious diseases*, ed 9, Philadelphia, PA, 2020, Elsevier.

Bourbeau P, Riley J, Heiter BJ, et al.: Use of the BacT/Alert Blood culture system for culture of sterile body fluids other than blood, *J Clin Microbiol* 36:3273–3277, 1998.

Carroll KC, Pfaller MA, Landry ML, et al.: *Manual of clinical microbiology*, ed 12, Washington, DC, 2019, ASM.

Chapin-Robertson K, Dahlberg SE, Edberg SC: Clinical and laboratory analyses of cytospin-prepared Gram stains for recovery and diagnosis of bacteria from sterile body fluids, *J Clin Microbiol* 30:377–380, 1992.

Everts RJ, Heneghan JP, Adholla PO, et al.: Validity of cultures of fluid collected through drainage catheters versus those obtained by direct aspiration, *J Clin Microbiol* 39:66–68, 2001.

Ince A, Rupp J, Frommelt L, et al.: Is "aseptic" loosening of the prosthetic cup after total hip replacement due to nonculturable bacterial pathogens in patients with low-grade infection? *Clin Infect Dis* 39:1599–1603, 2004.

Khatri G, Wagner DK, Sohnle PG: Effect of bone biopsy in guiding antimicrobial therapy for osteomyelitis complicating open wounds, *Am J Med Sci* 321:367–371, 2001.

Kim SH, Jeong HS, Kim YH, et al.: Evaluation of DNA extraction methods and their clinical application for direct detection of causative bacteria in continuous ambulatory peritoneal dialysis culture fluids from patients with peritonitis by using broad-range PCR, *Ann Lab Med* 32(2):119–125, 2012.

Levy PY, Fenollar F: The role of molecular diagnostics in implant-associated bone and joint infection, *Clin Microbiol Infect* 18:1168–1175, 2012.

National Kidney and Urologic Diseases: *Kidney disease statistics for the United States*, 2009.

Runyon B, Antillon MR, Akriviadis EA, et al.: Bedside inoculation of blood culture bottles with ascitic fluid is superior to delayed inoculation in the detection of spontaneous bacterial peritonitis, *J Clin Microbiol* 28:2811–2812, 1990.

Teitelbaum I, Burkart J: Peritoneal dialysis, *Am J Kidney Dis* 42:1082–1096, 2003.

Von Essen R, Holtta A: Improved method of isolating bacteria from joint fluids by the use of blood culture bottle, *Ann Rheum Dis* 45:454–457, 1986.

77

Quality in the Clinical Microbiology Laboratory

OBJECTIVES

1. Distinguish between the terms total quality management (TQM), continuous quality improvement (CQI), performance improvement (PI), quality assurance (QA), LEAN, Six Sigma, and individualized quality control program (IQCP).
2. Describe the quality program associated with the microbiology laboratory.
3. Identify acceptable guidelines for specimen collection and transport and give examples of unacceptable specimens.
4. State the purpose of the Standard Operating Procedure Manual.
5. Explain the requirements for laboratory personnel, use of reference laboratories, and elements of patient reports.
6. Define proficiency testing (PT) and outline the necessary steps to achieve successful results.
7. Design a log to check performance for instruments and media used in the microbiology laboratory.
8. Explain the requirements for antimicrobial susceptibility tests (ASTs).
9. Compare the maintenance of reference-quality control stocks in bacteriology, mycology, mycobacteriology, virology, and parasitology.
10. Outline a QA program for the microbiology laboratory to include all phases of infectious disease diagnosis and differentiate between external and in-house QA audit programs.
11. Describe daily monitoring activities by microbiologists and supervisors that result in providing quality care to the patient population.

Since the publication of the report "To Err is Human" by the Institute of Medicine, the endeavor for a safer and a more efficient health care delivery system has been in full force. The issue of quality in the medical laboratory has evolved over more than four decades after the publication of the recommendations for **quality control (QC)** in 1965. Just as microbial taxonomy has changed over the years, the approach to quality has evolved as well. QC is now seen as only one part of the total laboratory quality program. Quality also includes **total quality management (TQM)**, **continuous quality improvement (CQI) or performance improvement (PI)**, **individualized quality**

control program (IQCP), and **quality assurance** (QA). TQM, CQI, and PI are umbrella terms, encompassing the entire institution's quality program. TQM evolved as an activity to improve patient care by having the laboratory monitor its work to detect deficiencies and subsequently correct them. CQI, IQCP, and PI went a step further by seeking to improve patient care by placing the emphasis on preventing mistakes; CQI, IQCP, and PI advocate continuous training to guard against having to correct deficiencies. IQCP, however, goes one more step further, and allows a laboratory to determine an IQCP that may result in running QC less frequently, as long as the risk assessment demonstrates accuracy and supports the validity of the process.

The **LEAN methodology** concentrates on eliminating redundant motion, recognizing waste, and identifying what creates value from the client's perspective. The main objective for the medical laboratory is to deliver quality patient results at the lowest cost, within the shortest time frame, while maintaining client satisfaction. It involves five principles: value, value stream, flow, pull, and continuous improvement. The first principle is to define the value in the process from the client's perspective, which is what the patient knowingly pays for the attributes of service. Next, the value stream is identified for each process providing that value, challenging the wasted steps, and eliminating them. The next part involves ensuring the service flows continuously through the remaining value-added step. Then, it is all pulled together by introducing a continuous flow of events between all steps of the process where continuous flow is possible. The last principle is continuous improvement through management working toward perfection on an ongoing basis, so the number of steps and time is constantly under scrutiny. The scope of resources and the information needed to provide the service to the client needs to be monitored also. These principles can increase quality, throughput, capacity, and efficiency while decreasing cost, inventory, space, and lead time. Ultimately it will provide better patient care within the clinical laboratory.

Six Sigma is a relatively new concept compared with TQM. Six Sigma originated in 1986 from Motorola's drive to reduce defects by minimizing variation in processes through metrics measurement. The process focuses on CQIs for achieving near perfection by restricting the number of possible defects to fewer than 3.4 defects per million. Six Sigma projects follow a project methodology inspired by Deming's Plan-Do-Study-Act Cycle. The methodology is composed of five phases bearing the acronym **DMAIC:** define, measure, analyze, improve, control. The purpose is to aid in making precise measurements, identifying exact problems, and providing measurable solutions. When implemented correctly, Six Sigma can help organizations reduce operational costs by focusing on reducing defects, minimizing turnaround time, and trimming costs. The main difference between TQM and Six Sigma is the approach. TQM tries to improve quality by ensuring conformance to internal requirements, whereas Six Sigma focuses on improving quality by reducing the number of defects and impurities. Six Sigma is also fact-based, data-driven, and results-oriented, providing quantifiable and measurable bottom-line results, linked to strategy and related to customer requirements.

QC is associated with the internal activities that ensure diagnostic test accuracy. QA is associated with the external activities that ensure positive patient outcomes. Positive patient outcomes in the microbiology laboratory include:
- Reduced length of stay
- Reduced cost of stay
- Reduced turnaround time for diagnosis of infection
- Appropriate antimicrobial therapy
- Customer (physician or patient) satisfaction

CQI and PI, through well-thought-out programs of QC and QA, are part of the requirements for laboratory accreditation under Clinical Laboratory Improvement Amendments (CLIA, 1988).

IQPC provides a mechanism for the laboratory to review the preanalytical, analytical, and postanalytical phases of testing and create an individual QC process unique to the laboratory's testing and environment. An IQPC must include a risk assessment, QC, and quality assessment plan. An IQPC must assess the following:
- Specimen
- Test system
- Reagents
- Environment
- Testing personnel

CLIA does not require any specific types of tools or assessment be utilized if the laboratory demonstrates that the QC plan meets CLIA requirements. The medical laboratory director remains responsible for ensuring that the plan meets CLIA guidelines.

Quality Program

Laboratory quality is defined as accuracy, reliability, and timeliness of reported test results. The laboratory results must be as accurate as possible, all aspects of the laboratory operations must be reliable, and reporting must be timely to be useful in a clinical or public health setting. Each laboratory must establish and maintain written policies and procedures that implement and monitor quality systems for all phases of the total testing process (preanalytical, analytical, and postanalytical), as well as general laboratory systems. The medical laboratory director is primarily responsible for the QC and QA programs. However, all laboratory personnel must actively participate in both programs. Federal guidelines (CLIA, 1988) are considered minimum standards and are superseded by higher standards imposed by individual states or private certifying agencies, such as the College of American Pathologists (CAP) or The Joint Commission (TJC).

Using a set of standards established by the United States military for the manufacture and production of equipment, the International Organization for Standardization (ISO) established standards for industrial manufacturing. The ISO 9000 documents provide guidance for quality in manufacturing and service industries and can be broadly applied to many other kinds of organizations. ISO 9001:2000 addresses general quality management system requirements and applies to laboratories. There are two ISO standards that are specific to laboratories:
- ISO 15189:2007. Medical laboratories—requirements for quality and competence.
- ISO/IEC 17025:2005. General requirements for the competence of testing and calibration laboratories.

Another important international standards organization for laboratories is the Clinical and Laboratory Standards Institute, or CLSI. CLSI uses a consensus process involving many stakeholders for developing standards. CLSI has two documents that are very important in the clinical laboratory:
- QMS14-A: Quality Management System: Leadership and Management Roles and Responsibilities; Approved Guideline.
- QMS01-A4: Quality Management System: A Model for Laboratory Services; Approved Guideline—Fourth Edition.

The basic elements of a QC program are described in the following sections.

Specimen Collection and Transport

The laboratory is responsible for providing written policies and procedures that ensure positive identification and optimum integrity of a patient's specimen, from the time of collection or receipt of the specimen through completion of testing and reporting of results.

These guidelines and instructions should be available to health care providers for use when specimens are collected. The written collection instructions should be in detail and include the following:
- Test purpose and limitations
- Patient selection criteria
- Timing of specimen collection (e.g., before antimicrobials are administered)
- Optimal specimen collection sites
- Approved specimen collection methods
- Specimen transport medium criteria

- Specimen transport time and temperature
- Specimen holding instructions if it cannot be transported immediately (e.g., hold at 4°C for 24 hours)
- Minimum acceptable volume requirements where applicable
- Availability of test (onsite or sent to reference laboratory)
- Turnaround time
- Result reporting procedures

The collection instructions should include information on how a requisition should be filled out electronically or by hand, and the laboratory must include a statement indicating that the requisition must be filled out entirely. In addition to standard information, such as patient name, hospital or laboratory number, and ordering physician, other critical information includes (1) whether the patient is receiving antimicrobial therapy, (2) the suspect agent or syndrome, (3) immunization history (if applicable), and (4) travel history when certain microorganisms or parasites are suspected. The laboratory should also establish criteria for unacceptable specimens. Examples of unacceptable specimens include the following:

- Unlabeled, mislabeled, or incompletely labeled specimens
- Quantity not sufficient for testing (QNS)
- Use of an improper transport medium, such as stool for ova and parasites not submitted in preservative(s)
- Use of improper swab, such as use of wooden shaft or calcium alginate tip for viruses
- Inappropriate handling of specimen with respect to temperature, timing, or storage requirements
- Improper collection site for test requested, such as stool for respiratory syncytial virus
- Specimen leakage from transport container
- Sera excessively hemolyzed, lipemic, or contaminated with bacteria

The rejected specimen will be logged electronically or manually. A rejection of specimen report will be sent to the ordering clinician. The rejected specimens will not be returned. Sometimes, specimens not meeting the requirements may be accepted by the laboratory if the specimen is irretrievable or it has been acquired through an invasive procedure. If this happens, approval by the ordering physician and laboratory director must be secured with a disclaimer on the final report, indicating that the specimen was not collected properly, and the results should be interpreted with caution.

Standard Operating Procedure Manual

The requirement for a Standard Operating Procedure Manual (SOPM) is considered part of the QC program. The SOPM should define test performance, tolerance limits, reagent preparation, required QC, result reporting, and references. The SOPM should be written in the format of CLSI and must be reviewed and signed annually or biannually by the medical laboratory director who appears on the CLIA certificate; in addition, all changes must be approved and dated by the laboratory director. The SOPM

should be available in the work areas. It is the definitive laboratory reference and is used often for questions related to individual tests. Any obsolete procedure should be dated when removed from the SOPM and retained for at least 2 years.

Personnel

It is the medical laboratory director's responsibility to employ sufficient qualified personnel for the volume and complexity of the work performed. For example, published studies regarding staffing of virology laboratories suggest one technologist per 500 to 1000 specimens per year. Technical on-the-job training must be documented, and the employee's competency must be assessed twice in the first year and annually thereafter. Continuing education programs should be provided, and verification of attendance should be maintained in the employee's personnel file. CLIA has improved the regulations associated with personnel competency (CLIA subpart K:493.1235). Laboratory employee competency assessment must include the following: (1) Direct observation of test performance, to include patient preparation (if applicable), specimen handling, processing, and testing; (2) monitoring the recording and reporting of test results; (3) review of intermediate test results or work sheets, QC results, patient results, and preventative maintenance records; (4) direct observation of performance or instrument maintenance and function checks; (5) assessment of test performance through testing previously analyzed specimens and internal blind testing of samples or external patient samples; and (6) assessment of problem-solving skills. These competency assessments must be documented and completed by qualified personnel.

Reference Laboratories

Not all testing can be completed in one facility. A laboratory test that cannot be performed in-house and needs to be sent somewhere else is considered a reference laboratory test. The reference laboratory is a separate entity from the facility that collects and sends the specimen. It must be accredited or licensed. The referral laboratory's name, address, and licensure numbers should be included on the patient's final report.

Patient Reports

There should be an established system for supervisory review of all laboratory reports. This review involves checking the specimen workup to verify that the correct conclusions were reached, and no clerical errors were made in reporting results. Reports should be released only to individuals authorized by law to receive them (physicians and various midlevel practitioners). Clinicians should be notified about "panic values" immediately. Panic values are potentially life-threatening results; for example, positive Gram stain for cerebrospinal fluid (CSF) or a positive blood culture. Reference ranges must be included on the report where appropriate. All patient records should be maintained for at least 2 years. However, maintaining records for at least 10 years may be needed to support medical necessity in the event of a postpayment billing audit by the Centers for Medicare and Medicaid Services.

Proficiency Testing

Proficiency testing (PT) is a QA measure used to monitor the laboratory's analytical performance compared with its peers and reference standards. It provides an external validation tool and objective evidence of the laboratory competence for patients, as well as accrediting and oversight agencies. Laboratories are required to participate in a PT program for each analyte (test) for which a program is available; the laboratory must maintain an average score of 80% to maintain licensure in any subspecialty area. If a new regulated analyte is added, the medical laboratory must contact the PT agency to add that analyte as soon as possible. Laboratories must remain enrolled in the same PT program for one year before changing to a different program. The federal government no longer maintains a PT program, but some states, such as New York—as well as several private accrediting agencies, such as CAP—send out "blind unknowns." These unknowns are to be treated exactly as patient specimens, from accessioning into the laboratory computer or manual logbook through workup and reporting of results. The testing personnel and medical laboratory director are required to sign a statement when the PT is completed attesting to the fact that the specimen was handled exactly like a patient specimen. In this way, PT specimens establish the accuracy and reproducibility of a laboratory's day-to-day performance. The laboratory's procedures, reagents, equipment, and personnel are all checked in the process. Furthermore, errors on PT help point out deficiencies, and the subsequent education of the staff can lead to overall improvements in laboratory quality. When scores (evaluations) come back, critiques accompanying them should be discussed with the entire technical staff. Evidence of corrective action in the event of problems should be documented, including changes in procedures, retraining of personnel, or the purchase of alternative media and reagents.

Some laboratories have a system of internal PT in addition to those received from external agencies. When external audit is not available for a testing method, laboratories are required by law to set up an internal program to revalidate the test, at least semiannually. Internal PT samples can be set up by (1) seeding a simulated specimen and labeling it as an autopsy specimen so that no one panics if a pathogen is recovered, (2) splitting a routine specimen for workup by two different technologists, or (3) sending part of a specimen to a reference laboratory to compare and confirm the laboratory's result.

Performance Checks

Instruments

Instruments and equipment logs should contain the following information:
- Instrument name, serial number, and date of implementation in the laboratory.
- Procedure and periodicity of function checks with at least the frequency specified by the manufacturer; function checks must be within the manufacturer's established limits before patient testing is conducted.
- Acceptable performance ranges.
- Instrument function failures, including specific details of steps taken to correct the problems (corrective action).
- Date and time of service requests and response.
- Maintenance records as defined and with at least the minimum frequency specified by the manufacturer.

In addition, with the advances in technology, some instruments have on-board controls that are intended to be the same procedure as using external QC material. If the material represents a similar matrix to the patient samples, and the material goes through the exact same testing procedure, the on-board controls may be used to satisfy the previous need for external QC. It is the medical laboratory director's responsibility to ensure that the material used meets all regulatory requirements.

Instrument maintenance records should be retained in the laboratory for the life of the instrument. Specific guidelines regarding the periodicity of testing for autoclaves, biologic safety cabinets, centrifuges, incubators, microscopes, refrigerators, freezers, water baths, heat blocks, and other microbiology laboratory equipment can be found in a few of the references listed at the end of this chapter.

Commercially Prepared Media Exempt From Quality Control

The CLSI Subcommittee on Media Quality Control collected data over several years regarding the incidence of QC failures of commonly used microbiology media. Based on its findings, the subcommittee published a list of media that did not require retesting in the user's laboratory if purchased from a manufacturer who follows CLSI guidelines. The laboratory must inspect each shipment for cracked media or Petri dishes, hemolysis, freezing, unequal filling, excessive bubbles, clarity, and visible contamination. The manufacturer must supply written assurance that CLSI standards were followed; this verification must be maintained along with the laboratory's QC protocol.

User-Prepared and Nonexempt, Commercially Prepared Media

QC forms for user-prepared media should contain the amount prepared, the source of each ingredient, the lot number, the sterilization method, the preparation date, the expiration date (usually 1 month for agar plates and 6 months for tubed media), and the name of the preparer. Both user-prepared and nonexempt, commercially prepared media should be checked for proper color, consistency, depth, smoothness, hemolysis, excessive bubbles, and contamination. A representative sample of the lot should be tested for sterility; 5% of any lot is tested when a batch of 100 or fewer units is received, and a maximum of 10 units are tested in larger batches. A batch is any one shipment of a product with the same lot number; if a separate shipment of the same lot number of a product is received, then it is considered a different batch and needs to be tested separately.

Sterility is examined by incubating the medium for 48 hours under the environmental conditions and temperature routine used within the laboratory. Both user-prepared and nonexempt, commercially prepared media should also be tested with QC organisms of known physiologic and biochemical properties. Tables listing specific organisms to test for various media can be found in a few of the references listed at the end of this chapter.

Antimicrobial Susceptibility Tests

The goal of QC testing of antimicrobial susceptibility tests (ASTs) is to ensure the precision and accuracy of both the supplies and the microbiologists performing the test. The laboratory must check each lot number and shipment of antimicrobial agent(s) before, or concurrent with, initial use, using approved control organisms. Criteria regarding frequency of testing are the same regardless of the methodology, such as minimum inhibitory concentration (MIC) broth dilution or Kirby-Bauer (Chapter 11). Each new shipment of microdilution trays or Mueller-Hinton plates should be tested with CLSI-approved American Type Culture Collection (ATCC [Rockville, MD]) reference strains.

Reference strains for MIC testing are selected for genetic stability and give MICs within the midrange of each antimicrobial agent tested. Reference strains for Kirby-Bauer testing have clearly defined mean diameters for the respective zone of inhibition for each antimicrobial tested. ATCC numbers of reference strains are different for various AST methods. QC MICs and zone diameters are annually updated and published by the CLSI Subcommittee on Antimicrobial Susceptibility Testing. New tables should be obtained from the CLSI regularly.

Each susceptibility test system must also be tested with use (usually daily) for 20 consecutive days. If three or fewer MICs or zone of inhibition diameters per drug-reference strain combination are outside the reference range during the 20-day testing period, laboratories may switch to weekly QC testing. Thereafter, aberrant results obtained during the weekly testing must be vigorously investigated. If a source of error, such as contamination, incorrect reference strain used, or incorrect atmosphere of incubation is found, QC testing may simply be repeated. However, if no source of error is uncovered, 5 consecutive days of retesting must be

performed. If accuracy and precision are again acceptable, weekly QC testing may resume; if the problem drug/organism combinations are still outside the reference ranges, 20 days of consecutive testing must be reinitiated before weekly testing can be reinstated. Under no circumstances should any drug/organism combination be reported for a patient isolate if QC testing has failed.

Stains and Reagents

Containers of stains and reagents should be labeled as to contents, concentration, storage requirements, date prepared (or received), date placed in service (commonly called the "date opened"), expiration date, source (commercial manufacturer or user prepared), and lot number. All stains and reagents should be stored according to the manufacturer's recommendations and tested with positive and negative controls before use. Tables listing specific organisms to test for various stains or reagents can be found in several references at the end of this chapter. Outdated materials or reagents that fail QC even after retesting with fresh organisms should be discarded immediately. Patient specimens should not be tested using the lot number in question until the problem is resolved; in the case of a repeat failure, an alternative method should be used, or the patient's specimen should be sent to a reference laboratory.

Antisera

The lot number, date received, condition received, and expiration date must be recorded for all shipments of antisera. In addition, the antisera should be dated when opened. New lots must be tested concurrently with previous lots, and testing must include positive and negative controls. Periodicity of testing thereafter should follow the requirements of agencies that inspect an individual laboratory and may include with use, monthly, or semiannual checks.

Kits

Kits that have been approved by the US Food and Drug Administration (FDA) need to be tested as specified in the manufacturer's package insert. Each shipment of kits must be tested even if it is the same lot number as a previously tested lot, because temperature changes during shipment may affect the performance. Components of reagent kits of different lot numbers must not be interchanged unless otherwise specified by the manufacturer.

Maintenance of Quality Control Records

All QC results should be recorded and, when applicable, must include a review of the effectiveness of corrective actions taken to resolve problems, revision of policies and procedures necessary to prevent recurrence of problems, and discussion with appropriate staff. If temperature is adjusted or a biochemical test is repeated, the new readings within the tolerance limits should be listed. In many laboratories, the supervisor reviews and initials all forms weekly; the director then reviews each one monthly. QC records should be maintained for at least 2 years, except those on equipment, which must be saved for the life of each instrument.

Maintenance of Reference Quality Control Stocks

Stock organisms may be obtained from the ATCC, commercial vendors, or PT programs; well-defined clinical isolates may also be used. The laboratory should have enough organisms on hand to cover the full range of testing of all necessary materials, such as media, kits, and reagents.

Bacteriology

Nonfastidious, aerobic bacterial organisms can be saved up to 1 year on trypticase soy agar (TSA) slants. Long-term storage (less than 1 year) of aerobes or anaerobes can be accomplished either by lyophilization (freeze drying) or freezing at –70°C. Frozen, nonfastidious organisms should be thawed, re-isolated, and refrozen every 5 years; fastidious organisms should be thawed, re-isolated, and refrozen every 3 years. Stock isolates may be maintained by freezing them in 10% skim milk; trypticase soy broth (TSB) with 15% glycerol; 10% horse blood in sterile, screw-cap vials; or the Microbank commercially available system (Pro Lab Diagnostics, Round Rock, TX).

Mycology

Yeasts may be treated as nonfastidious bacterial organisms for maintaining stock cultures. Molds can be stored on potato dextrose agar (PDA) slants at 4°C for 6 months to 1 year. For longer-term storage, PDA slants may be overlaid with sterile mineral oil and stored at room temperature. Alternatively, sterile water can be added to an actively sporulating culture on PDA, the conidia (spores) can be teased apart to dislodge them from the agar surface, and the water can then be dispensed to sterile, screw-top vials. These vials should be capped tightly and stored at room temperature.

Mycobacteriology

Acid-fast bacilli (AFB) may be kept on Lowenstein-Jenson (LJ) agar slants at 4°C for up to 1 year. They may also be frozen at –70°C in 7H9 broth with glycerol.

Virology

Viruses may be stored indefinitely at –70°C in a solution containing a cryoprotectant, such as 10% dimethyl sulfoxide (DMSO) or fetal bovine serum.

Parasitology

Slides and photographs must be available for QC purposes. Trichrome and other permanent slides may be purchased from commercial vendors. Clinical slides may be preserved indefinitely by adding a drop of Permount and a coverslip. Clinical slides prepared in-house should be inspected periodically, because the preservation solution may deteriorate and crack over time.

Quality Assurance Program

Because QA is the method by which the overall process of infectious disease diagnosis is reviewed, any of the steps involved in the diagnosis of an infectious disease may be studied. These steps include the following phases:
- Preanalytical Phase
  - Ordering of test by the clinician
  - Processing of test by the clinician
  - Processing of test request by the clerical staff
  - Collection of specimen by health care providers or patients
  - Transport of specimen to the laboratory
  - Initial processing of specimen in the laboratory, including specimen accessioning
- Analytical Phase
  - Examination and workup of culture by the microbiologist
  - Interpretation of specimen results by the microbiologist
- Postanalytical Phase
  - Formulation of a written or printed report by the microbiologist
  - Communication of the microbiologist's conclusions to the clinician in written or printed format
  - Interpretation of report by the clinician
  - Institution of appropriate therapy by the clinician

Analytical testing (the work completed in the microbiology laboratory) is now seen as only one part of a continuing spectrum of steps that begins when the physician orders the test and ends when he or she receives the results and treats the patient.

QA audits are planned and conducted by examining the three phases of testing. The goal is to look at the proficiency with which the patient is served by the whole facility, including the laboratory. The outcome is to look at the consequences to the patient based on the work that was performed. QA audits involve an analysis of how the system works and how it can be improved.

Types of Quality Assurance Audits

One way to conduct a QA audit is for the laboratory to subscribe to an external interlaboratory QA program. Topics to be audited are selected nationally. Data are then collected for a specified period and then returned to the program provider for analysis. A summary is compiled and returned to the institution with a comparison with other facilities of similar size and scope of service. That way, an individual facility can compare its results with those of its peers, a process called **benchmarking.** QA audits in microbiology may include areas such as (1) blood culture use, (2) health care–associated infections, (3) cumulative susceptibility results, (4) antibiotic usage, (5) turnaround time for CSF Gram stains, (6) viral hepatitis test use, (7) laboratory diagnosis of tuberculosis, (8) blood culture contamination rates, (9) appropriateness of the ordering of stools for microbiology testing, and (10) sputum quality. Other laboratory-wide audits are also applicable to the microbiology laboratory, including error reporting, quality of reference laboratories, and effects of laboratory computer downtime. A facility that does not subscribe to an external program may select topics for audits through suggestions from the medical, nursing, or pharmacy staff; complaints from the medical or nursing staff; or deficiencies and/or observations noted in the laboratory.

Physicians may suggest an audit to measure the transcription accuracy of their orders by nursing unit clerical personnel. Nursing administrators may suggest an audit of contaminated urine cultures to assess the compliance of the nursing staff in instructing patients about proper urine culture collection techniques. Pharmacists may notice improper antibiotic use by the clinical staff—for example, a patient was not placed on the appropriate therapy after the pathogen was reported or the patient remains on antibiotic therapy to which his or her organism is resistant after the susceptibility report has been charted. Complaints from the medical or nursing staff can involve failure of the laboratory to conduct all the tests requested on the requisition, performance of the wrong test, or an unexpected delay in turnaround time of test results. All complaints to the laboratory must be documented. Corrective action and follow-up with the laboratory, medical, and nursing staff must also be documented.

Deficiencies or problems in the laboratory's performance should also be documented. If, for example, the laboratory notices a dramatic and unseasonable rise in the number of positive respiratory syncytial virus (RSV) direct antigen tests in the summer, and the problem is traced back to a QC problem that a new employee did not recognize, a QA audit might be indicated to study the outcome of the patients, including inappropriate treatment for RSV and failure to institute treatment for the true causative agent. Alternatively, microbiologists may notice they are receiving many ova and parasite (O&P) examinations and stool cultures on patients hospitalized for more than 3 days. Because current cost containment guidelines suggest that this is inappropriate, the microbiology laboratory personnel could undertake a study to determine the percentage of positive results and the number of patients who tested positive for *Clostridiodes difficile* cytotoxin, which is the more likely cause of diarrhea in patients hospitalized for more than 3 days. If the audit showed that none of the stool cultures or O&P examinations tested positive and no stools were analyzed for

C. difficile cytotoxin, then these findings would be presented to the medical staff. Some months after the medical staff in-service, the number of stool culture and O&P requests on patients hospitalized longer than 3 days would be reevaluated in the hope of a dramatic decrease in numbers of inappropriate tests.

Conducting a Quality Assurance Audit

Box 77.1 is an example of how an in-house QA audit may be conducted.

Continuous Daily Monitoring

Daily activities of microbiologists and supervisory personnel ensure that patients get the best quality care. These activities include (1) comparing results of morphotypes seen on direct examinations with what grows on the culture to ensure that all organisms have been recovered, (2) checking antimicrobial susceptibility reports to verify that profiles match those expected from a species, and (3) studying culture and susceptibility reports for clusters of patients with unusual infections or multidrug-resistant organisms. These and many other processes result in continual improvement to all test systems, ultimately resulting in quality patient care.

ⓔ Visit the Evolve site for a complete list of procedures, review questions, and case studies.

Bibliography

Anderson NL, Noble MA, Weissfeld AS, et al.: Quality systems in the clinical microbiology laboratory. In Sewell DL, coordinating, editors: *Cumitech 3B*, Washington, DC, 2005, ASM Press.

Centers for Medicare and Medicaid Services. *CLIA IQCP, What is an IQCP?* Accessed July 6, 2016. Available at: https://www.cms.gov/Regulations-and-Guidance/Legislation/CLIA/Downloads/CLIAbrochure13.pdf.

Clinical and Laboratory Standards Institute: *Quality management system: leadership and management roles and responsibilities; approved guideline QMS14-A*, Wayne, PA, 2015, Clinical and Laboratory Standards Institute.

Clinical and Laboratory Standards Institute: *Quality management system: a model for laboratory services; approved guideline QMS01-A4 — fourth edition*, Wayne, PA, 2015, Clinical and Laboratory Standards Institute.

Clinical and Laboratory Standards Institute: *Methods for dilution antimicrobial susceptibility tests for bacteria that grow aerobically; approved standard M7-A10*, Wayne, PA, 2015, Clinical and Laboratory Standards Institute.

Clinical and Laboratory Standards Institute: *Performance standards for antimicrobial disk susceptibility tests; approved standard M2-A12*, Wayne, PA, 2015, Committee for Clinical and Laboratory Standards Institute.

Clinical Laboratory Improvement Amendments (CLIA) Regulations. *Subpart K.* 2011;493:1235.

• BOX 77.1   **Quality Assurance Audit on STAT[a] Turnaround Times**

Background

After a complaint regarding turnaround time for STAT RSV direct antigen tests one winter, the microbiology laboratory at General Hospital has decided to audit its turnaround time. The medical staff indicated that it would like to turn the test around in 2.5 h (150 min) from the time of collection to the time the physician is notified; the medical staff feels that this will ensure the maximum patient benefits.

Study Design

All RSV requests for direct antigen testing were evaluated for a 3-month period to determine whether laboratory personnel were meeting this turnaround time.

Results

Month	REPORTS GIVEN IN <150 MINUTES		REPORT TIME EXCEEDING 150 MINUTES		COMBINED AVERAGES	
	Number of Specimens	Average Time	Number of Specimens	Average Time	Number of Specimens	Average Time
December	57	114 min	15	195 min	72	130 min
January	114	108 min	14	179 min	128	116 min
February	70	114 min	3	165 min	73	116 min

Analysis

In all, 273 reports were reviewed. The average reporting time for the 3-month period was under the acceptable 150 min. In December and January, 15 and 14 specimens, respectively, had turnaround times that exceeded 150 minutes, with an average of 195 min in December and 179 min in January; in February, 3 reports exceeded 150 min.

Conclusions

The overall (combined) average reporting time, although remaining within 150 min, could be improved. There was a dramatic drop in February after the medical staff complaint. This was undoubtedly a result of in-services given to courier and clerical staff regarding the need to transport and accession the STAT specimens quickly.

Recommendations

Because hospital-wide systems have been improved, appropriate follow-up would be to audit the STAT turnaround time for another test—for example, Gram stain of cerebrospinal fluid—in 3 to 6 months to verify that it also meets the 150-min turnaround time requirement.

[a]"Immediately"; derived from Latin *statim*.
RSV, Respiratory syncytial virus.

Daly DA: Quality assurance, quality control, laboratory records, and water quality. In Garcia LS, editor: *Clinical microbiology procedure handbook*, ed 3, Washington, DC, 2010, ASM Press.

International Organization for Standardization: *Medical laboratories—particular requirements for quality and competence; ISO 15189:2012(E)*, Geneva, Switzerland, 2012, International Organization for Standardization.

Leber AL: *Clinical microbiology procedure handbook*, ed 4, Washington, DC, 2016, ASM Press.

National Committee for Clinical Laboratory Standards: *Assessment of laboratory tests when proficiency testing is not available; approved guideline GP29-A2*, Wayne, PA, 2008, National Committee for Clinical Laboratory Standards.

National Committee for Clinical Laboratory Standards: *Assessments: laboratory internal audit program; approved guideline QMS15-A*, Wayne, PA, 2013, National Committee for Clinical Laboratory Standards.

National Committee for Clinical Laboratory Standards: *Development and use of quality indicators for process improvement and monitoring of laboratory quality; approved guideline QMS12-A*, Wayne, PA, 2010, National Committee for Clinical Laboratory Standards.

National Committee for Clinical Laboratory Standards: *Development of in vitro susceptibility testing criteria and quality control parameters; approved guideline M23-A3*, Wayne, PA, 2008, National Committee for Clinical Laboratory Standards.

National Committee for Clinical Laboratory Standards: *Methods for antimicrobial susceptibility testing of anaerobic bacteria; approved standard M11-A8*, Wayne, PA, 2012, National Committee for Clinical Laboratory Standards.

National Committee for Clinical Laboratory Standards: *Quality assurance for commercially prepared microbiological culture media; approved standard M22-A3*, Wayne, PA, 2004, National Committee for Clinical Laboratory Standards.

National Committee for Clinical Laboratory Standards: *Quality control of microbiological transport systems; approved standard M40-A2*, Wayne, PA, 2014, National Committee for Clinical Laboratory Standards.

National Committee for Clinical Laboratory Standards: *Quality management system: a model for laboratory services; approved guideline*

QMS01-A4, Wayne, PA, 2011, National Committee for Clinical Laboratory Standards.

National Committee for Clinical Laboratory Standards: *Quality management system: continual improvement; approved guideline QMS06-A3*, Wayne, PA, 2011, National Committee for Clinical Laboratory Standards.

National Committee for Clinical Laboratory Standards: *Quality management system: development and management of laboratory documents; approved guideline QMS02-A6*, Wayne, PA, 2013, National Committee for Clinical Laboratory Standards.

National Committee for Clinical Laboratory Standards: *Quality management system: qualifying, selecting, and evaluating a referral laboratory; approved guideline QMS05-A2*, Wayne, PA, 2012, National Committee for Clinical Laboratory Standards.

National Committee for Clinical Laboratory Standards: *Training and competence assessment; approved guideline QMS03-A3*, Wayne, PA, 2009, National Committee for Clinical Laboratory Standards.

National Committee for Clinical Laboratory Standards: *Using proficiency testing (PT) to improve the clinical laboratory; approved guideline GP27-A2*, Wayne, PA, 2007, National Committee for Clinical Laboratory Standards.

U.S. Department of Health and Human Services: Medicare, Medicaid and CLIA programs: regulations implementing the clinical laboratory improvement amendments of 1988 (CLIA). Final rule, *Fed Regist* 57:7002–7186, 1992.

Westgard S. *Quality Management Cocktail ISO, Lean, and Six Sigma*. Accessed July 6, 2016. Available at: www.westgard.com.

78

Infection Control

OBJECTIVES

1. Define and compare health care–associated infections and community-acquired infections.
2. List three factors that determine the likelihood that a given patient would acquire a health care–associated infection.
3. State the most common types of health care–associated infections and identify the risk factors that predispose patients to acquire each infection.
4. Explain the emergence of antibiotic-resistant microorganisms and their impact on health care.
5. Describe hospital infection control programs and outline the structure and responsibilities of the infection control committee in a medical facility.
6. Identify the means of transmission for microorganisms within a health care facility.
7. Interpret the role of the microbiology laboratory in an infectious disease outbreak.
8. Compare the two major ways to characterize microorganism strains involved in an outbreak.
9. Discuss techniques for isolation precautions used to prevent the spread of health care–associated infections.
10. Identify potential useful applications for surveillance cultures.
11. Explain the contribution of the environment to health care–associated and community-associated infections. In your explanation, discuss the importance of a multimodal approach to reducing these infections.
12. Discuss the role of federal influences on state-level health care–associated infections program initiatives and reporting activities.
13. Identify health care worker infection and illness reporting mandates.

It is estimated that between 1.75 and 3 million (5% to 10%) of the 35 million patients admitted annually to acute-care hospitals in the United States acquire an infection that was neither present nor in the prodromal (incubation) stage when they entered the hospital. These infections are called **health care–associated infections (HAIs).** HAI has replaced old confusing terms such as nosocomial, hospital-acquired, or hospital-onset infections. Treatment of HAI is estimated to add between $4.5 and $15 billion annually to the cost of health care and represents an enormous economic problem in today's environment of cost containment. The societal cost of HAIs in acute-care hospitals in the United States has been estimated at $96 to

$147 billion per year. In addition, many of these infections lead to the death of hospitalized patients (patient mortality) or, at minimum, additional complications (patient morbidity) and further antimicrobial chemotherapy.

Some of the earliest efforts to control infection followed the recognition in the 19th century that women were dying in childbirth from bloodstream infections caused by group A streptococcus *(Streptococcus pyogenes)* because physicians were spreading the organism by failing to wash their hands between examinations of different patients. Hand washing is still a key component of a modern **multimodal infection control** program. Moreover, the first recommendations for isolation precautions in US hospitals were published in the late 1800s, when guidelines appeared advocating placement of patients with infectious diseases in separate hospital facilities. By the late 1950s, the advent of HAI caused by *Staphylococcus aureus* finally ushered in the modern age of infection control. In the past four decades, we have learned that, in addition to hospitalized patients acquiring infections, health care workers (HCWs) are also at risk of acquiring infections from patients. Thus, present-day infection control and prevention programs have evolved to prevent the acquisition of infection by patients and caregivers. To be successful, a multimodal approach must be supported by the hospital administration (the C-suite) and involve all departments on an enterprise-wide basis.

In contrast, **community-acquired infection** is an infection contracted outside a health care setting or an infection present on admission. Community-acquired infections are often distinguished from HAIs by the types of organisms that affect patients who are recovering from a disease or infection. Community-acquired respiratory infections commonly involve strains of *Haemophilus influenzae* or *Streptococcus pneumoniae* and are usually more sensitive to antibiotic treatment.

The American Recovery and Reinvestment Act of 2009 was signed into law on February 17, 2009. The Recovery Act was designed to stimulate economic recovery in various ways, including strengthening the nation's health care infrastructure and reducing health care costs. Within the Recovery Act, $50 million was authorized to support states in the prevention and reduction of HAI. For example, 2014 funding supported state HAI infrastructure; antimicrobial stewardship; prevention of *Clostridioides difficile,* carbapenem-resistant Enterobacterales (CRE), and hemodialysis bloodstream infections; HAI data validation; and promotion of safe injection practices. Many have considered the federal funding a critical resource for the development and proper functioning of state HAI programs.

Usually HAI data reporting occurs on the state level, but federal reporting requirements also exist. Federal reporting of HAIs by hospitals is required under the Centers for Medicare and Medicaid Services (CMS) Inpatient Quality Reporting Program (IQR Program). The IQR Program, which began in 2010, was developed under the Medicare Prescription Drug, Improvement and Modernization Act of 2003. The Deficit Reduction Act added new requirements. Medicare-certified facilities ("subsection (d)" hospitals) are required to submit data on specific quality measures, including HAIs, to receive full reimbursement. The CMS has set a goal of reducing HAI conditions by 20% from 2014 through 2019. To reach its goal, CMS is assisting many hospitals through Hospital Improvement Innovation Networks. The networks collaborate with federal agencies, private partners, and patient advocacy organizations to make hospital care safer. Consequently, HAIs continued to decline according to the latest national scorecard released by the Agency for Healthcare Research and Quality (AHRQ). The overall rate decreased dramatically from 2010 through 2016, resulting in fewer deaths and significant cost savings. However, rates of certain HAI conditions, such as pressure ulcers, rose in recent years.

Incidence of Health Care–Associated Infections

The Centers for Disease Control and Prevention (CDC) has established the National Healthcare Safety Network (NHSN) program to monitor the incidence of HAI in the United States. Data collected in NHSN are used to improve patient safety at the local and national levels. In aggregate, the CDC analyzes and publishes surveillance data to estimate and characterize the national burden of HAIs. Regardless of a hospital's size or medical school affiliation, the rates of infections at each body site are consistent across institutions. The system currently serves more than 13,000 medical facilities. The CDC plans on expanding the NHSN to more than 17,000 facilities. As part of that plan, the CDC will continue its efforts to work with state and local health departments to assist with NHSN data collection and implementation of prevention strategies.

Facilities participating in the IQR Program are required to use the NHSN for reporting HAI data. Hospitals must enroll in the program and complete NHSN training to comply with these federal regulations. After HAI data are collected, they are publicly reported on a federal website called Hospital Compare.

Most HAIs are urinary tract infections (UTIs; 33%), followed by pneumonia (15%), surgical site infections (15%), and bloodstream infections (13%). The remaining 24% are other miscellaneous infections. On average, each HAI adds 5 to 10 days to the affected patient's hospital stay. Of individuals with hospital-acquired bloodstream or lung infections, 40% to 60% die each year. Likewise, patients with indwelling urinary catheters have a threefold increased chance of dying from urosepsis—a bloodstream infection that is a complication of a UTI—than those who do not have one.

Infection rates vary according to hospital type. Large, tertiary-care hospitals that treat the most seriously ill patients often have higher rates of HAI than do small, acute-care community hospitals; large medical school–affiliated (teaching) hospitals have higher infection rates than do small teaching hospitals. This difference in the risk of infection is probably related to several factors, including but not limited to the severity of illness, the frequency of invasive diagnostic and therapeutic procedures, and variation in the effectiveness of infection control programs. Within hospitals, the surgical and medical services have the highest rates of infection, whereas the pediatric and nursery services have the lowest. Moreover, within services, the predominant type of infections varies—that is, surgical site infections are the most common on the surgical service, whereas urinary tract or bloodstream infections are the most common on medical services or in the nursery.

Types of Health Care–Associated Infections

Most HAIs are endogenous in origin—that is, they involve the patient's own microbiota. Three principal factors determine the likelihood that a given patient will acquire an infection:

- Susceptibility to infection and/or immune status of the patient
- The virulence of the infecting organism
- The nature of the patient's exposure to the infecting organism

In general, hospitalized individuals have increased susceptibility to infection. Corticosteroids, cancer chemotherapeutic agents, and antimicrobial agents all contribute to the likelihood of HAI by suppressing the immune system or altering the host's normal microbiota to that of resistant microbes. Likewise, foreign objects, such as urinary or intravenous catheters, impair or physically circumvent the body's natural barriers to infection. Nonetheless, these medications or devices are necessary to cure the patient's primary medical condition. Finally, exerting influence over the virulence of the pathogens is not possible because it is not possible to immunize patients against HAI. Patients with serious community-acquired infections are commonly admitted to the hospital, and the disease may spread by either direct contact; by contact with contaminated food, water, medications, or medical devices (fomites); or by airborne transmission. Thus, the HAI may never be completely eliminated, only controlled.

Catheter-Associated Urinary Tract Infections

UTIs are the most common type of health care–associated infection reported to the NHSN. Among UTIs acquired in the hospital, approximately 75% are associated with a urinary catheter. Gram-negative rods produce most health care–associated UTIs, and *Escherichia coli* is the number one organism involved. Gram-positive organisms, *Candida* spp., and other fungi cause the remainder of the infections. The risk factors that predispose patients to acquire a health care–associated UTI include advanced age, female gender, severe underlying disease, and the placement of indwelling urinary catheters.

Ventilator-Associated Pneumonia (VAP)

The most common HAI pathogens that cause pneumonia include gram-negative rods, *S. aureus,* and *Moraxella catarrhalis. S. pneumoniae* and *H. influenzae,* which cause most community-acquired pneumonias, are not important etiologic agents in health care–associated infections except very early during the hospital course (first 2 to 5 days); these infections probably represent infections that were already incubating at the time of hospital admission. The risk factors that predispose patients to acquire a health care–associated lung infection include advanced age, chronic lung disease, large-volume aspiration (the microorganisms in the upper respiratory tract are aspirated into the lungs instead of being spit out or swallowed), chest surgery, hospitalization in intensive care units, and intubation (placement of a breathing tube down a patient's throat), or attachment to a mechanical ventilator (which controls breathing).

Surgical Site Infections

Approximately 4% of surgical patients develop surgical site infections; 50% of these infections develop after the patient has left the hospital, so this number is likely an underestimate of the true prevalence of infection. Gram-positive organisms (*S. aureus,* coagulase-negative staphylococci, and enterococci) cause most of these infections, followed by gram-negative rods and *Candida* spp. The risk factors that predispose patients to acquire a health care–associated wound infection include advanced age, obesity, infection at a remote site (that spreads through the bloodstream), malnutrition, diabetes, extended preoperative hospital stay, longer than 12 hours passing between preoperative shaving of the site and surgery, extended time of surgery, and inappropriate timing of prophylactic antibiotics (given to prevent common infections before they seed the surgical site). Surgical wounds are classified as clean, clean-contaminated, contaminated, or dirty, depending on the number of potentially contaminating organisms at the site. Bowel surgery is considered "dirty," for example, whereas surgery for a total hip replacement is considered "clean."

Central Line–Associated Bloodstream Infections

A central line–associated bloodstream infection is a serious infection that occurs when microbes enter the bloodstream through a central line. A central line is a tube that health care providers place in a large vein in the neck, chest, or arm to give fluids, blood, or medications or to do certain medical tests quickly. CLABSIs result in thousands of deaths each year and billions of dollars in added costs to the US health care system, yet these infections are preventable. The risk factors that predispose patients to acquire a CLABSI include age 1 year or younger or 60 years or older, malnutrition, immunosuppressive chemotherapy, loss of skin integrity (e.g., burn or decubiti [bedsore]), severe underlying illness, indwelling device (e.g., catheter), intensive care unit stay, and prolonged hospital stay.

Emergence of Antibiotic-Resistant Microorganisms

Antibiotic resistance is one of the biggest public health challenges in recent years. Each year in the United States, at least 2 million people get an antibiotic-resistant infection, and at least 23,000 people die. In most cases, antibiotic-resistant infections require extended hospital stays and costly and toxic alternatives. Fighting this threat is a public health priority that requires a collaborative global approach across sectors. Antibiotic resistance happens when microorganisms develop the ability to defeat the drugs designed to kill them.

Antibiotic resistance does not mean the body is becoming resistant to antibiotics; it is that organisms have become resistant to the antibiotics designed to kill them. The organisms that cause HAIs have changed over the years because of selective pressures from the use (and overuse) of antibiotics (Chapter 10). Risk factors for the acquisition of highly resistant organisms include prolonged hospitalization and prior treatment with antibiotics. In the preantibiotic era, most HAIs were caused by *S. pneumoniae* and group A *Streptococcus (S. pyogenes)*. In the 1940s and 1950s, with the advent of treatment of patients with penicillin and sulfonamides, resistant strains of *S. aureus* appeared. Then, in the 1970s, treatment of patients with narrow-spectrum cephalosporins and aminoglycosides led to the emergence of resistant aerobic gram-negative rods, such as specific species of *Klebsiella, Enterobacter, Serratia,* and *Pseudomonas.* During the late 1970s and early 1980s, the use of more potent cephalosporins played a role in the emergence of antibiotic-resistant, coagulase-negative staphylococci, enterococci, methicillin-resistant *S. aureus* (MRSA), and *Candida* spp. Similarly, the 1990s witnessed the emergence of beta-lactamase-producing, high-level gentamicin-resistant, and vancomycin-resistant enterococci (VRE). The 21st century has seen the emergence of vancomycin-resistant *S. aureus* (VRSA) and CRE, which include normal microbiota of the gastrointestinal tract that are highly resistant to antibiotics.

The patients' microbiome changes quickly after hospitalization from viridans streptococci, saprophytic *Neisseria* spp., and diphtheroids to potentially resistant microorganisms found in the hospital environment. The colonized nares, skin, gastrointestinal tract, or genitourinary tract can later serve as reservoirs for endogenously acquired infections. Moreover, if patients colonized with resistant microorganisms return to nursing homes in the community harboring these organisms, they can also transfer them to other patients. This further increases the pool of patients who harbor multidrug-resistant organisms when they, in turn, are hospitalized. These new patients contaminate the hospital environment and serve as potential reservoirs for spread to additional patients.

Hospital Infection Control Programs

Hospital or health care facility infection control programs are designed to detect and monitor HAIs and to prevent or control their spread. The major responsibilities for an infection control program include surveillance, environmental monitoring, continuous quality improvement, consultation, outbreak and isolation management, regulatory compliance, and education. Infection control programs are usually headed by an infection control professional. This person should possess knowledge of epidemiology statistics, patient care practices, occupational health, sterilization, disinfection, and sanitation, infectious diseases, microbiology, education, and management. To plan and coordinate these responsibilities, many programs include multidisciplinary support teams to carry out many of the functions. The infection control team is usually headed by an infection control practitioner (often a nurse or laboratory practitioner with special training), and should include a microbiologist, an epidemiologist (usually an infectious disease physician), the dietary manager, a pharmacist, the chief nursing officer, operating room manager (when applicable), and the director of environmental services.

The infection control practitioner collects and analyzes surveillance data, monitors patient care practices, and participates in epidemiologic investigations. Daily review of charts of patients with fever or positive microbiology cultures allows the infection control practitioner to recognize problems with HAIs and to detect outbreaks as early as possible. The infection control practitioner is also responsible for the education of health care providers in techniques such as hand washing, processing environmental surfaces, and isolation precautions, all of which collectively minimize the acquisition and spread of infections.

It is the infection control practitioner's job to identify all cases of an outbreak. The investigation of the cluster of cases during an outbreak involves its characterization in terms of commonalities, such as location in the facility (e.g., nursery, intensive care unit); identifying or excluding the role of a specific caregiver; and prior respiratory or physical therapy. Risk factors—including underlying diseases, current or prior antimicrobial therapy, and placement of a urinary catheter—are also assessed. This information helps the infection control committee determine the reservoir of the organism in the facility—that is, the place where it exists and how the organism is transmitted from its reservoir to the patient.

Microorganisms are spread in health care facilities through several modes:
- Direct contact—for example, in contaminated food or intravenous solutions
- Indirect contact—for example, from patient to patient on the hands of HCWs (MRSA, rotavirus)
- Droplet contact—for example, inhalation of droplets (>5 μm in diameter) that cannot travel more than 3 feet (pertussis)
- Airborne contact—for example, inhalation of droplets (>5 μm) that can travel large distances on air currents (tuberculosis)
- Vector-borne contact—for example, disease spread by vectors, such as mosquitoes (malaria) or rats (rat-bite fever); this mode of transmission is rare in hospitals within developed countries

Once the reservoir is known, the infection control practitioner can implement control measures, such as reeducation regarding hand washing (in the case of spread by HCWs) or hyperchlorination of air-conditioning cooling towers such as in the case of legionellosis (caused by the bacterium *Legionella pneumophila*).

Role of the Microbiology Laboratory

The microbiology laboratory supplies the data on organism identification and antimicrobial susceptibility profiles that the infection control practitioner reviews daily for evidence of HAI. Thus, the laboratory personnel must be able to detect potential microbial pathogens and then accurately identify them to species level and perform appropriate susceptibility testing. The microbiology laboratory staff should also monitor multidrug-resistant organisms by tabulating data on antimicrobial susceptibilities of common isolates and studying trends indicating emerging resistance. Significant or abnormal findings or trends in susceptibility profiles of isolates should be immediately reported to the infection control practitioner. If an outbreak is suspected, the laboratory works in tandem with the infection control committee by (1) saving all isolates, (2) culturing possible reservoirs (patients, personnel, or the environment), and (3) performing typing of strains to establish relatedness between isolates of the same species. Microbiology laboratories are also obligated by law to report certain isolates or syndromes to public health authorities. It is the responsibility of the laboratory to be familiar with the reporting requirements within the service area of the laboratory.

Characterizing Strains Involved in an Outbreak

The ideal system for typing microbial strains involved in outbreaks should be standardized, reproducible, sensitive, stable, readily available, inexpensive, applicable to a wide range of microorganisms, and field tested in other epidemiologic investigations. Standardization of methods is important so that results from one institution can be compared with those from another, facilitating a larger investigation if deemed necessary. Although no such perfect system is currently available, several methods are used to aid in typing epidemic strains. There are two major ways to type strains using either phenotypic traits or molecular typing methods.

Classic phenotypic techniques include biotyping (analyzing unique biologic or biochemical characteristics), the use of antibiograms (analyzing antimicrobial susceptibility patterns), and serotyping (serologic typing of bacterial or viral antigens, such as bacterial cell wall [O] antigens). Bacteriocin typing, which examines an organism's susceptibility to bacterial peptides (proteins), and bacteriophage typing, which examines the ability of bacteriophages (viruses capable of infecting and lysing bacterial cells) to attack certain bacterial strains, have been useful for typing *Pseudomonas aeruginosa* and *S. aureus,* respectively; these techniques, however, are not widely available.

Genotypic, or molecular, methods have largely replaced phenotypic methods as a means of confirming the relatedness of strains involved in an outbreak. Plasmid analysis and restriction endonuclease analysis of chromosomal DNA are widely used. Plasmids are extrachromosomal pieces of genetic material (nucleic acids) that self-replicate (reproduce) in tandem with the bacterial genome and are passed to newly replicated organisms during cell division. Plasmids may also be transferred from one bacterial cell to another by conjugation or transduction (Chapter 2). Plasmid analysis has often been used to explain the occurrence of unusual or multiple-antibiotic resistance patterns. It has been shown that plasmids or R factors (resistance genes carried on plasmids) can facilitate outbreaks when a specific plasmid is transmitted from one genus of bacteria to another. Plasmid profiles, patterns created when plasmids are separated based on molecular weight by agarose gel electrophoresis, can also be used to characterize the similarity of bacterial strains. Relatedness of strains is based on the number and size of plasmids, with strains from identical sources showing identical plasmid profiles. Plasmids themselves or chromosomal deoxyribonucleic acid (DNA) may also be typed by means of restriction endonuclease digestion patterns. Restriction enzymes recognize specific nucleotide sequences in DNA and produce double-stranded cleavages that break the DNA into smaller fragments. The fragments of various sizes are separated using gel electrophoresis based on molecular weight. The specific recognition sequence and cleavage site have been defined for a great many of these enzymes. Modifications of the basic restriction endonuclease technique have been developed to reduce the number of bands generated to fewer than 20 to make the gels easier to interpret. These include pulsed-field gel electrophoresis (PFGE) and hybridization of ribosomal ribonucleic acid (RNA) with short fragments of DNA. Plasmid restriction digests have been used to type *S. aureus* and coagulase-negative staphylococci, and PFGE is the preferred method for typing enterococci, enteric gram-negative rods, and other gram-negative rods.

Other molecular methods, such as polymerase chain reaction (PCR), are used in conjunction with these methods for strain typing. In addition to strain typing, susceptibility to some antibiotics can be predicted by PCR and sequencing of specific genetic loci within the bacterial genome. Advances in next generation sequencing (NGS), which allows a laboratory to sequence an entire microorganism genome in less than an hour, has the potential to revolutionize epidemiological studies. This will undoubtedly improve the speed associated with the identification of antibiotic-resistant bacterial infections or confirm results observed in culture-based assays.

Molecular methods (nucleic acid–based tests) are discussed in more detail in Chapter 8.

Preventing Health Care–Associated Infections

The CDC published guidelines in the 1970s specifying isolation precautions in hospitals. Techniques for isolation precautions included (1) HCWs washing their hands between caring for different patients; (2) isolation of infected patients in private rooms or placing patients with the same clinical syndrome in semiprivate rooms if private rooms are not available; (3) wearing of masks, gowns, and gloves when caring for infected patients; (4) bagging of contaminated articles, such as bed linens, before removing them from the room; (5) processing of all isolation rooms after the patient is discharged; and (6) placement of cards on the patient's door specifying the type of isolation and instructions for visitors and HCWs. Categories of isolation were also established that included (1) strict isolation for highly contagious diseases such as chickenpox, pneumonic plague, and Lassa fever; (2) respiratory isolation for diseases such as measles, *H. influenzae,* or *Neisseria meningitidis;* (3) enteric precautions for diseases such as amoebic dysentery, *Salmonella,* and *Shigella;* (4) contact isolation for patients infected with multidrug-resistant bacteria; (5) acid-fast bacilli (AFB) isolation for persons suspected of having a *Mycobacterium tuberculosis* infection; (6) drainage and secretion precautions for persons with conjunctivitis and burns; and (7) blood and body fluid precautions for individuals with acquired immune deficiency syndrome (AIDS). Over time, a system of disease-specific precautions was added to the category-specific ones, and hospitals were given the option of using one of the two systems. Disease-specific precautions were more cost-effective, in that only those precautions specifically necessary were used to interrupt the transmission of a single disease.

In 1996, the CDC developed a new system of standard precautions synthesizing the features of universal precautions (Chapter 4) and body substance isolation. Standard precautions are used in the care of all patients and apply to blood; all body fluids, secretions, and excretions except sweat, regardless of whether they contain visible blood; nonintact skin; and mucous membranes.

• **BOX 78.1** **Infection Control Measures for Standard Precautions**

- Health care workers (HCWs) should wash hands frequently using a plain soap except in special circumstances—for example, preoperatively or after handling dressings from patients on contact isolation.
- HCWs should wear gloves when touching blood, body fluids, secretions, excretions, and contaminated items.
- HCWs should wear a mask, gown, eye protection, or face shield as appropriate.
- Each hospital should ensure that it has adequate procedures for routine care, cleaning, and disinfection of environmental surfaces, beds, bed rails, and bedside equipment.
- Hospitals should handle, transport, and launder used linen soiled with blood, body fluids, secretions, and excretions in a manner that prevents skin and mucous membrane exposure and contamination of clothing, and that prevents the transfer of microorganisms to other patients or the environment.
- HCWs should take care to prevent injuries when using needles, scalpels, and other sharp instruments or devices.
- HCWs should use equipment, such as mouthpieces and resuscitation bags, instead of mouth-to-mouth resuscitation.
- HCWs should refrain from handling patient care equipment if they have exudative lesions or weeping dermatitis.
- Hospitals should place incontinent or nonhygienic patients in a private room.
- Hospitals should ensure that reusable equipment is properly sterilized.
- Hospitals should ensure that single-use items are discarded properly.

Modified from Healthcare Infection Control Practices Advisory Committee (HICPAC), 2007.

In addition, transmission-based precautions are used for patients known (or suspected) to be infected with pathogens spread by airborne or droplet transmission or by contact with dry skin or fomites. Box 78.1 lists infection control measures for standard precautions. Table 78.1 lists the infectious agents or syndromes along with the respective infection control measures for each transmission-based precaution. Many infection control practitioners find these guidelines substantially less cumbersome to implement than the old category- and disease-specific measures. Health care facilities, however, may modify these guidelines to fit their individual situations as long as their number of HAIs remains low.

Some of the potential agents of bioterrorism can be transmitted person to person (smallpox, pneumonic plague, and viral hemorrhagic fevers including Ebola) and some cannot (anthrax). The ones that can be easily transmitted have specific transmission-based precautions—that is, airborne precautions for smallpox, droplet precautions for patients with pneumonic plague, and contact precautions for individuals with one of the viral hemorrhagic fevers (Ebola, Marburg, and others).

Surveillance Methods

Most routine environmental cultures in a health care facility are now considered to be of little use and should not be performed unless there are specific epidemiologic implications. The decision to perform these cultures should be determined by the infection control team. However, certain surveillance cultures are still performed as a method of limiting outbreaks. These include culturing cooling towers or hot water sources for *Legionella* spp.; culturing water and dialysis fluids; endotoxin testing; culturing blood bank products, especially platelets; and surveillance cultures for VRE, MRSA or oxacillin-resistant *S. aureus*, and VRSA using rectal and oropharyngeal swabs. Physical rehabilitation centers often culture hydrotherapy equipment (whirlpools) quarterly to verify that cleaning methods are adequate; some centers perform such routine cultures more frequently.

Routine surveillance of air handlers, food utensils, food equipment surfaces, and respiratory therapy equipment is no longer recommended; neither is monitoring infant formulas prepared in-house nor items purchased as sterile. A better approach is for the infection control team to monitor patients for the development of an HAI that might be related to the use of contaminated commercial products. In the event of an outbreak or an incident related to suspected contamination, a microbiologic study would be indicated. However, most often, such infections are caused by in-use contamination, rather than contamination during the manufacturing process. Suspect lots of fluid and catheter trays should be saved, and the US Food and Drug Administration (FDA) should be notified if contamination of an unopened product is suspected.

Although some institutions still require preemployment stool cultures and ova and parasite examinations on food handlers, most now recognize that this is of limited value. It is much more important for food handlers to submit specimens for these tests if they develop diarrhea. Similarly, most hospitals no longer screen personnel routinely for nasal carriage of *S. aureus*. Although a significant percentage of the general population, including hospital personnel, are known to carry this organism, most individuals rarely shed enough organism to pose a hazard, and there is no simple way to predict which nasal carriers will disseminate staphylococci.

All steam and dry-heat sterilizers and ethylene oxide gas sterilizers should be checked at least once weekly with a liquid spore suspension test vial to verify complete sterilization.

Health care facilities that perform bone marrow transplantation or treat hematologic malignancies may also conduct surveillance cultures of severely immunocompromised patients who occupy laminar flow rooms. In these instances, the isolation of specific organisms may have predictive value for subsequent systemic infection. Air sampling for fungi during construction is also indicated, especially if patients

TABLE 78.1	Transmission-Based Precautions	
Type of Precaution	Specific Etiologic Agents or Syndromes	Infection Control Measures
Airborne	Measles Varicella Tuberculosis Smallpox	Place patient in private room that has monitored negative air pressure, 6–12 air changes per hour, and appropriate discharge of air outdoors or monitored HEPA filtration of room air before air is circulated to other areas of the hospital or cohorting of patients—that is, placing patients with the same infection in the same room, if private rooms are not available. Health care workers (HCWs) should wear respiratory protection when entering rooms of patients with known or suspected tuberculosis and, if not immune, for patients with measles or varicella as well. Transport patients out of their room only after placement of a surgical mask.
Droplet	Invasive *Haemophilus influenzae* type b infection, including meningitis, pneumonia, epiglottitis, and sepsis Invasive *Neisseria meningitidis* infection, including meningitis, pneumonia, and sepsis Diphtheria (pharyngeal) *Mycoplasma pneumoniae* Pertussis Pneumonic plague Streptococcal pharyngitis, pneumonia, or scarlet fever in infants and young children Adenovirus, influenza virus Mumps Parvovirus B19 Rubella	Place patient in private room without special air handling or ventilation or cohort patients. HCWs should wear mask when working within 3 feet of patient. Transfer patients out of their room only after placement of a surgical mask.
Contact	Gastrointestinal, respiratory, skin, or wound infections, or colonization with multidrug-resistant bacteria *Clostridiodes difficile* For diapered or incontinent patients: *Escherichia coli* O157:H7, *Shigella*, hepatitis A virus, or rotavirus Respiratory syncytial virus, parainfluenza virus, and enterovirus infections in infants and young children Skin infections such as diphtheria (cutaneous), herpes simplex virus (neonatal or mucocutaneous), impetigo, major abscesses, cellulitis, or decubiti, pediculosis (lice infestation), scabies (mite infestation), staphylococci furunculosis (boils) in infants and young children, zoster (disseminated or in the immunocompromised host) Viral hemorrhagic infections (Ebola, Lassa, or Marburg)	Place patient in a private room without special air handling or ventilation or cohort patients. HCWs should wear gloves when entering the patient's room. HCWs should wash hands with a special antimicrobial agent or a waterless antiseptic agent. HCWs should wear a mask and eye protection during activities that are likely to generate splashes of blood, body fluids, secretions, or excretions. HCWs should wear a gown during procedures likely to generate splashes. HCWs should ensure reusable equipment is properly sterilized. HCWs should ensure that single-use items are properly discarded.

Modified from Healthcare Infection Control Practices Advisory Committee (HICPAC), 2007.

are immunocompromised and are being treated near the construction site.

The US Pharmacopeia published requirements for monitoring of sterile compounding in hospital pharmacies. The laminar flow hoods, biologic safety cabinets, clean rooms, and donning areas must be monitored weekly or monthly so that intravenous or intrathecal products and drugs used in the operating room are made (compounded) under sterile conditions.

ⓔ Visit the Evolve site for a complete list of procedures, review questions, and case studies.

Bibliography

American Recovery and Reinvestment Act of 2009, Public Law 111-5, 42 U.S.C. § 241(a).

Banerjee SN, Emori TG, Culver DH, et al.: The national nosocomial infection surveillance system: secular trends in nosocomial primary bloodstream infections in the United States, 1980-1989, *Am J Med* 91(Suppl 3B):86S, 1991.

Centers for Disease Control and Prevention: Public health focus: surveillance, prevention and control of nosocomial infections, *Morb Mortal Wkly Rep* 41:783–787, 1992.

Centers for Disease Control and Prevention: *Healthcare-Associated Infections (HAIs): state-based HAI prevention*, 2015, Available at http://www.cdc.gov/HAI/state-based/. Accessed 16 November 2018.

Centers for Disease Control and Prevention: *Healthcare facility HAI reporting requirements to CMS via NHSN: current or proposed requirements*, 2014, Available at: http://www.cdc.gov/nhsn/PDFs/CMS/CMS-Reporting-Requirements.pdf. Accessed 16 November 2018.

Centers for Disease Control and Prevention: *National Healthcare Safety Network (NHSN)*, 2015, Available at: http://www.cdc.gov/nhsn/. Accessed 16 November 2018.

Centers for Disease Control and Prevention: *National Healthcare Safety Network (NHSN). About NHSN*, 2015, Available at: http://www.cdc.gov/nhsn/about.html. Accessed 16 November 2018.

Centers for Disease Control and Prevention: *National and state healthcare associated infections: progress report*, 2015, Available at: http://www.cdc.gov/HAI/pdfs/progress-report/hai-progress-report.pdf. Accessed 16 November 2018.

Coffin SE, Zaoutis TE: Healthcare-associated infections. In Long SS, Pickering LK, Prober CG, editors: *Principles and practice of pediatric infectious diseases*, ed 3, New York, NY, 2008, Churchill Livingstone.

Craven DE, Chroneou A, Zias N, Hjalmarson KI: Ventilator-associated tracheobronchitis: the impact of targeted antibiotic therapy on patient outcomes, *Chest* 135:521–528, 2009.

Craven DE, Steger KA, Barber TW: Preventing nosocomial pneumonia: state of the art and perspectives for the 1990s, *Am J Med* 91(Suppl 3B):44S–53S, 1991.

Edwards JR, Peterson KD, Andrus ML, et al.: The National Healthcare Safety Network (NHSN) report, data summary for 2006 through 2007, issued November 2008, *Am J Infect Control* 36:609–626, 2008.

Emori TG, Gaynes RP: An overview of nosocomial infections, including the role of the microbiology laboratory, *Clin Microbiol Rev* 6:428–442, 1993.

Garibaldi RA, Cushing D, Lerer T: Risk factors for postoperative infection, *Am J Med* 91(Suppl 3B):158S–163S, 1991.

Garner JS, Favero MS: *Guideline for hand washing and hospital environmental control, 1985*, Atlanta, 1985, Centers for Disease Control, pp PB85-923404.

Garner JS, Simmons BP: *CDC guideline for isolation precautions in hospitals*, Atlanta, 1983, Centers for Disease Control, pp PB85-923401.

Gastmeier P, Geffers C, Brandt C, et al.: Effectiveness of a nationwide nosocomial infection surveillance system for reducing nosocomial infections, *J Hosp Infect* 64:16–22, 2006.

Griffith JT, Rohde RE: Ebola: implications for the clinical laboratory, *Clin Lab Sci* 1–6, 2014, December, Available at: http://www.ascls.org/images/publications/journals/Ebola_virus_manuscript.pdf. Accessed 16 November 2018.

Guidelines for the management of adults with hospital-acquired: ventilator-associated, and healthcare-associated pneumonia, *Am J Respir Crit Care Med* 171:388–416, 2005.

Guidelines for the Prevention of Intravascular Catheter-Related Infections. Centers for Disease Control and Prevention. Available at: www.cdc.gov/mmwr/PDF/rr/rr5110.pdf.Accessed November 16, 2018.

Horan TC, Andrus M, Dudeck MA: CDC/NHSN surveillance definition of healthcare-associated infection and criteria for specific types of infections in the acute care setting, *Am J Infect Control* 36:309–332, 2008.

Hospital Infection Control Practices Advisory Committee: Guideline for infection control in healthcare personnel, *Am J Infect Control* 26:289, 1998.

Hospital Infection Control Practices Advisory Committee: Guideline for isolation precaution in hospitals, *Infect Control Hosp Epidemiol* 17:53–80, 1996.

Hospital Infection Control Practices Advisory Committee: Guideline for prevention of intravascular device-related infections, *Am J Infect Control* 24:262–277, 1996.

Hospital Infection Control Practices Advisory Committee: *Guideline for prevention of nosocomial pneumonia*, Atlanta, 1994, Centers for Disease Control and Prevention, pp PB95–176970.

Hospital Infection Control Practices Advisory Committee: Guideline for prevention of surgical site infection, *Infect Control Hosp Epidemiol* 20:247–280, 1999.

Hospital Infection Control Practices Advisory Committee: Recommendations for preventing the spread of vancomycin resistance, *Infect Control Hosp Epidemiol* 16:105–113, 1995.

Hospital Infections Program, National Center for Infectious Diseases, Centers for Disease Control and Prevention: Public health focus: surveillance, prevention, and control of nosocomial infections, *Morb Mortal Wkly Rep* 41(42):783–787, 1992.

Javis WR: Infection control and changing health-care delivery systems, *Emerg Infect Dis* 7:170–173, 2001.

Jewett JF, Reid DE, Safon LE, et al.: Childbed fever: a continuing entity, *J Am Med Assoc* 206:344–350, 1968.

Klevens RM, Edwards JR, Richards CL, et al.: Estimating healthcare-associated infections in US hospitals, 2002, *Public Health Rep* 122:160–166, 2007.

Marchetti A, Rossier R: Economic burden of healthcare-associated infections in US acute care hospitals: societal perspective, *J Med Econ* 16:1399–1404, 2013.

McGowan Jr JE, Weinstein RA: The role of the laboratory in control of nosocomial infection. In Bennett JV, Brachman PS, editors: *Hospital infections*, ed 3, Boston, 1992, Little, Brown.

Miller JM, Bell M: Epidemiologic and infection control microbiology. In Isenberg HD, editor: *Clinical microbiology procedures handbook*, ed 2, Washington, DC, 2004, ASM Press.

Mitchell-Hogan A, Rohde RE, Tille P, et al.: The changing role of the healthcare environment, *Clin Lab Sci* 29(1):44–48, 2016.

Nichols RL: Surgical wound infection, *Am J Med* 91(Suppl 3B):54S–64S, 1991.

Reagan J, Rohde RE, Mitchell-Hogan A, et al.: The legal landscape: HAI public reporting in the United States, *Clin Lab Sci* 29(1):39–43, 2016.

Rohde RE, Felkner M, Reagan J, et al.: Healthcare-associated infections (HAI): the perfect storm has arrived!, *Clin Lab Sci* 29(1):28–31, 2016.

Rubin R: Hospital-acquired conditions declining, *J Am Med Assoc* 320(4):331, 2018, https://doi.org/10.1001/jama.2018.10151.

Rutala WR, Weber DJ: *The Healthcare Infection Control Practices Advisory Committee (HICPAC): guideline for disinfection and sterilization in healthcare facilities*, 2008, Available at: http://www.cdc.gov/hicpac/pdf/guidelines/Disinfection_Nov_2008.pdf. Accessed 16 November 2018.

Siegel JD, Rhinehart E, Jackson M, Chiarello L. The Healthcare Infection Control Practices Advisory Committee. *2007 Guideline for Isolation Precautions: Preventing Transmission of Infectious Agents in Healthcare Settings.* Centers for Disease Control and Prevention. Available at: www.cdc.gov/ncidod/dhqp/pdf/guidelines/Isolation2007.pdf. Accessed November 16, 2018.

Stamm WE: Catheter-associated urinary tract infections: epidemiology, pathogenesis, and prevention, *Am J Med* 91(Suppl 3B):65S–71S, 1991.

Tille P, Rohde RE, Felkner M, et al.: The perfect storm: emerging trends and pathogens in healthcare, *Clin Lab Sci* 29(1):32–38, 2016.

U.S. Department of Health and Human Services Office of Disease Prevention and Health Promotion: *National action plan to prevent healthcare-associated infections: road map to elimination*, 2015, Available at: http://www.health.gov/hai/prevent_hai.asp#hai_plan. Accessed 16 November 2018.

US Pharmacopeial Convention, Inc: Pharmaceutical compounding—sterile preparations. In *United States pharmacopeia*, vol. 27. Rockville, MD, 2004, US Pharmacopeial Convention, Inc, (Suppl 1.

Wenzel RP, editor: *Prevention and control of nosocomial infections*, ed 3, Baltimore, 1997, Williams & Wilkins.

Wenzel RP, Edmond MB: The impact of hospital-acquired bloodstream infections, *Emerg Infect Dis* 7:174–177, 2001.

Wong ES, Hooton TM. *Guideline for Prevention of Catheter-Associated Urinary Tract Infections.* Centers for Disease Control and Prevention. Available at: www.cdc.gov/ncidod/dhqp/gl_catheter_assoc.html. Accessed November 16, 2018.

79

Sentinel Laboratory Response to Bioterrorism

OBJECTIVES

1. Define and give examples of a bio crime.
2. Distinguish between covert and overt assaults.
3. Define and give examples of select agents.
4. Site two laws that govern the possession of select agents.
5. List the government agencies that must be notified, by registration, before a laboratory may possess a select agent.
6. State the components of a biosecurity plan.
7. Summarize the standard operating procedures required for laboratories that maintain select agents.
8. Diagram and give a brief description of the Laboratory Response Network.
9. Identify responsibility of each hierarchical level through which an agent passes in its process of being defined as an agent of bioterrorism.
10. Outline the steps microbiology laboratories must follow if a select agent is isolated from a clinical specimen.
11. Explain the requirements for operation as a sentinel laboratory.
12. Name the government agencies responsible for the investigation and management of a bioterrorism event.
13. Given microbiologic characteristics, identify the most likely suspect agent of terror.

General Considerations

Bioterrorism may have started centuries ago; however, lack of proper documentation made it difficult for historians and microbiologists to differentiate natural epidemics from alleged biological attacks. The practice of clinical microbiology changed significantly after *Bacillus anthracis* was intentionally released into the United States postal system in October 2001. Before this release there were a few events in which microorganisms were used to intentionally harm the civilian population in the United States.

The first incident, in 1984, was a large community outbreak of salmonellosis caused by the intentional contamination of restaurant salad bars in The Dalles, Oregon. In this incident, a cult leader, Baghwan Sri Rajneesh, set out to influence the outcome of a local election by incapacitating voters. Cultures of *Salmonella enterica* serotype Typhi were grown at a laboratory within the cult's compound. Ultimately, 751 individuals fell ill; luckily there were no deaths. Another religious cult, Aum Shinrikyo, known for

the famous sarin gas attack in Tokyo in 1995, was developing biological weapons using *Clostridium botulinum* and *B. anthracis,* but with no proof of effectiveness. In 1996, an outbreak among laboratory workers took place and was caused by a microbiology technologist in Dallas, Texas, purposely contaminating muffins and donuts with *Shigella dysenteriae* type 2. Forty-five laboratory workers developed gastroenteritis; four individuals were hospitalized.

The event in October 2001 stunned the country. Although there had previously been sporadic instances of suspicious letters, those events proved to be hoaxes. This outbreak resulted from the delivery of weaponized anthrax spores in mailed letters or packages; ultimately there were 11 cases of inhalational anthrax and 11 of cutaneous disease. Five individuals died. The attacks prompted institutions to implement or modify bioterrorism readiness plans. The US government also reviewed the public health response and identified areas for improvement.

Bio Crime

A bioterrorism event, also known as a **bio crime,** is an intentional assault on a person, or group of people, using a pathogen or toxin. The assault may be overt or covert. An overt attack is announced. The letters sent to Senators Daschle and Leahy in 2001 are examples of an overt event; a note inside each envelope announced that the individual opening it had been exposed to *B. anthracis* spores. A covert attack is unannounced; the recipient receives no indication that a threat is present. The package sent to the journalist at American Media, Inc., is an example of a covert event; an environmental investigation of his office uncovered the anthrax spores after his death and the illness of a coworker.

Government Laws and Regulations

The bombings at the World Trade Center in 1993 and the federal building in Oklahoma City in 1995 led Congress to pass the Antiterrorism and Effective Death Penalty Act of 1996. Section 511 (d) restricts the possession and use of materials capable of producing catastrophic damage in the hands of terrorists by requiring their registration. A companion law, the Uniting and Strengthening America by Providing Appropriate Tools Required to Intercept and Obstruct Terrorism (USA PATRIOT) Act of 2001, prohibits any person to knowingly possess any biologic agent, toxin, or delivery system of a type or in a quantity that, under the circumstances, is not reasonably justified by prophylactic, protective, bona fide research, or other peaceful purpose. Later, the Public Health Security and Bioterrorism Preparedness and Response Act of 2002 required institutions to notify the Department of Health and Human Services (DHHS) or the United States Department of Agriculture (USDA) of the possession of specific pathogens or toxins called **select agents**. Therefore, clinical laboratories possessing any select agents must register with the Centers for Disease Control and Prevention (CDC), a branch of the DHHS. Violation of any of these statutes carries criminal penalties. The pathogens and toxins classified as select agents are listed in Box 79.1. The list is updated as needed.

Bioterrorism agents are divided into three categories: A, B, or C. **Category A agents** are considered those presenting the highest risk to public health and national security, because they are easily disseminated or transmitted from person to person and have high mortality rates. Category A includes pathogens such as *B. anthracis* and *Yersinia pestis*. **Category B agents** are moderately easy to disseminate and have moderate to low mortality rates. This category includes *Brucella* spp. and *Clostridium perfringens* toxin. **Category C** contains emerging pathogens that could be engineered for mass spread in the future. Additional information may be found in Appendix F of the fifth edition of the CDC and the National Institutes of Health (NIH) manual *Biosafety in Microbiological and Biomedical Laboratories* (BMBL). The publication contains national guidelines to promote the safety and health of workers in biological and medical laboratories.

Biosecurity

Biosecurity is the latest issue of concern for microbiology laboratory directors and managers. Laboratories must conduct a risk assessment and threat analysis to write a security plan. This plan must include physical security (e.g., electronic card key access and locked freezers and refrigerators), and data system (laboratory information system) security and security policies for personnel.

Most hospital clinical laboratories have decided not to store any select agents. Some commercial laboratories, on the other hand, store select agents for use as positive controls for comparison with suspect samples. These laboratories must write standard operating procedures (SOPs) for (1) the access of select agents; (2) specimen accountability; (3) the receipt of select agents into the laboratory; (4) the transfer or shipping of select agents from the laboratory; (5) the reporting of incidents, injuries, and breaches of security; and (6) an emergency response plan if security is breached or the isolate is unintentionally released during an accident. They must also register the agents with the CDC.

• BOX 79.1 List of Select Agents[a]

Viruses

Crimean-Congo hemorrhagic fever virus
Eastern equine encephalitis virus
Ebola viruses
Hendra virus
Herpesvirus 1 (Herpes B virus)
Lassa fever virus
Marburg virus
Monkeypox virus
Nipah virus
Reconstructed 1918 influenza virus
Rift Valley fever virus
South American hemorrhagic fever viruses (Junin, Machupo, Sabia, Flexal, Guanarito)
Tick-borne encephalitis complex viruses
Variola major virus (smallpox virus)
Variola minor virus (Alastrim)
Venezuelan equine encephalitis virus

Bacteria

Bacillus anthracis
Brucella abortus, Brucella melitensis, Brucella suis
Burkholderia (Pseudomonas) mallei
Burkholderia (Pseudomonas) pseudomallei
Clostridium botulinum
Francisella tularensis
Yersinia pestis
Rickettsiae
Coxiella burnetii
Rickettsia prowazekii
Rickettsia rickettsii

Toxins

Abrin
Botulinum toxins
Clostridium perfringens epsilon toxin
Conotoxins
Diacetoxyscirpenol
Ricin
Saxitoxin
Shiga-like ribosome inactivating proteins
Shigatoxin
Staphylococcal enterotoxins
T-2 toxin
Tetrodotoxin

[a]HHS and USDA Select Agents and Toxins, 7 CFR Part 331, 9 CFR Part 121, and 42 CFR Part 73.

Each clinical laboratory should have a bioterrorism response plan. The plan should include policies and procedures to be enacted when a suspicious isolate cannot be ruled out as a biothreat agent. If a laboratory has any questions about isolating, identifying, or submitting an organism that may be an agent of bioterrorism, laboratory personnel should call the state public health laboratory. The select agent must be either sent to a public health laboratory or destroyed within 7 days of identification. If the agent is autoclaved, its destruction must be documented using Animal and Plant Health Inspection Service (APHIS)/CDC Form 4, available at https://www.selectagents.gov/forms.html.

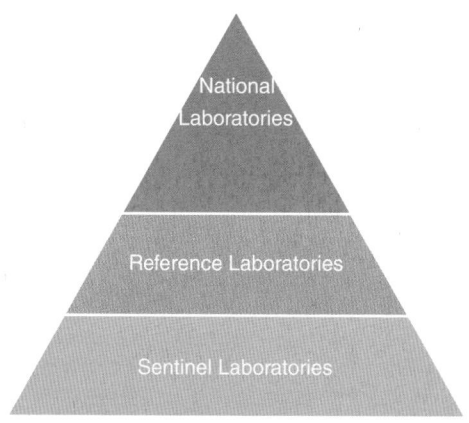

• **Fig. 79.1** Laboratory network for biologic terrorism.

Most of these laboratories are hospital-based clinical institutions and commercial diagnostic laboratories. **Reference laboratories** possess the required reagents and technology to perform confirmatory testing on pathogens. According to the CDC, reference laboratories are made up of more than 150 state and local public health, military, international, veterinary, agriculture, food, and water testing laboratories. In addition to laboratories in the United States, facilities located in Australia, Canada, the United Kingdom, Mexico, and South Korea serve as reference laboratories abroad. Confirmed bioterrorism agents are sent to a national laboratory. **National laboratories,** such as those at the CDC, US Army Medical Research Institute for Infectious Diseases, or the Naval Medical Research Center, are responsible for the definitive characterization of agents (Fig. 79.1).

Laboratory Response Network

Laboratory testing and communication between clinical and public health laboratories are critical when responding to a bioterrorism event. To address this issue, the CDC, in partnership with the Association of Public Health Laboratories and the Federal Bureau of Investigation (FBI), established the **Laboratory Response Network (LRN).** The LRN is a three-tier system. **Sentinel (formerly level A) laboratories** receive patient samples, rule out pathogens, and transfer suspicious specimens to reference laboratories. According to the CDC, the LRN works with the American Society for Microbiology (ASM) and state public health laboratory directors to ensure that private and commercial laboratories are part of the LRN. There are an estimated 2500 private and commercial laboratories serving in the sentinel capacity in the United States.

Role of the Sentinel Laboratory

The main role of sentinel microbiology laboratories is to determine whether a targeted agent is suspected in a human specimen. Detection and recognition of a possible bioterrorism event depend on the following:

- A laboratory having an active microbial surveillance and monitoring program
- Vigilant technologists looking for a disease that (1) does not occur naturally in a geographic region (e.g., plague in New York City); (2) is transmitted by an aerosol route of infection; and (3) is a single case of disease caused by an unusual agent (e.g., *Burkholderia mallei*)
- Good communication with infection control practitioners, infectious disease physicians, and local or regional public health laboratories

TABLE 79.1   Algorithm for Sentinel Laboratories for Likely Bioterrorism Agents[a]

Agent	Sentinel Laboratory Procedures	Comments
Bacillus anthracis	Colony: large, nonhemolytic, stands up like a beaten egg (Fig. 79.2) Gram stain: large, gram-positive rods (Fig. 79.3) Catalase: positive Motility: nonmotile Optional: use of the Red Line Alert Test (Tetracore, Inc.), cleared by the Food and Drug Administration, to rule out *B. anthracis* (see Chapter 15 for a more complete discussion of this test)	May be mistaken for *Bacillus megaterium*
Brucella spp.	Colony: small, nonhemolytic Gram stain: lightly staining tiny gram-negative coccobacilli Oxidase: positive Urease: positive Motility: nonmotile	May be mistaken for *Haemophilus* or *Francisella*
Francisella tularensis	Colony: pinpoint growth after 48 h Gram stain: pleomorphic, minute, faintly staining gram-negative coccobacilli Oxidase: negative Urease: negative Beta-lactamase: positive	May be mistaken for *Haemophilus* or *Actinobacillus*

Continued

TABLE 79.1	Algorithm for Sentinel Laboratories for Likely Bioterrorism Agents[a]—cont'd	
Agent	**Sentinel Laboratory Procedures**	**Comments**
Yersinia pestis	Colony: pinpoint growth on blood agar after 24 h Gram stain: gram-negative rods exhibiting bipolar staining Catalase: positive Oxidase: negative Urease: negative Indole: negative	Rapid systems may misidentify as *Shigella* spp., H2S-negative *Salmonella* spp., *Acinetobacter* spp., and *Yersinia pseudotuberculosis*
Clostridium botulinum	None	Send all specimens to reference laboratory; patient must get antitoxin immediately
Smallpox and hemorrhagic fever viruses	None	Smallpox can be mistaken for herpes virus if inoculated into routine tissue culture cells

[a]See individual chapters for a more detailed discussion of each organism.

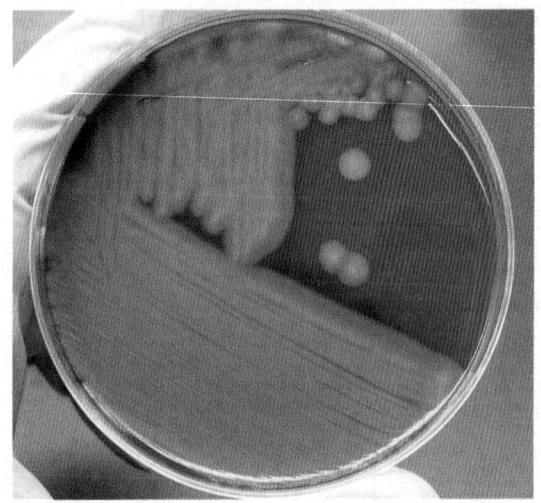

• **Fig. 79.2** Colony of *Bacillus anthracis*.

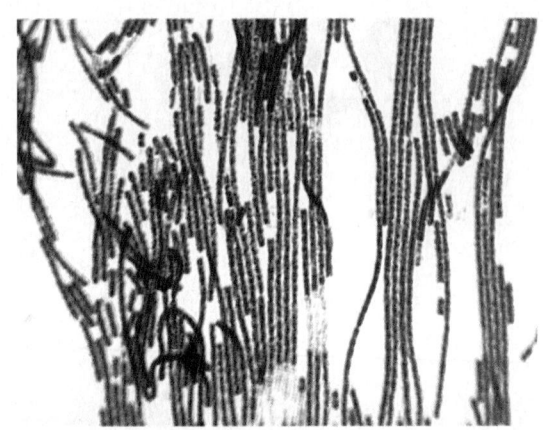

• **Fig. 79.3** Gram stain of *Bacillus anthracis*.

Sentinel laboratories must have a class II biologic safety cabinet, have copies of level A protocols containing the algorithms for ruling out suspicious microorganisms (Table 79.1), and participate in an applicable proficiency testing program such as the College of American Pathologist's Laboratory Preparedness Survey. Because sentinel laboratories rule out and refer microorganisms, proper knowledge of appropriate packaging and shipping is critical (Chapter 4); all specimens must be classified as infectious. Sentinel laboratories should never accept nonhuman specimens such as those from animals or the environment. Such specimens should be submitted directly to the nearest reference laboratory.

Rapid communication between LRN sentinel members and their reference public health laboratories is essential. Each sentinel laboratory must know how to contact public health officials 24 hours/day. Sentinel laboratories, however, do not make the determination that a bioterrorist event has occurred and do not notify law enforcement. The FBI has primary responsibility when a bioterrorism event occurs as outlined in Presidential Decision Directive 39. A bioterrorist event is first and foremost a criminal investigation. The Federal Emergency Management Agency (FEMA) has the lead role in consequence management. FEMA receives assistance from the Department of Defense (DOD), Department of Energy (DOE), USDA, Department of Transportation (DOT), DHHS, and Environmental Protection Agency (EPA). FEMA, for example, calls for the deployment of the National Pharmaceutical Stockpile by the CDC so victims may be appropriately treated. Early recognition is the key to saving lives, and sentinel laboratorians are on the front lines in the fight against bioterrorism.

Because sentinel laboratories are charged with ruling out possible bioterrorism agents and referring suspicious isolates to reference laboratories for confirmatory testing, each sentinel laboratory's bioterrorism response plan must include a telephone number and contact information for the reference laboratory.

Anthrax *(Bacillus anthracis)*
Brucella spp.
Botulinum toxin
BT readiness plan
Burkholderia spp.
Coxiella burnetii

Novel influenza viruses
Packing and shipping
Plague *(Yersinia pestis)*
Smallpox
Staphylococcal enterotoxin B
Tularemia *(Francisella tularensis)*

[a]Complete guidelines available at https://www.asm.org/index.php/science-skills-in-the-lab/sentinel-guidelines

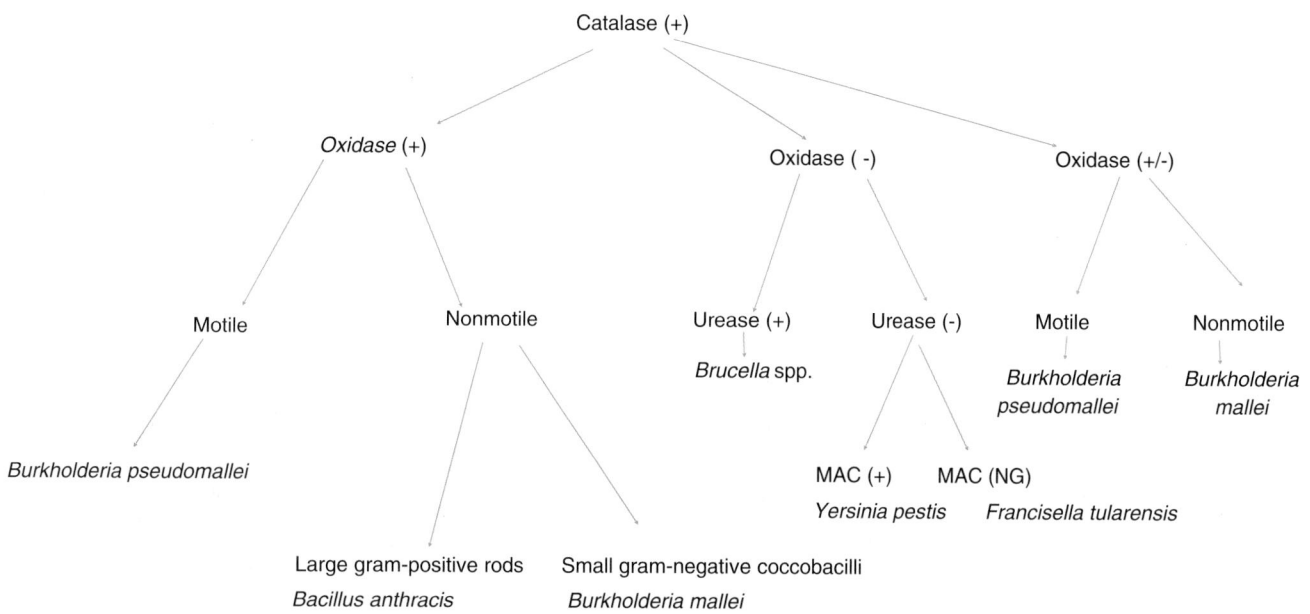

• **Fig. 79.4** Algorithm for the differentiation of bioterrorism agents.

A sentinel laboratory's key responsibility is to be familiar with likely agents involved in a bio crime; it must have SOPs to accomplish this task. To standardize the process nationwide, ASM has compiled a series of guidelines entitled "Sentinel level clinical laboratory guidelines for suspected agents of bioterrorism and emerging infectious diseases." Guidelines for individual bacteria listed in Box 79.2 may be accessed on the ASM website at https://www.asm.org/index.php/science-skills-in-the-lab/sentinel-guidelines. Algorithms for the identification of likely bioterrorism agents are provided in Table 79.1 and Fig. 79.4.

ⓔ Visit the Evolve site for a complete list of procedures, review questions, and case studies.

Bibliography

Barras V, Greub G: History of biological warfare and bioterrorism, *Clin Microbiol Infect* 20(6):497–502, 2014.
Centers for Disease Control and Prevention: Laboratory security and emergency response guidance for laboratories working with select agents, *MMWR (Morb Mortal Wkly Rep)* 51(RR19):1–6, 2002.
Hawley RJ, Eitzen Jr EM: Biological weapons—a primer for microbiologists, *Annu Rev Microbiol* 55:235–253, 2001.
Jernigan JA, Stephens DS, Ashford DA, et al.: Bioterrorism-related inhalational anthrax: the first 10 cases reported in the United States, *Emerg Infect Dis* 7:933–944, 2001.
Jorgensen J, Pfaller M, Carroll K, et al.: *Manual of clinical microbiology*, ed 11, Washington, DC, 2015, ASM Press.
Klietmann WF, Ruoff KL: Bioterrorism: implications for the clinical microbiologist, *Clin Microbiol Rev* 14:364–381, 2001.
Kolavic SA, Kimura A, Simons SL, et al.: An outbreak of *Shigella dysenteriae* type 2 among laboratory workers due to intentional food contamination, *J Am Med Assoc* 278:396–398, 1997.
Morse SA: Bioterrorism: laboratory security, *Lab Med* 32:303, 2001.
Sewell DL: Laboratory safety practices associated with potential agents of biocrime or bioterrorism, *J Clin Microbiol* 41:2801–2809, 2003.
Snyder JW: Role of the hospital-based microbiology laboratory in preparation for and response to a bioterrorism event, *J Clin Microbiol* 41:1–4, 2003.
Torok TJ, Tauxe RV, Wise RP, et al.: A large community outbreak of salmonellosis caused by intentional contamination of restaurant salad bars, *J Am Med Assoc* 278:389–395, 1997.
US Department of Health and Human Services/CDC and National Institutes of Health: In Chosewood LC, Wilson DE, editors: *Biosafety in microbiological and biomedical laboratories (BMBL)*, ed 5, Washington, DC, 2009, US Department of Health and Human Services.

Glossary

Abscess Localized collection of pus, a fluid in infected tissue that consists of white blood cells, bacteria, and dead tissue.

Abstriction Formation of spores in fungi by pinching off or constriction.

Accessioning Receipt of a specimen delivered to the laboratory, and the recording and assigning of a unique numerical identifier.

Accidental host A patient that becomes infected with a parasite that is not normally associated with the human as a host; a host that is not required as part of the parasitic life cycle.

Accolé forms See appliqué forms.

Accuracy Ability of a test under evaluation to match or be close to the value or the results of an accepted standard test.

Acidic dye (stain) A dye or stain that has a negative charge and binds to positively charged molecules. Generally, used for background staining in microbiology.

Acid-fast Characteristic of certain bacteria, such as mycobacteria, that involves resistance to decolorization by acids when stained by an aniline dye, such as carbolfuchsin.

Acquired immunity The body's specific response in the host to the infecting organism.

Acquired immunodeficiency syndrome (AIDS) Disease characterized by opportunistic infections and other complications that result due to immunodeficiency because of a viral infection with human immunodeficiency virus (HIV).

Acquired resistance When a microorganism that was initially susceptible to an antimicrobial agent becomes resistant to an agent by mutation or by acquisition of an antimicrobial-resistant genetic determinant.

Acridine orange A nonspecific cationic fluorescent dye that binds to all nucleic acids.

Acrodermatitis chronica atrophicans (ACA) A long-lasting, diffuse, red or bluish-red skin rash that is associated with third-state Lyme borreliosis.

Active immunization Activation of the immune system resulting in exposure to an antigen either by direct contact with the antigen in the environment or through artificial means.

Acute Occurs rapidly, generally with notable symptoms that may be severe.

Acute phase The physiological response of the human body soon after the onset of an infection or injury.

Acute sera Serum collected for antibody determination early during an illness when little or no antibody would have been produced.

Acute urethral syndrome Lower urinary tract infection that may be difficult to differentiate from cystitis.

Adiaspores Spores produced by the systemic fungus *Emmonsia* spp., which increase in size within the host but do not reproduce. These become walled or granulomatous in the lungs of the infected patient.

Aerial hyphae Fungal filaments (hyphae) that are found above the nutrient base or substrate.

Aerobe, strict or obligate Microorganism requiring the presence of ambient air, which contains 21% oxygen and a small amount of carbon dioxide (0.03%). Cannot live or grow in the absence of oxygen, or anaerobically.

Aerobic respiration The process of generating energy (adenosine triphosphate) with oxygen as the final electron receptor.

Aerosol Atomized particles suspended in air; in context of this textbook, microorganism suspended in air.

Aerotolerance test Culture that is used to identify a true anaerobe. A blood agar plate is inoculated and placed in an anaerobic environment; two chocolate plates are inoculated, and one is placed in a CO_2 incubator. Growth only on the blood agar and no growth on chocolate indicates that the organism is a true anaerobe.

Aerotolerant Anaerobes that do not use oxygen but are not killed by a small amount (5% O_2).

Affinity The strength of the binding of a single antigen-binding site on the antibody to the specific antigen.

Agar The most common solidifying agent used for microbiological media; it comes from the cell walls of Phaeophyta (brown algae), has the unique property of melting at high temperatures (≥95°C), and solidifies after the temperature falls below 50°C.

Agar dilution (antibiotic susceptibility testing) Agar plates containing a single antibiotic dilution used to determine antimicrobial susceptibility. Series of plates with doubling dilutions must include a plate without antibiotic for a growth control.

Agarose gel electrophoresis Separation of proteins based on molecular weight by electrical current–stimulated movement through a semisolid gel matrix.

Agglutination Aggregation or clumping of particles, such as bacteria when exposed to a specific antibody.

Alcohols (chemical disinfectant or antiseptic) 60% to 90% ethyl or isopropyl alcohol may be used as a chemical disinfectant on inanimate objects or an antiseptic on living tissue.

Aldehydes (chemical disinfectant) Formaldehyde, glutaraldehyde, and ortho-phthalaldehyde (OPA) used on surfaces such as floors. All but OPA require activation and produce strong fumes. OPA is sporicidal (kills endospores).

Aleurioconidia Hyphae where a cross wall divides the hyphae and the terminal cell differentiates into a spore.

Alopecia A medical condition that results in the loss of hair in patches or spots.

Amastigote A life cycle stage in some protozoans that is nonmotile and has no external flagella or cilia.

Ameboma Inflammatory granulomatous lesion because of amebic colitis in the bowel.

American Type Culture Collection (ATCC) Nonprofit organization that manages the commercial collection, storage, and distribution of microorganisms including fungi and bacteria as well as cell cultures for research and clinical diagnostics.

Amies medium Transport medium, with or without charcoal, that is a modification of Stuart medium (glycerol phosphate is replaced with an inorganic phosphate buffer) used for maintaining the viability of microorganisms.

Aminoglycosides Group of related antibiotics that contain an amino-modified glycoside that inhibit protein synthesis.

Amniotic Pertaining to the innermost fetal membrane forming a fluid-filled sac.

Amplicon Amplified nucleic acid product.

Anabolic (anabolism) Reactions that are synthetic in nature, generally requiring energy.

Anaerobe, strict or obligate Microorganism that grows only in complete or nearly complete absence of molecular oxygen. Atmosphere is generally composed of 5% to 10% hydrogen (H_2), 5% to 10% CO_2, 80% to 90% nitrogen (N_2), and 0% O_2.

Anaerobic respiration The process for energy generation in the absence of oxygen. Final electron acceptors may be organic or inorganic such as sulfate or nitrate.

Analyte specific reagent (ASR) Reagents, antibodies, nucleic acid probes, primers, proteins, etc., with specific properties or chemical activities provided by manufacturers for *in vitro* diagnostic use without predetermined performance characteristics. Each laboratory must determine their use and demonstrate appropriate performance characteristics. ASR is considered a medical device regulated by the US Food and Drug Administration (FDA).

Anamnestic response (secondary antibody response) More rapid production of antibodies in response to exposure to an antigen previously encountered.

Anamorph Asexual fungal form.

Anergy Absence of reaction to antigens or allergens.

Angiogenesis Forming new capillaries from preexisting ones.

Anicteric No jaundice.

Annealing The process of heating nucleic acids and then cooling to permit complementary sequences to pair during analytical processes.

Annelides Fungal organisms that form cells on the end of conidiophores or hyphae.

Annellophores Reproductive structure of a fungus that forms contiguous cells at the end.

Antagonism The interaction of two or more drugs (antimicrobials) that may interfere with or reduce the effectiveness of the treatment.

Anthroponotic A disease of humans that can be transmitted to other humans or animals.

Antibiogram A cumulative susceptibility report that tracks resistance or susceptibility of commonly isolated organisms to antimicrobials.

Antibiotic Substance produced by a microorganism that inhibits or kills other microorganisms.

Antibody (immunoglobulin) Substance (glycoprotein) formed in blood or tissues that interacts only with the antigen that induced its synthesis (e.g., agglutinin).

Antibody-mediated immunity See humoral immunity.

Antibody titer The measurement of an antibody in a serum sample. Determined by a serial dilution of the sample and expressed as the reciprocal of the highest dilution that demonstrates a positive result.

Anticoagulant Substance used to prevent clotting of specimens such as blood, bone marrow, and synovial fluid.

Anticodon A series of three nucleotides on the transfer RNA that is complementary and binds to the genetic code (triplet) on the messenger RNA.

Antigen Molecular structure that is capable of stimulating production of antibody.

Antigenic determinant See epitope.

Antigenic drift Minor changes that occur continuously over time as the virus replicates.

Antigenic shift Major changes that result in novel viral antigens.

Antimicrobial Chemical substance produced either by a microorganism or by synthetic means that is capable of killing or suppressing the growth of microorganisms.

Antimicrobial susceptibility testing (AST) Procedures used to detect *in vitro* resistance to antimicrobial agents. Procedures are based on serial dilutions or breakpoints for antimicrobials.

Antiparallel Used to describe the directionality of two molecules that are next to each other but that structurally run in opposite directions. This is used to describe the structure of DNA with a 5-prime phosphate to 3-prime hydroxyl on one strand, paired with a second strand that runs 3-prime hydroxyl to 5-prime phosphate.

Antiseptic A compound or chemical that is used on living tissue that stops or inhibits growth of microorganisms without necessarily killing them.

Antral puncture A surgical procedure used to drain or collect a specimen for diagnostic testing from the maxillary sinus.

Apical Anterior, narrowed ending of an anatomical structure of a microorganism.

Apical complex An anatomic structure that consists of cytoskeletal arrangements at the tip or narrowed end of a group of protozoans that functions to enable host cell penetration.

Apophysis Enlarged area or swelling of the sporangiophore immediately below the columella in a fungal organism.

Apoptosis Programmed cell death.

Appliqué forms (accolé forms) Trophozoite or ring stage of malaria that is attached to the outer periphery of the red blood cell; often appears like it is sitting on the outside of the cell rather than inside the cell.

Arboviruses Arthropod-borne viruses.

Arbitrary primed polymerase chain reaction (PCR) Amplification of multiple fragments within a nucleotide sequence that uses multiple short (6 to 10 nucleotides) oligonucleotide primers, not designed to amplify a specific known sequence.

Arthritis, septic Infection of synovial tissue and joint fluid of one or more joints; characterized by joint pain, stiffness, swelling, and fever.

Arthroconidium (plural Arthroconidia) Spore formed by septation of a hypha and subsequent separation of septa. Appear as square or rounded blocks.

Ascites Condition in which amounts of fluids increase and accumulate in the peritoneal cavity during infection or an inflammatory process.

Ascitic fluid Serous fluid in peritoneal cavity.

Ascocarp A large, saclike structure (fruiting body) that contains sexual spores of a fungus in the taxonomic group *Ascomycota*.

Ascospore Haploid asexual reproductive spores formed in the ascus of a fungus in the taxonomic group *Ascomycota*; usually form in groups of eight.

Aseptate Lacking septation or cellular cross walls; may also be referred to as coenocytic.

Aseptic meningitis Meningitis characterized by an increase in lymphocytes and other mononuclear cells in the cerebrospinal fluid; culture negative for most bacterial pathogens and is most often associated with viral or fungal pathogens.

Aspiration Inhalation of a fluid or solid.

Asaccharolytic Unable to break down carbohydrates.

Assimilation Utilization of nutrients. Assimilation tests are used to determine whether yeasts are able to grow with a carbohydrate or nitrate as a single source of energy; these tests are useful for biochemical identification of yeasts.

AST See antimicrobial susceptibility testing.

Atrophic rhinitis See ozena.

Auramine-rhodamine A basic dye that binds to the mycolic acid in acid-fast organisms and fluoresces at short-wave lengths.

Autochthonous Indigenous (originally occurring) inhabitant of a particular place or habitat.

Autoclave Instrument used to sterilize biohazardous trash and heat-stable objects using moist heat in the form of saturated steam under 1 atmosphere (15 pounds per square inch [psi]) of pressure with the two most common sterilization temperatures of 121°C and 132°C.

Autoinfection Infection that develops from a source within the host to another anatomical site. An example includes a parasite that is capable of migration to other areas of the body, causing damage.

Auxotroph Differing from an organism's wild type strain (prototroph) by an additional nutritional requirement that can utilize inorganic carbon sources (CO_2).

Average Nucleotide Identity (ANI) This is a comparative score between the genomic sequences of two organisms. An identity score of 95% or above is generally considered the same species, with a score below 75% as an unreliable identity between two genome sequences.

Avid The property of binding strongly, such as an antibody that strongly binds to an antigen.

Avidity Firmness of union of two substances; used commonly to describe the overall strength of binding between multiple binding sites (more than one) of an antibody to antigen.

Axial fibril Proteinaceous structure enclosed within a membrane sheath that wraps around a central core from the anterior to the posterior end of a microorganism.

Axial filament Multiple axial fibrils are the building blocks of an axial filament, which may also be referred to as an endoflagella.

Axoneme The central core of a motility organelle (cilia or flagella) in a eukaryotic microorganism; microtubule arrangement that consists of two central fibrils, surrounded by nine peripheral fibrils, referred to as a 9 + 2.

Axostyle A group of microtubules that begins at the base of a flagellum and runs the length of the body of a protozoan; may run the full length of the body and extend beyond, providing rigidity and assisting in the motility of the organism.

B

Bacillary angiomatosis Raised vascular lesions on the skin, organs, and mucous membranes associated with *Bartonella* spp. infections.

Bacille Calmette-Guérin (BCG) An attenuated strain of *Mycobacterium tuberculosis* used for immunization.

Back-up broth Supplemental or enrichment broth added to a routine culture to enhance the growth of an organism or group of organisms in the event there is no growth on the primary solid media used for isolation.

Bacteremia Presence of viable microorganisms (bacteria) in blood.

Bacterial vaginosis Noninflammatory condition in vagina characterized by foul-smelling vaginal discharge and presence of mixed bacteria.

Bactericidal Term used to describe a drug that kills microorganisms (bacteria).

Bacteriophage Virus that infects a bacterial cell.

Bacteriocins A protein that is produced by one type of bacteria that targets and kills other completing bacteria.

Bacteriostatic Term used to describe a drug that inhibits or slows the growth of a microorganism (bacteria) without killing it.

Bacterium (plural Bacteria) A single-celled prokaryotic microorganism.

Bacteriuria Presence of bacteria in urine.

Bartholinitis Inflammation of the Bartholin glands that are located posteriorly to the vagina, one on each side.

Base pair (bp) The formation of pairing of a nucleotide base on one strand of DNA, hydrogen-bonded to another nucleotide on a separate complementary strand of DNA.

Base sequence The order of nucleotides in a nucleic acid, either DNA or RNA.

Basic dye (stain) A dye or stain that has a positive charge and binds to negatively charged molecules on the outside surface of microorganisms.

Basidiospores Haploid asexual reproductive spores formed in the ascus of a fungus in the taxonomic group *Basidiomycota*; usually form in groups of four with two of each mating type.

Basidium (plural Basidia) Reproductive spore-producing structure of the fungi classified as a *Basidiomycota*.

Beta-lactamase Enzyme that is produced by a variety of microorganisms that breaks or disrupts the beta-lactam ring structure found in penicillins and/or cephalosporin.

Bifurcated Divided into two branches.

Binary fission The process of asexual reproduction, cellular division in prokaryotic cells. Cells may divide either longitudinally (along the long axis) or transversely (along the short axis), resulting in doubling of the cells.

Binomial nomenclature   Naming of microorganisms that contains two names by convention, the genus followed by the species.

Biocides   Chemicals that can be used to destroy all life forms are also considered sterilants. When used for shorter times, may be used as a disinfectant.

Biofilm   Well-organized mono- or polymicrobial microcolonies of microorganisms enclosed in a polymer matrix of protein and polysaccharides that are separated by water channels that remove wastes and deliver nutrients.

Biologic resistance   The natural (genetically determined) resistance of an organism to death or damage from a chemical or compound such as an antimicrobial.

Biological safety cabinet (BSC)   An enclosure used to prevent the acquisition or spread of infection by a relatively dangerous organism. These cabinets, also called *biosafety hoods*, vary in design according to the nature of the agents (BSC 1 to 4). The enclosures maintain a negative pressure and a laminar air curtain, both of which operate to prevent escape of organisms from the interior of the hood. Air that is exhausted may be passed through a high-efficiency bacterial filter that traps microorganisms or may be passed through a furnace that incinerates the organisms.

Bioluminescence   Light generation by living organisms.

Biopsy   Removal of tissue for diagnostic purposes (e.g., lymph node biopsy).

Biosafety Level 1 to 4 (BSL)   A specified set of practices or precautions used to prevent transmission of and infection by a microbial organism. Level 1 is considered the lowest level of precautions that can be used with microbial organisms that generally do not cause disease, all the way up to level 4, which is used for organisms considered exotic, highly contagious infectious agents that are typically fatal, and for which there are no current treatments or vaccines available to prevent infection.

Biotin   Small vitamin with two binding sites, one of which can bind covalently with amine or sulfhydryl chemical groups, leaving the other free to form a strong bond with the protein avidin, which, in turn, can be bound to an enzyme. The system is used as a chemical label for nucleic acid probes, antibodies, or other molecules for *in vitro* detection.

Biotype   Biologic or biochemical type of an organism. Organisms of the same biotype display identical biologic or biochemical characteristics.

Biphasic media   A microbiological culture system that contains both a liquid and a solid component.

Biseriate   Two layers, a mutalae and a phialide.

Blastoconidium   A spore formed by budding on hyphae, pseudohyphae, or on a single cell, as in yeasts.

Bleach   See hypochlorite solution.

Blepharitis   Inflammation of eyelids.

Blind passage   Serial passage (growth) of an infectious agent through either artificial media or an animal without any intermediate identification or characterization.

Blood-brain barrier   Layer of cells between the central nervous system and the capillaries of the circulatory system that is tightly packed and selectively permeable.

B lymphocytes (B cells)   Bone marrow–derived lymphocytes that, when activated (plasma cells) by specific antigens, produce antibodies in humoral immunity.

B memory cells   A type of lymphocyte that results from the activation of a B lymphocyte that has been exposed to an antigen to produce protective antibodies. The parent B lymphocyte activates multiples and divides, creating more active cells known as plasma cells and other B memory cells that will remain in the body for years, to respond to a secondary challenge by the original activating antigen.

Boil   An infection of the skin around a hair follicle or oil gland that appears red and swollen.

Boric acid   Preservative that can be used with urine specimens for transport.

Bothrium (plural Bothria)   Suction groove on the scolex of tapeworms.

Bradyzoite   A slow-growing form of a microorganism that is stationary (nonmotile) within the host tissue.

Branched DNA   A synthetic oligonucleotide structure that utilizes a primary probe or complementary target region that binds to the nucleic acid, with extender sequences that function to either capture a secondary target sequence that can be detected with a signal probe (amplifying the signal only) or used to then bind a set of primers, followed by amplification prior to detection.

Breakpoint   Level of an antibacterial drug achievable in the serum or body fluid. Organisms inhibited by this level of drug are considered susceptible.

Bright-field microscopy   See light microscopy.

Bronchial lavage   Similar to bronchial washings, but this term implies instillation of a larger volume of sterile physiological buffered saline before aspiration. Alveolar organisms may be present in the lavage.

Bronchial washings   Flushing of the lower respiratory tract with a sterile physiological buffered saline solution followed by aspiration from bronchial tree during bronchoscopy.

Bronchitis   Inflammation of mucous membranes of bronchi caused by infectious agents or chemical irritation.

Bronchiolitis   Inflammation, swelling, and narrowing of the smallest airways, bronchioles, in the lungs.

Bronchoscopy   Examination of bronchi through a bronchoscope: a tubular, illuminated instrument introduced through the trachea.

Brood capsule   Cyst of a tapeworm that is fluid filled, where the protoscolices (anterior heads) of the worm develop prior to being released.

BSC   See biological safety cabinet.

Bubo   Inflammatory enlargement of lymph node, usually in the groin, pelvic region, neck, or axilla.

Bubonic plague   Most common form of disease caused by *Yersinia pestis* that results in the formation of buboes.

Buccal capsule   Mouth or anterior oral opening of a nematode that connects to the esophagus.

Bud scar   Ring or indentation left on the surface of a mother cell where the bud or daughter cell developed and then detached.

Buffy coat   Layer of white blood cells and platelets between the plasma and the red blood cell mass when blood is centrifuged for separation.

Buffered formalin   A phosphate-buffered 10% formalin solution that is used as a fixative for a variety of tissues and parasites for microscopy.

Bulb   The esophageal bulb is at the posterior end of the esophagus that contains glands in nematodes.

Bulla (plural Bullae)   Large blebs or blisters, filled with fluid, in or just beneath the epidermal layer of skin.

Bursitis   Inflammation of a bursa, which is a small sac lined with synovial membrane and filled with fluid interposed between parts that move on each other.

Butt   Lower portion of artificial culture medium in a tube while the upper portion is distributed in the form of a slanted surface, leaving an air space between the slant and the opposite wall of the tube.

Butyrous   Butterlike consistency.

C

Calabar swelling   A transient nonerythematous swelling that is an allergic response to a microfilarial infection.

Calcofluor white   A fluorescent (white-blue) stain that binds to structures that contain cellulose and chitin. Predominantly used for visualizing fungi in tissues.

Calibrated loop   Bacteriologic loop that is calibrated to deliver a specified volume of fluid. Used as a means of semi-quantitating the number of microorganisms present in a urine culture.

CAMP test   A diffusible extracellular protein (CAMP factor) named after Christie, Atkins, and Munch-Peterson that is produced by specific organisms (e.g., group B streptococci) and acts synergistically with the beta-lysin of *Staphylococcus aureus* to cause enhanced lysis of red blood cells forming a flame-shaped ("campfire") pattern on blood agar.

Canaliculitis   Inflammation of the lacrimal (tear-secreting gland of the eye) canaliculi (narrow channels for nerves, veins, or capillaries).

Candle jar   A jar with a lid providing a gas-tight seal in which a small white candle is placed and lit after the bacterial culture plates have been placed inside. Candle will burn until the oxygen concentration has been lowered to the point at which it will no longer support the flame. Atmosphere of such a jar has a lower oxygen content than room air and a carbon dioxide content of about 3%.

Cannula   An artificial tube for insertion into a tube or cavity of the body.

CAPD   Chronic ambulatory peritoneal dialysis.

cAST   Commercial/computerized antibiotic susceptibility testing.

Capnophilic   Term used to describe microorganisms that demonstrate enhanced growth in an incubation atmosphere with increased carbon dioxide concentration.

Capsid   Protein layer or coat surrounding viral nucleic acid core.

Capsomere   Protein subunits of the viral capsid.

Capsule   Gelatinous material surrounding a microorganism's cell wall, usually composed of polysaccharides and protein.

Carbuncle   Enlarged cluster of red, swollen, and painful boils.

Carrier   A host that harbors a pathogenic organism but has no disease or damage because of the presence of the pathogen.

Caseous   Cheeselike; necrotic tissue, cells, and fluid accumulation.

Cat scratch disease (CSD)   Disease caused by *Bartonella henselae* that is transmitted by a bite, lick of an open wound, or scratch from a domestic or wild feline (cat).

Catabolic (catabolism)   Reactions that are degradative in nature; may result in the generation or formation of energy (ATP).

Catalase   Bacterial enzyme that breaks down peroxides, resulting in the formation of water and oxygen.

Catarrhal stage The first stage of whooping cough (*Bordetella pertussis*) that appears similar to a cold with a runny nose lasting 1 to 2 weeks.

Cathartics Medications that accelerate the rate of passing feces or defecation without softening.

Catheter Flexible tubular (rubber or plastic) instrument used for withdrawing fluids from (or introducing fluids into) a body cavity or vessel (e.g., urinary bladder catheter).

Cation A positive ion.

cDNA See complementary DNA molecule.

Cell culture *In vitro* cultivation and maintenance of eukaryotic cells in artificial growth medium.

Cell envelope Outer structure of a cell that includes the cell membrane, cell wall, and outer cell membrane, if present.

Cell line A cell culture that has specific characteristics that are maintained and that has been passed (subcultured) *in vitro*.

Cell line, continuous Line of tissue cells that is maintained in a specific phase of growth by serial passage (subculturing) of an established cell line.

Cell line, primary Preparation of a cell culture from a specific tissue by isolating the cells using mechanical or enzymatic methods and establishing the cell culture in a flask with appropriate artificial growth medium.

Cell-mediated immunity (CMI) or cellular immunity Human specific immune response carried out by special lymphocytes of the T (thymus-derived) class.

Cell membrane (cytoplasmic membrane) Contains the internal contents of the cell (cytoplasm or cytosol) from the environment. Serves as an osmotic barrier and controls which molecules enter and leave the cell.

Cellular arrangement Characteristic cellular arrangement that is identifiable for groups of microorganisms such as clusters, chains, pairs or tetrads, etc. Cellular arrangement is determined genetically by the means of cellular division.

Cellular immunity See cell-mediated immunity.

Cellular membrane See cytoplasmic membrane.

Cellular morphology Characteristic, repeating cellular shape that is generally monomorphic (single shape) and identifiable for specific microorganisms such as bacilli, cocci, vibrios, and spirillum.

Cellulitis Inflammation of the layers of the subcutaneous tissue.

Cell wall Outer layer of a cell that is present in some cells between the cell membrane and the internal contents. Imparts rigidity and structural integrity to the cell.

Central nervous system (CNS) The CNS consists of the brain and the spinal cord.

Central vacuole (body) form Commonly identified morphological form of the intestinal protozoan *Blastocystis hominis*, where a central vacuole encompasses most of the internal cell with a small ring of cytoplasm visible on the periphery.

Cephalic Referring to the head, or anterior structure, head-end of a parasite.

Cercariae Tailed, free-swimming larval stage of a trematode.

Cerebriform Appearance that is convoluted with brainlike folds. Term is used to describe fungal macroscopic colony morphology (topology).

Cereulide A heat-stable toxin that is produced by *Bacillus cereus* that causes nausea and vomiting (emetic).

Cervical Pertaining either to the neck or to the cervix of the uterus.

Chancre A painless genital ulcer generally associated with the primary stage in syphilis.

Charcot-Leyden crystals Slender crystals shaped like a double pyramid with pointed ends, formed from the breakdown products of eosinophils and found in feces, sputum, and tissues; indicative of an immune response that may have parasitic or nonparasitic causes.

Chemical disinfectant Chemicals that deactivate or kill some of the living organisms on inanimate surfaces. One of the most common is chlorine bleach.

Chemical hygiene plan All laboratories are required to have a chemical hygiene plan to protect the employees from exposure to health hazards and injuries, as well as processes and procedures for treatment when needed.

Chemical sterilant See biocides.

Chemotaxis Directed movement either toward or away from a chemical based on a concentration gradient.

Chemotaxonomic A method of classification that compares the biochemical make-up of cells to determine identity and relatedness, such as fatty-acid and protein profiles or cell wall composition.

Chemotherapeutic Chemical agent used to treat a disease; in microbiology typically, an infection caused by a bacteria, fungus, parasite, or virus. An antimicrobial, antifungal, antiviral, or antiparasitic agent.

Chlamydoconidia See chlamydospore.

Chlamydospore Thick-walled spore formed directly from a vegetative cell or hyphae that may be terminal or intercalary (in between).

Cholangitis Infection of the common bile duct.

Cholera A disease of the small intestine that results in severe fluid loss as a result of a bacterial infection, generally caused by strains of *Vibrio cholerae*.

Cholestasis Interference with the flow of bile from the liver.

Chorioamnionitis Infection in the uterus of the amnion and chorion fetal membranes during pregnancy.

Chorioretinitis Inflammatory process in the back of the eye involving the retina and the choroids.

Chromatoidal bar Aggregations of ribosomes that may be identified in the cyst of an amoeboid protozoan.

Chromatography Method of chemical analysis by which a mixture of substances is separated by fractional extraction or adsorption or ion exchange on a porous solid.

Chromogen An organism that can produce pigment during colonial growth is pigmented (e.g., *Flavobacterium* spp., yellow).

Chromogenic Giving rise to color, as chromogenic substrates for colored products of biochemical reactions or chromogenic bacteria that produce pigmented colonies.

Chromosome Structural organization of the deoxyribonucleic acid that carries the genetic code for an organism. Chromosome numbers vary from one organism to another and are double-stranded linear or circular molecules.

Chronic Condition that persists for a long period, resulting in slow pathogenesis or damage to the patient.

Chyluria Lymphatic rupture resulting in lymph fluid excreted into the urine.

Cilia Hairlike projections on the outside of eukaryotic cells. Cilia line the mucosal cells of the bronchi and trachea to move mucus and particles trapped in the respiratory tract, referred to as the mucociliary escalator. Also, present on protozoan, eukaryotic organisms as organelles for locomotion.

Clavate Club-shaped. Term used to describe macro- or microconidia of fungal organisms.

Cleavase An enzyme that is used in molecular diagnostics that is used to cleave an unpaired overlapping end of a synthetic oligonucleotide.

Clinical resistance The level of antibiotic resistance in an organism when the drug can no longer be effectively used for treatment.

Clonal expansion A process where a single cell multiplies and divides to produce activated clones of the specific cell. Term is used to describe the multiplication of T lymphocytes and B lymphocytes in the specific adaptive immune response.

Clone Group of cells or microorganism of identical genetic makeup derived from a single common ancestor.

Clue cell A vaginal epithelial cell that is coated with bacteria associated with bacterial vaginosis.

Coagglutination Agglutination of particulate antigens that aggregate with antigens with more than one specificity. An example is protein A–containing cells of *Staphylococcus aureus* coated with antibody molecules when exposed to corresponding antigen.

Coccidia Group of spore-forming protozoans.

Codon A set of three nucleotides.

Coenocytic hyphae See aseptate. May also be sparsely septated.

Coenurus Larval form of a tapeworm or cestode.

Coenurosis Infection caused by a larval form of a tapeworm or cestode.

Cold enrichment The incubation of a microbial culture in a temperature below body temperature (35°C to 37°C) to enhance the growth of a microorganism and eliminate the growth of contaminating organisms incapable of growth at the lower temperature.

Cold sterilization Use of chemicals (glutaraldehyde, OPA, or peracetic acid) to remove all life forms from inanimate surfaces without the use of heat.

Colitis Inflammation of the mucosa of colon.

Columella Structure on the top stipe of a reproductive fungal element that comes into direct contact with the sporangiospores inside the sporangia.

Colonial morphology Visible characteristics of microorganisms grown on artificial media. Some examples include shape, elevation, margins, texture, pigment, and more.

Colonization Growth of a microorganism in or on a human host without causing damage.

Colonizer See nonpathogenic.

Colony Macroscopically visible growth of a microorganism on solid artificial culture medium.

Colony-forming unit (CFU) Colony count.

Combination media Microbiological media that has two properties for the growth of microorganisms, such as selective and differential.

Commensal Microorganism living on or in a host but causing the host no harm.

Community-acquired Pertaining to outside the hospital, such as a community-acquired infection.

Competent Term used to describe cells or a microorganism that can take up nucleic acids from the external environment naturally or following chemical treatment.

Complement (system or proteins)   Set of serum proteins that are included in a catalytic cascade during immune activation. Proteins are cleaved into different fragments; each fragment has a specific function that differs from the original intact protein.

Complement fixation test (CF)   Antigen-antibody test based on fixation of complement in the presence of both elements and use of an indicator system to identify complement fixation.

Complementary   Term used to describe the ability of two molecules to bind together by pairing chemical and physical structure, such as complementary nucleic acid sequences.

Complementary DNA molecule (cDNA)   A DNA sequence that has been synthesized from an RNA molecule. In eukaryotic DNA technology, the cDNA is complementary to the RNA and does not include the introns that are found in the original DNA template used to transcribe the RNA. Remember, following transcription, eukaryotic RNA is processed and spliced, and introns are removed.

Complex   Commonly used to describe two or more species of organism that cannot be distinguished based on phenotypic, metabolic, or clinical presentation. Individual species may be referred to as molecular siblings.

Composite transposon   A composite transposon includes an internal gene or coding sequence for an antibiotic resistant or other virulence determinant, flanked on both sides by an insertion sequence.

Condylomata   A lesion on the skin that is elevated and irregular; resembles a wart.

Congenital   A disease or infection that existed before birth.

Conidia   Asexual spores in fungi.

Conjugation   The transfer of genetic material between bacteria by direct contact via tubular structures referred to as pili.

Conjunctivitis   Inflammation of the conjunctivae or membranes of the eye.

Constant region   Portion of the antibody that is identical within a specific isotype (e.g., IgG), and represents the C or carboxyl terminus of the glycoprotein that binds to immune cells.

Constitutive   An essential metabolic component or chemical such as an enzyme that is produced continuously independent of changing environment or nutritional conditions.

Continuous cell line   A group of cells that can be grown repeatedly in artificial culture while maintaining the original characteristics of the cell line.

Contrast   The ability to differentiate one item from another. Stains are used to add contrast to microorganisms to improve the ability to differentiate and increase the contrast of the organism in comparison to the background during microscopy.

Convalescent sera   Serum collected later in the course of an illness than the acute serum, usually at least 2 weeks after initial collection.

Convalescent stage   The period following an illness when an individual begins to improve or recover.

Copulatory bursa   A structure identifiable on some species of male helminths that is used to attach or hold the female worm by the male during sexual mating.

Coracidium   A ciliated larva of a helminth found in water that infects an intermediate host in the parasite life cycle.

Coremia   Clusters of conidiophores tied together; resembles a bundle of threads.

Corepressor   A molecule that combines with another repressor molecule, activating the repressor and preventing transcription of a specific genetic sequence.

Corrosive   A type of chemical that erodes another substance or material.

Coryneform   Club- or rod-shaped gram-positive bacterium.

Counter stain   See secondary stain.

CPE   See cytopathogenic (cytopathic) effect.

Creutzfeldt-Jakob disease   Debilitating prion-caused disease characterized by dementia, ataxia, delirium, stupor, coma, and death; has been transmitted by organ transplant.

Critical concentration   The concentration of a drug is the amount of drug required to prevent growth above the 1% threshold of the test population of tubercle bacilli.

Critical value (panic value)   A laboratory result that indicates a serious state or result for a patient, prompting immediate notification of the primary care provider.

Crossing point   See threshold cycle.

Cross-reaction   When an antibody for a specific antigen reacts with a similar antigen that is different from the immunogen the antibody is directed to.

Croup   See laryngotracheobronchitis. Inflammation of upper airways (larynx, trachea) with respiratory obstruction, often caused by virus infections in children.

Crush prep   See squash prep.

CSF   Cerebrospinal fluid.

Culdocentesis   Aspiration of fluid from the cul-de-sac by puncture of the vaginal vault.

Cut-off value   See threshold.

Cutting plates   Two large ventral platelike structures in the buccal capsule of a hookworm, *Necator* spp., used to aid in feeding.

Cycling probe technology   This technique uses an RNA probe between a reporter and a quencher molecule. The center RNA portion of the molecule is degraded by RNase H releasing the quencher from the reporter resulting in fluorescence. This continues in subsequent cycling with another probe binding and continuing through the reaction.

Cyst   A cyst may be a pocket of fluid within a tissue. A parasitic cyst is a reproductive stage of the organism that may be embryonated or unembryonated and is often resistant to the environment and may be the infective stage of the parasite.

Cysticercoids   Larval stage of a tapeworm.

Cysticercosis   Tissue infection caused by the larval stage (cysticercoid) of a tapeworm.

Cystitis   Inflammation of urinary bladder, most often caused by bacterial infection.

Cytoadherence   Some organisms can adhere or stick to other cells in biological organisms. Some species of malaria, for instance, will stick to the epithelial cells of the peripheral vessels in the human body.

Cytocentrifugation   Specialized centrifuge where the hydraulic forces of the liquid cause the fluid to move away from the sediment that is collected on an absorbent material, leaving the particulate matter and cellular debris in the center of the microscope slide.

Cytokine   Group of biochemicals that are released by specific cells during inflammation that influence other cells.

Cytopathic effect (CPE)   Visible effect or physical changes associated with a specific virus infection seen in cell culture.

Cytoplasm   Fluidlike portion of the cell that contains molecules or various particles and is enclosed within the cell membrane.

Cytoplasmic (cellular) membrane   Membrane that encloses the cytoplasm of the cell.

Cytosol   The fluid portion of the cytoplasm.

Cytostome   Opening in microorganisms that is an invagination or structure that functions in the uptake of nutrients; a primitive mouth.

Cytotoxic T cells (Tc)   Specific subset of T lymphocytes that targets and kills tumor cells or other human cells that are abnormal or infected with intracellular pathogens.

Cytotoxin   Toxin that produces cytopathic effects *in vivo* or in a tissue culture system.

D

Dacryoadenitis   Inflammation of the lacrimal (tear) glands.

Dacryocystitis   Inflammation of the lacrimal sac, due to a blockage in the tear duct.

Dark-field microscopy   Technique used to visualize very small microorganisms or their characteristics by a system that permits light to be reflected or refracted from the surface of objects being viewed. The background field appears dark and the microorganisms appear bright.

Deamination   The removal of an amine group from an amino acid resulting in a decrease in the pH of the medium.

Debridement   Surgical or other removal of dead or dying tissue. Typically used to remove the infecting organism and stop the spread of infection.

Decarboxylation   The removal of a carboxyl group from an amino acid, often resulting in the formation of CO_2. This reaction will only occur in an anaerobic environment in an acidic pH.

Decolorizer   Solution used during staining processes to remove excess stain. Different chemicals are used in different staining procedures.

Decontamination   Process of rendering an object or area safe for unprotected people by removing or making harmless biologic or chemical agents.

Decorticated   Removal of outer covering. Lacking the mammillated outer covering of a helminth egg.

Decubitus ulcer   A craterlike defect in skin and subcutaneous tissue caused by prolonged pressure on the area. This occurs primarily over bony prominences of the lower back and hips in individuals who are unable to care for themselves well and unable to roll or move periodically; also known as a pressure sore or bedsore.

Defensins   Molecules naturally produced by animals to defend against bacterial infections and disease.

Definitive host   Host in which the sexual reproduction of a parasite occurs; required in the parasite's life cycle.

Dematiaceous   See melanized.

Denaturation   Process by which the structure of a molecule is disrupted using heat and chemicals to break the bonds. The term is generally used to describe double-stranded DNA becoming single-stranded by heating or chemical means; also referred to as melting and separating the secondary through quaternary structures of protein folding using heat and chemical buffers.

Dendritic cells White blood cells that are distributed throughout the tissues of the body that are primary phagocytes, which digest and present antigens to specific immune cells.

Denticle Small extension where a conidium is attached.

Deoxynucleotide triphosphates (dNTPs) Basic structure of nucleic acids, a nucleotide that binds to deoxyribose to form the building blocks of deoxyribonucleic acid. The "N" stands for any of the nitrogenous bases.

Deoxyribonucleic acid (DNA) The molecule that contains the genetic code for most living things. Consists of a sugar-phosphate backbone, nitrogenous bases, and deoxyribose.

Dermatome Area of the skin attached to a single nerve.

Dermatophyte A cutaneous fungus that infects the hair, skin, or nails.

Dermis Layer of skin beneath the epidermis that is composed of dense connective tissue rich in blood and nerve supply.

Desquamation Shedding or scaling of skin or mucous membrane.

DFA test Direct fluorescent antibody test.

DIC See disseminated intravascular coagulation.

Dichotomous Branching in two directions.

Differential media Employ some factor (or factors) that allow colonies of one bacterial species or type to exhibit certain metabolic or culture characteristics that can be used to distinguish them from other bacteria growing on the same agar plate. Differential factors are generally visible differences based on metabolic capabilities that can be detected using dyes or indicators that change color with a change in pH or other chemical reaction.

Differential stain A stain that includes two dyes, one primary and one secondary that are sequentially used to stain a structure. Based on the process and affinity of the dyes, the stains attach to different components in a cell, providing a means to differentiate and identify specific organisms based on unique chemical properties or structures.

Digital microscopy An automated or semiautomated system that uses sophisticated software and unique technology that permits laboratories to acquire microscopic digital images of using a web-based interface. This interface allows images using a fully automated microscope to be viewed on a single screen.

Diluent Fluid used to dilute a substance or solute.

Dimorphic fungi Fungi with both a mold phase and a yeast phase.

Diploid cell line A cell line that contains two complete sets of genes or chromosomes that can be passed or subcultured for an extended period in cell culture.

Direct life cycle A parasitic life cycle where the organism remains in a single host type for the entire life cycle and can be transmitted directly between hosts.

Direct microscopic examination A microscopic examination directly from the specimen or sample, prior to any enhancement or growth techniques to isolate organisms from the specimen.

Direct smear A smear or spreading of a sample or specimen from the collection container, without further testing or alteration in the specimen or sample.

Direct transmission The acquisition of an infectious agent or microorganism by coming into direct contact with the microbial reservoir of the agent or organism.

Direct wet mount A preparation from clinical material suspended in sterile saline or other liquid medium on a glass slide and covered with a coverslip; used for microscopic examination to detect microorganisms in clinical material and to detect motility directly.

Disease An abnormal physiological state or condition where the patient demonstrates some type of damage or dysfunction.

Disinfectant Agent that destroys or inhibits microorganisms that cause disease on inanimate objects.

Disinfection The process of removing most of the microorganisms from the surface of an inanimate object or surface.

Disjuncture cell A cell that fragments or lyses to release a spore. After release of the spore, the cell appears as an empty cell.

Disk diffusion (antimicrobial susceptibility testing) A technique that uses small filter-paper disks impregnated with antibiotics. The disks are placed on artificial media that has been inoculated with a lawn of organism. The antimicrobial diffuses into the media and is tested for ability to inhibit the growth of the organism.

Disseminated intravascular coagulation Numerous small blood vessels become clogged with blood clots and bleeding occurs because of the depletion of coagulation factors.

Diurnal Normal day activity, where an organism has a regular day/night life cycle.

DNA See deoxyribonucleic acid.

DNA minor groove A location on double-stranded DNA in which the strand backbones are closer together on one side of the helix than on the other.

dNTPS See deoxynucleotides.

Donovan body Intracellular amastigotes inside tissue cells of the reticuloendothelial system.

Donovanosis A condition caused by *Klebsiella granulomatis* that causes a sexually transmitted disease also known as granuloma inguinale.

Droplet nucleus An aerosolized particle that contains a potentially infectious agent that generally travels three feet or less.

Duplex See hybrid.

Dx Diagnosis.

Dysentery Inflammation of the intestinal tract, particularly the colon, with frequent bloody stools (e.g., bacillary dysentery).

Dysesthesias Pain when touched.

Dysgonic Growing poorly (bacterial cultures).

Dysnomia Demonstrating difficulty recalling verbal or written material upon request.

Dyspareunia Persistent genital pain during sexual intercourse.

Dysuria Painful or difficult urination.

E

Ecchymosis Discoloration of the skin or bruising due to bleeding under the skin.

Echinulate Spines or spikey, rough looking.

Ectocyst Part of a hydatid cyst, the outermost layer.

Ectoparasite Organism that lives on or within the superficial layers of the skin without gaining access to internal organs.

Ectothrix Outside of hair shafts.

ECV See epidemiologic cutoff value.

Edema Excessive accumulation of fluid in tissue spaces.

Effacement Shortening, thinning, or destruction of epithelial cells.

Effusion Fluid escaping into a body space or tissue (e.g., pleural effusion).

Egg packet Diagnostic form of the tapeworm *Dipylidium caninum* found in the feces of infected individuals.

Electron microscopy Microscope that utilizes a beam of electrons to achieve magnifications more than 100,000 times.

Elementary body The infectious stage of *Chlamydia* or a cellular inclusion body of a viral disease.

ELISA Enzyme-linked immunosorbent assay.

Elution Process of extraction by means of a solvent.

EMB Eosin-methylene blue (agar plate).

Emetic toxin Preformed bacterial toxin that induces vomiting.

Empiric therapy Used to initiate therapy based on the physician determining the most likely organism causing a patient's clinical symptoms and then selecting an antimicrobial that, in the past, has worked against that organism in a hospital or geographic area.

Empyema Accumulation of pus in a body cavity, particularly empyema of the thorax or chest.

Encephalitis Inflammation of the brain.

Endocarditis A serious infection of the endothelium of the heart, usually involving leaflets of the heart valves where destruction or distortion of valves occurs because of the formation of vegetation that may lead to serious physiologic disturbances and death; also, an inflammation of the endocardial surface (much less common).

Endocervix Mucous membrane of the cervical canal.

Endocyst The layer within a hydatid cyst that is deepest within the structure.

Endocytosis Method by which a cell membrane extends and surrounds a particle or cell, then invaginates and engulfs the material in an internal vesicle or phagosome.

Endoflagella Axial filament or internal flagella found within a prokaryotic organism, spirillum, or spirochete.

Endogenous Developing from within; internal cause.

Endoparasite Parasite that lives inside the human body; penetration and reproduction within human organ systems causing damage.

Endophthalmitis Inflammation of internal tissues of the eye; may rapidly destroy the eye.

Endospore A spore that develops inside a bacterial cell during poor environmental conditions such as desiccation or lack of available nutrients; nonvegetative.

Endothelium Squamous epithelium lining of the blood vessels.

Endothrix Within the hair shaft.

Endotoxin Substance containing lipopolysaccharide complexes found in the cell wall of bacteria, principally gram-negative bacteria; believed to play an important role in many of the complications of sepsis such as shock, disseminated intravascular coagulation, and thrombocytopenia.

Enrichment media Used in cultures for the enhancement of growth of an organism. The media may be selective or contain specific nutrients or chemicals to increase the growth of an organism or group of organisms.

Enteric fever Typhoid fever; paratyphoid fever.

Enteroinvasive   Capable of invading the mucosal surface and sometimes the deeper tissues of the bowel.

Enterotoxin   Toxin affecting the cells of the intestinal mucosa.

Entropion   Folding inward of the eyelid.

Enzyme-based test   Biochemical test that measures the activity of an enzyme to identify a specific metabolic pathway that can be used to correlate with other laboratory results in an identification scheme. Phenotypic, generally based on a visible or measurable chemical reaction.

Enzyme-linked immunosorbent assay (ELISA)   An immunologic assay that uses an enzyme conjugated to antibodies to produce a visible endpoint.

Epidemiologic cutoff value   Distribution of the minimum inhibitory concentration that is used to separate bacterial populations into those with acquired resistance and the original population.

Epidemiology   The study of the occurrence and distribution of disease and factors that control presence or absence of disease.

Epidermis   Outermost layer of skin made of layered squamous epithelial cells.

Epididymitis   Inflammation of the epididymis characterized by fever and pain on one side of the scrotum; seen as a complication of prostatitis and cystitis.

Epifluorescence   The principle of fluorescent microscopy in which the excitation light is emitted from above.

Epigenetic   Influences on the expression of genes that are not controlled by genetic mechanisms.

Epiglottitis   Inflammation of the epiglottis, a structure that prevents aspirating swallowed food and fluids into the tracheobronchial tree; a serious infection because the swollen epiglottis may block the airway.

Epimastigote   Life cycle form of a *Trypanosoma* spp. that is found in the salivary glands of the vector.

Episome   Small genetic element that exists as an extrachromosomal circular molecule that replicates independently of the chromosome or while integrated in the chromosome.

Epithelium   Tissue composed of contiguous cells that forms the epidermis and lines hollow organs and all passages of the respiratory, digestive, and genitourinary systems.

Epitope   The molecule or chemical groups on an antigen recognized by the specific antibody.

Epizootic   A disease that is temporarily present in a given population of animals.

Erysipelas   An acute cellulitis caused by group A streptococci or *Erysipelothrix* spp.

Erysipeloid   Bacterial infection caused by *Erysipelothrix* spp., generally an acute dermatitis resembling erysipelas.

Erythema   Redness of the skin from various causes.

Erythema migrans   A bullseye-shaped rash associated with Lyme disease.

Erythema nodosum   Skin inflammation in the fatty layers that appear as tender, red, painful lumps.

Erythrasma   A minor, superficial skin infection caused by *Corynebacterium minutissimum*.

Eschar   A black, necrotic lesion associated with cutaneous anthrax.

Etiology (etiologic)   Cause or causative agent.

Eugonic   Growing luxuriantly (bacterial cultures) on artificial media.

Eukaryotic   Organisms with a true nucleus, in contrast to bacteria and viruses.

Exanthem   Skin eruption as a symptom of an acute disease, usually viral.

Exanthem subitum   Viral illness that appears with a high fever, sore throat, and a faint red rash.

Exfoliative toxin   Toxin that causes a blistering and peeling of the skin.

Exoantigen test   *In vitro* immunodiffusion test method for identifying fungal hyphae as *Histoplasma*, *Blastomyces*, or *Coccidioides*.

Exoerythrocytic cycle   Portion of the malarial life cycle occurring in the vertebrate host in which sporozoites, introduced by infected mosquitoes, penetrate the parenchymal liver cells and undergo schizogony, producing merozoites, which then initiate the erythrocytic cycle.

Exogenous   From outside the body.

Exotoxin   A toxin produced by a microorganism that is released into the surrounding environment.

Extension   PCR cycle, where the polymerase synthesizes or extends the new strand from the 3′ hydroxyl of the primer. Generally carried out at 72°C.

Exudate   Fluid that has passed out of blood vessels into adjacent tissues or spaces; high protein content.

F

Fab region   The region or fragment of the antibody that binds the epitope of an antigen.

Facialis   Of the face.

Facultative anaerobe   Microorganisms that are capable of growth under either anaerobic or aerobic conditions.

Fascia   Membranous covering of muscle.

Fastidious   An organism that requires a special nutritional or environmental condition for growth.

Favus   Superficial disease of the scalp caused by a dermatophyte.

Fc region   The Fc region of the antibody is the tail end or bottom of the Y-shaped molecule that binds to cells.

Febrile   Demonstrating a fever.

Feeding (viral cultures)   During the cultivation of viral cultures, periodic replacement of the nutritional fluid in the culture is termed feeding.

Fermentation   Anaerobic decomposition of carbohydrate that results in the production of acid, alcohol, and/or gas.

Fibrinolysin   The breakdown of fibrin clots due to enzymatic action.

Filamentous   Threadlike.

Filariform   The infective larval stage of roundworms for a human host.

Filtration   Method to remove contamination such as microorganisms from heat-labile liquids by pulling the solution through a cellulose acetate or cellulose nitrate membrane with a vacuum.

Fimbriae   Proteinaceous fingerlike surface structures of bacteria that provide for adherence to host surfaces. Also capable of antigenic variation in some microorganisms.

Fistula   Abnormal opening between two surfaces or between a viscus or other hollow structure and the exterior.

Flagella   Complex structures mostly composed of the protein flagellin that are responsible for bacterial motility.

Flammable   A material or chemical that can easily be set on fire.

Flatulence   The production of gas, often following the ingestion of food.

Floccose   Cottony, in tufts.

Flocculation test   A soluble antigen and antibody that generate an end-product that forms macroscopically or microscopically visible clumps.

Fluorescence microscopy   A microscope that uses various wavelengths of ultraviolet light and filters to excite and visualize fluorophores attached to antibodies or other molecules for the visualization of microorganisms directly or in tissues.

Fluorescent   Emission of light by a substance (or a microscopic preparation) while acted on by radiant energy, such as ultraviolet rays, as in the immunofluorescent procedure.

Fluorochrome   A dye that becomes fluorescent or self-luminous after exposure to ultraviolet light.

Fluorophore   A fluorescent molecule that can absorb light energy and then is elevated to an excited state that is released as fluorescence in the absence of a quencher.

Folliculitis   Inflammation or infection of a hair follicle.

Fomite (vehicle)   Any inanimate object that may be contaminated with disease-causing microorganisms and thus serves to transmit disease.

FTA   Fluorescent treponemal antibody.

FTA-ABS   Fluorescent treponemal antigen-antibody absorption: test; indirect fluorescent antibody stain used to detect antibodies directed against whole-cell antigens of *Treponema pallidum* (syphilis bacillus).

Fungemia   Presence of viable fungi in blood.

Fungus (plural Fungi)   Saprophytic eukaryotic organism that obtains nutrients from dead or dying organic matter.

FUO   Fever of unknown origin.

Furuncle   A fluid-filled or pus-filled enlargement at the base of an inflamed or infected hair follicle.

Fusiform   Spindle-shaped, as in the anaerobe *Fusobacterium nucleatum*.

Fusion protein (F protein)   A protein on the envelope of a virus that functions to assist in fusion of the viral envelope with the host cell membrane during entry to the host cell.

Fusoid   A structure that has a wide center and tapered at both ends; scientific term for spindle-shaped.

G

Gametocyte   A cell that divides through the process of meiosis, forming a haploid gamete.

Gametogony   The process or term used to describe the formation of gametes.

Gamma hemolysis   No hemolysis of red blood cells on artificial media.

Gamogony   Fission (dividing in half) resulting in the production of sporozoan gametes.

Gangrene   Death of tissue resulting from disease, injury, or failure of blood supply.

Gas-liquid chromatography (GLC)   A method for separating substances by allowing their volatile phase to flow through a heated column with a carrier gas and measuring the time required to detect their presence at the distal end of the column.

Gastric aspirate   Fluid aspirated from the stomach via a tube placed in the stomach by way of the nose or mouth.

Gastroenteritis   Inflammation of the mucosa of the stomach and intestines.

GC   Gonococcus.

Gene A sequence of nucleic acids that code for a functional product.

Gene expression The visible effect of a gene or phenotypic evidence.

Generalized transduction The movement of any genetic material from a host cell to another via a bacteriophage or virus.

Generation time The amount of time it takes a microorganism to divide into daughter cells.

Genetic code Nucleotide triplets on either DNA or RNA that correlate to a specific amino acid.

Genetic shift Major change in the nucleic acid of a virus. Often associated with influenza viruses that exchange RNA genome segments with another viral strain.

Geniculate Bent.

Genital primordium Genital swelling and opening apparent on a parasite.

Genogroups Viruses in a specific genus that are related.

Genome The entire genetic make-up in an organism.

Genome-to-genome distance A nucleotide sequence technique that uses calculations to determine the relatedness of organisms at the genetic level. The technique is representative of the previous manual DNA-to-DNA hybridization technology.

Genomospecies A species that can be differentiated using genetic or molecular sequences, not considered an actual recognized independent species.

Genomovars A variety of an organism that is genetically different but phenotypically indistinguishable.

Genotype Related to characteristics of an organism's genetic makeup; constituent nucleic acids.

Genotypic A characteristic that is determined by the genetic makeup or nucleic acid sequence and epigenetic mechanisms.

Germicide An agent that destroys germs; disinfectant.

Germ tube Tubelike process, produced by a germinating spore that develops into a regular, hyphal-like structure.

Giant cell See syncytia.

Glabrous Smooth fungal colonial morphology without aerial hyphae.

GLC Gas-liquid chromatography.

Goblet cell Cells found in the respiratory, gastrointestinal, or reproductive tracts. The cells are shaped like goblets with the cellular organelles located on one end with the opposite end containing numerous mucin-filled secretory vesicles.

Granulocytopenia Reduced number of granulocytic white blood cells in the blood.

Granuloma Aggregation and proliferation of macrophages to form small (usually microscopic) nodules; may be associated with a variety of infections, including tuberculosis, forming a hard granuloma or tubercle.

Granuloma inguinale Sexually transmitted disease caused by *Klebsiella granulomatis* that demonstrates a painless, inflammatory reaction in or near the genitals.

Granulomatous amebic encephalitis (GAE) A disease caused by free-living amebae that demonstrates as an acute or chronic infection that is often fatal.

Grocott methenamine silver stain (GMS) A histological silver stain, used to identify fungal structures in tissue.

Growth-based tests Microbiological tests that require an incubation period at a specified temperature and increased growth of the microorganism *in vitro*. Failure for the organism to grow results in an invalid test (end-product measurement) or negative test (nutritional or selective growth).

Growth medium Chemical formula of nutrients and vitamins required for the cultivation of microorganisms. May be liquid, solid, or semisolid media.

Guanidinium isothiocyanate Chemical compound that denatures proteins. Used in nucleic acid extractions to denature enzymes such as RNAse or DNAse that would damage or reduce the yield of the extraction.

Gumma A soft, painless, noninfectious granuloma-like lesion.

H

HAART See highly active antiretroviral therapy.

HACEK *Haemophilus, Aggregatibacter, Cardiobacterium, Eikenella,* and *Kingella.* The *Haemophilus* organisms in this group have been reclassified as *Aggregatibacter,* but the acronym remains unchanged in the clinical environment.

Halogens (chemical disinfectant) Nonmetal element with low melting and boiling points; may exist as gases, liquids, or solids. The chemicals generally kill microorganisms when used in disinfectants.

Halophilic Preferring high halide (salt) content; salt loving.

Hansen disease Leprosy, a disease caused by *Mycobacterium leprae.*

Haverhill fever A disease caused by the microorganism *Streptobacillus moniliformis,* also known as rat-bite fever.

Hemadsorption Ability of certain virally infected cells to bind erythrocytes; mediated by glycopeptide adherence molecules (induced by viral activities within the cell) on the cell's surface.

Hemagglutinin (HA) A glycoprotein found on the surface of a virus particle that participates in the attachment and entry of the virus into the host cell. Exists in multiple antigenic forms or serotypes.

Hemagglutination Agglutination of red blood cells caused by certain antibodies, virus particles, or high molecular weight polysaccharides.

Hematogenous Disseminated by the bloodstream.

Hematuria Blood in the urine.

Hemin (X-factor) Iron containing compound found inside red blood cells that is a required nutritional factor for some fastidious microorganisms.

Hemiparesis Paralysis on one side of the body.

Hemolysin A substance that lyses red blood cells.

Hemolysis, alpha Partial destruction of, or enzymatic damage to, red blood cells in a blood agar plate, leading to greenish discoloration about the colony of the organism producing the alpha hemolysin.

Hemolysis, beta Total lysis of red blood cells about a colony on a blood agar plate, leading to a completely clear zone surrounding the colony.

Hemolysis, gamma No hemolysis is seen with organisms classified as gamma-hemolytic.

Hemolytic uremic syndrome (HUS) Inflammation and damage to the small capillaries in the kidneys that leads to renal insufficiency and may result in death.

Hemoptysis Coughing up blood.

HEPA High-efficiency particulate air filter; used in biological safety cabinets to trap pathogenic microorganisms.

Herd immunity Immunity to an infectious agent in a high percentage of a given population of people that helps prevents spread of the disease.

Hermaphroditic An organism that can produce gametes of both male and female sexes.

Herpes Inflammation of the skin characterized by clusters of small vesicles (e.g., caused by herpes simplex); disease caused by herpes simplex virus.

Heterophile antibody Nonspecific, weak antibodies that are produced in a variety of infectious diseases and other medical conditions.

Heterotroph Organism that requires an external organic carbon source for energy production.

Hexacanth embryo A six-hooked embryo of a tapeworm.

Highly active antiretroviral therapy (HAART) Combination antiretroviral therapy of multiple drugs, generally three or more.

High-pressure liquid chromatography (HPLC) Similar to gas-liquid chromatography but capable of higher resolution because of increased pressure of liquid carrier that runs through the column.

Homogenization Mixing components so that the resulting mixture appears as a single component, or uniform.

Homologous recombination The act of a genetic sequence or fragment combining with another molecule by pairing with a similar sequence.

Horizontal gene transfer Genetic transfer from one organism to another, not through reproduction of the organism.

Hospital information system (HIS) Computer and software system used in a health care or hospital organization.

Howell-Jolly bodies Basophilic staining clusters of DNA found in red blood cells in the peripheral circulation.

HPLC High-pressure (or performance) liquid chromatography.

Household bleach See hypochlorite solution.

Human granulocytic anaplasmosis (HGA) Disease that is transmitted by a tick and caused by the bacterium *Anaplasma phagocytophilum.*

Human microbiome See microbiome.

Human monocytic ehrlichiosis (HME) Disease where the organism *Ehrlichia chaffeensis* infects human monocytes or macrophages.

Humoral immunity Antibody-mediated immunity.

HUS See hemolytic uremic syndrome.

Hutchinson triad Set of three clinical symptoms of deafness, blindness, and notched peg-shaped teeth associated with a diagnosis of congenital syphilis.

Hyaline Colorless, transparent.

Hyalohyphomycosis Fungal disease caused by hyaline or colorless fungal organisms.

Hybrid (duplex) Two nucleic acid strands that have complementary base sequences that have specifically bonded with each other and formed a double-stranded molecule.

Hybrid capture The use of a synthetic oligonucleotide or nucleic acid sequence to capture a complementary sequence in solution for amplification or quantitation in a molecular assay.

Hybridization Mixing of two molecular components, such as two nucleic acids or a protein and a nucleic acid under conditions where they interact and attach to each other indicating a reaction of identity, similarity, or complementation.

Hybridoma The product of fusion of an antibody-producing cell and an immortal malignant antibody-producing cell.

Hydatid cyst A large pouch generally filled with fluid and associated with an *Echinococcus* spp.

Hydatid sand Immature scolices of the tapeworm *Echinococcus* spp.

Hydrocele Fluid-filled sac within the scrotum.

Hydrogen peroxide (chemical disinfectant) A compound that is composed of hydrogen and water that is an effective disinfectant against a wide variety of microorganisms.

Hydrolysis Breakdown of a substrate by an enzyme that adds the components of water to key bonds within the substrate molecule.

Hyperalimentation Process by which nutrition (literally "extra nutrition") is provided; typically administered intravenously in subjects who are not able to absorb foods well from the gut because of disease of the bowel, in subjects in whom it is desirable to put the bowel "at rest" to promote healing, and in malnourished individuals to improve their nutritional status (e.g., before surgery); usually done over an extended period and requires the use of a special-access intravenous catheter such as a Hickman catheter.

Hyperemia Increased blood in a part, resulting in distention of blood vessels.

Hyperinfection Repeated reinfection by a parasitic worm that is already in the host.

Hypertonic Hyperosmotic fluid in comparison to another fluid that is separated by location or a membrane.

Hypertrophy Increased size of an organ resulting from enlargement of individual cells.

Hypha (plural Hyphae) Tubular cell making up the vegetative portion of mycelium of fungi.

Hypnozoites Dormant forms of malarial parasites that are found in the liver.

Hypochlorite solution (NaOCl) 5.25% to 6.15% disinfectant also referred to as household bleach.

Hypofunction Insufficient or decreased function.

Hypoperfusion Reduced blood flow.

Hypoxia Decreased oxygen content of tissues.

I

Iatrogenic Contraction of a disease or illness caused by a medical examination, procedure, or treatment.

Icteric Yellow coloration or pigmentation; jaundice.

Identification scheme Series of procedures or methods used to identify a microorganism. The extent of the identification scheme or work-up depends on the type of organism and its propensity to be the cause of a patient's infection or disease.

Idiotype The antigenic specificity of either a group of antibodies or T-cell receptor (TCR) produced from a population of cloned cells.

IFA Indirect fluorescent antibody; test that detects antibody by allowing an antibody to react with its substrate and adding a second fluorescein dye–labeled antibody that will bind to the first.

Ig, IgG, IgM, etc. Immunoglobulin, immunoglobulin G, immunoglobulin M, etc.

Immortalization See transformation.

Immunization See vaccination.

Immunodiffusion Detection of antigen or antibody by observing the precipitin line formed in a semisolid gel matrix when homologous antigens and antibodies are allowed to diffuse toward each other and react.

Immunofluorescence Microscopic method that uses a fluorescent dye linked (conjugated) to specific antibodies to determine the presence or location of an antigen (or antibody) by demonstrating fluorescence when the preparation is exposed to ultraviolet radiation.

Immunoglobulin (antibody) Synonymous with antibody; five distinct classes have been isolated: IgG, IgM, IgA, IgE, and IgD.

Immunoperoxidase stain Combination of an enzyme that catalyzes production of a colored product with an antibody to facilitate detection of certain antigens, particularly viral antigens.

Immunosuppression Depression of the immune response caused by disease, irradiation, or administration of antimetabolites, antilymphocyte serum, or corticosteroids.

Impetigo Acute inflammatory skin disease, caused by streptococci or staphylococci, characterized by vesicles and bullae that rupture and form yellow crusts.

Incineration Method of treating infectious waste. Hazardous material is burned to ashes at temperatures of 870°C to 980°C.

Inclusion bodies Microscopic bodies, usually within body cells; thought to be virus particles in morphogenesis.

Inclusion conjunctivitis Inflammation of the conjunctiva of the eye; may be caused by *Chlamydia* sp.

Indigenous flora See microbiota.

Indirect concentration wet mount The second part of the classic ova and parasite examination is a concentration step. Because many laboratories no longer do direct wet preps prior to concentration, this terminology has been used to distinguish a wet prep following concentration of the specimen.

Indirect life cycle A parasite that requires multiple hosts to complete the reproductive cycle.

Indirect microscopic examination A microscopic examination of an organism after cultivation on artificial media, not directly from the clinical specimen.

Indirect smear A smear of an organism placed on a microscope slide after cultivation of the organism on artificial media, not directly from the clinical specimen.

Indirect transmission The acquisition of an infectious agent or microorganism by coming into contact through an intervening living vector or nonliving fomite or vehicle of transmission that is not the reservoir.

Indirect wet prep A preparation of a clinical specimen that has been preserved to prevent infection or contamination killing the organisms. Associated with a concentration of a stool specimen in preservative for the identification of parasites.

Inducible A metabolic component or chemical such as an enzyme that is turned on or expressed only when required in changing environmental or nutrient conditions.

Induction The process of turning on the production of a metabolic component or chemical at the level of transcription or translation in response to changing environmental or nutrient conditions.

Induration Abnormal hardness of a tissue or part resulting from hyperemia or inflammation, as in a reactive tuberculin skin test.

Infection Invasion by and multiplication of microorganisms in body tissue resulting in disease.

Inflammation Generalized nonspecific immune response that is activated when cells within the body release chemical mediators resulting in vasodilation and increased circulation. The symptoms of inflammation include heat, redness, swelling, and pain.

Inhibitory quotient Ratio of the average peak achievable level of antibiotic in a body fluid from which an organism was isolated to the minimum inhibitory concentration of that organism.

Insertion sequence (simple transposon) Transposable element containing genes that encode the information required to move among plasmids and chromosomes.

***In situ* hybridization** Detection of nucleic acid of a pathogenic organism in tissue sections by separating the DNA into single-stranded molecules and allowing a labeled strand of homologous DNA to bind to the target. The target can be visualized by developing the label (i.e., enzymatic precipitate, fluorescence, or radiolabel).

Inspissation Process of making a liquid or semisolid medium thick by evaporation or absorption of fluid.

Integron A group of genes that move together as a cassette and includes the gene to produce the enzyme integrase that mediates the recombination event.

Integument Outer protective layer of a parasitic worm.

Intercalary Located in between two structures.

Interfacing Communicating between.

Intermediate host Required host in the life cycle in which essential larval development must occur before a parasite is infective to its definitive host or to additional intermediate hosts.

Intermittent carrier An individual colonized with a different strain of a potential pathogenic microorganism over time.

Intertriginous Location where two areas of skin rub or touch each other; folds of skin.

Intoxication Food poisoning caused by the ingestion of preformed toxins.

Intramuscular (intraperitoneal, intravenous) Within the muscle (peritoneum, vein), as in intramuscular injection.

Intracystic Inside the bladder or a cyst.

Intrinsic resistance Natural resistance to antimicrobials based on physiology; generally encoded in chromosomal sequence.

Invariant natural killer cells (iNKT cells) Special population of T cells that recognize lipid-based antigens.

Invasion When a microorganism can break through the primary and secondary immune defenses of the host.

In vitro Literally, within glass (i.e., in a test tube, culture plate, or other nonliving material). Refers to testing of a microorganism in a laboratory environment.

In vivo Within the living animal or human host.

Involution forms Abnormally shaped bacterial cells occurring in an aging culture population.

Iodine tincture Iodine in alcohol.

Ion-exchange chromatography Separation of components of a solution by chromatography based on the reversible exchange of ions in the solution with ions present in or on an external matrix.

Iso cytidine (iso C) Pyrimidine base that is an isomer of cytosine.

Iso guanosine (iso G) Purine base that is an isomer of guanine.

Isothermal amplification   Amplification of a nucleic acid sequence using a single temperature during the entire process.

Isotonic   Of the same osmolality of body tissues, red blood cells, bacteria, etc.

Isotype (antibody)   Five major types of antibodies found in the immune system based on heavy chain constant regions; IgG, IgM, IgE, IgE, and IgA.

K

Karyosome   Dense mass of chromatin material inside a nucleus.

Keratitis   Inflammation of the cornea.

KIA   Kligler iron agar (tube).

Kinetoplast   A mass of mitochondrial DNA that may be visible in some flagellated protozoans.

KOH   See potassium hydroxide stain.

Kohler illumination   Process of steps that ensures even illumination in bright-field microscopy.

Koplik spots   White spots or patches inside the oral cavity associated with the rubeola (measles) virus.

L

Labialis   Fluid-filled lesions or cold sores on the lips.

Laboratory developed tests (LDTs)   A diagnostic test that has been designed and developed in the laboratory. The laboratory must demonstrate the performance characteristics and clinical efficacy of the test.

Laboratory information system (LIS)   Computer system that is utilized within the laboratory that is capable of interfacing with instruments and the hospital computer system.

Lacrimal gland   Paired exocrine glands that secrete tears.

Lag phase   Period of slow microbial growth that occurs following inoculation of the culture medium. Organisms grow slow as they adjust to the changes in the nutrients, temperature, and osmotic pressure or other selective pressures in the medium.

Laked blood   Hemolyzed blood; hemolysis may be affected in various ways, but alternate freezing and thawing is a simple method.

Laminar flow   Nonturbulent flow of air in layers (flowing in a vertical direction in the case of a biosafety hood.)

Laryngitis   Inflammation of the larynx.

Laryngotracheobronchitis   Inflammation of the larynx, trachea, and bronchi.

Latent   An infectious disease that is capable of latency remains in a dormant state within the host without apparent signs or symptoms. Latent infectious agents can reactivate and become active infections.

Lateral gene transfer   Transfer of genetic material across from one cell to another, not due to normal cell growth and division. May be genetic transfer to another genus or species of microorganism or infectious agent.

Latex agglutination   Agglutination of latex particles coated with antibody molecules when exposed to the corresponding antigen.

LCR   Ligase chain reaction.

LDT   See laboratory developed tests.

Lectin   Naturally produced proteins or glycoproteins that can bind with carbohydrates or sugars to form stable complexes.

Legionnaires' disease   Febrile and pneumonic illness caused by *Legionella* spp.

Leishman-Donovan (L-D) body   Small, round intracellular form (called amastigote or leishmanial stage) of *Leishmania* spp. and *Trypanosoma cruzi*.

Lepromatous leprosy   Disseminated leprosy.

Leprosy   See Hansen disease.

Leukocytoclastic vasculitis   Inflammation of the small blood vessels that is immune mediated. May also be called hypersensitivity vasculitis.

Leukocytosis   Elevated white blood cell count.

Leukopenia   Low white blood cell count.

LGV   Lymphogranuloma venereum; the name for certain strains of *Chlamydia trachomatis* that cause a systemically expressed sexually transmitted disease.

Light microscopy (bright field)   Microscope that uses visible light for detection. Items appear dark on a bright background.

Limit of detection (LOD)   Lowest level an analyte can be detected in comparison to a negative sample.

Lipopolysaccharide   Carbohydrate-lipid complex; integral substance in gram-negative cell walls. Also known as endotoxin.

Liposome   Small, closed vesicle consisting of a single lipid bilayer.

Lipoarabinomannan (LAM)   A glycolipid that is a major cell wall component in *Mycobacterium tuberculosis*.

Liquid phase extraction   Nucleic acid purification completed by separating phases in solution and centrifugation. Often uses organic compounds for phase separation.

Livestock-associated infection (LAI)   Infectious disease acquired through contact with livestock.

LOD   See limit of detection.

Logarithmic phase   Period of maximal growth rate of a microorganism in a culture medium.

L-phase   Cells that form without cell walls.

LPS   Lipopolysaccharide; see endotoxin.

Lysis   Disintegration or dissolution of bacteria or cells.

Lysogenic   Refers to the life cycle of a virus capable of lysogeny.

Lysogeny   Viral genome integrated into that of its host bacterium resulting in replication of the virus through the replication and division of the host organism.

Lysosome   Internal cellular–membrane-enclosed vesicle that contains digestive enzymes.

Lysozyme   The enzyme, muramidase, produced in animals including humans that is capable of digesting cell wall components, peptidoglycan residues, in gram-positive and gram-negative bacteria.

M

MAC   *Mycobacterium avium-intracellulare* complex.

Macrophage   See monocyte.

Macroconidia   Large, usually multiseptate, club- or spindle-shaped fungal spores.

Macrodilution (antibiotic susceptibility testing)   Procedure is the same as determining minimum inhibitory concentration with a microdilution (0.05 to 0.1 mL of media) with a larger volume of media, usually 1 mL or greater.

Macules   Small, round, flat color changes in the skin.

Magnification   The measurement of enlargement for visualization of an object that can be completed using a microscope and various sets of lenses.

Maintenance medium   Viral maintenance media is a liquid formula that is placed over cell cultures to maintain growth of the cells without initiating rapid growth; rapid growth also results in rapid death, which is undesirable in cell culture.

Major histocompatibility complex   Large group of genes on the human chromosome that encodes for proteins on the surface of cells that play a role in recognition of self and nonself molecules.

Mammillated   Covering that is rough or lumpy.

Mass spectrometry   Method for determining composition of a substance by observing its volatile products during disintegration and comparing them with known standards.

Master mix   See reaction mix.

Mastoidectomy   Procedure that removes air from within the skull near the inner ear.

Matrix-assisted laser desorption ionization time-of-flight mass spectrometry (MALDI-TOF MS)   Ionization method that uses a matrix to absorb the laser energy, allowing the protein ions to escape.

Matrix protein   Viral structural proteins that attach the viral envelope to the viral core proteins and stabilize the virion structure.

MBC   Minimum bactericidal concentration.

McFarland standard   0.5 McFarland standard, which is commercially available, provides an optical density comparable to the density of a bacterial suspension of 1.5×10^8 CFU/mL.

Media, differential   Media that incorporates a substrate and indicator system so that organisms possessing certain enzymes are recognized.

Media, enrichment   Media that contain high levels of nutrients to enhance the growth of an organism or group of organisms.

Media, selective   Culture media that contain inhibitory substances or unique growth factors such that one organism or organisms being sought will grow and prevent the growth of other types of organisms.

Mediastinum   Space in the middle of the chest between the medial surfaces of the two pleurae.

Melena   Feces that contains blood; appears dark and has a sticky consistency.

Melioidosis   Disease caused by *Burkholderia pseudomallei*.

Melting temperature (Tm)   The temperature is a calculated value based on the number of purines and pyrimidines. When applied to a double-stranded DNA, 50% of double-stranded DNA becomes single-stranded. Formula 2°C (#A+#T) + 4°C (#G + #C)

Meningitis   Inflammation of the meninges, the membranes that cover the brain and spinal cord (e.g., bacterial meningitis).

Meningoencephalitis   Concomitant meningitis that occurs with encephalitis (inflammation of the brain parenchyma).

Mesophilic   An organism that prefers to grow in a temperature range generally between 20°C and 45°C.

Merogony   Parasitic protozoan asexual reproduction via duplication of the nucleus.

Meront   The form of a parasitic protozoan that undergoes reproduction or doubling of the nucleus and organelles of the cell.

Merozoite   Product of schizogonic cycle in malaria that invades red blood cells.

Mesenteric adenitis   Inflammation of mesenteric lymph nodes.

Mesentery   A fold of the peritoneum that connects the intestine with the posterior abdominal wall.

Metabolic profile   A series of biochemical reactions that are characteristic of a specific organism or group of organisms used for identification purposes.

Metacercariae   A tailless, encrusted larva of a trematode.

Metacestode larvae   Larval stage of a tapeworm found in an intermediate host.

Metacyclic   Infective cycle of a trypanosome outside of the host.

Metastatic   Spread of an infectious (or other) process from a primary focus to a distant one via the bloodstream or lymphatic system.

Metulae   Outer branch of a fungus that is directly attached to the conidia.

MHA-TP   Microhemagglutination test for antibody to *Treponema pallidum*.

MIC   Minimum inhibitory concentration.

Microaerobic   Requiring a partial pressure of oxygen less than that of atmospheric oxygen for growth. Refers to both capnophilic and microaerophilic organisms.

Microaerophilic   Microorganism that grows under reduced O_2 (5% to 10%) and increased CO_2 (8% to 10%).

Microarray   High throughput molecular diagnostic test that uses a solid surface coated with numerous nucleic acid sequences.

Microbiome   The total populations of varying microorganisms that live in or on a host and do not cause harm. Considered normal flora, microbiota or indigenous flora provide protection to the host from other potentially invading pathogens.

Microbiota   The microorganisms that are generally present as colonizers in and on the surface of living organisms. Considered normal or indigenous flora or resident microbiota. Prevent the colonization of the surfaces by other pathogenic microorganisms or infectious agents.

Microconidia   Small, single-celled fungal spores.

Microdilution (antibiotic susceptibility testing)   Determining the minimum inhibitory concentration of an antibiotic using a small media volume of 0.05 to 0.1 mL.

Microfilaria   Embryos produced by filarial worms and found in the blood or tissues of individuals with filariasis.

Microforms   Abnormally small yeast cells, ranging from 2 to 5 μm.

Microorganism-mediated resistance   Acquired antimicrobial resistance because of mutational genetic events, gene exchange, or both.

Miliary   Of the size of a millet seed (0.5 to 1.0 mm); characterized by the formation of numerous lesions of the above size distributed rather uniformly throughout one or more organs.

Minimum bactericidal concentration (MBC)   The minimum concentration of antimicrobial agent needed to yield a 99.9% reduction in viable CFUs of a bacterial or fungal suspension.

Minimum inhibitory concentration (MIC)   The minimum concentration of antimicrobial agent needed to prevent visually discernible growth of a bacterial or fungal suspension.

Miracidium   Free-swimming, ciliated larval stage of a fluke.

Mixed culture   More than one organism growing in or on the same culture medium and mixed within the colonies, as opposed to a single organism in pure culture or a pure colony.

Mobilome   The set of mobile genetic elements within an organism's genome.

Mode of action   Also known as mechanism of action; the biochemical interaction of the drug and the intended target.

Mode of transmission   The means in which an individual encounters an infectious agent or microorganism.

Molecular sibling   An organism that cannot be distinguished from another based on phenotypic, metabolic, and clinical presentations; it is recognized as a different species from its sibling based on molecular analysis.

Molecular weight size marker   These are commercially prepared prestained or unstained proteins or nucleic acid markers of known sizes that are applied to electrophoresis to monitor the separation of the molecules and are used as comparative size markers based on migration distance.

Monocistronic   Single gene or coding sequence.

Monoclonal antibody   Antibody that is derived from a single cell producing one antibody molecule type that reacts with a single epitope.

Monocyte   Mononuclear phagocytic cell present in the peripheral blood circulatory system that when activated by invasion of a foreign agent or microorganism, the cell moves toward the site of injury or infection and is a primary phagocyte known as a macrophage.

Monolayer   A confluent layer of tissue culture cells one cell thick.

Monomicrobic   Contains one single, specific organism.

Monozoic   An oocyst that develops into a single sporozoite.

Mordant   Chemical that combines with a dye or stain and fixes it within the material or cell.

Morphotype   Group of bacteria that is distinguishable from others based on physical characteristics.

Morulae   Cytoplasmic vacuoles containing enriched organisms.

MOTT   Mycobacteria other than *Mycobacterium tuberculosis*.

Mucociliary escalator   Ciliated cells that line the mucus membranes of the bronchi and trachea. Upward movement of cilia transfers infectious agents and particles trapped in mucus out of the lower lungs.

Mucopurulent   Term used to describe material containing both mucus and pus (e.g., mucopurulent sputum).

Mucosa   A mucous membrane.

Mucosa-associated lymphoid tissue (MALT)   Areas of focused lymphoid tissue and cells throughout the body and associated with mucous membranes such as in the lungs.

Mucosal surface phagocytes (M cells)   Macrophages and neutrophils that migrate to the mucosal surfaces.

Mucus   Thick, sticky, gelatinous chemical naturally produced by the body that lines the sinuses, nose, mouth, throat, esophagus, and lungs. Contains chemicals such as digestive enzymes (i.e., lysozyme) and antibodies that protect the body from infecting microorganisms; it lubricates the membranes to keep them from drying.

Multilocular   Multiple chambers.

Multiple myeloma   Malignancy involving antibody-producing plasma cells.

Multiplex PCR   A PCR reaction with more than one primer pair in the reaction mixture is used to amplify more than one target sequence, generally from multiple different organisms simultaneously.

Murein layer   The peptidoglycan layer that consists of protein and sugar within the cell wall of bacteria.

Murein sacculus   The entire composition of the peptidoglycan layer that surrounds the cell.

Mutagen   A chemical or radiation that is capable of causing mutations in nucleic acids.

Mutation   Change in the original nucleotide sequence of a gene or genes.

Mycelium   Mass of hyphae making up a colony or visible structure of a fungus.

Mycetoma   Chronic infection, usually of feet, caused by various fungi or by *Nocardia* or *Streptomyces*, resulting in swelling and sinus tracts; pulmonary mycetoma is a mass of fungal hyphae ("fungus ball") growing in a cavity formed during previous tuberculosis infection or other pathologic condition.

Mycolic acid   Long-chain fatty acids found in the cell walls of *Mycobacterium* spp.

Mycoses   Diseases caused by fungi (e.g., dermatomycosis, fungal infection of the superficial skin).

Mycotic aneurysm   Bacterial infection causing inflammatory damage and weakening of an arterial wall.

Myocarditis   Inflammation of the heart muscle.

Myositis   Inflammation of a muscle, sometimes caused by infection, as in pyomyositis.

N

NAD   See nicotinamide adenine dinucleotide.

Noncarriers   An individual that is not colonized with any potential pathogenic microorganism.

Nares   External openings of nose (i.e., nostrils).

Nasopharyngeal   Pertaining to the part of the pharynx above the level of the soft palate.

Natural killer cells (NK cells)   Type of lymphocyte (white blood cell) that is part of the innate or natural nonspecific immunity. The cells destroy tumor cells and virally infected cells.

Necrosis   Pathologic death of a cell or group of cells.

Necrotizing fasciitis   A very serious, painful infection involving the fascia (membranous covering) of one or more muscles; may spread widely in short periods since there is no anatomic barrier to spread in this type of infection.

Negative control   A standardized sample used in a diagnostic assay or test that is reproducible and consistently demonstrates a negative result in the assay.

Negative validation testing   Method used to compare a validation of a test to invalid data.

Negri bodies   Inclusion bodies found in nerve cells infected with the rabies virus.

Neonatal   First 4 weeks after birth.

Nephelometry   Measurement of turbidity where the photometer is placed at angles to the suspension, and the scattered light, generated by a laser or incandescent bulb, is measured.

Nested PCR   A PCR assay that involves the sequential use of two primer sets, with one set inside the other, amplifying internal sequence within the first amplicon.

Neuraminidase (NA)   Viral protein of influenza virus. Cleaves sialic acid residues in mucus, permitting the virus to attach, and assists in releasing the virus from infected cells.

Neurotrophic   Having a selective affinity for nerve tissue.

Neutrophil (PMN, polymorphonuclear cell)   A white blood cell that contains a multilobed nucleus. The cell is considered the first responder to any break or penetration of barriers to infection. The cell is a nonspecific phagocyte.

Next-generation sequencing (NGS)   High-throughput DNA sequencing that uses parallel processing of amplified DNA templates in separated chambers.

NGU Nongonococcal urethritis.

Nicotinamide adenine dinucleotide (NAD) Metabolic cofactor used in energy-generating pathways.

Nick translation Use of enzymes to break DNA and repolymerize small sections of the molecule, usually to label the DNA with a radioactive nucleotide.

Nocturnal Active during the nighttime.

Nomenclature Naming of microorganisms according to established rules and guidelines. Also, see binomial nomenclature.

Nonphotochromogen Slow-growing, non-pigmented mycobacteria independent of light conditions.

Nonseptate See aseptate.

Nonspecific immune defense mechanisms Physical or chemical attributes of the human structure or function that are not directed at a specific infectious agent. Considered part of the natural innate immune system.

Nontuberculous mycobacteria (NTM) All species of mycobacteria that do not belong to *Mycobacterium tuberculosis* complex.

Normal flora See microbiota.

Northern blot Separation of RNA using electrophoresis followed by transfer to a solid membrane surface and detected using a labeled complementary nucleic acid probe.

Nosocomial Pertaining to or originating in a hospital or other health care facility, for example, nosocomial infection also referred to as health care–associated or acquired infection.

Nucleic acid hybridization Process by which the single-stranded nucleic acid fragment or probe unites (hybridizes) with complementary DNA.

Nucleic acid probe Piece of labeled single-stranded DNA used to detect complementary nucleic acid in clinical material or a culture that specifically identifies the presence of the sequence in the material.

Nucleocapsid Virus nucleic acid core enclosed in the protein capsid coat.

Nucleoid Genetic material of a prokaryotic cell; generally, centrally located.

Nucleoprotein Protein complex with nucleic acid.

Nucleotide Contains a nucleoside (which is a sugar), a nitrogenous base, and a phosphate that make up the building blocks of nucleic acids.

Nucleus Membrane-bound structure that encloses the nucleic acid genome in eukaryotic cells.

Nutritive media Media that support the growth of a wide range of nonfastidious microorganisms and are considered nonselective.

O

Octal numbers Numbers used in computer databases to identify biochemical profiles of organisms and thus their identification.

O-F Oxidation-fermentation medium. Paired set of tubes that contains a carbohydrate. One tube is overlaid with oil to produce anaerobic conditions, and the other is left open to atmospheric oxygen. Differentiates an organism's ability to oxidize or ferment the carbohydrate.

Oil immersion Use of immersion oil to fill the space between the slide being studied and the special objective (oil immersion lens) of the microscope; this keeps the light rays from dispersing and provides good resolution at high magnification (total magnification of 1000×).

Oligonucleotide probe See probe.

Oncogenic Possessing the potential to cause normal cells to become malignant; causing cancer.

Oncosphere Larval form of a tapeworm found in the intermediate host.

Oncovirus Virus capable of causing cancer.

ONPG O-nitrophenol-β-galactopyranoside (β-galactosidase test).

Onychomycosis Infection of the nail and nail bed and surrounding tissue.

Oocyst A cyst that contains a diploid zygote from a protozoan.

O&P Ova and parasite examination. Includes three parts, a wet mount, concentration, and a smear that is permanently stained for detection and detailed identification of parasites from fecal samples.

Operator region Region of a sequence of genes or operons that lie within the promoter region and controls transcription by the binding of a regulatory protein.

Operculated ova Ova possessing a cap or lid.

Operculum The cap or lid of a parasitic egg or ovum.

Operon A set of genes in a prokaryotic cell that are controlled by one promoter and function as a set of products that work together.

Opportunistic infection An infection caused by an opportunistic pathogen.

Opportunistic pathogen Organism that does not normally cause disease or damage in a host, but under specific conditions or opportunities causes pathology or disease.

Opsonize (opsonization) To facilitate destruction of pathogens by phagocytic ingestion or lysis by complement through the action of coating antibodies or complement fragments.

Optical density A measurement of turbidity.

Oral cavity The oral cavity includes the mouth, the buccal mucosa (lining inside of the mouth), the palate (bony roof of the mouth), the tongue, and the floor of the mouth underneath the tongue.

Origin of replication Specific sequence on a segment of a chromosome where replication begins.

Orolabial Mouth and lips.

Osteomyelitis Inflammation of the bone and the marrow.

Otitis Inflammation of the ear from a variety of causes, including bacterial infection; otitis media is inflammation of the middle ear.

Otomycosis Fungal ear infection.

Ovum Female reproductive cell or egg.

Oxidation A metabolic pathway of the microorganism that involves use of oxygen as a terminal electron acceptor.

Oxidation-reduction potential Electromotive force exerted by a nonreacting electrode in a solution containing the oxidized and reduced forms of a chemical, relative to a standard hydrogen electrode; the more negative the value, the more anaerobic conditions are.

Oxidative phosphorylation Metabolic pathways that utilize oxygen to add phosphates to organic molecules resulting in energy rich molecules to fuel cellular processes.

Oxidizing (chemical) Chemical that can accept electrons from another chemical.

Ozena Chronic nasal drainage (rhinitis); may be accompanied with cellular destruction.

P

Palindromic sequence A sequence of a nucleic acid that reads the same in the forward and reverse direction.

Pandemic Epidemic over a wide geographic area, or even worldwide.

Papilla A bump or protrusion that extends from a plant, fungus, or tissue.

Papules A slightly elevated red rash that contains no fluid.

Paracentesis Surgical transcutaneous puncture of the abdominal cavity to aspirate peritoneal fluid.

Parafungal Organisms that resemble fungi but have characteristics of protozoans.

Parasite Organism that lives on or within and at the expense of another organism.

Paratenic Not required for the development or life cycle of the parasite.

Parenchymatous Soft cellular tissue.

Parenteral Route of administration of a drug other than by mouth; includes intramuscular and intravenous administration.

Paronychia An infection of the tissues surrounding the nails.

Par otitis Inflammation of the parotid gland, the largest of the salivary glands; mumps is the most common cause of this.

Paroxysm Rapid onset (or return) of symptoms; term usually applies to cyclic recurrence of malaria symptoms, which are chills, fever, and sweating.

Paroxysmal stage Stage of pertussis that is evident by violent coughing with a characteristic whooping sound.

Parthenogenesis A form of asexual reproduction in which growth and development occur without fertilization.

Passive immunization Immunization that is a result of passively providing either antibodies or cells from another immune individual.

Pasteurization Heating a substance to remove pathogenic organisms without removing all organisms within a food; extends the shelf life of the food.

Pathogen Microorganism that causes infection and/or disease.

Pathogenesis The process or development of disease.

Pathogenic Producing disease.

Pathogenicity The ability of an organism or infectious agent to produce disease.

Pathogenicity islands Stretches of DNA that contain genes associated with bacterial virulence and are absent in avirulent or less virulent strains of the same species.

Pathologic Caused by or involving a morbid condition, as a pathologic state.

Pauciseptate Few or sparsely septate cross walls.

PCR See polymerase chain reaction.

Peak level The highest concentration a drug or antimicrobial can reach in the patient's blood.

Peliosis Proliferation of small blood capillaries and spaces that fill with blood in a specific organ or tissue.

Penicillin-binding protein Enzymes essential for bacterial cell wall production, trans peptidases. When bound by penicillin, cell wall synthesis stops.

Penicillinase (β-lactamase) Enzyme produced by some bacterial species that inactivates the antimicrobial activity of certain penicillins (e.g., penicillin G).

Peptide nucleic acid probe (PNA) Synthetic nucleic acids that have replaced the negatively charged sugar-phosphate backbone of DNA with a neutral polyamide backbone.

Peptidoglycan Bacterial cell wall or murein layer that gives the bacterial cell shape and strength to withstand changes in environmental osmotic pressures.

Peracetic acid (chemical disinfectant) (0.23%) combined with hydrogen peroxide, effective for removal of contamination when organic material such as blood or body fluids are present.

Percutaneous Performed through the skin (e.g., percutaneous bladder aspiration).

Pericarditis Inflammation of the covering of the heart (pericardium).

Perineum The portion of the body bound by the pubic bone anteriorly, the coccyx posteriorly, and the bony prominences of the ileum on both sides.

Periodic acid–Schiff (PAS) stain Method of staining that relies on a specific reaction known as the Schiff reaction used to stain polysaccharides, glycogen, glycoproteins, and glycolipids in tissue or cells.

Periodicity A recurring cycle that has a specific pattern.

Periplasmic space Space between the inner cellular membrane and the outer membrane of a gram-negative microorganism.

Peritoneal cavity Space between the visceral and parietal layers of the peritoneum.

Peritoneum Large, moist, continuous sheet of serous membrane lining the abdominal pelvic cavity and the outer coat of the organs contained within the cavity.

Peritonitis Inflammation of the peritoneal cavity, most often caused by bacterial infection.

Pernicious anemia A decrease in red blood cells due the body's inability to absorb or a decrease in vitamin B_{12} (deficiency).

Persistent carrier An individual that is colonized with a single strain of a potential pathogenic microorganism for an extended period.

Persister cells Microbial cells that are deep within a bacterial biofilm that display reduced metabolism and a higher level of antibiotic resistance.

Personal protective equipment (PPE) Protective equipment that is worn to avoid infection, including gowns, gloves, mask, respirators, and other more advanced equipment based on the degree of infectious agent.

Pertussis Upper respiratory infection characterized by a sustained cough primarily caused by *Bordetella pertussis*.

Petechiae Tiny hemorrhagic spots in the skin or mucous membranes.

PFGE See pulsed-field gel electrophoresis.

Phaeohyphomycosis Term used to describe any infection caused by a dematiaceous organism.

Phagocyte A type of white blood cell that can engulf bacteria and other particles in the body and digest and remove them.

Phagocytosis Process of ingesting cells.

Phagolysosome A membrane-enclosed structure within a cell, following the fusion of a phagosome and lysosome, which functions in the digestion and removal of foreign materials.

Phagosome Internal vesicle that contains foreign material within a phagocytic cell.

Phase-contrast microscopy Technique for direct observation of unstained material in which light beams pass through the object to be visualized and are partially deflected by the different densities of the object. The light beams are deflected again when they impinge on a special objective lens, increasing in brightness when aligned in phase.

Phenolic (chemical disinfectant) Derivatives of carbolic acid (phenol) such as *ortho*-phenyl-phenol and *ortho*-benzyl-*para*-chlorophenol.

Effective in killing all types of microorganisms but is not considered sporicidal (it is unable to destroy endospores).

Phenotype Pattern of characteristics of an organism beyond the genetic level that includes readily observable features.

Phenotypic A characteristic that is observable.

Phialide Projection of a fungus that is directly attached to the conidia or reproductive spores.

Photo bleaching Fading or the permanent loss of fluorescence because of chemical damage to the fluorochrome.

Photochromogen Mycobacteria that produce pigment after exposure to light but whose colonies remain buff-colored in the dark.

Photometer Instrument that converts the light that impinges (strikes) the surface of a detector and converts the interaction to an electrical impulse, which can be quantified.

Phycomycosis Serious infection involving fungi, often beginning with necrotic lesions in the nasal mucus or palate but rapidly spreading to involve other tissues. Seen in immunocompromised patients.

Phylogeny Subdivision of biology that characterizes and separates organisms based on evolutionary relatedness.

PID Pelvic inflammatory disease.

Pili Structures in bacteria similar to fimbriae that participate in bacterial conjugation and transfer of genetic material.

Planktonic Free-living organisms that float in a liquid environment or body of water; organisms do not live attached to surfaces.

Plasma Fluid portion of blood; obtained by centrifuging anticoagulated blood.

Plasma cell An activated B cell that produces antibodies.

Plasmids Extrachromosomal DNA elements of bacteria carrying a variety of determinants that may permit survival in an adverse environment or successful competition with other microorganisms of the same or different species.

Plateau phase The final phase of PCR when no additional products are being produced and all the reaction components are used up.

Pleomorphic Having more than one form or shape, usually widely different forms, as in pleomorphic bacteria that microscopically may appear as both cocci and rods in the same sample.

Plerocercoid Larvae of tapeworms, generally the infective stage of an intermediate host.

Pleura The serous membrane enveloping the lung and lining the internal surface of the thoracic cavity.

Pleural empyema Foci or collection of pus and microorganisms in the pleural cavity.

PMN See neutrophil.

PNA See peptide nucleic acid probe.

Pneumolysin Bacterial cholesterol-dependent exotoxin that forms pores in the membranes of human cells inducing further cellular damage and cell lysis.

Pneumonia Inflammation of the lungs, primarily caused by infectious agents.

Pneumonic plague Respiratory form of an infection with *Yersinia pestis*.

Pneumothorax Introduction of air (usually inadvertently) into the pleural space, leading to collapse of the lung on that side.

Poisonous (chemical) Capable of causing serious illness and death.

Polar filament Filament or tubule in a spore or egg of a parasite that is used to penetrate a host cell.

Polar tubule See polar filament.

Polycistronic A nucleic acid sequence that encodes an mRNA, which contains more than one gene or cistron in a single molecule.

Polyclonal antibody Collection of antibodies made by multiple B cell lineages to the same antigen.

Polymerase An enzyme that makes a polymer of nucleic acid; DNA polymerase or RNA polymerase.

Polymerase chain reaction (PCR) A method for expanding small discrete sections of DNA by binding DNA primers to sections at the ends of the DNA to be expanded and using cycles of heat (to create single-stranded DNA) and cooler temperatures (to allow a DNA polymerase enzyme to create new sections of DNA between the primer ends).

Polymicrobic Contains more than one specific type or species of microorganism.

Polymorphic An organism with more than one life cycle form or cellular shape.

Polymorphonuclear cell See neutrophil.

Polyphasic taxonomy Classification of organisms using a complex analysis of the ribosomal ribonucleic acid (rRNA) sequences, whole genome sequences, epigenetics, and mass spectrometry. This includes mechanisms of control, regulation, transcription, and translational products.

Polysome A messenger RNA that contains multiple ribosomes all simultaneously translating proteins.

Polyvinyl alcohol (PVA) Used as a preservative for stool (fecal) specimens in clinical microbiology to maintain the structure of parasites.

Porin Membrane proteins or pores found in the outer membrane of gram-negative organisms.

Positive control A standardized sample used in a diagnostic assay or test that is reproducible and consistently demonstrates a positive result in the assay.

Post-herpetic neuralgia Burning pain in the nerves following shingles.

Posttranscriptional regulation Regulation of gene expression at the RNA level, prior to translation.

Posttranslational modification Modification of a protein following translation includes adding chemical groups such as phosphates, methyl groups, or others.

Post zone High antigen concentration that results in all antigen-binding sites of available antibodies bound to antigen preventing cross-linking or lattice formation.

Potassium hydroxide stain (KOH) A solution of potassium hydroxide that is used to break up the keratin in tissue cells releasing fungi, in order to visualize them microscopically.

PPD Purified protein derivative (skin test antigen for tuberculosis).

Precipitin test Detection of antigen by allowing specific antibody to diffuse through liquid or gel until an antigen-antibody complex forms; this complex is visualized as a line of precipitated material.

Precision Reproducibility of a test when run several times.

Prepuce Foreskin.

Prevalence Frequency of disease in a population at a given time.

Primary amebic meningoencephalitis (PAM) Fatal infection caused by the free-living ameba *Naegleria fowleri*.

Primary antibody response The first encounter with an antigen that results in the production of antibodies. The classic primary antibody response is predominantly IgM with low levels of IgG.

Primary culture   The initial culture from a specimen on a battery of media based on the site of infection used for additional testing for organism identification and antimicrobial susceptibility testing.

Primary plate reading   Examining the primary culture battery of media used for identification of an organism. Requires correlation of the morphological characteristics and biochemical characteristics of the isolates to direct Gram stains from the primary specimen and the site of infection.

Primary stain   The first stain that is applied to a microscopic smear of an organism in a complex differential stain followed with a decolorization of the smear and application of a secondary stain.

Primer extension   See extension.

Primers   A single-stranded nucleic acid sequence or oligonucleotide used for the initiation of DNA synthesis in an amplification assay. Two primers, a forward and a reverse, are required to complete the synthesis of a double-stranded amplicon.

Prion   Proteinaceous infectious agent associated with Creutzfeldt-Jakob disease and perhaps other chronic, debilitating central nervous system diseases.

Probe   A single-stranded nucleic acid sequence or oligonucleotide that is conjugated with a label and used to detect a specific nucleic acid sequence in a molecular assay by hybridizing to the complementary target.

Proboscis   Tubular appendage on the scolex of a tapeworm.

Procercoid   The first larval stage of a tapeworm that develops within a copepod.

Proctitis   Inflammation of the rectum.

Prodromal   Early manifestations of a disease before specific symptoms become evident.

Proglottid   Segments of the tapeworm containing male and female reproductive systems; may be immature, mature, or gravid.

Prognosis   Forecast as to the possible outcome of a disease.

Prokaryotic   Organisms without a true nucleus.

Promastigote   Life cycle stage of some flagellated protozoans that has a single anterior flagellum and lacks an undulating membrane.

Promoter   A region in a DNA sequence where initiation of transcription begins.

Prophylaxis   Preventive treatment (e.g., the use of drugs to prevent infection).

Prostatitis   Inflammation of the prostate gland, usually caused by infection, characterized by fever, low back or perineal pain, and at times urinary frequency and urgency; a common background factor for recurrent cystitis in males.

Prosthesis   An artificial part such as a hip joint or eye.

Protein A   A protein on the cell wall of strains of *Staphylococcus aureus* (Cowan strain) that binds the Fc portion of antibodies.

Prototroph   Naturally occurring or wild strain.

Prozone   High concentration of antibody versus antigen resulting in failure to cross-link; may result in false negatives.

Pseudohyphae   Extensions from yeast that are irregular, sausage-shaped cells with constrictions evident.

Pseudomembrane   Necrosis of mucosal surface simulating a membrane.

Pseudomembranous colitis (PMC)   Syndrome in the large bowel characterized by a layer of necrotic tissue and dead inflammatory cells often caused by the toxin of *Clostridioides difficile*.

Pseudopodia   Extension from an amoeboid cell that pulls the cell for movement.

Psittacosis   Zoonotic disease caused by *Chlamydia psittaci*.

Psychrophilic   Cold loving (e.g., microorganisms that grow best at low [4°C] temperatures).

Pulsed-field gel electrophoresis (PFGE)   Electrophoretic method that separates large fragments of nucleic acid though an agarose matrix with alternating pulses of current in an electrical field.

Pure colony   A single bacterial or fungal colony on artificial media that is a result of separation and arises from a single cell.

Purine   A double ring compound that is composed of carbon and nitrogen. The purines consist of adenine and guanine and are used in the synthesis of DNA and RNA, as well as other high-energy molecules ATP and guanosine triphosphate (GTP).

Purulent   Consisting of pus.

Pus   Product of inflammation, consisting of fluid and many white blood cells; often bacteria and cellular debris are also present.

Pustule   Containing purulent material consisting of necrotic inflammatory cells.

Pyelonephritis   Infection of the kidney and renal pelvis and the late effects of such infection.

Pyocin   Pigment produced by a bacterium that has antibacterial properties against other strains or species of bacteria.

Pyogenic   Pus-producing.

PYR test   The enzyme, l-pyroglutamyl-amino peptidase, hydrolyzes l-pyrrolidinyl-β-naphthylamide (PYR) to produce β-naphthylamine. When the β-naphthylamine combines with cinnamaldehyde reagent, a red color is produced.

Pyriform   Pear-shaped.

Pyrimidine   A single ring compound that is composed of carbon and nitrogen. The purines thymine and cytosine are used in the synthesis of DNA; uracil and thymine are used in the synthesis of RNA.

Pyridoxal   Active form of vitamin B_6.

Pyrogenic   Fever-inducing.

Pyrosequencing   Method that incorporates a luminescent signal (generation of a pyrophosphate) when nucleotides are added to the growing nucleic acid strand. The release of the pyrophosphate during extension is converted to ATP, which is then used in a chemical reaction to release a chemical signal for each nucleotide. The amount of light is proportional to the amount of the specific nucleotide.

Pyuria   Presence of eight or more leukocytes per cubic millimeter on microscopic examination of uncentrifuged urine.

Q

QC   Quality control.

Q fever   Disease caused by the organism *Coxiella burnetii*.

QNS   Quantity not sufficient.

Quaternary ammonium compounds (chemical disinfectant)   Quaternary ammonium compounds utilize cationic detergents to disrupt the cellular membranes of microorganisms and other organic cells.

Quencher   Molecule that can accept energy from a fluorophore and then dissipate the energy so that no fluorescence results.

Quenching   The transfer of the light energy to nearby molecules in the sample such as free radicals, salts of heavy metals, or halogens.

Quorum sensing   Bacteria produce a variety of molecules when they are multiplying. In this process, they release chemicals that are sensed by the organisms around them. Once they reach a critical mass, the signal up-regulates or down-regulates specific genes to enhance survival of the organism.

R

Radioisotope   Unstable molecule that emits detectable radiation (e.g., gamma rays, x-rays) for a known period (half-life). Can be incorporated into other compounds as a label for later detection by radiographic film exposure or by measurement in a scintillation-counting instrument.

Rapid-growing mycobacterium (RGM)   Growth is apparent sooner than 7 days after subculture to Lowenstein-Jensen medium.

Rat-bite fever   Zoonotic disease caused by *Streptobacillus moniliformis* or *Spirillum minus*.

Reaction mix   Also referred to as master mix.

Reagin   A nonspecific antibody that is produced in syphilis and hypersensitivity reactions.

Real-time PCR (RT-PCR)   A nucleic acid amplification method that uses the incorporation of a fluorescent signal into the amplicon for direct detection during the assay, in real time. May be qualitative or quantitative.

Recrudescence   Recurrence of symptoms.

Redia   Cylindrical larvae of a trematode.

Reiter syndrome   Autoimmune disease that arises following an infection.

Replication fork   The area of DNA synthesis where the two strands of a double helix are unwound, and active replication is in progress.

Reporter molecule   A dye or molecule attached to a probe to detect the specific target sequence.

Repression   The act of shutting off gene transcription, generally by an end-product feedback mechanism.

Repressor   A protein that binds to DNA or RNA, inhibiting the expression of a gene at the transcriptional or translational level.

Reservoir   Source, organism, environment, or place of origin from which an infectious agent may be disseminated; for example, humans are the only reservoir host for *Mycobacterium tuberculosis*.

Resident microbiota   See microbiota.

Resin   Plant product composed largely of esters and ethers of organic acids and acid anhydrides.

Resolution   The extent to which detail in the magnified object is maintained.

Resolving power   Characteristic of a microscope that is defined as the least distance between two objects that when magnified still allows the two objects to be distinguished from each other.

Restriction endonuclease   Enzyme that breaks nucleic acid (usually DNA) at only one specific sequence of nucleotides.

Restriction fragment length polymorphism (RFLP)   A technique that uses restriction endonucleases to produce fragments of nucleic acids that are separated by electrophoresis to identify the different patterns produced by the fragments or fingerprint of the organism.

Restriction site   Also referred to as recognition site or restriction endonuclease site.

Reticulate body   The metabolically more active form of elementary bodies of *Chlamydia* spp.

Reticuloendothelial system Macrophage system, which includes all the phagocytic cells of the body except for the granulocytic leukocytes.

Retroinfection Larva from an *Enterobius* spp. migrate into the anus increasing the level of infection.

Retrovirus An RNA virus that replicates by transcribing from RNA to DNA and then back to RNA. The initial replication enzyme is reverse transcriptase.

Reverse algorithm A method used to diagnose syphilis that begins and ends with a specific syphilis serology test, in place of beginning with a nonspecific screening test.

Reverse transcription Synthesis of DNA from RNA by using the enzyme reverse transcriptase.

Reverse transcription PCR (RT-PCR) A target sequence amplification reaction that begins with RNA and using a reverse transcription enzyme, synthesizes a complementary DNA sequence or amplicon.

RFLP See restriction fragment length polymorphism.

Rhabditiform larvae Nematode larvae that are passed from a definitive host.

Rheumatoid factor IgM antibodies produced by individuals against their own IgG.

Rhinitis Inflammation in the nasal cavity or nose.

Rhinoscleroma Granulomatous (forms masses of immune cells) bacterial infection of the nose.

Rhinorrhea Runny nose.

Ribonucleic acid (RNA) Nucleic acid molecule composed of adenine, guanine, cytosine, and uracil that is generally single stranded and includes messenger RNA (mRNA), transfer RNA (tRNA), ribosomal RNA (rRNA), noncoding RNA (ncRNA), microRNA (miRNA), small regulatory RNA (sRNA).

Ribosome Complex of RNA and proteins that bind mRNA and tRNA to process protein translation in a cell.

Ribotyping A molecular method that uses specific ribosome sequences to place organisms in taxonomic groupings.

Residual body Vesicles of indigestible material in macrophages removed from the cell by exocytosis.

Rhabditoid larvae See rhabditiform larvae.

Rhizoid Fine tubular growth from the stolon or hyphae of a fungus, that appears rootlike.

RNA See ribonucleic acid.

RNase Ubiquitous and stable enzymes that are capable of digesting RNA.

RNase H An enzyme, ribonuclease H, that degrades RNA when it is hybridized to a complementary DNA sequence.

Roseola A mild rash that may include fever caused by herpes viruses.

Rostellum Conelike protrusion from the scolex on the anterior end of a tapeworm. May be armed with hooklets or be unarmed (no hooklets).

RPR Rapid plasma reagin; nontreponemal test for antibodies developed in response to syphilis infection.

RT-PCR See real-time PCR or reverse transcription PCR.

Rugose Fungal colonial morphology characterized by furrows that radiate out from the center.

Saccharolytic Capable of breaking down sugars.

Safety data sheets (SDS) Previously known as material safety data sheets. Provided by manufacturers for chemicals and reagents that include health and safety precautions, storage,

and disposal, as well as emergency information if the material is hazardous.

Salpingitis Fallopian tube inflammation.

Sandwich hybridization Also referred to as a capture probe with a detection probe. The first nucleic acid probe is attached to a solid support and captures the target nucleic acid, followed by hybridization of the second detection probe for identification.

Saprophytic Organisms that obtain nutrients by living on dead organic matter.

SBT See serum bactericidal testing.

Scalded skin syndrome A systemic disease caused by *Staphylococcus aureus* exfoliative toxin (serine protease) producing strains that result in systemic peeling of the skin. Due to systemic damage, patients are highly susceptible to other secondary bacterial infections.

Schizogony Stage in the asexual cycle of the malaria parasite that takes place in the red blood cells of humans.

Schizonts Sporozoites are transmitted from the mosquito vector of the malarial parasite, which mature into schizonts. Schizonts feed on the hemoglobin in the red blood cells.

Schlichter test Synonym for the serum bactericidal level test.

Schüffner dots Round, generally uniform red dots observed in red blood cells infected with malarial species.

Sclerotia A hard mass of mycelium.

Sclerotic Hard, indurated.

Scolex (plural Scolices) Head portion of a tapeworm; may attach to the intestinal wall by suckers or hooklets.

Scotochromogen Pigmented *Mycobacteria* spp. independent of light or dark exposure.

Scutula A mass of hyphae and spores that form a cup-shaped structure.

SCV See small colony variant.

Sebum Oil secreted from the sebaceous glands of the skin to moisten the skin to prevent drying.

Secondary antibody response See anamnestic response.

Secondary stain Used in a differential staining technique. The second dye applied following a decoloration step. Part of staining methods that use two dyes, used to differentiate organisms based on specific structural characteristics.

Selective media Support the growth of one group of organisms but not another organism by adding antimicrobials, dyes, or alcohol or other inhibitory chemicals to a medium.

Semiconservative replication Replication of DNA that begins with two parent strands. Each strand is used as a template to create a complimentary daughter strand; this results in two duplexes that are composed of one parent and one daughter strand.

Semiquantitative culture (isolation) A technique that provides an approximate quantity of colony forming units by either using a calibrated loop or streaking for isolation and estimating colony count based on quadrants.

Semisolid media Bacterial media that contain a lower concentration of agar than solid media. Generally used to visualize the motility of organisms by observing the growth as it moves through the semisolid mixture.

Senescent Aging.

Sense strand The strand of nucleic acid in a double-stranded DNA molecule that encodes the translatable sequence in the 5 to 3 prime orientation.

Sensitivity Ability of a test to detect (the microorganism, nucleic acid, or other compound)

all true cases of the condition being tested for (patient displays signs and symptoms of infectious disease); absence of false-negative results. May also be referred to as analytical sensitivity. (Also see specificity.)

Sepsis A systemic inflammatory reaction caused by microorganisms in the bloodstream that may cause organ damage resulting in death.

Septate Having cross walls.

Septic shock Acute circulatory failure caused by toxins of microorganisms; often leads to multiple organ failure and is associated with a relatively high mortality.

Septicemia Systemic disease associated with presence of pathogenic microorganisms that are multiplying or their toxins are in the blood.

Septum (plural Septa) Single cross wall found in yeast or fungi.

Serology Study or diagnostics that utilizes serum and examines the interactions of antibodies and antigens.

Serosanguineous Like serous but with some blood present grossly.

Serous Like serum.

Serotype A strain of a microorganism that can be differentiated based on antigen types using specific antibodies.

Serpiginous A skin lesion that appears as a wavy line.

Serum Cell- and fibrinogen-free fluid remaining after whole blood clots.

Serum bactericidal testing (SBT) Lowest dilution of a patient's serum that kills a standard inoculum of an organism isolated from that patient; it is related to antibiotic level achieved in the patient's serum and the bactericidal activity of the drug.

Sessile Organisms that grow permanently attached to a substrate surface.

Sheath The outer covering present on some microfilariae, that is, the egg membrane. Unsheathed microfilariae rupture the egg membrane during development and are not sheathed.

Shell vial Small vials that contain a coverslip covered with a monolayer of cells. The cells are inoculated by centrifuging the sample, bringing the potential virus in close contact with the cells.

Shine-Dalgarno sequence Ribosomal binding site upstream of the start codon for protein translation in bacteria.

Shingles Reactivation of chicken pox. Develops a red rash that generally follows major nerve lines.

Sigma factor Accessory protein that is required and binds to the RNA polymerase to recognize the start site for transcription in bacteria.

Signal amplification A method in nucleic acid detection where the signal is enhanced using branched repeating structures and the target is not amplified.

Signs Observable and measurable physiological changes during an infection or disease.

Simple stain A single dye that is applied to a structure on a microscopic smear to improve contrast.

Simple transposon See insertion sequence.

Sinus Suppurating tract; paranasal sinus, hollows, or cavities near the nose (e.g., frontal and maxillary sinuses).

Sinusitis Inflammation of the mucous membranes of the sinuses.

Skin-associated lymphoid tissue (SALT) Immune surveillance-specific cells that are localized within the layers of the skin, including keratinocytes, Langerhans cells, and immunocompetent lymphocytes.

Skin colonizers Generally considered normal microbiota of the surface of the skin. Protect against invading pathogens and do not harm the host.

Slant See definition of "butt." The slant is the upper surface of the artificial solid medium in the tube and is exposed to air.

Slime layer Loose layer of extracellular polysaccharide and proteins that surround a bacterial cell.

Slow-growing mycobacteria (SGM) Require more than 7 days to produce colonies on solid media such as Lowenstein Jensen.

Small colony variant (SCV) Morphological variants of a microorganism that are generally slow-growing subpopulations of a bacterium. They are often resistant to antibiotics and have different phenotypic characteristics.

Sodium polyanethol sulfonate (SPS) Anticoagulant typically found in blood culture media.

Sodoku Zoonotic disease caused by the gram-negative bacterium *Spirillum minus*.

Solid phase extraction A method of extraction for nucleic acids from a sample that uses a solid support column constructed of fibrous or silica matrices, magnetic beads, or chelating agents to bind the nucleic acids.

Solid-phase immunosorbent assay (SPIA) ELISA test in which the captured antigen or antibody is attached to the inside of a plastic tube or microwell, or to the outside of a plastic bead, in a filter matrix, or some other solid support. Allows faster interaction between reactants and more concentrated visual products than ELISA tests performed in liquid.

Somatic Pertaining to the body (of a cell) (e.g., the somatic antigens of *Salmonella* spp.).

Somnolence Feeling drowsy and persistent sleepiness.

Southern blot Also referred to as Southern hybridization. Identification of specific genetic sequences by separating DNA fragments by gel electrophoresis and transferring them to membrane filters *in situ*. Labeled complementary DNA applied to the filter binds to homologous fragments, which can be identified by detecting the presence of the labeled DNA in association with bands of certain molecular size. Named after its discoverer, E.M. Southern.

Spargana White, wrinkled, and ribbon-shaped larvae of the parasite *Spirometra* spp.

Sparsely Small numbers.

Specialized transduction The movement of genetic material that is always connected to the same sequence in the genome from a host cell to another via a bacteriophage or virus.

Specific immune defense mechanisms Functions within the immune system that require a direct interaction and recognition of an antigen that results in the production of a targeted, specific immune response. May result in the production of immune memory.

Specificity Ability of a test to correctly yield a negative result (detect no microorganism, nucleic acid, or other compound) when the condition being detected, or the disease, is absent; absence of false-positive results. May also be referred to as analytical specificity. (Also see sensitivity.)

Spectrum of activity The type of microorganism or bacteria that an antimicrobial does and does not have the ability to affect by either slowing the growth or killing the microorganism.

Spikes A protein extension on a viral capsid or envelope that interacts with the receptor on the host cell that mediates binding and entry into the host cell.

Spiral groove Runs laterally across the posterior end of the parasite *Chilomastix mesnili*, giving the organism a curved posterior that assists the organism during movement.

Spongiform encephalopathies A degenerative brain disorder that is associated with prion disease, where the brain appears with holes like a sponge.

Sporangiophore The entire fungal reproductive structure, including the stalk, sporangium, and sporangiospores.

Sporangiospores Fungal spore that is produced and enclosed within a sporangium.

Sporangium A saclike structure produced at the tip of a long stalk, the sporangiophore.

Spore Reproductive cell of bacteria, fungi, or protozoa; in bacteria, may be inactive, resistant forms within the cell.

Sporocyst The zygote (diploid) stage of a parasite.

Sporogony The asexual reproductive process that results in the formation of sporozoites in parasites.

Sporont Sexual reproductive structure that is diploid but undergoes division known as sporogony for sporozoites.

Sporoplasm Structure of protoplasm that is used to form a spore in the Class Microsporidia.

Sporozoite Slender, spindle-shaped organism that is the infective stage of the malarial parasite; it is inoculated into humans by an infected mosquito and is the result of the sexual cycle of the malarial parasite in the mosquito.

Sputum Material discharged from the surface of the lower respiratory tract air passages and expectorated (or swallowed).

Squash (crush) prep Compressing a microscope slide on the top of another microscope slide that has a tissue or granular specimen and then spreading it with the secondary slide.

Standard precautions (universal precautions) Infection control guidelines used in the care of all patients; they apply to blood, body fluids, and secretions and excretions except sweat.

Start codon The first set of three nucleic acid bases at the beginning of an mRNA where translation of the protein begins.

Stat *Statim* (Latin); immediately.

Stationary phase Stage in the growth cycle of a bacterial culture in which the vegetative cell population equals the dying population.

STD Sexually transmitted disease.

Steatorrhea Excretion of large amounts of fat in the feces.

Sterile (sterility) Free of living microorganisms (the state of being sterile).

Sterilization Method that is capable of killing all life forms including endospores.

Stolon Horizontal stem of a plant or fungi that connects vertical growth of the organisms.

Stomatitis Inflammation of the mucous membranes of the oral cavity.

Stop codon A set of three nucleic acid bases on an mRNA that signals the termination of translation.

Strain typing Generally completed by molecular techniques to determine if an organism is identical to another organism or slightly different. Techniques include ribotyping, sequencing, Pulse Field Gel electrophoresis, and repetitive sequence-based PCR.

Streaking for isolation Technique used to separate microorganisms on artificial media to produce single isolated colonies from a single cell, to produce pure cultures or pure isolates for use in diagnostic testing.

Streptolysin O Oxygen-labile, immunogenic toxin produced by *Streptococcus pyogenes*, group A streptococci.

Streptolysin S Oxygen-stable, nonimmunogenic toxin produced by *Streptococcus pyogenes*, group A streptococci.

Stringency Condition that is described in molecular diagnostics that indicates a chemical and temperature environment that when high requires a specific match between two nucleic acid sequences close to 100%. Low stringency indicates a lower degree of complementation or match and allows flexibility in the interactions between two nucleic acid sequences.

Strobila Long chain of proglottids, or body of a tapeworm.

Struvite crystals Found in the urine of patients infected with ammonia-producing microorganisms. The crystals are composed of magnesium ammonium phosphate.

Stuart medium Semi-solid transport medium that minimizes growth of microorganisms while maintaining viability. Can be used for anaerobes and fastidious organisms such as *Neisseria* spp.

Subclinical Asymptomatic.

Subculture Passing a microorganism from a primary culture to additional artificial media for continued cultivation.

Substrate A substance on which an enzyme acts.

Substrate hyphae Filamentous structures that grow along the surface of the agar.

Substrate level phosphorylation The addition of a phosphate to an organic molecule, creating a high-energy bond that is processed during an intermediate step in a metabolic pathway.

Sulfur granule Small colony of organisms with surrounding clublike material; yellow-brown; resembles grain of sulfur.

Superantigen Molecules produced by microbes (viruses, bacteria, and perhaps parasites) that act independently to stimulate T-cell activities, including cytokine release. Among the most potent T-cell mitogens, superantigen stimulation can result in anergy, or alternatively, systemic immune system activation.

Superinfection Strictly speaking, superinfection refers to a new infection superimposed on another that is being treated with an antimicrobial agent. The new infecting agent is resistant to the therapy initially used and thus survives and causes persistence of the infection (now resistant to the treatment) or a new infection at a different site. The term is used to indicate persistence or colonization with a new organism without any evidence of resulting infection.

Superoxidized water (SOW) 144 mg/L of hypochlorous acid and chlorine, useful as an antiseptic or a disinfectant.

Suppuration Formation of pus.

Suppurative thrombophlebitis Inflammation of a vein wall.

Sympodial Branching of hyphae on two sides where one filament develops more strongly than the opposite. Branching is uneven as result.

Symptoms Something that is felt by an individual due to disease or illness that cannot be measured directly.

Synanamorph Fungi that have different asexual forms of the same fungus.

Syncytia Structure resulting from fusion of cell membranes of several cells to form a multinucleated cellular structure; usually the result of viral infection of the cells.

Syndrome Set of symptoms occurring together (e.g., nephrotic syndrome).

Synergism   Combined effect of two or more drugs, such as antimicrobials, that is greater than the sum of their individual effects.

Synovial fluid   Viscid fluid secreted by the synovial membrane; formed in joint cavities and bursa.

T

Tachypnea   Rapid breathing.

Tachyzoite   The trophozoite form of *Toxoplasma gondii* found in nerve and muscle tissue in the host.

TAE   See tris-acetate buffer.

Taq polymerase   Thermostable DNA polymerase that is used in PCR. Originally isolated from the microorganism *Thermus aquaticus*.

TBE   See tris-borate buffer.

T cells (T lymphocytes)   Lymphocytes involved in cellular immunity and activation of humoral immunity. Types of T cells include T helper, T suppressor, T regulatory, and cytotoxic T cells.

Target amplification   Nucleic acid technique used to copy a specific gene or sequence logarithmically using PCR.

Tegument   An asymmetric fibrouslike structure that surrounds the capsid of a virus and contains approximately 20 proteins. It is essential for initiation of viral replication.

Teichoic acids   Glycerol or ribitol phosphate polymers combined with various sugars, amino acids, and amino sugars that are in the cell wall of gram-positive bacteria.

Teleomorph   Sexual fungal form.

TEM   Transmission electron micrograph.

Temperature enrichment   Using a specific temperature that is either higher or lower than 37°C for the enhanced growth of a microorganism that is capable of growth above or below body temperature. This eliminates contaminating growth of organisms not capable of growth outside of normal body temperature. Used to cultivate most clinically relevant microorganisms.

Template   Template strand of DNA that is copied into a complementary RNA during transcription.

Tenesmus   Painful, unsuccessful straining in an attempt to empty the bowels due to a persistent feeling of needing to pass stool.

Therapy, antimicrobial   Treatment of a patient to combat an infectious disease.

Thermal cycler   A laboratory instrument that can be programmed to change temperatures; includes repeat cycling at specified times used to complete nucleic acid amplification reactions or PCR.

Thermolabile   Adversely affected by heat (as opposed to thermostable, not affected by heat).

Thoracentesis   Drainage of fluid from the pleural space.

Thoracic   Pertaining to the chest cavity.

Threshold   The portion of the curve in PCR where the signal begins to increase exponentially or logarithmically.

Threshold cycle (CT)   The amplification cycle number in which the fluorescent signal rises above background by 10× the standard deviation of the baseline fluorescence; also referred to as the crossing point (CP) or cycle quantification (CQ).

Thrush   A form of *Candida* infection that typically produces white plaquelike lesions in the oral cavity.

Time-kill studies   Process used to determine the effectiveness of an antimicrobial agent or disinfectant that compares the amount of time required to slow the growth or kill the infectious agent.

Tinea   Dermatophyte infection (tinea capitis, tinea of scalp; tinea corporis, tinea of the smooth skin of the body; tinea cruris, tinea of the groin; tinea pedis, tinea of the foot).

Tissue culture   See cell culture.

Titer   Level of a substance such as antibody or toxin present in material such as serum; reciprocal of the highest dilution at which the substance can still be detected.

T lymphocytes (T cells)   Thymus-derived lymphocytes important in cell-mediated immunity.

Tm   See melting temperature.

Tolerance   A form of resistance to antimicrobial drugs; of uncertain clinical importance. See tolerant.

Tolerant   Characteristic of an organism that requires a great deal more antimicrobial agent to kill it than to inhibit its growth.

Tonsillitis   Inflammation of the tonsils.

Toxic shock syndrome   A systemic disorder that may be fatal, caused by a bacterial toxin. It results in the release of biological mediators that result in low blood pressure, organ damage, and shock.

Toxins   A chemical or protein that is produced by an animal, plant, fungi, or microorganism that can cause disease.

TPI   *Treponema pallidum* immobilization test; a test for antibodies against the agent of syphilis that uses live treponemes.

Trichiasis   Curling or ingrowth of eyelashes.

Trachoma   Serious eye infection caused by *Chlamydia trachomatis*; often leads to blindness.

Transduction   Moving genetic material from one prokaryote to another via a bacteriophage or viral vector.

Transformation   (1) Process in which an organism takes up free DNA that is released into the environment when another organism dies and then lyses. (2) Process by which a virus changes a cell into a tumor or immortal cell line; a cancer-causing or transforming virus.

Transient bacteremia   Incidental and brief presence of bacteria in the bloodstream.

Transient colonizers   Microorganisms that are intermittently present on the surface of the human body or other animal. The organisms are capable of surviving for short periods on the surfaces but are unable to continue to multiply and reproduce for extended periods.

Transmission-based precautions   Infection control guidelines used for patients known or suspected to be infected with pathogens spread by airborne or droplet transmission or by contact with dry skin or fomites.

Transposon   Genetic material that can move from one genetic element to another (i.e., between plasmids or from a plasmid to a chromosome); so-called jumping genes.

Transposition   The movement of a transposon from one genetic element to another.

Transtracheal aspiration   Passage of needle and plastic catheter into the trachea to obtain lower respiratory tract secretions free of oral contamination.

Transudate   Similar to exudate but with low protein content.

Trench fever   Bacterial disease transmitted by lice.

Tris-acetate buffer (TAE)   Used in nucleic acid separation techniques, fragments migrate more rapidly due to conductivity than in tris-borate buffer, resulting in better resolution with small fragments.

Tris-borate buffer (TBE)   Used in nucleic acid separation techniques, fragments migrate more slowly than tris-acetate buffer, resulting in better resolution with larger fragments.

Trogocytosis   The transfer of membrane fragments on an antigen-presenting cell to a lymphocyte.

Trophozoite   Feeding, motile stage of protozoa.

Tropism   Preferred environment or destination; attraction to. In viral infection, preference for a tissue site (rabies viruses have a tropism for neural tissue).

Trough level   The lowest concentration for a drug or antibiotic in the bloodstream prior to the administering of another subsequent dose.

Trypomastigote   Life cycle in flagellated protozoans with a flagellum extending externally on the posterior end of the organism.

TSI   Triple sugar iron (agar tube).

TTA   Transtracheal aspiration.

Tubercle   Granuloma in the lung associated with *Mycobacterium tuberculosis* infection. See granuloma.

Tuberculoid leprosy   Localized leprosy.

Tularemia   Infectious disease caused by *Francisella tularensis*.

Turbidity   Density of the organism present in the liquid medium; at least 106 bacteria per milliliter of broth are needed for turbidity to be detected with the unaided eye. A spectrophotometer may be used to measure the turbidity using the optical density (OD) of the culture.

Tympanocentesis   Draining of fluid from the middle ear.

Type III secretion system   Found in many gram-negative pathogens and is responsible for secretion and injection of virulence-associated factors into the cytoplasm of host cells.

Type IV secretion systems (bacterial)   Bacterial devices that deliver macromolecular molecules such as proteins across and into cells.

Typhoid fever   Bacterial infection caused by *Salmonella enterica* subsp. *enterica*.

Typing   Methods of grouping organisms, primarily for epidemiologic purposes (e.g., biotyping, serotyping, bacteriophage typing, and the antibiogram).

Tzanck test   Stained smear of cells from the base of a vesicle examined for inclusions produced by herpes simplex virus or varicella-zoster virus.

U

Umbilicate   A bacterial or fungal colony demonstrating a depressed or sunken center.

Umbonate   A bacterial or fungal colony demonstrating a raised center.

Undulating membrane   Extension of the plasma membrane in protozoan flagellates that appears as a flap along the body for motility.

Uniserate   Single row or layer.

Universal precautions   See standard precautions.

Ureteritis   Inflammation of the ureter.

Urethritis   Inflammation of urethra, the canal through which urine is discharged (e.g., gonococcal urethritis).

Urosepsis   Sepsis (systemic response to organisms in the bloodstream) caused by a urinary tract infection.

Urticarial   Itchy, raised rash.

UTI   Urinary tract infection.

V

Vaccination The process of administering a vaccine, which is generally a part of a microorganism or virus, or an attenuated bacterial toxin or microorganism that will activate the individual's immune response, resulting in the production of specific antibodies to the vaccine.

Variable regions The variable region of an antibody consists of the amino terminus of both the heavy and light chain proteins of the antibody. The regions have variable amino acid sequences that differ from one antibody to another, to enable the antibodies to bind to different antigens.

VD Venereal disease.

VDRL Venereal Disease Research Laboratory; classic nontreponemal serologic test for syphilis antibodies. Uses cardiolipin, lecithin, and cholesterol as cross-reactive antigen that flocculates in the presence of "reaginic" antibodies produced by patients with syphilis. Best test for cerebrospinal fluid in cases of neurosyphilis.

Vector An arthropod or other agent that carries microorganisms from one infected individual to another.

Vegetation In endocarditis, the aggregates of fibrin and microorganisms on the heart valves or other endocardium.

Vegetative hyphae Filamentous structures that grow down into the agar and draw nutrients from the agar substrate.

Vehicle See fomite.

Ventral disk Rigid protein structure on the ventral (underside) side of a parasite used for attachment to host cells.

Verrucose Furrowed or convoluted topology of a fungal colony.

Verruga Small bump on the skin or mucous membrane generally associated with a human papillomavirus.

Vesicle A small bulla or blister containing clear fluid.

V-factor See nicotinamide adenine dinucleotide (NAD).

Villi Minute, elongated projections from the surface of intestinal mucosa that are important in absorption.

Villose Soft hairlike.

Vincent angina An old term, seldom used currently, referring to anaerobic tonsillitis. Also referred to as acute necrotizing ulcerative gingivitis, or trench mouth.

Viral inclusions Nuclear or cytoplasmic inclusions that are clumps of proteins indicating viral replication inside the infected cell.

Viral neutralization The process where specific antibodies bind to the viral receptor molecule, blocking the virus's ability to bind with the host cell receptor and neutralizing the virus by preventing it from infecting the cell.

Viremia Presence of viruses in the bloodstream.

Virion The complete viral particle, including nucleocapsid, outer membrane or envelope, and all adherence structures.

Viroid Infectious naked RNA, single stranded with no protein coat. Primarily these infect plants.

Virulence Degree of pathogenicity or disease-producing ability of a microorganism.

Virulence factors Attributes or characteristics that enhance the organism's ability to invade or cause disease.

Virus Infectious agent that requires a living cell to reproduce.

Visceral Deep within tissue or organs (viscera).

Viscus (plural Viscera) Any of the organs (viscera) within one of the four great body cavities (cranium, thorax, abdomen, and pelvis).

Vitox Commercial supplement used in the preparation of Modified Thayer Martin or New York City Medium for the isolation of *Neisseria* spp.

VP Voges-Proskauer: a biochemical test that detects the presence of acetoin in bacterial cultures.

W

Wayson stain Special stain that uses basic fuchsin and methylene blue to identify the bipolar staining of *Yersinia pestis*.

Weil-Felix reaction Agglutination test for the diagnosis of rickettsia infections.

Western blot Proteins of an organism are separated by gel electrophoresis and transferred to membrane filters. Antiserum (labeled antibody) is allowed to react with the filters, and specific antibody bound to its homologous antigen is detected.

White piedra External fungal infection of hair that presents with soft nodules.

Wilkins-Chalgren agar Anaerobic agar for the isolation and identification of *Prevotella* spp.

Workup See identification scheme.

X

Xenodiagnosis Method of diagnosis infection by allowing the insect vectors to feed on the patient and then examine the vector for the infecting agent.

X-factor See hemin.

Z

Ziehl-Neelsen Traditional hot acid-fast method of staining organisms that contain muramic or mycolic acid.

Zone edge test Penicillin (10-U) disk test performed on Mueller-Hinton agar to determine whether the organism produces beta-lactamase. A sharp edge is considered positive and a fuzzy edge is considered negative.

Zone of equivalence Concentration when antigen and antibody are in equal concentrations resulting in maximum interactions and measurable cross-linking.

Zoonosis (zoonotic infection) A disease of animals (not human) transmissible to humans (e.g., tularemia).

Zoosporogenesis Reproduction of zoospores.

Zygomycetes Group of fungi with nonseptate hyphae and spores produced within a sporangium.

Zygospores Thick-walled diploid fungal cell that arises from the fusion of two haploid gametes.

Index

A